Dr Ante Bilić
liječnik - stomatolog

Ante Bilić
11. 07. 81.

SODEMAN'S

PATHOLOGIC PHYSIOLOGY

Mechanisms of Disease

WILLIAM A. SODEMAN, Jr., M.D., F.A.C.P.

Professor and Chairman, Department of Comprehensive Medicine,
University of South Florida College of Medicine, Tampa, Florida

THOMAS M. SODEMAN, M.D., F.C.A.P., F.A.C.P.

Assistant Clinical Professor of Pathology,
East Carolina University School of Medicine,
Greenville, North Carolina; Associate Director,
Clinical Laboratories, Lenoir Memorial Hospital, Kinston,
North Carolina

SIXTH EDITION   *1979*

W. B. SAUNDERS COMPANY *Philadelphia / London / Toronto*

W. B. Saunders Company: West Washington Square
                          Philadelphia, PA   19105

                          1 St. Anne's Road
                          Eastbourne, East Sussex BN21 3UN, England

                          1 Goldthorne Avenue
                          Toronto, Ontario M8Z 5T9, Canada

Library of Congress Cataloging in Publication Data

Sodeman, William A 1936–

Sodeman's Pathologic physiology.

Includes bibliographies.

1. Physiology, Pathological.   I. Sodeman, Thomas M.,
   joint author.   II. Title.   III. Title: Pathologic
   physiology. [DNLM: 1. Pathology. QZ140.3 S679s]

RB113.S6 1979   616.07   78–1790

ISBN 0–7216–8473–4

Sodeman's PATHOLOGIC PHYSIOLOGY: Mechanisms of Disease   ISBN   0-7216-8473-4

Last digit is the print number: 9   8   7   6   5   4   3   2

CONTRIBUTORS

J. A. ABILDSKOV, M.D.
Professor of Medicine and Director, Nora Eccles Harrison Cardiovascular Research and Training Institute, University of Utah College of Medicine, Salt Lake City, Utah.

EZRA A. AMSTERDAM, M.D.
Associate Professor of Medicine and Director, Coronary Care Unit, Department of Cardiovascular Medicine, University of California School of Medicine and Sacramento Medical Center, Davis and Sacramento, California.

CHARLES E. BILLINGS, M.D., M.Sc.
Clinical Professor of Preventive Medicine, Ohio State University; Chief, Aviation Safety Research Office, NASA–Ames Research Center, Moffett Field, California.

GILES G. BOLE, M.D.
Professor of Internal Medicine, University of Michigan Medical School; Physician-in-Charge, Arthritis Division and Rackham Arthritis Research Unit, University of Michigan Medical Center, Ann Arbor, Michigan.

ROBERT J. BOLT, M.D.
Professor and Chairman, Department of Medicine; Director of Medical Services, University of California, Davis; Sacramento Medical Center, California.

GEORGE A. BRAY, M.D.
Professor of Medicine, UCLA School of Medicine; Director, Clinical Research Center, Harbor General Hospital, Los Angeles, California.

SAMUEL C. BUKANTZ, M.D.
Professor of Medicine, University of South Florida, College of Medicine; Chief, Division of Allergy and Immunology, VA Hospital and Tampa General Hospital, Tampa, Florida.

THOMAS WADE BURNS, M.D.
Professor of Medicine and Director, Division of Endocrinology, University of Missouri School of Medicine; Attending Endocrinologist, University of Missouri Medical Center; Consultant in Endocrinology, VA Hospital, Columbia, Missouri.

ANTHONY N. DEMARIA, M.D.
Associate Professor of Medicine and Director, Noninvasive Cardiology, Department of Cardiovascular Medicine, University of California School of Medicine and Sacramento Medical Center, Davis and Sacramento, California.

HAROLD T. DODGE, M.D.
Professor of Medicine, and Co-Director, Division of Cardiology, University of Washington School of Medicine, Seattle, Washington.

LEONARD S. DREIFUS, M.D., F.A.C.C.
Professor of Medicine and Physiology, Jefferson Medical College of the Thomas Jefferson University; Chief, Cardiovascular Division, Lankenau Hospital, Philadelphia, Pennsylvania.

LOUIS J. ELSAS, II, M.D.
Professor of Pediatrics and Director, Division of Medical Genetics, Department of Pediatrics, Emory University School of Medicine; Attending Physician, Grady Memorial Hospital, Emory University Hospital and The Henrietta Egleston Hospital, Atlanta, Georgia.

ALLAN J. ERSLEV, M.D.
Cardeza Research Professor of Medicine, Jefferson Medical College of Thomas Jefferson University; Attending Physician, Thomas Jefferson University Hospital, Philadelphia, Pennsylvania.

EDMUND BERNEY FLINK, M.D., Ph.D.
Professor of Medicine, West Virginia University School of Medicine; Attending Physician, West Virginia University Hospital, Morgantown, West Virginia.

THOMAS G. GABUZDA, M.D.
Professor of Medicine, Jefferson Medical College of Thomas Jefferson University; Chief, Department of Hematology, Lankenau Hospital, Philadelphia, Pennsylvania.

RAY W. GIFFORD, JR., M.D.
Head, Department of Hypertension and Nephrology, The Cleveland Clinic Foundation, Cleveland, Ohio.

ARTHUR C. GUYTON, M.D.
Chairman and Professor, Department of Physiology and Biophysics, University of Mississippi Medical Center, Jackson, Mississippi.

W. PROCTOR HARVEY, M.D.
Professor of Medicine, Georgetown University School of Medicine; Chief of Cardiology, George-

CONTRIBUTORS

town University Hospital; Consultant Cardiologist, Washington VA Hospital, Bethesda Naval Hospital and Walter Reed General Hospital, Washington, D.C.

FRANK L. IBER, M.D.
Professor of Medicine and Chief, Division of Gastroenterology, University of Maryland; Gastroenterologist in Chief, University of Maryland Hospital, Loch Raven VA Hospital and Ft. Howard VA Hospital, Baltimore, Maryland.

J. WARD KENNEDY, M.D.
Professor of Medicine, University of Washington School of Medicine; Chief of Cardiology, Seattle VA Hospital, Seattle, Washington.

JOHN H. KILLOUGH, M.D., Ph.D.
Associate Professor of Medicine and Associate Dean, Jefferson Medical College, Thomas Jefferson University; Attending, Thomas Jefferson University Hospital and Wilmington Medical Center, Philadelphia, Pennsylvania and Wilmington, Delaware.

JOSEPH B. KIRSNER, M.D., Ph.D.
Louis Block Distinguished Service Professor of Medicine, Former Deputy Dean for Medical Affairs, University of Chicago; Attending Physician, A.M. Billings Hospital, University of Chicago, Chicago, Illinois.

RICHARD F. LOCKEY, M.D.
Associate Professor of Medicine, Division of Allergy and Immunology, The University of South Florida College of Medicine; Assistant Chief, Allergy and Immunology, VA Hospital, Tampa, Florida.

DEAN T. MASON, M.D.
Professor of Medicine, Professor of Physiology, and Chairman, Department of Cardiovascular Medicine, University of California School of Medicine and Sacramento Medical Center, Davis and Sacramento, California.

W. K. C. MORGAN, M.D., F.R.C.P.(Ed.)
Professor of Medicine, University of Western Ontario; Medical Director, Sir Adam Beck Chest Unit, London, Ontario.

ROBERT M. NAKAMURA, M.D.
Adjunct Professor of Pathology, University of California, San Diego, La Jolla, California; Chairman, Department of Pathology, Green Hospital of Scripps Clinic, Scripps Clinic and Research Foundation, La Jolla, California.

WILLIAM W. PARMLEY, M.D.
Professor of Medicine, UCSF School of Medicine; Chief, Cardiovascular Division, Moffitt Hospital, San Francisco, California.

ANANDA S. PRASAD, M.D., Ph.D.
Professor of Medicine and Chief of Hematology, Wayne State University School of Medicine, Detroit, Michigan; Attending Physician, Detroit General Hospital and VA Hospital, Allen Park, Michigan.

JEAN H. PRIEST, M.D.
Associate Professor of Pediatrics; Assistant Professor, Division of Medical Genetics, Department of Pediatrics, Emory University School of Medicine; Attending, Grady Memorial Hospital, Atlanta, Georgia.

DOUGLAS SEATON, M.D., M.R.C.P.
Consultant Physician, Ipswich Hospital, Ipswich, England.

DANA LEROY SHIRES, JR., M.D., F.A.C.P.
Professor of Internal Medicine and Chief, Section of Nephrology, Department of Internal Medicine, University of South Florida College of Medicine; Consulting Nephrologist, Tampa General Hospital, Tampa VA Hospital and University Community Hospital, Tampa, Florida.

DAVID B. SKINNER, M.D.
Dallas B. Phemister Professor and Chairman, Department of Surgery, University of Chicago and University of Chicago Hospitals, Chicago, Illinois.

PHILIP J. SNODGRASS, M.D.
Professor of Medicine, Indiana University School of Medicine; Chief, Medical Service, V.A.M.C., Indianapolis, Indiana.

THOMAS M. SODEMAN, M.D.
Assistant Clinical Professor of Pathology, East Carolina University School of Medicine, Greenville, North Carolina; Associate Director, Clinical Laboratories, Lenoir Memorial Hospital, Kinston, North Carolina.

WILLIAM A. SODEMAN, JR., M.D., F.A.C.P.
Professor and Chairman, Department of Comprehensive Medicine, University of South Florida, College of Medicine, Tampa, Florida.

JOHN FREDERICK STAPLETON, M.D.
Professor of Medicine, Georgetown University School of Medicine; Medical Director, Georgetown University Hospital, Washington, D.C.

H. J. C. SWAN, M.D., Ph.D.
Professor of Medicine, UCLA School of Medicine; Director, Department of Cardiology, Cedars-Sinai Medical Center, Los Angeles, California.

MORTON N. SWARTZ, M.D.
Professor of Medicine, Harvard Medical School; Physician, Chief of Infectious Disease Unit, Massachusetts General Hospital, Boston, Massachusetts.

ROBERT C. TARAZI, M.D.
Vice-Chairman, Research Division, The Cleveland Clinic Foundation, Cleveland, Ohio.

ERNEST S. TUCKER, III, M.D.
Associate Clinical Professor of Pathology and Pediatrics, University of California School of Medicine, San Diego; Pathologist, Green Hospital, Scripps Clinic and Director, Scripps Immunology Reference Laboratory, Scripps Clinic and Research Foundation, La Jolla, California.

YOSHIO WATANABE, M.D., D.M.Sc., F.A.C.C.
Professor of Medicine, Fujita Gakuen University School of Medicine, Toyoake, Aichi, Japan.

DAVID W. WATSON, M.D.
Clinical Associate Professor of Medicine, University of California, Davis, Davis, California.

LOUIS WEINSTEIN, M.D., Ph.D.
  Visiting Professor of Medicine, Harvard Medical School; Physician and Director of the Clinical Services of the Division of Infectious Diseases, Peter Bent Brigham Hospital, Boston, Massachusetts.

JOAN WIKMAN-COFFELT, Ph.D.
  Assistant Professor of Medicine and Director, Cardiovascular Biochemistry, Department of Cardiovascular Medicine, University of California

School of Medicine, Davis and San Francisco, California.

CHARLES S. WINANS, M.D.
  Professor of Medicine, Section of Gastroenterology, University of Chicago Pritzker School of Medicine, Chicago, Illinois.

K. LEMONE YIELDING, M.D.
  Chief, Laboratory of Molecular Biology, Professor of Biochemistry, Associate Professor of Medicine, University of Alabama School of Medicine, Birmingham, Alabama.

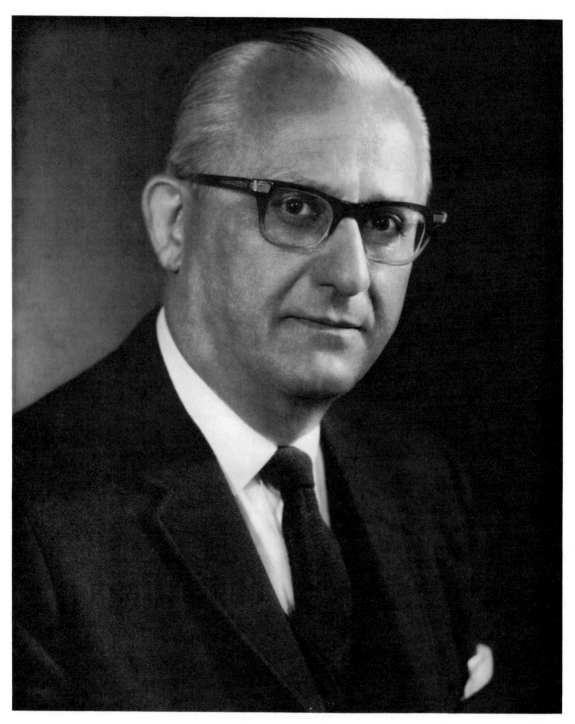

William A. Sodeman, Sr., M.D., F.A.C.P.

PREFACE

The 6th edition of *Pathologic Physiology* marks the 29th year of publication. Continuous updating of established chapters by their authors has stressed the ever changing atmosphere in medicine and the need for continuing education. In the core areas of biochemistry and immunology and in the sections on the lung, kidney, rheumatic disease, allergy, spleen, pancreas, gallbladder, and chemical agents of disease, new authors have contributed substantially to important changes in this edition. While much of the information has changed over 29 years, the basic goal of this text—to provide an understanding of the physiology of dysfunction as it appears in the clinical presentation of disease—remains the cornerstone of its construction. The editors and, we hope, the readers are deeply appreciative of the efforts of the authors to provide this logical link. The authors have been most gracious, diligent and resourceful in their efforts.

The editors are grateful to the W. B. Saunders Company and its efficient staff for their professional handling of the coordination and progression of the multiple stages of editorial revision. The editors wish to express special appreciation to Mr. John Hanley, whose support and efforts assured this orderly development. To the families of the authors, the editors offer a collective thanks for their understanding and patience during preparation time.

With the deepest gratitude, the editors express their thanks for faithful support and understanding through the many hours required in text preparation, reading and checking manuscripts to our families and in particular to our wives, M. Agnes Sodeman, Marjorie C. Sodeman, and Mary H. Sodeman.

WILLIAM A. SODEMAN, SR., M.D.
WILLIAM A. SODEMAN, JR., M.D.
THOMAS SODEMAN, M.D.

PREFACE
TO
THE
FIRST
EDITION

This volume, a collaborative effort by 25 authors, approaches problems of disease in the field of internal medicine from the standpoint of disturbed physiology. Unlike the usual text, which is devoted to discussions of etiology, pathology, symptoms and treatment, this work analyzes symptoms and signs and the mechanisms of their development. The monograph is not intended to take the place of standard texts on physiology or textbooks of medicine. It does not aim at the completeness of either, but does try to bridge the gap between them by presenting a clinical picture of disease seen as physiologic dysfunction. An attempt is made to promote understanding of how and why symptoms appear, so that the student or physician may have a reasonable explanation for the findings he elicits. Neurologic problems are considered only as they are related to the various disease groups. The same is true of metabolic disturbances and disorders of acid-base balance.

The Editor thanks the contributors for their ready cooperation in covering certain aspects of disease in which presentation of material is at times most difficult. He thanks the Saunders Company for their help and guidance, and also Miss Brent S. Robertson for her long hours of hard work and patience in reading and checking manuscripts.

WILLIAM A. SODEMAN, M.D.

CONTENTS

CONTENTS

Section IV. GASTROENTEROLOGY, ENDOCRINOLOGY,
AND METABOLISM

Section
I

SCIENTIFIC
FOUNDATIONS

Metabolic Biochemistry

Thomas M. Sodeman, M.D.

Characterization of the normal state and of the complex changes wrought by disease formulates the goal of biochemical research. Locked in the intricate interlinking pathways toward that goal are the sources of the structural elements of cells, their physiology, and their metabolic regulation. The protoplasm of the cell, contained by the cell wall and holding numerous organelles, consists of a mixture of water, minerals, and organic macromolecules. From these mixtures stem the physiologic characteristics of life. The study of these chemical mixtures, their components, synthesis, storage, interaction, and degradation forms the fundamentals of biochemistry. A clear understanding of biochemistry is essential. Most, if not all, of the pathologic processes to be discussed in this text involve either primary defects or secondary alterations in biochemical processes.

The biochemical processes of the body occur at a subcellular level and involve synthesis and catabolism of organic material, regulation of exchange of material, and conversion of chemical energy into usable forms. The chemical composition and ratio of compounds of cells is complex and varies between cell types. Oxygen, carbon, hydrogen, nitrogen, phosphorus, and sulfur contribute most of the structural mass of the cell and provide the elements for its intrinsic chemical physiology. Additional elements — for example, metals sodium and magnesium — are essential for life. Of known elements, only 19 appear to be absolutely essential. The task of unraveling the chemical nature of cell function and structure is formidable and is certain to lead to change in the understanding of even the most well established biochemical mechanisms.

The intent of this chapter is to review biochemical principles that govern biologic processes. It is assumed that basic organic chemical concepts of covalent bonds, bond angles, and the spatial relationships between atoms are familiar. The chemical and physical properties of biochemical compounds in most situations reflect the nature of the functional groups.

Fundamental groups of alcohols, aldehydes, ketones, amines and carboxylic acids are encountered throughout carbohydrate, lipid, and protein metabolism (Table 1–1). Alcohols are hydroxylated hydrocarbons and alkyl derivatives of water. In polyhydric forms they represent sugars and, as cyclic or ring forms, steroids. Aldehydes and ketones are composed of a carbonyl group ($-C=O$) with one or two alkyl groups attached. These organic configurations are also present in the polyhydric alcohols of sugars and other organic compounds. Amines are alkyl derivatives of ammonia and, as will be discussed, are essential elements in proteins. The carboxylic functional group consists of a carbonyl and hydroxyl group on the same atom. Functionally they form weak acids.

These functional groups and their activity in oxidation, esterification, reduction and other reaction modes provide many of the characteristics of organic compounds.

EQUILIBRIUM

Equilibrium is the process in which a forward reaction is equal to the reverse reaction. While there is no net change in reactants and products, turnover is occurring on either side of the reac-

TABLE 1-1 FUNCTIONAL GROUPS

Alcohol	$R{-}CH_2{-}OH$
Aldehyde	$R{-}C{=}O$ $\quad\ \ \|$ $\quad\ \ H$
Ketone	R $\quad\diagdown$ $\qquad C{=}O$ $\quad\diagup$ R
Amines	$R{-}NH_2$
Carboxylic acid	$R{-}COOH$

tion through equal change. A better term for the equilibrium in biologic processes is "steady state." This implies that a concentration of a substance can be held constant. The equilibrium or steady state is non-productive in the biologic system with regard to the thermodynamics of the system. No free energy is made available by the system. Biologic studies are more concerned with the initial state, routes, and rate of conversion in which energy changes occur. This is, essentially, the study of the kinetics of the reaction. Isolation of a single reaction in an in vitro system permits an understanding of interaction of the components and the thermodynamics that occur. In vivo study is more difficult because the components of a reaction, either reactants or products, are influenced by the complex pathways that yield or utilize them in the continuous biologic system. Under these circumstances, equilibrium becomes less important. The concentrations of many substances are held at rigid levels within the body. This steady state is controlled by reactions producing or utilizing the components. Feedback mechanisms that control enzymes and enzyme substrate induction represent some of the controls that assure availability of reactants and energy necessary for biologic processes. All chemical reactions to some degree are reversible; however, in biochemical pathways, the products of a reaction are usually utilized in the next step. This forces the reaction one way, resulting in irreversibility and non-equilibrium of reaction.

The reaction kinetics and steady state can be expressed mathematically and the influence of component concentrations, temperature and pressure can be analyzed to determine the dynamics of the reaction and interacting systems. The environmental demands on in vivo reactions are difficult to comprehend at the subcellular level. For this reason, reaction characteristics are more commonly thought of in terms of the changing concentrations of intermediates and the effects these may have in regulation of distant, though indirectly coupled, reactions. A patholog-

ic state may be derived from or result in the inability of regulatory influences to compensate for changes in biochemical interactions. Changes in the immediate kinetics of a reaction or distal reactions can result in the development of new steady states with accumulations or depletions of pathway components. Such effects can be seen in storage diseases, the inability to maintain sufficient glucose levels or the failure of normal trigger mechanisms to initiate the coagulation cascade in the absence or depression of key factors.

THERMODYNAMICS

Thermodynamics is the study of quantitative changes in energy as biologic reactions pass to equilibrium. It is not concerned with processes at equilibrium, as that is a terminal state in which free energy is zero. The energy produced within a system may take the form of heat, osmotic, mechanical, chemical, or electrical energy. Transfer of energy type from one form to another may be completed in biologic systems.

In the biologic system energy is primarily obtained by chemical linkage to oxidative reactions. The energy of a system can be considered in two parts. Entropic energy is that energy required internally by the system to maintain its molecular configuration. Enthalpic energy is the energy available externally for work (free energy). In the conversion of glucose in the presence of oxygen to yield carbon dioxide and water, 673,000 cal./mole of free energy are produced that may be transferred by chemical means to reactions requiring energy. In a reaction process some energy is lost as heat and may not be utilized in chemical reactions.

The difference in energy states of a substrate versus the product is a measure of the extent to which a reaction will proceed. Exergonic reactions, i.e., those that yield energy, may proceed spontaneously. Whether an exergonic reaction will spontaneously occur depends on the energy of activation of the reactants. Each molecule has an average level of energy that maintains its molecular configuration. For a reaction to occur spontaneously, a critical energy level or barrier must be reached so that bonding or exchange may occur between elements. When two atomic orbits merge, a more stable configuration occurs which will require less energy. Enzymes, through the formation of an enzyme–reactant complex, reduce the energy of activation and thus accelerate a reaction. Endergonic reactions, on the other hand, require large amounts of energy to proceed.

The energy requirement of reactions plays an important role in determining the availability of products and, therefore, in the control of subsequent reactions. In biologic systems there is both compartmentalization and linkage of reactions to assure the efficient availability of reaction products and energy necessary to activate or drive a reaction. Energy is usually supplied by chemical means and under strictly controlled mechanisms. The energy released in a reaction may contribute to further activation of the initial substrate or may provide energy for closely associated reactions. The product of the reaction may be sufficiently activated to reduce the energy requirements for the next step.

In the metabolic process, the mechanism of free energy transfer relies heavily on intermediate energy absorbers, for example, adenosine triphosphate (ATP). The advantage of energy absorbers lies in their universal activity which permits energy transfer in a wide variety of reactions. Throughout the biochemical pathways, ATP has an essential role in providing energy to endogonic processes. ATP is composed of a purine, ribose, and three phosphate groups. It carries a central position in relation to other organophosphates in its ability to yield and accept high energy phosphate. ATP has the stability necessary to function as an energy storehouse. The source for the high energy bond is provided in the respiratory chain oxidation in mitochondria, catabolism of substrates and from high energy storage depots like creatine phosphate in muscle. Upon hydrolysis ATP liberates 7.6 Kcal./mole of free energy. Three factors are involved in this release: a change in resonance energy; ionization released energy; and relief of electrostatic repulses. The prime reservoir of energy is in the body's macromolecules, which, through metabolic processes, provide high energy phosphates. Lipids are particularly effective in this process and provide the added advantage of osmotic stability in the cell.

ENZYMES

Enzymes are protein biocatalysts that reduce the necessary chemical energy for activation of a reaction. They are not consumed, and, therefore, only small quantities are required. In contrast to catalysts, they tend to be reaction-specific. Six functional classes of enzymes have been established and are outlined in Table 1–2.

TABLE 1–2 ENZYME CLASSIFICATION

Oxidoreductases
Transferases
Hydrolases
, Lyases
Isomerases
Ligases

Almost all biochemical reactions are enzyme catalyzed. Many enzymes require nonprotein cofactors or coenzymes in their reactions. Coenzymes are important in transferring groups between reactants and, unlike enzymes, are not reformed in the reaction. B-vitamins are a common structural part of coenzymes.

The three-dimensional structure of enzymes plays an important role in their function and stability. An enzyme, a relatively large molecule in comparison with the substrate, combines with a substrate, altering the enzyme configuration to bring functional or catalytic groups into place.

Enzyme aggregates resulting from association of subunits form a series of multiple molecular forms with similar enzymatic activity but structural differences. One form may dominate over others in a tissue. Clinically, multiple molecular forms are expressed in isoenzymes of dehydrogenases, phosphatases, transaminases, and protolytic enzymes.

Measurements of circulating enzymes have become routine in the practice of medicine as an indicator of cellular damage or genetic defects. Because of the small quantities present, enzymes are measured by their activity. This has given rise to a number of arbitrary units. Many of the enzymes in plasma have no physiologic function in the blood but represent release from cells and normal cellular degradation. Other enzymes exist in proenzyme forms; for example, coagulation factors and lipoprotein lipase which, upon activation, play critical roles in the body's homeostatic processes.

METABOLIC REGULATION

The regulation of metabolic processes is particularly controlled by enzyme activity. Control may be based on the amount of enzyme synthesized, enzyme inhibition, activation, degradation, and covalent modification of protein structure. Regulatory mechanisms also include the availability of substrates or cofactors, transport systems, and compartmentalization of reactions. Compartmentalization permits localization of reaction and independence from potentially influencing processes. It provides an orderly sequence for controlled enzymatic processes linking reactants and assures energy transfer. Compartmentalization does pose problems when reactants must be moved from one compartment to another. Translocation may require a converting process to change a metabolite to a permeable state or form for passage across a membrane and then similar processes for reconversion. Such a process would require two forms of enzymes physically separated.

Metabolic processes tend to maintain a steady state within cells despite short term changes within the environment. Chemical processes must occur at the right time and rate to meet the coordinated processes in a cell. Enzymes play a key role in this regulation. Many factors are involved in enzyme control. Among those not yet mentioned is control of synthesis by substrate induction, product repression or feedback repression, regulated enzyme degradation, and by hormonal and dietary influences. Secondary enzyme activation provides one method for regulation. In this process, a proenzyme is converted to an active form by a second enzyme. This provides a mechanism to concentrate an enzyme at an appropriate site ready for its physiologic demand. Examples can be seen in the coagulation process and in digestive enzymes. Knowledge of these regulatory processes is limited, but they are important in understanding the pathologic physiology of disease and the possible approaches to therapy. The ability to control enzymes may in the future open new avenues for therapeutics.

BIOLOGIC OXIDATION

Free energy in the cell ultimately lies in the oxidative reaction. In biologic systems this mostly involves the transfer of hydrogen and formation of water. Chemical oxidation is defined as the loss of electrons and reduction as a gain in electrons. The energy released in this process may be chemically conserved in high energy phosphates. This process of coupling of oxidation to high energy carriers is referred to as oxidative phosphorylation. When a coenzyme — for example, ATP or NAD — is reduced, a mechanism for reoxidation and regeneration is available in the cell. This system, the respiratory chain, provides an assemblage of enzymes in coupled reactions that can transport electrons and provide high energy bonds. It is compartmentalized in the mitochondria. These high energy bonds provide a mechanism to store energy formed in biologic oxidation.

The energy from oxidation of fatty acids, amino acids and carbohydrates is made available in the mitochondria through the respiratory chain. Numerous enzymes are involved in the oxidative process. Among these are oxidases, aerobic and anaerobic dehydrogenases, hydroperoxidases, and oxygenases. The respiratory chain transports reducing equivalents, hydrogen or electrons, for reaction with oxygen to form water. The order is arranged sequentially, with increasing tendency for free energy exchange or redox potential. The main mitochondrial chain (Fig. 1–1) is initiated by a NAD-linked dehydrogenase system and proceeds through flavoprotein and cytochrome systems to molecular oxygen. Metabolic pathways feed reducing equivalents (NAD or $FADH_2$) into the system. The terminal cytochrome system possesses many elements, starting with coenzyme Q, which links flavoprotein to cytochrome, and extends through cytochromes, C_1, C, A, and A_3. The respiratory chain provides three sites at which energy change is sufficient to permit coupling with ADP to form ATP. Each mole of NADH that enters the chain yields three moles of high energy phosphate, and each mole of $FADH_2$, two moles. The control of the respiratory process is the availability of substrate, ADP, and oxygen.

High energy bonds are not produced solely in the respiratory chain. Substrate phosphorylation involving the production of high energy bonds during metabolic oxidation sequences of glucose, lipid, and amino acids will be reviewed later in this chapter during specific discussions. Mechanisms are available to transfer to the mitochondria the NADH produced by glycolysis in the cytosol using substrate pair translocation systems.

The impact of both mitochondrial and substrate phosphorylation is to provide energy. With oxidation of glucose in the glycolytic process and citric acid cycle, six high energy phosphate bonds are produced and two are used. These represent phosphorylation at the substrate level. Linkage with the respiratory chain, with reoxidation of reduced coenzymes, yields 34 high energy bonds per cycle of glucose. Through these processes it is possible to account for 42 per cent of the free energy of glucose metabolism. Under anaerobic conditions, two high energy phosphate bonds are produced.

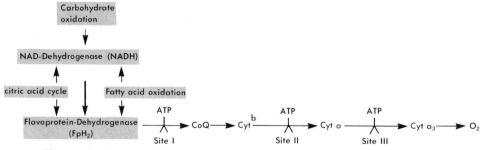

Figure 1–1 Mitochondrial respiratory chain for transport of reducing equivalents.

TABLE 1-3 CARBOHYDRATE

CLASSIFICATION

Monosaccharides— $C_nH_{2n}O_n$
Disaccharides — $C_n(H_2O)_{n-1}$
Oligosaccharides —
Polysaccharides — $(C_6H_{10}O_{5x})$

CARBOHYDRATE METABOLISM

Carbohydrate Structure

Carbohydrates may be defined as aldehyde or ketone derivatives or polyhydric alcohols and are divided into four major groups (Table 1–3). Monosaccharides, including trioses, tetroses, pentoses, hexoses, and heptoses, are physiologically important carbohydrates. The hexose sugars of glucose, fructose, galactose and mannose are common dietary components and provide a major energy source. D-ribose, a pentose sugar, is an essential component of nucleic acid. Disaccharides such as sucrose, maltose, and lactose are composed of two monosaccharides united by a glycosidic linkage and are common elements of the daily diet. Polysaccharides occur in the forms of starches, glycogen, and dextrins. Polysaccharides in the form of glucosaminoglycans (mucopolysaccharides) and glycoproteins (mucoproteins) are important structural components of the body. Glycoproteins are elements of blood groups and certain hormones.

Glycolysis

This process, the Embden-Meyerhof pathway, is a complex sequence in which glucose and other carbohydrates are metabolized to pyruvate or lactate. It is an extramitochondrial function, occurring in the cytosols of cells. A schematic outline of the glycolytic process is included in Figure 1–2. In the initial step, glucose is phosphorylated to glucose 6-phosphate in the presence of hexokinase or, in the liver, by glucokinase. The reaction is irreversible and is associated with an extensive heat loss. Glucose 6-phosphate is a major pivotal compound in carbohydrate metabolism. Processes involving synthesis and degradation of glycogen, both from glucose or citric acid components, and entry into the hexose monophosphate shunt involve this critical component. The third step in glycolysis involves an irreversible phosphorylation reaction which is followed by a splitting of the hexose molecule into two triose phosphate molecules. These trioses are interconvertible. The glycolysis pathway continues with oxidation of glyceraldehyde 3-phosphate and the addition of an inorganic phosphate in a NAD-dependent step. At steps 6 and 8, high energy phosphate bonds are produced. In the later step, the conversion of phosphenolpyruvate to pyruvate under the influence of pyruvate kinase, a third irreversible point occurs in the glycolytic pathway.

The outcome from this point depends on the availability of oxygen. Under hypoxic situations, the NADH produced in step 5 is available for conversion of pyruvate to lactate. Under aerobic conditions, the NADH is utilized in the mitochondrial respiratory chain and pyruvate is utilized in the citric acid cycle. Pyruvate enters the mitochondria via a transport system where, under the influence of a pyruvate dehydrogenase enzyme complex, it is converted irreversibly to acetyl-CoA. This complex involves thiamine pyrophosphate, lipoic acid, transacetylase, and two dehydrogenases. $FADH_2$ is produced in the reaction, to be oxidized later by NAD. Regulation of the process is by ATP, which acts through cyclic AMP (cAMP) to activate a phosphatase that dephosphorylates and activates the enzyme complex.

In addition to pyruvate's major role in supplying acetyl-CoA in the mitochondria, it also supplements the citric acid cycle intermediate, oxaloacetate. This is achieved by pyruvate carboxylase in the presence of ATP and CO_2 in an irreversible reaction. The process is regulated by acetyl-CoA.

Hexose Monophosphate Shunt

An alternate pathway for oxidation of glucose 6-phosphate is provided in the hexose monophosphate shunt (HMP) or pentose phosphate shunt (Fig. 1–3). This process occurs, like glycolysis, in the cytosol. Isolation of the shunt enzymes has demonstrated high levels in liver, red blood cells and adipose tissue and low activity in skeletal muscle. Through a series of enzyme reactions, glucose 6-phosphate undergoes dehydrogenation and decarboxylation to ribulose 5-phosphate and CO_2. Two NADP-dependent reactions are involved in accepting electrons. If three molecules of glucose 6-phosphate are metabolized in the HMP shunt, three pentoses are formed. By being rearranged through transketolase and aldolase reactions, one molecule of glyceraldehyde 3-phosphate and two molecules of glucose 6-phosphate can be reformed for final oxidation.

What, then, is the point of the alternate pathway? It appears to be a major source for NADPH. In the red blood cell, approximately 10 per cent of glucose 6-phosphate enters the shunt. The NADPH produced is linked by glutathione enzymes with peroxidase, which provides a mechanism for preventing accumulations of H_2O_2 that would cause oxidative denaturation of hemoglobin. In adipose tissue, NADPH is necessary for the synthesis of fatty acids and steroids. The pentose phosphate shunt also provides sugars for nucleotide and nucleic acid synthesis in the form of ribose 5-phosphate.

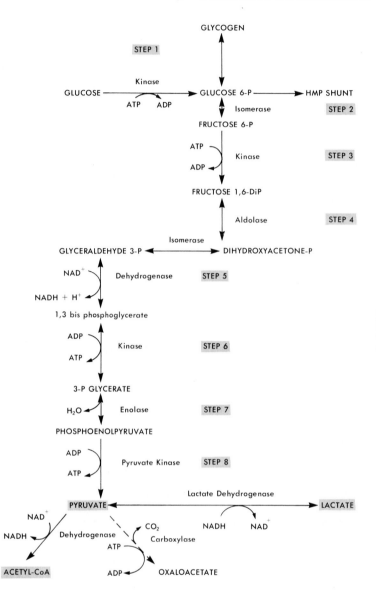

Figure 1–2 Embden-Meyerhof pathway for glycolysis is located in the cytosol and catalyzes the conversion of carbohydrates to pyruvate and lactate.

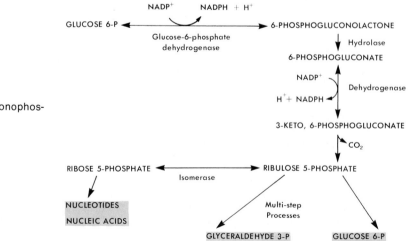

Figure 1–3 Hexose monophosphate shunt.

Glycogenesis

This process consists of the synthesis of glycogen. It may occur in all tissues, but is most prominent in liver and skeletal muscle. The steps include the phosphorylation of glucose to glucose 6-phosphate and then conversion to glucose 1-phosphate by a mutase enzyme. The glucose 1-phosphate then enters a cycle reacting with uridine triphosphate (UTP) and, under the influence of glycogen synthetase, is linked in a 1,4-glycosidic bond with a glucose residue. Through a series of successive linkages, a glycogen molecule is enlarged with branches occurring every 6 to 12 glucose residues. Control of glycogenesis is through the enzyme glycogen synthetase I, which is activated by synthetase phosphatase under the influence of glucose or insulin. Inactivation of glycogen synthetase is under the influence of ATP. Adenylate cyclase is stimulated to form $3'$ $5'$-cyclic AMP from ATP. This reaction, initiated by epinephrine, norepinephrine, or glucagon, increases cAMP, which activates a protein kinase that converts glycogen synthetase to its inactive form.

Glycogenolysis

This process consists of the breakdown of glycogen and is initiated by the action of the enzyme phosphorylase. The phosphorylase enzyme breaks the 1,4 linkage to yield glucose 1-phosphate. Once in the form of glucose 1-phosphate, enzymes exist to convert it in liver or kidney, but not muscle, to free glucose.

Separate distinct forms of phosphorylase exist in muscle and liver cells. In muscle, phosphorylase a activity in part is controlled via hormones through the basic cAMP sequence similar to that described for inactivation of glycogen synthetase. In this process cAMP activates an enzyme that condenses the inactive dimer, phosphorylase b, to the tetramer active form, phosphorylase a. Simple muscle contraction is also known to stimulate phosphorylase a independent of cAMP. Liver phosphorylase also exists in two forms in the cell. However, it is not influenced by cAMP, but rather is controlled by a specific phosphatase.

Gluconeogenesis

In addition to glycogenolysis, the process of gluconeogenesis can provide glucose in dietary carbohydrate restriction. In essence, the process is a reversal of glycolytic processes and involves the conversion of non-carbohydrates to glucose. As it is a reversal, gluconeogenesis activities are counterproductive to glycolytic processes.

Three irreversible steps occur in glycolysis that must be overcome to reverse the Embden-Meyerhof pathway. The first irreversible reaction is the conversion of phosphoenolpyruvate to pyruvate. This is accomplished by entry of pyruvate into the mitochondria, where it can be converted to oxaloacetate by pyruvate carboxylase. The mitochondria are not permeable to oxaloacetate. They are, however, permeable to malate that can be formed by reduction of oxaloacetate. Malate can be translocated by the dicarboxylate transport system to the cytosol for reaction with NAD and reduction to oxaloacetate. Under the influence of carboxykinase, oxaloacetate is converted to the glycolytic intermediate, phosphoenolpyruvate. A high energy GTP is necessary for this reaction.

The irreversible glycolytic reaction between fructose 1,6-bisphosphate and fructose 6-phosphate, and of glucose phosphorylation to glucose 6-phosphate is handled through enzymatic processes distinct from those in the glycolytic pathway. The enzymes for reversal of glycolysis are present in liver and kidney, but not in skeletal muscle.

Glucogenic amino acids, after transamination or deamination, provide members of the citric acid cycle or pyruvate that can be converted to glucose by gluconeogenesis. Similarly, lactate via pyruvate and glycerol activated by glycerokinase to glycerol 3-phosphate, enter the gluconeogenesis pathway. Gluconeogenesis in liver and kidney can then meet the body's needs for glucose in carbohydrate starvation once glycogen stores are exhausted.

Alternate Carbohydrate Metabolism

Glucose can be converted to glucuronic acid with intermediate formation of uridine diphosphoglucuronic acid. The latter is an important conjugant for hormones, drugs, and bilirubin. Glucuronic acid can be metabolized to xylulose and enter the pentose phosphate shunt.

Fructose, through multiple pathways, may enter at several steps in the glycolytic pathway for conversion to glucose. In man, a great deal of the fructose formed as a product of sucrose digestion is converted in the gastrointestinal wall to glucose. In the liver, it may be stored as glycogen. Fructose may also be metabolized by adipose tissue. Galactose formed by intestinal hydrolysis of lactose may be converted to glucose in the liver through a series of enzyme steps.

LIPIDS

Lipids are a heterogeneous group which, because of their high energy value, form an important dietary constituent. A classification of lipids is given in Table 1–4. The cornerstone of the lipid molecule is fatty acid. Natural fatty acids usually

TABLE 1–4 GENERAL CLASSIFICATION
OF LIPIDS

1. *Simple Lipids*
   Fats—fatty acid esters with glycerol
   Waxes—fatty acid esters with higher alcohols

2. *Compound Lipids*
   Phospholipids
   Glycolipids
   Aminolipids

3. *Derived Lipids*
   Hydrolysis products of other lipids

contain an even number of carbon atoms and may be saturated (no double bonds) or unsaturated (one or more double bonds). Common saturated fatty acids encountered in nature are acetic, palmitic, lignoceric, and butyric. Common unsaturated fatty acids are oleic, palmitoleic, linoleic, and arachidonic.

FATTY ACID OXIDATION

Triglycerides are esters of fatty acids and the alcohol, glycerol. The fatty acids at the three ester positions may vary, giving rise to a mixed acylglycerol. Less commonly they will all be of the same type. Hydrolysis of triglycerides occurs mostly in adipose tissue with the release of the fatty acid, which forms a complex with albumin in plasma. Glycerol, depending on the tissue availability of glycerokinase, may be reutilized or diffused out of the tissue for use elsewhere. Fatty acids circulating in plasma can be removed and undergo beta-oxidation to acetyl-CoA through a series of enzyme reactions in the mitochondria. To enter the mitochondria, fatty acids must first be converted to an acyl-CoA form by the action of thiokinase and ATP in microsomes or on the mitochondrial surface. This is the only step in β-oxidation of fatty acids that requires ATP. For long-chain fatty acids, a carnitine and its enzyme associated with the mitochondrial membrane, is essential for penetration of the acyl-CoA form through the mitochondrial wall. Short-chain fatty acid activation may occur directly within mitochondria, avoiding the carnitine step. Once in the mitochondria, acyl-CoA undergoes a series of dehydrogenase steps to remove two hydrogen atoms. The reduced coenzymes ($FADH_2$) and NADH) may enter the respiratory chain and provide ATP. The final enzymatic step in oxidation splits a two-carbon molecule of acetyl-CoA from the fatty acid chain. In the citric acid cycle, the acetyl-CoA can be further oxidized to Co_2 and water. β-oxidation yields considerably more energy than the oxidation of glucose. Fatty acids with odd numbers of carbon atoms yield the three-carbon propionyl-CoA on β-oxidation. This may be converted to succinyl-CoA and enter the citric acid cycle.

FATTY ACID SYNTHESIS

Two pathways are available for fatty acid synthesis. The mitochondrial system involves a reversal, with modifications, of β-oxidation. This system functions under anaerobic conditions and requires ATP, NADH, and NADPH. It adds acetyl-CoA units to existing long-chain fatty acids.

The principal site of fatty acid synthesis is the extramitochondrial system, which consists of a multienzyme functional unit that combines with acetyl-CoA to form acyl units. The malonyl-CoA is formed from acetyl-CoA in a separate reaction. Within this enzyme unit, the molecules are passed along as the reactions proceed. The initial steps involve a condensation of acetyl-CoA with malonyl-CoA, followed by reduction, dehydration, reduction, and the ultimate transfer of the saturated unit to the outer part of the enzyme complex. NADPH, derived primarily from the HMP shunt, acts as the hydrogen donor in both reductions. ATP, Mn^+ and HCO_3^- are also required. The process is repeated, adding acyl radicals until the 16-carbon unit of palmitate is formed. The acetyl-CoA used in both the mitochondrial and extra-mitochondrial systems is derived from carbohydrate and amino acid oxidation or by β-oxidation. The inability to transfer acetyl-CoA out of the mitochondria for fatty acid synthesis in the extramitochondrial system is overcome by transferring acetyl-CoA as a citrate with cleavage by ATP-citrate lyase in the cytosol to acetyl-CoA and oxaloacetate. Pyruvate may participate in fatty acid synthesis by providing acetyl-CoA in the mitochondria that may then be transferred out as citrate. The oxaloacetate formed may be converted to malate and provide NADPH; it may be utilized for glucose formation; or it may be transported into the mitochondria to function in the citric acid cycle.

LIPID METABOLISM

Nutritionally, lipid may be considered as essential or nonessential. The three essential long-chain unsaturated fatty acids that are of metabolic significance, and therefore must be supplied in the diet, are linoleic, linolenic and arachidonic acids. These essential fatty acids are important elements in the structural integrity of the cell and its organelles. The nonessential unsaturated fatty acids can be formed from the corresponding saturated fatty acid forms.

The level of free fatty acids (FFA) in plasma, resulting from lipolysis in adipose tissue, strongly influences metabolism in the liver and skeletal muscle.

TRIGLYCERIDES (TRIACYLGLYCEROL)

Triacylglycerols are synthesized in many tissues. The fatty acid portions of the molecule are provided by the synthesis pathways that have already been discussed. In the liver, kidney, intestines, and lactating mammary glands, glycerol can be provided by the action of glycerokinase, which, in the presence of ATP, forms glycerol 3-phosphate. In those tissues low in glycerokinase (adipose tissue and muscle), the glycerol 3-phosphate is derived from the Embden-Meyerhof pathway.

In triacylglycerol formation, fatty acids are activated to acyl-CoA by thiokinase, ATP, and CoA. The acyl-CoA and glycerol 3-phosphate combine in the presence of a transferase to form a diacylglycerol phosphate. Following a phosphohydrolase reaction, which removes the phosphate, a final acyl-CoA is added to form triacylglycerol.

Degradation of the molecule results from hydrolysis with the release of FFA and glycerol. This reaction is dependent on lipase (not lipoprotein lipase) and is not a simple reversal of synthesis. The fatty acid released upon hydrolysis may be reconverted into triacylglycerol or oxidized by β-oxidation for entry into the citric acid cycle. Depending on the availability of glycerokinase in tissue, glycerol may be reused or diffused into the plasma for transport to tissues with active glycerokinase.

Glucose availability in adipose tissue plays a key role in the level of FFA in plasma. By providing increased levels of glycerol 3-phosphate, glucose stimulates esterification with fatty acids and decreases the flow of fatty acids into the plasma pool. Glucose in adipose tissue may also be oxidized via the citric acid cycle or the HMP shunt, or may be converted to long-chain fatty acids. When carbohydrates are plentiful, adipose tissue tends to emphasize energy production and conversion to endogenous fatty acids for synthesis of acylglycerol. As carbohydrates are restricted, more glucose is conserved for glycerol 3-phosphate formation and esterification with free fatty acids; less glucose is diverted to energy production. However, lipolysis may exceed the rate of esterification despite the greater proportion of glucose being directed to glycerol 3-phosphate and plasma FFA increase. Energy is derived from oxidation of fatty acids rather than from glucose.

The activity of lipase is influenced by adrenocorticotropic hormone (ACTH), melanocyte-stimulating hormone (MSH), thyroid-stimulating hormone (TSH), growth-hormone (GH), epinephrine, and glucagon, all of which have a fat mobilization effect. This is thought to occur by activation of cAMP which, through a protein kinase, converts inactive lipase to an active form. Insulin and prostaglandins inhibit lipase by decreasing cAMP synthesis. In addition, insulin stimulates lipogenesis. Most of the studies of glucose and hormone effects on lipid metabolism have been carried out in experimental animals. The extent to which they will hold true in man is still not clear. Certainly, insulin has clinically demonstrated a corrective effect on fat metabolism in diabetics.

PHOSPHOLIPIDS

The phospholipid groups are defined in Table 1-5. In addition to fatty acids and alcohol, they contain a phosphoric acid residue and other compounds such as nitrogenous bases. A schematic diagram of their synthesis is presented in Figure 1-4. Phospholipids are synthesized from monoacylglycerol or intermediates of triacylglycerol. In the synthesis of lecithins or cephalins, the nitrogenous bases choline and ethanolamine are converted to active form by ATP and cytidine triphosphate. The phosphorylated base is then transferred to intermediate acylglycerol to form the appropriate phospholipid. Similarly, through transferase activity, inositol is added to acylglycerol molecules to form lipositol.

Cardiolipins are formed from an intermediate of lipositol by reaction with glycerol 3-phosphate. Phosphatidylserine is formed from phosphatidylethanolamine (cephalins) by direct reaction with serine. A plasmalogenic diacylglycerol is formed from dihydroxylacetone phosphate of the glycolytic pathway through the action of a transferase, NADPH-dependent reductase, and acyl-CoA. The sphingomyelins are phospholipids that contain a complex amino alcohol, sphingol, in place of glycerol. Sphingosine is formed from palmitol-CoA and serine through a series of enzyme reactions followed by reaction with choline and acyl-CoA. Cerebrosides contain the sphingosine fatty acid combination with a galactose moiety. These may further react with activated sulfate to yield sulfa-

TABLE 1-5 PHOSPHOLIPIDS

Phosphatidic acid	— cardiolipid
Phosphatidylcholine	— lecithin
Phosphatidylethanolamine	— cephalin
Phosphatidylinositol	— lipositol
Phosphatidylserine	— cephalin-like
Lysophospholipids	— lysolecithins
Plasmalogens	—
Sphingomyelin	—

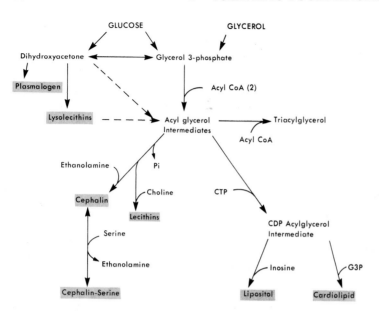

Figure 1–4 Biosynthesis of phospholipids.

tides. An alternate pathway for sphingomyelin synthesis is to form ceramide, a sphingosine-acyl derivative, and then add choline. Ceramide may also react with galactose and *N*-acetylneuraminic acid to form a ganglioside.

These numerous phospholipids play a vital role in the structural integrity of cells and biochemical pathways of many tissues, the details of which are beyond the scope of this review. Their clinical importance lies in inherited enzyme deficiencies which are associated primarily with accumulation. In the case of sulfatides, accumulations result in metachromatic-leukodystrophy, sphingomyelin in Niemann-Pick disease, and gangliosides in Tay-Sachs disease. Under normal circumstances, degradation involves the enzymatic hydrolysis into individual components with turnover at their own rates.

PROSTAGLANDINS

The prostaglandins are a series of 20-carbon (eicosanoic) acids derived from fatty acids. The basic structure, prostanoic acid, consists of two carbon chains bonded at the middle by a five-member ring. Variations in double bonds and functional groups give rise to 14 compounds divided into four divisions: A, B, E, and F. The prostaglandins exhibit hormone-like activity and appear to have potential therapeutic uses.

CHOLESTEROL

All steroids have a similar cyclic nucleus that resembles three phenanthrene rings to which a cyclopentane is added. The positions within the steroid nucleus have been internationally defined (Fig. 1–5). Cholesterol is based on this steroid nucleus. Most of cholesterol is synthesized in the body. Dietary cholesterol, however, does affect the production and plasma levels. Cholesterol synthesis involves the microsomal and cytosol fraction of the cell and occurs in such tissues as liver, adrenal cortex, intestine, and aorta. Synthesis can be broken down into three basic phases (Fig. 1–6).

The first phase is the formation of mevalonate, which uses a pathway involving condensation of

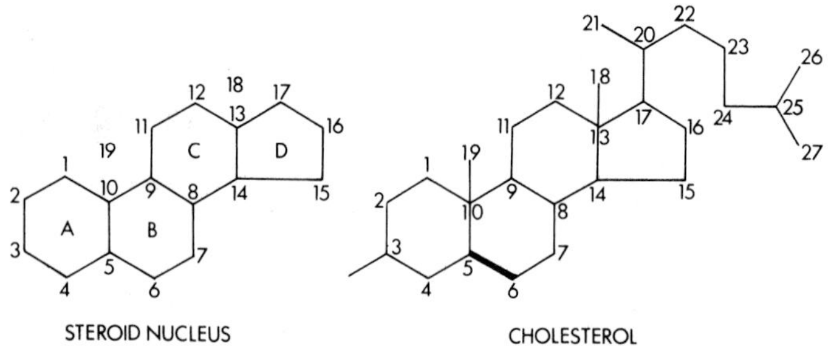

STEROID NUCLEUS   CHOLESTEROL

Figure 1–5 The steroid nucleus with standardized numbering for carbon atoms. The similarity of cholesterol can be seen.

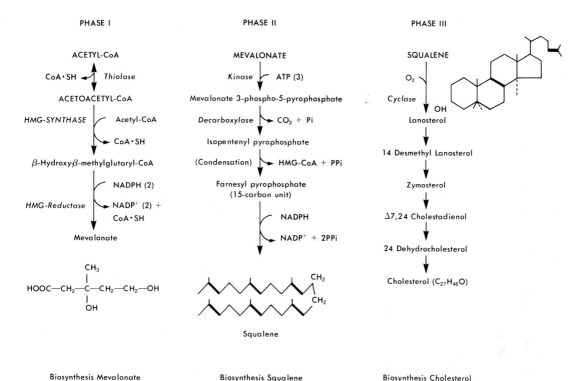

Figure 1-6 Biosynthesis of cholesterol involves three phases. First, the development of mevalonate. Second, the condensation to squalene. Third, the ring closure and modification to cholesterol.

acetyl-CoA molecules into a six-carbon structure. Reduction by NADPH yields mevalonate.

Phase two initially involves phosphorylation of mevalonate, and is followed by a series of steps involving decarboxylation, condensation of molecules, and a final reduction with the elimination of a pyrophosphate. The end-product is squalene, a 30-carbon unit.

The third phase of cholesterol synthesis involves the closure of squalene to form lanosterol, which has the familiar ring form structure of cholesterol. This phase appears to occur with squalene attached to a carrier protein. Through a series of changes to the side chains and steroid nucleus involving the loss of three methyl groups, cholesterol is formed. Cholesterol on the protein carrier may then be converted to bile acids or steroid hormones. Cholesterol is incorporated into very low density lipoprotein (VLDL) and low density lipoprotein (LDL) for transport in plasma.

Control of synthesis occurs early in the pathway through a feedback inhibition by cholesterol on the reductive enzyme forming mevalonate. Inhibition by cAMP has also been reported. Approximately one half the cholesterol eliminated from the body is excreted in feces after conversion to bile acids. The rest is lost as neutral steroids derived from cholesterol in the intestinal mucosa and converted to neutral steroids by bacteria in the lower intestine.

PLASMA LIPIDS

Dietary cholesterol is absorbed from the intestine, following which 80 to 90 per cent undergoes esterification with long-chain fatty acids. The esterified cholesterol is incorporated into chylomicrons and VLDL and transported via the lymphatics to plasma. Exogenous cholesterol will suppress endogenous production in liver but cannot eliminate it. Intestinal cholesterol synthesis is little affected by dietary cholesterol, since it seems to be controlled by bile acids. In a similar fashion, cholesterol causes feedback inhibition of its own synthesis. Equilibration of dietary cholesterol with plasma cholesterol takes several days.

Fatty acids in plasma are derived from lipolysis in adipose tissue and from the action of lipoprotein lipase on chylomicrons and VLDL. Carried by albumin, FFA are rapidly removed from circulation by tissues to be utilized in lipid synthesis pathways or to provide energy. In the fasting state, 25 to 50 per cent of energy is derived after β-oxidation of fatty acids and oxidation in the citric acid cycle.

Four major lipid-protein fractions are found in plasma: chylomicrons, VLDL, LDL, and HDL (Table 1-6). One or more apoproteins may be associated with the lipids. The apoproteins are grouped into four divisions: apo-A, B, C, and arginine-rich. The apoproteins associated with

TABLE 1–6

Lipoprotein	Apoprotein	Major Lipid
Chlomicron	B, CI II III	T
VLDL	B, CI II III Arg-rich	T
LDL	B	C
HDL	AI II, CI II III Arg-rich	P, C

T = triglyceride
C = cholesterol
P = phospholipid

the lipoprotein fractions are indicated in Table 1–6. A, B, C, and arginine-rich apoproteins contain carbohydrate components and represent glycoproteins. Elements of cholesterol, triglycerides, and phospholipids are present in each lipoprotein group; however, one or more may dominate over the other members. In Table 1–6 the dominant lipid component of each lipoprotein is listed.

Chylomicrons are formed in the gastrointestinal cell by incorporation of the apoprotein B synthesized by ribosomes with triglyceride, phospholipid, and cholesterol synthesized in the endoplasmic reticulum. Some portion of VLDL is also formed in the intestinal tract, although most is derived from the liver by incorporation of apoprotein and lipid in a similar fashion as chylomicrons in the intestine. Release from the cell in both processes is by reverse pinocytosis. The level of chylomicrons and, to a lesser extent, VLDL fluctuates with dietary levels of triglycerides. Apoprotein C is added to the chylomicrons and VLDL by transfer from HDL in the plasma.

Chylomicrons are rapidly cleared from plasma at the tissue interface by the action of lipase. About 80 per cent are removed by tissues other than liver. In fact, lipoprotein lipase, essential in clearing chylomicrons from plasma, is not found in significant quantities in hepatic tissue. The liver appears more important in processing lipoprotein remnants. Both phospholipids and apoprotein C–II are essential for lipoprotein lipase activity. In the extrahepatic tissue the triglyceride is hydrolyzed and fatty acids are released for endogenous use or into plasma. The apoprotein C on the chylomicron is transferred to HDL to be reused. A smaller, residual molecule on apoprotein B composed primarily of cholesterol and some triglyceride is taken up in the liver and further broken down. It has been suggested that a part of this remnant may form LDL. Most VLDL is produced in the liver as a transport vehicle for endogenously produced triglycerides. The VLDL produced in the liver, as well as that from the gastrointestinal tract, undergoes a similar degradation process to chylomicrons in extrahepatic tissues and the liver. In this case, the hepatic-processed remnant is the major source of body LDL. Evidence suggests that degradation of LDL occurs in fibroblasts. HDL is formed in the liver and intestine. Hepatic HDL is coated before release with the apoprotein C, while intestinal HDL acquires its apoprotein C by transfer from hepatic HDL.

The lipoproteins of endogenous sources are primarily hepatic in origin. Under normal circumstances, triglycerides are rapidly released from the liver. Carbohydrates encourage hepatic fatty acid and triglyceride synthesis. On carbohydrate restricted or high fat diets, increased levels of free fatty acids are found in plasma.

KETONES

Acetoacetate, β-hydroxybutyrate, and acetone represent a group of compounds known as ketone bodies. They are formed by mitochondrial enzymes in the *liver* under conditions involving a high rate of fatty acid oxidation. Acetoacetyl-CoA is the initial molecule in ketogenesis and is formed either as a final two-carbon element in β-oxidation or by condensation of two acetyl-CoA molecules. Acetoacetyl-CoA condenses with acetyl-CoA to form an intermediate that is enzymatically attracted to yield β-hydroxy-β-methylglutaryl-CoA and free acetoacetate. The carbons of the original acetyl-CoA are found in the acetoacetate molecule. β-hydroxybutyrate is formed by the action of a NADH-specific dehydrogenase enzyme on acetoacetyl-CoA. Acetoacetic and β-hydroxylbutyric acids are moderately strong acids that, in excessive amounts, deplete alkali reserves, resulting in clinical ketoacidosis.

Acetoacetate can be taken up in extrahepatic tissue and reactivated to acetoacetyl-CoA. Reactivation cannot occur in the liver. It can then be split by thiolase to acetyl-CoA and oxidized in the citric acid cycle. β-hydroxybutyrate can be reactivated by thiokinase and converted by dehydrogenation to acetoacetyl-CoA to be split and processed in the citric acid cycle. Acetone is formed spontaneously by decarboxylation of acetoacetic acid. Degradation is thought to occur by reversal of decarboxylase. Extrahepatic tissues utilize ketone bodies as energy substrates. They will be oxidized in preference to glucose and fatty acids. At approximately 70 mg./dl. the oxidation pathway becomes saturated, and further increases in ketones cause a rise in blood and urinary concentrations. In severely diabetic rats, studies suggest that ketonemia may also be increased by reduced catabolism, as well as by increased production.

CITRIC ACID CYCLE

The citric acid cycle, also known as the Krebs or tricarboxylic acid cycle, is an essential biochemical sequence providing the final pathway in carbohydrate, lipid, and amino acid oxidation (Fig. 1–7). It is an energy production system that, through a series of mitochondrial reactions, generates high-energy phosphate directly and through coupling with the respiratory chain.

Acetyl residues in an activated state associated with coenzyme A condense with a four-carbon molecule, oxaloacetate, and water in an essentially irreversible mode to form a six-carbon citrate molecule. The coenzyme bond is hydrolyzed in this process, and CoA is split away. Citrate then reacts with an iron-containing enzyme and, by dehydration and rehydration, forms isocitrate. Isocitrate undergoes a dehydrogenation with an NAD-dependent enzyme to form oxalosuccinate which, on decarboxylation, converts to α-ketoglutarate. The next reaction involves the irreversible oxidative decarboxylation in a series of steps associated with thiamine diphosphate, lipoate, NAD^+, FAD, and CoA similar to the process in converting pyruvate to acetyl-CoA. This process yields succinyl-CoA and a reduction of NAD to NADH. Succinyl-CoA is converted to succinate by splitting off CoA in the presence of inorganic phosphate. A high-energy phosphate (GPT) is produced in this step that can be transferred to ADP, forming ATP. Succinate, in the presence of flavoprotein-specific dehydrogenase, is converted to fumarate. Water is added to fumarate to yield malate, which is converted to oxaloacetate by malate dehydrogenase. In this step, a third molecule of NADH is produced. Two carbon atoms are lost

in one turn of the cycle, neither from the initial acetyl-CoA. Following a second revolution of the cycle, the initial two entry carbons will be lost as CO_2. The three molecules of NADH and one of $FADH_2$ produced by one turn of the citric acid cycle can be transferred to the respiratory chain. NADH will yield three high-energy phosphates and $FADH_2$ will yield two. Including the high energy bond produced in the cycle, a total of 12 phosphate bonds are formed.

The citric acid cycle provides a focal point for glucogenesis and fatty acid synthesis in the liver and kidney. In fatty acid synthesis, acetyl-CoA is transported out of the mitochondria after conversion to citrate and then is reconverted in the cytosol to acetyl-CoA for incorporation into fatty acids. Transamination and deamination of amino acids yields intermediates of the citric acid cycle or pyruvate. These may be converted to oxaloacetate which via malate may gain access to the cytosol and give rise to glucose by gluconeogenesis. Pyruvate may also give rise to acetyl-CoA for oxidation in the citric acid cycle or conversion to fatty acids.

AMINO ACIDS

Amino acids are the basic building blocks of proteins and are responsible for determining many of the properties of proteins. The general structural formula for amino acids is

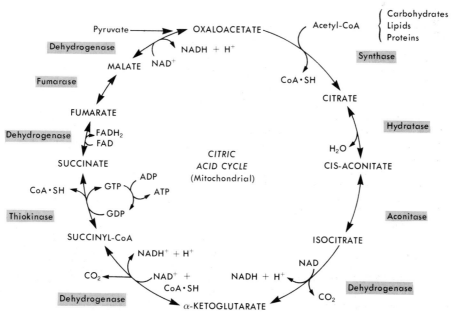

Figure 1–7 The citric acid cycle (Krebs cycle) provides a pathway for oxidation of carbohydrates, protein, and lipids.

TABLE 1–7 AMINO ACIDS

Classification	Names (trivial/symbolic/systematic)	
Non-polar hydrophobic	Alanine (Ala)	2-Aminopropanoic acid
	Leucine (Leu)	2-Amino-4-methylpentanoic acid
	Isoleucine (Ile)	2-Amino-3-methylpentanoic acid
	Phenylalanine (Phe)	2-Amino-3-phenylpropanic acid
	Valine (Val)	2-Amino-3-methylbutanoic acid
	Proline (Pro)	2-Pyrrolidinecarboxylic acid
	Methionine (Met)	2-Amino-4-(methylthio) butanoic acid
	Tryptophan (Trp)	2-Amino-3-(3-indolyl)propanoic acid
Neutral polarity	Serine (Ser)	2-Amino-3-hydroxypropanoic acid
	Threonine (Thr)	2-Amino-3-hydroxylbutanoic acid
	Tyrosine (Tyr)	2-Amino-3(4-hydroxyphenyl)propanoic acid
	Asparagine (Agn)	2-Amino-succinamic acid
	Glutamine (Gln)	2-Aminoglutaramic acid
	Cysteine (Cys)	2-Amino-3-mercaptopropanoic acid
	Glycine (Gly)	Aminoacetic acid
Positively charged	Lysine (Lys)	2,6-Diaminohexanoic acid
	Arginine (Arg)	2-Amino-5-guanidovaleric acid
	Histidine (His)	2-Amino-1H-imidazole-4-propanoic acid
Negatively charged	Aspartic acid (Asp)	Aminosuccinic acid
	Glutamic acid (Glu)	2-Aminoglutaric acid

$$\begin{array}{c} NH_2 \\ | \\ R-C-COOH. \\ | \\ H \end{array}$$ With the exception of two amino acids, those in proteins have the amino and carboxyl groups attached to the same alpha carbon. At pH 7.4 the amino group exists in a conjugated acid form ($R\text{-}NH_3^+$) and the carboxyl group in its conjugated base form ($R\text{-}COO^-$).

Only 20 of the many amino acids available in nature are involved in the protein structure. These 20 amino acids can be classified into subdivisions based on the charge or lack of charge of their R- group. These subdivisions consist of the non-polar or hydrophobic R- groups, uncharged (neutral) polar R- groups, positively charged R-groups, and negatively charged R- groups (Table 1–7). They may also be grouped on the basis of side chain molecular structure. Amino acids, with the exception of glycine, are optically active and may occur in levorotatory or dextrorotatory forms. In proteins, the levorotatory form is encountered. The characteristics of amino acids are due to the reactions of the functional side chain groups and the carboxyl and amino groups.

AMINO ACID CATABOLISM

Amino acids are versatile molecules that, upon catabolism, give rise to nitrogen, which can be converted to various nitrogenous products, and to carbon components, which may enter several pathways. Thirteen of the amino acids are gly-

TABLE 1–8 AMINO ACID CONVERTIBILITY

Glycogenic	Glycogenic-Ketogenic	Ketogenic
Alanine	Lysine	Leucine
Arginine	Tryptophan	
Cystine	Isoleucine	
Aspartate	Phenylalanine	
Glutamate	Tyrosine	
Glycine		
Histidine		
Hydroxyproline		
Methionine		
Proline		
Serine		
Threonine		
Valine		

cogenic. An additional five amino acids may be converted to either carbohydrates or ketones. One amino acid is solely ketogenic (Table 1–8).

In Figure 1–8 the entry points of the various amino acids into the citric acid cycle, glycolysis pathway and ketones are indicated. Eleven of the amino acids form acetyl-CoA — either directly, via pyruvate, or via acetoacetyl-CoA. Twelve amino acids are converted to citric acid cycle intermediates: five as α-ketoglutarate, three as succinyl-CoA, two as oxaloacetate, and two as fumarate. Certain amino acids' carbon skeletons can enter the citric acid cycle directly; others require extensive modification or cleavage for entry into the cycle. Those amino acids that form

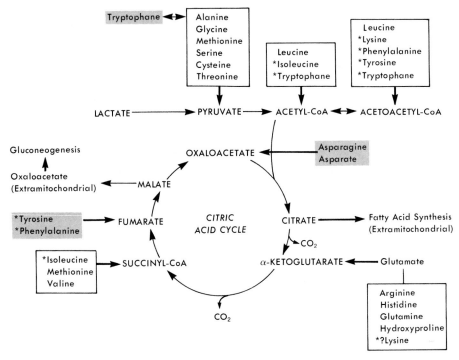

* = Both ketogenic and glycogenic.

Figure 1–8 Route for amino acid metabolism.

pyruvate have an option, by conversion to acetyl-CoA, to undergo complete oxidation in the citric acid cycle or, by conversion to oxaloacetic acid, to give rise to glucose.

Glycogenic amino acids, after removal of the amino group by transaminase or oxidative deamination reactions, provide a carbon skeleton that can be metabolized to citric acid cycle intermediates in the liver or kidney. All of them eventually form oxaloacetate in the mitochondrial citric acid cycle and are transported as malate or citrate to the cytosol for reconversion to oxaloacetate. Oxaloacetate in the cytosol is converted by decarboxylation, with GTP supplying high energy phosphate, to phosphoenolpyruvate, an intermediate in the glycolytic pathway. By modified reversal of glycolysis, glucose or glycogen may be formed.

Five amino acids listed in Table 1–8 are both glycogenic and ketogenic. This combined activity is derived from the fact that lysine, isoleucine, phenylalanine, and tyrosine are converted upon degradation to ketogenic acetyl-CoA or acetoacetyl-CoA and intermediate products of the citric acid cycle. Tryptophan can be converted to ketogenic by-products or directly to alanine, which is glycogenic.

Leucine yields neither pyruvate nor citric acid cycle intermediates during catabolism and, therefore, is not glucogenic. It is converted directly into acetyl-CoA. There is no metabolic pathway by which carbons of acetyl-CoA can give rise to new glucose. The carbons can, however, be incorporated into the glucose molecule. The acetyl-CoA can combine with oxaloacetate in the citric acid cycle to form citrate. During excessive production of amino acids, there is a large input into the citric acid cycle of intermediates, which increase the citrate concentration in the mitochondria. Transported from mitochondria to cytosol, citrate may be cleaved into oxaloacetate and acetyl-CoA. The acetyl-CoA is immediately available for fatty acid synthesis and the oxaloacetate is available for gluconeogenesis.

In catabolism of the amino acids, the amino group may be removed by amino transferases or transaminases and transferred to an alpha carbon of an α-keto acid. This yields an amino form of the ketoacid and the α-keto acid analogue of the amino acid (Fig. 1–9). Two common transaminases use α-ketoglutarate or pyruvate as the keto acid. When α-ketoglutarate is used, glutamate is produced. When pyruvate is used, alanine is formed. Glutamate and alanine may then serve as amino group donors for oxidative deamination to nitrogenous products or amino acid production. Transaminases all have a pyridoxal phosphate prosthetic group and are found in the mitochondria and cytosols of cells. They can act on most amino acids, and the reactions are reversible. These reactions are important for the concentration of cytoplasmic amino groups, primarily by

(1) α amino acid + α-Ketoglutarate $\xrightarrow{\text{transaminase}}$ α-keto acid + Glutamate

(2) Glutamate + NAD$^+$ $\xrightarrow{\text{Deaminase}}$ NADH + α Ketoglutarate + NH$_3$

(3) NH$_3$ + CO$_2$ + ATP + Ornithine cycle $\longrightarrow$ Urea + ornithine cycle

Figure 1–9 Generalized example of the process of transamination, deamination, and urea formation.

formation of glutamate which can then be transported into the mitochondria and undergo oxidative deamination. Most of the concentration of amino groups is centered around glutamate, which, through the action of glutamate dehydrogenase and the coenzyme NAD$^+$ or NADP$^+$ yields α-ketoglutarate and ammonia (NH$_3$) (Fig. 1–9). This reaction may occur both in the cytoplasm and the mitochondria and may accept amino groups from most amino acids. In the mitochondria, the reduced coenzyme may enter the respiratory chain.

UREA SYNTHESIS

Both endogenously produced ammonia from transamination and deamination in tissue and that formed by intestinal bacteria are toxic and must be eliminated from the body or modified. Intestinal ammonia is rapidly removed by the liver and may be reused for amino acid synthesis along with endogenous ammonia by reversal of deamination. The remainder is excreted as urea or uric acid. Only trace levels of ammonia are found in blood.

Besides reversal of deamination, ammonia may react with glutamic acid in an ATP-dependent

step to form glutamine. This is a major pathway in brain tissue for removal of ammonia. The glutamine formed in tissue may be transported to kidney and converted back to ammonia, where it plays a major role in acid-base balance, or to the liver, where glutamine may be hydrolyzed to yield ammonia for conversion to urea. Most ammonia is transported to the liver as glutamine.

The production of urea involves a cyclic pathway. Beginning in the mitochondria, ammonia condenses irreversibly with carbon dioxide in the presence of two ATP molecules to form carbamoyl phosphate (Fig. 1–10). In the next step, a carbamoyl group ($-\overset{\overset{\displaystyle O}{\|}}{C}-NH_2$) is donated to ornithine, forming citrulline, which diffuses into the cytosol. At this point, the second amino group is added. It is derived from aspartate and involves a condensation of aspartate and a carbamoyl group of citrulline to form argininosuccinate. ATP is again required in the reaction. The aspartate is formed by the action of aspartate transaminase on glutamate. Next, fumaric acid is cleaved from the argininosuccinate, forming arginine. The last step involves hydrolysis with cleavage of the guanidino group of arginine, reforming ornithine

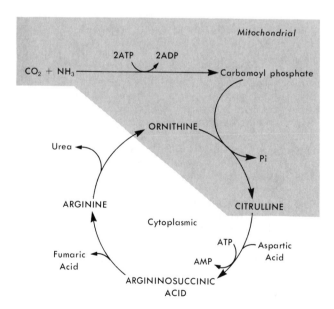

Figure 1–10 Urea synthesis.

TABLE 1–9 NUTRITIONALLY ESSENTIAL AMINO ACIDS

Arginine
Histidine
Isoleucine
Leucine
Methionine
Phenylalanine
Threonine
Tryptophan
Valine

and releasing urea ($C=O$ with two NH_2 groups). Urea formed in the liver is the major pathway of nitrogen excretion in man. It accounts for 95 per cent of the nitrogen eliminated by the kidney. The cycle costs three moles of ATP, ammonia, CO_2, and aspartate. Three of the amino acids involved do not occur in proteins; these are ornithine, citrulline, and argininosuccinate.

BIOSYNTHESIS OF AMINO ACIDS

As in the case of lipids, man can synthesize some amino acids, but not all. Thus, the latter are called *nutritionally essential amino acids* (Table 1–9). Ammonium ions serve as the nitrogen source for their synthesis. A series of multi-enzyme steps, many of which are complex, are required for the synthesis of nutritionally essential amino acids by bacteria or plants. These synthesis pathways differ, except for a few common points, from the degradation pathways. The biosynthetic pathways for nutritionally nonessential amino acids are, on the other hand, relatively short. They involve three basic methods: first, synthesis from intermediates of glycolysis, as occurs in formation of serine and glycine; second, the utilization of citric acid cycle intermediates, as occurs in the formation of alanine, glutamate, and aspartate; third, the utilization of other amino acids (Table 1–10). Regulation of synthesis is generally through feedback inhibition or enzyme synthesis repression.

Amino acids or portions of their structure contribute to the synthesis of many other products. These include hormones, coenzymes, porphyrins, vitamins, and pigments. The details of these many reactions are beyond the scope of this limited review; however, several examples of specific by-products will be listed. Glycine contributes both the α carbon and nitrogen atoms in the synthesis of porphyrins in hemoglobin. Methionine is a common precursor for formation of methylated molecules. Cysteine is involved in coenzyme A synthesis. Serine is an important fraction of some phospholipids. Tryptophan is the precursor of serotonin; tyrosine is the precursor of melanin, epinephrine, and norepinephrine. Arginine, glycine, and methionine are precursors of creatine, an important storehouse of energy in muscle. Creatinine, the anhydrous form of creatine, is formed by the irreversible nonenzymatic removal of water with the loss of phosphate.

PROTEINS

Proteins are formed by a series of amino acids that are linked by a covalent peptide bond (Fig. 1–11). In the simplest terms, the peptide bond is formed by reaction of an alpha amino group and alpha carboxyl group of separate amino acids with the loss of one mole of water. The uniqueness of

TABLE 1–10 NUTRITIONALLY NONESSENTIAL AMINO ACID SYNTHESIS

	Intermediate	Enzyme	Amino Acid
Citric acid	Oxaloacetate/glutamate	Transaminase	Aspartic acid
	α-ketoglutarate	Dehydrogenase	Glutamic acid
	Pyruvate/glutamate	Transaminase	Alanine
Glycolysis	3-Phosphoglycerate/glutamate	Transaminase	Serine
	Pyruvate/glyoxylate	Transaminase	Glycine
	$CO_2 + NH_3$	Synthetase	Glycine
Amino Acid	Serine	Transferase	Glycine
	Glutamic acid	Kinase/dehydrogenase	Proline
	Proline (protein bound)	Oxygenase	Hydroxyproline
	Methionine/serine	Transulfuration	Cysteine
	Phenylalanine	Oxygenase	Tyrosine
	Glutamic acid	Synthetase	Glutamine
	Aspartic acid	Synthetase	Asparagine

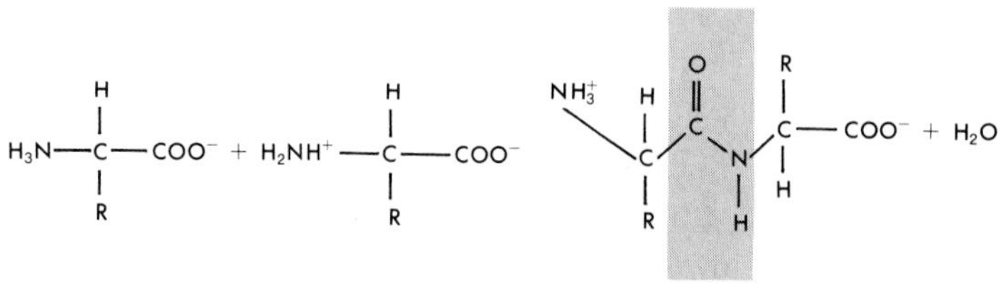

Figure 1–11 Simple formation of the peptide bond.

each protein lies in the arrangement of its amino acids. This explanation of peptide bond formation is not sufficient, however, in terms of the events in the cell. In the cell this reaction occurs on the ribosome and involves several forms of ribonucleic acid. Genetic information that establishes a protein's amino acid sequence is stored in the DNA nucleotide sequence. This information is transcribed and appears in the cytoplasm on messenger RNA (mRNA). The cell possesses the mechanism to translate information of mRNA into the sequence of amino acids. It does this through an adapter molecule, transfer RNA (tRNA), that recognizes the specific nucleotide sequence, as well as the counterpart amino acid. The process occurs on the ribosome. Since 20 amino acids are involved in protein formation, a similar number of distinct codes are available to identify them. These codes are carried by the nucleotides in mRNA and consist of a three-nucleotide codon providing the potential for 64 individual codes. Two of the 64 are "nonsense codons," which provide a signal to terminate the amino acid polymer. As there are 61 codons left for 20 amino acids, some amino acids have more than one codon. A single tRNA molecule possesses the proper anticodon for a given codon or codons in mRNA needed to recognize and provide an amino acid. Each amino acid added to the peptide chain requires its own tRNA. The tRNA differ from each other in their nucleotide sequences. The recognition by tRNA of its specific amino acid occurs through reaction with the enzyme, aminoacyl-tRNA synthetases. The synthetase enzymes are highly specific for a particular amino acid and tRNA. The reaction between the amino acid and enzyme occurs in the cytoplasm and requires ATP conversion to AMP. The endproduct is an aminoacyl-AMP-enzyme complex or activated amino acid. This amino acid-enzyme complex then recognizes its specific tRNA and attaches the amino acid at the 3′-hydroxyladenosyl terminus by an ester linkage. Once attached, the amino acid plays no role in the recognition of the steps to follow.

Transfer RNA can be thought of as a simple cross. At the top the amino acid is bonded at the ACC terminus; to the left, the thymidine-pseudouridine-cytidine loop binds to the ribosome surface; the base represents the nucleotide anticodon; and to the right there is a dihydrouracil loop. The ribosome contains two nucleoprotein subunits — a 60S unit and a 40S unit. The mRNA binds to the 40S ribosome under the influence of a protein initiation factor 3 (IF-3). Aminoacyl-tRNA interacts with GTP and initiation factor 2 (IF-2) to form a complex that, in the presence of initiation factor 1(IF-1), attaches the tRNA to the 40S ribosome. The initiation factors are released and the 40S ribosome particle merges with the 60S unit, hydrolyzing GTP and forming the 80S unit on which there are two binding sites for tRNA. The aminoacyl-tRNA entered initially at the P site, leaving the second, or A site, free. The next step involves the formation of a peptide bond and elongation of the peptide unit. The second amino acid in an activated state is carried by its tRNA to the A site, where it reacts with an elongation factor (EF-1) and GTP to form a complex. At this time, EF-1 and GDP are released. The amino acid at site A carries out a nucleophilic attachment on the esterified carboxyl group of the amino acid-tRNA at site P under the influence of a transferase. The aminoacyl residue is transferred from the P site tRNA to A site tRNA to form a dipeptide. The tRNA at site P is then discharged and, by the action of EF-2 and GTP, the tRNA at site A is relocated to the P site. Site A is now free for another amino acid-tRNA.

The initiation of the peptide chain begins when the amino acid methionine is brought into the ribosome as N-formylmethionyl-tRNA. Termination of the peptide chain is signaled by a nonsense codon on mRNA appearing at site A. As there is no tRNA that recognizes this, the peptide chain is complete. A releasing factor and enzyme then hydrolyze the bond between the peptide chain and tRNA at the P site. Once the protein is released, the ribosome dissociates to its subunits.

Considerable energy is used in peptide formation. The equivalent of four ATP molecules are required to activate the amino acids, and three GTP molecules are needed for attachment to the ribosome and translocation.

Simple proteins yield amino acids upon hydrolysis; conjugated proteins yield not only amino acids, but also organic components referred to as prosthetic groups.

Each protein has a characteristic three-dimensional shape or conformation that permits classification. The *primary structure* of a protein refers to the basic sequence of covalent linked amino acids. The *secondary structure* refers to the recurring arrangement along one dimension of the polypeptide chain. This is formed by disulfide or hydrogen bonds. Hydrogen bonds are formed by nitrogen and carboxyl oxygen of separate peptides sharing a hydrogen atom. A common secondary conformation is the α helix, which consists of a coiled backbone of peptide units. This permits maximal intrachain hydrogen bonding between coils of the helix. The helix has approximately 3.6 amino acids per turn, with hydrogen bonds between every fourth amino acid. The *tertiary structure* refers to the manner in which polypeptide chains bend and fold in three dimensions to form globular proteins. Weak associations or bonds are responsible for stabilizing this conformation. These are hydrogen bonds between peptide R- groups, hydrophobic interactions between non-polar R- groups, and ionic bonds between oppositely charged side chains. The *quaternary structure* refers to the configuration that develops when individual polypeptide chains group about each other.

The basic properties of the polypeptide are due to the nature of the R- side chains, the size of the amino acid polymer, its three-dimensional structure, and associated organic or inorganic molecules. The forces maintaining the confirmation of proteins can be interrupted by strong acids or bases, heat, heavy metal, and organic solvents. This process is referred to as denaturation.

Proteins may be classified by several methods. Common classifications group proteins as fibrous or globular, simple or conjugated, and by their relative solubility and antigenic properties. Examples of fibrous proteins are keratin, collagen, and elastin. In the clinical setting, solubility is used to separate proteins into albumin and globulins. More important are the collected ionic properties of the amino acids in proteins which permit electrophoretic separation into numerous fractions. For clinical purposes, these are grouped into five classes: albumin, α_1-globulins, α_2-globulins, β-globulins, and gamma globulins. Albumin consists of a single polypeptide chain in a globular form. It functions as a non-specific transport and provides considerable osmotic pressure. The main alpha$_1$ globulins are glycoproteins and high-density lipoproteins; the main alpha$_2$ globulins are haptoglobin, ceruloplasmin, prothrombin, glycoproteins, and VLDL. The major beta globulins are transferrin and LDL. The gamma globulins represent the immunoglobulins.

Proteins in the body are constantly broken down and resynthesized. This turnover is measured by the half-life of proteins, which is approximately 80 days for the average body protein. The average, weight-stable man degrades and synthesizes 400 gm. of protein a day. Most of the nitrogen metabolized in the body is contained in protein.

Although this discussion of polypeptide chains has referred primarily to protein, physiologically active free peptides exist. Two common ones are glutathione and bradykinin. In some cases, free peptides represent by-products of protein degradation.

PURINE AND PYRIMIDINE METABOLISM

Figure 1–12 shows the nitrogenous heterocyclic structures of purine and pyrimidine. In man there are three major pyrimidines — cytosine, thymine, and uracil — and two major purines — adenine and guanine. Humans can meet their need for these bases by endogenous synthesis and, therefore, need not rely on dietary sources.

Nucleotides are composed of a purine or pyrimidine base, to which a sugar is attached at N_1 or N_9 position. Free purine and pyrimidines and their nucleosides occur only in trace amounts in cells. Nucleotides are nucleosides phosphorylated on the hydroxyl groups of the sugar. These occur in significant amounts in cells. The pentose sugars incorporated in nucleosides are usually D-ribose or 2-deoxyribose bonded by a N-glycosidic bond. For example, the purine, adenine, plus a D-ribose sugar, yields adenine ribonucleoside, or adenosine; when phosphorylated, the result is adenosine monophosphate or adenylate. The abbreviations A, G, C, T, and U may be used to designate a nucleoside base. The prefix "D" is added to the nucleoside to indicate a deoxyribose sugar.

The synthesis pathway for purine in the cytosol is complex and involves the assemblage of the molecule from amino acids and carbon donors. Synthesis involves the phosphorylation of ribose 5-phosphate and ATP to 1-pyrophosphorylribosyl-5-phosphate (PRPP). Glutamine then adds nitrogen (N-9), which is followed by the addition of glycine to form N-7 and carbons 5 and 4 (C-5,4). This step requires ATP. Tetrahydrofolate carrier adds a formyl group at C-8. A second glutamine adds a nitrogen (N-3), again requiring ATP. Under the influence of a third ATP, the imidazole ring is closed, to be followed by a carboxylation reaction adding C-6 from CO_2. Aspartate provides N-1 and formul-tetrafolate provides C-2, completing the basic inosine monophosphate molecule. This molecule is then converted by amination or by oxidation and amination to guanosine monophosphate (GMP) or adenosine monophosphate

PURINE BASE   PYRIMIDINE BASE

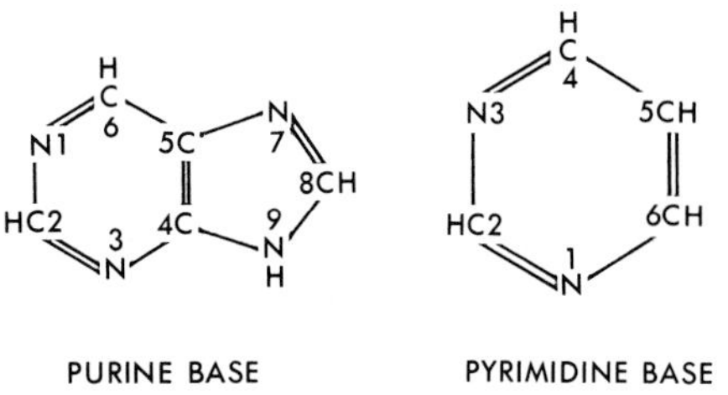

Figure 1–12 Structure of purine and pyrimidine bases, numbered by international system.

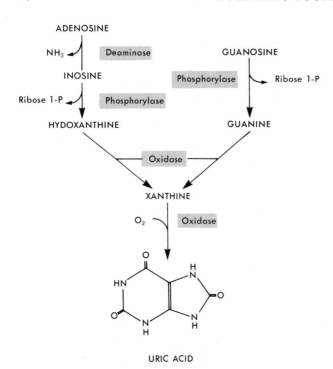

Figure 1–13 Formation of uric acid from purine nucleosides.

(AMP). The monophosphates can be converted to diphosphates or triphosphates by transfer of high energy groups.

Control of the purine synthesis is primarily directed by the availability of ribose 5-phosphate. Synthesis of ribose 5-phosphate depends on the availability of its substrate and feedback inhibition of the synthesis enzymes by purine. Salvage pathways are available in the body to convert free purine to nucleoside or to phosphorylate nucleotide to limit the loss of purine and to supply tissues that are incapable of purine synthesis. These salvage pathways also involve the interconversion of IMP, GMP, and deoxyribonucleotides to nucleosides.

Catabolism of purine involves conversion to uric acid. The purine nucleoside is acted upon by a phosphorylase to yield the free bases guanine or hypoxanthine. Both of these may be converted to xanthine, which, under the influence of xanthine oxidase, yields uric acid (Fig. 1–13).

The pyrimidine nucleotide synthesis requires PRPP, glutamine, CO_2 and aspartate. Thymidine also requires a tetrahydrofolate derivative. Unlike purine synthesis, the pyrimidine nucleus is formed separately from the PRPP and added later. Synthesis begins in the cytosol, with the carbamoyl phosphate of glutamine providing N-1 and CO_2 providing C-2. The step is ATP-dependent. The carbamoyl phosphate condenses with aspartate, which provides C-4, 5, 6, and N-3. Upon the loss of water a ring structure is formed. Through a series of reductase, transferase, and decarboxy-

lase steps, the molecule is altered, and ribose 5-phosphate is added to form uridine monophosphate (UMP). This molecule may undergo further phosphorylation and amination by glutamine to cytidine triphosphate, or a methyl group can be donated by tetrahydrofolate to form thymidine monophosphate (TMP). Synthesis is controlled by feedback repression, and derepression mechanisms. Purine and pyrimidine are synthesized in a coordinated manner.

Catabolism of pyrimidine occurs mainly in the liver, beginning with the hydrolysis and removal of the ribose-phosphate. Following a NADPH-dependent oxidation and hydration, the ring is broken. In the final step, uracil and cytosine form alanine, CO_2, NH_3, and thymine forms isobutyric acid, CO_2, and NH_3. Salvage mechanisms are not available for the free pyrimidine bases but are available for the conversion of nucleosides to nucleotides.

The structure and metabolism of nucleic acids are discussed in Chapter 2 and will not be introduced here except to express the fact that the chemical nature of DNA consists of monomeric units of nucleotides linked by 3′5′-phosphodiester bridge.

METABOLIC REGULATION

The numerous energy-producing pathways thus far discussed are strictly controlled to provide the necessary continuous flow of energy for cells. These pathways require a constant supply of substrates, enzymes, and cofactors that must be met by the complex transport systems and interconnecting sequences. Factors must be available at the appropriate time and concentration to meet the individual tissue needs and to assure an orderly metabolic process under a variety of nutritional states.

Some reactants in a metabolic pathway reach a steady state; others are at constant non-equilibrium. Unless controlled, the non-equilibrious reactions would rapidly deplete substrates and force equilibrium changes in earlier steady state substrates. Control of pathways can best be exercised at the non-equilibrium steps. Such control is possible by limiting the enzyme concentration in the reaction, by providing enzyme regulation through feedback or forward control, by controlling the availability of cofactors, and by hormone influence as inducers or repressors of enzyme synthesis.

Obviously, changes in substrate concentration and end-product removal also provide regulatory activity. Clearly the blood levels of carbohydrates, fatty acids, and amino acids influence the metabolic processes in tissues. Changes in dietary components can indirectly affect metabolic pathways through hormonal mechanisms. Glucocorticoids, glucagon, and epinephrine, for example, function as inducers of glucogenic enzymes, whereas insulin suppresses these enzymes. Insulin, on the other hand, stimulates glycogenesis, the HMP shunt, and lipogenesis. Since these hormones are responsive to blood glucose, indirect control occurs.

The major organs of the body are capable of carrying out the essential metabolic sequences of glycolysis, citric acid cycle, and lipid and protein processes. Individual characteristics of tissue do exist. For example, the liver is the major absorber from the gastrointestinal tract and plays a significant role in the metabolite distribution. Two thirds of the glucose molecules resulting from digestion are phosphorylated in the liver; the rest circulate to other tissues. Other carbohydrates are totally processed in the liver. Amino acids absorbed by the gastrointestinal tract enter the liver and, like glucose, have several options. Some may pass to other tissues for protein synthesis, or they may provide amino acids for protein synethesis in the liver. Amino acids, when in excess, may provide energy, glucose, fatty acids, or other elements, such as porphyrins. The liver also plays the only role in urea formation. Lipids enter the liver from the gastrointestinal tract, either via the portal tract or the systemic circulation. The glycerol fraction of lipids is capable of providing glucose, fatty acid fraction, lipoproteins, energy, cholesterol, and ketones.

Adipose tissue utilizes both blood glucose and fatty acids for energy and synthesis. It provides a storehouse for energy in the synthesis of lipids. Similarly, skeletal muscle utilizes both blood glucose and fatty acids to provide energy. Much of the glucose used is stored as glycogen, which provides energy by metabolism to pyruvate or lactate. In muscle carbohydrates supply less energy than do lipids.

Blood glucose levels are rigidly regulated. Glucose uptake in liver and extrahepatic tissue is related to the concentration in blood. At normal blood glucose levels, the liver produces glucose; at higher levels, production ceases, and a net uptake occurs in liver and extrahepatic tissues. Insulin plays a central regulatory role in this process. It increases uptake by extrahepatic tissues and probably also by hepatic tissue. It appears to increase transport across the cell membranes in addition to stimulating pathway elements. As indicated earlier in this chapter, glucocorticoids lead to gluconeogenesis, resulting in increased protein catabolism and, thus, amino acid uptake in the liver. In addition, it inhibits utilization of amino acids in extrahepatic tissue. Growth hormone decreases glucose uptake in muscle and mobilizes fatty acids from adipose tissue. The resultant hyperglycemia stimulates insulin. Adrenocorticotropic hormone (ACTH) can directly enhance the release of fatty acids from adipose tissue, but primarily has its effect through glucocorticoids. Epinephrine stimulates glycogen breakdown through its activity on hepatic and muscle phosphorylase. Glucagon, stimulated by hypoglycemia, activates phosphorylase in a manner similar to epinephrine, causing glycogenolysis. It also stimulates gluconeogenesis by its effects on proteins.

In carbohydrate restriction, blood glucose levels are maintained by glycogenolysis. As glucagon levels rise, insulin falls and lipolysis increases, causing fat mobilization. Fatty acids impair oxidation of gluconeogenesis and phosphofructokinase. Fatty acids increasingly provide energy for the body. If endogenous gluconeogenesis falls behind glucose utilization, fat mobilization further increases. Under these circumstances, glycerol provides an important source for glucose.

Lipogenesis is the conversion of glucose and intermediates to fat. In a diet high in carbohydrates, lipogenesis is stimulated and fatty acid oxidation is spared in preference to esterification. In high-fat diets or carbohydrate restriction, the reverse occurs, and FFA levels rise in plasma. The rate-limiting step in lipogenesis appears at the acetyl-CoA carboxylase step by feedback inhibition of acyl-CoA. In effect, if acyl-CoA is not being utilized, further fatty acid synthesis is inhibited. Insulin stimulates lipogenesis by increasing cellular glucose uptake, the production of glycerol 3-phosphate, and the availability of NADPH produced via the HMP shunt. It also inhibits lipolysis by depression of cAMP. The reverse occurs in insulin deficiency. The increased acetyl-CoA may result in increases in cholesterol. Glucocorticoids, ACTH, and epinephrine all increase lipolysis.

Acetyl-CoA is not glucogenic as are certain amino acids, lactate, and glycerol. It is true that acetyl-CoA from β-oxidation may enter the citric acid cycle and that its carbons may end up in glucose or glycogen molecules. However, there is no net conversion to glucose, since the molecule of acetyl-CoA incorporated into the cycle requires one molecule of oxaloacetate. No net change occurs. Similarly, there is no net conversion of fatty acids to amino acids. However, the reverse reaction may occur, with glucogenic amino acids

yielding fatty acids by the formation of either pyruvate or acetyl-CoA. Although fatty acids cannot increase glucose, glycerol released upon hydrolysis of triglycerides is readily converted to glucose in the liver and kidney, where there are high levels of glycerokinase. In the presence of ATP, glycerol 3-phosphate is produced for gluconeogenesis.

Lactate is formed by glucose oxidation in skeletal muscle under anaerobic conditions. It is also formed in erythrocytes, which lack a citric acid cycle. In the Cori-cycle, lactate formed in the skeletal muscle is transported to the kidney or liver, converted to pyruvate, and, by gluconeogenesis, processed to glucose.

REFERENCES

Conn, E. E., and Stump, P. K.: Outlines of Biochemistry, 3rd ed. John Wiley and Sons, New York, 1972.

Dickens, F., Randle, P. J., and Whelan, W. J.: Carbohydrate Metabolism and its Disorders, Vols. 1 and 2, Academic Press, New York, 1968.

Dickerson, R. E., and Geis, I.: The structure and Action of Proteins. Harper and Row, New York, 1969.

Dixon, M., and Webb, E. C.: Enzymes, 2nd ed. Academic Press, New York, 1964.

Harper, H. A., Rodwell, V. W., and Mayes, P. A.: Review of Physiological Chemistry, 16th ed. Lange Medical Publications, Los Altos, 1977.

Hoffman, W. S.: The Biochemistry of Clinical Medicine, 4th ed. Year Book Medical Publishers, Chicago, 1970.

Lehninger, A. L.: Biochemistry, 2nd ed. Worth Publishers, New York, 1975.

Mallette, M. F., Clagett, C. O., Phillips, A. T., and McCarl, R. L.: Introductory Biochemistry. The Williams & Wilkins Co., Baltimore, 1971.

McGilvery, R. W.: Biochemistry. W. B. Saunders Co., Philadelphia, 1970.

Montgomery, R., Dryer, R. L., Conway, T. W., and Spector, A. A.: Biochemistry: A Case-Oriented Approach, 2nd ed. The C. V. Mosby Company, St. Louis, 1977.

Newsholme, E. A., and Start, C.: Regulation in Metabolism. John Wiley and Sons, New York, 1973.

2

Molecular Biology

K. Lemone Yielding

GENERAL INTRODUCTION

Our present understanding of the chemistry of biologic processes has made it possible to approach human diseases and their management in terms of molecular derangements. For some years interests in "molecular" disease were concerned with the description of examples of genetically determined molecular defects such as hemoglobinopathies, enzyme deficiencies, storage diseases, and the like; but now the whole array of biologic processes involved in human diseases and their treatment should come into focus. These include all aspects of the function of the human organism as well as those for the variety of parasites which impose their effects. This chapter will summarize the basic principles and our current data base for considering diseases as problems in molecular biology.

Molecular biology is based on two simplifying premises: first, that biologic processes can be explained in chemical terms and, in fact, that knowledge of molecular structure can provide the basis for understanding function; second, that the reality of evolutionary design in biologic systems means that knowledge of complex systems in man or other higher organisms can be gained through study of simple organisms (and vice versa). The power of both premises is well illustrated by the substantial advances which have occurred in recent years. The progress in our understanding based on structure information is especially impressive in the area of nucleic acids and information transfer. Undeniably, the description of the structural details of DNA (and RNA) opened the way to tremendous advances in understanding of function. Structure analysis has not yet revealed the details of function for all classes of biomolecules because of the complexity of their three-dimensional structure and the complexity of their potential interactions in the cell. Progress continues at an impressive rate, however, to confirm the principle that function can be rationalized by knowledge of structure. This first premise carried into the study of disease would mean that diseases could be explained by identifying and studying relevant abnormal molecules and their deficient or aberrant functions, and that therapy should consist of appropriate molecular adjustments.

A major problem is in detecting primary and secondary events in view of the molecular *cascading* seen in biologic systems. Studies of inherited diseases have emphasized the principle of cascading and the distinction between primary and secondary molecular changes in disease, since a single primary molecular defect attributed to a single mutant gene can lead to complex diseases. Genetic diseases, therefore, have provided means for understanding disease mechanisms in all organ systems and thus represent nature's "laboratory" for the study of molecular disease mechanisms. Therapy, too, is complicated by the occurrence of both primary and secondary drug effects which are subject to the same cascading phenomenon described for disease perturbations. An increased understanding of biologic process coupled with identification of molecular drug targets should accelerate the development of new therapeutic approaches. Diseases provide the "natural" experiment for studying functional consequences of specific molecule changes and thus warrant most exhaustive study. Human disease studies have identified a variety of important biochemical concepts which were then tested and extended in simpler systems. The emphasis on molecular details must not lose sight of the fact, however, that the study of disease demands the integrated application of all disciplines within the medical and biologic sciences.

CHEMICAL PRINCIPLES AND BIOLOGIC SYSTEMS

Biology offers no exception to the full application of fundamental chemical and physical principles. A full description of a biologic process must include thermodynamics and kinetics of the process as well as details of molecular structures involved.

Thermodynamics is the consideration of (or accounting for) all forms of energy in a system. All differences between an initial and final state can be summarized by the expression ΔG (change in "free energy") $- \Delta H$ (change in enthalpy) $- T\Delta S$ (change in entropy as a function of temperature). Thus, any possibility for spontaneous change requires a decrease in free energy of the system through an increase in entropy (paraphrased as "disorder") and/or a decrease in enthalpy ("heat" or "available" energy). *Entropy* is an especially important term in biology because of the extensive (and energetically expensive) ordering of biomolecules in the face of the tendency of all systems of matter to become less ordered. Thus, cells must "live up-hill in a downhill world." It is clear that biologic systems cannot be completely "closed," since they must utilize energy from without to maintain their order as well as to achieve energetic events which must be expressed in terms of positive changes in enthalpy (or measurable energy).

Two very important principles operate. First, biologic systems and subsystems are tightly compartmentalized, with stringent preservation of order and function. Second, biologic subsystems are tightly *coupled*. Thus, degradative reactions in one system serve to energize and maintain other systems. This coupling is achieved through highly specific transfer of molecules between compartments and the generation and reaction of so-called "high energy" molecules which react with appropriate molecular partners to provide reactions that are highly favored energetically. Thus, while the free energy changes in one compartment are unfavorable, they will be coupled chemically with other favorable reactions.

Kinetics

Thermodynamics concerns only initial and final states. *Kinetics* is the study and description of both the route and the rate, and thus is concerned with the rate details of molecular changes.

The assignment of equilibrium conditions is based on the thermodynamics of the total system, but even at equilibrium molecular transformations are still occurring. Only *net* change is zero because the "forward" reaction(s) is equal to the "reverse" reaction(s) as dictated by the thermodynamics of the "initial" versus the "final" state(s). In biologic systems, dynamic "steady state" is a much more important concept than simple equilibrium. "Steady state" exists when *concentration(s)* remain constant with time ($dc/dT = 0$). This may be so because the sum of all processes which remove reactants is equal to all the processes which generate reactants.

Most biologic components may be considered within pseudo-steady state systems, since chemical concentrations are maintained so rigorously. The maintenance of these steady states in the face of continual fluctuations in the environment demands the most sensitive and effective regulatory mechanisms, of course. Recognition of biosystems as examples of steady state focuses attention on the importance of these control mechanisms, and emphasizes the role of molecular "turnover" and "degradation" as well as rates of formation in the determination of the functioning concentration of any biocomponent.

The intricate *cascading* and "interlocking" of biologic reaction sequences is widely evident and is the basis for the amplification of single molecular defects into complex disease states. It also accounts for "distant" adjustment in steady state concentrations through shifts in rates of precursor formation or product removal. The time required to achieve steady state in a reaction sequence depends on the individual rate constants of the contributing reactions and the volume or quantity ("pool size") of reactants involved. Thus, perturbation can result in a rapid appearance of shifts in concentration of small quantities of intermediates whose turnover is rapid, but may cause delayed and prolonged changes in the case of slow reactions. Thus, the rapidity of appearance of "disease" can be rationalized on kinetic grounds. The rapidity of change also dictates the type of regulatory mechanism which may be required. With a rapid oscillation, an immediate kinetic *stimulation* or *inhibition* of enzymes or of molecular transport may provide immediate compensation for the perturbation. Slower or prolonged changes in steady state may provoke or require readjustment in *concentrations* of such enzyme catalysts or transport mechanisms. Some aspects of biologic function do not achieve steady state in the strictest sense. Environmental insults, for example, may result in damage that cannot be compensated completely — despite all homeostatic mechanisms — with resultant progressive changes. These changes may be very slow or very rapid, depending on the kinetics of the systems involved.

Biologic systems are also complicated by the kinetics of cell division. For example, a sequence involving slow molecular turnover may not achieve steady state in a cell population that is dividing rapidly. Thus, without any differences in the natures or controls of any chemical processes, reactants may differ considerably in concentration between dividing and non-dividing cells owing to the differences in extent to which steady state is approached. Such non-steady state may provide an important regulatory distinction between such cells.

The study of chemical kinetics, therefore, must not ignore the importance of cell kinetics and the changes that occur during the cell cycle. This point is particularly significant when considering the response of cell populations to drugs and environmental insults. The kinetic distinctions between cells make it possible to exert control over specific cell populations (e.g., cancer cells) even when no qualitative distinctions can be made on the basis of their chemical processes!

The *rate limiting steps* for formation and removal of bioconstituents are important to assign because they define vulnerability to perturbations, and provide insight into disease as well as therapeutic manipulations. In looking at any change in steady state concentration, the following questions should be asked: (1) How critical is control of concentration, and is it primary or secondary to the biologic event in question? (2) What are *contributing processes and pathways*? (Where does it come from and where does it go?) (3) What are *rate limiting steps*? (4) Over what *volume* are perturbations distributed? (What is the "pool" size?) This determines the magnitude of a significant perturbation and the abruptness of change. (5) Over what *time course* does the perturbation appear? (6) How is the perturbation propagated? (7) Where is control normally exerted?

Catalysis is of extreme importance in biologic systems because reactions must proceed at useful rates, efficient foci for regulation must be available, and chemical product selection must be precise. Enzyme mechanisms, kinetics, and regulation therefore play central roles in the chemical reactions of cells.

The branching and cascading of chemical pathways provide a high level of complexity in biosystems so that consideration of a reaction in isolation is often meaningless. Thus, the concept of changes in steady state of an individual component must include all its secondary effects on other systems. The "concentration response curve" is often complex, owing to the interaction of multiple components at a control point. Many examples, therefore, of complex, cooperative, or high-order response curves are seen in biologic systems.

Kinetics in biosystems must therefore concentrate on several important issues: both chemical and cell kinetics; the concepts of steady state and coupling; the importance of rate limiting steps; pool sizes; enzyme catalysis and regulation; and the occurrence of complex dose-response curves.

MOLECULAR COMPONENTS AND PROCESSES

General Principles

Molecules are the basis for biologic processes. They provide information, structure, energy sources, energy transduction mechanisms, and waste disposal as well as a general millieu in which the cell must survive. The uniqueness of living systems is their high degree of complex order, which in turn must depend on a very complex and complete information system. This information system must be extraordinarily precise and must include self-replication and self-assembly mechanisms. All these features depend on specific molecular properties and can be described in such fundamental terms. In this brief discussion four major points will be considered.

The first point is that the very high degree of order in biomolecules has a strong dependence on the structural state of water (which constitutes most of the cell). Water, therefore, plays a dominant role in the determination of the cell's molecular properties. Water exists in a highly ordered state owing to its polarizability and resulting self-interactions by hydrogen bonding. Even at cell temperatures, water has a large amount of icelike structure comprised of orderly arrays of molecules in a lattice-like arrangement. This lattice may either be disrupted or stabilized by the insertion of non-water molecules, with substantial changes in entropy. Since the cellular concentration of water is better than 50 molar, these changes in entropy can represent a major driving force to accomplish seemingly unfavorable reactions. The enthalpy of interactions between solute and water is also important to consider, especially in the case of charged or polarizable molecules, but entropy changes are often the dominant factor in rationalizing the state of biomolecules. This is particularly true with respect to structure of a macromolecule, where individual moieties could either be inserted into the surrounding water layer or folded in a manner that excludes water. Water, therefore, determines whether or not biologic arrangements and biologic reactions can occur. In simple terms, the extreme ordering of some biologic molecules can occur because such ordering leads to an increase in disorder of the surrounding water molecules.

The second major point is that weak chemical interactions play large roles in biosystems. These weak interactions include hydrogen bonding; various charge phenomena, including "salt" and dipole bonding; and non-polar or hydrophobic interactions. Although each is of low energy, their combined totals of energy make them substantial factors in structure determination and serve to stabilize flexible macromolecules into useful shapes, to provide rapidly reversible responses of biomolecules to environmental changes, to generate specialized compartments or domains within cells, to provide for transport systems and molecular movement; and to generate the information exchange mechanisms on which all life depends. Specialized domains within the covalent macromolecular structure provide the "binding sites" for such weak interactions, with much of their binding energy resulting from water as the cell solvent.

The third general point to be established is that biologic systems function as complex information systems by virtue of their molecular composition. Informational content can be rationalized rather easily when it is recognized that all atoms and molecules are subject to highly specific interactions and are, in that sense, informational. Simple ions have a specific size, charge density, hydration shell, etc. that dictate the potential for interactions. Covalent molecules are highly specific in a three-dimensional sense and are, therefore, informational in a very specific way. The directed nature of covalent bonding and resulting three-dimensional specificity provide for the very important molecular templating, which is the basis for recognition and transmission. Sequential arrangements of molecular information bits in macromolecules, the complexity of temporal staging of information, and the interaction between two macromolecules of unique sequence all provide an extremely high order of discrimination. Each small molecule assumes a favored conformation that is based on its own structure in concert with its solvent domain and the influence of specific interactions with other molecules. In the case of a macromolecule, the total three-dimensional structure, although extremely complex, still depends on the state of each of its repeating units. Thus, when a change or interaction occurs, not only are the individual reactants involved, but rather distant changes in conformation and reactivity can be provided in the macromolecule. It is particularly intriguing to consider the details of the transduction of informational interactions either into a cascade of informational exchange, into messenger function, or into an energetic event. The conformational discriminations of molecules provide the basis for all these events. Thus, the individual information bits in biologic systems are arranged into a hierarchy: template interactions between small molecules based on three-dimensional molecular considerations and the directed nature of covalent bonds; more complex interactions resulting from arrangement of these information bits into a temporal framework within macromolecules; and interactions between such macromolecular arrangements and other macromolecules or small molecules to provide receptor-response loops.

The fourth general point to establish is that chemical reactivity in cells is tightly controlled through the operation of transfer reactions. Highly reactive chemical groups are transferred from donor to recipient in a controlled fashion that involves sequential steps of decreasing energy rather than the single burst of an exothermic reaction. Through the intervention of such transfer reactions, the chemical energy of oxidative reactions, for example, is used constructively to maintain cell processes and to promote reactions that may be unfavorable energetically. Any breakdown of this tight coupling, of course, is destructive to the cell. The whole of intermediary metabolism is concerned with the processes by which this type of control and type coupling is accomplished and regulated.

Structures of Macromolecules

Macromolecules play central roles in biologic systems. A remarkable feature of all macromolecules is their sequential covalent synthesis from a limited number of small precursors and their self-assembly or aggregation into very large structures. With each class of macromolecules the precursors are essentially the same for all life forms, with minor variations in structure that permit discrimination between organisms and between specific functions within the same organism.

Macromolecules serve a variety of functions within living systems, including: information storage and retrieval; structural integrity; formation of barriers to interface with the environment and between cell compartments; storage of chemical energy; and a variety of effector roles such as catalysis, energy transduction (chemical, thermal and mechanical), and molecular transpositions to provide secretion and transport. Their three-dimensional structures are derived from the unique secondary and tertiary weak binding of these assembled building blocks, driven energetically by their interactions with each other and, especially, with solvent. The tendency toward self-assembly is often strong, accounting for the aggregation and assembly into supramolecular structures (organelles, membranes, enzyme complexes, etc.). The self-assembly process is spontaneously driven by these molecular interactions and often can be demonstrated in isolated systems. Macromolecular defects may derive from fundamental precursor and assembly problems, from details of minor structural variations, or from the excesses and deficiencies which result purely from kinetic alterations either in formation or turnover.

Table 2–1 presents a summary of the major classes of macromolecules in biologic systems.

TABLE 2–1 MACROMOLECULES IN BIOLOGIC SYSTEMS

	DNA	RNA	Proteins	Glycogen	Mucopolysaccharides (Glycosaminoglycans)	Hetero-Oligosaccharides
Primary Structure Repeat (Backbone)	Deoxyribose polyphosphate ester of purine and pyrimidine glycosides.	Ribose polyphosphate ester of purine and pyrimidine glycosides.	Peptide bond.	Repeating glycoside of glucose (glucosyl-glucose).	Disaccharide repeating unit comprised of an amino sugar and a uronic acid in glycosidic linkage. All but hyaluronic acid also have O- or N- sulfate groups.	Glycoside residues attached through glycoside linkage to secreted polypeptides, cell wall lipids, and structure and secretory proteins.
Type of Structure	Linear, non-branching.	Linear, non-branching.	Linear with complex 3-D constraints.	Linear and branched.	Linear chains, variable in length linked covalently to a polypeptide core.	Often highly branched.
Type of Secondary and Tertiary Interactions	Template interactions are key to biologic role; these complementary self-interactions (intra- and inter-chain ring stacking and H-bonding of purines and pyrimidines) provide highly ordered helical structures which are packaged into manageable cellular units by specific binding to proteins.	Same potential as DNA, but less extensive.	H-bonding of peptide unit; non-covalent interactions between side chains (H-bonding, hydrophobic, charge); covalent bonds between side chains spontaneously (s-s) or enzymically. Supramolecular aggregation is common.	Minimal.	Extensive hydrophilic and electrostatic interactions.	May be highly specific (e.g., antigenic templating).
Synthesis and Assembly	Templated sequential addition of primary repeat with occasional postsynthetic (e.g., methylation) of specific bases. Segmental repair or segmental resynthesis also occurs.	Same as DNA with more extensive post synthetic modification by degradation of chain termini and addition of homogeneous repeating sectors.	Templated sequential addition of amino acids. Postsynthetic modifications include segmental hydrolysis, addition of non-peptide moieties, oxidation and reduction, and condensation.	Sequential addition of glucose units to growing chain; transfer of chain sectors within growing chain to form branch points (enzyme rather than template directed).	Sequential addition and modification in situ of monosaccharide units—directed by specificity of enzymes (not templated).	Sequential addition dictated by specific enzymes and growing chain termini.
Precursors Required in Addition to Enzymes	Deoxy purine and pyrimidine nucleotides. Deoxyribose moiety and thymine are unique to DNA.	Ribose, purine and pyrimidine nucleotides (uracil is unique to RNA).	Amino acids, tRNA, mRNA, and ribosomes; residues for postsynthetic modification.	UDP glucose.	Polypeptide chain; UDP monosaccharide unit; phosphoadenosine phosphosulfate.	Growing chain termini and appropriate activated glycoside residue.
Size	Immense.	Small to very large.	Small to very large.	Variable and heterogeneous.	Extremely variable; aggregates in excess of 10^6 mol. wt.	Highly variable.
Functions	Primary information storage and transcription.	Information transfer and translation.	Protean—structural, effector, transport, barrier, buffer, regulatory, receptor.	Storage.	Constitute "ground substance" and modulate the solvation and reaction environment of all tissues.	Lubricant; membrane integrity, recognition processes (e.g., antigenantibody, peptide hormones); regulation of molecular turnover.
Turnover	Primary stability is essential to life; limited segmental turnover occurs through damage and repair.	Some are very stable (e.g., ribosomal RNA) while some species turn over rapidly.	From very stable to very labile. Related to inherent (thermodynamic) stability. Final degradation of backbone is largely non-specific.	Rapid, tightly regulated.	Requires action of specific hydrolytic enzymes to control appropriate concentrations; otherwise, molecules are very stable.	Requires specific hydrolytic enzymes.

Each is comprised of characteristic repeating units arranged in some unique primary sequence. Each possesses some secondary structural characteristic which derives from the nature of the intramolecular ordering around this primary sequence, and each is characterized by a characteristic set of teritiary and quarternary interactions between the primary bits of information or repeating units and between these units and other macromolecules or small molecules. The tertiary and quaternary interactions of these macromolecules are dictated by the primary structure in concert with interactions with the medium and are unique for each molecule under a given set of conditions. For each molecule, the biologic properties depend, of course, on these three-dimensional structural characteristics as well as their primary chemical reactive property. Some macromolecules are characterized by their chemical inertness or stability; others by their dynamic reactive properties.

Unique binding sites for small molecules on macromolecules provide effector functions essential to the chemical processes of cells as well as the direct communication link between the environment and cell effector functions. Thus, macromolecules represent the receptors at which drugs and other biologically effective signals interact (usually reversibly and often weakly) to provoke substantial biologic consequences.

The major classes of macromolecules — nucleic acids, proteins, carbohydrates and lipids — will be discussed chiefly in terms of their roles in information storage, transfer, and utilization; structure formation; and effector functions. As emphasized above, all molecules are informational in nature, but nucleic acids represent the primary information system of the cell. Proteins play a major role in determining the structural properties of the cell, and although all constituent molecules are an integral part of the cell structure, carbohydrates and lipids contribute particularly to the structure of membrane barriers and to the intercellular matrix. Proteins play the major role in effector functions and primary communication with the environment. The important structural roles of complex polysaccharides and lipids and their participation in regulation and recognition must also be noted. All of these macromolecular constituents interact in forming the cell mass and dictating total cell function.

The detailed study of each set of macromolecules provides a unique challenge to the modern investigator. In each instance, studies involve several approaches. First, primary structure analysis by destructive sequence determination is well advanced and, in principle, solvable for any protein. This has resulted from (1) the ability to cleave massive proteins enzymatically into unique smaller units by selective backbone hydroly-

sis using enzymes and (2) from the ability to hydrolyze the backbone chemically by sequential cleavage from the end of the molecule, with identification of each repeating unit. The technology is fully automated and widely available. The limiting step for these procedures is still the availability of pure material, but microtechniques have reduced drastically the quantity of material required. Such primary sequence analysis for nucleic acids is also well advanced, and, although each gene of interest is comprised of at least three times as many primary repeating units as the corresponding gene product, this technology is now within the grasp of the modern molecular biologist. Effective sequence analysis for complex polysaccharides is assisted by advanced chromatographic and mass spectroscopic techniques and through the availability of specific glycosidases with which the terminal sugar at each successive hydrolytic step can be identified and hydrolyzed.

The study of primary sequences in situ within macromolecules is also of considerable value in identifying structure–function relationships in macromolecules. Although the sequence analysis for nucleic acids has been cumbersome, the complementary nature of polynucleotides makes it quite practical to identify short informational sequences within the macromolecule simply by the construction of an appropriate complementary probe. It is entirely practical, for example, to identify a gene by the complementary binding of an isolated messenger molecule. The added technology of synthesizing DNA sequences from messenger molecules by means of reverse transcriptase followed by amplification through cloning permits study of these sequences in different genetic surroundings (see below). The major approach for the identification of unique sequences within a large protein molecule has involved the use of the specific antibodies. This is complicated, however, by the fact that these unique sequences often are involved in extensive tertiary structure of the protein, which may modify considerably the ability of an antibody to bind. Moreover, antibody specificity is directed at tertiary as well as primary structure.

Identification of specific binding sites responsible for biologic properties (e.g., enzyme substrate site, antigen combining site, drug "receptor" site, etc.) is a problem of sequence identity as well as of surface topography, and is complicated by the fact that moieties which are adjacent in the folded, active configuration of a macromolecule may be quite distant from each other in the primary sequence. Furthermore, most site-binding is reversible, and may involve quite low concentrations of ligand and receptor. Identification of these moieties can be approached by chemical ablation or perturbation of the macromolecular structure, modification of ligand structure, affinity labeling, and photoaffinity labeling. Physical studies of the complexes in situ and the use of appropriate model compounds also have proved valuable. Reversible structure perturturbations also provide a valuable approach to the study of macromolecular structure and function. This is particularly interesting from the viewpoint of studying mechanisms of biological regulation, since regulation is effected through reversible perturbations in structure (and function). High-resolution electron microscopy in recent years has also made it possible to view directly specific macromolecules within cellular structures and thus to achieve an increased understanding of molecular structure. All major classes of macro-molecules now appear to be accessible to this technology.

One of the most intriguing approaches to the study of biomolecular structure and function has been the construction of model compounds of pre-cursor molecules with modeling of the biologic processes for which these molecules are responsible. The construction, for example, of the lipid bilayer membrane and the insertion of model peptides which serve either as channels or as transport carriers has provided a very incisive approach to the understanding of membrane function. The construction of sequences of collagen and elastin have also been used in studies of mechanisms for tissue calcification and offer promise for solution of this intriguing and important biologic problem. The construction of unique protein sequence and topographic models represents a complex and challenging synthetic problem for the chemist.

The "genetic experiment" (either that provided by nature or by the investigator) has been especially useful. The study of the structures and function of mutant gene products has long been a major source of progress in understanding structure–function relationships and the nature of biologic regulation. Until recently, the major genetic experiment was limited to spontaneous or induced mutations, which are random in nature and often complex in expression. It is now possible to isolate the messenger RNA for a particular gene and use a sepcific enzyme to copy this gene to form the corresponding DNA sequence. The recent breakthrough in plasmid technology now also makes it possible to clone this DNA sequence within a lower organism so that, potentially, quantities of this gene could be constructed for use in appropriate biologic studies. The whole technology of the construction of these genes and their potential insertion into other cells, of course, has created a tremendous amount of interest and controversy, but in terms of the medical sciences, represents one of the major breakthroughs in our capacity to study, understand, and modify disease processes.

Thus, macromolecules can be studied by the specific approaches of destructive analysis, analysis in situ — either of a non-destructive sort or through perturbation effects — and through the appropriate construction of models for the study of specific functional aspects.

Nucleic Acids

The roles of nucleic acids in providing the stable storage form for information in cells as well as the templating mechanisms for information read-out (transcription, translation, replication, reverse transcription, repair) are well known and need not be discussed in great detail here. These macromolecules, in providing two-dimensional copies of all the information in an organism to be translated into both time-dependent events and three-dimensional structures are necessarily immense in size and present special problems in environmental vulnerability and stability, fidelity of copying and translation, cellular packaging, and mechanisms for precise regulation. These problems are solved through special structural features and cellular processes, which will be summarized briefly.

The nucleic acids illustrate one of the basic premises of molecular biology, i.e., that knowledge of molecular structure can lead to an understanding of function. The double-helical structure of DNA deduced by Watson and Crick led to confirmation of the two-dimensional read-out nature of cellular information storage and retrieval, to an understanding of the stable nature of and replicative mechanism for the information system, and to a precise understanding of the chemical nature of genetic variability and mutations. Nucleic acids have both sequence specificity and three-dimensional specificity and provide the basis not only of the primary information system, but for the interaction of regulators so that biologic expression can be modulated. DNA is the most stable of the nucleic acids and usually represents the stable master copy of information within the cell; RNA is an intermediate expression or vector of information (messenger) and also provides a read-out mechanism for translation. There are, however, exceptions to this generalization in that some viruses consist of RNA rather than DNA.

The structures of RNA and DNA are paraphrased in Figure 2–1. The basic backbone of nucleic acids is a monotonous repeating unit of a sugar phosphate ester which provides stability, and whose polyanionic nature assures an extended structure of the polymer for ease in reading and modulation. The information bits consist of unique sequential arrangements of purine and pyrimidine bases, attached by glycosidic bond to the backbone, which provide a reading mechanism through the "templating" action of specific intramolecular interactions of weak hydrogen

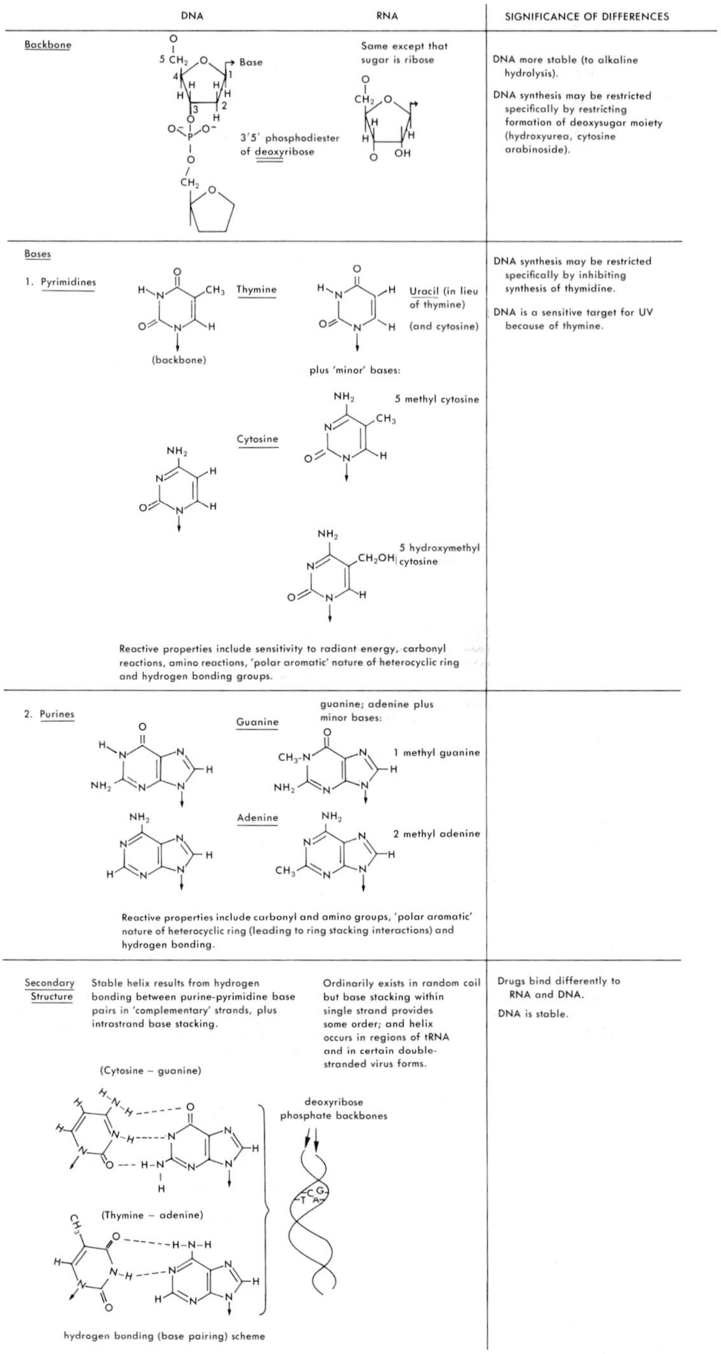

Figure 2–1 Diagram of primary and secondary aspects of DNA and RNA structure (with abbreviated structural formulas—Emphasis on 3D arrangement).

bonding and ring-stacking. The specific reactive properties of the bases also account for modifications known to impair or change function. For example, the bases are susceptible to modification by alkylating drugs, formation of various adducts, simple chemical cleavage of the glycosidic bond, or modification by absorption of radiant energy. Their specific functions and interactions may also be disrupted by binding of various aromatic heterocyclic drugs which show avidity for ordered sequences of purines and pyrimidines. This is particularly true for binding to the "core" of purine and pyrimidine base pairs in double-stranded DNA

In addition to their common features, DNA and RNA also show several important differences. First, there is a single copy of DNA made for each chromosome at each cell replication, whereas RNA may be synthesized in multiple copies. Second, DNA is much larger than RNA and thus represents a larger "target" for various insults. Both these factors combine with the critical role of DNA to make the cell particularly vulnerable to DNA damage. Third, the deoxysugar and thymine are unique to DNA and represent specific loci where DNA synthesis can be regulated — a point of considerable importance to chemotherapy. At the same time, the deoxysugar makes the DNA backbone more stable chemically by protecting it against alkaline hydrolysis. Its double helical structure also lends stability, as well as providing a complementary strand for use in replication and repair. The large target size of DNA also accounts for the major lethal effects of ionizing radiation, whereas UV irradiation kills cells largely because of the efficient and specific capture of radiant energy by the pyrimidines in DNA, with formation of dimers and consequent disruption of its information role.

The packaging of nucleic acids into three-dimensional structures serves primary functional and regulatory roles as well as solving cell logistic problems in handling such large molecules. The nature of "packaging" is related directly to the molecular details of function. For DNA and mRNA reading, sequential access to each of the information bits is required, and extensive three-dimensional structuring probably is not concerned with primary function. The highly structured state of DNA is more likely involved with determining which sequences will be expressed, when, and at what rates. DNA is packaged in a highly ordered fashion around basic protein "cores" interspersed with regions of extended DNA structure. In addition, a large number of acidic proteins as well as RNA molecules are associated with DNA to form cellular chromatin. The cellular "structuring" of DNA, therefore, involves the binding of a variety of proteins and RNA. Ribosomal RNA is also packaged with a number of specific proteins to serve its biologic

function. Transfer RNA, in contrast, assumed specific three-dimensional configurations by virtue of intramolecular interactions to provide specific recognition sites for the enzymes concerned with amino acid activation and for interaction with ribosomal units and with mRNA for translation. Thus, although nucleic acid information is basically two-dimensional in nature, three-dimensional structural considerations are of great importance within the total context of biologic function and regulation.

The structure of nucleic acids results in a number of types of predictable interactions with other molecules, as shown by the examples in Table 2–2. The backbone provides a repetitious, charged, hydrophilic domain for electrostatic binding. The purine and pyrimidine bases contribute a variety of reactive sites (amino and carbonyl groups, heterocyclic rings) and participate in ring-stacking interactions and hydrogen bonding. The highly ordered hydrophobic core of helical DNA is especially suited for hydrophobic and ring-stacking interactions. Thus, DNA, for example, can participate in interactions ranging from electrostic to hydrophobic and can react covalently as well. Strong binding of specific ligands often involves two or more of these interaction modes to provide highly cooperative and specific attachment. In the cell, accessibility is determined by the structural state of the polynucleotide, i.e., to what extent available sites are blocked by "natural" ligand binding or by complex "packaging." The biologic consequences are difficult to predict quantitatively, therefore, because of this variability in binding and because of the compensatory mechanisms that a cell may employ.

Based on the realization that the information responsible for a cell's characteristics is encoded in the sequence of DNA, it follows simply that a qualitative change in a DNA locus by removal, addition, or change in a nucleotide base information bit can result in a mutation or change in cell properties. Since the sum total of an organism's properties depends also on the dynamic interplay of all its systems, normal information expression also requires correct quantitative balance between the different elements of expression, particularly in highly complex organisms which go through a precisely timed sequence of differentiation and cell cycling. When the genetic load is disrupted by a change in chromosomal number, gross errors in differentiation occur (for example, the various human abnormalities associated with the occurrence of extra chromosomes; see Chapter 3). It is also noteworthy that changes in the information content of the cell can result from the imposition of external genetic material, such as that resulting from virus infections which may simply disrupt cell functions or may cause heritable changes in cell properties such as neoplastic transformation. The steps in-

TABLE 2–2 INTERACTION OF CHEMICAL AGENTS WITH NUCLEIC ACIDS

Type of Interaction	Drug	Nucleic Acid Structural Site(s) Involved	Effects on DNA Properties and Function	Clinical Use
Covalent	Alkylating agents nitrogen mustard, such antibiotics as mitomycin, etc.	Adds to N-7 position of guanine	Inhibits cell replication; also mutagenic	Cytotoxic agent
	Certain reactive aromatic hydrocarbons (fluorenylacetamide, for example)	Adds to N-8 position of guanine	Mutagenic, carcinogenic	
	Hydrazine and hydroxylamine	Reacts with C==O groups	Mutagenic	
	Nitrous acid	Reacts with NH_2 groups	Mutagenic	
Non-Covalent	Polyamines (spermine, spermidine)	Backbone (PO_4)	Stabilizes	
	Basic proteins (histones)	Backbone(PO_4)	Stabilizes	
	Acidic proteins	Specific base sequences	Regulation of structure and function	
	Ions	Backbone, and polar groups of bases	Backbone binding stabilizes, base binding disrupts DNA helix	
	Hydrocarbons	Stacks with purine bases	Mutagenic, carcinogenic	
	Heterocyclic drugs and antibiotics			
	1. Actinomycin	Ring-stacking (intercalation) and charge interaction with backbone (minor groove)	Inhibits RNA synthesis, and to a lesser extent DNA synthesis	Cytotoxic
	2. Streptomycin	Ribosomal RNA	Inhibits protein synthesis	Antibiotic
	3. Aminoquinoline antimalarial drugs	Ring-stacking and charge interaction with backbone	Stabilizes DNA helix, inhibits DNA synthesis and repair; inhibits RNA synthesis poorly	Antiparasitic
	4. Acridines (including quinacrine)	Ring-stacking and charge interaction with backbone	Same spectrum of action as aminoquinolines	Antiparasitic
	5. Furocoumarins	?	Photosensitivity	Vitiligo therapy
	6. Adriamycin	Ring-stacking (intercalation)	Inhibits replication	Cytotoxic
	7. Ethidium	Ring-stacking (intercalation)	Inhibits replication	Antiparasitic

volved in information storage and processing in nucleic acids are summarized in Table 2–3. These processes are especially pertinent to biologic regulation and can be exploited to explain disease processes or used for therapeutic applications. Sites for regulation are also indicated in Table 2–3.

DNA replication is a tightly controlled and precisely ordered process in which each strand of double helical DNA serves as a template for the synthesis of a new DNA strand for distribution to daughter cells. For the complex eukaryotic cell, replication is initiated at specific starting points, and each replicating unit (replicon) is copied on a precise time schedule in which chromosomal organization is maintained. Each parent strand and its complementary newly synthesized daugh-

ter strand is packaged into a new chromosome, and these are segregated into the daughter cells by a precise process of mitosis or meiosis in which each genetic locus is preserved. There can be exchange of information segments between identical sectors of chromosomes (crossing over) during both meiosis and mitosis, which serves to give a random assortment of differences in genetic markers carried on different members of a pair of chromosomes. Mitosis and meiosis differ only in the number of chromosomal doublings and the final distribution of chromosomal copies. For mitosis a simple doubling occurs, with daughter cells identical to the parents in chromosomal number. Meiosis produces cells (terminal germ cells) with half the parent number of chromo-

TABLE 2-3 INFORMATION STORAGE AND PROCESSING

Processes	Steps Required	Enzyme (and possible sites for regulation)

DNA Synthesis	1. Precursor synthesis
	  a. synthesis of purines and pyrimidines (thymine uniquely)
	  b. formation of nucleoside
	  c. phosphorylation to form nucleotides
	  d. reduction of ribonucleotides to deoxyribonucleotides
	2. Synthesis (formation of polydeoxyribose PO_4 backbone in *templated* sequential replicative process to form new duplex)
	3. Condensation of helical DNA and association with proteins to form chromatin and packaging into chromosomes
		1. Enzymes for precursor synthesis (thymidylate synthetase and kinase and ribonucleotide reductase are unique to DNA)
		2. Replicases (template and primer requiring polymerases to form information sequences)
		3. Ligases – to join short segments into total sequences and to restore nicks.
		4. Enzymes acting on secondary and tertiary structure – "unwinding," and "winding" enzymes
		5. Nucleases – 'editing' removal of mismatched bases in replication; nicking actions to provide DNA access for normal functions and repair; DNA turnover (cell death) and foreign DNA; "restriction"
		6. Modification enzymes – methylation of specific bases as control points for expression and in control of restriction DNAases

DNA Repair	1. Recognition of damage (surveillance) 2. Removal and synthesis and/or exchange of limited DNA sequences	1. Specific endonucleases 2. Exonucleases 3. Polymerases 4. Ligases 5. Recombinational enzymes
RNA Synthesis (Transcription)	1. Precursor synthesis (same as for DNA except uracil in lieu of thymine and ribonucleotides are not reduced) 2. Synthesis – templated sequential polymerization with release of RNA product and restoration of DNA duplex. 3. Processing of RNA transcript and transposition to site of function (sequences of bases are removed and poly A is added).	1. Enzymes of precursor biosynthesis pathways 2. Transcriptase (including factors for initiation which may include enzymes "unwinding" or "rewinding" of DNA template). 3. RNAases and polyadenylating enzymes (processing of mRNA)

Peptide Synthesis (Translation)	1. Formation and assembly of constituents of translation complex
	  a. template (messenger) transcription
	  b. formation of ribosomes
	    1) transcription of unique RNA (ribosomal)
	    2) synthesis of specific proteins
	    3) ordered aggregation (assembly)
	  c. transcription of specific tRNA molecules
	    1) synthesis
	    2) modification of specific nucleotides
	    3) folding into specific 3D structure
	  d. activation of amino acids (attachment to appropriate tRNA molecules)
	2. Sequential (templated) formation of peptide backbone
	3. Assembly (spontaneous) of secondary and tertiary structure
		1. All enzymes for RNA transcription (above)
		2. amino acid activating enzymes
		3. tRNA modification enzymes
		4. Peptide synthetase
		5. Transcriptase

Modification of Translation Products (Protein)	1. Synthesis or absorption of various non-protein moieties 2. Attachment of chemical groups to specific protein side chains 3. Modification of translated primary structure (oxidation, reduction, hydroxylation of side chains; hydrolytic removal of sections of primary sequence	1. Biosynthetic enzymes for non-protein moieties 2. Specific transferases for attaching non-protein moieties. 3. Hydroxylases, oxidoreductases for amino acid side chains. 4. Proteases (specific)
Reverse Transcription	Precursor synthesis (deoxyribonucleotides) Templated (RNA) synthesis of DNA	Reverse transcriptase
Discriminating Protein Regulatory and Effector Functions (Binding, Catalysis, etc.)	1. All steps for specific protein synthesis and modification 2. Signals reception (small molecule binding) 3. Protein response (conformational change) 4. Effector function (catalysis, transport, regulation)	1. All enzymes for protein synthesis and modification. 2. All enzymes for synthesis and modification of signal molecule.

somes through final segregation of single chromosomal copies into daughter cells during a reductive division. It is significant that final
chromosomal segregation for diploid organisms
such as man produces a cell with no redudancy of
information and thus no opportunity to recover
information lost during the division processes.
For either mitosis or meiosis, failure to segregate
chromosomes correctly (non-disjunction) can result in disruption in chromosomal number and
size, with resultant impairment of biologic function.

Lack of precision and appropriate control of
DNA replication and the attendant cell processes
of mitosis and meiosis are obviously detrimental
and provide the basis for disease. For example,
the growth of neoplastic tissues, the proliferation
of pannus in the joints in rheumatoid arthritis,
keloid formation, and psoriasis may all represent
excessive or inappropriate cell proliferation. Conversely, depression of the bone marrow and ulceration of the intestinal mucosa consequent to the
administration of a variety of toxic drugs or in
the course of irradiation represent examples of
inadequate replication and proliferation of cells.
Furthermore, disruptions in chromosomal size
and number, presumably from non-disjunction or
unequal exchange of chromosomal segments,
have devastating consequences for human development. Replicative processes and chromosomal
integrity also provide important targets for damage by a variety of environmental hazards.

An understanding of the specific structures and
processes involved in replication also provides
the rational basis for regulation. Thus, limitation
of the synthesis of thymidine by folic acid antagonists and certain fraudulent nucleotides or
inhibition of reductive formation of deoxyribose
nucleotides by hydroxyurea or cytosine arabinoside restricts replication at the precursor level.
The process of DNA copying by the DNA polymerase can be interfered with by a variety of
drugs and antibiotics which interact with the
DNA template, such as daunomycin and adria-
mycin, bleomycin, ethidium bromide, various antimalarials, mitomycin, nitrogen mustard and
other alkylating agents, and to some extent actinomycin D. Subsequent to DNA synthesis the
segregation process for the newly synthesized
DNA in mitosis can be blocked by the administration of specific mitotic inhibitors such as vincristine or colchicine which interact with the specialized contractile proteins responsible for mitotic
segregation of chromosomes. At the present time
it is not clear what the signal is in a cell for the
start of DNA synthesis and cell division, and no
exploitation of this mechanism has been possible
for therapeutic purposes. However, cells can be
stimulated to divide in-vitro by the administration of certain agents such as phytohemagglutin-

in and pokeweed mitogen, illustrating the potential for regulation of this process.

The central information role of DNA is protected by several important homeostatic mechanisms.
First, an "editing" process operates during replication to excise mismatched bases in the new
strand through a nuclease action which accompanies the polymerase. Even more interesting
are the mechanisms which operate to restore the
fidelity of information within preformed DNA.
The best understood mechanism is that of excision repair or *repair synthesis* in which modified
single-stranded segments of DNA are excised and
resynthesized complementary to the intact
strand. This process is called into action following
a variety of environmental insults, including UV
or ionizing irradiation, chemical modification of
bases, and thermal damage. The actions of a
number of specific enzymes have been identified
which recognize specific modifications and introduce a break in the damaged DNA strand. The
actual excision, resynthesis, and rejoining processes appear to be common to multiple types of
damage, but are subdivided into "long gap" and
"short gap" processes ranging from only a few to
as many as 2000 bases. Since the information is
intact in the complementary strand, these processes can be accomplished with high fidelity. Repair can also be accomplished following replication. New strand synthesis opposite the damaged
site is either interrupted to result in a single
strand gap or results in errors either during replication or in the daughter cell. Repair of the damaged region can also be accomplished after replication by a recombinational process to retrieve
information from another chromosome. Damage
at a locus involving both DNA strands is either
not repairable or must involve an error-prone
process, since neither strand has a complete information copy. Hence, the potent effects of neu-
tron irradiation, which introduces double strand
breaks, or multifunctional alkylating agents can
be rationalized partly on the grounds of lack of repair.

It has also been recognized that persistence of
unrepaired lesions can serve to provoke an error-
prone inducible "repair" process stressing the importance of regulation in this important system.
DNA repair processes (and their regulation) appear to represent, therefore, important homeostatic mechanisms by which the cell preserves
the integrity of its basic information system. The
possibility also exists that this is the means by
which the cell can undergo biologic variations by
modification of limited regions of DNA without
the necessity for undergoing cell division. Predictably, disease can result from defects in these
repair mechanisms since the stability of the information systems for somatic cells may be compromised. Such stability is particularly pertinent

to cancer and aging, and it is significant that several repair defects have been identified in human cells in association with increased cancer susceptibility. Human repair defects are summarized in Table 2–4.

Thus, xeroderma pigmentosum, Fanconi's anemia, ataxia telangiectasia, and Down's syndrome are all associated with increased risk of malignancy and have been shown to be defective in one or more repair mechanisms. In addition, it has been reported that the increased aging associated with progeria may also be correlated with a defect in cellular DNA repair. Repair systems may also be exploitable therapeutically for modifying the sensitivity of cancer cells to irradiation and alkylating agents, since such therapy works by introducing repairable lesions into cellular DNA.

The orderly read-out of stored information in the cell occurs through the processes of transcription (synthesis of a messenger RNA) followed by translation of this messenger into protein structure. Transcription represents the appropriate and timely templating of the information strand of the helical DNA into a single strand of messenger RNA, which is the vector for cytoplasmic expression. Studies with model systems in simple organisms have revealed that transcription is a tightly controlled process in which messenger RNA is made appropriate to the needs of the cell. For each gene, transcription must start at a precise initiation point and continue in a sequential fashion to the end of the gene. The details of the control of this process in cells, particularly mammalian cells, are not yet worked out, but it is clear that the initiation process involves both negative and positive control factors and that more than one gene may be controlled coordinately, possibly because a single large messenger is transcribed for several genes (polycistronic messengers). Transcription may be repressed by

the binding of some recognition molecule to the initiation region on DNA, so that it cannot occur unless an appropriate signal in the form of a small molecule interacts with this repressor to impede its binding. This permits small molecules to turn on transcription. In a similar fashion, small molecules may serve to turn off transcription if the DNA binding repressor binds more tightly in response to the small molecular signal. These processes of induction and repression are illustrated in Figure 2–2 and are essential to the understanding of enzyme induction and enzyme repression, both of which offer potential for exploitation in therapy. The control of virus infection and expression is also effected through such mechanisms.

When RNA is transcribed, not only is the unique messenger sequence synthesized, but additional RNA at each end of the messenger is included. These sequences, therefore, must be processed or eliminated before the message is translated by the cytoplasmic machinery. These steps of post-transcriptional messenger RNA processing have received considerable emphasis in recent years. The roles for the excess RNA synthesized have not been established, but the cell obviously makes a large investment in energy in order to synthesize these polynucleotide sequences and then to process them following the initial step of transcription.

Transcription offers several potential sites for regulation (and therapeutic manipulation). First, limitation in the unique RNA precursors required for transcription can be accomplished by metabolic blockade or by use of fraudulent nucleotides which compete for incorporation. Second, induction and repression may be accomplished either by the use of the appropriate small molecular signal, usually a product for the gene action in question or a related system, or by the use of fraudulent small molecules which serve to

TABLE 2–4   HUMAN DEFECTS IN DNA REPAIR

Xeroderma pigmentosum	Most have decreased excision of UV photoproducts Variants are deficient in postreplicative repair	Extreme UV sensitivity with high frequency of cancer in UV exposed areas; severe variants have CNS defects.
Ataxia telangiectasia; Bloom's syndrome	Decreased excision repair of ionizing radiation damage; Increased radiation sensitivity; Decreased chromosomal stability (Bloom's syndrome also sensitive to UV)	Increased cancer susceptibility; Immunodeficiency Cerebellar ataxia telangiectasia
Fanconi's anemia	Decreased excision repair following UV and ionizing radiation	Increased cancer susceptibility
Progeria	Cultured cells show decreased capacity to rejoin x-ray strand breaks	Premature aging

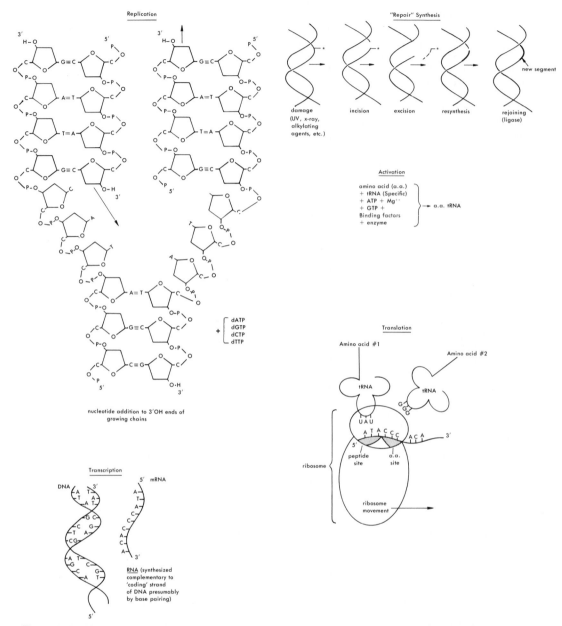

Figure 2–2 Diagrammatic sketch (with abbreviated chemical formula) to follow fate of DNA and RNA structure through replication, repair, transcription, and translation.

mimic their action. Third, the templating function of DNA may be interfered with by the binding of specific agents, such as actinomycin D, that bind to the DNA template and prevent copying. Fourth, the action of the RNA polymerase itself may be blocked (in bacteria) by such agents as the antibiotic rifamycin. Fifth, the processes by which the very large precursor messenger RNA is modified to provide the final messenger may also be subject to regulation, although the mechanisms involved have not been elucidated.

Translation is the process of converting the linear information sequence in the mRNA transcript into a protein molecule which in turn provides a three-dimensional biologic structure. The molecular structures involved directly in this complex process are: RNA derived from processing of the initial mRNA transcript; ribosomes, comprised of RNA and a large number of specific proteins; and "charged" transfer RNA from which all the correct amino acids are transferred sequentially into the growing peptide chain, based on the complementarity between a coding triplet in each tRNA and a triplet sequence within the mRNA. This complex sequence of events depends on a number of processes characteristic of the cascading nature of biologic events, providing multiple points for potential regulation. mRNA must be synthesized (in the appropriate amount and at the right time), processed to remove the non-coding sequences, transported out along the endoplasmic reticulum, and attached to ribosomes. Ribosomes are assembled in the cell from specific species of RNA (rRNA) and a large number of specific proteins, thus requiring transcription of rRNA, the appropriate mRNAs, and the complete processes concerned with translation as well as the proper cell milieu for self-assembly. The availability of tRNAs, charged with appropriate amino acids requires: tRNA transcription, processing, and correct formation of three-dimensional structure; availability of an amino acid pool; action of a series of specific "amino acid activating" enzymes which act to place the correct amino acid on each tRNA for subsequent transfer to the new protein. Finally, the peptide transfer reaction itself, which occurs on the ribosome, requires simultaneously specific three-dimensional interactions between the ribosome, each tRNA, the growing peptide chain, and the enzyme(s) that catalyze the transfer reaction. Thus, translation may be interrupted through changes in any of the structures of processes involved, and it is not surprising that a variety of antibiotics, such as streptomycin, chloramphenicol, puromycin, and cycloheximide, inhibit translation.

The action of interferon is particularly intriguing. These specific proteins are synthesized by mammalian cells in response to the presence of virus nucleic acids, and they appear to interfere specifically with the process of translation of virus messengers without interfering with host messenger. Since interferon production is host-specific but not virus-specific, it can be stimulated in host cells by the administration of synthetic polynucleotides as well as virus nucleic acids, and thus represents a potential means of controlling virus infections. The role of hormones and various other biologic regulators in modifying the process of translation is also under intensive investigation.

Post-translational events are also important to the process of formation of biologically active proteins. In addition to the spontaneous folding into tertiary structure described below, covalent modification occurs through: addition of non-protein moieties onto amino acid side chains (including: nucleotide, PO_4, carbohydrate, lipids, and various prosthetic groups; hydroxylation; ester formation; oxidation (reduction) of side chains; cross-linking between side chains; and proteolysis with removal of amino acid sequences from the primary structure. All these processes produce specific structure changes that relate to biologic function and must be considered as potential regulation (and disease) loci.

Information storage and processing in nucleic acids are important keys for the understanding and control of human diseases. It is especially significant that most of our present knowledge was acquired in a brief period of less than 25 years.

Proteins

Proteins constitute the work molecules for biologic systems. They provide structural integrity and specificity, appropriate solution properties and barrier functions (buffers and the like) as well as specific effector roles, such as transport, energy transduction, and catalysis and regulation. They are in the strictest sense informational molecules in that their unique three-dimensional structures provide the basis for all their discriminating interactions and functions. Proteins are especially well suited for biologic diversity because of the endless number of structures that can be generated from sequences of the 20 amino acids available. The most important insight into protein structure and function is the recognition that the primary covalent sequence of amino acids dictates the most favorable secondary structure (hydrogen bonding between peptide bonds in the chain), and tertiary structure (interactions between amino acid side chains) based on the lowest (and most favorable) free energy state of the protein and its surrounding medium. Because of this important governing thermodynamic principle, the read-out of two-dimensional information encoded in nucleic acids into a two-dimensional protein sequence is transformed into a unique three-dimensional structure. Furthermore, the association of protein into aggregates (quaternary structure) or other more complicated macrostructures, such as virus coats, ribosomes, membranes, etc., can also occur spontaneously according to the same governing principle. Current technology has made it quite feasible to learn the primary sequence of any protein so that the structure-function relationships can be established.

Individual amino acids in a protein chain may be viewed as serving two types of roles. First, they determine the unique reactivity required for the discriminating functions of proteins; second, they provide the structural basis for interacting with the environment and determining three-dimensional protein structure and stability. Therefore, modifying a protein (for example, by genetic "error") may either interfere with its functional and regulatory capacity or change its structural stability or both. Defects in red blood cells provide excellent examples of these different defects. Sickle hemoglobin, because of a single amino acid change (glutamate → valine), shows a tertiary structure lability, so that, although it can still bind O_2, its tertiary structure in the deoxygenated state is so distorted that it forces gross deformity of the red blood cells. A variety of other hemoglobin defects, in contrast, have a decreased capacity to bind O_2. Certain mutants for glucose-6-PO_4 dehydrogenase in the red cell show substantial changes in catalytic properties. This also illustrates an excellent example of the seemingly remote biologic effects that may result from an enzyme deficiency due to perturbation of interrelated steady state systems. The ultimate result of this enzyme deficiency is red blood cell fragility, apparently because the decreased reduction of NADP by glucose-6-PO_4 restricts availability of reduced gluthathione for reduction of methemoglobin. Pyruvate kinase deficiency associated with hemolytic anemias appears to result from a defect in enzyme stability which is expressed as the cell ages. It may well be that some instances of apparent complete enzyme absence may instead represent highly labile though potentially active enzyme, a point of considerable therapeutic interest.

Certain toxic effects also may be explained on the basis of modifications of protein structure, either in terms of functional capacity or of structural integrity. Thus, amino acid-specific reagents, such as heavy metals and thiols which react with -SH groups in proteins, or reactive organophosphates which react with "active" serines in enzyme catalytic sites, would be expected to have extensive biologic consequences. Modification of the protein environment can also be important in biologic systems. Cryoglobulins, for example, precipitate as the temperature is lowered because of the change in water structure, which in turn promotes protein aggregation. Another physical effect on proteins results from their natural tendency to unfold at interfaces owing to their content of both hydrophobic and hydrophilic groups. This is an important concept to consider, for example, in the construction of heart-lung machines and prosthetic heart valves or arteries, or during the infusion into the blood of chemical agents in order to prevent denaturation of blood elements and resulting toxic effects.

Protein secondary structure results from all the backbone rotations around the peptide bond, stabilized by hydrogen bonding between peptide units. When rotation is free and intrachain hydrogen bonding is not impeded by excessively bulky side chains or is made impossible by the occurrence of an amino acid in the sequence, a regular helix results. The pitch of this helix is dictated by the nature and size of each side chain. Non-helical regions may be stabilized in folded configurations (so-called "pleated sheet") which may be interspersed between helical regions in a large polypeptide. The regularity of a helical region results in a high degree of cooperativity in its structure stability. Furthermore, the sequential occurrence of repeated sequences within a polypeptide can extend such cooperative stability and a high order of structure over an immense molecule (e.g., collagen, elastin). Although the classic helix and pleated sheet account for most protein secondary structure, much attention is now directed at certain "non-classic" configurations of peptides, involving especially repeated sequences of polypeptides to generate unique biologic functions, such as ion channels, ion carriers, elastomeric properties, calcification, etc. It is particularly exciting that modeling of biologic functions of proteins can now be done both through theoretic calculations and through chemical synthesis of appropriate polypeptide sequences — now made possible through advanced protein technology.

Protein tertiary structure results from all the interactions of the side chains to generate the final three-dimensional structure. The role of water structure is a most important consideration, since the so-called "hydrophobic" interactions of the amino acid side chains are the most important quantitatively in protein tertiary structure. Such interactions derive their stability from the fact that removal of hydrophobic groups from solution results in a considerable increase in entropy of the water structure stability; thus, protein denaturation and renaturation depend on both thermodynamic and kinetic considerations. The protein, once formed, may be extremely stable even when the surrounding medium is changed, because the energy of activation for a structure transition is high owing to the combined effects of its many weak interactions or because of the imposition of covalent restraints in the form of the covalent disulfide bonds. Conversely, a protein may become quite labile or refuse to renature because of transport into an environment different from the site of synthesis or if its structure is modified following synthesis. A good example of the latter mechanism of post-translational modification is insulin. Proteolytic removal of a portion of the backbone of the precursor, proinsulin, prior to secretion removes its ability to renature following denaturation. Such proteolysis, in addition to providing biologically active structures at the time and site of need, also provides a limitation on their stability and turnover. Other pertinent examples are clotting factors, the complement system, digestive enzymes, and various kinins. In contrast, some of the effector and regulatory roles of proteins would require that structure transitions be rather freely reversible in the course of their function.

Quaternary structure is a special, though not separable, aspect of protein tertiary structure which serves to generate higher order structures through aggregation of individual protein molecules. This may result simply in multichain proteins (e.g., hemoglobin, gammaglobulin, a variety of enzymes, collagen) or in aggregates between proteins and other molecules. Not only is such aggregation critical to the formation of functional complexes and supramolecular structures, but provoked changes in these structures are a powerful mechanism for biologic regulation.

Protein tertiary structures provide specific domains for discriminating interactions with other molecules so that proteins may serve their various effector roles and may interact with specific molecule signals from the environment. Moreover, the transitions which occur in tertiary structure serve to provide basic mechanisms for effector roles and for responses to the binding of molecular signals.

Non-protein moieties in proteins also deserve special consideration, since they impart important properties and functions for structural and effector proteins. The covalent attachment of carbohydrate (via serine, threonine, and arginine covalent bonds) provides special binding properties such as immunologic specificity, cell recognition, and, perhaps, aspects of cell communication related to regulation. The process of attachment of carbohydrate to proteins in the Golgi apparatus may also serve an important secretory role. Transport lipoproteins have attracted clinical attention since the recognition of specific diseases, such as Tangier disease, in which abnormal lipid deposits in tissues result from deficient transport (for review, see Chapter 30). Lung surfactant is a lipoprotein which normally maintains the unique properties of the gas exchange surfaces of the lung and may provide major insight into understanding and treating lung disease. Lung surfactant appears to be deficient in hyaline membrane disease of the newborn and is a critical target for study in a variety of pulmonary diffusion difficulties (see Chapter 16). Lipoproteins also serve a variety of other functions such as the construction of membranes and cell organelles, and the lipid as well as the protein moieties provide extensive means of varying structure. The recent discovery of the many effects of prostaglandins has emphasized how potent lipid-protein interactions may also be in regulating biologic systems. A variety of specific small prosthetic molecules, such as heme, pyridoxal, nucleotides, metals, and even PO_4, also provide regulatory and functional properties for catalytic and carrier proteins and illustrate one of the ways minor dietary substances can influence biologic function.

The description and management of diseases in terms of deficiencies or abnormalities of proteins provide an interesting challenge to medical science, the approach to which will require thorough understanding of protein structure and function.

Specific Functional Classes of Proteins. A complete description of all classes of proteins is not feasible within this chapter. However, a brief classification will be useful to focus our attention on specific discussions of disease mechanisms which will follow in later chapters.

ENZYMES. Enzymes must serve three structural roles. First, structure must provide highly specific domains for recognition and binding of substrates and coenzymes. This is a demanding information role for this class of protein molecules which accounts for the specificity and selectivity for all the chemical reactions that make up a biologic system. Since such substrate or catalytic sites may be made up by the precise three-dimensional positioning of a few amino acid side chains from different (even distant) parts of the primary sequence, the entire amino acid structure of the protein participates in their generation. The complete description of a catalytic site is a demanding problem which requires, therefore, complete knowledge of three-dimensional structure and the identification of substrate molecule in situ. Although a variety of techniques are available for tentative identification of participating amino acid residues, only x-ray crystallography at present can solve the complete structure.

Second, enzyme structure must provide the chemical mechanisms for the extraordinary efficiency of enzyme catalysis. The understanding of enzyme mechanisms and their structural bases is a demanding and unsolved problem in molecular biology which could ultimately serve as the basis for generating molecular substitutes for deficient enzymes.

Third, enzyme structure must provide for all the discriminating interactions (communication) between enzymes and their environment and for the appropriate response patterns to these environmental signals. The binding sites for such regulatory molecules or signals, termed allosteric sites, are analogous to the substrate sites in their structure and specificity and reversible changes in enzyme conformational structure provoked by their binding provides the response mechanisms. In many instances the regulatory binding sites may be provided by separate protein subunits which are aggregated with the catalytic subunit to provide a coordinated regulatory and effector complex. Coordination of enzyme function also results from specific aggregates of enzymes which are responsible for sequential or interdependent functions. Isoenzymes (isozymes) are minor structural variants of the same protein which occur in different cell types or at specific stages of differentiation resulting from differential expression of redundant genes which are not identical. The fact that active enzymes (and other proteins) are often assembled from subunits amplifies this variability since the final active molecule can be composed of either or both structural forms of each subunit. For example, lactic dehydrogenase is composed of four identical chains which exist in two structural forms. The tetrameric enzyme exists in either pure form or as the predictable mixtures of the three hybrid aggregates, depending on the relative tissue concentrations of the different chains. The biologic functions of isoenzymes are still a matter for study, but their description is often useful diagnostically since it permits identification of the cell type of origin of, for example, an abnormal enzyme level in blood.

The consequences of a single genetic defect in enzyme structure may be expressed principally in terms of substrate binding, catalytic action, regulation, or stability, or through changes in all these properties due to the interdependence of protein structure and function.

OTHER PROTEINS WITH SPECIAL BINDING DOMAINS. Most protein functions depend on specialized binding properties exemplified by enzymes. The differences which exist between groups of proteins can be described in terms of the fates of the protein and its bound ligand(s). With enzymes, the primary substrates are modified chemically and the protein molecule is reusable. With transport proteins, the ligand is released unchanged either through some environment-provoked non-destructive change in transport protein conformation or through shifts in concentration gradients so that the transport process can be repeated. Thus, protein (peptides) can serve to translocate other molecules through reversible binding processes. A special binding and transport mechanism for peptides has also been defined through the generation of specific transmembrane ion channels through which specific ions can move. The gating for such movement results simply from reversible shifts in peptide conformation. In the case of proteins responsible for host defense (such as antibodies, complement, inflammation peptides, clotting factors, etc) irreversible changes are provoked by ligand binding which provide host protection by removing the ligand or by generating a new molecular structure from the binding protein. Protein hormones are a special class of binding proteins which bind specific target molecules in cells and cell surfaces to signal appropriate metabolic processes. Peptides and polypeptides with hormonal action vary in size from the tripeptide hypothalamic releasing factors to thyroglobulin (MW~600,000) which serves as the storage form from which active thyroid hormone is released. Hormone receptors for non-protein hormones are also highly specific receptor proteins which serve to bind hormones in target cells and promote their interactions with their ultimate targets.

The role of peptides and proteins in pharmacologic action also deserve special mention. It has been recognized for many years that many drug actions depend on specific receptors presumed to be protein in nature. The identity of such receptors and how they serve as effectors are central to the final understanding of drug action. Pharmacologically active peptides are especially intriguing. The extraordinary potencies of certain exogenous peptide toxins have long been recognized and provide mechanisms for a number of important disease processes (e.g., tetanus, botulism and "food poisoning," diptheria, mushroom poisoning, etc.). Such peptide toxins have also been used as probes for studying mechanisms of drug action. Recently, the recognition of endogenous peptides with pharmacologic actions has added a new dimension to studies of drug actions in the central nervous system, suggesting that such phenomena as sleep, pain perception, emotional level, etc., may be under control of peptide regulators. Even structural proteins have specialized binding domains which lead to stable structural aggregates that provide structure and barrier functions against the environment and may serve specific roles in such processes as calcification.

These brief comments illustrate that the provision of specific three-dimensional binding sites by protein structures play a central role in the success of biologic systems. The high specificity of the binding processes meets the demanding information needs of living systems and the structural changes in the protein and/or the bound ligand serve the large variety of effector roles required. The protein molecule may act, therefore, as a signal, or as a transducer of a molecular signal into some biologic response.

Structural Proteins

Collagens, the most abundant proteins in the body, provide the fibrous network that supports all cellular and supracellular structures. Collagen fibers are built up by aggregation of collagen molecules, each of which is comprised of a rigid supercoil of three α-chain molecules tightly wound together. The remarkable ordering, strength and stability of collagen, as well as its biologic variations, can be related to its unique structural features. The different types of collagen are provided by five types of α-chains which differ either in primary gene sequence or from post-translational modification. All α chains are homologous in the sense that they are comprised of repeating tripeptides with the formula -x-y-Gly-, in which 42 per cent of x and y residues are proline + hydroxyproline, and 22 per cent are alanine. The repeating tripeptide structure assures the long range regularity required for fiber assembly and stability.

The biosynthesis of collagen and the assembly of fibers for unique functions require at least eight sequential processes of post-translational modification. The mRNA for each type of α-chain codes for a procollagen molecule which has additional unique sequences at both the initial and terminal ends of the chain. After translation there is hydroxylation of prolyl and lysyl residues followed by addition of sugar moieties to specific hydroxylysyl groups. Chain association and disulfide bonding then occur, followed by the highly ordered process of triple helix formation and secretion from the cell. The secreted procollagen molecules are then converted into collagen by proteolytic cleavage followed by aggregation into fibers. Fibers are then stablized to provide the tensile strength by enzymic formation of intra and interfiber crosslinks through oxidation and condensation of lysine side chains.

This highly ordered sequence of events offers several opportunities for genetic defects and for pharmacologic and toxic intervention. Defects in the genes for α chain formation lead to specific excesses or deficiencies of collagen types (Ehlers-Danlos type IV; osteogenesis imperfecta). Changes in post-translational mechanisms result in hydroxylysine deficiency (Ehlers-Danlos type VI); deficiencies in proteolysis of procollagen to collagen (Ehlers-Danlos type VII); deficient cross-linking due to lysyl oxidase deficiency (Ehlers-Danlos type V) or unknown or secondary mechanism (Marfan's syndrome, homocystinuria, Menke's kinky hair syndrome). The roles of post-translational changes in collagen structure in aging and degeneration are also of great interest. Structural stability provided by collagen molecules can now be discussed in terms of molecular properties. The additional roles of collagen in such processes as calcification, ion sequestering, and transport are also problems of current interest.

Elastin is a fibrous extracellular protein of remarkable properties which imparts the normal elastic and resilient character exhibited by tissues. The precursor of all fibrous elastin, tropoelastin, has a molecular weight of 72,000, and four amino acids, alanine, glycine, proline, and valine, comprise 80 per cent of all its 850 amino acids. There are some 38 lysine residues from which specific crosslinks are formed to yield stable elastomeric fibers. The complete structure has not been determined, but the partial sequence is characterized by repeating runs of sequential polypeptides which may account for long range order in the fiber and the resulting elastomeric properties. The assignment of specific defects in elastin and its post-translational processing and stability to specific disease mechanisms must await more detailed structural knowledge. The importance of maintaining tissue elastic properties is self evident. In addition, the observations that elastin can serve as a matrix for calcification is highly relevant to formation of atheriosclerotic plaques as well as normal calcified tissues.

Keratin is a mixture of structure proteins which provide the "barrier" functions of cornified skin, hair, and nails. The "low sulfur" component is wound into superhelices to form fibrils which are imbedded in an amorphous matrix. These proteins collectively must then account for the extraordinary properties of the integumental system.

Membrane proteins are of great interest in terms of membrane stability as well as dynamic functions. Basement membranes are collagenous in nature. Cell membranes contain both integral (structural) and peripheral (adherent) proteins which account for specific properties. Integral proteins are characterized by one or more of two unique structural properties. First, they are amphipathic, i.e., they are comprised of both hydrophobic and hydrophilic domains to facilitate interaction with both the lipid membrane and the aqueous environment. Second, they often have essential non-protein substituents. For example, glycophorin of red cell membranes is composed of 60 per cent carbohydrate residues. The proteolipid of myelin is exceedingly rich in fatty acids probably bound by ester linkages. These non-protein moieties serve unique functional roles and are responsible for immunologic specificity and cell recognition. A cancer cell presumably is different, either qualitatively or quantitatively, since it displays altered antigenicity as well as loss of contact or density inhibition. Integral membrane proteins apparently have lateral mobility, but are oriented across the membrane in a highly organized manner. Peripheral or adherent membrane proteins have highly specific interaction sites for membrane attachment and also account for specific properties. Some of these proteins attach reversibly to account for regulation (e.g., peptide hormones). Both integral and "peripheral" proteins may also serve such effector roles as catalysis and transport.

Although *nuclear proteins* usually are thought of specifically in terms of their information role, they may also be classified as structural proteins. Quantitatively, basic proteins (histones) are the major class and provide the core around which the polyanionic DNA is wound into a stable and organized package. Part of the nuclear "package" is also comprised of acidic proteins, which also may serve more specific regulatory and catalytic roles in genetic expression. The nuclear proteins are also important determinants for interactions of drugs and hormones owing to the imposed constraints on DNA structure and availability as well as through provision of specific protein receptors.

Complex Carbohydrates

Complex carbohydrates serve important structural and functional roles. The intercellular matrix and surface properties of all tissues are maintained by the acid mucopolysaccharides. This is a group of related heteropolysaccharides containing acidic monosaccharides, usually glucuronic acid, alternating with an acetylated amino sugar. In addition, either or both substituents may be sulfated. These occur as free polysaccharides or in combination with specific proteins to form mucins or mucoproteins. The synthesis of these large molecules from regular repeating units depends on repetitious enzyme processes: coupling sequentially the appropriate precursors; addition of sulfates to sulfated mucopolysaccharides; attachment to protein moieties in the case of mucins; and formation of non-covalent aggregates. There is considerable microheterogeneity in size, ratios of repeating units, extent of modification (sulfation), and loci and extent of protein attachment since synthesis and secretion depend on these several independently functioning enzyme steps rather than a template or messenger process. Degradation and turnover for mucopolysaccharides appears to be the important control for limiting the amounts of mucopolysaccharides in tissues. This is a critical issue because of the extraordinary stability of these repetitious polymers. In contrast to proteins, which denature readily in the environment and can be degraded by any of a number of peptidases with wide specificity, mucopolysaccharides are stable in solution and require an arsenal of some 40 highly specific hydrolytic enzymes (contained mostly in lysomes) for their stepwise degradation. Thus, deficiencies of these lysosomal hydrolases result in tissue accumulations of their substrates, often referred to as "storage" diseases. (see Chapter 3).

Lipids

In addition to serving as the storage and transport forms for metabolic fuel, lipids provide structural components for membranes and cell surfaces, and are concerned with cell recognition devices at cell surfaces. The molecular details of the latter two classes of functions and the chemical structures required are complex issues of great current interest. A complex lipid consists of long-chain fatty acids esterified (or in either linkage) to a backbone of glycerol, glycerol phosphate or sphingosine. Both glycerol phosphate and sphingosine, in turn, may be attached to various additional head groups with large differences in polarity and size. These include simple and modified carbohydrate residues, ethanolamine, choline, and amino acids. Thus, the fatty acids provide a variable non-polar structure and the head groups provide extensive ranges of specificity for polar interactions and three-dimensional recognition sites. These structures are ideally suited for construction of membranes, therefore, and for dictating specific interactions at cell surfaces.

The simple lipids, which include sterols, carotenes, and prostaglandins as important members, are also important biologically and are characterized by their abilities to interact with a non-polar environment. Owing to the unique specificities of their interactions and their high affinities for membranous structures, they can be extremely potent biologically, as evidenced by effects of prostaglandins and steroid hormones. For some actions (e.g., steroid hormones), biologic action involves not only cell membrane penetration, but also attachment to specific cytoplasmic receptors with transport into the nucleus.

ASSEMBLY OF COMPLEX BIOLOGIC STRUCTURES

The state of knowledge about macromolecules combined with the current sophistication of electron microscopy provides promising background information on such complex structures as cell membranes, cell organelles, and parasites. The principle of "self assembly" demonstrated for tertiary and quaternary structure of proteins, based on the structures of the component molecules, also operates for more complex systems, as shown by the reassembly in-vitro of previously disrupted virus capsules, ribosomes, bacterial flagellae, and membrane components of animal cells.

Membranes

The discriminating barrier, transport, and regulatory functions of biologic membranes are essential for the properties of living cells, and the structural basis for their functions is under intensive investigation. Membranes do not appear to be simple barriers but complex aggregates of macromolecules which show structural variability depending on functional requirements. Thus, a myelin sheath, while similar to the plasma membrane of a liver cell, will also display distinct chemical differences. The concept that a membrane in any site is a dynamic complex of individually synthesized macromolecules is important to the question of assembly, stability, turnover, and function, and the structures of the individual component molecules are of critical interest. The lipid bilayer has served as a useful experimental model for the structural features of a membrane, particularly because molecules may be intruded into its structure and serve there as the "catalytic" or "carrier" units. For example, simple models for ion transport by both carrier and channel mechanisms can be demonstrated using peptide antibiotics which bind specific ions. A wide variety of genetic defects in amino acid, sugar phosphate, and ion transport result from specific defects in membrane function. Similarly, membranes are clearly important end organs for the action of specific drugs and hormones, as well as for acute toxic diseases and more chronic processes such as demyelination or chronic renal disease. Unfortunately, our knowledge of membrane structure still does not allow mechanistic discussions, but this will be an area of active discovery in the next few years. Genetic diseases may again serve as important study systems to identify the biochemical basis for function in much the same way as in intermediary metabolism.

Cell Organelles

A detailed discussion of organelles is beyond the scope of this chapter, but a few cogent points should be made for ribosomes, mitochondria and lysosomes as examples of the potential of the molecular approach.

Ribosomes, complex aggregates of RNA and specific proteins, are the site of protein synthesis as outlined above and therefore are rate-limiting for many biologic processes. They display self-assembly from experimentally disrupted molecular components and are the site of action of several antibiotics and other drugs. Abnormal or "mutant" ribosomes occur in microorganisms but probably preclude survival in higher forms, although the possibility that they may provide disease mechanisms cannot be excluded. In animal cells, the endoplasmic reticulum to which the ribosomes are attached is also a major concentration of a variety of enzymes which serve such varied functions as drug metabolism and detoxification.

Mitochondria are complex organelles with extensive responsibility for metabolic and energy support of the cell. They consist of membranous structures into which are incorporated a variety of catalytic and structural macromolecules. In addition, mitochondria contain DNA and can acccount for the phenomenon of cytoplasmic inheritance, since they carry the information for synthesizing some of their own components. Mitochondria apparently are self-replicating structures but there is a complex interplay between them and the nucleus, since some of their components are also dictated by nuclear DNA and are synthesized in the cytoplasm. Their structure and self-assembly are further complicated by the fact that their stability varies considerably from tissue to tissue (half-life of three days in liver and 30 days in brain); moreover, their various components show different turnover rates. At least one disease appears to represent a defect in mitochondrial morphogenesis (central core myopathy), and experimentally the resistance of malaria to certain chemotherapeutic agents seems to bear an inverse relationship to frequency of mitochondrial bodies in the parasites.

Lysosomes are of special interest as examples of the important role of compartmentalization of biologic function. These organelles contain a rather extensive variety of degradative enzymes and represent potential "suicide packages." On release, these enzymes are involved in digestion of phagocytosed or pinocytosed material, self-resorption in the event of cell death, and maintaining the normal steady-state concentrations of a variety of tissue components. "Storage diseases" result from deficiencies of lysosomal function, and tissue disruption can occur from excessive lysosomal activation as might occur as a consequence of chemical toxicity.

MOLECULAR BASIS FOR BIOLOGIC REGULATION

One of the most remarkable features of a living system is the precision with which its numerous chemical processes are integrated and regulated appropriately in response to signals from the environment. To this end, both simple and direct mechanisms exist as well as rather extensive and complex systems such as the endocrine glands. Based on an understanding of the structure and function of macromolecules and cell organelles these control phenomena may now be discussed in terms of molecular interactions. The result of perturbing a particular biochemical process depends on the nature of the process, what its role is in each system involved, whether it plays the rate-limiting role, and whether there are other compensating or amplifying mechanisms involved. It is also clearly important whether the perturbation is temporary or chronic.

Regulation of Nucleic Acid Directed Process

Control of nucleic acid structure and function provides the over-all control for biologic function. Regulatory interaction with these macromolecules, which are outlined above, can result from a variety of chemical agents. In addition to the direct binding of small molecules (e.g., hormones, drugs) to nucleic acids, specificity is amplified by the occurrence of specific receptor proteins which bind regulatory molecules and then interact with specific sites on DNA as receptor-ligand complexes to initiate, stimulate, or inhibit nucleic acid processes. Thus, much of the specificity and effectiveness of nucleic acid regulation depends on the discriminating binding of proteins.

Regulation of Membrane Function

The compartmentalization of cellular function dictates membrane functions as important regulatory loci. The descriptions of the molecular details of membrane transport and barrier functions are unfolding rapidly and will provide the basis for understanding such regulations. Specific ionophores which can direct transport of specific ions as well as the gating mechanisms for ion channels have already been recognized and have great potential for regulatory intervention. Furthermore, identification of specific membrane binding sites provides a molecular basis for regulation and cell communication which can be exploited both for our basic biologic understanding and potentially for therapeutic manipulation.

Regulation of Protein Function

The effector roles of proteins plus the precise discrimination provided by protein binding sites make this class of macromolecules ideal for monitoring small molecular "signals" from the environment. The strength of such molecular signals (extent of binding) depends simply on their concentration in the milieu. The simplest type of regulation is through competition at the functional site (for example, at the catalytic site of an enzyme or transport site of a membrane) by fraudulent "substrates." Methotrexate, an analogue of folic acid and a powerful inhibitor of dihydrofolate reductase, a rate-limiting enzyme for thymine (and therefore DNA) synthesis, is an example of such a competitive inhibitor which binds even tighter than the normal substrate. The search for useful competitive inhibitors is a straightforward process based simply on knowledge of substrate structure. For example, allopurinol was developed as a xanthine oxidase competitive inhibitor so that uric acid production could be reduced in gout. By blocking terminal formation of the highly insoluble uric acid, the much more soluble and excretable hypoxanthine becomes the terminal product. Fraudulent substrates also may be metabolized. For example, ingested glycols are oxidized to highly insoluble oxalic acid by alcohol dehydrogenase with catastrophic results, because the normal substrate is not available to saturate the enzyme. Similarly, drugs may compete at receptor sites for a natural "regulator" and either produce blockade of normal function or may themselves provoke a response. Table 2–5 lists several examples of well-known competitive inhibitors which have relevance to clinical medicine.

Many proteins also have specific sites, other than the effector or functional sites, which serve as sensors for monitoring the environment through binding a variety of specific regulatory substances. The consequence of such binding is a change in tertiary structure, with resulting change in functional properties. A regulator can thus serve to stimulate or inhibit a reaction and it need not bear any structural similarity to the substrate for the protein. This provides the molecular mechanism for appropriate regulation of a system by end product (feedback inhibition), cross-linked control between collateral systems, as well as hormonal and drug control. It also represents another type of macromolecular defect which could lead to disease, i.e., defective regulator binding sites with resulting inadequate or inappropriate control. This regulation by binding at nonsubstrate sites has been discussed exten-

TABLE 2–5   EXAMPLES OF COMPETITIVE INHIBITORS

Drug	Enzyme or Receptor	Reaction or Natural Substrate Inhibited	Examples of Clinical Use
Neostigmine	Acetylcholinesterase	Acetylcholine	Myasthenia gravis; Glaucoma
Atropine	Parasympathetic nerve endings (cholinergic endings)	Acetylcholine	Parasympathetic blockade
Guanethidine	Adrenergic endings	Catecholamines	Hypertension
Methyldopa	Dopa decarboxylase	Dopa, 5 —OH tryptophan	Hypertension
Ganglionic blocking drugs	Ganglionic receptor	Acetylcholine	Hypertension
Neuromuscular blocking agents (curare, etc., succinylcholine)	Neuromuscular junction	Acetylcholine	Anesthesia (muscle relaxation), spastic disorder
Antihistamine	"Histamine receptors"	Histamine	Allergy
Isocarboxazid (Marplan) Nialamide (Niamid) Phenelzine sulfate (Nardil) Tranylcypromine (Parnate)	Monoamine oxidase	Epinephrine, norepinephrine, dopa	Depressive disorders
Tetraethylthiuram disulfide (Antabuse)	Aldehyde dehydrogenase	NAD, acetaldehyde	Alcoholism
Ethanol	Alcohol dehydrogenase	Methanol → formaldehyde and glycol → oxalic acid by alcohol dehydrogenase	Methanol and glycol poisoning
Clomiphene	Estrogen receptor site	Estradiol	Infertility
Allopurinol	Xanthine oxidase	Xanthine, hypoxanthine	Gout

sively as "allosteric" regulation. The additional fact that the enzymes thus regulated are usually composed of subunits also tends to promote cooperative binding of the regulator and substrate molecules with the result that the system may be very sensitive to small concentration changes over a critical range. This type of regulation, then, results from the detection of small changes in the environment through discriminating binding by proteins and consequent changes in the three-dimensional structure on which their functional properties depend.

Therapeutically, allosteric regulation offers extensive potential for exploitation. For example, fraudulent feedback inhibitors can be employed to turn off metabolic pathways (as with certain nucleic acid precursors in cancer therapy) or abortive inhibitors can be used which bind but do not inhibit and therefore release a system from normal inhibition.

The simplest type of protein regulation involves detection by the enzyme or other effector molecule of changes in concentration of a small molecular signal. There are also secondary or remote mechanisms involved in regulation. For example, some proteins are modified covalently by specific enzymes to produce more stable changes in structure and function, with the primary regulatory signal operating on the modifying enzyme. The concept of a so-called "secondary messenger" in regulatory processes has also become quite important, although the choice of terms leads to some confusion with the "messenger" role of RNA. This concept, so beautifully established with cyclic AMP, interposes an additional, strictly regulatory enzyme between the environmental signal and the target enzyme(s) with the resulting regulatory enzyme product serving as the final enzyme stimulator or inhibitor. Thus, adenyl cyclase is stimulated or inhibited by a variety of drugs or metabolic products in its catalysis of cyclic AMP production. The levels of the cyclic AMP, in turn, are responsible for the regulation of an extensive array of biologic processes, with consequent amplification and orchestration of the environmental stimulus into function. It is particularly interesting that this mechanism has already been used to rationalize the defect in regulation of the kidney tubule in pseudohypoparathyroidism. A thorough understanding of such secondary regulation mechanisms is of great importance both for understanding diseases and for therapy.

Protein structure may also be modified in less specific ways by changes in the solvent environment. For example, the sickling of red blood cells due to hemoglobin S can be antagonized by urea, which is thought to modify protein structure by increasing solubility of hydrophobic groups through changes in water structure.

While function is the major consideration in the types of regulation discussed above, the influence of such changes on the structural stability of proteins is also very important.

Regulation of the Concentration of Proteins

The steady-state concentration of a protein or other macromolecule is the sum of all the processes involved in formation and breakdown. Regulation, then, depends on which step is rate limiting.

Enzyme induction, or environment-stimulated increase in enzyme level, and enzyme repression, a converse decrease in level, and enzyme repression, a converse decrease in level, were first elucidated in bacteria and are outstanding examples of mechanistic biology. The models for these processes, as illustrated in Figure 2–3, show transcription to be the rate-limiting process and assume protein stability to be relatively unimportant in these short-lived organisms. Classically, enzymes are induced by substrate and repressed by end products, so that function is linked to metabolic need. In higher organisms, control signals such as hormones must also be included, and, most importantly, all aspects of synthesis and breakdown must be considered. Thus, in addition to transcriptional control, translation, and assembly of final tertiary and quaternary structure (including any covalent modifications, or additions of nonprotein moieties), protein stability and consequent turnover are important. Each potential control point provides a locus for malfunction, and each offers a possible site for therapeutic manipulation. It is also clear that regulation may be imposed through secondary effects much in the same way as allosteric regulation (secondary messenger, and so on).

There has been considerable speculation about whether inherited deficiency diseases might become treatable based on gene transfer by plasmids. In fact, much less drastic methods may be applicable if the defect is not a complete deletion of the gene but one of depressed level since correction might be achieved through alterations in the regulation machinery or structure of the macromolecule.

Several diseases are already explicable based on faulty control of protein levels. For example, delta-aminolevulinic acid synthetase is excessive in porphyria, and chemical induction by drugs such as barbiturates results in disease exacerbation. Thalassemia appears to result from depressed (and unbalanced) levels of one of the two types of hemoglobin chains which normally must be available in equal amounts for normal assembly of the protein. Polycythemia results from overactivity of erythropoiesis.

The ability of drugs to perturb steady-state levels of enzymes by interacting at any of the control points is important therapeutically in explaining

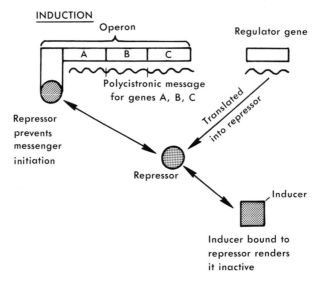

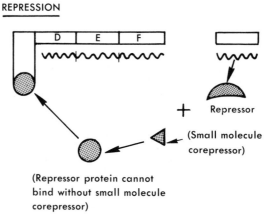

Figure 2–3 Model scheme for induction and repression of protein synthesis operating at the level of RNA transcription.

drug toxicity, and for developing insight into such regulatory effects. The ability of barbiturates to induce glucuronyl transferase and mixed-function oxidases has found application in treatment of both congenital jaundice of Crigler-Najjar syndrome and physiologic jaundice of the newborn. It is also well known that tolerance to drugs may be induced through the mechanism of increasing levels of metabolizing enzymes and that "cross tolerance" may be observed (for example, the tolerance to alcohol evoked by barbiturates and vice versa).

Therapeutic approaches based on regulation of macromolecular levels are limited chiefly by our lack of information about specific disease defects and about mechanisms for producing the appropriate perturbations. Our knowledge about both these points is increasing rapidly, however, and it is clear that this type of thinking will dominate therapeutics. Cancer chemotherapy illustrates how regulatory principles can be applied when the chemical objective is clear and many of the mechanisms are known. Since the problem is one of uncontrolled cell growth, therapy is aimed at preventing cell proliferation and viability, both of which are ultimately dependent on DNA directed processes. A summary of current chemotherapy reveals that DNA synthesis is inhibited by limiting precursors; by fraudulent feedback inhibition; competitive inhibition; and by interference with the DNA template through simple or covalent drug binding and the destructive effects of radiation. The ultimate aim of chemotherapy to spare normal cells, of course, can be realized only through sufficient knowledge of regulation in both populations of cells.

COMMENTS ON THE MOLECULAR BASIS FOR DISEASE

In order to understand the consequence of molecular derangements in terms of disease, it is clearly essential to define the full role(s) for the molecule involved. For example, an enzyme deficit (or toxic damage) could result in a deficiency state in the case of a synthetic enzyme; an excess of some cell component if it is a degradative enzyme; seemingly remote or widespread effects if it is a regulatory enzyme; or no expression of disease if compensating regulatory mechanisms are called into play or if there is no current demand for the particular biologic role played. Thus, a pseudocholine esterase deficiency is not expressed unless the individual is given the appropriate toxic drug; Hurler's and Hunter's syndromes result from defects in normal mucopolysaccharide degradation and turnover, and patients with McArdle's syndrome cannot synthesize glycogen normally. Certain other defects prevent normal cross-linking of metabolic pathways; for example, in galactosemia, galactose cannot be converted to glucose. The disturbance, however, results from accumulation of the substrate rather than from a metabolic deficiency. Diseases also result from excesses, as pointed out in the example of acute intermittent porphyria. In all instances, there may also be far-reaching consequences of a defect resulting from the secondary regulatory roles served by enzyme products. An excellent example of this is the adrenogenital syndrome, in which the molecular defect is hydroxylation of the 11-position of the steroid nucleus to form active adrenal corticoids. These individuals not only show severe adrenal insufficiency but also are severely masculinized, because the normal hydroxysteroid product is not present to regulate (inhibit) early steps in steroid biogenesis, with resultant overproduction of androgens.

It is also interesting to consider the kinetics of disease development and recovery in terms of perturbation of steady-state concentrations of molecules. Whereas some alterations are manifested immediately owing to rapid achievement of new steady states, others develop slowly even over the course of many years, either through cumulative defects (arterioscleroses, for example) or through slow achievement of a new steady state owing to low rates of synthesis and turnover.

REFERENCES

Ashwell, M., and Work, T. S.: The biogenesis of mitochondria. Ann. Rev. Biochem., 39:251, 1970.

Bornstein, P.: The biosynthesis of collagen. Ann. Rev. Biochem., 43:567, 1974.

Brady, R. O.: Sphingolipidosis. Ann. Rev. Biochem., 47:687, 1978.

Burgess, R. R.: RNA polymerase. Ann. Rev. Biochem., 40:711, 1971.

Cozzarelli: The mechanism of action of inhibitors of DNA synthesis. Ann. Rev. Biochem., 46:641, 1977.

Dorfman, A., and Matalon, R.: The mucopolysaccharidoses. In J. B. Stanbury, J. B. Wyngaarden, and D. S. Fredrickson, (Eds.) The Metabolic Basis of Inherited Disease, 3rd ed., McGraw-Hill Book Co., New York, 1972, p. 1218.

Drake, J. W., and Baltz, R. H.: The Biochemistry of mutagenesis. Ann. Rev. Biochem., 45:11, 1976.

Fessler, J. H., and Fessler, L. I.: Biosynthesis of procollagen. Ann. Rev. Biochem., 47:129, 1978.

Gerduschek, E. P., and Haselkorn, R.: Messenger RNA. Ann. Rev. Biochem., 38:647, 1969.

Goldberg, I. H., and Friedman, P. A.: Antibiotics and Nucleic acids. Ann. Rev. Biochem., 40:775, 1971.

Goulian, M.: Biosynthesis of DNA. Ann. Rev. Biochem., 40:855, 1971.

Hanawalt, P. C., and Setlow, R. B. (Eds.): Molecular Mechanisms for Repair of DNA. Plenum Press, 1975.

Heath, E. C.: Complex polysaccharides. Ann. Rev. Biochem., 40:29, 1971.

Holzer, H., and Duntzl, W.: Metabolic regulation by chemical modification of enzymes. Ann. Rev. Biochem., *40*:345, 1971.

Kivirikko, K. I., and Risteli, L.: Biosynthesis of collagen and its alterations in pathological states. Med. Biol., *54*:159, 1976.

Korn, E. D.: Cell membranes: Structure and synthesis. Ann. Rev. Biochem., *38*:263, 1969.

Kornfeld, R., and Kornfeld, S.: Comparative aspects of glycoprotein structure. Ann. Rev. Biochem., *45*:217, 1976.

Lark, K. G.: Initiation and control of DNA synthesis. Ann. Rev. Biochem., *38*:569, 1969.

Lengyel, P., and Soll, D.: Mechanism of protein biosynthesis. Bacteriol. Rev., *33*:264, 1969.

Lindahl, U., and Hook, M.: Glycosaminoglycans and their binding to biological macromolecules. Ann. Rev. Biochem., *47*:385, 1978.

McKibbin, J. M.: Fucolipids. J. Lipid Res. *19*:131, 1978.

Miller, E. J.: The collagen of joints. *In* The Joints and Synovial Fluid. L. Sokoloff (Ed.), Academic Press, New York, 1978, p. 205.

The Molecular Basis of Life — An Introduction to Molecular Biology. Readings from *Scientific American*. W. H. Freeman, San Franciso, 1968.

Perry, R. P.: Processing of RNA. Ann. Rev. Biochem., *45*:605, 1976.

Pestka, S.: Inhibitors of ribosome functions. Ann. Rev. Biochem., *40*:697, 1971.

Revel, M., and Groner, Y.: Post-transcriptional and translational controls of gene expression in eukaryotes. Ann. Rev. Biochem., *47*:1079, 1978.

Schimke, R. T., and Doyle, D.: Control of enzyme levels in animal tissues. Ann. Rev. Biochem., *39*:929, 1970.

Singer, S. J.: The molecular organization of membranes. Ann. Rev. Biochem., *43*:805, 1974.

Urry, D. W.: Basic aspects of calcium chemistry and membrane interaction: on the messenger role of calcium. Ann. N. Y. Acad. Sci., *307*:3, 1978.

Urry, D. W.: Molecular perspectives of vascular wall structure and disease: the elastic component. Perspectives Biol. Med., *21*:265, 1978.

Urry, D. W.: Non-classical helical states and diverse biological functions of sequential polypeptides. Int. J. Quantum Chem., Quantum Biol. Symp., *5*:51, 1978.

Watson, J. D.: Molecular biology of the gene, 2nd ed. W. A. Benjamin, Menlo Park, 1970.

Whelan, W. T., (Ed.): MTP International Review of Science. Biochemistry, Series 1. Biochemistry of Carbohydrates. Butterworth, London, 1975.

Wu, R.: DNA Sequence Analysis. Ann. Rev. Biochem., *47*:607, 1978.

3

Medical Genetics

Louis J. Elsas, II, and Jean H. Priest

INTRODUCTION

The field of medical genetics has increased man's understanding of the pathologic physiology of inherited human disease and his ability to predict and prevent these disease processes. Cellular engineering, mass screening, environmental engineering, genetic counseling, and prenatal diagnosis are some clinical realities that have resulted over the last decade through the application of this body of information.

The mechanisms and recurrence risks for pathologic processes caused by the interaction of multiple genes and the environment provide accurate figures and alternatives to families seeking counseling for such common anomalies and diseases as cleft palate, pyloric stenosis, spina bifida, hypertension, early onset heart disease, and duodenal ulcer. Other diseases caused by a single mutant gene of large effect conform to mendelian patterns of inheritance. Pedigree analysis provides information about recurrence risks and genetic mechanisms for subsequent offspring and may lead to an understanding of the molecular mechanisms that produce the disease. Testing lipid phenotypes in pedigrees from a large population of early onset heart disease led to the identification of three genes that were found to account for 54 per cent of all myocardial infarctions occurring before age 60.

The chromosome is now recognized as the nuclear structure responsible for the physical transmission of genetic information. Abnormalities in chromosome structure or number are associated with numerous clinical syndromes. New techniques using Giemsa banding and fluorescent staining now make possible the identification of individual chromosomes and their subparts. Translocations, deletions, and inversions can now be confirmed and related to abnormal phenotypes. Using combinations of pedigree analysis, biochemical analysis, cell fusion, and chromosome analysis, over 200 human genes have been localized to specific chromosomes.

Progress has been made in characterizing catalytic and structural proteins and relating their function and variation to genetic control. The assumption of A. E. Garrod that an abnormal gene product resulted in impaired cellular metabolism and produced an "inborn error of metabolism" has been verified and extended in many disorders.

The molecular concepts derived from microbial systems by Watson and Crick for the biochemical transmission of genetic information through deoxyribonucleic acid (DNA); by Jacob and Monod for the regulation of gene expression; and by Nirenberg for the translation of triplet codons in nucleic acids to specific amino acids in a peptide chain have found application in human disease. Single amino acid changes occur in sickle hemoglobin and can be explained by a single base pair substitution (point mutation) in the DNA triplet codon. These and other observations in genetic regulation and variation of hemoglobin chain synthesis and structure provide direct evidence that the genetic concepts derived from microbial systems apply to man. The genetic axiom "one gene — one enzyme" now extends to "one gene — one polypeptide."

The "inborn errors of metabolism" include defects of structural proteins, subunits of functioning proteins, transport proteins, proteins regulating gene expression, proteins involved with coenzyme function, and proteins involved in the repair of DNA itself. Replacement of abnormal enzymes, deficient enzyme products, or coenzymes; addition of inducers or feedback inhibi-

49

tors; restriction of toxic precursors, or by-products; and replacement of the deficient genes themselves are therapeutic maneuvers being studied or used to treat this group of disorders.

The disciplines of population genetics, biochemical genetics, and cytogenetics align in studying, defining, counseling, and treating inherited pathologic processes.

This chapter will review basic mendelian genetics as a necessary prerequisite to the principles of human genetics. Three general categories of genetic disorders will then be discussed: (1) diseases caused by multiple genes and the environment; (2) diseases associated with chromosomal abnormalities; and (3) diseases caused by single genes of large effect. All genetic diseases cannot be discussed in this chapter, and examples are used arbitrarily to illustrate a category of a presumed pathophysiologic mechanism.

MENDELIAN INHERITANCE

MENDEL'S EXPERIMENTS

Although Rabbi Simon ben Gamaliel (Talmud of Maimonides, A.D. 100) excused brothers of "bleeders" from circumcision, it was not until 1900 that Mendel's laws of 1860 were accepted and a formal study of patterns of inheritance in man begun. In 1975, 2336 traits were catalogued in patterns conforming to mendelian inheritance. All of these diseases are caused by single genes of large effect.

It is important to begin our discussion of pathologic physiology with Mendel's principles of inheritance. Mendel's observations were made while experimenting with *Pisum sativum* or garden pea plant between 1856 and 1865. He selected 34 varieties of true-breeding plants and studied discontinuous characters such as the length of the stem, the position of the flowers relative to the stem, the seed color, and the coat texture. Since the flower could fertilize itself and be protected from outside artifact, Mendel could cross hybrids derived from true breeders and thus make quantitative calculations of those disparate characteristics which appeared in subsequent generations. In one such experiment, the texture of the seed coat was either wrinkled or smooth. When he crossed true-breeding plants containing wrinkled seeds with plants containing smooth seeds, he found that in the F_1 generation only smooth-coated seeds were present. When he self-fertilized these smooth-seeded (F_1) plants, he found 25 per cent (1/4) true-breeding smooth plants, 25 per cent (1/4) true-breeding wrinkled plants, and 50 per cent (2/4) smooth, impure breeders, which, when self-fertilized, reproduced the same 1:2:1 ratio.

Phenotype

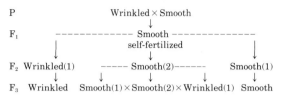

He recognized that the wrinkled coat was transmitted from the F_1 to the F_2 generation in an unchanged state, although it was not phenotypically evident in the F_1 hybrid plant. To explain the disappearance of this hereditary trait in the F_1 hybrid and its predictable recurrence, he recognized that the physical expression (phenotype) differed from the genetic constitution (genotype), which must be composed of two transmissible characters (genes). Mendel's *first law* stated that a unit of genetic information was transmissible unchanged from generation to generation (gene). His *second law* stated that alternate forms of this gene (later called an allele) must segregate during gamete formation and recombine independently in the offspring to provide this 1:2:1 ratio. From the phenotypic expression of these discontinuous traits, the concepts of dominance and recessivity were derived. In the F_1 hybrid derived from two pure-breeding strains, that allele which is expressed is dominant (smooth, S). The unexpressed allele is recessive (wrinkled, w). The genotypes in this experiment can now be written:

Genotype

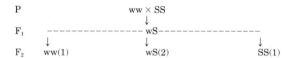

To test the relationship of transmission between two different discontinuous traits, Mendel designed another set of experiments. He compared the textures of the seeds with their internal color. If he crossed true-breeding plants having smooth seeds and yellow interiors with plants having wrinkled seeds and green interiors, all the F_1 hybrids were smooth and yellow. When this hybrid was self-fertilized, he found a ratio of 9 smooth-yellow seeds, 3 smooth-green, 3 wrinkled-yellow, and 1 wrinkled-green out of a total of 16. These ratios (9/16; 3/16; 1/16) were the product of the probability that either trait would appear independent of the other. Thus, for the two dominant traits (smooth seeds with yellow interiors), there was a 3/4 × 3/4 probability, or 9/16. For the recessive traits (wrinkled seeds with green interior), the probability was 1/4 × 1/4, or 1/16. Mendel recognized that the texture of the seed and the color of its interior were independent traits which were not allelic. Thus, his *third law* stated that nonallelic traits do not segregate but assort randomly and recombine with the product of their independent probabilities.

Because the botanists of Mendel's time were observing continuous rather than discontinuous traits, his concepts of a unit of inheritance lay dormant until 1900, when they were rediscovered independently by several different geneticists. By 1902, his observations had been applied in a pedigree analysis of man to explain the patterns of recurrence of brachydactyly. It should be remembered that the concepts of dominance and recessivity were derived from phenotypes and not from biochemical or molecular mechanisms of inheritance. However, the analyses of pedigrees using mendelian concepts are used to predict recurrence risks and to offer insights into the abnormal genetic mechanisms producing disease, even when the biochemical mechanisms are unknown.

AUTOSOMAL DOMINANT INHERITANCE

This pattern of inheritance is the most common mode of monogenic transmission in man, although recessive traits are becoming more prevalent as new metabolic disorders are discovered through modern screening techniques. Most autosomal dominant traits exhibit distinct phenotypic abnormalities, making them relatively easy to detect. From mendelian concepts, one can predict the pedigree pattern for expression of a single dominant gene.

Consider the mating A in Figure 3–1. The heterozygote is affected and, by definition, expresses the dominant trait. If such a parent mates with a homozygous normal, on the average, one half the progeny will be affected heterozygotes and one half will be normal. In mating B, two affected heterozygotes mate. Their alleles segregate during gamete formation and recombine randomly. It could be predicted that one fourth of their offspring would be affected homozygotes, one half affected heterozygotes, and one fourth normal homozygotes. Seventy-five per cent (3/4) of the offspring from this mating would be affected by the dominant trait. A schematic pedigree representing an autosomal dominant pattern of inheritance is indicated in Figure 3–2. Since the heterozygote expresses this trait, there is parent-to-offspring transmission, and a vertical pattern of abnormal individuals is produced. Since the mutant gene is located on an autosome, there is an approximately equal distribution of males and females. On the average, 50 per cent of a patient's offspring are affected.

Important in genetic counseling is the fact that each individual pregnancy has a genetic risk for the given disorder independent from any previous pregnancy. In autosomal dominant patterns of inheritance, if an individual does not express a dominant trait, he cannot transmit it to subsequent generations. This reassuring fact must be

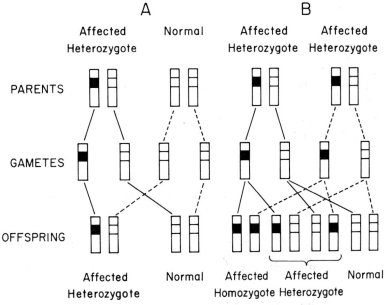

Figure 3–1 Schematic representation of the transmission of an autosomal dominant phenotype. *A* and *B* represent separate matings.

tempered against the difficulty in differentiating the disease from other similar diseases, the age at which the abnormal phenotype is expressed, and the spectrum of expression. For example, the fact that a child of a patient with familial colonic polyposis (an autosomal dominant trait) does not demonstrate polyps by sigmoidoscopy at age 5 years does not mean that polyps will not occur later in life or that they are not present in regions beyond the view of the sigmoidoscope.

In 1975, 1218 dominant traits were catalogued, including acute intermittent porphyria, Huntington's chorea, hemorrhagic telangiectasia, Marfan syndrome, hypertrophic subaortic stenosis, polycystic kidney disease, neurofibromatosis, hereditary nephritis with deafness, familial polyposis, brachydactyly, tuberous sclerosis, and so on. Despite our current lack of knowledge regarding the basic defect in many of these disorders, the dominant pattern of inheritance suggests several mechanisms for their expression and molecular control. In a dominant trait the heterozygote expresses the mutant allele. Thus, the mutant gene product could interfere with the function of the normal gene product by producing an abnormal subunit in a protein complex, rendering the complete complex less effective. Examples of this concept would be dysfibrinogenemia or abnormalities in structural proteins such as collagen in Marfan syndrome or the dominant forms of Ehlers-Danlos syndrome. Dominant mutant alleles might produce proteins which interfere with the regulation of gene expression (repression or

feedback control) as in acute intermittent porphyria. These concepts will be considered in more detail later when *inborn errors of metabolism* are discussed.

AUTOSOMAL RECESSIVE INHERITANCE

From the scheme represented in Figure 3–3, one can predict the pattern of inheritance for an autosomal recessive trait. In mating A, a normal homozygote marries a phenotypically normal carrier of an autosomal recessive trait. In accordance with mendelian principles, the heterozygote does not express the trait. The offspring of such a mating are all phenotypically normal, although, on the average, 50 per cent (1/2) are heterozygotes. The mating in Figure 3–3, labeled B, is the more common situation requiring genetic counseling for an autosomal recessive trait. Here, two phenotypically normal parents carry an autosomal recessive mutation and produce an affected child. A recurrence of this phenomenon can be predicted from Mendel's hybridization experiments. On the average, a 1:2:1 ratio of homozygous normal:heterozygous:homozygous abnormal is expected and produces the classic ratio of 3 phenotypic normals to 1 affected. A schematic pedigree conforming to these predictions is outlined in Figure 3–4.

Several differences from the autosomal dominant pedigree outlined in Figure 3–2 are obvious. There is no parent-to-offspring transmission of the phenotypic trait, but siblings are affected, and a horizontal pattern as compared to the verti-

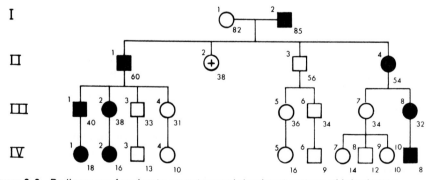

Figure 3–2   Pedigree conforming to an autosomal dominant pattern of inheritance.

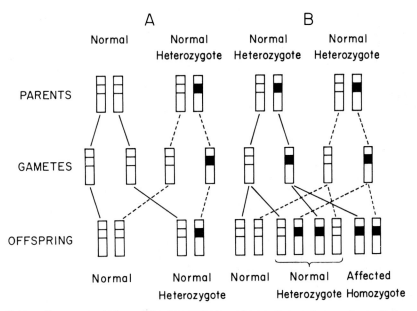

Figure 3–3 Schematic representation of the transmission of an autosomal recessive trait. *A* and *B* represent separate matings.

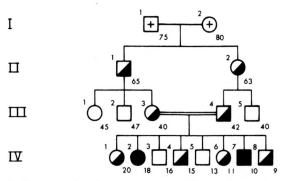

Figure 3–4 Pedigree conforming to an autosomal recessive pattern of inheritance.

cal pattern of dominant inheritance is produced. Twenty-five per cent rather than 50 per cent recurrence in siblings is seen. Since recessive traits are rare in the population, consanguineous matings are more likely to produce the affected homozygote. Subjects III–3 and III–4 are first cousins and their consanguineous mating is indicated by the horizontal double bar.

In recessive traits with identifiable biochemical abnormalities heterozygotes can be detected by appropriate studies, although they are phenotypically normal under normal environmental conditions. High-risk populations such as adult Jews of eastern European origin are screened for the asymptomatic heterozygous Tay-Sachs disease genotype. The partially closed symbols represent phenotypically normal heterozygotes detectable by biochemical tests. Unlike the situation for the dominant traits, a phenotypically unaffected member in this pedigree cannot be assured that he has no greater risk than the general population for transmitting the disorder. The risk of having an affected offspring is based on the product of the probability that the unaffected member carries the mutant gene, that he will marry a carrier, and that both mutant genes will be transmitted to the offspring. If heterozygotes can be detected by biochemical means, more precise information can be given. Suppose patient IV–1 (Fig. 3–4) seeks counseling regarding recurrence risks and is found to carry the mutant gene for Tay-Sachs disease by biochemical testing. Her mate is then tested. If he carries the mutation, the risk of producing a phenotypically affected child is 25 per cent ($1/2 \times 1/2 = 1/4$). If her mate is normal, all their children will be unaffected, although each has a 50 per cent risk of being a carrier. Since these recessive traits are located on autosomes, males and females are affected equally.

In 1975, 947 diseases of man were classified as autosomal recessive traits. Most of the inborn errors of metabolism are included in this category.

X-LINKED INHERITANCE

In both the previous patterns of inheritance, the mutant gene was located on one of the 22 autosomes of man. Let us now consider a mutation residing on the X chromosome. In Figure 3–5A, a female carrying an X-linked mutation marries a normal male. The expectations of such a mating are that 50 per cent of the female offspring and 50 per cent of the male offspring will inherit the maternal X chromosome containing the mutant gene. If the mutant allele is recessive to the normal allele, the carrier female will not express the trait, but the male, who has only one X chromosome, is hemizygous for the trait and

has no normal allele. He, therefore, would express the disorder. The prediction is that one half of the sons will be affected and the other half will be unaffected and unable to transmit the mutation. One half of the daughters will be heterozygotes and carry the mutation and one half will be homozygous normal, but all will be phenotypically normal.

Let us turn now to the critical mating (Fig. 3–5B). The mutation is located on the X chromosome of an affected male; all his daughters will inherit this X chromosome containing the mutation, but none of his sons can inherit this disorder because they must all receive his Y chromosome. The pattern of inheritance for an X-linked trait is illustrated by the pedigree in Figure 3–6. Heterozygotes for X-linked traits are indicated by a symbol with a darkened inner circle. If the trait is recessive, only hemizygous males are affected phenotypically. Since maternal uncles of affected males are commonly affected, an oblique pattern of inheritance is seen. Subject II–1 is an affected male and does not transmit the trait to any of his sons. Both his daughters are carriers and the trait reappears in his grandson, subject IV–2. On the average, half the sons of a carrier female are affected and half the daughters are carriers. A homozygous affected female may appear in a pedigree for an X-linked recessive trait if a hemizygous affected father marries a heterozygous carrier female, or rarely if the X chromosome containing the normal allele is inactivated during lyonization, leaving only cells with the mutant X-chromosome (see later, the Lyon Hypothesis). In 1975, 171 diseases of man were catalogued as X-linked recessive traits.

If the X-linked trait depicted in Figure 3–6 were familial hypophosphatemic rickets, heterozygous females would have abnormally low tubular reabsorption of phosphate and perhaps rickets. This is a dominant X-linked trait. If the trait is rare twice as many females are affected as males, presumably because there is twice the risk for a female to inherit the mutant X chromosome. If the trait is common, as in Xga blood groups, the ratio of females to males is less than twofold (see Hardy-Weinberg Equilibrium). Direct parent-to-offspring transmission is seen. The progeny of subject II–1 provide a critical test of this hypothesis. In this situation, neither of his sons (III–1, III–3) but all his daughters (III–2, III–4) are affected. If such a critical mating were not present, an X-linked dominant trait might be mistaken for an autosomal dominant. Prediction and prevention in this disease is critical. Treatment with oral phosphates and vitamin D should be instituted before weight-bearing age to preserve normal bone growth. An accurate pedigree analysis is therefore imperative to aid in prediction, early diagnosis, and prevention.

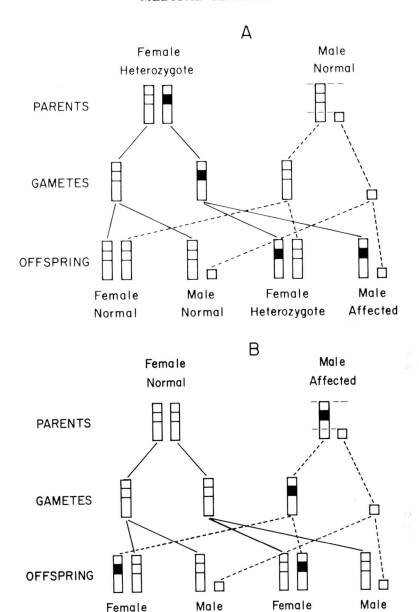

Figure 3–5 *A,* Schematic representation of X-linked transmission: Maternal heterozygote. *B,* Schematic representation of the critical mating in X-linked transmission: Paternal hemizygote.

There are many problems in analyzing pedigrees for "mendelizing phenotypes." Mendelian inheritance may be simulated by environmental mechanisms. Women with phenylketonuria may produce retarded children with microcephaly and other congenital anomalies even though the children are genotypically heterozygotes. The retardation presumably is caused by the effect of high concentrations of phenylalanine on the developing fetus. Phenocopies may be produced by intrauterine infections. Rubella virus may produce a syndrome of deafness and chorioretinal degeneration simulating Usher syndrome, an autosomal recessive trait. Environmentally-caused diseases may masquerade as mendelian traits. At least one instance is known of a mother affected by the rubella syndrome who produced a child with a similar syndrome. Recessive traits which usually

LEGEND:

☐ Normal male
◯ Normal female
◉ Heterozygous female, Phenotypically normal or abnormal
■ Hemizygous male, Phenotypically abnormal
+ Deceased
I Generation
¹◯₂ Superscript = position in pedigree
      Subscript = age in years

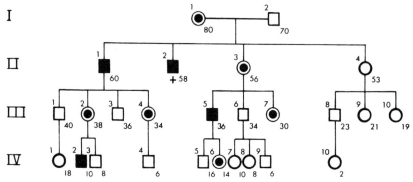

Figure 3–6 Pedigree conforming to an X-linked pattern of inheritance. If heterozygous females are phenotypically normal, the trait is recessive, as in hemophilia A. If she is phenotypically affected, the trait is dominant, as in familial hypophosphatemic rickets.

are not clinically manifest may produce disease under unusual stressful circumstances. When heterozygotes for sickle cell hemoglobin (AS) are subjected to lowered atmospheric pressure, such as in nonpressurized aircraft flights, a "sickle crisis" may occur. Similarly, if the genetic determinant used in a pedigree analysis of sickle cell disease is erythrocyte sickling upon in-vitro exposure to sodium metabisulfite, a dominant rather than recessive pattern of inheritance would emerge. Despite these semantic problems, pedigree analysis and mendelian classification aid in establishing a probable genetic cause, in predicting high-risk individuals, and in suggesting basic genetic mechanisms. The problems raised by phenotypic expression will be solved by more precise information concerning the mutant gene product.

THE HARDY-WEINBERG LAW: FREQUENCY OF GENES IN A POPULATION

In 1908, Hardy, an English mathematician and Weinberg, a German physician, independently developed a mathematical formulation for determining the frequency of genotypes in a population. This Hardy-Weinberg Law, which is quite simply the binomial expansion, states that given two alleles, p and q, then $p + q = 1$. Therefore, for a population at equilibrium were mutation rates are small, where marriage is random, and where selection is minimal:

$$p^2 + 2pq + q^2 = (p + q)^2 \text{ and}$$

$p^2 =$ frequency of homozygotes for the p allele

$2pq =$ frequency of heterozygotes for p and q alleles

$q^2 =$ frequency of homozygotes for the q allele.

From this relationship one can see that heterozygotes for rare autosomal recessive traits are relatively common. For instance, phenylketonuria may occur in only (1/10,000) one in every ten thousand live births. Therefore:

$$q^2 = 1/10,000$$

$$q = 1/100$$

Since $p + q = 1$

then $p = 1 - 1/100 = 99/100$

The frequency of heterozygotes in the population is given by the expression:

$$2 \, pq = 2 \times \frac{99}{100} \times \frac{1}{100}$$

which is approximately

1/50 or 2%

Thus 2 per cent of the population carry the gene for PKU, even though the disease occurs in only 0.01 percent. The relatively high frequency of heterozygotes also enables one to see why saving homozygous affected individuals and enabling them to reproduce will not alter the gene frequency perceptibly in several centuries.

Another use of the Hardy-Weinberg Law enables an understanding of why females affected by X-linked dominant traits have twice the frequency of affected males. Affected males can have only one genotype since they are hemizygous. From the Hardy-Weinberg equation, their population frequency is given by the expression, "q". Females who are affected may be either heterozygous ($2pq$) or homozygous (q^2). Thus, the ratio of the frequency of females to males expressing an x-linked dominant trait is

$$\frac{\text{female}}{\text{male}} = \frac{(2pq + q^2)}{q}$$

If the disorder is rare the frequency of a homozygous affected female (q^2) is negligible and the expression becomes

$$\frac{\text{female}}{\text{male}} = \frac{2pq}{q} = 2p/1$$

where p is nearly one and females have a 2/1 ratio to males. If the trait is common, then q^2 cannot be ignored and this ratio becomes smaller.

MULTIFACTORIAL GENETIC DISORDERS

Although Mendel's hybridization studies were quantitated using discontinuous traits, he also made some observations on traits that blended into a continuum between the parental phenotypes. He recognized that when purple-petaled and white-petaled plants were crossed, an intermediate mauve color was found in the hybrid. When this F_1 hybrid was self-fertilized, a range of color from purple to white was produced in the progeny. These observations seemed to contradict the concept of single gene effects, but Mendel suggested that flower petal color was determined by more than a single gene and that the expressed color resulted from a blending of these genes. Such common conditions as diabetes, schizophrenia, cleft palate, extremes in intelligence quotient and height, club foot, spina bifida, and pyloric stenosis recur in populations and families with frequencies suggesting some genetic influences. Falconer interpreted these observations in the following manner: (1) there are both heritable and environmental influences acting upon the final phenotypic expression; (2) the hereditary component is polygenic and represents a continuum of genetic expression within the population; and (3) the small affected fraction of the population exceeded a threshold liability produced by both a larger number of "risk genes" and the environmental influences to produce the disease (Fig. 3–7). These hypotheses meet certain predicted conditions:

1. If these traits are not monogenic in causation, they will not conform to a mendelian pattern of recessive or dominant inheritance. Therefore, if one looked at the recurrence in first-degree relatives, one would *not* expect to find either a 25 per cent recurrence (autosomal recessive) or a 50 per cent recurrence (autosomal dominant) but rather some other calculable increased risk over the general population. There should be a marked reduction in its recurrence from the first-degree relatives to the second-degree relatives, but still some definable increased risk over the general population. This contrasts sharply with either recessive or dominant inheritance. In mendelian recessive traits, one would expect no increased risk to second-degree relatives, barring consanguinity.

2. A second condition tests the recurrence of traits in monozygous and dizygous twins. In either recessive or dominant monogenic traits, the phenotype must be present in both monozygotic twins (100 per cent concordance). In these forms of inheritance, the recurrence rates in dizygous twins are the same as in first-degree relatives. In a multifactorial trait, one would expect an increased incidence in monozygous twins, but not 100 per cent concordance because of different nongenetic influences. The increased incidence found in dizygous twins should reflect this environmental effect. The recurrence rate found in first-degree relatives should be the same in dizygous twins.

3. One might expect that the more severe the disease expression, the greater the recurrence, since more "risk genes" must be present.

4. One might also expect that, if the disease is more frequent in one sex, then the sex with the lower incidence figure would have a higher threshold and would require more "risk genes" to manifest disease.

TABLE 3–1 MULTIFACTORIAL INHERITANCE OF CLEFT LIP
WITH OR WITHOUT CLEFT PALATE

| | Incidence in General Population (Per cent) | Mono-zygous Twin | Relatives Affected (Per cent) | | | | |
| | | | First Degree | | Second Degree | | Third Degree |
Condition			(Siblings)	(Children)	(Aunts and Uncles)	(Nephews and Nieces)	(First Cousins)
Overall recurrence risk for cleft lip ± cleft palate	0.1	40 (400X)	4.4 ± 0.7	3.3 ± 1.2 (40X)	0.7 ± 0.1	1.1 ± 0.5 (9X)	0.4 ± 0.1 (4X)
Bilateral cleft lip + palate	--	--	6.0		--		--
Unilateral cleft lip − palate	--	--	2.5		--		--
Two affected siblings	--	--	12.0		--		--

Data taken from Carter, C. O.: Hosp. Pract., 5:45, May, 1970.
Blanks (−−) indicate insufficient data.
Numbers in parentheses followed by X (400X) indicate the increased risk relative to the general population.

5. Finally, one might anticipate that in families in which more than a single sibling is affected, the recurrence risks for a third affected offspring would be greater, since, again, more of the "risk genes" must be present in the parents and the probability of liability gene transmission is increased.

Carter's data for cleft lip with or without cleft palate satisfy these criteria. Other known familial causes of cleft lip and palate were excluded, i.e., cleft lip and palate with lower lip mucous pits (Van der Woude syndrome, an autosomal dominant trait; trisomy 13, oral-facial-digital syndrome; and so on). Table 3–1 gives the combined data from four different studies in populations with cleft lip. The general incidence of cleft lip is 0.1 per cent. Monozygous twins were both affected in 40 per cent of cases, whereas in dizygous twins both were affected in only 4 per cent. Neither of these values would be consistent with a monogenic disorder. The first-degree relatives had a fortyfold increased frequency over the general population. The second-degree relatives had a ninefold increase, and the third-degree relatives had a fourfold increase. When a more severe form of the disease was present, such as bilateral cleft lip with cleft palate, a higher recurrence risk figure for first-degree relatives was found (6 per cent). When the milder form of the disease, unilateral cleft lip without cleft palate, was present, a lower recurrence risk of 2.5 per cent was found. When two siblings were affected, the recurrence risk for a third affected individual within that family rose to 12 per cent. These data can be explained on the basis of a continuously distrib-

uted liability produced by multiple genes and the environment, with a threshold beyond which the disease is manifest (Fig. 3–7).

Several other relatively common disorders of man conform to a multifactorial mode of inheritance (Table 3–2). In some instances, the environmental influences are greater than the heritable component. For example, Carter reminds us that Laplanders and the American Indians swaddle their infants with legs extended and adducted. In both these groups, the incidence of dislocation of the hip is higher than the negligible incidence in certain Asiatic groups such as the Chinese, whose infants are held on a back sling with hips flexed and abducted. The incidence in a population in which neither of these environmental extremes is present is approximately 0.2 per cent. At least two genetic factors (acetabular dysgenesis and familial joint laxity) and at least two environmental factors (breech positioning at birth and swaddling) have been described which adversely affect the incidence and recurrence risk figures for dislocation of the hip. A twenty-five-fold increase over the incidence in the general population is found in first-degree relatives of patients with congenital dislocation of the hip. There is only a threefold and twofold increased risk to second- and third-degree relatives, respectively. In pyloric stenosis, a sex predilection has been demonstrated. Although pyloric stenosis occurs more commonly in males than in females (0.5 vs. 0.1 per cent), the recurrence risk to the sons of affected fathers is ten times the general population risk. In keeping with the postulates for a mulifactorial mode of inheritance, the female

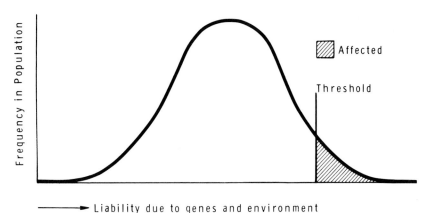

Figure 3–7 Multifactorial inheritance. The continuous distribution of liability to develop a multifactorial disease is determined by many genes and the environment. A threshold of liability indicates the limit beyond which disease is expressed.

may require more "risk genes" before manifesting the trait if perhaps hormonal influences protect her. If an increased number of "risk genes" is required for her to express the disease, a recurrence risk should be higher in her hormonally unprotected male offspring. Sons of females with pyloric stenosis have a two-hundredfold increased incidence relative to the general population. Carter has determined that in the London area, the incidence of spina bifida cystica is ap-

proximately 0.2 per cent. The recurrence is 2 per cent in families in which one member has been affected. After two children in a family are affected, the risk rises to 12.5 per cent.

These kinds of data are useful in relating recurrence risk figures to families, but the concept of a continuous distribution and "multifactorial" disease should not inhibit attempts to find specific causes within these heterogeneous groups. The "continuous" expression of an enzyme function in

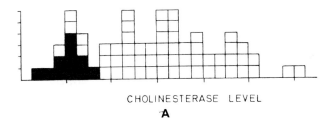

CHOLINESTERASE LEVEL

A

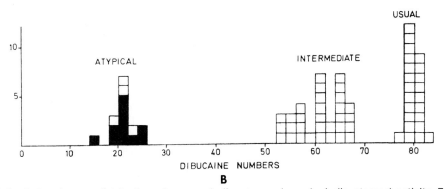

B

Figure 3–8 *A,* Continuous distribution of serum cholinesterase (pseudocholinesterase) activity. Each square represents one individual. Suxamethonium-sensitive individuals are marked in black. *B,* Distribution of dibucaine numbers (per cent inhibition) on identical serum specimens. Discrimination of three phenotypes is evident. (From Harris, H., et al.: Acta Gent. (Basel), *10*:1, 1960.)

TABLE 3–2 MULTIFACTORIAL INHERITANCE—EMPIRICAL DATA FROM FAMILIES
WITH CONGENITAL MALFORMATIONS

Condition	Incidence in General Population (Per cent)	Increased Risk Relative to General Population			
		Relatives			
		Monozygous Twin	First Degree	Second Degree	Third Degree
Dislocation of hip (Females)	0.2	200X	25X	3X	2X
Pyloric stenosis (Males)	0.5	80X	10X (Males)	5X	1.8X
Pyloric stenosis (Females)	0.1	--	200X (Males)	20X	1.8X
Spina bifida cystica	0.2	--	10X	--	--
Talipes equinovarus	0.1	300X	25X	5X	2X
Ankylosing spondylitis (Males)	0.02	--	35X	10X	3X
Early-onset ischemic heart disease (Males)	0.15	--	6X	--	--

Blanks (--) indicate insufficient data.
Numbers in parentheses followed by X (200X) indicate the increased risk relative to the general population.
Data compiled from Carter, C. O.: Hosp. Pract., 5:45, May, 1970, and Falconer, D. S.: Ann. Hum. Genet., 29:51, August, 1965.

population studies may be related to multiple genotypes in that population. Harris clearly demonstrated the continuous distribution of serum cholinesterase (pseudocholinesterase) activity if serum hydrolytic activity alone were the genetic determinant (Fig. 3–8A). Only a small portion of the population (closed squares) was functionally defective and no mendelian pattern was delineated. When other characteristics of the gene products were examined, such as resistance to dibucaine, three phenotypes become evident: "usual," "intermediate," and "atypical" (Fig. 3–8B). This trimodal distribution then suggested mendelian rather than multifactorial inheritance in which "usual" was homozygous normal, "intermediate" was heterozygous, and "atypical" was homozygous abnormal. The discriminant, "dibucaine resistance," resolved the genetic control mechanisms for this enzyme function into a mendelian pattern. Since this earlier description, other parameters of resistance, inheritance, and separation of isozymes have demonstrated at least two loci for pseudocholinesterase activity and 10 genotypes to account for the continuous polygenic distribution in the population. Environmental factors such as liver disease, general nutrition, and renal glomerular integrity contribute further to the "multifactorial" pattern of enzyme activity originally found.

CYTOGENETICS

Another mechanism for disease in man results from chromosomal abnormalities of two general types. There may be a numerical variation from the normal number or the normal number may be present but gross structural abnormalities of individual chromosomes may exist. Chromosomal aberrations have been known to occur in plants and animals for a long time, but only in the past 20 years have human cytogenetic techniques advanced sufficiently to demonstrate that such aberrations occur in humans as well.

THE CHROMOSOMES

In man, the normal chromosome number, 46, was definitively established by 1956. There are 22 pairs of autosomes, which are identical in both sexes, and one pair of sex chromosomes. The latter two chromosomes have a similar appearance in the female, XX, but are dissimilar in the male, one being like the X chromosome of the female and the other, Y, being smaller. The chromosomes appear in metaphase as double structures, the *chromatids*, which lie adjacent to each other and are connected at a constriction called the *centromere*. An analysis of the chromosomes has permitted their classification based on length and shape, the latter being determined by position of the centromere. A chromosome is called metacentric when its centromere is approximately in the middle, the chromatid arms being about equal in length. The centromere may be toward one end, making the arms on opposite sides of the centromere unequal, one arm longer than the other. *Acrocentric* chromosomes are those with position of the centromere very close to one end. Satellites

TABLE 3-3 MORPHOLOGIC CHARACTERISTICS OF HUMAN METAPHASE CHROMOSOMES

Groups	Chromosome Number	Characteristics
A	1, 2, 3	#1 is longest, metacentric, #2 is 2nd longest, submetacentric, #3 is 3rd longest, metacentric
B	4, 5	Relatively long chromosomes; more submetacentric
C	6 to 12, and X	Medium length, metacentric and submetacentric; X is one of the longer chromosomes in this group
D	13 to 15	Acrocentric chromosomes; longer than G group; have satellites
E	16 to 18	Smaller than above groups: #16 is metacentric, #17 and #18 submetacentric #18 is shorter than #17
F	19, 20	Four small metacentric chromosomes that look like the letter X.
G	21, 22, Y	Short acrocentrics; have satellites; Y is similar but may be slightly longer, long arms closer together and with secondary constriction and no satellites

Data compiled from references cited in bibliography under CHROMOSOMAL GENETICS—General.

can be present on acrocentric chromosomes. These are DNA staining regions on the distal short arm that are separated from it by a secondary constriction (non-staining area) (Fig. 3–9).

The autosomes are divided into seven groups, A to G, depending on their length and position of the centromere. They are numbered from 1 to 22, primarily in order of decreasing length (Table 3–3). The X chromosome by length is placed between chromosomes 7 and 8, but without detailed measurements cannot be differentiated by standard staining techniques from other larger members of the C group. The Y is small and acrocentric and usually cannot be differentiated easily from those in group G. The earlier techniques made it possible to group chromosomes in a satisfactory way, but only within groups A and E was it possible to separate individual pairs (Fig. 3–10).

During the early 1970s, newer banding techniques increased the cytogeneticist's ability to distinguish individual chromosomes. Q-banding (quinacrine banding) is produced by quinacrine stain and fluorescence microscopy. G-banding (Giemsa banding) is produced by various pretreatments, usually trypsin, of chromosomes on slides, followed by a stain, usually Giemsa. R-banding (reverse banding) comes out the other way around — non-staining bands by Q- and G-techniques are positively stained by R- technique (Fig. 3–11). Note that since the ends of most chromosomes do not stain by Q- and G- but do stain by R-banding, the latter is useful to detect small terminal deletions or translocations. However, Q- and G- techniques are the two used most commonly for diagnosis of the chromosome abnormalities discussed later in this chapter. The X chromosome is easily identified by its characteristic

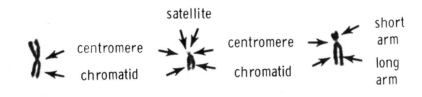

Figure 3–9 Types of human metaphase chromosomes.

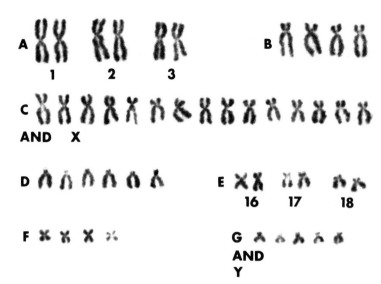

Figure 3–10 Normal male karyotype using standard staining techniques. Forty-six chromosomes are arranged in seven groups (A to G). Note that the X chromosome cannot be differentiated from the C group; the Y is very similar to the others of the G group. Only pairs 1, 2, 3, 16, 17, and 18 can be identified within the groups.

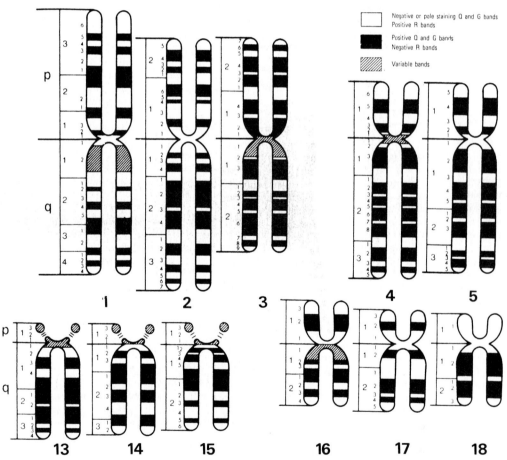

Figure 3–11 A diagrammatic representation of chromosome bands based on the patterns observed in different cells stained with the Q-, G-, or R-band technique. Regions and bands are numbered consecutively from the centromere outward along each chromosome arm. In designating a particular band, four items are required: chromosome number, arm symbol, region number, and band number within that region. (Modified from Paris Conference, 1971, Standardization in Human Cytogenetics.)

Illustration continued on opposite page

banding pattern; the Y chromosome is identified by bright fluorescence on long arms after Q-banding.

One additional technique, called C-banding (centromere banding), stains the centromere regions of all human chromosomes except the Y; it shows positive C-banding on the long arms. The chromosome regions stained by this technique are thought to contain DNA with highly repeating base sequences. This type of DNA has been equated with genetic inactivity, and therefore variations in size of C-banded chromosome regions occur in normal individuals and are termed C-band polymorphisms. Q-band polymorphisms also occur normally, particularly in the regions of acrocentric chromosome short arms and satellites. Both types of polymorphisms show mendelian inheritance; in any chromosome pair heterozygous for the polymorphism, one member is identified as paternal and one as maternal by morphologic study. This important principle is illustrated in more detail in Figure 3–12. Normal variation in length of the Y chromosome occurs in the Q-banded region of its long arm. Each son has his father's Y with respect to this length characteristic.

MITOSIS AND MEIOSIS

The many cells of the body are derived from division of preceding cells; hence, it is essential that we review briefly mitosis, meiosis, and the cell cycle. The non-dividing state of a cell is termed *interphase*. During a portion of this time, termed the (S) period, semiconservative DNA replication occurs and chromatids are doubled. The time after mitosis (M) and before (S) period is termed (G_1), for gap-1; the time after synthesis of DNA and before the next mitosis is termed (G_2), for gap-2 (Fig. 3–13). RNA and protein synthesis occur during all of interphase. The doubled chromatids do not separate until next mitosis.

During interphase the chromosomes are extended; however, as the cell enters prophase of mitosis, they condense and become discrete. In *metaphase,* the next stage, chromosomes are independently oriented (not paired) on the equatorial plate. Duplicated chromatids are held together at the centromere, which is also the attachment point of the chromosome to some of the spindle fibers. During the next stage, *anaphase,* the doubled chromatids move apart, pulled by spindle fibers to each pole of the dividing cell.

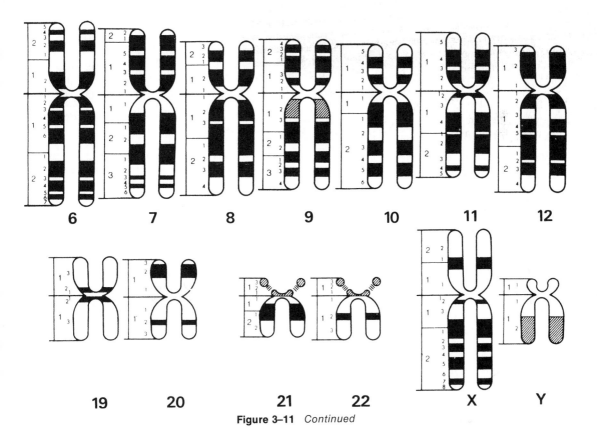

Figure 3–11 *Continued*

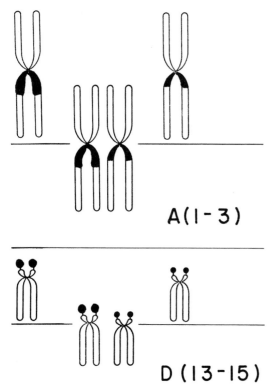

A (1 - 3)

D (13 - 15)

Figure 3–12 *Upper.* C-band polymorphism for the A group chromosome #1 is illustrated. To the left is one parental #1 with a longer C-band; to the right is one #1 with a shorter C-band from the other parent. In the upper middle is the heterozygous pair #1 in the child, one identifiable member from each parent.

Lower. Q-band polymorphism for a D group chromosome is illustrated. To the left is one parental D chromosome (say, #13) with a large satellite. To the right is a D (#13) from the other parent, with a smaller satellite. In the lower middle is the heterozygous D (#13) pair in the child, one identifiable member from each parent.

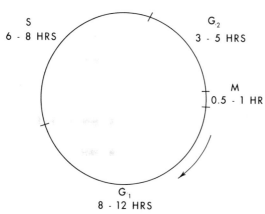

Figure 3–13 Diagram of the cell cycle of most cultured mammalian diploid cells. The approximate length of each part of the cycle is indicated in hours. Direction of progression is indicated by the arrow. Terminology is explained in the text.

Each chromatid is now called a chromosome. During *telophase* the nuclear membrane forms about each set of chromosomes and the cell divides into two daughter cells. Thus a newly formed cell nucleus contains the same number and kinds of chromosomes as the cell it came from. This paired number of chromosomes in each cell is called *diploid*.

During formation of germ cells, a modification of the process just described occurs called *meiosis*. The chromosomes, instead of remaining independent as in mitosis, line up in pairs during metaphase of the first meiotic division, termed meiosis I. One of each pair goes to each daughter cell, giving rise to the haploid number. In meiosis II, chromatids separate, as in a mitotic division, and the haploid number is again distributed to each daughter cell. Reduction of the diploid number of chromosomes to haploid is essential in sexual reproduction since fertilization will again join two haploid sets from father and mother to reestablish the diploid.

CHROMOSOMAL ABNORMALITIES

The normal diploid number of chromosomes in man is 46 in all the somatic cells. In gametes, however, the haploid number is 23 and includes one of each pair. One could suspect that a variation in chromosome number or gross structure would add or subtract many genes from the individual cell and lead to an abnormality. One must bear in mind, however, that some structural changes may occur as normal variations in man without any significant phenotypic expression. Gross chromosomal abnormalities are associated with a number of clinical disorders. The relationship of chromosomal abnormalities to the disease state in terms of the precise pathophysiologic mechanisms is not known.

Before considering specific syndromes associated with chromosomal abnormalities, it is necessary to review a cytogenetic shorthand first standardized in 1971 and now in common usage. A brief synopsis of this is presented, using only the common terms or terms used in this chapter. (Table 3–4 summarizes some nomenclature symbols.) The karyotype is written by noting total number of chromosomes followed by the sex chromosomes. For example, 46,XY is the normal male and 46,XX is the normal female karyotype.

In considering numerical aberrations, 45,X indicates a total number of 45 chromosomes with only one X; 47,XXY indicates a total of 47, two X chromosomes and a Y; 47,XY,+D indicates a male with trisomy of one of the D group chromosomes; 47,XX,+18 indicates a female with 47 chromosomes due to trisomy of number 18; 45,XY,−C indicates a male with 45 chromosomes, the missing one being of the C group.

Chromosomal mosaics are shown by separating

TABLE 3–4 NOMENCLATURE SYMBOLS

A–G	the chromosome groups
1–22	the autosome numbers
X,Y	the sex chromosomes
diagonal (/)	separates cell lines in describing mosaicism
plus sign (+) or minus sign (−)	when placed immediately before the autosome number or group letter designation indicates that the particular whole chromosome is extra or missing; when placed immediately after the arm, structural, or other designation indicates an increase or decrease in length
(?)	questionable identification of chromosome or structure
(*)	chromosome or structure explained in text or footnote
:	break – no reunion, as in terminal deletion
::	break and join
→	from-to
ace	acentric
cen	centromere
del	deletion
dic	dicentric
dup	duplication
end	endoreduplication
h	secondary constriction or negatively staining region
i	isochromosome
inv	inversion
inv (p−q+) or inv (p+q−)	pericentric inversion
mar	marker chromosome, unknown origin
mat	maternal origin
mos	mosaic
p	short arm of chromosome
pat	paternal origin
q	long arm of chromosome
r	ring chromosome
rcp	reciprocal translocation
rec	recombinant chromosome
s	satellite
t	translocation
ter	terminal or end
pter	end of short arm
qter	end of long arm
tri	tricentric
repeated symbols	duplication of chromosome structure

the several cell lines by a diagonal slash. For example, 45,X/46,XY indicates a chromosome mosaic with two cell lines: one has 45 chromosomes and a single X; the other is normal with 46 chromosomes and XY. The mosaic karyotype, 46,XY/47,XY,+21 indicates a mosaic with one normal male cell line and another with one additional number 21.

In defining structural abnormalities, the short arm of a chromosome is designated with a small "p"; the long arm with a "q." A minus sign (−) after a symbol is used to designate decrease in chromosome material. Therefore, 46,XY,5p− indicates a male with 46 chromosomes, but chromosome 5 has a deletion of the short arm. The karyotype 46,XX,22q− shows a female with normal chromosome number, but a deletion of the long arm of chromosome 22. A plus sign (+) after a symbol is used to designate increase in chromosome material. Therefore, 13p+ indicates increase in length of the short arm of chromosome 13. An isochromosome for X long arm is designated 46,X,i(Xq) in an individual who also has one normal X. A ring X chromosome is written 46,X,r(X) in an individual who also has one normal X.

Translocations are indicated by the letter "t" followed by parentheses that include the chromosomes involved. One type of translocation is used as an example and is designated 45,XX,−14,−21,+t(14q21q); the individual is a female with 45 chromosomes. One chromosome 14 and one 21 are missing. The long arms of these two chromosomes are united in a translocation (t).

Chromosome abnormalities may lead to a number of consequences. (1) They have been associated with fetal loss since spontaneously aborted fetuses have a variety of chromosomal defects. The incidence can be as high as 50 per cent in the first trimester, falls to as high as 15 per cent in the second trimester, and is about 1 to 2 per cent in the last trimester of pregnancy. (2) Various types of congenital malformation syndromes, most of them associated with mental retardation, result from chromosomal abnormality. Surveys of newborn infants report the incidence of viable major chromosome defects to be about 5 per 1000 consecutive births, equally distributed between sex chromosome and autosomal abnormalities. (3) Neoplasia is associated with aneuploidy, and a specific chromosomal abnormality (22q−) occurs

TABLE 3–5 CLASSIFICATION OF CHROMOSOMAL ABNORMALITIES

1. Numerical
   A. Polyploidy
   B. Aneuploidy
      (1) Autosomal
      (2) Sex chromosomal
2. Structural
   A. Translocations
   B. Deletions
   C. Isochromosomes
   D. Ring chromosomes
   E. Inversions

in chronic granulocytic leukemia. Chromosomal abnormalities will be discussed in relation to two major groups, numerical and structural (Table 3–5), although these groups can overlap to some extent.

NUMERICAL ABNORMALITIES OF THE CHROMOSOMES

Polyploidy

This term refers to an abnormal number of chromosomes in multiples of the haploid number, 23. As mentioned previously, the diploid state, 46 is normal for somatic cells. Triploidy is a form of polyploidy in which 69 chromosomes are present, three of each chromosome instead of the normal pair (Fig. 3–14). Triploidy is considered to be abnormal because it is found in spontaneously aborted fetuses and rarely in live-born infants. In either case it is associated with severe congenital malformations. In tetraploidy, 92 chromosomes, four of each individual chromosome are present. Tetraploidy occurs normally in some tissues such as liver.

Aneuploid States

Aneuploidy is the term applied to an increase or decrease in the normal (euploid) number of chromosomes, but not involving a full haploid set.

The aneuploid state may involve autosomes, sex chromosomes or sometimes both. In *trisomy*, a form of aneuploidy with 47 chromosomes, one chromosome of a pair is present three times instead of two. Clearly described congenital malformation syndromes are associated with complete autosomal trisomies as summarized in Table 3–6.

In *monosomy*, only one chromosome is present in a particular chromosome pair instead of two. Only a few viable cases of full autosomal monosomy are reported, for G group or number 21 chromosome. Monosomy for the X chromosome is well known, however, and is the basis for Turner syndrome. Other aneuploid states may occur that are more complex; some involve trisomy of two chromosomal pairs, producing a karyotype with 48 chromosomes. An example is the combination of both Down syndrome and Klinefelter syndrome in the same individual (48,XXY,+21).

Nondisjunction

During nuclear division chromosomes or chromatids normally separate or disjoin from each other. Meiotic nondisjunction (failure of disjunction) can occur in the gonads of chromosomally normal males or females as illustrated in Figure 3–15, resulting in trisomic offspring after fertilization. If the chromosomes of a pair do not separate in meiosis I, one daughter cell will contain

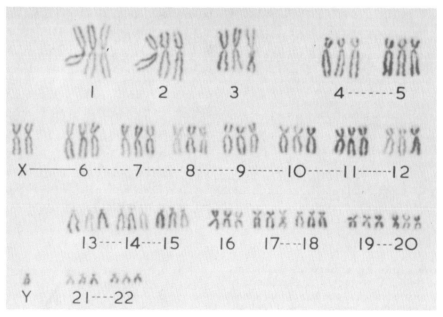

Figure 3–14 A karyotype of a spontaneously aborted fetus, 69,XXY. All autosomes are present in triplicate; the sex chromosomes consist of two X chromosomes and a Y. Because no banding is used here, the assignment of numbers, X, and Y is by centromere position and length. Only numbers 1, 2, 3 and 16 are known with certainty. (Courtesy of Professor Paul E. Polani.)

TABLE 3-6 THE FULL TRISOMY SYNDROMES

Trisomic Chromosome	Brief Clinical Description
8	General dysmorphy of bones; abnormalities of vertebrae and iliac bones; brachymesophalangy; syndactyly; club foot; limitation of joint movement; macrocephaly; mental retardation.
13	Sloping forehead; colobomas; microphthalmia or anophthalmia; arrhinencephaly; cleft lip and palate; cardiac defects; polydactyly; prominent heels; flexion of fingers; apneic spells; seizures; hemangiomas; retarded development.
18	Prominent occiput; small head; small palpebral fissures; flat nasal bridge; small mandible; short sternum; flexed fingers; syndactyly; retarded development; small hypothenar muscles; renal abnormality; rockerbottom feet; hypertonic.
21	Small head; slanting palpebral fissures; epicanthal folds; speckling of iris; flat nasal bridge; large tongue; short neck; cardiac defects; short stature; broad, short hands; incurved 5th finger; single flexion crease 5th finger; palmar single transverse lines; gap between toes 1 and 2; plantar furrow; hypotonia; hyperextensible joints; frequent infections; mental retardation.
22	Small head; antimongoloid slant of eyes; preauricular skin tags; small chin; cardiac defects; finger-like thumbs; hypotonicity; retarded development; characteristic facies.

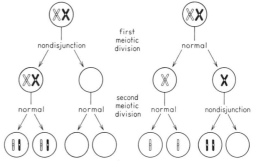

Figure 3-15 Nondisjunction occurring at the first and second meiotic divisions. Nondisjunction at meiosis I produces gametes containing both members of the pair of chromosomes concerned, or neither member. Nondisjunction at meiosis II produces gametes containing (or lacking) two identical chromosomes both derived from the same member of the pair. (From Thompson, J. S., and Thompson, M. W.: Genetics in Medicine, 2nd ed. W. B. Saunders Co., Philadelphia, 1973.)

both members. Recall that in some individuals these two members can be distinguished by their polymorphisms, or normal variations in morphology. Therefore a misdivision in meiosis I is characterized by the presence of two different-looking members of the pair, as shown at the left in Figure 3-15. If the meiotic I division is normal, but nondisjunction occurs in meiosis II, only one type of polymorphic chromosome for any given pair will be present in duplicate, since chromatids of the same chromosome fail to separate in meiosis II (shown at the right in Figure 3-15). This morphologic distinction between a meiotic I and II nondisjunctional error can be used to pinpoint the error in any individual case of trisomy.

Factors leading to the production of nondisjunction are not completely understood. In Down syndrome, incidence of the condition increases with the advancing age of the mother. Similar maternal age effect is noted also in other forms of autosomal trisomy. A possible explanation for these observations is that at birth the female already has a lifetime's supply of oocytes. They have entered prophase of meiosis I and remain arrested prior to metaphase of meiosis I until ovulation many years later. The longer this time, the greater the opportunity for damage from infection, drugs, or other environmental factors. The delay in completion of first (reductional) division of meiosis I is greater in older than younger women. Therefore, a meiotic I error might be predicted in an older woman who produces a trisomic child. Figure 3-16 illustrates proof of meiotic I error in such a situation. The chromosome polymorphisms have been quantitated by a technique using densitometry to record differences in Q-banding along chromosomes number 21 from a Down syndrome child (upper), father (middle), and older mother (lower). These are strip chart recorder tracings that record differences in intensity of fluorescence on the Y coordinant and differences in length of the chromosome on the X coordinant. In chromosome 21 the polymorphic area is in the region of short arm, which on these tracings is to the left. In this analysis the problem is to assign or match up the three trisomic chromosomes of the child at the top with the parental chromosomes below. It is fairly easy to see — and computer analysis has proved — that the child has three different-looking chromosomes number 21, two of which are from the mother and one from the father. If you refer again to Figure 3-15 you will note that this situation is found in a meiotic I error. Since this error is in the older

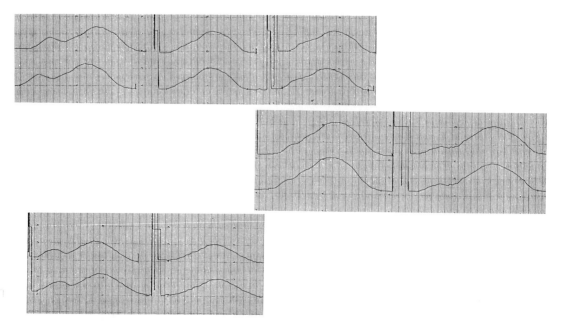

Figure 3–16   Densitometric strip chart recorder tracings of chromosomes 21 from Down syndrome index case (top), father (middle), and mother (below). See text for detail.

mother and not the father, our initial prediction is upheld in this example.

Autosomal Aneuploidy

Trisomy 21 and Down Syndrome. In 1959, Lejeune and his colleagues were the first to find that patients with Down syndrome had an extra chromosome belonging to group G. This additional chromosome is now accepted as number 21 by its characteristic banding pattern. Recent studies suggest that trisomy for the proximal part of subband 21q22 (see Fig. 3–11) is responsible for the clinical syndrome. Production of an enzyme, superoxide dismutase (soluble), is also mapped to this same region on chromosome 21. Thus far, although activity of this enzyme in 21 trisomy is dose-related (in other words, is 1.5 times the level found in diploid individuals), its relationship to clinical symptoms in Down syndrome is not understood. Mapping of human chromosomes and

the significance of this important area of study will be discussed again a little later.

In the past a majority of Down syndrome cases were age-dependent, associated with advancing age of the mother. Maternal meiotic nondisjunction is postulated to be a cause for these trisomic individuals. Exceptions to maternal age dependence were soon studied in more detail. Some had the following characteristics: (1) there was a familial occurrence; (2) mothers were younger; (3) affected children had 46 instead of 47 chromosomes, but one was abnormal; (4) one clinically normal parent, more frequently but not exclusively the mother, had 45 chromosomes and one of these was the same unusual chromosome. It became apparent from study of this parent that the abnormal chromosome was a translocation of chromosome 21 to a D chromosome, usually number 14; in addition, the parent was missing a separate 21 and a separate number 14, making the total chromosome complement "balanced." The affected child had the 14/21 translocation, one separate 14 and two separate 21s producing separate 21 and a separate number 14, making the total chromosome complement "balanced." The affected child had the 14/21 translocation, one separate 14 and two separate 21s producing clinical symptoms identical to 21 trisomy. Figure 3–17 illustrates segregation of the involved chromosomes in meiosis of a 14/21 balanced carrier mother. If an ovum receives both a separate 21 and the 14/21 translocation, fertilization by a normal haploid sperm would result in a zygote with translocation Down syndrome.

Another type of Down syndrome is due to translocation of one chromosome 21 to another 21. In this situation a balanced 21/21 carrier who transmits the translocation in meiosis, could only produce Down syndrome offspring following fertilization by a normal haploid gamete. Carrier

state for translocation of 21 to other chromsomes is also reported as a cause of Down syndrome offspring.

Translocation Down syndrome accounts for only about 5 per cent of all cases. Somewhat under 5 per cent are mosaics for 46/47,+21 and have milder clinical symptoms. The remainder are 47,+21 trisomics, either maternal age-dependent or age-independent. Now most genetic clinics are reporting an incidence of about 85 per cent age-independent Down syndrome among cases ascertained by clinical symptoms after birth. Thus by far the greatest number of individuals with clinical Down syndrome have 21 trisomy for reasons still unknown. Penrose has postulated an autosomal recessive inheritance for 21 trisomy, but many individual pedigrees do not support this hypothesis. Maternal irradiation, delayed fertilization, and infection are other postulated causes. Reproduction of an individual who is already trisomic is referred to as secondary (inevitable) nondisjunction and is known to result in trisomic offspring. It is possible that a reservoir of undetected 46/47,+21 mosaics in the general population could serve as a continuing source for trisomic Down syndrome.

Other Autosomal Trisomy Syndromes. Lejeune and his co-workers also described a syndrome from full trisomy of chromosome 8. The clinical features are summarized in Table 3–6. Patau and others reported patients with retarded development and a very striking constellation of severe congenital malformations usually incompatible with life; the cause was trisomy of chromosome 13 (Table 3–6). As in the situation of Down syndrome, the clinical picture can also be produced by translocation of a chromosome 13 to another chromosome, most frequently another member of the D group. A slightly more common type of congenital malformation was described by Edwards and his co-workers. In this, there is trisomy of chromosome 18, the smallest member of the E group. These patients again have characteristic clinical symptoms (Table 3–6), and there is a predominance of females. Another syndrome of congenital defects has now been established by banding analysis to be due to 22 trisomy.

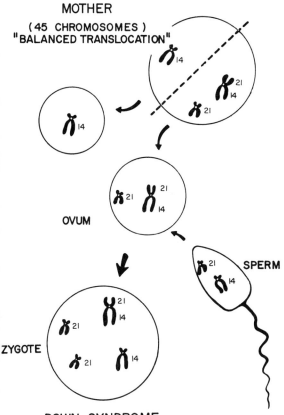

DOWN SYNDROME
TRANSLOCATION TYPE

Figure 3–17 The mechanism for production of a 14/21 translocation Down syndrome (see text for detailed explanation). It should be noted that only the split of the primary oocyte producing Down syndrome of the translocation type is shown. Other splits of the oocyte would result in viable offspring with normal chromosomes or with the "balanced" carrier state.

Sex Chromosomal Aneuploidy

Determination of Sex. The primitive gonad is bipotential and can develop into either an ovary or a testis depending upon the type of sex chromosomes. In humans the Y chromosome is male determining and promotes testicular development from the medullary portion of the primitive gonad. In the presence of two X chromosomes, the cortex of the primitive gonad develops into an ovary. Importance of the Y chromosome is underlined by the fact that an XXY individual is a

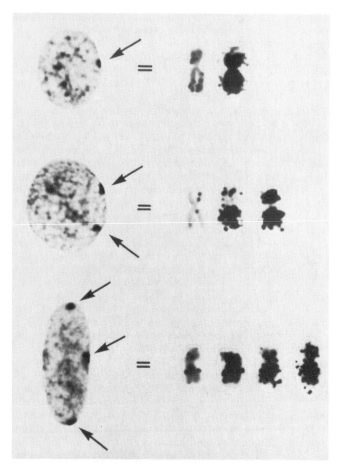

Figure 3–18 Three cell nuclei from XX, XXX, and XXXX individuals are shown. These demonstrate the number of X bodies designated by the arrows. Alongside each nucleus are the X chromosomes from metaphases after labeling with tritiated thymidine. Note that all X chromosomes in excess of one are late-labeling. (Photograph supplied through the courtesy of Professor Paul E. Polani.)

male despite the presence of two X chromosomes. In fact, XXXY and XXXXY individuals are also phenotypic males despite the additional X chromosomes. On the other hand, a 45,X individual is phenotypically female, but one with failure of ovarian differentiation, and has Turner syndrome. The suggestion is that a second X chromosome is necessary for the primitive gonad to develop into a normal ovary.

Sex Chromatin. Some years before modern techniques of human chromosome analysis were developed, Barr and Bertram in 1949 discovered the presence of a condensed chromatin mass in cell nuclei of females. A similar body was not present in cell nuclei of males. Female sex chromatin (Barr body; X body) usually appears as a plano-convex condensation of chromatin about 1μ in diameter along the nuclear membrane (Fig. 3–18, top). More recently (1970) bright fluorescence on the Y chromosome long arm was shown to give a bright spot in interphase, termed the male sex chromatin (Y body) (Fig. 3–19A and Fig. 3–20A). Quinacrine stain and fluorescence microscopy are required for its examination.

Studies of female and male sex chromatin are very useful to screen for the number of X or Y chromosomes, respectively, present in an individual. In clinical practice, smears of the buccal mucosa are readily available, and these are usually studied.

An X body is seen in at least 15 to 20 per cent of readable buccal smear nuclei of the normal female. Its presence indicates two X chromosomes in the cell, one of which is "inactivated" or condensed to form the female sex chromatin. An X body is not seen in normal males (XY) or in patients with classic Turner syndrome (45,X). The XXX female has some cells with two X bodies, and the XXXX individual has some cells with three X bodies (Fig. 3–18, middle and lower). Thus the rule follows: number of X chromosomes is 1+n, where n is the number of X bodies.

Condensed chromatin of the X body is associated not only with genetic inactivity and greater condensation of chromosomal DNA, but also with late onset and completion of DNA replication within S period of the cell cycle. If tritiated thymidine is supplied to cells late in the S period,

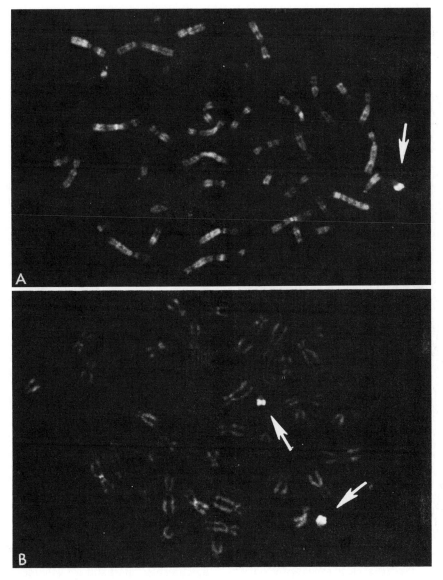

Figure 3–19 Metaphase chromosomes stained with quinacrine mustard (QM). *A.* This photomicrograph shows the Y chromosome in a normal male, 46,XY. *B.* This photomicrograph shows two fluorescent Y chromosomes in a male with 47,XYY.

late replicating X chromosomes will incorporate preferentially the tritium label. They will appear heavily labeled with exposed silver grains in photographic emulsion applied over metaphases on microscope slides, a technique called autoradiography (illustrated in Fig. 3–18).

A Y body (male sex chromatin) is seen in at least 50 per cent of readable buccal smear nuclei of normal males. Its presence indicates one Y chromosome in the cell; individuals with 47,XYY have two Y bodies (Figs. 3–19 and 3–20). Thus the rule follows: number of Y chromosomes is n,

where n is the number of Y bodies. Variation in size of the fluorescent segment on the Y chromosome occurs normally and accounts for the overall variability in length of the Y. Rarely the limits of normal variation are such that no fluorescent spot is seen in interphase in a normal XY individual with a small Y. This situation merely points out the fact that sex chromatin analysis is only a screening procedure for chromosomal sex. Chromosome analysis is the definitive way to identify genetic sex.

Lyon Hypothesis. Observations on female sex

72 I — SCIENTIFIC FOUNDATIONS

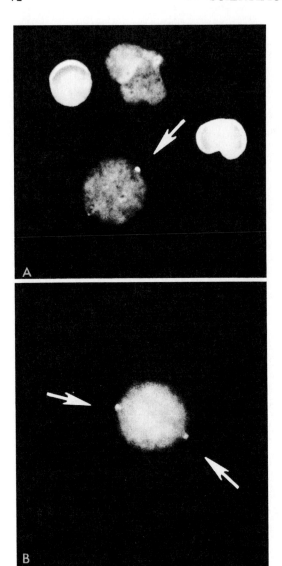

Figure 3-20 Peripheral blood lymphocytes stained with quinacrine mustard. *A.* This photomicrograph shows a single Y body (*arrow*). *B.* This photomicrograph shows two Y bodies (*arrows*) in a patient with 47,XYY chromosomes.

chromatin along with other biologic studies on the genetics of mice led Mary Lyon to make the hypothesis that only one X chromosome is active in each cell during interphase. The second X chromosome, if we may use an analogy from sports, "takes to the sidelines" as an inactive condensed chromatin body. Furthermore, any additional X chromosome also becomes inactive and appears as an X body. This helps to explain why additional X chromosomes do not have the same devastating effects which the presence of extra

autosomes have in Down syndrome and the other autosomal trisomies.

Basic features of the Lyon hypothesis are that: (1) in the female, all or most of one X chromosome is genetically inactive and forms the Barr body; (2) decision about whether maternally derived X chromosome (X^M) or paternally derived (X^P) is inactive is made early in embryonic life and is random in each cell; and (3) all cells subsequently have the same inactive X chromosome, either (X^M) or (X^P). Therefore these cells and all their descendants have the same active X chromosome, (X^M) or (X^P).

The Lyon hypothesis clarifies some confusing clinical and biologic problems pertaining to quantitative gene expression. Why does the male with only one X chromosome have the same amount of gene product for genes carried on the X chromosome as a female who has two X chromosomes? The level of glucose-6-phosphate dehydrogenase (G6PD), an enzyme with wide tissue distribution in the body, is controlled by an X-linked gene and is equivalent in normal males and females. Levels of coagulation Factor VIII (antihemophilic globulin) are also equivalent in normal men and women. The mechanism for this "dosage compensation" can be understood in light of the Lyon hypothesis if one of the two X chromosomes of the female is inactive.

Occasionally a heterozygous female for the hemophilia trait has a bleeding disorder manifested by reduced circulating Factor VIII. Why is this X-linked recessive trait expressed? The Lyon hypothesis provides one explanation. Since inactivation of one X chromosome is initially a random event, occasionally almost all X chromosomes containing the normal allele for Factor VIII could be inactivated; most cells, then, would express the mutant allele.

Turner Syndrome (Gonadal Dysgenesis). This syndrome is a form of primary hypogonadism in phenotypic females who have gonadal dysplasia, amenorrhea, short stature, and lack of secondary sex characteristics. A variety of congenital defects, including webbing of the neck and coarctation of the aorta may accompany this syndrome. Nipples are widely spaced on the chest, and pigmented nevi are frequently present on the skin. Lymphedema has been described in the early weeks of life. The syndrome is accompanied by high gonadotropin excretion in urine and low urinary estrogens, as would be expected in primary gonadal failure. Many of these individuals are X body negative and cytogenetic studies have shown that their karyotype is 45,X.

The number of patients with Turner syndrome is believed to be only a small fraction of the total number of conceptions with the 45,X karyotype. Studies show that this karyotype occurs frequently in spontaneously aborted fetuses. The frequency with which it is found suggests that most of such conceptuses are aborted and only less than 10 per cent survive to be born and show Turner syndrome.

Interesting associations with Turner syndrome are the clinical accompaniment of Hashimoto's thyroiditis and the even more frequent finding of circulating antibodies to thyroglobulin. These associations may be more common in patients with isochromosome X, described in the next paragraph. The question is raised whether development of antibodies is the consequence of the chromosomal abnormality or whether the reverse might be true. A high incidence of thyroid antibodies has been found in families of these patients,

suggesting that the tendency to autoantibody formation in parents might be related to chromosomal abnormalities of the children.

In contrast to the majority of patients with Turner syndrome, a minority were found to be X chromatin positive, with a normal number of chromosomes. In some of these patients, the 44 autosomes were all normal, as would be expected, and a single normal-appearing X chromosome was present. The other X was a structurally abnormal isochromosome. This chromosome is believed to arise as a result of misdivision through the centromere as illustrated in Figure 3–21. In this situation an isochromosome composed of two X long arms shows a characteristic banding pattern

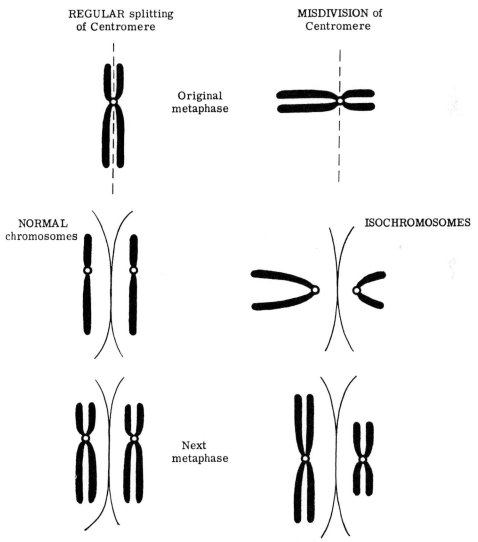

REGULAR splitting of Centromere

MISDIVISION of Centromere

Original metaphase

NORMAL chromosomes

ISOCHROMOSOMES

Next metaphase

Figure 3–21 The mechanism for production of an isochromosome. (From Hamerton, J. L. (ed.): Chromosomes in Medicine. William Heinemann Medical Books, Ltd., London 1962.)

since both arms are mirror images of each other. Isochromosomes for the X short arm apparently do not survive; banding studies do not confirm their existence. It is clear, however, that X chromosomes can break in different places, forming partial isochromosomes, X duplications, or X-X translocations. (Structural abnormalities of chromosomes are described again in the next section.) In the decision as to which X chromosome makes an X body at the time of inactivation, an abnormal X usually becomes the inactive one. X long arm isochromosomes are longer than a normal X and produce a morphologically larger Barr body.

Instances of Turner syndrome with one normal X and a deleted X have been described. The deleted X is termed Xp- or Xq- depending on site of the deletion. A ring X, termed r(X), is usually considered a form of X deletion since intact opposite ends of chromosomes do not normally form rings. Therefore, terminal deletions are assumed to exist but often are difficult to prove, even with banding. Deleted X chromosomes form morphologically smaller X bodies.

Turner mosaics are described with reasonable frequency. Among these are: 45,X/46,XX; 45,X/46,XY; 45,X/47,XXX; 45,X/47,XYY; and some with three cell lines, as 45,X/46,XX/47,XXX. Number of Barr bodies per cell and percentage of X body positive cells in buccal smear may be

useful in screening for these mosaics. All examples of Turner syndrome other than 45,X may be termed Turner variants. They have varying degrees of involvement with features of the syndrome, although gonadal dysgenesis and short stature usually are present. The exact role of X chromosome in determining stature is not presently settled. Turner variants with a cell line containing a Y chromosome are at risk for gonadal tumors and therefore the cytogenetic diagnosis is critical for their management.

Originally, it was felt that 45,X Turner syndrome had its origin in meiotic nondisjunction (Fig. 3–22), but another explanation for occurrence of the chromosomal abnormalities found in Turner syndrome has its basis in the relative frequency of mosaic types. This hypothesis suggests that nondisjunction occurs soon after formation of the zygote rather than before. If one X in a cell division of a 46,XX line fails to enter a daughter cell, subsequent cell development could be 45,X/46,XX; if chromatids of one X in a 46,XX cell separate but move to the same daughter cell, subsequent cells could be 45,X/47,XXX or 45,X/46,XX/47,XXX; if the Y in a 46,XY cell is not included in a daughter cell the result would be 45,X or 45,X/46,XY; and so forth. Mosaicism need not necessarily occur if one cell line is lost, particularly if the abnormal cell division occurs very early in development of the zygote. Absence of a

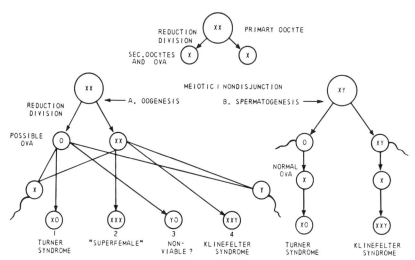

Figure 3–22 Meiotic division and nondisjunction. In normal meiotic division of a primary oocyte, each of the secondary oocytes and ova contains one X chromosome. For simplification, the polar bodies are ignored. The same process in spermatogenesis leads to X or Y chromosome-containing sperm. A. In meiotic I nondisjunction involving oogenesis, an ovum with no X chromosomes and another with both X chromosomes are shown. In each instance, the result of fertilization by an X-containing sperm and the result of fertilization by a Y-containing sperm are depicted. The possible combinations could lead to Turner syndrome, an XXX "super-female," or Klinefelter syndrome. The YO offspring has not yet been shown for humans and is nonviable in the Drosophila. B, meiotic I nondisjunction is shown occurring in spermatogenesis. Each possible sperm is shown fertilizing a normal ovum.

clear maternal age effect associated with Turner syndrome gives support for the idea that some cases are due to somatic nondisjunction.

Multiple X Females. The normal female has two X chromosomes, but females with more than two X chromosomes have been described. The triple-X female (47,XXX) has two X bodies. Although the first patient with this disorder had amenorrhea and gonadal dysgenesis, subsequently no consistent clinical picture has been defined. Some are fertile and produce clinically normal children. Renal malformations occur with some regularity.

Tetra-X females (48,XXXX) with three X bodies, and penta-X females (49,XXXXX) with four X bodies have also been described (see Fig. 3–18, middle and lower).

Klinefelter Syndrome. This syndrome is one of the common forms of primary hypogonadism and infertility in the male. It occurs about once in every 400 live male births and does not appear to be a usual cause of spontaneous abortion. The condition was described in 1942 in phenotypic males who had small, firm testes, azoospermia, and elevated levels of gonadotropin in urine. Gynecomastia occurs in 40 to 50 per cent of the cases, and mental abnormalities occur in about 25 per cent. Its association with some degree of mental retardation is evident, in that as many as 1:100 inmates in some institutions for the mentally retarded have Klinefelter syndrome. In the mid 1950s it was first discovered that these individuals were X chromatin positive. Soon after the application of cytogenetic techniques, it was found that these patients had a karyotype of 47,XXY. Now it can be shown that both X and Y body are present in the same cell. Several mosaic varieties of Klinefelter syndrome such as 46,XY/47,XXY, and 46,XX/47,XXY have been described. The syndrome in some of these patients is incomplete.

One origin of the abnormal karyotype is nondisjunction in meiosis (Fig. 3–22). Pedigree studies using color vision and other X-linked genes as markers indicate maternal or paternal origin for the nondisjunction. Another theoretic mechanism is mitotic nondisjunction.

Additional varieties of Klinefelter syndrome have 48,XXXY and 49,XXXXY chromosomes. The clinical picture of hypogonadism is present, but there may be greater degree of mental retardation. The 49,XXXXY patients may have several additional features, including radioulnar synostosis and more severe hypogonadism, with hypoplasia of the penis and scrotum.

XYY Individuals. In 1965, a syndrome was described in males with two Y chromosomes. These men were tall and showed antisocial aggressive behavior. Many were incarcerated because of crimes of a violent nature. Recent studies have shown that the incidence of this karyotype is not as infrequent as was originally thought. In surveys of newborn infants the incidence is about 1 per 1000 consecutive newborns. Also, many of these individuals do not manifest the aggressive behavior problems noted in earlier studies.

STRUCTURAL ABNORMALITIES OF THE CHROMOSOMES

Although total number may be normal, the chromosomes may be abnormal in structure (see Table 3–5). Structurally abnormal chromosomes have already been considered in connection with Turner syndrome, since structural abnormalities of the X (isochromosome, deletion, ring, translocation) can produce some clinical features resembling complete absence of an X. Structural abnormalities of autosomes, with or without change in total number, can produce clinical features of full or partial trisomies or monosomies, or deletion syndromes.

Translocations

If a separated chromosomal fragment becomes attached to another chromosome, it is said to be translocated. Sometimes parts of two different chromosomes exchange places with each other, producing a reciprocal translocation. If the translocated pieces are large enough, the chromosomes involved will be morphologically altered and can be recognized as abnormal. If, however, the translocated pieces are very small, they may be difficult to recognize under the microscope. Small but clinically significant translocations may be undetected for this reason. Translocations can be balanced or unbalanced genetically, examples being the 14/21 and 21/21 translocations already discussed in connection with Down syndrome. Recall that total chromosome number can also be changed by this type of translocation, usually referred to as centric fusion or Robertsonian.

Deletions

A number of syndromes associated with the deletion of a piece of chromosome have now been reported (Table 3–7). A well characterized one is 5p- syndrome or cri du chat syndrome first described by Leujeune and others in 1963. The major feature of this disorder is a characteristic mewing cry like that of a cat. The peculiar cry results from abnormal development of the larynx, and this feature is lost as the infant grows older. Some cases are due to translocation, and under these circumstances one parent may be a carrier.

A brief summary of the clinical findings in other deletion syndromes is presented in Table 3–7. Note the overlap between different syndromes as well as characteristic features.

TABLE 3–7 THE DELETION SYNDROMES

Chromosome Deletion	Characteristic Clinical Findings
4p-	Midline scalp defect
	Colobomas
	Ptosis of eye lids
	Preauricular dimple or sinus
	Beaked nose
	Cleft palate
	Carplike mouth
	Hypospadias (males)
	Small birth weight
	Sacral dimple or sinus
	Oblique nail striations
	Severe psychomotor retardation
	Seizures
	Delayed bone maturation
5p-	Small head
	Hypertelorism
	Narrow ear canals
	High palate
	Heart disease
	Hypotonia
	Cry like a cat
	Poor muscular development
13q-	Microcephaly, arrhinencephaly
	Colobomas, microphthalmia
	Micrognathia
	Congenital heart disease
	Imperforate anus
	Hypospadias, bifid scrotum
	Hand and foot anomalies
	Psychomotor retardation
18q-	Small head, asymmetric face
	Hypertelorism
	Hearing loss, narrow ear canals
	Maxillary hypoplasia
	High palate
	Heart and renal malformations
	Failure to thrive
	Proximally placed thumbs
	Abnormal toe implantation
	Hypotonia, mental retardation
21q-	Antimongoloid slant of eyes
	Prominent nasal bridge
	Micrognathia
	Skeletal malformations
	Growth retardation, psychomotor retardation
	Hypertonia
22q-	Epicanthal folds
	Microcephaly
	High palate
	Syndactyly of toes
	Psychomotor retardation
	Hypotonia

Inversions

Inversions can result from two breaks along the course of a chromosome and realignment after a 180-degree reversal of the order of the chromosome. If the breaks are on the same side of the centromere, a paracentric inversion occurs and the realignment does not change the shape of the chromosome. If the breaks occur on opposite sides of the centromere, a pericentric inversion occurs; if the segments are unequal in size, position of the centromere may be altered.

CHROMOSOMES AND NEOPLASIA

Leukemia

In 1960, Nowell and Hungerford reported the association of a G-group chromosomal abnormality with chronic myelogenous leukemia. One chromosome had lost almost half of the distal long arm. This finding was believed to be a deletion, although translocation of the missing piece to another larger chromosome could not be ruled out. The abnormality was called a Ph[1] chromosome, or Philadelphia chromosome, after the place of first report (Fig. 3–23). This was the first time a specific chromosomal abnormality was associated with a specific malignant condition. The Ph[1] chromosome is now shown to be a deleted chromosome 22 (22q-), and the missing piece may be translocated to another chromosome, frequently a number 9.

In the acute phase of chronic myelogenous leukemia additional chromosome abnormalities may occur, the most common change being addition of a second Ph[1] (22q-) chromosome. An additional C group chromosome may appear, most frequently a number 8. In other acute leukemias the gains and losses of whole chromosomes are also nonrandom.

Solid Tumors

Nonrandom chromosomal abnormalities occur in some animals exposed to chemical and viral mutagenic agents. Thus far the search for similar associations in human tumors is not conclusive. Some hypotheses have been put forward to account for chromosome changes in neoplastic tissues: (1) the specific karyotypic changes are related to specific inducing agents; (2) malignancy represents an imbalance between genes concerned with the expression or suppression of malignancy, this imbalance being reflected at the chromosomal level by nonrandom chromosome changes.

Chromosome Breakage Syndromes

Several inherited diseases associated with chromosomal breaks have stimulated a great deal of interest in recent years, particularly since they are also associated with leukemia, lymphoma, or solid tumor formation. Bloom syndrome is a rare autosomal recessive disorder characterized by a sun-sensitive telangiectatic skin, erythema, low birth weight, stunted growth, and increased chromosome breakage. There are also chromosome rearrangements, some consisting of quadriradial figures (pairing of somatic chromosomes) that are

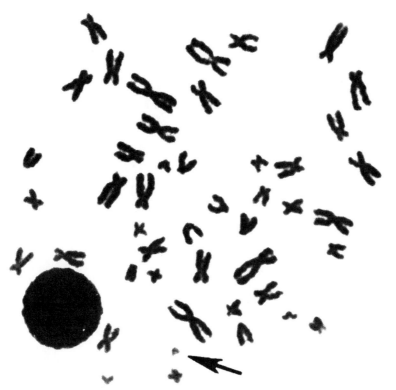

Figure 3-23 Photomicrograph of a metaphase from a patient with chronic myelogenous leukemia, 46,XY,Gq-. The Gq- is shown by an arrow. Banding studies show the abnormal chromosome to be a 22 (see text).

thought to represent cytologic evidence for somatic crossing-over. Leukemia is the more common neoplasm in this disorder.

Fanconi anemia is another disease with autosomal recessive inheritance and chromosome breakage, as well as pancytopenia, skin pigmentation, congenital malformations of the skeleton, hypogonadism, and increased risk of leukemia.

Ataxia-telangiectasia (Louis-Bar syndrome) is also associated with chromosomal instability and neoplasia. In this disorder there is progressive cerebellar ataxia, multiple telangiectasia of skin and eye, and recurrent sinopulmonary infections. The inheritance is autosomal recessive.

In the three genetic disorders just mentioned, chromosomal instability has been documented by direct cytogenetic observation in individuals homozygous or heterozygous for the responsible genes. In a fourth genetic disorder, xeroderma pigmentosum, chromosome breaks and rearrangements are less obvious but nevertheless appear to be present, particularly in skin cultures at later subcultures. The inheritance is autosomal recessive and affected individuals are prone to multiple skin cancers in areas exposed to sunlight. Cul-

tured cells from affected individuals are shown to be defective in DNA repair.

In all the disorders just mentioned, the critical question is whether a cell with chromosomal rearrangements could become the start of a malignant cell line.

CHROMOSOME MAPPING

The goal of human gene mapping is to determine chromosomal location of all known specific genes. In general terms, the accomplishments of this endeavor would provide a better understanding of how genes function and would be a prerequisite for genetic engineering. The classic method of mapping human genes has been to follow the pattern of inheritance of individual single gene traits through many generations of a family to learn what traits are linked or associated with one another on a single chromosome. Sometimes the exact chromosome could be identified, particularly if it were an X, and in a few cases the linear order of genes and some estimate of their distance apart could be determined by this method.

Newer cytogenetic techniques permitted identification of chromosome polymorphisms, and these could in turn be used as markers to locate genes coding for specific traits or enzymes. Another method, deletion mapping, has been useful to some extent because if part of a chromosome is absent so will products of the missing genes be absent.

Nevertheless, family studies in human populations are extremely difficult because families are relatively small, generation time is long, and controlled sexual breeding is not possible. The techniques of somatic cell hybridization have greatly increased our ability to map chromosomes, such that every chromosome now has at least one assignment and some chromosomes have many. This method allows fusion of two genetically different parent cells.

The experience to date with chromosomes in hybrid cells, particularly human–other animal cell crosses, shows that there is loss of parental chromosomes. If the loss of particular human chromosomes can be correlated with absence of specific gene functions, a step is taken toward gene localization. In human–mouse cell hybridization one problem has been the rapid and uncontrolled loss of human chromosomes. This problem can be approached statistically as shown in Table 3–8. In this example, the expression of an enzyme (peptidase A) is correlated with presence of human chromosome 18. Different hybrid cell cultures were each grown from single mouse–man hybrid cells, termed cloning, and each cloned culture was analyzed for presence (+) or absence (−) of peptidase A activity and of particular human chromosomes. Concordant cloned cultures show presence or absence of chromosome and enzyme expression, respectively, while discordant cultures show presence of one and absence of the other. Ideally all clones are concordant and none discordant if enzyme expression is correlated with a particular chromosome. In this example, for chromosome 18 there are 27 concordant and 1 discordant, the closest fit in this data set. The discordant clone was classified as enzyme (−) and chromosome 18 (+), but in the particular culture only a small percentage of cells were chromosome (+) in spite of cloning, and the enzyme activity was difficult to measure. (Experiments are rarely if ever perfect!)

Results of human chromosome mapping can be summarized by locating symbols for the gene products on the chromosome diagrams presented in Figure 3–11. If exact chromosome location is known, the symbol is placed next to the appropriate band region. At present, the relatively full chromosomes (which include 1, 2, 6, 9, 15, and the X) are not necessarily shown to be the ones having fewest viable rearrangements. A problem is limitation in the kinds of gene products that can be measured in hybrid cell cultures. Another prob-

TABLE 3–8 CORRELATION OF PEPTIDASE A EXPRESSION WITH PRESENCE OF HUMAN CHROMOSOMES

Human Chromosome	Number of Concordant Clones* +/+ or −/−	Number of Discordant Clones* +/− or −/+
1	21	7
2	19	9
3	21	7
4	14	14
5	18	10
6	16	12
7	19	9
8	16	12
9	17	11
10	23	5
11	20	8
12	15	13
13	20	8
14	−	−
15	−	−
16	18	10
17	19	9
18	27	1
19	15	13
20	17	11
21	18	10
22	13	15
X	22	6
Y	17	11

*Presence (+) or absence (−) of enzyme activity is placed to the left of diagonal line (/) and presence (+) or absence (−) of human chromosome to the right.

lem is: How do we determine precisely which chromosomes or chromosome regions we need most? Are they the regions with least polymorphism? Are they the chromosomes with fewest viable rearrangements? A better understanding of gene expression in the whole organism is needed before correlation of specific gene products with phenotype can be made.

MOLECULAR BASIS FOR INHERITANCE

The basic unit of inheritance first postulated by Mendel must have at least three properties. It must control a specific function in the organism. It must replicate and transmit this function from one generation to the next. It must mutate and produce variations in this function. This basic unit of inheritance should be present in all cells of the organism. The physical basis for these properties is satisfied by the chromosome. Reduction division seen during meiosis and gamete formation, recombination during zygote formation, chromo-

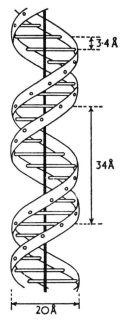

Figure 3–24 The double helical model of DNA as proposed by Watson and Crick. Each helical strip is composed of deoxyribose linked by phosphate bonds at 3 and 5 position. Paired bases joined by hydrogen bonding provide a loose association between the two chains. Each full turn of the double helix (34 Å) contains 10 base pairs. (From Watson, J. D., and Crick, F. H. C.: Nature, *171*:737, 1953.)

some replication preceding mitosis, and phenotypic aberrations associated with abnormal chromosomes satisfy these requirements.

Watson and Crick, in 1953, first pointed out that deoxyribonucleic acid (DNA) was a biochemical contained in bacteria and in the cell nucleus of mammals and satisfied the requirements at a molecular level. Since the concepts of the inborn errors of metabolism relate to primary defects in gene structure and the function of their protein products, a brief review of the structure of DNA and of the regulation of gene expression is useful. The Watson-Crick model for DNA proposed that it consisted of two antiparallel polynucleotide chains coiled around a common axis to form a double helix (Fig. 3–24). A continuous chain is formed, consisting of alternating molecules of deoxyribose joined at their 3 and 5 position by phosphate. The two single strands appear like the banisters of a spiral staircase. The steps or horizontal bars represent a paired purine and pyrimidine, loosely bound by hydrogen bonds. Guanine (G) is paired with cytosine (C), and adenine (A) with thymine (T). This complementary base pairing must be purine with pyrimidine, and only adenine pairs with thymine and only guanine

with cytosine. The double-helical model, with its base pairs oriented internally and joined by noncovalent bonds, provides a molecular method of replication. Each strand can unwind, separate, and serve as a template for replication of a new thread derived from substrates in the cell. A single strand of DNA permits only the insertion of that base complementary to it on the new strand of DNA as it grows alongside the original strand. This semiconservative model for replication of the DNA molecule was confirmed by Meselson and Stahl (Fig. 3–25). The original parent molecule of DNA dissociates, and each strand directs the synthesis of a new strand complementary to itself. Thus, the first generation daughter molecules contain one original and one newly synthesized helical strand. In the second generation, one half the molecules are composed of two new strands and one half contain an original and a newly formed strand. In microbial systems, purified DNA polymerase can use a primer single strand of DNA and replicate by matching one of the four deoxyribose triphosphates (GTP, ATP, CTP, or TTP) with the complementary base on the primer strand. The chain grows by adding appropriate bases at the 3' hydroxy group and releasing pyrophosphate. DNA replication in chromosomes of higher organisms is more complex and less well understood. Autoradiographic studies indicate that several points along the chromosome may replicate. The SU40 nucleotide sequences are now clarified and parallel use of the same nucleotide sequences for different peptide messages has become evident. In addition, the role of histones and other proteins in the complex chromosome have poorly understood functions relative to replication and transcription.

The double helix model provides several possibilities for error or mutation. For instance, the base might exist in its tautomeric form and, during replication, pair with a new base not complementary to the original strand. This erroneous base would then direct the insertion of a new base complementary to itself in the second and subsequent generations. Mutations are produced also by chemicals which are structurally similar to the bases. Bromodeoxyuridine is structurally similar to thymine but pairs with guanine rather than adenine. If this pyrimidine analog were incorporated into the DNA strand, guanine would replace adenine in subsequently formed strands. Many other mutagenic agents are known such as acridine dyes, nitrogen mustards, nitrous acid, and ultraviolet light. Ultraviolet light increases the incidence of interaction between bases on the same strand. These dimers (thymine-thymine) are excised in one process (dark repair). Using the other DNA strand as a template, new bases are then inserted. Abnormalities in this repair mechanism are reflected in man by the disease xeroderma pigmentosum. In this autosomal recessive

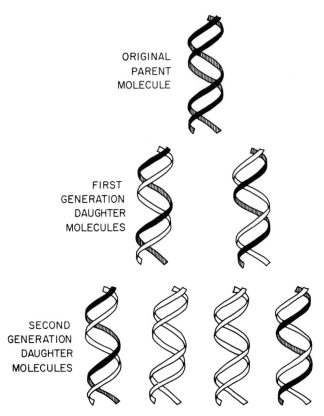

ORIGINAL
PARENT
MOLECULE

FIRST
GENERATION
DAUGHTER
MOLECULES

SECOND
GENERATION
DAUGHTER
MOLECULES

Figure 3–25 Model for semiconservative DNA replication. Solid, black helical strands represent original DNA molecules; open, white strands represent DNA freshly synthesized from the media. In the first generation, there is a 1:1 ratio of old to freshly synthesized strands. In the second generation, only 2 of 8 or one fourth are original strands. (From Meselson, M., and Stahl, F. W.: Proc. Nat. Acad. Sci., *44*:671, 1958.)

trait, an endonuclease necessary to initiate repair is defective, and thymine-thymine dimers are not excised at a normal rate.

The DNA molecule can replicate and undergo variation. How does it relate to the organ or cell function? It is probable from studies of bacteria and from a few examples in mammalian systems that the amino acid sequence of a polypeptide chain is determined by the sequence of bases on a single strand of DNA. The operational scheme by which genetic information coded on a single DNA strand is transcribed to messenger RNA and translated into a sequence of amino acids on a growing peptide chain is outlined in Figure 3–26. The mechanisms involved are detailed in another chapter, but the events will be summarized briefly here.

There are three classes of ribonucleic acid (RNA) which enable DNA to direct the synthesis of polypeptides. Messenger RNA (mRNA) is formed upon a template of single-stranded DNA. Messenger RNA is a single-stranded nucleic acid similar to DNA but contains ribose rather than deoxyribose, and uracil (U) instead of thymine (T). Messenger RNA associates with a second class of stable RNA, ribosomal RNA in the cytoplasm. Amino acids in the cytoplasm are activated by "activating enzymes" and "recognized" by a third class of RNA, soluble or transfer RNA (sRNA). Soluble RNA has an additional recognition site which binds to complementary bases on the mRNA strand. Each amino acid has a specific sRNA which attaches to its carboxy end and to the mRNA-ribosomal complex at the complementary site on the mRNA template. The sequence of amino acids is determined by the mRNA strand and the amino acids are covalently bound at their carboxy terminal. The length of this peptide is determined by punctuation marks in the genetic code. This dogma has become more complicated when viral genomes are studied. Processing including splicing of mRNA in the middle to form functional peptides is present and controlled by as yet unknown mechanisms. However, for practical purposes we may consider that a sequence of DNA results in the production of a peptide chain which may have one of many functions.

Various control mechanisms between DNA and its expression as a polypeptide chain have been postulated from microbial systems. The operon model of Jacob and Monod is indicated in Figure 3–27. In their negative control hypothesis, a repressor protein prevents the structural genes from producing mRNA by binding to a site on the DNA

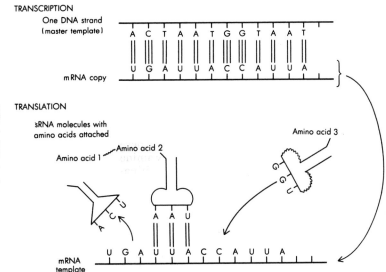

TRANSCRIPTION

One DNA strand (master template)

A C T A A T G G T A A T

U G A U U A C C A U U A

mRNA copy

TRANSLATION

sRNA molecules with amino acids attached

Amino acid 1   Amino acid 2   Amino acid 3

A A U

U G A U U A C C A U U A

mRNA template

Figure 3–26 A model for the transcription and translation of DNA into proteins. (From Hartman, P. E., and Suskind, S. R.: Gene Action. Foundations of Modern Genetics Series, Prentice-Hall, Inc., Englewood Cliffs, 1965.)

molecule called an operator. In the presence of an inducer, the repressor protein is inactivated and does not bind to the operator, and the structural genes in the operon are transcribed. Ptashne has isolated a protein from bacteria with characteristics predicted for a repressor substance, including the ability to bind to genetically competent DNA. Other models of positive control systems have been postulated.

There is indirect evidence for the existence of these working models of protein biosynthesis and DNA regulation in mammalian cells, although no operon *per se* has been defined. Evidence of general regulation of gene expression is derived from cultured liver cells, some of whose enzymes are induced by cortisol. When cells are stimulated with cortisol, there are more enzymes produced and new nuclear RNA species (mRNA) are found. The process of induction is prevented by inhibiting DNA transcription with actinomycin D before adding coprtisol. These data are interpreted to in-

dicate that cortisol induces the transcription of normally repressed genes. There are many controls not only at transcription but also at the translational and post-translational events. Mammalian protein biosynthesis differs from microbial systems, since mammalian cells have a nuclear membrane not present in microbial systems. Newly formed messenger RNA must cross this nuclear membrane to associate with ribosomes located in the cytoplasm. It is probable that many nuclear RNA species are prevented from reaching the sites of protein synthesis in the cytoplasm by selectivity across this potential barrier. It is known that RNA species complementary to DNA are present in a wider variety in the nucleus than in the cytoplasm of mammalian cells, even though nuclear RNA is degraded more rapidly. Regulatory mechanisms may exist not only at the transcription of messenger RNA from DNA but also at levels of nuclear membrane transport, at translation of mRNA into peptides, and with the interaction of

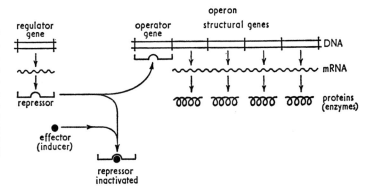

Figure 3–27 The operon model for the negative regulation of mRNA synthesis. Normally a regulator gene produces a repressor protein which binds to an operator portion of DNA, preventing other genes in the operon from transcribing mRNA. An inducer inactivates the repressor protein, allowing expression of structural genes. (From Davidson, J. N.: The Biochemistry of the Nucleic Acids. 5th ed. Methuen and Co., New York, 1965.)

the peptides with others to form functioning proteins.

A precise definition of the mRNA code for specific amino acids became possible following the discovery by Nirenberg that polyphenylalanine is formed when an artificial mRNA, polyuridylic acid, is added to bacterial ribosomes. The genetic code described in microbial systems probably functions in higher organisms including man (Fig. 3–28). The essential features of the genetic code are that each amino acid is dictated by a sequence of three bases (triplet codons). These triplet codons are arranged in a linear fashion and do not overlap, so that one group of three specifies one amino acid, the next group of three specifies a second amino acid, and so on. The four bases of an mRNA strand (UCAG) can occur in 64 different triplet sequences. Sixty-one triplet combinations are known to specify one of the 20 amino acids. There are three triplet codons which do not specify amino acids but act as punctuation and result in termination (term) of the growing polypeptide chain. These so-called "termination codons" are UAA, UAG, and UGA. Most of the amino acids have more than one code word and therefore the genetic code is said to be degenerate. Thus, the process of gene expression in mammalian cells proposes a sequence of events by which single strands of nuclear DNA transcribe their triplet codons to messenger RNA. Messenger RNA proceeds through the nuclear membrane and associates with cytoplasmic ribosomal complexes. Specific "activated" amino acids bound to sRNA are then added in a linear fashion to form polypeptide chains. A large amount of post-translational changes occur in mammalian polypeptides, such as cutting and splicing to form immunoglobulins. Thus, more than one gene may produce a single functional polypeptide. These polypeptide chains must interact with each other, with different peptide chains and with the environment to form functioning proteins which may be expressed in a variety of cellular, metabolic processes.

HEMOGLOBIN VARIANTS: A HUMAN MODEL OF MOLECULAR DISEASE

The first direct evidence that gene mutations result in altered human proteins came from observations in sickle cell anemia. This disease occurs in a small percentage (1 to 2 per cent) of black

Second base

First base	U		C		A		G		Third base
U	UUU	Phe	UCU	Ser	UAU	Tyr	UGU	Cys	U
	UUC		UCC		UAC		UGC		C
	UUA	Leu	UCA		UAA	term.	UGA	term	A
	UUG		UCG		UAG	term	UGG	Try	G
C	CUU	Leu	CCU	Pro	CAU	His	CGU	Arg	U
	CUC		CCC		CAC		CGC		C
	CUA		CCA		CAA	Gln	CGA		A
	CUG		CCG		CAG		CGG		G
A	AUU	Ile	ACU	Thr	AAU	Asn	AGU	Ser	U
	AUC		ACC		AAC		AGC		C
	AUA		ACA		AAA	Lys	AGA	Arg	A
	AUG	Met	ACG		AAG		AGG		G
G	GUU	Val	GCU	Ala	GAU	Asp	GGU	Gly	U
	GUC		GCC		GAC		GGC		C
	GUA		GCA		GAA	Glu	GGA		A
	GUG		GCG		GAG		GGG		G

Figure 3–28 Codon assignments. (Modified from Woese, C. R.: The Genetic Code. Harper and Row, New York, 1967.)

populations. It is expressed by severe anemia, infarctions of various organs such as the kidney and lungs, susceptibility to bone infections, and death, frequently in the second decade of life. Erythrocytes subjected to low oxygen tensions became elongated, filamentous, and sickle shaped. Sickling of the erythrocytes can be demonstrated in 8 per cent of the black population of the United States, and this may occur in the absence of disease. These individuals are said to have sickle trait. Neel suggested that individuals with the sickle trait were heterozygous and those expressing disease were homozygous for an abnormal gene. Family studies further supported this hypothesis. In 1949, Pauling demonstrated that normal hemoglobin and hemoglobin S differed in their electrophoretic properties. Red cells from normal individuals contained only hemoglobin A, but cells from patients with sickle cell trait contained both hemoglobin A and the abnormal sickle hemoglobin (hemoglobin S). A third abnormal hemoglobin, hemoglobin C, was discovered by Itano and Neel. In family studies, this hemoglobin was also determined by a single gene, and heterozygotes for this gene had both hemoglobin A and hemoglobin C in their red blood cells. Homozygotes for the mutant C gene formed only hemoglobin C but clinically had only a mild anemia. That the two mutations were allelic became evident when patients with both mutant hemoglobins were found (double heterozygotes). Since the two hemoglobins were readily differentiated by electrophoresis, pedigree analysis of the two mutations (hemoglobin C and hemoglobin S) could be made. When one parent was a double heterozygote (SC) while the other was normal (AA), offspring were produced with either hemoglobin C trait (AC) or sickle cell trait (AS). No offspring were doubly heterozygous (SC) or homozygous normal (AA). Thus, hemoglobin S, C, and A segregated during meiosis and were presumably alleles.

A molecular basis for these pedigrees became evident when the structure of the variant hemoglobins was determined. Normal hemoglobin A was found to contain four polypeptide chains, two alpha (α_2) and two beta (β_2) chains, each with a characteristic amino acid sequence. The α-chain contained 141 amino acids, the β-chain 146 amino acids, and their precise sequences have been established. The nature of the difference between hemoglobin A and hemoglobin S was determined by Ingram in 1957 when he found that one amino acid in the β polypeptide chain at position 6 was occupied by glutamic acid in hemoglobin A and by valine in hemoglobin S. This position was subsequently found to be occupied by a lysine residue in hemoglobin C (Table 3–9). In all three of these β polypeptide chains, the sequence of the other 145 amino acids was identical. Thus, not only were the mutations occurring at the same locus, but at the same amino acid position of the chain. In molecular terms, the gene is defined as that sequence of DNA which produces a functional polypeptide. The mutations for S and C hemoglobin occur within the gene at identical codon sites (point mutations) and are homoallelic. The messenger RNA triplet codon, GAA, and its complementary DNA codon, CTT, are the code for glutamic acid (Table 3–9). A single base change from A to U produces GUA, the codon for valine and hemoglobin S. The substitution of A in the first position for G results in AAA, the genetic codon for lysine and hemoglobin C. These observations provide strong support for the concept that genetic mutations in mammals represent changes of bases in the DNA sequence of a particular gene.

Structure-function relationships between normal hemoglobin A, hemoglobin S, and hemoglobin C provide some insight into how a single base substitution can result in the expression of a systemic disease. Perutz and Mitchison observed that deoxygenated sickle cell hemoglobin is less soluble in aqueous solutions than deoxygenated normal hemoglobin. These observations suggested a molecular mechanism for the sickling phenomenon. Murayama demonstrated that substitution of valine for glutamic acid at the 6th position in the two β chains of tetrameric hemoglobins allowed intermolecular hydrophobic bonding and molecular stacking between hemoglobin molecules. Perutz and Lehmann suggested that the 6th position of the β polypeptide chain of hemoglobin occupies the surface of the tertiary structure and that normally the polar group (glutamic acid) adheres to a complementary site on its neighboring hemoglobin molecule. In the absence of this polar group, linear aggregates of hemoglobin S occur. In homozygotes for sickle cell disease, the intracellular concentration of hemoglobin S is high and leads to intermolecular stacking. Deoxy-

TABLE 3–9 MUTANT CODONS THAT COULD PRODUCE OBSERVED VARIANTS IN HUMAN HEMOGLOBIN

Variant Hemoglobin	Amino Acid (Position 6)	mRNA Triplet	DNA Triplet
A	Glutamic	GAA	CTT
S	Valine	GUA	CAT
C	Lysine	AAA	TTT

genated red blood cells sickle in the venous circulation, increase blood viscosity, impede the circulation of the venous capillaries, block smaller blood vessels, and form thrombi leading to tissue infarction. The sickled red cells are less well able to withstand the stresses of the circulation and have a shorter survival time leading to hemolytic anemia. A pathologic structural-functional relationship is also seen in patients homozygous for hemoglobin C. These patients have only mild hemolysis as compared to the severe fatal disease produced by hemoglobin S. Substitution of another polar amino acid, lysine, in the 6th position of the β-chain (hemoglobin C) does not produce intermolecular stacking and high viscosity, although a tendency to gel is observed under reduced oxygen tension. It is still not clear how a lysine substitution produces this functional defect in hemoglobin C.

Over 100 different variants of the α or β chains of hemoglobin have been identified. The functional expression of these mutant gene products depends on the charge and location of the amino acid substitution, the resultant conformational change in the tetrameric hemoglobin molecule, and the interaction of these polypeptides with their four prosthetic heme groups. Genetic control of the rate of protein synthesis is reflected by observations on variations in the rate of hemoglobin synthesis. Impaired enzyme function may be caused by a reduction in the rate of protein synthesis, either absolute or relative, rather than by structural changes. The *thalassemias* represent a group of chronic hemolytic anemias caused by a reduction in the rate of α- or β-chain synthesis. Homozygotes for β-chain thalassemia manifest severe hemolytic anemia from birth and have a deficiency of normal β-chain production and consequently of normal tetrameric hemoglobin A ($\alpha_2\beta_2$). Other normal polypeptide chains δ or γ are produced in excess. The resultant red cells contain both increased amounts of hemoglobin F ($\alpha_2\gamma_2$) and A_2 ($\alpha_2\delta_2$), are deformed, and are subject to increased hemolysis. There are several reviews on this subject.

INHERITED METABOLIC DISORDERS

PROTEINS AS MUTANT GENE PRODUCTS

Few mutant proteins other than the hemoglobin peptide chains have had adequate analysis of amino acid sequence to demonstrate single amino acid substitutions. Most inherited metabolic diseases of man are characterized by the functional derangement imposed on the organism by its mutant gene products. A. E. Garrod first introduced the term "inborn error of metabolism" and described four diseases: alkaptonuria, albinism, cystinuria, and pentosuria, which conformed to mendelian patterns of inheritance and presumably resulted from a block in a major metabolic pathway. He noted that when protein or other precursors of homogentisic acid were administered orally to patients with alkaptonuria, the urinary excretion of homogentisic acid increased. He theorized that this "block-in-reaction sequence" was under genetic control, since pedigree analyses were consistent with an autosomal recessive mode of inheritance. The enzyme defect in alkaptonuria was not discovered until 50 years later, when homogentisic acid oxidase activity was found missing in the liver and kidneys of patients affected with alkaptonuria. Garrod's concepts have been extended from the "one gene — one enzyme" to "one gene — one polypeptide" or "one cistron — one functional polypeptide."

Variations in human proteins do not usually produce a functional impairment. A number of normally functioning protein variants including hemoglobins, phosphoglucomutase, lactate dehydrogenase, red cell acid phosphatase, and haptoglobin have been discovered during routine electrophoretic surveys in various normal populations. The vast array of "structural" gene loci in normal individuals has been described in detail by Harris. Using electrophoretic surveys, he has described the considerable protein polymorphism present in normal populations. He has classified the genetic control of these multiple molecular forms into three categories: (1) there may be several gene loci coding for structurally distinct polypeptide chains of a protein; (2) there may be only one gene locus, but many different alleles at this locus; and, finally, (3) there may be secondary "post-translational" modifications of the basic protein. When the mutant gene product results in functional derangement, an inborn error of metabolism exists. The functional defect may be expressed by many different pathogenic mechanisms. The mutant protein may transport substrates across the plasma membrane, catalyze a reaction in a metabolic pathway, interact with other proteins to affect hemostasis, provide active coenzymes from precursor vitamins, excise thymine dimers from normal DNA, and so on. The severity of the clinical pathologic condition produced will depend on the degree of alteration and the metabolic role of the mutant gene product.

The discussion of inherited pathologic physiology will be subdivided into categories according to the metabolic role played by the mutant gene product in the intact organism (Table 3–10). These categories include diseases caused by defective proteins which normally would (1) catalyze plasma membrane transport; (2) catalyze major metabolic pathways with disease caused by accumulation of toxic precursors; (3) catalyze a major pathway with disease caused by over-

TABLE 3-10 CLASSIFICATION OF INHERITED METABOLIC DISORDERS BY DEFECTIVE PROTEINS

Proteins Act As Follows:
1. Catalyze plasma membrane transport.
2. Catalyze major cellular metabolic pathways—
  a. Disease is caused by accumulation of toxic precursors;
  b. Disease is caused by toxic by-products from a normally minor pathway;
  c. Disease is caused by deficiency of end-product;
  d. Disease is caused by overproduced intermediates through loss of feedback control.
3. Circulate in blood and provide and maintain various functions (clotting; metal transport; immunity; oxygen transport).
4. Produce or bind coenzymes involved in specific enzymatic reactions.
5. Catalyze the removal of potentially toxic pharmacologic or environmental agents.
6. Maintain structural integrity of organs (collagen, membrane proteins).

---

production of toxic by-products from a minor pathway; (4) catalyze a needed product in the pathway with disease caused by a deficiency of this product; (5) catalyze products in the major pathway which act as feedback inhibitors and cause disease by overproduction of products; (6) circulate in the blood and have many different functions (clotting, metal binding, immunity, oxygen transport); (7) catalyze the production of specific coenzymes involved in a major pathway; (8) catalyze the removal of potentially toxic pharmacologic or environmental agents; and (9) maintain structural integrity of organs and cells (Table 3–10).

INHERITED DISORDERS CAUSED BY DEFECTIVE MEMBRANE TRANSPORT

The jejunal epithelium and the proximal renal tubular epithelium have cells which have differentiated for the transport of essential substrates from outside the cell to its interior. This transport step shares several characteristics with enzymes, such as saturation, steric specificity, energy dependence, competitive and noncompetitive inhibition, and concentrative ability. Direct evidence for the existence of substrate-specific permeases has been obtained from microbial systems. In man, evidence for their existence is obtained from pedigree analysis of inherited diseases in which this transport function is defective and can be studied. Most of these inherited transport defects have been defined in the intestine or kidney. Table 3–11 lists some inborn errors of membrane transport, the tissues affected, substrates malabsorbed, and the proposed mode of inheritance.

TABLE 3-11 SOME DISEASES CAUSED BY PLASMA MEMBRANE TRANSPORT MUTATIONS

Disease	Tissues Affected	Malabsorbed Substrate	Mode of Inheritance	Clinical Expression
Cystinuria	Kidney ± gut	Cystine ± lysine, arginine, ornithine	Autosomal Recessive	Renal lithiasis (cystine)
Hartnup disease	Gut + kidney	Neutral amino acids	Autosomal Recessive	Nicotinic acid deficiency (pellagra)
Blue diaper syndrome	Gut	Tryptophan	Autosomal Recessive	Hypercalcemia
Methionine malabsorption	Gut	Methionine	Autosomal Recessive(?)	Mental retardation, white hair, failure to thrive
Glucose-galactose malabsorption	Gut + kidney	Glucose and galactose	Autosomal Recessive	Refractory diarrhea
Renal glycosuria	Kidney	Glucose	Autosomal Recessive	Benign glycosuria
Hypophosphatemic rickets	Kidney	Phosphate	X-linked Dominant	Rickets
Congenital chloridorrhea	Gut	Chloride	Autosomal Recessive	Diarrhea, alkalosis
Hereditary spherocytosis	Erythrocyte	Sodium	Autosomal Dominant	Hemolytic anemia
B_{12} malabsorption	Ileum	B_{12}	Autosomal Recessive	Juvenile pernicious anemia

Garrod first recognized the familial occurrence of cystine stone formation, which he ascribed to a block in metabolic reaction sequence. In 1951, Dent and Rose suggested that cystinuria was caused by an error in the renal tubular transport mechanism for cystine, arginine, ornithine, and lysine. These four dibasic amino acids were found in excess in affected patients' urine. An autosomal recessive mode of inheritance was confirmed by Harris. Rosenberg defined three different forms of cystinuria. Types I, II, and III were distinguished by comparing, in a pedigree analysis, differences in dibasic amino acid transport across the gut in homozygous affected individuals, and in heterozygotes by variations found in urinary excretion of the dibasic amino acids. These three genetically distinct types of cystinuria were subsequently demonstrated to be allelic. Type II–III double heterozygotes expressed the clinical phenotype and produced offspring who were either Type II or Type III heterozygotes, but none were normal nor clinically affected. Disease is caused by malabsorption of cystine in the proximal renal tubule. When the urine contains greater than 30 mg. of cystine per 100 ml., cystine crystallizes and forms stones. Cystinuric homozygotes and double heterozygotes excrete over 600 mg. of cystinine in 24 hours. Cystinuria is the most common cause of bladder calculi at birth and may account for 5 per cent of all nephrolithiasis. It is most commonly expressed during the third and fourth decades of life. The urine from members of an affected family should be screened for asymptomatic stone formation. Cystine is more soluble in dilute urine and in an alkaline pH. Stone formation may be decreased by maintaining water diuresis and a urinary pH above 7.5. Renal stones once formed may be dissolved by the administration of D-penicillamine (β,β-dimethylcysteine), which forms soluble penicillamine-cystine disulfides.

Renal stone formation is but one of many clinical manifestations produced by heritable defects in membrane transport permeases. In Hartnup disease, malabsorption of the neutral amino acids by the intestinal mucosa may have no ill effects. However, if the defect is severe and enough tryptophan is malabsorbed, intracellular nicotinamide deficiency may result. The disease is then expressed as a pellagra-like syndrome with ataxia, sun-sensitive rashes, and dementia. Treatment consists of administration of the deficient vitamin, niacin. In familial glucose-galactose malabsorption, severe osmotic diarrhea occurs in infants from the inability of their jejunal mucosa to transport glucose and other sterically similar monosaccharides. Direct evidence for the genetic control of intestinal glucose transport was obtained by in-vitro studies of jejunal biopsy material. As seen in Figure 3–29, epithelial cells from an affected homozygote were unable to accumulate glucose over a 60-minute incubation period, whereas cells from her clinically normal brother and normal controls concentrated glucose to levels 15 times that in the extracellular space. Biopsies from both parents demonstrated partial impairment of this transport function. These data indicate that the proband is homozygous for the glucose transport mutation; that her brother is homozygous for the normal allele; and that both parents and her half-sister are heterozygotes, each carrying one mu-

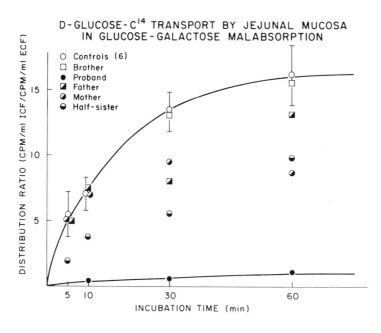

D-GLUCOSE-C¹⁴ TRANSPORT BY JEJUNAL MUCOSA IN GLUCOSE-GALACTOSE MALABSORPTION

○ Controls (6)
□ Brother
● Proband
◪ Father
◑ Mother
◕ Half-sister

DISTRIBUTION RATIO (CPM/ml ICF/CPM/ml ECF)

INCUBATION TIME (min)

Figure 3–29 Jejunal mucosa from the affected proband (●) is unable to accumulate glucose, whereas normals (○) and her brother (□) concentrate to levels 15 times more. Both parents and a half-sister (◑◪◕) accumulate intermediate amounts of glucose, indicating a partial transport defect and identifying them as heterozygotes for the mutant gene. Distribution ratio is calculated from the ratio of counts per minute per milliliter of intracellular space to counts per minute per milliliter of extracellular space (CPM/ml ICF:CPM/ml ECF).

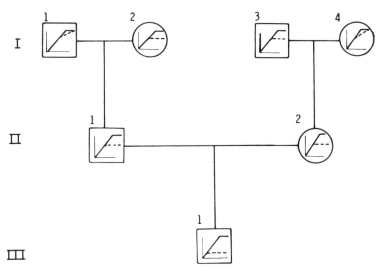

Figure 3–30 Autosomal recessive inheritance of renal glycosuria. The results of renal glucose titration are inscribed within the pedigree symbols. Broken lines (– – –) represent observed deviation from the theoretic curve (—). The proband (III-1) expresses severe Type A glycosuria and his parents (II-1, II-2) and grandparents (I-2-, I-3) have milder forms. Grandparents (I-1 and I-4) have normal curves.

tant and one normal allele. The osmotic diarrhea induced by ingested glucose is prevented by substituting fructose as the dietary carbohydrate source. This monosaccharide has a different steric configuration and membrane transport requirements. In familial glucose-galactose malabsorption, absent intestinal glucose transport is shared by a partial defect in the kidney. In *renal glycosuria,* the kidney tubule is unable to reabsorb glucose, but this genetic defect is not expressed by the intestine. In one family, renal glucose transport was quantitated using in-vivo titration techniques, and an autosomal recessive mode of inheritance was defined (Fig. 3–30). Heterogeneity for renal glucose transport is evidenced by the different types of abnormal curves found in other families with familial glycosuria. In contrast to glucose-galactose malabsorption, renal glucose malabsorption produces no ill effects unless iatrogenic disease arises from a misdiagnosis of diabetes mellitus.

Defective accumulation of phosphate, vitamins, sodium, and chloride may result from other heritable membrane transport mutations. The changes resulting from these defects vary. In familial hypophosphatemic rickets, the best genetic determinant of this X-linked dominant trait is defective phosphate reabsorption by the proximal renal tubule. If this is the initiating event, it is postulated that hypophosphatemia results, hydroxylation of cholecalciferol (vitamin D) is impaired, calcium absorption is reduced, and bone resorption occurs to maintain normal serum phosphate levels. In addition, shortened lower body segments, rickets in children, and osteomalacia in adults may result. In congenital chloridorrhea, adults may manifest malabsorption of chloride by the colon, resulting in watery diarrhea, hypochloremia, and decreased renal chloride filtration. Bicarbonate ion is reabsorbed in the absence of tubular chloride to maintain a normal electropotential gradient. Increased bicarbonate reabsorption by the kidney tubule results in continued metabolic alkalosis. In hereditary spherocytosis, impaired erythrocyte membrane permeability to sodium results in a shortened survival of the erythrocyte and hemolytic anemia. This condition is inherited as an autosomal dominant trait with parent-to-offspring transmission. In vitamin B_{12} malabsorption, juvenile pernicious anemia results. This autosomal recessive trait is seen in children with normal gastric acid secretion in whom intrinsic factor can be demonstrated, but who cannot transport vitamin B_{12} across the intestinal epithelial cell.

INHERITED DISORDERS RESULTING FROM PRECURSOR ACCUMULATION

The most commonly described inborn error of metabolism results from a metabolic block in a major pathway and the accumulation of toxic precursors. One such disease is alkaptonuria, a defect in homogentisic acid oxidase activity. This enzyme normally catalyzes the conversion of homogentisic acid to maleylacetoacetic acid in the ox-

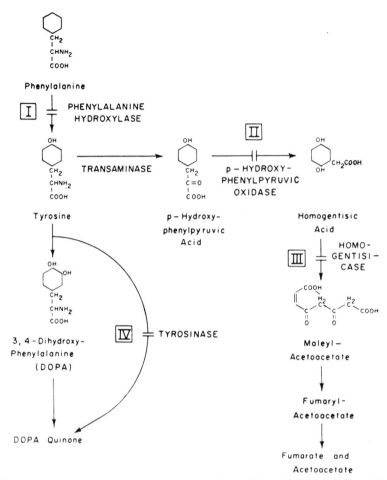

Figure 3–31 The normal metabolic pathway for phenylalanine. *I,* The deficiency of phenylalanine hydroxylase results in phenylketonuria. *IV,* The deficiency of the enzyme tyrosinase results in albinism. *II* and *III* represent deficiencies of enzymes which lead to tyrosinosis and alkaptonuria. (From Hsia, D. Y.: Inborn Errors of Metabolism. Year Book Medical Publishers, Inc., Chicago, 1959.)

idative catabolic pathway of tyrosine (Fig. 3–31). Virtual absence of this enzyme in kidney and liver results in the accumulation of homogentisic acid in tissues and excretion into the urine. Homogentisic acid accumulation in cartilaginous tissue is associated with premature arthritis and provides this tissue with the characteristic dark tinge caused by its oxidation. The disease is not usually manifest until after 30 years of age, and whether tissue deposition could be delayed or prevented with restricted phenylalanine and tyrosine intake is unknown.

An array of storage diseases have been delineated, in which glycogen, sphingolipids, cystine, or mucopolysaccharides are found in excess in tissues. The deposition of these compounds presumably results from a block in their normal metabolic pathway. The precise mechanisms by which intracellular storage of these compounds produces clinical manifestations are not as yet clear.

In classic galactosemia, a defect in galactose-1-phosphate uridyl transferase results in accumulation of the hexose monophosphate, galactose-1-phosphate and its precursor galactose. Because different errors exist in this catabolic pathway, the pathogenesis of disease in this disorder is somewhat better understood. Galactose-1-phosphate accumulates in liver, kidney, and brain and produces cirrhosis, renal tubular malabsorption, and mental retardation. The molecular mechanism by which galactose-1-phosphate accumulation interferes with normal cellular function is not clear, although the hexosemonophosphate has been postulated to be a "phosphate sink" preventing adequate production of ATP and other physiologically necessary high-energy phosphate bonds. In another defect in galactose utilization, galactokinase deficiency, galactose is accumulated in the blood and tissues but galactose-1-phosphate is normal or reduced. In this disorder, cataracts are manifest without impairment of kidney, liver, or brain. Cataract formation in both classic galactose-1-phosphate uridyl transferase deficiency and galactokinase deficiency presumably results from excessive accumulation of galactose and conversion in the lens by aldose reductase in the presence of triphosphopyridine nucleotide to galactitol. This poorly effluxed alcohol is trapped in the lens, creates an osmotic gradient, and produces degeneration of lens fibers. The pathologic condition created by both enzyme defects can be ameliorated if detected early and if dietary restriction of nonessential galactose-containing sugars is instituted.

Maple syrup urine disease or branched-chain α-keto acidemia results from defective decarboxylation of the branched-chain α-keto acids. The reaction sequence is indicated in Figure 3–32. Isoleucine, leucine, and valine, the branched-chain amino acids, are reversibly transaminated to their branched-chain α-keto acid derivatives,

α-keto-β-methyl valeric, α-keto isocaproic, and α-keto isovaleric acids. Subsequent decarboxylation of all three of these organic acids to their coenzyme A derivatives is blocked in maple syrup urine disease. The α-keto acids and their branched-chain amino acid precursors accumulate in tissue and blood and are excreted in the urine. Racemers of these branched-chain α-keto acids impart a fragrant odor of maple syrup to the patient's urine. The enzyme defect is expressed in leukocytes isolated from the peripheral blood and in fibroblasts cultured from patient's skin. Analogous to α-ketoglutarate decarboxylation, three different enzyme proteins are involved in branched-chain α-keto acid decarboxylation. These include a thiamine-dependent α-keto acid decarboxylase; a lipoyl-containing transacylase; and a flavoprotein, lipoamide oxidoreductase. Four soluble cofactors are involved in the over-all reaction: thiamine pyrophosphate (Thp~p); reduced coenzyme A (CoASH); Mg^{++}; and oxidized nicotinamide adenine dinucleotide (NAD+). The complex of these three enzymes and cofactors which decarboxylate α-keto isocaproic acid, α-keto-β-methyl valeric acid, and α-keto isovaleric acid resides in

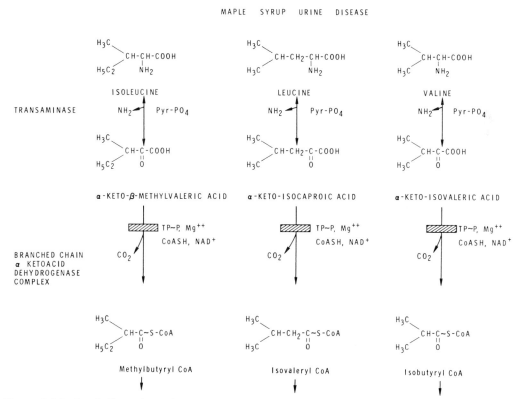

Figure 3–32 Catabolic pathway for branched-chain amino acids. Bar ■ represents block in maple syrup urine disease. ThP ~ P, CoASH, Mg^{++} and NAD+ are soluble cofactors involved in the oxidative decarboxylation of α-keto acids. At least three proteins are also involved.

inner mitochondrial membrane. It is not surprising that at least four different forms of the disease have been described, since there are many different molecular sites which could produce a block in this reaction. In the "classic" form, keto acid decarboxylase activity is absent in the white cells and fibroblasts obtained from homozygous affected patients. Severe central nervous system depression may occur during the first few days of protein ingestion, and apnea and coma result. If infants survive this initial insult, permanent neurologic damage may persist. Quantitatively different reductions in parental (obligatory heterozygotes) decarboxylase activity by cultured fibroblasts were seen in one family. Thus, different non-complementing mutant gene products may commonly result in absent function producing affected double heterozygotes. The "intermittent" form is differentiated from the classic phenotype by its later onset in childhood, by its episodic remitting and non-progressive course, and by leukocyte and fibroblast enzyme activity in homozygotes which retain up to 20 per cent of activity. Environmental insults such as protein ingestion and infections induce intermittent episodes characterized by branched-chain α-keto acidemia and death, if the stress persists. In reported cases, only one parent, usually the father, has reduced α-keto acid decarboxylase activity in peripheral leukocytes. An "intermediate" variant is characterized by persistent branched-chain α-keto aciduria, mild non-progressive psychomotor retardation, hyperuricemia, and reduced enzyme activity in leukocytes and fibroblasts. Leukocyte activity is 15 to 20 per cent of normal, and fibroblast activity 42 to 47 per cent of normal. Both parents have greater than normal activity in cultured fibroblasts, and homozygotes do not respond to thiamine administration. A fourth phenotype characterized by branched-chain amino aciduria and delayed development responded dramatically to oral thiamine. Thus, at least one variant of maple syrup urine disease has been defined, in which the administration of large amounts of cofactor involved in the keto acid decarboxylase step augmented defective enzyme function.

The pathologic physiology in all four variants is presumably caused by the effects of α-keto isocaproic acid on myelin formation and central nervous system mitochondrial oxidation. Examination of the myelin suggests that changes in myelin formation do not occur before birth. The acute reversible aspects of the disease support this concept, since normal development will occur in affected children who are treated during the neonatal period with diets restricted in branched-chain amino acids. High concentrations of α-keto isocaproic acid inhibit decarboxylation of pyruvic acid, protein synthesis, and amino acid transport by neural tissue in various animal systems. The severity of these insults is related to the tissue concentrations of α-keto isocaproic acid which determine reversibility or continued interference in function. This disease process is caused by the toxic effects of these immediate precursors, accumulated as a result of defects in the major decarboxylation pathway of branched-chain α-keto acids. However, more complex effects of this impaired enzyme have recently been recognized. Hypoglycemia and hypoalaninemia may be sequelae of decreased enzyme in skeletal muscle. α-Keto isocaproic acid utilization and conversion to alanine by skeletal muscle is a major source of gluconeogenesis by liver to maintain whole-body glucose homeostasis.

INHERITED DISEASES CAUSED BY PRODUCTS OF MINOR PATHWAYS

The precursor in the metabolic block of a major pathway may not be the immediate cause of the disease. Instead by-products of an alternate minor pathway may cause the disease. The activity of such a pathway is normally minimal, but is enhanced by abnormal precursor accumulation. For example, cataracts in *galactosemia* are caused not by galactose or galactose-1-phosphate. Rather, the increased concentration of galactose in lens fibers results in excessive amounts of non-diffusible galactitol produced as a result of an alternate pathway through aldose reductase. A second example is *phenylketonuria*. A deficiency in phenylalanine hydroxylase results in the accumulation of phenylalanine. It is, however, the deaminated by-product of phenylalanine, phenylpyruvic, which produces the characteristic ferric chloride reaction in the urine and metabolic acidosis. Since a moderate elevation of phenylalanine alone is not toxic, these by-products in high concentrations may interfere with central nervous system processes. Although mental retardation and demyelination are consequences of the untreated disease, the basis for their pathogenesis remains an enigma.

A third example is *hyperoxaluria*, which is characterized by the excretion of large amounts of oxalic acid, nephrolithiasis, nephrocalcinosis, and early renal failure. The stones are formed from calcium oxalate, a nonessential end product of glycine degradation. This disorder is caused by excessive biosynthesis of oxalic acid, which is formed from glycine through the irreversible oxidation of glyoxilic acid. Two causes for excessive accumulation of glyoxilic acid and its insoluble by-product, oxalic acid, have been postulated. In Type I, a defect in the soluble enzyme glycolic acid α-ketoglutarate carboligase blocks conversion of glyoxilic acid to α-OH-β-ketoadipic (one of six alternate routes for glyoxilic acid) and results in accumulation of glyoxilic acid and conversion to oxalic acid. In Type II, Williams described excessive D-glyceric aciduria as well as hyperoxaluria and found deficient D-glyceric acid oxidase in the leukocytes of affected patients and of the mother but not of the father. These authors postulate that a deficiency in this enzyme reduces conversion of glyoxilic acid to glycolic acid. Both types lead primarily to excesses of glyoxilic acid by blocking normal dissimilation and secondarily to increased biosynthesis of oxalic acid normally present but in smaller amounts. These examples then represent inborn errors of metabolism, the manifestations of which are caused not by the precursor in the metabolic block but by the overproduction of by-products from the accumulating precursor.

INHERITED DISEASES CAUSED BY DEFICIENCIES OF END-PRODUCT

A pathologic condition may result from a mutant gene product which reduces the intracellular concentration of essential end products in its pathway. *Albinism* represents a group of disorders caused by impaired production of melanoprotein from tyrosine. A specialized cell, the melanocyte, is the source of pigment in hair, skin, and eyes. Hydroxylation of L-tyrosine to 3,4-dihydroxy-phenylalanine (DOPA) and its subsequent oxidation to dopa-quinone utilize the same enzyme, tyrosinase (Fig. 3–31). Non-enzymatic reactions then occur in the melanocyte, resulting in polymerization of dopa-quinone derivatives and reaction with a specialized protein to form melanoprotein. Melanocytes are present in albinism but do not contain melanin. Many different clinical forms of albinism exist with different genetic patterns of inheritance. Classic oculocutaneous albinism (Type I) is expressed as diffuse hypopigmentation of the hair, skin, fundus oculi, and iris. It is inherited as an autosomal recessive trait. Melanocytes are present but are presumably deficient in tyrosinase. The disease expression therefore is due to a deficiency of the end-product melanin, which normally acts as a sunscreen and protects cells from light energy. In albinism, instead of tanning, affected individuals burn on exposure to light. Exposed skin has an increased tendency to develop malignant melanomas. Photophobia, nystagmus, and visual impairment result from melanin deficiency in the eye.

Defective formation of thyroid hormone represents another group of inborn errors of metabolism in which deficiency of the product of the enzyme pathway results in expression of disease. Several different enzymatic defects have been described which produce a deficiency of functioning thyroid hormone. These include (1) an iodide transport defect; (2) iodide organification defects; (3) a defect in the coupling of iodotyrosyl to form thyroxine; (4) failure to synthesize normal thyroglobulin; and (5) failure to dehalogenate organic iodide. Mental retardation or cretinism is caused by a deficiency in the end product, thyroid hormone.

Congenital adrenal hyperplasia results from an inherited, relative or absolute, loss in one of the enzymes which produces normal hormonal steroids from cholesterol. When this block in the normal biosynthetic pathway results in insufficient production of salt-retaining mineralocorticoids and anti-inflammatory glucocorticoids, persistent loss of sodium in the urine, vomiting, dehydration, hypotension, shock, or sudden death may occur. At least five different enzyme deficiencies in this pathway have been described including 21-hydroxylase, 11-hydroxylase, 3 β-hydroxysteroid dehydrogenase, 17-hydroxylase, and 18-hydroxylase. Salt wasting may occur in all except the 11-hydroxylase deficiency, in which salt retaining hormones 11-deoxycortisol and 11-deoxycorticosterone are formed in excess and protect the organism against deficient aldosterone production. An autosomal recessive pattern of inheritance is presumed for these disorders.

INHERITED DISEASES CAUSED BY LOSS OF FEEDBACK INHIBITION

In the preceding section, it was shown that deficiency of essential end-products in the major metabolic pathway produces abnormalities directly. In the pathogenesis of some heritable disorders, loss of regulation in a metabolic pathway produces the disease state. The failure to synthesize thyroxine results in mental retardation. The total phenotype is due not only to deficient hormone but also to loss of feedback inhibition of hypothalamic thyrotropin releasing factor, excess secretion of TSH, and the formation of excessive thyroid parenchyma. The goiter expressed in familial hypothyroidism results from the loss of end-product inhibition of TSH regulatory control mechanisms.

In the adrenogenital syndrome, particularly in 11-hydroxylase deficiency, the end-product deficiency may not in itself produce the entire syndrome. A precursor, 11-deoxycorticosterone, is accumulated in one group (the 11-hydroxylase deficiencies), conserves renal sodium, and may even produce hypertension. However, another pathologic process in this disorder is masculinization. Normally, cortisol and corticosterone regulate hypothalamic-pituitary ACTH secretion by acting as depressants on corticotropin-releasing factor. Corticotropin-releasing factor acts to stimulate synthesis and release of ACTH. When cortisol production is reduced, as in 21-hydroxylase deficiency, this negative feedback control is lost, more ACTH is produced, and excessive androgenic steroids in the pathway are formed. Levels of ACTH, 17-ketosteroids, and potent androgens such as testosterone are elevated in plasma and tissues. This pathologic process occurs during intrauterine development and may cause clitoromegaly or ambiguous genitalia in the female infant, macrogenitosomia in the male, and virilization with epiphyseal closure in both. The whole process is reversed by providing exogenous cortisol in physiologic amounts, returning feedback inhibition to the hypothalamic-pituitary-ACTH axis.

One of the most important recent advances in genetics is the understanding of early onset coronary heart disease and its relationship to regulation of cholesterol biosynthesis. In a combined biochemical and genetic analysis in 500 survivors of myocardial infarction, Goldstein, Motulsky and Brown found that over half had a monogenic trait producing one of three plasma lipid phenotypes: familial hypercholesterolemia; familial hypertriglyceridemia; combined hyperlipidemia. Ten per cent had familial hypercholesterolemia, but 1/500 persons in the general population are affected by this autosomal dominant trait. Subsequent studies using cultured skin fibroblasts, lymphocytes, and cultured aortic smooth muscle cells from homozygous and heterozygous patients with familial hypercholesterolemia demonstrated at least three genetically distinct defects in low-density lipoprotein-cholesterol (LDL-cholesterol) binding and pinocytosis by plasma membrane (Fig. 3–33). The extracellular complex of LDL-cholesterol regulates its own plasma membrane receptor and thus protects the cell from overaccumulation of cholesterol and its esters. Subsequently, within the cell free cholesterol suppresses the rate-limiting enzyme in cholesterol biosynthesis, hydroxymethyl glutaryl CoA reductase (HMGCoA reductase). Thus, phenotypically affected heterozygotes with partially reduced membrane binding functions have increased intracellular cholesterol esters and a two- to threefold increase in plasma cholesterol levels. These abnormalities are associated with atherosclerosis and myocardial infarc-

tions between age 35 and 45 years. Homozygous affected individuals occur in the population rarely, with an estimated frequency of 1/1,000,000. By comparison, they have little or no LDL-cholesterol binding and/or invagination, a sixfold or greater elevation in plasma cholesterol, and myocardial infarctions between the ages of 5 and 15 years. Since heterozygotes express early onset heart disease, familial hypercholesterolemia is an autosomal dominant trait.

In *acute intermittent porphyria,* partial impairment of an enzyme in the heme biosynthetic pathway results in loss of feedback regulation of δ-aminolevulinic acid synthetase. Acute intermittent porphyria is characterized by hepatic overproduction of porphyrin precursors δ-aminolevulinic acid and porphobilinogen. Increased activity of hepatic δ-aminolevulinic acid synthetase has been described in patients affected with this disorder. Family studies in 600 patients from Sweden describe direct parent-to-offspring transmission, with both sexes equally affected. This indicates an autosomal dominant pattern of inheritance. A dominant mutation with increased enzyme activity led to the hypothesis that the gene mutation involves regulation of an operator gene repressed by normal biosynthesis of heme. Granick found that hepatic δ-aminolevulinic acid synthetase is an inducible enzyme. Studies in intact animals and cultured liver cells indicate that both carbohydrate and heme act to repress δ-aminolevulinic acid synthetase production. Marver and Schmid have demonstrated a primary partial impairment of the enzyme uroporphyrinogen synthetase. This defect interferes with heme biosynthesis, which in turn results in loss of feedback inhibition of δ-aminolevulinic acid synthetase and overproduction of δ-aminolevulinic acid and porphobilinogen. Acute intermittent porphyria is characterized by intermittent episodes of severe abdominal pain, psychoses, and paralysis.

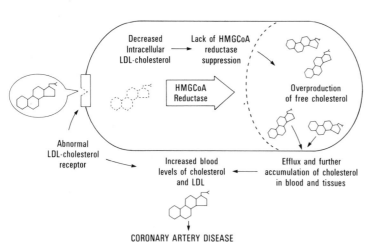

Figure 3–33 Schematic Model in Familial Hypercholesterolemia. Pathogenesis of early onset heart disease results from genetically determined impairment in the number and function of plasma membrane low density lipoprotein (LDL)-cholesterol binding sites. Heterozygotes have partial impairment with adult onset of disease expression, whereas affected children who are homozygous have absent binding sites and express coronary disease before puberty.

Photosensitivity is not present nor is there excessive excretion of preformed porphyrins. A number of factors are known to provoke acute attacks in patients with this disorder including steroids, barbiturates, infections, female sex hormones, and starvation. All these agents increase heme protein production and further reduce available free heme to act as negative control in the biosynthesis of δ-aminolevulinic acid synthetase. During attacks, the urine contains excessive amounts of porphobilinogen, which on standing in an acid pH will polymerize to form porphyrins and other dark reddish pigments. There is no quantitative correlation between acute clinical episodes, increased enzyme activity, and excessive production of porphobilinogen. Other hepatic porphyrias, hereditary coproporphyria, and variegate porphyria also are inherited in an autosomal dominant pattern, have excess porphyrin production, and presumably are caused by enzyme impairment distal to uroporphyrinogen synthase in the heme biosynthetic pathway.

In an inborn error of pyrimidine biosynthesis, *orotic aciduria*, a single rare mutant gene produces a deficiency of two enzyme functions: orotic acid phosphoribosyl transferase (O-PRT) and orotidine-5'-phosphate decarboxylase (ODC). This block results in the accumulation and excretion of a relatively insoluble pyrimidine nucleotide precursor, orotic acid, and reduced synthesis of its mononucleotide product, uridylic acid. Orotic acid is found in the urine of affected children and produces needle-shaped crystals and obstructive urinary tract symptoms when affected individuals become dehydrated. Children also manifest megaloblastic anemia and psychomotor retardation, presumably caused by "pyrimidine deficiency." A deficiency of this end-product, uridylic acid (uridine-5'-monophosphate), results in overproduction of orotic acid, since it acts as a feedback inhibitor of carbamyl phosphate synthetase and aspartate transcarbamylase, initial enzymes in the biosynthetic pathway of uridylic acid production. If the feedback inhibitor uridine is provided, reduction in the rate of orotic acid overproduction is seen in patients and in cells cultured from their skin. Uridine replacement also improves the anemia and growth retardation.

Another inborn error of nucleotide feedback control is exemplified by defects in purine biosynthesis. The enzyme hypoxanthine-guanine-phosphoribosyltransferase (HGPRTase) acts to catalyze the formation of the mononucleotides inosinic and guanylic acid from hypoxanthine and guanine using phosphoribosyl pyrophosphate (PRPP). Defects in this enzyme result in reduced feedback inhibition of the de-novo synthesis of uric acid, increased cellular concentrations of PRPP, and marked overproduction of uric acid. Patients affected with complete HGPRTase defi-

ciency have severe mental retardation, chorea, spasticity, and a bizarre compulsion to self-mutilation. They also exhibit hyperuricemia, urinary uric acid stones, and clinical gout. The gene is located on the X chromosome. Female heterozygotes demonstrate mosaicism for HGPRTase activity in fibroblasts cultured from their skin. Approximately half their cells are unable to incorporate tritiated hypoxanthine into nucleic acids (HGPRTase deficient), while the other half have normal enzyme activity. These observations support the Lyon hypothesis for early random and continued X-inactivation. The mechanism by which HGPRTase deficiency interrupts normal brain biochemistry and function is unknown. Two possibilities exist: that an important purine nucleotide is deficient or that an abnormal purine intermediate is overproduced. Neither of these possibilities is confirmed, but uric acid is clearly overproduced and this aspect of the disease can be classified as an inherited defect resulting in loss of feedback control of de-novo purine biosynthesis.

INHERITED DISEASE ASSOCIATED WITH DEFICIENT OR ABNORMAL CIRCULATING PROTEINS

A wide variety of genetically controlled proteins circulate in the blood. In some, changes in concentration, structure, or function may have no effect on the organism as a whole; in others, such changes may have distinctly deleterious results. Perhaps the best known of this group are disorders of immunoglobulin production. In fact, the field of immunogenetics encompasses not only the control of immunoglobulins, but the complete immune reaction, which includes circulating complement, various regulatory enzymes, leukocytes, and lymphocytes as well. These concepts are discussed in a later chapter. Reduction in the concentration of thyroxine-binding globulin, a protein controlled by a locus on the X chromosome, reduces the serum protein-bound iodide but does not alter metabolic function. Dominantly inherited variants of the iron-binding protein, transferrin, have been described but none of these structural mutations have a known effect on iron metabolism. On the other hand, a recessively inherited *atransferrinemia* has been described in which there is a transferrin deficiency with a refractory hypochromic anemia. In *Wilson disease*, reduction in circulating ceruloplasmin, a polyamine oxidase which is induced by and binds 95 per cent of serum copper, is associated with copper deposition in almost all tissues of the body. The deposition of copper in liver, brain, eyes, and kidney results in cirrhosis, extrapyramidal tract degeneration, pathognomonic corneal Kayser-Fleischer rings, and renal tubular dysfunction. Removal of copper from these organs with chelating agents such as penicillamine will prevent impairment and in some instances improve organ malfunction. Although reduction in circulating ceruloplasmin remains the best genetic determinant of affected homozygotes, approximately 2 to 3 per cent of patients with phenotypic Wilson disease have chemically and functionally normal ceruloplasmin. The basic mutant gene product and the relationship between tissue copper and reduced levels of ceruloplasmin still remain unsolved.

The hemostatic mechanism in man is provided by several different factors under genetic control. In *classic hemophilia A,* an X-linked recessive trait, hemizygous males have diminished functional antihemophilic globulin (Factor VIII, AHG). *Vascular hemophilia* or Von Willebrand disease is an autosomal dominant trait in which there is also a deficiency of Factor VIII. It is interesting that the more serious coagulation defect (classic hemophilia A) more commonly has detectable immunologic AHG which is hemostatically defective, whereas "vascular" hemophilia A (Von Willebrand disease) has no immunoreactive material but the disease is characterized by a less severe defect in hemostasis. Hemophilia B or *Christmas disease* is a defect in Factor IX (plasma thromboplastin component) and, like Factor VIII, deficiency is also transmitted in an X-linked recessive pattern. Studies in families in which classic hemophilia A and hemophilia B were segregating showed that the two disorders were clearly nonallelic.

Several families have been reported with hemostatic defects expressed as mild prolongation of blood and plasma coagulation times and by the presence of *abnormal fibrinogens.* These dysfibrinogenemias are inherited in an autosomal dominant pattern when prolonged prothrombin time is used as the genetic determinant. Several different abnormal fibrinogens have been described. Ratnoff and Bennett tabulated these variants. Most abnormal fibrinogens are immunologically distinct. Affected individuals have two populations of fibrinogen, normal and mutant. Mammen suggested that a substitution of a strongly basic amino acid (arginine) for serine in Fibrinogen-Detroit changed the conformational site for active polymerization and resulted in interference with the clotting properties of the normal fibrinogen which was also present. Another disorder, *congenital afibrinogenemia,* has been described. In this disorder, there is absent coagulation of blood in the affected individuals, and parents have mild coagulation defects. This disorder is inherited as an autosomal recessive trait. The dominant pattern of inheritance in dysfibrinogenemia and the expressed coagulation defects in "afibrinogenemic" heterozygotes indicate that in both disorders the mutant gene product (fibronogen) is altered, so that it interferes with the product of its normal allele and results in phenotypic expression.

Congenital a-beta-lipoproteinemia is an autosomal recessive disease characterized by the absence of circulating low-density lipoprotein. This disease is expressed by abnormal red blood cell structure (acanthocytes); steatorrhea; diffuse central nervous system abnormalities (cerebellar, posterior column, peripheral nerve); and engorgement of upper intestinal absorptive cells with triglycerides when fat is present in the diet. The genetic effect is now known to be a block in either the secretion or synthesis of apoprotein B, which is a component of both LDL and VLDL. Patients affected by this disease have reduced plasma cholesterol, all of which is bound to high-density lipoprotein (HDL). HDL-cholesterol is not taken up by normal fibroblasts, and fails to suppress HMG CoA-reductase or stimulate cholesterylester formation (Fig. 3–33). The pathologic processes in red cell membranes and central nervous system may reflect a deficiency of these membranal sterols.

INBORN ERRORS CAUSED BY REDUCED COENZYME BINDING OR PRODUCTION

Renewed interest in cofactor interaction with enzymes has resulted from the immediate therapeutic effects of administering supraphysiologic doses of vitamins whose coenzyme products augment defective enzyme pathways. Rosenberg defined the "vitamin dependent inborn errors" as genetic disturbances leading to specific biochemical abnormalities, affecting one reaction catalyzed by a vitamin and responding only to pharmacologic amounts of that vitamin. This definition thus clearly differentiates vitamin dependency from vitamin deficiency, which affects many pathways, responds to physiologic amounts of the vitamin, and is acquired. Frimpter first demonstrated decreased cystathionase activity in the liver from patients with *cystathioninuria.* When liver homogenates were incubated with its coenzyme, pyridoxal phosphate, activity was markedly increased. He also showed that cystathionine excretion in patients was lowered significantly by the administration of large amounts of vitamin B_6. Vitamin B_6 is phosphorylated to pyridoxal-5' phosphate or pyridoxamine-5'-phosphate by specific kinases requiring adenosine triphosphate. These phosphorylated compounds act as coenzymes for a large number of apoenzymes which regulate the catabolic pathways for fatty acids, amino acids, and glycogen. Since cystathionase activity alone was impaired in cystathioninuria, a vitamin deficiency was unlikely. Frimpter's work suggested that the mutation in cystathioninuria altered that portion of the specific apoenzyme which bound its active coenzyme, pyridoxal phosphate. Other inborn errors of metabolism demonstrating vitamin B_6 dependency include infantile

Figure 3–34 Inborn errors of metabolism expressing vitamin dependency could arise from any of the four mechanisms represented. (Adapted from Rosenberg, L. E.: New Engl. J. Med., *281*:145, 1969, with permission of author.)

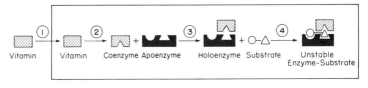

Vitamin   Vitamin   Coenzyme Apoenzyme   Holoenzyme Substrate   Unstable Enzyme-Substrate

(1) Defective Transport of Vitamin into Cell

(2) Defective Conversion of Vitamin to Coenzyme

(3) Defective Formation of Holoenzyme

(4) Unstable Enzyme-Substrate Complex Resulting in shortened biologic half-life

convulsions, pyridoxine-responsive anemia, xanthurenic aciduria, and homocystinuria. In homocystinuria, B_6 apparently stabilizes the mutant cystathionine synthase and increases its biologic half-life (Step 4, Fig. 3–34).

Only two reactions in mammalian systems have demonstrated a requirement for B_{12} coenzymes. The best example from man comes from studies of vitamin B_{12} responsive *methylmalonic aciduria.* This disorder arises from impairment in the conversion of methylmalonyl CoA to succinyl CoA. The reaction is catalyzed by the enzyme methylmalonyl CoA-mutase and its coenzyme 5′-deoxyadenosylcobalamin, a vitamin B_{12} derivative. Metabolic ketoacidosis accompanied by coma and shock was a common finding during the early weeks of life in six patients described. Other findings included hypotonia, hepatomegaly, osteoporosis, neutropenia, and thrombocytopenia. The appearance of long-chained ketones, including butanone and hexanone in the urine; intermittent hyperglycinemia and glycinuria; and the excretion of large amounts of the unusual organic acid methylmalonic acid characterized the biochemical phenotype. Biochemical studies in-vitro revealed that peripheral blood leukocytes and cultured skin fibroblasts from affected patients were unable to convert methylmalonic acid to succinic acid. Normal levels of tissue and plasma vitamin B_{12} were found. When 1-mg. doses of hydroxycobalamin were given to one child with this disease, methylmalonic acid excretion fell and white blood cell utilization of methylmalonate rose. Continued administration of these large doses of vitamin B_{12} lowered this child's sensitivity to valine, methionine, threonine, and isoleucine, precursors of methylmalonic acid. If fibroblasts were grown in tissue culture media containing physiologic concentrations of vitamin B_{12}, very low intracellular concentrations of the active coenzyme 5′-deoxyadenosylcobalamin were produced. However, when the cells were grown in medium with 10,000-fold increases of vitamin B_{12}, 5′-deoxyadenosylcobalamin rose to normal levels. Methylmalonate CoA mutase activity and its ability to bind coenzyme was normal in fibroblast homogenates from two patients, indicating that

the apoenzyme was normal and had a normal affinity for its coenzyme. A primary genetic defect was thus postulated in the production of the coenzyme 5′-deoxyadenosylcobalamin from its precursor, vitamin B_{12} (Step 2, Fig. 3–34). Using cell fusion and complementation techniques, at least four genetically different B_{12}-responsive forms of methylmalonic aciduria have been defined in the transport and conversion of B_{12} to its active cofactors.

In these metabolic disorders, defects occur in the binding or the production of coenzymes involved in the major catalytic reaction. Only a few of the vitamin dependency syndromes have been adequately evaluated at the molecular level, but many possible abnormalities exist (Fig. 3–34): the vitamin may not be (1) transported into a specialized cell; (2) converted to its active coenzyme; or (3) bound to its apoenzyme to form a holoenzyme. Finally (4) vitamins or their coenzyme products may stabilize normal or mutant enzyme complexes in supraphysiologic (greater than necessary to prevent deficiency states) concentrations. This latter mechanism producing vitamin responsivity has been postulated in thiamine-responsive maple syrup urine disease and pyridoxine-responsive homocystinuria. Therapeutic importance of this type of pathologic physiology is evident. In certain instances, administration of high concentrations of the precursor vitamin may augment the defective coenzyme or enzyme pathway and provide the individual with some protection against the toxic precursor or deficient product resulting from the altered pathway. In at least one reported case of B_{12}-responsive methylmalonic aciduria, a fetus was diagnosed prepartum, and the mother and her fetus were treated with massive doses of B_{12}. The child at birth was prevented from developing methylmalonic acidemia.

DISEASES CAUSED BY ENZYMES REGULATING DRUG METABOLISM

Some inherited disorders are not expressed until the organism is stressed by the administration of certain drugs. Such a disorder might arise if a mutant gene product did not remove a potentially toxic drug. A well-known example of this disorder is *serum cholinesterase* deficiency. As described previously, this enzyme hydrolyzes choline esters, notably the muscle relaxant succinyldicholine. Different types of mutant gene products can be analyzed in pedigrees by their resistance to inhibitors. A silent allele has also been described which results in the complete loss of enzyme activity in the homozygous condition. Immunochemical studies suggest that this "silent allele" produces a true absence of the total enzyme protein, whereas other mutant alleles produce products which differ only in their kinetic properties for the binding of cholinesterase and various inhibitors. The abnormal enzymes, however, have similar immunochemical properties, electrophoretic mobilities, and molecular size. Pedigree analyses suggest ten different phenotypes from three alleles at one locus (E_1). A second locus (E_2) has been described for this protein when examined by starch gel electrophoresis. The (E_2) locus is characterized by an isozyme with a fifth subunit (C_5) which is seen in approximately 10 per cent of European people. The functional attributes of this electrophoretic variation are as yet unknown. Individuals who are homozygous for an atypical allele or doubly heterozygous for the atypical silent allele are unable to hydrolyze succinyldicholine, a drug used to induce transient muscular paralysis during surgery. Normally, it is removed in minutes, but in affected individuals the drug persists in its pharmacologically active form for a prolonged period of time.

The use of a pedigree and biochemical analysis in the diagnosis and prevention of this disorder in a family is illustrated in Figure 3–35 (compare with Figure 3–8). The 19-year-old proband (III–1)

PSEUDOCHOLINESTERASE DEFICIENCY

(Pedigree Mi)

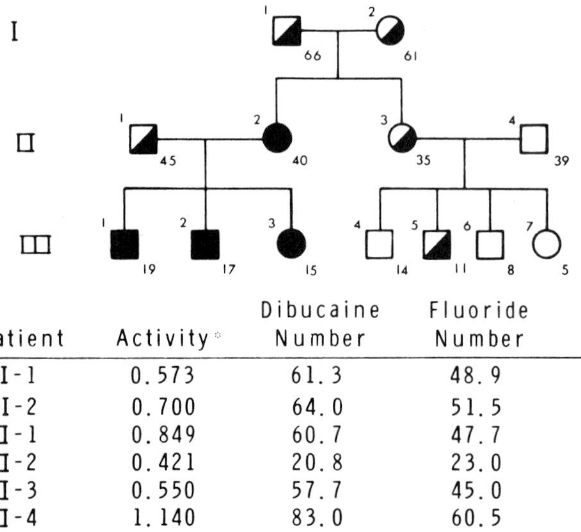

Patient	Activity*	Dibucaine Number	Fluoride Number	Probable Genotype
I-1	0.573	61.3	48.9	UA
I-2	0.700	64.0	51.5	UA
II-1	0.849	60.7	47.7	UA
II-2	0.421	20.8	23.0	AA
II-3	0.550	57.7	45.0	UA
II-4	1.140	83.0	60.5	UU
III-1	0.394	18.8	26.6	AA
III-2	0.391	12.4	23.2	AA
III-3	0.418	9.8	17.3	AA
III-4	1.054	81.2	64.6	UU
III-5	0.922	59.0	52.0	UA
III-6	1.070	80.3	63.8	UU
III-7	1.140	78.8	62.8	UU
(Normal)	(0.6-1.2)	(77-83)	(57-68)	(UU)

*µmoles benzoylcholine hydrolyzed / min / ml

Figure 3–35   An example of combined pedigree and biochemical analysis in a family with pseudocholinesterase deficiency. Members represented by closed symbols are sensitive to succinyldicholine. "A" is atypical and "U" is the usual allele. Dibucaine and fluoride numbers indicate per cent inhibition of hydrolytic activity. (Assays were performed through the courtesy of B. N. LaDu, M.D., Ph.D.)

is a healthy football player who had a molar tooth extracted. During surgery, succinyldicholine was administered and he remained paralyzed for six hours. A family history indicated that his mother had a similar respiratory arrest four years earlier following hysterectomy. Serum from the mother (II–2), proband, and siblings (III–2, III–3) had reduced hydrolytic activity as well as resistance to dibucaine and fluoride consistent with the homozygous atypical genotype (AA). This initial family history evaluation suggested direct parent-to-child transmission of an autosomal dominant trait which was contrary to the usual recessive mode of inheritance for serum cholinesterase deficiency. Serum from the clinically normal father (II–1) had normal enzyme activity but increased resistance to dibucaine and fluoride, suggesting that he was heterozygous (AU). This finding provided evidence for an autosomal recessive mode of inheritance. The mother and siblings were advised to avoid drugs of this type in the future. The normals and heterozygotes were reassured that they were not sensitive.

Another group of inborn errors caused by drug administration resulted from the observations of Hockwald that American blacks develop an acute hemolytic anemia after receiving synthetic antimalarial drugs such as primaquine. This abnormal hemolytic response to the drug was caused by a deficiency of the enzyme glucose-6-phosphate dehydrogenase (G6PD), which normally catalyzes the oxidation of glucose-6-phosphate to 6-phospho-gluconate with reduction of the coenzyme NADP to NADPH. This is the first step in the oxidation of glucose via the pentose shunt pathway, which serves to maintain the intracellular concentration of reduced coenzyme NADPH and glutathione. It is postulated that the interaction of primaquine with mutant G6PD results in failure to maintain reduced NADPH, diminution of reduced glutathione, fragility of red cell membrane, and hemolysis. Other drugs can produce these hemolytic crises; these include the sulfonamides, antimalarials, and fava beans (favism). Different mutant G6PD proteins occur in blacks, Mediterranean, and Middle Eastern populations. They are all X-linked recessive traits. Of 21 variants described, six are associated with hemolytic disease and presumably have specific properties which render red blood cells unstable. Female heterozygotes may be sensitive to these drugs, depending on lyonization effects and the quantitative impairment in G6PD.

Another inherited disease produced by drugs was found after isoniazid (INH) was introduced for tuberculosis therapy. Initial studies revealed two distinct groups of individuals with different rates of removal of INH from the plasma. Evans demonstrated that six hours after a 40 mg. per kg. dose, a group of subjects known as "slow inactivators" had plasma INH concentrations above 4 μg. per ml., whereas the "rapid inactivators" had levels below 3 μg. per ml. Rapid inactivators had a higher proportion of the drug in the urine in an acetylated form as compared to slow inactivators, who excreted the drug unchanged. Acetylation of INH occurs in the liver as a consequence of the enzyme acetyl-coenzyme A transferase. The activity of this enzyme is much greater in the livers of rapid inactivators as compared to slow inactivators. This enzyme is also concerned with the acetylation of drugs such as sulfamethazine and sulfadiazine. This pathologic physiology has some significance in the use of the drug for the treatment of tuberculosis. Slow inactivators of INH are more likely to develop peripheral neuropathy after prolonged administration, but this rare complication of INH treatment can be prevented by the simultaneous administration of pyridoxine. Rapid inactivators may require higher doses to provide adequate circulating levels of the unacetylated active form. It is presumed from pedigree analyses that slow inactivators are homozygous for a "slow allele" and that rapid inactivators are either heterozygous or homozygous for the "rapid allele."

All three of the above examples of genetically determined enzyme defects are related to the metabolism of drugs and emphasize again the interrelationships of genetic and environmental factors in the pathogenesis of disease. Since the underlying genetic differences are brought out by drugs, these and several conditions of a similar nature have been called pharmacogenetic disorders. Wider application of this concept would include the effects of life styles on genetically susceptible individuals. Thus, persons heterozygous for α-1-antitrypsin deficiency would develop emphysema if exposed to dust or cigarette smoke. Persons who have decreased negative feedback control for arylhydrocarbon hydroxylase may develop lung cancer if exposed to carcinogenic hydrocarbons. Individuals with high levels of pepsinogen may be prone to duodenal ulcer. The broader term now used for the interplay of genetic susceptibility and the environment is *ecogenetics*.

DISEASES CAUSED BY ABNORMAL STRUCTURAL PROTEINS WHICH MAINTAIN STRUCTURAL INTEGRITY OF ORGANS

Collagen is a protein which constitutes the principal structural element of vertebrate connective tissue. Collagen fibers are formed by a series of metabolic processes as outlined in Figure 3–36. At least five genetically distinct collagen α chains are translated, hydroxylated, assembled into a triple helix, glycosylated, cleaved, extruded into the extracellular space, and cross-linked by several processes. These functions are catalyzed by sever-

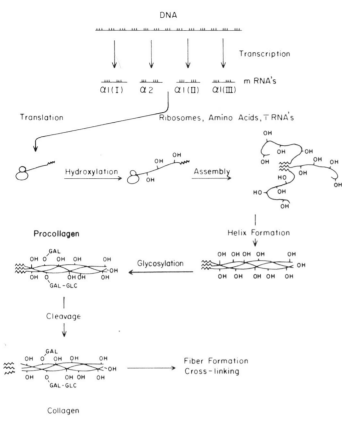

Figure 3–36 Collagen biosynthetic pathway. Processes of transcription, translation, hydroxylation of lysyl and prolyl residues, assembly and glycosylation occur within cells. Procollagen cleavage and extrusion from the cell occur in association with cell membranes. Fiber formation and crosslinking occur extracellularly. Formation of monomeric collagen is depicted. (From Miller, E. J., and Matukas, V. J.: Fed. Proc., *33*:1197–1204, 1974.)

al enzymes including prolyl and lysyl hydroxylases, monosaccharide transferases, procollagen peptidase, and lysyl oxidase. The presence of hydroxylysine and hydroxyproline in the finished product are unique to this protein.

Many disorders of man have been proposed as caused by abnormalities in collagen. A partial list might include: pseudoxanthoma elasticum, Marfan syndrome, cutis laxis, osteogenesis imperfecta, Ehlers-Danlos syndrome, chondrodystrophy, interstitial nephritis, and so on. All these diseases are heterogeneous, but recent advances have provided evidence for specific defects in a group of disorders clinically classified as Ehlers-Danlos syndrome. The composite clinical disorder is characterized by joint laxity; hyperextensible, friable skin; retinal detachment; small cornea; vertebral anomalies; and abnormal atrophic scar formation. At least seven subtypes have been defined on the basis of genetic and phenotypic differences. The first to be defined and evaluated at biochemical and genetic levels is Type VI, characterized by hydroxylysine-deficient collagen and impaired lysyl hydroxylase in cultured skin fibroblasts (Figure 3–37). This enzymatic defect was found partially impaired in skin cultured from both parents, confirming an autosomal recessive pat-

tern of inheritance. Studies on the enzyme, a microsomal oxygenase, indicate that Vitamin C is a principal physiologic reductant. The patient identified in Figure 3–37 responded to 4 grams per day of Vitamin C with increased urinary hydroxylysine production, increase in corneal size, decrease in bleeding time, and improved muscle tone.

Collagen is the most obvious protein involved in maintaining structural integrity of organs. However, several proteins are involved in maintaining cellular structure. For instance, intermolecular stacking of S-hemoglobin produces the sickling phenomenon of sickle cell anemia; abnormal spectrin may produce the spherocytes of hereditary spherocytic anemia; and the absence of β-lipoprotein the increased sphingomyelin-to-lecithin ratio seen in acanthocytic red cells of patients with abetalipoproteinemia.

APPLICATIONS TO MANAGEMENT OF INHERITED DISEASE

Although knowledge in the field of human genetics has grown rapidly, our concern as physicians has been to find applications for this knowledge even in its present sketchy state. Table 3–12

Ehlers Danlos Syndrome (TYPE VI)

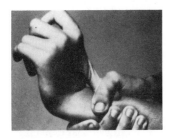

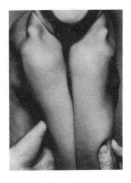

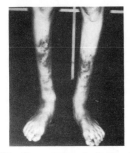

	Skin Hydroxylysine (*Residues/1000*)	HOLYS HOPRO
Patient (JDH)	0.5	0.011
Controls (25)	5.1 ± 0.7	0.061 ± 0.009

Figure 3–37 Composite photograph of an eight-year-old boy with hydroxylysine deficient collagen describing hyperflexibility of finger and shoulder joints and abnormally friable skin with scorbutic scar formation. His cultured skin fibroblasts had less than 10 per cent of normal collagen lysyl hydroxylase activity.

represents a composite of both factual and speculative approaches to the management of inherited diseases. These therapeutic approaches have been categorized according to the level of recognition of the pathogenic mechanisms. Thus, if all we recognize at present is an abnormal phenotype as in Down syndrome, muscular dystrophy, or spina bifida, therapeutic approaches are limited to genetic counseling regarding the recurrence risks and to rehabilitation of the patient. In some instances the clinical phenotype may be expressed in cultured fetal cells or in amniotic fluid, and

TABLE 3–12 THERAPY OF INHERITED DISEASE

Level of Recognition	Treatment

1. Clinical Phenotype	1. Genetic Counseling
	  a. Antenatal diagnosis
	  b. Rehabilitation

2. Impaired Reaction Sequence
  a. Toxic precursor
  b. Deficient product
  c. Deficient coenzyme
  d. Sensitivity to environment
	2. Environmental Engineering
	  a. Restriction
	  b. Replacement
	  c. Vitamin administration
	  d. Exposure prevention

3. Defective Gene Product
  a. Enzyme
  b. Structural protein
  c. Regulation
	3. Cellular Engineering
	  a. Replacement
	  b. Prevention of structural changes
	  c. Provision of inducer, repressor, or feedback inhibitor

4. Mutant DNA	4. Genetic Engineering
	  a. Transformation
	  b. Transduction

more precise counseling such as antenatal diagnosis can be offered. There are over 200 different disorders currently monitorable by these techniques — some only through indirectly associated findings such as increased amniotic fluid α-fetoprotein in fetuses with open neural tube anomalies or hereditary nephrosis. Another example would be the diagnosis of a male fetus in the case of X-linked recessive disorders, where the mother is a known or at-risk carrier of an incurable disorder such as Duchenne pseudohypertrophic muscular dystrophy. In many other disorders specific enzyme defects are demonstrable in cultured amniotic fluid cells and provide more precise criteria for the probable phenotype of the fetus. Genetic counseling will become more precise as techniques of antenatal diagnosis improve. At this level of recognition, treatment of the affected individual must also be considered. Let us assume that a patient with phenylketonuria was not detected early enough in life to prevent mental retardation. Dietary restriction, controlled educational programs, and specific training may potentiate the patient's remaining capabilities such that he can take part in our complex society. If the homozygous affected patient happens to be a reproductive-aged female, control of her blood phenylalanine to normal levels during conception and pregnancy may prevent the otherwise absolute risk to her offspring of having microcephaly and mental retardation as a result of maternal phenylketonuria.

Many inborn errors of metabolism are detected by the presence of abnormal concentrations of potentially toxic precursors in an impaired reaction sequence and can be treated before the disease is clinically manifest. The best example of this is the statewide screening of newborn infants for elevated blood phenylalanine levels to diagnose phenylketonuria. Treatment of this group of disorders involves a form of environmental engineering in which the potentially toxic precursor, phenylalanine, is restricted in the diet to prevent manifestations of the clinical phenotype. The sequelae of many other disorders such as hypothyroidism, galactosemia, maple syrup urine disease, and homocystinuria are similarly preventable through mass screening (non-selective) of all newborns. Early retrieval, diagnosis, and treatment before the third week of life are also prerequisites of such a preventive program. In other diseases such as Hartnup disease, the pellagra-like symptoms are preventable by the administration of the deficient end-product, nicotinic acid. In vitamin dependency syndromes such as vitamin responsive methylmalonic aciduria, the administration of massive amounts of the vitamin precursor will increase the deficient coenzyme and ameliorate the blocked reaction sequence and clinical problems attendant to the untreated condition. Such

approaches during the third trimester of pregnancy have prevented newborn manifestations of methylmalonic acidemia by treating the mother with mg. quantities of B_{12} per day. Environmental engineering may also be provided in circumstances in which an individual has a mutant gene product reflected only under stressful environmental conditions. The group of pharmacogenetic disorders is a good example of this situation in which patients are sensitive to the administration of primaquine (G6PD deficiency) or succinyldicholine (pseudo-cholinesterase deficiency). Prediction and prevention can be effected through pedigree analysis and chemical evaluation of "high-risk" members. Speculation in this area grows as we analyze the complex alleles of circulating blood proteins such as the α_1-antitrypsin. Fagerhol has pointed out that functional defects in antitrypsin activity and protein phenotypes may be associated with increased susceptibility to pulmonary disease, cirrhosis, and clotting disorders. As more knowledge is collected relating the structural and functional defects of this group of proteins and as populations are screened for their protein genotype, physicians may offer specific suggestions concerning the best type of environment in which an individual should live. For instance, a presymptomatic patient with α_1-antitrypsin deficiency and a protein genotype of ZZ (deficient) or MZ (40 per cent activity) may be advised to live in a rural rather than urban area to retard the development of lung disease resulting from the polluted environment. Patients in families where high serum group I pepsinogen is linked to duodenal ulcer may develop life styles amenable to preventing ulcer disease. Similarly, children in families with high blood levels of LDL and cholesterol may be treated with 7-ketosterol analogs to bypass the LDL-cholesterol receptor, suppress HMG CoA reductase, reduce cholesterol biosynthesis, and prevent atherosclerosis.

In some of the inborn errors alluded to previously, the defective gene product has been defined as a functional or regulatory impairment of cell metabolism. At this level of recognition, therapy can be considered in terms of cellular engineering in which the objective is the replacement of a defective enzyme. This concept is not novel, since we all recognize the value of insulin or antihemophilic globulin in inherited disorders such as diabetes mellitus or hemophilia A. However, the administration of specific enzymes involved in intracellular function remains at present in the area of research. Purified enzymes can be enclosed in semipermeable inert nylon microspherules to protect the enzyme from immune host response. Catalase has been injected intravenously to revert the abnormal biochemical phenotype in acatalasemic mice, and urease has raised the blood ammonia in dogs. If the enzyme is lysosomal or cytoplasmic, its eventual deposition in liver may provide function to the organism in which this enzyme is deficient. Purified α-1,4-glucosidase from *Aspergillus niger* has reduced liver glycogen in patients dying from glycogen storage disease, Type II. Similarly, glucocerebrosidase enclosed in liposomes or autologous red blood cell ghosts has alleviated organomegaly in Gaucher disease. In other instances, the defective gene product may be a structural protein whose molecular structure is recognized. The administration of cyanate and carbamyl phosphate to patients with sickle cell disease is a form of cellular engineering aimed at correcting the molecular aggregation of sickle hemoglobin and is under study. In some disorders, the defective enzyme function may be inducible. Thus, in hepatic glucuronyl transferase deficiency, sodium phenobarbital has enhanced this enzymatic pathway and the perinatal utilization of bilirubin. Steroid hormones may also be effective inducers of some enzymes. In one patient with Type III glycogen storage disease, a double enzyme deficiency involving amylo-1,6-glucosidase and glucose-6-phosphatase was described. A fourfold increase in glucose-6-phosphatase activity occurred upon administration of triamcinolone. Repression of an overactive pathway may also become a form of genetic engineering. In orotic aciduria the administration of uridine represses the initial step of this pathway and reduces the formation of insoluble orotic acid.

Transplantation has become a reality in several heritable disorders. Kidney transplants in Fabry disease have provided ceramide trihexosidase, and reduced deposition of ceramide trihexoses in other organs. Thymus transplants in DiGeorge syndrome and marrow transplants in agammaglobulinemia have literally cured these disorders in the immune mechanisms.

Finally, the most intriguing aspect of therapy in inherited disease of man involves the recent approaches to gene insertion into mammalian cells. Although many of the fundamental genetic and regulatory processes of mammalian cells remain unknown, transduction using bacterial viruses and transformation using cell fusion techniques have demonstrated science's ability to introduce new functional genes into mammalian cells. The recently simplified methods of recombination have made transduction a real possibility in many disorders, including insertion of the gene for insulin into diabetics. Although transformation *per se* has not been used in mammalian cells derived from humans, Harris' group demonstrated that by fusing a chick red blood cell whose nucleus carries the gene for inosinic acid pyrophosphorylase with a mouse fibroblast A_9 cell which was deficient in this enzyme function, transformation of the mutant mouse cell line was accomplished. Transduction has been utilized in one human disease, galactosemia. Merril's group produced a λ-phage (λpgal) lysogenic for *E. coli* which carried part of the bacterial galactose operon coding for α-D-galactose-1-phosphate uridyl transferase (UDP-Gal-1-P). This λ-phage will infect cultured fibroblasts derived from the skin of patients lacking this enzyme function (galactosemia) and return UDPGal-1-P activity. The infected fibroblasts retained this activity for at least eight population doublings (40 days in culture) and manufactured new λ-specific RNA. Whether other side-effects from λ-pgal infection will be seen in intact mammals is currently under investigation. Although these new developments do not provide practical genetic engineering, it is now clear that science has provided means by which genes can be transferred and inserted into mammalian cells. These basic tools will provide answers to many questions concerning gene function and perhaps in the future, a method for treating inherited disorders.

GLOSSARY OF GENETIC TERMS

Acrocentric — Chromosomes with the centromere close to one end.

Alleles — Alternate forms of a gene.

Aneuploid (aneuploidy)—Deviation from the basic diploid number or from exact multiples of the basic (haploid) number in a chromosome series.

Arm (chromosome) — The portion located on either side of the centromere of a metaphase chromosome.

Autosome — Any non-sex chromosomes (22 pairs in humans).

Balanced translocation—Rearrangement of chromosomal material, without genetic effect.

Break (chromosome) — Interruption in staining of the chromosome arm, with displacement in the alignment of the portions on either side of the interruption.

Cell cycle (cell life cycle)—The cycle in the life of a cell which includes progression through mitosis (M) and interphase.

Centromere — (*also kinetochore* or *primary constriction*) — A non-staining area on a chromosome, separating the chromosome arms; the point of attachment of the chromosome to the mitotic spindle.

Chromatid — One of two structurally distinguishable (by light microscopy) longitudinal subunits of a metaphase chromosome.

Chromatin—Areas of a cell nucleus that stain with a DNA stain. (See also *Sex chromatin.*)

Cis — Two genes on the same chromosome are cis to each other or coupled.

Cistron — The gene considered on a functional basis as defined by the cis-trans complementation test. Two mutants in the same cistron do not complement; two mutants in different cistrons do.

Codon — A triplet of three bases in a strand of DNA which codes for a specific amino acid.

Complementation — Interaction of two cytoplasmic products to produce a normal phenotype.

Crossing-over — The exchange of genetic material between members of a pair of homologous chromosomes that leads to the formation of recombinants.

Deletion (chromosome) — Absence of part of a chromosome.

Diploid—Possessing two genomes. In man somatic cells normally contain the diploid number of chromosomes: 46 (2n).

Discontinuous traits — Two clearly different phenotypes which do not blend with one another.

Dominant — The phenotype expressed in the F_1 heterozygote resulting from a cross between two true-breeding strains. The dominant allele determines the phenotype expressed by a heterozygote.

Endoreduplication (endopolyploidy) — The result of a partial mitosis involving doubling of chromosome number without division of nucleus or cytoplasm.

End-product repression — Repression of synthesis of the messenger RNA from the operon for an anabolic (synthetic) pathway caused by the accumulation of an end-product of the pathway.

Episome — A piece of DNA which can remain separate from the rest of the genome or can become integrated into it. A type of plasmid.

F_1 — The first filial generation (the progeny) of a cross between two individuals.

Fragment (chromosome) — A portion of a chromosome without a centromere.

Feedback inhibition — Inhibition of an enzyme in an anabolic pathway by an allosteric effect of an end-product or derivative of the end-product in this pathway.

Frameshift mutation — A mutation arising from the insertion or deletion of a nucleotide pair.

Gap (chromosome) — Interruption in staining of a chromosome arm, without disturbance of alignment of the portions on either side of the interruption.

Gene — (a) Classic mendelian definition: The fundamental biologic unit of heredity transmitted from generation to generation unchanged;

   (b) Molecular definition: Unit of function of a cistron. One gene codes for one polypeptide chain.

Genome — One copy of each allele.

Genotype—The genetic constitution of an individual.

Haploid — A haploid cell contains one copy of a genome. The normal gamete contains only one member of each chromosome pair and is therefore haploid. In man, the haploid chromosome number (n) is 23.

Hemizygote—An individual possessing only one allele at a given locus. Since human males have only one X chromosome, they are said to be hemizygous with respect to X-linked genes.

Heterochromatin (heterochromatization; heterochromatic) — Nuclear areas that stain "differently" with DNA stains.

Heterogeneity — The result of a trait whose phenotypic expression is produced by a number of different genetic mechanisms.

Heterokaryon — Cell with two or more genomes of different types.

Heterozygote — An individual who has two different alleles for a given gene.

Homozygote — An individual possessing a pair of identical alleles for a given gene.

Hyperdiploidy (hypodiploidy) — More (or less) than the diploid number of chromosomes — a form of aneuploidy.

Isochromosome — A chromosome consisting of identical arms on either side of the centromere.

Karyotype — A systematized arrangement of chromosomes.

Linkage — Association of genes on one chromosome.

Locus — A cluster of genes located in a linkage group.

Map distance (genetic distance) — The distance between two genes equal to the number of progeny recombinant for them divided by the total number of progeny.

Meiosis—That form of cell division in the formation of gametes producing the haploid chromosome number (n) from a diploid cell (2n).

Metacentric — Chromosomes with the centromere located in the center, making the two arms on either side of it equal in length.

Missense mutation — A change in a gene resulting in the incorporation of an incorrect amino acid into its product.

Monosomic (monosomy) — One chromosome pair contains 1 instead of 2 chromosomes.

Monozygotic — Twins derived from a single fertilized ovum (identical twins).

Mosaic — An individual or tissue with at least two cell lines, differing in genotype or karyotype, derived from a single zygote.

Mutant — An altered gene, or an individual bearing such an altered gene.

Mutation — An alteration in genetic material that is transmitted from one generation to the next.

Nonsense mutation — A change in a gene resulting in the formation of one of the "stop" codons in place of a codon for a particular amino acid and leading to formation of a partial protein that is terminated at the site of the mutation.

Operon — A genetic unit consisting of an operator and the cistrons whose actions it controls.

Phenocopy — An individual whose appearance is produced by an environmental effect, but whose phenotype is similar to one produced by a genetic effect.

Phenotype — The physical constitution of an individual. This includes physical, biochemical, and physiologic makeup of an individual as determined by his genotype and the environment in which he develops.

Pleiotropy — The situation in which a single gene or gene pair produces multiple effects.

Point mutation — A change in a single base pair.

Polyploidy — The designation for the occurrence of chromosome numbers in multiples of the basic haploid number (n), other than the diploid number (2n), e.g., triploidy (3n), tetraploidy (4n), and so on.

Proband — Same as *propositus*.

Propositus — Also called index case, or proband; the family member who first draws attention to a pedigree of a particular trait.

Protein polymorphism — The occurrence of two or more different forms of the same protein.

Recessive — That phenotype which is *not* expressed in the F_1 heterozygote resulting from a cross between two true breeding strains. In classic genetics this term can only be used when the F_1 heterozygote is phenotypically identical to that of one of the homozygotes. In human genetics "recessive" refers to a gene which is expressed only when homozygous.

Recombination — The formation of new combinations of linked genes by crossing-over between them.

Ring (chromosome) — Attachment of opposite ends of a chromosome to form a ring.

Satellite — DNA staining structure on the distal end of a chromosome arm and separated from it by a secondary constriction.

Secondary constriction — A non-staining area on a chromosome arm.

Segregation — The separation of alleles and chromosomes during meiosis.

Sex chromatin, female (Barr body, X body)—A characteristic area in the interphase nucleus, composed of X-chromosome material that stains heavily with a DNA stain.

Sex chromatin, male (Y body) — A characteristic area in the interphase nucleus composed of Y-chromosome material that fluoresces brightly.

Sex chromosomes — XX in human female; XY in human male: 1 pair is normally present in each individual.

Silent allele — An allele which has no detectable product, presumably produced by a nonsense mutant.

Somatic — Pertaining to cells other than germ cells.

Tetraploid — The quadruple basic number in a chromosome series (4n).

Trans — Two genes on different chromosomes are trans to each other, or in repulsion.

Transcription, RNA — The process by which new RNA is made from a DNA template.

Transduction — A form of recombination in bacteria in which a bacteriophage serves as the DNA vector.

Transformation — The form of recombination in bacteria in which naked DNA serves as the vector.

Translation — The process by which genetic information contained in DNA is carried by mRNA from the nucleus to the cytoplasm and affects amino acid sequences in the synthesis of proteins.

Translocation—The transfer of a piece of one chromosome to another chromosome.

Triploid — The triple basic number in a chromosome series (3n).

Trisomy — The state of having one extra chromosome per cell. Instead of the usual pair of homologous chromosomes, there are now three.

X-linked — Genes on the X chromosome or traits determined by such genes are X-linked.

REFERENCES

GENERAL GENETICS

Bergsma, D. (ed.): Birth Defects. Atlas and Compendium. The National Foundation. The Williams and Wilkins Co., Baltimore, 1973.

Carter, C. O., David, P. A., and Laurence, K. M.: A family study of major central nervous system malformations in South Wales. J. Med. Genet., *5*:81, 1968.

Carter, C. O., and Evans, K. A.: Inheritance of congenital pyloric stenosis. J. Med. Genet., *6*:233, 1969.

Carter, C. O.: Genetics of common disorders. Br. Med. Bull., *25*:52, 1969.

Carter, C. O.: Multifactorial genetic disease. Hosp. Pract., *5*:45, 1970.

Cavalli-Sforza, L. L., and Bodmer, W. F.: The Genetics of Human Populations. W. H. Freeman and Company, San Francisco, 1971.

Edwards, J. H.: The simulation of mendelism. Acta Genet. (Basel), *10*:63, 1960.

Falconer, D. S.: The inheritance of liability to certain diseases, estimated from the incidence among relatives. Ann. Human Genet., *29*:51, 1965.

Goodman, R. M. (ed.): Genetic Disorders of Man. Little, Brown & Co., Boston, 1970.

Harris, H., Whittaker, M., Lehmann, H., and Silk, E.: The pseudocholinesterase variants. Esterase levels and dibucaine numbers in families selected through suxamethonium sensitive individuals. Acta Genet. (Basel), *10*:1, 1960.

Haws, D. V., and McKusick, V. A.: Farabee's brachydactylous kindred revisited. Bull. Johns Hopkins Hosp., *113*:20, 1963.

King, K. C.: A Dictionary of Genetics, 2nd ed. Oxford University Press, New York, 1974.

Lubs, H. A., and dela Cruz, F. (eds.): Genetic Counseling. Raven Press, New York, 1977.

McKusick, V. A.: Human Genetics. Prentice-Hall, Inc., Englewood Cliffs, New Jersey, 1964.

McKusick, V. A., and Claiborne, R. (eds.): Medical Genetics. HP Publishing Co., Inc., New York, 1973.

McKusick, V. A.: Mendelian Inheritance in Man: Catalogs of Autosomal Dominant, Autosomal Recessive, and X-linked Phenotypes, 4th ed. Johns Hopkins Press, Baltimore, 1976.

Mendel, G.: Versuche über Pflanzenhybriden. Leipzig, Engelmann, 1901. Translated in J. Heredity, *42*:1, 1951.

Mulvihill, J. J., Miller, R. W., and Fraumeni, J. F. (eds.): Genetics of Human Cancer. Progress in Cancer Research and Therapy, Vol. 3. Raven Press, New York, 1977.

Riccardi, V. M.: The Genetic Approach to Human Disease. Oxford University Press, New York, 1977.

Smith, D. W.: Recognizable Patterns of Human Malformation. Genetic, Embryologic and Clinical Aspects, 2nd ed. W. B. Saunders Co., Philadelphia, 1976.

Thompson, J. S., and Thompson, M. W.: Genetics in Medicine, 2nd ed. W. B. Saunders Co., Philadelphia, 1973.

CHROMOSOMAL GENETICS

General

DuPraw, E. J.: DNA and Chromosomes. Holt, Rinehart and Winston, Inc., New York, 1970, Ch. 9.

Ford, E. H. R.: Human Chromosomes. Academic Press, New York and London, 1973.

Hamerton, J. L., Canning, N., Ray, M., and Smith, S.: A cytogenetic survey of 14,069 newborn infants. I. Incidence of chromosome abnormalities. Clin. Gen., *8*:223, 1975.

Makino, S.: Human Chromosomes. Igaku Shoin Ltd., Tokyo, 1975.

Ohno, S., Klinger, H. P., and Atkin, N. B.: Human oögenesis. Cytogenetics, *1*:42, 1962.

Paris Conference (1971): Standardization in Human Cytogenetics. Birth Defects: Original Article Series, *VIII*:7, The National Foundation, New York, 1972. *Or* Paris Conference (1971): Standardization in human cytogenetics. Cytogenetics, *11*:313, 1972.

Paris Conference (1971), Supplement (1975): Standardization in Human Cytogenetics. Birth Defects: Original Article Series, *XI*:9, The National Foundation, New York, 1975.

Priest, J. H.: Medical Cytogenetics and Cell Culture. Lea and Febiger, Philadelphia, 1977.

Schwarzacher, H. G., Wolf, U., and Passarge, E. (eds.): Methods in Human Cytogenetics. Springer-Verlag Inc., New York, 1974.

Yunis, J. J. (ed.): Human Chromosome Methodology. Academic Press, New York and London, 1974.

Chromosome Banding

Arrighi, F. E., and Hsu, T. C.: Localization of heterochromatin in human chromosomes. Cytogenetics, *10*:81, 1971.

Bobrow, M., Pearson, P. L., Pike, M. C., and El-Alfi, O. S.: Length variation in the quinacrine-binding segment of human Y chromosomes of different sizes. Cytogenetics, *10*:190, 1971.

Caspersson, T., Lomakka, G., and Zech, L.: The 24 fluorescence patterns of the human metaphase chromosomes — distinguishing characters and variability. Hereditas, *67*:89, 1971.

Craig-Holmes, A. P., Moore, F. B., and Shaw, M. W.: Polymorphism of human C-band heterochromatin. I. Frequency of variants. Am. J. Hum. Genet., 25:181, 1973.

Dutrillaux, B., and Lejeune, J.: Cytogenétique humaine. — Sur une nouvelle Technique d'Analyse du Caryotype humain. C. R. Acad. Sci. (Paris), 272:2638, 1971.

Seabright, M.: A rapid banding technique for human chromosomes. Lancet, ii:971, 1971.

Sex Chromatin

Barr, M. L., Bertram, L. F., and Lindsay, H. A.: The morphology of the nerve cell nucleus, according to sex. Anat. Rec., 107:283, 1950.

Goad, W. B., Robinson, A., and Puck, T. T.: Incidence of aneuploidy in a human population. Am. J. Hum. Genet., 28:62, 1976.

Lyon, M. F.: Sex chromatin and gene action in the mammalian X-chromosome. Am. J. Hum. Genet., 14:135, 1962.

Mittwoch, U.: Sex Chromatin. J. Med. Genet., 1:50, 1964.

Pearson, P. L., Bobrow, M., and Vosa, C. G.: Technique for identifying Y chromosomes in human interphase nuclei. Nature, 226:78, 1970.

Priest, J. H.: Medical Cytogenetics and Cell Culture. Sex Chromatin. Lea & Febiger, Philadelphia, 1977, Ch. 10.

Congenital Defect Syndromes

Allderdice, P. W., Davis, J. G., Miller, O. J., Klinger, H. P., Warburton, D., Miller, D. A., Allen, F. H., Abrams, C. A. L., and McGilvray, E.: The 13q-deletion syndrome. Am. J. Hum. Genet., 21:499, 1969.

Becker, K. L., Hoppman, D. L., Albert, A., Underdahl, L. O., and Mason, H. L.: Klinefelter's syndrome. Arch. Int. Med., 118:314, 1966.

Beratis, N. G., Kardon, N. B., Hsu, L. Y. F., Grossman, D., and Hirschhorn, K.: Parental mosaicism in trisomy 18. Pediatrics, 50:908, 1972.

Borgaonkar, D. S., Mules, E., and Char, F.: Do the 48, XXYY males have a characteristic phenotype? Chem. Genet., 1:272, 1970.

Caldwell, P. D., and Smith, D. W.: The XXY (Klinefelter's) syndrome in childhood: detection and treatment. J. Pediatr., 80:250, 1972.

de Grouchy, J.: Chromosome 18: a topologic approach. J. Pediatr., 66:414, 1965.

Edwards, J. H., Harnden, D. G., Cameron, A. H., Crosse, V. M., and Wolff, O. H.: A new trisomic syndrome. Lancet, i:787, 1960.

Ford, C. E., Jones, K. W., Polani, P. E., de Almeida, J. C., and Briggs, J. H.: A sex-chromosome anomaly in a case of gonadal dysgenesis (Turner's syndrome). Lancet, i:711, 1959.

Grace, E., Drennan, J., Colver, D., and Gordon, R. R.: The 13q- syndrome. J. Med. Genet., 8:351, 1971.

Hook, E. B.: Behavioral implications of the human XYY genotype. Science, 179:139, 1973.

Hsu, L. Y. F., Shapiro, L. R., Gertner, M., Lieber, E., Hirschhorn, K.: Trisomy 22: a clinical entity. J. Pediatr., 79:12, 1971.

Jacobs, P. A., Baikie, A. G., Court Brown, W. M., MacGregor, T. N., Maclean, N., and Harnden, D. G.: Evidence for the existence of the human "super female." Lancet, ii:423, 1959.

Jacobs, P. A., and Strong, J. A.: A case of human intersexuality having a possible XXY sex-determining mechanism. Nature, 183:302, 1959.

Kakati, S., Zihill, M., and Sinha, A. K.: An attempt to establish trisomy 8 syndrome. Humangenetik, 19:293, 1973.

Klinefelter, H. F., Reifenstein, E. C., and Albright, F.: Syndrome characterized by gynecomastia, aspermatogenesis without A-Leydigism, and increased excretion of follicle-stimulating hormone. J. Clin. Endocrinol., 2:615, 1942.

Lejeune, J., Gautier, M., and Turpin, R.: Étude des chromosomes somatiques de neuf enfants mongoliens. C. R. Acad. Sci. (Paris), 248:1721, 1959.

Lejeune, J., Lafourcad, J., Berger, R., Vialette, J., Boeswill-

wald, M., Seringe, P., and Turpin, R.: Trois Cas de Deletion Partielle des Bras Courts d'un Chromosome 5. C. R. Acad. Sci. (D.) (Paris), 257:3098, 1963.

Lemli, L., and Smith, D. W.: The XO syndrome: a study of the differential phenotype in 25 patients. J. Pediatr., 63:577, 1963.

Miller, O. J., Breg, W. R., Warburton, D., Miller, D. A., de Copoa, A., Allderdice, P. W., Davis, J., Klinger, H. P., McGilvray, E., and Allen, F. H.: Partial deletion of the short arm of chromosome No. 4 (4p-): clinical studies in five unrelated patients. J. Pediatr., 77:792, 1970.

Patau, K., Smith, D., Therman, E., Inhorn, S. L., and Wagner, H. P.: Multiple congenital anomalies caused by an extra autosome. Lancet, i:790, 1960.

Penrose, L. S., and Smith, G. F.: Down's Anomaly. Little, Brown & Co., Boston, 1966.

Polani, P. E., Hunter, W. F., and Lennox, B.: Chromosomal sex in Turner's syndrome with coarctation of the aorta. Lancet, ii:120, 1954.

Sinet, P.-M., Couturier, J., Dutrillaux, B., Poissonnier, M., Raoul, O., Rethore, M.-O., Allard, D., LeJeune, J., and Jerome, H.: Trisomie 21 et superoxyde dismutase-1 (IPO-A). Exp. Cell Res., 97:47, 1976.

Smith, D. W., Patau, K., Therman, E., Inhorn, S. L., and DeMars, R. I.: The D₁ trisomy syndrome. J. Pediatr., 63:326, 1963.

Telfer, M. A., Baker, D., Clark, G. R., and Richardson, C. E.: Incidence of gross chromosomal errors among tall criminal American males. Science, 159:1249, 1968.

Telfer, M. A., Richardson, C. E., Helmken, J., and Smith, G. F.: Divergent phenotype among 48,XXXX and 47,XXX females. Am. J. Hum. Genet., 22:326, 1970.

Tuncbilek, E., Halicioglu, C., and Say, B.: Trisomy-8 syndrome. Humangenetik, 23:23, 1974.

Turner, H. H.: A syndrome of infantilism, congenital webbed neck, and cubitus valgus. Endocrinology, 23:566, 1938.

Warren, R. J., and Rimoin, D. L.: The G deletion syndromes. J. Pediatr., 77:658, 1970.

Warren, R. J., Rimoin, D. L., and Summitt, R. L.: Identification by fluorescent microscopy of the abnormal chromosomes associated with the G-deletion syndromes. Am. J. Hum. Genet., 25:77, 1973.

Wertelecki, W., and Gerald, P. S.: Clinical and chromosomal studies of the 18q- syndrome. J. Pediatr., 78:44, 1971.

Fetal Wastage

Bhasin, M. K., Foerster, W., and Fuhrmann, W.: A cytogenetic study of recurrent abortion. Humangenetik, 18:139, 1973.

Carr, D. H., and Gedeon, M.: Four familial translocations ascertained through spontaneous abortions. Hum. Genet., 31:93, 1976.

de la Chapelle, A., Schröder, J., and Kokkonen, J.: Cytogenetics of recurrent abortion or unsuccessful pregnancy. Int. J. Fertil., 18:215, 1973.

Kajii, T., Ohama, K., Niikawa, N., Ferrier, A., and Avirachan, S.: Banding analysis of abnormal karyotypes in spontaneous abortion. Am. J. Hum. Genet., 25:539, 1973.

Kim, H. J., Hsu, L. Y. F., Paciuc, S., Cristian, S., Quintana, A., and Hirschhorn, K.: Cytogenetics of fetal wastage. N. Engl. J. Med., 293:844, 1975.

Chromosomes and Neoplasia

German, J.: Oncogenic Implications of Chromosomal Instability. *In* McKusick, V., and Claiborne, R. (eds.): Medical Genetics. HP Publishing Co., Inc., New York, 1973, Ch. 4.

Harnden, D. G.: Cytogenetics of Human Neoplasia. *In* Mulvihill, J. J., Miller, R. W., and Fraumeni, J. F. (eds.): Genetics of Human Cancer. Progress in Cancer Research and Therapy, Vol. 3. Raven Press, New York, 1977, Ch. 8.

Hecht, F., and McCaw, B. K.: Chromosome Instability Syndromes. *In* Mulvihill, J. J., Miller, R. W., and Fraumeni, J. F. (eds.): Genetics of Human Cancer. Progress in Cancer Research and Therapy, Vol. 3. Raven Press, New York, 1977, Ch. 9.

Nowell, P. C., and Hungerford, D. A.: Chromosome studies in human leukemia. II. Chronic granulocytic leukemia. J. Nat. Cancer Inst., 27:1031, 1961.

O'Riordan, M. L., Robinson, J. A., Buckton, K. E., and Evans, H. J.: Distinguishing between the chromosomes involved in Down's syndrome (trisomy 21) and chronic myeloid leukaemia (Ph¹) by fluorescence. Nature, 230:167, 1971.

Rowley, J. D.: Are Nonrandom Karyotypic Changes Related to Etiologic Agents? In Mulvihill, J. J., Miller, R. W., and Fraumeni, J. F. (eds.): Genetics of Human Cancer. Progress in Cancer Research and Therapy. Vol. 3. Raven Press, New York, 1977, Ch. 10.

Chromosome Mapping

Creagan, R., Tischfield, J., McMorris, F. A., Chen, S., Hirsch, M., Chen, T. R., Ricciuti, F., and Ruddle, F. H.: Assignment of the genes for human peptidase A to chromosome 18 and cytoplasmic glutamic oxaloacetate transaminase to chromosome 10 using somatic cell hybrids. Cytogenet. Cell Genet., 12:187, 1973.

Davidson, R. L., and delaCruz, F. (eds.): Somatic Cell Hybridization. Raven Press, New York, 1974.

McKusick, V. A.: The mapping of human chromosomes. Sci. Am., 224:104, 1971.

McKusick, V. A., and Ruddle, F. H.: The status of the gene map of the human chromosomes. Science, 196:390, 1977.

Pardue, M. L., and Gall, J. G.: Molecular hybridization of radioactive DNA to the DNA of cytological preparations. Proc. Nat. Acad. Sci., U.S.A., 64:600, 1969.

Ruddle, F. H., and Kucherlapati, R. S.: Hybrid cells and human genes. Sci. Am., 231:36, 1974.

Third Annual International Workshop on Human Gene Mapping. Baltimore, 1975. Cytogenet. Cell Genet., 16, 1976.

MOLECULAR BASIS FOR INHERITANCE

Braunitzer, G., Hilse, K., Rudloff, V., and Hilschmann, N.: The hemoglobins. Advanced Protein Chem., 19:1, 1964.

Celma, M. L., Dhar, R., Pan, J. and Weissman, S. M.: Comparison of nucleotide sequence of messenger RNA for the major structural protein of SV40 with the DNA sequence encoding the amino acids of the protein. Nucleic Acids Research, 4: 2549, 1977.

Cleaver, J. E.: Defective repair replication of DNA in xeroderma pigmentosum. Nature, 218:652, 1968.

Crick, F. H. C.: The genetic code. Proc. Roy. Soc. B, 167:331, 1967.

Granner, D. K., Hayashi, S. L., Thompson, E. B., and Tomkins, G. M.: Stimulation of tyrosine aminotransferase synthesis by dexamethasone phosphate in cell culture. J. Molec. Biol., 35:291, 1968.

Hartman, P. E., and Suskind, S. R.: Gene Action, 2nd edition, Prentice-Hall, Inc., Englewood Cliffs, New Jersey, 1969.

Ingram, V. M., and Stretton, A. O.: Genetic basis of the thalassaemia diseases. Nature, 184:1903, 1959.

Ingram, V. M.: Gene mutations in human haemoglobin: the chemical difference between normal and sickle cell haemoglobin. Nature, 180:326, August 10, 1957.

Itano, H. A., and Neel, J. V.: A new inherited abnormality of human hemoglobin. Proc. Nat. Acad. Sci. (U.S.A.), 36:613, 1950.

Jacob, F., and Monod, J.: Genetic regulatory mechanisms in the synthesis of proteins. J. Mol. Bio., 3:318, 1961.

Jacob, F., and Monod, J.: On the regulation of gene activity. Cold Spring Harbor Symposia on Quant. Biol., 26:193, 1961.

Kornberg, A.: Enzymatic synthesis of DNA. John Wiley and Sons, Inc., New York, 1962.

Krieg, D. R.: Specificity of chemical mutagenesis. Progr. Nucleic Acid Res., 2:125, 1963.

Lehmann, H., and Carrell, R. W.: Variations in the structure of human haemoglobin with particular reference to the unstable haemoglobins. Brit. Med. Bull., 25:14, 1969.

Meselson, M., and Stahl, F. W.: The replication of DNA in *Escherichia coli*. Proc. Nat. Acad. Sci. (U.S.A.), 44:671, 1958.

Miller, O. J., Allerdice, P. W., Miller, D. A., Breg, W. R., and Migeon, B. R.: Human thymidine kinase gene locus: assignment to chromosome 17 in a hybrid of man and mouse cells. Science, 173:244, 1971.

Murayama, M.: Structure of sickle cell hemoglobin and molecular mechanism of the sickling phenomenon. Clin. Chem., 14:578, 1967.

Neel, J. V.: The inheritance of sickle cell anemia. Science, 110:64, 1949.

Neel, J. V.: The inheritance of sickling phenomenon with particular reference to sickle cell disease. Blood, 6:389, 1951.

Nirenberg, M. W., and Matthaci, J. H.: The dependence of cell-free protein synthesis in *E. coli* upon naturally occurring or synthetic polyribonucleotides. Proc. Nat. Acad. Sci. (Wash.), 47:1588, 1961.

Pauling, L., Itano, H. A., Singer, S. J., and Wells, I. C.: Sickle cell anemia, molecular disease. Science, 110:543,1949.

Perutz, M. F., and Lehmann, H.: Molecular pathology of human haemoglobin. Nature, 219:902, 1968.

Perutz, M. F., and Mitchison, J. M.: State of haemoglobin in sickle-cell anaemia. Nature, 166:677, 1950.

Prescott, D. M.: The structure and replication of eukaryotic chromosomes. In Prescott, D. M., Goldstein, L., and McConkey, E. (Eds.): Advances in Cell Biology. Vol. 1. Appleton-Century-Crofts, New York, 1969, pp. 57–117.

Ptashne, M.: Specific binding of the λ-phage repressor to λ-DNA. Nature, 214:232, 1967.

Speyer, J. F.: The genetic code. In Taylor, J. H. (Ed.): Molecular Genetics. Part II. Academic Press, Inc., New York, 1967, pp. 137–191.

Stamatoyannopoulos, G.: The molecular basis of hemoglobin disease. Ann. Rev. Genet., 6:47, 1972.

Sullivan, D. T.: Molecular hybridization used to characterize the RNA synthesized by isolated bovine thymus nuclei. Proc. Nat. Acad. Sci. (U.S.A.), 59:846, 1968.

Watson, J. D.: The Double Helix. Atheneum Publishers, New York, 1968.

Watson, J. D.: Molecular Biology of the Gene. 2nd edition. W. A. Benjamin, Inc., New York.

Watson, J. D., and Crick, F. H. C.: Genetical implications of the structure of deoxyribose nucleic acid. Nature (London), 171:964, 1953.

Weatherall, D. J.: Genetics of the thalassaemias. Brit. Med. Bull., 25:24, 1969.

Woese, C. R.: The present status of the genetic code. Progr. Nucleic Acid Res. and Molec. Biol., 7:107, 1967.

INHERITED METABOLIC DISORDERS

General References

Bondy, P. K., and Rosenberg, L. E. (eds.): Duncan's Diseases of Metabolism, 7th ed. W. B. Saunders Co., Philadelphia, 1974.

Gardner, L. I.: Endocrine and Genetic Diseases of Childhood, 2nd ed. W. B. Saunders Co., Philadelphia, 1975.

Garrod, A. E.: Inborn errors of metabolism (Croonian Lectures). Lancet, 2:1, 73, 142, 214, 1908.

Harris, H.: The Principles of Human Biochemical Genetics, 2nd ed. American Elsevier Publishing Co., Inc., New York, 1975.

Nyhan, W. L. (ed.): Heritable Disorders of Amino Acid Metabolism. John Wiley and Sons, Inc., New York, 1974.

Stanbury, J. B., Wyngaarden, J. B., and Fredrickson, D. S. (eds.): The Metabolic Basis of Inherited Disease, 3rd ed. McGraw-Hill Book Co., New York, 1972.

Membrane Transport

Bolis, L., Hoffman, J. F., and Leaf, A.: Membranes and Disease. Raven Press, New York, 1976.

Christensen, H. N.: Biological Transport. 2nd ed. W. A. Benjamin, Reading, Mass., 1975.

Crane, R. K.: Intestinal absorption of sugars. Physiol. Rev., 40:789, 1960.

Crawhall, J. C., Scowen, E. F., and Watts, R. W.: Further observations on use of D-penicillamine in cystinuria. Br. Med. J., 1:1411, 1964.

Dent, C. E., and Rose, G. A.: Amino acid metabolism in cystinuria. Q. J. Med., *20*:205, 1951.

Elsas, L. J., and Rosenberg, L. E.: Familial renal glycosuria: a genetic reappraisal of hexose transport by kidney and intestine. J. Clin. Invest., *48*:1845, 1969.

Elsas, L. J., Hillman, R. E., Patterson, J. H., and Rosenberg, L. E.: Renal and intestinal hexose transport in familial glucose-galactose malabsorption. J. Clin. Invest., *49*:576, 1970.

Elsas, L. J., Busse, D., and Rosenberg, L. E.: Autosomal recessive inheritance of renal glycosuria. Metabolism, *20*:968, 1971.

Evanson, J. M., and Stanbury, S. W.: Congenital chloridorrhea or so-called congenital alkalosis in diarrhea. Gut, *6*:29, 1965.

Goldberg, L. S., and Fudenberg, H. H.: Familial selective malabsorption of vitamin B_{12}. Re-evaluation of an in vivo intrinsic-factor inhibitor. N. Engl. J. Med., *279*:405, 1968.

Harris, H., Mittwoch, U., Robson, E. B., and Warren, F. L.: Phenotypes and genotypes in cystinuria. Ann. Hum. Genet., *20*:57, 1955.

Jacob, H. S., and Jandl, J. H.: Increased cell membrane permeability in the pathogenesis of hereditary spherocytosis. J. Clin. Invest., *43*:1704, 1964.

Milne, M. D., Crawford, M. A., Girao, C. B., and Loughridge, L. W.: The metabolic disorder in Hartnup disease. Q. J. Med., *29*:407, 1960.

Pardee, A. B.: Crystallization of a sulfate-binding protein (permease) from Salmonella typhimurium. Science, *156*:1627, 1967.

Rosenberg, L. E., Downing, S., Durant, J. L., and Segal, S.: Cystinuria: biochemical evidence for three genetically distinct diseases. J. Clin. Invest., *45*:365, 1966.

Rosenberg, L. E.: Genetic Heterogeneity in Cystinuria. *In* Nyhan, W. L. (ed.): Amino-Acid Metabolism and Genetic Variations. McGraw-Hill Book Co., Inc., New York, 1968.

Schoen, E. J., and Reynolds, J. B.: Severe familial hypophosphatemic rickets. Normal growth following early treatment. Amer. J. Dis. Child., *120*:58, 1970.

Scriver, C. R., and Hechtman, P.: Human Genetics of Membrane Transport with Emphasis on Amino Acids. *In* Harris, H., and Hirschhorn, K. (eds.): Advances in Human Genetics, Plenum Press, New York, 1970, pp. 211–274.

Winters, R. W., Graham, J. B., Williams, T. F., McFalls, V. W., and Burnett, C. H.: A genetic study of familial hypophosphatemia and vitamin D resistant rickets with a review of the literature. Medicine, *37*:97, 1958.

Major Metabolic Pathways

Biglieri, E. G., Herron, M. A., and Brust, N.: 17-hydroxylation deficiency in man. J. Clin. Invest., *45*:1946, 1966.

Bongiovanni, A. M.: The adrenogenital syndrome with deficiency of 3 beta-hydroxysteroid dehydrogenase. J. Clin. Invest., *41*:2086, 1962.

Bowden, J. A., and Connelly, J. L.: Branched chain alpha-ketoacid metabolism. II. Evidence for the common identity of alpha-ketoisocaproic acid and alpha-keto-beta-methylvaleric acid dehydrogenases. J. Biol. Chem., *243*:3526, 1968.

Brown, M. S., Anderson, R. G. W., and Goldstein, J. L.: Mutations affecting the binding, internalization, and lysozomal hydrolysis of low density lipoprotein in cultured human fibroblasts, lymphocytes and aortic smooth muscle cells. J. Supramol. Struct., *6*:85, 1977.

Childs, B., Grumbach, M. M., and Van Wyk, J. J.: Virilizing adrenal hyperplasia: a genetic and hormonal study. J. Clin. Invest., *35*:213, 1956

Dancis, J., Hutzler, J., and Rokkones, T.: Intermittent branched-chain ketonuria, variant of maple-sugar-urine disease. N. Engl. J. Med., *276*:84, 1967.

Dancis, J., Hutzler, J., and Cox, R. P.: Enzyme defect in skin fibroblasts in intermittent branched-chain ketonuria and in maple syrup urine disease. Biochem. Med., *2*:407, 1969.

Fitzpatrick, T. B., Seiji, M., and McGugan, A. D.: Melanin pigmentation. N. Engl. J. Med., *265*:328, 374, and 430, 1961.

Fujimoto, W. Y., and Seegmiller, J. E.: Hypoxanthine-guanine phosphoribosyltransferase deficiency: activity in normal, mutant, and heterozygote-cultured human skin fibroblasts. Proc. Natl. Acad. Sci. (U.S.A.), *65*:577, 1970.

Gabrilove, J. L., Sharma, D. C., and Dorfman, R. I.: Adrenocortical 11 beta-hydroxylase deficiency and virilism first manifest in the adult woman. N. Engl. J. Med., *272*:1189, 1965.

Goldstein, J. L., and Brown, M. S.: Familial hypercholesterolemia: a genetic regulatory defect in cholesterol metabolism. Am. J. Med., *58*:147, 1975.

Granick, S., and Urata, G.: Increase in activity of gamma-aminolevulinic acid synthetase in liver mitochondria induced by feeding of 3,5-dicarbethoxy-1,4-dihydrocollidine. J. Biol. Chem., *238*:821, 1963.

Griffin, R. F., and Elsas, L. J.: Classic Phenylketonuria: diagnosis through heterozygote detection. J. Pediatr., *86*:512, 1975.

Hsia, D. Y.: Galactosemia. Charles C Thomas, Springfield, Ill., 1969.

Huguley, C. M., Jr., Bain, J. A., Rivers, S. L., and Scoggins, R. B.: Refractory megaloblastic anemia associated with excretion of orotic acid. Blood, *14*:615, 1959.

Kalckar, H. M., Braganca, B., and Munch-Petersen, A.: Uridyl transferases and the formation of uridine diphosphogalactose. Nature, *172*:1038, 1953.

Kinoshita, J. H., Futterman, S., Satoh, K., and Merola, L. O.: Factors affecting the formation of sugar alcohols in ocular lens. Biochem. Biophys. Acta., *74*:340, 1963.

Koch, J., Stokstad, E. L., Williams, H. E., and Smith, L. H.: Deficiency of 2-oxo-glutarate: glyoxylate carboligase activity in primary hyperoxaluria. Proc. Natl. Acad. Sci. (U.S.A.), *57*:1123, 1967.

LaDu, B. N., Zannoni, V. G., Laster, L., and Seegmiller, J. E.: The nature of the defect in tyrosine metabolism in alcaptonuria. J. Biol. Chem., *230*:251, 1958.

Marver, H. S., and Schmid, R.: The Porphyrias. *In* Stanbury, J. B., Wyngaarden, J. B., and Frederickson, D. S. (eds.): The Metabolic Basis of Inherited Disease. McGraw-Hill Book Co., Inc., New York, 1970.

Menkes, J. H., Hurst, P. L., and Craig, J. M.: New syndrome: progressive infantile cerebral dysfunction associated with an unusual urinary substance. Pediatrics, *14*:462, 1954.

Menkes, J. H.: Maple syrup disease: investigations into the metabolic defect. Neurology, *9*:826, 1959.

Meyer, U. A., and Marver, H. S.: Intermittent acute porphyria: clinical demonstration of a genetic defect in porphobilinogen metabolism. Clin. Res., *19*:398, 1971.

Meyer, U. A., and Schmid, R.: Intermittent acute porphyria: the enzymatic defect in brain dysfunction in metabolic disorders, F. Plum (ed.). Research Publication, Assoc. Nerv. Ment. Dis., *53*:211, 1974.

Motulsky, A. G.: Current concepts in genetics: the genetic hyperlipidemias. N. Engl. J. Med., *294*:823, 1976.

O'Brien, W. M., LaDu, B. N., and Bunim, J. J.: Biochemical, pathologic and clinical aspects of alcaptonuria, ochronosis and ochronotic arthropathy. Review of world literature (1584–1962). Am. J. Med., *34*:813, 1963.

Rosenbloom, F. M., Henderson, J. F., Caldwell, I. C., Kelley, W. N., and Seegmiller, J. E.: Biochemical bases of accelerated purine biosynthesis de novo in human fibroblasts lacking hypoxanthine-guanine phosphoribosyl-transferase. J. Biol. Chem., *243*:1166, 1968.

Schulman, J. D., Lustberg, T. J., Kennedy, J. L., Museles, M., and Seegmiller, J. E.: A new variant of maple syrup urine disease (branched-chain ketoaciduria): clinical and biochemical evaluation. Am. J. Med., *49*:118, 1970.

Seiji, M., Fitzpatrick, T. B., Simpson, R. T., and Birbeck, M. S.: Chemical composition and terminology of specialized organelles (melanosomes and melanin granules) in mammalian melanocytes. Nature, *197*:1082, 1963.

Silberberg, D. H.: Maple syrup urine disease metabolite

studies in cerebellum cultures. J. Neurochem., *16*:1141, 1969.

Stanbury, J. B., and DeGroot, L. J.: The clinical chemistry and pathologic physiology of thyroid tissue. Clin. Chem., *13*:542, 1967.

Tschudy, D. P., Perlroth, M. G., Marver, H. S., Collins, A., Hunter, G., Jr., and Rechcigl, M., Jr.: Acute intermittent porphyria: the first "over-production disease" localized to a specific enzyme. Proc. Natl. Acad. Sci. (U.S.A.), *53*:841, 1965.

Visser, H. K., and Cost, W. S.: A new hereditary defect in the biosynthesis of aldosterone: urinary C_{21}-corticosteroid pattern in three related patients with a salt-losing syndrome, suggesting an 18-oxidation defect. Acta Endocrinol., *47*:589, 1964.

Waisman, H. A.: Induced Phenylketonuria in Experimental Animals — Opportunities and Limitations. *In* Anderson, J. A., and Swaiman, K. F. (eds.): Phenylketonuria and Allied Metabolic Diseases. U.S. Dept. of Health, Education and Welfare, Children's Bureau, Washington, 1967, pp. 21–31.

Waldenström, J., and Haeger-Aronsen, B.: The porphyrias: a genetic problem. Progr. Med. Gen., *5*:58, 1967.

Welland, F. H., Hellman, E. S., Gaddis, E. M., Collins, A., Hunter, G. W., Jr., and Tschudy, D. P.: Factors affecting the excretion of porphyrin precursors by patients with acute intermittent porphyria. I. The effect of diet. Metabolism, *13*:232, 1964.

Williams, H. E., and Smith, L. J., Jr.: L-glyceric aciduria. A new genetic variant of primary hyperoxaluria. N. Engl. J. Med., *278*:233, 1968.

Circulating Proteins

Beck, E. A., Charache, P., and Jackson, D. P.: A new inherited coagulation disorder caused by an abnormal fibrinogen (fibrinogen Baltimore). Nature, *208*:143, 1965.

Elsas, L. J., Hayslett, J. P., Spargo, B. H., Durant, J. L., and Rosenberg, L. E.: Wilson's disease with reversible renal tubular dysfunction. Ann. Intern. Med., *75*:427, 1971.

Fagerhol, M. K., and Laurell, C.-B.: The Pi system: inherited variants of serum alpha₁-antitrypsin. *In* Steinberg, A. G., and Bearn, A. G. (eds.) Progress in Medical Genetics, 7th ed., Grune & Stratton, New York, 1970.

Forman, W. B., Ratnoff, O. D., and Boyer, M. H.: An inherited qualitative abnormality in plasma fibrinogen: fibrinogen Cleveland. J. Lab. Clin. Med., *72*:455, 1968.

Harris, H.: Genes and isozymes. Proc. Roy. Soc. Lond., *174*:1, 1969.

Heilmeyer, L., Keller, W., Vivell, O., Keiderling, W., Betke, K., Wohler, F., and Schultze, H. E.: Congenital transferrin deficiency in a seven-year old girl. German Med. Monthly, *6*:385, 1961.

Holtzman, N. A., Naughton, M. A., Iber, F. L., and Gaumnitz, B. M.: Ceruloplasmin in Wilson's disease. J. Clin. Invest., *46*:993, 1967.

Iterschhorn, R.: Adenosine deaminase deficiency and immunodeficiencies. Fed. Proc., *36*:2166, 1977.

Levy, R. I., Fredrickson, D. S., and Laster, L.: The lipoproteins and lipid transport in a-beta-lipoproteinemia. J. Clin. Invest., *45*:531, 1966.

Mammen, E. F., Prasad, A. S., Barnhart, M. I., and Au, C. C.: Congenital dysfibrinogenemia: fibrinogen Detroit. J. Clin. Invest., *48*:235, 1969.

Prichard, R. W., and Vann, R. L.: Congenital afibrinogenemia: report on a child without fibrinogen and review of the literature. Am. J. Dis. Child., *88*:703, 1954.

Rapaport, S. I., Patch, M. J., and Moore, F. J.: Antihemophilic globulin levels in carriers of hemophilia. Am. J. Clin. Invest., *39*:1619, 1960.

Ratnoff, O. D., and Bennett, B.: The genetics of hereditary disorders of blood coagulation. Science, *179*:1291, 1973.

Robertson, J. H., and Trueman, R. G.: Combined hemophilia and Christmas disease. Blood, *24*:281, 1964.

Stites, D. P., Hershgold, E. J., Perlman, J. D., and Fudenberg, H. H.: Factor VIII detection by hemagglutination inhibition: hemophilia A and Von Willebrand's Disease. Science, *171*:196, 1971.

Coenzyme Function

Danner, D. J., Lemmon, S. K., and Elsas, L. J.: Substrate specificity and stabilization by thiamine pyrophosphate of rat liver branched chain α-ketoacid dehydrogenase. Biochem. Med., *19*:27, 1978.

Danner, D. J., Wheeler, F. B., Lemmon, S. K., and Elsas, L. J.: In vivo and in vitro response of human branched chain α-ketoacid dehydrogenase to thiamine and thiamine pyrophosphate. Pediatr. Res., *12*:235, 1978.

Elsas, L. J., and Danner, D. J.: Effect of Thiamine on Normal and Mutant Human Branched Chain Alpha-Ketoacid Dehydrogenase. *In* Gubler, L. J., Fujiwara, M., and Dreyfus, P. (eds.) Thiamine. John Wiley and Sons, New York, 1974, pp. 335–353.

Elsas, L. J., Pask, B. A., Wheeler, F. B., Perl, D. P., and Trusler, S.: Cofactor resistant maple syrup urine disease. Metabolism, *21*:929, 1972.

Erbe, R. W.: Inborn errors of folate metabolism. N. Engl. J. Med., *293*:753, 807, 1975.

Frimpter, G. W.: Cystathioninuria: nature of the defect. Science, *149*:1095, 1965.

Frimpter, G. W.: Cystathioninuria. *In* Nyhan, W. L. (ed.): Amino Acid Metabolism and Genetic Variation. New York, McGraw-Hill Book Co., 1967, pp. 315–323.

Haggard, M. E., and Lockhardt, L. H.: Megaloblastic anemia and orotic aciduria. A hereditary disorder of pyrimidine metabolism responsive to uridine. Am. J. Dis. Child., *113*:733, 1967.

Longhi, R. L., Fleisher, L. D., Tallan, H. H., and Gaull, G. E.: Cystathioninine beta-synthase deficiency: A qualitative abnormality of the deficient enzyme modified by Vitamin B₆ therapy. Pediatr. Res., *11*:100, 1977.

Mahoney, M. J., and Rosenberg, L. E.: Inherited defects of B₁₂ metabolism. Am. J. Med., *48*:584, 1970.

Morrow, G., and Barness, L. A.: Combined vitamin responsiveness in homocystinuria. J. Pediatr., *81*:946, 1972.

Rosenberg, L. E.: Vitamin Responsive Inherited Diseases Affecting the Nervous System. *In* Plum, F. (ed.): Brain Dysfunction in Metabolic Disorders. Raven Press, New York, 1974.

Rosenberg, L. E.: Inherited amino-acidopathies demonstrating vitamin dependency. N. Engl. J. Med., *281*:145, 1969.

Scriver, C. R.: Vitamin responsive inborn errors of metabolism. Metabolism, *22*:1319, 1973.

Scriver, C. R., Clow, C. L., MacKenzie, S., and Delvin, E.: Thiamine-responsive maple syrup urine disease. Lancet, *1*:310, 1971.

Pharmacogenetics

Bell, J. C., and Riemensnider, D. K.: Use of serum microbiologic assay technique for estimating patterns of isoniazid metabolism. Am. Rev. Tuberc., *75*:995, 1957.

Evans, D. A., Manley, K. A., and McKusick, V. A.: Genetic control of isoniazid metabolism in man. Br. Med. J., *2*:485, 1960.

Harris, H., Robson, E. B., Glenn-Bott, A. M., and Thornton, J. A.: Evidence for non-allelism between genes affecting human serum cholinesterase. Nature, *200*:1185, 1963.

Hockwald, R. S., Arnold, J., Clayman, C. B., and Alving, A. S.: Status of primaquine: toxicity of primaquinine in Negroes: report to Council on Pharmacy and Chemistry. J.A.M.A., *149*:1568, 1952.

Jenne, J. W.: Partial purification and properties of the isoniazid transacetylase in human liver. Its relationship to the acetylation of P-aminosalicylic acid. J. Clin. Invest., *44*:1992, 1965.

Kirkman, H. N.: Glucose-6 phosphate dehydrogenase variants and drug-induced hemolysis. Ann. N.Y. Acad. Sci., *151*:753, 1968.

Structural Proteins

Elsas, L. J., Miller, R. L., and Pinnell, S. R.: Inherited human collagen lysyl hydroxylase deficiency: ascorbic acid response. J. Pediatr., *92*:378, 1978.

Jacob, H. S., Ruby, A., Overland, E. S., and Mazia, D.: Abnormal membrane protein of red blood cells in hereditary spherocytosis. J. Clin. Invest., *50*:1800, 1977.

McKusick, V. A.: Heritable Disorders of Connective Tissue, 4th ed. C. V. Mosby Co., St. Louis, 1972.

Miller, M. J., and Matukas, V. J.: Biosynthesis of collagen. Fed. Proc., *33*:1197–1204, 1974.

Pinnell, S. R., Krane, S. M., Kenzora, J. E., and Glimcher, M. J.: A heritable disorder of connective tissue. Hydroxylysine-deficient collagen disease. N. Engl. J. Med., *286*:1013, 1972.

MANAGEMENT OF INHERITED DISEASE

Acosta, P. B., and Elsas, L. J.: Dietary Management of Inherited Metabolic Disease: Phenylketonuria, Galactosemia, Tyrosinemia, Homocystinuria, Maple Syrup Urine Disease. ACELMU Publishers, 1350 Carolyn Drive, Atlanta, Georgia, 1976.

Boyer, S. H., Siggers, D. C., and Krueger, L. J.: Caveat to protein replacement therapy for genetic disease: immunological implications of accurate molecular diagnosis. Lancet, Sept. 23, 1973, p. 654.

Brady, R. O., Gal, A. E., and Pentcher, P. G.: Evolution of enzyme replacement therapy for lipid storage disease. Life Sci., *15*:1235, 1974.

Brock, D. J. H.: Biochemical and cytological methods in the diagnosis of neural tube defects. Progr. Med. Genet., *II*:1, 1977.

Cerami, A., and Manning, J. M.: Potassium cyanate as an inhibitor of the sickling of erythrocytes in vitro. Proc. Natl. Acad. Sci., *68*:1180, 1971.

Childs, B., and Simopoulous, A. P. (Chairpersons): Genetic Screening Programs, Principles, and Research. Assembly of Life Sciences, National Research Council, Washington, D.C., 1975.

Elsas, L. J., Priest, J. H., Wheeler, F. B., Danner, D. J., and Pask, B. A.: Maple Syrup Urine Disease; Coenzyme function and prenatal monitoring. Metabolism, *23*:569, 1974.

Fagerhol, M. K.: Quantitative studies on the inherited variants of serum alpha₁-antitrypsin. Scand. J. Clin. Lab. Invest., *23*:97, 1971.

Fagerhol, M. K.: The serum alpha₁-antitrypsin polymorphism. Abstract in symposium delivered at the 4th International Congress of Human Genetics, Paris. Excerpta Medica: International Congress Series, No. 233, p. 3, Amsterdam, 1971.

Fratantoni, J. C., Neufeld, E. F., Uhlendorf, B. W., and Jacobson, C. B.: Intrauterine diagnosis of the Hurler and Hunter syndromes. N. Engl. J. Med., *280*:686, 1969.

Gillette, P. N., Petersen, C. M., Lu, Y. S., and Cerami, A.: Sodium cyanate as a potential treatment for sickle-cell disease. N. Engl. J. Med., *290*:654, 1974.

Howell, R. R.: Genetic disease: the present status of treatment. Hosp. Pract., *7*:75, 1972.

Hug, G., and Schubert, W. K.: Lysosomes in type II glycogenosis. Changes during administration of extract from Aspergillus niger. J. Cell Biol., *35*:C1, 1967.

Huntley, C. C., and Stevenson, R. E.: Maternal phenylketonuria. Course of two pregnancies. Obstet. Gynec., *34*:694, 1969.

Kerr, G. R., Chamove, A. S., Harlow, H. F., and Waisman, H. A.: "Fetal PKU": the effect of maternal hyperphenylalaninemia during pregnancy in the rhesus monkey (*Macaca mulatta*). Pediatrics, *42*:27, 1968.

Kraus, L. M., and Kraus, A. P.: Carbamyl phosphate mediated inhibition of the sickling of erythrocytes in vitro. Biochem. Biophys. Res. Comm., *44*:1381, 1971.

Lauer, R. M., Mascarinas, T., Racela, A. S., and Diehl, A. M.: Administration of a mixture of fungal glucosidases to a patient with type II glycogenosis (Pompe's disease). Pediatrics, *42*:672, 1968.

Lubs, H. A., and Lubs, M. L.: Genetic Disorders. *In* Burrow, G. N., and Ferris, T. S. (eds.): Complications During Pregnancy. W. B. Saunders, Co., Philadelphia, 1975.

Marion, J. P., Danner, D. J., Ballou, W. R., Marion, R., and Elsas, L. J.: Testing for the Tay-Sachs gene in the Atlanta Jewish population. South. Med. J., *70*:833, 1977.

Merril, C. R., Geier, M. R., and Petricciani, J. C.: Bacterial virus gene expression in human cells. Nature, *233*:398, 1971.

Milunsky, A., Littlefield, J. W., Kanfer, J. N., Kolodny, E. H., Shih, V. E., and Atkins, L.: Prenatal genetic diagnosis (three parts). N. Engl. J. Med., *283*:1370, 1441, 1498, 1970.

Moses, S. W., Levin, S., Chayoth, R., and Steinitz, K.: Enzyme induction in a case of glycogen storage disease. Pediatrics, *38*:111, 1966.

Nadler, H. L., and Gerbie, A. B.: The role of amniocentesis in the intrauterine detection of genetic disorders. N. Engl. J. Med., *282*:596, 1970.

Nalbandian, R. M. (ed.): Molecular Aspects of Sickle Cell Hemoglobin. Charles C Thomas, Springfield, Ill., 1971.

Philippart, M., Franklin, S. S., Gordon, A.: Reversal of an inborn sphingolipidosis (Fabry's disease) by kidney transplantation. Ann. Int. Med., *77*:195, 1972.

Rabovsky, D.: Molecular biology: gene insertion into mammalian cells. Science, *174*:933, 1971.

Schwartz, A. G., Cook, P. R., and Harris, H.: Correction of a genetic defect in a mammalian cell. Nature (New Biol.), *230*:5, 1971.

Scriver, C. R.: Treatment of inherited disease: realized and potential. M. Clin. North Am., *53*:941, 1969.

Watson, C. J., Bossenmaier, I., Cardinal, R., and Petryka, Z. J.: Repression by hematin of porphyrin biosynthesis in congenital erythropoietic porphyria. Proc. Natl. Acad. Sci. (U.S.A.), *71*:278, 1974.

Yaffe, S. J., Levy, G., Matsuzawa, T., and Baliah, T.: Enhancement of glucuronide-conjugating capacity in a hyperbilirubinemic infant due to apparent enzyme induction by phenobarbital. N. Engl. J. Med., *275*:1461, 1966.

4

Dynamics of Immune Response, Immunocompetence, Immunodeficiency, and Tumor Immunology

Ernest S. Tucker, III
and Robert M. Nakamura

DYNAMICS OF THE IMMUNE RESPONSE AND IMMUNOCOMPETENCE

INTRODUCTION

Immunology has become the Rosetta stone of modern medicine. It has helped to explain and "demystify" many puzzling diseases. The importance of the immune response in protecting and preserving a normal state of health is well known. By contrast, the role of the immune response and immune reactions in the pathogenesis of disease is now increasingly apparent. Indeed, because of these conflicting biologic and pathologic activities, immunologic responses and reactions sometimes appear as enigmas.

Our present knowledge of the intricacy and complexity of the immune response has been growing greatly since the turn of the century. In the last decade, there have been giant steps in this accumulation of knowledge. We are rapidly approaching a point where the biochemical and cellular details of the immune response will be so well known that we will be able to "map"

an individual's potential for immune reactivity to a wide range of chemical and biologic factors. This application of knowledge will cause the enigmas to be less puzzling. We should soon be able to understand exactly how the protective aspects of the immune response become subverted to those which are damaging and destructive.

Immunology today can be likened to a large octopus with tentacles which extend into many areas of biology and medicine. At the center of the discipline there is a body of facts and observations, theories and hypotheses which can be considered as the current "dogma" of the science. In Chapters 4 and 5, this body of knowledge will be presented, emphasizing the main points and principles which have now been well confirmed and are basic to a critical understanding of immunology. There will be an occasional excursion from this centerpiece in order to highlight or emphasize a point of information and to show its application to a specific problem in the clinic or the laboratory.

Embryologists and developmental biologists have shown the evolution of adaptive systems from the simple to complex multicellular organisms. It has been observed that the phenomenon of enzyme induction in bacteria is similar to the induction of antibody in a higher organism. In the bacterium, adaptive enzyme induction occurs when there is a limitation of available substrate material for energy metabolism or other vital functions. This substrate limitation induces a genetic activation which leads to the formation of a specific group of proteins possessing enzymatic activity that will allow the bacterium to metabolize and assimilate the substrate. In the case of an antibody response, we will see later that there is also a genetic activation followed by elaboration of the specific antibody protein which reacts with the initiating antigen. In this context the immune response appears to be an adaptive response predetermined by the genetic makeup of the organism. As an adaptive mechanism, it is an important determinant of the organism's ability to survive and prosper. Without the ability to mount an immune response, an organism would readily succumb to any of a variety of lethal factors.

In higher organisms such as vertebrates, the immune response is of great complexity and diversity. However, in lower organisms, such as the primitive unicellular and multicellular forms, one does not encounter the specifically reactive cells and molecules that characterize the immune response of higher animals. At the primitive level, reaction of the organism to hazardous factors is by less specific means. Commonly the organism simply moves away to avoid a noxious agent. At other times, an offending material may phagocytosed and digested, thus inactivating its potential harmful effect. In the higher organisms, such non-specific forms of protection persist, but they are enhanced by more specific and potent humoral and cellular components of the immune response. The complexity, diversity and specificity of the immune response afford a greater margin of protection. Those reactions of higher organisms which correspond to primitive forms are due to the biochemical and cellular factors of the general inflammatory response.

The inflammatory response is notably augmented by the immune response. This augmentation occurs because of specific antibody and reactive lymphocytes which amplify host mediator systems to destroy or inactivate pathogenic factors. It provides considerable protection for the host, but, as mentioned, also can lead to damage of the host's tissues. The conditions of health operate to maintain a delicate balance between these potentially opposing forces. This interplay has been explored extensively in recent years, and we now understand many intricacies of its operation.

A MODEL OF THE IMMUNE SYSTEM

The structure and function of the immune system can best be understood by referring to a simplified model. The model which has been selected is one of a simple servomechanism. Self-regulating or homeostatic systems are characteristic of many biologic systems. They are readily understood in our modern world of cybernetics and computers which causes us to think in terms of servo-regulated systems.

The specific model we will follow is illustrated in Figure 4–1. It has the following components: an input signal; a central unit for processing the signal; an output produced by the central unit; and a feedback loop that links the output to the input signal. We can find many examples of analogous mechanical systems, such as a thermostatically-controlled central heating system or a computer-controlled machine or device. In biologic systems, examples are equally numerous, e.g., the simple neurogenic reflex arc and the control mechanisms that regulate respiratory and cardiovascular activity.

In our model, each of the immune components is identified by analogy with those of the servo-regulatory system. The stimulating antigen, immunogen, is identified as the input signal or stimulus. The lymphatic tissues and cells are designated as the central processor. Antibodies and specifically reactive T-lymphocytes are the output of the lymphatic tissues. A feedback loop is created by reactivity of the antibodies and reactive T-lymphocytes with the immunogen. The feedback effect is negative, since the result of antibody or reactive T-lymphocyte combining with immunogen is to neutralize or inactivate, thus diminishing its input to the system.

The pathway or direction followed by the input signal or immunogen to arrive at the lymphatic tissues (central processing apparatus) is called the afferent limb; the pathway of the output signal of antibody and reactive T-lymphocytes from the lymphatic tissues is designated as the efferent limb.

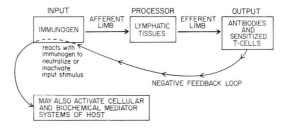

A MODEL OF THE IMMUNE SYSTEM DEPICTING
INTERRELATIONS OF THE MAJOR COMPONENTS
Figure 4–1

By frequent reference to the model throughout the coming presentations, the reader will be able to maintain a perspective for understanding the general way in which the immune system operates. Each upcoming section will provide important details about the major components of the immune system. At the conclusion, the reader should be able to arrange the information so as to see with clarity the functional interrelationships of the components.

IMMUNOGENS AND ANTIGENS

In our model, the input signal is designated as the stimulating antigen or immunogen. In earlier literature, the term "antigen" was used as an inclusive one to indicate any substance which could elicit an immune response as well as react with the antibody or lymphocytes produced. Recent studies have necessitated a redefinition of terms in order to clarify those substances that elicit an immune response. The term "immunogen" is now the one preferred to designate a substance or material that will stimulate an immune response in a sensitive and immunocompetent host animal. *Immunogen* is considered as the special class of antigens denoting those which are capable of immune stimulation. Other types of *antigen* may exhibit reactivity with antibodies or sensitized lymphocytes but do not produce a stimulatory effect.

To be considered an immunogen, an antigen must be shown to elicit an immune response in some animal. The immune response may occur either as antibody production or as proliferation of specifically reactive T-lymphocytes. It is now known that each of the different populations of cells leading to production of antibody or sensitized lymphocytes react only with specific sites on the entire immunogen. These reactive sites on the immunogen molecule are called *determinants*. As illustrated in Figure 4–2, a single im-

munogen molecule may possess many different antigenic determinants along its molecular structure. Each of these determinants possesses a specific chemical composition and physical configuration which impart a unique molecular configuration to the determinant. As will again be mentioned later, each of these different determinants reacts with a different B- or T-lymphocyte within the tissues of a responsive animal. The ability of a particular B- or T- lymphocyte to react with a specific immunogenic determinant is regulated by the genome of the animal through the production of specific recognition molecules on the surface membranes of the lymphocytes.

The names now used to denote the structure of immunogenic determinants are the terms *haptenic determinant* and *carrier determinant*. These are used to designate two general classes of such molecular configurations found along the surface of immunogens. Carrier determinants are the structural areas which occur along the integral part of the molecule and depend on the folding and arrangement of the polymeric chains that comprise the macromolecule. By contrast, haptenic determinants are chemical groupings which usually project from the integral structure of the molecule and exist as discrete and sharply defined chemical groupings, such as side chains or groups which have been chemically linked at particular points along the molecular surface. The illustrations of these determinants as shown in Figure 4–2 will aid in understanding the differences between these two types of structure. A simple analogy which also helps in understanding the differences is to think of the haptenic determinants as spines which project from a leaf of a cactus while carrier determinants are folds of the leaf itself.

It is apparent that naturally occurring immunogens and antigens possess a variety of determinants so that the total immune response to an immunogen is quite varied and diverse. Indeed, we find that there are individual and separate antibodies as well as populations of reactive T-lymphocytes formed in response to each different determinant. Stated in another way, we find in the blood of an animal who had developed an immune response that there are different populations of antibodies and sensitized T-lymphocytes, each reactive with a different individual antigenic determinant. This explains the considerable heterogeneity of the immune response to an immunogen and the great diversity and heterogeneity when comparing the immune response to similar immunogens in different animals.

Antigens that function as immunogens have certain physical-chemical characteristics. One of these is the over-all three-dimensional size and

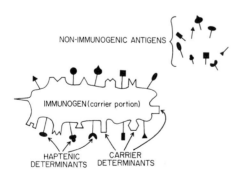

NON-IMMUNOGENIC ANTIGENS

IMMUNOGEN (carrier portion)

HAPTENIC   CARRIER
DETERMINANTS DETERMINANTS

DIAGRAM ILLUSTRATING DIFFERENCE BETWEEN
AN IMMUNOGEN AND NON-IMMUNOGENIC ANTIGENS

Figure 4–2

shape of the molecule, which is best expressed in terms of molecular weight. In general, macromolecules of small size—that is, with molecular weights less than 6000 daltons—usually do not behave as immunogens. Those ranging in size from 6000 to 30,000 daltons are often poor immunogens and require the use of adjuvants. Larger macromolecules, especially those above the molecular weight range of >35,000 to 40,000 daltons, are usually good immunogens.

The chemical structure of the molecule is also important; e.g., non-polar lipid molecules are poor immunogens compared to those with molecular polarity. The route of administration affects the degree of response to a particular immunogen. An immunogen that is administered and then becomes sequestered or trapped does not have access to lymphocytes; consequently it will not stimulate a response. Selection of the responding animal is also important because genetic factors determine the responses different animals give to the same immunogen. Instances frequently occur where a given animal or species is unresponsive to a particular immunogen while another may produce a marked response. Some molecules can be made immunogenic by being chemically linked or coupled to a larger macromolecule. In such instances, the coupled chemical becomes the haptenic determinant and the substrate macromolecule provides the carrier determinants.

Another consideration in establishing whether a substance is an immunogen is if it can cause the crosslinking of specific receptors on lymphocyte membrane surfaces at the time of initial recognition contact. As we will note again in a later section, such crosslinking activates enzyme systems in the cell, leading to blast transformation and subsequent cell multiplication. Some immunogens have similar repeating haptenic determinants that are closely spaced and produce crosslinking on direct contact with the recognition lymphocyte. However, most immunogens require a type of modification, called *processing*, before they are able to react effectively with the receptors on lymphocytes. This processing occurs within monocytes and histiocytes. The sequence of events in processing (Fig. 4–3) begins with phagocytosis of the antigen, followed by intracellular breakdown of the immunogenic molecule into smaller antigenic determinants which are then coupled with a material from the cell similar to ribonucleic acid (RNA). The processed antigen then moves to the cell surface, where contact with recognition lymphocytes occurs. Processed antigen is thus put in a form that is reactive with the lymphocyte receptors. Contact with the receptors causes the activation sequence leading to lymphocyte proliferation and differentiation.

The reaction of recognition lymphocytes with the processed antigen is now known to be more complex than a simple one-to-one stoichiometric relationship between antigen and responding lymphocyte. In the past few years it has been discovered that there are populations of lymphocytes that provide a helper function to augment production of antibody or sensitized lymphcytes and others that exhibit a suppressor effect. It has been found that these helper and suppressor cells arise from sub-populations of T-lymphocytes and are relatively specific in their reactivity with individual immunogens. More recently, these helper and suppressor cells have been found to secrete soluble factors of molecular size around 50,000 daltons which appear to be the active substances that evolve either a helper or suppressor effect depending on the cell of origin. These cells will be discussed later; they are mentioned here in order to emphasize the complexity of immunogen initiation of the immune response.

The investigative studies that have shown the action of helper and suppressor cells have

Figure 4–3

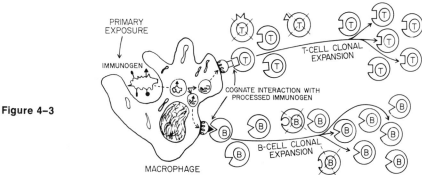

SCHEMATIC ILLUSTRATION OF EVENTS IN THE PRIMARY IMMUNE RESPONSE SHOWING STIMULATION OF VIRGIN T AND B LYMPHOCYTES BY REACTION WITH PROCESSED IMMUNOGEN

also demonstrated that, in general, B-cells recognize and react with haptenic determinants of an immunogen while T-cells preferentially react with the carrier determinants (see Fig. 4–6). Experiments with immunogens of varied haptenic and carrier determinants have also shown that in many instances where T- or B-cell reaction occurs with a haptenic determinant, the subsequent differentiation to a plasma cell with production of antibody or differentiation of specifically reactive T-lymphocytes *does not occur in the absence* of a concomitant helper T-cell reaction with the carrier determinants.

DEVELOPMENT AND MATURATION OF LYMPHOCYTIC TISSUES

The immune response of an animal to an immunogen depends on normally developed and functioning lymphocytic cells which possess the genetically determined receptors for reacting with the particular immunogen. Thus, normal immune functions (immunocompetence and immunoresponsiveness) depend on the full development and maturation of lymphocytic tissues. Investigations in experimental embryology have shown that the earliest appearance of specific cells destined to become the mature lymphocytic tissues occurs during the first trimester in the primitive yolk sac. Later, during the second and third trimesters, these primitive cells are found in the fetal liver and spleen. Finally, they accumulate in the marrow of the long bones. These are primitive stem cells that not only give rise to immature lymphocytes but also produce other important cell lines of the blood, including the erythrocytic, myelocytic, and megakaryocytic cell types (Fig. 4–4). The production of primitive lymphocytes from these stem cell foci appears to occur as the re-

sult of certain stimuli of normal differentiation and development which have not yet been identified nor their specific mode of action defined. These primitive lymphocytes then undergo further differentiation which causes them to segregate into two major types. One type has a high affinity for localization in the thymus. After release from the marrow foci of primitive stem cells, they enter the circulation and "home" to the thymus through a mechanism of specific attraction not yet fully understood. These cells are designated as "primitive" or "immature" T lymphocytes because of this affinity for thymic localization.

Another type of immature lymphocyte moves from the stem cell foci to other areas in the bone marrow in humans and many other vertebrates. In the chicken, these cells localize preferentially in a structure of the hind gut known as the bursa of Fabricius. These immature lymphocytes are referred to as "B-cells" or bursal-equivalent cells because of their tendency to localize in the bone marrow foci in the human and other vertebrates or the bursal structure in chickens.

The immature T- and B-lymphocytes undergo a period of maturation and differentiation in the tissues where they have homed. After they become mature cells, they emerge and enter the circulation, disseminating throughout the body to populate the peripheral lymphatic tissues, which include the lymph nodes, lymphoepithelial tissues, spleen, and the recirculating pool of lymphocytes in blood and lymphatic channels (Fig. 4–4). The cell surfaces of mature T- and B-lymphocytes have specific recognition molecules which enable them to react with specific immunogens.

The majority of these T- and B-lymphocytes show a pattern of constant recirculation through the lymphatics and the peripheral

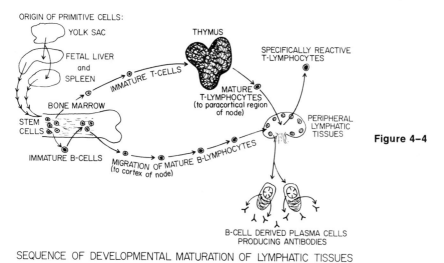

Figure 4–4

SEQUENCE OF DEVELOPMENTAL MATURATION OF LYMPHATIC TISSUES

blood so that there is a continuing change of the cell population at all times. In the lymphatics, specifically the lymph nodes and spleen, there is a preferential accumulation of the different cell types in specific anatomic areas. The B-lymphocytes accumulate in the cortical areas of lymph nodes and tend to recirculate about the cortical sinuses while T-lymphocytes predominate in the paracortical zones of lymph nodes. In the spleen, the small pencillar arteries found in the center of the lymphatic aggregates are surrounded by a cuff of cells which are predominantly T-lymphocytes. The B-lymphocytes tend to cluster eccentric to this zone and occasionally show follicle formation. The T- and B-lymphocytes in the circulating blood re-enter the lymph nodes across specialized vascular structures known as the *postcapillary venules* (Fig. 4–5). These venules possess a type of endothelial cell which exhibits a high profile and is called *high endothelium*. Postcapillary high endothelial venules predominate in the junctional zone between the cortex and paracortex of the lymph nodes. By traversing these structures, the T- and B-lymphocytes can rapidly re-enter the lymph nodes from the circulation and circulate through the sinuses of the node, exiting along the medullary sinuses into draining lymphatic channels. They then enter subsequent nodes in the chain and eventually return to the blood by way of drainage through the thoracic duct.

The second section of this chapter, which deals with immunodeficiency, will emphasize that failure of development and normal maturation of the lymphocytes at any point in the sequence can lead to a deficit of immune function. Some defects may be partial and selective, causing only minor impairment. Others may be of critical importance to survival. Defects that often lead to a lethal outcome are those associated with a significant impairment of T-lymphocyte function, either alone or in combination with a B-lymphocyte deficiency.

The events of differentiation and maturation of T-and B-lymphocytes are not as well known in the human as in some experimental animals. There is a strong presumption, however, that the sequence of events is similar. In the mouse, immature T-lymphocytes possess varied membrane receptors for different biochemical factors. These include thymic hormone receptors, beta adrenergic receptors, and others. When maturation is complete, the T-lymphocyte has lost many of these receptors and emerges with fewer receptors for biologic factors but has newly formed receptors for immunogen which develop during maturation. A similar change in membrane receptors is thought to occur in the maturation of B-lymphocytes.

Mature T- and B-lymphocytes have specific recognition molecules on their cell membranes which bind to specific immunogenic determinants. These molecules are different in T- and B-lymphocytes and differ in specificity between individual lymphocytes of either T or B type. An individual lymphocyte carries recognition molecules only for a specific individual determinant, usually one quite different from the specificity of its neighbors. This high degree of selectivity and specificity has been of great interest to geneticists because it appears to represent almost complete genetic (allelic) exclusion within each individual lymphocyte. Each lymphocyte appears to be programmed with a specific membrane receptor to respond only to certain determinant structures; the vast remainder of genetic information in each cell appears to be suppressed or excluded by mechanisms not yet understood.

Figure 4–5

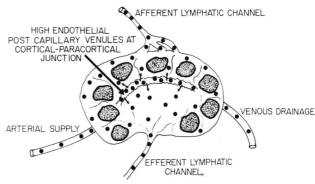

DIAGRAM OF LYMPH NODE CIRCULATION SHOWING LOCATION OF HIGH ENDOTHELIAL POST CAPILLARY VENULES WHERE LYMPHOCYTES TRANSIT DIRECTLY INTO NODE FROM BLOOD CIRCULATION

It has been established that the genes which determine the ability of an animal to respond to various immunogens are contained within the gene complex known as the *histocompatibility gene loci.* In the mouse these genes are designated as located in the H-2 region, in the human the designation of the histocompatibility loci is given by the abbreviation HLA (Human Leukocyte Antigens). In the human and the mouse there are different regions along these genetic loci which determine an individual's capacities for an immune response; these regions are specifically designated as the *immune response genes* or IR genes. Within the IR genes are specific loci which code for recognition of individual immunogenic determinants. As indicated above, only a single locus becomes expressed in the form of a membrane receptor for each individual lymphocyte of either T or B type. When the mechanisms of this selective allelic exclusion become understood, a significant advance in understanding gene function will have been made.

The identification and chemical structure of the specific receptors on membranes of T- and B-lymphocytes has attracted considerable interest. It has been clearly determined that the receptor molecules on mature B-lymphocytes are identical with the particular immunoglobulin which the cell will form after differentiating to a plasma cell. Immunoglobulins are the specific antibody products of the immune response by B-lymphocytes. Their chemistry and structure will be covered in more detail later, but it should be pointed out here that there are five major classes designated by letters of the alphabet preceded by the prefix Ig: thus, the designations IgG, IgM, IgA, IgD, and IgE. Each of the immunoglobulin classes is made by a different B-lymphocyte and each individual immunoglobulin made will vary with the stimulating immunogen.

It has been found that those B-lymphocytes which have not reached full maturity exhibit a change in the type of immunoglobulin receptor on the cell surface initially from IgM then to IgD until they reach final maturity, where the immunoglobulin receptor is identical with the type and specificity which the B-lymphocyte will secrete on stimulation. For example, a B-lymphocyte that will ultimately secrete immunoglobulin of IgG type in response to a bacterial antigen may at first be found to possess a receptor of the IgM type, which then shifts to IgD and finally to IgG. It should be emphasized, however, that at any point in this maturation sequence, should antigen contact occur, the cell will be stimulated to proliferation with secretion of the specific IgG immunoglobulin as genetically determined. There is some experimental evidence favoring the view that less mature

cells possessing IgM and IgD receptors function as latent cells in the initial primary response and as memory cells in the secondary immune response. These responses will be discussed in more detail later.

The membrane receptors on T-cells are not immunoglobulin but they do possess a similar high degree of specificity for the immunogen. As with B-cells, T-cells also exhibit a wide range of receptor specificities from cell to cell, each having different reactivity with a different immunogen. The receptors on T-lymphocytes appear to be genetically determined in the same way as the immunoglobulin receptors on B-cells. Experimental studies aimed at identification of the chemical structure of the T-cell receptor have shown the receptor to occur in close physical association with the HLA antigens on the cell surfaces. This close surface association corresponds to the close relationships of the loci within the genome. Aside from data indicating that the T-cell receptor is a glycoprotein, there is as yet no information as to its structural configuration. Presumably the amino acid sequence varies considerably in order to accommodate a wide range of cellular reactivity with different immunogenic molecules.

The membrane and intracellular biochemical events that occur following immunogen contact with the lymphocyte receptors lead to a marked change in cellular activity. In B-lymphocytes, the binding of antigen results in a phenomenon called "capping." This phenomenon results in movement of the antigen to concentrate in one area on the cell membrane. Following this, the B-cell exhibits increased synthetic metabolic activity accompanied by cellular enlargement and increase in nuclear size, a change which is described as *blast transformation.* Soon after blast transformation occurs, the cells enter the mitotic cycle and undergo division. This leads to an increase in the number of specific lymphocytes identical to the original. This proliferative increase is called *clonal expansion* (Fig. 4–3). T-cells undergo a similar increase in numbers as a consequence of immunogen stimulation.

As T- and B-lymphocytes increase in numbers following the first exposure to immunogen, some of them continue differentiation into specialized effector cells; others remain as memory cells which will respond to subsequent immunogen exposure. Some B-lymphocytes continue differentiation to form plasma cells, which manufacture and secrete antibody. T-cells, on the other hand, differentiate to form sub-classes of reactive cells. Some T-cells become either helper or suppressor cells; others become antigen reactive sensitized cells. Some of these latter cells can directly fix to antigens on tissue cells and cause death; some respond to antigen by the production of soluble factors, known as *lym-*

phokines, which promote cellular infiltrative reactions in tissue. The type of T-lymphocyte which kills on direct contact with tissue is called a *killer (K) T-lymphocyte.* These will be discussed in detail in Chapter 5.

CHARACTERISTICS OF THE IMMUNE RESPONSE

Attention is now directed to the sequence of events which comprise the steps in the immune response from initial immunogen exposure to production of antibody or reactive lymphocytes. It was previously emphasized that both T- and B-lymphocytes are in constant recirculation through the lymphatic tissues, lymph, and blood. Many studies have shown that the lymphocytes in the peripheral blood are approximately 80 per cent T-lymphocytes, while approximately 15 to 20 per cent are B-cells. The total number of lymphocytes circulating each day has been estimated at 10 to 12 times the number found in the blood at any given time. T-lymphocytes also circulate through the extravascular interstitial tissue of organs such as skin, kidney, ovary, uterus, testis, and others; B-lymphocytes do not. As mentioned earlier both T- and B- lymphocytes re-enter lymph nodes directly from the blood by way of the high endothelial postcapillary venules near the junction of cortex and paracortex in the lymph node (see Fig. 4–5).

Immunogen exposure may occur in a variety of ways. It can result from ingestion and absorption across the gastrointestinal tract, from inhalation and absorption along the mucosa of the respiratory tract, as a result of infection, or as a consequence of direct inoculation by injection or a penetrating wound. Some antigens may be absorbed directly across the skin barrier. Following entry of antigen into the tissues or circulation, non-specific inflammatory and cellular reactions occur, leading to clearance, degradation. or sequestration of the antigens in the tissues. Phagocytic cells, especially polymorphonuclear lymphocytes, tissue macrophages, and cells of the reticuloendothelial system, are the main participants in this phagocytic encounter with immunogen. The majority of antigens may be effectively eliminated by this first encounter. It is during this reaction that the antigen becomes "processed," as was discussed previously (Fig. 4–3).

The processed antigen is released to the surface of the phagocyte (macrophage), where contact with recognition lymphocytes occurs (Fig. 4–3). Some processed antigen is also released into the circulation and may randomly contact and interact with specific recognition lymphocytes either in the circulation or in the lymphatic tissues. Lymphocytes that react on this first exposure to immunogen follow the proliferative sequence of events already described and may differentiate further to give rise to a limited amount of antibody production, formation of specifically reactive T-cells, or formation of abundant memory cells. The responding cell may be either T or B type or both, depending on the immunogen characteristics and recognition by virgin lymphocytes. The antibody response from the first encounter is mainly of the IgM class and is formed in much smaller quantity than that produced following subsequent immunogen exposure. This initial antibody production does not appear to depend on T-helper cells. There is evidence that it is of IgM type because those receptors on recognition lymphocytes are more easily crosslinked by direct contact with small antigenic determinants and do not require facilitation by helper T-cells.

All the events that occur on the first encounter with antigen are described together as the *primary immune response.*It usually requires a period of four to seven days to become fully developed following antigen exposure. The actual tissue sites of the cellular reaction are determined by the point of antigen contact. T-cells traversing the tissues may encounter either native or processed immunogens at their site of entry; B-lymphocytes and other T-lymphocytes encounter antigen in regional lymph nodes after drainage from the site of entry. This contact in the local lymph nodes leads to cellular reactivity and proliferation. The sequence of changes observed in such a stimulated lymph node reflect those cellular events of proliferation and differentiation. In the early phase, the lymph node appears hypercellular and exhibits a change which has been called sinus plugging. All the sinuses within the paracortical region initially appear engorged with cells, followed by engorgement of the cortical zone and the medullary sinuses. Later, as the cell engorgement declines in the paracortex, hyperplasia of follicles appears in the cortical area. Cells in the paracortex during this engorgement are quite large and deeply basophilic, with prominent large nuclei characteristic of the blast transformation preceding the proliferative increase in cells. At this time, the lymph node becomes grossly enlarged and may become tender because of pressure and stretching on the surrounding tissues. After five to seven days, plasma cells can be found in the medullary sinuses accompanied by immature cells which appear to be blast forms of plasma cells. Increases in antibody concentration can be detected in the draining lymph as well as in the peripheral circulation. The plasma cells do not leave the node but remain in the sinuses and secrete antibody into the lymph fluid leaving the node. In the spleen, similar cellular responses occur in the malpighian follicles, where the lymphocytes are arranged in clusters. The increase in lymphocytes may, in addition to the activation and enlargement of the histiocytes along splenic sinusoids, cause splenic enlargement. Such enlargement is commonly encountered when there is massive intravascular antigenic exposure, as occurs with sepsis.

After the first encounter and response to immunogen, an individual is said to be sensitized and possesses a certain level of specific antibody to the initiating immunogen as well as a certain population of reactive T-lymphocytes. There are also increased numbers of recognition lymphocytes of either T or B type or both, depending on the nature of the primary reaction. The individual is thus in a condition of heightened responsiveness and will have increased reactivity on subsequent exposure to the same or similar immunogen. The over-all effect of the first exposure is to increase the numbers of specific recognition lymphocytes, thereby increasing the potential level of immune response even to a small dose of the immunogen encountered at a later time.

The *secondary immune response* occurs in a sensitized individual. It has also been called the anamnestic response, a term derived from the Greek word meaning to recall or recollect. In the secondary response, the biochemical and cellular events parallel those of the primary response but occur faster and in much greater quantity. There are also some qualitative differences, however, as regards the classes of antibody formed. In the secondary response, IgG is the major class of antibody, whereas in the primary response IgM predominated. Also, the important role of helper and suppressor cells in the regulation of the secondary immune response is becoming understood. In experimental studies, it has been shown that some animals who fail to respond to a particular immunogen do so because of the effects of suppressor cells. In other instances, it has been shown that failure of response is due to lack of a helper T-cell effect. The studies demonstrating these points have also shown that T-cells principally react with the carrier determinants of an antigen, whereas B-cells react with the haptenic (Fig. 4–6). In animals sensitized to the haptenic

determinants but not to the carrier determinants, an effective secondary immune response failed to develop. It has been further shown that the carrier effect could be substituted by a phenomenon called the *allogeneic effect*. These studies were done by cell transfer experiments of lymphocytes from an allogeneic donor strain to the sensitized animal. The allogeneic cells appear to exhibit an augmentation of B-cell response similar to that of the carrier-specific T-helper cells.

The cellular and tissue changes of the secondary response are similar to those of the primary, but even greater cellular proliferation and engorgement of lymph nodes with marked hyperplastic activity in follicles of the cortex is found. The medullary sinuses of the nodes become engorged with large blast cells as well as abundant plasma cells synthesizing and secreting antibody. Because of the marked cellularity, lymph nodes become enlarged and tender.

The secondary immune response is also reflected in the increase of peripheral lymphocyte count and specific antibody in the circulation. These are the products of the immune response, and their measurement can provide pertinent clinical information regarding the immunocompetence and immunoresponsivness of an individual. The ability to produce a substantial secondary immune response indicates immunocompetence and normal functioning of the entire immune system since both T- and B-lymphocytes participate in that response.

IMMUNOGLOBULINS

Referring to the model of the immune system, note that antibody is one of the major products of the immune response. Antibodies are now called immunoglobulins. In man and other higher veterbrates, immunoglobulins are designated by an alphabetic letter according to their particular class. They were first identified among the gamma globulins in electrophoretic studies by

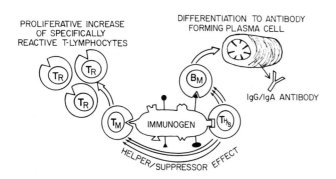

Figure 4–6

SCHEMATIC ILLUSTRATION OF EVENTS IN THE SECONDARY IMMUNE RESPONSE SHOWING DIFFERENTIAL STIMULATION OF T AND B MEMORY CELLS AND HELPER AND SUPPRESSOR T-LYMPHOCYTES

Tiselius and Kabat in the 1930s. Little was known about their molecular structure or their physical, chemical, and biologic characteristics until the work of the investigators since the 1950s. Today there is considerable information about the immunoglobulins of man and many other species.

As mentioned, in man and other higher animals there are five different classes of immunoglobulins. These have been separated according to their chemical structure and designated by the prefix Ig followed by the letter of the alphabet denoting the class, i.e., IgG, IgA, IgM, IgE, and IgD. The alphabetic class designation derives from the Greek letters assigned to the larger polypeptide chains, known as heavy or H chains, which make up part of the structure of each immunoglobulin. For example, it was determined that those molecules designated as IgG all possess H chains whose amino acid composition and antigenicity is similar and these chains are designated as gamma (γ) for IgG (μ for IgM, α for IgA, ϵ for IgE, and δ for IgD).

The basic structure of immunoglobulins is now well known, thanks to the intensive and illuminating research of the past two decades. Porter and Edelman were recently awarded the Nobel Prize for their work in the determination of the structure of immunoglobulins. The basic unit of immunoglobulin structure is epitomized by that of immunoglobulin IgG. Each molecule of IgG has been shown to contain four polypeptide chains: two identical longer chains designated as heavy or H chains and two identical shorter polypeptide chains designated as light or L chains. They are held together in a three-dimensional configuration by inter- and intrachain disulfide bonds. Each of the polypeptide chains, both heavy and light,

has been shown to exhibit a constant region and a variable region in each molecule. The constant regions of the heavy chains are the same for all molecules of a given immunoglobulin class made by a single individual (isotypes). The constant region of the light chains is the same for either of two classes of light chain molecules, designated either kappa (κ) or lambda (λ), in a given individual. The variable regions of both heavy and light chains differ among immunoglobulins in a single individual. These variable regions contribute to the structure of the antigen binding site in the antibody molecule. It appears that the variability is directly related to the specificity for antigen binding.

A schematic illustration of the structure of IgG is provided in Figure 4–7. The constant and variable regions referred to above and the general location of the interchain disulfide bonds are shown. The molecule is also divided into other major parts, shown in the diagram as the Fab portion and the Fc portion. The Fab portion contains those parts of heavy and light chains structurally arranged to form the two antigen binding sites, hence the term, *Fragment Antigen Binding (Fab)*. The Fc portion of the molecule is composed of the two segments of each heavy chain, including the interchain disulfide bond. As indicated in the diagram, the proteolytic enzyme, pepsin, will cleave the immunoglobulin molecule just above the inter-H-chain disulfide bond to yield peptide fragments from the Fc region and a divalent fragment, the F(ab')$_2$ fragment. Papain, by contrast, cleaves the molecule below that disulfide bond, yielding intact Fc fragment and univalent Fab fragments.

The Fc portion of the immunoglobulin molecule accounts for biologic activities other than antigen

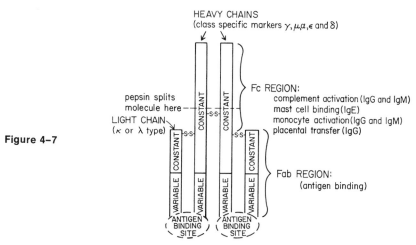

Figure 4–7

DIAGRAMMATIC ILLUSTRATION OF IgG(7S) IMMUNOGLOBULIN MOLECULE SHOWING MAJOR STRUCTURAL COMPONENTS AND REACTIVE SITES (IgA, IgE and IgD have similar structure)

binding. These include complement fixing activity (exhibited by IgM and IgG), specific transfer across the placental barrier (IgG), specific attachment to the cell membranes of basophils and mast cells (IgE), and fixation to cell membrane receptors of lymphocytes, monocytes, and macrophages (IgG). The importance of these different biologic activities will become apparent in the discussions of immunologic tissue injury in Chapter 5.

All the immunoglobulins have a basic unit of structure similar to IgG and exhibit similar physical-chemical characteristics. As noted earlier, their amino acid composition causes them to be relatively basic when compared to other serum proteins. They migrate with the gamma and slow beta globulin fractions on electrophoresis. Each basic unit possesses two sites for antigen binding and thus is considered to be bivalent. The molecular weight of the intact molecule of IgG is approximately 150,000 daltons. This results in a sedimentation coefficient of 7S in the ultracentrifuge on density gradient analysis. Each of the H chains has a molecular weight of approximately 50,000 daltons; each L chain is approximately 25,000 daltons. The immunoglobulins IgG, IgE, and IgD typically exhibit the four-chain, 7S structure, whereas IgA and IgM occur as polymers of the 7S units, thus exhibiting larger size and higher sedimentation coefficients. IgA may occur as a monomer similar to the IgG basic unit, but also occurs as a dimer and trimer with sedimentation coefficients ranging up to 13S. IgM normally occurs as a pentamer comprised of five 7S units linked together by a disulfide glycopeptide chain known as J chain. IgM has a high sedimentation coefficient of 19S. J chain also provides the link for IgA polymeric forms. The J chain is synthesized by all plasma cells, even those that do not produce polymeric forms of immunoglobulin. The polymeric forms of IgA and IgM are schematically illustrated in Figure 4–8. Because of their large size with increased numbers of antigen binding sites, they are of higher valence than the 7S molecules. Because of this, they are much more efficient in binding antigen in reactions such as agglutination and immune complex formation.

It was mentioned that immunoglobulins are produced by plasma cells which differentiate from immunogen-stimulated B-lymphocytes. The class and specificity of the immunoglobulin produced by each individual plasma cell differ according to the stimulating immunogen that selectively reacts with the immunoglobulin receptors present on the surface of the particular virgin or memory recognition B-lymphocyte. The marked degree of diversity in immunoglobulin response arises from the diverse recognition lymphocytes in a given individual. Antibodies will be produced to the many different determinants of a single

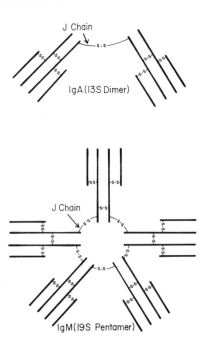

POLYMERIC STRUCTURES OF
IMMUNOGLOBULINS IgA AND IgM
Figure 4–8

immunogen, which will usually be of different classes and sub-classes as well as having differing antigen reactivities. Because of such heterogeneity there will be a wide range of antibody reactivity in a given antiserum for the different determinants. Some of the antibodies will have a high affinity and bind strongly to some of the antigen determinants; others will be of low affinity and will bind weakly. In general, larger immunogens with an abundance of heterogeneous determinants elicit an extremely heterogeneous antibody response, while a more homogeneous response occurs to immunogens of uniform composition. Indeed, a highly purified immunogen of uniform structure with determinants of identical or closely similar arrangement may produce an antibody response restricted to a single class of immunoglobulin with a limited range of reactivity. Commonly, however, most immunogens are quite heterogeneous and result in a polymorphic response.

In man and other veterbrates, the relative concentration of immunoglobulins in the circulation shows IgG to predominate, with average serum values in the human adult around a mean of 1200 mg./dl., while IgM values are around 125 mg./dl., IgA around 210 mg./dl. and IgE between 40 and 100 ng./dl. IgD is usually present in trace quantities. The finding of normal levels of serum immunoglobulins generally indicates a normal state of immunocompetence and immunoresponsivness.

The role of antibodies in the context of the model of the immune system is to neutralize or inactivate immunogen or to react and bind to antigenic molecules similar to the immunogen. Neutralization or inactivation of immunogen occurs as a result of the binding of antibodies to determinants in the antigen molecule. This binding covers critical reactive sites of the antigen and may result in biologic neutralization, or it can lead to the formation of immune complexes. Such complexes are cleared from the body by the reticuloendothelial system or may activate biochemical and cellular systems in the host which destroy the antigen. The net result is the elimination or suppression of the biologic hazard of the antigen, thus providing protection for the host.

Antigen binding is considered the primary biologic activity of antibodies. Other secondary biologic activities result from the activation of cellular and biochemical systems in the host. These secondary effects augment those of the primary. Those secondary biologic activities which were listed earlier are discussed here in further detail. Activation of the complement system is an activity exhibited by immune reactants with antibodies of the immunoglobulin classes IgM and IgG. The classic pathway of complement activation follows the formation of immune complexes in the circulation and tissues as well as formation of immune complexes along cell membranes. The effect of such activation is to yield molecules and fragments which cause chemotaxis of neutrophils into tissues, spasmogenic activity due to release of vasoactive cellular factors, immune adherence and opsonization, and instability with lysis of lipoprotein membranes of various cells and microorganisms. This array of effects produced by immune activation of the complement system is similar to that of the inflammatory response. Their protective value lies in the inactivation and destruction of hazardous biologic factors and microorganisms that may invade tissues during the course of an infection, injury, injection, or exposure. As will be discussed in the next chapter, these factors are responsible for tissue destruction in certain forms of immune injury.

The specific affinity of immunoglobulin IgE for the cell membranes of circulating basophils and tissue mast cells has now been well established. The IgE molecule binds through a structural area in the Fc portion of the molecule. This binding produces a state of sensitization of the basophil or mast cell. Subsequent exposure to antigen (allergen) which contacts the surface IgE results in loss of granules (degranulation) of those cells. Tissue reactions then occur due to the release of potent vasoactive factors from those granules. It is this sequence of events which occurs in those clinical disorders commonly called acute anaphylactic, atopic, or reaginic hypersensitivity.

Another secondary biologic activity of IgG is the ability to transfer specifically across the placental membrane. This depends on a specific structural site in the Fc portion of the molecule. IgG also fixes to membranes of lymphocytes, monocytes, and macrophages. This binding occurs through specific receptors for structural sites in the Fc portion of IgG. It appears to underlie tissue reactions ranging from phagocytosis to contact destruction of cells and foreign material. It is a mechanism for a broad range of cell recognition reactions covered in detail in Chapter 5.

SPECIFICALLY REACTIVE T-CELLS

The formation of increased numbers of T-cells specifically reactive for certain immunogens and antigens accounts for the other major output component of the immune response. The formation of such reactive cells parallels those events described in antibody production. The specifically reactive T-cells can be thought of as analogous to specific antibody. The sites for interaction (binding) with antigen are cell membrane receptors in contrast to the structural binding sites in molecules of antibody. The chemical composition and structure of such antigen binding sites in T-cells are not the same as those of immunoglobulins.

Two major classes of specifically reactive T-cells have now been described, although the pace of current investigative work suggests that others will no doubt be discovered and described in the near future. Those currently in central focus are called regulatory T-cells (helper or suppressor) and effector T-cells. The latter are distinguished by a response on contact with antigen, causing either synthesis and release of biologically active factors (lymphokines) or cell death on contact with cell-linked antigens. Regulatory T-cells function by helping or suppressing B-cells antibody response or T-cell effector response. Some of the points made earlier regarding the primary immune response should be reemphasized for T-cells. It was noted that clonal proliferation ensues following the initial interaction of immunogen and virgin recognition T-and B-lymphocytes. It was emphasized that recognition T-lymphocytes generally recognize and react with the carrier determinants of an immunogen. Clonal expansion of T-lymphocytes yields a greater number of specifically reactive cells. The individual thus has a greater capacity for response on subsequent exposure to immunogen. This is the same state of affairs observed with B-cell clonal expansion.

Regulatory activity by T-lymphocytes was initially discovered through some animal experiments already mentioned. Such regulatory T-cells in humans have been observed in in-vitro test systems, and they parallel the experimental animal findings. There is now agreement that such cells are important in the immune response in humans, although, as in the animal studies, the details of the mechanisms of regulation are not fully known. Most recently, it has been shown that there are soluble factors formed by both helper and suppressor T-cells which are specifically reactive with antigen and closely associated with histocompatibility antigens of the cell membranes. Earlier studies indicated a necessity for close proximity of the regulatory T-cells to the specifically responding effector T- or responding B-cell in order to achieve an effect, whether it was helper or suppressor. Regulatory T-cells have been observed to affect activities of both T- and B-cells, as emphasized in the illustration of Figure 4–6.

In experimental studies, the sensitivity of suppressor cells to low doses of x-irradiation and cytotoxic agents, such as cyclophosphamide, has been noted and applied in experiments on suppressor cell function. This point has not been clearly confirmed in humans, but there is strong suspicion that a similar sensitivity may exist. Also, it has been recently shown that some T-lymphocyte regulatory cells have receptors for an Fc structure of IgG and others have receptors for the Fc of IgM. Those with Fc gamma (IgG) receptors appear to have a helper function; those with Fc mu (IgM) have been associated with suppressor activity.

Effector T-cells are key participants in immunologic reactions known under such various labels as delayed hypersensitivity, cell-mediated immunity, tuberculin-type hypersensitivity, and cellular hypersensitivity. All these terms designate the sequence of events following interaction of antigen and specifically reactive T-cells which commonly lead to lymphocytic infiltrates and granuloma formation in tissues. Many experimental studies by various investigators in the past two decades have clarified the basic mechanisms of T-cell tissue reactions. There are two principal pathogenic sequences, and either may destroy the antigen or damage the tissue where the reaction occurs. One reaction sequence occurs when an effector T-lymphocyte migrating through the tissue reacts with antigen. Following contact with antigen, intense biochemical activity occurs in the cell, resulting in protein and nucleic acid synthesis and later leading to cell division. Before division, however, there is a secretory phase, with the production of numerous low molecular weight biochemical substances which are secreted into the local tissue from the cytoplasm of the activated lymphocyte(s). These substances, called *lymphokines*, have been found in both experimental and clinical studies to exhibit a wide range of biologic activities. They principally have an effect on other cells, producing activation, chemotaxis, or inhibitory changes. These effects on cells cause the succession of events of monocyte/macrophage recruitment (chemotaxis) into tissue, followed by phagocytosis

of antigen with formation and release of digestive enzymes that destroy antigen and produce tissue necrosis.

The other principal mode of T-cell effector activity is cell killing. It occurs when the reactive antigen is part of or closely linked to a cell membrane in close association with histocompatibility antigens. In this sequence the T-lymphocyte reactive with the antigen makes contact with antigen on the cell and thereby comes in close contact with the cell, inducing a biochemical effect that causes death of the antigen-bearing cell. This killing is presumed to be due to a cytotoxic factor from the T-lymphocyte. Such a cell is called a killer (K) T-cell. These K-cell reactions will be covered in more detail in Chapter 5.

IMMUNOLOGIC MEMORY

The concept of memory in the immune system implies a capacity for recall recognition of an immunogen due to previous exposure. This capacity resides in recognition lymphocytes, which arise from the clonal expansion folllowing an intial exposure to the immunogen. It is now recognized that the phenomenon of immunologic memory is a direct function of the increased numbers of recognition lymphocytes formed following the first immunogen exposure. During the primary response, the clonal proliferation of stimulated T- or B-lymphocytes produces progeny with reactivity identical to the original. This substantially increases the numbers of reactive cells in comparison to the original population. Some of the progeny continues differentiation to form plasma cells and specific antibody or form populations of effector and regulator T-lymphocytes. Most of the progeny do not undergo further differentiation but exist as copies of the original recognition lymphocytes within the tissues and circulating lymphocyte pool. Because of this increase in recognition cells, subsequent exposure to the immunogen causes a much greater response as measured by serum antibody production or numbers of specifically reactive T-lymphocytes. They appear to have developed more rapidly and in greater quantity. This rapidity, however, is more apparent than real, because the increased numbers of recognition cells react in greater numbers to form the differentiated cell types that produce antibody and reactive lymphocytes. The quantity and apparent speed of the response is a function of the sensitivity of the assay systems used to detect antibody and reactive cells. Current data do not show that the time interval between immunogen exposure and cellular response is substantially different for individual lymphocytes in either the primary or secondary immunologic responses. The phenomenon of immunologic memory thus is mainly quantitative. It provides the important condition of increased numbers of reactive cells. This augments the immune response necessary to assure host protection against the many hazardous factors we constantly contact. Primary immunization and booster stimulation in medical practice provide the needed increase in reactive cells that give a potent anamnestic host response when infection or exposure to toxins or other dangerous biologic materials occurs.

IMMUNODEFICIENCY

CLASSIFICATION OF IMMUNODEFICIENCY DISORDERS

Immunodeficiency diseases comprise an interesting group of disorders which demonstrate

TABLE 4–1 CLASSIFICATION OF PRIMARY IMMUNODEFICIENCY DISORDERS*

I. B-Cell (Antibody) Immunodeficiency Diseases
X-linked congenital hypogammaglobulinemia
X-linked immunodeficiency of IgG and IgA with hyper IgM
Common variable immunodeficiency
Selective IgA deficiency
Selective IgM deficiency
Selective deficiency of IgG subclasses

II. T-Cell (Cellular) Immunodeficiency Diseases
Congenital thymic hypoplasia
Chronic mucocutaneous candidiasis

III. Combined B-Cell and T-Cell Immunodeficiency Diseases
Severe combined immunodeficiency diseases
Cellular and antibody immunodeficiency with abnormal immunoglobulin synthesis (Nezelof's syndrome)
Wiskott-Aldrich syndrome (immunodeficiency with eczema and thrombocytopenia)
Immunodeficiency with short-limbed dwarfism
Immunodeficiency with enzyme deficiency
  (a) adenosine diaminase deficiency
  (b) nucleoside phosphorylase deficiency

IV. Phagocytic Dysfunction
Chronic granulomatous disease
Glucose-6-phosphate dehydrogenase deficiency
Myeloperoxidase deficiency
Chediak-Higashi syndrome
Job's syndrome
Tuftsin deficiency

V. Complement Abnormalities and Immunodeficiency Diseases
C1q, C1r and C1s deficiency
C2 deficiency
C3 deficiency
C5 dysfunction

*(Modified from Ammann, A. J., and Fudenberg, H. H.: Chap. 26, p. 334. Basic and Clinical Immunology. (H. H. Fudenberg, et al., Eds.). Lange Medical Publications, Los Altos, CA, 1976, p. 334).

TABLE 4–2 EXAMPLES OF SECONDARY IMMUNODEFICIENCY SYNDROMES

I. T-Cells (Cellular) Immunodeficiency
Malignant diseases such as Hodgkin's disease, chronic infections, e.g., leprosy, sarcoidosis
Aging
Intestinal lymphangiectasia (obstruction of lymph flow)

II. B-Cell (Antibody) Immunodeficiency
Lymphomas (decreased antibody synthesis)
Nephrotic syndrome (increased loss and catabolism of immunoglobulins)
Multiple myeloma, macroglobulinemia (increased abnormal and defective immunoglobulins and decreased synthesis of normal immunoglobulins and antibody)

defective function of some portion of the immune system. These diseases may be broadly categorized as either disturbances in the synthesis of various components of the immunologic system or as abnormalities of their catabolism and include the endogenous breakdown or external loss of these components. Four major aspects of the immune system are involved in the defense against various viral, bacterial, and microbial infections. These systems consist of: (1) B-cell, or antibody-mediated, immunity; (2) T-cell, or cell-mediated, immunity; (3) phagocytic mechanism; and (4) the complement system. Each of these systems can act independently or in conjunction with one or more of the others. The immunodeficiency disorders can be classified under five major categories (Table 4–1): (1) antibody, or B-cell, deficiency diseases; (2) cellular, or T-cell, immunodeficiency diseases; (3) combined B- and T-cell immunodeficiency diseases; (4) diseases with a phagocytic dysfunction; and (5) complement abnormalities and immune deficiency diseases.

The immunodeficiency diseases may be categorized into those which are *primary*, resulting from a failure of proper development of the humoral and/or cellular immune systems. Often excluded from the primary group of immunodeficiency diseases are hypercatabolic disorders and disorders of the complement system. The *secondary*, or acquired, immunodeficiency diseases may occur in patients in association with a variety of diseases and include immunodeficiency states associated with intestinal lymphangiectasia, protein-losing enteropathy, x-irradiation, immunosuppressive and cytotoxic drugs, lymphoreticular malignancies, etc. Some examples of secondary immunodeficiency syndromes are listed in Table 4–2.

PRIMARY B-CELL IMMUNODEFICIENCY DISEASES

The stem cell differentiates and gives rise to a population of precursor B-cells, which can be

TABLE 4–3   LYMPHOCYTE SURFACE MARKERS

Surface Marker	T-Cell	B-Cell
(1) Rosettes with sheep erythrocyte (E)	+	−
(2) Antithymocyte heteroantisera	+	−
(3) Easily detectable surface immunoglobulin	−	+
(4) Anti-B-cell heteroantisera	−	+
(5) Complement receptors (EAC rosettes)	−	+
(6) IgG Fc receptor		
(a) IgG coated erythrocyte rosettes	±	+
(b) Aggregated IgG	−	+

found in the marrow and spleen. The cells acquire an ability to express surface immunoglobulin. Fully mature B-cells can synthesize immunoglobulin and express it on the surface; they differentiate into cells capable of secreting antibody in response to an antigenic stimulation. The B- and T-cells are identified by certain surface markers, as listed in Table 4–3. The classic B-cell is identified by surface Ig and Fc and complement receptors. The mature, small B-lymphocyte is itself only a precursor for the plasma cells that appear on antigenic stimulation (Fig. 4–9). The deficient humoral immune system can result from the failure of these terminal stages of differentiation despite the presence of normal-appearing small B-lymphocytes.

Deficient T-helper function also can decrease and compromise the humoral response. Production of IgA, IgG, and IgE appears to require T-helper function. IgM production is less dependent on T-cell help. The development of mature T-cells is due to the precursor lymphoid cells, which mature under the influence of the thymus. Prethymic cells may migrate to the intact thymus gland and differentiate into an immunocompetent T-cell under the influence of thymic hormones. The thymus plays a definite role in the normal maturation of the T-cells.

There are four types of primary panhypogammaglobulinemia involving all classes of immunoglobulins (including IgG, IgA, IgM, IgD, and IgE) which will be discussed below:

1. Transient Hypogammaglobulinemia of Infancy

This is a relatively benign condition. Babies are born with mostly maternal gamma globulins

MATURATION OF B-CELLS

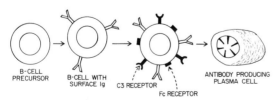

B-CELL PRECURSOR   B-CELL WITH SURFACE Ig   C3 RECEPTOR   Fc RECEPTOR   ANTIBODY PRODUCING PLASMA CELL

Figure 4–9

which have passed through the placenta. The adopted maternal gamma globulin is naturally catabolized during the first six months of life, and normally the infant's own immunoglobulin system becomes competent. Some children may have a prolonged physiologic depression of the initiation of gamma globulin synthesis which may last two or three years. The number of B-lymphocytes with surface immunoglobulin or complement receptors remains normal. The affected child is susceptible to bacterial respiratory infections and bronchitis. Between 1.5 to 2.5 years of age, immunoglobulin production usually becomes normal. These children have an excellent prognosis and rarely require treatment. With any low levels of IgG, treatment with immune serum globulin may be indicated. This disorder should be distinguished from the more serious immunoglobulin defects with a poor prognosis.

2. X-Linked Hypogammaglobulinemia

This syndrome was first recognized by Bruton in 1952 and is characterized by a deficiency of B-lymphocytes that results in failure of production of immunoglobuin of all classes. This is a pure B-cell deficiency in which normal cellular immunity is present with a very low concentration of circulating immunoglobulins. The disorder is X-linked, and usually only males are affected. The serum concentration of IgG is usually below 100 mg./dl. and IgA, IgM, and IgD are commonly undetectable. The B-cell immunoglobulin-producing cells usually are absent in the bone marrow, blood, lymphoid tissue, and mucosal tissue. The lymph nodes show paucity of germinal centers and plasma cells.

During the first few months of life, the infants are protected by the placental transfer of the maternal IgG antibody. After the maternal placentally-transferred IgG has been catabolized, these patients are susceptible to severe recurrent infections with common bacteria, including pharyngitis, otitis media, pneumonia secondary to streptococci, *Staphylococcus aureus*, *Hemophilus* influenza, and *Neisseria* meningitis. The diagnosis usually is made by demonstration of panhypogammaglobulinemia, diminished number of circulating surface-bearing immunoglobulin containing B-cells, and family history of other males with the disease in the mother's family. The treatment consists of periodic injections of immune gamma globulin.

3. Sex-Linked Hypogammaglobulinemia with Normal or Increased IgM

In this disorder, IgG and IgA are deficient, whereas IgM levels are normal to increased. B-cells bearing IgM type antibodies can be demonstrated. The thymic-dependent system is normal, and the immunologic abnormalities indicate an arrest in the development of B-cells from the IgM- to the IgG-producing cells. Most of the cases of this sex-linked recessive disorder are males. There is also a high incidence of neutropenia, thrombocytopenia, hemolytic anemia, and B-cell lymphomas.

An acquired form of this abnormality may be a consequence of congenital rubella infection, transcobalamin II deficiency, and hypogammaglobulinemia. Transcobalamin II deficiency has been found to be associated with a panhypogammaglobulinemia, and is a transport protein involved in vitamin B_{12} metabolism. This disease is inherited as an autosomal recessive trait. Megaloblastic anemia, granulocytopenia, and thrombocytopenia can be found. B- and T-cells are demonstrated by their surface markers, although antibody production is low to absent. The hematologic and immunologic abnormalities can be corrected by administration of large amounts of vitamin B_{12}.

4. Common Variable, Unclassifiable Immunodeficiency

This is the most common type of panhypogammaglobulinemia in which both sexes are affected. In this disease, the degree of immunoglobulin deficiency is less marked than in the X-linked form. The clinical onset is usually delayed until late childhood or adulthood. There is a great variation in the time of onset, clinical manifestation, and the degree of disordered T-cell cellular immunity. There has also been a high associated incidence of other immunologic abnormalities, such as systemic lupus erythematosus, hemolytic anemia, and thrombocytopenia purpura.

Four different types of defects have been identified in these common variable immunodeficient patients:

(1) Absence of B-cells.

(2) B-cells are present in a resting state with decreased antibody production. The B-cells are unresponsive to T-cell mitogenic signal in the presence of antigen.

(3) B-cells are present, and these cells are responsive to the T-cell signal in the presence of antigen. IgE is synthesized but not secreted. In this case, there is a defect with failure of glyco-

sylation and of the heavy chain of the immunoglobulin, which suggests that the secretion defect is due to a failure of incorporation of carbohydrate into the immunoglobulin molecule.

(4) Normal B-cells which are suppressed by humoral factors or suppressor T-cells. Experiments have reported that T-cells from some patients with common variable immunodeficiency actually suppressed normal lymphocyte synthesis of Ig after pokeweed mitogen stimulation in culture. Since T-cells are involved in modulating the terminal differentiation of B-cells to immunoglobulin-secreting cells, some patients with common variable immunodeficiency probably have an abnormality of T-cell regulators which is responsible for perpetuating hypogammaglobulinemia.

SELECTIVE IMMUNOGLOBULIN DEFICIENCY DISORDERS

There are possibly six combinations of the deficits of the three major immunoglobulins. In addition, subclass deficiencies of IgG have been found.

Selective Deficiency of IgA

Selective deficiency of serum IgA is the most common primary immunodeficiency in humans and the incidence is four to seven in 1000 patients. Autosomal dominant and recessive inheritance have been reported. Serum IgA levels are usually below 5 to 10 mg./dl. The IgA-producing cells are decreased, and secretory IgA and the external secretions are low to absent. Free secretory component is usually found. In many cases the IgM levels in the external secretion in IgM-producing cells, and external secretory sites are increased. The defect appears to be at the level of the terminal differentiation of B-cells to plasma cells.

IgA deficiency is a result of a variety of genetic defects and can be produced by a congenital rubella virus, cytomegalovirus, or *Toxoplasma gondii* infection. The selective IgA deficiency has a striking association with autoimmune diseases, non-tropical sprue, or ataxia telangiectasia.

Ataxia telangiectasia is associated about 80 per cent of the time with an IgA deficiency. Recently, a deficiency of secretory component has been described in a patient with chronic intestinal candidiasis. The serum levels of IgA were normal, but neither IgA nor secretory component could be demonstrated in external secretions. There is no satisfactory treatment for IgA deficiency. Patients with a serum IgA deficiency who receive blood transfusions can develop an anaphylactoid reaction, since IgA is often recognized as a foreign protein in transfused blood. In patients with sensitivity to IgA, blood or plasma depleted of IgA must be given to avoid the allergic reaction.

Selective IgM Deficiency

The selective IgM deficiency is the second most common selective immunodeficiency disorder. In most cases the IgM serum levels are below 20 mg./dl. Many of these patients have recurrent infections with septicemia, meningitis, gastrointestinal disorders, atropic skin diseases, and lymphoreticular malignancies. Because IgM has a short half-life, replacement therapy to raise IgM level is difficult.

IgG Subclass Deficiency

Selective deficiencies of different combinations of IgG-1, IgG-2, IgG-3, and IgG-4 have been reported. Total IgG level in these cases may be normal or slightly decreased. Diagnosis is usually indicated by a restricted heterogeneity of the electrophoretic mobility of the IgG or the lack of antibody production against certain antigens. It requires the quantitative measurement of IgG subclasses. The patient should be treated with immune serum globulin which contains all the subclasses of IgG.

PRIMARY T-CELL DISORDERS

Very few pure T-cell cellular disorders are seen. The majority of the T-cell immunodeficiency disorders are associated with some aberration in the humoral immune system to form antibodies. This is in concert with the observation that most antigens such as proteins and haptens require both the T- and B-cells for normal antibody production. Thus, a complete absence of T-cells will result in a defect of antibody production to all T-cell-dependent antigens. Many of the immunodeficiencies may initially be classified primarily as a T-cell or B-cell defect. However, when followed for a prolonged time, the immunodeficiency becomes severe and may eventuate in combined T- and B-cell deficiency. The patients with a T-cell immunodeficiency are susceptible to a variety of infectious agents, such as virus, bacteria, and protozoa, which usually result in intracellular types of infections.

Congenital Thymic Aplasia (DiGeorge's Syndrome)

The diagnosis of congenital thymic aplasia, or DiGeorge's syndrome, usually is made shortly after birth, since these patients present with congenital heart disease and hypoparathyroidism. Clinically, the patient shows hypocalcemia, which appears within 24 hours after birth and is frequently associated with tetany.

DiGeorge's syndrome results from interference with normal embryonic development at approximately 12 weeks' gestation. The thymus and parathyroid glands develop from the epithelial evaginations of the third and fourth pharyngeal pouches. In many patients with DiGeorge's syndrome the thymus is not completely absent but is hypoplastic or in an abnormal location. The terms "complete" and "partial" DiGeorge's syndrome are used to describe various degrees of immunodeficiency found in such patients. The complete absence of the thymus could result in a definite defect in the humoral antibody system, whereas the patient with a partial thymus gland would show primary manifestations of a T-cell deficiency. The peripheral lymphocyte count is low and the number of circulating T-cells is low or absent at the time of birth. The studies of B-cell immunity are difficult to interpret since IgG in fetal serum at birth represents maternal transfer of gamma globulin. IgM and IgA are normally present in very small amounts in newborns.

The congenital heart disease associated with DiGeorge's syndrome may require immediate corrective surgery. Calcium is administered to correct the hypocalcemia, and vitamin D and parathyroid hormone are used to treat hypoparathyroidism. Fetal thymus transplant at less than 14 weeks' gestation is the treatment of choice to correct the T-cell abnormality. The fetal thymus transplant has been successfully used in cases of DiGeorge's syndrome, with rapid reconstitution of T-cell immunity. The mechanism of reconstitution of T-cell immunity with the fetal transplant may be due to a humoral factor within the thymus, since one patient with DiGeorge's syndrome has been reconstituted with implantation of fetal thymus in a millipore chamber.

Fresh blood transfusions with live leukocytes should not be given to patients with a T-cell immune defect because of a possible graft versus host reaction. The blood products should first be irradiated (3000 R).

Chronic Mucocutaneous Candidiasis with and without Endocrinopathy

The majority of these patients have only minor defects in T-cell immunity. They usually have a chronic *Candida* infection of the skin and mucous membranes associated with idiopathic endocrinopathy. The etiology of the disease is not well-defined. There may be a basic autoimmune disorder associated with the T-cell defect. A wide variety of endocrine abnormalities have been seen, including hypoparathyroidism, Addison's disease, and diabetes. The total lymphocyte count and lymphocyte response to phytohemagglutinin and other mitogens and the total number of T-cells are normal. Delayed-hypersensitivity skin tests to a variety of antigens are normal, but the hallmark of the disease is an absent delayed-hypersensitivity skin test response to Candida antigen in the presence of severe Candida infection. B-cell immunity is intact in patients with chronic mucocutaneous candidiasis, and immunoglobulin levels usually are normal to elevated.

Specific treatment of the endocrinopathy is indicated. A combination of antifungal drugs such as amphotericin and transfer factor obtained from a Candida-positive donor may result in eradication of the chronic Candida infection. Prolonged remissions have been observed.

PRIMARY T- AND B-CELL DISORDERS

Severe Combined Immunodeficiency

There are two major forms of severe combined immunodeficiency disease. Each is inherited in a distinctive pattern. The X-linked recessive form was previously termed the X-linked lymphopenic agammaglobulinemia. The autosomal recessive form was initially termed the Swiss type of autosomal recessive lymphopenic agammaglobulinemia. Both disorders are characterized by a complete absence of T- and B-cell immunity, and the patients rarely survive beyond one year of age because of poor resistance to infections. The etiology of severe combined immunodeficiency disease is not known. It is commonly believed that the disorder is a result of a defect in the stem cell differentiation with absence of normal development of immunocompetent T- and B-cells. However, recent evidence suggests there may be other etiologic factors. Patients with deficiency of the enzyme adenosine deaminase have demonstrated laboratory and clinical manifestations of a severe combined T- and B-cell immunodeficiency.

The majority of patients with severe combined T- and B-cell immunodeficiency become symptomatic before 6 months of age with recurrent respiratory infections, Candida infections of the skin and mouth, and diarrhea. There are a certain number of infants with mild combined immunodeficiency disease who appear quite normal at six to nine months of age and who may not demonstrate an increased incidence of infection. Patients suspected of having such an immunodeficiency should never be immunized with live attenuated viral vaccine, since there is complication of paralytic polio or fatal encephalitis following immunization with live polio, live measles, or mumps vaccine. *Pneumocystis carinii* and progressive vaccinia are frequent complications.

The T-cell abnormalities are present at birth with lymphopenia; and other findings are a decreased number of T-cells, absence of peripheral blood lymphocyte response to PHA and allogeneic cells, and absent thymus shadow. Adenosine deaminase deficiency may be seen in severe combined immunodeficiency, although the majority

of this group of patients have normal enzyme levels. Studies of B-cell immunity are abnormal, with an absence of antibody response following immunization. Biopsy of lymph node and skin will show depletion of T- and B-dependent areas. Biopsy of colonic mucosa will demonstrate an absence of plasma cells.

The treatment of choice for patients with severe combined immunodeficiency is a histocompatible bone marrow transplant. Because of the inheritance of histocompatibility antigens, the most favorable donors are the patient's siblings. Patients who lack a histocompatible donor have been treated with fetal thymus or fetal liver transplant. Both forms of therapy have resulted in successful reconstitution of T-cell immunity. In most cases B-cell immunity has remained absent and has required the use of regular gamma globulin administration. All patients should be treated immediately following diagnosis with regular injections of gamma globulin.

Cellular Immunodeficiency with Abnormal Immunoglobulin Synthesis (Nezelof's Syndrome)

Patients with this disorder demonstrate the following features: (a) susceptibility to viral, bacterial, fungal, and protozoal infections; (b) abnormally depressed T-cell function; and (c) a varying degree of antibody immunodeficiency with various levels of specific immunoglobulins. The disease is sporadic, has no genetic pattern, and is found in both males and females.

The primary defect is a T-cell deficiency, and the B-cell abnormalities are the result of failure of normal T- and B-cell interaction. As discussed above, a complete absence of T-cells will result in B-cell abnormalities with defective antibody production to many antigens.

The immunologic defect in these cases has been treated with fetal thymus transplantation and transfer factor, and thymosin has been used with partial success in the reconstitution of T-cell immunity.

Wiskott-Aldrich Syndrome

Patients with Wiskott-Aldrich syndrome show thrombocytopenia, which may be present at birth. The disorder is inherited and sex-linked recessive. The primary defect may be in the macrophages, although the patients demonstrate T- and B-cell abnormalities. The macrophages and immune lymphocytes are unable to process polysaccharide antigen normally. The consequence is an inability to form antibody against polysaccharide-containing organisms such as *Hemophilus* influenza, pneumococcus, and coliform bacillus. As patients become older they manifest a gradual loss of both T- and B-cell functions.

The patients show complications of thrombocytopenia with bleeding, ecchymosis, and petechiae. Anemia is frequently present, and a Coombs'-positive hemolytic anemia may be seen. Infants with Wiskott-Aldrich syndrome may be protected during the first five to six months of life by maternal antibody. Subsequently they experience recurrent viral and bacterial infections, with eczema of the skin. These patients have an increased incidence of lymphoreticular malignancies compared to the normal control population.

Studies of the T-cell function during early infancy may be normal. Varying degrees of T-cell and B-cell dysfunction may be seen with progression of the disease. The patient shows an absence of blood group IgM isoagglutinins, and no antibody response is seen following immunization with a polysaccharide antigen such as typhoid. Often there is a normal to elevated level of serum IgG, decreased serum IgM, and elevated IgA and IgE levels.

Treatment consists of platelet transfusions and antibiotics for thrombocytopenia and infections. The immune defect has been treated with bone marrow transplantation with moderate restoration of T- and B-cell immunity; however, the thrombocytopenia was not corrected. Transfer factor has been reported to be successful in treatment of some patients; however, the disease usually progresses in spite of transfer factor administration.

Immunodeficiency with Ataxia Telangiectasia

By four years of age patients with ataxia telangiectasia usually develop characteristic symptoms of ataxia, telangiectasia, and recurrent sinopulmonary infections. Telangiectasia usually is present by two years of age and is seen on the bulbar conjunctiva, the ears, and over the bridge of the nose. This disorder is inherited as an autosomal recessive. The disease may involve a primary immunologic defect with secondary involvement of other organs resulting from a viral or autoimmune disease.

About 80 per cent of patients with ataxia telangiectasia lack both serum and secretory IgA. In a majority of the cases, both IgA and IgE may be absent. Antibody to IgA may develop in these patients similar to selective serum IgA immunodeficiency. In these patients, circulating IgA bearing lymphocytes are present. Cell-mediated immunity is usually impaired, and the thymus gland is hypoplastic. There is lymphopenia, with depressed response of T-cells to mitogen and allogeneic cells.

The immune defects in ataxia telangiectasia resemble those of the congenitally nude mouse with selective IgA deficiency. In these nude mice

the IgA deficiency and the T-cell defect were corrected with thymic allografts. Thus, the primary T-cell defect in ataxia telangiectasia could result in IgA and IgG deficiency by failure to facilitate normal development or suppression of B-cell maturation. Therapy primarily has consisted of gamma globulin treatment for the B-cell defects. Transfer factor and thymus transplantation have been done on a limited number of patients.

Immunodeficiency with Short-Limbed Dwarfism

This immunodeficiency exists as three distinct syndromes. The most severe form (Type I) is associated with severe combined immunodeficiency disease. Type II is associated with cellular immunodeficiency, and Type III is associated with antibody immunodeficiency. The severity of the immunologic defects varies in each disorder. All three show similar skeletal abnormalities, and these disorders appear to be inherited in an autosomal manner. In short-limbed dwarfism associated with severe combined immunodeficiency, the patients become ill in infancy with viral, bacterial, fungal, or protozoal infections. Patients with short-limbed dwarfism and cellular immunodeficiency are susceptible to recurrent respiratory tract infections.

Individuals with short-limbed dwarfism and antibody deficiency remain well for five to six months of life and then experience recurrent bacterial infections following a course similar to that of patients with congenital hypogammaglobulinemia.

Treatment is dependent upon the form of immunodeficiency present. Short-limbed dwarfism associated with combined immunodeficiency is best treated with a histocompatible bone marrow transplant. Short-limbed dwarfism with cellular immunodeficiency could be treated with a compatible bone marrow transplant, although fetal thymus transplantation has been attempted with limited success. The short-limbed dwarfism with antibody deficiency may be treated with regular gamma globulin injections.

Immunodeficiency with Enzyme Deficiency

Two forms of enzyme deficiency exist in association with immunodeficiency. The first to be discovered was adenosine deaminase deficiency, which is associated with both T- and B-cell immunodeficiency. The second was nucleoside phosphorylase, which is associated with a T-cell immunodeficiency. Adenosine deaminase and nucleoside phosphorylase are enzymes necessary for the catabolism of the purine adenosine. Adenosine deaminase catalyzes the conversion of adenosine to inosine, and nucleoside phosphorylase catalyzes the conversion of inosine to hypoxanthine. The exact mechanism by which a deficiency of the enzyme results in the immune defect is not known. It is postulated that the immunodeficiency is the result of pyrimidine starvation secondary to accumulation of adenine nucleotides. Other possibilities are that elevated adenosine results in altered immune function as well as the suppressive effects of accumulated adenosine on lymphocyte functions. The mode of inheritance of these enzyme defects is autosomal recessive. The carrier state can be shown in both sexes by decreased adenosine deaminase or nucleoside phosphorylase activity.

The degrees of immunodeficiency may be variable. Patients with adenosine deaminase deficiency may have severe combined immunodeficiency or partial defects in T- and B-cell immunity or in B-cell and T-cell immunity alone. These patients usually become symptomatic after the first six to 12 months.

The diagnosis of immunodeficiency with enzyme deficiency may be best established by enzyme assays of red cells. White blood cells and tissue are also deficient in the enzyme. An intrauterine diagnosis of adenosine deaminase has been made using cultured amniotic cells. Patients with nucleoside phosphorylase deficiency are unable to form uric acid. A rapid diagnosis of immunodeficiency with nucleoside phosphorylase may be made by measuring the serum or urine uric acid, which is extremely low.

The treatment of patients with immunodeficiency and enzyme deficiency varies with the severity of the defect. Bone marrow transplantation utilizing a histocompatible donor has been accomplished in several patients.

DISORDERS OF THE COMPLEMENT SYSTEM

There are a few significant defects in the complement system that may lead to a state of susceptibility to infection. The genetically-determined abnormalities of the complement system have been described and can be classified into:

(1) Defects in inhibitors which result in spontaneous consumption of complement components.

(2) Synthesis of defective complement molecules.

(3) Absence of a complement component.

Hereditary angioedema is caused by defective synthesis of C 1 esterase inhibitor. In normal persons, the C 1 esterase inhibitor blocks the activity of C 1s and therefore is capable of suppressing the progression of the complement sequence beyond C 1. Patients with hereditary angioedema suffer from episodic triggering of the complement system and develop angioedematous reactions in tissues, particularly those of the upper respiratory tract. Recurrent attacks of edema usually involve the skin, gastrointestinal tract, and respiratory mucosa, and involvement of the larynx can be very serious. Hereditary angioedema may exist in two genetic variants. In one type, there is an absence of the C 1 esterase inhibitor; the other variety may involve the formation of a non-functional C 1 esterase molecule.

Patients with C 3 deficiency may have repeated infections with pyogenic bacteria. The C 3 deficiency leads to an absence of complement-mediated immunoadherence and opsonization as well as defective activation of the latter components of complement. C 3 deficiency may occur in different ways, such as failure of synthesis of C 3 and absence of C 3 inactivator leading to hypercatabolism of C 3. Patients with a defect in C 3 catabolism as a result of abnormal activity of C 3 inactivator may suffer from recurrent pyogenic infections. Treatment consists of replacement of C 3 with normal plasma.

Familial C 5 dysfunction has been described in patients with Leiner's syndrome who suffer from generalized seborrheic dermatitis, severe diarrhea, and recurrent bacterial infections, usually of the gram-negative variety. Autosomal recessive C 2 deficiency may be associated with diseases such as systemic lupus erythematosus. In these individuals the biologic functions of the complement system may be impaired.

PHAGOCYTIC DISORDERS

Phagocytic disorders can be divided into extrinsic and intrinsic defects. The extrinsic disorders may be secondary to: (1) deficiency of antibody and complement factors; (2) suppression of the phagocytic cells by immunosuppressive agents; (3) interference of phagocytic function by corticosteroids; and (4) suppression of circulating neutrophils by autoantibodies.

Intrinsic phagocytic disorders are related to enzymatic deficiencies within the metabolic pathway necessary for killing the bacteria. They include chronic granulomatous disease with a deficiency of NADPH or NADH oxidase, myeloperoxidase deficiency, and glucose–6–phosphate dehydrogenase deficiency.

Chronic Granulomatous Disease (CGD)

The major immunologic features include: (1) susceptibility to infection with unusual organisms of low virulence such as *Staphylococcus albus* and *Serratia marcescens*; (2) it is a sex-linked inheritance, and female variants occur; (3) onset of symptoms occurs by two years of age, with pneumonia, draining lymphadenitis, and splenomegaly; and (4) diagnosis is established by quantitative nitro-blue tetrazolium test and quantitative killing curve of bacteria.

The chronic granulomatous disease is inherited as a sex-linked disorder with manifestations appearing in the first two years of life. A rare female variant of this disease has been described. The enzymatic deficiency in chronic granulomatous disease is felt to be either NADH or NADPH oxidase. In the female variant, glutathione peroxidase is believed to be deficient. With the enzymatic deficiency, the intracellular metabolism of the neutrophils and monocytes is abnormal, with decreased oxygen consumption and decreased utilization of glucose by the hexose monophosphate shunt with decreased production of hydrogen peroxide and diminished iodinization of bacteria and decreased superoxide anion production. The net result is decreased intracellular killing of certain bacteria and fungi. These individuals are susceptible to the so-called organisms which have low virulence for normal individuals; such organisms have a catalase enzyme and will destroy the hydrogen peroxide which may be present in the cell.

The recommended test for diagnosis of chronic granulomatous disease is the quantitative nitro-blue tetrazolium (NBT) test. This test is based on the fact that normal leukocytes reduce the NBT dye at a normal rate during in-vitro phagocytosis of particles such as latex. The leukocytes of patients with CGD show no nitro-blue tetrazolium dye reduction, whereas carriers may have normal or reduced nitro-blue tetrazolium reduction noted mainly in the polymorphs and the monocytes. Patients with CGD are unable to kill certain bacteria at a normal rate. The peripheral white count usually is elevated, even if the patient does not have active infection. Cell immunity is normal and complement factors may be elevated. There are two variants of the disease. One is the female variant of chronic granulomatous disease associated with deficient glutathione peroxidase; the other is associated with a deficient glucose–6–phosphate dehydrogenase.

Chediak-Higashi Syndrome

This disease is a multisystem autosomal recessive disorder. The symptoms include recurrent bacterial infection with a variety of organisms, hepatosplenomegaly, partial albinism, central nervous system abnormalities, and a high incidence of lymphoreticular malignancy.

The characteristic abnormality is a giant cytoplasmic granular inclusion in white blood cells and platelets which is observed on routine peripheral blood smears. There may be an abnormal neutrophil chemotaxis with abnormal intracellular killing of organisms, which also include streptococci and pneumococci as well as organisms found in chronic granulomatous disease. The killing defect consists of delayed killing time.

Oxygen consumption, hydrogen peroxide formation, and hexose monophosphate shunt activity are normal. There is no treatment other than specific antibiotic therapy for the infecting organism.

Job's Syndrome

Job's syndrome was originally described as a disease of recurrent "cold" staphylococcal abscesses of the skin, lymph nodes, or subcutaneous tissue. Also, the patient studied did not have abnormal immunologic tests. There have been reports that Job's syndrome may be a variant of chronic granulomatous disease. Treatment consists of appropriate antibiotic therapy, and the prognosis is uncertain.

Tuftsin Deficiency

Tuftsin deficiency has been reported as a familial deficiency of phagocytosis stimulating tetrapeptide which is cleaved from apparent immunoglobulin molecules in the spleen. Two families with a deficiency have been described. Tuftsin also appears to be absent in patients who have been splenectomized. Gamma globulin therapy was found to be beneficial in the two families reported.

SECONDARY IMMUNE DEFICIENCY DISEASES

Depressed immune functions occur quite frequently as a consequence of various disease states. The secondary immunodeficiencies are frequently observed in certain infections, malignant conditions (especially those involving the lymphoid system), loss of proteins from the body, drug therapy, aging, and debilitating diseases. The secondary immunodeficiency may affect both the humoral and cellular immune systems. Examples of certain disorders primarily associated with a T- or B-cell defect are shown in Table 4–2. In many cases both the T-cell and B-cell systems may be suppressed to a variable degree.

In certain infections such as rubella, there may be a decrease in the immune function. Many lymphoproliferative disorders are accompanied by a secondary immunodeficiency state. This includes multiple myeloma, Waldenström's macroglobulinemia, and other lymphoproliferative diseases. These disorders have often been called monoclonal gammopathies because excessive amounts of monoclonal types of immunoglobulins are produced. Patients with multiple myeloma frequently suffer recurrent infections and have an unusual susceptibility to various bacterial and fungal infections. The antibody synthesis against exogenously administered antigen is markedly decreased. Patients with Hodgkin's disease develop

munodeficiency of the cellular
le the humoral immune func-
ally normal. It has been dis-
is a serum factor involved
lipoprotein which acts as an
factor. Patients who have ac-
tive chronic hepatitis B infections have also been
known to possess a serum factor which suppresses cellular immune function.

Patients with chronic lymphocytic leukemia
develop deficiency of both T- and B-cell immune
systems. Both immune systems are essentially
normal in acute lymphocytic leukemia. In the
latter phases of these lymphoreticular malignant
conditions, defective defense host mechanisms
allow recurrent infections.

Patients with nephrotic syndrome have low
serum levels of albumin and gamma globulin because excessive amounts of these proteins are lost
in the urine. Protein losses from the intestinal
tract during certain acute and chronic diseases of
the bowel may lead to hypogammaglobulinemia
and intestinal lymphangiectasia. Both serum
proteins and lymphocytes are lost in the stool.

DIAGNOSIS AND LABORATORY
EVALUATION OF IMMUNODEFICIENCY
DISORDERS

The Clinical Manifestations of the
Immunodeficient Patient

Recurrent infection is the hallmark of the immunodeficient patient. The following types of infection may suggest an immunologic defect:

(1) Recurrent infection caused by bacteria of
high grade virulence.

(2) Those caused by low grade virulence or unusual organisms.

(3) Those caused by fungi and unusual reactions to vaccines.

The nature of the immune deficiency determines the spectrum of infections which may be
encountered. The primary T-cell deficiencies
demonstrate an unusual susceptibility to intracellular infections, which may be caused by
viruses, fungi, and certain bacteria such as tuberculosis. B-cell deficiencies allow infections by organisms which are largely disposed by opsonization, and such bacteria are pneumococci,
staphylococci, and streptococci.

In the evaluation of patients suspected of immunodeficiency diseases one should obtain a detailed history. Some of the important points to be
investigated are:

(1) History of allergy and tests completed in
past.

(2) Prior surgery, particularly T & A and ap-
pendectomy. Results of pathologic examination
on excised tissue may help in the assessment of
the immune system.

(3) Radiation therapy to thymus or nasopharynx.

(4) Sites of infections and organisms recovered; age at onset of infections.

(5) Previous immunizations and reactions.

(6) Prior gamma globulin treatment.

(7) Family history of collagen diseases, endocrine disorders, tumor, or early death.

Evaluation of the T-Cell Deficiency

Generally, a T-cell deficiency is indicated by
increased susceptibility to infection by fungi,
viruses, atypical acid fast organisms, and some of
the so-called lower grade pathogens. Various organisms which are involved include *Candida albicans*, vaccinia and mumps virus, mycoplasma,
and *Pneumocystis carinii*. *Pneumocystis carinii* is
frequently involved and produces pulmonary lesions in patients with a combined B- and T-cell
deficiency. In these patients the pneumonia
shows characteristic accumulations of foamy,
pink-staining exudate containing many Pneumocystis organisms. The following tests are used for
the evaluation of the T-cell system:

(1) Absolute lymphocyte count.

(2) Delayed type skin reaction.

(3) Lymphocyte stimulation test.

(4) Migration inhibitory factor test.

(5) Examination of circulating lymphocytes for
T-cell markers.

(6) Radiologic evidence of normal lymphoid
tissues.

Skin tests for delayed hypersensitivity to common antigens may be of little help in young children who have not had the opportunity to develop
a cell-mediated immune reaction to the antigens.
However, a negative skin test to Candida antigens in children suffering from infection with
this fungus has a diagnostic usefulness. Morphologic analysis of the small lymphocytes in the
peripheral blood and the deep cortical areas of
biopsy lymph nodes provides some information
about the adequacy of the T-cell system.

Evaluation of the B-Cell System

The deficiency of the B-cell system is generally
indicated with frequent bouts of infections with
pathogenic organisms causing otitis media, pneumonia, meningitis, and other infections. Such organisms include pneumococcus, streptococcus,
hemophilus, meningococcus, and hepatitis virus.
A variety of immunologic tests are available for
quantitation of the immunoglobulin levels. The
antibody tests for humoral immunity can be divided into two groups: (a) tests for the presence of
immunoglobulin and existing antibodies to common antigens; and (b) tests for antibody formation following active immunization. The immunoglobulin levels can be quantitated by various

techniques, including radial immunodiffusion, immunofluorescence, and other immunoprecipitin techniques. There should be some caution in the evaluation of immunoglobulin levels in adult sera as they may vary greatly from individual to individual. The measurements may not be reliable in the case of quantitation of various monoclonal gamma globulins owing to the nature of the specificity of the antisera and the various standards used. Absence or low serum levels of one or more immunoglobulins may have three possible causes:

(1) Absence or decreased number of B-cells in circulation of lymphoid tissue.

(2) A defect in the immunoglobulin secretion by B-cells.

(3) An increased rate of immunoglobulin catabolism.

Tests which can be carried out to distinguish between the various possibilities involve the immunofluorescent staining of the membrane of the various lymphocytes to analyze the B-cell population in the circulation as well as in the lymph nodes. In addition, one can look for the presence of germinal centers and plasma cells in the lymph nodes.

Tests for T-Cell Function

1. **Absolute Lymphocyte Count.** The count in normal children usually is above 2000/cu. mm. during the first four years of life. The lymphocyte count during maturation is an average of 2500, with a lower limit of 1000/cu. mm. Normal infants should show a count greater than 1500 small lymphocytes/mm.

2. **Delayed Type Skin Reactions.** Five different antigens may be employed: Trichophytin, Candida, streptokinase-streptodornase, mumps, and purified protein derivative (PPD). Most normal persons show a positive response to one or more antigens. The most consistently positive antigen is Candida, which shows a positive delayed skin reaction in 80 to 95 per cent of normal persons seven months of age or older. If skin reactions to the above panel of delayed-hypersensitivity antigens are negative, sensitivity tests to 2–4 dinitrochlorobenzene may be indicated.

3. **Lymphocyte Stimulation Test.** This test is an in-vitro test useful in the diagnosis of thymic dysplasia in infants whose absolute lymphocyte count appears within the normal range. In this test a pure lymphocyte fraction obtained from peripheral blood is cultured with phytohemagglutinin (PHA). Lymphocytes from normal persons will show 50 per cent or more conversion to blast forms, whereas cells from individuals with thymic abnormalities demonstrate little or no transformation of lymphocytes in culture.

4. **Migration Inhibitory Factor Test.** The sensitized thymus-derived T-lymphocytes in the presence of antigen release a number of factors, one of which inhibits the migration of macrophages from capillary tubes. Production of the migration inhibitory factor (MIF) is a good in-vitro indicator of the presence of cell-mediated immunity.

5. **Examination of Circulating Lymphocytes for T-Cell Markers (Table 4–3).** Human T-lymphocytes have a surface receptor for sheep erythrocytes that provides a reliable marker for the identification of T-cells. This reaction is temperature-dependent, requiring reduced temperature and prolonged incubation at 4° C. E-rosette formation requires viable lymphocytes and has been shown to be dependent on a surface receptor.

The method of enumerating peripheral E-rosettes involves isolation of lymphocytes on a Ficoll-Hypaque gradient to remove human erythrocytes and adding an excess ratio of sheep erythrocytes to lymphocytes; then incubating overnight at 4° C. and resuspending and counting cells with more than three or more adherent red cells/lymphocytes. The presence of peripheral blood lymphocyte forming E-rosettes in normal adults varies between 65 and 78 per cent.

Antithymocyte serum, the antisera to T-cells, has been developed by immunization of animals with human thymus cells and human or monkey thymus cell suspensions. Extensive absorption with erythrocytes, immunoglobulin and B-cells, such as B-cell chronic lymphatic leukemia or cultured B-cell lines and human fetal embryonic liver cells, is required to render such antisera specific for human T-cells. If the absorbed antiserum is used in immunofluorescence tests, approximately 80 per cent of peripheral blood lymphocytes are identified as T-cells. Recent studies have demonstrated a subpopulation of T-cells with a surface receptor for the Fc portion of the IgG. This group of T-cells with Fc receptors may represent T-helper cells.

6. **Radiologic Evidence of Normal Lymphoid Tissue of Thymus and Pharynx.**

7. **Lymph Node Biopsy.** A depletion of paracortical lymphoid cells indicates a T-cell defect.

Tests for B-Cell Function

A. Tests for Presence of Immunoglobulins and Existing Antibodies to Common Antigens. 1. SCHICK TEST. If an individual has been previously immunized with diphtheria toxoid and his humoral immune system is normal, the Schick test will be negative. A positive Schick test in such cases is presumptive evidence of IgG deficiency.

2. A AND B ISOHEMAGGLUTININS. Isohemagglutinins are present normally after about one year of age and are primarily of the IgM class. The absence of isohemagglutinins is presumptive evidence of IgM deficiency. The isoagglutinin titer in first two years of life is low.

3. IMMUNOELECTROPHORESIS. To determine

qualitative levels of immunoglobulins IgG, IgM, and IgA. The sera of newborns show a normal absence of IgM and IgA.

4. QUANTITATIVE IMMUNOGLOBULIN DETERMINATIONS. IgG concentration of 200 mg./100 ml. is considered the lower adult threshold value. IgA deficiency shows less than 5 mg./100 ml. of serum.

5. QUANTITATION OF IgG SUBCLASSES. Patients with normal levels of immunoglobulins may have a history of recurrent pyogenic infection which is associated with selective IgG subclass deficiencies.

6. RECTAL MUCOSAL BIOPSY EXAMINATION. A biopsy may be taken for routine histology and immunofluorescent localization of IgG, IgM, and IgA immunoglobulins. Infants over one month of age will have many plasma cells in the lamina propria of the rectal mucosa. This is a good screening test for evidence of antibody production in suspected humoral immune deficiency cases.

7. CIRCULATING B-LYMPHOCYTES FOR SURFACE IMMUNOGLOBULINS (TABLE 4–3). The presence of easily detectable surface immunoglobulin as determined by vital staining with immunofluorescent antisera to IgG heavy chain determinants has been applied to identify B-cells. To avoid some of the problems related to Fc receptors, reagents using Fab and $(Fab')_2$ digest of antisera are used. Careful attention to temperature during the staining procedure is observed, and incubation of cells at 37° C. and washing before staining with immunofluorescent conjugates has been reported to detect lymphocytes with stable surface Ig. The dominant surface Ig determinants on B-cells in normal individuals are IgM and IgD. Many B-cells carry both of these determinants. The significance of the strong representation of IgD, besides its minor contribution to serum Ig, has suggested that it may be important in the clonal maturation of B-cells or in triggering further events affecting B-cell response. The number of circulating B-cells with easily detectable surface Ig in peripheral blood of normal adults has ranged from 8 to 15 per cent.

B-cells have a surface receptor for the third component of complement and have been utilized as a means of detecting B-cells in suspension. The most widely applied method demonstrates complement receptors using sheep erythrocytes sensitized with purified IgM antibodies and reacted with complement. These EAC cells can then be demonstrated to adhere to B-lymphocytes to form rosettes through the complement surface receptor. Peripheral blood lymphocytes in normal individuals with EAC receptors also have surface Ig markers. Many B-cells have receptors for the Fc portion of the IgG and may be identified by using IgG coated erythrocytes or fluorescent-tagged aggregated IgG. Such a receptor is also present on monocytes and some T-cells. Since some B-cells apparently lack Fc receptor, application of this technique as a lymphocyte marker probe is limited. The identification of a population of lymphoid cells that have Fc IgG receptor but lack other B-cell and T-cell markers has raised the question whether there may be a third population of lymphoid cells. The cell responsible for lymphoid cell-mediated antibody-dependent cytotoxicity has been shown to have Fc receptors without other identifying surface markers.

B. Tests for Antibody Formation Following Active Immunization. 1. DIPHTHERIA, PERTUSSIS, AND TETANUS (DPT) VACCINATION. A standard dose is given weekly for three successive weeks. Following immunization with diphtheria toxoid, one can administer a Schick test. A positive Schick test is seen in agammaglobulinemia.

2. ACTIVE IMMUNIZATION WITH TYPHOID VACCINE. Typhoid immunization can be given once a week for three weeks. Typhoid O and H agglutinins can be easily determined in the clinical laboratory. The anti-H titer after three injections will be 160 or greater, and patients with an antibody deficiency may have a titer of less than 1:5.

TUMOR IMMUNOLOGY

TUMOR ANTIGENS

Cancer can be defined as a disease which can be triggered and influenced by a wide variety of factors such as viruses, genes, and chemical and physical agents. The factors involved in a particular tumor may be single or multiple.

It is well established that the existence of specific antigens on tumors induced by chemical, physical, or viral agents may elicit an immunologic response in the host. Antigens associated with the tumor which can be qualitatively, quantitatively, or temporally different from normal cells are called *tumor-associated antigens (TAA)*. Antigens present in tumor cells but absent in normal cells have been called *tumor-specific antigens (TSA)*. Antigens which are able to induce an immune response or resistance to tumor growth in the autochthonous host have been called *tumor-specific transplantation antigens (TSTA)*. The majority of the tumors, including those induced by chemical carcinogens and viruses as well as spontaneously arising tumors, carry antigens that elicit an immune response in the host.

During carcinogenesis there is often a retrogressive dedifferentiation, normally repressed in the mature normal cell, which leads to increased expression of the genetic information. This process leads to increased formation of fetal or embryonic components of the cell. With the advent of sensitive immunologic assay methods, there has been increasing evidence that extremely small amounts of fetal antigens may be present in normal adult persons. With development of a tumor, there is a reversion of the cell to the embryonic form, and the fetal antigens are formed in increasing amounts. Therefore, the quantitative measurement of fetal antigens is useful — practically diagnostic — in the characterization of certain tumors that produce large quantities of these antigens. The embryonic or fetal antigens are more correctly referred to as *tumor-associated phase-specific antigens (TAPSA)*, since such antigens are found in high concentration in fetal and tumor tissues, and in very low concentration in normal adult tissues.

The tumor cells, when compared to their normal counterparts, may show:

(1) Deletion of normal surface cell antigens.

(2) Membrane alteration with changes in composition and immunochemical reactivity.

(3) Formation of tumor-specific antigens (TSA).

(4) Retrogressive dedifferentiation with formation of tumor-associated phase-specific antigens (TAPSA) or fetal antigens.

Deletion of Normal Surface Cell Antigens

An early loss of the blood group antigens A, B, and H has been shown in many human epithelial cancers, such as squamous cell carcinoma of the cervix, head, and neck. Tests for the presence or absence of A, B, and H antigens on histologic sections of tumor have been used for early immunologic diagnosis of carcinoma. The exact mechanism leading to deletion of normal surface antigens in tumor cells is unknown. One postulated mechanism is that the cell surface may combine with the carcinogen to form a neoantigen, leading to antibody production; the resulting autoantibody causes the deletion of the surface antigen.

Membrane Alterations of Tumor Cells

When compared to their normal counterparts, the surface membranes of tumor cells demonstrate many physicochemical and immunochemical differences. Surface membrane changes in tumor cells definitely involve a difference in the distribution and density of normal membrane macromolecules. Tumor cells are more susceptible than normal cells to agglutination by plant agglutinins, such as Concanavalin A and wheat germ agglutinins. In addition, there are alterations in the lipid and glycoprotein composition of tumor cell membranes.

Tumor-Specific Antigens (TSA) and Tumor-Specific Transplantation Antigens (TSTA)

Tumors may be induced experimentally by chemical or physical agents and viruses. Individually distinct antigens are expressed in tumors induced by chemical or physical agents so that cross-immunization is rarely possible, even in the presence of tumors of similar morphology induced by the same carcinogen. In contrast to the virus-induced tumor, each new tumor has unique properties of its own antigenic specificity. On the other hand, tumors induced by the same virus in different species may display identical tumor antigens, which are related and specific for the virus-induced tumor. Individually specific neoantigens may be shown in several tumors of one host induced by the same carcinogen. The absence of immunologic cross reactivity in certain tumor antigens induced by chemical carcinogens such as methylcholanthrene has been proved. The neoantigens of chemically induced tumors are best demonstrated by in-vitro serologic techniques such as immunodiffusion and immunofluorescence.

There are two major categories of tumor-associated antigens in virus-induced neoplasms: (1) the virus-specific antigens; and (2) the newly formed antigens which were not present in normal cells before neoplastic transformation. Virus-induced tumors have been shown to have individually specific antigens in addition to the common antigens coded by the virus. Antigens belonging in the second category may arise as a product of specific interaction of the viral genome with the host genome, resulting in uncovering of normal or preexisting cell products such as fetal embryonic antigens.

Two categories of tumor antigens have been distinguished: (1) those that form part of the cell surface; and (2) those that do not. Those that do not form a part of the cell surface are exemplified by certain viral-related antigens of the DNA viruses. They may be products of viral genes, although not incorporated into virus particles, and may continue to be produced within tumor cells that no longer release infectious virus. The group-specific antigens of RNA oncogenic viruses provide another example; in this case the antigens are components of the virus particle and are not known to play any part in the rejection of tumor cells. The group-specific antigens are located intracellularly and elicit an immune response which can be demonstrated serologically. The antigens responsible for rejection reactions and relevant to immunotherapy are at the cell surface, where they make the cell vulnerable to attack by humoral and cellular immune responses. These cell-surface antigens are called TSTA because the usual techniques for their demonstration involve transplantation of tumor cells from one host organism to another. There is a common belief that a distinction could be made between chemically-induced tumors and virus-induced tumors, since chemically-induced tumors possess unique TSTA and virus-induced tumors share a TSTA common to all tumors. This difference is relative rather than absolute, and thus individually distinct TSTA may be a characteristic of tumors generally. This feature of individually distinct TSTA is often overlooked in virus-induced tumors with a viral-related cross reacting antigen.

One of the best examples for the existence of a human tumor virus is the Epstein-Barr virus (EBV), which is a DNA virus. EBV is closely associated with infectious mononucleosis, Burkitt's lymphoma, and nasopharyngeal carcinoma, and is believed to be the etiologic agent in infectious mononucleosis. Current evidence has been obtained for the presence of the EBV genome in tumor biopsies of Burkitt's lymphoma and nasopharyngeal carcinoma. On the other hand, the EBV genome has not been found in a variety of other lymphoproliferative diseases.

There is some indirect evidence that cervical carcinoma may result from Herpes simplex virus type II infection. Preliminary studies for Herpes simplex viral genome in cervical cancer biopsies with nucleic acid hybridization have produced both positive and negative results.

RNA tumor viruses have been demonstrated in association with mouse mammary carcinoma, mouse leukemia, and mammary carcinoma in Rhesus monkeys. The hypothesis for the viral etiology of human breast cancer stems from the various studies of mouse mammary cancer. The evidence for etiologic association of an RNA tumor virus in human breast cancer is still incomplete. A recognizable virus has not been isolated from human breast cancer tissue, and the virus-like particles that have been isolated from human milk have not been shown to have biologic tumor-inducing activity.

There are experimental data to support the concept that RNA viruses may be involved in the pathogenesis of human leukemia. However, there is no convincing evidence that viral particles seen with the electron microscope are regularly present in leukemic cells. In addition, the virus-like particles have been noted in normal patients.

Phase-Specific Fetal Antigens Associated with Human Tumors

Trace amounts of fetal antigens and the probable regression of gene activity at a given phase in the adult differentiated cell can be detected in normal adult tissue. Many of the fetal antigens which can be considered as phase-specific gene products appear in malignant tumors in larger amounts than in normal tissue. The tumor cells can arise from either: (1) a transformation of normal cells, with a retrogressive dedifferentiation of phase-specific gene products; or (2) undifferentiated cell populations which express significant amounts of the fetal phase-specific gene product.

In Table 4–4 are listed some of the more common fetal and placental antigens associated with human tumors. The fetal antigens which can be transported across the cell membranes are significant, since immunologic tests for the quantitation of such antigens are useful as tumor markers.

TABLE 4–4   FETAL AND PLACENTAL ANTIGENS ASSOCIATED WITH HUMAN TUMORS

Antigen	Fetal Tissue of Origin	Principal Type of Tumors
I. Fetal Antigens		
(1) Alpha-fetoprotein (AFP)	Liver	Hepatomas, teratomas
(2) Carcinoembryonic antigen (CEA) and subspecies CEA-S	GI tract	GI tract and variety of other tumors
(3) α_2H-ferroprotein	Liver	Leukemia, Hodgkin's disease
(4) Fetal sulfoglycoprotein	GI tract	Stomach cancer
(5) B-oncofetal antigen	Fetal organs	All types of carcinoma
(6) γ-fetoprotein (γFP)	GI tract, spleen, thymus	Many different tumors
(7) Pancreatic oncofetal antigen	Pancreas	Pancreatic tumors
II. Placental Antigens		
(1) Human chorionic gonadotropin (HCG)	Trophoblasts	Choriocarcinoma, teratocarcinoma
(2) Placental alkaline phosphatase	Placenta	Various tumors

Alpha-fetoprotein has a high binding affinity to estrogen and may play a role in hormonal regulation. There is some evidence that AFP has immunoregulatory properties with a suppressive effect on antibody synthesis. This phenomenon has been demonstrated in-vitro to a T-cell-dependent antigen in both the primary and secondary antibody response. The exact physiologic role for most of the other fetal proteins is not well known. However, certain fetal proteins such as CEA and AFP are tumor markers, and assays for the antigens are useful to monitor the tumor growth as discussed below.

IMMUNE RESPONSE TO TUMOR

It is generally accepted that cell-mediated and humoral immune responses play a major role in host–tumor relationships. Histologic evidence of immune response to the tumor is indicated by infiltration of several types of mononuclear inflammatory cells, including lymphocytes and histiocytes, and increased cellularity of the regional lymph nodes. The ability of the host to distinguish the tumor-associated antigens as well as foreign antigens and to respond to them forms the basis of the classic immunologic surveillance theory of host defense against neoplasia. Immune cells play a significant role in these host defense mechanisms against neoplasia.

The cell-mediated immune mechanisms play a significant role in tumor rejection responses. The tumor-specific immune responses can be monitored in-vitro by employing a cytotoxicity test, demonstrating the cytotoxic or cytostatic effects of sensitized lymphocytes by determining their capacity to inhibit the growth of tumor cells in culture. In-vitro studies have shown that immunocompetent cells can destroy tumor cells. At least four distinct reactions against tumor cells have been described:

1. Lysis of Tumor Cells by Activated T-cells (Fig. 4–10)

The contact of a sensitized T-lymphocyte with a target cell results in selective destruction and

LYSIS OF TUMOR CELLS BY ACTIVATED T CELLS

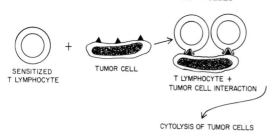

Figure 4–10

LYSIS OF TUMOR CELLS BY ANTIBODY AND COMPLEMENT

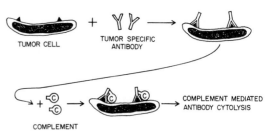

Figure 4–11

increased permeability of the plasma membrane of the target cells.

2. Lysis of Tumor Cells in the Presence of Antibody and Complement (Fig. 4–11)

This is the classic reaction of lysis of cells with antibody and complement. The binding of complement components requires suitable aggregation of surface-bound immunoglobulin; such aggregation requires close apposition of several molecules of the membrane tumor antigens.

3. Antibody Dependent Cellular Cytotoxicity (ADCC) of Tumor Cell

ADCC is mediated by non-immune and nonspecific effector cells that lack T-cell or B-cell markers. The effector cells are called K, or killer cells. They initiate lysis of the tumor cells bound with sensitizing antibody to specific tumor antigens. The cytotoxicity is mediated by nonimmune mononuclear cells attacking antibody-sensitized target cells through the Fc receptors (Fig. 4–12). Free immune complexes can inhibit the K cell function, presumably by binding to the Fc receptors. There may be competition for these receptors between free immune complexes and target-bound antibodies. Very low dilutions of antiserum insufficient to induce complement-dependent lysis may still be effective in inducing ADCC. There is evidence to demonstrate that the effector cells are neither T-cells nor the classic B-cells.

4. Lysis of Tumor Cells by Armed Macrophages

Peritoneal macrophages can become specifically cytotoxic after incubation with either immune lymphoid cells or cell-free supernatant from cultures consisting of sensitized lymphocytes and specific macrophage arming factor (SMAF) (Fig. 13). The SMAF is believed to be smaller than the intact immunoglobulin and has a specific recognition site for the target cells. The type of lympho-

ANTIBODY DEPENDENT CELLULAR CYTOTOXICITY OF TUMOR CELLS

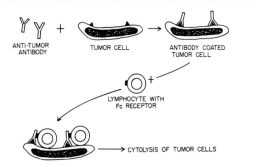

Figure 4-12

cyte involved in the generation of SMAF has not been definitely characterized. This phenomenon has been primarily demonstrated in experiments with mice.

IMMUNE SURVEILLANCE, IMMUNODEFICIENCY, AND CANCER

Immune surveillance is the mechanism whereby the host mounts an immune response against antigens expressed by the tumor. By somatic mutation or other equivalent processes, the immune system is able to recognize and eliminate foreign patterns of antigens arising in the body. The concept of immune surveillance suggests that a mutant cell which is potentially responsible for neoplastic transformation develops neoantigens and elicits an immunologic host response. The immunologic response monitored against this antigen is sufficient so that a clone of immunocompetent cells can appear and eliminate the abnormal mutants.

It is generally accepted that some form of an immune surveillance mechanism occurs continuously, but there is considerable controversy as to whether the surveillance mechanism requires immunologic rejection rather than elimination by nonimmunologic mechanisms. The evidence for an immune surveillance system is as follows: (1) after renal transplantation, patients taking immunosuppressive drugs develop an increased incidence of tumor; (2) stimulation of immune reactivity by specific immunization or non-specific methods causes a decreased incidence of tumor after infection with certain oncogenic viruses; and (3) there is increased incidence of both lymphoreticular and solid tumors in patients with immunodeficiency diseases.

The increased incidence of cancer with old age has been cited as an example of the association of human malignancy with impaired immunologic status and thus as evidence supporting the concept of immunosurveillance. Observed exceptions to the increased incidence of cancer with old age are germ cell tumors of the testes, which occur mostly in young men, and nodular sclerosing Hodgkin's disease, which is seen mostly in young women.

It is well established that the incidence of malignancy is greatly increased in patients with congenital immunodeficiency diseases in comparison with the general population. The incidence of cancer is roughly 10 per cent for patients with Wiskott-Aldrich syndrome, common variable immunodeficiency, or ataxia telangiectasia, and is about 5 per cent for patients with Bruton type agammaglobulinemia or severe combined immunodeficiency.

If the concept of immunosurveillance is valid, one would predict an excess of cancer in patients with impaired immunity secondary to other diseases. In patients with respiratory sarcoidosis and lepromatous leprosy, a depressed T-lymphocyte function has been demonstrated, although there is no evidence that leprosy is associated with increased risk of malignancy. On the other hand, the

LYSIS OF TUMOR CELLS BY MACROPHAGES AND SPECIFIC MACROPHAGE ARMING FACTOR

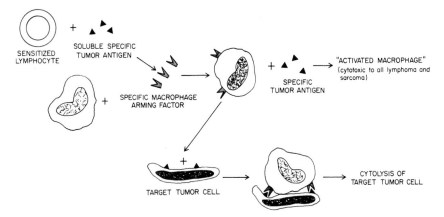

Figure 4-13

risk of developing cancer in patients with respiratory sarcoidosis was found to be greater than in the general population.

Recipients of renal transplants constitute the largest group of patients receiving immunosuppressive drugs over a prolonged period. Renal transplant patients showed an increased incidence of lymphoma 35 times that of the general population, and the tumors were mostly reticulum cell sarcomas. Risk of skin cancer was four times higher than normal, and the risk of other types of cancer was slightly higher than expected. It has been postulated that Herpes virus infection in a setting of prolonged antigenic stimulation may be responsible for the increased incidence of lymphoid malignancy and epithelial tumors of the skin, lip, and cervix in patients on immunosuppressive therapy. It is well known that the majority of transplant recipients showed evidence of infections with Herpes virus, especially cytomegalovirus. The evidence for Herpes virus etiology for other cancers is weaker than it is for the EBV and Burkitt's lymphoma; however, serologic evidence points to the association of the EBV with nasopharyngeal carcinoma and Herpes simplex type II with cervical carcinoma. It is of interest that cervical carcinoma is among the few non-lymphoid malignancies occurring with greater frequency among transplant patients than in the general population.

The immune surveillance theory has been challenged with the observation that malignancies in individuals with immunodeficiency are usually in the lymphoreticular system. Schwartz has proposed that the defect in immunity does not involve a failure of surveillance against neoplastic cells but that the disordered immune system in immunodeficient patients is unable to terminate the lymphoproliferative response to antigenic stimulation and the subsequent formation of lymphoreticular tumors.

In transplant patients the majority of the tumors (60 per cent) were reported to be of lymphoid origin, and the frequency was even higher in patients who were congenitally T-cell deficient. This is *not* consistent with the immune surveillance concept, which states that neoplastic cells should appear spontaneously in the body and be rejected by the immune system. There is no increased incidence of mammary carcinoma, which is a common tumor, in immunodeficient patients. Skin, lip, and cervical cancers are the only epithelial tumors that show a slightly increased incidence in transplant patients. It is suspected that these epithelial tumors are of viral origin. Thus, patients with defective T-cell systems are more susceptible to virus infections and virus-related tumors.

MECHANISMS OF TUMOR ESCAPE AND IMMUNOLOGIC ENHANCEMENT

There are numerous factors which can facilitate the escape of tumor cells from the immune surveillance mechanism. Some of the important considerations are as follows:

(1) Modulation of the cell-surface antigenic structure with alteration of the host immune response.

(2) Rapid turnover of antigenic cell-surface antigens with release of large amounts of free tumor-associated antigens and immune complexes.

(3) Production of tumor cell-specific antibody and host tissue enzymes which inactivate suppressor lymphoid cells.

(4) Rapid growth of the malignant cells, with formation of a large tumor mass.

(5) Development of a varying tumor cell population which is less immunogenic to the host.

(6) Appearance of suppressor cells which dampen host immune response against the tumor cells.

(7) Immunosuppressive agents responsible for neoplastic transformation.

(8) Immune deficiencies in the host.

Many serum factors which include antigen-antibody complexes, antigens, and antibody capable of blocking the cytotoxic effect of sensitized cells, can provide important escape mechanisms. The nature of blocking serum factors and the mechanism of blocking have been only partially elucidated. Blocking may occur by binding of serum factors to antigens, thus preventing cellular recognition by specific lymphoid effector cells. The degree of blocking produced by immune complexes is critically related to their physical configuration. The most effective complexes are small and soluble, because large complexes are readily removed from the circulation by the reticuloendothelial cells. Small complexes with a molecular weight of less than 1,000,000 are stable and are potent inhibitors of effector cells in antibody-dependent cytotoxicity.

Proposed mechanisms for the ability of serum factors to suppress host immune response against neoplastic cells have been categorized as afferent, central, or efferent inhibition, depending on which portion of the immune system is blocked.

1. Afferent Blockade. Antibodies or antibody parts of immune complexes bind to antigenic determinants on the tumor and mask the antigenic sites, thus preventing recognition by the host immune cells.

2. Efferent Blockade. The antigenic sites of the tumor are masked by antibody and/or immune complexes, which prevents recognition and destruction of the tumor cells by immune effector cells. Soluble antigens and antigen-antibody complexes may bind to recognition sites of the immune effector cells and interfere with the ability of these cells to recognize the target tumor cells.

3. Central Blockade. Tolerogenic soluble serum factors and/or suppressor cells could induce a state of tolerance and prevent a tumor destructive immune response.

The afferent blockade is an important mechanism for enhancing tumor growth in-vivo. The effector mechanism is a plausible explanation for blocking in-vitro with the use of hyperimmune antisera. Enhancement is often achieved with a single injection of antiserum, yet the binding of antibody to tumor cells is a transient phenomenon. The masking hypothesis is difficult to explain with the observation that very small quantities of antiserum are sufficient to induce enhancement. It seems more plausible that enhancement may be the result of an effector cell inhibition or central blockade.

IMMUNOLOGIC EVALUATION AND DIAGNOSIS OF CANCER

There are several approaches to the immunodiagnosis of cancer, as shown in Table 4–5. A popular approach is the detection of tumor-associated antigens. Several of the various assays may seem promising, although the usefulness, sensitivity, and specificity of most of the assays remain to be determined.

The tumor-associated antigens may be found in larger quantities in tumor cells than in normal cells. To be useful for immunodiagnosis, the tumor antigens should be common to a variety of tumors, at least of the same histologic type, and appear and persist in circulation or in biologic fluids. Common antigens in tumors have been identified and classified in the following categories:

1. Virus-Induced or Associated. Tumors induced by the same virus may share some of the same common tumor-associated antigens even when they differ in morphologic appearance.

2. Fetal or Embryonic Antigens. Such antigens are present on normal fetal cells and in a variety of tumors, regardless of etiology.

3. Tissue Antigens. Normal tissue antigens may be expressed in larger amounts in tumor cells and some of these may be specific for the organ from which the tumor is derived.

Assays for Tumor-Associated Antigens

Circulating antigens potentially useful for immunodiagnosis of cancer may be divided into categories of fetal antigens, hormones, and miscellaneous. A useful test would have the features of a high specificity with high sensitivity, with a definite quantitative difference from normal to benign cases. Currently, many of the tumor cell markers are useful for following patients known to have tumor, but have not been proved useful for early detection of cancer patients prior to metastatic lesions.

The fetal and placental antigens suggested for possible diagnostic application are listed in Table 4–4. CEA is present in non-malignant adult tissue and normal plasma. The use of serum CEA assays to differentiate between patients with tumors and patients with benign diseases depends on relative concentrates of CEA in tumor tissue versus other non-tumor tissues, and the destruction of the barrier to leakage of CEA into the plasma. Many of the studies of patients with benign gastrointestinal diseases and cancer patients with localized disease have demonstrated a large percentage of false-positives, and many patients with localized GI cancer do not have elevated CEA values. More recently, a subspecies assay for CEA, called CEA-S, has been developed. The assay for CEA-S detected a higher proportion of patients with GI cancer and had a very low incidence of false-positive/negative results in non-cancer patients. Currently, CEA and CEA-S assays are most useful in monitoring patients with cancer known to produce CEA substances and to indicate prognosis.

Alpha-fetoprotein (AFP) has been found to be present in small amounts in normal serum. Serum AFP assays are useful in the differential diagnosis and serve to monitor patients with hepatoma, choriocarcinoma, and testicular tumors. More recently, serum and amniotic fluid AFP assays have been useful for the detection of neural tube defects of the fetus in pregnancy.

Investigations on the various other tumors associated with fetal antigens are currently under

---

TABLE 4–5 IMMUNODIAGNOSIS OF CANCER

I. DETECTION OF TUMOR ASSOCIATED ANTIGENS ON TUMOR CELLS, AND IN PLASMA AND BIOLOGICAL FLUIDS
II. IMMUNE COMPETENCE OF CANCER PATIENTS
III. IMMUNE RESPONSE TO TUMOR ASSOCIATED ANTIGENS
    A. Humoral Immunity
    B. Cell Mediated Immunity

way; however, their practical usefulness has not been sufficiently documented.

Certain hormones have been reported to be useful as tumor markers. Human chorionic gonadotropin (HCG) and human placental lactogen (HPL) may be ectopically produced by a small proportion of tumor arising in areas outside the reproductive tract. HCG assays have been useful in monitoring choriocarcinoma and certain testicular tumors known to produce HCG. Pro-ACTH (adrenocortical trophic hormone) may be useful in the diagnosis of lung cancer, and a high percentage of patients with lung cancer have demonstrated elevated serum ACTH in preliminary studies.

Tests for Immune Competence in Immunodiagnosis of Cancer

There is a correlation between general immunocompetence and the level of specific tumor immunity with extent of disease and prognosis in patients in a wide variety of malignancies. The changes in levels of general immunocompetence and specific tumor immunity will parallel the changes in the clinical status of the patient with cancer. In almost every type of human cancer tested, patients who have a poor, depressed immune competence have a worse prognosis than patients demonstrating a normal immune system.

Immunocompetence declines markedly with advancing disease, and the patient becomes more immunodeficient. Progressive tumor growth with resulting immunodeficiency has been observed in Hodgkin's disease, leukemia, lymphomas, and in a wide variety of solid epithelial tumors such as carcinomas of the breast, lung, colon, head and neck. In Hodgkin's disease there is often a depressed cell-mediated immune reaction, whereas in chronic lymphocytic leukemia, humoral antibody response is impaired while the cell-mediated immunity is slightly depressed. Cell-mediated immunity and inflammation may be markedly suppressed in various solid tumors, whereas the antibody response is only mildly impaired.

The depression of the immune competence of cancer patients may be useful diagnostically. In the normal or benign disease population decreased immune competence may have diagnostic implications. It has been demonstrated that immune functions which are impaired in cancer patients include delayed hypersensitivity responses, peripheral blood lymphocyte counts, lymphocyte blastogenic responses, T-lymphocyte levels, B-lymphocyte levels, serum immunoglobulin levels, complement levels, primary and secondary antibody responses, specific anti-tumor levels, in-vivo delayed hypersensitivity to tumor antigens, and in-vitro lymphocyte cytotoxicity to target cells.

Immune response and various nonimmunologic host defense mechanisms can be evaluated in cancer patients by a variety of techniques, as enumerated in Table 4–6. Cellular immunity can be evaluated in many ways: for example, the delayed hypersensitivity skin test; measurement of the lymphocyte blastogenic response to mitogens or antigens; and the production of migration and inhibitory factor. Measurements as simple as lymphocyte and monocyte counts in the peripheral blood may be useful and may correlate with prognosis.

Humoral immunity can be quantitated by measuring immunoglobulin levels, isoantibody titers, complement levels, primary antibody response to antigens such as typhoid or keyhole limpet hemo-

---

TABLE 4–6   ASSAYS FOR IMMUNE COMPETENCE IN TUMOR PATIENTS

I. Cellular Immunity
    (1) Skin tests for delayed hypersensitivity
        (a) Tests for previous sensitization with recall antigens (e.g., Candida, streptokinase – streptodornase, trichophytin, mumps)
        (b) Primary sensitization (e.g., dinitrochlorobenzene)
    (2) Quantitation for circulating T- and B-lymphocytes
        (a) E-rosette assay for T-lymphocytes
        (b) Immunofluorescent assays for B-lymphocytes
    (3) Lymphocyte function
        (a) Total WBC and total lymphocyte count
        (b) Response to mitogens, PHA, Con A, and pokeweed
        (c) Production of lymphokines
    (4) Macrophage function

II. Humoral Immunity
    (1) Quantitative immunoglobulins
    (2) Isoantibody levels (blood group isoagglutinins)
    (3) Serum complement level
    (4) Primary antibody response to typhoid, keyhole limpet hemocyanin
    (5) Secondary antibody response to antigens such as tetanus and diphtheria

cyanin, and secondary response to antigens such as tetanus and diphtheria.

Immune Response to Tumor-Associated Antigens

There have been several human studies involving immune response to specific tumor-associated antigens. The tests for delayed hypersensitivity reactions to extracts of tumors have been done in a manner similar to the tests for the common bacterial-fungus antigens. Routine hypersensitivity skin test reactions have been observed in patients with the following tumors: leukemia; colon cancer; breast carcinoma; carcinoma of the lung; and cancer of the cervix. Skin test reactivity to leukemia-associated antigens has been shown to correlate with the clinical status of the patient. In general, delayed hypersensitivity skin tests to the specific tumor-associated antigens correlate with the clinical state and are useful for monitoring response to therapy. Because of the possible hazard of inoculation of cancer antigen into patients who do not have cancer, the potential usefulness of such skin tests for cancer screening and diagnosis is limited.

Cell-mediated cytotoxicity assays may have a possible application in immunodiagnosis. The lymphocytes removed from patients with cancer can exhibit in-vitro growth of the tumor cells or may demonstrate cytotoxic inhibition of the cultured tumor cells. Such assays are performed primarily in the larger diagnostic cancer centers, primarily on a clinical investigation basis.

Leukocyte migration inhibition assays have been performed with the use of patient cells reacted with the extract of the tumor tissue. Reactivity to common tumor-associated antigens has been observed by this method in patients with breast cancer, malignant melanoma, lymphoma, and leukemia. Further, the leukocyte migration assay has been reported to show good correlation with delayed-hypersensitivity skin test reactions.

Potential fruitful approaches which remain to be developed are useful tests for the detection of antibodies to tumor-associated antigens. Antibodies to common tumor antigens have been described in melanoma and osteosarcoma. The specificity of the reactions in melanoma and osteosarcoma must be studied further. This approach is very sensitive and can be useful for the early diagnosis of cancer.

IMMUNOTHERAPY

There are many problems associated with current methods of immunotherapy. The human tumor antigens have not been well defined in terms of location, such as cytoplasmic or surface, their immunogenicity, cross reactivity with normal tissue antigens, and interaction with host immune surveillance systems. The approaches to enhance the normal immune system to combat and contain the growth of cancer have been: (1) increasing cell mediated immunity; (2) augmenting antibody mediated immunity; and (3) stimulating the general immunocompetence with use of specific and nonspecific reagents.

There are seven major approaches to immunotherapy listed in Table 4–7.

Active Non-specific Immunotherapy

This mode of therapy usually involves use of adjuvants such as BCG or *C. parvum* to increase the general immunocompetence with augmentation of cell-mediated and humoral response. These

TABLE 4–7 APPROACHES TO IMMUNOTHERAPY OF CANCER*

Approach	Mechanism of Action
(1) Active-non-specific	Increase general immunocompetence Activate macrophages
(2) Immunorestorative	Restore immunocompetence
(3) Active specific	Increase specific cell-mediated-humoral antitumor immunity
(4) Adoptive	Transfer tumor immunity from immune cells
(5) Passive	Transfer humoral tumor-specific antibodies, cytotoxic, deblocking, opsonizing, antibody-dependent cellular cytotoxicity or drug- or isotope-transporting antibody
(6) Local	Locally active macrophages kill tumor cells by bystander effect of delayed hypersensitivity; induce specific tumor immunity
(7) Combination of above	

*(Modified from Hersh, et al.: Immunotherapy of cancer. *In* Cancer, A Comprehensive Treatise, Vol. 6, p. 425. Plenum Press, New York, 1977.)

non-specific adjuvant reagents may have one or more of the following immunologic effects: increase in general immunocompetence; augmentation of cell mediated or humoral responses; expansion of T-lymphocyte population and activation of the macrophages; or enhancement of the reticuloendothelial system. This approach has been used in the therapy of many tumors, such as melanoma, leukemia, colon cancer, lung carcinoma, and breast carcinoma, with variable degrees of success.

Immunorestoration

Certain agents such as levamisole and thymosin have been used to restore cell-mediated responsiveness. Levamisole is a chemical agent which probably acts through a cyclic nucleotide or prostaglandin system in lymphocytes and helps restore cell-mediated responsiveness in sensitized hosts.

In patients who are immunodeficient and immunosuppressed, the administration of thymic hormones has been known to increase the percentage of peripheral circulating E-rosette T-cell types of lymphocytes. The possibility of thymic factors which can augment cell-mediated response of cancer patients has been shown to enhance in-vitro cell function. Preliminary results have demonstrated some clinical improvement in tumor patients; however, further studies are needed to determine the true therapeutic benefits.

Active Specific Immunotherapy

This mode of therapy includes immunization with tumor cells or antigens. The tumor cells may be modified with virus or chemicals prior to immunization to enhance specific cell-mediated and humoral immunity in the host. Specific stimulation of immunity has been attempted by:

1. Unmodified Cancer Cells or Cell Surface Antigens as Immunogens. Allogeneic cancer cells as immunogen have been used in the immunotherapy of human leukemia. The human leukemia cells were irradiated to prevent cell division and injected periodically into recipients previously induced into remission of acute lymphocytic leukemia by chemotherapy. Concurrent with the tumor vaccine, BCG was administered. The immunotherapy with both irradiated allogeneic cells of BCG was synergistic, whereas either modality alone was ineffective.

2. Treatment of Cancer Cells with Neuraminidase. This is based on the hypothesis that enzymatic removal of sialic acid residues from cancer cell membranes increases their immunogenicity and facilitates immunospecific rejection. The efficacy of this treatment has not been established.

3. Virus-Modified Cancer Cells. Virus infections of cells may produce strongly immunogenic viral antigens on the cell surface which enhance the immunogenicity of weak tumor specific antigens. The immune response is not directed to the virus alone, because rejection of subsequent tumor challenge is tumor-specific. These studies have been extended to humans with malignant disease on a limited basis. No therapeutic benefits have been noted in patients with osteogenic sarcoma given influenza virus-infected autologous or allogeneic tumor cells.

4. Chemically Modified Membranes on Cancer Cells. Chemicals can be coupled to tumor cell membranes and enhance the cell mediated cytotoxicity in experimental animal tumor models. Most of the experimental work has been in animal models using substances such as 2-4-dinitrophenol. This approach is still in the early stages of clinical experimentation for treatment of human tumors.

Adoptive Immunotherapy

This mode of therapy utilizes transfer of cells or cell products from a specifically immunocompetent donor to a tumor-bearing recipient. The therapy may involve transfer of T-lymphocytes, transfer factor, or immune RNA extracted from sensitized lymphocytes.

1. Transfusion of Normal T-lymphocytes. Often in cancer patients, the T-lymphocytes are depressed primarily or secondarily, and the therapeutic infusion of normal T-cells will initiate or augment an antitumor response. One major obstacle of adoptive immunotherapy is overcoming the histocompatibility antigen difference. Without HLA matching, the donor cells will not survive and a severe graft-versus-host reaction may occur in an immunosuppressed recipient.

2. Transfusion of Sensitized T-lymphocytes. The transfusion of allogeneic sensitized T-lymphocytes in the form of leukocyte transfusion was one of the first methods used in immunotherapy of human cancer. The donors and recipients should be matched with respect to the ABO blood group and HLA antigens. This mode of therapy has been only partially successful in humans.

3. Treatment with Transfer Factor. Transfer factor has been used to activate the immune response in cancer patients and other immunodeficient diseases. The small molecular weight transfer factor derived from sensitized T-lymphocytes can program recipient lymphocytes to develop certain aspects of specific cellular immunity such as T-cell mediated cytotoxicity. Transfer factor therapy has been used in cases of human malignant melanomas resulting in prolongation of life span and an interval of time for clinical recurrence of the tumor.

4. Transfer of Immune RNA. RNA is extracted from sensitized donor immune lymphocytes and injected into the recipient host. Experimental studies have shown that immunotherapy with immune RNA is more effective in inhibiting tumor growth if administered at a period when there is small tumor mass with growth in the early stages. This mode of therapy is not very effective when immune RNA is given to an animal with a well-established growing tumor. This approach in humans is still in the early stages of clinical investigation, and the mechanism of action and beneficial effects have yet to be determined.

Passive Immunotherapy

This refers to transfer of antitumor antibodies from an immune donor to a recipient host with tumor. The use of tumor-specific antibodies has been applied with some success in experimental animal models. However, studies with immunotherapy with antibodies in man have not been adequately tested. Most of the reported studies in man have not been very successful. There has been hesitation on the part of oncologists, since it is possible to enhance the growth of the tumor by administration of tumor antibodies by blocking specific cell-mediated immunity.

A better approach currently being used is to couple cytotoxic agents such as organic chemicals and radioactive substances to specific antibodies and use such reagents to kill tumor cells selectively.

Local Immunotherapy

This method refers to the injection of active-non-specific or adoptive immunotherapeutic reagents directly into tumor in order to induce local killing and enhance specific tumor immunity of the general host immune system.

Combinations of the above modes of immunotherapy have been used with variable results. In general, one can summarize by stating that immunotherapy by itself has not been found to be very effective in most cases. Immunotherapy has demonstrated some benefit when administered in conjunction with cancer chemotherapy.

REFERENCES

DYNAMICS OF THE IMMUNE RESPONSE AND IMMUNOCOMPETENCE

Bach, F. H., and Good, R. A.: Clinical Immunobiology. Academic Press, New York, 1972, 1974, 1976, Vols. 1–3.

Coutinho, A., and Möller, G.: Thymus-independent B-cell induction and paralysis. Adv. Immunol., 21: 114–227, 1975.

Dickler, H. B.: Lymphocyte receptors for immunoglobulin. Adv. Immunol., 24: 167–207, 1976.

Dupont, B., Hansen, J. A., and Yunis, E. J.: Human mixed-lymphocyte culture reaction: genetics, specificity, and biological implications. Adv. Immunol., 23: 108–187, 1976.

Fudenberg, H. H., Sites, D. P., Caldwell, J. L., and Wells, J. V.: Basic and Clinical Immunology, 2nd ed. Los Altos, Lange Medical Publications, 1978.

Gell, P. G. H., Coombs, R. R. A., and Lachmann, P. J.: Clinical Aspects of Immunology, 3d ed. Blackwell Scientific Publications, Oxford, 1975.

Golub, E. S.: The Cellular Basis of the Immune Response: An Approach to Immunobiology. Sinauer Assoc., Sunderland, Mass., 1977.

Good, R. A.: Structure-function relations in the lymphoid system. Clin. Immunobiol., 1: 1–26, 1977.

Hobart, N. J., and McConnell, I.: The Immune System: A Course on the Molecular and Cellular Basis of Immunity. Blackwell Scientific Publications, Oxford, 1975.

Humphrey, J. H., and White, R. G.: Immunology for Students of Medicine, 3d ed. Blackwell Scientific Publications, Oxford, 1970.

Hunsicker, L. G., Wintroub, B. U., and Austen, K. F.: Humoral amplification systems in inflammation. Clin. Immunobiol., 1: 179–192, 1972.

Ishizaka, K.: Cellular events in the IgE antibody response. Adv. Immunol., 23: 1–70, 1976.

Kabat, E. A.: Structural Concepts in Immunology and Immunochemistry. Holt, Rinehart & Winston, New York, 1976.

Katz, D. H.: Lymphocyte Differentiation, Recognition and Regulation. Academic Press, New York, 1977.

Katz, D. H.: Genetic controls and cellular interactions in antibody formation. Hosp. Pract., Feb. 1977, pp. 85–99.

Nakamura, R. M.: Immunopathology: Clinical Laboratory Concepts and Methods. Little, Brown & Co., Boston, 1974.

Rocklin, R. E.: Products of activated lymphocytes. Clin. Immunobiol., 3: 195–219, 1976.

Roitt, I.: Essential Immunology, 3d ed. Blackwell Scientific Publications, Oxford, 1977.

Rosenthal, A. S.: Immune Recognition: Proceedings of the 9th Leukocyte Culture conference. Academic Press, New York, 1975.

Schreiner, G. F., and Unanue, E. R.: Membrane and cytoplasmic changes in B-lymphocytes induced by ligand-surface immunoglobulin interaction. Adv. Immunol., 24: 38–150, 1976.

Shreffler, D. C., and David, C. S.: The H-2 major histocompatibility complex and the immune response region: Genetic variation, function, and organization. Adv. Immunol., 20: 125–190, 1975.

Spiegelberg, H. L.: Biological activities of immunoglobulins of different classes and sub-classes. Adv. Immunol., 19: 259–289, 1974.

Warner, N. L.: Membrane immunoglobulins and antigen receptors on B and T lymphocytes. Adv. Immunol., 19: 67–200, 1974.

GENERAL—IMMUNODEFICIENCY

Ammann, A. J., and Fudenberg, H. H.: Immunodeficiency diseases. In Fudenberg, H. H., et al. (Eds.): Basic and Clinical Immunology. Lange Medical Publishers, Los Altos, 1976, p. 334.

Bergsma, D., Good, R. A., Finstad, J., and Paul, N. W.: Immunodeficiency in Man and Animals. Birth Defects: Original Article Series, Vol. XI, No. 1, National Foundation. Sinauer Associates, Sunderland, Mass., 1975.

Clough, J. D.: Immunodeficiency states relevant to infection. Cleveland Clin. Q., 42: 49, 1975.

Fudenberg, H. H., Stites, D. P., Caldwell, J. L., and Wells, J. V.: Basic and Clinical Immunology. Lange Medical Publishers, Los Altos, 1976.

Litwin, S. D., Christian, C. L., and Siskind, G. W.: Clinical Evaluation of Immune Function in Man. Grune & Stratton, New York, 1976.

Nakamura, R. M.: Immunopathology: Clinical Laboratory Concepts and Methods. Little, Brown & Co., Boston, 1974.

SPECIAL TOPICS

Ammann, A. J.: T cell and T-B cell immunodeficiency disorders. Pediatr. Clin. North Am., *24*: 293, 1977.

Babior, B. M.: Oxygen-dependent microbial killing by phagocytes. N. Engl. J. Med., *298*: 659, 1978.

Bankhurst, A. D., Hastain, E., Husby, G., Diaz-Jouanen, E., and Williams, R. C.: Human lymphocyte subpopulations defined by double surface markers. J. Lab. Clin. Med., *91*: 15, 1978.

Bortin, M. M., and Rimm, A. A.: Severe combined immunodeficiency disease. Characterization of the disease and results of transplantation. J.A.M.A., *238*: 591, 1977.

Douglas, S. D.: Analytic review: disorders of phagocytic function. Blood, *35*: 851, 1970.

Goldman, A. S., and Goldblum, R. M.: Primary deficiencies in humoral immunity. Pediatr. Clin. North Am., *24*: 277, 1977.

Goldstein, A. L., Cohen, G. H., Rossio, J. L., Thurman, G. B., Brown, C. N., and Ulrich, J. T.: Use of thymosin in the treatment of primary immunodeficiency diseases and cancer. Med. Clin. North Am., *60*: 591, 1976.

Johnson, S. M., Asherson, G. L., Watts, R. W. E., North, M. E., Allsop, J., and Webster, A. D. B.: Lymphocyte purine 5'-nucleotidase deficiency in primary hypogammaglobulinaemia. Lancet, 168, Jan. 22, 1977.

Levin, A. S., Spitler, L. E., and Fudenberg, H. H.: Transfer factor therapy in immune deficiency states. Ann. Rev. Med., *24*: 175, 1973.

Moretta, L., Mingari, M. C., Webb, S. R., Pearl, E. R., Lydyard, P. M., Grossi, C. E., Lawton, A. R., and Cooper, M. D.: Imbalances in T cell subpopulations associated with immunodeficiency and autoimmune syndromes. Eur. J. Immunol., 7:696, 1977.

Rosen, F. S.: Primary immunodeficiency. *In* Litwin, S. D., Christian, C. L., and Siskind, G. W. (Eds.): Clinical Evaluation of Immune Function in Man. Grune & Stratton, New York, 1976.

Sandman, R., Ammann, A. J., Grose, C., and Wara, D. W.: Cellular immunodeficiency associated with nucleoside phosphorylase deficiency. Immunologic and biochemical studies. Clin. Immunol. Immunopathol., 8: 247, 1977.

Schulof, R. S., and Goldstein, A. L.: Thymosin and the endocrine thymus. *In* Stollerman, G. H. (Ed.): Advances in Internal Medicine. Year-Book Medical Publishers, Chicago, 1977, Vol. 22.

Stobo, J. D.: Surface markers for lymphocyte subpopulations. J. Lab. Clin. Med., *91*: 9, 1978.

Stoop, J. W., Zegers, B. J. M., Hendrickx, G. F. M., Siegenbeek van Heukelom, L. H., Staal, G. E. J., deBree, P. K., Wadman, S. K., and Ballieux, R. E.: Purine nucleoside phosphorylase deficiency associated with selective cellular immunodeficiency. N. Engl. J. Med., *296*:651, 1977.

Townes, A. S., and Postlethwaite, A. E.: Lymphocyte surface markers in human disease. *In* Stollerman, G. H. (Ed.): Advances in Internal Medicine, Vol. 22. Year-Book Medical Publishers, Chicago, 1977, p. 97.

Wara, D. W.: Laboratory diagnosis of immunodeficiency disease. Pediatr. Clin. North Am., *24*: 329, 1977.

GENERAL TUMOR IMMUNOLOGY

Becker, F. F. (Ed.): Cancer: A Comprehensive Treatise. Vol. I – III. Plenum Press, New York, 1975–1977.

Byers, V. S., and Levin, A. S.: Tumor immunology. *In* Fudenberg, H. H., et al. (Eds.): Basic and Clinical Immunology. Lange Medical Publishers, Los Altos, 1976, p. 334.

Harris, J. E., and Sinkovics, J. G.: The Immunology of Malignant Disease, 2nd ed. C. V. Mosby Co., St. Louis, 1976.

Holland, J. F., and Frei, E. (Eds.): Cancer Medicine. Lea & Febiger, Philadelphia, 1973.

Smith, R. T.: Possibilities and problems of immunologic intervention in cancer. N. Engl. J. Med., *287*: 439, 1972.

TUMOR ANTIGENS

Franchimont, P., and Zangerle, P. F.: Present and future clinical relevance of tumour markers. Eur. J. Cancer, *13*: 637, 1977.

Friedman, J. M., and Fialkow, P. J.: Cell marker studies of human tumorigenesis. Transplant. Rev., *28*: 17, 1976.

Metzgar, R. S., and Mohanakumar, T.: Tumor-associated antigens of human leukemia cells. Semin. Hematol., *15*: 139, 1978.

Miller, G.: Human cancer viruses. *In* Stollerman, G. H. (Ed.): Advances in Internal Medicine. Year-Book Medical Publishers, Chicago, 1976, Vol. 21, p. 189.

Prevost, J. M.: Oncogenic viruses: implications for human diseases (Part I). Eur. J. Cancer, *12*: 327, 1976.

Prevost, J. M.: Oncogenic viruses: implications for human diseases (Part II). Eur. J. Cancer, *12*: 499, 1976.

Schwartz, M. K.: Detection of tumor-associated antigens in plasma or serum. *In* Bach, F. H., and Good, R. A. (Eds.): Clinical Immunobiology. Academic Press, New York, 1976, Vol. 3, p. 405.

Spiegelman, S.: Viruses and human cancer. *In* Brown, E. B. (Ed.): Progress in Hematology. Grune & Stratton, New York, 1975, Vol. 9, p. 305.

Tomasi, Jr., T. B.: Structure and function of alpha-fetoprotein. Ann. Rev. Med., *28*: 453, 1977.

IMMUNE SURVEILLANCE, IMMUNODEFICIENCY AND CANCER

Hersh, E. M., Mavligit, G. M., and Gutterman, J. U.: Immunodeficiency in cancer and the importance of immune evaluation of the cancer patients. Med. Clin. North Am., *60*: 623, 1976.

Kamo, I., and Friedman, H.: Immunosuppression and the role of suppressive factors in cancer. *In* Klein, G. (Ed.): Advances in Cancer Research. Academic Press, New York, 1977, Vol. 25, p. 271.

Louie, S., and Schwartz, R. S.: Immunodeficiency and the pathogenesis of lymphoma and leukemia. Semin. Hematol., *15*: 117, 1978.

Moller, G., and Moller, E.: The concept of immunological surveillance against neoplasia. Transplant. Rev., *28*: 3, 1976.

Shearer, W. T., and Fink, M. P.: Immune surveillance system: its failure and activation. *In* Brown, E. B. (Ed.): Progress in Hematology. Grune & Stratton, New York, 1977, Chap. 10, p. 247.

IMMUNE RESPONSE TO TUMOR

Benacerraf, B.: Suppressor T-cells and suppressor factor. Hosp. Pract., *13*: 65, 1978.

Evans, R., and Alexander, P.: Mechanism of immunologically specific killing of tumour cells by macrophages. Nature, *236*: 168, 1972.

Leventhal, B. G., Mirro, Jr., J., and Yarbro, G. S. K.: Immune reactivity to tumor antigens in leukemia and lymphoma. Semin. Hematol., *15*: 157, 1978.

Piessens, W. F., and Moloney, W. C.: Immunological aspects of acute leukemia in man. Eur. J. Cancer, *12*: 511, 1976.

Roubinian, J. R., and Talal, N.: Neoplasia, autoimmunity and the immune response. *In* Stollerman, G. H. (Ed.): Advances in Internal Medicine. Year-Book Medical Publishers, Chicago, 1978, Vol. 23, p. 435.

MECHANISMS OF TUMOR ESCAPE AND IMMUNOLOGIC ENHANCEMENT

Baldwin, R. W., and Price, M. R.: Tumor antigens and tumor-host relationship. Ann. Rev. Med., *27*: 151, 1976.

Kamo, I., and Friedman, H.: Immunosuppression and the role of suppressive factors in cancer. *In* Klein, G. (Ed.): Advances in Cancer Research. Academic Press, New York, 1977, Vol. 25, p. 271.

Prehn, R. T.: Do tumors grow because of the immune response of the host? Transplant. Rev., *28*: 34, 1976.

Shearer, W. T., and Fink, M. P.: Immune surveillance system: its failure and activation. *In* Brown, E. B. (Ed.): Progress in Hematology. Grune & Stratton, New York, 1977, p. 247.

IMMUNOLOGIC EVALUATION AND DIAGNOSIS OF CANCER

Franchimont, P., and Zangerle, P. F.: Present and future clinical relevance of tumour markers. Eur. J. Cancer, 13: 637, 1977.

Gold, P.: Immunologic diagnostic techniques. In Holland, J. F., and Frei, E. (Eds.): Cancer Medicine. Lea & Febiger, Philadelphia, 1973, p. 349.

Herberman, R. B.: Immunologic approaches to the diagnosis of cancer. Cancer (Suppl.), 37: 549, 1976.

Herberman, R. B.: Immunologic tests in diagnosis of cancer. Am. J. Clin. Pathol., 68: 688, 1977.

Hersh, E. M., Mavligit, G. M., and Gutterman, J. U.: Immunodeficiency in cancer and the importance of immune evaluation of the cancer patient. Med. Clin. North Am. 60: 623, 1976.

Hersh, E. M., Mavligit, G. M., and Gutterman, J. U.: Immunological evaluation of malignant disease. Diagnosis, prognosis, and management. J.A.M.A., 236: 1739, 1976.

Martin, F., Martin, M. S., and Bourgeaux, C.: Fetal antigens in human digestive tumors. Eur. J. Cancer, 12: 165, 1976.

Nakamura, R. M., Plow, E. F., and Edgington, T. S.: Current status of carcinoembryonic antigen CEA and CEA-S assays in the evaluation of neoplasms of the gastrointestinal tract. Ann. Clin. Lab. Sci., 8: 41, 1978.

Reynoso, G.: Biochemical tests in cancer diagnosis. In Holland, J. F., and Frei, E. (Eds.): Cancer Medicine. Lea & Febiger, Philadelphia, 1973, p. 335.

IMMUNOTHERAPY

Gutterman, J. U.: Cancer systemic active immunotherapy today — prospects for tomorrow. Cancer Immunol. Immunotherap., 2: 1–9, 1977.

Harris, J. E., and Sinkovics, J. G.: The Immunology of Malignant Disease, 2nd ed. C. V. Mosby Co., St. Louis, 1976.

Hersh, E. M., Mavligit, G. M., Gutterman, J. U., and Richman, S. P.: Immunotherapy of human cancer. In Becker, F. F. (Ed.): Cancer: A Comprehensive Treatise. Plenum Press, New York, 1977, Vol. 6, p. 425.

Oettgen, H. F.: Immunotherapy of cancer. N. Engl. J. Med., 297: 484, 1977.

Sell, S., and Mendelsohn, J.: Transfer of specific immunity with RNA. Arch. Pathol. Lab. Med., 102: 217, 1978.

5

Mechanisms of Immunologic Disease and Autoimmunity

ROBERT M. NAKAMURA
AND ERNEST S. TUCKER, III

MECHANISMS OF IMMUNOLOGIC DISEASE

INTRODUCTION

Advances in knowledge of the immune response and immune reactivity achieved over the past two decades have been accompanied by a more complete understanding of the different pathways of immune tissue injury. In the first part of this chapter these varied pathogenic mechanisms will be examined. The second part will deal with the concepts of autoimmunity and will discuss patterns of autoimmune reactions encountered in human disease.

In considering immunologic tissue injury, an important central point should be emphasized: namely, that the tissue damage results from the immune activation of cellular and biochemical mediator systems of the host. The combination of the immune reactants produces only minimal direct effects, but as a trigger mechanism it sets the destructive factors into play.

The different types of immune reactivity were briefly described in Chapter 4. Antibodies and effector T-lymphocytes were noted to participate in quite different pathogenic sequences, all of which lead to a common effect of direct neutralization or inactivation of antigen or indirect inactivation due to cellular and biochemical mediators. From extensive experimental studies in animals, each of the major mechanisms of immune injury has been studied and each step in the pathogenic sequences has been thoroughly defined. Based on these experimental studies, clinical investigators have extended our under-

standing of the mechanisms of human disease by applying data from comparative and somewhat parallel studies in animals. Because of this approach, immunologic factors are now recognized in many human diseases and disorders that previously were of obscure etiology and pathogenesis. This has also led to new modes of therapy.

In the section on autoimmunity, it will be seen that the different forms of autoimmune disease correlate with the type of immune response in a given disorder. Some autoimmune diseases exhibit both T-cell-dependent and antibody-dependent injury, but others are not associated with a clearly defined pathogenesis. The question of an immune response to one's own tissues remains an enigma. We are now much closer to an understanding of the autoimmune phenomenon than before, but we still lack the needed information to know with assurance all the factors in autoimmunity. The discussion will indicate that the puzzle is not how we develop an immune response to our own tissues as antigens but rather how we develop and normally maintain a state of unresponsiveness. Key answers will no doubt be forthcoming from current and future research. With such knowledge we will gain substantial insight into the control and regulation of immunoresponsiveness.

BASIC PATTERNS OF IMMUNE INJURY

The different types of immune injury are related to the major forms of immune reactivity: those which are antibody-dependent and those which are dependent on effector T-cells. Table 5–1 gives a general classification of immune injury. There

TABLE 5–1 TYPES OF IMMUNOLOGIC INJURY

Type of Reaction	Onset	Antibody	Principal Cell	Site of Reaction	Biochemical Mediator(s)
Antibody Dependent:					
1. *Anaphylactic* (Atopic, reaginic)	Rapid (Seconds to minutes)	IgE	Basophil/Mast Cell	Varies with antigen portal of entry	Histamine, Serotonin, SRS-A (Slow reacting substance of anaphylaxis)
2. *Complement Mediated*					
a. *Immune Complex* (or tissue reactive antigen-antibody)	Intermediate (30 min. to 2 hours)	IgM/IgG	Neutrophil	Varies with tissue localization of complexes or site of reaction with tissue constituents	Complement-Chemotactic Factors Neutrophil Lysosomal Hydrolytic Enzymes
b. *Immune adherence* (Phagocytic Reaction)	Intermediate (Minutes to hours)	IgM/IgG	R-E Cells	Vascular Sinuses of Reticulo-Endothelial System	Complement—C3b
3. *Cytotoxic* (Natural Killer Cell Reaction)	Intermediate	IgG	Mononuclear Natural Killer Cell	Varies with tissue localization of target cell	Killer-Cell Factor
T-Cell Reactions:					
1. *Granulomatous*	Prolonged (Delayed) (18–48 hrs.)	None	Effector T-Cell and Monocyte/Macrophage	Varies with tissue localization of antigen	Soluble lymphokines from antigen stimulated T-cell
2. *Killer T-Cell Reactions*	Prolonged (18–48 hrs.)	None	Effector T-Cell (Killer T-Cell)	Varies with tissue location of target cell	Killer cell factor

are three major types of antibody-dependent injury; these are designated as anaphylactic, complement-dependent and cytotoxic. Each of these is associated with a certain class of immunoglobulin, a certain type of cell, and specific biochemical mediators. In each instance the immune reaction triggers those factors of the pathogenic sequence leading to destructive tissue reactions. Fortunately, these reactions are limited by inhibitors and inactivators that suppress the cellular and biochemical reactions at critical points.

Effector T-lymphocytes mediate two other major forms of immune injury. One of these is called the granulomatous hypersensitivity reaction. It follows antigen contact with an effector T-cell circulating through the tissue which synthesizes and releases biochemical factors that recruit other cells into the tissue to produce the lesion. This type of reaction is the more common and most characteristic of the delayed hypersensitivity lesions. The other type of T-cell-dependent reaction is called the cytotoxic or killer (K) cell reaction. It occurs less frequently and involves antigens on cell surfaces which are closely linked to histocompatibility antigens. In the immune reaction, the killer T-lymphocyte comes into contact with antigen on the target cell. It produces killing through release of a biochemical substance.

Each of these forms of immunologic injury will be considered in detail sufficient to enable the reader to understand the different mechanisms which are operative. Through this approach, an understanding of immune mechanisms can be gained that will aid in the differential analysis of complex clinical problems.

ANAPHYLACTIC INJURY

Anaphylactic disorders are common. It has been estimated that they affect one person in 20 in the U.S. They have been widely studied in the experimental laboratory and in clinical investigations. They are known by a variety of synonyms and pseudonyms bestowed through the years by many investigators. Some of these terms are: atopy or atopic reactions; reaginic hypersensitivity; P-K (Prausnitz-Kustner) reactivity; and, now, most are called IgE-mediated hypersensitivity.

The sequence of biochemical and cellular events in anaphylactic hypersensitivity is much better understood than it was a decade ago. Initially, the susceptible immunoresponsive host becomes sensitized by developing a significant antibody response of IgE (also called homocytotropic antibody) on exposure to the stimulating immunogen. The types of immunogens initiating these reactions include a variety of environmental substances such as pollens, animal dander, fungi and

molds, food substances, and plant materials. The IgE which is formed disseminates throughout the circulation to become selectively and uniquely attached to the cell membranes of basophils in the circulation and mast cells in the tissues. The attachment occurs through a structural area in the Fc part of the antibody molecule to a specific receptor in the mast cell membrane. The mast cells and basophils have a high affinity for IgE. The dissociation constant of IgE on the cell membrane is quite low, indicating that it is firmly attached. There is a relative abundance of these IgE molecules bound along the membrane and they are located close to each other physically. When the IgE becomes attached, the individual cells are said to be sensitized, and the individual is now in a sensitive state for reactivity on subsequent exposure to the allergen (antigen) (Fig. 5-1).

A second or subsequent exposure can occur via many routes, such as inhalation, ingestion, or injection. The allergen (antigen) must move across membrane and tissue barriers in order to come to the surface of sensitized basophils in the circulation or mast cells in the tissues. When this close encounter occurs with an allergen of sufficient size to react with the antigen binding sites of two closely adjacent IgE molecules, it produces a "bridging" effect. This "bridging" effect results in distortion of the cell membrane, followed by activation of various enzyme systems and leading to degranulation of the cells. After degranulation, there is release from the granules of potent biochemical factors which cause profound physiologic reactions in the surrounding local tissues. These factors include histamine, serotonin, and a potent vasoactive acidic lipid known as slow-reacting substance of anaphylaxis (SRS-A). There is also released a factor that is chemotactic for eosinophils, eosinophil chemotactic factor (ECF-A). The vasoactive factors cause an increase in blood flow and increase in capillary permeability, resulting in marked local edema of the tissues. These factors also cause constriction of smooth muscles, especially of bronchi and bronchioles, and stimulate secretions of mucous glands. These varied effects account for the sudden tissue changes characteristic of local and systemic anaphylactic reactions (Fig. 5-1).

The particular tissue site of reaction depends on the portal of entry (route of exposure) of the allergen. Allergens which are inhaled make contact with mast cells by crossing the mucous membranes of the nose and sinuses and lower respiratory tract. The local effects in those tissues are characterized by a marked increase in mucus secretion, with congestion and edema of the mucous membranes. The effect on bronchi and bronchiolar smooth muscle causes constriction with impairment of air flow, severely restricting pulmonary exchange and usually associated with the

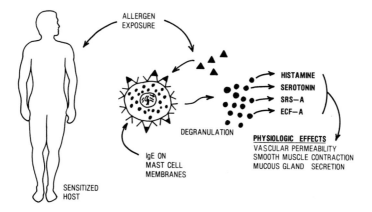

PATHOGENIC EVENTS IN ANAPHYLAXIS

Figure 5–1

sudden onset of wheezing respirations. Clinical problems such as chronic sinusitis and rhinitis as well as acute chronic and bronchial asthma are representative of anaphylactic hypersensitivity disorders.

The ingestion of allergens in food substances or oral medications can cause local and diffuse reactions in the gastrointestinal tract. Such exposure may produce symptoms of acute onset, commonly in the form of intestinal hypermotility, dyspepsia, colicky pain, and a sensation of fullness and bloating. These symptoms occur because of the local release of the pharmacologic mediators by the immune reaction along the submucosa of the gastrointestinal tract. Allergens may also be absorbed into the circulation from the gastrointestinal tract and disseminate throughout the body, resulting in generalized systemic reactions and/or localized reactions in the skin and viscera. In the skin, the acute reactions can present as edematous papules or larger urticarial lesions. Chronic skin reactions often occur in the form of maculopapular rashes and eczema. Acute systemic reactions can occur following the injection of an allergen, such as a drug or vaccine, in individuals with marked sensitivity. The condition of acute anaphylaxis can lead to shock, respiratory insufficiency, and death unless there is immediate treatment. Such profound systemic reaction is due to the massive intravascular release of pharmacologic mediators from the circulating basophils. The beta-adrenergic agent, epinephrine, must be administered quickly after the onset of symptoms to prevent death.

Because such disorders are common, they should always be suspected when there is a clinical history of a recurrent symptom complex or a chronic persistent disorder with intermittent episodes of acute severity. Such individuals will often have high serum levels of IgE related to their increased IgE response. In the U.S., normal levels of serum IgE range around 100 ng./dl., but in sensitive individuals levels in excess of 700 to 1000 ng./dl. are not uncommon. Sensitivity to specific allergens usually is detected by skin test reactivity to small doses of the allergen or by measurement of IgE reactive with specific allergens by a laboratory technique called RAST and PRIST procedures. Identification of sensitivity to certain allergens can be followed by immunotherapy and other measures to control the severity of the reactions.

COMPLEMENT-DEPENDENT INJURY

Another major type of antibody-mediated immunologic injury is that involving activation of the complement system as an effector. This form of injury follows immune reactions of antigen and antibody where the antibody is of the IgG or IgM class. These are the only two classes of immunoglobulins that activate the complement system as immune reactants. Immune complexes formed by IgG, IgA, and IgD do not exhibit complement activating effects, and, indeed, among the four sub-classes of IgG, only sub-classes IgG-1 and IgG-3 exhibit substantial complement activation.

The conditions of sensitivity in complement-dependent disorders are that the individual has been exposed to the antigen previously and has produced an antibody response of IgM and/or IgG. Subsequent exposure to the reactive antigen then results in immune complex formation which initiates activation of the complement system. The antigens in this form of hypersensitivity are often from infections with microorganisms, such as bacteria, fungi, and viruses; from injections or inoculations in the course of immunization or blood transfusion; or from drug therapy.

The steps in the activation of the complement

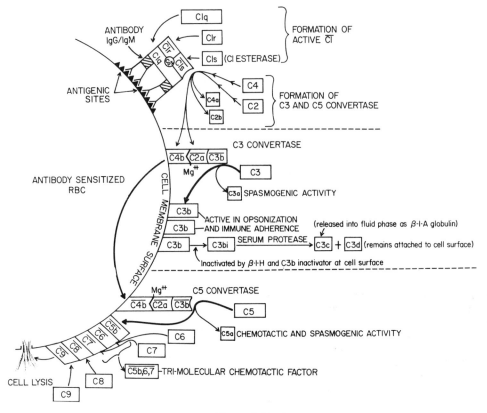

CLASSICAL PATHWAY OF COMPLEMENT ACTIVATION

Figure 5–2

system initiated by such immune reactions are called the classical pathway of complement activation. This sequence of steps is illustrated in Figure 5–2. The classical complement pathway will be contrasted with the alternative pathway which involves non-immune activation of the complement and serum properdin systems, illustrated in Figure 5–3.

In the classical pathway, the immune complex formed must be of a certain physical size that provides a macromolecular surface upon which the activation (fixation) of the components can occur. A system usually employed for complement assays is sheep erythrocytes sensitized with an IgM rabbit antibody (hemolysin) to which is added a source of complement, usually human serum. The immune reactants "fix" along the cell membrane, which provides the structural surface upon which activation occurs. As a result of binding to antigen, there is a steric change in the antibody molecules which exposes hidden structural sites in the Fc portion of the molecules to which attaches the initial reacting component of complement, Clq. It has been shown that binding of a single molecule of IgM, because of its poly-

meric structure, or two closely adjacent molecules of IgG will provide the binding site for Clq. Following the attachment of Clq, the rest of all the eleven proteins that comprise the nine components of the complement system become sequentially activated. At different steps in the activation sequence, molecular fragments are generated that exhibit a variety of biologic activities. These play a major role as mediators of the tissue effects of these reactions.

Following binding of Clq, activation of Clr and Cls occurs which, in the presence of calcium, forms a trimolecular complex designated altogether as the *activated $\overline{C1}$ complex*. The esterase activity of C1 shows a specific substrate affinity for components C2 and C4. Each of these components is cleaved by C1 esterase, each yielding two fragments, designated a and b. The 4b fragment combines with the 2a fragment in the presence of magnesium and binds to other sites on the cell membrane. This enzymatic complex is called C3 convertase ($\overline{C4b2a}$). It has enzymatic activity which cleaves C3, yielding fragments C3b and a small peptide fragment known as C3a. The C3b fragment may then bind to specific receptors at

MODES OF ALTERNATIVE PATHWAY ACTIVATION AND SUPPRESSION

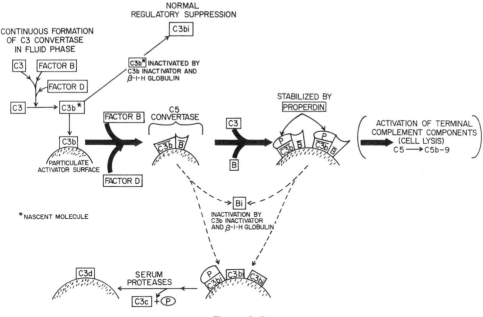

Figure 5–3

other sites on the cell membrane, where it shows biologic activities such as immune adherence and opsonization for phagocytosis.

The residual C3b molecules remain with the C4b2a complex to form a trimolecular enzyme called C5 convertase ($\overline{C4b2a3b}$) with high substrate affinity for complement component C5. C3b is also a link between the classical and alternative pathways of complement activation. As we will see later, it also participates in activation of the alternative pathway sequence. The C3a fragment is released into the fluid phase and exhibits an activity designated as spasmogenic. This describes its pharmacologic activity of causing smooth muscle contraction through the release of granule factors from basophils and mast cells. Previously this fragment was thought to have chemotactic activity, but recent studies have shown that activity only with the C5a cleavage fragment, which is produced later in the activation sequence.

The trimolecular C5 Convertase ($\overline{C4b2a3b}$) cleaves C5 into a and b fragments. The C5a fragment is released into the fluid phase, and it shows both chemotactic and spasmogenic activities as previously mentioned. The C5b fragment attaches to the cell membrane, providing a point for subsequent attachment to the remainder of the terminal components of the complement system, C6, C7, C8, and C9. This terminal assembly leads to cell membrane disequilibrium, resulting in hemolysis or breakdown of the lipoprotein membrane. As a transient product, the trimolecular

complex, C5b,6,7, may dissociate from the cell surface into the fluid phase as another factor chemotactic for neutrophils and monocytes.

Activation of the alternative pathway is illustrated in Figure 5–3 and can be contrasted with the classical pathway. It now appears that there is a continuous ongoing activation of the alternative pathway by the association of complement C3, properdin factor B (C3 proactivator), and properdin factor D (C3 proactivator convertase). This complex produces enzymatic cleavage of C3, yielding a continuous low level production of C3b. The C3b generated in this manner is a nascent molecule with a short life, since it normally is inactivated by the C3b inactivator enhanced by beta-1-H globulin in the blood. However, in the presence of certain types of surfaces, which can be designated as activator surfaces, the nascent C3b molecule becomes bound to the activator surface and is protected from inactivation. On the activator surface, further reaction with factor B and factor D yields an enzymatic complex composed of C3b and activated factor B ($\overline{C3b,B}$) along the surface. This enzymatic complex possesses C5 cleaving activity and is called the C5 convertase of the alternative pathway. As shown in Figure 5–3, this convertase can be stabilized by the molecule, properdin. It acts as the trigger molecule for activating the terminal complement components just as in the classic pathway leading to cell lysis or disruption of the lipoprotein membrane surface of the activator.

The extent of activation of the alternative

pathway is limited by the access of C3b inactivator and beta-1-H globulin to C3b molecules on the surface. On certain surfaces, the integrity of the $\overline{C3b,B}$ complex is protected because of restrictions due to the cell surface properties. In other instances where there is no cell surface restriction, the inactivators rapidly cleave C3b and B to inactive molecules, which in turn are further cleaved by serum proteases to inactive polypeptides. In contrast to earlier studies where it seemed that a specific activator triggered activation of the alternative pathway, it now appears that the alternative pathway is continuously activated at a low level and is normally under regulatory suppression by C3b inactivator and beta-1-H globulin. Augmentation occurs in the presence of a particulate activator surface that binds and protects the C3b from the serum inactivators. Surfaces which behave as particulate activators include bacterial cell walls, polysaccharides, aggregated immunoglobulins, and rabbit erythrocytes. Sheep erythrocytes, lacking the restrictive surface properties, are poor activator surfaces for the alternative pathway.

Returning to the specifics of complement-dependent reactions, the pathogenic sequence of immune complex injury is illustrated in Figure 5–4. It can be seen that formation of the immune complex in a sensitized individual is followed by entrapment of the complex in the tissue. This provides the focus for development of the lesion. Complement activation occurs on the immune complex in the tissue, yielding chemotactic factors that specifically attract the neutrophils.

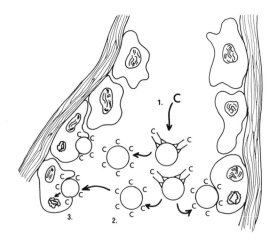

PATHOGENIC SEQUENCE IN COMPLEMENT DEPENDENT CYTOTOXICITY

1. COMPLEMENT ACTIVATION BY ANTIGEN—ANTIBODY REACTIONS ON ERYTHROCYTE SURFACE
2. COMPLEMENT (C3b) ON CELL SURFACE
3. PHAGOCYTOSIS AND INTRACELLULAR DESTRUCTION OF ERYTHROCYTE FACILITATED BY COMPLEMENT (C3b) ON CELL SURFACES

Figure 5–5

Once in the tissue, the neutrophils release destructive hydrolytic enzymes from their lysosomal granules. The degradative action of these enzymes produces the necrotic destructive lesion at the site of immune complex localization. Some examples of disseminated immune complex disease in humans include systemic lupus erythematosus, various forms of acute and chronic glomerulonephritis, polyarteritis nodosa, and disorders associated with a variety of infectious and neoplastic diseases.

Another second type of complement-dependent cell destruction occurs due to immune adherence. When there is immune activation of complement along a cell surface which generates abundant C3b, the C3b molecules attach to the cell surface. They act as specific receptors which facilitate rapid phagocytic clearance of the coated cells from the circulation by the phenomenon described as immune adherence. This causes the C3b covered cells to attach to receptors on reticuloendothelial cells as shown in Figure 5–5. Phagocytosis occurs and is followed by intracellular destruction of the engulfed cell or particle. When the cells affected are erythrocytes, chronic severe reactions of this type can lead to profound anemia and are incorrectly termed hemolytic. "Phagocytic anemia" would be a more appropriate diagnostic term. If leukocytes or platelets are the target cells, they are cleared from the circulation in a similar manner. Commonly these reactions are due to an immune reaction with antigens intrinsic to or linked to the cell surface.

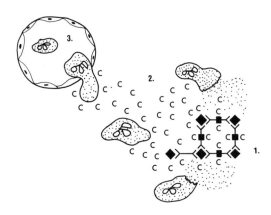

IMMUNE COMPLEX TISSUE INJURY PATHOGENIC SEQUENCE:

1. COMPLEMENT ACTIVATION BY ANTIGEN—ANTIBODY COMPLEX LODGED IN TISSUE
2. COMPLEMENT CHEMOTAXIS OF NEUTROPHILS INTO TISSUE SITE OF IMMUNE REACTION WITH RELEASE OF DESTRUCTIVE LYSOSOMAL ENZYMES
3. MIGRATION OF NEUTROPHIL FROM BLOOD VESSEL DUE TO CHEMOATTRACTION

Figure 5–4

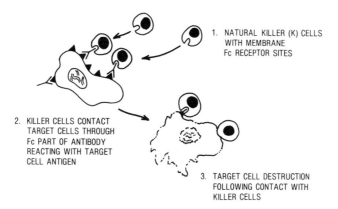

1. NATURAL KILLER (K) CELLS
   WITH MEMBRANE
   Fc RECEPTOR SITES

2. KILLER CELLS CONTACT
   TARGET CELLS THROUGH
   Fc PART OF ANTIBODY
   REACTING WITH TARGET
   CELL ANTIGEN

3. TARGET CELL DESTRUCTION
   FOLLOWING CONTACT WITH
   KILLER CELLS

MECHANISM OF ANTIBODY DEPENDENT
KILLER (K) CELL DESTRUCTION OF TARGET CELL

Figure 5–6

ANTIBODY-MEDIATED KILLER CELL CYTOTOXICITY

In recent years another mechanism of antibody-dependent cell injury has been described. It is called antibody-dependent cytotoxicity or natural killer (K) cell destruction. The sequence of events in this form of tissue injury is illustrated in Figure 5–6. It can be seen that a target cell which possesses antigens along the cell surface, either as part of the cell membrane or linked to the cell membrane, can bind antibody through the Fab region along the surface. Following this, the small mononuclear (natural killer) cells of the circulation which have a receptor site for the Fc portion of IgG come close to the antibody-coated target cell and contact the cell by receptor binding with the Fc portion of the antibody molecules. This cell contact then is followed by release of a biochemical factor that kills the target cell, which undergoes fragmentation and dissolution. In this reaction, the specificity derives from the antigen-antibody reaction, whereas the killer cell (K cell) effect is essentially non-specific. It is attracted to the target antigens by reaction of its Fc receptor with the antibody molecule bound to cell antigens. This mechanism of destruction appears to be due to release of a biochemical factor via an energy- and calcium-dependent reaction dependent on microtubule function in the K cell.

As a mode of tissue injury, these K cell reactions appear to be of importance in conditions where cells develop virus-associated, drug induced or tumor-associated antigens closely linked to HL-A antigens on the cell membranes. It also promises to provide the basis for an important therapeutic approach to the specific immunologic treatment of neoplasms.

T-CELL REACTIONS— GRANULOMATOUS INJURY

The forms of immune injury so far discussed have involved reactions of antigen with antibody, a product of B-cells. We will now consider those reactions which are dependent on T-lymphocyte activation and response. T-cells in these reactions serve as both reacting cells and as effector cells.

In the type of T-cell-dependent reaction resulting in the formation of a granuloma, the T-cell reacts with the stimulating antigen through specific receptors on the cell surface. Consequent to this contact, the T-lymphocyte is stimulated to increased metabolic activity and exhibits nuclear enlargement with cytoplasmic basophilia, a change described as blast transformation. Along with the increased metabolic activity there is production of many soluble biochemical factors that cause certain physiologic and biologic effects (Fig. 5–7). These factors are called *lymphokines*, and they are the primary mediators of this reaction sequence. Their activities include stimulation and activation of blood monocytes, causing their transformation to macrophages, a chemotactic effect on monocytes to specifically attract them into tissue, and a migration inhibition effect which limits motility of monocytes and macrophages once they have arrived at the tissue site. These lymphokines mediate the cellular events which produce a characteristic histopathologic lesion known as a granuloma. This sequence of events is illustrated in Figure 5–8. It shows diagrammatically the initial contact of effector T-lymphocyte with antigen, followed by synthesis and release of lymphokines, then by recruitment of monocytes from the circulation due to the chemotactic effect of the lymphokines, and finally transformation of monocytes into macrophages

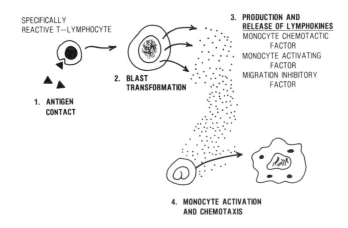

SPECIFICALLY
REACTIVE T—LYMPHOCYTE

3. **PRODUCTION AND**
   RELEASE OF LYMPHOKINES
   MONOCYTE CHEMOTACTIC
   FACTOR
   MONOCYTE ACTIVATING
   FACTOR
   MIGRATION INHIBITORY
   FACTOR

2. **BLAST**
   TRANSFORMATION

1. **ANTIGEN**
   CONTACT

4. **MONOCYTE ACTIVATION**
   AND CHEMOTAXIS

EVENTS OF T—LYMPHOCYTE DEPENDENT
REACTION FOLLOWING ANTIGEN CONTACT

Figure 5–7

with increased activity in cytoplasmic digestive vacuoles. Often, the individual macrophages cluster and fuse around a central site of antigen concentration, which may show focal necrotic change due to leakage of proteolytic enzymes. These events give rise to the typical appearance of a granuloma, with multinucleate giant cells surrounding a central area of necrotic change bounded by a mantle of mononuclear cells. Such a necrotic or cellular granuloma is a characteristic lesion of delayed hypersensitivity reactions. It is often observed in certain infectious diseases where there is antigen persistence with marked

T-cell reactivity, as in tuberculosis and in fungus and viral infections.

T-LYMPHOCYTE CYTOTOXICITY REACTION

A variant of immune injury produced by T-lymphocytes in a role as effector cells is called cytotoxic or killer (K) cell infiltrative reactions. This type occurs as a result of contact by the effector lymphocyte with histocompatibility-linked antigens on the surface of target cells. The sequence of events is illustrated in Figure 5–9.

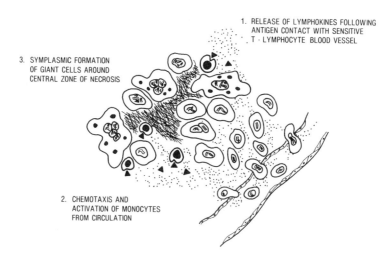

1. RELEASE OF LYMPHOKINES FOLLOWING
   ANTIGEN CONTACT WITH SENSITIVE
   T - LYMPHOCYTE BLOOD VESSEL

3. SYMPLASMIC FORMATION
   OF GIANT CELLS AROUND
   CENTRAL ZONE OF NECROSIS

2. CHEMOTAXIS AND
   ACTIVATION OF MONOCYTES
   FROM CIRCULATION

EVENTS IN THE DEVELOPMENT OF T—LYMPHOCYTE
DEPENDENT HYPERSENSITIVITY GRANULOMATOUS LESION

Figure 5–8

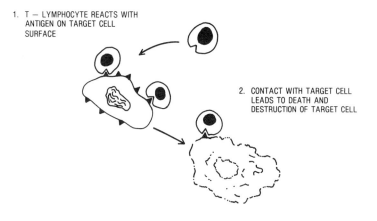

1. T — LYMPHOCYTE REACTS WITH
   ANTIGEN ON TARGET CELL
   SURFACE

2. CONTACT WITH TARGET CELL
   LEADS TO DEATH AND
   DESTRUCTION OF TARGET CELL

EVENTS IN CYTOTOXIC T—LYMPHOCYTE REACTION

Figure 5–9

Cell contact of the T-lymphocyte produces killing through a mechanism similar to that discussed above under antibody-dependent natural killer cell cytotoxicity. The principal difference in the mechanism is that the T-cell contacts the antigen directly, rather than through antibody linkage as in that form of injury. The killing effect appears to be due to release of a biochemical factor from the T-lymphocyte. It is energy-dependent and related to the integrity of microtubule function of the killer T-cell. Close contact with the target cell appears necessary to initiate the killing reaction. Some examples of such tissue reactions in human disease are the acute phase of homograft rejection, autoimmune tissue lesions, viral infections, and some forms of dermatitis.

Both the granulomatous and cytotoxic forms of T-cell reactivity can occur together, although one usually predominates as the primary form of the reaction. The site of lesions in these immunologic diseases as well as others depends on the localization of the immune reactants. This is usually determined by the portal of entry of the antigen, which often induces a local tissue reaction limited to the entry site or which also enters the circulation and becomes widely disseminated, with lesions throughout the body. The potential for dissemination of the reaction gives many variations of clinical patterns in immunologic disease. These patterns may vary considerably, even though there is a final common sequence of injury.

AUTOIMMUNITY

DEFINITIONS

Autoimmunity can be defined as a failure of an organism to recognize its own tissue, and includes any immune response to the host's own tissue, whether it is humoral (e.g., circulating autoantibodies) or cellular (e.g., delayed hypersensitivity). Autoimmunity is a concept which may explain the pathogenesis of a number of diseases and is a major immunologic phenomenon in clinical medicine.

The body is endowed with mechanisms to distinguish self from non-self. However, as discussed below, there are many pathways for the breakdown of the control mechanisms underlying self-recognition. Such breakdowns result in an autoimmune response. Autoantibodies which react with the tissue antigens of the host may or may not cause tissue injury and produce disease. The term "autoimmune disease" has been generally assigned to those conditions in which an immune mechanism of injury has contributed to the pathogenesis of the disease. In certain of the diseases, such as organ-specific autoimmune thyroiditis, the autoimmune response is the major factor in initiating the tissue injury. However, there are many other diseases in which the immunologic response is notably secondary to the initial tissue injury. Detection of autoantibodies may be of equal value in the diagnosis of the latter group of diseases. Autoimmunity may play a role in a wide range of clinical situations, including aging, response to viral and other microbial infections, organ-specific immunologic diseases, and generalized systemic immunologic diseases such as systemic lupus erythematosus.

The term autoallergic is often used interchangeably with autoimmune. The term allergy was originated by von Pirquet in 1906 to describe an altered reaction to repeated injections of heterologous gamma globulin to diphtheria toxin. Thus, allergy is often used to mean harmful altered reactions secondary to immune mechanisms. Today, the term allergy is most commonly applied to diseases characterized by hypersensitivity reactions, such as hay fever and asthma, which are mediated by cytophilic IgE antibodies. Hypersensitivity has been used to describe immune reactions similar to allergy and also to describe nonimmunologic reactions, such as nonimmune hypersensitivity to drugs.

Autoimmunity which is observed in clinical and experimental circumstances can be defined as an apparent termination of the natural unresponsive state to self. Immunologic tolerance is the result of an active physiologic process and is not simply the lack of immune response. There are two types of immunologic tolerance. One results in a central unresponsive state characterized by an irreversible loss of competent lymphocytes; the other is a peripheral inhibition, where competent cells are present but are suppressed. A definition of unresponsiveness is the inability to make a detectable immune response to an antigenic challenge, as distinguished from so-called tolerance, which is a term commonly used in transplantation immunology in addition to nonimmunologic events to describe endurance without ill-effects of substances such as endotoxins or a drug. However, for the purposes of this chapter, the terms unresponsiveness and tolerance will be used interchangeably, since the discussion will be confined to immune mechanisms.

CONCEPT OF UNRESPONSIVE STATE OR TOLERANCE AND RELATION TO AUTOIMMUNITY

Currently it is believed that a person becomes unresponsive to his own tissue antigens during fetal development and that the natural unresponsive state develops as a result of direct contact between the self-constituents and receptor sites on the surface of lymphocytes reactive to these antigens. This is a phenomenon which was first predicted by Burnet, who developed the clonal selection theory, which proposed that the contact of antibody-forming cells with their respective antigens during fetal or early postnatal life led to destruction or inactivation with elimination of the corresponding clones. Since then, many investigators have artificially induced an unresponsive state to a wide variety of antigens during the newborn period when an immature immune system was present.

The mode of induction of the natural unresponsive state is probably by two mechanisms: (a) the clones are immunocompetent cells capable of reacting to self-antigens and are eliminated by a mechanism of the clonal theory of Burnet; and (b) antigen-producing cells are made unresponsive by early exposure to self-antigen. The clonal selection theory was not easily reconciled with the observations on the experimental induction of autoimmunity. Weigle and co-workers have shown that injections of cross reacting thyroglobulins of other species in the absence of adjuvant elicited formation of autoantibodies against thyroglobulin and experimental thyroiditis. It became clear that the T- and B-cells interact in the production of autoantibodies and that the mechanisms of induction of the unresponsive state at the cellular level of the T- and B-cells are different.

In the cellular aspects of unresponsiveness, the cells involved are macrophages, B-cells, T-cells, and antibody-producing B-cells from the bone marrow. The evidence for direct cooperation between the T- and B- lymphocytes is well confirmed. When specific antigen-sensitive cells interact for production of antibodies, specifically reactive T-cells and B-cells must both interact. Although macrophages play a major role in the establishment of the unresponsiveness, they appear to be non-specific and under genetic control.

Both T- and B-lymphocytes can become unresponsive or tolerant. However, the kinetics of tolerance in these two lymphocyte populations differ greatly. Many autoantigens, such as thyroglobulin, protein hormones, and solubilized membrane antigens, circulate in limited concentrations in the body fluids. With limited concentrations of these self-components, the unresponsive state is maintained only in the T-cells, not in the B-cells. The natural unresponsive state is maintained to antigens such as native thyroglobulin because of the lack of T-cell helper signal, and autoantibody production is *not* initiated (Fig. 5–10).

On the other hand, high doses of antigen can induce unresponsiveness in both T- and B-lymphocytes. This was shown experimentally with injection of human gamma globulin in mice. Experiments in mice have shown that thymocytes become tolerant to human gamma globulin within 24 hours of exposure and that this tolerance lasts for 100 days. By contrast, B-cell tolerance requires an induction period between 15 and 21 days. The long latent period between exposure and tolerance to human gamma globulin in mice may indicate a relative resistance of the bone marrow cells to tolerance or a requirement for thymic cell–bone marrow interaction before tolerance can be induced. Even with high doses of antigen, the unresponsive state of B-lymphocytes is often incomplete, and some antibody of low affinity can still be formed. In the case of thyroglobulin and the involvement in thyroiditis, only

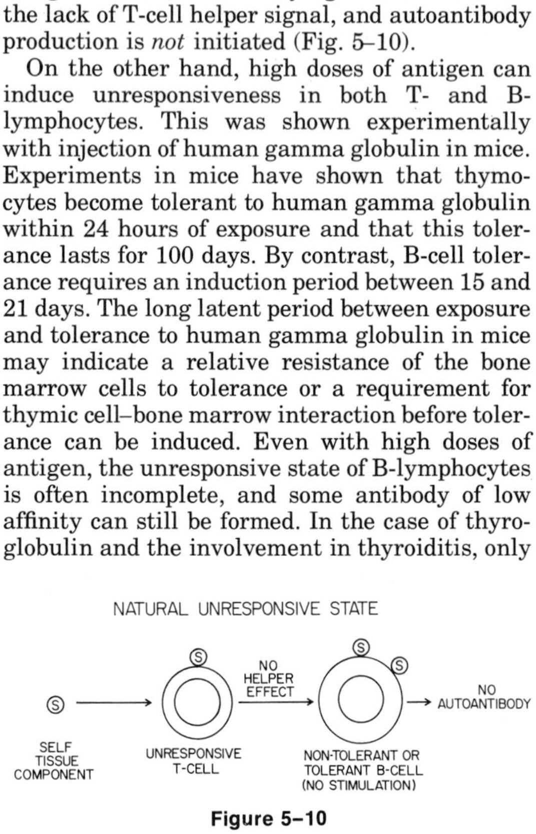

NATURAL UNRESPONSIVE STATE

Figure 5–10

the T-lymphocytes may be tolerant, leaving B-lymphocytes able to respond to autoantigens suitably presented to them with T-lymphocyte help. Mechanisms allowing the requirement for specific T-lymphocytes responding to autoantigens to be bypassed are discussed later in this chapter. Tolerance to autoantigen based on the selective unresponsiveness of T-lymphocytes can be easily bypassed by various viral or microbial infections and other events.

In contrast to the unresponsive state to thyroglobulin and thyroiditis, neither T- nor B-cells appear to be unresponsive to basic protein, and specific antigen-binding cells to basic protein were detected in both T- and B-cell populations. By deleting either the T- or B-cells from these populations as specifically-bound basic proteins, it was demonstrated that T-cells, not antibody, were responsible for induction of experimental allergic encephalitis.

Recent studies have demonstrated the existence of antireceptor or anti-idiotypic antibodies, which may arise as a result of various T-cell bypass mechanisms described below. These antireceptor or anti-idiotypic antibodies may block the expression of an immune response and produce a tolerance-like situation to self-antigen. When an animal makes an immune response to a given antigen, autoantibodies directed to the antibody made as the result of the antigenic stimulus also may be produced. The idiotypic determinants characteristic of a given antibody may also be present on lymphocytes with receptor for the antigen. Thus, the autoantibody to the idiotype may block or suppress the immune response to a given antigen, and the loss of the control mechanism could lead to expression of an autoimmune response to self-antigens.

GENETIC FACTORS IN AUTOIMMUNITY

The genetic basis of immunologic regulation is an important area of research today. A group of genes located within the major histocompatibility locus (MHC) play important roles in immunologic regulation. The differences and susceptibility to various viruses and the intensity of the cellular immune response of graft-versus-host reaction is also controlled within the cluster of genes located within the major histocompatibility region. Genetically-determined cell surface antigens termed Ia are important immunologic factors involved in antigen recognition, cellular interaction, and cellular cooperation. Much evidence suggests that genes associated with the major histocompatibility locus in man (HLA) may be important in the immune regulation and in the pathogenesis of autoimmunity. Many autoimmune disorders have been found to be associated with a particular HLA haplotype. The majority of the associations are with the second locus

genes, and this may be close to the immune response (Ir) genes in man. The association of HLA antigens has been found to be marked in cases of ankylosing spondylitis, in which as many as 90 percent of patients are found to possess HLA-B27 antigens. It should be noted that the association does not imply that the disease is caused by possession of the HLA-B27 antigen. Certain autoimmune diseases, particularly the organ-specific disorders, such as idiopathic Addison's disease, Grave's disease, chronic active hepatitis, and Sjögren's syndrome, occur more frequently in individuals who have HLA-B8. Other diseases, such as multiple sclerosis and rheumatoid arthritis, appear to be associated with lymphocyte-defined genetic loci whose products on the cell membranes are responsible for mixed lymphocyte reactivity.

Autoimmunity and autoimmune diseases are frequently associated with genetic and viral factors that interact with the immune system and influence regulation. Genetically-determined lymphocyte membranes in man determine the magnitude of response and mixed lymphocyte reactions, and may be closely associated in the development of autoimmunity. Although the exact mechanisms by which genetic factors and autoimmunity are related are unclear, it is likely that the immune response (Ir) genes, lymphocytic surface antigen, and possible receptors for specific viruses are involved. Viruses and other infectious agents are often associated with autoimmunity. Many virus buds from cell surfaces can incorporate normal membrane constitutents as part of their viral envelope. Such combinations of viral and host tissue antigens may become immunogenic and give rise to autoimmune responses.

GENERAL THEORIES AND MECHANISMS OF AUTOIMMUNITY

Autoimmunity arises when there is a disordered regulation and interaction of T- and B-cells in response to antigenic stimulation. The T- and B-cell interaction may be imbalanced as a consequence of genetic, viral, and environmental mechanisms acting singly or in combination. A central mechanism in this concept involves a disturbance of the delicate balance between the suppressor and helper activity of regulatory T-cells. Either an excess of T-cell activity or a deficiency of suppressor activity could lead to development of autoimmunity. The autoimmune state could probably arise by several mechanisms:(1) A bypass of either T-cell specificity or the need for T-cells in the presence of competent B-cells; (2) a stimulation of competent T-cells and/or B-cells in case of sequestered self-antigens; and (3) a loss of suppressor activity preventing autoantibody to self-antigens. Depending on the disease, any one

TABLE 5–2   TYPES OF REACTIONS INVOLVING BYPASS OF T-CELL
SPECIFICITY IN THE PRESENCE OF COMPETENT B-CELLS

1. Binding of foreign haptens as drugs to host tissue.
2. Infections by viruses and bacteria which alter host autoantigens.
3. Exposure to altered or cross reacting antigens, i.e., enzyme degradation, virus, and bacterial infections
4. Stimulation of competent B-cells by bacterial lipopolysaccharide (LPS).
5. Non-specific stimulation of helper T-cell activity with adjuvant.
6. Graft-versus-host reaction (non-specific stimulation of helper T-cell activity with allogeneic cells).

or combination of these possibilities may play a role involving a host of mediators in the autoimmune state and may result from a humoral response, a cellular response, or a combination of both.

T-Cell Bypass Mechanism of Autoimmunity

Most autoantigens, such as thyroglobulin, protein hormones, and soluble membrane antigen, circulate in very low doses. Prolonged exposure to these would produce selective tolerance in T-lymphocytes, leaving B-lymphocytes able to bind autoantigens and to be stimulated by autoantigens presented to them with appropriate T-lymphocyte help. Under such circumstances, the requirements for T-lymphocytes responding to autoantigenic determinants can be bypassed (Fig. 5–11).

In Figure 5–11 one can note that in the normal state the T-cell is tolerant and the B-cell is competent; no autoantibody is formed because the absence of the T-cell helper signals the presence of the autoantigen. On the other hand, the autoantigens will form immunogenic units with an-

AUTOIMMUNITY FOLLOWING ADMINISTRATION OF DRUG HAPTEN

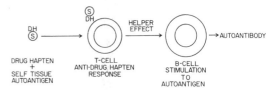

Figure 5–12

tigens that are able to initiate the T-cell helper signal to stimulate the existing immunocompetent B-cell. Among the helper determinants are viruses or bacteria and drugs. Any procedure that non-specifically activates lymphocytes, such as adjuvants or graft-versus-host reaction with allogeneic cells, can stimulate production of autoantibodies by the bypass of T-cell specificity.

The types of autoimmune reactions involving bypass of T-cell specificity in the presence of competent B-cells are listed in Table 5–2.

Autoimmunity Following Administration of Drugs. Some autoimmune manifestations following drug administration are remarkably specific. Thus, in patients treated with alpha methyldopa, Coombs'-positive autoimmune hemolytic anemias are not uncommon. Often the autoantigen in the body is IgG directed against the E antigen of the Rh series. The production of antinuclear factors in a syndrome like systemic lupus erythematosus is relatively frequent in patients treated with procainamide and hydralazine. There often is a coupling of drug or metabolite to an autoantigen which initiates a host T-lymphocyte reaction against the antigenic determinants of the drug; subsequently, autoantibodies are formed through a T-cell helper effect (Fig. 5–12). In some patients, following administration of hydantoin, there is generalized lymphoid hyperplasia and plasmacytosis with production of a variety of antibodies with specificity for erythrocytes. In such cases it is believed that hydantoin derivatives become attached to the surface of lymphoid cells and modify their major histocompatibility antigen complex in such a way that autologous T-lymphocyte recognizes them as foreign and reacts to them. There is also another situation in which nitrofurantoin treatment can

T-CELL BYPASS MECHANISM OF AUTOIMMUNITY

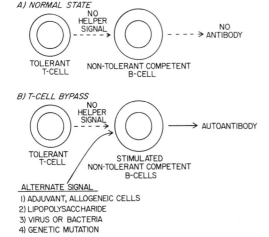

Figure 5–11

result in a wide variety of autoantibodies, including some with specificity for human albumin. A lupus-like syndrome with pulmonary reactions has been described in patients treated with nitrofurantoin.

Virus Infections. Virus infections can elicit autoantibody formation by two mechanisms. First, the viral antigens and autoantigens may become associated to form immunogenic units. Viral antigens stimulating host T-lymphocytes could then function as helper determinants, thereby stimulating B-lymphocyte responses to autoantigens. Second, some viruses such as the Epstein-Barr (EB) virus stimulate proliferation of the B-lymphocyte cell line with autoantibody production. There are two ways in which viral and host antigens can form immunogenic units. Host antigens can be incorporated in the envelopes of some viruses, and viral antigens can appear on the surfaces of infected host cells (Fig. 5–13). The viral antigens also may form complexes with and modify histocompatibility antigens or other membrane constituents such as the contractile protein actin. The modified viral antigens could stimulate T-cell helper effect and elicit autoantibody formation (Fig. 5–14).

In man, infection with viruses such as influenza, measles, varicella, and herpes simplex has often resulted in autoimmune manifestations such as platelet and red cell autoantibodies. The development of cold autoagglutinins after mycoplasma pneumonia infection probably occurs by a T-cell bypass mechanism. Following infectious mononucleosis, many patients' sera often react against several autoantigens. These include autoantibodies against nuclei, lymphocytes, erythrocytes, and smooth muscle. In addition, cross reactive heterophile antibodies may be noted following infectious mononucleosis and

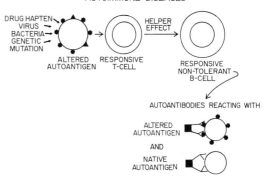

AUTOANTIBODY FORMATION IN CERTAIN ORGAN SPECIFIC AUTOIMMUNE DISEASES

Figure 5–14

other infections. The autoantibody is produced by a mechanism similar to that observed in altered self-component with virus or bacteria.

There has been much speculation about the possibility of an oncornavirus being involved in the pathogenesis of human systemic lupus erythematosus.

Degradation and Alteration of Autoantigens. Tissue damage with alteration of host antigens may play a role in eliciting autoimmune reactions. Partial degradation can expose antigenic determinants that are not available in the native molecules, and these can react with T-lymphocytes to induce autoimmunity. Many bacterial, viral, and parasitic infections are associated with transient positive tests for antiglobulin of the rheumatoid factor type, and among the underlying mechanisms are either partial degradation or alteration of immunoglobulin.

Adjuvant and Bacterial Infections. Immunologic adjuvants are non-specific B-lymphocyte stimulators, such as lipopolysaccharide or purified protein derivatives (Fig. 5–15). These immunologic adjuvants may induce autoimmune responses. It is possible that infections such as pertussis or other bacterial infections with liberation of products with adjuvant activities could produce polyclonal lymphocyte activation and autoimmunity. In rheumatic fever there is cross reaction of some determinants of the organism with the host tissue. Other determinants of the same molecule or complexes could be recognized by host T-lymphocytes and function as helper determi-

INTERACTION OF VIRUS, VIRAL ANTIGENS AND SELF-TISSUE ANTIGENS TO FORM IMMUNOGENIC UNITS

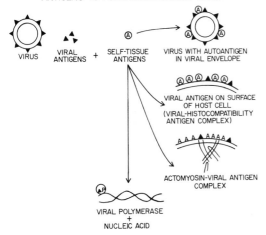

Figure 5–13

AUTOIMMUNITY FOLLOWING ADJUVANT AND ALLOGENEIC CELL STIMULATION

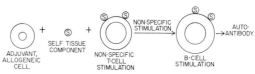

Figure 5–15

nants. Antibody to cardiolipin and cold autoantibodies to erythrocytes in syphilis and antibody to myocardial antigens in rheumatic fever can result from chronic infections or repeated injections of bacteria.

Graft-versus-host Reaction (Allogeneic Cells). The primary event in graft-versus-host reaction (GVH) is the response of donor T-lymphocytes to the major histocompatibility complex on lymphoid and hematopoietic cells of the recipient. A major effect is the stimulation of lymphoid tissue in the recipient, with development of lymphoreticular hyperplasia with germinal center enlargement and plasmacytosis. There is proliferation of recipient B-lymphocytes under the influence of a donor T-lymphocyte signal (Fig. 5–15).

In a normal person, autoantibody formation does not occur because T-lymphocytes are unable to react to autoantigens. However, when lymphocytes are non-specifically stimulated, as in the graft-versus-host reaction, there is an allogeneic effect leading to the production of antibodies which normally require T-lymphocyte help (Fig. 5–15). In this mechanism, the need for carrier-specific T-lymphocytes in the immune response can be bypassed; hence, the graft-versus-host reaction results in the formation of autoantibodies. This mechanism has been shown to result in autoantibodies in various experimental animal models such as glomerulonephritis and Coombs'-positive autoimmune hemolytic anemia.

Autoimmune Thyroiditis and Organ-specific Autoimmune Diseases. The classic example of the mechanism of T-cell specificity bypass mechanism is thyroiditis. Overwhelming evidence in studies of experimental thyroiditis as well as human thyroiditis has shown that the major factor in intiating tissue injury is the humoral autoantibody response.

It was previously thought that thyroglobulin was a sequestered antigen; however, various experiments subsequently showed that thyroglobulin was a semi-sequestered antigen present in the circulation in very small amounts after birth and that it was able to equilibrate between the intra- and extravascular compartments. In these organs, which are frequently associated with autoimmune diseases, it is felt that extremely low concentrations of self-antigen, such as thyroglobulin, are in circulation and that these concentrations are sufficient to maintain tolerance only at the level of the T-cells, not at the level of the B- or bone marrow cells. This is not a completely healthy condition since the unresponsiveness at the thymus level is adequate to inhibit any antibody response; however, it superimposes upon this a situation such as virus transformation or genetic mutation. This permits the thymus cells to react with the altered portion, the self-antigen, and the interaction takes place with the immuno-

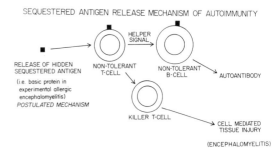

Figure 5–16

competent bone marrow cells, and the autoimmune process is initiated (Fig 5–14).

The mechanism involved in thyroiditis may operate in the organ-specific diseases such as primary adrenal gland atrophy, parathyroid hypoplasia, primary ovarian atrophy, etc. These organs release extremely small concentrations of self-antigens during the development of the natural unresponsive state, and tolerance is developed at the T-cell level and not at the B-cell level.

Sequestered Antigen Release Mechanism of Autoimmunity

It was formerly believed that many autoantigens are secluded from immunocompetent cells in the body; however, many antigens formerly thought to be secluded such as thyroglobulin protein hormones, now are known to circulate in small amounts — approximately 100 nanograms/ml. in the case of thyroglobulin. Cell membrane constituents such as major histocompatibility antigens are likewise known to circulate in low doses. However, there may well be segregation of some antigens in normal persons. An example is the ocular lens, which is segregated from blood vessels and lymphatics; its constituents do not normally elicit immune responses. The basic protein of myelin probably is effectively secluded from immunocompetent cells. In normal human adults neither T- nor B-cells appear to be tolerant to basic protein, and specific binding cells to basic protein can be detected in both T- and B-cells. This can explain the observation that T-cells and the cellular (delayed sensitivity) mechanism are the primary mechanism of injury in experimental allergic encephalitis (Fig. 5–16).

Loss of Suppressor Cell Activity in Autoimmunity

Several investigators have hypothesized that T-cells are involved in controlling B-cells by suppressing B-cell-dependent synthesis of autoantibody. As shown in Figure 5–17, the T-lymphocytes can inhibit autoimmune responses

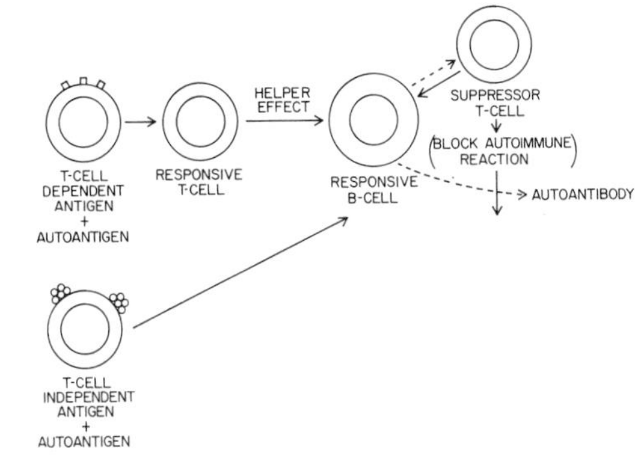

SUPPRESSOR T-CELLS IN THE PREVENTION OF AUTOIMMUNE REACTIONS

Figure 5-17

and provide a general mechanism for preventing or delaying them. Evidence has accumulated that the population of T-lymphocytes with suppressors and helper effects is distinct. The major evidence for suppressor control is that antibody is made at a fairly steady rate that is not influenced by injecting more antigen; injection of antilymphocyte serum causes a large temporary rise in the number of autoantibody secreting cells, and tolerance to many self-components may be maintained by active suppressor mechanisms.

With a loss of suppressor cell activity by aging, immune deficiency syndromes (i.e., thymic hypoplasia), or by other disease mechanisms, the self-reactive B-cells are permitted to proliferate, with resultant production of autoantibody and autoreactive lymphocytes (Fig. 5-18).

Experimental evidence to support the concept of loss of suppressor T-cell activity in development of autoimmune reactions is as follows: (1) Following early thymectomy, a strain of leghorn chickens developed a form of autoimmune thyroiditis more severe than that which occurs spontaneously (2) Spleen cells from old New Zealand Black mice (NZB) when transplanted to young NZB mice depleted of T-cells by antilymphocyte serum will

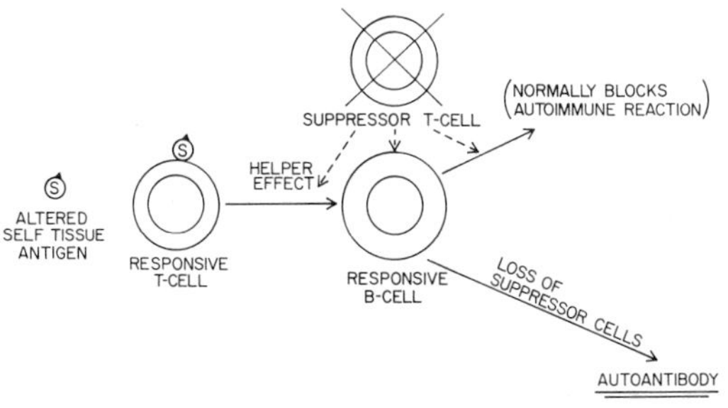

Figure 5-18

induce a persistent Coombs'-positive hemolytic anemia.

SUMMARY OF MECHANISMS OF AUTOIMMUNITY

One can see that numerous mechanisms may initiate an autoimmune response. The autoimmune reaction is the result of disruption of the normal pathways of interaction of T- and B-cells with autoantigens. Autoimmunity may arise whenever there is a state of immunologic imbalance in which B-cell activity is excessive and suppressor T-cell activity is diminished. This imbalance may occur as a consequence of genetic, viral, and environmental mechanisms acting singly or in combination. Manipulation of autoantigens in a way to stimulate helper T-functions, such as the use of adjuvants, immunogenic carriers, or cross reactive antigens, also induces the autoimmune phenomenon. Furthermore the decrease in normal suppressor cell activity caused by aging, cancer, or by other disease mechanisms, may permit self-reactive cells to proliferate, resulting in the production of autoantibody and autoreactive lymphocytes.

CLASSIFICATION AND EVALUATION OF AUTOIMMUNE DISEASES

Classification of Human Autoimmune Diseases

The autoimmune disorders can be broadly separated into three main groups: organ-specific, non-organ-specific, and diseases with non-organ-specific autoantibodies but with lesions restricted to one or only a few organs (Table 5-3).

Organ-specific Autoimmune Diseases. These disorders are characterized by chronic inflammatory changes in a specific organ. The autoantibodies in this group of diseases exhibit specificity for antigens of the diseased organ. Such autoantibodies may demonstrate species specificity, and familial clustering of diseases within this group occurs with remarkable frequency. Examples of this group are: (1) Hashimoto's autoimmune thyroiditis; (2) primary hypothyroidism; (3) thyrotoxicosis (Grave's diseases); (4) chronic atrophic gastritis; (5) primary adrenal atrophy; (6) post-rabies vaccination encephalomyelitis; and (7) autoimmune hemolytic anemia.

The pathogenic mechanism in autoimmune thyroiditis probably involves a bypass of T-cell specificity to initiate production of autoantibodies. It has been postulated that a deficiency in T-cells may be the key factor in initiating the whole process, and ultimately all categories of cells may be involved.

In thyrotoxicosis, there is human thyroid-

TABLE 5-3   ANTIBODIES IN VARIOUS AUTOIMMUNE DISEASES*

Diseases	Antigen Involved	Methods for Detection of Antibody
Organ-Specific, Endocrine Autoimmune thyroiditis, primary myxedema, thyrotoxicosis	Thyroglobulin	Immunofluorescent test (IFT) (indirect)—methanol-fixed human thyroid Passive hemagglutination Latex agglutination
	Cytoplasmic microsome	IFT (indirect)—unfixed human hyperplastic thyroid tissue Passive hemagglutination Complement fixation
Thyrotoxicosis	Thyroid cell surface antigen	Bioassay—mouse thyroid stimulation in vivo Radioimmunoassay with inhibition of TSH on human thyroid tissue receptor
Addison's disease	Adrenal cell cytoplasm	IFT (indirect) on unfixed human adrenal cortex
Parathyroid	Parathyroid cytoplasmic antigen	IFT (indirect) human parathyroid gland
Early-onset diabetes	Islet cell	IFT on human or guinea pig pancreas
Non-Organ-Specific Diseases Lupus erythematosus	Nuclear antigens	
Dermatomyositis		
Periarteritis nodosa		
Scleroderma		
Rheumatoid arthritis	Altered gamma globulin	Latex agglutination (rheumatoid factor) Rose test, sheep cell agglutination
	Rheumatoid arthritis precipitin	Immunodiffusion
Sjögren's syndrome		
Polymyositis		
Other collagen diseases		
"Autoimmune" liver diseases		

*(From Nakamura, R. M., and Tucker, E. S.: *In* Henry, J. B. [Ed.]: Clinical Diagnosis by Laboratory Methods, 16th edition. W. B. Saunders Company, Philadelphia, 1978, Chap. 35.)

TABLE 5–3 ANTIBODIES IN VARIOUS AUTOIMMUNE DISEASES (*Continued*)

Diseases	*Antigen Involved*	*Methods for Detection of Antibody*
Alimentary Tract Diseases		
Atrophic gastritis	Parietal cell microsomes	IFT (indirect) — human or mouse gastric mucosa substrate
Pernicious anemia	Intrinsic factor	Radioactive vitamin B_{12} binding assay
Sjögren's syndrome	Salivary duct cells	IFT (indirect) — unfixed human salivary gland
Ulcerative colitis	Colon, lipopoly-saccharide	IFT (indirect) — human or rat colon
Celiac disease	Reticulin	IFT (indirect) — rat kidney, liver
Crohn's disease	Reticulin	IFT (indirect) — rat kidney, liver
Liver Diseases		
Chronic aggressive hepatitis	Smooth muscle (actin)	IFT (indirect) — rat gastric mucosa, human cervical tissue
	Liver/kidney microsomal	IFT (indirect) — rat kidney and liver
Primary biliary cirrhosis	Mitochondrial	IFT (indirect) — rat kidney, unfixed
Other		
Myasthenia gravis	Skeletal or heart muscle	IFT (indirect) — rat skeletal muscle and calf thymus
	Acetylcholine receptor	Radioimmunoassay
Goodpasture's syndrome	Glomerular and lung basement membrane	IFT (direct) — biopsy of patient's kidney IFT (indirect) — patient's serum on human kidney substrate Radioimmunoassay on serum
Pemphigus vulgaris	Prickle cell desmosomes	IFT (direct and indirect) — human skin Peroxidase-labeled antibody
Bullous pemphigoid	Epithelial base-ment membrane	IFT (direct and indirect) — human skin Peroxidase-labeled antibody
Cicatricial pemphigoid	Epithelial base-ment membrane	IFT (direct) on biopsy of mucous membrane — indirect on human skin
Dermatitis herpetiformis	Reticulin	IFT (indirect) — rat kidney, liver
Autoimmune hemolytic anemia	Red cell	Coombs' antiglobulin test (direct and indirect)
Central nervous system		
Demyelinating diseases (i.e., multiple sclerosis)	Myelin	IFT (indirect) — mammalian spinal cord

stimulating immunoglobulin which is probably an anti-TSH receptor with a thyroid stimulating activity that acts longer than TSH. These antibodies can be either human-specific or cross reactive with other species, and they closely mimic TSH. The thyroid stimulating antibodies initiate the transduction process which results in stimulation of adenyl cyclase with increased thyroid hormone release.

Non-organ-specific Autoimmune Diseases. These diseases are characterized by widespread pathologic changes in many different organs and tissues throughout the body. Furthermore, the associated serum autoantibodies often lack organ and species specificity, and experimental lesions are not readily produced; however, similar diseases arise spontaneously in certain inbred animal strains. Examples of this group are: (1) systemic lupus erythematosus; (2) rheumatoid arthritis; and (3) various other connective tissue disorders such as progressive systemic sclerosis (scleroderma).

In the group of non-organ-specific autoimmune diseases, the primary mechanism of injury is by immune complexes. In systemic lupus erythematosus, the pathogenic complex is the DNA-anti-DNA complex. The factors involved in production of anti-DNA antibody are probably complex, with an abnormal imbalance and interaction of viral and genetic and immunologic factors.

Disorders with Non-organ-specific Autoantibodies with Lesions Restricted to One or Few Organs. By definition, these diseases combine the features of both organ-specific and non-organ-specific categories. Examples of this group are: (1) primary biliary cirrhosis; and (2) chronic aggressive hepatitis.

The autoimmune liver disorders are characterized by the production of non-organ-specific and non-species-specific antibodies, such as antimitochondrial and anti-smooth muscle cell antibodies. The relationships of these antibodies to immune injury and the lesion are unknown. The levels of the antibodies do not correlate with the severity or duration of the disease. There is evidence that the mechanisms of immunologic injury in liver disorders involve primarily a cellular immune mechanism via the suppressor cell and cytotoxic effector cell functions. In addition, there are humoral immunoregulatory factors which modulate the cellular functions of the immune system in the pathogenesis of the immunologic liver disorders.

Clinical Observations Which Indicate Autoimmune Pathogenesis

Autoimmune disorders are frequently associated with malignancies, immune deficiency syndromes, and aging. Possible autoimmune pathogenesis in a given disease is indicated when one observes: (1) the existence of autoantibodies; (2) amyloid deposits of denatured gamma globulin; (3) hypergammaglobulinemia with elevation of various immunoglobulins; (4) vasculitis, serositis, and glomerulonephritis, which suggest an immune complex disease; and (5) existence of other diseases, such as endocrinopathies, known to be associated with autoimmune disorders.

General Laboratory Tests

The most commonly used tests for the diagnosis of autoimmune disorders involve the detection of circulating antibodies. Tests for cellular sensitivity are done in the larger centers primarily on an investigative basis.

Immunofluorescence, enzyme-labeled antibody, and radioimmunoassay methods utilize primary antigen-antibody binding reactions and, because of their high sensitivity, are preferred for the detection of circulating and tissue-bound antibodies and antigens.

Tests that involve secondary antigen-antibody preparations, such as complement fixation, agglutination, and precipitation in agar gel, may not be as sensitive as immunofluorescence or radioimmunoassay in some circumstances, but may be technically more suitable for the identification of certain autoantibodies.

The indirect immunofluorescence test (IFT) and the more recently developed peroxidase-labeled antibody method are the most widely used immunohistochemical procedures for the detection of serum autoantibodies in the clinical laboratory. Both methods can be used to demonstrate: (1) autoimmune antibodies in serum; (2) tissue localization and fixation of autoantibody; and (3) deposition of antigen-antibody complexes in kidney, vessels, and other tissues.

In addition to tissue autoantibody detection, numerous other methods have proved useful in the evaluation of patients with suspected autoimmune disorders. These include various assays for cell-mediated immunity that have potential usefulness in studying patients with autoimmune thyroiditis, certain liver diseases, and rheumatoid arthritis. Still other, less cumbersome, methods are frequently employed, such as: (1) rheumatoid factor; (2) immune complexes in serum or joint fluid; (3) quantitation of serum immunoglobulins; (4) immunoelectrophoresis of serum and other body fluids; (5) cryoglobulins; (6) complement assays; and (7) biopsy of kidney, vessel, or joint for immunofluorescence localization of antibody and immune complexes.

Interpretation of Serum Autoantibody Levels. In general, the level of antibody is high in patients with autoimmune disorders and low in apparently healthy persons. A very high titer of autoantibody is significant, but a low or absent titer of autoantibody does not rule out the possibility of an autoimmune disorder. For example, in severe thyroiditis, at the height of the disease the gland may act as an immunoadsorbent and remove circulating antibody. In addition, thyroglobulin may be released into the circulation during the acute stage, neutralizing circulating autoantibody. Therefore, the level or titer of a given antibody must be interpreted in relation to the stage or treatment of a particular disease.

When adults are tested for rheumatoid factor and the antibodies to nuclear, parietal cell, thyroglobulin, thyroid epithelial cell, reticulin, mitochondrial, and smooth muscle, the incidence of autoantibodies in the general adult population to one or more antigens at a level of 1:10 titer or greater varies from approximately 21 to 27 per cent, with higher incidence in females. The incidence of certain autoantibodies increases with advancing age. Fifty per cent of subjects over 60 years old demonstrated low titers of one or more autoantibodies.

The antinuclear, antiparietal cell, and antithyroid antibodies are age- and sex-dependent, with an increasing incidence in females and older persons. On the other hand, the incidence of smooth muscle antibody and rheumatoid factor do not correlate with age and sex. The incidence of smooth muscle antibody and rheumatoid factor are similar in males and females.

Autoimmunity and Neoplasia

Autoimmune reactions to damaged or altered tissue may facilitate malignant degeneration with adoptive loss of cellular components. Human cancer and autoimmunity may be related since:

(1) Certain autoimmune diseases may be considered precancerous and are associated with a higher incidence of cancer than occurs in the control population;

(2) The host immune response to the invading cancer may initiate immunologic injury with formation of non-metastatic distant lesions.

There may be a step-by-step developmental sequence from normal immunologic regulation through autoimmunity and benign lymphoproliferation, leading ultimately to lymphoid neoplasia. Considerable evidence from studies in humans and animals suggests that autoimmunity, monoclonal immunoglobulin production, and malignant lymphocytic and plasma cell proliferation may be related events. There is a clear association between autoimmunity and the lymphoma that occurs in Sjögren's syndrome. Sjögren's syndrome represents a lymphocytic attack on the salivary and lacrimal glands, and the disease is associated with rheumatoid arthritis in almost 50 per cent of cases. The Sjögren's sicca syndrome often is benign, leading to progressive oral and ocular dryness. However, some patients exhibit an aggressive course, with lymphocytic infiltrates with lymphadenopathy. The term "pseudolymphoma" has been applied to this condition, and some of these patients develop malignant lymphomas without necessarily passing through the pseudolymphoma state. The lymphomas are often highly undifferentiated and may be associated with hypogammaglobulinemia and loss of antibodies.

Recently a pathologic entity termed "immunoblastic lymphadenopathy" has been described, and this entity has been confused with Hodgkin's disease. The lymph node shows immunoblastic proliferation in the B-lymphocyte plasma cell series, with proliferation of small vessels and deposits of amorphous interstitial material. The cellular proliferation is considered benign; however, the clinical course has a poor prognosis. Many of the patients show hypersensitivity reaction to drugs, and this entity supports the concept that there is uncontrolled immunoblastic proliferation following an antigenic stimulus, and a true neoplasm may develop.

REFERENCES

MECHANISMS OF IMMUNOLOGIC DISEASE

Adkinson, N. F., Jr., and Lichtenstein, L. M.: Assessment of allergic states: IgE methodology and the measurement of allergen-specific IgG antibody. Clin. Immunobiol., 3:305–344, 1976.

Cuatrecasas, D. and Greaves, M. F.: Receptors and Recogniton (Series A, #1 and #2)., John Wiley & Sons, New York 1976.

Cunningham-Rundles, W. F.: The reticuloendothelial system. Clin. Immunobiol., 3:289–302, 1976.

Crowle, A. J.: Delayed hypersensitivity in the mouse. Adv. Immunol., 20:197–259, 1975.

Fudenberg, H. H., Sites, D. P., Caldwell, J. L., and Wells, J. V.: Basic and Clinical Immunology, 2nd Ed. Lange Medical Publications, Los Altos, 1978.

Gell, P. G. H., Coombs, R. R. A., and Lachmann, P. J.: Clinical Aspects of Immunology, 3rd Ed. Blackwell Scientific Publications, Oxford, 1975.

Götze, O. and Müller-Eberhard, H. J.: The alternative pathway of complement activation. Adv. Immunol., 24:1–26, 1976.

Hobart, N. J., and McConnell, I.: The Immune System: A Course on the Molecular and Cellular Basis of Immunity. Blackwell Scientific Publications, Oxford, 1975.

Holborow, E. J., and Reeves, W. G.: Immunology in Medicine. Grune & Stratton, New York. 1977.

Humphrey, J. H., and White, R. C.: Immunology for Students of Medicine, 3rd Ed. Blackwell Scientific Publications, Oxford, 1970.

Kirkpatrick, C. H., and Reynolds, H. Y.: Immunologic and Infectious Reactions in The Lung. Marcel Dekker, Inc., New York, 1976.

Lichtenstein, L. M.: Allergy. Clin. Immunobiol., 1:243–268, 1972.

Nakamura, R. M.: Immunopathology: Clinical Laboratory Concepts and Methods. Little, Brown & Co., Boston, 1974.

Nussenzweig, V.: Receptors for immune complexes on lymphocytes. Adv. Immunol., 19:217–254, 1974.

Pangburn, M. K., and Muller-Eberhard, H. J.: Complement C3 convertase: cell surface restriction of beta-1-H control and generation of restriction on neuraminidase-treated cells. Proc. Natl. Acad. Sci., 5:2416–2420, 1978.

Perlmann, P.: Cellular immunity: antibody-dependent cytotoxicity (K-cell activity). Clin. Immunobiol., 3:107–130, 1976.

Pinsky, C. M.: Cell-meditaed immunity: in-vivo testing. Clin. Immunobiol., 3:97–104, 1976.

Roitt, I.: Essential Immunology, 3rd Ed. Blackwell Scientific Publications, Oxford, 1977.

Sell, S.: Immunology, Immunopathology and Immunity, 2nd Ed. Harper & Row, Hagerstown, 1975.

Schreiber, R. D., Pangburn, M. K., Lesavre, P. H., and Müller-Eberhard, H. J.: Initiation of the alternative pathway of complement: recognition of activators by bound C3b and assembly of the entire pathway from six isolated proteins. Proc. Natl. Acad. Sci., 75:August, 1978.

Thaler, M. S., Klausner, R. D., and Cohen, H. J.: Medical Immunology. J. B. Lippincott Co., Philadelphia, 1977.

AUTOIMMUNITY — GENERAL

Burnet, F. M.: Autoimmunity and Autoimmune Disease. F. A. Davis & Co., Philadelphia, 1972.

Burnet, F. M.: Immunology, Aging, and Cancer. Medical Aspects of Mutation and Selection. W. H. Freeman, San Francisco, 1976.

Gell, P. G. H., Coombs, R. R. A., and Lachmann, P. J.: Clinical Aspects of Immunology. Blackwell Scientific Publications, London, 1975.

Miescher, P. A., and Müller-Eberhard, H. J.: Textbook of Immunopathlogy, 2nd Ed. Grune & Stratton, New York, 1976.

Nakamura, R. M.: Immunopathology: Clinical Laboratory Concepts and Methods. Little, Brown & Co., Boston, 1974.

Talal, N.: Autoimmunity: Genetic, Immunologic, Virologic, and Clinical Aspects. Academic Press, New York, 1977.

GENETICS AND AUTOIMMUNITY

Bach, F. H.: The major histocompatibility complex and its relationship to autoimmune disease. *In* Talal, N. (Ed) : Autoimmunity: Genetic, Immunologic, Virologic, and Clinical Aspects. Academic Press, New York 1977, p 3.

Gill, T. J., Cramer, D. V., and Kunz, H. W.: The major histocompatibility complex — comparison in the mouse, man and the rat. A review. Am. J. Pathol., 90:737, 1978.

Sasazuki, T., McDevitt, H. O., and Grumet, F. C.: The association between genes in the major histocompatibility complex and disease susceptibility. Ann. Rev. Med., 28:425, 1977.

TOLERANCE

Allison, A. C.: Self-tolerance and autoimmunity in the thyroid. N. Engl. J. Med., 295:821, 1976.

Allison, A. C., and Denman, A. M.: Self-tolerance and autoimmunity. Br. Med. Bull., 32:124, 1976.

Weigle, W. O.: Immunologic unresponsiveness. Hosp. Prac., 6:121, May 1971.

Weigle, W. O.: Immunologic tolerance and immunopathology. Hosp. Prac., 12:71, June 1977.

MECHANISMS AND CONCEPTS OF PATHOGENESIS

Allison, A. C.: Autoimmune diseases: Concepts of pathogenesis and control. *In* Talal, N. (Ed.): Autoimmunity: Genetic, Immunologic, Virologic, and Clinical Aspects. Academic Press, New York, 1977, Chap. 4.

DeHeer, D. H., and Edgington, T. S.: Cellular events associated with the immunogenesis of anti-erythrocyte autoantibody responses of NZB mice. Transplant. Rev., 31:116, 1976.

Galbraith, R. M., and Fudenberg, H. H.: Autoimmunity in chronic active hepatitis and diabetes mellitus. Clin. Immunol. Immunopathol., 8:116, 1977.

Gershwin, M. E., and Steinberg, A. D.: The pathogenetic basis of animal and human autoimmune disease. Sem. Arthritis Rheumatol., 6:125, 1976.

Sell, S.: Immunopathology. Teaching monograph. Am. J. Pathol., 90:215, 1978.

Stobo, J. D., and Loehnen, C. P.: Immunoregulation and autoimmunity. Proc. Mayo Clin., 51:479, 1976.

Talal, N.: Disordered immunologic regulation and autoimmunity. Transplant. Rev., 31:240, 1976.

LABORATORY TESTS IN EVALUATION OF HUMAN AUTOIMMUNE DISEASES

Nakamura, R. M., Chisari, F. V., and Edgington, T. S.: Laboratory tests for diagnosis of autoimmune diseases. *In* Stefanini, M. (Ed.):Progress in Clinical Pathology. Grune &. Stratton, New York. 1975.

Nakamura, R.M., and Tan, E. M.: Recent progress in the study of autoantibodies to nuclear antigens. Human Pathol., 9:85, 1978.

Rose, N. R.: Laboratory diagnosis of the autoimmune diseases. *In* Prier, J. E., Bartola, J., and Friedman, H. (Eds.): Modern Methods in Medical Microbiology. Systems and Trends. University Park Press, Baltimore, 1976, p. 127.

AUTOIMMUNITY AND NEOPLASIA

Burnet, F. M.: Immunology, Aging, and Cancer. Medical Aspects of Mutation and Selection. W. H. Freeman, San Francisco, 1976.

Lukes, R. J., and Tindle, B. H.: Immunoblastic lymphadenopathy. N. Engl. J. Med., 291:1, 1975.

Roubinian, J., and Talal, N.: Neoplasia, autoimmunity and the immune response. Adv. Int. Med., 23:435, 1978.

Talal, N.: Recent clinical and experimental developments in Sjögren's syndrome. West. J. Med., 50:122, 1975.

CARDIORENAL AND RESPIRATORY SYSTEMS

6

Integrated Dynamics of the Circulation and Body Fluids

ARTHUR C. GUYTON

It would be pointless to review in this chapter all the details of hemodynamics, such as the interrelationships between pressure, resistance, and flow, or the problems of blood viscosity, or the differences between streamline and non-streamline blood flow, because these are found in every textbook of medical physiology. On the other hand, the integrative aspects of hemodynamics are extremely important to the clinician and, yet, are rarely written. It is these aspects that will be covered in this chapter.

Basic Philosophy of the Circulatory System

The purpose of the circulatory system is to provide transport for nutrients, excreta, and other substances to and from the cells. To do this there are two major groups of hemodynamic systems. One of these is geared to provide a continuous pressure level in the arterial tree and the other to control blood flow in each individual section of the circulation in accord with local needs. It will be the aim of this chapter to show how the different circulatory mechanisms operate together to provide continuous automatic function of the circulation and how dysfunction can lead to circulatory inadequacy.

BASIC FACTORS IN OVER-ALL CIRCULATORY FUNCTION AND REGULATION

Figure 6–1 depicts the basic factors in over-all function of the circulation and also shows their interrelationships. First, let us describe the six factors located around the periphery of the diagram in Blocks 1 through 6, beginning with arterial pressure. (1) When the arterial pressure increases, this causes the renal output of water and electrolytes also to increase. (2) Increased loss of water and electrolytes from the kidneys reduces the extracellular fluid volume. (3) This reduction of extracellular fluid volume causes a similar decrease in blood volume. (4) The decrease in blood volume decreases the circulatory filling pressure (the tightness with which the circulation is filled with blood). (5) Decreasing this factor decreases venous return and cardiac output. (6) The decrease in cardiac output obviously decreases arterial pressure.

Thus, one sees that an initial increase in arterial pressure causes a series of events which in turn tend to reduce the arterial pressure back toward

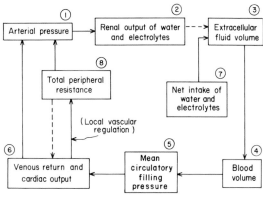

Figure 6–1 The major hemodynamic factors of circulatory function and their interrelationships.

169

normal. Conversely, a decrease in arterial pressure will cause exactly opposite effects, this time raising the diminished pressure back toward normal.

As one studies this circuit of Figure 6–1 (Blocks 1 through 6) he sees that it is a negative feedback hemodynamic mechanism that tends always to return the functional variables of the circulation back toward their normal levels. It is negative feedback loops such as this one that provide most control functions in the body. This specific hemodynamic negative feedback loop of Figure 6–1 is the most basic control loop of the circulatory system. Furthermore, complete understanding of this mechanism can help to explain many clinical circulatory abnormalities, as we shall see in subsequent pages.

Effects of Water and Electrolyte Intake. The two inside blocks of Figure 6–1 also deserve special mention. Block 7 shows that one's intake of water and electrolytes also plays a major role in over-all control of the circulation, obviously counterbalancing renal output of water and electrolytes.

Effect of Total Peripheral Resistance and Autoregulation. Block 8, total peripheral resistance, has two very significant effects on circulatory regulation: (1) An increase in total peripheral resistance tends to increase arterial pressure, but (2) an increase in total peripheral resistance also tends to decrease venous return and cardiac output. The second one of these two effects is often forgotten; many times its effect to reduce arterial pressure is more potent than the direct effect of the resistance to increase arterial pressure. For instance, when the total peripheral resistance increases because of venous constriction, the tendency to decrease cardiac output is much greater than the tendency to increase arterial pressure. Therefore, in this instance, the arterial pressure actually decreases instead of increasing because of the greatly decreased cardiac output. This interplay between the positive and negative effects of total peripheral resistance on pressure is mentioned here merely to illustrate one of the falsities that has crept into much understanding of circulatory hemodynamics, namely, a widespread impression that total peripheral resistance and arterial pressure are always directly related to each other.

It is also noted in Block 8 that an increase in cardiac output can increase total peripheral resistance, as illustrated by the dark arrow going from Block 6 to Block 8. This effect is frequently overlooked in schemes of circulatory function. It results from the ability of tissues to control their own local blood flows, which will be discussed later in this chapter. When the cardiac output becomes too great, blood flows through the tissues in excessive amounts, and the tissues attempt to return their flows back to normal. As a result, the local blood vessels constrict, thereby increasing total peripheral resistance. Conversely, whenever the cardiac output falls too low and blood flow in the tissues diminishes, the local vasculature dilates. This effect of cardiac output on vascular resistance is called *autoregulation*. As a result of it, there is a tendency for the total peripheral resistance to change in the same direction as the change in cardiac output. The effect, however, is not an instantaneous one. A small part of it occurs within the first minute or so, still more within the next hour, and much more over a period of days and weeks, as will be discussed later in this chapter in relation to local blood flow regulation.

With this rapid introduction to the major functional factors in circulatory control, now let us turn to one of the more specific circulatory functions.

LOCAL BLOOD FLOW AND ITS REGULATION

Every clinician is familiar with the ability of local tissues to protect their own blood flows. For instance, if a femoral artery suddenly becomes occluded, within 60 to 90 seconds collateral blood vessels open to supply blood to the leg. Then, during the next several weeks to several months, the collaterals become progressively larger, until finally blood flow is almost as adequate as before, particularly in very young persons.

On the other hand, exactly the opposite effects occur when blood flow to the tissues becomes too great. Some degree of acute constriction of the blood vessels occurs within the first minute or so, and this is followed gradually over days, weeks, and months by actual decrease in vascular dimensions.

Mechanisms of Local Blood Flow Regulation: Role of Oxygen

Different tissues have different mechanisms for control of local blood flow, depending on their special local needs. However, the majority of the tissues control local blood flow in relation to their need for oxygen. This is particularly true of all types of muscle—skeletal, cardiac, and smooth — which together make up approximately one half the body. Diminished oxygen delivery causes up to fourfold increase in blood flow within seconds to minutes; then, additional vasodilatation occurs during the ensuing half hour to hour.

In some tissues this effect of oxygen lack to control local blood flow is overshadowed by other more potent local factors for controlling blood flow. For instance, in the brain the factor that plays the most potent role is usually carbon dioxide, an increase in carbon dioxide causing increased blood flow and thereby providing increased removal of the excess carbon dioxide from the brain tissue. However, when the brain becomes moderately or extremely hypoxic, vasodilatation occurs as a result of the hypoxia in exactly the same way as it occurs in muscle.

Possible Vasodilator Substances Released in Response to Oxygen Deficiency. The basic mechanism by which decreased oxygen delivery to the tissues causes vasodilatation is still unknown. Some research workers believe that diminished oxygen in the tissues causes some humoral vasodilator factor to be released into the tissue fluids and that this in turn actively dilates the local vessels. The substance that has received widest attention in recent years has been *adenosine,* one of the breakdown products of adenosine triphosphate that is released in small quantities into the tissue fluid in hypoxic states. Other possible vasodilator substances that have been suggested include potassium, osmotic substances of any nature, adenosine triphosphate, carbon dioxide, lactic acid, histamine, and others. All these can indeed cause vasodilatation in large enough quantities, but to date none of them has been absolutely proved to be the major cause of the dilatation that occurs in hypoxia.

Possible Vasodilatation Caused By Oxygen Deficiency Per Se. More recently, experiments have shown that the vasodilating effect of tissue hypoxia could result from simple decrease of oxygen itself in the tissues rather than from the presence of vasodilator substances. Absence of oxygen prevents formation of significant quantities of ATP and other high-energy compounds in the smooth muscle cells of the vascular walls, so that the strength of contraction of these cells is diminished in exactly the same way that the strength of contraction of skeletal muscle is also diminished in hypoxia. Obviously, this could easily cause local vasodilatation when too little oxygen is available to the tissues.

Long-term Changes in Blood Vessels During Prolonged Ischemia or Hypoxia. In animals kept for months at high altitudes, the actual sizes and numbers of vessels in the tissues increase, causing a phenomenon called "increased vascularity." Furthermore, return of these animals to normal altitudes causes the vascularity to return toward normal. Essentially the same effects also occur when the tissues are made ischemic because of large artery obstruction. Unfortunately, the causes of these changes in vascularity are not yet known, but the vascularity changes themselves help to maintain proper delivery of oxygen and other nutrients to the tissues.

Other Normal and Pathologic Factors in Local Blood Flow Regulation. In the skin, local blood flow is controlled almost entirely by the body temperature control mechanism, acting mainly by means of nervous constriction or dilatation of the skin vessels.

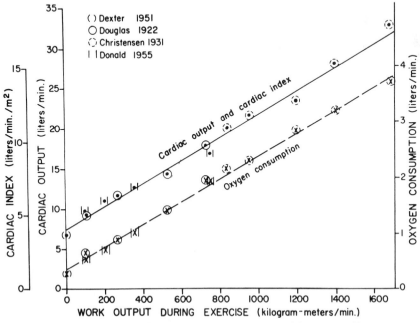

Figure 6–2 Relationship between cardiac output and work output *(solid curve)* and between oxygen consumption and work output *(dashed curve)* during exercise. (Reprinted from Guyton, A. C., et al.: Circulatory Physiology: Cardiac Output and its Regulation. 2nd ed. W. B. Saunders Co., Philadelphia, 1973.)

In the kidneys, blood flow is controlled primarily by the renal excretory loads, especially by the presence of excess sodium and other electrolytes in the plasma; it is also possible that some of the end-products of metabolism help to control renal blood flow. Only when the kidneys become extremely hypoxic does the hypoxia mechanism play any significant role in renal blood flow regulation.

Finally, any pathologic state that causes a direct shunt from the arteries to the veins increases the local blood flow and contributes to the overall control of the circulation. Thus, either minute pathologic arteriovenous fistulae or major A-V fistulae will both increase blood flow.

Local Blood Flow Regulation During Increased Tissue Activity. The local blood flow regulating mechanisms also respond to increased cellular activity. To give an example, Figure 6–2 shows the effect of progressive increase in work output during exercise on both oxygen consumption and cardiac output, illustrating that as tissue metabolism increases (indicated by increasing oxygen consumption), blood flow through the entire body also increases (indicated by the increasing cardiac output). Other examples in which increased tissue activity causes vascular dilatation include (1) increased metabolism of the tissues caused by thyrotoxicosis, (2) increased tissue activity caused by excessive catecholamines, and (3) increased metabolism caused by fever. Therefore, the increased local blood flows and increased cardiac outputs observed in these conditions can all be ascribed to the increased activities in the local tissue cells themselves.

CARDIAC OUTPUT: HEMODYNAMIC FACTORS AND ITS REGULATION

When one thinks of cardiac output regulation, he almost immediately thinks of the heart, but under normal conditions 90 to 95 per cent of cardiac output regulation is determined by peripheral circulatory factors, and not more than 5 to 10 per cent by the heart itself. On the other hand, when the heart becomes diseased and is then unable to provide adequate pumping capacity, the limiting factor in cardiac output regulation becomes the heart.

Role of the Heart in Cardiac Output Regulation

Even under resting conditions the normal human heart is capable of pumping between 10 and 15 liters of blood per minute, although it actually pumps only 5 to 6 liters. The simple reason for this difference is the following: only this smaller amount of blood flows into the heart from the veins, and, however much pumping ca-

pacity the heart may have, it can never pump more blood than flows into it. The normal heart merely keeps the input veins pumped almost dry, which can be illustrated by injecting a contrast medium into any of the peripheral veins and noting the slitlike character of the veins where they empty into the thorax.

Effect of the Nervous System on the Heart's Pumping Capacity. In dog studies, maximal sympathetic stimulation of the heart can increase the pumping capacity of the heart about 70 to 100 per cent. On the other hand, maximal vagal stimulation can stop the heart for a few seconds until the ventricles begin to beat at a very slow rate, driven by a ventricular pacemaker. After the ventricles have thus "escaped" from the vagal stimulation, the maximum pumping capacity of the heart is reduced to about 50 per cent of normal. Therefore, the total range of nervous control of heart pumping is probably between −50 per cent and +100 per cent.

Effect of Cardiac Hypertrophy on Heart Pumping Capacity. In athletes who train for endurance, the maximum cardiac output can be increased 50 to 100 per cent by the training procedure. At least part of this effect is caused by cardiac hypertrophy. Likewise, from study of certain disease conditions, such as left-to-right shunts, in which the heart must pump greatly increased amounts of blood indefinitely, one can also come to the conclusion that heart hypertrophy can increase the heart's pumping capacity as much as 100 per cent.

Cardiac Reserve. The difference between the heart's pumping capacity and the actual amount of blood pumped by the heart under resting conditions is called the "cardiac reserve." Thus, if the heart of an exceedingly well-trained athlete is capable of pumping 30 liters per minute but under resting conditions pumps only 5 liters, the cardiac reserve is 25 liters. Expressing this as a percentage, which is the usual method, this person has a cardiac reserve of 500 per cent above normal.

Role of Peripheral Circulation in Cardiac Output Control

If the peripheral blood vessels were rigid tubes, the peripheral circulation would play essentially no role in cardiac output regulation, because whenever the heart should pump increased quantities of blood into a peripheral vessel an equal amount of blood would be returned instantaneously to the input side of the heart. However, the fact that the peripheral vessels are highly distensible prevents this instantaneous increase in venous return. Instead, the extra blood pumped by the heart at first simply distends the arterial tree. Then it is allowed to flow through the small tissue vessels into the veins and, finally, back again to the heart only at the will of the tissues. Consequently, it is frequently said that cardiac output is controlled by venous return and that venous return is controlled by the tissues. This means simply that whatever amount of blood is allowed to flow through the small vessels of the tissues into the veins and thence into the heart is also the amount of blood that the heart pumps.

Cardiac Output Regulation as the Sum of Local Blood Flow Regulations.   The factors that control local blood flow in the peripheral circulation change from minute to minute in accord with the needs of the tissues, as already discussed, and these effects simultaneously alter venous return and cardiac output. Therefore, another way of looking at normal cardiac output regulation is simply to state that it is the sum of all the local blood flow regulations. If return of blood to the heart from any single tissue increases, cardiac output increases by approximately a similar increment.

This principle is illustrated very forcefully when one studies the effects of an arteriovenous fistula on circulatory function, as illustrated in Figure 6–3. This figure shows an instantaneous increase in cardiac output resulting from opening the fistula. The primary effect is to allow direct flow of blood from the arteries into the veins, and the surge of blood returning to the heart instantaneously increases the cardiac output. Within another few seconds, the nervous reflexes further compensate for the fistula by causing blood reservoirs to constrict throughout the body, thereby making still more blood available to be pumped by the heart. Then, during the next several days, renal retention of water and salt (for reasons discussed earlier in this chapter in relation to Figure 6–1) causes the blood volume to increase slightly, making even more blood available to the heart. Thus, within two to three days, there is full compensation to opening the A-V fistula, and *the cardiac output is increased by an amount exactly equal to the fistula flow,* if the heart does not go into failure.

Role of Blood Volume and "Mean Circulatory Filling Pressure" in Cardiac Output Regulation.   Another non-cardiac factor that even normally plays a supporting role in cardiac output regulation (and under certain abnormal conditions plays the major role) is the blood volume and its ability to fill the circulatory system, as measured by the "mean circulatory filling pressure." When the blood volume is increased, the quantity of blood in each vessel in the body tends also to increase. Therefore, the pressure in each vessel becomes slightly greater than normal. The algebraic sum of these pressures, weighted in proportion to the capacitances of the respective vascular segments, is the mean circulatory filling pressure. Unfortunately this has never been measured in the human being, but it is probably near that observed in the dog, 7 mm. Hg. This is also the average pressure in the peripheral circulation that tends to push blood toward the venous input side of the heart. Both mathematically and experimentally, it has been demonstrated that ve-

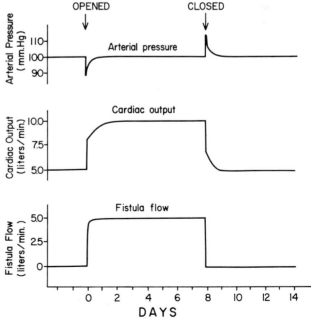

Figure 6–3 Effect of suddenly opening and suddenly closing an A-V fistula, showing changes in fistula flow, cardiac output, and arterial pressure.

nous return increases directly in proportion to an increase in mean circulatory filling pressure. On the other hand, the right atrial pressure exerts a back pressure to reduce flow of blood into the heart. Putting both these factors together, one finds that *return of blood to the heart is directly proportional to the mean circulatory filling pressure minus the right atrial pressure.*

EFFECT OF VASCULAR CAPACITY ON FILLING PRESSURE. The capacity of the circulatory system itself is another factor that helps to determine the mean circulatory filling pressure. Obviously, the greater the capacity, the greater must be the blood volume to create the same degree of filling pressure. Furthermore, the capacity of the circulatory system can be changed by nervous stimulation, hormonal effects, fever, and so forth. Some of these factors will be discussed later in the chapter in relation to blood volume regulation, but it is very clear that the tightness with which the circulatory system is filled with blood is determined by the ratio of the blood volume to the capacity of the system itself. Therefore, from the point of view of control of the circulation, one needs to think in terms of mean circulatory filling pressure and not in terms of blood volume itself.

Role of Mean Circulatory Filling Pressure in Circulatory Shock and in Heart Failure. There are two very important applications of the concept of circulatory filling pressure to clinical medicine — one to help explain circulatory shock and the other to explain one of the compensations in congestive heart failure. In circulatory shock, the blood volume is usually greatly decreased, but shock can also result from excessive dilatation of the vasculature, which simply increases the capacity of the system. That is, either decreased blood volume or increased vascular capacity decreases the mean circulatory filling pressure below its normal value and correspondingly can reduce venous return and cardiac output. In the early stages of some types of shock, such as hemorrhagic shock, the pumping capacity of the heart actually increases far above normal because of reflex nervous stimulation of the heart. Yet, despite this, the venous return is still too low, and the cardiac output cannot rise above the venous return; hence, the patient is in circulatory shock despite massive pumping effort by the heart. Thus, the concept of mean circulatory filling pressure is an exceedingly important one in understanding abnormal control of the circulation in circulatory shock.

In congestive heart failure, the primary abnormality occurs in the heart itself, but even a very weak heart can often pump normal cardiac output if it is constantly primed with excessive amounts of blood entering the right atrium. In severe congestive heart failure, the kidneys function very poorly, causing diminished urinary output and consequent increase in extracellular fluid volume and blood volume. As a result, the mean circulatory filling pressure sometimes rises to as high as 20 to 30 mm. Hg, which is three to four times the normal value. This excessive pressure plays a significant role in pushing extra quantities of blood toward the heart, often compensating completely for the weak heart, so that cardiac output is normal. This is an example in which one hemodynamic factor, an increase in blood volume and mean circulatory filling pressure, opposes another factor, decreased pumping ability of the heart, to afford almost normal delivery of blood to the tissues despite a severe abnormality in the circulation. Unfortunately, though, there often comes the time when the heart becomes so weak that, whatever the increase in blood volume and mean circulatory pressure, the heart still cannot pump enough blood to supply the tissues adequately. Therefore, kidney function never returns to normal, and fluid continues to be retained indefinitely. This obviously leads to the state of *decompensation.*

Quantitative Method for Assessing Respective Roles of the Heart and Peripheral Circulation in Cardiac Output Regulation

Figure 6–4 presents a graphic procedure that can be used to determine the relative hemodynamic roles of the heart and of the peripheral circulation in cardiac output regulation. Note first the curve labeled "cardiac output curve." This illustrates the effect of increasing right atrial pressure on cardiac output, showing that as the pressure rises from about −4 mm. Hg up to 6 mm. Hg the cardiac output rises from zero to a plateau level of about 13 liters per minute.

The curve labeled "venous return curve" shows the effect on venous return of increasing right atrial pressure. As the right atrial pressure rises to approach approximately 7 mm. Hg (the mean circulatory filling pressure), the venous return falls to approach zero.

Now, let us see what happens when the two curves interact with each other. First, let us assume that the right atrial pressure is 7 mm. Hg. At this pressure, the cardiac output is 13 liters per minute and venous return is zero. Therefore, blood will be pumped rapidly out of the right atrium, and the right atrial pressure will decrease. Venous return will increase upward along the venous return curve while cardiac output will decrease downward along the cardiac output curve. As long as there is greater cardiac output than venous return, the blood volume in the heart will be decreasing and the right atrial pressure will be falling. But when the right atrial pressure reaches that point at which the two curves cross each other, venous return and cardi-

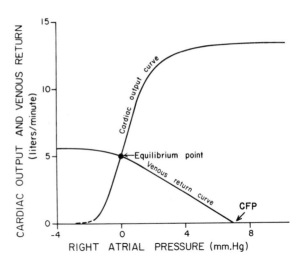

Figure 6–4 Interrelationship between cardiac output and venous return, showing (1) that the ability of the heart to pump blood can be expressed by *cardiac output curves,* (2) that the ability of blood to flow into the heart can be expressed by *venous return curves,* and (3) that the actual operating conditions of the circulation are expressed by the equilibrium point at which the two curves cross. The point labeled CFP represents the mean circulatory filling pressure of the system. (Modified from Guyton, A. C., et al.: Circulatory Physiology: Cardiac Output and Its Regulation. 2nd ed. W. B. Saunders Co., Philadelphia, 1973.)

ac output become equal, and the right atrial pressure also becomes stable. Therefore, this point is called an "equilibrium point," depicting the steady-state operational condition of the circulation. In Figure 6–4, which represents the normal condition of the circulation, the equilibrium point shows a cardiac output of approximately 5 liters per minute and a right atrial pressure of approximately 0 mm. Hg (with reference to atmospheric pressure).

Analysis of Sequential Events Following Acute Heart Failure.   We can now use the principle of equating venous return and cardiac output curves to analyze the sequence of events following an acute heart attack. In Figure 6–5 the two dark curves represent the same normal curves as those in Figure 6–4. Immediately after the heart attack, assuming that the attack occurs within seconds, the peripheral circulation has not yet been changed at all. However, the strength of the heart has been reduced to the long-dashed curve of the figure. This equates with the normal venous return curve at point B, showing that instantaneously the cardiac output falls to 2 liters per minute while the right atrial pressure rises to 4 mm. Hg. At this low cardiac output, the person is likely to faint and is certain to become very weak.

EFFECT OF CIRCULATORY REFLEXES. Within seconds the cardiovascular reflexes become active, and they change both the venous return curve and the cardiac output curve to the small-dashed curves. The venous return curve is changed because sympathetic stimulation tightens the blood vessels around the blood, thereby increasing the mean circulatory filling pressure, and in turn promoting greater tendency for blood to flow from the peripheral vessels to the heart. The cardiac function curve is increased because sympathetic stimulation increases the strength of contraction of the undamaged portions of the

heart. These sympathetic reflexes begin to act within two to three seconds and reach full development in 30 seconds to one minute. Therefore, the cardiac output rises by the end of this time from point B to the new equilibrium point, C, which represents a cardiac output of 3.5 liters per minute and an atrial pressure of 5.5 mm. Hg.

EFFECT OF HEART RECOVERY AND FLUID RETENTION.   During the next week, the strength of the heart improves because of (a) increase in collateral circulation to the ischemic areas of the heart, (b) some degree of hypertrophy of the undamaged heart muscle, and (c) stiffening of the infarcted portion of the myocardium to reduce aneurysmal bulging of this area. Simultaneously, the low cardiac output causes the kidneys to retain water and salt for a variety of different reasons, thereby increasing the mean circulatory filling pressure still further and further elevating the venous return curve. Therefore, the respective venous return and cardiac output curves become those represented by the dot-dashes, and the new equilibrium point becomes point D in Figure 6–5. By this time, the cardiac output has returned to normal, and renal output of water and salt is again in balance with the intake of water and salt. However, in the meantime, the body has accumulated fluid, the blood volume has increased a small amount, and the right atrial pressure has not risen to 6 mm. Hg. Yet, despite the fact that the pumping capacity of the heart is only one half normal, the cardiac output has returned essentially to normal. This demonstrates again the importance of the peripheral circulatory system in long-range control of cardiac output.

Cardiac Output in Abnormal States

Figure 6–6 illustrates the effects of different abnormal states on cardiac output. One can read-

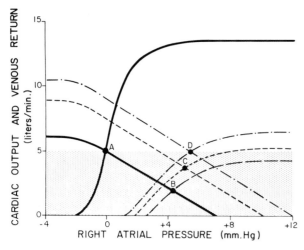

Figure 6–5 Use of cardiac output and venous return curves to analyze changes in cardiac output and right atrial pressure following acute onset of cardiac failure, showing complete cardiac output compensation at equilibrium point D after a week or more of recovery. (Reprinted from Guyton, A. C., et al.: Circulatory Physiology: Cardiac Output and Its Regulation. 2nd ed. W. B. Saunders Co., Philadelphia, 1973.)

ily understand most of the different factors that decrease the cardiac output in such states as myocardial infarction, hemorrhagic shock, traumatic shock, valvular heart disease, and cardiac shock. On the other hand, the factors that increase the cardiac output above normal are not so readily understood.

High Output States. Each one of the high output states illustrated in Figure 6–6 is associated with reduced total peripheral resistance. For instance, in beriberi, the total peripheral resistance is often reduced to as low as 50 per cent of normal, and in patients with A-V shunts the total peripheral resistance occasionally is reduced to as low as 30 to 40 per cent of normal. In anemia, blood viscosity is greatly reduced and, also, diminished delivery of oxygen to the tissues causes vasodilatation; thus, two different effects decrease the

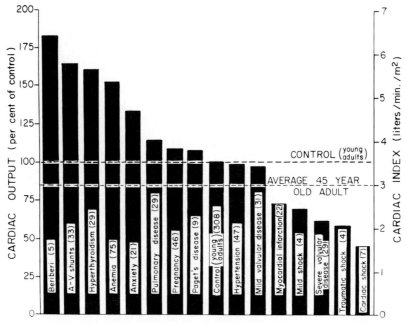

Figure 6–6 Cardiac output in different pathologic conditions. The figures in parentheses represent number of patients from which the average values were obtained. (Constructed from data in National Academy of Sciences: Handbook of Circulation. W. B. Saunders Co., Philadelphia, 1959.)

total peripheral resistance. In pulmonary disease, diminished delivery of oxygen to the tissues can dilate the peripheral vessels and, also, increased metabolism because of extra respiratory effort dilates the blood vessels in the respiratory muscles; both these effects reduce the total peripheral resistance. And, finally, in pregnancy and in Paget's disease, increased vascular shunting in both these conditions decreases total peripheral resistance.

Thus, in none of these high cardiac output conditions can one ascribe the high output to excess pumping capacity of the heart. Instead, one finds the total peripheral resistance to be decreased and the cause of the increased cardiac output to be increased venous return. Indeed, in many of these conditions, the pumping capacity of the heart is actually reduced rather than increased.

One might suspect hyperthyroidism and anxiety to be exceptions to this rule that high output is caused by peripheral factors, because the heart becomes hyperactive in both these states. However, increasing heart activity by pacing it with a pacemaker at a high rate in a normal resting person or in an animal does not significantly alter cardiac output, even though this procedure does indeed increase the pumping capacity of the heart itself. Therefore, at present, there is no proved condition in which higher than normal cardiac output is caused by increased pumping capacity of the heart itself. The increased pumping capacity merely increases the cardiac reserve, not the cardiac output.

Low Output Caused by Cardiac Insufficiency. The above principles illustrate once again that so long as the heart has unused cardiac reserve, the cardiac output is controlled almost entirely by factors in the peripheral circulation. However, when the cardiac reserve approaches zero, and particularly when the cardiac pumping capacity actually falls below the needs of the body's tissues, the heart does then become the limiting factor in the control of cardiac output. This is illustrated in Figure 6–6 by the cardiac outputs in patients with myocardial infarction, severe valvular heart disease, and cardiac shock. All these conditions impose limits on the amount of blood that the heart can pump. Note also that in these conditions the peripheral tissues lose their ability to control their own local blood flows because the heart does not supply enough blood flow to allow this luxury. Therefore, the flows in the respective tissues will no longer be distributed according to the needs of the tissues. As a consequence, one would expect some tissues to deteriorate more than others. The one most notably affected is usually the kidneys, which can cause death of the person even if all the other tissues do survive.

VENOUS PRESSURE, ITS REGULATION, AND ITS ABNORMALITIES

Venous pressure regulation is inextricably tied to the regulation of cardiac output, which one can see by referring to both Figures 6–4 and 6–5. At the same time that venous return interacts with the cardiac pumping capacity to determine cardiac output it also determines right atrial pressure, which is the central venous pressure. In general, increased pumping capacity of the heart is associated with reduced central venous pressure, whereas diminished pumping capacity is associated with elevated central venous pressure. Also, any peripheral circulatory factor that increases venous return is associated with increased central venous pressure, and any factor that reduces venous return is associated with diminished central venous pressure. However, when factors affect both the heart and the peripheral circulation simultaneously, the central venous pressure is then determined by a balance between the two respective factors; the only way to determine this balance accurately is by use of some quantitative method, such as the graphic method illustrated in Figures 6–4 and 6–5.

Mean Circulatory Filling Pressure as the Upper Limit to Central Venous Pressure. Referring again to Figure 6–4 one will note that as the right atrial pressure rises to approach the mean circulatory filling pressure, venous return approaches zero. Therefore, the upper limit to which the central venous pressure can rise is the mean circulatory filling pressure. The normal value for this filling pressure in the dog (it has never been measured in human beings) is 7 mm. Hg. However, when the venous return and cardiac output fall below normal, nervous reflexes can increase the filling pressure up to levels as high as 18 to 20 mm. Hg. Therefore, if the normal heart is weakened slowly enough for the reflexes to develop completely, cardiac output will decrease to zero only when the right atrial pressure rises to a maximum value of 18 to 20 mm. Hg.

In pathologic conditions that cause retention of body fluids and consequent increase in blood volume, the mean circulatory filling pressure, even without reflex stimulation, can be as high as 20 to 30 mm. Hg — in congestive failure, for instance. Therefore, progressive deterioration of the heart under these conditions can cause the central venous pressure to rise to maximum values of 20 to 30 mm. Hg, or perhaps even higher for short periods of time because of superimposed action of sympathetic reflexes.

Peripheral Venous Pressure versus Central Venous Pressure. Unfortunately, the peripheral venous pressure does not always correlate well with central venous pressure. The reason for this is that veins are frequently compressed in their courses to the heart, and the pressure beyond each compression point must rise enough to overcome the compression before the blood vessel will open enough to allow blood flow. The peripheral venous pressure, therefore, is more often a measure of the degree of venous compression than a measure of the central venous pressure. For this reason, to obtain meaningful venous pressure measurements, it is usually necessary to pass a catheter into a central vein. The tip of this catheter need not pass all the way into the right atrium, however, because the negative intrathoracic pressure keeps the central veins widely open so that central venous pressure measured anywhere inside the thoracic cavity will be within 1 mm. Hg of the right atrial pressure itself.

When the central venous pressure rises above 6 to 10 mm. Hg, the pressure in many or most of the peripheral veins then becomes great enough to overcome external compression on the veins. When this happens, the peripheral veins remain filled essentially all the time, and the resistance between the peripheral veins and the central veins becomes very slight. Therefore, now, the pressure measured in the peripheral veins becomes nearly equal to the pressure in the central veins (except for hydrostatic pressure difference). Furthermore, pressure waves generated in the right atrium as a result of cardiac pumping are now transmitted with ease along the veins. This accounts for the obvious pulsation of the veins in the neck in congestive heart failure.

Hydrostatic Reference Level for Measuring Venous Pressure. Extremely minute changes in central venous pressure can have marked effects on the output of the heart, which can be understood by referring to the cardiac output curve in Figure 6–4. In this figure, an increase in right atrial pressure from 0 to 1 mm. Hg is shown to increase the cardiac output approximately 30 per cent. Therefore, all central venous pressures must be measured at a very exact hydrostatic pressure level to be meaningful. Different reference levels have been suggested, such as one third the thickness of the chest behind the sternum, 10 cm. anterior to the back, and so forth. However, physiologic studies have shown that there is one point in the heart at which the central venous pressure changes less than 1 mm. Hg, regardless of the position of an animal. This is the very midpoint of the tricuspid valve. A basic physiologic reason for the constancy of pressure at this point is the following: Whenever the pressure at the tricuspid valve rises above its normal control value, the right ventricle fills more than normally and automatically pumps the increased quantity of blood out of the right ventricle; this obviously decreases

the tricuspid pressure back toward normal. Conversely, decreased pressure at the tricuspid valve decreases the filling of the ventricle so that less blood is pumped; therefore, the pressure rises once again back to its normal control value at the tricuspid valve level.

Thus, a physiologic hydrostatic reference point for measurement of venous pressure is the midpoint of the tricuspid valve. However, if the venous pressure is always measured with the patient in precisely the same position from one time to another and from one patient to another, any of the hydrostatic reference points — such as 10 cm. in front of the patient's back — will usually serve adequately. One of the most unforgivable mistakes, however, is to refer the measured pressure to the level of the catheter tip when the pressure is measured by a transducer at the external catheter end, because it makes no significant difference where the tip of the catheter lies in the central veins; the hydrostatic column of blood inside the veins beyond the tip of the catheter compensates for changes in position of the catheter tip, still making it essential that the pressure be measured in relation to the tricuspid valve.

ARTERIAL PRESSURE AND HEMODYNAMIC FACTORS IN ITS REGULATION

Fortunately, our bodies possess a large number of arterial pressure control mechanisms, no one of which can regulate arterial pressure under all conditions, though the total consortium of these mechanisms performs admirably. Eight of the best known arterial pressure control systems are described in the following sections. Three of these are strictly hemodynamic controls: the stress relaxation, the capillary-fluid shift, and the renal-body fluid mechanisms. The last of these is a crucial one in the long-term control of arterial pressure.

1. The Baroreceptor Reflex. An increase in arterial pressure stretches the *baroreceptors* (also called pressoreceptors) located in the carotid sinuses, in the arch of the aorta, and in other large central arteries. Signals from these are transmitted to the brain stem and thence back to the peripheral blood vessels to dilate them and also to the heart to decrease its pumping activity; both these effects reduce the arterial pressure back toward normal.

2. The Chemoreceptor Reflex. A decrease in arterial pressure decreases blood flow to the *chemoreceptors* in the carotid and aortic bodies. The decreased flow decreases the available oxygen to the chemoreceptors and also enhances the build-up of carbon dioxide in these receptors. Both these effects stimulate the chemoreceptors, causing them also to transmit signals by way of the brain stem to the blood vessels and the heart, this time raising the arterial pressure back toward normal.

3. The Central Nervous System Ischemic Response. When the arterial pressure is reduced below approximately 60 mm. Hg, the brain stem becomes ischemic and elicits the so-called central nervous system ischemic response. This sends powerful signals through the sympathetic nerves to the blood vessels to cause vasoconstriction and to the heart to enhance its pumping activity, thus bringing the arterial pressure back up to a level that will prevent brain ischemia.

4. Stress Relaxation. When the arterial pressure rises above normal because of an acute increase in blood volume, such as immediately following massive blood infusion, the pressure frequently is increased in all or most of the other vessels of the circulation as well as in the arteries. The smooth muscle cells of all the vessels gradually become stretched, a phenomenon called "stress relaxation." This increases the capacity of the vascular tree, thereby decreasing the mean circulatory filling pressure, decreasing cardiac output, and decreasing arterial pressure back toward normal. Conversely, when the pressures in all the respective vessels fall acutely to a level below normal, the blood vessels slowly contract around the blood and return the pressure back upward toward normal.

5. The Renin-Angiotensin-Vasoconstrictor Mechanism. Decrease in arterial pressure below normal causes the kidneys to release renin. The renin in turn enzymatically splits angiotensin from renin substrate in the plasma proteins. The angiotensin then causes peripheral vasoconstriction. The vasoconstriction causes a direct effect to increase total peripheral resistance and thereby returns the arterial pressure back upward toward normal.

6. The Aldosterone Pressure Regulating Mechanism. Decrease in arterial pressure increases aldosterone secretion. This occurs to a slight extent because angiotensin stimulates the adrenal cortex, but most of the effect probably occurs because of other not yet understood effects of decreased arterial pressure acting either directly or indirectly on the adrenal glands. The increased aldosterone in turn causes the kidneys to retain salt, which then has several indirect effects to cause the kidneys also to retain water. The increased water and salt increase the extracellular fluid volume, which increases blood volume, which increases cardiac output, which in turn increases arterial pressure back toward normal.

7. The Capillary-Fluid Shift Mechanism. Increase in arterial pressure is frequently accompanied by an increase in capillary pressure, especially after an acute increase in blood volume.

When this occurs, excess fluid begins to filter from the capillaries into the tissue spaces thereby reducing the blood volume, reducing cardiac output, and reducing arterial pressure back toward normal. This effect also operates in the opposite direction when the capillary pressure falls below normal.

8. The Renal-Body Fluid Pressure Regulating Mechanism. A decrease in arterial pressure has a direct effect on the kidneys to reduce renal output of water and salt. This results primarily from (a) decreased glomerular filtration rate caused by decreased glomerular pressure, and (b) increased tubular reabsorption caused by reduced peritubular capillary pressure. The result is retention of water and salt in the body and consequent progressive increase in extracellular fluid volume and blood volume as the person ingests additional quantities of water and salt. The increase in blood volume increases cardiac output and thereby returns the arterial pressure back toward normal. This mechanism is essentially the important hydrodynamic feedback control system illustrated at the outset of this chapter in Figure 6–1.

Interaction of Different Pressure Control Systems — The Concept of Feedback Gain

The greatest problem in understanding arterial pressure regulation has been to understand how all the different pressure regulating mechanisms interact with each other and under what conditions different mechanisms are important. To understand this, it is first necessary to explain the concept of feedback gain in control systems.

Let us assume that the normal arterial pressure is 100 mm. Hg and that some abnormal factor suddenly increases this pressure to 180 mm. Hg. The baroreceptors become stretched, and within seconds the baroreceptor reflux returns the arterial pressure to about 110 mm. Hg. Thus, 70 mm. Hg compensation occurs, and there is still 10 mm. Hg abnormality. The ratio of these two values, 70/10, is a mathematical measure of the ability of the control system to control arterial pressure; this ratio is also the feedback gain of the system. In this case the feedback gain is 70 divided by 10, or a gain factor of 7.

To give another example, if the arterial pressure is increased above its control value by sudden closure of a large arteriovenous fistula, the kidneys begin to excrete more water and salt than the net intake of these. Consequently, the body fluid volumes decrease, cardiac output decreases, and arterial pressure returns to normal. Furthermore, the arterial pressure will not stop falling until urinary output of water and salt returns exactly to equal the intake, which means that the arterial pressure must return all the way back to its control value and not merely a certain proportionate way. Therefore, the correction is some finite value, and the final abnormality is zero. A finite value divided by zero is infinity. Therefore, the renal-body fluid feedback mechanism for control of arterial pressure has a feedback gain of infinity when allowed long enough time to respond fully.

In a similar manner, we can derive gains for the eight well-known arterial pressure control mechanisms. The values for these are approximately the following when each is operating under optimal conditions:

CNS ischemic response	11.0
Baroreceptor reflex	7.0
Chemoreceptor reflex	4.0
Stress relaxation mechanism	2.8
Capillary-fluid shift mechanism	2.5
Renin-angiotensin-vasoconstrictor mechanism	1.6
Aldosterone, body fluid pressure control mechanism	1.0
Renal-body fluid pressure control mechanism	∞

Response Time-Courses of Respective Arterial Pressure Control Mechanisms. Figure 6–7 illustrates approximate response time-courses of the different pressure control mechanisms. Note that the time scale is approximately a logarithmic one, beginning with seconds and then extending to minutes, hours, and days. The three nervous

feedback mechanisms — the baroreceptor, the chemoreceptor, and the CNS ischemic effects — all begin to act within seconds and reach full gains within 30 seconds to a minute. Therefore, these are the mechanisms that are most important for control of arterial pressure from second to second or from minute to minute. They are the mechanisms that prevent sudden death following rapid bleeding and that prevent fainting when a person stands up. Each of the three nervous pressure control mechanisms operates in a different pressure range. The baroreceptors function most effectively at pressures between 80 and 180 mm. Hg, the chemoreceptors between 40 and 100 mm. Hg, and the CNS ischemic response mainly below 60 mm. Hg. The extreme gain of the CNS ischemic response at very low pressures causes it to resist strongly any final decrease of pressure below about 30 mm. Hg. It causes the sympathetic nervous system to become stimulated to its maximum, causing the heart to beat very forcefully and causing the highest possible degree of sympathetic constriction of the peripheral vessels. Therefore, this mechanism is frequently called the "last-ditch stand" against final circulatory collapse.

At least three non-nervous pressure control mechanisms begin to operate within minutes and continue to operate perhaps for hours or days. These are the stress relaxation mechanism, the renin-angiotensin-vasoconstrictor mechanism, and the capillary-fluid shift mechanism. None of them has a major amount of gain, but when

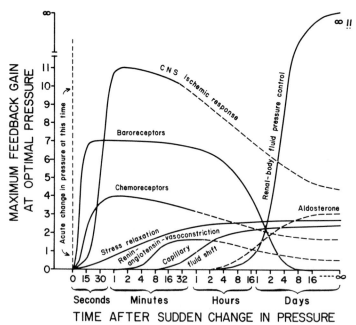

Figure 6–7 Response time-courses of the major arterial blood pressure regulating mechanisms. This figure also shows approximate feedback gains of these mechanisms at different times after their responses have been initiated. Note especially the infinite gain that occurs in the renal-body fluid-pressure control mechanism at infinite time. (Preprinted from projected publication by Guyton, A. C., et al.: Arterial Pressure Regulation and Hypertension. Philadelphia, W. B. Saunders Co.)

added to the gains of the other mechanisms they play very significant roles in maintaining normal arterial pressure temporarily in such conditions as slow bleeding, dehydration, and loss of the nervous controls of the circulation.

Finally come the long-term controls of arterial pressure, which are based primarily on retention of water and salt by the kidneys. The aldosterone mechanism has a finite gain while the direct renal-body fluid pressure control mechanism has infinite gain if given adequate time to come to full equilibrium, which in practice is several weeks. Because of this infinite gain, the renal-body fluid pressure control mechanism is the one that under long-term conditions dominates arterial pressure control for reasons that will be discussed in more detail in the following section.

Importance of Infinite Gain in the Renal-Body Fluid Pressure Control Mechanism and Its Significance in Long-term Arterial Pressure Regulation

When two or more control systems attempt to control the same factor at the same time, the contribution of each of the systems toward the final level of control is determined by the ratio of their gains. Note in Figure 6–7 that, at infinity time, the renal-body fluid pressure control system has infinite gain while all the others have finite gains. Therefore, the ratio of the renal-body fluid pressure control system gain to all the others is infinity divided by some finite value, which is still infinity. Consequently, the long-term arterial pressure level calculates to be determined almost entirely by the renal-body fluid pressure control system. Let us explain this mechanism more fully.

Renal output of water and electrolytes is highly dependent upon arterial pressure. This effect is illustrated in Figure 6–8 by the curve labeled "Normal renal output curve." This curve was determined in dogs by infusing sodium chloride solution at increasing rates for several days to several weeks while also recording the effect on mean arterial pressure and on urinary output. As illustrated, a very slight increase in arterial pressure is associated with a tremendous increase in renal output of both water and salt. And, conversely, a very slight decrease in arterial pressure is associated with a marked decrease in output. Only part of the increase in urinary output is caused by the rise in pressure itself. However, other simultaneous effects also increase the output, which is the cause of the extremely steep curve in Figure 6–8. For instance, during fluid loading, the rate of secretion of renin by the kidneys decreases, and this greatly increases the excretion of both salt and water. Likewise, fluid loading is usually associated with a decrease in aldosterone, which also allows increased urinary

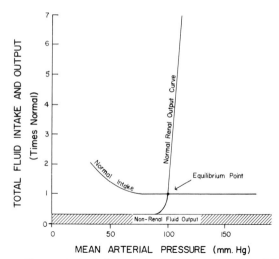

Figure 6–8 Relationship between mean arterial pressure and (1) normal fluid intake (curve labeled "normal intake") and (2) normal fluid output (curve labeled "normal renal output curve"). The point at which these two curves cross, called the "equilibrium point," depicts the pressure at which the arterial pressure will stabilize in the long-term steady-state condition. (Preprinted from projected publication by Guyton, A. C., et al.: Arterial Pressure Regulation and Hypertension. W. B. Saunders Co., Philadelphia.)

output. And, finally, fluid loading is often associated with decreased sympathetic activity, this also acting as still another factor to increase urinary output. Regardless of all the causes of the extreme steepness of the relationship between urinary output and arterial pressure, one can readily understand its importance for long-term control of arterial pressure. That is, whenever the arterial pressure rises above normal, this is generally associated with a tremendous increase in urinary output, which in turn causes the pressure to fall back toward normal. Conversely, a decrease in arterial pressure causes fluid retention, which increases the pressure also back toward normal.

Equilibration between Fluid Intake and Fluid Output. Also shown in Figure 6–8 is a curve labeled "normal intake" showing that at normal arterial pressures the intake of water and salt by a normal person remains essentially constant. Only when the pressure is very low is this not true, presumably because ischemia of the thirst center in the brain causes some increase in fluid intake.

It is axiomatic that the rate of fluid intake must over an extended period of time equal the rate of fluid output. This occurs where the two curves in Figure 6–8 cross each other at the point labeled *equilibrium point*. If ever the arterial pressure rises too high, then one would expect the urinary output also to become excessive. As a consequence, the rate of fluid loss from the body becomes greater than fluid intake. Over an extended period of time this will cause the arterial pressure to fall and also cause the renal output of fluid to decrease until total fluid output again equals fluid intake. When this has been achieved, the arterial pressure becomes stabilized. Conversely, if the pressure falls too low, the fluid intake becomes greater than the output; the body fluids build up until the intake and output again become equal and the pressure stabilized.

If one will think for a few moments about the meaning of the diagram in Figure 6–8, he will see that the renal-body fluid pressure control mechanism has the capability of stabilizing the arterial pressure to a very precise level. This is the result of the infinite gain feature of this control mechanism. That is, this system continues to modify the fluid volume until the precise pressure point is reached, which is what is meant by infinite gain.

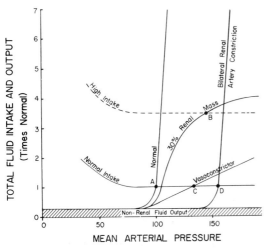

Figure 6–9 Fluid intake and fluid output curves under different conditions. The long-term level at which the arterial pressure will stabilize is determined by (1) the fluid intake curve under which the animal is operating and (2) the fluid output curve under which it is operating. Point A depicts the arterial pressure under normal conditions. Point B depicts the arterial pressure when the renal mass has been reduced to only 30 per cent of normal and there is also a high level of fluid intake. Point C depicts the long-term arterial pressure level when the animal or person is under the long-term influence of a vasoconstrictor substance and there is simultaneously a normal fluid intake. Point D depicts the long-term arterial pressure level when there is a normal fluid intake and simultaneously both renal arteries are constricted. (Preprinted from projected publication by Guyton, A. C., et al.: Arterial Pressure Regulation and Hypertension. W. B. Saunders Co., Philadelphia.)

Effect of Changes in Renal Function or in Fluid Intake on the Arterial Pressure Level. Figure 6–9 illustrates two fluid intake curves representing two levels of fluid intake and four different renal output curves, each representing a different state of kidney function. The normal renal output curve and the normal intake curve cross each other at point A. Therefore, the arterial pressure normally will stabilize only at point A. At any other point, there will be either a negative or positive fluid balance which will continue until the pressure returns to point A.

To the far right in the figure is a renal output curve labeled "Bilateral renal artery constriction." This is the curve recorded when both renal arteries are constricted, and it is also the curve recorded in rats that have spontaneous hypertension. Note that this output curve crosses the intake curve at point D. Therefore, so long as the kidneys operate in this state (and there is also normal intake of fluid), the only steady-state arterial pressure level that can be achieved is that represented by point D, or a level of approximately 155 mm. Hg. At any other pressure level besides this, there will be either a positive or negative fluid balance which will continue until the pressure returns to this level.

Now, note the curve labeled "Vasoconstrictor." When a vasoconstrictor substance circulates in the body, it not only constricts the arterioles in the limbs, splanchnic areas, and so forth; it constricts the renal arterioles as well. As a consequence, the renal output curve decreases to the one shown in the figure. This curve crosses the normal intake curve at point C. Therefore, the arterial pressure, over any extended period of time will stabilize at point C.

Finally, note the curve labeled "30%" renal mass." This curve crosses the normal intake curve at a pressure slightly greater than 100 mm. Hg. In other words, so long as the intake of fluid remains normal, the arterial pressure will hardly be changed from normal even though 70 per cent of the kidney mass has been removed. In fact, animal experiments show that simple removal of kidney mass will rarely raise the arterial pressure more than 10 mm. Hg so long as fluid and salt intake remain normal. Instead, the animal always goes into uremia before a significant rise in pressure occurs. On the other hand, if the animal is simultaneously loaded with a high intake of water and salt, then the arterial pressure does rise markedly. This is illustrated by point B in Figure 6–9 where the high intake curve crosses the low renal mass curve, showing an arterial pressure of approximately 140 mm. Hg. Thus, when there is decreased renal mass, the arterial pressure is determined to a great extent by the rate of water and salt intake. On the other hand, in a normal animal, the intake of water and salt has very little effect on the arterial pressure. This can be understood by noting the point at which the high intake curve crosses the normal renal output curve; this crossing point occurs at an arterial pressure level of approximately 105 mm. Hg, which represents hardly any rise in arterial pressure.

To summarize, the level at which the arterial pressure stabilizes is determined by the point at which the fluid output curve crosses the intake curve. At any other pressure level besides this, there will be either a positive or negative fluid balance which will continue until the pressure returns to the stable level dictated by the point where the two curves cross. However, if ever either of these two curves itself changes, then the pressure also will change accordingly.

Determinants of the Long-term Level of Arterial Pressure. From the above discussion one sees that there are only two basic factors that in the long run determine the arterial pressure level. These are the fluid intake curve and the fluid output curve as illustrated in Figures 6–8 and 6–9. However, one will understand that anything that affects the shape or quantitative level of either of these two curves can also affect the long-term level of arterial pressure. Since the intake of fluid remains relatively constant from one person to another and from day to day, the factor that most often sets the arterial pressure level is the characteristics of the output curve. Most clinicians already know the different factors that can shift this curve to high pressure levels, but let us list a few of these:

(1) Certain types of kidney disease, especially pathologic constriction of the renal vasculature. Also, thickening of the glomerular membrane, which tends to decrease the rate of glomerular filtration, will elevate the long-term arterial pressure level.

(2) Excessive reabsorption of electrolytes and fluid by the tubules. This occurs especially in the presence of excess steroids.

(3) Constriction of the renal vasculature as a result of circulating hormones. Hypertension of this type is illustrated by the hypertension that occurs in patients with pheochromocytomas and in patients with reninomas. In the first instance the catecholamines cause marked constriction, especially of the afferent arterioles of the kidneys. In the second instance, the renin causes formation of angiotensin II, which in turn constricts the arterioles of the kidneys — perhaps a little more constriction of the efferent arterioles than of the afferent arterioles.

(4) Sympathetic stimulation of the kidneys, which constricts the renal arterioles and results in a tendency toward diminished formation of glomerular filtrate.

(5) Changes in electrolyte intake, which in turn alter the urinary volume output by the kidneys.

To summarize, any factor that alters the shape or quantitative level of either the fluid intake curve or the fluid output curve as depicted in Figures 6–8 and 6–9 is a determinant of the long-term arterial pressure level.

Lack of Correlation in Many Instances Between Arterial Pressure on the One Hand and Cardiac Output, Total Peripheral Resistance, or Blood Volume on the Other Hand. For years, investigators have argued the importance of total peripheral resistance, cardiac output, blood volume, and extracellular fluid volume in the regulation of the long-term level of arterial pressure. However, one will note that not any of these factors has a direct effect to change either the normal fluid intake curve or the normal renal output curve as illustrated in Figures 6–8 and 6–9. Therefore, none of these four factors is a *primary* determinant of the long-term steady-state level of arterial pressure. To give an example, a change in cardiac output obviously can cause a temporary change in arterial pressure. But if this altered arterial pressure then causes the fluid output to become unequal to the fluid intake, the total peripheral resistance, blood volume, and/or cardiac output will automatically be altered as needed until that level of arterial pressure is achieved which will once again bring intake and output into balance.

Therefore, total peripheral resistance, blood volume, and cardiac output are nothing more than *dependent variables* in the system.

It is exceedingly important to understand the difference between the *determinants* of the long-term arterial pressure level and the dependent variables because a change in a determinant will always of necessity alter the long-term pressure. On the other hand, a change in one of the dependent variables will simply throw the system out of balance temporarily, but the system will automatically readjust the dependent variables until the arterial pressure comes back exactly to where it was. Therefore, it is mainly fruitless to argue whether or not one of the dependent variables correlates with arterial pressure. For instance, in the type of hypertension that occurs immediately after a massive transfusion, the total peripheral resistance is at first greatly reduced while cardiac output is greatly elevated. On the other hand, in hypertension caused by a pheochromocytoma, the total peripheral resistance is greatly increased while the cardiac output is often reduced. Thus, these factors are nothing more than manipulated pawns in the regulation of arterial pressure.

CAPILLARIES AND CAPILLARY EXCHANGE

The body has roughly 50 billion capillaries, and their total cross-sectional area is a thousand or more times the total cross-sectional area of the aorta. It is rare that any cell of the body lies more than 30 to 50 microns from the nearest capillary. These facts bespeak the functions of the capillaries, namely, to deliver nutrients or humoral agents to the cells and to remove excreta from the cells.

The principal means for capillary exchange of both water and nutrients between the blood and the interstitial fluid is by the process of *diffusion.* In fact, diffusion is so great through the capillary walls that water molecules diffuse in each direction many times as rapidly as the blood itself flows in the capillaries. Therefore, there is constant mixing of most of the constituents of the interstitial fluids with those of the blood.

Dynamic Equilibrium at the Capillary Membranes

Figure 6–10 illustrates a capillary in juxtaposition to its surrounding tissues. It also shows colloid osmotic pressures and hydrostatic pressures on each side of the capillary membrane. It is the dynamic equilibrium at this capillary membrane that prevents excessive quantities of fluid from filtering through the capillary membranes into the interstitial spaces. This can be explained as follows.

Since plasma proteins leak through the capillary membrane only to a slight extent, their concentration in the blood remains relatively high, causing a normal plasma colloid osmotic pressure of about 28 mm. Hg in the human being. The plasma protein that does leak into the interstitial spaces creates an average interstitial fluid colloid osmotic pressure of about 5 mm. Hg, varying

from as little as 1 to 2 mm. Hg in some tissues with only slightly porous capillary membranes, such as in the brain, to as high as 20 mm. Hg in tissues with extremely porous membranes, as in the liver. The colloid osmotic pressure of the plasma is so much greater than that of the interstitial fluid that it creates a continual pressure for movement of fluid from the interstitial spaces into the capillaries. In Figure 6–10 this difference between the two colloid osmotic pressures is shown to be 28 minus 5, or 23 mm. Hg, that is, a *net* colloid osmotic absorptive pressure of this amount.

On the other hand, the average capillary pressure in the capillaries, as measured in several different ways, averages about 17 mm. Hg. This value is considerably lower than the 25 mm. Hg so often taught in the past. This hydrostatic pressure tends to force fluid outward through the capillary membrane. Yet, when it competes with the 23 mm. Hg colloid osmotic absorptive pressure attempting to move fluid inward, one finds 6 mm. Hg more absorptive pressure than hydrostatic pressure tending to force fluid outward. Therefore, under normal circumstances, there is a net absorptive capability of the capillaries, which can create a *negative* pressure (less than atmospheric pressure) in the interstitial spaces averaging about −6 mm. Hg. On studying Figure 6–10 once again, a hydrostatic pressure of −6.5 mm. Hg is shown in the tissue spaces rather than the theoretic value of −6. The extra 0.5 mm. Hg is caused by the pumping action of the lymphatics, which causes a minute trickle of fluid to flow from the tissue spaces into the lymph vessel and thereby creates slightly more negative pressure in the

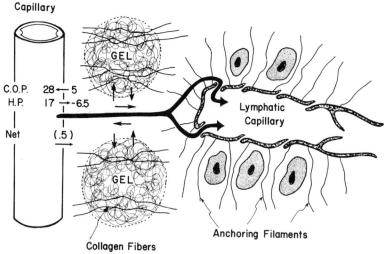

Figure 6–10 Capillary, tissue fluid, and lymph vessel relationships, illustrating dynamics at the capillary membrane, net outflow of fluid from the capillaries into the lymph vessels, and diffusional exchange of fluid and dissolved substances within the free fluid of the interstitial spaces and between the free fluid and the gel fluid.

interstitial spaces than can theoretically be accounted for by the colloid osmotic and hydrostatic forces at the capillary membrane.

If we now add separately the colloid osmotic and the hydrostatic forces on the two sides of the membrane, we find a colloid osmotic pressure difference of 23.0 mm. Hg (28 minus 5) attempting to cause absorption and a hydrostatic difference of 23.5 mm. Hg (17 minus −6.5) attempting to force fluid outward from the capillaries. Summing these values there is a net *filtration pressure* averaging about 0.5 mm. Hg at the capillary membrane. This 0.5 mm. Hg represents a continual state of nonequilibrium at the membrane, and it causes net filtration of fluid out of the capillaries into the tissue spaces, thereby providing the small trickle of fluid that flows into the lymph vessels. The lymph vessels in turn transport the fluid back into the circulation, so that a steady state develops, with neither loss of fluid out of the circulation nor gain of fluid.

LYMPHATIC DRAINAGE FROM THE TISSUES

In a sense, the lymphatic system is older than the venous system because at lower phylogenetic levels of animalhood whole blood is discharged directly from small blood vessels into the tissue spaces; the blood cells, along with other tissue fluid constituents, are then drained into lymphatic type vessels that pump the mixture back toward the heart. In higher animals some of these early vessels have remained relatively unchanged and have become the lymph vessels; others have changed into a less porous tubular system that comprises the capillaries and veins. The lymph vessels still perform the same function that they did in the lower animals, namely, they drain any excess fluid, cells, and debris that collect in the interstitial spaces.

Determinants of Lymph Flow

The rate of lymph flow is determined by four major factors: (1) pumping action of the lymph vessels themselves, (2) pumping effect of tissue motion, (3) pumping action at the tips of the terminal lymphatic capillaries, and (4) the pressure of fluid in the tissue spaces.

Lymphatic Valves and Pumping Action of the Lymph Vessels. The lymph vessels undergo continual rhythmic contraction, this occurring in all lymph vessels from the lymph capillaries up to the thoracic duct itself. Also all lymph vessels larger than the lymph capillaries have valves which are all oriented toward the point of discharge from the lymphatic system into the circulation at the junctures of the jugular and subclavian veins. Because of this orientation of the valves, contraction of a section of a lymph vessel will propel fluid toward the circulation but never backward toward the tissues. Combining this valve function with the natural rhythmic contraction of lymph vessels, the larger lymph vessels can pump against a pressure head of at least 15 to 20 mm. Hg.

Lymphatic Pumping Caused by Tissue Motion. Obviously, any tissue motion that compresses the lymph vessels from the outside can also compress fluid from one lymph vessel segment to another, but only in the direction that the valves are oriented. Therefore, tissue motion provides another propelling force to cause flow in the lymph vessels.

The Terminal Lymphatic Capillary Pump. Lymphatic contraction or compression also causes lymphatic pumping at the very tips of the lymphatic capillaries, which can be understood by referring again to Figure 6-10. The endothelial cells lining the lymphatic capillary are shown in this figure to overlap each other. At the point of overlap, the cells are not attached to each other, but instead, their inner edges can flap to the interior. Therefore, if the pressure outside the capillary is greater than that inside, fluid can push the flaps open and move to the interior. On the other hand, if the capillary is compressed or if it contracts so that the pressure inside becomes greater than that on the outside, any attempt of the fluid to escape from the capillary will close the flaps. Thus, the junctures between the endothelial cells are actually valves, allowing fluid to move into the lymphatic capillary but not in the outward direction.

Other structures important to terminal lymphatic pumping are the *anchoring filaments*. These are shown attached to the outside surfaces of the endothelial cells. They extend into the surrounding tissues where they are held tightly between the cells by the hyaluronic acid gel that fills the intercellular space. When the tissues are compressed, the cells compress the lymphatic capillary and cause fluid to move away from the capillary toward the larger lymphatics. Then, when the tissues recoil because of the tissue turgor, the anchoring filaments pull the lymphatic capillary to an open position. Experiments indicate that this creates a negative pressure inside the capillary and causes fluid to flow from the surrounding tissue areas into the lymphatic capillary. Once filled, another cycle of compression of the capillary will again force fluid into the larger lymph vessels. Thus, tissue motion of any type creates actual sucking at the very tips of the terminal lymphatic capillaries, and it is this sucking action that keeps the trickle of fluid flowing from the tissue spaces into the lymphatic system and from there back into the blood circulation.

Recent motion pictures have shown that even the terminal lymphatic capillaries undergo rhythmic contraction several times a minute, presumably caused by myofibrillae in the cytoplasm of the endothelial cells themselves. Obviously, this contraction also aids in the suction pump action of the terminal lymphatic capillaries. It is still a question whether this rhythmic motion is strong enough to be of significant value in comparison with the tissue motion itself.

Effect of Interstitial Fluid Pressure on Lymph Flow. Though the large lymph vessels can pump against a pressure head of 15 to 20 mm. Hg, the suction pump at the tips of the vessels seems to be a relatively weak one, having in most tissues a suction limit of about -7 mm. Hg. In other words, if the interstitial fluid pressure falls below -7 mm. Hg, lymph flow becomes essentially zero despite full pumping by the terminal suction pump.

When the interstitial fluid pressure rises above -7 mm. Hg, the lymphatic suction pump begins to function, and the rate of lymph flow increases almost linearly until the interstitial fluid pressure rises to equal atmospheric pressure. The normal rate of lymph flow from a typical peripheral tissue at a normal interstitial fluid pressure of approximately -6.5 mm. Hg is about 0.1 ml. of lymph per 100 grams of tissue per hour, illustrating the extremely slow trickle of fluid that normally flows in the lymphatics. However, when the interstitial fluid pressure rises to approach 0 mm. Hg (atmospheric pressure level), lymph flow increases 10- to 50-fold, now delivering as much as 1 to 5 ml. per 100 grams of tissue per hour.

INTERSTITIAL FLUID DYNAMICS AND EDEMA

There is a very common misbelief that the interstitial spaces are large, baggy chambers filled with freely mobile fluid. Even though the interstitial fluid spaces do represent about one sixth of the total tissue by volume, this concept is still far from the truth. Instead, the interstitial compartment is highly structured, filled primarily with two types of structural elements: (1) collagen fibers and (2) a gel matrix composed mainly of hyaluronic acid. The amount of freely mobile fluid in normal tissue spaces is probably a fraction of 1 per cent.

Figure 6–10 illustrates two gel masses lying between a blood capillary and a lymphatic capillary and also surrounded by tissue cells. Actually, this diagram is very out of proportion because it shows a large free fluid space between the two gel bodies, whereas in normal tissues this space is nothing more than minute sluices along the cell surfaces. This figure also shows two types of fluid mobility that occur within the interstitial spaces. The large arrows show a net trickle of fluid from the capillary through the tissue free fluid sluice and thence into the lymphatic capillary. The small arrows illustrate diffusion of substances into and out of the blood capillary and also back and forth between the free fluid space and the gel. Thus, continual dynamic equilibria exist between the different fluid compartments of the tissues.

Interstitial Pressures — Interstitial Fluid Pressure, Solid Tissue Pressure, and Total Tissue Pressure. In an earlier section of this chapter we have already pointed out that the normal *interstitial fluid pressure* in the free fluid of the interstitial spaces is about -6.5 mm. Hg, which is caused by the terminal lymphatic suction mechanism and by a tendency for the colloid osmotic pressure of the plasma to cause absorption of fluid from the tissue spaces through the capillary walls.

However, another type of pressure also occurs in the interstitial spaces. This is pressure exerted by the solid elements of the tissues and is called *solid tissue pressure.* When fluid is removed from the free fluid spaces by capillary osmosis or by lymphatic pumping, the decreased pressure in the free fluid immediately sucks fluid from the gel into the free fluid, and this fluid also is removed. Therefore, suction occurs in the entire interstitial space. In consequence, the walls of the interstitial spaces crowd toward each other — only to be held apart by the positive solid tissue pressure exerted by the solid structures in the spaces.

The solid structures in the interstitial spaces that exert solid tissue pressure are mainly the collagen fibers plus the reticulum of the hyaluronic acid gel. At present we do not know how much of the solid tissue pressure is caused by the gel and how much by the collagen and other fibers. However, the sum of these pressures must be great enough to oppose the negative suction effect of the interstitial fluid pressure, and it must also be great enough to overcome any other compressional forces that exist on the tissues, such as pressure exerted by a blood pressure cuff, pressure caused by turgor of the skin, pressure caused by compression points on the surface of the body, and so forth. When the skin and other tissues exert zero turgor and there is no compression from outside the body, the algebraically averaged solid tissue pressure must exactly equal the negative interstitial fluid pressure. If the fluid pressure is -6.5, then the solid tissue pressure must be 6.5. If we assume that skin elasticity causes the skin to press against the tissue with a pressure of another 2 mm. Hg, then the solid tissue pressure would be 8.5 mm. Hg.

Finally, one can sum the interstitial fluid pressure and the solid tissue pressure to determine still another quantity, the *total tissue pressure,* which is the pressure acting on any surface in a tissue by the summated effects of both the fluid and the solid elements. Assuming an average interstitial fluid pressure of -6.5 mm. Hg and a solid tissue pressure of 8.5 mm. Hg, then the total tissue pressure would be 2.0 mm. Hg.

Significance of the Different Types of Tissue Pressure. Because the above three different types of tissue pressure all exist in the tissue spaces, and because different methods for measuring tissue pressure measure different ones of these pressures, major confusion has developed regarding the true tissue pressure and its significance. However, if one will follow the logic of the above discussion, one can readily see that each of the different types of tissue pressure has its own peculiar significance, as follows:

Interstitial fluid pressure is the pressure that promotes fluid movement (a) from one part of a tissue to another part, (b) through the pores of a capillary membrane, or (c) from the tissue spaces into the lymphatics. In other words, interstitial fluid pressure relates to the fluids themselves and the forces that cause their mobility in the tissues.

Solid tissue pressure is pressure caused by contact points between solid elements of the tissues. Therefore, the greater the solid tissue pressure, the greater will be the forces exerted by these contact pressure points and, therefore, also the greater will be the distortional forces caused in the tissues. It is solid tissue pressure that causes the shapes of cells to be irregular, causes at least part of the folding of the fibers in the tissue spaces, and distorts such structures as capillaries, and so forth.

Interstitial fluid pressure and solid tissue pressure can be summated with each other by any structure that is capable of summating forces over a spatial domain. For instance, if fluid is compressing a capillary at one point and a fiber is compressing the capillary at a slightly different point, the elastic coefficient of the capillary membrane allows it to summate these two compressional forces even though they are not acting at precisely the same point. This is also true of cell membranes and of any other solid surface in a tissue. Therefore, total tissue pressure can act on any solid surface in a tissue. One of the most important of these solid surfaces is the blood vessels. Thus, the compressional force of the tissues against the blood vessels is equal to the total tissue pressure and is not equal to either the interstitial fluid pressure or the solid tissue pressure alone except when one of these is zero.

If we recognize, in accord with the discussion in the above section, that interstitial fluid pressure, solid tissue pressure, and total tissue pressure usually are very different from each other, the importance of distinguishing them becomes clear. In clinical medicine the two that are especially important are the interstitial fluid pressure, which is related primarily to the problem of interstitial fluid edema, and total tissue pressure, which is related primarily to the problem of blood vessel collapse.

Measurement of the Different Types of Tissue Pressure. MEASUREMENT OF TOTAL TISSUE PRESSURE. Methods are now available for measuring both interstitial fluid pressure and total tissue pressure. From these two values one can calculate the algebraically averaged solid tissue pressure.

The time-honored method for measuring tissue pressure has been to insert a minute needle into the tissue, then to inject about 1 cu. mm. of fluid at the tip of the needle, and, finally, to measure the pressure in this minute bolus of injected fluid using an extremely low compliance pressure measuring device. When pressure is measured in this manner, it gives a value of 1 to 3 mm. Hg, which is equal to the total tissue pressure. One might ask why this method measures total tissue pressure rather than interstitial fluid pressure, particularly since fluid is at the tip of the needle. The answer to this is that the fluid injected into the tissue temporarily displaces the solid tissue elements, so that the solid tissue pressure at this point is temporarily zero. Therefore, so long as the small bolus of fluid remains at the tip of the needle, its surface with the tissue is pressed against by the total tissue pressure, so that the pressure measured is total tissue pressure, not interstitial fluid pressure. If, however, one waits 30 seconds to several minutes after injecting the bolus of fluid and then records the pressure, it will likely be extremely erratic, depending upon whether the tip of the needle has become occluded with tissue and upon many other factors. Sometimes it still measures the positive value and sometimes it measures values as low as -20 to -30 mm. Hg (particularly when there is motion in the tissues and a ball-valve action develops at the tip of the needle). Therefore, this method can be used for measuring total tissue pressure only so long as the bolus of fluid is still present at the tip of the needle. Unfortunately, it usually cannot measure the true interstitial fluid pressure, which develops in the spaces surrounding the tip of the needle after a few minutes is allowed for absorption of the bolus of fluid. Further proof that this method measures total tissue pressure is afforded by pressures measured in minute flaccid balloons implanted in the tissues. These balloons, because of their continuous surface structure, certainly measure total tissue pressure, and they too measure a pressure of 1 to 3 mm. Hg in most tissues.

MEASUREMENT OF INTERSTITIAL FLUID PRESSURE. To measure interstitial fluid pressure, some device must be inserted into the tissue that can remain there long enough for the fluid in the interstitial spaces to come to equilibrium with the fluid in the device. The method that has been used most successfully thus far has been to implant a small hollow but porous capsule, 0.5 to 2.0 cm. in diameter, in the tissue. Over a period of days, the fluid inside the capsule comes to equilibrium with the fluid in the surrounding spaces. When pressure is measured inside this capsule, it is found to average about −6.5 mm. Hg in most tissue and allowed to come to equilibrium for with tight capsules such as the kidneys, which give higher pressure.

Unfortunately, the implanted capsule method often cannot be used in clinical patients, although it has been applied in a few instances in human beings. A newer method has been developed that gives an indication of the interstitial fluid pressure but probably does not measure its true value in all instances. This is a wick method in which a small wick of cotton protruding from the tip of a 1-mm. Teflon tube is inserted into the tissue and allowed to come to equilibrium for about one half hour. A low displacement manometer connected to the Teflon tube then records a pressure of about −2 to −5 mm. Hg, a less negative pressure than that usually measured with the perforated capsule. However, the fact that this method does measure a negative pressure demonstrates that other methods besides the porous capsule method can also be used for measuring negative interstitial fluid pressure. Furthermore, the wick method can be applied to the human being, though the problem of bleeding around the inserted wick is likely to nullify the validity of the pressure measurements. Those who have employed this method thus far in human beings have used it primarily for determining *changes* in interstitial fluid pressure rather than for measuring true value of the pressure.

Regulation of Interstitial Fluid Pressure

The interstitial fluid pressure remains reasonably constant most of the time and remains at a subatmospheric pressure level in essentially all external soft tissues. This regulation of the interstitial fluid pressure is achieved in the following way. If the pressure becomes too great, lymph flow increases. The lymph flow in turn drains some of the excess fluid from the interstitial spaces and reduces the pressure. However, the pressure is reduced even more in still another way, as follows: The increased lymph drainage carries increased quantities of protein away from the interstitial spaces, thereby reducing the interstitial fluid colloid osmotic pressure. When this happens, the still high colloid osmotic pressure of the plasma causes osmotic reabsorption of fluid from the interstitial spaces into the blood. This second effect normally accounts for nine tenths or more of the reabsorption of excess fluid from the usual tissue space, while the lymphatic drainage mechanism accounts for less than one tenth. In severe edematous states, on the other hand, the lymphatic drainage mechanism becomes progressively more important, sometimes outdoing the osmosis mechanism because of the extreme rates of lymph flow that occur at high interstitial fluid pressures.

Regulation of Interstitial Fluid Volume

Obviously, the regulation of interstitial fluid volume is also closely related to the regulation of interstitial fluid pressure, because whenever the interstitial fluid volume increases, the tissue spaces expand, and correspondingly the interstitial fluid pressure increases. The same sequence as that described above for interstitial fluid pressure regulation ensues once more: namely, increased pressure increases lymph flow, decreases tissue fluid colloid osmotic pressure, increases capillary osmotic absorption of fluid from the tissue spaces, and thereby returns interstitial fluid volume back toward normal. Therefore, all these factors operate together in a simple but extremely important basic control system to keep the interstitial fluid pressure, protein concentration, and fluid volume all regulated to very exact levels.

Physiologic Basis of Edema

Positive Interstitial Fluid Pressure as Cause of Edema. In several thousand measurements of interstitial fluid pressure using the perforated capsule technique and encompassing both non-edematous and edematous tissues, it has been found that loose areolar subcutaneous tissues will invariably be edematous if the interstitial fluid pressure is positive — that is, above atmospheric pressure; on the other hand, the tissues will be non-edematous if the pressure is negative (less than atmospheric pressure). Therefore, whether or not edema exists in these tissues seems to be determined by a simple factor: whether the interstitial fluid pressure is above atmospheric pressure or less than atmospheric pressure.

The Normally "Dry" State of the Interstitial "Free" Fluid Compartment. The fluid in the interstitial fluid compartment exists in two states: (1) a "free" state in which the fluid flows freely and (2) a "gel" or "non-mobile" state, Figure 6–11 illustrates the volumes of interstitial fluid in both of these states at the different interstitial fluid pressures. At a normal pressure of −6.5 mm. Hg

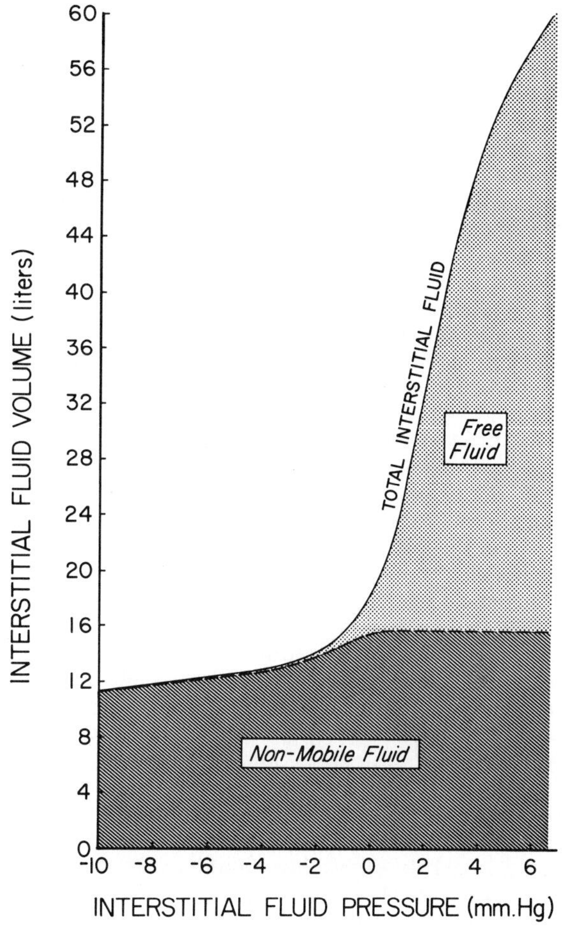

Figure 6–11   Changes in total interstitial fluid volume, free fluid volume, and non-mobile fluid volume (gel fluid) in the tissue spaces as the interstitial fluid pressure rises from a negative value of −10 up to a positive value of 7 mm. Hg. Note the rapid appearance of free fluid in the interstitial spaces as the interstitial fluid pressure crosses from the subatmospheric pressure range into the supra-atmospheric pressure range. (Reprinted from Guyton, A. C., Granger, H. J., and Taylor, A. E.: Physiol. Rev., 51:527, 1971.)

there is essentially zero free fluid, as shown in the figure, whereas, on the other hand, there are approximately 12 liters of non-mobile gel fluid in the adult human being.

Thus, in the normal interstitial fluid spaces, the interstitial fluid volume is regulated to essentially zero free fluid. Furthermore, whenever any significant amount of free fluid begins to develop in the tissues, the lymphatic and capillary osmotic mechanisms normally return this free fluid to the circulatory system almost immediately. Thus, in effect, the mechanisms for regulating interstitial fluid volume normally maintain an almost completely "dry" state in the *free* fluid portion of the interstitial spaces. The fluid that does exist in the interstitial spaces is almost entirely that fluid which is bound in the form of a gel.

Character of the Interstitial Fluids in Edema — Pitting Edema.   Note also in Figure 6–11 the changes in both free fluid and non-mobile fluid volumes when the interstitial fluid pressure rises. The non-mobile fluid volume increases

about 30 per cent as the interstitial fluid pressure rises from −6.5 mm. Hg up to zero — that is, before frank edema occurs. This is caused by the natural tendency of the gel reticulum to expand and thereby to pull fluid into the gel. However, when the free interstitial fluid pressure rises above zero, the gel has by then expanded to its limit, so that thereafter the non-mobile gel fluid volume does not increase further. Instead, above this very critical level of zero pressure the free interstitial fluid volume increases drastically.

The sudden increase in *free* fluid volume as the interstitial fluid pressure rises above atmospheric pressure accounts for the pitting phenomenon observed in most forms of extracellular fluid edema. Free fluid is highly mobile in the tissue spaces, whereas the gel fluid is almost completely non-mobile. Therefore, in the normal state of the interstitial spaces, pitting does not occur. On the other hand, when vast amounts of free fluid develop, the fluid can be made to flow freely from one sector of the tissues to another. Thus, pressure with a finger on an edematous area will move fluid from the point of compression, and a pit will remain for a few seconds to a minute or more after the finger is removed — that is, until the fluid has time to flow back into the pitted area.

The high mobility of free fluid in edema also explains several other clinical phenomena, such as the continual weeping of wounds in edematous tissues and the failure of wounds to heal in edematous tissues. It explains, too, at least part of the dependent nature of edema. For instance, if a person has generalized edema, fluid can actually flow through the tissues from the top side of the body to the low side, such as from one breast to the other in a patient lying on her side. Obviously, another cause of dependent edema is high pressure in the dependent capillaries.

Role of Gel in the Interstitial Spaces. Although very little research has been performed on the functional importance of gel in interstitial spaces, the gel probably has at least three very valuable functions. One of these is to prevent dependent edema even in the normal person. Measurements of fluid flow in free fluid versus fluid flow through hyaluronic gel have shown a difference of several hundred thousandfold. In other words, the fact that the tissue spaces normally are filled with gel and not with free fluid prevents the fluid from flowing from the upper parts of the body to the lower parts. With one sixth of our body composed of interstitial fluid, one can readily understand that if the fluid were not in a gel state, both legs would almost certainly be perpetually edematous.

Second, the non-mobile nature of the gel prevents spread of infection in the tissues. Indeed, some bacteria are extremely pathogenic simply because they secrete hyaluronidase to dissolve the gel and allow movement of the local fluids with consequent spread of the bacteria.

Third, the gel probably is important to keep the formed elements of the tissues separated at appropriate distances from each other. Since most nutrients are transported from the capillaries to the cells and most excreta from the cells to the capillaries by the process of diffusion, it is essential that appropriate avenues be maintained for adequate diffusion through the spaces. If the cells should be crowded completely upon each other, enough space would not be available for the diffusion process, and one would expect outlying cells to be deficient in certain nutrients. For instance, glucose will not diffuse through cells because it becomes trapped inside cells. Therefore, it is essential that glucose diffuse *between* cells if it is to reach those cells far removed from the capillaries. Fortunately, such substances diffuse in tissue gel almost equally as rapidly as in free fluid. On the other hand, the diffusion process operates most efficiently for short distances of diffusion. Therefore, it is important that the mechanism for controlling interstitial fluid volume maintain the volume only at a certain level — not too little, not too much. This is accomplished by the mechanism that maintains the tissue fluid compartment normally dry of free fluid and limits the volume to the gel fluid.

Tissue Nutrition in Edema. One of the major problems in edema is nutrition of the tissue cells, because expansion of the tissue spaces increases the distances required for diffusion. Every physician becomes cognizant of this when treating varicose ulcers of the leg, because it is almost impossible for these to heal in a continuously edematous leg. Also, nutrition of essentially any tissue of the body can be compromised at least to some extent by edema. Indeed, functional measurements in the heart have even shown that an edematous myocardium has considerably decreased pumping capability.

Role of Capillary and Lymphatic Dynamics in Causation of Edema. The roles of the capillaries and the lymphatics in causing edema are so well known that they require only transient mention at this point. There are basically four dynamic abnormalities that can cause edema: (1) high capillary pressure, (2) low plasma colloid osmotic pressure, (3) increased permeability of the capillaries, and (4) blockage of the lymphatics. All these tend to increase the interstitial fluid pressure, and when this pressure rises above the atmospheric pressure level, edema occurs. Increased permeability of the capillaries increases the tendency for edema in three ways: (a) by allowing more rapid leakage of fluid into the tissue spaces; (b) by decreasing the effectiveness of the proteins to cause colloid osmotic pressure at the capillary pores (that is, the proteins leak through the pores rather than creating colloid osmotic pressure); and (c) by buildup of protein in the interstitial spaces and loss of protein from the blood, thus causing greatly enhanced tissue colloid osmotic pressure as well as reduced plasma colloid osmotic pressure. Although the literature frequently refers to all three of these as being important, one can show mathematically that only the last of the three is usually of real significance, namely, increased tissue colloid osmotic pressure and decreased plasma colloid osmotic pressure because of protein leakage. Long before the other two can possibly become important, this last effect will have killed the patient because of massive edema and volume depletion.

Safety Factors Against Edema

Fortunately, the human being has tremendous capability for resisting the development of edema. For instance, the capillary pressure in a usual tissue must rise to approximately two times normal before edema will appear, or the colloid osmotic pressure of the plasma must fall from the normal level of 28 mm. Hg to below 10 mm. Hg before edema will occur. From the previous discussion of interstitial fluid dynamics and of edema, one can readily understand how these tremendous safety factors come about.

Basically, edema cannot occur until the interstitial fluid pressure rises above atmospheric pressure, and there are three different mechanisms that come into play to prevent this from occurring. These are the following:

1. The normal negative interstitial fluid pressure of approximately −6.5 mm. Hg must be lost before edema can occur. Therefore, the mechanisms discussed above for maintenance of the normal negative interstitial fluid pressure constitute the first safety factor.

2. When the interstitial fluid pressure begins to rise, lymph flow increases rapidly, increasing an average of 20- to 25-fold by the time the interstitial pressure rises from its normally negative value up to the level of atmospheric pressure. This greatly enhanced lymph flow constitutes a second safety factor against edema. Approximately 7 mm. Hg excess filtration pressure is required across the capillary membrane to form the amount of lymph that can be carried away by this high level of lymph flow.

3. When the lymph flow increases, the rapid movement of fluid through the interstitial spaces toward the lymph vessels washes protein out of the interstitial spaces. This decreases the colloid osmotic pressure in the interstitial fluid from the normal value of about 5 mm. Hg down to approximately 1 mm. Hg. Therefore, the plasma colloid osmotic pressure becomes 4 mm. Hg more effective for absorbing fluid from the tissue spaces. This adds another 4 mm. Hg of safety factor.

Adding the above safety factors, 6.5 + 7.0 + 4.0, one finds a total safety factor of approximately 17.5 mm. Hg. This explains the necessity for the colloid osmotic pressure to decrease from the normal value of 28 down to 10 mm. Hg. before edema will occur. It also explains the doubling of capillary pressure required before edema occurs, an increase from 17 to 34 mm. Hg, or a safety factor of 17 mm. Hg. Finally, recent experiments have also shown that edema can be used in a normal arm exposed to an external vacuum greater than 18 mm. Hg but cannot be caused by a vacuum less than 18 mm. Hg.

There obviously is a clinical state one might call "pre-edema," which means a state in which much of the safety factor has been dissipated even though the edema state itself has not yet been reached.

BLOOD VOLUME AND ITS REGULATION

Hemodynamic Factors. The basic hemodynamic mechanisms for blood volume regulation can be understood by combining the discussions from previous sections of this chapter. First, referring again to Figure 6–1, one notes that an increase in blood volume increases cardiac output, which increases arterial pressure, which increases urinary output, which decreases extracellular fluid volume, which finally returns the blood volume back toward normal. All steps of this mechanism have been proved in individual physiologic experiments. Also, in animals with the nervous system completely destroyed, infusion of several hundred milliliters of saline causes approximately a tenfold increase in urinary output within less than one minute. This increase continues, but with progressive decrement, for an hour or more until the urinary output gradually dwindles back to its control value. In the meantime, essentially all the excess saline infused is recovered in the urine.

Hormonal Factors. Two different hormones have been especially implicated in blood volume regulation, antidiuretic hormone and aldosterone. However, when either of these two hormones is infused for as long as a month into an animal at rates several times as high as the normal secretory rate, it is rare that the blood volume will change more than a few per cent, and the extracellular fluid volume also usually will change no more than 5 to 15 per cent. The only instance in which these volumes do change excessively occurs when the heart fails as a secondary result of the hormone administration, in which case excessive quantities of fluid do then accumulate, but because of the heart failure rather than because of the hormone itself.

This brings up the question of what these two hormones actually control if it is not volume. Recent studies have demonstrated that ADH is mainly concerned with control of the sodium concentration in the extracellular fluid and aldosterone with the control of potassium concentration. When both the thirst and ADH mechanisms are blocked, sodium concentration varies very widely depending on the intake of salt and/or water. And when excess quantities of ADH are secreted, the sodium concentration decreases markedly. The mechanism of this effect is the following: The ADH causes an initial retention of water by the kidneys, but this in turn sets into play a number of different effects, including a slight rise in arterial pressure, that cause a secondary increase in urinary output containing large amounts of salt. Consequently, the sodium concentration of the extracellular fluids decreases while the water content of the body increases slightly.

In the case of aldosterone, it has been taught so frequently that aldosterone controls body sodium that it is difficult to understand why aldosterone actually is far more effective in the control of extracellular fluid potassium than in the control of extracellular fluid sodium. Aldosterone does indeed cause excessive renal tubular reabsorption of sodium but also excessive secretion of potassium. When the sodium is reabsorbed, the ADH and thirst mechanisms automatically increase the body water as well and therefore bring the sodium concentration back to the normal level. Also, the extracellular fluid volume increases, and this activates a secondary increase in urinary output to cause loss of both the extra water and sodium, which is the mechanism called "aldosterone escape." As a result of this effect aldosterone fails to affect sodium concentration measurably. Therefore, the only remaining major effect of aldosterone on the extracellular fluid is its effect on the potassium concentration rather than on either the sodium concentration or the total extracellular fluid volume.

Nervous Factors.   Dilatation of the atria of the heart initiates potent nervous vasodilating reflexes to the kidneys and also transmits signals to the neurohypophysis to diminish the secretion of antidiuretic hormone. Both these effects increase the output of urine. Therefore, it is frequently said that the atrial receptors are "volume receptors" that detect increases in blood volume and in turn help to rectify the abnormality. However, this mechanism seems to be important in volume regulation only transiently, because the high atrial pressures occurring in heart failure do not cause continued excessive urinary output, as the mechanism would suggest.

Relationship Between Blood Volume Regulation and Interstitial Fluid Volume Regulation

Retention of fluid by the kidneys does not mean that the fluid will necessarily remain in the blood, because extracellular fluid is partitioned between the plasma compartment of the blood and the two interstitial fluid compartments, the free fluid compartment and the gel compartment. Under normal circumstances, in the absence of edema, the free fluid compartment volume of the interstitial spaces is essentially zero, and it is only the gel compartment with which we are concerned. When extra amounts of fluid are available, the recoil effect of the gel reticulum causes the gel to absorb moderate amounts of the extra fluid. On the other hand, in dehydration states fluid is pulled out of the gel and returned to the circulation either by capillary osmosis or through the lymphatics. Therefore, there is a dynamic equilibrium between the plasma volume and the interstitial gel volume.

Measurements have shown that infusion of a balanced electrolyte solution into the circulatory system of a nonedematous person will cause approximately two thirds of the fluid to enter the gel compartment of the tissue spaces and the remainder to stay in the blood. Therefore, in the pre-edema state, retention of water and salt by the kidneys increases both blood volume and interstitial fluid volume. Conversely, dehydration decreases both of these; indeed, severe dehydration can cause circulatory shock.

Tissue Compliance Change in Edema.   An entirely different effect occurs once the edema stage is reached, that is, once the interstitial fluid pressure rises above atmospheric pressure level. Referring again to Figure 6–11, one notes that the total interstitial fluid volume now increases extremely rapidly with very little additional rise in the interstitial fluid pressure. This is in contrast to a marked rise in pressure occurring with only a small volume increase in nonedematous tissues. The reason for this difference is that the gel in the normal tissue spaces is in a compacted state, and the volume cannot change without simultaneous marked changes in the negative pressure that causes the compaction. On the other hand, once the interstitial fluid pressure rises into the positive pressure range, there is not a significant restraining force to prevent outward stretching of the tissue spaces. The only major restraining force is the skin, and measurements show that the skin exerts less than one twenty-fifth as much restraining force on changes in the interstitial fluid volume as do the elastic compaction forces of the gel. To express this another way, in the negative interstitial fluid pressure range, the compliance of the tissue space is slight, whereas in the positive interstitial fluid pressure range the looseness of the skin and other tissue elements allows the compliance to increase 25-fold.

Therefore, once the interstitial pressure rises to a positive value, tremendous quantities of free fluid begin to collect in the tissue spaces, and this fluid collects despite extremely little additional rise in interstitial fluid pressure.

Safety Valve Function of the Interstitial Fluid Spaces for Blood Volume.   The significance of edema to the circulatory system probably has escaped most physiologists and clinicians alike. The ability for tremendous quantities of fluid to collect rapidly in tissue spaces when the blood volume rises above a certain critical level is actually an important safety valve for the circulatory system. Were it not for this, it would be impossible to infuse more than 1 to 3 liters of electrolyte solution into a normal patient without killing him, which one can demonstrate any time he wishes by simply infusing several liters of fluid intravenously at a rate too rapid for the fluid to transude out of the capillaries into the interstitial spaces. Pressures throughout the system rise to extreme values and can cause rupture of vessels, arrhythmias of the heart, and typical signs of acute cardiac failure.

Therefore, the edema mechanism is an important safety valve for blood volume control in the human being. Furthermore, this "safety valve" functions at a very exact capillary pressure level — at exactly that capillary pressure at which the total safety factor against edema has been dissipated.

Significance of Blood Volume Measurements and of Mean Circulatory Filling Pressure

Because it is very easy to measure blood volume by injecting any type of indicator material that will stay in the circulatory system and then measuring the degree of dilution of the indicator, blood volume measurements are frequently made; yet they are rarely of great significance. The reason for this is elementary: blood volume is automatically adjusted to fit the capacity of the circulatory system itself, and even such oddities as varicose veins can change both the capacity of the circulatory system and the blood volume markedly. Likewise, a state of vasoconstriction, as occurs in patients with pheochromocytomas, can greatly reduce the capacity of the circulation. Or vasodilatation, as caused by block of the sympathetic nervous system, can increase the capacity of the system.

The tightness with which the blood volume fills the circulatory system is measured by the mean circulatory filling pressure, and this can change as a result of a change in either blood volume or circulatory capacity. From our earlier discussion of cardiac output regulation, it is clear that it is not blood volume per se that affects venous return and cardiac output but, instead, the mean circulatory filling pressure. Therefore, alteration of the mean circulatory filling pressure, whether it be caused by a change in blood volume or change in capacity of the system, has essentially the same effect on the circulation regardless of the cause.

Consequently, the factor that needs to be measured, so far as the dynamics of the circulation are concerned, is not blood volume but, instead, mean circulatory filling pressure. In animals, in which it is possible to stop the heart and to bring pressures to equilibrium throughout the system, it is possible to measure this pressure, the normal value for which is 7 mm. Hg. In human beings, this measurement has never been achieved. In the meantime, one can understand why blood volume measurements are much less useful in ex-

plaining hemodynamic function of the circulation than are such functional measurements as arterial pressure and cardiac output.

Relationship Between Right Atrial Pressure and Blood Volume

Every clinician is very familiar with the fact that an increase in right atrial pressure, as occurs in heart failure, is usually associated with increased blood volume. This can readily be understood on the basis of the hemodynamics already discussed in this chapter. When the heart fails and the right atrial pressure increases, venous return immediately decreases, thereby reducing cardiac output, arterial pressure, and urinary output. Consequently, the body fluid volumes begin to increase and continue to increase until the mean circulatory filling pressure has risen enough to oppose the negative effect of right atrial pressure on venous return. When this has been achieved, a new steady state will have been reached. But, in the meantime, since the mean circulatory filling pressure has been greatly increased — for instance, an increase in right atrial pressure of 6 mm. Hg will cause almost a 6 mm. Hg rise in mean circulatory filling pressure, from the normal value of 7 up to 13 mm. Hg—one can readily understand how this is associated with an increase in blood volume.

In acute conditions, an increase in mean circulatory filling pressure of 1 mm. Hg is associated with an increase in blood volume a little over 2 per cent. However, in chronic conditions, in which the phenomenon of stress relaxation allows slow stretching of the circulatory system, a rise in mean circulatory filling pressure of 1 mm. Hg is associated with as much as 5 per cent increase in blood volume. Therefore, in patients with long-standing congestive heart failure, in which the mean circulatory filling pressure is sometimes as high as 25 mm. Hg, the blood volume can occasionally increase to as much as 50 to 100 per cent above normal.

PULMONARY CIRCULATION

Many of the same hemodynamic principles that apply to the systemic circulation also apply to the pulmonary circulation, but this is not entirely true. For instance, the pulmonary system is a low pressure system, for which reason it has correspondingly thinner arterial and arteriolar vasculature, as well as less smooth muscle in the vessel walls. This is very fortunate, because the pulmonary vasculature receives the same stroke volume output from the right heart that the entire systemic arterial tree receives from the left heart. The high degree of distensibility of the pulmonary arteries, despite their short length, is of major advantage in allowing the pulmonary vascular tree to absorb the large thrust of blood with each heart beat. Also, because of very low pulmonary vascular resistance from the arteries to the veins, only about one tenth that of the systemic circulation, there is marked runoff of blood from the pulmonary arteries to the left atrium even before systole is complete, which decreases the quantity of blood that must be accommodated in the pulmonary arterial tree. These two factors acting together cause the pulmonary arterial pulse pressure to be only about 14 mm. Hg, in contrast to 40 mm. Hg in the aorta.

Effect of Alveolar Hypoxia on Local Vascular Resistance. There are three important exceptions to the usual rule that blood flow is distributed indiscriminately to all alveoli. The first of these exceptions occurs when some alveoli are ventilated to a lesser extent than others. If the poorly ventilated alveoli were perfused with blood to the same extent as the other alveoli, the oxygen levels in the poorly ventilated alveoli would become depressed, thereby creating hypoxia in the adjacent blood vessels. However, the effect of hypoxia on these vessels is exactly opposite to its effect on systemic vasculature, causing in this instance vasoconstriction instead of vasodilatation. The vasoconstriction reduces the perfusion of the affected alveolar walls and thereby shunts blood flow to other alveoli that are better ventilated. Unfortunately, though, this mechanism is a weak one — that is, it does not have a very high feedback gain. Therefore, it is not as important a mechanism as one might wish it to be to control distribution of blood flow to the respective alveoli.

Pulmonary physiologists have also pointed out that hypoxia occurring in all of the alveoli at the same time can sometimes cause enough vasoconstriction of the total pulmonary vasculature to elevate pulmonary arterial pressure significantly. Occasionally, the rise in pulmonary arterial pressure is enough to cause right heart failure with corresponding reduction in cardiac output. Oxygen therapy often aids this condition, presumably by decreasing the pulmonary vascular resistance.

Effect of Atelectasis on Local Blood Flow. The second condition in which unequal distribution of alveolar blood flow occurs to a significant extent is atelectasis. When a bronchus is blocked, the alveoli beyond the block begin to collapse within minutes, and whole segments of the lung can become collapsed over a period of hours. The mechanical collapse of the alveoli causes the solid tissues between the alveoli to close tightly around the local blood vessels, in some cases actually kinking the vessels. As a result, in total atelectasis as much as 80 per cent of blood flow is usually shunted to the normal lung tissue. This may be a very fortunate effect because it ensures that essentially all the blood flow passing through the lungs will flow in juxtaposition to ventilated alveoli and will bypass the nonventilated alveoli.

Effect of Hydrostatic Pressure on Local Blood Flow in the Lung. Still a third hemodynamic factor that causes non-uniform blood flow in the pulmonary circulation is the different hydrostatic levels of the different parts of the lung. When a person is in a standing position, the apex of his lung lies as much as 10 to 15 cm. above the midlevel of the heart, which means that the pulmonary arterial pressures are only barely high enough to pump blood through the apical vessels. Indeed, only the systolic pressure is high enough, so that blood flows through the apical vessels in spurts synchronized with cardiac systole. At the base of the lung, on the other hand, located some 10 cm. below the level of the heart, the pulmonary vessels are subjected not only to normal pulmonary vascular pressure but also to an additional 7 mm. Hg hydrostatic pressure. Therefore, both the diastolic and systolic pressures are considerably elevated in the base of the lung, and blood flows through this region continuously throughout systole and diastole. This difference creates another problem, namely, that in the standing, quiet state the base of the lung is overperfused while the apex is underperfused. This effect is partially compensated by the fact that the base of the lung is, for mechanical reasons, ventilated to a greater extent than is the apex. Fortunately, during exercise, when the fullest functional capacity of the lungs is needed, the pulmonary pressures rise throughout the lungs, and all portions now reach almost optimal ventilation-perfusion ratios.

Pulmonary Edema

Capillary dynamics in the lungs obey almost exactly the same principles as those discussed earlier for the systemic circulation, but a few differences are important.

Normal Mechanism for Keeping the Alveoli "Dry." To keep the alveoli in their normal "dry" state — that is, filled with air rather than with fluid — the pulmonary interstitial fluid pressure is almost certainly negative in the same way that it is in peripheral tissues. Indirect measurements indicate this pressure to be about −8 mm. Hg. Negative pressure in the interstitial spaces of the lungs obviously would keep the alveolar membrane pulled tightly against the capillaries and their supporting structures. It would also provide an absorptive force for causing absorption of any stray fluid that might occur in the alveoli, thus returning the alveoli to their normal dry state.

On the other hand, if the interstitial fluid pressure of the lungs should ever rise into the positive range, one would expect pulmonary edema to result in the same way that edema results in peripheral tissues.

Safety Factor Against Pulmonary Edema. The safety factor against edema in the lungs is greater than in systemic tissues. The pulmonary capillary pressure must be increased acutely to approximately 30 mm. Hg, or to about 2 mm. Hg greater than the colloid osmotic pressure of the blood, before pulmonary edema will ensue. Since the normal pulmonary capillary pressure in the human being is about 7 mm. Hg, the safety factor against pulmonary edema can be calculated to be approximately 23 mm. Hg, which compares with 18 mm. Hg in the systemic circulation. An acute increase in pulmonary capillary pressure above 30 mm. Hg will cause a proportionately increased rate of fluid transudation into the lungs (based on studies in dogs), and when the pressure is raised acutely to 50 mm. Hg it can cause lethal pulmonary edema in as little as one half hour.

Role of Lymphatics in Chronic Pulmonary Edema. In chronic pulmonary edema, still another safety factor occurs. Even a few weeks of elevated left atrial pressure causes great overgrowth of the pulmonary lymphatics, increasing their lymph carrying capacity sometimes as much as six- to tenfold. Therefore, one would expect that pulmonary capillary pressure would have to rise much higher than the 30 mm. Hg required in acute conditions before pulmonary edema would occur. This corresponds to the finding in many catheter laboratories that patients with chronic mitral stenosis frequently have chronic elevations of pulmonary capillary pressure in the 35 to 45 mm. Hg pressure range without evident pulmonary edema.

Alveolar Membrane Leakage and Alveolar Fluid in Pulmonary Edema. Another primary difference between pulmonary edema and systemic edema is that the limiting boundary of the pulmonary interstitial spaces, the alveolar membrane, is a very thin and weak one-cell layer membrane. Therefore, in contrast to the skin on the surface of the body, the alveolar membrane cannot withstand significant amounts of positive pressure in the interstitial spaces of the lungs. Evidence at present indicates that these alveolar membranes begin to break when the interstitial fluid pressure rises above approximately 1 to 2 mm. Hg positive pressure. When this happens, fluid in the interstitial spaces of the lungs simply flows immediately into the alveoli. Therefore, only very early pulmonary edema can be confined to the interstitial spaces; if this edema develops to any significant extent, a major share of the edema fluid immediately flows through the broken alveolar membranes into the alveoli themselves.

ARTERIAL PULSATION

The clinically important features of arterial pulsation are so well understood by most clinicians that they deserve little comment at this point. However, it is important to review a few simple principles.

Arterial Elasticity and Net Stroke Volume as Determinants of Arterial Pulse Pressure. The basic determinants of arterial pulse pressure are twofold: (1) the elasticity of the arteries; and (2) the net stroke volume output of the heart, which is defined as the stroke volume of the heart minus the volume runoff through the small vessels during the period of systole. In other words, the greater the net gain of blood volume in the arterial tree between the beginning of systole and the end of systole, the greater also will be the arterial pulse pressure. Also, the higher the volume elasticity coefficient of the arterial vessels — that is, the less the distensibility — the greater will be the pulse pressure.

Obviously, a large number of other factors can affect one or both of these two basic determinants of the pulse pressure. These include the presence or absence of arteriosclerosis, the degree of active vasoconstriction or vasodilatation of the arterial tree, and the sizes of the arteries themselves, all of which affect the volume elasticity coefficient of the arterial system. Factors that can affect the net stroke volume output include cardiac output, heart rate, and degree of peripheral vasodilatation. That is, stroke volume output is equal to cardiac output divided by heart rate, and net stroke volume output is stroke volume diminished by the amount of blood runoff during systole.

Diminished Peripheral Pulsation. The clinical habit of feeling the peripheral pulse can be a highly valuable art, even to the extent that a few clinicians can estimate arterial pressure quite accurately by feeling the radial artery, although, in general, this art is no longer developed significantly by most clinicians. Only two features of the peripheral arterial pulse are noted by the usual clinician — the pulse frequency pattern and the intensity of pulsation.

The significance of diminished intensity of the peripheral pulse is illustrated in Figure 6–12, which shows a recorded arterial pulse curve from the dorsalis pedis artery before and after stimulation of the sympathetic nerves. Note that the pulse pressure diminished markedly following the vasoconstriction and that the mean pressure level also diminished. This figure demonstrates that there is a high degree of correlation between the intensity of peripheral arterial pulsation and tissue perfusion. Consequently, the clinical dictum that diminished pulsation means diminished tissue perfusion is indeed a well-founded one, al-

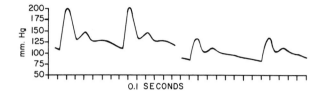

Figure 6-12 Pressure contour in the dorsalis pedis artery recorded, first, under normal conditions and, second, during stimulation of the sympathetic nerves supplying the femoral artery. (Modified from Alexander, R. S., and Kantrowitz, A.: Surgery, *33*:42, 1953.)

though, of course, this also has its exceptions, especially when collateral vessels have taken over the function of a normally pulsatile artery.

Some physiologists have claimed that arterial pulsation per se plays a significant role in maintenance of peripheral perfusion. However, this is still a very doubtful concept and has been both supported and denied by different investigators. The only value of peripheral arterial pulsation that has thus far been proved beyond doubt is its capability, in at least some instances, to promote lymph flow. In a completely pulseless tissue, lymph flow is greatly diminished, particularly when an animal is under the influence of anesthesia such as sodium pentobarbital that can block lymph vessel vasomotion.

The Hemodynamic Anomaly of Pulsus Alternans. Pulsus alternans is a condition in which the arterial pulse alternates — usually every other heart beat: first strong, then weak, then strong, and continuing in this alternating pattern. Thus far, it has never been appropriately explained. It is mentioned here because several basic studies of circulatory hemodynamics have recently offered a possible explanation. One of these was a computer study in which the systemic circulation and the pulmonary circulation were simulated mathematically to operate in a complete circuit. In performing different experiments with the simulation, several conditions were found in which typical pulsus alternans occurred. One of these was abnormality of ventricular re-

sponse to changes in atrial pressure. When the computer was programmed so that a very minute change in atrial pressure would cause marked change in ventricular output, the left ventricle would first pump an excessively large quantity of blood into the systemic circulation during one heart beat, but during the next heart beat the right ventricle would pump an excessively large quantity into the lungs, the blood volume oscillating back and forth between the pulmonary circulation and the systemic circulation. It was also possible to cause oscillation of the blood volume between the central circulation of the chest region and the more peripheral circulation. Furthermore, the system frequently would be working completely normally and would then be thrown into pulsus alternans by some transient event that occurred in the simulated circulation. This is completely in accord with typical findings in the clinical catheter laboratory, when a sudden event related to the catheterization procedure itself often can throw a person into pulsus alternans.

This phenomenon and its possible explanation have been discussed here because, if the explanation is correct, the phenomenon is strictly a hemodynamic problem resulting from resonance within the mechanical system itself, not too unlike the resonance that occurs in the pipe of a pipe organ, with pressure waves reflecting back and forth from one end of the pipe to the other.

REFERENCES

Berne, R. M., and Rubio, R.: Regulation of coronary blood flow. Adv. Cardiol., *12*:303, 1974.

Bevegard, B. S., and Shepherd, J. T.: Regulation of the circulation during exercise in man. Physiol. Rev., *47*:178, 1967.

Bishop, V. S., and Stone, H. L.: Quantitative description of ventricular output curves in conscious dogs. Circ. Res., *20*:581, 1967.

Braunwald, E.: Regulation of the circulation. I. N. Engl. J. Med., *290*:1124, 1974.

Braunwald, E.: Regulation of the circulation. II. N. Engl. J. Med., *290*:1420, 1974.

Coleman, T. G., and Guyton, A. C.: Hypertension caused by salt loading in the dog. III. Onset transients of cardiac output and other circulatory variables. Circ. Res., *25*:153, 1969.

Duling, B. R., and Berne, R. M.: Propagated vasodilatation in the microcirculation of the hamster cheek pouch. Circ. Res., *26*:163, 1970.

Fishman, A. P., and Hecht, H. H. (eds.): The Pulmonary Cir-

culation and Interstitial Space. University of Chicago Press, Chicago, 1969.

Genest, J., Koiw, E., and Kuchel, O.: Hypertension. McGraw-Hill Book Co., New York, 1977.

Goetz, K. L., Bond, G. C., and Bloxham, D. D.: Atrial receptors and renal function. Physiol. Rev., *55*:157, 1975.

Gregg, D. E.: Coronary Circulation in Health and Disease. Lea and Febiger, Philadelphia, 1950.

Guyton, A. C., and Coleman, T. G.: Quantitative analysis of the pathophysiology of hypertension. Circ. Res., *24*(Suppl. 1):*1*, 1969.

Guyton, A. C., Coleman, T. G., Cowley, A. W., Jr., Manning, R. D., Jr., Norman, R. A., Jr., and Ferguson, J. D.: A systems analysis approach to understanding long-range arterial blood pressure control and hypertension. Circ. Res., *35*:159, 1974.

Guyton, A. C., Jones, C. E., and Coleman, T. G.: Circulatory Physiology: Cardiac Output and Its Regulation, 2nd Ed. W. B. Saunders Co., Philadelphia, 1973.

Guyton, A. C., Taylor, A. E., and Granger, H. J.: Circulatory Physiology II. Dynamics and Control of the Body Fluids. W. B. Saunders Co., Philadelphia, 1975.

Herd, J. A.: Overall regulation of the circulation. Ann. Rev. Physiol., 32:289, 1970.

Jones, C. E., Crowell, J. W., and Smith, E. E.: A cause-effect relationship between oxygen deficit and irreversible hemorrhagic shock. Surgery, 127:93, 1968.

Korner, P. I.: Circulatory adaptations in hypoxia. Physiol. Rev., 39:687, 1959.

Lundgren, O., and Jodal, M.: Regional blood flow. Ann. Rev. Physiol., 37:395, 1975.

Patel, D. J., Vaishnav, R. N., Gow, B. S., and Kot, P. A.: Hemodynamics. Ann. Rev. Physiol., 36:125, 1974.

Rowell, L. B.: Human cardiovascular adjustments to exercise and thermal stress. Physiol. Rev., 54:75, 1974.

Stainsby, W. N.: Local control of regional blood flow. Ann. Rev. Physiol., 35:151, 1973.

Starling, E. H.: The Linacre Lecture on the Law of the Heart. Longmans Green and Co., London, 1918.

Yoffey, J. M., and Courtice, F. C. (eds.): Lymphatics, Lymph, and Lymphomyeloid Complex. Academic Press, Inc., New York, 1970.

7

Systemic Arterial Pressure*

ROBERT C. TARAZI, AND RAY W. GIFFORD, JR.

The pressure in arteries and veins was first measured in 1733 by Stephen Hales, who inserted a cannula into an artery and into a vein of a mare and noted the rise of the blood column in a tube. The arterial column rose approximately 8 feet, whereas the venous column rose only 12 inches. Since that time, tubes have been successfully inserted into various segments of the circulation of conscious unrestrained subjects and the pressure determined by sensitive manometers with high frequency of response. Thus, a map could be drawn of pressure variations along the circulatory circuit and of its fluctuations with different phases of the cardiac cycle (Fig. 7–1). The marked drop of pressure observed at the systemic arteriolar level led to a subdivision of the circulation into a "high-pressure" (resistance) segment and a "low-pressure" (capacitance) segment. The first is thought to be mainly concerned with flow distribution and regulation, and the second with priming of the cardiac pump and control of its output and possibly with regulation of intravascular volume. Important as these subdivisions are, the essential unity of the circulation must not be forgotten. A greater transmission of pressure from arteries to capillaries (as by arteriolar vasodilatation) may increase capillary ultrafiltration and reduce intravascular volume while concomitantly increasing venous return. Conversely, venoconstriction may, under certain conditions, relocate blood to the cardiopulmonary area, enhance cardiac output, and thus influence

arterial pressure. Blood pressure in capillaries, veins, and the lesser circulation is discussed elsewhere in this text and will be referred to here only insofar as it influences systemic arterial pressure.

Left ventricular contraction provides a phasic output of energy for the circulation; during systole, the intraventricular pressure rises from an average of 8 mm. Hg to about 120 mm. Hg under normal conditions. Blood is ejected into the aorta when the intraventricular pressure forces open the semilunar valves; during that portion of the cycle, systolic pressure is practically equal in the ventricle and aorta. At the end of systole, the heart muscle relaxes, and as intraventricular pressure falls steeply, the semilunar valve is closed. While blood is running from the arterioles into capillaries and veins, the large arteries, which had absorbed part of the energy of systole, now recoil on the diminishing volume of blood left by ventricular ejection, so that arterial pressure falls gradually during diastole. Thus, the arterial pressure pulse results from the ejection of a small volume of blood into a partly filled container of limited distensibility. This ejection distends at first only the proximal portion of the aorta, but the pressure wave generated is then rapidly transmitted to the rest of the arterial tree, with a velocity inversely proportional to the distensibility of the vessels involved. Since compliance of the arterial tree is less far out from the central aorta, the pulse wave velocity increases the farther it travels. When the wave reaches the main branching sites, but especially the precapillary resistance barrier, it is reflected back. Summation of the advancing waves with reflected waves may alter pulse tracings to a greater or lesser

---

*Many concepts and mechanisms described in this chapter are related to general concepts discussed in Chapter 6.

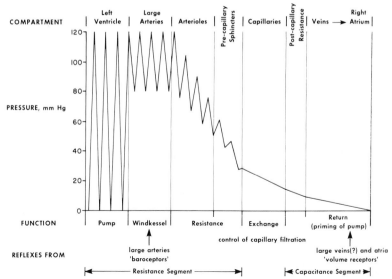

Figure 7–1 Functional subdivisions of the systemic circulation and pressure variations in its different segments. (After Folkow and Neil.)

extent, depending on the particular artery considered, the speed of wave transmission, and the degree of peripheral vasoconstriction at that time. Particularly obvious is the peaking of pulse waves in the femoral arteries when the size of the wave often becomes greater than in more central vessels, and phasic backflow may occur. Conditions stiffening arterial walls such as hypertension or sclerosis will also increase pulse wave velocity.

Pulse wave velocity must not be confused with the velocity of blood flow. The actual volume of blood yielded by the heart will have moved only a few centimeters by the time the pressure wave has reached the distal ends of the arterial system. Blood movement can be likened to the result of pushing a series of billiard balls: applying force on a ball at one end displaces another at the other end. As total surface area of the vasculature increases with repeated branching of the vessels, blood flow velocity decreases; simultaneously, the pulse wave velocity increases. This explains why the velocity of the pressure pulse is approximately 15 times that of blood flow in the aorta but may be as great as 100 times the velocity of blood flow in the distal arteries.

DETERMINATION OF ARTERIAL PRESSURE AND DEFINITION OF TERMS

Arterial pressure can be determined either directly (intra-arterial insertion of a needle or tube connected to a manometer) or indirectly, usually by auscultation over an artery to which pressure is applied proximally (sphygmomanometer). The choice of method will depend on purpose; the accuracy of determinations does not depend on the method used as much as on the attention given to seemingly minor but really quite important details.

Direct Method

The pressure determined in this way depends on the type of manometer to which the intra-arterial cannula is connected. The older U-tube mercury manometer has so much inertia that it cannot rise and fall rapidly and therefore simply oscillates around a mean level of pressure. To record faithfully rapidly changing pressures, manometers with higher frequency responses are currently used with optimal damping to ensure a uniform output throughout the range of frequencies expected. The records obtained are illustrated in Figure 7–2. The difference between the highest (systolic) and lowest (diastolic) pressure of a cycle is called the pulse pressure (PP). An integrated mean for the pressure developed throughout a whole cardiac cycle can either be recorded by electronically damping the response of the recording system or be determined by planimetry. The *mean arterial pressure* (MAP) thus obtained reflects the average pressure pushing blood through the systemic circulation and is therefore used to calculate peripheral resistance (see later discussion); it is not equal to the arithmetic mean of the systolic and diastolic pressures but depends in part on the heart rate and relative

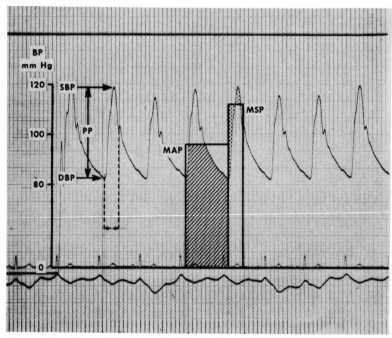

Figure 7–2 The line defining mean arterial pressure (MAP) can be drawn so that the area added (blank) is equivalent to the area subtracted (blank) from the whole cardiac cycle. Similarly, mean systolic pressure (MSP) can be estimated by adding an area (stippled) equivalent to that subtracted (stippled) from the ventricular ejection period only (from onset of pulse to incisure).

duration of systole and diastole; a close approximation is obtained as follows: MAP = DBP + ⅓ PP. The *mean systolic pressure* (MSP) is determined by integrating the area under the systolic part of the cycle; again, the following calculation yields a close approximation in most conditions: MSP = DBP + 0.8 PP. Its main use is in calculations of cardiac work and tension-time indices; it is closely related to myocardial oxygen consumption, since pressure work is more costly to the heart than volume work.

Indirect Method

The instrument universally used is the sphygmomanometer; the arterial pressure is usually measured in man at the brachial artery with the subject seated or lying down, with the arm slightly flexed and at heart level. Time should be allowed for recovery from recent exercise or excitement; clothing should not constrict the arm and the patient should be put as much at ease as possible. A cloth-covered rubber bag is placed firmly and snugly around the upper arm with its lower edge about an inch above the antecubital space. The bag should be 20 per cent wider than the diameter of the limb on which it is to be used (12 to 14 cm. for the average adult but wider for obese patients) and should be long enough (25 to 30 cm.) to encircle the limb almost completely. There should be no bulging or displacement of the bag when inflated. The air pressure inside the bag is determined by a mercury manometer or by an aneroid manometer calibrated against a mercury manometer. While the brachial or radial pulse is palpated, the bag is inflated to a pressure 30 mm. Hg higher than that required to obliterate the pulse. The pressure is then gradually reduced at a rate approximately 2 to 3 mm. Hg per second while a stethoscope, which is applied firmly but with as little pressure as possible over the previously palpated brachial artery, is employed. As the pressure in the bag falls, a series of sounds—the Korotkoff sounds—are heard as follows:

Phase I: Sudden appearance of a clear, sharp, snapping sound that grows louder.
Phase II: Sound is softened and becomes prolonged into a murmur.
Phase III: Sound again becomes crisper and increases in intensity.
Phase IV: Distinct abrupt muffling of the sound.
Phase V: The point at which sounds disappear.

It is universally agreed that the first appearance of vascular sounds (phase I) indicates the breakthrough of the pulse wave and gives the systolic pressure. In contrast, the best index of diastolic pressure is still a subject of controversy. The American Heart Association recommended phase IV in 1967 but then chose phase V in 1969. Part of the controversy is due to individual differences regarding ease or dependability in recognition of "muffling" as opposed to "disappearance" of a sound. Numerous studies have shown that phase V corresponds more closely to the direct intra-arterial diastolic pressure; however this may be only an empiric coincidence. There is no logical connection in the laws of physics between phase V and diastolic pressure, whereas the abrupt muffling of the arterial sound (phase IV) signals that blood flow is no longer impeded during diastole by the cuff pressure. In practice, there is usually little difference between the two phases, but they may become widely separated when arterial flow is increased. In such cases it is best to note both phases, so that blood pressure is recorded as, for example, 128/88/76. The first figure represents the systolic (phase I); the second, the diastolic (phase IV); and the third, phase V pressure.

Sometimes, particularly in some hypertensive patients, the usual sounds heard over the brachial artery when the cuff pressure is high disappear as the pressure is reduced and then reappear at a lower level. This early, temporary disappearance of sound is called the *auscultatory gap* and occurs during the latter part of phase I and phase II. Because this gap may cover a range of 40 mm. Hg, one can seriously underestimate the systolic pressure or overestimate the diastolic pressure, unless its presence is excluded by first palpating for disappearance of the radial pulse as the cuff pressure is raised.

When all sounds have disappeared, the cuff should be deflated rapidly and completely. One to two minutes should elapse for the release of blood trapped in the veins before further determinations are made.

An important sign to be looked for actively, especially in patients with some indication of cardiac dysfunction, is *pulsus alternans*. This is detected by noting that after the first sounds are heard and as pressure is reduced, their rate suddenly doubles, strong sounds alternating with weak sounds. It is an important sign of left ventricular failure and should be carefully distinguished from arrhythmia (irregular intervals between sounds) or respiratory variations of arterial pressure; the degree of alternans (interval between phase I and level of doubling of the sounds) and the heart rate at the moment should be carefully noted. The wider the alternans and the slower the heart rate at the time, the more seriously must this sign be viewed; minor degrees of alternation are not uncommon with marked tachycardia.

Blood pressure can also be determined during sphygmomanometry in three other ways. The first, the *palpatory,* involves palpating the radial pulse and noting the pressure at which it returns, after it has been obliterated by elevation of the pressure in the cuff above the pressure in the brachial artery. This method is not used extensively for several reasons. In the first place, only the systolic pressure can be determined, and, in general, it is inaccurate, being too low by approximately 5 to 10 mm. of mercury. However, the method is useful, in part at least, in assuring from the absence of the radial pulse that the brachial pulse is exceeded, a point that cannot always be settled by the auscultatory method.

The second is the *oscillometric.* In the Pachon type oscillometer two rubber bags are contained in the cuff, and the pressure in these bags is transmitted to a recording manometer. The mechanism is so arranged that when the column of blood reaches the lower cuff, the pulsation is reversed on the record. The entrance of the column of blood into the artery under the second cuff and the reversal of the record signal the systolic pressure. As the pressure is further reduced, the oscillations become greater and greater until they suddenly diminish markedly in size. This point is commonly taken as the diastolic pressure, but the precise point on the record at which the change occurs is not always evident.

The third method depends on a Doppler effect and is gaining in importance and popularity, especially in pediatric practice and for patients with peripheral vascular disease. A narrow ultrasound beam is directed toward any peripheral artery; when pressure in the sphygmomanometer cuff exceeds the systolic level, the artery collapses; then, as pressure within the cuff is gradually lowered the empty artery begins to receive blood flow intermittently and then continuously. The effects of these variations on reflected ultrasound can be recognized by auscultation or recorded after suitable amplification.

Slight differences in pressure between both arms are not uncommon on repeated determinations; however, meaningful comparisons can be made only by simultaneous determinations of blood pressure on both sides. Care must be taken to utilize cuffs appropriate to each arm's size; significant differences are reproducible and usually greater than 10 mm. Hg. They usually are due to some obstruction in arterial supply to the arm with the lower pressure.

The blood pressure may be taken in other parts of the body, particularly in the leg. When this is done, the patient rests in the horizontal position and the cuff is placed around the thigh, the sound being elicited over the artery in the popliteal space by application of the diaphragm of the stethoscope there. A special wide "thigh-cuff" should be used, wrapped firmly, but not tightly, with the compression bag over the posterior aspect of the midthigh. The systolic pressure thus recorded in the thigh is higher by 10 to 40 mm. Hg than that in the arm, but the diastolic is essentially the same. This difference is mainly spurious (uncomfortable position, difficulty of proper compression), although a minor part may be related to the effect of reflected pulse waves. It is accentuated in aortic insufficiency (Hill's sign), but more importantly it disappears or becomes reversed (arm pressure > thigh pressure) in coarctation of the aorta or obstruction at the aortic bifurcation and sometimes in abdominal aortic aneurysms.

Correlation Between Direct and Indirect Methods

Cuff readings are closely related to direct measurements, although levels are on the average 5 mm. Hg too low for the systolic and 8 mm. Hg too high for the diastolic (taken as phase IV). Actually, the disappearance of sounds (phase V) often coincides with diastolic pressure measured directly but it is less easy to define in some cases than phase IV and admits of wider variations. One of the most important factors affecting the accuracy of indirect recordings is the size of cuff used and its proper application to ensure adequate and even compression of the artery. The smaller the cuff in relation to the arm circumference, the higher the recorded pressure and the greater the error.

In both methods, the relation of the arm and manometer to the "heart level" is crucial; lowering or raising the arm from that level will increase or reduce recorded pressure because of hydrostatic factors involved, hence the importance of keeping the arm level with the fourth intercostal space whenever blood pressure is determined while the subject is sitting or standing.

BASIC FACTORS DETERMINING ARTERIAL PRESSURE

Pressure, Flow, and Resistance

Blood flow through vessels depends on two factors — the pressure head driving it and the resistance it meets. The relationship between these factors is defined by some basic hydrodynamic laws developed by Newton, Hagen, Poiseuille, and others. Translated into clinical terms, these laws have become essential for the understanding of arterial pressure variations in health and disease.

As just stated, the flow of any liquid along a tube is associated with a pressure gradient along that tube dependent on the rate of flow and on the resistance it meets. Because resistance (R) cannot

be measured directly, it is calculated as the ratio of the pressure gradient (ΔP) to the rate of flow (F):

$$R = \Delta P/F \qquad (1)$$

The rate of flow of liquids within cylindrical vessels can be mathematically deduced from Newton's principles on laminar movement of fluids. If the liquid is of uniform viscosity and its flow streamlined and nonpulsatile, then

$$F = \frac{\Delta P \times r^4}{1 \times v} \times \frac{\pi}{8} \qquad (2)$$

(r = radius of vessel, l = its length, and v = the fluid viscosity; $\frac{\pi}{8}$ is a constant, arising from calculus derivations).

Strictly speaking, these conditions are not met in the circulation, but despite the obvious differences, this fundamental law (Poiseuille) is largely valid for hemodynamic studies. The calculations derived from it are very useful in assessing the relative parts played by blood flow and peripheral resistance in changes of arterial pressure. The clinical equivalents of F, ΔP and R (formula 1) in the systemic circulation are cardiac output (CO), mean arterial pressure (MAP), and total peripheral resistance (TPR), respectively. Cardiac output and mean arterial pressure are determined directly and TPR is calculated as their ratio.* Rearranging the terms in (1) leads to the basic equation describing the relationship of arterial pressure, cardiac output, and peripheral resistance

$$MAP = CO \times TPR \qquad (3)$$

It is important to realize the approximations and simplifications involved in this formula and the consequent reservations involved in its application to the intact organism. An example of simplifications in the use of MAP as the equivalent of ΔP: the marked difference between systemic arterial and central venous pressure as well as the relatively small fluctuations of the latter allows

---

*Resistance can be calculated from either cardiac output or from cardiac index (CI = CO/body surface area); since cardiac output is related to body size while MAP is not, the latter approach is preferable. In either case, resistance can be expressed in arbitrary units, PRU (peripheral resistance units) = $\left(\dfrac{\text{mm. Hg}}{\text{L./min./M.}^2}\right)$, or in fundamental units of force. For the latter, pressure in mm. Hg is converted to dynes/cm.² (1 mm. Hg = 1333 dynes/cm.²) and flow to cm.³/sec. (1 L. = 1000/60 cm.³/sec.); the calculated resistance is then expressed in dynes sec./cm.⁵ This can be achieved practically by multiplying PRU by 80.

its disregard in calculations of resistance in the systemic circulation. This simplification naturally is not possible for the pulmonary circulation; in calculations of pulmonary vascular resistance, pulmonary wedge pressure or the left atrial pressure must be subtracted from the mean pulmonary arterial pressure.

The main reservation relates to the understanding and evaluation of changes in total peripheral resistance; the simplicity of this formula must not lure one into simplistic interpretations of that calculated value. A first caveat: Total peripheral resistance is the composite of the vascular resistance of each organ. Resistances to flow obey the same laws as electric resistances for combinations of series and of parallel arrangements. Therefore, a change in TPR does not necessarily indicate that similar quantitative or even similar directional changes are occurring in all individual vascular territories. The second caveat concerns the relationship of ΔTPR to vasoconstriction and dilatation. Within the usual physiologic limits of blood viscosity and assuming a constant vascular length in the same individual, variations in resistance will usually result from active, passive, or structural changes of vessel diameter. Since the radius is magnified to the fourth power in equation 2, flow and pressure are markedly affected by relatively small changes in vessel size. The temptation is strong to translate immediately ΔTPR into an index of peripheral arteriolar vasoconstriction. Although this may frequently be correct, one must not fail to recognize the important role that large and small arteriovenous shunts, precapillary sphincters, passive arterial variations, structural changes, and collateral vessels may sometimes play in these changes.

Factors Determining Pulse Pressure

Aside from forces regulating the average level of arterial pressure, a number of factors determine the width of pulsations around the mean. This discussion concerns those factors affecting central pulse pressure rather than the local variations already mentioned, resulting from reflected waves and altered distensibility of various peripheral portions of the arterial tree.

The aorta and its main branches take up a relatively large volume of blood under pressure during systolic ejection; during diastole, the pressure energy thus stored is gradually used to press blood onward. This "Windkessel function" helps transform an intermittent input to a more even outflow (Wiggers). The factors determining pulse pressure will therefore relate mainly to (1) quantity of blood ejected per beat (stroke volume); (2) compliance of the aorta and large vessels; and to a lesser degree (3) speed of ejection of blood. The aortic wall is not a perfectly elastic material and

its viscous components imply that the more rapidly blood is ejected, the greater its resistance to stretch and therefore the larger the rise in pulse pressure.

Obviously, the larger the stroke volume, the wider the pulse pressure; the causes of increased stroke volume are usually evident (aortic insufficiency, complete heart block, various high output states). In contrast, conditions associated with diminished aortic compliance are not often clinically evident but are suspected from the resultant systolic hypertension and wide pulse pressure. The effects of altered compliance can be readily appreciated from the physical definition of the term:

Vascular compliance (or volume distensibility) =

$$\frac{\text{Increased in volume } (\Delta V)}{\text{Increase in pressure } (\Delta P)}$$

Translated into clinical terms,

$$\text{Aortic compliance} = \frac{\text{Stroke volume}}{\text{Pulse pressure}}$$

from which follow:

(a) Stroke volume = Pulse pressure × Aortic compliance

(b) $\text{Pulse pressure} = \dfrac{\text{Stroke volume}}{\text{Aortic compliance}}$

If compliance were constant, stroke volume could be deduced from pulse pressure, and cardiac output could then be calculated by multiplying pulse pressure by heart rate. Unfortunately, variables are too great for useful interpretations of the formula.

It is readily seen that decrease in compliance will result in wider pulse pressure per ml. of blood ejected. Compliance decreases slightly as arterial pressure increases or with sympathetic stimulation; it is markedly reduced by loss or fragmentation of aortic elastic and muscular tissue, as occurs with age or extensive atheromatous involvement with secondary medial fibrosis or intimal calcification. Reduction of aortic distensibility per se leads to a slight decline in diastolic and a marked rise in systolic pressures (isolated systolic hypertension). Diastolic hypertension cannot therefore be ascribed to reduced aortic compliance alone. The wide pulse pressure found in many subjects with diastolic hypertension poses a special problem. In experimental models, with aortic distensibility held constant, increasing peripheral resistance will be associated with declining pulse pressure. Inordinate rise of systolic pressure in patients with diastolic hypertension therefore reflects either a large stroke volume or, more frequently, a secondary loss of large vessel distensibility.

Effect of Age and Environmental Factors on Arterial Blood Pressure

Definition of a "normal" arterial blood pressure is so closely linked to the concept of hypertension that it is better to postpone it to that section. For now, it is sufficient to point out the often wide variations in both systolic and diastolic pressures encountered from moment to moment in the same subject. Most are related to such obvious causes as body movement, position, pain, emotional stress, and the like. Under ordinary conditions, blood pressure measured even after a few minutes' rest in the doctor's office (casual pressure) is markedly higher than that recorded under basal conditions. Smirk defined "basal pressure" as the one recorded in the morning 10 to 12 hours postprandially; after an additional half hour rest in a warm room, repeated recordings are obtained over 30 to 45 minutes in a monotonous, silent atmosphere to the lowest attainable levels. Home blood pressures recorded by the patient himself or by a lay relative often approximate basal levels. The difference (casual minus basal) is called "supplemental pressure." Although the basal pressure might statistically be more closely related to the clinical consequences of hypertension, it has found little clinical acceptance. Most epidemiologic and clinical experience has been derived from studies of casual pressure.

Age, Sex, and Body Build. Until adulthood is reached, the age factor may make a remarkable difference (Fig. 7–3); subsequent changes with age vary in different populations and from subject to subject. In some, pressure does not rise with age; in others the rate of rise is quite marked. Studies in Wales suggest that the rate of rise in Western populations, at least, correlates with the initial level of blood pressure. Young men tend to have higher pressures than young women, but between ages 35 and 45, the curves for systolic pressure cross and women's pressures subsequently rise more steeply with age than men's. There is no evidence that menopause is associated with a unique hypertension. Obese subjects tend to have higher blood pressure that cannot be accounted for by a systematic error due to increased arm circumference.

Posture and Exercise. With standing, pulse pressure narrows as the systolic drops slightly and the diastolic rises by about 5 mm. Hg, so that mean arterial pressure does not vary by more than ±5 to 10 mm. Hg. Changes in arterial pressure with dynamic exercise (cycling, walking) are proportional to the severity of exercise; it may reach 200/100 when exercise becomes strenuous.

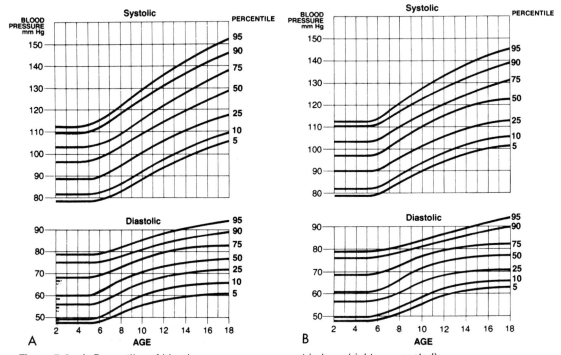

Figure 7–3 *A*, Percentiles of blood pressure measurement in boys (right arm, seated).
B, Percentiles of blood pressure measurements in girls (right arm, seated). (With permission, Report of the Task Force on Blood Pressure Control in Children. Pediatrics, *59*:803, 1977.)

Static exercise, e.g., sustained contraction of forearm muscles, is associated with an abrupt reflex rise in pressure proportional to the muscular tension developed.

Variations With Daily Activities. The size of these variations as recorded by automatic recorders is quite impressive, averaging in one study 24 mm. Hg (range 15 to 40) for systolic and 14 mm. Hg (5 to 20) for diastolic in normotensive subjects. Arterial pressure falls profoundly during sleep but is most unstable in REM (rapid eye movement) sleep. Relation of pressure variations to nocturnal cardiovascular accidents is still conjectural.

SOME ASPECTS OF ARTERIAL PRESSURE REGULATION

Arterial blood pressure is only one aspect in a highly integrated cardiovascular control system. Accordingly, to understand its disturbances one should consider the cardiovascular system as a whole, including not only cardiac performance and peripheral resistance, but also the indirect effect of capacitance vessels on blood flow and the ways in which hemodynamic functions can be modified by sympathetic neural activity and hormonal factors. Control of circulatory pressure must be closely associated with control of the volume distending the circulation, and arterial pressure reflects, in part, this relationship between container (blood vessels) and content (blood volume). Hence, the mechanisms regulating the size and distribution of extracellular fluids must be considered along with factors controlling hemodynamic functions.

Hemodynamic Aspects

Physical bases of mean arterial and pulse pressure have already been discussed. Arterial pressure can be regulated by variations of either cardiac output or peripheral resistance or both.

Interrelationship Between Output and Resistance. In acute studies, cardiac response to changes in peripheral resistance is to increase output for a decrease in peripheral resistance and to decrease output for an increase in resistance. Thus, any effect on pressure is at least attenuated. This relationship underlines the importance of peripheral factors in determining cardiac output (given normal myocardial contractility) by controlling the flow of blood from arteries to veins. Conversely, primary changes in output lead to reciprocal changes in peripheral resistance, tending to maintain pressure constant. This relationship is probably mediated principally through baroreceptor reflexes (see later discussion).

Chronic changes in blood flow unrelated to local needs of tissues have been associated with a different type of long-term readjustment. In such cases, a persistent inappropriate increase of cardiac output is thought to induce a progressive constriction of local vessels over a period of days or months until finally blood flow through the tissues returns to near normal. Return of output to normal is associated with increased peripheral resistance (Fig. 7–4). This sequence of events has been termed total body autoregulation; the term is an extrapolation to the whole organism from a phenomenon first described in local isolated circulation. Local regulation of blood flow to the needs of the tissues depends on (a) concentration of local metabolites and (b) myogenic response of vessel wall to stretch (Bayliss mechanism).

The total circulation is affected by these local tissue factors but also by multifaceted neural, humoral, and structural influences. Whether extrapolation to that situation of the term "autoregulation" is justified has been hotly debated. Obviously the term means different things to different investigators; for some, development of collateral vessels is a phenomenon of long-term flow regulation. Whatever its exact mechanism, the concept supposes that regulation of flow to the needs of the tissues has been disassociated from and has superseded pressure regulation. As regards regional circulations (renal, cerebral, etc.), maintenance of blood flow despite pressure varia-

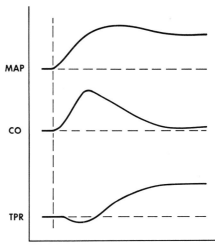

Figure 7–4 Diagrammatic illustration of the results of a sustained increase in cardiac output (CO) unrelated to peripheral demands; as output rises, mean arterial pressure (MAP) increases while total peripheral resistance (TPR) remains unchanged or even decreases slightly. Within a few weeks, however, TPR increases and cardiac output returns toward normal; MAP remains elevated because of the persistent increase in resistance.

tions (within limits) has been well established. For the systemic circulation as a whole, "autoregulation" has been invoked both to describe and explain the transition of a "high flow–normal or low resistance" pattern to a "normal flow–high resistance" situation.

This concept is particularly important in relation to current theories regarding hypertension. The transition from high output to high resistance has been described in many experimental hypertensions; the present debate centers on whether it is an obligatory step in the initiation and evolution of most forms of hypertension. In many situations, both in man and animals, it has been shown that a high output hypertension can persist for a long time without apparent secondary rise of TPR. More important, prevention of the initial rise in cardiac output did not in many instances prevent the development of increased resistance and hypertension. Thus, even when present, the evolution from a high output to a high resistance state may not necessarily mean "autoregulation"; it may depend on many factors including neural or humoral mechanisms as well as the effects of structural changes on resistance vessels and cardiac performance.

Blood Vessels and Arterial Blood Pressure. All systemic vessels — arteries, veins, and capillaries—participate each in its way in arterial blood pressure regulation. The following classification of blood vessels is based on the functional characteristics of each segment (Folkow):

1. "Windkessel" vessels (aorta and its large branches) damp the pulsatile output from the left ventricle and help steady the blood flow to the periphery; their main effect is on pulse pressure.

2. Resistance vessels (small arteries and arterioles) furnish most of total resistance to flow and regulate the distribution of cardiac output. Their high intrinsic (myogenic) tone is continuously modified by physical, chemical, and neural influences. As flow is proportional to the fourth power of the radius, seemingly minor changes in diameter may exert a powerful influence on blood pressure (Poiseuille).

3. Exchange vessels (capillaries) are guarded by precapillary sphincters and postcapillary resistance vessels (venules and small veins). Diffusion, filtration, and reabsorption occur through the capillary walls, but the capillaries themselves have no active influence on this exchange. The net fluid transfer between plasma and interstitial fluid, given normal plasma oncotic pressure, depends on the ratio of precapillary to postcapillary resistance which is controlled by sphincters and resistance vessels at either end of the capillaries. Changes in this ratio affect primarily blood volume and indirectly arterial pressure. A fall in pressure at the arteriolar end will favor intravascular shift of fluid and thus help to some degree in restoring arterial pressure. Conversely, venoconstriction will favor capillary filtration and reduction of plasma volume.

4. Capacitance vessels (veins) add little to peripheral resistance but accommodate the larger portion of blood volume and thus play an important role in circulatory regulation. They are well supplied by sympathetic nerves and may react differently from resistance vessels to nervous and humoral stimuli. To ascribe a role to veins in regulation of arterial pressure may look paradoxic, but cardiac output depends on venous return. Venoconstriction resulting from sympathetic stimulation will not significantly alter peripheral resistance but will lead to decreased venous capacity. This will enhance a translocation of blood out of systemic veins into the cardiopulmonary area, raise cardiac output, and thus help prevent or correct falls in arterial pressure due to blood loss or excessive peripheral pooling.

Intravascular Volume and Arterial Pressure

The vascular circuit just described is obviously not a homogeneous system; each of its subdivisions has its own pressure/volume characteristics. The arterial segment has limited distensibility and is maintained at high pressure and low volume; it is thought to contain about 20 per cent of the total blood volume. Although the capillary bed is of considerable length, it contains only 5 per cent of the total blood volume. Capillary pressure is determined by the balance of constriction between precapillary arterioles and postcapillary venules. The venous side of the circulation is a low pressure, highly distensible compartment which contains about 75 per cent of the intravascular volume.

Both the arterial and venous compartments are importantly affected by sympathetic vasomotor outflow but, characteristically, these effects are different. Neural influences alter arterial capacity and volume but little, but small changes in that segment will affect arterial pressure directly. In contrast, sympathetic vasomotor activity plays a large role in determining venous capacity, but the contribution of veins to total peripheral resistance is small. More important is their control of venous return and influence on cardiac output. In that respect and within certain limits, the distribution of intravascular volume may be more important than its magnitude; thus it is possible to have, on the one hand, a large blood volume, venous pooling, low central blood volume, and low cardiac output or, on the other, a small blood volume, diminished venous capacity, a disproportionately high central blood volume, and a normal or even increased cardiac output.

The potential of vascular adaptability is such that changes in blood volume are not normally reflected to any important degree in arterial pressure variations unless the change is acute or excessive (hemorrhage). Conditions marked by hypervolemia (polycythemia vera) are not necessarily associated with hypertension. This efficacy of adaptation implies that important disturbances in regulation may lead to only subtle changes in pressure/volume relationships. On the other hand, arterial pressure becomes quite sensitive to blood volume changes when neural reflexes are interfered with. A small blood loss that would normally be well tolerated may lead to profound hypotension if suffered by a patient treated with neural blocking agents. Conversely, fluid retention and plasma volume expansion will nullify an initial good response to such hypotensive agents as ganglion blockers, guanethidine, reserpine, and similar drugs.

Factors regulating blood volume are beyond the scope of this discussion; they include renal excretory mechanisms, balance between interstitial and intravascular component of extracellular fluid volume, and neurohumoral control mechanisms (see appropriate sections).

Principles of Vascular Control

The inherent myogenic activity of vessel walls is responsible for a *basal vascular tone* which is locally regulated by the vasodilator action of tissue metabolites. Superimposed on this, neurogenic mechanisms exert a "remote" control to adjust the circulation to the requirements of the body as a whole. Various circulating hormones add their excitatory or inhibitory influences.

Vascular innervation is not restricted to arteries; all vessels except capillaries are innervated. Arterioles are supplied by two sets of nerves — sympathetic vasoconstrictors (alpha-adrenergic) and other vasodilator fibers. Sympathetic nerve fibers reach the vessels either from plexuses along their walls or through somatic nerve trunks. This distribution is important, for strip-

ping the greater vessels of their nerve supply will not affect the smaller vessels. The more important neural influence on the arterial side is vasoconstriction; similarly, the overriding effect of sympathetic stimulation on veins is alpha-adrenergic venoconstriction. Thus, the main effects of sympathetic stimulation are increases in resistance and enhancement of venous return.

Vasodilator fibers are less widespread and not tonically active. Beta-adrenergic receptors are found in arteries and probably in veins; their functional importance is debated. Cholinergic sympathetic vasodilator nerves supply only the larger resistance vessels of skeletal muscle and are activated mainly when the animal is alerted (defense reaction); as most other regions are vasoconstricted, the muscles may thus be provided with near maximum blood supply. Parasympathetic vasodilator nerves supply some specialized tissues such as salivary glands and external genitalia.

Hormonal influences include circulating epinephrine (from adrenal medulla), which stimulates both alpha- and beta-receptors, so that it usually causes a redistribution of blood flow; myocardium, muscle, and liver receive more blood at the expense of other circuits (kidney, skin, gastrointestinal tract) which are vasoconstricted. Angiotensin is discussed later. Many other "vasoactive agents" are known (prostaglandins, histamine, serotonin, vasopressin); specialized reviews should be consulted for details of their effects. Particular note, however, should be made of prostaglandins, a ubiquitous series of compounds synthesized in a variety of tissues from essential unsaturated fatty acids, predominantly arachidonic acid. Recent work has led to growing awareness of the importance of these acids as local hormones, meaning that they are involved principally in the modulation of regional circulation in the tissues where they are formed. Whether circulating prostaglandins have any important systemic effect is open to question. Various series of prostaglandins (PG) have been identified with differing actions on veins, arteries,

TABLE 7-1 SIMPLIFIED SCHEME OF PROSTAGLANDIN SYNTHESIS AND ACTIONS

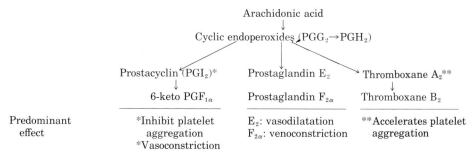

Predominant effect	*Inhibit platelet aggregation *Vasoconstriction	E$_2$: vasodilatation F$_{2\alpha}$: venoconstriction	**Accelerates platelet aggregation

and platelets (Table 7–1). The net balance on vascular flow may well depend on the balance of the different compounds formed.

Finally, especially in the context of blood pressure regulation, it is important to remember that salt-water equilibrium profoundly affects the activity and responsiveness of smooth muscles. Changes in sodium gradient across cell membrane may enhance constriction (if extracellular sodium is increased) or relaxation (if sodium is depleted.) The role of other ions, such as potassium, calcium, and magnesium, has been studied extensively in-vitro and in-vivo (Haddy). In actual practice however, the situation is more complex than can be discerned through controlled experiments. Salt and water equilibrium involves changes in volume (intra- and extravascular) as well as in ion gradients. Changes in serum electrolytes usually involve more than one; Haddy has pointed out the synergistic effect of some common combinations. Thus a reduction in serum potassium would enhance the effect of a simultaneous rise in serum calcium to increase myocardial contractility and induce vasoconstriction. To cite a practical example, this particular combination is frequently produced by hemodialysis; its effect on arterial pressure is counterbalanced by the simultaneous loss of fluid and modulated by the humoral and neurogenic responses to hypovolemia. Thus, even in relatively simple situations, the control of arterial pressure remains a multifactorial process.

Neural Reflexes and "Central" Reactions

Neural circulatory reflexes act mainly to stabilize arterial pressure at the levels set for a particular subject. They help buffer the impact of stimuli by raising arterial pressure when it is lowered or decreasing it when it rises. When neural activity is impaired by drugs or disease, arterial pressure may fluctuate widely between hypertension in the supine position and hypotension and fainting on standing.

Like all neural reflexes, they comprise an afferent and an efferent limb joined through a center (the vasomotor center). They are activated from sensory receptors in different parts of the circulation; the most important are located in the carotid sinus and aortic arch. These stretch receptors are sensitive to expansion or deformation of the arterial wall and respond more to a pulsatile than to an equivalent steady pressure (the term *baroreceptor* is inaccurate because they do not respond to pressure *per se*). Fibers from the carotid sinus travel cephalad in the glossopharyngeal nerve; those from the aortic arch employ the vagus. The carotid sinus reflex is normally the more powerful, possibly because it guards the blood supply to the central nervous system. But other sensitive vascular areas, e.g., the mesenteric, can also induce compensatory blood pressure responses in anesthetized animals with cut sinus nerves and vagi (Heymans).

The stretch receptors are activated when arterial pressure rises and the consequent impulses inhibit the tonic activity of the vasomotor center. This latter term is applied to a group of neurons located in the upper medulla and lower pons which maintain normally a slow rate of firing to essentially all sympathetic vasoconstrictor fibers. Baroreceptor impulses normally exert an inhibitory influence on the center; when blood pressure tends to fall, their activity is reduced, thus liberating the vasomotor center. The consequent increase in sympathetic discharge helps restore pressure to normal. The vasomotor center influences the heart as well as the peripheral vessels, so that increase or reduction of cardiac activity (chronotropic and inotropic) parallels the increase or decrease in vasoconstrictor impulses. Efferent impulses travel along the two components of the autonomic system — sympathetic and parasympathetic. Of these the sympathetic is of greater importance because of its wider distribution to the peripheral vasculature and in the heart, going to both atria and both ventricles. Vagal fibers supply mainly the sinoatrial and atrioventricular nodes and the atria; there is evidence, however, of some parasympathetic influence on ventricular function as well.

These reflexes play a major role in circulatory adjustments to postural changes (see discussion of hypotension). Both sides of the reflex are demonstrated in responses to the Valsalva maneuver (a sustained increase in intrathoracic pressure obtained by blowing against some resistance for 20 to 30 seconds). During the period of straining, venous return is sharply curtailed and cardiac output decreased, so that systolic pressure falls. Resultant reflex sympathetic stimulation increases heart rate and limits fall in diastolic pressure. When straining is suddenly stopped, blood rushes into the thorax and the resurgent cardiac output is thrust into an arterial system whose outflow resistance has been increased. This results in a brief overshoot of arterial pressure; the opposite reflex readjustment then leads to bradycardia and a decline of pressure to prestrain levels.

These sequential variations with the Valsalva maneuvers usually are classified into four phases (Fig. 7–5): phase 1 is a brief rise in pressure with onset of straining; phase 2 is the reduction in pulse pressure and increase in heart rate; phase 3 is further drop in pressure as straining is suddenly stopped and the resultant increased pulmonary vascular capacity momentarily reduces return to the left ventricle further; phase 4 refers to the overshoot in arterial pressure and reflex brady-

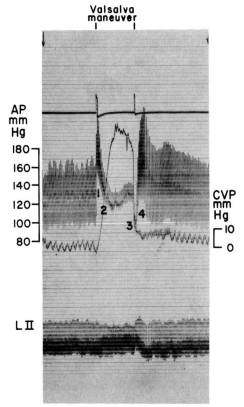

Figure 7–5 Response to a Valsalva maneuver performed for 20 seconds. From above downward are shown (a) signal indicating beginning and end of straining; (b) arterial pressure (AP) showing four phases: *1*, initial rise with onset of straining; *2*, the fall in pulse pressure as venous return is temporarily diminished; *3*, a further fall in pressure with the first deep breaths on cessation of strain; and *4*, the pressure overshoot as an increased left ventricular output is now thrown in a constricted vascular bed; (c) central venous pressure (CVP) tracing showing the marked increase during straining; (d) electrocardiogram (lead II), which shows the slowing in heart rate with phase 4 after its increase during phase 2.

cardia. These responses, however, depend not only on the integrity of neural reflexes but also on the degree of volemia and on cardiac compensation. In heart failure, blood pressure actually rises during straining, and phase 4 is abolished ("square wave" response).

The effectiveness of this system in controlling excessive pressure fluctuations immediately raises the question of its inability to prevent hypertension. This failure is related to the fact that the receptors eventually adapt to whatever pressure level they are exposed to if this pressure is maintained long enough (Fig. 7–6). This resetting of baroreceptors not only prevents the reflex from functioning as a long-term control system but

may also act in reverse, increasing the difficulties of initiating antihypertensive therapy.

Apart from reflexes originating from the "high-pressure" circuit, there are also sensory endings in the thorax from the "low-pressure" segment, the fibers from which are vagal in location. They respond to shifts in blood volume or rather to distention in vessel walls related to such shifts. Recent experiments suggest that vagal fibers originating in the cardiopulmonary region exert, like the carotid and aortic baroreceptors, a tonic inhibition of the vasomotor center. Further, vagal afferents from the cardiopulmonary region also play an important role in blood volume regulation. Stimulation of cardiac receptors, especially in the left atrium, leads to increased excretion of water and sodium related in various degrees to renal vasodilatation as well as to reduction of ADH, inhibition of renin release, and possibly stimulation of a blood-borne diuretic agent. Translated into clinical terms, left atrial and pulmonary congestion should lead to reduction of plasma volume; conversely, a drop in cardiopulmonary volume leads to vasoconstriction and to retention of water and salt.

Reflexes mediated through vagal afferents are depressor; pressor reflexes can arise from the heart and from larger vessels. The latter are carried through afferent sympathetic fibers. The sympathetic cardiac afferents can lead to reflex increases in myocardial contractility, heart rate, and peripheral resistance. They may be important in some types of paroxysmal hypertension.

Of less importance for arterial pressure control are chemoreceptor reflexes. They are not very effective in the normal pressure range, but in hypertensive states diminished arterial oxygen concentration excites the carotid and aortic bodies, thus reflexly elevating arterial pressure.

It is evident that there are many inputs to the central nervous system. The net effect on cardiovascular function and arterial pressure depends on central integration of this information. Review of recent studies by Mancia, et al., suggests that the carotid sinus reflex dominates when the carotid sinus, cardiopulmonary, and carotid chemoreflexes interact. The cardiopulmonary receptors appear to become more effective in pressure regulation only when input from the carotid baroreceptors is decreased or when chemoreceptors are activated.

"Central Reactions." In contrast to the feedback system of baroreceptor reflex, these reactions do not serve to control arterial pressure. The circulatory response to hypothalamic stimulation is a marked blood pressure rise with profound inotropic and chronotropic excitation of the heart. It represents a full mobilization of the organism for fight or flight. It is mentioned here because its frequent repetition or its possible evolution into a conditioned reflex, has been pro-

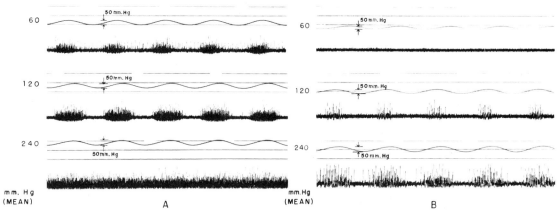

Figure 7–6   Neurogram from carotid sinus nerve of normotensive (A) and renal hypertensive dog (B); at a mean arterial pressure of 60 mm. Hg, nerve activity was clearly present in dog A but absent in the hypertensive animal. At 240 mm. Hg MAP, firing was continuous in A but still intermittent in B, suggesting that the normal range of baroreceptor response had been shifted upward in the hypertensive animal. (After McCubbin, J., et al.: Baroreceptor function in chronic renal hypertension. Circ. Res., *4*:205, 1965, by permission of The American Heart Association, Inc.)

posed as a possible cause for hypertension. Conversely, the "playing dead" reaction (profound bradycardia, hypotension, and fainting occurring in some animals when cornered) may be analogous to some cases of emotional fainting in patients. In these conditions, the muscle cholinergic vasodilator system is markedly activated.

The Kidney and Blood Pressure Regulation

There are two aspects of the close relationship existing between systemic arterial pressure levels and renal function. The first relates to the excretory function of the kidney; diminished excretion of salt and water in the face of maintained intake leads to hypervolemia and hypertension to achieve greater filtration and a new equilibrium between intake and output.

The second mechanism is related to a more "active" process, a renal pressor system capable of raising pressure directly when activated. Although these two mechanisms are often associated, they can also be disassociated in both clinical and experimental situations. This is discussed at greater length under Mechanisms in Hypertension; at this point only the *renal pressor system* will be described.

The importance of this system in regard to hypertension is that its end product, angiotensin II, is the most potent pressor substance known and also a stimulator of aldosterone. The system itself is really two enzyme systems in series (Fig. 7–7). In the first reaction, a proteolytic enzyme of renal origin called *renin* reacts with a circulating alpha-2-globulin (renin substrate or angiotensinogen) to release the decapeptide angiotensin I.

This serves as substrate for converting enzyme which, by releasing two amino acids, produces the octapeptide, angiotensin II; the converting enzyme is present in plasma and tissues and there is evidence to suggest that in some species the major conversion of angiotensin I to II occurs in the lung. Angiotensin II is inactivated by plasma and tissue angiotensinases. Renin not only is active in circulating blood but is also stored in arterial walls; the importance of this local storage and possible later activation is yet to be determined. Still under investigation too is a phospholipid renin inhibitor system dependent on a renal phospholipase and a circulating phospholipid inhibitor.

Angiotensin I has no direct effect on arterial pressure, whereas only nanogram amounts of angiotensin II can produce substantial elevations. Information currently available suggests that the plasma concentration of angiotensin II is usually less than 100 picograms per ml. Because of difficulties in measuring circulating angiotensin, current information concerning the renal pressor system comes from studies of plasma renin activity (PRA); it should be emphasized that the methods widely used provide an estimate of the activity of renin but do not measure it directly.

Source of Renin — The Juxtaglomerular Apparatus.   Renin comes from the kidney — hence the term renal pressor system. It is formed and stored in the juxtaglomerular (JG) apparatus, or complex, at the vascular pole of the glomerulus. At this point the macula densa portion of the distal tubule is in close proximity to the afferent and efferent arterioles. The JG complex is composed of granular cells in the afferent arterioles, the macula densa and the polkissen, a group of cells

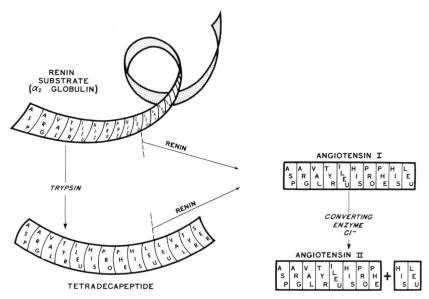

Figure 7–7 Renin-angiotensin system. (After F. M. Bumpus. *In* Page, I. H., and McCubbin, J.: Renal Hypertension. Year Book Medical Publishers, Chicago, 1969.) The normal amino acid sequence of angiotensin II is essential for its biologic action; recently, analogs obtained by substitution of some amino acids have been shown to block, through competitive inhibition, various effects of the octapeptide. They are therefore very useful tools for investigation (? treatment) of some types of hypertension.

in the triangle formed by the afferent and efferent arteriole and the distal tubule. The complex is richly innervated by sympathetic nerve fibers.

Renin seems to be primarily located in the granular cells of the afferent arteriole; experimentally there is a close relationship between the granularity of these cells and their renal renin content. The role of the macula densa in renin production has not yet been exactly defined. However, its cells are in close contact with JG cells and their cytologic characteristics are distinct from those of other cells in the distal tubule, suggesting a difference in function at this site. The strategic location of the JG apparatus between an arteriole and a tubule seems particularly suited for a system apparently related to both arterial pressure and sodium excretion.

It was first assumed that the factor stimulating *renin release* was renal ischemia but this was later disproved, since release could be stimulated by alterations in sodium balance that do not produce ischemia and by reductions in perfusion pressure too small to decrease renal blood flow significantly. Two concepts regarding the mechanism of renin release were then developed, the intrarenal baroreceptor hypothesis and the macula densa theory. According to the first, the renal afferent arterioles and JG cells respond to changes in stretch which could be secondary to changes in intravascular volume or in arterial pressure. For others, the macula densa is a primary sensing

element responding to changes in the sodium load reaching it. Neither theory can explain all experimental observations and it seems possible that both types of receptor exist and that they influence each other. In addition to these intrarenal mechanisms, sympathetic nerves and circulating humoral agents may play important modifying roles.

A common denominator for the many stimuli that affect renin release is "effective blood volume"; its apparent correlates in clinical situations include serum sodium as well as actual blood volume. Rapid reduction of intravascular volume expansion turns off the stimulus for does the reduction produced by a low-sodium diet or diuretic drug treatment. Conversely, plasma volume expansion turns off the stimulus for renin release and reduces PRA. So predictable are these responses that dietary sodium restriction and intravenous sodium chloride infusion are used as standard tests of the renal pressor system. These maneuvers alter both blood volume (and extracellular fluid volume) and sodium balance; under normal conditions both stimuli act in the same direction on renin release. Under experimental conditions the two stimuli can be dissociated and it would seem that changes in intravascular volume predominate over changes in serum sodium in determining PRA. That is not to say that serum sodium plays no role in influencing renin release. On the contrary, this has been clearly shown in animal experiments utilizing renal perfusion techniques with which it is possible to vary sodium concentration of the perfusate without varying that of the whole body. Hyponatremia increased renin release and hypernatremia diminished it. It has been suggested that the reason why diuretic drugs increase PRA is not only because they decrease plasma volume but also because they diminish sodium transport by macula densa cells. In this connection, changes in serum potassium must be taken into account in the interpretation of renin data. Hypokalemia may stimulate and hyperkalemia may inhibit PRA, independent of associated alterations in either aldosterone secretion or sodium balance.

Though it is not essential for renin release, the sympathetic nervous system may alter it directly or indirectly. The role of arterial baroreceptors in the control of renin release is debatable; however, cardiopulmonary receptors appear to exert a tonic restraint on renin release by reflex inhibition of sympathetic outflow to the kidney. Conditions associated with rise in PRA are usually those associated with increased sympathetic activity (upright posture, hypovolemia). Both alpha- and beta-adrenergic blocking drugs have been shown to diminish PRA. As well as manipulations of sodium intake, upright posture is frequently used as a clinical test of renin release. Patients with idiopathic orthostatic hypotension sometimes fail to show the expected increase of PRA with standing.

Pressor Effects of the Renin-Angiotensin System. Though angiotensin II is the most powerful vasoconstrictor agent, its direct effect on resistance vessels might not be its most important contribution to arterial pressure regulation except in special cases. Possibly of greater significance for circulatory control are its effects on aldosterone secretion and sympathetic functions.

Infusions of even small subpressor doses of angiotensin lead to marked increase in aldosterone secretion. The resultant fluid retention and increase in sodium stores set the stage for blood pressure elevation, water retention by increasing extracellular fluid volume, and sodium retention by increasing vascular responsiveness to vasoconstrictor agents.

On the other hand, angiotensin has major effects on sympathetic nervous activity. It enhances activity through a direct stimulatory action on the vasomotor center; the area postramus is one place where blood-brain barrier against angiotensin breaks down. Peripherally, it enhances sympathetic nerve effects by diminishing neuronal norepinephrine uptake, thus allowing a greater concentration of the neurohormone to reach vascular receptor sites. Angiotensin is also a potent stimulus for catecholamine release from the adrenal medulla. Thus, it is obvious that no matter how potent a vasoconstrictor angiotensin

may be in its own right, it has the potential for affecting arterial pressure in many other ways. Its effects on nerve function are suggesting that angiotensin may eventually prove to be an important modulator of neural activity.

Renal Pressor System and Hypertension. It is obvious by now that "renin" has emerged as a very complex system as regards both its control mechanisms and the extent of its effects. Assessment of its participation in hypertension is therefore *not* easy. It has been attempted along two lines, both of which are applicable to man; their value and limitations for investigation, diagnosis, and therapy must therefore be clearly outlined. The first consists of determination of plasma renin activity (PRA) or, less frequently, of one or the other of its components (renin concentration or angiotensin II). Valuable as they are, estimates of peripheral plasma renin activity (PRA) cannot be expected to define all disturbances of this system. A normal PRA does not rule out the possibility of important minor variations in circulating angiotensin II. Conversely, an elevated PRA can be found in normotensive states such as hepatic cirrhosis or the nephrotic syndrome, showing that there is more to any hypertension than the renal pressor system. The number of factors affecting renin release make it clear that reported levels of renin activity cannot, therefore, be interpreted out of context. They can be evaluated correctly only in relation to clinical setting, posture of patient at time of sampling, level of arterial pressure, sodium balance (24-hour urinary sodium), serum electrolytes, and some estimate of intravascular volume.

The second approach is to determine the effect on arterial pressure of interference at different points with the renin-angiotensin cascade (Table 7–2). Thus, beta-adrenergic blockers have been used to reduce renin release; inhibitors of the converting enzyme diminish or prevent the formation of angiotensin II while angiotensin antagonists compete with it for binding to end-organ receptors. This approach is useful in that it attempts to define more or less directly the functional importance of the renin system. However, each agent used has other actions besides its effect on "renin" and may elicit counteractions which cloud the picture. Beta blockade has important hemodynamic and possible central nervous system effects; converting enzyme inhibition leads to increased bradykinin levels because that same converting enzyme is responsible for bradykinin degradation. Angiotensin antagonists come closer to the goal but some have significant agonistic effects and all do not interfere equally with all actions of angiotensin.

The renal pressor system has been implicated in malignant hypertension, renovascular hypertension, and the hypertension induced by oral contraceptives. In most other hypertensions, there is no clear evidence of its participation. In

TABLE 7–2 AGENTS INTERFERING WITH THE RENAL PRESSOR SYSTEM

| Renin Cascade | Interference | | |
	Agent	Action	"Caveats"
Angiotensinogen			
(1) Renin	(1) β-blockers	interfere with renin release	hemodynamic and CNS effects
Angiotensin I / CE	(2) converting enzyme (CE) inhibitors	competitive antagonism of CE	increased bradykinin
Angiotensin II — end organs	(3) angiotensin antagonists	competitive inhibition	(a) agonist effect (b) unequal action on different receptors
Angiotensin III			
Inactive fragments			

primary aldosteronism, aldosterone alone is increased while PRA is suppressed. Animal studies have suggested that excess renin may cause vascular injury; the lesions are those of arteriolar necrosis and might be related to changes seen in accelerated hypertension. There is no evidence to date that "renin" is related to the common atherosclerotic complications of hypertension.

Each type of hypertension is discussed separately, so that we will refer here only to that related to the use of oral contraceptive agents. The estrogen component of these medications increases renin substrate, and although renin itself is not necessarily increased, more angiotensin is formed, and circulating angiotensin is usually increased. Hypertension however occurs only in a few of the women so treated; its exact nature has not yet been determined, nor its relationship to possible genetic predisposition, association with sympathetic disturbance, or dependence on fluid retention. Clinical studies with blockers of the renal pressor system might give some of the answers needed. Practically however, when treatment is discontinued, the components of the renal pressor system return to normal levels and the hypertension disappears.

HYPERTENSION*

Hypertension means elevated arterial pressure, either systolic or diastolic or both, as is

*See also Chapter 6.

often the case. Diastolic elevation had been considered the hallmark of hypertension while systolic blood pressure was thought to be more variable and its elevation inconsequential. Recent evidence has shown both assumptions to be false; diastolic pressure levels vary as much as the systolic, and systolic hypertension is associated with increased morbidity and mortality. The close relation between mean systolic pressure and myocardial oxygen requirements shows that systolic hypertension is not hemodynamically insignificant; it imposes a costly load on the heart and seems as closely related to cardiac hypertrophy as diastolic hypertension, if not more so. The basic mechanisms of systolic hypertension have been reviewed and this discussion will deal with what is called diastolic hypertension, although systolic pressure is elevated as well.

Hypertension by itself is not a diagnosis. It is the result of a number of diseases and disturbances — some serious and progressive, others transient — and it can be classified in many ways. The following is modified from Pickering:

1. By kind
   a. Systolic hypertension
   b. Diastolic hypertension
2. By degree
   a. Nonmalignant
   b. Malignant
3. By cause
   a. Primary or unexplained — essential hypertension
   b. Secondary hypertension

A list of causes is given in Table 7–3.

TABLE 7-3 AN ETIOLOGIC CLASSIFICATION OF HYPERTENSION

I. *Arterial Hypertension (elevation of systolic and diastolic blood pressures)*
   A. Essential hypertension
      1. Labile (intermittent)
      2. Established ("fixed")
   B. Renal hypertension
      1. Kidney disease
         a. Glomerulonephritis
         b. Chronic pyelonephritis
         c. Congenital polycystic kidneys
         d. Obstructive uropathy
         e. Diabetic glomerulosclerosis
         f. Interstitial nephritis due to analgesics, gout, hypercalcemia
         g. Connective tissue diseases, periarteritis nodosa, scleroderma, lupus erythematosus
         h. Renal tumor
         i. Renal amyloidosis
         j. Radiation nephritis
         k. Hereditary nephritis
      2. Renal arterial disease
         a. Fibrous dysplasias
         b. Atherosclerotic disease
         c. Embolic obstruction
         d. Traumatic arterial dissection or occlusion
      3. Compression of kidney
         a. Perinephritis
         b. Perirenal hematoma, usually post-traumatic
   C. Endocrine hypertension
      1. Catecholamine excess: pheochromocytoma
      2. "Steroid" hypertension
         a. Mineralocorticoid excess
            (1) Primary aldosteronism
            (2) Functional enzymatic block leading to adrenal hyperplasia (e.g., 11-hydroxylase deficiency in adrenogenital syndrome, 17-hydroxylase deficiency, androgen-induced hydroxylase deficiency in masculinizing tumors)
            (3) Iatrogenic: Excess DOC or fluorinated steroid administration
         b. Glucocorticoid excess—various causes of Cushing syndrome (adrenal, pituitary, ectopic ACTH syndromes, ovarian tumors)
      3. Oral contraceptives
      4. Condition associated with hypertension
         a. Acromegaly
         b. Thyroid disorders
            (1) Myxedema
            (2) Thyrotoxicosis, usually a cause of systolic, not diastolic, hypertension
   D. Neurogenic hypertension
      1. Anxiety states (?)
      2. Intracranial disease
         a. Increased intracranial pressure
         b. Encephalitis
         c. Diencephalic syndrome
         d. Lead encephalopathy
      3. Disturbances in vasomotor center
         a. Bulbar poliomyelitis
         b. Disturbances in vascular supply
      4. Spinal cord and peripheral nerves
         a. Transection of the cord, transverse myelitis
         b. Polyneuritis
         c. Porphyria
   E. Hypertension of coarctation of the aorta
   F. Hypertension of toxemia of pregnancy
      1. Preeclampsia
      2. Eclampsia
II. *Systolic Hypertension*
   A. Caused mainly by an increased stroke output of the left ventricle
      1. Complete heart block
      2. Aortic regurgitation
      3. Patent ductus arteriosus
      4. Thyrotoxicosis
      5. Arteriovenous fistula
      6. Paget's disease of bone
   B. Caused mainly by a decreased distensibility of the aorta
      1. Arteriosclerosis of aorta
      2. Coarctation of aorta

Definition of Hypertension

To speak of elevated arterial pressure begs the question of what constitutes "normal" pressure levels. Mathematical limits can be defined by population surveys (means, standard deviations) but the absence of a demonstrable cause for deviation from the norm in the vast majority of cases has led to a re-examination of basic concepts regarding the nature of hypertension. Put simply, the question is, is there a natural dividing line between normal and raised arterial pressure, or is hypertension a purely quantitative alteration of a biophysical measurement (pressure)? In the first case, hypertension would be a specific disease leading to pressure elevation; in the second, it would be a simple quantitative deviation from normal with no specific point at which the disease can be said to begin.

The controversy is not yet completely settled. One school of thought (Platt and co-workers) is that hypertension is a specific disease entity. Two groups exist — those whose pressures do and those whose pressures do not increase with age — and the difference between them is determined by monogenic inheritance. Pickering and co-workers have argued very strongly that arterial pressure is a biophysical characteristic, like height, whose frequency distribution curves show no natural subdivision into separate groups and which is governed by a graded multifactorial or polygenic inheritance. Arguments are based on complicated statistical analysis of population surveys but also fundamentally, we think, on the persistent failure to uncover "the fault" that would explain essential hypertension.

A very important benefit from these discussions has been the attention drawn to the quantitative aspects of hypertension. Whatever its basic nature, there is no doubt about the importance of the actual level of pressure. Perhaps in no other disease does the quantitative deviation of a single variable so influence the course and complications of the disorder. Studies by life insurance companies have shown an impressive relationship between mortality and blood pressure levels extending over the whole range of arterial pressures, with no sudden break at any point. Aside from specific characteristics of diseases associated with hypertension, high blood pressure has consequences of its own. Many are closely related to the level of pressure itself and are prevented or reversed by adequate pressure control. These would include left ventricular failure, hypertensive encephalopathy, and the malignant phase. Fibrinoid necrosis can occur in any form of hypertension, with the possible exception of aortic coarctation, if the pressure is high enough. The relationship with pressure is less clear-cut for other complications; atherosclerotic complications are more frequent in hypertensive patients but may develop in normotensive subjects. In this case the duration of hypertension may be more important than its level. Although strokes are prevented to a certain extent by control of arterial pressure, myocardial infarction does not seem to be.

General Pathophysiologic Aspects in Hypertension

The number of unrelated diseases associated with hypertension indicates that there must be a variety of ways to produce a chronic rise of blood pressure. These are called pressor mechanisms. In a sense, this term is a misnomer because, with the exception of pheochromocytoma, the physiologic abnormalities associated with hypertension have not been shown to be causal. Although these abnormalities represent distinct aberrations of a number of cardiovascular control systems, the degrees to which they participate in arterial pressure elevation are not known. There is a real difference between recognizing the "cause" of a particular hypertension and describing its mechanism.

Hypertension is a disease of regulation; the mosaic theory proposed by Page in 1949 stressed the multifactorial response of the body to environmental influences. A disturbance of one factor will lead to automatic involvement of others, so that a whole new set of relationships may be established, often making it very difficult to decide which came first.

Some of these secondary alterations may be responsible for what might be termed *post-causal* hypertension, meaning persistence of hypertension even after removal of its primary cause. This can be shown experimentally in hypertension produced by renal arterial constriction; removal of the ischemic kidney will reduce blood pressure only if performed within a certain time after the provoking maneuver; if nephrectomy is delayed, hypertension will not be relieved. A clinical counterpart of this situation might be surmised when removal of apparently primary causes (e.g., adrenocortical tumor, pheochromocytoma, renal arterial stenosis) fails to relieve the patient of his hypertension. It is, however, very difficult in man to ascertain whether one is not dealing with the coexistence of two separate causes for the hypertensive disease, e.g., renal arterial stenosis in a patient with essential hypertension.

Of the possible factors helping to perpetuate hypertension, three are of particular interest.

1. The vulnerability of the renal vessels to increased pressure loads, leading to development of arteriolar nephrosclerosis.

2. The structural adaptation of vessel walls to hypertension; the thickened wall amplifies the luminal reduction produced by even normal stimuli (Folkow).

3. Resetting of baroreceptors: the fact that carotid sinus reflexes are active in hypertensive patients led to questioning why they did not prevent hypertension. McCubbin, et al., showed in dogs with chronic renal hypertension that there is a shifting upward in response of baroreceptors, i.e., an adaptation resetting the reflex to operate normally at higher pressure levels (Fig. 7–6). Once developed, this resetting may well militate for a time against attempts at reducing arterial pressure.

SECONDARY HYPERTENSION

The mechanisms responsible for a secondary hypertension are not completely known in all cases. The following is a summary of some of the main types. A certain degree of overlapping is unavoidable and this section should be read along with that on essential hypertension.

Renal Hypertension*

One of the important results of recent studies has been the differentiation of hypertensive states associated with renal disease into two types — one related, at least initially, to activation of some pressor mechanism, and the other related to loss of renal substance and possibly of an antipressor effect. The first is exemplified by

---

*See also Chapter 14.

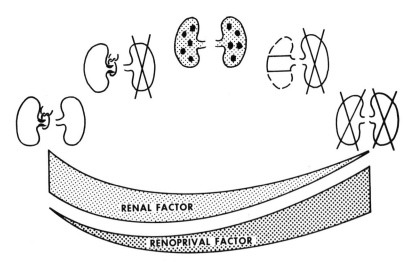

Figure 7–8 Renal and renoprival mechanisms in various types of "renal" hypertension; at one extreme is the renal mechanism activated by critical narrowing of one renal artery, the other remaining intact. At the other, removal of both kidneys leads to a renoprival volume-dependent state. In between these two extremes, both renal and renoprival factors participate in different combinations in the development of hypertension, depending on amount of renal tissue lost and on impairment of circulation through the remainder. (Modified from Tarazi, R. C., et al.: Pathol. et Biol. *16*:547, 1968.)

unilateral renal arterial stenosis and the second by the anephric state. In a schematic form that admits of many exceptions, the first type is characterized in man by elevated plasma renin activity (especially in recent hypertension), low plasma volume, and indices of increased neurogenic activity. The second type is marked by a positive correlation between blood volume and arterial pressure and very low or absent circulating renin; neurogenic activity fluctuates inversely with the degree of volemia. Patients with bilateral renal disease show varying mixtures of these two extremes, with either the "renal" or "renoprival" element predominating according to the type or stage of the lesion (Fig. 7–8).

Renovascular Hypertension. A large body of knowledge has been accumulated concerning this type of hypertension since the classic experiments of Goldblatt in dogs. Essential to proper evaluation of experimental studies is the realization of the extent of differences that may result from variation in techniques, timing of observations, and animal species used. More relevant perhaps to clinical situations is the extent of interference with the kidneys. Clipping of one renal artery is different from bilateral clipping; again, unilateral narrowing of a renal artery leaving the contralateral kidney intact differs in hemodynamic and humoral results from unilateral clipping with contralateral nephrectomy. Essential to the difference is the degree of fluid retention associated with bilateral maneuvers; the greater the retention, the lower the PRA and the smaller the response to angiotensin antagonists.

This interaction of volume factors with the renal pressor system does not negate the role of either.

Studies in man have shown that cardiac output was elevated in many patients with renovascular hypertension, but also that this increase was not alone responsible for the maintenance of their hypertension. Total peripheral resistance was raised in patients with both normal and elevated outputs; successful surgical repair or nephrectomy was associated with reduction in resistance more often than with reduction in output. This common participation of varying degrees of increased output and resistance in the maintenance of renovascular hypertension in man corresponds to recent experimental studies in rats and dogs. Although the early rise of arterial pressure following clipping of renal arteries or cellophane wrapping of the kidney is primarily due to increased cardiac output, later stages are characterized by a delayed rise in peripheral resistance with a return of output toward normal. The change in hemodynamic pattern with time has been related to autoregulatory mechanisms discussed earlier in this chapter.

The increase of output and initiation of hypertension following renal arterial clipping have been related to fluid retention consequent on the reduction in renal perfusion pressure. However, no change in blood volume was noted in the initial stages of perinephritic hypertension in dogs when cardiac output was rising; indeed, in both man and dogs with chronic renovascular hypertension plasma volume is slightly reduced. The

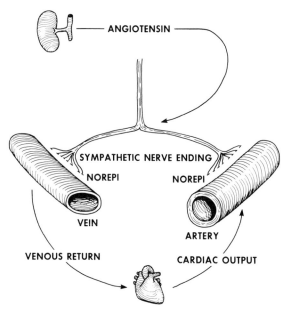

Figure 7–9 Diagram of possible ways by which angiotensin may raise arterial pressure, apart from a direct vasoconstrictor effect. It may act centrally (stimulation of vasomotor center) or peripherally (inhibiting re-uptake of norepinephrine (norepi) by sympathetic nerve endings, thus potentiating its action); arterial pressure is raised by a combination in different proportions of increased peripheral resistance (arteriolar constriction) and increased cardiac output (venoconstriction enhancing venous return).

combination of lower intravascular volume and increased cardiac output suggested an increased tone of the capacitance vessels shifting blood toward the heart. This is presumably related to enhanced sympathetic activity by angiotensin, since the latter has little, if any, direct effect on veins. Simultaneous stimulation of arterioles directly or indirectly (Fig. 7–9) helps set the stage for increased peripheral resistance. Once established, hypertension may be perpetuated by the development of secondary factors obscuring the initial disturbance (see later discussion).

It is generally agreed that the renal pressor system plays an important role in the early stages of renovascular hypertension; its participation in the chronic stage is much more debatable. This is probably because of the number of factors involved in any hypertension of sufficient duration. Doubts regarding the role of "renin" in this condition are based in part on the normal PRA in long-term renal arterial clip experiments. However, a normal PRA does not negate the possibility that angiotensin II may be marginally increased; further, the effects of the renal pressor system may be amplified by any degree of fluid retention. As regards clinical situations, it is im-

portant to recall that conclusions from animal studies might not apply unreservedly to man.

Control of hypertension has been achieved in some patients by unilateral nephrectomy or surgical correction of long-standing renal arterial stenosis. To decide which patients will respond to these measures, PRA determinations or evaluation of BP response to angiotensin antagonists might be useful if properly evaluated (see above). Peripheral plasma renin activity is not infrequently elevated in patients with renal arterial stenosis and seems to be directly related to the height of diastolic arterial pressure. This is important to remember, since these patients in a hospital setting often have mild labile hypertension and a finding of normal PRA does not mean that the hypertension is non-renal. Because peripheral PRA is inconsistently elevated in renovascular hypertensive subjects, measurements in renal venous blood have been advocated. Results have been correct in a majority of instances; they are based on the likelihood that in unilateral renal arterial stenosis the affected kidney will produce, either spontaneously or in response to adequate stimulation, more renin than the unaffected kidney.

Hypertension and Renal Parenchymal Disease. This type of hypertension is so often complicated by the features attendant on diminished kidney function that acceptable studies of its mechanism in man have been very difficult to obtain. Furthermore, the time course of renal decompensation can be compressed into a few days or extended over several years, so that hypertensive mechanisms may be quite different from one case to the other. Whether the diseased kidneys are still present or have been removed is another important factor; in some instances the characteristics of hypertension are radically altered by bilateral nephrectomy, even though the removed organs had practically no excretory function left.

The dependence of arterial pressure on volume expansion characterizes the hypertension associated with loss of renal tissue. In contrast with the slight plasma volume contraction seen in essential and renovascular hypertension is the direct correlation between arterial pressure and intravascular volume found in many patients with renal parenchymal disease (Fig. 7–10). In each patient, however, the hypertensive features will depend on the individual proportion of the renal and renoprival elements outlined earlier.

The hypertension of acute glomerulonephritis has been related to hypervolemia with consequent circulatory congestion, high ventricular filling pressure, and increased cardiac output, the total peripheral resistance remaining inappropriately normal in the face of increased blood flow.

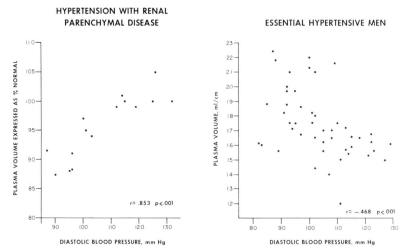

Figure 7–10 Contrasting relationship of intravascular volume and arterial pressure in essential hypertensive men and patients with renal parenchymal disease. (After Tarazi, R. C., et al.: Arch. Int. Med., *125*:835, 1970. Copyright 1970, American Medical Association.)

In patients with end-stage kidney disease, two varieties of hypertension may be seen. The first and more common is volume-dependent; the height of the arterial pressure is related to the degree of volemia and can be controlled by diuretics (if still effective) or by dialysis; PRA is not elevated. The second group of patients do not respond well to dehydration or the usual vasodilators; their hypertension seems to depend on continued activation of the renal pressor system and is markedly reduced (or made easier to manage) by nephrectomy.

Hemodynamic findings in the hypertension of renal parenchymal disease are quite variable because of the number of complicating factors present, such as degree of anemia, fluid balance, myocardial status, and so on. However, when conditions are strictly controlled, the increase in pressure is found to depend on an absolute or relative increase in total peripheral resistance. It differs from essential hypertension in the absence of a preferential redistribution of blood flow to the muscles. Brod, et al., who reported these findings, interpret them as a definite qualitative difference from the "patterns of persistent stress or preparedness to exercise characteristic of essential hypertension."

Coarctation of the Aorta

The hypertension associated with coarctation of the aorta is an experiment of nature of considerable hemodynamic interest. It has demonstrated that the body can adjust peripheral resistance differently in organs above and below the coarctation so as to provide all of them with a normal blood flow. Unfortunately, the mechanism of this precise adjustment has not yet been determined, although it offers the best possible example for autoregulation of blood flow.

Although the renal arteries usually are below the aortic constriction, there is no unequivocal evidence for activation of a renal pressor mechanism. The hypertension is probably related to the mechanical obstruction. Cardiac output in coarctation is usually increased; the ejection of a large stroke volume into an aorta with decreased capacity and relatively limited runoff accounts for the large pressure found in vessels above the area of constriction. As output and rate of ejection are increased with exercise, so is the systolic blood pressure, often to alarming levels, even in patients who have near normal blood pressure at rest. By diminishing this increase of cardiac output with intravenous propranolol, blood pressure rise with exercise is attenuated despite the significant increase in total peripheral resistance induced by the drug.

The importance of adaptive changes to hypertension can be seen in the occasional complications that follow surgical repair. When the obstruction is removed, vessels below the coarctation are suddenly exposed to higher pressures than they are used to; concomitantly baroreceptor reflexes are activated by the drop of pressure in their area. The result may be a hypertensive crisis with arteriolar necrosis in the lower body parts.

Pheochromocytoma

Most interesting and unusual is the hypertensive state associated with pheochromocytoma, a tumor of the medullary portion of the adrenal gland. It is one of the rare types in which the actual pressor mechanism is known. The tumors contain large amounts of epinephrine and norepinephrine in varying proportions. Hypertension may be persistent but is often paroxysmal. Symptoms result from release of the hormones from the tumor, causing sudden rapid rises in blood pressure, tachycardia, anxiety, headache, perspiration, nausea, and epigastric and precordial pain. All symptoms do not always appear but it would be a most unusual patient who would not have at least one or two. Norepinephrine produces no tachycardia and does not affect the cardiac output. Epinephrine does both and produces hypermetabolism and hyperglycemia as well. Variations in the clinical picture depend in large part on these variables, but there are exceptions. The only definitive means of making the diagnosis are biochemical tests showing increased catecholamine excretion; these include determination of urinary vanillylmandelic acid (VMA), metanephrines, and catecholamines either during a hypertensive period or following a provocative test. Intravenous histamine (0.025 mg.) may bring on an attack and is probably still the more reliable provocative agent as regards both blood pressure response and urinary excretion of catecholamine metabolites. Adrenergic blocking agents such as phentolamine or dibenzyline will reduce the elevated pressure. Phentolamine is especially useful for hypertensive episodes; dibenzyline is preferred for medical treatment if tumors are inoperable. Beta-adrenergic blockers may be needed to control tachycardia or ventricular irritability induced by excess catecholamines. Since beta blockade would leave α-mediated vasoconstriction unopposed, beta blockers should be given only under cover of α-adrenergic blocking agents.

Primary Aldosteronism (Conn's Disease)

The frequency of this condition as a cause of hypertension is not known. It is certainly a more frequent cause than is pheochromocytoma; however, it is less common than autopsy findings of small adrenocortical nodules might suggest. It results from autonomous hypersecretion of aldosterone by small single or multiple tumors of the adrenal cortex zona glomerulosa; sometimes only bilateral hyperplasia is found, with no strictly defined tumor (see Chapter 32). Its importance stems from the possibility of specific therapy or surgical cure for this type of hypertension.

The diagnosis is suggested by finding hypokalemia and inappropriate kaliuresis (>30.0 mEq. daily urinary potassium excretion with a serum potassium <3.5 mEq./L.) in a hypertensive patient with no history of recent diuretic therapy; the clinical picture is otherwise very similar to essential hypertension. The specific endocrine derangement is indicated by (1) low plasma renin activity that cannot be stimulated by low sodium intake (thus excluding secondary aldosteronism), and (2) more specifically, increased aldosterone excretion that cannot be suppressed by high sodium intake (thus reflecting the abnormality in regulation). Adrenal venography has been recommended for localization of the lesion.

The metabolic abnormalities in primary aldosteronism are better understood than the mechanism of its hypertension. Increased aldosterone excretion leads to sodium and water retention; stimulation of potassium-for-sodium exchange in the distal tubule leads to hypokalemia from excessive potassium loss in the urine. Increase in extracellular sodium and relative expansion of plasma volume probably account for the suppression of plasma renin activity, since administration of spironolactone can stimulate it. The classic hemodynamic pattern of this hypertension includes hypervolemia, increased cardiac output, and an elevated total peripheral resistance. But this can be modified by excessive rises in blood pressure or by coincident essential hypertension; in such cases plasma volume and cardiac output may be reduced to low normal levels.

There are other causes of hypertension due to *mineralocorticoid excess*, all sharing the same pattern of suppressed plasma renin activity and easily induced hypokalemia (Fig. 7–11). Some result from excess administration of sodium-retaining steroids or steroid-like substances (e.g., licorice) and simply require discontinuing the drug or readjusting its dose. Others are due to enzymatic blocks (congenital or acquired) in hydroxylation of adrenal steroids at the 11 or 17 position. These blocks interfere with the production of cortisol and hence with its negative feedback control over ACTH production. The resultant excessive ACTH drive leads to adrenal hypersecretion of mineralocorticoids and consequent hypertension. Treatment consists of ACTH suppression by dexamethasone. Still other cases result from disordered hormonal production by adrenal and extra-adrenal tumors.

ESSENTIAL HYPERTENSION

By far the commonest type, essential hypertension still remains a diagnosis by exclusion, reached only by ruling out the various causes of elevated arterial pressure. It is characterized by a strong hereditary element and a long natural course, so that in early phases the subject appears normal except for the high blood pressure.

All the mechanisms discussed earlier have been at one time or another linked with essential hypertension. It is obviously very difficult in slowly developing asymptomatic processes to differentiate primary factors from secondary reactions. Until now no animal model exists for essential hypertension; the relation of genetic strains

SIMPLIFIED SCHEME OF MINERALOCORTICOID HYPERTENSIONS

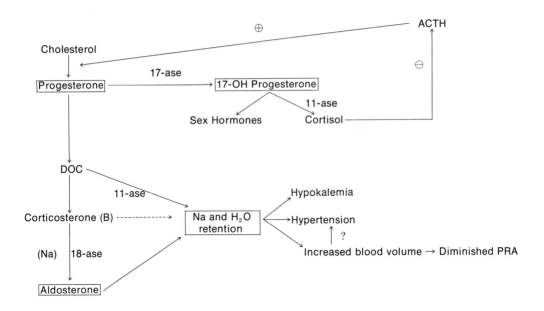

Key:
⊕ Positive stimulus
⊖ Negative feedback
11-ase, 17-ase = 11 beta or 17 alpha-hydroxylase
PRA = plasma renin activity

(a) 11 beta-hydroxylase deficiency leads to decreased cortisol; the increased ACTH drive leads to hypertension secondary to DOC excess and to accumulation of 17 OH-products increasing androgenic hormones.
(b) 17 alpha-hydroxylase deficiency leads to decreased cortisol and therefore to increased ACTH drive, but sex hormones are usually absent owing to lack of 17 hydroxylation; hypertension is related to increased DOC and corticosterone as sodium retention decreases their conversion to aldosterone.
(c) Combined DOC, corticosterone, and aldosterone excess occurs in adrenocortical tumors, especially if malignant, and in disordered ACTH drive (ectopic); cortisol is usually also increased in these cases.
(d) In primary aldosteronism, only aldosterone is increased.
(e) Iatrogenic hypertension usually results from excess DOC or fluorinated cortisol derivatives with unrestricted salt intake.

Figure 7–11.

of spontaneously hypertensive rats to the human disease is still conjectural. Another difficulty is the lack of homogeneity resulting from lack of precision in diagnosis; there are probably different subgroups still included, for want of a better definition, under the over-all term of "essential or idiopathic hypertension."

Hemodynamic Characteristics

The main development in this area concerns the relationship between fixed and labile essential hypertension. Well-established essential hypertension is associated with a normal cardiac output and elevated peripheral resistance. The elevated resistance seems to be uniformly distributed in practically all vascular territories except

in the kidney, where it may be more intense, and in the skeletal muscular system, where it is slightly less marked. This pattern was likened by Brod to a constant preparedness for exercise or response to unspecified stress. Within this general framework a certain gradation has been described wherein a progressive reduction of resting cardiac output occurred with development of progressive cardiac involvement in the course of the disease. Even before cardiac decompensation occurred, cardiac output was reduced (and total peripheral resistance further increased) in hypertensive patients with definite left ventricular hypertrophy.

Contrasting with the above findings, an increasing number of studies from laboratories in the United States and Europe have established that a large proportion of patients with intermittent, usually mild elevations of arterial pressure (borderline hypertension) have increased cardiac output and normal, near normal, or subnormal values of total peripheral resistance. The suggestion is that this pattern of "increased output-normal resistance" is the beginning phase leading to increased resistance and fixed hypertension. It is not yet evident from information available whether increase in cardiac output represents an early stage in the development of hypertension or a qualitatively different hemodynamic type of the disease. Although a normal or low cardiac output is most frequent among established essential hypertensives and a high output is common in borderline hypertension, exceptions *do* occur in both conditions. The answer must await longitudinal clinical studies of labile hypertensive subjects.

The reason for the increased output in borderline hypertension is not clear; oxygen consumption is normal for that level of output in contrast with other idiopathic high output states. Resting heart rate, although slightly faster than normal, is not faster than that in other forms of hypertension. This finding reawakened interest in the old suggestion that an "augmented force" of the heart beat could play a role in the genesis of hypertension; but an increase in output might as well represent a normal cardiac response to constriction of the capacitance vessels and central redistribution of blood. Similarities with hemodynamic findings in renovascular hypertension are obvious; however, the mechanisms involved in essential hypertension are still purely conjectural.

In these considerations of increased output, it must be remembered that in the final analysis, hypertension is the result of failure of the peripheral circulation to adapt to systemic flow. Indeed, some abnormality in peripheral circulatory adjustment is demonstrable even in patients with "normal total peripheral resistance." Although correctly said to be "within normal range," their resistance is abnormally high for their cardiac output, as is shown by comparison with normotensive subjects with equivalent levels of output. The abnormality is clearly revealed during muscular exercise.

In the absence of cardiac failure, response to dynamic exercise in hypertensive patients is much the same as in normal subjects. Cardiac output increases proportionately to oxygen uptake, and peripheral resistance falls. This fall is never to normal levels, so that blood pressure remains high; although the heart responded normally, the extent of reduction in peripheral resistance was not commensurate with the rise in output, especially in young subjects. The anomaly of peripheral reactions in hypertension is also shown in the pattern of response to stressful interviews. The resultant increase of blood pressure was due to increased cardiac output in 80 per cent of normal subjects, whereas most hypertensive patients responded by an increase in total peripheral resistance.

Neurogenic Factors

The obvious effects of emotional factors on arterial pressure have led to many assumptions regarding the role of *psychogenic factors* in essential hypertension. It has been suggested that frequent psychogenic rises in blood pressure may culminate finally in fixed hypertension. The corticohypothalamic "defense reaction" not only may be activated by manifest threats but is also said to occur whenever "alertness" is raised. Repeated increases in arterial pressure would lead to structural adaptation (hypertrophy) of the arterioles, which in turn would amplify the vasoconstrictive effects of even normal nerve traffic or circulating substances. Various alterations found in essential hypertension — namely, altered regional blood flow, modest increase in basal heart rate, and decrease in plasma volume — have been likened to the pattern of "preparedness to exercise."

Despite its attractiveness, this hypothesis still remains to be proved, since there is no firm evidence that psychogenic stimuli result in chronic sustained hypertension. These stimuli are difficult to quantitate and nerve traffic cannot yet be measured directly in man. Studies showing excessive pressure rise in hypertensive patients in response to stressful experiences do not differentiate between increased sympathetic outflow from vasomotor centers and increased vascular responsiveness to normal outflow. The problem is complicated by the possible influence of such ill-defined factors as personality traits. Pavlov noted that it is easier to produce a neurotic state in "sanguine" than in "melancholic" dogs. Promising studies are being conducted in the area of conditioned blood pressure control and the effects of reticular formation on baroreceptor activity.

The hypertension produced in laboratory animals by sino-aortic denervation does not bear any real resemblance to essential hypertension. It is accompanied by wide swings of blood pressure and marked tachycardia; the pressure falls to normal levels when the animal is quiet or asleep and is unusually sensitive to neural blocking agents. Apart from rare cases of polyneuritis involving the ninth cranial nerve, disturbances of baroreceptor mechanism probably do not have a causative role in essential hypertension. Secondary resetting of their threshold and/or diminished sensitivity of the reflex due to functional or structural changes in the carotid arteries might theoretically play a minor role in its maintenance.

The striking antihypertensive effectiveness of drugs that suppress adrenergic functions is still one of the main evidences that neural factors operate in some way to maintain hypertension. A clinically applicable way to estimate their importance is to determine the immediate pressure response to an intravenous injection of a ganglion blocker. The pressure reduction obtained in essential hypertensive subjects correlated significantly with pre-injection diastolic pressure and total peripheral resistance. Again, the higher the pressure and the resistance, the smaller the plasma volume, so that intravascular volume was inversely related to sympathetic activity. At the present time there is no way of knowing whether intravascular volume is reduced because increased sympathetic tone has reduced vascular capacity or whether increased sympathetic outflow is a compensatory response to a reduced plasma volume.

An important aspect developed over the past decade is the close and reciprocal interaction between the renal pressor and sympathetic nervous systems. The potentiating action of angiotensin on the cardiovascular effects of the sympathetic nervous system has already been discussed. On the other hand, sympathetic hyperactivity may help trigger the renin-angiotensin system by restricting blood flow to the kidney (a part of the "defense reaction"). Thus, whether a neurogenic or a hormonal factor is the initial event, both may inter-react to maintain a more sustained neurohumoral drive on the cardiovascular system (Folkow and Neil). The clinical relevance of these relationships is underlined by the experience that renovascular hypertension can be effectively treated by drugs that suppress adrenergic activity.

Extracellular Fluid and Blood Volume

There now seems little question that plasma volume is quite regularly altered in various forms of hypertension. It is reduced in essential hypertension in relation to the level of diastolic pressure and peripheral resistance, so that the higher the resistance, the lower the volume. Since extracellular fluid volume is usually normal in this condition, the reduction in plasma volume probably reflects a subtle abnormality in the distribution of fluid between its intravascular and interstitial compartments. Hypertension accompanying renal arterial disease or pheochromocytoma is also characterized by reduced plasma volume.

In contrast, plasma volume is modestly expanded in primary aldosteronism, although not as consistently as is usually suggested. The more striking abnormality is the positive correlation between total blood volume and arterial pressure

found in patients with renal parenchymal disease (see Renal Hypertension). Finally, a subgroup of essential hypertension has been described with plasma volume either expanded or inappropriately normal for height of diastolic pressure. This group possibly represents the same type of hypertension as is being tentatively characterized by various investigators as having increased extracellular fluid volume, increased exchangeable sodium, and hyporeninemia with no evidence of primary aldosteronism.

The clinical relevance of volume studies is not limited to diagnostic considerations. As indicated above, pressure responsiveness to ganglion blockers is inversely related to degree of volemia, hence the greater sensitivity of patients with low plasma volume (spontaneous or diuretic-induced) to neural blocking drugs. Conversely, pressure response to these drugs is attenuated or lost when hypervolemia develops, as it often does during their administration. The increase in plasma volume during treatment results from diminished tone of capacitance vessels with resultant transfer of fluid from the interstitial to the intravascular compartment and is accentuated by actual fluid retention. This "false tolerance" to the neural blocking drugs is reversed and pressure control is restored by adequate volume depletion with diuretics.

Renal Pressor System

At the present time there is no indication of any gross abnormality of this system in nonmalignant essential hypertension. Plasma renin levels usually are within normal range but occasionally can be quite low and unresponsive to the usual stimuli used to increase circulating renin. Laragh and co-workers have classified essential hypertensive subjects into low, normal, and high renin categories, suggesting that the first depend more on volume factors and the latter two on renin mechanisms. An attractive hypothesis links these observations with those on volume factors in the following scheme. Essential hypertension could be viewed as being of two sub-types: one with normal-to-high PRA, contracted plasma volume, and probably increased sympathetic drive; the second with low PRA, expanded plasma volume, and particular responsiveness to diuretic therapy. However it is not yet clear whether this subdivision describes different sub-types or only extremes at either end of a graded spectrum of variations. Exceptions do occur; levels of PRA are influenced by age, and long-term studies are needed to determine whether some of these differences are not simply time-dependent.

In the majority of subjects with essential hypertension aldosterone secretion correlates normally with urinary sodium excretion. In some, however, discrepancies between levels of plasma renin activity and aldosterone excretion have been described, especially under the stimulus of sodium deprivation. The role of this hormonal imbalance is still not clear.

Malignant hypertension — of whatever origin—is associated with marked secondary aldosteronism: high plasma renin activity; hyponatremia; hypokalemia; and great rises of aldosterone excretion. Activation of the renin-angiotensin system in this condition has been viewed as partly responsible for the intensification of the vascular disease and of hyponatremia.

In summary, this review of pathophysiologic mechanisms in essential hypertension has revealed multifactorial disturbances. Any of the numerous changes that occur in hypertension cannot be considered alone; the complexity of relationships and practical impossibility to differentiate primary from secondary factors explain the failure of finding a "single" cause of essential hypertension.

Alterations with Antihypertensive Therapy

Recent developments have led to concerted efforts for control of hypertension; this is often achieved by drug therapy which introduces marked alterations in mechanisms regulating arterial pressure. Better understanding of these alterations will help accurate evaluation of problems in the increasing number of treated hypertensive subjects.

Attempts at lowering arterial pressure set in motion a number of counter-reactions; further, all antihypertensive drugs in common use have one or more actions which tend to thwart their own effectiveness. Thus, sympatholytics as well as vasodilators can cause fluid retention and plasma volume expansion. During treatment with beta blockers, peripheral resistance can increase and thus limit the reduction in blood pressure. Conversely, treatment with many vasodilators reduces peripheral resistance but reflexly increases cardiac output. Both diuretic agents and vasodilators increase plasma renin activity, which may antagonize their antihypertensive effects although this has not been established. Thus, hypertension remains a multifactorial problem not only in its initiation and in its maintenance but also in its response to therapy.

The clinical implications of these observations are twofold: (1) Studies of the physiologic characteristic of any hypertension may be misleading if made while patients are on antihypertensive therapy or too soon after it is stopped. (2) Antihypertensive agents sometimes fail simply because one pressor mechanism has been substituted for another. Most patients with moderate or severe hypertension will require a combination of

drugs; the choice must be based on a consideration of the mechanisms involved and balanced in order to minimize the counteractions anticipated from each of its components.

HYPOTENSION

General Considerations and Definition of Terms

Low systemic arterial pressure impairs tissue perfusion; however, the pressure level at which blood flow is critically diminished will vary, depending on the extent and rate of reduction in blood pressure, local condition of the vessels, and adequacy of compensating mechanisms. Hence, a numerical definition of hypotension raises the same problems of "normalcy" as a numerical definition of hypertension. Some normal subjects have arterial pressures below 90/60 mm. Hg with no apparent cause and no sign of ill-effect. The brain can apparently be adequately perfused, even in the upright position, by systolic pressures as low as 60 mm. Hg or less. The symptoms of diminished vitality, easy fatigue, or dizziness that have been sometimes loosely ascribed to hypotension (systolic below 100 mm. Hg) are just as frequently found in normotensives or in hypertensive patients.

A low arterial pressure level by itself is not necessarily a pathologic finding; in fact, chronic "hypotension" in the absence of associated disease may be a favorable condition because of the diminished cardiovascular load. Pathologic hypotension is the level at which blood flow to vital organs (brain, heart, kidneys) is impaired. Obviously perfusion will be more easily impaired by acute hypotension than by a chronic reduction in arterial pressure that may allow time for more effective compensatory adjustments of blood flow. The effects of hypotension may be subdivided into (a) those resulting directly from impaired organ perfusion, e.g., fainting due to cerebral ischemia; and (b) those due to activation of compensatory mechanisms, e.g., sweating and tachycardia from sympathetic stimulation secondary to decreased baroreceptor activity. The resulting clinical picture will therefore vary markedly with the cause of hypotension, its time course, the pattern of blood flow alteration, the activation of compensatory mechanisms or their failure, and any pre- or coexisting disease.

Postural Hypotension. This is characterized by a marked fall in arterial pressure with dizziness and possibly syncope on standing but a quite adequate circulation and pressure when lying down (Fig. 7–12).

Though acute hypotension (postural, cardiac, or reflex) is one of the commonest causes of syn-

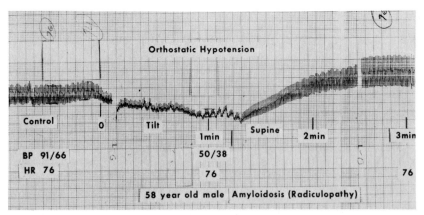

Figure 7–12 Intra-arterial pressure record of a patient with postural hypotension due to loss of sympathetic nerve function; note the rapid (as opposed to sudden) reduction in pressure from the beginning of head-up tilt and the unchanged heart rate despite the fall in pressure. As soon as the patient is returned to the horizontal position, arterial pressure begins to rise to even hypertensive levels; this tilt-back overshoot occurs following head-up tilt in patients with organic or drug-induced sympathetic dysfunction and has been related to liberation of catecholamines.

cope, the two terms are not synonymous. *Syncope* refers to a sudden, transient loss of consciousness; it is indeed very frequently due to hypotension and impaired cerebral perfusion but might in other instances result from biochemical derangements like hypoglycemia or reflect cerebral dysfunction as in the cerebral type of carotid sinus syndrome. Most fainting spells (vasovagal attacks or vasodepressor syncope) occur when the subject is standing and are associated with a fall in arterial pressure. They differ from "postural hypotension" in that they may occur when the subject is in the supine position, an extra-provocative factor is usually present (emotional disturbance, sight of blood, pain, hot weather), and signs of vagal activity (slowing pulse, nausea) are evident. Whereas all symptoms associated with postural hypotension quickly disappear as soon as the patient lies or falls down, the vasovagal disturbance clears much more slowly. Vasodepressor syncope is characterized by a sudden reduction in peripheral vascular resistance

(Fig. 7–13), venoconstriction rather than dilation, and little change in cardiac output. There is no evidence for excessive plasma volume contraction.

Shock. Despite its lack of precision, this term does evoke an impressive and readily recognizable picture and will certainly continue to be used clinically. It describes a condition of marked weakness, a variable degree of mental torpor with weak rapid thready pulse, cold clammy skin, and unobtainable or very low arterial pressure by usual method of examination. Many of these signs may not necessarily be found; arterial pressure may occasionally be relatively normal, especially if the patient was previously hypertensive. In some cases central pressure obtained by arterial cannulation may be high while brachial pressure is clinically unobtainable owing to marked peripheral vasoconstriction. Mentation may be unexpectedly clear if peripheral and renal vasoconstriction are intense enough to secure adequate cerebral blood flow. Instead of being cold

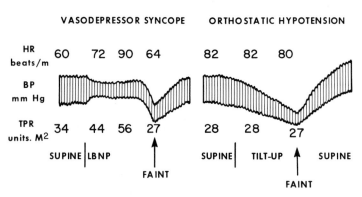

Figure 7–13 Semidiagrammatic illustration of hemodynamic events in vasodepressor syncope and in orthostatic hypotension due to loss of sympathetic activity. In the former, the drop in blood pressure occurs suddenly after a normal response to tilt (simulated in this case by lower body negative pressure, LBNP); heart rate and total peripheral resistance increase before they suddenly drop. In contrast, arterial pressure is gradually reduced to hypotensive levels in patients with sympathetic paralysis (see Fig. 7–12), with no change in either TPR or heart rate; note also the post-tilt overshoot of the arterial pressure.

and clammy, the skin may be dry and hot in cases of bacteremic shock. However, despite these variations, the picture is usually readily recognizable; the basic fault is a gross impairment of tissue perfusion due to marked reduction in cardiac output. The subject is much too extensive to be covered in this chapter; it is important, however, to underline its differences from other types of hypotension and to realize that in any hypotension, the body suffers not from the fall in arterial pressure per se but from the reduced blood flow that hypotension produces or signifies.

Chronic Hypotension. Chronic hypotension with vague or nonspecific symptoms may be associated with a variety of diseases such as aortic stenosis, adrenocortical insufficiency, malabsorption syndrome, severe cardiac failure, and constrictive pericarditis. The clinical picture is dominated by the primary disease of which hypotension is only a sign. Some of these conditions may be associated with postural hypotension also. In contrast with such secondary forms of hypotension, an idiopathic, chronically low arterial pressure is not really a pathologic condition. Indeed, statistical studies would suggest enhanced longevity for apparently healthy people with idiopathic hypotension.

Pathophysiology of Postural Hypotension

Adjustment to Postural Changes. The pressure in a column of fluid depends on its specific gravity and the vertical distance from the point of measurement to the reference level; hence, the pressure at the bottom of a U tube will obviously be higher than that at the top. However, the pressure head required to drive fluid through a system of horizontal tubes will not be altered by the addition to that system of an unyielding U tube dipping below the line of flow. Similarly, if blood vessels were rigid tubes, standing up would not affect arterial or venous blood pressure at the heart's level and cardiac output would not change. The intravascular pressures in the feet would be markedly increased by an amount equal to their distance below the phlebostatic or zero point, but the arteriovenous gradient would not be altered, since arterial and venous pressures would be affected to the same extent.

Vessels, however, are not rigid impermeable tubes. As we stand, the pull of gravity pools blood in distensible veins below the heart and plasma is lost to interstitial fluid as capillary pressure and ultrafiltration increase. Diminished venous return reduces cardiac output and unless compensatory mechanisms perform adequately the subsequent fall in arterial pressure will result in impaired cerebral perfusion and loss of consciousness. Fortunately, adjustment mechanisms normally are quite effective and arterial pressure is maintained (see page 198). Even with passive head-up tilt, which exaggerates the effect of gravity by minimizing the support derived from contraction of the lower limb muscles, mean arterial pressure varies only by ± 10 mm. Hg.

This stability is due to an almost instantaneous reflex increase in sympathetic vasomotor outflow (see Neural Reflexes). Obviously vasoconstriction must occur in the resistance vessels to offset the effect of reduction in output and in the capacitance vessels to diminish pooling and help hasten venous return. As part of this sympathetic stimulation, heart rate increases slightly. The same reflexes are involved in bleeding or when mechanical factors hinder venous return (e.g., recumbency in late pregnancy).

Associated with this increased sympathetic activity, catecholamine concentration is increased in plasma and urine. The increase in epinephrine is due to reflex sympathetic stimulation of the adrenal medulla, and the increase in norepinephrine is mostly due to increased activity of the sympathetic vasomotor nerves. Other hormones are also involved in the response to upright posture; renin and aldosterone secretion are increased and there is even some evidence that antidiuretic hormone may be released, probably in response to reduced tension on intrathoracic volume receptors. Plasma renin activity was found to be elevated within a few minutes of upright tilt, but its rise lagged behind the reflex increase in pulse rate and diastolic blood pressure. Renin release is markedly affected by sympathetic nerve activity and circulating catecholamines and may be impaired in some patients with autonomic nerve disease or during treatment with adrenergic blocking drugs; however, increased catecholamine production is not an indispensable prerequisite for adequate stimulation of renin and aldosterone in the upright posture.

Whatever the reflex effects on resistance vessels, the capillary vessels in the feet during standing must still contend with a pressure exceeding 100 mm. Hg, far above the maximum colloid osmotic pressure of plasma proteins. Plasma loss by diffusion could thus be enormous; this is prevented by contraction of precapillary sphincters, thus effectively shutting off filtration from a large number of dependent capillary beds. In addition, counterpressures develop in dependent areas to prevent overdistention of veins and help balance some of the rise in capillary pressure. Intramuscular tissue pressure increases with muscular contraction. Lower limb veins are compressed when leg and thigh muscles contract, and blood is pushed upward; as the muscles relax, backward flow of blood is prevented by intravenous valves. By interrupting the column of blood in the veins at different points, valves also prevent transmission of the full weight of that column to small dependent venules. Thus, "muscular pumping" helps lower both venous pressure and effective capillary filtering pressure; when interfered with, the incidence of fainting is increased. This may happen in normal subjects standing motionless at attention, or tilted passively and then supported in the upright position, or in patients with incompetent venous valves and dilated varicose veins.

Cerebral Circulation. The oxygen requirements of the central nervous system are fairly constant, and cerebral blood flow must therefore be kept constant if consciousness and life are to be preserved. The cerebral vessels are remarkably unresponsive to the usual neural and hormonal stimuli; the constancy of flow is secured by local autoregulatory mechanisms dependent on local production of carbon dioxide and local oxygen needs. Arterial Pco_2 is the most powerful regulator of cerebral flow; doubling Pco_2 approximately doubles cerebral flow, whereas a decrease in oxygen saturation to about 75 per cent increases flow approximately 40 per cent. However, the vasodilator effect of oxygen deficiency increases at very low saturations. This close adaptation of cerebral flow to neuronal metabolic needs ensures an impressively constant flow over wide ranges of arterial pressure down to quite low levels (50 to 60 mm. Hg mean pressure). Thus, whenever widespread sympathetic vasoconstriction develops (shock, hemorrhage, or upright posture), the cerebral vasculature is not materially affected by it but blood is redistributed toward the brain (and heart) from other constricted vascular beds. Moreover, since cerebral vessels and cerebrospinal fluid are enclosed within a rigid cavity, variations in cerebrospinal fluid or extravascular pressure with standing parallel very closely the variations in intravascular pressure, thus increasing the stability of the cerebral circulation. The stability of cerebral flow despite marked fluctuations in arterial pressure may explain why antihypertensive therapy is very rarely associated with cerebral damage, even when transient hypotension develops. As soon as blood pressure is increased beyond a minimal level (as by lying down), cerebral blood flow is rapidly restored to near normal.

Pathophysiologic Classification. Orthostatic hypotension is characterized by a fall of at least 20 mm. Hg in both systolic and diastolic pressure on assumption of the standing position; in severe cases the patient cannot even stand up, since simple sitting leads to severe reduction in blood pressure. Severe hypotension may also develop in positions other than standing; women in late pregnancy may faint when lying on their backs, and patients with atrial myxoma or pedunculated intra-atrial thrombus may faint on sitting up.

TABLE 7–4   HEMODYNAMIC RESPONSES IN ORTHOSTATIC HYPOTENSION

	Normal	Oligemia or Diminished Venous Return	Idiopathic Orthostatic Hypotension	
			Early	Advanced
1. *Standing Up*				
Blood pressure	Little change: mean arterial pressure varies by <10 mm. Hg	Reduction in both systolic and diastolic pressures, sometimes quite marked		
Heart rate	Increased by about 15%	Marked increase	Slight increase	No change
Cardiac output	Reduced, usually 10 to 20%	Reduced to varying degree	Reduced, usually >25%	Reduced >25%
Total peripheral resistance	Increased by 15 to 20%	Marked increase	Slight increase may occur	No increase
2. *Phenylephrine*				
Blood pressure	Increased, depending on dose	Normal response	Response > normal because of denervation hypersensitivity	
Heart rate	Slowed with blood pressure rise	Normal response	Response may be normal	No change despite rise in blood pressure
3. *Valsalva Maneuver Overshoot (Phase IV)*				
	Rise in diastolic pressure averages 25 to 35% of control	Normal or increased	Absent	Absent and return from phase III may be quite slow

These types of postural hypotension are due to impaired ventricular filling and diminished cardiac output.

Orthostatic hypotension is the commonest form of postural hypotension; the blood pressure in the supine position may be reduced, normal, or even elevated. The patient may feel and look quite normal when lying down or some circulatory disorder may be apparent, e.g., rapid pulse and low arterial pressure as in hemorrhage or adrenocortical insufficiency. However, whatever the cause of the orthostatic fall in pressure, the clinical picture on standing is common to all (Table 7–4). The patient feels dizzy, weak, and faint; ataxia, blurring of vision, or occasionally some dysar-thria develops, and unless he lies down rapidly, he may become unconscious. All symptoms, including syncope, clear up rapidly in the supine position.

Postural hypotension may have different causes (Table 7–5) that essentially can be linked to either of two basic mechanisms. In the first group, cardiac output is so reduced that, despite reflex sympathetic stimulation, arterial pressure falls (sympathicotonic type). The second group is characterized by failure of the barostatic mechanism at some point along the reflex arc; hence, there are no or inappropriately few signs of sympathetic activity. Reflexes may be interfered with by disease or simply slowed by such factors as

TABLE 7–5   POSTURAL HYPOTENSION

I. *Diminished Cardiac Output*
  A. Interference with venous return and cardiac filling at the muscular, venous, or cardiac level:
    1. Poor muscular pumping mechanism:
      a. Muscular atrophy
      b. Poor postural adjustment in young asthenic persons standing at strict attention
      c. Passive tilting
    2. Venous disease:
      a. Incompetent valves
      b. Varicose veins
      c. Obstruction (e.g., late pregnancy)
    3. Cardiac: Tamponade, constrictive pericarditis, atrial myxoma, ball valve thrombus
  B. Absolute or relative depletion of intravascular volume:
    1. Relative: Due to dilatation of capacitance vessels by drugs (e.g., nitrites) or disease (e.g., venous angiomatosis)
    2. Absolute:
      a. Hemorrhage, internal or external
      b. Excessive loss of fluid by diuresis, vomiting, diarrhea
      c. Increased capillary permeability with loss of fluid in interstitial spaces
      d. Urinary salt wasting due to selective hypoaldosteronism
  C. Diminished myocardial performance:*
    1. Myocarditis, severe coronary arterial disease
    2. Postural arrhythmias with excessively slow or extremely rapid heart rate
    3. Outlet obstruction as in aortic or pulmonary stenosis (usually leads to exercise rather than orthostatic hypotension)

II. *Impaired Peripheral Resistance*
  A. Arteriolar:
    1. Disease: Relatively rare (e.g., amyloidosis), and then usually associated with neural involvement as well
    2. Arteriolar vasodilators as nitrites or nitroprusside
  B. Neurologic dysfunction:
    1. Lesion in afferent limb: Tabes dorsalis, rarely in polyneuritis
    2. Lesion in central nervous sytem:
      a. Some forms of chronic idiopathic hypotension; possible relationship to Shy-Drager syndrome
      b. Parkinsonism either isolated or part of a more extensive degenerative disease
      c. Cerebral arteriosclerosis
      d. Syringomyelia, various myelopathies, Wernicke's syndrome, tumors
      e. Drugs (e.g., meprobamate)
    3. Lesion in efferent sympathetic limb: (parasympathetic may be affected but is not responsible for hypotension)
      a. Some forms of chronic idiopathic hypotension
      b. Polyneuritis (e.g., diabetes, porphyria)
      c. Myelopathies
      d. Iatrogenic:
        (1) Postsympathectomy
        (2) Neural blocking drugs
          (a) Ganglion blocking agents, adrenergic blockers
          (b) Monoamine oxidase inhibitors
          (c) L-dopa
III. *Undetermined or Mixed Mechanisms*
  A. Adrenocortical insufficiency: Possibly related to cardiac dysfunction and aggravated by fluid loss; reactions of resistance and capacitance vessels said to be normal
  B. Diabetic acidosis
  C. Pheochromocytoma (distinctly uncommon)

*Note: Cardiac failure as such is *not* a cause of orthostatic hypotension; in fact, patients in congestive failure tolerate head-up tilt very well, possibly because of their hypervolemia.

aging, prolonged recumbency, physical exhaustion, or starvation. The commonest cause of orthostatic hypotension, however, is inhibition of sympathetic reflexes by drugs that interfere with ganglionic transmission or with norepinephrine liberation at the nerve endings or that block alpha-adrenergic receptors (see Table 7–5). The effects of bed rest on sympathetic activity are particularly important to note, since even short periods of inactivity may aggravate orthostatic hypotension due to other causes. By the same token, repeated head-up tilting may reduce the postural fall in pressure produced by some neurologic lesions.

Clinical differentiation of various types is not always easy. When present, signs of associated disease or history of drug intake give helpful clues, but determination of the mechanism involved and localization of the lesion require a stepwise, reasoned approach. Causes listed as Group I are usually readily differentiated from those in Group II-B by the intensity of sympathetic activity in the first group and its relative absence in the second (Table 7–5). Clinical signs of increased sympathetic drive include pallor, sweating, and tachycardia; hemodynamic studies may document the simultaneous increase in peripheral resistance, diminution in forearm blood flow, and venoconstriction. The absence of these signs despite the fall in arterial pressure characterizes neurogenic hypotension (Table 7–5). However, although the absence of tachycardia during hypotension indicates an inadequate neural response, its presence does not necessarily exclude a neurogenic lesion. Thus, heart rate may increase in early idiopathic hypotension before cardiac nerves are involved or in hypotension due to lumbar sympathectomy. The same remarks apply to pallor and sweating. Failure of peripheral resistance to increase is particularly significant. The picture in vasodepressor syncope is quite different; here the pulse actually slows and peripheral resistance suddenly falls as the patient faints (Fig. 7–13).

LOCALIZATION OF DEFECT IN THE BARORECEPTOR ARC (GROUP II-B). Lesions in the efferent limb will be characterized by loss of pressure responses to all reflex pressor maneuvers, whatever the origin of the reflex—baroreceptor as in the Valsalva maneuver, pain as in cold pressor test, or psychologic as in stressful mental arithmetic. These stimuli will not raise blood pressure as they normally should, because the final common neural pathway is not functioning. However, arteriolar responsiveness to norepinephrine infusion will be intact or indeed exaggerated (denervation hypersensitivity) in contrast with the impaired responsiveness found in purely arteriolar lesions. Similarly, loss of reflex sweating (warming contralateral limb) despite the presence of responsive sweat glands suggests an efferent or

central sympathetic defect. In many but not all cases of efferent limb dysfunction, the cardiac nerves (sympathetic and parasympathetic) are involved; if the heart is functionally denervated, its rate will be higher than expected and fixed, unresponsive to atropine injections, carotid sinus stimulation, or increase in arterial pressure by phenylephrine. If neural involvement is not far advanced (early idiopathic postural hypotension) or is localized (as following lumbar sympathectomy), demonstration of reflex cardiac slowing will indicate that afferent nerves, medullary centers, and parasympathetic efferent nerves are intact.

Pathophysiologic localization of central lesions is more difficult; reflex pressor responses are also interfered with. Some help may be derived from the presence of other neural signs (rigidity, parkinsonism, nystagmus, alterations of deep reflexes, and so on) but especially from demonstration of intact peripheral sympathetic innervation. This is most readily achieved by showing increased toe or finger blood flow with local anesthesia of the corresponding nerves. Lesions of afferent baroreceptor nerves may be suspected when orthostatic reflexes are absent (hypotension and unchanged heart rate during head-up tilt), in contrast with normal pressor responses to cold stimulus and mental arithmetic, normal peripheral blood flow response to nerve blockade, and intact vagal supply to the heart (increased rate following atropine injection). The loss of baroreceptor sensitivity may be demonstrated by absence of reflex bradycardia when blood pressure is raised and lack of pressor response to maneuvers lowering arterial pressure.

Idiopathic Orthostatic Hypotension

This syndrome affects men more frequently than women; it is a slowly progressive condition marked by obvious neural autonomic involvement (postural hypotension, loss of sweating, fixed heart rate), subtle neurologic signs (pupillary abnormalities, generalized hyperreflexia, disturbed bladder regulation), and usually intact sensation and mental faculties. Association with parkinsonism is particularly frequent and may be very disabling. In many instances, the disease may represent variants of the syndrome described by Shy and Drager but not all forms are necessarily related to the same pathologic alterations. Some may be due to involvement of sympathetic nerves and others to degeneration of preganglionic spinal neurons. The initial description of the syndrome by Bradbury and Eggleston stressed the triad of postural hypotension gradually increasing in severity, anhidrosis slowly spreading to involve most of the body surface, and impotence. Plasma and urinary catecholamines are usually decreased. Responses of the renin-angiotensin-aldosterone system were impaired in some patients and reported as normal in others. In our experience, abnormalities in PRA were not helpful in localization of the lesion. Plasma volume is often contracted, and because of reduced sympathetic support cardiac performance becomes overly dependent on changes in pre-load.

Cerebrovascular Disease and Hypotension

A sudden fall in systemic blood pressure can cause focal neurologic impairment, especially in patients with atherosclerotic narrowing or occlusion of intracranial vessels or of the carotid or vertebral arteries. On the other hand, cerebrovascular disease may itself cause hypotension and fainting, so that determination of which event came first may be very difficult. The question is particularly relevant in antihypertensive therapy; it is our opinion that hypotension has been grossly overrated as a cause of strokes. Though hypotensive episodes were very frequent in the heroic days of ganglion blocking therapy, the incidence of permanent neurologic damage was not particularly increased. This impression is supported by the rarity of cerebral infarction in pa-

tients with idiopathic orthostatic hypotension, many of whom are elderly and subject to frequent hypotensive spells.

Postural hypotension is more common in patients with cerebrovascular disease than in normal controls. Central interference with the baroreceptor reflex may be one cause; pressor response to the Valsalva maneuver is often blunted and may be completely absent in elderly patients with cerebral atherosclerosis. Patients may easily faint while coughing or when straining at stool or during micturition, possibly because of reflex failure of vasoconstriction in the face of diminished venous return rather than because of laryngeal or vesical reflexes. However, anatomic interference with baroreceptor arc may not be the only factor; a study of such patients showed barely adequate reflexes so that systemic blood pressure could be adequately maintained unless an additional factor such as a sedative drug or prolonged rest was added. Recumbency even for relatively short periods such as a night's rest reduces sympathetic activity; hypotension is therefore aggravated in the early morning hours. Prolonged recumbency adds the additional stress of blood volume contraction.

REFERENCES

Folkow, B., and Neil, E.: Circulation. New York, Oxford University Press, 1971.

Genest, J., Koiw, E., and Kuchel, O. (eds.): Hypertension: Physiopathology and Treatment. New York, McGraw-Hill Book Co., 1977.

Mancia, G., Lorenz, R. R., and Shepherd, J. T.: Reflex Control of Circulation by Heart and Lungs. In Guyton, A. C., and Cow-

ley, A. W. (eds.): Cardiovascular Physiology II, Volume 9. Baltimore, University Park Press, 1976, pp. 111–144.

Page, I. H., and McCubbin, J. W.: The physiology of arterial hypertension. In Hamilton, W. F., and Dow, P. (eds.): Handbook of Physiology, Vol. III. Circulation. Washington, D.C., American Physiological Society, 1965, pp. 2163–2208.

8

Mechanisms of Cardiac Contraction: Structural, Biochemical, and Functional Relations in the Normal and Diseased Heart

DEAN T. MASON,
JOAN WIKMAN-COFFELT,
EZRA A. AMSTERDAM,
AND ANTHONY N. DEMARIA

The clinician has appreciated for many years that major improvements in the understanding and management of heart disease attend advances in knowledge of the fundamental mechanisms making up and governing contraction of cardiac muscle in normal and pathologic states. Although a complete detailed elucidation of the contractile process is not yet available and controversy remains concerning certain of its aspects, intensive investigation in the past decade has provided a considerable body of new information which has permitted formulation of the events involved in myocardial contraction in health and disease. These advances have been stimulated by contributions from members of several disciplines, including the clinical investigator, physiologist, pharmacologist, biochemist, and anatomist, through the development of a multiplicity of improved techniques and their application to experimental biologic systems and to patients.

The purpose here is to present the status of this field and the progress that has recently taken place, particularly at the level of the myocardial cell, in enhancing the clinical understanding of the mechanisms and regulation of contraction of the normal and diseased heart. The discussion that follows is intended to provide an over-all integrated conceptual view of the various principal characteristics of the myocardium relating to the complex phenomenon of cardiac contraction. Attention is focused on the subcellular organizational structure of heart muscle and the biochemical processes which control the energy system within the myocardium. Proceeding from this anatomic and metabolic background, the mechanism linking electrical excitation of heart muscle with activation of its contractile machinery is considered, and the molecular biochemical basis of the contractile process itself is analyzed. Finally, the function of the normal and failing heart is assessed in terms of its muscle mechanical properties. Emphasis will be placed on the clinical meaning of the events constituting cardiac contraction in order to translate important, newly perceived basic concepts into improved principles and practical information applicable to evaluation and care of the patient with cardiovascular disease.

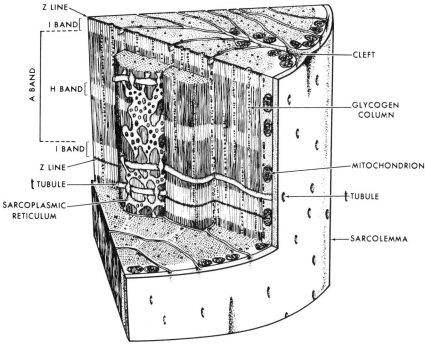

Z LINE
I BAND
A BAND
H BAND
I BAND
Z LINE
t TUBULE
SARCOPLASMIC RETICULUM

CLEFT
GLYCOGEN COLUMN
MITOCHONDRION
t TUBULE
SARCOLEMMA

Figure 8–1 Three-dimensional cross-sectional view of a single myocardial cell or fiber. (Reproduced with permission from Wikman-Coffelt, J., et al.: *In* Mason, D. T. (Ed.): Congestive Heart Failure, Yorke Medical Books, New York, 1976.)

MYOCARDIAL ULTRASTRUCTURE

Sophisticated delineation of the microanatomic features of heart muscle has now become possible with the recent development and utilization of modern methods in the examination of cardiac morphology. These studies have shown clearly that there is a definite relationship between the fine spatial architecture of heart muscle (Fig. 8–1) and the contractile mechanism of the functioning ventricle. Thus, a subcellular structural basis has been established for myocardial mechanical activity and cardiac pump performance in which the fundamental individual contractile component is recognized to be the *sarcomere*.

Myocardial Cell and Myofibrils

The gross musculature of the ventricles is traditionally described as being encircled by superficial, middle and deep muscle bundles which arise and insert at the fibrous skeleton of the valve annuli. In the past, the separate nature of these three layers was emphasized, whereas the view currently proposed by Grant holds that the spiral bundles may represent more of a transitional continuum with outer and inner fibers at right angles to those in the midwall. Under the light microscope, the muscle bundles are composed of individual branching striated muscle cells or fibers, approximately 50μ long and 15μ wide, oriented in the same direction within a given bundle (Fig. 8–2). In turn, the muscle fiber contains multiple parallel rows of longitudinal *myofibrils* which traverse the entire length of the cell. Each myofibril consists of several of the basic contractile units, sarcomeres, which are joined serially, end to end, in a single line (Fig. 8–2, *B*).

Sarcomere and Myofilaments

Further delineation of myocardial morphology or ultrastructure requires the resolution and magnification powers of the electron microscope (Fig. 8–3). The sarcomeres themselves are composed of specific arrangements of two sets of overlapping *myofilaments* of contractile proteins: *thick filaments* of myosin molecules and *thin filaments* of actin molecules (Fig. 8–2, *C*). It is the biochemical and biophysical interactions that occur at precise sites between these strands of actin and myosin aggregates that ultimately produce contraction with generation of force and shortening of heart muscle. Within an individual myocardial cell, the sarcomere bodies of neighboring myofibrils lie next to each other with their ends adjacent, so that the banded organization of contractile proteins inside the sarcomere imparts a cross-striated appearance to the muscle fiber.

A. MUSCLE CELL (FIBER)

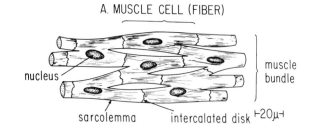

B. MYOFIBRIL

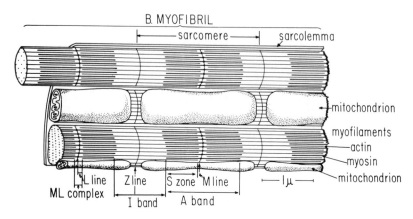

C. SARCOMERE at L_{max}

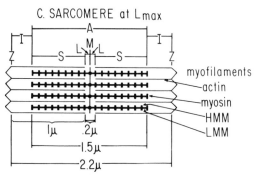

Figure 8–2 *A,* Myocardial structure viewed under light microscope showing synctium of cells or fibers. Since the interculated disks (derivatives of the cell's superficial sarcolemma-transtubular membrane system) represent true cell-to-cell junctions, the myocardium comprises a functional but not a true anatomic syncytium. *B,* Ultrastructure of longitudinal section of an individual fiber schematized from electron microscope demonstrating parallel myofibrils composed of serially connected sarcomeres in register with sarcomeres of adjacent fibrils. Horizontal rows of mitochondria are situated throughout the cell. *C,* Diagrammatic representation of a sarcomere at L_{max} (resting length at which active tension becomes maximal) showing overlapping arrangement of thick (myosin) and thin (actin) myofilaments. *S* = S zone (area of actin-myosin overlap); *HMM* = heavy meromyosin; *LMM* = light meromysin.

The relative densities of the cross bands identify the location of the contractile proteins within the sarcomere (Figs. 8–2, *C* and 8–3). The myosin filaments are indicated by the broad dark *A band* of constant length (1.5 μ in the center portion of the sarcomere); the stationary myosin units are held to each other by linkages at the midpoint of their filaments, shown by the dark M line. Sur-

rounding the myosin units are the sliding actin filaments of constant length (1.0 μ) attached at either end of the sarcomere at the dark Z line, which also connects adjacent sarcomeres at this point. The Z bands and intercalated disks have an important generative function in the production of new sarcomeres (Legato, 1970). From the light *I band* of variable dimension, the actin fila-

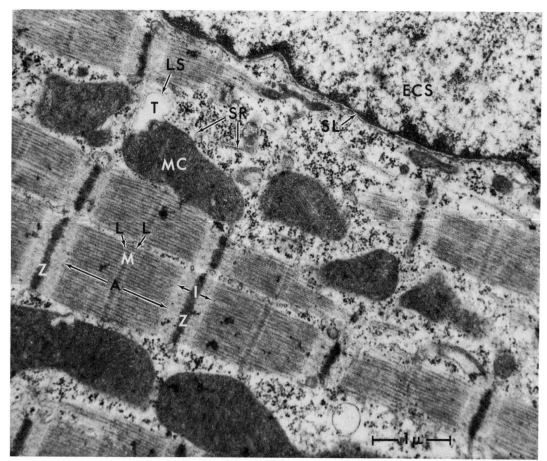

Figure 8–3 Electron micrograph of longitudinal section of canine right ventricle showing characteristic bands *(A and I)* and lines *(Z, M, and L)* of sarcomere substructure. Individual sarcomeres are delineated by dark Z lines. *MC* = mitochondrion; *SL* = sarcolemma; *T* = sarcotubule; *LS* = lateral sac of sarcoplasmic reticulum *(SR); ECS* = extracellular space.

ments run centrally to be largely covered by the fixed myosin framework. Under physiologic conditions, over-all sarcomere length (Z to Z distance) varies during the cardiac cycle between 1.5 and 2.2 μ, depending on the degree of end-diastolic fiber stretch and the extent of shortening during contraction. Immediately lateral on both sides of the M line is a thin light L line; this central area is the ML complex or pseudo-H zone. In acutely overstretched skeletal muscle and to a lesser degree in myocardium, a pathologic wide H zone appears, indicating partial disengagement of the thick and thin filaments. In contrast, slippage and malalignment of myofibrils appear to be the principal morphologic alterations in chronic excessive dilation of the ventricle (Spotzitz and Sonnenblick, 1976). Alterations in molecular composition and physical structure of the contractile proteins and myofilaments themselves are not found in heart failure.

Contractile Proteins: Thin Filaments

Concerning the two primary contractile proteins of the sarcomere, the *actin* and *myosin* chains possess distinct structural and functional properties (Wikman-Coffelt, et al., 1976) (Fig. 8–4). The thin filament is principally constituted by two helical chains of globular actin molecules (Figs. 8–4, 8–5). As observed in cross section of the sarcomere, each thin filament is surrounded by three thick filaments and each thick filament is encompassed by six thin filaments (Fig. 8–4, *B*). Although actin enhances the enzymatic action of myosin ATPase to more active actomyosin ATPase, there is no enzymatic participation of actin itself in the contractile mechanism. Instead, the physiologic role of actin is its ability to combine reversibly at specific binding sites on the thin filament with the myosin cross bridges, one myosin head attaching to each active actin site.

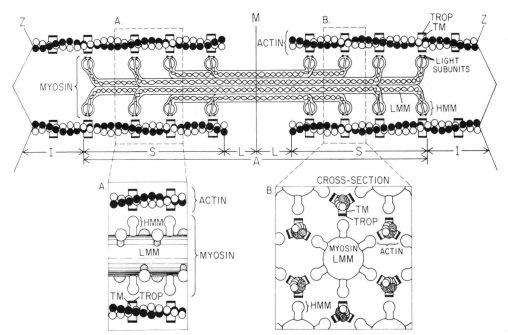

Figure 8–4 Diagrammatic representation of the contractile proteins of heart muscle during relaxation, indicating the relative longitudinal configurations and positions of actin and myosin filaments and modulatory proteins, tropomyosin (*TM*) and troponin (*TROP*), as viewed by electron microscopy. Each thick filament is composed of horizontal aggregations of myosin molecules with long shafts (light meromyosin; *LMM*) and cross-bridge heads (heavy meromyosin: *HMM*) containing light subunits regulating myosin ATPase activity which interact with myosin-binding sites on actin of the thin filament during contraction. Inserts *A* (horizontal view) and *B* (cross section) indicate three-dimensional orientation of actin-myosin relationships within the S zone, demonstrating hexagonal lattice of six thin filaments arranged around each thick filament, and each thin filament surrounded by three thick filaments.

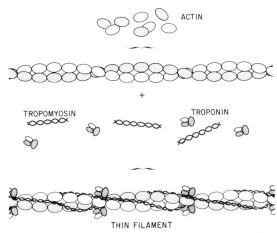

Figure 8–5 Representation of the components of a thin filament. *A*, Depolymerized globular actin; *B*, polymerized fibrous actin, tropomysin, and troponin; *C*, the reconstituted thin filament composed of fibrous actin with tropomyosin alongside the actin grooves and troponin at each turn of the double helix of actin.

Thus, according to the sliding filament theory of contraction offered by Huxley, formation of cross bridges between active sites of actin and myosin causes inward movement of the thin filament centrally along the fixed thick filament framework. In this contractile process, the lengths of the two filaments remain unchanged while the sarcomere shortens.

In addition to the two primary contractile proteins, actin and myosin, two regulatory proteins, *tropomyosin* and *troponin,* are located along the thin actin filament (Fig. 8–4). Tropomyosin and troponin are not contractile proteins as such but rather they serve a modulatory role in the contractile mechanism of inhibiting the actin-myosin interaction. Tropomyosin molecules lie in elongated chains longitudinally along the paired actin strands of the thin filament. Troponin is attached at regular intervals to tropomyosin, coinciding with the grooves of the actin double-helix. During relaxation of cardiac muscle, troponin in consort with tropomyosin prevents cross

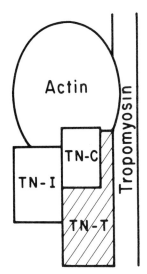

Figure 8–6 Representation of the three subunits of troponin (TN) showing their relation to the other proteins of the thin filament. (Reproduced with permission from Wikman-Coffelt, et al., *In* Mason, D. T. (Ed.): Congestive Heart Failure, Yorke Medical Books, New York, 1976.)

ing myosin with the result that no interaction takes place; a single tropomyosin molecule traverses seven actin molecules thereby masking the actin sites for interaction with myosin. *Troponin I,* like tropomyosin, has the ability to regulate the interaction between actin and myosin. *Troponin T* serves to bind the troponin complex to tropomyosin. *Troponin C* binds available Ca^{++} for initiation of contraction and deactivates the inhibitory action of troponin I. Thus troponin C-Ca^{++} becomes a derepressor, exerting a conformational change which forces tropomyosin into the helical groove of actin, thereby exposing the actin sites for interaction with myosin. Recent evidence indicates that phosphorylation of troponin I plays an important role in the contraction process, since this subunit is phosphorylated by myocardial *cyclic AMP-dependent protein kinase.*

bridge reaction between actin and myosin. As demonstrated by Ebashi, troponin contains the receptor protein for the specific binding of calcium in the contractile system. Although calcium is considered in the broad sense as the activator of mechanical contraction, this action actually functions as the specific inactivator of the troponin-tropomyosin complex's inhibition of actin-myosin linkage formation. Two further protein subcomponents complete the troponin structure (Fig. 8–6): a tropomyosin-binding protein and an actin-myosin interaction inhibitor.

For further clarification, the assembly of proteins (actin, tropomyosin and troponin) which comprise the thin filament is depicted in Figure 8–5. During polymerization, depolymerized globular actin (Fig. 8–5, *A*) is converted to the fibrous form, resulting in a double helix with seven actin molecules to a turn (Fig. 8–5, *B*). Conversion of depolymerized actin to polymerized actin occurs with the addition of ATP and calcium. As also shown in Figure 8–5, *B*, tropomyosin is a long linear molecule composed of two subunits with a double helical conformation. The reconstituted polymerized thin filament is represented in Figure 8–5, *C*. Troponin is a globular molecule, affixed near the end of each tropomyosin molecule, consisting of three subunits termed troponin I, C, and T (Fig. 8–6). As indicated, the reaction between actin and myosin is controlled by troponin and tropomyosin. During contraction, actin is *turned on* and reacts with myosin. In contrast, during relaxation actin is *turned off,* thus repuls-

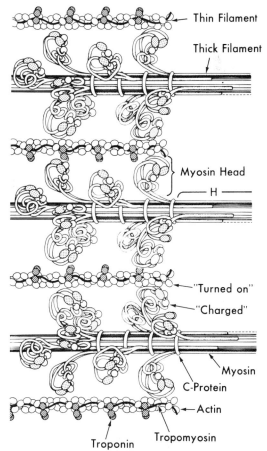

Figure 8–7 Diagrammatic representation of alternating myofilaments in longitudinal view in a portion of a lateral section of thick filaments. H = midzone ML band of the thick filaments. (Reproduced with permission from Wikman-Coffelt, et al.: *In* Mason, D. T. (Ed.): Congestive Heart Failure, Yorke Medical Books, New York, 1976.)

Contractile Proteins: Thick Filaments

The thick filament is composed of staggered parallel clusters of a few hundred myosin molecules (Fig. 8–4), each characterized by an elongated rodlike core of interwoven paired helical coils *(light meromyosin)* with globular lateral endings

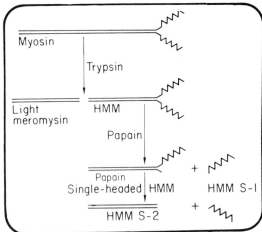

Figure 8–9 Separation of the components of whole myosin by cleavage with proteolytic enzymes. Trypsin produces the two major fragments: light meromyosin and heavy meromyosin (HMM). Papain digestion results in division of heavy meromyosin into its S_2 and S_1 fragments. (Reproduced with permission from Wikman-Coffelt, J., et al.: *In* Mason, D. T. (Ed.): Congestive Heart Failure, Yorke Medical Books, New York, 1976.)

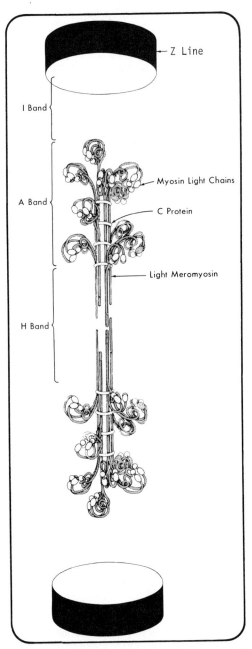

Figure 8–8 Three-dimensional view of a single thick filament containing several pairs of myosin molecules. (Reproduced with permission from Wikman-Coffelt, J., et al.: *In* Mason, D. T. (Ed.): Congestive Heart Failure, Yorke Medical Books, New York, 1976.)

or heads *(heavy meromyosin)*. The globular projection contains the principal functional component of myosin: the cross bridge of the thick filament which interacts with actin of the thin filament to produce contraction (Fig. 8–4). Further, each globular cross-bridge is paired with light myosin subunits at their termination. These light subunits *(light chains)* of heavy meromyosin are thought to influence the level of enzyme activity of *myosin adenosine triphosphatase* (ATPase) in the remaining portion of the heavy meromyosin *(heavy chains)*, as well as to influence the intensity of the actin-myosin linkage itself. Myosin ATPase splits the terminal phosphate bond off ATP and thereby liberates the energy for the contractile process.

The ultrastructure of interdigitating thick and thin filaments is illustrated in Figure 8–7 as they appear in longitudinal section. Three thick and four thin filaments are shown, tropomyosin is in the groove of the double helix of actin molecules, and troponin is located at every seventh actin molecule. The thick filaments are composed of bundles of myosin molecules, each consisting of a central strand with lateral terminating heads that spiral outward from the core of the cylinder. These myosin molecules are grouped sequentially so that the myosin heads spiral along both A band sections of the filament. Only the small midzone (ML complex or H zone) of the filament is without myosin heads. With actin turned on during contraction (Fig. 8–7), the myosin heads establish cross-bridge contact with actin, and enzymatic activity in the myosin heads takes place. Figure 8–8 provides a three-dimensional view of

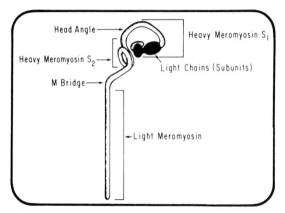

Figure 8–10 Representation of the configuration of one of the two heavy chains of whole myosin. The myosin heavy chain is comprised of light meromyosin and heavy meromyosin (HMM). The M bridge is between light and heavy meromyosin, and the head angle between heavy meromyosins S_1 and S_2. In addition, two myosin light chains are bound within the heavy chain myosin head (HMM S_1). (Reproduced with permission from Wikman-Coffelt, J., et al.: *In* Mason, D. T. (Ed.): Congestive Heart Failure, Yorke Medical Books, New York, 1976.)

a single thick filament with several pairs of myosin aggregates.

The manner by which the nature and nomenclature of the myosin fragments of the whole myosin oligomere have been established is represented in Figure 8–9. The proteolytic enzyme, trypsin, hydrolyzes whole myosin at the *hinge region* (M bridge) to produce two fragment pairs, light meromyosin and heavy meromyosin. Heavy meromyosin is separated by papain digestion into its two components: *heavy meromyosin S_1 and S_2* (Fig. 8–9). Figure 8–10 delineates the configuration of one (220,000 molecular weight) of the two heavy chains comprising whole myosin. The *myosin head* (heavy meromyosin S_1) contains two light chains wrapped within this segment; and it is specifically this heavy chain S_1 component in which the ATPase activity of myosin is contained and the site of myosin which forms the cross-bridge with actin. Heavy chain S_2 meromyosin forms a tight helix, whereas meromyosin S_1 is elliptically shaped (Fig. 8–10). Light meromyosin constitutes the backbone of the thick filaments. Movement of the heavy meromyosin S_1 head, by changing the degree of its *head angle* (Fig. 8–10), results in pushing the thin filaments together during contraction.

Superficial Membrane System

In addition to the sarcomere contractile apparatus which occupies approximately one half the myocardial fiber, there are other important specialized subcellular constituents. The individual myocardial fibers are covered by the *sarcolemma* membrane, of which the *intercalated disks* and *transverse tubular system* are derivatives of major significance (Figs. 8–1, 8–3, 8–11). The intercalated disks are situated at intercellular junctions between the terminal sarcomeres of the cell, thereby locking fibers together at their ends. In the ventricular myocardium, deep invaginations at frequent intervals of the sarcolemma from the fiber surface vertically into the interior of each cell constitute the complex transtubular network or T system. The intercalated disks and transverse tubular membranes provide pathways for rapid transmission of the depolarizing impulses which electrically excite adjacent fibers and the intracellular membrane–sarcomere contractile system. In addition to contributing a vehicle for excitation, the transtubular system provides a comprehensive extension of the extracellular

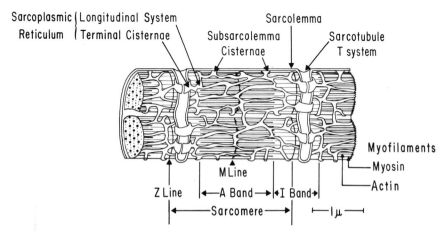

Figure 8–11 Longitudinal diagram of myocardial ultrastructure reconstructed from electron micrographs showing relationships between the superficial (sarcolemma and wide T system) and intracellular (sarcoplasmic reticulum) membranes of the cardiac fiber.

space throughout the cell so that transmembrane cation transport of sodium, potassium, and calcium accompanying depolarization, repolarization, excitation-contraction coupling, and relaxation occurs quickly and synchronously within myocardial fibers. Furthermore, the T system furnishes a conduit for ready entry and egress of metabolites and other substances between the interstitial medium and the sarcoplasm, and access is afforded to cardiovascular drugs, such as digitalis and antiarrhythmic agents, for their action on intracellular membranes and related enzyme systems in the vicinity of the contractile apparatus within the entire fiber, even if the drugs do not actually cross the membrane in clinically meaningful doses.

Sarcoplasmic Reticulum

An extensive intracellular tubular membrane system, the *sarcoplasmic reticulum* (Figs. 8–1, 8–3, 8–11), complements the transtubular T system structurally and functionally in support of the process of excitation-contraction coupling and mechanical relaxation. The T-tubular system is in contact with the extracellular environment and runs a vertical pathway through the width of the sarcomere I bands. The sarcoplasmic reticulum is entirely within the cell and its general orientation is at right angles to the T system, so that the sarcotubular structure courses longitudinally in the A band region (actin-myosin crossbridge area) along the rows of sarcomeres with multiple branching interconnections. *Lateral sac cuff modifications (terminal cisternae)* of the narrow sarcoplasmic reticulum (longitudinal L system) occur at its point of contact with the wider T system in the lateral I band on one side of the Z line. The sarcotubular lateral sacs store calcium; the intracellular transport of calcium from this area is important in linking membrane excitation with troponin of the contractile apparatus. Also, lateral sacs abut the intercalated disks and sarcolemma to provide each of the specialized membranes with a complete system for excitation-contraction coupling. An interesting exception is the Purkinje cell, which has no transverse tubular system (Legato, 1970). Perhaps dissimilarities in the electrical and contractile responses of different types of cardiac cells to pharmacologic agents are, in part, the result of variations in the extent and nature of development of the transtubular network and inherent modifications in the characteristics of the superficial membranes.

Mitochondria

The final myocardial substructure to be considered is the *mitochondrion,* which contains the aerobic biochemical systems of the fiber (Figs. 8–1, 8–3, 8–11). The mitochondria, located between the myofibrils, are abundant in accordance with the heart's high requirements for oxygen, and they constitute nearly 30 per cent of the myocardial cell. The mitochondria, situated near the A bands and thus myosin ATPase, are the metabolic power plants in which oxygen and appropriate substrates are utilized to produce ATP, the final direct energy source for myocardial contraction and other biochemical reactions. In the cytoplasm or sarcoplasm, glycogen granules are stored and the process of anaerobic glycolysis is operative. Morphologically, the mitochondrion is surrounded by a membrane from which there are numerous cristae infoldings on which the process of oxidative phosphorylation takes place. In addition, the mitochondrial membranes are capable of accumulating calcium, which might serve as an internal buffer against abnormal rises of sarcoplasmic calcium during diastole and perhaps might represent a mechanism influencing myocardial compliance or a source of activator calcium.

MYOCARDIAL METABOLISM

The principal biochemical processes which relate to the ultimate contractile function of the ventricle include those involved in regulation of energy metabolism, contractile machinery of the sarcomere, the muscle relaxing system, electrical and transport activity of the membranes, and protein synthesis within the fiber. It is emphasized that these chemical mechanisms are interrelated, and alterations in any one of them may influence activity in the other pathways. For conceptual purposes, the sequence of reactions important in myocardial energy metabolism is substrate availability and energy production, storage, and utilization.

Energetics

Normal heart muscle is uniquely dependent on *aerobic* metabolism for its energy supply. To satisfy this obligatory need, the myocardium requires the delivery of a continuous supply of large quantities of oxygen via the coronary circulation. The oxygen demand of the heart is considerably greater than for other organs and, since myocardial oxygen extraction is nearly maximal at body rest, increases in oxygen need are primarily accomplished by elevations of coronary blood flow. *Myocardial oxygen consumption* of the ventricle is principally determined by three hemodynamic-related variables: (1) intramyocardial systolic tension (primarily governed by systolic pressure and ventricular volume); (2) contractility; and (3) heart rate (Fig. 8–12). In addition to these three major determinants, external work or ventricular

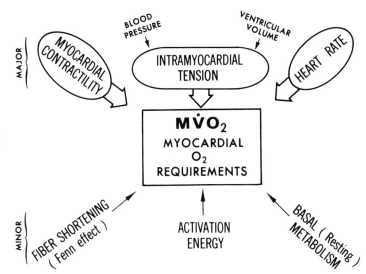

Figure 8–12 Major and minor determinants of myocardial oxygen consumption (MV̄O₂).

shortening *(Fenn effect),* energy of activation-relaxation, and basal diastolic energy requirements contribute to a relatively minor degree to over-all myocardial oxygen requirements (Fig. 8–12). In considering the effects of an intervention on myocardial oxygen consumption, such as with the administration of digitalis or nitroglycerin, it is important to appreciate that the final result quantitatively is dependent on the entire hemodynamic functional status of the heart, an interplay among the more important factors regulating oxygen utilization, and the summation of their individual actions.

Oxidative Phosphorylation. Since ATP is the immediate energy source for the contractile apparatus and biochemical reactions elsewhere in the cell, myocardial energy metabolism is normally directed toward aerobic production of ATP in the mitochondria by substrate oxidation (dehydrogenation of citric acid intermediates requiring nicotinamide adenine dinucleotide), with discharge of carbon dioxide in the *Krebs cycle,* consequent transport of hydrogen and its electrons through the respiratory chain of flavoproteins and cytochromes (resulting in oxygen consumption and making of water), and *oxidative phosphorylation* in which inorganic phosphate acquires a high-energy bond and combines with adenosine diphosphate (ADP) to form ATP (Fig. 8–13). Schwartz has shown depressed mitochondrial energy production in the severely failing myocardium, whereas respiratory function in the mitochondria is increased in the hypertrophied heart prior to failure. Although abnormalities in mitochondrial energy metabolism may contribute to myocardial dysfunction in heart failure, these biochemical aberrations generally are not considered causative of failure due to chronic hemodynamic overload.

The predominant substrate fuel for myocardial ATP synthesis consists of the circulating *free fatty acids,* consumption of which accounts for the majority of oxygen extracted by the heart. Concerning other primary substrates, normally *blood glucose* is used preferentially in the postprandial state. Circulating lactate is also an important fuel, particularly when its blood concentration is evaluated by prolonged skeletal muscle exercise. Blood pyruvate, like glucose, lactate, and free fatty acids, is readily taken up by the myocardium in proportion to its arterial blood concentration. Blood-borne ketone bodies and even amino acids may serve as substrates in certain abnormal conditions. Conversion of the substrate fuels into acetyl-coenzyme A is necessary for their entry into the citric acid cycle for aerobic ATP production. Concerning blood glucose as substrate in myocardial energy systems, after the substance is transported across the sarcolemma-transtubular membranes and metabolized to glucose-6-phosphate under the influence of insulin, it may be stored as glycogen or undergo anaerobic glycolysis to pyruvate in the sarcoplasm. In normal conditions, pyruvate is oxidized to acetyl-coenzyme A and undergoes aerobic metabolism in the citric acid cycle within the mitochondria. In the absence of hypoxia, the heart does not produce lactate.

Anaerobic Glycolysis. The importance of *anaerobic glycolysis* as a source of energy varies with the state of oxygenation of the myocardium. Normally, glycolysis is of considerably less significance, since this entire process results in only two ATP molecules for each molecule of glucose,

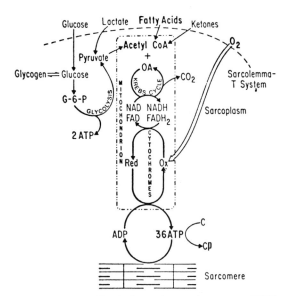

Figure 8-13 Metabolic pathways for energy (ATP) production shown diagrammatically within the cardiac cell. *NAD* = nicotinamide adenine dinucleotide; *FAD* = flavin adenine dinucleotide; *NADH* = reduced NAD; *FADH$_2$* = reduced FAD; *Ox* = oxidation; *Red* = reduction; *CP* = creatine phosphate; *C* = creatine; *G-6-P* = glucose-6-phosphate. See text for further explanation.

whereas each glucose molecule provides 36 molecules of ATP in the aerobic pathways (Fig. 8–13). When myocardial oxygen delivery falls, there is increased glycolysis, although this is an ineffective process alone for maintaining energy supply, and ATP levels decline. Also, less pyruvate enters the citric acid cycle during enhanced glycolytic metabolism in myocardial hypoxia. Consequently, in the heart relatively deprived of oxygen, pyruvate is reduced to *lactate,* and lactate is not extracted; thereby, the hypoxic myocardium may produce more lactate than it consumes, with the result that coronary sinus blood will contain more lactate than systemic arterial blood. In contrast, lactate concentration is greater in arterial blood than in the coronary venous effluent in the normally metabolizing heart owing to myocardial lactate extraction for aerobic synthesis of ATP. By selective catheterization of the coronary sinus, Gorlin has shown that detection of abnormal myocardial lactate metabolism or balance provides a useful biochemical means for the objective identification of myocardial ischemia in patients with coronary artery disease. Furthermore, when the abnormality is not present at rest in patients with angina pectoris, it can often be revealed by increasing the mechanical and metabolic activity of the heart by the performance of exercise, by increasing heart rate with a pacemaker catheter, or by administration of isoproterenol.

Creatine Phosphate. In regard to myocardial energy storage, *creatine phosphate* functions as a limited reservoir of high-energy phosphate to maintain ATP. Thus, following the cleavage of ATP by myofibrillar ATPase to ADP and inorganic phosphate in the contraction reaction and by the additional myocardial ATPases in other biochemical processes requiring energy utilization, ADP is replenished with a high-energy phosphate from creatine phosphate or by oxidative phosphorylation to re-form ATP. Creatine phosphate is resynthesized by oxidative phosphorylation. Although creatine phosphate serves as a ready source of auxiliary chemical energy for ADP, it is relatively small in quantity, even in the normal heart. In chronic heart failure, ATP levels are not depleted, although creatine phosphate is often diminished, but this reduction follows rather than precedes abnormal contractile performance.

Protein Synthesis

The mechanisms of protein synthesis in the heart are generally the same as those in other organs. Protein synthesis in the myocardium provides a continuously operative system for renewal of fiber structure and enzymatic machinery, as well as a rapidly responsive compensatory mechanism for ventricular hypertrophy induced by cardiac mechanical stress. ATP is consumed in the process of protein synthesis, which consists of the stages of: (1) *replication* in the nucleus (DNA-controlled synthesis of DNA by *DNA polymerase*); (2) *transcription* in the nucleus in which nucleoli are centers of RNA activity (RNA synthesis by *RNA polymerase* on the chromosomal template); and (3) *translation* involving three types of RNA in the sarcoplasm (formation of specific proteins on ribosomal RNA, directed by messenger RNA containing the genetic code, from amino acids carried by transfer RNA).

Excessive intramyocardial tension appears to be the transducer that couples mechanical systolic overload with increased protein synthesis. Increased muscle mass resulting from chronic elevation of hemodynamic burden is due to hypertrophy rather than hyperplasia of myocardial fibers, although there is some proliferation of connective tissue cells. Activation of all stages of protein synthesis occurs rapidly after hemodynamic stress, with increases in DNA in connective tissue cells and elevations of RNA synthesis and incorporation of amino acids into proteins in myocardial cells. For example, even the creation of acute mild pulmonic stenosis in dogs is a potent stimulus for RNA and protein synthesis within 24 hours after pulmonary banding, resulting in substantially increased weight of the hypertrophied right ventricle with correspondingly increased myosin content.

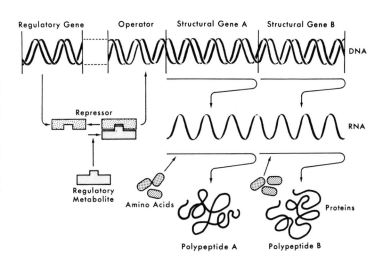

Figure 8–14 Diagram of two genes under one operator constituting a genome and the regulatory gene codes for the repressor, which in turn has the ability to repress or induce transcription of the genome, depending on the presence of certain metabolites in the system. (Reproduced with permission from Wikman-Coffelt, J., et al.: In Mason, D. T. (Ed.): Congestive Heart Failure, Yorke Medical Books, New York, 1976.)

Transcription. Transcription is the process by which genetic information, stored in nuclear DNA, is transferred to RNA. The result is the formation of nucleotide polymers containing triplet codons corresponding to those found in DNA. The regulation of the transcription system involving a repressor is depicted in Figure 8–14. In the transcription process of gene control, a regulatory gene directs the synthesis of a specific protein; the repressor binds to a metabolite or hormone and serves as the regulatory signal. This binding can either activate or inactivate the repressor, depending on whether the system is repressive or inductive. The repressor in its active state binds the genetic operator and prevents production of messenger RNA from the associated structural gene. In contrast, in an inductive system, the operator remains repressed until the regulatory metabolite complexes with and prevents function of the repressor. With this model of gene control

applied to the myosin system via the transcription process, the cell possesses the ability to respond rapidly to new environmental stress, such as excessive ventricular hemodynamic burden leading to myocardial hypertrophy. Further, the rapid elevation in RNA synthesis that occurs (for example, in the right ventricle with pulmonic stenosis) may be aided by the availability of an additional factor that acts as an inducer at the transcriptional level.

Translation. Translation is the cellular process through which information that has been transcribed to RNA is utilized to produce proteins (Fig. 8–15). Protein synthesis takes place on cellular particles called ribosomes that travel along the instruction tape of messenger RNA reading the genetic message. The process of translation is divided into three stages: (1) initiation; (2) elongation; and (3) termination. Before the sequence of translation is discussed, it is ben-

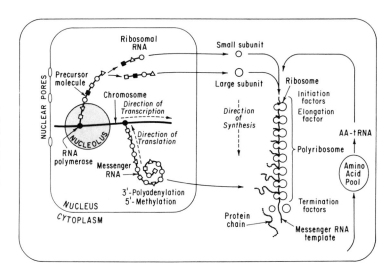

Figure 8–15 Diagram of transcription in the cytoplasm. The transcription of ribosomal RNA is restricted to the nucleolus. The two ribosomal RNA molecules (28S and 18S RNA) are derived from the larger parent precursor molecule, which separates into the two.

eficial to examine the three different types of RNA involved in the process and the respective role of each type of RNA.

Ribosomal RNA (rRNA) is one of the three major types of RNA manufactured during the process of transcription. This type of RNA is transcribed from genes located on chromosomes found in the nucleolus. Initially, a precursor RNA molecule is formed and later cleaved to form an 18S and a 28S RNA subunit. The 28S subunit combines with several types of proteins, moves out of the nucleus, and eventually forms the 60S component of the ribosomes. Likewise, the 18S subunit combines with protein, as well as with a smaller 5S RNA molecule, and thus forms the 40S component of the ribosome. The many different proteins that compose the ribosome are in equilibrium with a pool of free ribosomal proteins in the cytoplasm of the cell. Present evidence indicates that the turnover rate varies for each of these proteins.

Messenger RNA (mRNA) is the second of the three types of RNA made in the nucleus and transported to the cytoplasm for production of a protein such as myosin. The mRNA molecules for myosin heavy chains have been purified. It appears that both mRNA and its carrier protein are complexed to the smaller ribosomal subunits when they reach the cytoplasm (Fig. 8–15). When mRNA was purified from the cytoplasm of various cells, it was found to be characterized by its long stretches of polyadenylic acid, one of the four nucleotides comprising RNA. Unlike rRNA and tRNA, mRNA has little tertiary structure and is thus very susceptible to ribonuclease cleavage.

Transfer RNA (tRNA) is the third type of RNA molecule. It is the smallest of the three. Several tRNA varieties have been sequenced, and it has been found that the molecule has an over-all clover-leaf configuration with about 80 per cent of its nucleotides paired. Each amino acid has specific tRNA varieties to which it binds. Further, each amino acid also has a specific aminoacyl-tRNA synthetase enzyme that is responsible for mediating this binding reaction. Certain regions of these individual tRNA molecules contain the anticodon that can match up with the corresponding mRNA codon. This system provides the capacity for accurate recognition between amino acid and code of the mRNA to insure the proper placement of each amino acid in precise sequences in the formation of a specific polypeptide chain.

Specific Protein Synthesis. Protein synthesis is initiated by the complexing of mRNA to the 40S particle of the ribosome. This event is followed by the combination of the 40S particle with the associated mRNA to the larger 60S subunit of the ribosome. To begin translation of the mRNA tape, various soluble initiation factors are required. Certain of these factors, along with guanosine 5'-triphosphate (GTP) and the correct concentration of magnesium (Mg^{++}) and ammonium (NH_4^+) ions, provide the conditions for the binding of the first tRNA-associated amino acid to the initiating codon of the mRNA.

The complete ribosome contains two binding sites for tRNA. One site, located on the 40S ribosomal subunit, is designated the aminoacyl-tRNA binding site; the other site on the subunit is referred to as the peptidyl-tRNA binding site. Present evidence indicates that the specific tRNA associated with amino acid formylmethionine is required for the initiation of translation. It appears that the structure of this molecule enables it to move directly from the aminoacyl site to the peptidyl site on the ribosome, despite the fact it has only one amino acid bound to it. This translocation reaction allows the binding of a new tRNA and associated amino acid to the recently vacated 30S site of the ribosome. It is believed that the hydrolysis of GTP provides the energy needed in this translocation reaction. Two soluble factors, aminoacyl transferase I and II, along with sulfhydryl compounds and Mg^{++} and NH_4^+, also play a role in this translocation.

The peptide bond formation necessary to bind the two separate amino acids is catalyzed by peptidyl synthetase, located in the 60S ribosomal subunit, and does not require soluble initiation factors or GTP. By continuing the cycle of tRNA binding, peptide bond formation and translocation, it is possible to form peptides containing specific amino acid sequences governed by the code provided by the mRNA (Fig. 8–16).

Protein synthesis is concluded when the ribosome reads a terminator codon located on the mRNA. The terminator codon, in conjunction with certain releasing factors, dissociates the ribosome into its original 40S and 60S subunits and provides for the release of the protein and mRNA. Interestingly, it is possible for several ribosomes to read a single mRNA molecule simultaneously. In this situation, the group of ribosomes is referred to as a polyribosome.

Myosin Synthesis. Increase in myosin synthesis is accompanied by augmentation of myosin ATPase activity in certain situations, such as in the stressed ventricle in the presence of mild pulmonic or mild aortic stenosis. At the same time, in these specific hemodynamic situations, the proportion of myosin heavy chains to myosin light chains is increased. In other studies it has been shown that myosin heavy chains have a turnover rate that is twice that of myosin light chains. A phenomenon such as the disparate turnover rates of light and heavy chains of myosin may be the result of regulation at the level of translation or transcription.

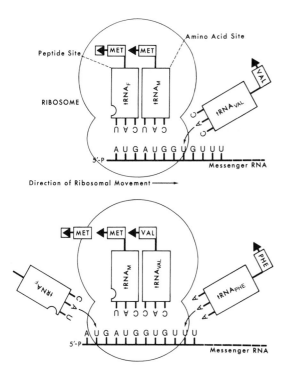

Figure 8–16 Diagram of translation occurring on the messenger RNA complexed to the ribosome. The process of translation begins at the 5′ end of the messenger RNA. The transfer RNA molecules are shuttling amino acids to the peptide site to form the growing peptide chain. (Reproduced with permission from Wikman-Coffelt, J., et al.: In Mason, D. T. (Ed.): Congestive Heart Failure, Yorke Medical Books, New York, 1976.)

It is possible that a type of regulation at the translation level described for hemoglobin occurs in myosin synthesis: a selective translation of α or β chains depending on the presence of messenger-specific translational factors. The greater turnover rate of myosin heavy chains may be due to greater affinity or availability of translational factors for the messenger for myosin heavy chains.

Conversely, the greater synthesis of myosin heavy chains in comparison with that of light chains may be due to control at the transcriptional level. As shown in Figure 8–14, each of the myosin chains may be under different genetic control, so that an activator of one gene would not necessarily be a potent activator of other genes. Gene amplification, which constitutes multiple copies of certain genome sequences, occurs in mammalian tissues. The possibility exists that there is redundance of genes for myosin chains.

Gene duplication facilitates speedy transcription when certain molecules are in great demand, such as occurs with ribosomes. This allows for several simultaneous transcriptions of the same type of molecule at one time. Thus it is speculated that there may be various degrees of gene duplication of the myosin chains (Fig. 8–14), with each of the light and heavy chains having its code in a separate genome controlled by its own operator.

As shown by Meerson, Rabinowitz and Nair, and others, activation of all stages of protein synthesis occurs rapidly following acute stress, with increased DNA in connective tissue cells and elevations of RNA and incorporation of amino acids into proteins in myocardial cells. With chronic hemodynamic overload, however, there is some diminution of these processes. It is currently considered that alterations in protein synthesis, as in energy metabolism, do not exert a causative role in heart failure but may contribute to it.

Cyclic AMP (cAMP)

Another important biochemical system in heart muscle is that involved with the intracellular regulatory substance cyclic AMP *(adenosin monophosphate)*, discovered by Sutherland. Cyclic AMP is synthesized in the sarcoplasm from ATP by stimulation of the enzyme adenylate cyclase of the plasma sarcolemma and transtubular membranes. The activity of adenylate cyclase is enhanced by beta-adrenergic receptor stimulation located also in the plasma membranes. It has been suggested that the positive inotropic action of several cardiovascular agents is mediated by activation of this process leading to increased cAMP formation: catecholamines by stimulation of the beta receptor; and glucagon, thyroid hormone, and tolbutamide by direct action on adenylate cyclase. Furthermore, the increased contractility produced by aminophylline has been attributed to the drug's ability to inhibit phosphodiesterase, an intracellular enzyme which inactivates cAMP. The mechanism through which cAMP increases myocardial glycogenolysis has been established (cyclic nucleotide stimulation of protein kinase causes phosphorylation of phosphorylase kinase from ATP which, in turn, activates the phosphorylase enzyme degrading glycogen). Concerning the significance of cAMP in the modulation of cardiac contraction, recent evidence suggests that myocardial cAMP-dependent protein kinase phosphorylates protein components in sarcoplasmic reticulum governing calcium transport and in troponin itself, thereby influencing the effects of calcium in the contractile reaction. Concerning the heart failure state, adenylate cyclase activity is not altered, but its stimulation by certain cardiovascular agents may be impaired.

Norepinephrine

Examination of the biosynthesis of *myocardial norepinephrine* is important in the consideration of mechanisms governing mechanical performance of heart muscle, since this hormone is the neurotransmitter directly linking cardiac sympathetic activity with beta receptor stimulation, resulting in elevated contractility and heart rate. The sympathetic nervous system normally exerts a major regulatory role in the augmentation of cardiovascular function in response to increased metabolic demands of the peripheral tissues, such as during physical exercise. The rich sympathetic innervation of heart muscle permits the heart to produce the majority of its own norepinephrine requirements. In the terminals of sympathetic nerves, norepinephrine is synthesized through a series of steps from tyrosine, in which *tyrosine hydroxylase* is the rate-limiting enzyme. The neurotransmitter is stored in the nerve ending in granules which protect it from enzymatic destruction by monoamine oxidase in the neuronal cytoplasm. In response to sympathetic impulses, norepinephrine is released to activate myocardial beta receptors. Importantly, in the failing heart the activity of tyrosine hydroxylase is markedly reduced, thus resulting in severe decrease of myocardial norepinephrine. The depression of norepinephrine appears to be the result of disturbed metabolic function in the neuron rather than actual loss of neural tissue. While this defect deprives the dysfunctioning ventricle of an adaptive mechanism for increasing its contractility, the depletion of myocardial norepinephrine is not responsible for the intrinsic weakness of the failing muscle. In heart failure, there is supersensitivity of myocardial beta receptors to circulating norepinephrine, and blood levels of this hormone are elevated because of its increased synthesis in the peripheral vasculature and the adrenal medulla; thereby, this supporting mechanism is restored, in part, to the failing heart.

It is apparent that a number of highly important biochemical processes are operative in the intact ventricle. Their complete integrity of function and proper integration are essential for normal mechanical and hemodynamic performance of the heart. Although aberrations have been identified in certain of these systems in the failing myocardium, the current view is that abnormalities in myocardial energy metabolism, protein synthesis, AMP reactions, and norepinephrine production may contribute by encroaching on compensatory mechanisms but do not play the primary causative role in the onset of congestive heart failure induced by chronic hemodynamic overload. A more promising probability is that the biochemical defect or constellation of abnormalities resides in the mechanism of excitation-contraction coupling and the function of the contractile proteins.

EXCITATION-CONTRACTION COUPLING AND THE CONTRACTILE PROCESS

Electrical Excitation

The electrical event constituting excitation of the myocardial fiber involves *depolarization* of the cell by rapid ingress of sodium into the sarcoplasm (*phase 0 spike* of the *action potential*) (Fig. 8–17), followed by egress extracellularly of an equal amount of potassium (repolarization of the action potential). Depolarization and repolarization do not require ATP energy. Instead, the rapid Na^+ influx constituting complete phase 0 depolarization is a passive process which appears to be governed by activated Na^+ carriers (electrostatically controlled fast membrane channels or pores). The rate of rise of the spike action potential determines *conduction velocity;* relative to the surface ECG, phase 0 depolarization in the ventricles is denoted by the QRS complex, in the atria by the P wave, and collectively by the PR interval in the sinoatrial node-atria-atrioventricular node.

Although the *repolarization* period is signified by three stages (phases 1, 2, and 3), the mechanism is accomplished most quickly during *phase 3* by rapid K^+ efflux from the fiber (Fig. 8–17). More germane to the present discussion of the subcellular events involved in cardiac contraction, gradual inward Ca^{++} current occurs via slow calcium channels during the *phase 2* action potential plateau (Fig. 8–17), resulting in Ca^{++} move-

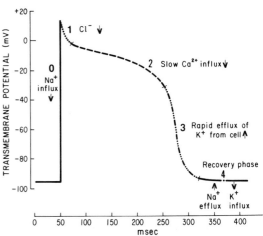

Figure 8–17 Diagram of ventricular muscle fiber action potential correlating phasic voltage changes with flux of cations in and out of the cell during the cardiac cycle.

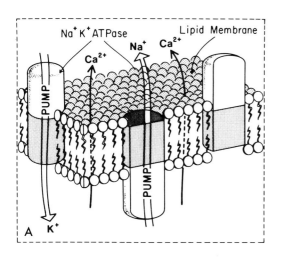

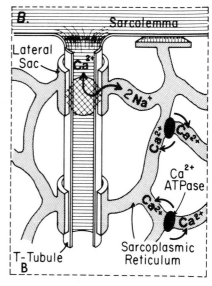

Figure 8–18 *A*, Diagram of the transtubular cell membrane comprised of phospholipids interspersed with the $Na^+ - K^+$ ATPase pump proteins operative during diastole (phase 4) establishing the increased extracellular Na^+ and increased intracellular K^+ gradients. *B*, The transtubular cell membrane proteins mediating the $Na^+ - Ca^{++}$ exchange system are shown associated with the sarcoplasmic reticulum. The T-tubules mediate such exchange between the sarcoplasmic reticulum and the extracellular space during phases 2 (Ca^{++} entrance) and 4 (Ca^{++} exit) of the electrophysiologic cycle.

ment into the cell which is important in the process of excitation-contraction coupling. Simultaneous relatively slow egress of K^+ appears to take place during phase 2. The entire repolarization period constitutes the action potential *duration* which governs the *refractory period* of heart muscle, and is represented for the ventricles on the surface ECG by the QT interval.

During diastole, following repolarization, the *phase 4* recovery portion of the electrophysiologic cycle ensues in which the depolarization entered-Na^+ leaves the cell and the repolarization egress-K^+ returns into the fiber (Fig. 8–17). These cation exchanges during mechanical relaxation require the active energy-utilizing transport mechanism of the *transtubular $Na^- $-$K^+ATPase$ pump* (Fig. 8–18, *A*). In addition, the phase 2 entered-Ca^{++} is removed from the fiber during the resting period by a sarcolemma Na^+-Ca^{++} exchange transport system (Fig. 8–18, *B*). Schwartz, Langer, and Repke have proposed the sarcolemma-transtubular membrane sodium-potassium pump ATPase enzyme as the pharmacologic receptor for *digitalis*, and the increased calcium influx responsible for the positive inotropic effect of the glycoside may result from the drug's interference with this enzyme pump. There appears to be reduction of membrane sodium-potassium ATPase activity in heart failure.

Mechanical Activation

When the stimulating impulse from the cardiac pacemaker arrives at the surface of the myocardial cell (Fig. 8–19, *A*), an orderly sequence of events is initiated in which *calcium* movement is the chief component linking electrical excitation of the fiber with *mechanical activation* of the contractile machinery in the sarcomere. Excitation of the individual cell proceeds as the depolarization wave spreads throughout the entire fiber along the sarcolemma and its interior transtubular membrane system (Fig. 8–19, *B*). When the depolarizing current in the transtubular system reaches the intimately apposed cisternae calcium depots of the sarcoplasmic reticulum, ionic calcium release is triggered from the lateral sacs into the sarcoplasm (Fig. 8–19, *C*). Together with an apparently smaller but crucial quantity of ionic calcium influx across the sarcolemma-transtubular membrane occurring during phase 2 of the transmembrane action potential, this discharged calcium immediately diffuses to the sarcomeres, where it binds to the specific troponin C calcium-receptor protein (Fig. 8–6) on the thin myofilaments in the overlap region (A band) between the thick and thin filaments (Fig. 8–7).

Mechanical activation is then achieved by the binding of activator-calcium to troponin C which

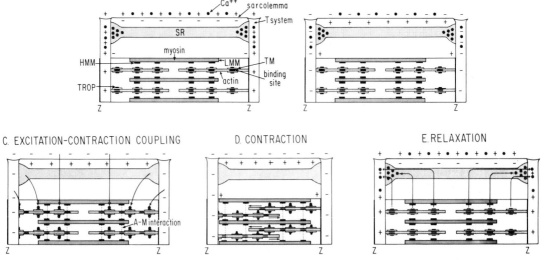

A. REST   B. EXCITATION

C. EXCITATION-CONTRACTION COUPLING   D. CONTRACTION   E. RELAXATION

Figure 8–19 Diagrammatic sequence of subcellular events underlying the phases of the cardiac cycle. *A,* At rest, extracellular calcium (solid dots) is concentrated in the interstitial medium around the sarcolemma and in the T system, and intracellular calcium (solid dots) is sequestered in the lateral sacs of the sarcoplasmic reticulum (*SR*). *B,* With electrical excitation, complete depolarization of the fiber occurs by rapid influx of sodium during Phase O of the spike action potential, resulting in positive intracellular voltage. *C,* Excitation-contraction coupling is triggered by excitation, resulting in release of intracellular calcium from the SR and entry of extracellular calcium during Phase 2 of the action potential, with delivery of calcium (arrows) to troponin of the contractile apparatus within the sarcomeres. Calcium binding to troponin derepresses troponin (*TROP*)–tropomyosin (*TM*) inhibition of myosin linkage with specific binding site on actin. Thereby, actin-myosin (*A-M*) interaction initiates contraction. *D,* The process of contraction takes place by sequential making and breaking of A-M interconnections, with consequent sliding of actin centrally (arrows) along the fixed myosin filaments, producing force development and sarcomeric shortening. *E,* Relaxation occurs with removal of calcium by SR (arrows), with calcium returned extracellularly and sequestered in SR lateral sacs. Repolarization takes place by potassium efflux with re-establishment of negative intracellular voltage which, in diastole, is maintained with sodium extrusion and potassium return by sarcolemma-T membrane pump ATPase activity.

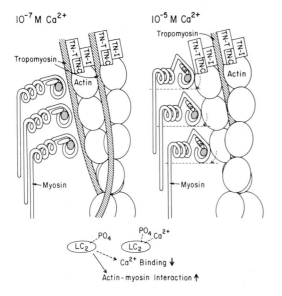

Figure 8–20 Diagram of the molecular events of the modulator and contractile proteins constituting excitation-contraction coupling. The resting state is shown in the left panel, with the troponin-tropomyosin complex blocking myosin head contact with actin. However, with greater calcium delivered to troponin C (right panel), troponin C-Ca^{++} binding overcomes troponin I-tropomyosin inhibition of actin-myosin interaction. Thus, the long tropomyosin strand is pushed deep into the groove between the paired chains of fibrous actin molecules, so that the active sites of the actin molecules become exposed to the myosin heads. Thereby, mechanical activation is initiated by the formation of actin-myosin linkages. The myosin head is brought into contact with the actin active site by tightening of the heavy meromyosin S$_2$ coil and by increasing the hinge angle between light meromyosin and heavy meromyosin S$_2$. Myosin ATPase hydrolysis of ATP causes the head angle between heavy meromyosin S$_1$ and S$_2$ to increase, leading to a swivel motion of the myosin head (curved arrows) with the actin chain propeled toward the sarcomere center (direction of the curved arrows). At the bottom of the figure, the increased intensity of the actin-myosin reaction caused by phosphorylation (PO$_4$) of the myosin light chain C$_2$ (LC$_2$) is shown (left-side LC$_2$). Such LC$_2$ phosphorylation decreases LC$_2$ Ca^{++} binding affinity; in agreement is that LC$_2$-Ca^{++} binding diminishes LC$_2$ phosphorylation (right-side LC$_2$).

overcomes the troponin I-tropomyosin complex inhibition of actin and myosin interaction, with the result that actin-myosin electrostatic cross bridges are formed. Delineation of the precise mechanism of activation involved is shown in Figure 8–20. Thus Ca^{++} binding to troponin C produces structural alteration of the troponin C protein which is transmitted through troponin I to tropomyosin, so that tropomyosin moves deeper into the groove of the double helix of actin molecules. In this manner, these configurational changes of the troponin-tropomyosin complex free the actin binding sites to link directly with the myosin heads, thereby allowing actomyosin ATPase activity to occur with initiation of the active state of the contractile process. The temporal course of the entire *excitation-contraction coupling* process takes place relatively quickly as indicated clinically by the average 0.06-second delay between the beginning of the scaler electrocardiographic QRS complex and the onset of isovolumic ventricular contraction.

Contractile Mechanism

The onset of contraction takes place with development of force and contractile element shortening by the *cyclic interaction* of *actin-myosin linkages* pulling the thin filaments along the immobile thick filaments towards the center of the sarcomeres (Fig. 8–19, *D*). It is believed that the electrostatic links are next broken as myosin binds another ATP (Fig. 8–21). Thus, a repetitive sequence of making and breaking cross linkages is established as the actin filament slides past the myosin filament during the entire course of ventricular contraction. For shortening of the sar-

comere to occur, each actin-myosin cross-bridge must perform sequentially as shown in Figure 8–22. It is thus necessary for the myosin head to attach to actin, swivel, detach and then reattach to the next actin binding site at a point further laterally on the thin filament. The result is a rowing motion of the myosin heads pulling the thin filaments together centrally and causing their overlap with decreasing distance between Z lines; thereby producing sarcomere, myofilament, muscle fiber, and ultimately ventricular shortening.

The structural features of whole myosin, relationships of myosin heavy chains within the thick filament, and the movement of a myosin heavy chain during contraction are shown in Figure 8–23. Both the light meromyosin backbone (tail region) and the proximal lateral heavy meromyosin S_2 portion form a tight helix; the terminal lateral myosin head extension, heavy meromyosin S_2, is elliptically shaped (Fig. 8–23, *A*). The thick filament is formed by myosin molecules stacked in series, joined only by the light meromyosin tail portions, with the M bridge being the hinge region of the single spaced heavy meromyosin spiralling outward (Fig. 8–23, *B*); the midportion of the thick filament is without heavy meromyosin (Fig. 8–23, *C*). With binding of ATP and cation to the myosin head in the active state, the bridge angle increases and the heavy meromyosin S_2 coil tightens to bring the myosin head in contact with actin; with ATP hydrolysis by myosin ATPase in the myosin head, the head angle (junction between meromyosins S_1 and S_2) increases so that inward swivel of the myosin head occurs, thus propeling the actin filament toward the center of the sarcomere (Fig. 8–23, *D*).

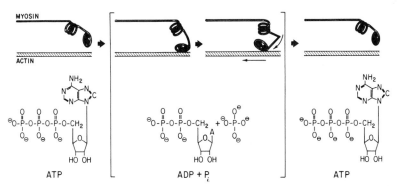

Figure 8–21 Diagram depicting the biochemical activity of myosin ATPase and the molecular alterations so produced of myosin and actin constituting the active state of the contractile process. In the top panel, a single myosin head and single actin filament are shown, with the sequence of events proceeding from left-to-right (thick arrows). In the left panel, myosin, actin, and the chemical structure of ATP are shown in the resting state. In the left-center panel, mechanical activation occurs with formation of an actin-myosin linkage. In the right-center panel, the contractile process is initiated by myosin ATPase hydrolysis of ATP to ADP and inorganic phosphate (Pi); this biochemical reaction results in increased swivel of the myosin head (curved arrow) thus pushing the actin filament in the direction (straight arrow) of the center of the sarcomere, thus causing sarcomere shortening. In the right panel, the myosin head detaches from actin and ATP is reproduced.

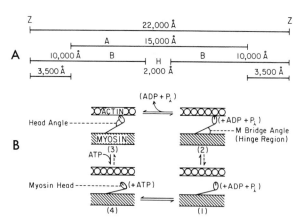

Figure 8–22   Panel *A* shows the spacing of the myofibrillar proteins within the resting sarcomere. A = thick filament; B = two thin filaments; H = central H zone; Z = two Z lines. Panel *B* shows the sequence of the process of activation of myosin. Diagrammed are the configurational changes that occur in heavy meromyosin due to the binding of ATP and cation to the myosin head with hydrolysis of ATP by myosin ATPase, resulting in subsequent sliding of the actin filaments. Frames 2 through 4 represent progressive phases of the active state and the resting state is in frame 1.

Figure 8–24, *A* is a three-dimensional model of a sarcomere in the relaxed state in which the thick filament is shown with two of the six thin filaments that surround it. On contraction, the thin filaments move centrally, thereby closing the area of the H band (Fig. 8–24, *B*). Thus, this sequence in Figures 8–24, *A* to 8–24, *B* demonstrates the systolic movement of the thin filaments, bringing the Z lines attached to the distal end of the thin filaments closer together after a sequence of ATP hydrolytic cycles takes place in the myosin heads during the active state. The Z lines are the terminal ends of the sarcomere and thus demark the zone of contact between the sarcomeres in series. From these observations, it is apparent that when the sarcomeres shorten during contraction, the whole cardiac fiber in turn shortens. The proteins that comprise the Z lines are bound tightly to the outer ends of the fibrous actin molecules.

The decrease in distance between the Z lines of a single sarcomere upon contraction results in the partial or total disappearance of the I bands, depending on the degree of shortening. Shortening may terminate when myosin is in contact with the Z lines (Fig. 8–24, *B*). However, systolic shortening may terminate before myosin reaches the Z lines, or, conversely, contraction may continue to the extreme extent of compressing the thick filaments into a wavy pattern and causing the thin filaments to slip past one another in the H band region.

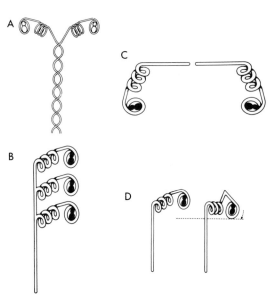

Figure 8–23   Panel *A* = whole myosin molecule showing the two different types of light chains in the myosin heads associated with the remainder of myosin: the heavy chains constituting heavy meromyosins S_1 and S_2 and light meromyosin. Panel *B* shows serial stacking of the myosin heavy chains in which the tail region (light meromyosin) of one myosin heavy chain complexes with the tail regions of the adjacent myosin heavy chains. Panel *C* represents the tail-to-tail repulsion of two myosin heavy chains at the sarcomere center H zone. The right side of panel *D* delineates the movement of the head angle of a single myosin head (arrow) to the distance indicated by the horizontal broken line and tightening of the heavy meromyosin S_2 coil during the active state; the left side of panel *D* represents the myosin chain configuration in the resting state.

Mechanical Relaxation

The phase of the excitation-contraction activating coupling process in which calcium is delivered to the contractile apparatus does not require ATP energy. The contractile reaction involving myosin ATPase utilizes the great majority of total myocardial energy which varies according to the muscle loading conditions and contractile state. Following development of the full active contractile state, the active process of relaxation ensues, with calcium departing from the sarcomere and rapidly binding to the sarcoplasmic reticulum (Fig. 8–19, *E*). The cation is then pumped back into the lateral sacs by *sarcotubular calcium pump ATPase* (relaxing factor) (Fig. 8–18, *B*), the total energy needed for relaxation being relatively small.

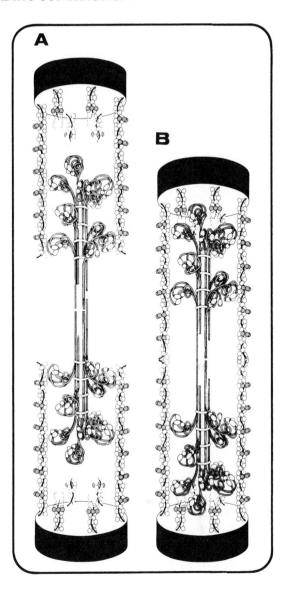

Figure 8–24 Three dimensional view of a complete thick filament surrounded at each of its ends by six thin filaments, two of which are shown in full length. The lateral limits of the sarcomere are shown by the disc-like Z lines to which the lateral ends of the thin filaments are attached. In panel A, the sarcomere is in the relaxed state with the central ends of the thin filaments extending only up to the beginning of the central H zone. In panel B (active state of complete contraction), the central ends of the actin filaments from both sides of the sarcomere are in contact, thereby entirely closing the H zone. In addition, the movement of the thin filaments towards the middle of the sarcomere during systole decreases the distance between the two Z lines; this process underlies cardiac muscle shortening during contraction (Reproduced with permission from Wikman-Coffelt, J. et al.: *In* Mason, D. T. (Ed.): Congestive Heart Failure, Yorke Medical Books, New York, 1976.)

Concerning calcium dynamics, essentially no sarcoplasmic calcium is present during diastole, and the quantity of available calcium stored intracellularly is insufficient in itself to activate subsequent systole. Myocardial cells are not able to contract in a calcium-free external medium and, unlike skeletal muscle, some extracellular calcium is indispensable for contraction. The total amount of calcium provided to the sarcoplasm from internal and external sources is normally sufficient to activate all myosin molecules of the thick filament, with contraction taking place when a critical threshold of sarcoplasmic calcium concentration is reached. The greater the rate and quantity of calcium delivered to troponin, the faster the rate and number of activated interactions between actin and myosin, with consequent more rapid rate of tension development, greater maximum tension, and increased contractility.

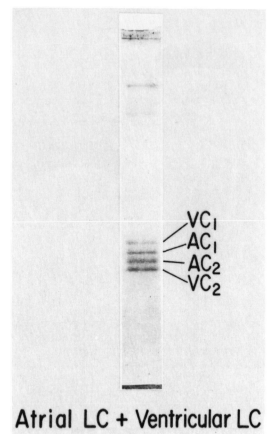

Atrial LC + Ventricular LC

Figure 8–25 One-dimensional slab gel electrophoresis of canine atrial light chains (AC), one (AC$_1$) and two (AC$_2$), and ventricular light chains (VC), one (VC$_1$) and two (VC$_2$). Four separate bands are evident, indicating the heterogeneity of these four light chains (LC).

Myosin ATPase Activity

One of the most intriguing aspects of contractile protein performance relates to the elucidation of the molecular alterations of myosin determining the degree of myosin ATPase activity, since increased rate of myosin ATPase hydrolysis of ATP during the active state stimulates the intensity of actin-myosin linkages and thereby correlates directly with a greater degree of cardiac contractility. In this regard, the function of the two myosin light chains contained within the coil of a single myosin head, meromyosin S$_2$ (Fig. 8–10), is of particular importance. Until recently, the concept was entertained that both light subunits simply suppressed the activity of myosin ATPase within the head of the myosin heavy chains. Very recent heavy and light chain dissociation and reassociation studies have shown that the function of the myosin light chains is considerably more complex, with each light subunit

possessing quite different properties. These two light chains are designated C$_1$ (28,000 molecular weight) and C$_2$ (18,000 MW). The larger light chain (C$_1$) is variable in structure among different species, is also altered during the hypertrophy process in the same species, and influences myosin ATPase activity; the smaller light chain (C$_2$) binds calcium, becoming more firmly attached to the myosin head with such Ca^{++} binding, and the C$_2$ light subunit spans the distance from the actin linkage site to the hinge angle of heavy meromyosin S$_2$ (Fig. 8–10).

Present evidence indicates that the presence of light chain C$_1$ is required for myosin ATPase activity, apparently increasing or decreasing the enzyme's function, depending on the C$_1$ light subunit's features in different chronic situations. In contrast, the light chain C$_2$ does not influence myosin ATPase function; instead, it undergoes phosphorylation, with the result that the phosphorylated light chain C$_2$ enhances the intensity of the actin-myosin interaction. Whereas the phosphorylated C$_2$ light chain increases the turnover rate of actin-myosin linkages, there exists an inverse relation between such phosphorylation and the Ca^{++} binding affinity of the C$_2$ light chain protein (Fig. 8–20). Thus both myosin light chains are capable of substantially influencing cardiac contractility in disparate manners favorably or unfavorably in consort, or may have opposing effects on contractile state, depending on the chronic circumstances.

Importantly, concerning canine myosin light chains, the immunologic properties on electrophoresis (Fig. 8–25) and the degree of Ca^{++}-stimulated myosin ATPase function differ markedly between atrial and ventricular myocardium. Furthermore, among different animal species, ventricular myosin light chains evaluated by radioimmunoassay against antimyosin ventricular light chains are immunologically distinct (Fig. 8–26) and the levels of ventricular myocardial ATPase activity (Fig. 8–27) vary considerably. In general, the smaller animals (rat, guinea pig, cat, rabbit) with greater basal metabolic rate normally demonstrate higher ventricular myosin ATPase activity at greater optimal pH than larger species (dog, sheep, human) (Fig. 8–27).

As alluded to above, greater concentrations of Ca^{++} delivered to the contractile proteins during the active state increase both the number and maximum turnover rate of actin-myosin cross-bridge formation, thus elevating both contractile force and contractility. Influencing these phenomena are apparently both Ca^{++} binding and phosphorylation of troponin and myosin, as well as interrelationships between myosin ATPase activity and cross-bridge linkage. Elevation of myosin ATPase activity increases both the number and intensity of actin-myosin connections, depending on the number of available Ca^{++}-turned

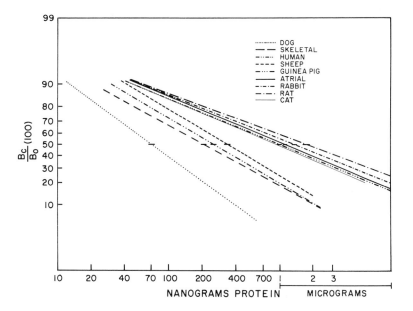

Figure 8–26 Homologous radioimmunoassay of myosin against antimyosin of ventricular light chains from different animal species, demonstrating limited species cross-reactivity and disparate antigenic sites of cardiac myosin light chains among the various species. Concerning the smaller versus the larger animals, considerable differences in the immunologic and structural properties of the ventricular light chains were observed.

on actin molecules. Phosphorylation of troponin I decreases calcium sensitivity of troponin C-Ca^{++} derepressor activity. This derepressor activity of troponin C is regained in the presence of elevated Ca^{++} concentrations, while in consort there is increased phosphorylation of myosin light chain C$_2$-Ca^{++} binding affinity. In addition, myosin light chains may play a role in enhancing Ca^{++} sensitivity of troponin C. Furthermore, Ca^{++}

binding of myosin heavy chains may enhance myosin ATPase activity. At present, using purified enzyme systems, acute changes in myosin ATPase activity have not been demonstrated; instead, all changes in myosin ATPase activity seen experimentally have been produced by animal preparations of chronic ventricular hemodynamic overload or have occurred in animals with chronic primary contractility disturbance.

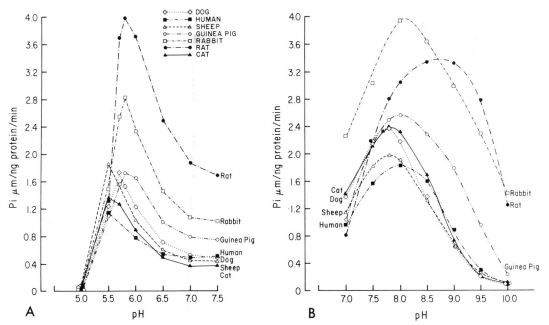

Figure 8–27 Optimal pH curves of Ca^{++}-activated (panel A) and K$^+$-activated myosins (panel B) of different animal species. The smaller animals demonstrated greater myosin ATPase activity and higher optimal pH values than the larger animal species.

Cardiac Hypertrophy and Failure

Although the induction of ventricular hypertrophy may result from different factors, including pressure overload, volume overload, hormonal influences, exercise, hypoxia and primary disturbances of contractility, development of hypertrophy caused by all these conditions is characterized by a common initial mechanism of protein synthesis. The stress engendered by these stimuli causes activation of the genetic apparatus of the myocardial cell, resulting in enhancement of nucleic acid and protein synthesis as well as induction of new genetic expressions. Thus myocardial cellular hypertrophy results from these biochemical sequences, thereby providing prolonged adaptation for the heart.

Ventricular pressure or volume overload leads to *increased wall tension* and stretch of muscle fibers, thus resulting in increased end-diastolic sarcomere length, which in turn activates the growth process of myocardial cellular hypertrophy. Present evidence suggests that this genetic activation mechanism appears to be preceded by changes in *tissue* PO_2 *and* PCO_2 and an alteration in the *phosphorylation potential* secondary to the increased workload demand. Elevation of myocardial norepinephrine induced by tension and muscle stretch may also play a role in the activation of the early ventricular hypertrophy process. Therefore, the common final pathway in the hypertrophy process may be mediated via norepinephrine released from sympathetic nerve endings in the myocardium by increased wall tension. This neurotransmitter may, in turn, trigger the biochemical process of hypertrophy; thus *norepinephrine* has been considered a myo-cardial cellular hypertrophy hormone and perhaps the hypertrophying factor itself. Thereby the increased levels of norepinephrine may elicit rises in *cAMP,* thus increasing *RNA polymerase* activity, resulting in elevated *protein synthesis* and thus myocardial hypertrophy. In this regard, RNA polymerase has been shown to increase during early stages of cardiac hypertrophy; this enzyme is activated by cAMP, which in turn leads to increases in RNA; as the result, protein content is augmented.

Since an increase in muscle mass accompanies hypertrophy, ventricular systolic stress is lessened. In this manner the hypertrophy process compensates for an excessive hemodynamic load by producing more sarcomeres and, in some types of hypertrophy, improves cardiac function to normal. A new principle described herein is the concept of physiologic versus pathologic ventricular hypertrophy in response to disparate settings. *Physiologic hypertrophy* is signified by normal or augmented contractile state with concomitant levels of myosin ATPase activity, in contrast to *pathologic hypertrophy* characterized by depressed contractility and diminished myosin ATPase function.

Biochemical and mechanical alterations of cardiac performance, myosin ATPase activity and contractility, respectively, which distinguish physiologic from pathologic ventricular hypertrophy, are dependent on at least four principal variables: (1) *degree of stress;* (2) *duration of stress;* (3) *nature of inciting stimulus;* and (4) *species, age, and health* of the animal studied. *Hyperthyroidism* affords a useful experimental model of physiologic hypertrophy in which left ventricular weight is considerably increased, as

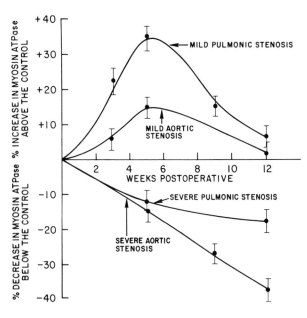

Figure 8–28 Comparison of disparate canine myosin ATPase function (K+-activated enzymatic V_{max} values) from hemodynamically stressed ventricles under different degrees and durations of right and left ventricular outflow obstruction.

well as are myosin ATPase activity and hemodynamic and mechanical indices of contractility. Concerning experimental examples of *chronic hemodynamic overload* in dogs, mild right or left ventricular outflow obstruction causes sustained increases in myosin ATPase and inotropic function for several weeks in the stress-hypertrophied ventricle prior to eventual depression of such activity (Fig. 8–28). In contrast, severe canine pulmonic or aortic stenosis results in immediate progressive declines in myosin ATPase activity and contractility in the stressed hypertrophied ventricle (Fig. 8–28). Thus differential responses of physiologic versus pathologic hypertrophy in the stressed ventricle are produced by chronic right or left ventricular pressure overloading, the type of hypertrophy being dependent on the severity and duration of the hemodynamic burden.

The primary disorder or combination of abnormalities responsible for *depressed contractile state* of the hypertrophied ventricle with the development of heart failure appears to result from defective *excitation-contraction coupling* and/or dysfunction of the *contractile proteins.*

Enhancement of the rate and quantity of calcium influx from external sources appears to be an important mechanism for increasing myocardial contractility such as with digitalis. Negative inotropic drugs diminish this calcium influx, and Briggs has shown their reduction of sarcotubular calcium pump ATPase. Concerning depressed contractility in heart failure, there may be abnormal transport of calcium by the sarcoplasmic reticulum as evidenced by its impairment of calcium uptake, binding, release, and pump ATPase activity as demonstrated by Schwartz, Gertz, Chidsey, and others. Chidsey has suggested a maldistribution of myocardial intracellular calcium in chronic hemodynamic overload in which depressed sarcoplasmic function leads to increased mitochondrial sequestration of calcium, with total intracellular calcium being unaltered. Katz has shown that the early decline of contractility in myocardial ischemia, with attendant intracellular acidosis due to lactate production, results directly from hydrogen ion inhibition of calcium binding to troponin. In the final phase of ischemic heart disease, exhaustion of ATP supply for myosin ATPase leads to the development of irreversible ventricular contracture, whereas decreased contractility in the earlier stage of ischemia due to disturbed excitation-contraction coupling may be reversible with reperfusion of the myocardium with oxygenated blood.

In regard to dysfunction of the contractile proteins in heart failure, attention has been focused on abnormal energy utilization. Thus the activity of myofibrillar ATPase is reduced in the failing myocardium as demonstrated by Alpert, Sonnenblick, Luchi, and others. Diminished activity of this enzyme in heart failure reduces the intensity of interaction between actin-myosin linkages and thereby lowers contractile state. The failing heart does not appear to be inefficient in its conversion of chemical energy to mechanical work. Additional considerations are that dysfunction of hypertrophied muscle may be related to changes in myofibril arrangement and quantitative differences in the generation of subcellular constituents. Furthermore, it is likely that in circumstances in which there is divergence of results and views concerning the causative, contributory, or coincidental nature of certain biochemical abnormalities in the pathogenesis of depressed mechanical function and contractility in the failing myocardium, these dissimilarities reflect basic differences in the types of heart failure studied: acute or chronic, mild or severe, experimental or human, idiopathic, drug-induced, ischemic, or volume or pressure overload.

Finally, concerning the *myosin molecular alterations* causing the kinetic disorders of diminished myosin ATP hydrolysis, thereby less intense actin-myosin interaction, responsible for *reduced contractility* of pathologic hypertrophy resulting in the decreased contractile force of abnormal cardiac function, reduced myosin ATPase activity appears to be due either to structural alterations in the myosin light chain C_1 governing myosin ATPase function or in the active site of the myosin head heavy chains containing myosin ATPase. These molecular alterations in heavy and light chain myosins may be due to pathologic hypertrophy-induced changes in specific isoenzymes regulating the synthesis of the different myosin subunit proteins during the course of cardiac hypertrophy. Consistent with this concept that the activity of myosin ATPase is gradually altered by new protein biosynthesis during the hypertrophy process by production of new specific myosin subunit isoenzymes are the electrophoretic (Fig. 8–25) and radioimmunoassay findings documenting major diversity of light chain structure between canine atrial and ventricular myosins concordant with considerable differences of myosin ATPase activity in these two areas. Also consistent with this view are the dissimilarities of light chain structure (Fig. 8–26) and disparities of myosin ATPase activity (Fig. 8–27) from ventricles of different animal species. Furthermore, there is increased protein synthesis of myosin light compared to heavy chains in the stressed hypertrophied left ventricle of dogs with chronic aortic stenosis; and even disparate synthesis of light and heavy chains occurs between the normal canine ventricles resulting in twice the number of light chains per heavy chains in the right ventricle than in the left.

The possibility also exists that myosin ATPase activity may be adversely affected by a charge modification of the light myosin C_1 subunit during pathologic hypertrophy. At the present time,

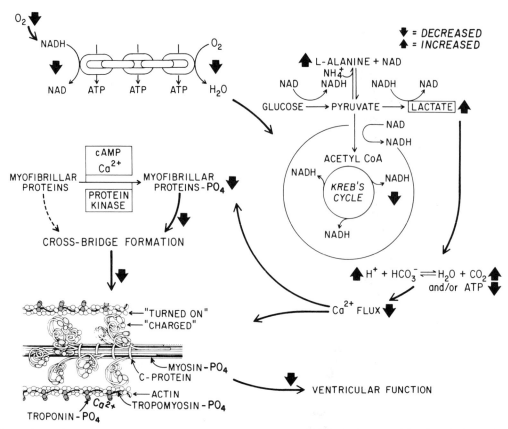

Figure 8–29 Postulated mechanism whereby myocardial contractility is depressed in chronic hemodynamic overload. Reduction in myocardial PO_2 is followed by depression of the cytochrome oxidase system, decreased ATP production, an increase in NADH, and depression of oxidative Krebs cycle integrity. The result is tissue acidity as documented by increased myocardial tissue pCO_2. Under these conditions intracellular Ca^{++} concentrations may decrease (impaired excitation-contraction coupling) and phosphorylation of myofibrillar proteins diminishes. Reduced intracellular Ca^{++} concentration and diminished light chain phosphorylation may lead to reduced cardiac contractility by diminishing the availability and intensity of actin-myosin interactions.

relevant abnormalities of myosin light chain C_2 have not been detected concerning negative inotropic changes during cardiac hypertrophy. Thus, the decrease in contractility related to depressed myosin ATPase function with pathologic hypertrophy appears to be due to the synthesis of modified isoenzymes leading to myosin molecular abnormalities and/or due to charge aberrations of myosin. In addition, contractility may also be depressed by reducing myocardial tissue pH (acidity) and also by the extent of contractile protein phosphorylation (Fig. 8–29), both mechanisms which may adversely affect the intensity of actin-myosin interactions.

MYOCARDIAL FUNCTION

Preload

The force of contraction of the myocardium is controlled by two fundamental mechanisms in-

herent in the contractile machinery of the sarcomere: (1) extent of diastolic stretch (*preload*) of the myofilaments, and (2) *contractility* (contractile or inotropic state) related to the intensity of biophysical and biochemical interactions between the myofilaments. Concerning the first mechanism, the length of the sarcomere at end diastole governs the degree of overlap of the movable actin and fixed myosin contractile filaments and thereby determines the number of interaction sites between the heavy meromyosin heads and actin active sites. Since the myosin filament is 1.5 μ long, with all but 0.2 μ of its center containing reactive spines, and the actin filament is 1.0 μ long, the optimal sarcomere length at which each of the possible actin-myosin cross bridges can be established is 2.2 μ (Fig. 8–30) as shown by Sonnenblick in heart muscle and by Huxley in skeletal muscle.

In heart muscle, Sonnenblick has shown that the extent of diastolic overlap of actin and myosin

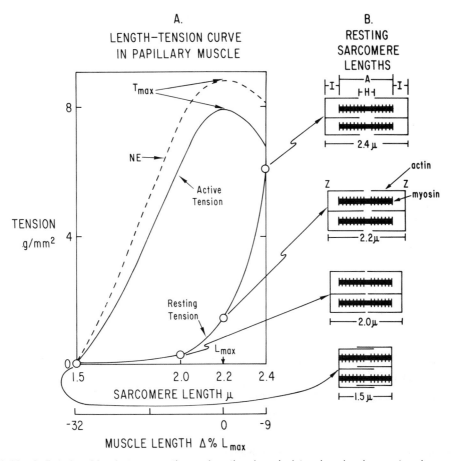

Figure 8–30 *A,* Relationships between active and resting (passive) tension development and sarcomere and papillary muscle length of the feline right ventricle. The active tension curve is elevated by increased contractile state induced by norepinephrine (*NE*). T_{max} = maximal active tension at L_{max}. *B,* Diagrammatic resting sarcomere lengths showing relation between actin and myosin filaments at different preloads.

filaments between sarcomere lengths of 1.5 to 2.2 μ is directly related to the force of contraction, the strongest contraction occurring at the maximum overlap of 2.2 μ initial sarcomere length and the weakest at 1.5 μ with the minimum overlap. This relationship between sarcomere resting length and developed force is the ultrastructural basis for the *length-active tension curve* of isolated cardiac muscle (Fig. 8–30) and the *Frank-Starling principle* of the *ventricular function curve* of the intact heart (Fig. 8–31), relating end-diastolic volume to performance characteristics of the heart (stroke volume, cardiac output, or stroke work). In the normal left ventricle the upper limit of normal end-diastolic pressure of 12 mm. Hg corresponds to the optimal 2.2 μ individual sarcomere length, while the resting muscle length at which the maximum developed tension occurs (L_{max}) on the length-active tension curve represents the optimal sarcomere length. Thus, a wide spectrum of initial sarcomere lengths ranging from 1.5 to 2.2 μ is operative on the ascending

limb of the ventricle function and length-tension curves. Normally the heart works at an intermediate point, usually on the upper portion, of the steep ascending limb of its function curve; thereby, the ventricle can improve its systolic performance by augmenting end-diastolic volume.

Active tension declines in skeletal muscle at sarcomere lengths greater than 2.2 μ, since thick and thin filament overlap diminishes, resulting in fewer actin-myosin linkages when the muscle is acutely overstretched. The relative disengagement of the actin filament from the myosin band is indicated by the abnormal central H zone and expanded I band representing the areas of non-overlap of filaments (Fig. 8–30, *B*). Thus, in acutely overstretched skeletal muscle and to a lesser extent cardiac muscle, sarcomere lengths greater than 2.2 μ are observed on the descending limb of the length-active tension curve. However, the predominant finding on the descending limb of the ventricular function curve of the chronic-

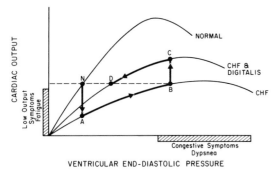

Figure 8–31 Ventricular function curves relating cardiac performance characteristics to extent of preload in the normal state, congestive heart failure (*CHF*), and CHF treated with digitalis. Points N through D represent in sequence: normal contractile state (*N*), depression of contractility (*A*), Frank-Starling compensation (*B*), increase in contractility toward normal with digitalis (*C*), and less utilization of preload compensation which digitalis allows (*D*). Although points N, D and B represent equal cardiac output on the vertical axis, each requires a progressively greater end-diastolic pressure indicated by the horizontal axis. The excessive end-diastolic pressures causing pulmonary congestion and the reduced levels of cardiac performance resulting in low cardiac output symptoms are represented by the cross-hatched areas. (Reproduced with permission from Mason, D. T., et al.: *In* Yu, P. N., and Goodwin, J. F. (Eds.): Progress in Cardiology. Lea and Febiger, Philadelphia, 1972.)

ally overdistended heart is slippage of myofibrils, with attendant distortion of orderly vertical register alignment of sarcomeres, rather than excessive elongation of individual sarcomere units with removal of paracentral filament binding sites.

Heart muscle also exhibits a *length-passive tension curve* which determines its *diastolic compliance* and *distensibility* characteristics (Fig. 8–30, *B*). Thus, passive tension is generated upon stretch of the myocardium in its resting state. In the intact ventricle, this length-passive tension curve is represented by the relation between end-diastolic pressure and end-diastolic volume. Cardiac muscle exhibits considerable resting tension as it is stretched to lengths approaching the physiologic limit of sarcomere length of 2.2 μ or 12 mm. Hg in the intact ventricle. This increase in passive tension contributes to total tension of the myocardium during systole, as does the greater effect of consequent rise in active developed tension at greater muscle lengths, thereby strengthening the force of contraction. The heart becomes extremely stiff when it is overstretched beyond the length corresponding to the apex of its ventricular function curve, reulting in marked elevations of end-diastolic pressure without improvement in ventricular performance. Clinically, alterations in compliance of the whole ventricle occur in certain chronic cardiac dis-

orders. Compliance is reduced in idiopathic hypertrophic cardiomyopathy, myocardial fibrosis, and excessive pressure loading in aortic stenosis. In chronic volume overloading the entire diastolic pressure-volume curve is displaced to the right, usually with reduced *functional distensibility* at the ventricle's elevated operating end-diastolic pressure.

Contractility

Concerning contractility, this second important basic functional variable of the myocardium which allows intrinsic control of its strength of contraction can be defined mechanically as the unique quality of heart muscle to alter its contractile force and velocity independent of fiber length. As is the case for the Frank-Starling principle, changes in myocardial contractility have a specific subcellular foundation. Although skeletal muscle exhibits a length-active tension relationship similar to heart muscle, skeletal muscle does not possess the physiologic regulatory mechanism of acutely variable contractility characteristic of heart muscle. Whereas length-induced changes in contractile force are determined quantitatively by the number of operative active sites between actin and myosin, the cellular basis of variable myocardial contractility is dependent on alterations in the qualitative nature (intensity and rapidity) of these cyclic force-generating sites between the contractile proteins.

Recently it has been considered by Katz and Brady that the process of actin-myosin interaction at constant myofilament overlap governing contractility appears to comprise two biophysical-chemical components: (1) *activation rate* of actin-myosin binding sites (rate at which activator calcium is delivered to modulator troponin, thereby preventing troponin-tropomyosin inhibition of actin-myosin reactive sites); and (2) *interaction rate* between actin-myosin molecules at the activated binding sites (rate of energy release and conversion of chemical to mechanical energy in the contractile process). These subprocesses are conceived as having two specific mechanical correlates quantifying contractility: (1) peak rate of tension rise or peak dT/dt (binding activation rate controlled by excitation-contraction coupling) and (2) peak rate of contractile element shortening or V_{max} (binding interaction rate regulated by the level of myosin ATPase activity). Furthermore, maximum systolic tension of heart muscle is determined by the number of actin-myosin interactions as governed by myofilament overlap and quantity of calcium bound to troponin.

Afterload

In addition to the fundamental intrinsic preload and contractility mechanisms of the myocardium regulating contractile force, there are two further independent properties of heart muscle determining cardiac performance which are largely under extrinsic autonomic control. The first of these is the *afterload* imposed on the muscle in order to shorten in an isotonic contraction of isolated muscle and to deliver stroke volume during ejection in the intact heart. Ventricular afterload is the myocardial wall tension during ejection defined by the *Laplace relation,* in which tension is directly equated with the product of ventricular systolic pressure and radius and wall stress is inversely related to wall thickness. Herein, *wall tension* is considered in terms of total force per unit of ventricular circumferential length (thus independent of wall thickness), whereas *wall stress* is force per unit of cross-sectional wall area (thus reduced by wall thickness). Thus, afterload is largely related to aortic pressure, which, in turn, is principally modulated by *aortic impedance* (instantaneous rate of pressure to flow change) to left ventricular ejection. Aortic impedance is predominantly determined by the *arterial compliance* (relation of pressure to flow) in the large arteries, and by *total peripheral vascular resistance* (the clinical equivalent of impedance) which is controlled by the rate of run-off from the systemic arteriolar beds.

In addition, afterload (tension) is a function of ventricular size (preload); a large ventricle must meet a higher afterload than a smaller ventricle at the same level of aortic and ventricular systolic pressures. Thus, when end-diastolic volume is increased, the ventricle generates more systolic tension to develop the same pressure for opening the aortic valve and to eject the same stroke volume. For the dilated ventricle to deliver an increased stroke volume in relation to the elevation of end-diastolic volume, it also moves up the ascending limb of its ventricular function curve, resulting in further rise in systolic tension (afterload).

Heart Rate

The final independent property of cardiac muscle normally governing ventricular performance is the *heart rate*. The frequency of contraction is primarily controlled by the autonomic nervous system through unequal reciprocal changes in activity of its parasympathetic and sympathetic components. Thus, like afterload which is largely determined by changes in peripheral vascular resistance and in turn is regulated by adrenergic activity and regional metabolic factors, the heart rate is also principally controlled by means extrinsic to the ventricle. Concerning the role of heart rate in the regulation of cardiac output which is the product of heart rate and stroke volume, normally the frequency of contraction is very important in rapid adjustments of cardiac

output, while chronic alterations in cardiac output are more the result of changes in stroke volume governed by the ventricular loading conditions and contractile state.

Dyssynergy

When considering cardiac function in certain clinical heart disorders, it is important to add a fifth factor which adversely affects ventricular performance: abnormal temporal sequence or *dyssynergy* of ventricular contraction as demonstrated by Gorlin. The normal pattern of left ventricular contraction takes place in a coordinated manner, with integrated inward movement of the ventricular wall during ejection (Fig. 8–32, A). However, intraventricular conduction defects may cause a disorderly contraction sequence which in itself decreases cardiac function. More importantly, dyssynergy of contraction is also produced by localized disturbances in muscle function. Thus, segmental abnormalities of ventricular contraction occur commonly in coronary artery disease, and dyssynergy per se may contribute greatly to impaired cardiac function, in addition to the regional abnormalities of contractility and compliance accompanying the deranged wall movement (Figs. 8–32 B, C and D). Increased systolic compliance as occurs in ventricular aneurysm and dyssynergy each disturbs ventricular function in terms of the Frank-Starling relation by producing an adverse effect

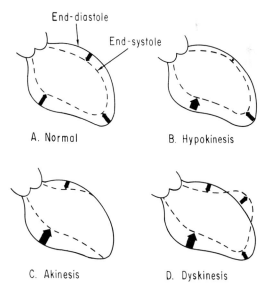

Figure 8–32 Localized patterns of left ventricular (*LV*) dyssynergy. The direction and extent of internal wall movement from end-diastole to end-systole are shown by the arrows. *RAO* = right anterior oblique view. (Reproduced with permission from Mason, D. T., et al.: *In* Yu, P. N., and Goodwin, J. F. (Eds.): Progress in Cardiology. Lea and Febiger, Philadelphia, 1972.)

analogous to decline in preload, as has been shown in specialized papillary muscle preparations with increased series elasticity and muscles contracting asynchronously in tandem.

Evaluation of Contractility

From the foregoing discussion concerning the regulation of myocardial contraction it is apparent that the function of the heart is normally determined by the interplay among its preload, contractility, afterload, and heart rate. The terms *cardiac function* and *ventricular performance* are used in the general sense to refer to the integrated action of all these determinants and not necessarily only to the single determinant, contractility itself. The contractile state and function of the heart can be evaluated by two general approaches: (1) its *pump (hemodynamics)*, and (2) its *muscle (mechanics)* performance characteristics. In the traditional approach of pump analysis the standard hemodynamic variables of cardiac output, stroke volume, systolic ejection rate, and ventricular end-diastolic pressure and the more complex measurements of ventricular end-diastolic volume, ejection fraction, stroke work, stroke power, and ventricular mass are studied in the basal state and also evaluated within the background of the Frank-Starling principle of end-diastolic length changes (usually estimated clinically as end-diastolic pressure) relative to systolic performance (ventricular function curve segments in response to interventions such as intravascular volume expansion). In addition, cardiac contractility and function have recently been evaluated by the second approach in terms of muscle mechanics which describe the force, velocity, and length characteristics of the myocardium.

Length-Active Tension Curve. An understanding of the property of contractility and its assessment by mechanical and hemodynamic techniques can be achieved by consideration of the mechanics of contraction in isolated muscle. During *isometric contraction,* contractile state can be evaluated by the relative position and shifts of the length-active tension curve (isometric force-length relation) utilizing papillary muscle preparations (Fig. 8–30, *A*). The length-active tension curve is obtained by stretching the muscle, electrically stimulating it at a fixed length, and determining the active tension it produces while contracting isometrically; this procedure is carried out throughout a series of muscle lengths to establish the entire curve for a given contractile state. In the study of the inotropic effect of a pharmacologic agent, the entire technique is repeated after bathing the muscle with the drug to assess the new level of contractility. An upward displacement of the ascending limb of the curve indicates qualitatively that an increase in con-

tractility has occurred (Fig. 8–30, *A*) and a downward shift identifies a directional decrease in contractility. Thus, alterations of the entire *length-isometric tension curve* signify changes in *inotropism,* while movements along a given stationary curve denote variations in fiber length. Depressed length-tension curves are observed in muscles taken from failing hearts. Concepts gained from studies of the myocardial length-tension mechanical relationship can be extended to the clinical evaluation of cardiac function by hemodynamic means. Thus, the systolic force-resting length framework of analysis of the inotropic and preload properties of isolated cardiac muscle also applies to the assessment of these properties in the intact ejecting heart employing Frank-Starling ventricular function curves (Fig. 8–31).

Force-Velocity Curve. A more precise conceptual analysis of myocardial mechanical properties and contractility is provided by consideration of muscle models containing functionally different components: the *contractile element* (CE), *series elastic* component (SE), and *parallel elastic* component (PE) (Fig. 8–33). As originally proposed by Hill in skeletal muscle and extended to cardiac muscle by Abbott and Mommaerts, Sonnenblick, Brady, Hefner, and Parmley, the CE develops force and shortens when activated (CE *active state*) and represents the intensity of interaction between the cyclic binding sites of the myofilaments; the CE is freely extensible at rest. The SE and PE are conceived as passive inert springs with different stress-strain characteristics. The SE is thought to reside in the myofilaments and cell membranes, while the PE is considered to be in the supporting connective tissue structures. According to the 3-component model shown (Maxwell adaptation of Hill model), the SE is in series with the CE, and the PE is connected alongside the CE and SE. Diastolic ten-

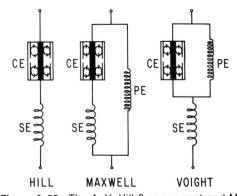

Figure 8–33 The A. V. Hill 2-component and Maxwell and Voight 3-component modifications of mechanical models of heart muscle. *CE* = contractile element; *SE* = series elastic element; *PE* = parallel elastic element.

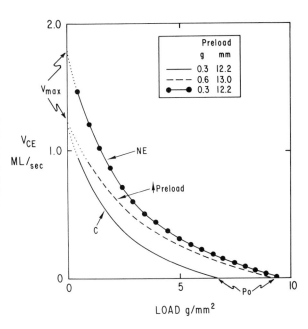

Figure 8–34 Force-velocity relationship in feline right ventricular papillary muscle in control state (C), after increasing initial muscle length (preload), and with augmentation of contractility by norepinephrine (NE) at control initial muscle length. V_{CE} = contractile element velocity expressed in muscle lengths (ML) per second. V_{max} = maximal V_{CE} at zero load obtained by extrapolation of force-velocity curve. P_O = maximal isometric force.

sion (preload) results from stretching the stiff PE. During isometric contraction after electrical stimulation, the rate of CE shortening (V_{CE} occurs at the same rate the nonlinear, more distensible SE spring elongates (V_{SE}, leading to the generation of active tension without change in muscle length.

In heart muscle preparations allowing *isotonic contraction,* the muscle shortens when the force developed equals the load (afterload) against which it is contracting. During isotonic contraction, tension is constant while the muscle shortens. Since the SE is stationary at the onset of muscle shortening, the initial peak fiber shortening rate *(FSR)* is equal to V_{CE} for the total load encountered (tension or force exerted). By repeating a series of isotonic contractions over a wide range of different loads and graphing the relationship between systolic load and V_{CE} (peak FSR), an inverse *force-velocity curve* is obtained in which V_{CE} declines as force increases (Fig. 8–34). Maximum V_{CE} (V_{max}) is obtained by extrapolation of the curve to zero load. Maximum force (P_O), which is directly related to preload, is achieved at the load at which no fiber shortening takes place (at zero V_{CE}). Since alterations in contractile state change V_{max}, while variations in preload directly affect P_O but are generally held not to influence V_{max}, V_{max} is considered an independent numerical index of contractility, with the value directly related to inotropic state (Fig. 8–34). Thus, the maximum rapidity of unloaded CE cyclic interactive sites (activity of myosin ATPase) is envisaged as being uninfluenced by sarcomere length or number of linkage sites. Some workers prefer that V_{max} estimated by force-velocity curve extrapolations be considered an empirical index of contractile state because of possible influence on this value by instantaneous changes in CE length, active state, internal viscosities, and muscle model uncertainties, although these concerns have been refuted by others. It is important that from consideration of the force-velocity-initial and shortening length relationship, both *peak external work* (product of force and extent of muscle shortening) and *power* (product of force and FSR) are dependent on preload and contractility.

Contractile element velocity can also be determined from isometric contractions of isolated ventricular papillary muscles. Since V_{SE} equals V_{CE} during isometric systole, V_{CE} can be determined from the rate of SE elongation which is defined as the rate of tension development (dT/dt) related to the SE modulus or stiffness factor (dT/dl). The *SE modulus* is described as the product of a constant (K) and muscle tension (T), plus the constant C; C is disregarded because of its relatively small value. From these considerations, V_{CE} is calculated from the equation (dT/dt)/(KT), in which K is 32/muscle length at body temperature. A force-velocity curve is obtained by plotting the relationship of instantaneous V_{CE} to simultaneous tension throughout the course of a single contraction.

The concepts developed from study of isolated cardiac muscle mechanics have recently been extended to the assessment of contractility and performance of the intact heart experimentally and in patients. In the investigation of left ventricular mechanics, the development of chamber force and tension are related to the velocity and extent of contractile element and fiber shortening. The approach utilizing muscle mechanics provides a

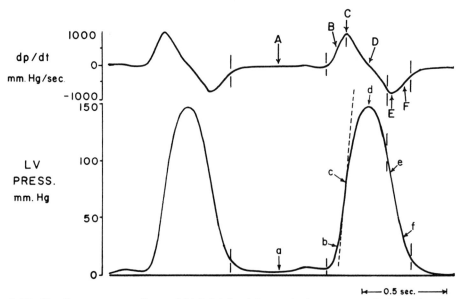

Figure 8–35 Simultaneous recordings of high-fidelity left ventricular pressure (*LV*) and its first derivative (*dp/dt*) in a patient with an aortic valve prosthesis. The various portions of the first derivative and corresponding segments of the pressure recording from which they were continuously computed are labeled. During ventricular filling when rate of change of ventricular pressure is minimal, dp/dt is flat at a level near zero (segment A). With the onset of isovolumic contraction, dp/dt rises slowly and then rapidly (segment B) to reach the peak dp/dt (point C), the maximal rate of pressure rise, indicated by slope of the diagonal broken line. Peak dp/dt usually occurs at the instant of opening of the semilunar valves, thus at peak isovolumic ventricular pressure. During early and middle phases of ventricular ejection, dp/dt descends to the baseline, and during late ejection, as intraventricular pressure decreases, dp/dt becomes negative (segment D). The rate of decrease of ventricular pressure is maximal at point E during isovolumic relaxation (segment F). Left ventricular pressure was recorded by direct needle puncture. (Reproduced with permission from Mason, D. T.: Am. J. Cardiol., 23:516, 1969.)

means for the quantitative analysis of the principal determinants of cardiac performance including the numerical evaluation of contractile state. Although the pump characteristics of cardiac output, mean systolic ejection rate and ejection fraction indirectly reflect the extent and velocity of fiber shortening respectively, hemodynamic variables are influenced by alterations in loading in addition to changes in contractility. In the application of the principles of muscle mechanics to the ventricle as a whole, its integrated function is described in terms of representative or average values of force, velocity, and length of the entire ventricle. The methods for evaluation of the mechanics of ventricular contraction have been developed along two different lines: the properties of (1) *isovolumic* and (2) *ejection* phases of systole.

Isovolumic Indices. Concerning the techniques for assessment of the mechanics of isovolumic ventricular contraction, an important method is determination of the rate at which intraventricular pressure rises or the first derivative of ventricular pressure *(dp/dt)* (Fig. 8–35). *Peak dp/dt* itself is a valid and sensitive measure for the study of ventricular inotropic state in intrapatient studies when loading conditions are con-

stant. Thus, with ventricular loading stable, peak dp/dt itself correlates directly with the contractile state of the ventricle in the study of interventions in single patients. However, peak dp/dt is a complex function also directly dependent on the preload or left ventricular end-diastolic pressure (LVEDP) and afterload (arterial diastolic pressure in the case of peak dp/dt). An increase in LVEDP causes an elevation of instantaneous dp/dt throughout the course of isovolumic contraction including peak dp/dt, whereas a rise in arterial diastolic pressure elevates only peak dp/dt. Since changes in loading conditions of the ventricle ordinarily occur in response to most physiologic and pharmacologic interventions in individual patients and in the basal state among different patients, usually it is not possible precisely to evaluate changes in ventricular contractile state by the determination of peak dp/dt alone.

The recognition that dp/dt is influenced by preload and afterload variations has led to the development of contractility indices in which dp/dt is modified by certain hemodynamic and mechanical variables which minimize or cancel the changes in dp/dt caused by inconstant loading. Thus, by relating these loading-related correction factors to dp/dt, it is possible to employ dp/dt in the assessment of contractility despite concurrent alterations in loading. One approach which is useful in intrapatient studies is the examination of the time interval from the onset of ventricular contraction to maximum dp/dt *(time-to-peak dp/dt)* in relation to peak dp/dt itself (Fig. 8–36). Alterations in contractility produce opposite changes between time-to-peak dp/dt and peak dp/dt, while variations in loading result in directionally similar changes in these two variables. Although directionally opposite changes between time-to-peak dp/dt and peak dp/dt indicate a qualitative alteration of contractility, large concomitant changes in LVEDP or arterial diastolic pressure might obscure alterations in inotropic state analyzed in this manner. In the presence of changes in LVEDP without associated variations of arterial diastolic pressure, alterations in contractility can be studied using the ratios: peak dp/dt to integrated systolic isovolumic tension (IIT), peak dp/dt to peak isovolumic pressure (PIP), peak dp/dt to maximum isovolumic ven-

tricular tension (MIT), peak dp/dt to LVEDP, and (peak dp/dt)/PIP related to left ventricular end-diastolic circumferential fiber length. As with peak dp/dt, these ratios are dependent on arterial diastolic pressure.

When LVEDP is nearly constant and arterial diastolic pressure varies, the relation of dp/dt to peak common developed isovolumic pressure (CPIP) or *(dp/dt)/CPIP* correlates directly with contractile state independent of afterload variations (Fig. 8–37). The relation between dp/dt and simultaneously developed pressure during the course of isovolumic contraction can also be applied in the assessment of basal contractile state among different patients. Thus, dp/dt determined at the developed isovolumic ventricular pressure of 50 mm. Hg common to each of the different ventricles corrects for differences in arterial diastolic pressure. Since the preload of the different ventricles varies widely, dp/dt at common developed isovolumic pressure of 50 mm. Hg is modified by relating it to left ventricular end-diastolic volume index (LVEDVI). This ratio (dp/dt_{CPIP})

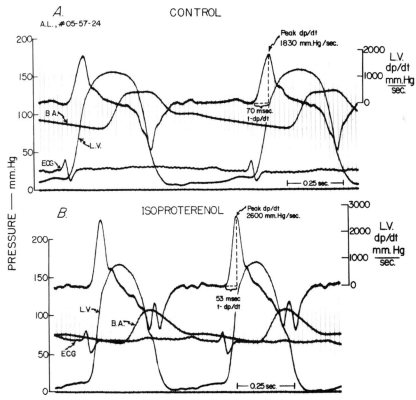

Figure 8–36 Simultaneous recordings of the high-fidelity left ventricular pressure, its first derivative, and brachial arterial pressure (*B.A.*) during the control period (*A*) and after increasing contractility with isoproterenol (*B*) in a patient with an aortic valve prosthesis. The interval from the onset to peak dp/dt (t-dp/dt) is indicated. Left ventricular pressure was recorded by direct needle puncture. (Reproduced with permission from Mason, D. T.: Am. J. Cardiol., 23:516, 1969.)

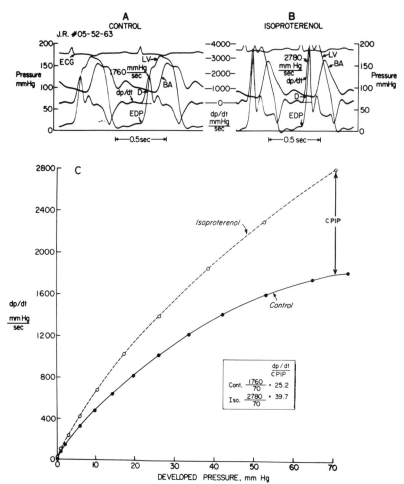

Figure 8–37 *A* and *B*, Simultaneous recording of high-fidelity left ventricular (*LV*) pressure, its first derivative (*dp/dt*), the brachial arterial pressure (*BA*), and electrocardiogram during the control period (*A*) and during isoproterenol (*B*). EDP = LV end-diastolic pressure; *D* = peak isovolumic LV pressure. The numerical values of dp/dt indicated are at the highest common developed isovolumic pressure (*CPIP*). *C*, Relation between LV dp/dt and developed isovolumic pressure at 5-msec. intervals throughout isovolumic systole of the contractions shown in *A*, during the control period (*Cont.*), and *B*, during isoproterenol (*Iso.*). The arrows indicating CPIP of both curves are the points at which the ratios of (dp/dt)/CPIP shown in the insert were calculated. (Reproduced by permission of the American Heart Association, Inc., from Mason, D. T., et al.: Circulation, *44*:47, 1971.)

/LVEDVI is analogous to V_{CE} corrected for its preload-dependence at an isopressure point on the pressure-velocity curve to be described.

It has recently been shown that the contractile state can be quantified clinically by determination of *ventricular pressure-velocity curves* from high-fidelity recordings of isovolumic ventricular systolic dp/dt and pressure (Fig. 8–38). This new method is based on force-velocity concepts derived from study of isometric myocardial mechanics discussed earlier in isolated muscle and, from a single beat, provides segments of isovolumic pressure-V_{CE} curves related to the entire force-velocity relationship. In the intact heart during isovolumic contraction, alterations in ventricular geometry are small and thus V_{CE} can be

assumed essentially equivalent to V_{SE}. In the calculation of isovolumic ventricular V_{SE}, and thereby V_{CE}, knowledge of tension is not necessary; only the value of isovolumic pressure is required, since pressure is essentially the only independent variable, and chamber radius and wall thickness cancel in the equation for isovolumic V_{SE}. Therefore, isovolumic V_{CE} in ejecting beats can be determined entirely from isovolumic ventricular pressure (IP) and corresponding dp/dt by use of the equation for isovolumic V_{SE}: $(dp/dt)/(32 \times IP)$ expressed in muscle lengths (ML) per second.

The isovolumic pressure-velocity curve can be constructed from an individual contraction by relating instantaneous V_{CE} to simultaneous total isovolumic pressure from the closure of the atrioventricular valve to the opening of the semilunar valve (Fig. 8–38). Extrapolation of the pressure-velocity descending limb to zero pressure allows estimation of maximum V_{CE} or V_{max}. In practice, the segment of the pressure-velocity curve is averaged from several beats. Like V_{max} obtained from isometric and isotonic contractions in isolated papillary muscle, ventricular V_{max} is related directly to contractile state and is independent of physiologic variations in left ventricular end-diastolic volume and pressure; some dependence is reported with very large preload increases. This practical method of determining pressure-velocity relations in the assessment of contractility obviates the complex angiographic techniques for the calculation of tension. Importantly, ventricular pressure-velocity and tension-velocity curves of a given beat extrapolate to identical values of V_{max}.

The pressure-velocity method of assessing left ventricular contractile state can be applied both in studies of interventions in individual patients and in the evaluation of basal contractility in different patients, since V_{max} is expressed in terms of muscle units and is independent of loading and wall thickness. Utilizing this method in patients with primary and secondary ventricular hypertrophy, a spectrum of decreasing inotropic state has been demonstrated between those without failure and those with failure (Fig. 8–38). Although determination of V_{max} from isovolumic pressure and its dp/dt has been thought to require a truly isovolumic portion of systole, recent evidence indicates

that mitral insufficiency itself has little to no effect on V_{max} obtained from pressure-velocity curves. Abnormal ventricular compliance and dyssynergy such as occur in coronary artery disease have been considered conditions in which the pressure-velocity method is not applicable in the study of contractility. Recent work, however, has demonstrated that when SE stiffness is altered or dyssynergy produced, the determination of V_{max} extrapolated from the isovolumic pressure-velocity relation remains valid. V_{max} does not appear to be influenced by regional myocardial necrosis itself, since maximum velocity is sensitive only to the intensity of operative binding sites between myofilaments. Although compliance variations, altered temporal contraction sequence, non-isovolumic systole, and segmental necrosis may considerably affect loaded V_{CE} prior to aortic valve opening, the accompanying slope change of the pressure-V_{CE} curve is such that the extrapolation to V_{max} is essentially undisturbed. Therefore, in these particular conditions there may be marked disparity between ventricular hemodynamic performance and contractility assessed as V_{max}. In addition to V_{max}, certain other properties of the isovolumic total pressure velocity relation are useful in evaluating contractility such as peak measured V_{CE} (V_{pm}), which is a finite value not requiring extrapolation (Fig. 8–38).

The isovolumic *total pressure*-velocity method for the evaluation of contractile state is based on the two-component Hill model in which CE and SE are connected in series. It has been suggested that

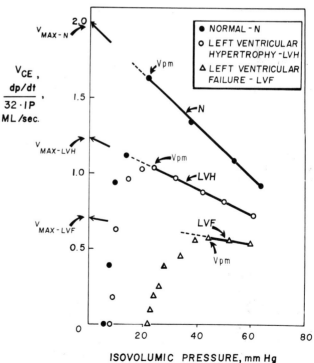

Figure 8–38 Representative comparison of the pressure-velocity relation during isovolumic systole of the left ventricle in a normal patient, in a patient with aortic stenosis with left ventricular hypertrophy in the absence of failure, and in a patient with aortic stenosis with left ventricular hypertrophy and failure. The diagonal broken lines indicate extrapolation of the isovolumic segments to V_{max} at zero load. Vpm = peak measured V_{CE}. IP in the V_{CE} equation and pressure on the horizontal axis are total isovolumic pressure. (Reproduced with permission from Mason, D. T., et al.: *In* Alpert, N. R. (Ed.): Ventricular Hypertrophy. Academic Press, New York, 1971.)

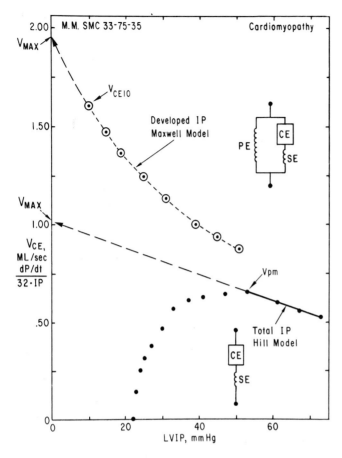

Figure 8–39 Left ventricular (*LV*) pressure-velocity relation during isovolumic contraction obtained by the use of total instantaneous isovolumic pressure, as IP, in the calculation of instantaneous V_{CE} (2-component Hill model) and on the abscissa for LVIP (closed dots and solid lines) compared to the isovolumic pressure-velocity relation determined by employment of developed instantaneous isovolumic pressure in the V_{CE} equation (3-component Maxwell model) and on the abscissa for LVIP (open circles and broken lines). The extrapolations to V_{max} are shown by the long broken lines and arrows. The appropriate muscle models are shown. The two pressure-velocity curves were obtained from the same LV beat in a patient with a cardiomyopathy. *Vpm* = peak measured V_{CE} using total IP; $V_{CE}10 = V_{CE}$ at 10 mm. Hg developed IP. (Reproduced with permission from Mason, D. T., et al.: *In* Yu, P. N., and Goodwin, J. F. (Eds.): Progress in Cardiology. Lea and Febiger, Philadelphia, 1972.)

the PE component should also be considered during isovolumic contraction by subtracting LVEDP from total isovolumic pressure to obtain developed isovolumic pressure for use in the V_{CE} equation and on the abscissa of the pressure-velocity curve (Fig. 8–39). With the isovolumic *developed pressure*-velocity curve obtained by utilization of the three-component model, V_{CE} is infinitely high at very small developed isovolumic pressures and, therefore, the first point on the descending pressure-velocity limb is usually arbitrarily taken at 10 mm. Hg. It is also possible to estimate right ventricular contractility by application of this developed pressure-V_{CE} approach, since this method allows description of a descending limb at relatively low isovolumic pressures. In contrast, the onset of the total pressure-V_{CE} descending curve is delayed until development of full active state of the ventricle (Fig. 8–39); thus the total IP-V_{CE} method may not be applicable in beats with relatively small amplitudes of isovolumic pressure. Comparing the degree of sensitivity to contractility and preload of the principal contractility indices employing isovolumic dp/dt, the order of decreasing inotropic and loading sensitivities is peak dp/dt, (dp/dt)/CPIP, total and then developed pressure V_{CE} methods, with peak dp/dt at the top of

the spectrum being very sensitive to inotropism but still somewhat responsive to loading, while developed pressure V_{CE} on the bottom is not altered by large changes in end-diastolic volume but is relatively insensitive to contractility. Contractility indices designed to obviate loading influences become inherently less sensitive to contractility.

Ejection Indices. The systolic ejection techniques applied to analysis of ventricular force-velocity properties and contractile state examine fiber shortening rate or circumferential fiber shortening velocity (V_{CF}) to determine V_{CE} according to the principles of isotonic mechanics elucidated in isolated muscle (see earlier discussion). One approach to the analysis of V_{CF} in intrapatient studies is the cinegraphic method of determining rate of change of epicardial dimensions by measurement of the velocity of movement, frame by frame, of roentgenopaque markers which were previously sutured to the ventricle's surface at therapeutic operation. Other techniques for the study of external border motion are the measurement of epicardial segmental velocity as determined noninvasively by radar-kymography and invasively by the movement of branch points of coronary arteries during angiography.

A more promising approach to the evaluation of V_{CE} and contractility during ejection is the study of endocardial wall motion. Angiographic study of instantaneous tension-velocity-length relations during ejection provides determination of V_{CF} at peak midwall tension (T) at which V_{SE} is zero; thereby, V_{CF} *at peak T* equals V_{CE} at peak tension. Thus, a single V_{CE}-tension relation is established which identifies a point on the force-velocity curve of the ventricle, similar to the manner in which a point is determined on the isotonic force-velocity curve of papillary muscle by determination of peak FSR at peak T from a single isotonic contraction. The electromagnetic velocity catheter in the ascending aorta has also recently been used in determining instantaneous V_{CF} related to corresponding tension in the ejecting ventricle. Ventricular V_{CE} at peak T correlates well with cardiac function, and V_{CE} values less than 1.30 circumferences per sec. indicate depressed contractility. Although loading dependent and not V_{max}, V_{CE} at peak T is applicable in nonisovolumic contractions and does obviate the need for the SE constant. It has been shown that *mean V_{CF}*, determined angiographically as the relation of extent of internal wall shortening (end-diastolic volume minus end-systolic volume, corrected for end-diastolic volume) to duration of ejection, provides a good correlation with the more difficult calculation of V_{CE} at peak T. Furthermore, V_{CF} determined by echocardiographic measurements of left ventricular endocardial dimensions relates closely to mean V_{CF} calculated by angiographic means.

SUMMARY

The hemodynamic function of the heart as a pump is dependent on the mechanical properties of its myocardium in which the sarcomere is the basic subcellular contractile unit. The contractile apparatus of the sarcomere consists of four protein aggregates: the primary interactng actin and myosin molecular chains and the modulator proteins troponin and tropomyosin, which inhibit actomyosin reaction. Resting sarcomere length controls the extent of myofilament overlap which determines the number of actin-myosin binding sites, the subcellular basis for the Frank-Starling principle. The intensity of interaction between thick and thin filaments regulates contractility.

Excitation throughout the myocardial fiber takes place by the rapid spread of the depolarization wave along the network of sarcolemma cell membrane invaginations constituting the transverse tubular system. Excitation-contraction coupling is achieved by delivery of calcium from the sarcoplasmic reticulum and from outside the cell to troponin. The combination of calcium with troponin activates the contractile process by releasing troponin-tropomyosin inhibition of actin-

myosin binding. Contraction occurs by myosin ATPase-regulated cyclic interactions between the actin-myosin linkages with the development of force (dp/dt) and shortening (V_{CE}). ATP energy for operation of the contactile machinery is produced in surrounding mitochondria by oxidative phosphorylation of circulating free fatty acids and glucose.

Concerning translation of the physicochemical mechanisms mediating contraction to mechanical variables, it is envisaged that peak systolic tension measures the number of active actin-myosin binding sites (muscle length) and that peak dp/dt (maximum rate of ventricular pressure rise) and V_{max} (maximum velocity of contractile element shortening) are properties expressing contractility which are related to two different processes: activation rate of actin-myosin binding or activity of sarcotubular calcium transport (peak dp/dt) and interaction rate of actin-myosin binding turnover or activity of myosin ATPase (V_{max}). Abnormalities in sarcotubular and myosin enzymatic activity are currently considered the most likely biochemical defects to account for depressed contractility in the failing myocardium.

Myocardial mechanical properties and contractile state can be assessed in isolated papillary muscle during isometric (length-active tension curve) and isotonic (force-velocity curves) contractions. Concepts developed from study of heart muscle can be extended to the evaluation of the intact ventricle. Cardiac function is normally governed by four determinants: preload (end-diastolic volume), afterload (systolic tension), contractility (inotropic state), and heart rate, to which dyssynergy is included as a fifth factor in certain types of heart disease. Ventricular function and contractility can be assessed in terms of pump (hemodynamics) and muscle (mechanics) performance of the heart. Concerning analysis of myocardial mechanics in the intact heart, contractility can be quantified by isovolumic indices utilizing dp/dt and ejection indices employing V_{CF} (circumferential fiber shortening rate).

When systolic pressure or volume overloading or a primary defect in contractility is imposed upon the heart, there are three principal *compensatory mechanisms* available for the direct support of cardiac function and its fundamental goal of maintaining normal cardiac output at rest: (1) the Frank-Starling principle, (2) ventricular hypertrophy, and (3) the sympathetic nervous system. Deleterious symptoms necessarily accompany the operation of these compensatory mechanisms in their primary role of sustaining basal stroke volume, and these symptoms (dyspnea due to ventricular dilation, angina pectoris resulting from hypertrophy and tachycardia subsequent to adrenergic activity) limit the extent to which the adaptive systems can be employed. In *compensated* heart failure (Classes I, II, and III Cardiac

Functional Classification of the New York Heart Association), these reserve mechanisms achieve normal basal cardiac output from the dysfunctioning ventricle at the expense of increased ventricular end-diastolic, pulmonary, and systemic venous pressures. With bodily exertion, further elevations of these pressures occur, with attendant dyspnea and reduced response of cardiac output with fatigue (Class II). In patients with more advanced depression of ventricular performance, there are symptoms of congestion and fatigue even with ordinary physical activity (Class III), although the resting cardiac output may be normal. Finally, *decompensated* congestive heart failure (Class IV) evolves with chronic low cardiac output causing resting fatigue and oliguria, despite maximum use of compensatory mechanisms with resultant persistent congestive symptoms at rest. Thus, in the decompensated failing heart, marked impairment of contractility exceeds the capacity of preload, hypertrophy, and adrenergic protection for supporting basal cardiac output at normal levels. It is pointed out that the standard clinical functional classification of congestive heart failure is more coupled to symptoms consequent to secondary factors (compensatory mechanisms) in this condition rather than to the crucial hemodynamic variable (cardiac output) and the fundamental cause (depressed contractility) of decompensation.*

*The authors gratefully acknowledge the secretarial assistance of Leslie J. Silvernail and Yolanda Valentine and medical artistry of Kathryn Marr.

REFERENCES

MYOCARDIAL ULTRASTRUCTURE

Braunwald, E., Chidsey, C. A., Pool, P. E., Sonnenblick, E. H., Ross, J., Jr., Mason, D. T., Spann, J. F., and Covell, J. W.: Congestive heart failure: Biochemical and physiological considerations. Ann. Intern. Med., 64:4, 1966.

Braunwald, E., Ross, J., Jr., and Sonnenblick, E. H.: In Braunwald, E., et al. (Eds.): Mechanisms of Contraction of the Normal and Failing Heart. Little, Brown and Co., Boston, 1976.

Carney, J. A., and Brown, A. L., Jr.: Human cardiac myosin: electron microscopic observations. Circ. Res., 17:336, 1965.

Cole, H. A., and Perry, S. V.: The phosphorylation of troponin I from cardiac muscle. Biochem. J., 149:525, 1975.

Davies, R. E.: Molecular theory of muscle contraction: calcium-dependent contractions with hydrogen bond formation plus ATP-dependent extensions of part of myosin-actin cross-bridges. Nature (London), 199:1068, 1963.

Ebashi, S., and Endo, M.: Calcium ion and muscle contraction. In Butler, J. A. V., and Noble, N. (Eds.): Progress in Biophysics and Molecular Biology. Pergamon Press, New York, 1968, p. 123.

Grant, R. P.: Notes on the muscular architecture of the left ventricle. Circulation, 32:301, 1965.

Hanson, J., and Lowy, J.: Molecular basis of contractility in muscle. Br. M. Bull., 21:264, 1965.

Haugaard N., Haugaard, E. S., Lee, N. H., and Horn, R. S.: Possible role of mitochondria in regulation of cardiac contractility. Fed. Proc., 28:1657, 1969.

Huxley, H. E.: Structural arrangements and contraction mechanism in striated muscle. Proc. Roy. Soc. London (Biol.), 160:442, 1964.

Katz, A. M.: Contractile proteins of the heart. Physiol. Rev., 50:63, 1970.

Katz, A. M.: Physiology of the Heart. Raven Press, New York, 1977.

Legato, M. J.: Sarcomerogenesis in human myocardium. J. Mol. Cell. Cardiol., 1:425, 1970.

Ross, J., Jr., Sonnenblick, E. H., Taylor, R. R., Spotnitz, H. M., and Covell, J. W.: Diastolic geometry and sarcomere lengths in the chronically dilated canine left ventricle. Circ. Res., 28:49, 1971.

Spiro, D., and Sonnenblick, E. H.: Structural conditions in the hypertrophied and failing heart. In Mason, D. T. (Ed.): Congestive Heart Failure. Yorke Medical Books, New York, 1976, pp. 13–24.

Wikman-Coffelt, J., Fenner, C., Salel, A. F., Kamiyoma, T., and Mason, D. T.: In Mason, D. T. (Ed.): Congestive Heart Failure. Yorke Medical Books, New York, 1976, pp. 53–75.

Wilkinson, J. M., Perry, S. V., Cole, H. A., and Trayer, I. P.: The regulatory proteins of the myofibril. Separation and biological activity of the components of inhibitory-factor preparations. Biochem. J., 127:215, 1972.

MYOCARDIAL METABOLISM

Alpert, N. R., Hamrell, B. B., and Halpren, W.: Mechanical and biochemical correlates of cardiac hypertrophy. Circ. Res., 35:(Suppl. 2) 71, 1974.

Braunwald, E.: Control of myocardial oxygen consumption: physiologic and clinical correlations. Am. J. Cardiol., 27:416, 1971.

Chidsey, C. A., Braunwald, E., Morrow, A. G., and Mason, D. T.: Myocardial norepinephrine concentration in man: Effects of reserpine and of congestive heart failure. N. Engl. J. Med., 269:653, 1963.

Cohen, L. S., Elliott, W. C., Rolett, E. L., and Gorlin, R.: Hemodynamic studies during angina pectoris. Circulation, 31:409, 1965.

Coleman, H. N., Sonnenblick, E. H., and Braunwald, E.: Myocardial oxygen consumption associated with external work: the Fenn effect. Am. J. Physiol., 217:291, 1969.

Cooper, G., Gunning, J. F., Harrison, C. E., and Coleman, H. N.: Contractile and energetic behavior of hypertrophied and failing myocardium. In Mason, D. T. (Ed.): Congestive Heart Failure. Yorke Medical Books, New York, 1976, pp. 97–110.

Covell, J. W., Braunwald, E., Ross, J., Jr., and Sonnenblick, E. H.: Studies on digitalis. XVI. Effects on myocardial oxygen consumption. J. Clin. Invest., 45:1535, 1966.

Covell, J. W., Chidsey, C. A., and Braunwald, E.: Reduction of the cardiac response to postganglionic sympathetic nerve stimulation in experimental heart failure. Circ. Res., 19:51, 1966.

Epstein, S. E., Skelton, C. L., Levey, G. S., and Entman, M.: Adenyl cyclase and myocardial contractility. Ann. Intern. Med., 72:561, 1970.

Katz, A. N.: Effects of ischemia on the contractile process of heart muscle. In Mason, D. T. (Ed.): Congestive Heart Failure. Yorke Medical Books, New York, 1976, pp. 77–84.

Kramer, R. S., Mason, D. T., and Braunwald, E.: Augmented sympathetic neurotransmitter activity in the peripheral vascular bed of patients with congestive heart failure and cardiac norepinephrine depletion. Circulation, 38:629, 1968.

Laks, M. M., Morady, F., Garner, D., and Swann, H. J. C.: Temporal changes in canine right ventricular volume, mass, cell size, and sarcomere length after banding the pulmonary artery. Cardiovasc. Res., 8:106, 1974.

Lindenmayer, G. E., Sordahl, L. A., Harigaya, S., Allen, J. C., Besch, H. R., and Schwartz, A.: Some biochemical studies on subcellular systems isolated from fresh recipient human cardiac tissue obtained during transplantation. Am. J. Cardiol., 27:277, 1971.

Lindenmayer, G. E., Sordahl, L. A., and Schwartz, A.: Re-evaluation of oxidative phosphorylation in cardiac muscle from normal animals and animals in heart failure. Circ. Res., 23:439, 1968.

Mason, D. T.: Autonomic nervous system and regulation of cardiovascular performance. Anesthesiology, 29:670, 1968.

Mason, D. T.: The Failing Heart. Disease-a-Month Series, Year Book Medical Publishers, Chicago, January 1977.

Meerson, F. K., and Pomointisky, V. D.: The role of high-energy phosphate compounds in the development of cardiac hypertrophy. J. Mol. Cell. Cardiol., 4:571, 1972.

Meerson, F. Z., Alekhina, G. M., Aleksandrov, P. N., and Bazardjan, A. G.: Dynamics of nucleic acid and protein synthesis of the myocardium in compensatory hyperfunction and hypertrophy of the heart. Am. J. Cardiol., 22:337, 1968.

Morkin, E., and Ashford, R. P.: Myocardial DNA synthesis in experimental cardiac hypertrophy. Am. J. Physiol., 215:1409, 1968.

Nair, K. G., Cutiletta, A. F., Koide, R., and Rabinowitz, M.: Biochemical correlates of cardiac hypertrophy. Circ. Res., 23:451, 1968.

Namm, D. H., and Mayer, S. E.: Effects of epinephrine on cardiac cyclic 3′,5′-AMP, phosphorylase kinase and phosphorylase. Molec. Pharmacol., 4:61, 1968.

Opie, L. M.: Metabolism of the heart in health and disease, Parts 1 to 3. Am. Heart J., 76:865, 1968; 77:100 and 383, 1969.

Pool, P. E., Covell, J. W., Levitt, M., Gibb, J., and Braunwald, E.: Reduction of cardiac tyrosine hydroxylase activity in experimental congestive heart failure. Circ. Res., 20:349, 1967.

Pool, P. E., Spann, J. F., Jr., and Buccino, R. A.: Myocardial high energy phosphate stores in cardiac hypertrophy and heart failure. Circ. Res., 21:365, 1967.

Rabinowitz, M., and Zak, R.: Mitochondria and cardiac hypertrophy. Circ. Res., 36:367, 1975.

Rabinowitz, M., Nair, K. G., and Zak, R.: Cellular and subcellular basis of cardiac hypertrophy. Med. Clin. North Am., 54:211, 1970.

Rall, T. W., Sutherland, E. W., and Berthet, J.: The relationship of epinephrine and glucagon to liver phosphorylase. IV. Effect of epinephrine and glucagon on the reactivation of phosphorylase in liver homogenates. J. Biol. Chem., 224:463, 1957.

Schwartz, A., Sordahl, L. A., Entman, M. L., Allen, J. C., Reddy, Y. S., Goldstein, M. A., Luchi, R. J., and Wyborny, L. E.: Abnormal biochemistry in heart failure. In Mason, D. T. (Ed.): Congestive Heart Failure. Yorke Medical Books, New York, 1976, pp. 25–44.

Sobel, B. E., Henry, P. D., Robison, A., et al.: Depressed adenyl cyclase activity in the failing guinea pig heart. Circ. Res., 24:507, 1969.

Spann, J. F., Jr., Buccino, R. A., Sonnenblick, E. H., and Braunwald, E.: Contractile state of cardiac muscle obtained

from cats with experimentally produced ventricular hypertrophy and heart failure. Circ. Res., 21:341, 1967.

Spann, J. F., Jr., Chidsey, C. A., Pool, P. E., and Braunwald, E.: Mechanism of norepinephrine depletion in experimental heart failure produced by aortic constriction in the guinea pig. Circ. Res., 17:312, 1965.

Vogel, J. H. K., and Chidsey, C. A.: Cardiac adrenergic activity in experimental heart failure assessed with beta receptor blockade. Am. J. Cardiol., 24:198, 1969.

Wikman-Coffelt, J., Fenner, C., Coffelt, J. R., Salel, A., Kamiyama, T., and Mason, D. T.: Chronological effects of mild pressure overload on myosin ATPase activity in the canine right ventricle. J. Mol. Cell. Cardiol., 7:219, 1975.

Wikman-Coffelt, J., Fenner, C., McPherson, J., Zelis, R., and Mason, D. T.: Alterations of subunit composition and ATPase activity of myosin in early hypertrophied right ventricles of dogs with mild experimental pulmonic stenosis. J. Mol. Cell. Cardiol., 7:513, 1975.

Wikman-Coffelt, J., and Mason, D. T.: Mechanism of decreased contractility in chronic hemodynamic overload. In Mason, D. T. (Ed.) Advances in Heart Disease, I. Grune & Stratton, New York, 1977, pp. 491–504.

Wikman-Coffelt, J., and Mason, D. T.: The contractile proteins of cardiac muscle: myosin function in the normal and hemodynamically overloaded heart. In Mason, D. T.: Advances in Heart Disease, II. Grune & Stratton, New York, 1978.

Wikman-Coffelt, J., Parmley, W. W., and Mason, D. T.: The cardiac hypertrophy process: analysis of factors determining pathologic versus physiologic development. Circ. Res., in press.

Wikman-Coffelt, J., Walsh, R., Fenner, C., Kamiyama, T., Salel, A., and Mason, D. T.: Effects of severe hemodynamic pressure overload on the properties of canine left ventricular myosins. Mechanism by which myosin ATPase activity is lowered during chronic increased hemodynamic stress. J. Mol. Cell. Cardiol., 8:263, 1976.

Wikman-Coffelt, J., Zelis, R., Fenner, C., and Mason, D. T.: Studies on the synthesis and degradation of light and heavy chains of cardiac myosin. J. Biol. Chem., 248:5206, 1973.

Zak, R., Martin, A. F., Reddy, M. K., and Rabinowitz, M.: Control of protein balance in hypertrophied cardiac muscle. Circ. Res., 38:Suppl. 1, 146, 1976.

EXCITATION-CONTRACTION COUPLING AND THE CONTRACTILE PROCESS

Banerjee, S. K., Flink, I. L., and Morkin, E.: Enzymatic properties of native and N-ethylmaleimide-modified cardiac myosin from normal and thyrotoxic rabbits. Circ. Res., 39:319, 1976.

Beeler, G. W., Jr., and Reuter, H.: Membrane calcium current in ventricular myocardial fibers. J. Physiol. (London), 207:191, 1970.

Besch, H. R., Allen, J. C., Glick, G., and Schwartz, A.: Correlation between the inotropic action of ouabain and its effects on subcellular enzyme systems from canine myocardium. J. Pharmacol. Exp. Ther., 171:1, 1970.

Chandler, B. M., Sonnenblick, E. H., Spann, J. F., and Pool, P. E.: Association of depressed myofibrillar adenosine triphosphates and reduced contractility in experimental heart failure. Circ. Res., 21:717, 1967.

Conway, G., Heazlitt, R. A., Montag, J., and Mattingly, S. F.: The ATPase activity of cardiac myosin from failing and hypertrophied hearts. J. Mol. Cell. Cardiol., 7:817, 1975.

Draper, M., Taylor, N., and Alpert, N. R.: Alteration in contractile protein in hypertrophied guinea pig hearts. In Alpert, N. R. (Ed.): Cardiac Hypertrophy. Academic Press, New York, 1971, p. 315.

Fabian, F., Mason, D. T., and Wikman-Coffelt, J.: Calcium binding properties of cardiac and skeletal muscle myosins. F.E.B.S. Letter, 81:381, 1977.

Fuchs, F., Gertz, E. W., and Briggs, F. N.: The effect of quinidine on calcium accumulation by isolated sarcoplasmic reticulum of skeletal and cardiac muscle. J. Gen. Physiol., *52*:955, 1968.

Gertz, E. W., Hess, M. L., Lain, R. F., and Briggs, F. N.: Activity of the vesicular calcium pump in the spontaneously failing heart lung preparation. Circ. Res., *20*:477, 1967.

Harigaya, S., and Schwartz, A.: Rate of calcium binding and uptake in normal animal and failing human cardiac muscle. Circ. Res., *25*:781, 1969.

Higuchi, M., Stewart, D., Mason, D. T., Ikeda, R., and Wikman-Coffelt, J.: Immunological, electrophoretic and kinetic properties of cardiac myosins from various species. Comp. Biochem. Physiol., *60*:495, 1978.

Hoffman, B. F., and Cranefield, P. F.: Physiological basis of cardiac arrhythmias. Am. J. Med., *37*:670, 1964.

Huxley, H. E.: Mechanism of muscular contraction: Recent structural studies suggest a revealing model for cross-bridge action at variable filament spacing. Science, *164*:1356, 1969.

Ito, Y., and Chidsey, C. A.: Intracellular calcium and myocardial contractility. IV. Distribution of calcium in the failing heart. J. Mol. Cell. Cardiol., *4*:507, 1972.

Katz, A. M., and Brady, A. J.: Mechanical and biochemical correlates of cardiac contraction. Mod. Conc. Cardiovasc. Dis., *40*:39, 45; 1971.

Katz, A., and Tada, M.: The "stone heart": A challenge to the biochemist. Am. J. Cardiol., *29*:578, 1972.

Langer, G. A., and Serena, S. D.: Effects of strophanthidin upon conduction and ionic exchange in rabbit ventricular myocardium: relation to control of active state. J. Mol. Cell. Cardiol., *1*:65, 1970.

Long, L., Fabian, F., Mason, D. T., and Wikman-Coffelt, J.: A new cardiac myosin characterized from the canine atria. Biochem. Biophys. Res. Comm., *76*:626, 1977.

Luchi, R. J., Kritcher, E. M., and Thyrum, P. T.: Reduced cardiac myosin adenosine triphosphate activity in dogs with spontaneously occurring heart failure. Circ. Res., *24*:513, 1969.

Mason, D. T., Vera, Z., DeMaria, A. N., Lee, G., Awan, N. A., and Massumi, R. A.: Treatment of tachyarrhythmias. *In* Mason, D. T. (Ed.): Cardiac Emergencies. Williams & Wilkins Co., Baltimore, 1978.

Nayler, W. G., and Merrillees, N. C. R.: Cellular exchange of calcium. *In* Harris, P., and Opie, L. H. (Eds.): Calcium and the Heart. Academic Press, New York, 1971, pp. 24–65.

Pool, P. E., Chandler, B. M., Spann, J. F., Jr., Sonnenblick, E. H., and Braunwald, E.: Mechanochemistry of cardiac muscle. IV. Utilization of high-energy phosphates in experimental heart failure in cats. Circ. Res., *24*:313, 1969.

Repke, K.: Effect of digitalis on membrane ATPase of cardiac muscle. *In* Drugs and Enzymes. Proceedings of 2nd International Pharmacology Meeting. Pergamon Press, New York, 1965, pp. 65–87.

Schwartz, A.: Calcium and the sarcoplasmic reticulum. *In* Harris, P., and Opie, L. H. (Eds.): Calcium and the Heart. Academic Press, New York, 1971, pp. 66–92.

Sordahl, L. A., Wood, W. G., and Schwartz, A.: Production of cardiac hypertrophy and failure in rabbits with Ameroid clips. J. Mol. Cell. Cardiol., *1*:341, 1970.

Sulakhe, P. V., and Dhalla, N. S.: Excitation-contraction coupling in the heart. VII. Calcium accumulation in subcellular particles in congestive heart failure. J. Clin. Invest., *50*:1019, 1971.

Swynghedauw, B., Leger, J. J., and Schwartz, K.: The myosin isozyme hypothesis in chronic heart overloading. J. Mol. Cell. Cardiol., *8*:915, 1975.

Thomas, L. L., and Alpert, N. R.: Functional integrity of the SH_1 in myosin from hypertrophied myocardium. Biochim. Biophys. Acta, *481*:680, 1977.

Wikman-Coffelt, J., Fenner, C., Walsh, R., Salel, A., Kamiyama, T., and Mason, D. T.: Comparison of mild versus severe pressure overload on the enzymatic activity of myosin in the canine ventricles. Biochem. Med., *14*:139, 1975.

Wikman-Coffelt, J., Walsh, R., Fenner, C., Kamiyama, T., Salel, A., and Mason, D. T.: Activity and molecular changes in left ventricular and right ventricular myosin during right ventricular volume overload. Biochem. Med., *14*:33, 1975.

MYOCARDIAL FUNCTION

Abbott, B. C., and Mommaerts, W. F. H. M.: A study of inotropic mechanisms in the papillary muscle preparation. J. Gen. Physiol., *42*:533, 1959.

Brady, A. J.: Active state in cardiac muscle. Physiol. Rev., *48*:570, 1968.

Braunwald, E., Ross, J., Jr., Gault, J. H., Mason, D. T., Mills, C., Gabe, I. T., and Epstein, S. E.: Assessment of cardiac function. Ann. Intern. Med., *70*:369, 1969.

Brutsaert, D. L., Claes, V. A., and Sonnenblick, E. H.: Velocity of shortening of unloaded heart muscle and the length-tension relation. Circ. Res., *29*:63, 1971.

Bunnell, I. L., Grant, C., and Greene D. G.: Left ventricular function derived from the pressure-volume diagram. Am. J. Med., *39*:881, 1965.

Capone, R. J., Mason, D. T., Amsterdam, E. A., and Zelis, R.: The effect of mitral regurgitation and ventricular aneurysm on Vmax calculated from pressure-velocity data during "isovolumic" systole. Circulation, *44(Suppl. II)*:96, 1971.

Cooper, R. H., O'Rourke, R. A., Karliner, J. S., Peterson, K. L., and Leopold, G. R.: Comparison of ultrasound and cineangiographic measurements of the mean rate of circumferential fiber shortening in man. Circulation, *46*:914, 1972.

Covell, J. W., Ross, J., Jr., Sonnenblick, E. H., and Braunwald, E.: Comparison of the force-velocity relation and the ventricular function curve as measures of the contractile state of the intact heart. Circ. Res., *19*:364, 1966.

DeMaria, A., Bonanno, J. A., Amsterdam, E. A., Massumi, R. A., Zelis, R., and Mason, D. T.: Radarkymography. *In* Weissler, A. M. (Ed.): Noninvasive Techniques in Cardiac Evaluation. New York, Grune & Stratton, 1974, pp. 275–300.

DeMaria, A., Kamiyama, T., Peng, C. L., Mason, D. T., Amsterdam, E. A., Massumi, R. A., and Zelis, R.: Alterations of ventricular function and myocardial contractility indices induced by ventricular asynchrony. Clin. Res., *21*:414, 1973.

DeMaria, A. N., Neumann, A. L., and Mason, D. T.: Echographic evaluation of cardiac function. *In* Mason, D. T. (Ed.): Congestive Heart Failure. Yorke Medical Books, New York, 1976, pp. 91–224.

Dodge, H. T., and Baxley, W. A.: Left ventricular volume and mass and their significance in heart disease. Am. J. Cardiol., *23*:528, 1969.

Falsetti, H. L., Mates, R. E., Greene, D. G., et al.: Vmax as an index of contractile state in man. Circulation, *43*:467, 1971.

Forrester, J. S., Diamond, G., Parmley, W. W., and Swan, H. J. C.: Early increase in left ventricular compliance after myocardial infarction. J. Clin. Invest., *51*:598, 1972.

Frank, M. J., and Levinson, G. E.: An index of the contractile state of the myocardium in man. J. Clin. Invest., *47*:1615, 1968.

Fry, D. L., Griggs, D. M., Jr., and Greenfield, J. C., Jr.: Myocardial mechanics: Tension-velocity-length relations of heart muscle. Circ. Res., *14*:73, 1964.

Gaasch, W. H., Battle, W. E., Oboler, A. A., Banas, J. S., Jr., and Levine, H. J.: Left ventricular stress and compliance in man with special reference to normalized ventricular function curves. Circulation, *45*:756, 1972.

Gabe, I. T., Gault, J., Ross, J., Jr., Mason, D. T., Mills, C. J., Shillingford, J. P., and Braunwald, E.: Measurement of instantaneous blood flow velocity and pressure in conscious man with a catheter-tip velocity probe. Circulation, *40*:603, 1969.

Gault, J. H., Ross, J., Jr., and Braunwald, E.: Contractile state of the left ventricle in man: Instantaneous tension-velocity-length relations in patients with and without disease of the left ventricular myocardium. Circ. Res., *22*:451, 1968.

Gleeson, W. L., and Braunwald E.: Studies on the first derivative of the ventricular pressure pulse in man. J. Clin. Invest., *41*:80, 1962.

Glick, G., Sonnenblick, E. H., and Braunwald, E.: Myocardial force-velocity relations studied in intact unanesthetized man. J. Clin. Invest., 44:978, 1965.

Gordon, A. M., Huxley, A. F., and Julian, F. G.: Variation in isometric tension with sarcomere length in vertebrate muscle fibres. J. Physiol., 184:170, 1966.

Grossman, W., Brooks, H., Meister, S., et al.: New technique for determining instantaneous myocardial force-velocity relation in the intact heart. Circ. Res., 28:290, 1971.

Grossman, W., Hayes, F., Paraskos, J. A. Saltz, S., Dalen, J. E., and Dexter, L.: Alterations in preload and myocardial mechanics in the dog and in man. Circ. Res., 31:83, 1972.

Herman, M. V., and Gorlin, R.: Implications of left ventricular asynergy. Am. J. Cardiol., 23:538, 1969.

Hill, A. V.: The heat of shortening and the dynamic constants of muscle. Proc. Roy. Soc. London, Series B, 126:136, 1938.

Karliner, J. S., Gault, J. H., Eckberg, D. E., Mullins, C. B., and Ross, J., Jr.: Mean velocity of fiber shortening. A simplified measure of left ventricular myocardial contractility. Circulation, 44:323, 1971.

Levine, H. J.: Clinical Cardiovascular Physiology. Grune & Stratton, New York, 1976.

Levine, H. J., and Britman, M. A.: Force-velocity relations in intact dog heart. J. Clin. Invest., 43:1383, 1964.

Levine, H. J., McIntyre, K. M., Lipana, J. G., and Bing, O. H. L.: Force-velocity relations in failing and nonfailing hearts of subjects with aortic stenosis. Am. J. Med. Sci., 259:79, 1970.

Mason, D. T.: Usefulness and limitations of the rate of rise of intraventricular pressure (dp/dt) in the evaluation of myocardial contractility in man. Amer. J. Cardiol., 23:516, 1969.

Mason, D. T., and Braunwald, E.: Studies on digitalis. IX. Effects of ouabain on the nonfailing human heart. J. Clin. Invest., 42:7, 1963.

Mason, D. T.: Regulation of cardiac performance in clinical heart disease: interactions between contractile state, mechanical abnormalities and ventricular compensatory mechanisms. Am. J. Cardiol., 32:437, 1973.

Mason, D. T.: Afterload reduction and cardiac performance: physiologic basis of systemic vasodilators as a new approach in treatment of congestive heart failure. Am. J. Med., 65:106, 1978.

Mason, D. T., and Braunwald, E.: Hemodynamic techniques in the investigation of cardiovascular function in man. In Gordon, B. (Ed.): Clinical Cardiopulmonary Physiology. 3rd ed. New York, Grune and Stratton, 1969, p. 153.

Mason, D. T., Braunwald, E., Covell, J. W., Sonnenblick, E. H., and Ross, L. L.: Assessment of cardiac contractility: The relation between the rate of pressure rise and ventricular pressure during isovolumic systole. Circulation, 44:47, 1971.

Mason, D. T., Miller, R. R., and DeMaria, A. N.: Cardiac catheterization in the clinical assessment of heart disease and ventricular performance. In Mason, D. T. (Ed.): Congestive Heart Failure. Yorke Medical Books, New York, 1976, pp. 225–271.

Mason, D. T., Sonnenblick, E. G., Ross, J., Jr., Covell, J. W., and Braunwald, E.: Time to peak dp/dt: A useful measurement for evaluating the contractile state of the human heart. Circulation, 32(Suppl. 2):145, 1965.

Mason, D. T., Spann, J. F., Jr., and Zelis, R.: Quantification of the contractile state of the intact human heart. Maximal velocity of contractile element shortening determined by the instantaneous relation between the rate of pressure rise and pressure in the left ventricle during isovolumic systole. Am. J. Cardiol., 26:248, 1970.

Mason, D. T., Spann, J. F., Jr., Zelis, R., and Amsterdam, E. A.: Alterations of hemodynamics and myocardial mechanics in patients with congestive heart failure: Pathophysiologic mechanisms and assessment of cardiac function and ventricular contractility. Prog. Cardiovasc. Dis., 12:507, 1970.

Mason, D. T., and Zelis, R.: Clinical quantification of cardiac contractility by mechanical properties of isovolumic systole. In Besse, P., and Bricaud, H. (Eds.): Left Ventricular Performance in Man. Expansion Scientifique, Paris, 1975, pp. 9–22.

Mason, D. T., Zelis, R., Amsterdam, E. A., and Massumi, R. A.: Clinical determination of left ventricular contractility by hemodynamics and myocardial mechanics. In Yu, P. N., and Goodwin, J. F. (Eds.): Progress in Cardiology. Lea and Febiger, Philadelphia, 1972, pp. 121–154.

Mason, D. T., et al.: Comparison of the contractile state of the normal, hypertrophied, and failing heart in man. In Alpert, N. R. (Ed.): Ventricular Hypertrophy. Academic Press, New York, 1971, pp. 433–444.

McCullagh, W. H., Covell, J. W., and Ross, J., Jr.: Left ventricular dilatation and diastolic compliance changes during chronic volume overloading. Circulation, 45:943, 1972.

McDonald, I. G.: Contraction of the hypertrophied left ventricle in man studied by cineradiography of epicardial markers. Amer. J. Cardiol., 30:587, 1972.

Mehmel, H. C., Krayenbuehl, H. P., and Wirz, P.: Isovolumic contraction dynamics in man according to two different muscle models. J. Appl. Physiol., 33:409, 1972.

Mirsky, I., Ghista, D., and Sandler, H.: Cardiac Mechanics: Physiological, Clinical, and Mathematical Considerations. John Wiley & Sons, New York, 1974.

Mitchell, J. H., Hefner, L. L., and Monroe, R. G.: Performance of the left ventricle. Am. J. Med., 53:481, 1972.

Parmley, W. W., Chuck, L., and Sonnenblick, E. H.: Relation of Vmax to different models of cardiac muscle. Circ. Res., 30:34, 1972.

Peterson, K. L., Uther, J. B., Shabetai, R., and Braunwald, E.: Instantaneous left ventricular tension-velocity relations obtained with an electromagnetic velocity catheter in the ascending aorta. Clin. Res., 20:173, 1972.

Rackley, C. E., Dodge, H. T., Coble, Y. D., and Hay, R. E.: A method for determining left ventricular mass in man. Circulation, 29:666, 1964.

Rackley, C. E., Russell, R. O., Moraski, R. E., Mantle, J. A., Field, B. J., and Smith, M.: Catheterization evaluation of cardiac function in acute and chronic coronary artery disease. In Mason, D. T. (Ed.): Congestive Heart Failure. Yorke Medical Books, New York, 1976, pp. 273–290.

Ross, J., Jr., Covell, J. W., Sonnenblick, E. H., and Braunwald, E.: Contractile state of the heart characterized by force-velocity relations in variably afterloaded and isovolumic beats. Circ. Res., 18:149, 1966.

Ross, J., Jr., Gault, J. H., Mason, D. T., Linhart, J. W., and Braunwald, E.: Left ventricular performance during muscular exercise in patients with and without cardiac dysfunction. Circulation, 34:597, 1966.

Russell, R. O., Jr., Frimer, M., Porter, C. M., and Dodge, H. T.: Left ventricular power in heart disease. Am. J. Cardiol., 23:136, 1969.

Salel, A. F., Kamiyama, T., Peng, C. L. Mason, D. T., Amsterdam, E. A., Massumi, R. A., and Zelis, R.: Pressure-velocity curves in the evaluation of right ventricular contractility. Circulation, 46(Suppl. 2):216, 1972.

Sarnoff, S. J., and Mitchell, J. H.: Control of function of heart. In Hamilton, W. F., and Dow, P. (Eds.): Handbook of Physiology. Vol I, Section 2. American Physiological Society, Washington, D.C., 1962, pp. 489–532.

Siegel, J. H., and Sonnenblick, E. H.: Isometric time-tension relationships as an index of myocardial contractility. Circ. Res., 12:597, 1963.

Sonnenblick, E. H.: Implications of muscle mechanics in the heart. Fed. Proc., 21:975, 1962.

Sonnenblick, E. H.: Instantaneous force-velocity-length determinants in the contraction of heart muscle. Circ. Res., 16:441, 1965.

Sonnenblick, E. H.: Contractility of cardiac muscle. Circ. Res., 27:479, 1970.

Sonnenblick, E. H., Ross, J., Jr., Spotnitz, H. M., Covell, J. W., and Spiro, D.: The ultrastructure of the heart in systole and diastole: Changes in sarcomere length. Circ. Res., 21:423, 1967.

Taylor, R. R., Ross, J., Jr., Covell, J. W., and Sonnenblick, E. H.: A quantitative analysis of left ventricular myocardial function in the intact, sedated dog. Circ. Res., 21:99, 1967.

Urschel, C. W., Covell, J. W., Sonnenblick, E. H., Ross, J., Jr., and Braunwald, E.: Myocardial mechanics in aortic and mitral valvular regurgitation: the concept of instantaneous impedance as a determinant of the performance of the intact heart. J. Clin. Invest., 47:867, 1968.

Urschel, C. W., Henderson, A. H., and Sonnenblick, E. H.: Model dependency of ventricular force-velocity relations: importance of developed pressure. Fed. Proc., 29:719, 1970.

Wolk, M. H., Keefe, J. F., Bing, O. H. L., Finkelstein, L. J., and Levine, H. J.: Estimation of Vmax in auxotonic systoles from the rate of relative increase of isovolumic pressure: (dP/dt)KP. J. Clin. Invest., 50:1276, 1971.

Yang, S. S., Bentivoglio, L. G., Maranhao, V., and Goldberg, H.: Cardiac Catheterization Data and Hemodynamic Parameters. F. A. Davis Co., Philadelphia, 1972.

Yeatman, L. A., Jr., Parmley, W. W., and Sonnenblick, E. H.: Effects of temperature on series elasticity and contractile element motion in heart muscle. Am. J. Physiol., 217:1030, 1969.

Yeatman, L. A., Jr., Parmley, W. W., Urschel, C. W., and Sonnenblick, E. H.: Dynamics of contractile elements in isometric contractions of cardiac muscle. Am. J. Physiol., 220:534, 1971.

Zelis, R., Amsterdam, E. A., and Mason, D. T.: "Isometric" Vmax as an index of contractility independent of series elastic and fiber shortening: Implications concerning pressure-velocity data in myocardial fibrosis, valvular regurgitation, ventricular aneurysm and ventricular septal defect. Circulation, 44(Suppl. II):89, 1971.

9

Cardiac Output, Cardiac Performance, Hypertrophy, Dilatation, Valvular Disease, Ischemic Heart Disease, and Pericardial Disease

HAROLD T. DODGE, AND J. WARD KENNEDY

CARDIAC OUTPUT

The measurement of cardiac output by what is now known as the Fick principle was first applied in animals at the end of the last century. Since this method requires sampling of mixed venous blood from the pulmonary artery or right ventricle, its application to man followed the development of right heart catheterization in the 1940s. The indicator dilution method for determining cardiac output was developed by Stewart in 1897 and by Hamilton in 1929 and became widely applied in the 1950s. Both the direct Fick and indicator dilution methods have become standard techniques in cardiac catheterization laboratories and have recently been brought into limited use in intensive and coronary care units for the serial measurement of cardiac output during the course of severe illness. More recently, the development of sensitive thermistor probes has allowed modification of the indicator dilution method to the thermodilution method, in which warm or cool saline instead of a dye is used as an indicator. The development and wide application of angiocardiography have provided another method for measurement of the output of the heart by analysis of the change in volume (stroke volume) of the left ventricle during the cardiac cycle. Quantitative angiocardiographic methods for measuring left ventricular stroke volume and minute output are particularly useful in evaluating ventricular performance in patients with heart disease, as will be discussed later.

In addition to the above methods for directly measuring cardiac output in man there have also been many methods devised to estimate cardiac output indirectly. These include analysis of arterial pulse waves; the ballistocardiogram; systolic time intervals using electrocardiographic, phonocardiographic, and carotid pulse wave data; ultrasonic echocardiography; and, most recently, the development and application of instruments for measuring blood flow velocity with ultrasound by the Doppler shift principle. Although some of these methods are useful in predicting directional changes in cardiac output during the course of illness, they all appear to be less accurate than the direct Fick and indicator dilution methods.

Fick Method

This method depends upon a knowledge of the quantity of oxygen entering the system measured as the oxygen consumption as determined from samples of expired air and the difference in oxygen content between venous and arterial blood. Since venous blood from different parts of the body has a variable oxygen content, it must be mixed to obtain a sample that represents total body venous oxygen content. When blood passes through the right ventricle, adequate mixing occurs. The mixed venous sample for Fick cardiac output determination is therefore obtained from the pulmonary artery through a right heart catheter. Occasionally, a right ventricular sampling site is utilized when the pulmonary artery cannot be entered. The arterial sample may be obtained from any convenient peripheral artery in the absence of a right-to-left cardiac shunt. When a shunt is present, the sample must be obtained upstream from the shunt.

The formula for determining cardiac output (CO) is as follows:

$$\text{Cardiac output} = \frac{\text{Oxygen Consumption}}{\text{Arteriovenous oxygen difference}}$$

A typical value for oxygen consumption in an average-sized adult male at rest is 240 ml. per minute. The normal resting arteriovenous oxygen difference is in the range of 40 ml. of O_2 per liter of blood. Substituting into the formula,

$$CO = \frac{240}{40} = 6.0 \text{ L./minute}$$

Errors in the measurement of oxygen consumption and oxygen content of arterial and venous blood result in a total error of the method of 8 to 10 per cent. In applying the method, the chief limitations are the necessity of right heart catheterization and the cooperation of the patient to obtain a representative sample of expired air that can be used for measuring oxygen consumption.

Indicator Dilution Method

The indicator dilution technique is preferred over the direct Fick method in many laboratories because it eliminates the need for right heart catheterization. A known quantity of indicator (I), usually indocyanine green, is injected into the venous circulation and the resultant time-concentration curve is determined by continuous withdrawal of arterial blood through a densitometer.

$$\text{Cardiac output} = \frac{I}{\bar{C} \cdot t}$$

where $\bar{C}$ represents the mean concentration of the indicator during the time (t) from the appearance to disappearance of the indicator as determined from the time-concentration curve. The validity of the method depends on two assumptions: (1) that there is complete mixing of indicator prior to sampling and (2) that the indicator concentration curve with respect to time represents only the first passage of the indicator past the sampling site. Since recirculation of indicator distorts the terminal portion of the primary curve to a greater or lesser extent, depending upon the injection and sampling sites and the status of circulatory dynamics, various methods have been developed to separate the primary curve from the recirculation curve. These methods are based on the assumption that the fall of concentration in the primary curve follows an exponential time course that can be determined by relating the logarithm of the concentration to time. The time-concentration curve is plotted on a semilogarithmic graph, and the initial portion of the primary curve is identified and then extrapolated as a straight line to zero. This process eliminates the recirculation component of the curve and thus defines the primary curve. An adequate portion of the primary curve must be obtained to permit this extrapolation. From the primary curve, values for $(\bar{C})$ and (t) are determined. Small special-purpose computers are now available to separate the primary and recirculation curves and give immediate cardiac output results.

The thermo-dilution technique is similar to the indicator dilution technique described above but has the advantage that there is no significant recirculation of the indicator since the temperature difference of the injectate and the blood is lost into tissue prior to recirculation. In general, there is good agreement between the results of the Fick, indicator dilution, and thermo-dilution methods for determining cardiac output in man. The development of a balloon tipped, flow directed thermo-dilution catheter that can be inserted into the pulmonary artery without fluoroscopic control has greatly facilitated the use of the thermo-dilution cardiac output technique. This method is now widely used as an aid in the care of critically ill cardiac patients.

Normal Cardiac Output

Since the cardiac output is a fundamental measurement of cardiac function, it has been the subject of extensive study in normal animals and man, at rest and during various stresses, and in patients with all types of heart diseases. This subject is well reviewed by Wade and Bishop (1962). Cardiac output is best expressed in terms of body size, and, in general, body surface area is used instead of body weight. The term cardiac index is used to refer to the cardiac output per square meter of body surface area. It is frequently convenient to express the output of the heart per beat as stroke volume or the cardiac index per beat as stroke index. The resting cardiac index in normal man is approximately 3.3 L. per min. per $M.^2$, with a low value of about 2.8 L. per min. per $M.^2$ Cardiac output decreases with age at the rate of approximately 25 ml. per min. per $M.^2$ per year after early adulthood. Assuming a resting heart rate of 70 beats per minute, the normal stroke index is 46 ml.

Regulation of Cardiac Output

The cardiac output normally increases under the stimulus of muscular exercise up to five times the resting value, depending somewhat upon the age and physical training of the individual. There are many factors which make possible such large changes of flow, some of which will be described below.

The return of venous blood to the right heart is regulated in such a manner that the venous return equals the systemic output of the left ventricle. Venous return to a great extent is regulated by alterations in the tone of the venous capacitance vessels which contain most of the blood volume. Increases or decreases in venous tone therefore have a marked effect on the filling of the right atrium and ventricle and thereby on the output of the left ventricle. Increases or decreases of circulating blood volume also cause respective changes of venous return and cardiac output if not compensated for by changes in venous tone. Cardiac output may increase for a short time with increases in blood volume as occurs with overtransfusion, but compensatory increased volume of venous capacitance vessels soon reduces the right ventricular filling volume, pressure, and output. In patients with chronic heart failure, circulating blood volume is chronically increased owing to retention of sodium and water by the kidneys, and venous tone is increased. As a result, an increased volume of blood is present in the central circulation, which elevates the filling volume and pressure of the two ventricles to maintain cardiac output through the Frank-Starling mechanism. Accordingly, venous return is a major factor in the control of cardiac output in both health and disease and is determined by the blood volume and the capacity and tone of the venous bed.

Autonomic Control of Cardiac Output

The autonomic nervous system has a major controlling influence on cardiac output by its ef-

fect upon heart rate, myocardial contractility, and vasomotor tone. In general, parasympathetic tone is greater than sympathetic tone when an individual is at rest. Maximal stimuli to increase sympathetic tone occur during heavy exercise and under severe psychologic stress. Increased parasympathetic tone occurs with vomiting, occasionally in response to severe pain, and with vigorous carotid sinus massage. Sympathetic nerve stimulation has a positive inotropic and chronotropic effect on the heart, resulting in increased heart rate and increased myocardial contractility, which results in increased force, extent, and velocity of myocardial fiber shortening. This causes an increase in stroke volume, provided that venous return is adequate to maintain filling of the right ventricle. In contrast to this, increased parasympathetic tone decreases the heart rate and little or no effect on contractility of the ventricles. Peripheral vasculature tone increases with sympathetic stimulation, and this results in increased venous return to the right heart, increased ventricular filling pressure, and increased stroke volume. The effects of increased sympathetic tone — i.e., increased heart rate, increased myocardial contractility, and increased venous return — all combine to increase cardiac output.

Peripheral Oxygen Requirement

In general, cardiac output varies according to the requirement of the peripheral tissues for oxygen. Control of regional circulation is maintained so that cardiac output is shunted to the particular organ in need of oxygen. For example, during physical exertion blood flow is preferentially increased to the working muscles and reduced to the splanchnic bed and kidneys. When there is a marked reduction in cardiac output, as in some patients with heart failure, there is reduced blood flow to the skin, muscle, and splanchnic vascular beds. As the cardiac output drops further, renal and finally cerebral blood flow falls. Regulation of regional blood flow therefore plays an important role in maintaining the tissue oxygen needs of the body during various activities and under many different conditions.

Vascular Resistance

The peripheral vasculature of the systemic circulation and, to a lesser extent, of the pulmonary circulation is under autonomic nervous system and hormonal control. The vascular resistance, therefore, will vary depending on the hemodynamic state of the patient. Systemic vascular resistance becomes chronically elevated in idiopathic or renal vascular hypertension.

In chronic mitral stenosis, pulmonary vascular resistance is chronically elevated. It is frequently important to determine the systemic and/or pulmonary vascular resistance.

The resistance of a vascular bed can be calculated if the flow and pressure drop across the bed are known. For these calculations, mean pressures are utilized and the values are reported in dynes-second centimeters^{-5} (dsc.$^{-5}$). In order to calculate resistance in dsc.$^{-5}$, pressure measured in mm. Hg must be converted into dynes per cm.^{2} by multiplying by 1332. Liters per minute are converted to ml. per sec. by multiplying further by 0.06, yielding a conversion factor of 80. Therefore:

$$\text{Resistance in dsc}^{-5} = \frac{\text{Mean pressure (mm. Hg)} \times 80}{\text{Flow (L./min.)}}$$

Systemic vascular resistance (SVR) is calculated as follows:

$$\text{SVR} = \frac{\text{Mean arterial pressure} \times 80}{\text{Cardiac output (L./min.)}}$$

Total pulmonary artery resistance is calculated in a similar manner. In some instances it is useful also to measure the pulmonary vascular resistance (PVR) in order to separate the components of total pulmonary resistance which results from the pulmonary vasculature from that component resulting from left atrial pressure. This is, of course, most useful in evaluating patients with left atrial hypertension such as occurs with mitral stenosis or left ventricular failure. Pulmonary vascular resistance is determined by using the pulmonary flow and the difference between the mean pulmonary artery (Pa mean) and mean left atrial pressure (LA mean).

$$\text{PVR} = \frac{(\text{Pa mean} - \text{LA mean}) \times 80}{\text{Pulmonary flow (L./min.)}}$$

Normal values for systemic, total pulmonary, and pulmonary vascular resistance are listed in Table 9–1 as reported by Barratt-Boyes (1958). As is apparent from these values, total pulmonary resistance is mostly the result of left atrial pressure, not resistance in the pulmonary vasculature. In other words, about two thirds of right heart pressure work goes into filling the left heart under normal resting conditions.

Therapeutic Control of Cardiac Output

In situations of high or low cardiac output due to disease, the physician often attempts to control the cardiac output with drugs or by

TABLE 9–1 NORMAL VALUES— INTRACARDIAC PRESSURES

	Systolic	Diastolic	Mean
Right Atrium	3–7	0–2	0–6
Right Ventricle	15–30	0–5	–
Pulmonary Artery	15–30	6–12	9–17
Left Atrium	–	–	5–12
Left Ventricle	100–140	2–12	–
Vascular Resistance			
Systemic	1130±178 dsc.⁵		
Total Pulmonary	205± 51 dsc.⁵		
Pulmonary Vascular	67± 23 dsc.⁵		

(Adapted from data in Barratt-Boyes, B. G., and Wood, E. H.: J. Lab. Clin. Med., *51*:72, 1958.)

other maneuvers. In several different circumstances, cardiac output is abnormally high, as in febrile patients, conditions of increased metabolism such as thyrotoxicosis, arteriovenous shunts, severe anemia, or ineffective oxygen carrying capacity of hemoglobin as in carbon monoxide poisoning. In all these conditions, cardiac output returns toward normal with correction of the abnormality that caused the elevated output.

In conditions of abnormally low cardiac output, the physician often is faced with a more difficult problem. Low cardiac output due to inadequate venous return as a result of inadequate blood volume is easily treated with transfusion or fluid replacement. Low cardiac output due to bradycardia may be successfully treated with drugs or an artificial pacemaker. When cardiac output is inadequate because of poor myocardial contraction, sympathomimetic drugs or digitalis glycosides may be used to increase myocardial contractile force. At times, venous filling pressure may be artificially elevated above normal levels by the administration of saline or plasma in an attempt to increase cardiac output. Unfortunately, the depressed cardiac output such as occurs in advanced myocardial failure often remains low in spite of current therapeutic methods.

Recently, work by several investigators has shown that chronic reduction of peripheral vascular resistance or ventricular afterload may be achieved by various arterial and venous dilating drugs such as sublingual and topical nitroglycerin, sublingual or oral isosorbide dinitrate, oral hydralazine, and nitroprusside given by continuous infusion. Additional vasodilating agents are also currently being evaluated for this purpose. These vasodilating agents, which are now often referred to as "ventricular unloading drugs," result in increased cardiac output with no increase in cardiac work by reducing systemic vascular resistance. When applied to patients with advanced heart failure and/or cardiogenic shock, these agents have resulted in reduced mortality and improved medical management of heart failure.

CARDIAC CATHETERIZATION

The technique of cardiac catheterization merits brief mention in a text of pathologic physiology because much of what is known of altered cardiac function in various disease states has been gained through the use of this technique. Cardiac catheterization was first carried out by Forssmann in 1929 when he passed a catheter into his own right atrium. It was André Cournand and colleagues who introduced the use of this important technique for the study of normal and pathologic physiology. Today, all chambers of the heart and much of the venous and arterial vasculature are regularly catheterized for purposes of blood sampling, pressure recording, and the injection of radiographic contrast material for angiographic visualization. The usual sites of catheter insertion include the veins of the antecubital fossa, the femoral vein, and the brachial and femoral arteries. Large vessels may be entered safely with the percutaneous Seldinger technique. This method involves needle puncture of the vessel with insertion of a flexible guide wire over which the catheter is inserted. When smaller vessels are entered, a small incision with isolation of the vessel for cannulation is required.

Catheterization of the right atrium, ventricle, and pulmonary artery is performed by advancing a catheter from a large peripheral vein through these chambers under fluoroscopic guidance. The development of a flow directed balloon tipped catheter by Swan and Ganz now permits right heart catheterization without fluoroscopy. The large arteries, aorta, and left ventricle are catheterized in a manner similar to that used in the right heart by passing the catheter retrograde from an insertion site in a large artery — usually the brachial or femoral artery. Specially designed catheters are used to selectively cannulate the left and right coronary arteries for purposes of coronary angiography. The left atrium is the cardiac chamber least accessible to the cardiologist. It is usually catheterized by the transseptal technique in which, with the aid of a long needle, a catheter is passed across the interatrial septum from right-to-left atrium. Occasionally, the left atrium is catheterized retrograde across the mitral valve from the left ventricle. In the hands of an experienced cardiac catheterization team, the risk of

death resulting from these procedures is between one and two per thousand.

Intracardiac Pressure Recordings

Recording pressure in the various chambers of the heart and the great vessels is often a major goal of cardiac catheterization. This is usually accomplished by attaching a fluid-filled catheter to a pressure transducer. The electrical output of the transducer is amplified, displayed on an oscilloscope, and recorded on paper or magnetic tape. The system is calibrated and the zero level of the transducers is set at the level of the midthorax. Normal pressures for the various cardiac chambers are given in Table 9–1. At times, it is more convenient to limit catheterization to the right side of the heart. When this is the case, an estimate of pulmonary venous pressure and left atrial pressure can be obtained by passing an end-hole catheter out into a terminal pulmonary artery. When "wedged" in this position, the catheter records the pressure transmitted back across the pulmonary capillary bed from the pulmonary veins. This pressure is termed the pulmonary wedge or pulmonary capillary pressure. The mean pulmonary wedge pressure will generally be within 2 mm. Hg of the mean left atrial pressure, unless pulmonary venous obstruction is present.

In the last several years, various types of catheters have been developed which contain a pressure transducer at the distal tip. These catheter tip manometers are capable of recording pressures more accurately in the heart because they are free from the hydraulic damping effects, time delays, and motion artifacts which distort pressures recorded through fluid-filled catheters. These improved pressure recording systems have allowed the detailed analysis of the rapid pressure changes which occur in the right and left ventricle during early systole and early diastole. The maximum rate of rise of the left ventricular pressure, generally referred to as LV dp/dt, has been used as an index of left ventricular myocardial performance. Catheter tip manometers make it possible to record LV dp/dt with sufficient accuracy to permit their use for evaluating myocardial contractility in man. Multiple variables influence the LV dp/dt, including heart rate, filling pressure (preload), aortic diastole pressure (afterload), myocardial inotropic state, and left ventricular diastolic volume. Because of these many influences, LV dp/dt is more useful in evaluating changes of myocardial performance in a single patient than in comparing the myocardial performance in one patient with that of another.

Various types of valvular abnormalities due to congenital and rheumatic heart disease can now be treated surgically, so that it has become important to evaluate precisely the severity of valve stenosis or incompetence or both. Congenital aortic, pulmonary, and postrheumatic mitral and aortic valve stenosis are the most common types of valvular stenosis, although the other cardiac valves may become stenotic on either a congenital or rheumatic basis. Cardiac catheterization is required to measure the pressure on each side of a stenotic valve, so that the pressure gradient across the valve can be determined. Figure 9–1 is taken from the simultaneous recording of left ventricular and aortic pressure in a patient with aortic stenosis. The high-fidelity left ventricular pressure was obtained with a catheter tip manometer. The shaded area represents the gradient across the stenotic aortic valve. The mean gradient can be obtained by dividing the shaded area by the duration of the valve gradient. Figure 9–2 is taken from simultaneous pressure recordings in the left atrium and left ventricle in a patient with mitral stenosis. The left ventricular pressure was recorded through a fluid-filled catheter and there is some oscillation in the pressure during diastole, indicating an underdamped pressure manometer system. The diastolic gradient across the mitral valve is represented by the shaded area. In these two examples, large pressure gradients are present across these stenotic valves, but since the pressure gradient is

a function of both valve orifice size and flow across the valve, the severity of valvular stenosis is best determined by calculation of the cross-sectional area of the valve. This can be done by utilizing the formulas developed by Gorlin and Gorlin. These relate the gradient in pressure across the valve during the period of valve flow and rate of flow across the valve to the area of the valve orifice. Empirical correction factors have been introduced based upon surgical and postmortem observations.

The basic formula is as follows:

$$\text{Valve orifice} = \frac{\text{Valve flow}}{(K)\ \sqrt{\text{Pressure gradient}}}$$

In the case of the mitral valve the valve flow is measured per diastolic second, whereas when calculating the area of the aortic valve orifice the flow is determined per systolic second. The pressure gradient is the mean difference in pressure across the valve during diastolic filling for mitral stenosis and systolic ejection for aortic stenosis. The K values are 31.0 and 44.5 for the mitral and aortic valves respectively. When there is no valvular incompetence or intracardiac shunt, the flow across the valve is equal to the cardiac output. When valvular incompetence is also present, the flow across the valve is increased and must be taken into account if an accurate valve area is to be obtained. Usual-

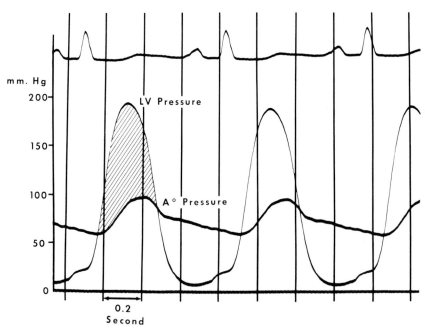

Figure 9–1 Left ventricular and central aortic pressure in a patient with tight valvular aortic stenosis. The shaded area indicates the pressure gradient across the valve during systole.

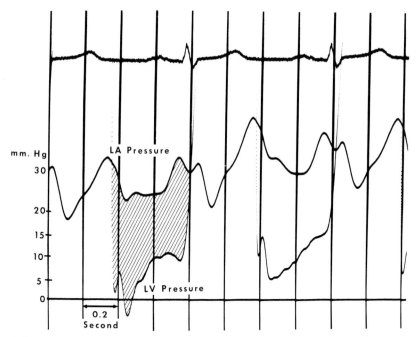

Figure 9-2 Left ventricular and left atrial pressure in a patient with mitral stenosis. Only the lower portion of the left ventricular pressure is seen. The shaded area indicates the pressure gradient across the mitral valve during diastole.

ly the mitral valve orifice is constricted to less than 1.2 cm.^{2} or the aortic valve to less than 1.0 cm.^{2} before symptoms develop that are significant enough to consider surgical correction.

Intracardiac Shunts

Cardiac catheterization techniques are used to locate and quantify intracardiac shunts. This is generally done by determining the oxygen content of blood samples from the appropriate cardiac chambers and great vessels. Frequently, the cardiac catheter will pass through the intracardiac defect or abnormal venous or arterial channel directly, demonstrating its presence. The introduction of a dye, radiopaque contrast media, or hydrogen gas may also be used to detect or demonstrate abnormal blood flow.

Left-to-Right Shunts

Abnormal shunting of blood occurs most commonly from the systemic to the venous circulation and is identified by demonstrating oxygenated blood entering the venous circulation. Conditions in which this occurs include patent ductus arteriosus; aorticopulmonary window; atrial septal defect; ventricular septal defect; and anomalous pulmonary venous drainage to the vena cava, coronary sinus, or right atrium. Occasionally, left-to-right shunts may develop following birth, as with the rupture of a sinus of Valsalva aneurysm into the right heart or the development of a ventricular septal defect following infarction of the interventricular septum. Arteriovenous fistulae may be congenital or acquired and result in a functional arteriovenous shunting of blood.

In general, these defects are easy to recognize at cardiac catheterization by sampling blood from the appropriate sites on the right side of the heart. An increase in oxygen saturation or content occurs at the level of the shunt, thus localizing it anatomically. By comparing the oxygen content of mixed venous blood proximal and distal to the level of the shunt, the volume of the shunt can be calculated utilizing the Fick principle. As shown below, these formulas yield a value for systemic blood flow and pulmonary blood flow. The difference between the two is the shunt flow. The ratio of pulmonary to systemic flow is often used to express the severity of the shunt. For example, if the pulmonary flow is 10 L. per min. and the systemic flow is 5 L. per min., the magnitude of the shunt would be 2:1.

In the case of a ventricular septal defect and in the absence or right-to-left shunting; for example,

$$\text{Pulmonary blood flow} = \frac{O_2 \text{ consumption (ml./min.)}}{\text{Systemic arterial } O_2 \text{ content} - \text{Pulmonary arterial } O_2 \text{ content}}$$

$$\text{Systemic blood flow} = \frac{O_2 \text{ consumption (ml./min.)}}{\text{Systemic arterial } O_2 \text{ content} - \text{Right atrial } O_2 \text{ content}}$$

$$\text{Left-to-right shunt flow} = \text{Pulmonary blood flow} - \text{Systemic blood flow}$$

In the case of an atrial septal defect, the mixed venous O_2 content needs to be obtained from samples taken in the inferior and superior venae cavae. In this situation,

$$\text{Mixed venous } O_2 \text{ content} = \frac{\text{SVC } O_2 + 2 \text{ IVC } O_2}{3}$$

The 2:1 ratio is employed because of the large blood flow in the IVC relative to that in the SVC. In resting subjects the oxygen content of IVC blood is higher than that of SVC samples because of the contribution of renal venous blood, which has a relatively high oxygen content.

Cyanotic Heart Disease

The term cyanotic heart disease is used to refer to patients with systemic arterial oxygen desaturation due to a cardiovascular abnormality. Cyanosis is generally the result of the shunting of systemic venous blood into the systemic arterial circulation and occurs in such conditions as tetralogy of Fallot, single ventricle, truncus arteriosus, tricuspid atresia, and transposition of the great vessels.

For right-to-left shunting to occur across a patent ductus, ventricular septal defect, or atrial septal defect, the pressure on the right side of the defect must be higher than on the left side at least at some time during the cardiac cycle. Occasionally, right-to-left shunting only occurs during exercise and may be noted by exertional cyanosis. Right-to-left shunting occurs across a patent ductus either because it is located distal to a coarctation of the aorta or because of the presence of pulmonary hypertension of such severity that the total pulmonary resistance is greater than the systemic resistance. In this situation, there may be differential cyanosis, with cyanosis greater in the lower extremities. When right-to-left shunting occurs in patients with ventricular septal defect it is associated with either pulmonary hypertension due to increased pulmonary vascular resistance or pulmonary stenosis of the valvular or infundibular type. Pulmonary stenosis and ventricular septal defect are most often seen as features of the tetralogy of Fallot, the other two features

being right ventricular hypertrophy and dextroposition of the aorta with overriding of the interventricular septum, so that the aorta communicates more or less directly with the right ventricular outflow tract. Atrial septal defect is less often associated with a right-to-left shunt. When this occurs, pulmonary hypertension has resulted in right ventricular failure and elevation of right atrial pressure to a level higher than the pressure in the left atrium. In the combination of atrial septal defect and tricuspid stenosis, right-to-left shunting at the atrial level will occur without pulmonary stenosis or right ventricular failure.

The calculation of right-to-left shunt is similar to the calculation of left-to-right shunts except that pulmonary venous blood must be either sampled or assumed to be 98 per cent saturated. If the patient is breathing oxygen, it can be assumed that the sample is fully saturated. Pulmonary blood flow (PBF) is then determined by the following formula:

$$\text{PBF} = \frac{O_2 \text{ consumption}}{\text{Pulmonary venous } O_2 - \text{Pulmonary artery } O_2}$$

The systemic flow is calculated as follows:

$$\text{SF} = \frac{O_2 \text{ consumption}}{\text{Systemic arterial } O_2 - \text{Mixed venous } O_2}$$

The mixed venous O_2 should be obtained proximal to the shunt, since a bidirectional shunt may be present. The magnitude of right-to-left shunt is determined by subtracting the pulmonary blood flow from the systemic blood flow. When a bidirectional shunt is present, the effective pulmonary blood flow (Eff Pul BF) must be determined. This is the quantity of blood that picks up oxygen while circulating through the lungs and is determined by the following formula:

$$\text{Eff Pul BF} = \frac{O_2 \text{ consumption}}{\text{Pulmonary venous } O_2 - \text{Mixed venous } O_2}$$

A bidirectional shunt may then be calculated as follows:

$$\text{Right-to-left shunt} =$$
$$\text{Systemic flow} - \text{Effective pulmonary flow}$$

Left-to-right shunt =
    Pulmonary flow — Effective pulmonary flow

The validity of flow values determined by these methods depends upon rapid and accurate sampling of blood in the various cardiac chambers and vessels concerned. Blood entering the right atrium from the superior vena cava, inferior vena cava, and coronary sinus varies considerably in its O_2 content. The inferior vena cava blood has a high O_2 content owing to a large component of renal venous blood, whereas the blood draining the coronary circulation has a very low O_2 content. The atrium does not mix the blood well, so that blood flows in a laminar fashion through the atrium and into the right ventricle. Better mixing occurs here, so that the blood entering the pulmonary artery is usually relatively homogeneous. The non-mixing of blood in the right atrium and vena cava results in the possibility of sampling errors and in resultant inaccurate shunt flow calculations. Rapid sampling and duplicate measurements can, however, give good estimates of flow which are of value in the clinical evaluation of patients.

Frequently, a left-to-right shunt is associated with pulmonary hypertension. When the pulmonary vascular resistance reaches systemic levels, right-to-left shunting develops and surgical correction of the defect becomes hazardous, if not impossible. In the presence of pulmonary hypertension due to cardiac shunts, great care must be taken in calculating blood flow and pulmonary artery pressure so that accurate pulmonary resistance values can be obtained. In borderline cases it may be useful to measure pulmonary flow and pressure before and during oxygen administration. If pulmonary vascular resistance falls with oxygen administration, surgical correction may be possible, whereas failure of a drop in pulmonary artery pressure suggests that pulmonary vascular resistance is fixed and not due in part to anoxia.

LEFT VENTRICULAR VOLUME AND MASS

There are now four methods of determining left ventricular chamber volumes in man: (1) indicator dilution; (2) radiographic contrast angiocardiography; (3) isotope angiography; and (4) echocardiography. With the indicator dilution methods, an indicator is injected into the left ventricle and sampled immediately above the aortic valves with a sensor which responds rapidly to changes in the concentration of the indicator. The indicator dilution curves show a steplike decrease in indicator concentration, with the change of concentration per beat

being a function of the volume of the left ventricle at end-diastole and the dilution with each stroke (stroke volume). End-diastolic volume (EDV) is computed as follows:

$$EDV = \frac{\text{Stroke volume}}{\left(1 - \frac{Cn}{Cn - 1}\right)}$$

where stroke volume is determined by the standard indicator dilution method for measuring cardiac output and $\frac{Cn}{Cn - 1}$ is the ratio of beat-to-beat changes of concentration of indicator in the aorta. The accuracy of the volume determination is dependent on complete mixing of indicator in the left ventricle, a concentration of dye in the aorta which is equivalent to that in the ventricle, and a sufficiently high-frequency response of the system for indicator detection to determine accurately indicator concentration and ventricular washout as a step function. Various indicators have been used and include dyes, saline, and cold saline with appropriate indicator detection systems. These methods have the advantage of requiring a small volume of indicator which does not in itself cause physiologic changes, and measurements can be repeated frequently. In general, the indicator dilution methods have given larger end-diastolic and residual volumes than the angiocardiographic methods. This difference may be related to uneven mixing of the indicator.

Left ventricular chamber volumes can also be determined from angiocardiograms and cineangiocardiograms taken in biplane as well as single plane projections (Fig. 9–3). The methods most generally used assume that the left ventricle can be represented by an ellipsoid reference figure, with volume computed as

$$V = 4/3 \, \pi \, abc$$

where a equals the major semidiameter and b and c equal the two minor semidiameters. The differences in methods used for computing volume by various laboratories are due to differences in the methods applied for determining the chamber dimensions. It has been demonstrated that in most subjects the two minor semidiameters (b and c) are similar. Accordingly, chamber volume can be computed from films taken in a single projection by assuming that b and c are equal, and the formula for computing volume becomes

$$P = 4/3 \, \pi \, ab^2$$

When the time of filming is recorded together with the electrocardiogram and left ventricular pressure, as shown in Figure 9–4, the computed volumes can be related to time within the cardiac cycle to construct a left ventricular volume

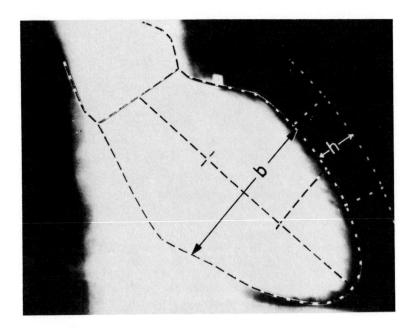

Figure 9–3 Angiocardiogram with the left ventricle and a segment of left ventricular wall outlined. Wall thickness is indicated by *h* and semidiameter by *b*. (From Dodge, H. T.: Determination of left ventricular mass. Radiol. Clin. North Am., 9:459, 1971.)

curve as shown in Figure 9–5. From this volume curve, end-diastolic, end-systolic, and stroke volumes can be determined. The portion of the end-diastolic volume ejected with systole $\left(\dfrac{SV}{EDV}\right)$ has been termed the systolic ejection fraction. From the slopes of the ejection and filling limbs, the rates of ventricular ejection and filling, respectively, can be computed. In addition, the angiocardiographic methods provide information on ventricular shape and dimensions, permit visualization of focal contraction abnormalities as seen in ischemic heart disease, and also provide information on wall thickness. When added to chamber dimensions, the latter has made it possible to compute left ventricular mass as follows:

Vol. LV chamber + Wall =

$$4/3\pi\,(a + h)\,(b + h)\,(c + h)$$

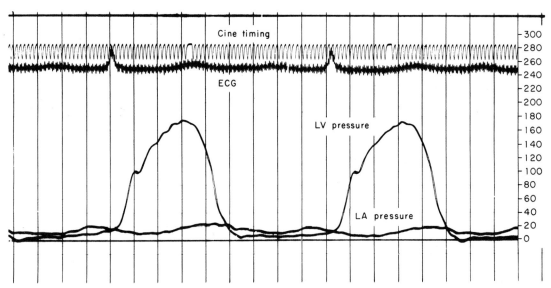

Figure 9–4 Recording of time of cine filming (65 frames per second) with respect to the ECG and left ventricular and atrial pressure in a patient with mitral stenosis.

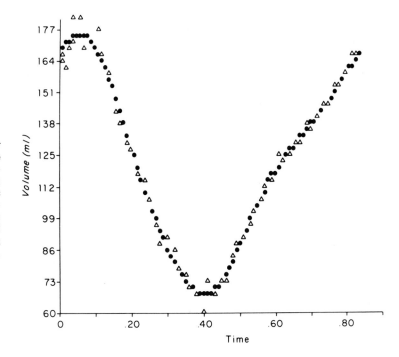

Figure 9-5 Left ventricular volumes computed from cine films taken at 65 frames per second are plotted as triangles with respect to time within the cardiac cycle. From these computed volumes a volume curve has been generated, as shown by the solid circles, through the use of a curve-fitting computer program.

LV mass (g.) = [(Vol. chamber + wall) − Vol. chamber] 1.050

where a, b, and c equal chamber semidiameters as previously defined, h equals wall thickness, and 1.050 is the specific gravity of heart muscle. Normal values for left ventricular chamber volumes, ejection fraction, wall thickness, and mass are given in Table 9–2.

With the rapid development of nuclear medicine techniques in cardiology, several methods for determining cardiac chamber volumes and left and right ventricular systolic ejection fraction have become available. The most useful are those utilizing a gamma scintillation camera (Anger camera) to record radioactivity in the heart chambers. Activity can be observed following the intravenous bolus injection of the radionuclide as it passes through the right heart, pulmonary circulation, and left heart chambers.

This "first pass" technique has the advantage of sequential observation of the four cardiac chambers so that overlapping of the chambers is avoided. With the "first pass" technique, the radioactive material is in the heart for only a short time, so the resolution of the gamma camera images is limited by low radioactivity counting rates. The blood pool method, currently favored by many laboratories, utilizes radioactive agents which are bound to red blood cells or albumin, so that the tracer remains in the intravascular compartment. The patient is monitored by an electrocardiogram, which is linked to the gamma camera so that the radionuclide images of the heart can be timed with the cardiac cycle. In this manner, a high resolution image of the cardiac chambers can be developed over several hundred heart beats for each phase of the cardiac cycle, as illustrated in Figure

TABLE 9-2 NORMAL VALUES IN ADULTS AND CHILDREN

	End-Diastolic Volume (ml./M²)	Stroke Volume (ml./M²)	End-Systolic Volume (ml./M²)	Ejection Fraction (SV/EDV)	Wall Thickness (mm.)	Left Ventricle Mass (g./M²)
ADULTS	70±20	45±13	24	0.67±0.08	10.9±2.0	92±16
CHILDREN AND INFANTS						
Less than 2 Years of Age	42±10	28.6	13.4	0.68±0.05		96±11
More than 2 Years of Age						
(3 to 16 Years)	73±11	44±5	27±7	0.63±0.05		86±11

(From Dodge, H. T.: Determination of left ventricular volume and mass. Radiol. Clin. North Am., 9:459, 1971.)

EJECTION
FRACTION

R—WAVE
SYNCHRONOUS
EQUILIBRIUM
IMAGES

^{99m}Tc—RBC

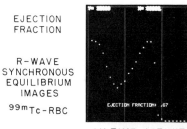

LV TIME ACTIVITY

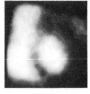

END DIASTOLIC IMAGE   LV AND BKG REGIONS

Figure 9–6 This figure illustrates the technique of isotope angiography for the determination of left ventricular ejection fraction. In the lower left panel is the end-diastolic image of the heart in the left anterior oblique view. In the right lower panel the region of the left ventricle has been identified and to the right a background region (BKG) from which background radiation levels are determined. Cardiac images are developed by collecting scintillation information in 0.04-second windows over several hundred cardiac cycles by interfacing the gamma camera-computer with the electrocardiogram. In the upper panel, the time activity from the left ventricular region of interest is displayed, and the computed ejection fraction is presented. In this case, the time activity curve is normal and the ejection fraction is 67 per cent.

9–6. This usually requires two to six minutes of imaging, during which time the patient must remain in a constant hemodynamic state and at relatively unchanging heart rate.

These radionuclide techniques for imaging the cardiac chambers have been termed isotope angiography. Advances in technology have been rapid in this field, such that it is likely that several types of standard radiographic contrast angiography will be replaced by this safer, non-invasive method in the near future. Like radiographic contrast angiography, isotope angiography requires expensive imaging equipment and subjects the patient to ionizing radiation. Expense and minimal radiation hazard will limit its use.

Echocardiography is a technique which utilizes pulsed high frequency sound to determine the position and motion of cardiac structures. Like radionuclide techniques, the field of ultrasound has developed rapidly and now has many clinical applications. In cardiology, ultrasound first became clinically useful for the evaluation of mitral valve abnormalities because the an-

terior leaflet of the mitral valve formed a large, relatively flat surface for the reflection of sound waves. Early use of this technique was also applied for the evaluation of pericardial effusions because the presence of fluid between the posterior left ventricular wall and lung gave an easily recognizable echo-free space. As equipment improved and experience increased, many other structures of the heart have been usefully evaluated by echocardiography, including left atrial and left ventricular chamber dimensions. The change in these dimensions during the various phases of the cardiac cycle has allowed investigators to estimate left ventricular volume, stroke volume, and ejection fraction from echocardiograms. The thickness of the posterior left ventricular wall can also be estimated by echocardiography, so that an estimate of left ventricular muscle mass can also be made if one assumes that wall thickness is uniform in its distribution. Although echocardiographic measurements of left ventricular dimensions are useful, the current single probe technique does not provide a view of the long axis of the ventricle, so that the length-area method for calculating volumes described above is not applicable to echocardiographic data. Newer techniques utilizing dimensions recorded simultaneously from multiple echo transducers have produced images that visualize a larger portion of the left ventricle. It is likely that this technique or others currently under development will provide much more quantitative information about left ventricular function than is possible at present. Echocardiography has the great advantage of being entirely non-invasive and almost entirely without hazardous side-effects. Unfortunately, the transmission of ultrasound is very poor through lung tissue. In about one third of older adults, lung tissue between the heart and chest wall prevents a satisfactory echocardiographic examination.

LEFT VENTRICULAR PUMP FUNCTION

The left ventricular end-diastolic volume in the normal adult of average size is in the range of 120 to 130 ml. Approximately two thirds of this end-diastolic volume is ejected with systole. Values for this ejection fraction which are greater than 0.5 are usually accepted as normal (see Table 9–2).

In the presence of lesions that place a chronic volume overload on the left ventricle, the ventricle dilates but the relationship between stroke volume and end-diastolic volume remains much as in the normal; namely, greater than one half the end-diastolic volume is ejected with systole. The left ventricular stroke volume with very severe aortic and/or mitral value insufficiency may approach, but rarely exceeds, 300 ml. With lesions that place a chronic pressure overload on the left ventricle, as is observed with aortic valvular stenosis, the left ventricle hypertrophies with a thickened wall, but end-diastolic volume and ejection fraction are similar to those observed in normal subjects. This is in contrast to the ventricular dilatation and reduced ejection fraction observed with acute pressure loads. Ventricular hypertrophy very likely provides the mechanism whereby the ventricle with a chronic pressure overload functions at a normal volume and with a normal ejection fraction.

With myocardial disease the left ventricle dilates inappropriately for the stroke volume, so that the residual volume is increased and the ejection fraction reduced. In patients with severe myocardial disease, ejection fractions of less than 0.10 are occasionally observed. Even in the presence of mechanical overloads such as those imposed by valvular heart disease, the relationship of stroke volume and end-diastolic volume as expressed by the ejection fraction has proved to be of value in assessing myocardial function.

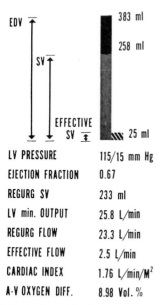

LV PRESSURE	115/15 mm Hg
EJECTION FRACTION	0.67
REGURG SV	233 ml
LV min. OUTPUT	25.8 L/min
REGURG FLOW	23.3 L/min
EFFECTIVE FLOW	2.5 L/min
CARDIAC INDEX	1.76 L/min/M^2
A-V OXYGEN DIFF.	8.98 Vol. %

Figure 9–7 Left ventricular pressure, volume, and cardiac output data from a patient with severe mitral valve insufficiency. The end-diastolic volume, stroke volume, and effective stroke volume, or forward flow, are as indicated. (Adapted from Dodge, H. T., and Baxley, W. A. In Gordon, B. L. (ed.): Clinical Cardiopulmonary Physiology, 3rd ed. Grune and Stratton, Inc., New York, 1969. By permission of Grune and Stratton, Inc.)

The difference between left ventricular stroke volume, as determined by the angiocardiographic method and forward flow, or effective cardiac output per stroke, as measured by the Fick or indicator dilution methods, provides a method for quantifying the volume of regurgitant flow in patients with aortic and/or mitral valve insufficiency and shunt flow in patients with ventricular septal defect. An example of findings in a patient with mitral insufficiency is shown in Figure 9–7. Patients with severe valvular insufficiency may have regurgitant volumes per stroke in the range of 250 ml. which may be in excess of 80 per cent of the left ventricular stroke volume. Left ventricular minute outputs in such patients may be as large as 25 to 30 liters per minute.

From the slopes of the ejection and filling limbs of ventricular volume curves the rates of ventricular ejection and filling respectively can be determined. Figure 9–8 shows a curve of ventricular filling and ejection rates calculated from a ventricular volume curve in a patient with ischemic heart disease. The maximum rates of filling and ejection are usually similar, and in the normal resting subject are in the range of 500 ml. per second. With severe aortic and/or mitral valve insufficiency, peak-ejection and filling rates approach 1500 ml. per second. Peak values as low as 200 ml. per second are observed in patients with mitral stenosis, aortic stenosis, or severe myocardial disease.

Chronic disease is often associated with altered left ventricular distensibility. Figure 9–9 shows the left ventricular end-diastolic pressure-volume relationships of patients with chronic heart disease. End-diastolic volumes of as much as four times normal are observed with filling pressures that are within the normal range. With the increased distensibility, the ventricle functions at a large volume with little or no increase in filling pressure or pulmonary venous pressure. This is important because pulmonary venous hypertension secondary to an elevated ventricular filling pressure is associated with dyspnea. In general, patients with more distensible left ventricles are those with chronic volume overloads or longstanding chronic myocardial disease.

Reduced ventricular distensibility is often observed with thick-walled hypertrophied left ventricles as occurs with aortic valve stenosis or hypertrophic subvalvular aortic stenosis. Here the filling pressure may be elevated in the presence of a normal ventricular end-diastolic volume. Some patients with ischemic heart disease also have elevated filling pressures with normal end-diastolic volumes.

The functional characteristics of the left ventricle as a pump in performing pressure-volume

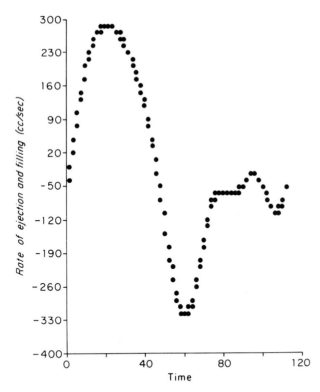

Figure 9-8 Rate of left ventricular ejection and filling with respect to time within the cardiac cycle as determined from the first derivative of a left ventricular volume curve. The positive values are during ejection and negative values during ventricular filling. Zero time is the onset of QRS of the ECG.

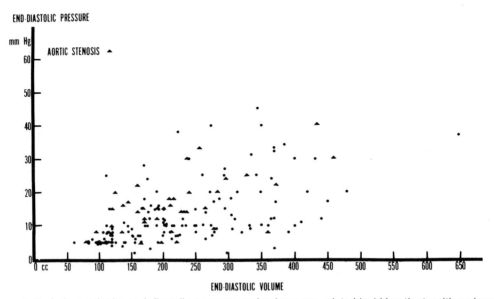

Figure 9-9 Left ventricular end-diastolic pressure and volume are related in 144 patients with various types and durations of heart diseases. Patients with aortic valvular or subaortic stenosis are designated by the triangles. From Dodge, H. T., and Baxley, W. A., Hemodynamic Aspects of Heart Failure. Am. J. Cardiol., 22:24, 1968.

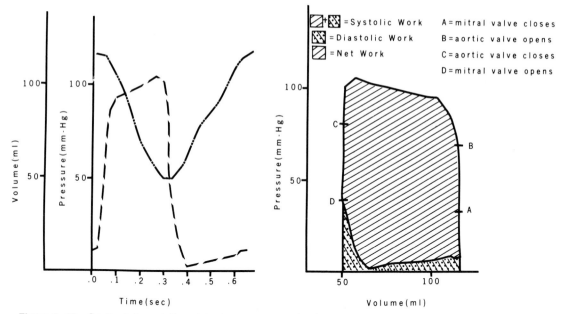

Figure 9–10 On the left are left ventricular pressure and volume curves plotted with respect to time after the QRS of the electrocardiogram. On the right, a pressure-volume curve has been constructed, with work values as indicated by the shaded areas. Mitral valve closure is delayed within the isovolumic contraction period because of an elevated left atrial pressure due to mitral stenosis. The mitral valve opens early in the isovolumic relaxation period also because of an elevated left atrial pressure from mitral stenosis.

work can be determined from the ventricular pressure-volume relationships as shown in Figure 9–10. By relating pressure and volume with respect to time a pressure volume curve is constructed, with pressure on the vertical axis and volume on the horizontal axis. The height of the curve is determined by the systolic pressure, location on the horizontal axis by the end-diastolic volume, and the excursion along the horizontal axis by the stroke volume. The superior and inferior portions of the curves represent pressure-volume relationships during systole and diastole respectively. The shape of the curve is altered by mechanical defects such as aortic or mitral insufficiency, which shorten or abolish the isovolumic contraction and/or relaxation period. Differences in locations and shapes of pressure-volume curves as determined from patients with various heart diseases are illustrated in Figure 9–11.

Left ventricular systolic work is determined from the pressure-volume relations during systole and is illustrated by the area beneath the systolic portion of the curve in Figure 9–10, or

$$\text{Systolic work} = \int_{V_d}^{s} P d V$$

where V_s and V_d are the end-systolic and end-diastolic volumes respectively and P is the ven-

tricular systolic pressure. Systolic stroke work values as much as three to four times normal are observed with severe mitral and aortic valve insufficiency. Values as much as four to five times normal occur when severe valvular insufficiency is associated with ventricular hypertension from aortic stenosis.

The level of work expended in distending the diastolic left ventricle can be determined from the pressure-volume relationships of the left ventricle during diastole. This is illustrated by the area beneath the pressure-volume curve of Figure 9–10, or

$$\text{Diastolic work} = \int_{V_s}^{V_d} P d V$$

where P and V are the pressure and volume respectively during diastole. With left ventricular failure and an elevated left ventricular filling pressure, increased work is performed in distending the diastolic left ventricle. This work is performed by the left atrium and right ventricle and is the physiologic basis for the left atrial dilatation and right ventricular dilatation and hypertrophy observed with chronic left ventricular failure.

The difference between the systolic work and diastolic work values has been termed net work and is represented by the area enclosed by the

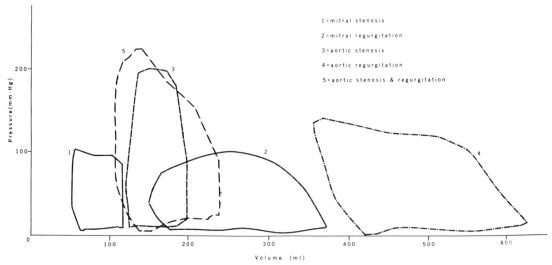

Figure 9–11 Examples of left ventricular pressure-volume curves from patients with different types of heart diseases (mitral stenosis, mitral regurgitation, aortic stenosis, aortic regurgitation, and aortic stenosis and regurgitation). The curve from the patient with mitral stenosis shows well-defined isovolumic contraction and relaxation periods, a normal stroke volume, and relatively normal stroke work. The relatively larger stroke work values in the other patients can be roughly estimated by comparing the areas beneath the systolic limbs of the pressure-volume curves. The patients with aortic regurgitation, mitral regurgitation, and aortic stenosis and regurgitation have greatly elevated stroke work values with large stroke volumes as is evident by the excursion of the curves along the horizontal or volume axis. The abnormality in shape and location of these curves is evident. Patients with valvular insufficiency have a shortening or absence of isovolumic contraction and relaxation periods. Patients with aortic valve stenosis have elevated systolic pressures. Patients with large stroke volumes have elevated end-diastolic volumes.

pressure-volume loop shown in Figure 9–10. In considering the left ventricle as a pump, the net work is then the energy delivered as pressure-volume work in systole less the energy expended in distending the left ventricle as pressure-volume work during diastole. With increasing left ventricular failure, net work is decreased relative to systolic and diastolic work. This is illustrated in Figure 9–12, which shows a pressure-volume curve from a patient with a

left ventricular end-diastolic volume of 525 ml. and pressure of 20 mm. Hg. Systolic work is 37.5 gram-meters per stroke. Diastolic work is nearly 30 per cent of this, and net work is only 26.5 gram-meters per stroke.

The most accurate method for computing left ventricular systolic and net work values is from ventricular pressure and volume curves as described above. However, left ventricular stroke work (LVSW) may also be estimated from

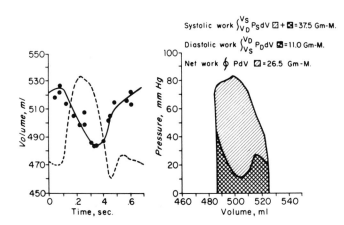

Systolic work $\int_{V_D}^{V_S} P_S dV$ ▨ + ▩ = 37.5 Gm-M.

Diastolic work $\int_{V_S}^{V_D} P_D dV$ ▩ = 11.0 Gm-M.

Net work $\oint PdV$ ▨ = 26.5 Gm-M.

Figure 9–12 Left ventricular pressure, volume, and pressure-volume curves from a patient with ischemic heart disease and left ventricular failure. The various pressure-volume work components are designated and described in the text. (Adapted from Dodge, H. T., and Baxley, W. A.: Hemodynamic aspects of heart failure. Am. J. Cardiol., 22:24, 1968.)

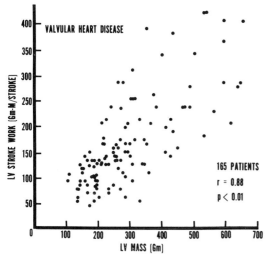

Figure 9-13 Relationship of left ventricular stroke work and mass in 165 patients with valvular heart disease. (From Dodge, H. T., and Baxley, W. A.: Left ventricular volume and mass and their significance in heart disease. Am. J. Cardiol., *23*:528, 1969.)

stroke volume (SV) and left ventricular systolic pressure (LVSP) as follows:

$$LVSW = SV\ (\overline{LVSP} - LVEDP)$$

where $\overline{LVSP}$ equals the mean left ventricular systolic pressure during ejection and LVEDP is left ventricular end-diastolic pressure.

Ventricular power is the rate at which work is performed and can be calculated from the systolic pressure-volume relationships of the left ventricle as $P \times dV/dt$, where P is instantaneous pressure and dV/dt the instantaneous rate of ejection. Peak power values in the range of 500 gram-meters per second are observed in normal resting human subjects and values in excess of four times this in patients with severe aortic and/or mitral valve disease.

In chronic heart disease left ventricular hypertrophy is observed as a response to chronic pressure and/or volume overloads and also in association with chronic left ventricular dilatation. In patients with valvular heart disease and as shown in Figure 9-13, where left ventricular weight is related to left ventricular stroke work, the extent of hypertrophy is directly related to the workload. The manner in which the heart hypertrophies differs, however, depending on whether the increased work is a result of a pressure or volume overload. With compensated volume overloads, the wall shows only a small amount of thickening as end-

diastolic volume is increased, and the ratio of left ventricular mass to end-diastolic volume is close to 1.0. With pressure overloads, the wall thickness is considerably increased, with end-diastolic volume being relatively normal so that the ratio of left ventricular mass to end-diastolic volume is greater than 1.0. It has been shown that in compensated valvular heart disease and with either pressure or volume overloads, the wall thickness is increased in proportion to chamber dimensions and systolic pressure, so that systolic wall stress or force per unit of cross-sectional area of ventricular wall remains relatively normal.

Left ventricular hypertrophy is also observed in the presence of chronic left ventricular dilatation, even when left ventricular stroke work is diminished, as occurs in patients with myocardial disease. In Figure 9-14 left ventricular end-diastolic volume is related to left ventricular mass and, as can be seen, increase in left ventricular weight is roughly proportional to that of volume. Significant ventricular dilatation is regularly associated with ventricular hypertrophy in man with chronic heart disease. The stimulus to hypertrophy is very likely the increased wall force that occurs with the increased chamber dimensions and reduced wall thickness that accompany ventricular dilatation.

The above observations on increased left ventricular mass in the presence of chronic work overloads and ventricular dilatation are consistent with a growth of myocardium in patients with chronic heart disease. In experimental animals with left ventricular dilatation and hy-

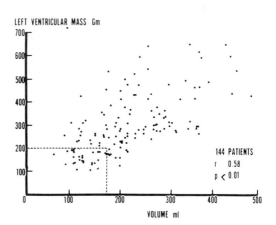

Figure 9-14 Relationship of left ventricular end-diastolic volume and mass in 144 patients with various types of heart diseases. (From Dodge, H. T., and Baxley, W. A.: Hemodynamic aspects of heart failure. Am. J. Cardiol., *22*:24, 1968.)

pertrophy from an induced chronic volume overload, maximal sarcomere lengths have been shown to be unchanged from the 2.2 μ observed in the normal left ventricle. This together with the observations of increased myocardial mass in man with chronic heart disease suggests that growth of new myocardium and sarcomeres is an important adaptive mechanism in chronic heart disease and that the Frank-Starling mechanism may not be important in these chronic adjustments. There is currently a controversy concerning the contractile state of myocardium which is hypertrophied in response to pressure and volume overloads. Some groups have reported normal and others depressed contractility when expressed per unit of myocardium.

MYOCARDIAL PERFORMANCE

Myocardial performance can be more directly evaluated in the intact heart through an analysis of wall forces and motion. The forces present within the myocardium of the chamber walls are a function of the chamber pressure, dimensions, and wall thickness. A method for computing these forces for the left ventricle is to assume that the ventricle can be represented as a thin-walled ellipsoid of revolution and to apply the Laplace expression:

$$\frac{T_1}{R_1} + \frac{T_2}{R_2} = P$$

where T_1 and T_2 are mean wall tensions in the meridional and circumferential directions respectively and R_1 and R_2 are the associated principal radii of curvature. P is chamber pressure. Tension is expressed in force per linear cm., if dimensions are expressed in terms of cm., and can be considered as the force acting per cm. of slits in the wall placed perpendicular to the principal radii of curvature. The wall forces also can be expressed in terms of stress (σ) or force per unit area (cm.^{2}) by dividing tension by wall thickness (h). The Laplace expression then becomes

$$\frac{\sigma_1}{R_1} + \frac{\sigma_2}{R_2} = \frac{p}{h}$$

where σ_1 and σ_2 equal wall stress in the directions of the principal radii of curvature. Wall stress or force per unit area is expressed in the same units as those used for chamber pressure. The largest wall force values are in the circumferential direction.

Because of the above relationships between chamber pressure, wall thickness, and wall stress, wall stress increases more rapidly than chamber pressure as chamber dimensions increase and wall thickness decreases, as occurs when the diastolic left ventricle is acutely distended. During systole, chamber dimensions decrease and wall thickness increases so that wall stress decreases relative to chamber pressure. As described previously, in compensated heart disease associated with chronic pressure or volume overloads, wall thickness is increased so that wall stress values are similar to those found in normal subjects. In subjects with left ventricular failure, large wall stress values are frequently present, indicating that myocardial hypertrophy has not been adequate to compensate for the increase in dimensions and decrease of wall thickness as the chamber has dilated.

The relationship of wall stresses in the directions of the principal chamber axes to wall motion expressed in terms of change of these axes during systole has provided a method for expressing myocardial performance of the intact ventricle in terms of force, extent, and velocity of shortening. This has been used to apply knowledge concerning the relationships of force to the extent and velocity of myocardial contraction as determined in in-vitro studies to the intact ventricle of experimental animals and man.

In-vitro studies of contractile characteristics of myocardium indicate that the myocardial contractile state can be evaluated independently of preload or the Frank-Starling effect from an analysis of myocardial force and velocity of contraction relationships. With this approach to evaluate myocardial contractility, a model to represent the contractile apparatus of the myocardium is assumed. This model consists of a contractile element (CE), a series elastic element (SE), and, for a three-component model, a parallel elastic element. Myocardial contractility is expressed in terms of velocity of contraction of the contractile element (VCE) with respect to force to determine force-VCE relationships. These force-velocity relationships, when extrapolated to zero force, provide a measure of VCE under zero load which has been termed V_{max}. Some studies indicated that V_{max} is independent of fiber length, or the Frank-Starling effect. However, there is controversy concerning the validity of this concept when applied to isolated heart muscle preparations and even more controversy when applied to evaluate the myocardial contractile state of the intact ventricle of experimental animals and man. For a further discussion of these concepts refer to the section on heart muscle and its dynamics (Chapter 8).

The preceding studies and concepts are the basis for evaluation of myocardial contractile state of the intact ventricle in experimental animals and man from high-fidelity ventricular pressure data recorded during the isovolumic contraction period and from studies of ejection phase dynamics. During the isovolumic period, if one assumes no change of cardiac dimensions and wall thickness,

$$VCE = \frac{(dp/dt)}{(K \times P)}$$

where K is equal to the elastic modulus of the series elastic element and P the corresponding isovolumic pressure. VCE extrapolated to zero pressure provides a measure of V_{max}, an index of myocardial contractility. If a three-component model with a parallel elastic component is assumed, developed pressure (DP) is substituted for P in the above equation. DP is computed as P less the initial or end-diastolic pressure. The expression (dP/dt) / K × DP is said to be less sensitive to changes of preload and to provide a more precise index of myocardial contractile state.

Indices of myocardial contractile state as determined from the ventricular ejection phase include the velocity of ventricular circumference change (VCF), VCF at peak wall stress which is equivalent to VCE, peak VCE and VCE extrapolated to zero load, or V_{max}. These computations require knowledge of chamber dimensions, pressure and wall thickness, and instantaneous changes of these parameters during systole. The reader is referred to the section on heart muscle and its dynamics for a further discussion of the theoretical basis for these concepts and their application to evaluate the myocardial contractile state (see Chapter 8).

HEMODYNAMICS OF HEART FAILURE

Cardiac enlargement, increased ventricular filling pressure, and a low cardiac output at rest, or relative to the demands of some stress such as exercise, are features of heart failure. Basically, the clinical picture of heart failure is the result of a decreased ability of the heart to contract, an increased pressure-volume load, a combination of increased load and depressed contractility, or occasionally interference with venous return to the heart as occurs with constrictive pericarditis. Figure 9–7 illustrates an example of failure resulting from a large volume overload due to mitral regurgitation. In man with chronic heart disease and ventricular failure there is compensation for the decreased myocardial contractility and increased mechanical pressure and volume loads by cardiac dilatation (Frank-Starling mechanism) and by cardiac hypertrophy as previously described. It is often difficult to determine precisely when in the course of chronic

heart disease these mechanisms for compensation become inadequate to maintain cardiac output and heart failure develops. In fact, these mechanisms of chamber dilatation and hypertrophy can be viewed as early manifestations of cardiac decompensation as they represent the initial adjustments of the diseased heart. Because there are limits to the extent of cardiac dilatation and hypertrophy that occur in disease, once these compensatory mechanisms develop there is a diminished capacity of the heart to adjust to further increases in mechanical loads or further decreases of myocardial contractility.

A fundamental mechanism by which the ventricles maintain stroke volume in response to acute increases of systolic pressure (afterload), volume overload, or depression of contractility is through chamber dilatation, which has been termed the Frank-Starling mechanism. The increased fiber length which occurs with chamber dilatation is associated with an increased force and extent of contraction. Figure 9–15 shows what have been termed ventricular function curves. With normal myocardial function, chamber volume enlargement is associated with increases of stroke work and stroke volume along a theoretically normal curve. With depressed myocardial function, lower stroke volume and stroke work are generated from a given end-diastolic volume, and stroke volume is maintained through ventricular dilatation. A depressed systolic ejection fraction, as is observed in man with myocardial disease, is a numerical expression of a depressed ventricular function curve, since it indicates inappropriate chamber enlargement with a low stroke volume and large residual volume relative to end-diastolic volume. Drugs that have a positive inotropic effect elevate a depressed ventricular function curve.

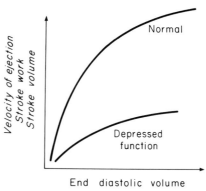

Figure 9–15 Schematic representation of a normal and a depressed ventricular function curve as defined by the relationship of parameters as given on the horizontal and vertical axes.

With acute increases of ventricular end-diastolic volume there is an eventual leveling off of the ventricular function curves, so that further increases in volume result in no further increase in stroke work or stroke volume. Indeed, under some conditions a descending limb of the function curves has been demonstrated. With ventricular dilatation, ventricular diastolic pressure is increased and filling pressure is often used as an index of diastolic volume or preload in determining ventricular response to a changing preload. In man with heart failure due to acute myocardial infarction it has been shown that little increase or even a fall of stroke volume occurs with elevation of left ventricular end-diastolic pressure beyond 22 to 25 mm. Hg.

As described previously, chronic increases of ventricular chamber volume or work load are associated with ventricular hypertrophy. There is a question concerning the role of the Frank-Starling mechanism in the adjustments to chronic increases of ventricular volume and pressure loads, and hypertrophy may be the dominant response to chronic loads.

Measures of ventricular pump performance in addition to stroke volume relative to end-diastolic volume (ejection fraction) can be used to assess myocardial performance in chronic heart disease. These are stroke work, ventricular ejection rate, or peak power. As with stroke volume, none of these parameters has significance for evaluating myocardial performance unless the measure is related to ventricular end-diastolic volume. In the presence of myocardial disease, depressed values relative to volume are observed. This is illustrated in Figure 9–16, in which stroke power normalized for end-diastolic volume is related to the ejection fraction.

There is a problem with using stroke work relative to volume to assess myocardial performance in chronic heart disease. As described previously, the adjustment to chronic systolic pressure over-load is ventricular hypertrophy rather than dilatation. Accordingly, stroke work relative to chamber volume is high in compensated pressure overload states and decreases with myocardial failure, but it still may be high relative to the stroke work/end-diastolic volume relationships observed in other types of heart disease. As a result stroke work/end-diastolic volume does not appear to provide a very useful index for evaluating myocardial performance in chronic heart disease.

With ventricular failure, abnormally low values for ventricular performance are also obtained by analysis of ventricular pressure changes during isovolumic contraction (dp/dt) and of wall force and motion relationships. The velocity of circumference change relative to end-diastolic circumference (VCF) is depressed. Derived values for peak VCE, VCE at peak stress, and V_{max} are also depressed.

ISCHEMIC HEART DISEASE

Ischemic heart disease results from an inadequate supply of oxygenated blood to the myocardium. For practical purposes this disease is due to atherosclerotic occlusive disease of the large extramural coronary arteries, although disease of these vessels occasionally results from other pathologic processes such as embolization, fibromuscular disease of the arteries, and arteritis of variable etiology. Atherosclerosis, although usually diffusely distributed in the proximal portions of the coronary arteries, tends to cause localized areas of stenosis or occlusion. The localized distribution of highly stenotic or occlusive lesions results in regional areas of ischemic or infarcted myocardium. Myocardial functional abnormalities are therefore usually of a segmental or regional distribution in patients with ischemic heart disease. When myocardial damage becomes

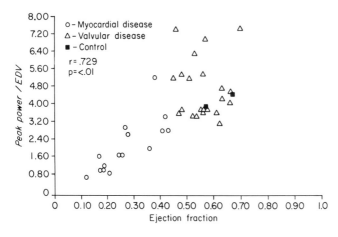

Figure 9–16 A significant correlation is demonstrated for the relationship of left ventricular peak power normalized for end-diastolic volume and ejection fraction in 39 subjects with various types of heart diseases as coded. The subjects indicated as "control" had no demonstrable disease affecting the left ventricle. (From Gensini, G. G. (ed.): The Study of the Systemic, Coronary and Myocardial Effects of Nitrates. Courtesy of Charles C Thomas, Publisher, Springfield, Illinois.)

very extensive due to multiple sites of high-grade stenosis or occlusions of coronary arteries, the entire left ventricle may exhibit reduced contraction. In order to evaluate left ventricular performance in ischemic heart disease it is necessary to study the extent and severity of regional contraction abnormalities.

Selective Coronary Arteriography

Selective coronary arteriography, which was developed by Mason Sones in the late 1950s, is required to define precisely the presence and severity of coronary atherosclerosis. This method is carried out by the insertion of a catheter into the right brachial or a femoral artery and selectively cannulating each coronary orifice. Three to 7 ml. of radiographic contrast material is injected over 1 to 3 seconds, while the image is recorded with a high-gain image intensifier cineangiographic system. High quality cineangiograms of the coronary arteries currently have a resolution of between 75 and 100 line pairs per inch. The right coronary artery is studied in at least two views, and a minimum of three views of the left coronary artery are filmed. Stenosis in these vessels can be easily appreciated and its severity graded relatively accurately. Pharmacologic agents such as nitroglycerin may be given and the studies repeated in order to evaluate the presence of coronary artery spasm. Selective coronary arteriography is also carried out in conjunction with other catheterization techniques in the evaluation of older patients with valvular heart disease, since valvular and coronary heart disease may co-exist. Selective coronary arteriography is a safe procedure when carried out by experienced teams. Reports from experienced laboratories indicate that mortality from these procedures rarely occurs, except in very ill patients with disease of the left main coronary artery or with advanced atherosclerosis of all three major coronary arteries. Over-all mortality resulting from the procedure is between one and two deaths per thousand studies.

Most angiographers grade lesions by the percentage of greatest diameter narrowing as seen on multiple views of the vessel as compared with nearby segments of normal appearing vessel. Despite many limiting factors, this method of clinically reading coronary arteriograms has been effective in selecting patients for coronary artery surgery. Lesions of greater than 70 per cent stenosis of major proximal coronary vessels are considered to be hemodynamically significant. This statement implies that lesions of this severity limit coronary blood flow and result in myocardial ischemia and angina pectoris. Gould and co-workers have studied the flow and pressure gradients across adjustable coronary occluders on the circumflex coronary arteries of dogs. They have shown that in the resting animal coronary flow is not reduced until an 80 to 85 per cent stenosis is applied. When coronary flow is greatly increased with coronary vasodilating drugs to mimic severe exercise, coronary blood flow is reduced by a stenosis of 40 to 50 per cent. These observations indicate that coronary flow reserve, or the ability to increase coronary flow across a stenosis, begins to be limited with mild coronary stenosis but an actual decrease in resting flow requires severe narrowing of the vessel.

In patients with ischemic heart disease, coronary arterial stenoses are usually multiple, may be located serially along a vessel, and may be connected in parallel through the presence of collateral vessels. Additionally, the hemodynamic effect of a particular atherosclerotic lesion depends not only on the severity of stenosis but on its length and shape. For example, an irregular lesion which causes increased turbulence of blood flow will have greater pressure loss across it than a smooth lesion which permits more laminar flow. A great deal remains to be learned about the proper physiologic evaluation of coronary atherosclerotic lesions.

Evaluation of regional contraction abnormalities is difficult because it requires that all aspects of the left ventricle including its apex, free wall, anterior and posterior surfaces, and septum be visualized and studied. At this time angiocardiography is the best method available for visualizing the left ventricle and for the detailed evaluation of segmental abnormalities of left ventricular contraction. The evaluation of left ventricular function in patients with ischemic heart disease is best carried out in conjunction with selective coronary arteriography. Indications for study include angina pectoris, symptoms of heart failure, or persistent chest pain following recovery from a myocardial infarction. Occasionally, patients with heart failure of uncertain etiology are also studied in this manner. Left ventricular angiocardiography may be carried out in single or biplane views with direct or cine filming techniques. In most situations single plane cineangiocardiography is adequate for clinical purposes, although biplane methods are preferable. One method for evaluating ventricular segmental contraction abnormalities is by analysis of end-diastolic and systolic films. This may be carried out by tracing the outline of the opacified chamber and constructing a line from the apex of the left ventricle to the center of the aortic valve. By superimposing systolic and diastolic outlines, the symmetry and extent of contraction can be assessed.

Regional contraction abnormalities can be conveniently divided into five types:

I. *Normal:* The entire ventricular wall moves

inward appropriately toward the geometric center of the ventricle. Occasional patients with small volumes and normal ejection fractions have ventricles that appear asymmetrical at end-systole due to distortion of the cavity shape by the papillary muscles.

II. *Borderline Abnormal:* The ventricle demonstrates a minor degree of contraction asymmetry involving less than 25 per cent of the wall.

III. *Localized Akinesis or Hypokinesis:* More than 25 per cent but less than 75 per cent of the ventricular wall has diminished or absent contraction.

IV. *Localized Dyskinesis:* More than 25 per cent of the ventricular wall demonstrates paradoxic outward motion during systole.

V. *Diffuse Akinesis or Hypokinesis:* More than 75 per cent of the ventricular surface has diminished or absent contraction.

Selective coronary arteriograms usually demonstrate that the coronary vessels which supply an akinetic or dyskinetic region have severe stenosis or total occlusion. Often, however, severely stenotic or occluded coronary vessels supply areas of myocardium which appear to contract normally. Severe coronary artery disease is not, therefore, necessarily associated with areas of abnormal myocardial contraction, at least in the resting subject. Generally, there has been a good correlation between definite electrocardiographic evidence of myocardial infarction and regional contraction abnormalities as assessed by left ventricular angiocardiography. The opposite, however, is not true. Frequently, a severe myocardial contraction abnormality may be present and the electrocardiogram does not definitely localize an infarct to that region of the heart. Electrocardiography, selective coronary arteriography, and left ventricular angiography are all necessary to evaluate fully the patient with ischemic heart disease. Each method yields information not available from the others and together they give a rather complete picture of the left ventricle, its blood supply, electrical integrity, and contractile function.

Ventricular Performance in Ischemic Heart Disease

The incidence of significant segmental contraction abnormalities in patients with ischemic heart disease varies with the patient group submitted to angiocardiographic studies. Patients with angina pectoris without a history or electrocardiographic evidence of prior myocardial infarction often have a normal contraction pattern. Not infrequently, however, these patients have a modest reduction in ejection fraction and an elevation of diastolic pressure. Under the stress of tachycardia induced with right atrial pacing, the end-diastolic pressure often becomes abnormally elevated, and abnormal contraction patterns may appear, or become more marked. Diastolic pressure rise is especially likely to occur in those in whom pacing induces anginal pain. Exercise in this group of patients is also associated with the development of regional contraction abnormalities, decreased ejection fraction, and with increased left ventricular end-diastolic pressure and subnormal increase in cardiac output.

The majority of patients who have suffered a myocardial infarction and have associated electrocardiographic evidence of myocardial scar will have a segmental area of abnormal left ventricular contraction. It has been postulated that akinesis of more than 25 per cent of the ventricular myocardium must result in either ventricular dilatation or reduction in stroke volume. This theory rests upon estimates of the limits of contractile element shortening which can occur under physiologic conditions. Quantitative assessment of the extent of segmental contraction abnormality in large groups of patients suggests that this theory is essentially correct. When more than 25 to 30 per cent of the left ventricular wall is akinetic or dyskinetic, ventricular dilatation and reduced ejection fraction are usually present. The left ventricular end-diastolic pressure is also elevated in most of these patients. Major contraction abnormalities (Type IV or V) are nearly always associated with a history of heart failure and a resting ejection fraction below 40 per cent.

Methods are now available which permit more precise analysis of segmental left ventricular performance in patients with coronary artery disease. Such studies are performed from analysis of chamber margins or regional wall thickening from each frame of cineventriculagrams taken at 60 frames per second or higher rates. Normal standards for extent and timing of wall motion have been established for these techniques and are used as a basis for determining the frequency and extent of segmental wall motion abnormalities in patients with coronary disease. Such studies have demonstrated that most patients with greater than 70 per cent narrowing of a coronary artery have segmental abnormalities of extent or timing of contraction in the region of the left ventricle supplied by the narrowed coronary artery. These abnormalities often are not detected by subjective analysis of the cine films, nor by the more common form of analysis of an end-diastolic and an apparent end-systolic film. In fact, the more detailed types of analyses have demonstrated that even in the normal there may be no one cine film that represents maximum inward contraction for all segments of the ventricle. In patients with ischemic heart disease, abnormalities of timing of wall motion and differences in timing of wall motion of different regions of the left ventricle are very common and often quite marked. Delayed maximum inward motion and accordingly relaxation is particularly common. Whether the abnormalities of timing of wall motion are manifestations of myocardial weakness, damage, ischemia, or delayed timing of depolarization is unknown. The asynchronous segmental wall motion and delayed inward motion and relaxation do undoubtedly contribute to the reduced ventricular systolic performance and perhaps to the increased wall stiffness in diastole observed in patients with ischemic heart disease. There are commonly segments with hyperkinesia to compensate for segments which are hypokinetic, so that, although substantial regions of the ventricle are hypokinetic, over-all ventricular diastolic volume and ejection fraction may be normal. Figure 9–17 illustrates the application of a technique for analysis of segmental extent and timing of

wall motion in a patient with coronary artery disease.

Left ventricular myocardial hypertrophy is frequently present in patients with ischemic heart disease. This appears to be closely related to a history of congestive heart failure and the presence of left ventricular dilatation. There is a close correlation between the increase in left ventricular diastolic volume and the increase in myocardial mass. However, the degree of myocardial hypertrophy relative to diastolic volume is less in ischemic heart disease than in patients with valvular heart disease. This is probably due to the fact that these patients usually do not have an increased volume or pressure load on the left ventricle. In addition, the lesser degree of left ventricular hypertrophy in ischemic heart disease

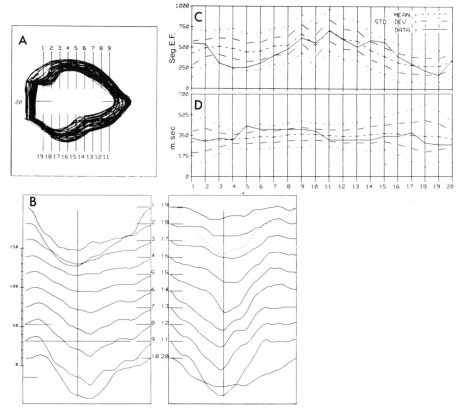

Figure 9–17 The left ventricular chamber margins for systole and diastole of one heart beat have been digitized from a cineventriculogram filmed at 60 frames per second in the anteroposterior projection, stored in computer memory, and played back with the long axes superimposed as shown in panel A. Segmental border motion is determined along each of the numbered hemiaxes, also shown in panel A, and displayed with respect to time by the solid line curves in panel B. The chamber volume curve is illustrated by the dotted curves in panel B. In panels C and D the segmental ejection fractions (fractional motion toward the long axis) and time from QRS to maximum inward segment motion, respectively, are illustrated by the solid lines and related to normal values. Mean normal values with one and two standard deviations from the mean are designated by the dotted and dashed lines. It is evident that this patient has hypokinesia of segments 3–7, hyperkinesia of segments 14 and 15, and delayed time to maximum inward segment motion in segments 5–8.

may be related to shorter duration of disease or an expression of inadequate coronary arterial blood supply.

It is of interest that the electrocardiogram is relatively insensitive in detecting the presence of left ventricular hypertrophy in patients with ischemic heart disease. It should be remembered that ventricular hypertrophy as estimated from angiocardiograms or as determined from left ventricular weight at autopsy does not separate normal myocardial tissue from fibrous tissue and scar and is therefore subject to variable error in estimating actual muscle mass, depending upon the extent of ischemic damage present. The presence of considerable fibrosis and scarring may account for the disparity between electrocardiographic and angiocardiographic evidence of ventricular hypertrophy.

Mitral Regurgitation in Ischemic Heart Disease

Mild mitral regurgitation is frequently present in patients with ischemic heart disease. It is often intermittent and associated with the presence of congestive heart failure, or it may be present only during episodes of myocardial ischemia. Mitral regurgitation in ischemic heart disease may be the result of papillary muscle dysfunction, dilatation of the mitral annulus secondary to left ventricular dilatation, or papillary muscle rupture.

The two papillary muscles of the left ventricle receive their blood supply from terminal branches of the anterior descending and posterior descending coronary arteries. Since the terminal portions of these muscles are free in the ventricular cavity they are directly subjected to intercavity pressure. The combination of these two factors may explain why these small muscles are especially vulnerable to ischemia and infarction. The papillary muscles must contract in concert with the ventricle so that the mitral valve is held in a competent position across the mitral orifice throughout systole. Failure of these muscles to contract will result in prolapse of the mitral valve into the left atrium during the later portion of systole, as indicated in Figure 9–18. Clinically, this will result in a mid- or late systolic ejection murmur which is characteristic of papillary muscle dysfunction. When left ventricular dilatation is extensive, the papillary muscles are pulled down and laterally away from the mitral valve. If the muscles contract with systole in a normal manner, the mitral valve will be held down in the ventricle in an incompetent position throughout systole, as illustrated in Figure 9–18 B. This situation will usually result in a blowing pansystolic murmur. This type of regurgitation frequently disappears when treatment for congestive heart failure results in reduction in

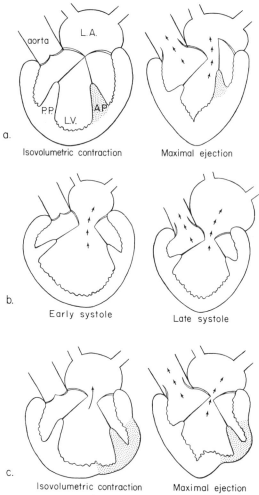

Figure 9–18 The mechanism of mitral regurgitation secondary to ischemia or infarction of the anterior lateral papillary is shown in diagrammatic form (a). During isovolumic contraction and early systole the mitral valve is competent, but during the maximal ejection period the anterior valve leaflet prolapses into the left atrium and mitral regurgitation results.

The mechanism of mitral regurgitation secondary to left ventricular chamber dilatation is shown in (b).

The mechanism of mitral regurgitation which results from infarction of the papillary muscle and the underlying left ventricular wall is shown in (c). In this example the infarcted left ventricular wall is aneurysmal and bulges out during systole. (Adapted from Burch, G. E., DePasquale, N. P., and Phillips, J. H.: Am. Heart J., 75:399, 1968. Copyright 1968, American Medical Association.)

left ventricular volume. It is of interest that patients with long-standing left ventricular dilatation of any cause often develop mitral regurgitation. At surgical or postmortem examination some of these patients are found to have a dilated mitral annulus and normal valve leaflets, indicating that mitral incompetence has resulted from enlargement of the mitral annulus secondary to ventricular dilatation. It is not certain how often mitral regurgitation is due to displacement of the papillary muscle by a dilated ventricular cavity and how often annular dilatation plays an important role in the production of valve incompetence.

Quantitative angiocardiographic assessment of patients with ischemic heart disease indicates that in those patients with mitral regurgitation there is evidence of extensive ventricular dilatation, with the left ventricular end-diastolic volume greater than 150 ml. per M.^{2} in the majority of cases. In addition, these patients nearly always give a history of prior myocardial infarction and congestive heart failure. Left ventricular contraction patterns are also nearly always distinctly abnormal. These findings are not consistent with isolated ischemia or infarction of one or the other papillary muscle but are indicative of more widespread damage of the left ventricular myocardium. A number of recent studies have been carried out in an attempt to create papillary muscle dysfunction in dogs. One or both papillary muscles have been injected with sclerosing material and in another study the base of a papillary muscle was ligated. In those animals in which damage was confined to the papillary muscle, mitral regurgitation did not result. When the underlying left ventricular wall was also injured, mitral valve incompetence developed. These animal studies and clinical experience in man suggest that mitral regurgitation in ischemic heart disease is the result of extensive ischemia or infarction of the papillary muscle and the underlying ventricular wall, as seen diagrammatically in Figure 9–18C.

In rare instances, mitral regurgitation develops acutely during the early phase of recovery from myocardial infarction as a result of rupture of a papillary muscle. When the entire muscle body ruptures, the resultant regurgitation is of severe proportions, and pulmonary edema, shock, and death occur rapidly in nearly all instances. Immediate support of the circulation and replacement of the mitral valve is now possible and will undoubtedly result in a few survivals in this group of patients. At times, only one or two heads of the papillary muscle with their attached chordae tendineae rupture. In these instances, the regurgitation which results is less severe, and survival with or without surgical treatment may be possible.

Rupture of the Interventricular Septum

The development of an interventricular septal defect is an unusual and serious complication of acute myocardial infarction. In most such cases there is the sudden development of a systolic murmur associated with heart failure and often systemic arterial hypotension. Septal rupture usually occurs during the first six days following myocardial infarction in patients who have extensive transmural infarction of the anterior or posterior wall which also involves the interventricular septum. The prognosis in these patients remains poor despite attempts at surgical repair because of the extensive myocardial damage usually present.

Ventricular Aneurysms

Angiocardiographic studies have shown that small areas of the left ventricular wall which bulge paradoxically with ventricular systole are common in patients who have had a transmural myocardial infarction. Large ventricular aneurysms which are apparent on simple chest x-ray and fluoroscopy are less common and probably occur in 3 to 10 per cent of patients who survive transmural myocardial infarction. Large ventricular aneurysms have a profound effect on left ventricular dynamics because as they expand with systole they accept a volume load from the contractile portion of the ventricle. However, the volume load is rarely marked and does not approach the levels of volume load observed in patients with moderate or severe aortic or mitral valve insufficiency. Patients with large ventricular aneurysms usually develop congestive heart failure, probably as a result of the loss of a substantial portion of contractile muscle as well as the mechanical effects of the aneurysm. Since most ventricular aneurysms are lined with mural thrombi they are also associated with an increased incidence of systemic embolization. In addition, recurrent ventricular arrhythmias are common in these patients. Surgical resection of large ventricular aneurysms is indicated for heart failure which is resistant to medical treatment and in patients who have had systemic embolization which cannot be controlled with anticoagulants. Occasionally, aneurysms have been resected for recurrent episodes of ventricular tachycardia with apparent success. The risk and success of aneurysm resection depends on the functional capacity of the remaining myocardium.

VALVULAR HEART DISEASE

Diseases of various types affect the cardiac valves and result in valvular stenosis, regurgitation, or a combination of these lesions. Rheumatic endocarditis remains the main cause of chronic valvular deformity and resultant dysfunction, despite the reduction in the incidence of rheumatic fever that has occurred since the introduction of effective antibiotics in Western countries. Rheumatic fever and especially virulent forms of rheumatic valvular disease continue to be a major health problem in the developing countries. In recent years there has been an increasing appreciation of other etiologic factors responsible for valvular heart disease. It is now known, for example, that many cases of isolated aortic stenosis result from congenital bicuspid malformations of the valve. Many causes of pure mitral regurgitation are also recognized, including congenital abnormalities, dysfunction and rupture of the papillary muscles, rupture of chordae tendineae, mitral annular dilatation, myxomatous degeneration of the valve leaflets, and prolapse of the mitral valve. Bacterial endocarditis continues to be an important cause of mitral, aortic, and tricuspid valve destruction, although changes in the clinical and bacteriologic picture have resulted from the widespread use of antibiotics.

Mitral Stenosis

Mitral stenosis for practical purposes is due to rheumatic heart disease, although a congenital form of the disease and obstruction of the valve orifice due to left atrial myxoma do occur. The valve becomes thickened and there is fusion of the valve commissures. Calcification of the valve leaflets and mitral annulus is often present. The chordae tendineae are thickened, shortened, and fused to a variable degree. Generally, the valve orifice will be reduced to 1.2 cm.^{2} or less in cross-sectional area before significant symptoms develop. The major effect of mitral valve obstruction is a chronic increase in left atrial and pulmonary venous pressure. This increased pressure is transmitted back to the pulmonary capillaries and pulmonary artery. There is resultant interstitial edema and marked thickening of the alveolar walls. The small muscular pulmonary arteries and arterioles develop marked muscular hypertrophy and there is reduction in the lumen of these vessels. As one would suspect from these anatomic changes in severe mitral stenosis there may be elevation of pulmonary artery pressure which is greater than can be accounted for by the elevation in pulmonary venous and left atrial pressure, indicating increased resistance across the pulmonary vascular bed. This increased pulmonary vascular resistance may at times rise to systemic levels with resultant severe pulmonary artery hypertension.

The major symptom in mitral stenosis is exertional dyspnea. As the disease advances, dyspnea at rest and marked fatigue develop. Right heart failure and functional tricuspid regurgitation often occur, and peripheral edema and ascites may then become prominent.

The lungs in mitral stenosis become fibrotic and noncompliant. There is abnormal distribution of alveolar perfusion and ventilation which results in functional shunting of blood through the lungs. The upper lobes have increased perfusion whereas flow to the bases is reduced. This feature of mitral stenosis can often be appreciated on upright chest radiographs.

Despite the marked anatomic changes that occur in the lungs of patients with severe mitral stenosis, pulmonary artery hypertension and increased pulmonary vascular resistance are reversible following surgery which successfully relieves mitral valve obstruction. Recent studies in patients immediately following mitral valve replacement have shown that the pulmonary artery pressure and calculated pulmonary vascular resistance fall rapidly within the first few days following valve replacement. Studies done several weeks later indicate that further reduction in vascular resistance occurs with time. The reversibility of pulmonary vascular resistance in mitral stenosis is in contrast to the irreversible nature of the high pulmonary vascular resistance that develops in some patients with congenital heart disease with left-to-right shunts.

The left atrium in mitral stenosis becomes increased in volume and the atrial wall becomes hypertrophied. In a recent study of 25 patients, atrial volume ranged from 44 to 288 ml. per M.^{2}, the average volume being more than three times the normal value. Occasional patients have been seen who have giant left atria, but marked left atrial enlargement is usually associated with mitral regurgitation. The maximum volume of the atrium is not linearly related to the severity of mitral stenosis, since other factors such as the duration of disease and the severity of rheumatic involvement of the atrial myocardium are factors in determining atrial volume. As long as sinus rhythm persists, atrial contraction plays an important role in forcing blood through the obstructed mitral orifice into the left ventricle. Unfortunately, the majority of patients with mitral stenosis eventually develop atrial fibrillation. Presumably this is the result of chronic atrial hypertension and dilatation, although the exact mechanisms are not clear. Atrial fibrillation has three deleterious effects: (1) it reduces left ventricular filling; (2) it usually results in an increase in heart rate, with resultant decrease in the diastolic portion of the cardiac cycle; and (3) it allows stagnation of blood in the dilated left atrium and its appendage. For cardiac output to be maintained in the face of atrial fibrillation left atrial pressure must increase to compensate for loss of atrial contraction and reduced diastolic filling time. This increase in atrial pressure may result in the development of left atrial thrombi which then often embolize with devastating consequences. Control of the heart rate in patients with atrial fibrillation and anticoagulant therapy are, therefore, major therapeutic measures in this disease.

Mitral stenosis is unique among acquired disease of the left side of the heart because it protects rather than stresses the left ventricle. Studies of the left ventricle indicate that in the majority of cases the ventricular volume and mass are normal. In an occasional advanced case, however, actual atrophy of the ventricular myocardium may occur. Despite normal diastolic volume, the left ventricular stroke volume often is reduced. This combination of reduced stroke volume and normal diastolic volume results in a reduced ejection fraction in about one third of patients with mitral stenosis, with half of these having an ejection fraction below 40 per cent. It is not clear at this time whether this reduced ejection fraction is indicative of myocardial dysfunction or whether it is merely an expression of reduced filling volume and pressure (preload).

Right ventricular hypertrophy accompanies the development of pulmonary hypertension in patients with mitral stenosis. Since the right ventricle is unaccustomed to developing high pressures, it often dilates, and functional tricuspid regurgitation frequently occurs. Venous hypertension, congestive hepatomegaly, peripheral edema, and ascites then follow. Sustained pulmonary hypertension occasionally causes dilatation of the pulmonary artery and annulus of the pulmonary valve, with resultant pulmonary valvular insufficiency. Since associated aortic valve insufficiency is commonly present in patients with mitral stenosis, the differentiation of aortic from pulmonary valve insufficiency requires cardiac catheterization and angiocardiography. Both tricuspid and pulmonary valve insufficiency can be expected to become less prominent or disappear entirely following successful valve repair or replacement.

Since mitral stenosis commonly occurs in young women, the disease is often complicated by pregnancy. During pregnancy, there is an increase in both blood volume and cardiac output. Although these changes may be accommodated by patients with other types of heart disease of modest severity, they are poorly tolerated by the patient with mitral stenosis. Not uncommonly, in fact, the first symptoms of heart disease leading to the diagnosis of mitral stenosis occur during pregnancy. Reducing activity and the control of blood volume with low-sodium diet and diuretics are generally successful in bringing these patients through pregnancy and delivery. Occasionally, these measures are not adequate and mitral commissurotomy is required during the second trimester.

Surgical Considerations. Mitral commissurot-omy can be performed with or without the aid of cardiopulmonary bypass. This operation, as it is performed today, is highly successful in the majority of cases in relieving mitral valve obstruction at least temporarily. The operation can be carried out with low mortality (1 to 4 per cent) in functional class II and III patients, but carries a considerably higher mortality in class IV patients. Most cardiac surgery centers therefore recommend that this operation be carried out on patients with mitral stenosis when they become significantly disabled by symptoms of their disease. It is best to operate on patients well before they have developed severe limitation, since the operative mortality increases greatly and the benefits of surgery are reduced. If valve replacement is contemplated because of heavy valve calcification and/or associated mitral regurgitation, surgery should be delayed longer, since operative mortality is greater and long-term results are less favorable with this procedure.

Mitral Regurgitation

Mitral regurgitation may occur as a "pure" lesion or may be associated with mitral stenosis. When it is associated with stenosis it is nearly always due to rheumatic heart disease, whereas "pure" mitral regurgitation may be the result of many different diseases.

Pure mitral regurgitation resulting from papillary muscle dysfunction and papillary muscle rupture has been discussed in the section on ischemic heart disease. Other causes of mitral regurgitation are ruptured chordae tendineae, mitral annular dilatation and displacement of the papillary muscle due to ventricular dilatation, dysfunction of the mitral valve apparatus due to endocardial fibrosis, and postrheumatic deformity of the valve. Congenital clefts of the mitral valve occur and are often associated with atrial septal defects of the primum type. Myxomatous degeneration of the valve leaflets also occurs.

In the past, mitral regurgitation was thought to be a benign condition. Although considerable mitral regurgitation may be well tolerated for years, there is no question that it can cause left ventricular failure and death. The hemodynamics of left ventricular ejection are greatly altered in mitral regurgitation. Normally during the isovolumic phase of systole the myocardial fibers develop tension without shortening. When the intracavitary pressure reaches the pressure in the aorta, the aortic valve opens and ejection occurs. In the presence of mitral regurgitation, the isovolumic phase of systole is greatly shortened, or eliminated, since ejection into the left atrium occurs as soon as left ventricular pressure exceeds left atrial pressure.

Angiographic studies of patients with pure mitral regurgitation have shown that there is left ventricular dilatation which is linearly related to the severity of valvular regurgitation. There is also left ventricular hypertrophy, although this is less than that seen with aortic regurgitation of similar magnitude. The systolic ejection fraction is generally in the normal range in patients with mitral regurgitation of rheumatic etiology, but is nearly always depressed when regurgitation is due to ischemic heart disease or congestive cardiomyopathy. Chronic mitral regurgitation is frequently present in idiopathic hypertrophic subaortic stenosis, but is usually of mild to moderate severity and results from displacement of the papillary muscles by the distorted hypertrophied ventricle rather than from disease of the mitral leaflets or annulus. The left ventricle has a normal or increased ejection fraction in contrast to the depressed ejection fraction seen with other types of cardiomyopathy.

The left atrium is always enlarged in patients with chronic mitral regurgitation and is generally larger than in patients with mitral stenosis, as shown in Table 9–3. In a small number of cases it reaches giant proportions (greater than 300 ml. per M.^{2}). The maximum atrial volume is a poor guide to the severity of mitral regurgitation, but the change in atrial volume during the cardiac cycle is increased in mitral regurgitation and has been shown to be related to the severity of regurgitation. The large cyclic change in atrial volume is not dependent on atrial contraction, since it occurs passively early in diastole. Only the small increment of left atrial emptying which results from atrial contraction is lost when atrial fibrillation develops in these patients.

Pulmonary artery pressure is variable in mitral regurgitation and is dependent on the severity of valvular regurgitation and, more importantly, on the compliance of the left atrium and the pulmonary venous bed. Most often left atrial

volume is moderately increased and the atrial wall relatively stiff, so that there is a large systolic pulse pressure or "V" wave seen in the left atrial pressure tracing. This large "V" wave plus a variable increase in pulmonary vascular resistance results in elevation of the pulmonary artery and right ventricular pressure. In some cases of chronic mitral regurgitation, however, the left atrium is unusually large and distensible. This large baglike structure absorbs the regurgitant volume from the left ventricle with little increase in pressure. In these circumstances, severe mitral regurgitation may be present with normal pulmonary artery pressure. When mitral regurgitation develops acutely, such as occurs with ruptured chordae tendineae, a small non-compliant left atrium is suddenly subjected to a large pressure and volume load. The left atrial "V" wave may be extremely high (in the range of 60 to 80 mm. Hg) and pulmonary artery pressure is likewise greatly elevated. This combination of events often results in the sudden onset of pulmonary edema.

Surgical treatment of pure mitral regurgitation requires cardiopulmonary bypass with open repair of the valve or prosthetic replacement. Valve clefts and fenestrations may be repaired directly or patched with pericardium or fabric. Best results are obtained when the valve is normal and the annulus is enlarged or when there is chordal rupture. When there is considerable loss of valve substance or the valve is thickened and inflexible, replacement is required.

Combined Mitral Stenosis and Regurgitation

Rheumatic involvement of the mitral valve frequently distorts the leaflets and supporting structures so that a combination of stenosis and regurgitation results. Scarring is usually severe in these cases and heavy calcification is frequently present. The symptoms and clinical features will depend on whether stenosis or regurgitation is the dominant hemodynamic lesion.

Abnormalities in atrial and ventricular function and anatomy are generally midway between those seen in either pure stenosis or regurgitation alone. Quantitation of the severity of regurgitation in a series of these patients showed that regurgitation flows of more than 5.0 liters per min. per M.^{2} occurred only when valve stenosis was absent.

The presence of both stenosis and regurgitation is of therapeutic importance because surgical treatment usually requires valve replacement, with its attendant mortality and postoperative morbidity. These cases should therefore be treated with conservative medical management until they reach functional class III status.

TABLE 9–3 LEFT ATRIAL VOLUME IN MITRAL VALVE DISEASE

	Number of Cases	Mean	1 SD	Range of Volume
Maximum LA Volume (ml.M.^{2})				
Normal	22	35	9	22–50
Mitral Stenosis	25	117	57	44–288
Mitral Stenosis and Regurgitation	27	180	106	84–594
Mitral Regurgitation	27	183	116	63–547
LA Volume Change (ml./M^2)				
Normal	22	18	7.4	5–30
Mitral Stenosis	25	14	9	1–45
Mitral Stenosis and Regurgitation	26	23	11	4–50
Mitral Regurgitation	27	46	27	12–124

(By permission of the American Heart Association, Inc.)

Several patients have now been evaluated with quantitative angiographic or echocardiographic techniques before and after clinically successful mitral valve surgery. After surgical treatment for mitral stenosis, there is the expected reduction in left atrial and right heart pressures with increase in resting cardiac output. Left ventricular volume and mass show little change following surgery, since they are usually normal in these patients preoperatively. In patients with mitral regurgitation, successful surgical correction usually results in a reduction in left atrial and right-sided pressures. Left ventricular volume is reduced toward normal, but there is little regression in left ventricular muscle mass. In patients with reduced left ventricular pump function as measured by a low preoperative ejection fraction, there is often a further decline in ejection fraction following surgery. In patients with normal ventricular function prior to surgery, some remain normal and others have a reduced ejection fraction after surgery. The fall in ejection fraction in some patients after surgery indicates that it is probably due to an increase in left ventricular afterload, which occurs when the mitral valve becomes competent and no longer allows ejection of blood from the left ventricle into the low-pressure left atrium. These studies suggest that patients with mitral regurgitation should be treated surgically prior to the development of left ventricular dysfunction.

AORTIC VALVE DISEASE

Aortic stenosis is most often the result of rheumatic endocarditis and is frequently associated with mitral valve disease. When aortic stenosis occurs as an isolated lesion and there is no history of prior rheumatic fever the disease is likely to be the result of a congenital malformation of the valve. It is now known from autopsy studies that bicuspid and other malformations of the aortic valve are common congenital cardiac abnormalities. It is the gradual thickening, fibrosis, and calcification of these abnormal valves which eventually result in isolated calcific aortic stenosis in middle and later life.

Aortic stenosis in its pure form uncomplicated by a valvular incompetence presents a systolic pressure load on the left ventricle. This pressure load develops gradually as the valve stenosis becomes more severe and ventricular hypertrophy progresses at a rate adequate to maintain normal cardiac output. Severe aortic valve obstruction may be present for a prolonged period, during which time the patient remains asymptomatic. Eventually, owing to either further valve narrowing or decrease in myocardial performance, the cardiac output cannot increase adequately to

meet the demand of exercise. The patient then develops exertional dyspnea and may also experience angina pectoris, lightheadedness, or actual syncope. Finally, with further deterioration in myocardial function, congestive heart failure develops.

Evaluation of patients who have exertional lightheadedness or syncope has shown that hypotension develops with physical exertion and at that time symptoms appear. This hypotension which occurs with upright exercise is the result of limited ability to increase cardiac output. The available blood flow is preferentially shunted to the low resistance bed of the working leg muscles, with resulting hypotension and cerebral ischemia. The same phenomenon can be observed in patients with tight mitral stenosis, although syncope is uncommon.

Angina pectoris often occurs in patients with aortic stenosis. Since aortic stenosis occurs most commonly in middle-aged men, associated atherosclerotic heart disease may be the cause of the anginal syndrome. When aortic obstruction is severe, however, angina pectoris frequently occurs in the presence of normal coronary arteries. Angina results from inadequate oxygen supply to the myocardium. In aortic stenosis this is due to a combination of factors including increased myocardial oxygen consumption resulting from increased pressure work, left ventricular hypertrophy, and reduced coronary artery perfusion pressure. The reduction in coronary perfusion pressure occurs because of low aortic root pressure and elevated left ventricular chamber pressure during systole and to some extent in the later portion of diastole.

When syncope and/or angina are present in a patient with aortic stenosis there is a high risk of sudden death, which often is associated with physical exertion. It is probable that this is secondary to exertional hypotension resulting in reduced coronary arterial blood flow, myocardial ischemia, and the development of ventricular fibrillation. Patients with tight aortic stenosis and symptoms of angina pectoris and/or syncope require urgent evaluation and surgical correction.

Myocardial Function in Aortic Stenosis

Prior to the onset of myocardial failure the left ventricle responds to a pressure load by hypertrophy without chamber dilatation. The left ventricle in aortic stenosis therefore has normal volume and hypertrophy of the left ventricular myocardium including the wall, trabeculae, and papillary muscles. Ventricular ejection fraction is usually maintained in the normal range. The left ventricular systolic pressure may be as high as 300 mm. Hg, although it is usually in the range of 200 mm. Hg. This results in a large pressure gradient across the stenotic valve. The aortic pressure is low, has a small pulse pressure, and is slow rising with an anacrotic notch.

Despite a normal end-diastolic volume and ejection fraction, the filling pressure may be significantly elevated before the onset of congestive heart failure. This is the result of vigorous left atrial contraction ejecting blood into the thick-walled noncompliant left ventricle. The elevation of end-diastolic pressure is, therefore, a poor indication of left ventricular myocardial failure in these patients.

In patients with aortic stenosis who have developed congestive heart failure the left ventricle often shows moderate chamber dilatation, reduced stroke volume, reduced ejection fraction, and marked elevation in left ventricular end-diastolic pressure. As the myocardium progressively weakens, the pressure generated in the chamber is reduced and the flow and pressure gradient across the valve fall. If only the pressure gradient is measured during cardiac catheterization and the flow and valve orifice are not determined, the severity of valve stenosis may not be fully appreciated.

Treatment of Aortic Stenosis.   Once severe aortic stenosis has resulted in significant dyspnea, angina, syncope, or congestive heart failure, surgical treatment for relief of aortic valve obstruction must be considered. In an occasional case it may

be possible to relieve the stenosis by plastic repair of the valve, but the vast majority of cases require valve replacement.

The evaluation of patients by quantitative angiocardiographic techniques before and after surgery indicates that there is a reduction in left ventricular systolic pressure work, a decrease in end-diastolic pressure, and little change in end-diastolic volume. Patients with a low ejection fraction before surgery usually have an increase in ejection fraction toward normal after surgery. Figure 9–19 presents the pressure-volume diagram in a patient with aortic stenosis without myocardial failure before and following successful homograft aortic valve replacement. The difference in the area enclosed by the two loops represents the reduction in pressure-volume work following surgery. The end-diastolic volume is unchanged despite a fall in the diastolic pressure. Studies of left ventricular mass before and one year following surgery suggest that myocardial hypertrophy regresses substantially following successful surgical treatment.

Aortic Regurgitation

Unlike aortic stenosis, aortic regurgitation is a disease of many causes, rheumatic heart disease being the major one. Other causes include syphilitic aortitis, congenital malformations of the aor-

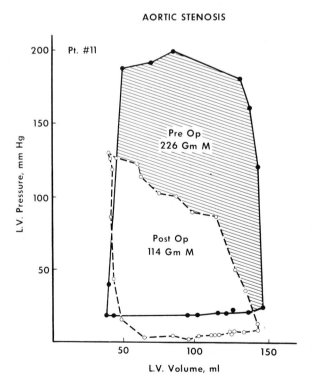

AORTIC STENOSIS

Pt. #11

Pre Op
226 Gm M

Post Op
114 Gm M

L.V. Pressure, mm Hg

L.V. Volume, ml

Figure 9–19 Left ventricular pressure-volume diagrams constructed from cardiac catheterization and angiocardiographic data acquired before and after successful aortic valve replacement for severe aortic stenosis. The area beneath the systolic portion of each loop represents the pressure-volume systolic stroke work of the left ventricle. Preoperatively, systolic work was 226 gram-meters per beat; following aortic valve replacement, systolic work fell to 114 gram-meters per beat. The shaded area indicates the reduction in work as a result of surgery. (Adapted from Kennedy, J. W., Twiss, R. D., Blackmon, J. R., and Merendino, K. A.: Hemodynamic studies one year after homograft aortic valve replacement. Circulation, Suppl. II to Vols. 37 and 38, p. 110, 1968. By permission of the American Heart Association, Inc.)

tic valve often associated with a high ventricular septal defect, Marfan's syndrome with ascending aortic dissection, aneurysm with aortic annular dilatation and cusp rupture secondary to chest wall trauma. When bacterial endocarditis involves the aortic valve severe regurgitation often results. Hypertension of a severe degree occasionally causes mild aortic regurgitation which is reversible when the blood pressure is lowered.

Aortic regurgitation, when severe, places a large volume load on the left ventricle. Since the large stroke volume is ejected into the high resistance systemic circulation, a component of pressure overload also occurs in this disease in contrast to the pure volume overload seen in mitral regurgitation. The stroke volume is greatly increased and its forceful ejection from the ventricle results in a wide pulse pressure and often in an elevation in aortic systolic pressure. The leaking aortic valve results in retrograde flow in the aorta during diastole and a fall in aortic diastolic pressure. The impressive peripheral vascular findings in this disease, which include pistol-shot pulses, pulsating capillaries in the nail beds, and systolic head bobbing, are expressions of widened arterial pulse pressure and/or retrograde diastolic flow in large arteries.

The clinical course of patients with chronic aortic regurgitation is usually a long one, with many years of hemodynamically significant regurgitation tolerated without symptoms. When congestive heart failure finally develops, the downhill course is rapid.

Left ventricular enlargement is a major feature of this disease with both hypertrophy of the myocardium and an increased chamber volume. As in mitral regurgitation, the ventricular diastolic volume is increased in direct proportion to the volume of regurgitation and in extreme cases may reach nearly 800 ml. (Fig. 9–20). The total left ventricular stroke volume is greatly increased, with the forward or systemic stroke volume remaining in the normal range until left ventricular failure develops. Total left ventricular stroke volume including forward and regurgitant fractions may reach 300 ml. or more, with total output approaching 30 liters per minute. This level of ventricular output occasionally seen in these patients at rest is about the same as that achieved by a well-trained healthy young man during maximum exercise. The limits of left ventricular output, therefore, seem to be quite similar in health and in the individual with a compensated left ventricle and severe aortic regurgitation. However, the large minute outputs observed with aortic valve insufficiency are primarily a result of the large stroke volume, whereas the increased outputs observed with exercise are primarily achieved by an increased heart rate. With aortic regurgitation, left ventric-

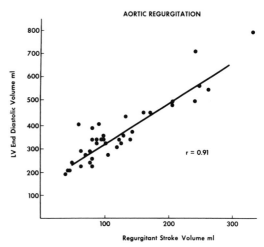

Figure 9–20   The relationship between the left ventricular end-diastolic volume and the regurgitant stroke volume in 38 patients with pure aortic regurgitation. There is a linear relationship between the severity of regurgitation and the ventricular end-diastolic volume. (From Kennedy, J. W., Twiss, R. D., Blackmon, J. R., and Dodge, H. T.: Quantitative angiocardiography, III. Relationship of left ventricular pressure, volume and mass in aortic valve disease. Circulation. *38*:838. 1968. By permission of The American Heart Association, Inc.)

ular mass may be very large, approaching 1000 grams in severe cases, and averaged 425 grams in 38 cases studied by quantitative angiocardiography. This condition produces the largest left ventricles seen in clinical medicine.

Left ventricular filling pressure is dependent on the severity of aortic regurgitation, the left ventricular myocardial compliance, and the heart rate. When aortic regurgitation is very severe, the pressures in the aorta and left ventricle may equilibrate during the end of diastole usually at a level of 30 to 40 mm. Hg. This is most likely to occur if the patient has bradycardia. In Figure 9–21, the left ventricular and aortic pressures are seen in a man with severe aortic regurgitation and sinus bradycardia at a rate of 54 per minute. At end-diastole, the pressure in the aorta is 48 mm. Hg and 35 mm. Hg in the left ventricle. Following right atrial pacing at a rate of 82 per minute, the end-diastolic pressure in the aorta became normal at 75 mm. Hg and fell to 10 mm. Hg in the left ventricle. This change in heart rate also resulted in a reduced left ventricular end-diastolic volume and regurgitant flow per beat but no significant change in the volume of aortic regurgitation per minute. This effect of heart rate on ventricular filling pressure accounts for the fact that some patients with aortic regurgitation have dyspnea and angina at rest but have little exercise limitation.

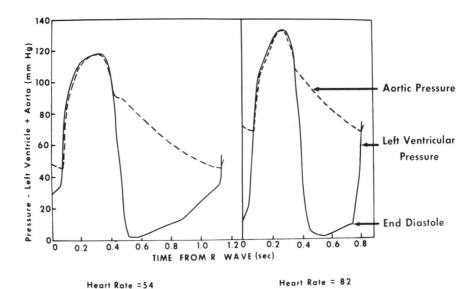

Figure 9–21   Left ventricular and aortic pressure in a patient with severe aortic regurgitation and sinus brady-cardia heart rate 54 (left panel) and during right atrial pacing at heart rate 82 (right panel). With pacing, the aortic pressure during diastole has increased, whereas the left ventricular end-diastolic pressure has decreased to a normal level. (From Judge, T. P., Kennedy, J. W., Bennett, L. J., et al.: The quantitative hemodynamic effects of heart rate in aortic regurgitation. Circulation, *44*:355, 1971.)

Angina is relatively common in aortic regurgitation, although not as frequent as in aortic stenosis. Left ventricular oxygen consumption is increased in aortic regurgitation because of the associated pressure-volume overload and the ventricular hypertrophy. In addition, the pressure gradient between the aortic root and the intramyocardial and subendocardial coronary vessels is reduced as a result of low aortic diastolic pressure and elevated left ventricular filling pressure. The occurrence of angina pectoris is therefore easily explained in this disease. When aortic regurgitation occurs in middle age, coronary atherosclerosis is also likely to be a contributing factor as a cause of angina, especially when aortic regurgitation is not severe. Patients with syphilitic aortitis may get calcification and obstruction of one or both of the coronary ostia, which will account for an occasional case of angina in this form of the disease.

When congestive heart failure develops in patients with aortic regurgitation there is either further dilatation of the ventricle, decrease in the total left ventricular stroke volume, or both, so that the ejection fraction falls, the ventricular filling pressure increases, and pulmonary vascular congestion develops. With marked left ventricular dilatation, functional mitral regurgitation occurs owing to enlargement of the mitral annulus or displacement or excessive lengthening of the papillary muscles. The development of

mitral regurgitation results in a further decrease of forward output and this combination of valvular defects is poorly tolerated.

Bacterial endocarditis of the aortic valve often results in the sudden development of severe aortic regurgitation due to fenestration, tearing, or rupture of one or more valve cusps. The sudden pressure-volume overload imposed on the normal left ventricle is poorly tolerated and there is extreme elevation of ventricular filling pressure and acute dilatation of the chamber. Pulmonary edema may develop suddenly and immediate surgery is often required as a life-saving measure. If the patient survives without surgical treatment, the left ventricle gradually dilates and the myocardium hypertrophies as the left ventricle adjusts to the chronic pressure-volume overload.

Treatment of Aortic Regurgitation. Medical treatment is useful in controlling congestive heart failure. The primary form of treatment is valve repair or replacement. Patients should be disabled by symptoms before valve replacement is recommended. Risk of surgery in aortic regurgitation varies with the cause of the disease, age of the patient, and myocardial function. In good-risk patients without myocardial failure the surgical mortality is in the range of 5 per cent — somewhat lower than the risk in patients with aortic stenosis.

Studies of patients before and after successful valve replacement for severe aortic regurgitation indicate that the end-diastolic volume is greatly reduced following surgery, although it may not return completely to normal. The filling pressure and pressure-volume work are also decreased toward normal and left ventricular hypertrophy regresses but does not become normal. When ventricular function is depressed prior to surgery, as indicated by a low preoperative ejection fraction, it remains abnormal in many patients following surgical correction, suggesting that when better surgical therapy is available valve replacement should be performed at an earlier stage of this disease.

Combined Aortic Stenosis and Regurgitation

The combination of aortic stenosis and regurgitation results from thickened deformed valve leaflets which cannot open or close properly. The disease is most often due to rheumatic endocarditis but also is the frequent result of a congenitally malformed valve. The clinical and hemodynamic pictures are dependent on whether stenosis or regurgitation is the predominant lesion. Very severe aortic regurgitation does not occur in the presence of significant valve obstruction, so that the marked peripheral vascular signs of aortic regurgitation are less prominent or absent. Surgical treatment is indicated when the patient is disabled by symptoms, and valve replacement is nearly always required.

Combined Aortic and Mitral Valve Disease

When disease of both the mitral and aortic valves is present, one lesion may alter the effects of the other and the over-all hemodynamic picture. The most detrimental combination of valve lesions is aortic stenosis and mitral regurgitation because aortic valve obstruction increases the severity of mitral regurgitation and decreases systemic flow. When both aortic and mitral stenosis occur together, the left ventricle is protected from pressure load by limited filling and may fail to undergo the usual hypertrophy. Because of decreased flow, the murmurs of both lesions will be diminished, particularly that of aortic stenosis, and the diagnosis may be difficult to make at the bedside. Proper surgical treatment requires that obstruction at both valves be relieved.

In patients with valvular heart disease, tricuspid valve disease is usually associated with mitral valve disease. Tricuspid regurgitation is most often functional and secondary to pulmonary hypertension and right ventricular dilatation. Such functional tricuspid regurgitation usually regresses when mitral valve disease has been adequately treated surgically and there is no residual left ventricular failure to elevate pulmonary vascular pressures. Occasionally, the tricuspid valve is structurally abnormal owing to involvement by the rheumatic process with organic tricuspid stenosis, tricuspid regurgitation, or both. In this situation, the tricuspid valve may require valvuloplasty or replacement. Other types of tricuspid valve disease include congenital tricuspid stenosis and atresia, Ebstein's anomaly of the tricuspid valve, and tricuspid valve insufficiency from endocardial fibrosis of the right heart as occurs in the carcinoid syndrome.

THE CARDIOMYOPATHIES

The term cardiomyopathy is used to refer to a group of diseases which involve the myocardium directly. The term primary myocardial disease has been used to refer to the subgroup of cardiomyopathies which are idiopathic and the term secondary myocardial disease used to designate the group in which causative factors are known. Although there is no uniform agreement on terminology, Fowler has suggested that cardiomyopathy is a satisfactory term for this entire group of diseases. Further classification into idiopathic and secondary cardiomyopathy seems sensible and should avoid confusion. A classification from Fowler is given in Table 9–4. The list of secondary cardiomyopathies is long but the number of cases represented by that group is quite small, being less than 25 per cent in the experience of most cardiology services.

The true incidence of the various cardiomyopathies is not well known because of the tendency to diagnose ischemic heart disease when obvious congenital and rheumatic heart disease are not present. When carefully looked for, various types of cardiomyopathy are frequently recognized. It must be remembered that the specific incidence will vary considerably depending on the particular population of patients concerned. It is known that idiopathic cardiomyopathy is more frequent among indigent patient populations than in individuals from higher socioeconomic groups. Recent animal experiments suggest that exercise in the face of active myocarditis due to virus infection or Chagas' disease is associated with an increase in myocardial damage. Nutritional deficiency has a similar detrimental influence. These studies offer a possible explanation for the high incidence of these diseases in indigent populations.

Idiopathic Cardiomyopathy

There are two general categories of diseases in the idiopathic group — obstructive and nonobstructive. The obstructive cardiomyopathies are

TABLE 9–4 CLASSIFICATION OF
CARDIOMYOPATHIES

Idiopathic Cardiomyopathy
  Nonobstructive cardiomyopathy
    Alcoholic cardiomyopathy
    Postinfectious cardiomyopathy (when infectious
      agent cannot be identified)
    Familial cardiomyopathy
    Peripartal cardiomyopathy
    Cardiomyopathy without identifiable antecedent
      illness
  Obstructive cardiomyopathy
    Familial
    Nonfamilial

Secondary Cardiomyopathy
  Myocarditis
    Viral: Coxsackie B, Coxsackie A, echo virus, in-
      fluenza virus, infectious mononucleosis
    Rheumatic
    Septic (including bacterial endocarditis)
    Diphtheritic
    Syphilitic
    Chagas' disease
    Trichinosis
    Allergic
    Toxic
    Uremic
    Toxoplasmic
  Neuromuscular and neurologic disorders
    Progressive muscular dystrophy; pseudohyper-
      trophic and facioscapulohumeral muscular dys-
      trophy
    Friedreich's ataxia
    Myotonic muscular dystrophy
  Connective tissue diseases: rheumatoid disease, der-
    matomyositis, scleroderma, disseminated lupus
    erythematosus
  Mucopolysaccharidosis (e.g., Hurler's syndrome,
    Hunter's syndrome)
  Sarcoidosis
  Amyloid disease
  Primary and metastatic tumors
  Metabolic disorders
    Glycogen storage disease
    Nutritional deficiency
      Beriberi
      Kwashiorkor
    Thyrotoxicosis
    Myxedema
    Hemochromatosis
    Nutritional cirrhosis

(From Fowler, N. O.: Progr. Cardiovasc. Dis., *14*:113–
128, 1971. By permission of Grune & Stratton, Inc.)

very different from the nonobstructive in their
hemodynamic manifestations and will be discussed first.

Obstructive Cardiomyopathies. The obstructive
cardiomyopathies, known as idiopathic hypertrophic subaortic stenosis (IHSS), have been well
studied since the classic report of Braunwald and
colleagues in the early 1960s. The unusual dynamic character of the obstruction has been defined and rational methods of medical and surgical treatment have been developed. A familial
incidence has been recognized in about 30 per
cent of cases, but the etiology remains obscure.

This disease has been recognized from infancy
to old age but is usually seen in young adults. It is
manifest by palpitations, angina, or effort or post-
exertional syncope and is associated with a high
incidence of sudden death. Symptoms of pulmonary congestion and congestive heart failure develop late in the disease. Physical examination
reveals a systolic ejection murmur at the lower
left sternal border and an intact aortic second
sound. There is an associated murmur of mitral
insufficiency in about 50 per cent of cases. The
ejection murmur increases in intensity with
standing, during the Valsalva maneuver, or following the administration of amyl nitrite or nitroglycerin. The beat following a premature contraction is characterized by an increase in the
systolic pressure gradient and in the intensity of
the ejection murmur and by a reduced arterial
pulse pressure. Treatment with digitalis may
cause an increase in the murmur and a worsening of symptoms and is contraindicated in this
disease. Hemodynamic studies reveal a pressure
gradient between the left ventricular inflow tract
and outflow tract. The pressure gradient is increased by the drugs and maneuvers noted above
and is often decreased by the administration of a
beta blocking drug such as propranolol.

Left ventricular angiocardiography usually reveals generalized left ventricular hypertrophy
with marked hypertrophy of the papillary muscles. The basal portion of the interventricular
septum is greatly hypertrophied, although this
may be difficult to appreciate by angiography.
The end-diastolic volume of the left ventricle is
usually normal but the end-systolic volume is
smaller than normal with almost complete obliteration of the apical portion of the ventricle,
which may appear as a finger-shaped cavity.
Quantitative angiocardiographic evaluation reveals an increased ejection fraction and marked
increase in left ventricular mass. The coronary
arteries often appear to be unusually large.

Left ventricular end-diastolic pressure is
usually elevated and may be extremely high
while left ventricular dp/dt is elevated as well.
The high filling pressure in combination with an
elevated ejection fraction and LV dp/dt suggest
that the myocardium is noncompliant but retains
normal or has increased contractility.

Surgical exploration reveals a normal aortic
valve and localized hypertrophy of the basal portion of the interventricular septum just below the
aortic valve. This area of the septum may be
fibrotic and there is often considerable thickening
of the endocardium. It appears, therefore, that
outflow obstruction develops in this disease be-

cause the anterior leaflet of the mitral valve is pulled into apposition with the hypertrophied interventricular septum during systole. The actual site of obstruction is often difficult to visualize by angiography.

Echocardiography has become accepted as a useful non-invasive technique for the diagnosis of IHSS (idiopathic hypertrophic subaortic stenosis). The echocardiogram usually demonstrates asymmetric thickening of the basal portion of the interventricular septum as compared with the thickness of the posterior left ventricular wall in a ratio of $\geq$ 1.3:1. In addition, the anterior leaflet can be shown to move anteriorly toward the septum during systole instead of posteriorly, as in normals. The echo recording often shows the anterior leaflet echoes joining the echoes of the septum, suggesting that at least a portion of the valve contacts the septum during mid- or late systole. This is strong evidence that the outflow obstruction present in IHSS occurs as a result of this phenomenon. Some patients only have asymmetric septal hypertrophy (ASH), without abnormal motion of the mitral valve or other evidence for obstruction. ASH is often found in asymptomatic family members of patients with IHSS, suggesting that ASH may be a genetic marker of the disease.

From the above description it can be appreciated that conditions which reduce end-diastolic volume or increase the contractile state of the left ventricle will tend to increase the subvalvular pressure gradient. These include inotropic drugs such as isoproterenol and digitalis glycosides, reduced venous return to the left heart as induced by postural changes, the Valsalva maneuver or loss of blood volume, and reduced left ventricular afterload as induced with nitroglycerin or amyl nitrite. Beta blocking drugs are specific for this disease in that they can be shown to reduce or eliminate the outflow obstruction in many of these cases. When severe obstruction is present that does not respond to beta blockade, surgical treatment with excision of the hypertrophied muscle of the outflow tract may be beneficial.

Nonobstructive Cardiomyopathies. The majority of idiopathic cardiomyopathies are of the nonobstructive type. In the United States they are found most often in patients with high alcohol consumption or women in the immediate pre- or postpartum periods. Although alcohol administration has been shown to reduce ventricular contractility, the actual etiologic role of alcohol in the production of chronic progressive cardiomyopathy is not known. Peripartum cardiomyopathy is also not well understood, although it is most common in poorly nourished individuals, suggesting the importance of nutritional factors.

In years past, it was thought that most cases of chronic heart disease were either of valvular eti-

ology or due to chronic myocarditis. When the high incidence of ischemic heart disease in Western countries became appreciated, chronic myocarditis became an unusual diagnosis. Although there are well-documented cases of acute viral or bacterial myocarditis having progressed to produce chronic myocardial failure, in general there is complete recovery. In fact, it is extremely unusual to see patients with cardiomyopathy in whom one can obtain a history suggesting an infectious etiology. Therefore, although the concept that chronic cardiomyopathy is due to either prior or continuing low-grade myocarditis is appealing, there is little evidence to support this view.

Most patients with nonobstructive cardiomyopathy present with symptoms and signs of heart failure, but occasionally arrhythmias are the presenting complaint. Chest pain is unusual. The heart is large and all four chambers are frequently involved. Auscultation reveals a prominent atrial and/or ventricular gallop sound and there may be no murmur. When a murmur is present it is due to functional mitral and/or tricuspid regurgitation.

Cardiac catheterization usually reveals elevated atrial pressures with large "a" waves. The end-diastolic pressure is elevated in both ventricles and the pulmonary artery pressure is elevated secondary to the elevation of the left heart filling pressure. The cardiac output is low and the arteriovenous oxygen difference may be greatly elevated. Left ventricular dp/dt is depressed.

Angiocardiography reveals dilated cardiac chambers. The left ventricle has an increased diastolic volume and poor stroke volume, yielding a low ejection fraction, usually below 40 per cent. In severe cases, the ejection fraction may be as low as 10 per cent. The papillary muscles are not prominent but the left ventricular free wall is generally hypertrophied to a modest degree. Left ventricular mass is elevated and is generally equal to the diastolic volume of the left ventricle, yielding a left ventricular mass to end-diastolic volume ratio of about one.

Occasionally, there is a restrictive hemodynamic pattern seen in these patients with marked elevation in venous pressure and high plateau diastolic pressures seen in all cardiac chambers as is found in constrictive pericarditis. At times, it may be difficult to distinguish this disease from constrictive pericarditis without the aid of pericardial and myocardial biopsy. The restrictive form of the disease is seen most often in patients who either have myocardial infiltration with amyloid or hemochromatosis or have marked thickening and fibrosis of the endocardium. A form of extreme endomyocardial fibrosis is prevalent among natives of Uganda. In this condition, there is dense fibrosis of endocardium and myocardium with involvement of the papillary muscles resulting in mitral regurgitation. The etiology of this disease remains obscure.

Secondary Cardiomyopathies

Cardiomyopathy may be associated with a large number of specific disease entities, as shown in Table 9–4. Myocardial involvement as is seen with most of these diseases has hemodynamic features similar to those observed with the non-obstructive cardiomyopathies described above. There is loss of myocardial contractile force with ventricular dilatation, high filling pressure, low ejection fraction, and low cardiac output. When there is myocardial infiltration there is a tendency toward reduced myocardial compliance and a restrictive filling pattern. Exceptions are the cardiomyopathies associated with thyrotoxicosis and beriberi, in which cardiac output is elevated.

Specific cardiomyopathies are associated with certain neuromuscular diseases, including Friedreich's ataxia and the muscular dystrophies. In Friedreich's ataxia there is progressive myocardial fibrosis and obliterative disease of the small coronary arteries which is not due to atherosclerosis. The basis for the relationship between the neuromuscular disease and the cardiomyopathy is not apparent at this time.

Unfortunately, the majority of patients with cardiomyopathy represent difficult therapeutic problems. Cardiomyopathies due to specific infections and those due to a specific nutritional or metabolic abnormality may often be treated specifically. Patients with obstructive cardiomyopathy usually respond favorably to therapy with drugs or surgery. The majority of patients with the non-obstructive types of cardiomyopathy will have a favorable clinical response to non-specific measures such as bed rest, digitalis, diuretics, and unloading therapy. Not infrequently, the response is dramatic and clinical improvement continues for a number of years. However, these diseases are usually progressive, and response to therapy becomes less satisfactory as the disease progresses.

PERICARDIAL DISEASE

The pericardium, a fibrous sac surrounding the heart, consists of an outer parietal and inner visceral portion lined by a serous surface and normally contains a small amount of serous fluid. It has been demonstrated to have a function in limiting acute dilatation of the heart and possibly serves to isolate the heart from the lungs and to inhibit the spread of infection from the lungs to the heart. These functions do not seem to be very important in that surgical removal of the pericardium is unassociated with abnormalities of heart function, although there may be some increase in the size of the cardiac silhouette on x-ray examination. Disease of the pericardium is manifest through pain, pericardial effusion, or pericardial constriction of the heart.

Pericardial pain is associated with inflammation or other conditions that irritate the pericardium. The most common cause of pericardial pain is acute pericarditis, but pain also occurs with irritation from leakage of blood into the pericardium, as may be associated with trauma, perforation of the heart, or dissecting aneurysm. The pain is substernal or precordial in location and, in contrast to the pain accompanying myocardial infarction, is accentuated by respiratory movements and occasionally by swallowing. The patient is often more comfortable when sitting and leaning forward. The pain may radiate to the neck, left shoulder, arm, or back. Studies have demonstrated that pain sensation arises from the inferior portion of the parietal pericardium and is transmitted via the phrenic nerves. However, pericardial pain has been relieved by stellate ganglion block, suggesting that at least some pericardial pain fibers travel with the sympathetic nerves.

Pericarditis

The most frequent cause of acute pericarditis is so-called acute idiopathic or non-specific pericarditis. Pericarditis also occurs in association with a large number of other diseases and conditions which include myocardial infarction, postmyocardial infarction and post-thoracotomy syndrome; specific bacterial, viral, and fungal infections; neoplasms, uremia; certain drug sensitivity reactions; and connective tissue disorders such as rheumatic fever and lupus erythematosus. The pain is often severe and may simulate the pain of myocardial infarction. Inflammatory disease of the pericardium is usually accompanied by systemic signs associated with inflammation such as fever and leukocytosis. On auscultation there is usually a pericardial friction rub, which is a scratchy type sound, often with three separate components associated with atrial systole, ventricular systole, and ventricular diastole. There are often electrocardiographic changes which are characterized by an ST current of injury directed downward and to the left in the direction of the cardiac apex, probably a result of diffuse epicardial injury. Over a period of days, and as the ST subsides, the T wave characteristically becomes abnormal and directed up toward the right shoulder, away from the cardiac apex. Pericarditis is usually associated with pericardial effusion, which is manifest as an increase in the size of the heart on x-ray examination and occasionally by evidence of pericardial tamponade.

Pericardial Effusion

Whether pericardial effusion is associated with pericardial tamponade depends on the rate and volume of fluid accumulation within the pericardium. Acute effusions and/or bleeding of 200 to 300 ml. within the pericardium may result in tamponade. When pericardial fluid accumulates slowly, the pericardial sac enlarges, so that more than a liter may be present with no evidence of tamponade.

Large pericardial effusions are usually observed with the more chronic forms of pericarditis and, in contrast to acute pericarditis, pain is slight or absent. Pericardial effusion is also common in myxedema and congestive heart failure. The pressure-volume characteristics of the pericardium are such that substantial amounts of fluid may accumulate with little increase in pressure. However, a volume is reached at which pressure begins to rise rapidly with further small increases in volume.

On examination, the patient with pericardial effusion characteristically shows an increase in the area of cardiac dullness to percussion with a quiet precordium and distant heart sounds. The cardiac silhouette is enlarged, often with a water-bottle type configuration. Low voltage is often present on the electrocardiogram.

With pericardial tamponade there is interference with diastolic filling of the heart, resulting in an elevated filling pressure. A characteristic hemodynamic feature of pericardial tamponade is elevation of right and left atrial pressure and the diastolic pressure in the right and left ventricles to similar levels, as is observed in constrictive pericarditis (Fig. 9–22). This feature is often helpful in differentiating pericardial tamponade from left ventricular failure which is associated with higher filling pressures on the left side of the heart. Dyspnea is usually present, but orthopnea absent unless tamponade is severe. Arterial hypotension also occurs with severe tamponade.

Pulsus paradoxicus is a classic finding in pericardial tamponade and is recognized by a rise and fall of systemic systolic arterial pressure of more than 8 to 10 mm. Hg in the recumbent subject during quiet respiration. There have been a number of explanations for this phenomenon. It appears to be related to increased filling of the right heart with reduced filling of the left heart during inspiration. Because in pericardial tamponade there is a restriction of diastolic volume of the entire heart, an increase in diastolic volume of the right ventricle, as occurs during inspiration, must be associated with a reduced diastolic volume of the left heart. An increased pulmonary blood volume is also suggested as contributing to reduced filling of the left ventricle during inspiration. It should be appreciated that pulsus paradoxicus is not a specific finding for pericardial tamponade but also may occur with any condition associated with larger than normal respiratory changes of intrathoracic pressure and with heart failure.

The differentiation of pericardial effusion and tamponade from generalized cardiac enlargement is a rather common clinical problem. Demonstration of pericardial fluid by echocardiog-

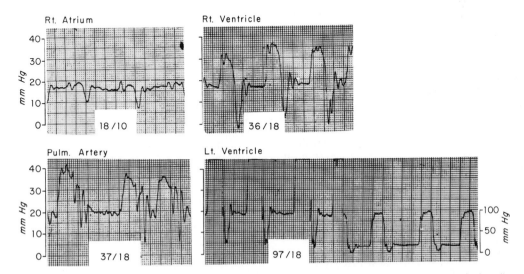

Figure 9–22 Pressures from a patient with constrictive pericarditis. The similarity of pressures during diastole in the right atrium, pulmonary artery, and right and left ventricles is shown. Both right and left ventricular diastolic pressures show a characteristic early diastolic dip followed by a diastolic plateau.

raphy or of a wide margin between the cardiac chamber and the external surface of the cardiac shadow by a radioisotope blood pool scan, by angiocardiography, or by filming following the introduction of carbon dioxide into the venous circulation is often helpful. The demonstration of fluid by pericardiocentesis, of course, establishes the diagnosis of pericardial effusion. Examination of the fluid may also be helpful in establishing an etiologic basis for pericardial effusion and pericarditis.

The treatment for pericardial tamponade is removal of pericardial fluid. This results in a prompt relief of symptoms due to the tamponade.

Constrictive Pericarditis

Constrictive pericarditis occurs when pericardial fibrosis and thickening result in restriction of diastolic feeling of the heart. In this condition the visceral and parietal layers of the pericardium are adherent and may be greatly thickened and densely fibrotic with areas of calcification. Pericardial constriction is known to occur with or following infection of the pericardium with tuberculosis, pyogenic organisms, certain viral diseases, and with acute idiopathic pericarditis. It also occurs with neoplastic involvement of the pericardium, with certain connective tissue disorders such as lupus erythematosus, following radiation therapy, and following hemopericardium from a variety of causes. However, in most patients it is not possible to establish a cause.

The laboratory and clinical findings are consequences of the restricted diastolic filling which results in venous pressure elevation. Because the entire heart is encased in this sac, filling pressures are usually elevated to similar levels on the two sides of the heart, so that right and left atrial, right and left ventricular diastolic, pulmonary wedge, and pulmonary artery diastolic pressures are nearly equal. This is illustrated in Figure 9–22. Other features of the pressure tracings characteristic of constrictive pericarditis are as follows: (1) a rapid fall of ventricular pressure in early diastole resulting in an early diastolic dip followed by a flat diastolic plateau (see right and left ventricular pressures in Figure 9–22); (2) a rapid descent of right atrial pressure with the onset of ventricular filling (y descent) which often results in a right atrial pressure curve that has a "w" or "m" configuration. Right ventricular and pulmonary artery systolic pressures are usually only modestly elevated, with the right ventricular diastolic pressure one third or more of the systolic pressure, also as shown in Figure 9–22. These pressure findings are not absolutely diag-

nostic of constrictive pericarditis and occasionally occur with chronic myocardial failure and fibrosis. However, with left ventricular failure the filling pressure is usually higher on the left side of the heart and right ventricular and pulmonary artery systolic pressures are usually higher than is observed with constrictive pericarditis. Stroke volume is small, but, unless constriction is severe, the cardiac index is only slightly reduced and increases with exercise through an increase in heart rate. The cardiac chamber volumes are characteristically normal or reduced. A thickened wall of the heart due to pericardial thickening can usually be demonstrated by angiocardiography or by positioning a cardiac catheter against the wall of the right atrium at the time of cardiac catheterization, so that the distance from the endocardium to the external surface of the right atrium can be visualized.

Patients with constrictive pericarditis may have an elevated venous pressure for long periods prior to the development of other symptoms or signs such as edema and exertional dyspnea. Edema often appears as ascites and in longstanding cases may be complicated by cardiac cirrhosis of the liver. Weeping of plasma with plasma proteins into the gastrointestinal tract as a result of venous pressure elevation may contribute to hypoproteinemia which is observed in severe cases of long duration. In spite of an elevated venous pressure and edema, orthopnea is usually absent and pulmonary edema is unusual.

On examination, patients with constrictive pericarditis have findings associated with an elevated systemic venous pressure and peripheral edema. Pleural effusion is often present. The area of cardiac dullness and the cardiac silhouette on x-ray examination are of normal size or only moderately enlarged. Heart sounds may be distant, and a pericardial knock sound in early diastole resembling a third heart sound is often present. A paradoxic pulse is occasionally observed. The electrocardiogram commonly has low voltage and flat or abnormally directed T waves. Atrial fibrillation is present in approximately one third of patients. On chest x-ray or fluoroscopic examination approximately 50 per cent of patients with constrictive pericarditis have pericardial calcification.

In patients with constrictive pericarditis and edema, symptomatic improvement is observed following diuresis induced by one of the diuretic drugs. However, surgical removal of the constricting pericardium is the definitive therapy. Unfortunately, pericardiectomy for constrictive pericarditis is associated with a significant mortality, which is in the range of 5 to 10 per cent, and occasionally with incomplete relief or recurrence of constriction.

REFERENCES

GENERAL

Conn, H. L., and Horwitz, O.: Cardiac and Vascular Diseases. Lea and Febiger, Philadelphia, 1971.

Friedberg, C. K.: Diseases of the Heart, 3rd ed. W. B. Saunders Co., Philadelphia, 1966.

Hurst, J. W.: The Heart, 4th ed. McGraw-Hill Book Co., New York, 1978.

Zimmerman, H. A.: Intravascular Catheterization, 2nd ed. Charles C Thomas, Springfield, Illinois, 1966.

CARDIAC OUTPUT, PRESSURE MEASUREMENTS, AND CARDIAC CATHETERIZATION

Barratt-Boyes, B. G., and Wood, E. H.: Cardiac output and related measurements and pressure values in the right heart and associated vessels, together with an analysis of the hemodynamic response to the inhalation of high oxygen mixtures in healthy subjects. J. Lab. Clin. Med., 51:72, 1958.

Brandfonbrener, M., Landowne, M., and Shock, N. W.: Changes in cardiac output with age. Circulation, 12:557, 1955.

Burch, G. E., and DePasquale, N. P.: Cardiac performance in relation to blood volume. Am. J. Cardiol., 14:784, 1964.

Donald, K. W., Bishop, J. M., and Wade, O. L.: Effect of nursing positions on cardiac output of man with a note on the repeatability of measurements of cardiac output by the direct Fick method and with data on subjects with normal cardiovascular system. Clin. Sci., 12:199, 1953.

Dow, P.: Estimations of cardiac output and central blood volume by dye dilution. Physiol. Rev., 36:77, 1956.

Fegler, G.: The reliability of the thermo-dilution method for determination of the cardiac output and the blood flow in central veins. Q. J. Exp. Physiol., 42:254, 1957.

Fry, D. L., Noble, F. W., and Mallos, A. J.: An evaluation of modern pressure recording systems. Circ. Res., 5:40, 1957.

Gorlin, R., and Gorlin, S. G.: Hydraulic formula for calculation of the area of the stenotic mitral valve, other cardiac valves and central circulatory shunts. Am. Heart J., 1:41, 1951.

Hamilton, W. F., Riley, R. L., Attah, A. M., Cournand, A., Fowell, D. M., Himmelstein, R. P., Wheeler, N. C., and Witham, A. C.: Comparison of Fick and dye injection methods of measuring cardiac output in man. Am. J. Physiol., 153:309, 1948.

Kinsmann, J. M., More, J. W., and Hamilton, W. F.: Studies on the circulation. Injection method; physical and mathematical considerations. Am. J. Physiol., 89:322, 1929.

Mandel, D.: A Practice of Cardiac Catheterization. Chapter 13. Blackwell Scientific Publications, Oxford and Edinburgh, 1968.

Reeves, J. T., Grover, R. F., Filley, G. F., and Blount, S. G., Jr.: Cardiac output in normal resting man. J. Appl. Physiol., 16:276, 1961.

Samet, P., Bernstein, W. H., and Levine, S.: Transseptal left heart dynamics in 32 normal subjects. Dis. Chest, 47:633, 1965.

Selzer, A., and Sudrann, R. B.: Reliability of the determination of cardiac output in man by means of the Fick principle. Circ. Res., 6:485, 1958.

Shapiro, G. G., and Kravetz, L. J.: Damped and undamped frequency responses of underdamped catheter manometer systems. Am. Heart J., 80:226, 1970.

Stewart, G. N.: Researches on the circulation time and on the influences which affect it. J. Physiol., 22:169, 1887.

Swan, H. J., Marcus, H. S., and Allen, H. N.: Cardiac flow, volumes and pressure. In Conn, H. L., and Horwitz, O. (Eds.): Cardiac and Vascular Diseases. Lea and Febiger, Philadelphia, 1971, pp. 54–73.

Swan, H. J. C., Ganz, W., Forrester, J., Marcus, H., Diamond, G., and Chonette, D.: Catheterization of the heart in man with the use of a flow-directed balloon-tipped catheter. N. Engl. J. Med., 283:445, 1970.

Thomassen, B.: Cardiac output in normal subjects under standard basal conditions. The repeatability of measurements by the Fick method. Scand. J. Clin. Lab. Invest., 9:365, 1957.

Visscher, M. B., and Johnson, J. A.: The Fick principle: Analysis of potential errors in its conventional application. J. Appl. Physiol., 5:635, 1953.

Wade, O. L., and Bishop, J. M.: Cardiac Output and Regional Blood Flow. F. A. Davis Co., Philadelphia, 1962.

Yanof, H. M., Rosen, A. L., McDonald, N. M., and McDonald, D. A.: A critical study of the response of manometers to forced oscillations. Phys. Med. Biol., 8:407, 1963.

LEFT VENTRICULAR VOLUME, MASS, AND PUMP FUNCTION

Bartle, S. H., and Sanmarco, M. E.: Comparison of angiocardiographic and thermal washout techniques for left ventricular volume measurement. Am. J. Cardiol., 18:235, 1966.

Borer, J. S., Bacharach, S. L., Green, M. V., Kent, K. M., Epstein, S. E., and Johnson, G. S.: Real time radionuclide cineangiography in the noninvasive evaluation of global and regional left ventricular function at rest and during exercise in patients with coronary artery disease. N. Engl. J. Med., 296:839–844, 1977.

Bove, A. A., and Lynch, P. R.: Measurement of canine left ventricular performance by cineradiography of the heart. J. Appl. Physiol., 29:877, 1970.

Bristow, J. D., Van Zee, B. E., and Judkins, M. P.: Systolic and diastolic abnormalities of the left ventricle in coronary artery disease. Circulation, 42:219, 1970.

Bunnell, I. L., Grant, C., and Greene, D. G.: Left ventricular function derived from the pressure-volume diagram. Am. J. Med., 39:881, 1965.

Burns, J. W. Covell, J. W., Myers, R., and Ross, J., Jr.: Comparison of directly measured left ventricular wall stress and stress calculated from geometric reference figures. Circ. Res., 28:611, 1971.

Davila, J. C., and Sanmarco, M. E.: An analysis of the fit of mathematical models applicable to the measurement of left ventricular volume. Am. J. Cardiol., 18:31, 1966.

Dodge, H. T.: Determination of left ventricular volume and mass. Radiol. Clin. North Am., 9:459, 1971.

Dodge, H. T., and Baxley, W. A.: Left ventricular volume and mass and their significance in heart disease. Am. J. Cardiol., 23:528, 1969.

Dodge, H. T., Hay, R. E., and Sandler, H.: An angiocardiographic method for directly determining left ventricular stroke volume in man. Circ. Res., 11:739, 1962.

Dodge, H. T., Sandler, H., Ballew, D. W., and Lord, J. D., Jr.: The use of biplane angiocardiography for the measurement of left ventricular volume in man. Am. Heart J., 60:762, 1960.

Dodge, H. T., Sandler, H., Baxley, W. A., and Hawley, R. R.: Usefulness and limitations of radiographic methods for determining left ventricular volume. Am. J. Cardiol., 18:10, 1966.

Falsetti, H. J., Mates, R. E., Greene, D. G., and Bunnell, I. L.: V_{max} as an index of contractile state in man. Circulation, 43:323, 1971.

Feigenbaum, H.: Echocardiography, 2nd ed. Philadelphia, Lea and Febiger, 1976.

Gault, J. H., Covell, J. W., Braunwald, E., and Ross, J., Jr.: Left ventricular performance following correction of free aortic regurgitation. Circulation, 42:773, 1970.

Gault, J. H., Ross, J., Jr., and Braunwald, E.: Contractile state of the left ventricle in man. Circ. Res., 22:451, 1958.

Graham, T. P., Jr., Jarmakani, M. M., Canent, R. V., Capp, M. P., and Spach, M. S.: Characterization of left heart volumes and mass in normal children and in infants with intrinsic myocardial disease. Circulation, 38:826, 1968.

Graham, T. P., Jr., Jarmakani, M. M., Canent, R. V., Jr., and Morrow, M. N.: Left heart volume estimation in infancy and childhood. Circulation, 43:895, 1971.

Gramiak, R., and Wang, R. C.: Cardiac Ultrasound. St. Louis, C. V. Mosby Co., 1975.

Grant, C., Greene, D. G., and Bunnell, I. L.: Left ventricular enlargement and hypertrophy. Am. J. Med., 39:895, 1965.

Greene, D. G., Carlisle, R., Grant, C., and Bunnell, I. L.: Estimation of left ventricular volume by one-plane cineangiography. Circulation, 35:61, 1967.

Holt, J. P.: Estimation of the residual volume of the ventricle of the dog heart by two indicator dilution techniques. Circ. Res., 4:187, 1956.

Hood, W. P., Jr., Rackley, C. E., and Rolett, E. L.: Wall stress in the normal and hypertrophied human left ventricle. Am. J. Cardiol., 22:550, 1968.

Hood, W. P., Jr., Thomson, W. J., Rackley, C. E., and Rolett, E. L.: Comparison of calculations of left ventricular wall stress in man from thin-walled and thick-walled ellipsoidal models. Circ. Res., 24:575, 1969.

Hugenholtz, P. G., Kaplan, E., and Hull, E.: Determination of left ventricular wall thickness by angiocardiography. Am. Heart J., 78:513, 1969.

Hugenholtz, P. G., Wagner, H. R., and Sandler, H.: The in-vivo determination of left ventricular volume: comparison of the fiberoptic-indicator dilution and the angiocardiographic methods. Circulation, 37:489, 1968.

Jarmakani, M. M., Graham, T. P., Jr., Canent, R. V., and Capp, M. P.: The effect of corrective surgery on left heart volume and mass in children with ventricular septal defect. Am. J. Cardiol., 27:254, 1971.

Jarmakani, M. M., Graham, T. P., Jr., Canent, R. V., Spach, M. S., and Capp, M. P.: Effect of site of shunt on left heart-volume characteristics in children with ventricular septal defect and patent ductus arteriosus. Circulation, 40:411, 1969.

Karliner, J. S., Gault, J. H., Eckberg, D., Mullins, C. B., and Ross, J., Jr.: Mean velocity of fiber shortening. A simplified measure of left ventricular myocardial contractility. Circulation, 44:323, 1971.

Kasser, I. S., and Kennedy, J. W.: Measurement of left ventricular volumes in man by single plane cineangiocardiography. Invest. Radiol., 4:83, 1969.

Kennedy, J. W., Baxley, W. A., Figley, M. M., Dodge, H. T., and Blackmon, J. R.: Quantitative angiocardiography. The normal left ventricle in man. Circulation, 34:272, 1966.

Levine, J. H., McIntyre, K. M., Lipana, J. G., and Bing, O. H. L.: Force velocity relations in failing and nonfailing hearts of subjects with aortic stenosis. Am. J. Med. Sci., 259:79, 1970.

Mason, D. T., Spann, J. F., Jr., and Zelis, R.: Quantification of the contractile state of the intact left ventricle. Maximal velocity of contractile element shortening determined by the instantaneous relation between the rate of pressure rise and pressure in the left ventricle during isovolumic systole. Am. J. Cardiol., 26:248, 1970.

Mirsky, I.: Left ventricular stresses in the intact human heart. Biophys. J., 9:189, 1969.

Rackley, C. E., Dear, H. D., Baxley, W. A., Jones, W. F., and Dodge, H. T.: Left ventricular chamber volume, mass and function in severe coronary artery disease. Circulation, 41:605, 1970.

Rackley, C. E., Dodge, H. T., Coble, Y. D., Jr., and Hay, R. E.: A method for determining left ventricular mass in man. Circulation, 29:666, 1964.

Rapaport, E., Wiegand, B. D., and Bristow, J. D.: Estimation of left ventricular residual volume in the dog by a thermodilution method. Circ. Res., 11:803, 1962.

Ross, J., Jr., and Sobel, B. E.: Regulation of cardiac contraction. Ann. Rev. Physiol., 34:47, 1972.

Ross, J., Jr., Sonnenblick, E. H., Taylor, R. R., Spotnitz, H. M., and Covell, J. W.: Diastolic geometry and sarcomere lengths in the chronically dilated canine left ventricle. Circ. Res., 28:49, 1971.

Sandler, H., Dodge, H. T., Hay, R. E., and Rackley, C. E.: Quantitation of valvular insufficiency in man by angiocardiography. Am. Heart J., 65:501, 1963.

Sandler, H., and Dodge, H. T.: Left ventricular tension and stress in man. Circ. Res., 13:91, 1963.

Sandler, H., and Dodge, H. T.: The use of single plane angiocardiograms for the calculation of left ventricular volume in man. Am. Heart J., 75:325, 1968.

Schelbert, H. R., Verba, J. W., Johnson, A. D., Brock, G. W., Alazraki, N. P., Rose, F. J., and Ashburn, W. L.: Nontraumatic determination of left ventricular ejection fraction by radionuclide angiocardiography. Circulation, 51:902–909, 1975.

Swan, H. J. C., and Beck, W.: Ventricular non-mixing as a source of error in the estimation of ventricular volume by the indicator-dilution method. Circ. Res., 8:989, 1960.

Taylor, R. R., Covell, J. W., and Ross, J., Jr.: Left ventricular function in experimental aorto-caval fistula with circulatory congestion and fluid retention. J. Clin. Invest., 47:1333, 1968.

Turina, M., Bussmann, W. D., and Krayenbuhl, H. P.: Contractility of the hypertrophied canine heart in chronic volume overload. Cardiovasc. Res., 3:486, 1969.

Urschel, C. W., Covell, J. W., Sonnenblick, E. H., Ross, J., Jr., and Braunwald, E.: Myocardial mechanics in aortic and mitral valvular regurgitation. The concept of instantaneous impedance as a determinant of the performance of the intact heart. J. Clin. Invest., 47:867, 1968.

HEMODYNAMICS OF HEART FAILURE

Baxley, W. A., Jones, W. B., and Dodge, H. T.: Left ventricular anatomical and functional abnormalities in chronic postinfarction heart failure. Ann. Intern. Med., 74:499, 1971.

Braunwald, E., Frahm, C. J., and Ross, J., Jr.: Studies on Starling's law of the heart. V. Left ventricular function in man. J. Clin. Invest., 40:1882, 1961.

Braunwald, E., Ross, J., Jr., and Sonnenblick, E. H.: Mechanism of contraction of the normal and failing heart. N. Engl. J. Med., 277:794, 853, 910, 962, 1012; 1967.

Chatterjee, K., Swan, H. J. C.: Vasodilator therapy in acute myocardial infarction. Mod. Concepts Cardiovasc. Dis., 43:119, 1974.

Cohn, J. N., Khatri, I. M., and Hamosh, P.: Diagnostic and therapeutic value of bedside monitoring of left ventricular pressure. Am. J. Cardiol., 23:107, 1969.

Cohn, J. W., Mathew, K. J., Franciosa, J. A., and Snow, J. A.: Chronic vasodilator therapy in the management of cardiogenic shock and intractable left ventricular failure. Ann. Int. Med., 81:777–780, 1974.

Dodge, H. T., and Baxley, W. A.: Hemodynamic aspects of heart failure. Am. J. Cardiol., 22:24, 1968.

Patterson, S. W., Piper, H., and Starling, E. H.: The regulation of the heart beat. J. Physiol., 48:465, 1914.

Rapaport, E., and Scheinman, M.: Rationale and limitations of hemodynamic measurements in patients with acute infarction. Mod. Concepts Cardiovasc. Dis., 38:55, 1969.

Russell, R. O., Jr., Porter, C. M., Frimer, M., and Dodge, H. T.: Left ventricular power in man. Am. Heart J., 81:799, 1971.

Russell, R. O., Jr., Rackley, C. E., Pombo, J., Hunt, D., Potanin, C., and Dodge, H. T.: Effects of increasing left ventricular filling pressure in patients with acute myocardial infarction. J. Clin. Invest., 49:1539, 1970.

Sarnoff, S. J., and Bergland, E.: Ventricular function. I. Starling's law of the heart studied by means of simultaneous right and left ventricular function curves in the dog. Circulation, 9:706, 1954.

ISCHEMIC HEART DISEASE

Barnard, P. M., and Kennedy, J. H.: Postinfarctional ventricular septal defect. Circulation, 32:76, 1965.

Bashour, F. A.: Mitral regurgitation following myocardial infarction. The syndrome of papillary mitral regurgitation. Dis. Chest, 48:113, 1965.

Baxley, W. A., Jones, W. B., and Dodge, H. T.: Left ventricular anatomical and functional abnormalities in chronic postinfarction heart failure. Ann. Intern. Med., 74:499, 1971.

Bristow, J. D., Bruce, E. V., and Judkins, M. P.: Systolic and diastolic abnormalities of the left ventricle in coronary artery disease. Studies in patients with little or no enlargement of ventricular volume. Circulation, 42:219, 1970.

Burch, G. E., DePasquale, N. P., and Phillips, J. H.: The syndrome of papillary muscle dysfunction. Am. Heart J., 75:399, 1968.

Daggett, W. M., Burwell, L. R., Lawson, D. W., and Austen, W. G.: Resection of acute ventricular aneurysm and ruptured interventricular septum after myocardial infarction. N. Engl. J. Med., 283:1507, 1970.

Dumesnil, J. G., Ritman, E. L., Fry, R. L., Gau, G. T., Rutherford, B. D., and Davis, G. D.: Quantitative determinations of regional left ventricular wall dynamics by roentgen videometry. Circulation, 50:700, 1974.

Effler, D. B., Favaloro, R. G., Groves, L. K., and Loop, F. D.: The simple approach to direct coronary artery surgery. J. Thorac. Cardiovasc. Surg., 62:503, 1971.

Effler, D. B., Groves, L. K., and Favaloro, R.: Surgical repair of ventricular aneurysm. Dis. Chest, 48:37, 1965.

Falsetti, H. L., Geraci, A. R., Bunnell, I. L., Greene, D. G., and Grant, C.: Function of left ventricle and extent of coronary lesions: failure of correlation in cineangiographic studies. Chest, 59:610, 1971.

Gould, K. L., and Lipscomb, K.: Effects of coronary stenoses on coronary flow reserve and resistance. Am. J. Cardiol., 34:48–55, 1974.

Hamilton, G. H., Murray, J. A., and Kennedy, J. W.: Quantitative angiocardiography in ischemic heart disease. The spectrum of abnormal left ventricular function and the role of abnormally contracting segments. Circulation, 45:1065, 1972.

Herman, M. V., Heinle, R. A., Klein, M. D., and Gorlin, R.: Localized disorders in myocardial contraction. N. Engl. J. Med., 277:222, 1967.

Miller, G. E., Cohn, K. E., Kerth, W. J., Selzer, A., and Gerbode, F.: Experimental papillary muscle infarction. J. Thorac. Cardiovasc. Surg., 56:611, 1968.

Rackley, C. E., Dear, H. D., Baxley, W. A., Jones, W. B., and Dodge, H. T.: Left ventricular chamber volume, mass and function in severe coronary artery disease. Circulation, 41:605, 1970.

Schrinert, G., Falsetti, H. L., Bunnell, I. L., Dean, D. C., Gage, A. A., Grant, C., and Green, D. G.: Excision of akinetic left ventricular wall of intractable heart failure. Ann. Intern. Med., 70:437, 1969.

Selzer, A., Gerbode, F., and Kerth, W. J.: Clinical hemodynamic and surgical considerations of rupture of the ventricular septum after myocardial infarction. Am. Heart J., 78:598, 1969.

Sharma, B., Goodwin, J. F., Raphael, M. J., Steiner, R. E., Rainbow, R. G., and Taylor, S. H.: Left ventricular angiography on exercise. A new method of assessing left ventricular function in ischemic heart disease. Br. Heart J., 38:49, 1976.

Stewart, D. K., Dodge, H. T., and Frimer, M.: Quantitative Analysis of Regional Myocardial Performance in Coronary Heart Disease. In Cardiovascular Imaging and Image Processing: Theory and Practice, 1975. Society of Photo-optical Instrument Engineers, Bellingham, Washington, 72:217, 1976.

Stinson, E. B., Becker, J., and Shumway, N. E.: Successful repair of postinfarction ventricular septal defect and biventricular aneurysm. J. Thorac. Cardiovasc. Surg., 58:20, 1969.

Swithinbank, J. M.: Perforation of the interventricular septum in myocardial infarction. Br. Heart J., 21:562, 1959.

MITRAL VALVE DISEASE

Arvidsson, H.: Angiocardiographic observations in mitral valve disease, with special reference to the volume variations in the left atrium. Acta Radiol., Suppl. 158, p. 1, 1958.

Blackmon, J. R., Rowell, L. B., Kennedy, J. W., Twiss, R. D., and Conn, R. D.: Physiologic significance of maximal oxygen intake in "pure" mitral stenosis. Circulation, 36:497, 1967.

Braunwald, E.: Mitral regurgitation: physiological, clinical and surgical considerations. N. Engl. J. Med., 281:425, 1969.

Braunwald, E., and Awe, W. C.: Syndrome of severe mitral regurgitation and normal left atrial pressure. Circulation, 27:29, 1963.

Braunwald, E., Braunwald, N. S., Ross, J., Jr., and Morrow, A. G.: Effects of mitral valve replacement on the pulmonary vascular dynamics of patients with pulmonary hypertension. N. Engl. J. Med., 273:509, 1965.

Dalen, J. E., Matloff, J. M., Evans, G. L., Hoppin, F. G., Bhardnaj, P., Harken, D. E., and Dexter, L.: Early reduction in pulmonary vascular resistance after mitral valve replacement. N. Engl. J. Med., 277:387, 1967.

DeSanctis, R. W., Dean, D. C., and Bland, E. F.: Extreme left atrial enlargement. Circulation, 29:14, 1964.

Ellis, L. B., and Harken, D. E.: Closed valvuloplasty for mitral stenosis. N. Engl. J. Med., 270:643, 1964.

Friedberg, C. K.: Diseases of the Heart, 3rd ed., Chapter 27. W. B. Saunders Co., Philadelphia, 1966.

Friedman, W. F., and Braunwald, E.: Alterations in regional pulmonary blood flow in mitral valve disease studies by radioisotope scanning. Circulation, 24:363, 1966.

Gerami, S., Messmer, B. J., Hallman, G. L., and Cooley, D. A.: Open mitral commissurotomy, results of 100 conservative cases. J. Thorac. Cardiovasc. Surg., 62:366, 1971.

Hawley, R. R., Dodge, H. T., and Graham, T. P.: Left atrial volume and volume changes in heart disease. Circulation, 34:989, 1966.

Hessel, E. A., Kennedy, J. W., and Merendino, K. A.: A reappraisal of nonprosthetic reconstructive surgery for mitral regurgitation based on an analysis of early and late results. J. Thorac. Cardiovasc. Surg., 52:193, 1966.

Kennedy, J. W., Yarnall, S. R., Murray, J. A., and Figley, M. M.: Quantitative angiocardiography: IV. Relationships of left atrial and ventricular pressure and volume in mitral valve disease. Circulation, 41:817, 1970.

Manhas, D. R., Hessel, E. A., Winterscheid, L. C., Dillard, D. H., and Merendino, K. A.: Repair of mitral incompetence secondary to ruptured chordae tendineae. Circulation, 43:688, 1971.

Merendino, K. A., Thomas, G. I., Jesseph, J. E., Herron, P. W., Winterscheid, L. C., and Vetto, R. R.: The open correction of rheumatic mitral regurgitation and/or stenosis: with special reference to regurgitation treated by posteromedial annuloplasty utilizing a pump oxygenator. Ann. Surg., 150:5, 1959.

Oleson, K. H.: The natural history of 271 patients with mitral stenosis under medical treatment. Br. Heart J., 27:349, 1962.

Osmundson, P. J., Callahan, J. A., and Edward, J. E.: Ruptured mitral chordae tendineae. Circulation, 23:42, 1961.

Roberts, W. C., Braunwald, E., and Morrow, A. G.: Acute severe mitral regurgitation secondary to ruptured chordae tendineae: clinical, hemodynamic and pathologic considerations. Circulation, 33:58, 1966.

Row, J. C., Bland, E. F., Sprague, H. B., and White, P. D.: The course of mitral stenosis without surgery. Ann. Intern. Med., 52:741, 1960.

Sanders, C. A., Armstrong, P. W., Willerson, J. T., and Dinsmore, R. E.: Etiology and differential diagnosis of acute mitral regurgitation. Prog. Cardiovasc. Dis., 14:129, 1971.

Sanders, C. A., Scannell, J. G., Hawthorne, J. W., and Austen, W. G.: Severe mitral regurgitation secondary to ruptured chordae tendineae. Circulation, 31:506, 1965.

AORTIC VALVE DISEASE

Anderson, F. L., Tsagaris, T. J., Tikoff, G., Thorne, J. L., Schmidt, A. M., and Kuida, H.: Hemodynamic effects of exercise in patients with aortic stenosis. Am. J. Med., 46:872, 1969.

Angell, W. W., Stenson, E. B., Ibur, A. B., and Shumway, W. E.: Multiple valve replacement with fresh aortic homograft. J. Thorac. Cardiovasc. Surg., 56:323, 1968.

Barratt-Boyes, B. G., and Roche, A. H. G.: A review of aortic valve homografts over a six and one-half period. Ann. Surg., 170:483, 1969.

Duvoisin, G. E., Wallace, R. B., Ellis, F. H., Anderson, M. W., and McGoon, D. C.: Late result of cardiac valve replacement. Circulation (Suppl. II), 37–38:1175, 1968.

Glancy, D. L., and Epstein, S. E.: Differential diagnosis of type and severity of obstruction to left ventricular outflow. Prog. Cardiovasc. Dis., 14:153, 1971.

Judge, T. P., Kennedy, J. W., Bennett, L. J., Wills, R. E., Murray, J. A., and Blackmon, J. R.: The quantitative hemodynamic effects of heart rate in aortic regurgitation. Circulation, 44:355, 1971.

Kennedy, J. W., Twiss, R. D., Blackmon, J. R., and Dodge, H. T.: Quantitative angiocardiography: III. Relationships of left ventricular pressure, volume and mass in aortic valve disease. Circulation, 38:838, 1968.

Morrow, A. G., Roberts, W. C., Ross, J., et al.: Obstruction to left ventricular outflow. NIH Clinical Staff Conference. Ann. Intern. Med., 69:1285, 1968.

Najafi, H.: Aortic insufficiency. Clinical manifestations and surgical treatment. Am. Heart J., 82:120, 1971.

Roberts, W. C.: The structure of the aortic valve in clinically isolated aortic stenosis. Circulation, 42:91, 1970.

Rotman, M., Morris, J. J., Behar, V. S., Peter, R. H., and Kong, Y.: Aortic valve disease — comparison of types and their medical and surgical management. Am. J. Med., 51:241, 1971.

Segal, J., Harvey, W. P., and Hufnagel, C.: A clinical study of 100 cases of severe aortic insufficiency. Am. J. Med., 21:200, 1956.

Shean, F. C., Austen, W. G., Buckley, M. J., Mundth, E. D., Scanwell, J. G., and Daggett, W. M.: Survival after Starr-Edwards aortic valve replacement. Circulation, 44:1, 1971.

Spangnuolo, M., Kloth, H., Taranta, D., Doyle, E., and Pasternack, B.: Natural history of rheumatic aortic regurgitation: criteria predictive of death, congestive heart failure and angina in young patients. Circulation, 44:368, 1971.

Wagner, H. R., Hugenhaltz, P. G., and Sandler, H.: Congenital aortic stenosis, compensating mechanisms in pure pressure overload. Circulation (Suppl. VI), 37–38:199, 1968.

THE CARDIOMYOPATHIES

Abelmann, W. H.: Experimental infection with *trypanosoma cruzi* (Chagas' disease). A model of acute and chronic myocardiopathy. Ann. N. Y. Acad. Sci., 153:137, 1969.

Adalman, A. G., McLoughlin, M. J., Merquis, Y., Auger, P., and Wigle, E. D.: Left ventricular cineangiographic observations in muscular subaortic stenosis. Am. J. Cardiol., 24:689, 1969.

Akbarian, M., Yankopoulos, N. A., and Abelmann, W. H.: Hemodynamic studies in beriberi heart disease. Am. J. Med., 41:197, 1966.

Alexander, C. S.: Idiopathic heart disease. I. Analysis of 100 cases with special reference to chronic alcoholism. Am. J. Med., 41:213, 1966.

Alexander, C. S.: Idiopathic heart disease. II. Electron microscopic examination of myocardial biopsy specimens in alcoholic heart disease. Am. J. Med., 41:229, 1966.

Bashour, F. A., McConnell, T., Skinner, W., and Hanson, M.: Myocardial sarcoidosis. Dis. Chest, 53:413, 1968.

Braunwald, E., Lambrew, C. T., Rockoff, S. D., Ross, J., Jr., and Morrow, A. G.: Idiopathic hypertrophic subaortic stenosis. I. A description of the disease based upon an analysis of 64 patients. Circulation, 30:3, 119; 1964.

Burch, G. E., and DePasquale, N.: Alcoholic cardiomyopathy. A review. Am. J. Cardiol., 23:723, 1969.

Burch, G. E., and Giles, T. D.: Alcoholic cardiomyopathy. Concept of the disease and its treatment. Am. J. Med., 50:141, 1971.

Chambers, R. J., Beck, W., and Schrire, V.: Ventricular dynamics in Bantu cardiomyopathy. Am. Heart J., 78:493, 1969.

Fowler, N. O.: Differential diagnosis of cardiomyopathies. Progr. Cardiovasc. Dis., 14:133, 1971.

Frank, S., and Braunwald, E.: Idiopathic hypertrophic subaortic stenosis. Clinical analysis of 126 patients with emphasis on natural history. Circulation, 37:759, 1968.

Goodwin, J. F.: Congestive and hypertrophic cardiomyopathies. Lancet, 1:731, 1970.

Hamby, R. I.: Primary myocardial disease. A prospective clinical and hemodynamic evaluation in 100 patients. Medicine, 49:55, 1970.

James, T. N.: Observations on the cardiovascular involvement including the cardiac conduction system in progressive muscular dystrophy. Am. Heart J., 63:48, 1962.

Lerner, A. M.: Virus myopericarditis. Ann. Intern. Med., 59:1068, 1968.

Mattingly, T. W.: The clinical and hemodynamic features of

primary myocardial disease. Trans. Am. Clin. Climat. Assoc., 70:132, 1958.

Mitchell, J. A., and Cohen, L. S.: Alcohol and the heart. Current Concepts Cardiov. Dis., 39:109, 1970.

Perloff, J. K., deLeon, A. C., Jr., and O'Doherty, D.: The cardiomyopathy of progressive muscular dystrophy. Circulation, 33:625, 1966.

Perloff, J. K., Lindgren, K. M., and Groves, B. M.: Uncommon or commonly unrecognized causes of heart failure. Progr. Cardiovasc. Dis., 12:409, 1970.

Popp, R. L., and Harrison, D. C.: Ultrasound in the diagnosis and evaluation of therapy of idiopathic hypertrophic subaortic stenosis. Circulation, 40:905, 1969.

Shaw, P. M., Gramiak, R., Kramer, D. H., and Yu, P. N.: Determinants of atrial and ventricular gallop sounds in primary myocardial disease. N. Engl. J. Med., 278:753, 1968.

Wagner, P.: Beriberi heart disease. Physiologic data and difficulties in diagnosis. Am. Heart J., 69:200, 1965.

PERICARDIAL DISEASE

Berglund, E., Sarnoff, S. J., and Isaacs, J. P.: Ventricular function: Role of the pericardium in regulation of cardiovascular hemodynamics. Circ. Res., 3:133, 1955.

Bradley, E. C.: Acute benign pericarditis. Am. Heart J., 67:121, 1964.

Capps, J. A.: Pain from the pleura and pericardium. J. Nerv. Ment. Dis., 23:263, 1943.

Conn, H. L., Jr., and Horwitz, O. (Eds.): Cardiac and Vascular Diseases. Lea and Febiger, Philadelphia, 1971, p. 1326.

Cooley, J. C., Clagett, O. T., and Kirklin, J. W.: Surgical aspects of chronic constrictive pericarditis. A review of 72 operative cases. Ann. Surg., 147:488, 1958.

Dalton, J. C., Pearson, R. J., and White, P. D.: Constrictive pericarditis. A review and long-term follow-up of 78 cases. Ann. Intern. Med., 45:445, 1956.

Dressler, W.: The post-myocardial infarction syndrome. Arch. Intern. Med., 103:28, 1959.

Drusin, L. M.: Post-pericardiotomy syndrome: A six year epidemiologic study. N. Engl. J. Med., 272:597, 1965.

Effer, D. B.: Chronic constrictive pericarditis treated with pericardiectomy. Am. J. Cardiol., 7:62, 1961.

Engle, M. A., and Ito, T.: The postpericardiotomy syndrome. Am. J. Cardiol., 7:73, 1961.

Gimlette, T. M. D.: Constrictive pericarditis. Br. Heart J., 21:9, 1959.

Guntheroth, W. G., Morgan, B. C., and Mullins, G. H.: Effect of respiration on venous return and stroke volume in cardiac tamponade. Circ. Res., 20:381, 1967.

Harrison, E. C., Crawford, D. W., and Lau, F. Y. K.: Sequential left ventricular function studies before and after pericardiectomy for constrictive pericarditis. Am. J. Cardiol., 26:319, 1970.

Harvey, W. P.: Auscultatory findings in diseases of the pericardium. Am. J. Cardiol., 7:15, 1961.

Hurst, J. W.: The Heart Arteries and Veins. McGraw-Hill Book Co., 4th ed. New York, 1978.

McKusich, V. A.: Chronic constrictive pericarditis. Some clinical and laboratory observations. Bull. Johns Hopkins Hosp., 90:3, 1952.

Portal, R. W., Besterman, E. M. M., Chambers, R. J., Sellors, T. H., and Somerville, W.: Prognosis after operation for constrictive pericarditis. Br. Med. J., 1:563, 1966.

Shobetai, R., Fowler, N. O., Fenton, J. C., and Masangkay, M.: Pulsus paradoxus. J. Clin. Invest., 44:1882, 1965.

Weissbein, A., and Heller, F. N.: A method of treatment for pericardial pain. Circulation, 24:607, 1961.

Wood, P.: Chronic constrictive pericarditis. Am. J. Cardiol., 7:48, 1961.

Yu, P. N. G., Lovejoy, F. W., Jr., Joos, H. A., Nye, R. E., Jr., and Mahoney, E. B.: Right auricular and ventricular pressure patterns in constrictive pericarditis. Circulation, 7:102, 1953.

10

Congestive Heart Failure

H. J. C. SWAN AND WILLIAM W. PARMLEY

INTRODUCTION

The general term congestive heart failure is used to designate a common series of syndromes seen in the clinical practice of medicine. These syndromes consist of the symptoms and physical signs associated with (1) failure of the left ventricle as a pump, (2) failure of the right ventricle as a pump, (3) pulmonary venous hypertension, and (4) systemic venous hypertension. Although these factors may be present alone or in combination in a given patient, and are frequently interrelated from the standpoint of mechanism, it is relevant to separate the general mechanics and consequences of failure of the left ventricle as a pump from those of failure of the right ventricle as a pump. For example, the usual consequences of failure of the left ventricle as a pump are an increase in pulmonary venous pressure with the associated symptoms of dyspnea and the findings of rales in the lung fields or of pleural effusion. However, pulmonary congestion and edema may also be a consequence of alteration of pulmonary capillary permeability by the direct effects of toxic gases or of central nervous system damage. The symptoms associated with failure of the right ventricle usually include ankle edema, abdominal swelling, and right subcostal pain which may be accompanied by the findings of peripheral edema, an enlarged liver, ascites, and increased jugular venous pulsation and pressure. Systemic venous congestion with the symptoms and signs of right heart failure may be due to failure of the right ventricle associated with chronic obstructive lung disease in association with normal left ventricular function or indeed might occur in the absence of primary disease of the heart itself as a consequence of primary pericardial disease with or without effusion.

DEFINITION OF HEART FAILURE

Perhaps it is appropriate to consider initially a rather broad physiologic definition of heart failure rather than the more specific clinical syndromes. Warren and Stead indicated that heart failure is that state which results from the inability of the heart to pump sufficient blood to the body tissues to meet ordinary metabolic demands. Indeed, when the heart is unable to meet the normal resting metabolic needs of the body tissue, ventricular stroke volume is usually profoundly decreased. Minor or moderate depressions of ventricular performance do not usually result in this alteration because compensating mechanisms become operative. One of the primary compensatory mechanisms available to the body to improve cardiac performance is to increase the heart rate and thus the frequency of emptying of the left ventricle. In the majority of mammalian species in which cardiac output increases under conditions of increased demand, the principal mechanism operates by increasing heart rate with a relatively unchanged level of stroke volume.

Using the current convention for the expression of flow values in the cardiovascular system in terms of body surface area (BSA), the normal stroke volume in a younger subject averages approximately 60 ml. per beat per $M.^2$ At a rate of 60 beats per minute, this results in a cardiac output of 3.6 L. per min. per $M.^2$, and during severe exercise at a heart rate of 180 beats per minute, a cardiac index of 10.8 L. per min. per M.^{2} may be achieved in the absence of any changes in stroke volume. Although small changes in stroke volume do occur, this is a secondary mechanism in the control of cardiac output. In patients with seriously reduced cardiac performance, one of the principal hemodynamic alterations is that the left ventricle may eject as little as 20 ml. per beat per M.^{2} or one third of normal stroke volume. However, a sinus tachycardia at a rate of 120 beats per minute will result in a cardiac index of 2.4 L. per min. per M.^{2}, which usually is adequate to meet resting metabolic needs.

In addition, partly as a consequence of the reduction in total cardiac output and the associated reduction of renal blood flow, the circulating blood volume increases. This, along with other factors, results in an enhanced filling pressure in the chambers of both right and left ventricles. An increased filling pressure results in a larger end-diastolic volume with a greater degree of fiber stretch. Thus, the performance of the heart may be enhanced secondarily for any given level of intrinsic contractile state by a greater fiber stretch — an additional mechanism to improve the function of the heart as a pump. However, as a consequence of the increased left ventricular diastolic pressure, there is increased pressure upstream in the left atrium and therefore in the pulmonary veins and capillaries which is transmitted into the pulmonary arteries. This results in an increase in pulmonary artery systolic, mean, and diastolic pressures. Hence, the right ventricle must do more work and progressively encounters greater difficulty in overcoming its outflow resistance, and a similar process of failure affects the right ventricle with the manifestations of systemic venous congestion. As a result, the common sequence of clinical congestive heart failure is a reduced left ventricular stroke volume accompanied by tachycardia and an increased left ventricular filling pressure, which tend to partly restore cardiac output and hence tissue perfusion but with an increase in myocardial oxygen needs, which are a direct function of both heart rate and left ventricular filling pressure (preload).

However, an important penalty for this compensation is the congestive changes in the lungs with increases in pulmonary arterial pressure and increased systemic venous pressure with congestive changes and edema. As a further generalization, it should be recognized that neither ventricle of the heart in the nonhypertrophied state is able to sustain significant acute increases in afterload.

This chapter will consider the general and specific mechanisms underlying failure of the heart as a pump with particular reference to the field of ischemic heart disease, in which important new

information is developing. The content is also related to our current ability to alter systematically the physiologic determinants of myocardial performance and thus to place the treatment of heart failure on a more rational and hence more effective basis.

NORMAL CARDIAC PERFORMANCE

It is necessary to review briefly certain characteristics of cardiac performance in the normal heart for a comparative background. During ventricular contraction, in association with shortening of the myocardial sarcomere, the volume and the shape of both ventricles alter. The principal shortening occurs in the free wall of each cardiac chamber, with lesser degrees of shortening occurring in the ventricular septum and in the base-to-apex dimension. The right and left ventricles differ in their geometric contraction characteristics. The right ventricle ejects its content by approximating the free wall to the right ventricular aspect of the ventricular septum. In contrast, the thicker-walled left ventricle contracts in a more circumferential manner, changing from an ellipsoid configuration during diastole to a narrow truncated cone during systole. This change in ventricular volumes between systole and diastole is the process by means of which blood is expelled from the ventricle. Since ventricular volumes are frequently dramatically altered in patients with heart failure, quantitative emphasis will be placed on the consideration of ventricular volumes and their change. Data pertaining to the accompaniments of normal cardiac function are included in Table 10–1.

Left Ventricular Ejection

The following pertains to the ejection characteristics of the left ventricle. The normal left ventricle has a volume of approximately 90 ml. per M.^{2} at end diastole (EDV). During contraction it ejects approximately two thirds of its content or 60 ml. per M.^{2} into the aorta — the stroke volume (SV) — and at end systole it cotains a residual volume of 30 ml. per M.^{2} (ESV). As a convenient measure of the pumping function of the left ventricle, the ratio of ejected or stroke volume to the end-diastolic volume — the ejection fraction (EF) — may be readily calculated: EF = SV/EDV. Utilizing the above data, the normal ejection fraction is approximately 0.66, and may vary from 0.60 to approximately 0.78. Deviations outside this range usually are abnormal. Note that this expression (EF) of ventricular performance will take into account abnormal valve leakage as

TABLE 10–1 NORMAL VALUES FOR CARDIAC PERFORMANCE AT REST

Cardiac index (L./min./M.^{2})	3.6
Heart rate (beats/min.)	60-90
Stroke index (ml./M.^{2})	60
Stroke work index (gm.-meters/M.^{2})	60
End-diastolic volume (ml./M.^{2})	90
End-systolic volume (ml./M.^{2})	30
Ejection fraction	0.67
LV end-diastolic pressure (mm. Hg)	<12
LV max dp/dt (mm. Hg/sec.)	1500
Segmental wall motion (% inward movement)	
Apical	30%
Anterior	50%
Inferior	40%

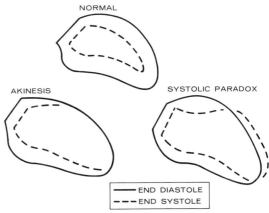

Figure 10–1 Normal and abnormal ventricular contraction patterns. The ventricular contours are shown as might be seen in a cineangiogram obtained in the right anterior-oblique projection. The solid line indicates the contour of the ventricular chamber at end diastole, and the dotted line indicates the position of the ventricular wall at end systole. Normally, the inward movement of the ventricular wall is uniform, involving all portions of the ventricle to approximately the same degree. In patients with diffuse cardiac disease, there is failure of contraction in all dimensions. In patients with localized cardiac disease, as shown in the two lower figures, there may be failure of movement of the affected portion of the ventricular wall, which is either scarred or stiffened (left). In certain instances the affected area may actually bulge during systole (right), providing not only a failure of contribution to contraction but a fundamental mechanical disadvantage.

well as the magnitude of forward blood flow. Thus, it is possible to describe the performance of the ventricle in patients with valvar incompetence in terms of the magnitude and proportion of volume ejected during ventricular contraction. Since EDV − ESV = total volume ejected, regurgitant volume (RV) is equal to (EDV − ESV) − SV, where SV=forward stroke volume.

The ejection fraction must not be confused with measures of the contractile state of the myocardium. Although it is possible to determine the instantaneous rate of volume change and thus arrive at an interpretation of ventricular function more closely related to the rate of sarcomere shortening, the ejection fraction accounts for only the ability of the heart to discharge its contents without relation to the time course or energetics of that process. The ejection fraction is one practically useful measure of pump function in the description of the heart in normal and abnormal states. Although the contractile state is usually depressed when the EF is reduced, normal values for EF may be found in the presence of a reduced contractile state, particularly when afterload falls.

Ventricular Contraction Patterns

Contraction of the ventricular wall is essentially a uniform process in the normal heart. The different elements and regions of the ventricular wall are displaced over a basically similar time course, occurring simultaneously for practical purposes over the whole mass of ventricular muscle. Normal end-systolic contraction, expressed as 1 minus the ratio of the end-systolic diameter to end-diastolic diameter for anterior, inferior, and apical segments, is given in Table 10–1. In the presence of certain abnormalities of intraventricular conduction, myocardial disease, or sequential underperfusion of the ventricle, this synchronous contraction may not be maintained. Under

such circumstances, specific elements of the myocardium may contract at a time later than the normally contracting myocardium, may not contract at all, and, under certain circumstances, may actually bulge or paradox during contraction of the remainder of the ventricle (Fig. 10–1). Each of these abnormalities of ventricular wall motion is mechanically inefficient and metabolically costly to the ventricle.

In addition to the process of contraction, the cardiac ventricles also are subjected to geometric changes associated with ventricular filling. Following ventricular systole, the sarcomeres of the myocardium lengthen to their resting position, thus markedly reducing the tension in the myocardial wall. This reduction in tension immediately results in passive changes in the internal dimensions of the ventricular cavity, particularly associated with the tendency of connective tissue and supportive elements to return to a position of least energy. This may result in diastolic suction when, following relaxation of the contractile elements, the heart develops a negative intracavity pressure and tends to "suck" blood into its cavity. However, this mechanism plays a small part in

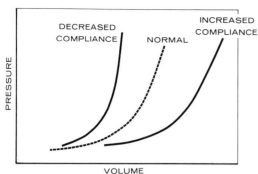

Figure 10–2 Passive pressure-volume relationship of the ventricles. The dotted line in the center indicates the general relationship between pressure and volume. As volume is increased initially, there is but a small rise in pressure. As volume increase continues, the rise in pressure is greater. Each of the solid lines indicates the alteration in pressure-volume relationships in decreased compliance *(left)* and increased compliance *(right)*. This can be considered as a greater or lesser degree of stiffness of the ventricle in relation to the filling volume. Ventricular compliance is a dynamic phenomenon, and this property can change rapidly.

filling of the ventricles, which is accomplished from the atria and great veins by reason of a slightly positive pressure within the vascular system relative to that external to the ventricle. The passive pressure-volume curve — representative of ventricular compliance — is concave to its pressure axis, so that blood is accepted in relatively large volumes from a low end-systolic volume, with very little change in filling pressure (Fig. 10–2). However, if filling is prolonged, the pressure will rise at an increasingly rapid level as the stiffer part of the ventricular pressure-volume curve is reached. Little attention has been paid to the passive pressure-volume relationships of the ventricle, yet they are all important in the concepts of heart failure. In normal human cardiac dynamics, the end-systolic volume of 30 ml. per M.^{2} is achieved at a filling pressure of between 0 and 3 mm. Hg. Addition of 60 ml. per M.^{2} (equivalent to the succeeding stroke volume) results in an increase in intraventricular pressure to between 8 and 12 mm. Hg at end diastole.

Thus, it is possible to describe the complete cardiac cycle in volumetric and pressure terms (Fig. 10–3). If we commence our consideration at the beginning of systole with an end-diastolic pressure of 12 mm. Hg and an end-diastolic volume of 90 ml. per M.^{2}, the intramyocardial tension rapidly increases until the intraventricular pressure equals that in the aortic root. No net volume change occurs, although a slight distortion of the ventricular wall accompanies the

movement of the mitral valve leaflets posterior into the left atrium. When the pressure in the ventricle reaches and exceeds that in the aortic root, ejection commences. In the normal heart, between one half and two thirds of the stroke volume is discharged from the ventricle during the first third of systole, whereas the flow into the aorta during the last third of systole is between 10 and 20 per cent of the total. The rates of change of dimension and volume follow a similar time course. For this reason, the normal heart has considerable adaptability at high heart rates, and even with considerable shortening of the duration of ventricular systole is still able to eject a great part of its content. However, when failure of the heart as a pump supervenes, the proportionate ejection of blood from the ventricle is more evenly distributed across the duration of ventricular systole, and the reserve capabilities of the ventricle are thus curtailed.

At the end of ventricular systole, the volume content of the ventricle has been reduced by the stroke volume and has returned to its end-systolic volume of 30 ml. per M.^{2} Following reduction of intramyocardial tension as a result of sarcomere relaxation, the pressure in the ventricle drops to between 0 and 3 mm. Hg. At this point, the pressure in the atrium is sufficient to open the atrioventricular valve and allow for the maxi-

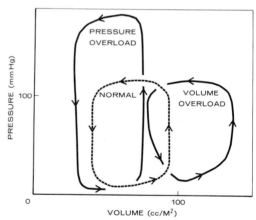

Figure 10–3 Pressure-volume relationships for the normal and abnormal ventricle. The dotted line indicates the normal pressure-volume loop (see text for details). With pressure overload and concentric hypertrophy there may be a reduction in end diastolic volume. However, greater work is performed in the generation of pressure for ejection of blood from the ventricle. In the presence of volume overload, there is an increase in all dimensions of the ventricle, so that the end-diastolic volume is substantively increased. The volume ejected is also increased, and the end-systolic volume is greater than normal in proportion to the magnitude of volume overload and the degree of compensation of the ventricle.

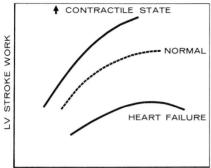

Figure 10–4 The relationship between left ventricular performance and left ventricular filling pressure (Frank-Starling relationship). Normally, an increased end-diastolic pressure is accompanied by a substantive increase in performance *(dotted line)*. In the presence of an enhanced contractile state in the same heart, the levels of performance are proportionately greater. In the presence of heart failure, the performance is less and when a critical level of diastolic pressure is reached, further increments of pressure are associated with a small reduction in performance.

mal rate of filling of the ventricle, which in the normal heart follows a similar time course as systole. Thus, approximately half of ventricular filling occurs in the first third of ventricular diastole, with a barely measurable increase in intraventricular pressure. The volume rate of filling of the ventricle is progressively reduced as ventricular pressure rises according to the passive compliance characteristics of the myocardial wall until end diastole, at which time atrial contraction adds a final increment of stroke volume to the ventricle. When atrial contraction has been completed, and the atrioventricular valves have commenced to float into their presystolic position, ventricular systole commences, and the cycle is repeated. The contraction pattern of the free wall of the ventricle is fundamentally uniform, with the greatest degree of shortening in the free wall and the least degree of shortening in the long axis and septal dimensions.

In addition, mechanisms of fundamental importance in the control and modification of normal or abnormal cardiac function include the tripartite relation between function and contractile state and presystolic fiber length — the Frank-Starling relationship (Fig. 10–4). The importance of these factors in the normal heart has already received consideration and will be discussed only in the context of heart failure per se. However, a central theme of critical importance in heart failure is a consideration of the factors which control myocardial oxygen consumption.

MYOCARDIAL OXYGEN CONSUMPTION

Since the report of Evans and Matsuoka in 1915, it has been generally appreciated that myocardial oxygen uptake is directly related to mean arterial pressure but is affected much less by changes in cardiac output. This generalization that pressure-work is much more costly than flow-work has been the framework upon which most of the subsequent studies of oxygen consumption have been performed. Furthermore, this concept has direct relevance to the pathophysiology of congestive heart failure and its effective therapy.

Fundamental studies in recent years by Sarnoff, Sonnenblick, Braunwald and associates have greatly enhanced our appreciation of the quantitative aspects of myocardial oxygen consumption. The important determinants of myocardial oxygen consumption are listed in Table 10–2 and are divided for convenience into those of major and minor importance. The subsequent discussion will focus on the relative importance of each of these determinants. The oxygen consumption of the beating heart ranges from about 8 to 15 ml. per min. per 100 grams myocardium, whereas the oxygen consumption of the noncontracting heart is approximately 2 ml. per min. per 100 grams. Thus, the basal requirements for oxygen are approximately 20 per cent of the total needs and are required for the normal metabolic processes in the myocardium which are not associated with contraction.

Tension-Time Index

The initial observations that pressure-work was a major determinant of oxygen consumption were extended by Sarnoff and associates, who demonstrated under carefully controlled conditions in the dog that there was a close relationship between the product of developed intraventricular pressure and the time for which it was maintained and the measured myocardial oxygen consumption. This concept of a "tension-time

---

TABLE 10–2 MYOCARDIAL OXYGEN CONSUMPTION

Major Determinants:
    Heart rate
    Tension development
    Contractile state
    Basal
Minor Determinants:
    Activation
    Depolarization
    Direct metabolic effect of catecholamines

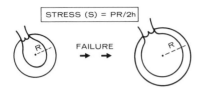

VENTRICULAR PRESSURE, ——————— P : SAME
RADIUS, ————————————————— R : INCREASED
WALL THICKNESS, ———————————— h : SAME OR DECREASED
WALL STRESS, ———————————— S : INCREASED
MYOCARDIAL O$_2$ CONSUMPTION, MVO$_2$: INCREASED

Figure 10–5 Relation of cardiac size to wall stress and to myocardial oxygen consumption. In heart failure, the end-diastolic volume (related to radius) is increased. Even when the wall thickness and internal pressure remain unchanged, the wall stress is increased in accordance with the law of Laplace. Hence, the myocardial oxygen consumption is increased.

index" has been of fundamental importance in relating the alterations in oxygen consumption that occur with changes in intraventricular pressure. Subsequently, the importance of wall tension rather than intraventricular pressure was emphasized. Since wall tension, according to the Laplace relation, is a direct function of the radius and intraventricular pressure, wall tension will be increased at the same intraventricular pressure if the heart dilates. Thus, in the enlarged failing heart, wall tension will be increased and myocardial oxygen consumption augmented, although there may be no change in ventricular pressure (Fig. 10–5). This fact further emphasizes the therapeutic importance of reducing the size of the failing heart. This may be accomplished by a reduction of circulating blood volume with diuretics or by inotropic stimulation as with digitalis, which can empty the ventricle more effectively and thus reduce the intraventricular volume.

Despite the obvious importance of the tension-time index as a determinant of myocardial oxygen consumption, it was observed in conscious dogs that myocardial oxygen consumption correlated poorly with the tension-time index during exercise or sympathetic stimulation. Similarly, the administration of inotropic agents, such as isoproterenol, often produced little change or even a decrease in the tension-time index, while oxygen consumption was greatly augmented. In a series of studies by Sonnenblick and associates, it became apparent that the velocity of contraction of the myocardium (as an index of the contractile state of the heart) was also a major determinant of myocardial oxygen consumption. Thus, when the tension-time index was maintained relatively constant, oxygen consumption was greatly augmented by changes in contractile state produced by paired electrical stimulation, norepinephrine, or an increase in calcium concentration. At the present time, therefore, it would appear that any intervention which increases the contractility of the myocardium will also increase myocardial oxygen consumption.

Initially, however, this fact did not appear compatible with data which showed that digitalis glycosides did not increase myocardial oxygen consumption, despite an increase in contractile state. This apparent discrepancy was resolved by Covell and associates, who noted that when digitalis was given to the nonfailing heart, there was little or no change in end-diastolic volume, whereas myocardial oxygen consumption was increased. When digitalis was given to the failing heart, however, oxygen consumption was essentially unchanged. This occurred because of a reduction in ventricular volume which reduced wall stress according to the Laplace relation. Thus, the increase in oxygen consumption produced by the positive inotropic effects of digitalis was offset by the decrease in oxygen consumption produced by a reduction in heart size and myocardial wall tension.

The minor determinants of myocardial oxygen consumption listed in Table 10–2 are of much less importance. For example, it has been estimated that the depolarization process requires only about 0.04 ml. oxygen per min. per 100 grams when the heart is stimulated at a frequency of approximately 100 beats per minute. This amounts to approximately 0.5 per cent of the total oxygen consumed by the normal working heart. The direct metabolic effect of catecholamines on the nonbeating heart was determined by administering isoproterenol to the arrested canine heart. The subsequent increase in basal oxygen consumption was relatively minor, being of the order of 5 to 10 per cent of that occurring when the same hearts were contracting.

PERFORMANCE OF THE HEART AS A MUSCLE

The performance of the heart *as a pump* is usually designated in terms of pressure and flow. Since the performance of the heart *as a muscle* is generally designated in terms of shortening and wall stress, the relationship between intraventricular pressure and wall stress is of importance. From the Laplace relation (T=PR), it is apparent that the wall tension (T) is dependent not only on intraventricular pressure but also on the size of the heart, or more specifically on the radius of curvature and thickness of the particular portion of the wall under consideration. Since the normal left ventricle approximates a truncated ellipsoid, there are at least two radii of curvature at any point on the wall which help determine the stress existing at that point on the ventricle. No attempt will be made in this discussion to present complex formulae which adapt the Laplace relation to an ellipsoid ventricle. Rather, the purpose here is to identify those factors of importance. Thus, if one assumes the heart to be a simple sphere with radius, R, and wall thickness, h, a simplified version of the Laplace formula states that wall stress, S, is related to pressure, P, by the formula $S = PR/2h$ (Fig. 10–5).

This relationship is exemplified in the variation of wall thickness in the normal left ventricle. For example, the apex of the left ventricle has a relatively thin wall, as compared to the free lateral wall. This occurs because the radius of curvature of the apex is proportionately shorter, so that less muscle mass is needed in order to maintain a constant relationship between wall stress and intraventricular pressure. In the free lateral wall of the ventricle, the radius of curvature is greater, and thus a thicker wall is needed in order to maintain the appropriate relationship between wall stress and intraventricular pressure.

Ventricular Hypertrophy

The Laplace relationship is also fundamental to the understanding of the pathophysiology of various forms of heart disease. For example, when a heart undergoes hypertrophy secondary to arterial hypertension, the necessity to produce an increased intraventricular pressure is met by thickening of the wall. From the Laplace relationship, it should be noted that if intraventricular pressure and wall thickness increase proportionately (at a constant radius), wall stress will tend to remain the same. It has been noted in experimental models of hypertrophy, however, that hypertrophied muscle may actually generate less force per cross-sectional area than normal muscle. If this is the case, wall thickness must increase proportionately more than intraventricular pressure in order to generate the appropriate pressure.

The Laplace relation also offers some explanation as to why the left ventricle may hypertrophy, although there is no increase in arterial pressure. When heart failure and cardiac dilatation occur, there is increased wall stress in the free wall of the left ventricle, although there may be no change in intraventricular pressure. This increase in both diastolic and systolic wall stress serves as a stimulus to hypertrophy, without an increase in arterial systolic pressure. A mandatory consequence of cardiac dilatation is also an increase in myocardial oxygen needs. Additionally, there may be nonreversible structural changes in chronic dilatation, such as fiber slippage, increased connective tissue content, and so on, which explain the failure of the heart to again return to its original size after the causative factors are removed.

For example, in patients with aortic insufficiency who undergo aortic valve replacement, those patients whose hearts return toward normal size also have an improvement in cardiac function, while those patients whose hearts remain enlarged (presumably because of irreversible structural changes) have little improvement in cardiac function. Although heart size may increase to enormous proportions following dilatation, there is no concomitant increase in sarcomere length. Instead, sarcomere lengths tend to remain close to their optimum length of 2.2 microns. This presumably can occur both because of the addition of sarcomeres in series and because of fiber slippage, which allows the heart to expand considerably but keeps sarcomeres at a reasonably optimal length. In patients with cardiac dilatation, a beneficial therapeutic intervention generally tends to reduce heart size, with a concomitant reduction in oxygen consumption. This effect is most often produced by salt restriction or diuretics, which reduce intravascular volume, and/or by digitalis, which increases contractile force and allows the heart to empty more completely and return to a smaller size. Reduction of afterload by vasodilator drugs also enhances cardiac emptying and can reduce heart size.

It is appropriate now to examine the specific functional aspects of the heart in "failure." As stated in the introduction, for the purposes of this discussion, failure of the left ventricle as a pump means that it is unable to sustain the metabolic needs of the body under ordinary circumstances. Every heart can be subjected to a level of stress at which cardiac insufficiency can occur. A combination of cardiac pacing and alpha constrictor drugs such as angiotensin would be able to increase ventricular afterload and the frequency of cardiac contraction to such a degree that even the most healthy heart would be unable to sustain this workload. Since an older person or a deconditioned younger one may develop dyspnea at low workloads, cardiac insufficiency must be considered in relation to the imposed workload. For example, acute, severe ("malignant") hypertension will produce evidence of failure in a heart with normal myocardium and normal coronary arteries. Relief of the hypertension with appropriate drugs will permit the heart to function normally.

Cardiac failure is the term usually applied to an inadequacy of blood flow to sustain the metabolic requirements of the body in the resting state at the optimal level of tissue oxygen tension. When the volume of blood delivered to the tissues of the body is decreased by reason of cardiac disease, a first-order compensatory mechanism available to the body tissues is their ability to extract a greater quantity of oxygen from the available blood flow. Thus, in spite of a reduced cardiac output, sufficient oxygen can be supplied to the tissues to meet resting metabolic needs. However, any increase in oxygen demand cannot be met at optimal levels of oxygen tension, and either local metabolic acidosis occurs or, more commonly, oxygen need is reduced by limitation of activity.

CORONARY CIRCULATION

One organ system deserving particular consideration is the coronary circulation. In the absence of occlusive disease of the epicardial coronary arteries, the coronary circulation is autoregulatory. It appears to function at an abnormally low Po_2 (20 to 23 mm. Hg), and there is a very effective extraction of oxygen from the incoming arterial blood. The coronary blood flow varies directly and almost linearly with myocardial oxygen consumption, since there is no reserve available to cardiac muscle by any further widening of the arterial venous oxygen difference. The thermodilution method of Ganz permits the study of rapid changes in the coronary circulation in man, and, in particular, the response to acute intervention. In subjects with normal coronary vessels, the mean coronary sinus blood flow was 122 ml. per min. — values similar to those reported for other methods. Blood flow in patients with epicardial occlusive coronary artery disease was not different at rest. However, during activity, normal subjects can increase coronary blood flow to a much greater degree. Although drugs, heart rate, and cardiac arrhythmias cause important changes, the highest resting levels and the greatest increases in coronary blood flow have been determined in subjects in whom a pressure load either existed or was imposed on the left ventricle. In heart failure, coronary blood flow is usually normal.

COMMON UNDERLYING MECHANISMS IN CLINICAL CARDIAC FAILURE (TABLE 10–3)

Increased Metabolic Demands

If the metabolic demand of the body is such that normal tissue metabolism cannot proceed without an increased blood flow, "heart failure" may be said to be present, in spite of a normal

TABLE 10–3 FACTORS IN THE CAUSATION OF HEART FAILURE

A. Increased metabolic (output) demand
   1. Anemia, thyrotoxicosis, fever, beriberi
   2. A-V fistula, Paget's disease, left-to-right shunts
B. Increased left ventricular work
   1. Coarctation of aorta, aortic stenosis, subaortic stenosis
   2. Hypertension: primary, secondary
C. Compromised ventricular contraction
   1. Pericarditis, endomyocardial fibrosis
   2. Cardiomyopathies: infiltrative, idiopathic
D. Coronary artery disease
   1. Ischemia, infarction
   2. Fibrosis, scar, aneurysm
E. Disorders of filling
   1. Mitral, tricuspid stenosis
   2. Pericardial disease, cardiac tamponade
F. Volume overload
   1. Aortic incompetence, mitral incompetence
   2. Transfusion
G. Intrinsic depression of contractile state
   1. Acute myocarditis
   2. Cardiomyopathy
H. Arrhythmias
   1. Tachyrhythmias — sinus, atrial, nodal, ventricular
   2. Bradyrhythmias — sinus, partial or complete A-V block

ejection fraction, normal stroke volume, and normal cardiac work. The recognized causes include, as an example, severe anemia, in which the quantity of oxygen delivered to the tissues is compromised by the quantity of hemoglobin available in the bloodstream. Since the body tissues require a relatively constant oxygen delivery, the cardiac output must increase in a direct relationship to the reduction in hemoglobin. When hemoglobin levels of 5 grams per 100 ml. or less are present, the cardiac output increases to values of 10 to 14 L. per min. to maintain tissue oxygen needs. This stress, which increases both cardiac frequency and stroke volume, may produce severe alterations of left ventricular filling pressure and signs of pulmonary congestion. Other examples of high output failure are severe fevers, beriberi, Paget's disease, and arteriovenous fistulas, by way of which large quantities of blood may pass directly from the arterial bed to the venous circulation without participating in metabolic exchange at a tissue level. In thyrotoxicosis, there is an increased metabolic demand at the tissue level, but also a direct cardiac effect.

Large left-to-right shunts may occur within the heart itself in certain forms of congenital heart disease. These include interatrial communications, ventricular septal defect, aorticopulmonary window, and patent ductus arteriosus. Since the vascular resistance in the pulmonary circulation is normally much less than in the systemic circulation, relatively large volumes of blood may flow into the lungs and not participate in systemic tissue perfusion. Although heart failure may occur in young patients with ventricular septal defect or patent ductus arteriosus, these common lesions usually are sustained for many years without the development of heart failure. This is due to a peculiar autoregulatory mechanism by means of which a reduction in systemic vascular resistance will deviate more of the output of the left ventricle to the systemic circulation during times of increased systemic metabolic need without an additional increase in cardiac work.

Mechanical lesions which increase left ventricular work include coarctation of the aorta, aortic stenosis (supravalvar, valvar, and subvalvar), hypertrophic subaortic stenosis, and systemic hypertension. Although hypertension is fundamentally a disease of the systemic arterial bed, its consequences upon the heart are highly significant and it is one of the two most common causes of heart failure. Hypertension imposes a workload which is usually, but not always, gradual in development and allows for compensatory hypertrophy to take place. Although the cardiac ventricles are effective and adaptable volume pumps, continued increases in afterload present even the hypertrophied heart with a formidable burden. In the presence of compromised coronary circulation due to obstructive atherosclerosis, the more moderate degrees of afterload increase may not be tolerated, and heart failure develops.

Mechanical Lesions Compromising Ventricular Contraction

These lesions include adherent pericardium, constrictive pericarditis, infiltrative cardiomyopathies, primary myocardiopathies, familial cardiomyopathy, and the multiple forms of endocardial and endomyocardial fibrosis. In these disease states, there is a major increase in the viscous resistance within the ventricular wall. The tension developed by contraction must overcome this additional burden before appropriate changes in ventricular geometry can result in expulsion of blood from the left ventricle.

Coronary Artery Disease

The commonest cause of left ventricular dysfunction is the reduction of blood flow to areas of the myocardium consequent upon occlusive coronary vascular disease. Atherosclerotic vascular disease may affect one or all of the epicardial arteries, but the intramyocardial vessels usually are spared. As a consequence, there is a limitation of blood flow to the myocardium, and ischemia results.

If this is due to a lesion in the larger coronary vessels (proximal occlusive disease), heart failure

may occur owing to the nonfunction of a large number of contractile elements. In patients with severe proximal three-vessel (or left main) disease, acute global myocardial ischemia with ventricular paralysis is now recognized as a cause of sudden death in the absence of cardiac arrhythmia. Other effects of coronary atherosclerosis include myocardial infarction, large scar formation, and patchy areas of localized intramyocardial fibrosis, associated with focal infarction, arrhythmias, and depression of ventricular function. This disease process, the commonest form of heart disease afflicting Western man, is characterized by chest pain of cardiac origin — angina pectoris — which is usually stress-related. This symptom is caused by myocardial ischemia, which also results in transient depression of ventricular function toward, if not reaching, those levels of performance considered ordinarily to be heart failure. Patients with coronary artery disease who ultimately exhibit chronic heart failure have, in addition to myocardial ischemia, severe focal or general destruction of myocardium characterized by previous myocardial infarction. Occasionally, patients who are relatively insensitive to cardiac pain under conditions of appropriate stress can exhibit severe primary depression of cardiac function with pulmonary edema and without previous myocardial damage.

Disorders of Ventricular Filling

The primary cause of inadequate left ventricular filling is stenotic disease of the mitral valve. This condition *per se* does not produce left ventricular failure. However, long-standing "pure" mitral stenosis will result in changes in the geometry and distensibility characteristics, in the submitral valve structures, and in the left ventricle. There is stiffening in the submitral endocardium and a "small" left ventricular cavity with markedly decreased compliance characteristics.

Volume Overload Associated With Valvar Incompetence

In the presence of incompetence of the aortic or mitral valve, the left ventricle is called upon to discharge a volume equivalent to the sum of that needed by the body tissues and, in addition, that which regurgitates through the incompetent valve. The autoregulatory characteristics of the systemic arterial bed, in which a demand for increased blood flow results in a reduction in peripheral resistance, automatically result in a relative increase in forward cardiac output proportionate to shunt or regurgitant flow. Then, relatively large volumes can be handled by the left ventricle, provided that the demand is not acute and that the contractile state of the myocardium remains adequate. If the mechanical burden increases acutely or gradually, a state is reached in which even a hypertrophied heart with normal contractility is unable to perform adequately, and forward blood flow declines. Not infrequently, the mechanical lesion may worsen (increasing regurgitation) or the contractile state may become depressed.

Intrinsic Depression of Myocardial Contractile State

It has been difficult to prove a functional deficit of chemical substrate or sarcomere function in cases of heart failure. Nevertheless, conditions such as acute myocarditis, cardiomyopathy, and heart failure of old age may be associated with insignificant demonstrable anatomic changes. The nature of spontaneous remission as well as the responses to inotropic agents indicates, however, that a true depression of contractile state may be the primary factor occasionally, and a phenomenon secondary to other factors frequently.

Primary Arrhythmias

Severe tachy- or bradyarrhythmias may in themselves cause cardiac failure. Also, uncoordinated ventricular activity and loss of atrial contraction are of major significance, particularly when ventricular compliance is decreased.

Mutiple Factors

Anemia and congenital heart disease and valvular and coronary disease underline the interrelation of multiple factors as causes of heart failure. The significant issue here is a comprehension of the adequacy of the heart to sustain its function and recognition of the additive nature of adverse factors as each reaches a critical value. Thus, a young patient may tolerate aortic valve stenosis for many years only to succumb to a small myocardial infarction, which may itself result in minimal symptoms. A patient with mild mitral stenosis will exhibit heart failure on the first attack of atrial fibrillation with a rapid ventricular response.

BIOCHEMICAL AND MECHANICAL ALTERATIONS IN HEART FAILURE

The myocardium, unlike skeletal muscle, is dependent almost exclusively on aerobic metabolism and cannot develop any appreciable oxygen debt. Because of its large number of mitochondria, the heart is fundamentally suited to function in an aerobic manner. Normally, the myocardium can adapt itself to a wide number of substrates and is capable of utilizing almost all nutritional substances that come to it via the coronary circulation. These include glucose, pyruvate, lactate, free and esterified fatty acids, acetate, ketone bodies, and amino acids. Thus, in a postprandial state, the myocardium uses primarily glucose, lactate, and pyruvate, with a respiratory quotient approaching 1.0. During fasting conditions, the arterial concentrations of free fatty acids and ketones are much higher, and the heart will utilize these substrates, with a reduction in the respiratory quotient toward 0.8. When glucose is metabolized via the glycolytic and citric acid cycles, 36 of the 38 moles of ATP formed per mole of glucose oxidized are produced as a result of aerobic mitochondrial activity. This emphasizes the importance of aerobic oxidation of glucose in terms of energy production in the form of ATP.

When any portion of myocardium becomes anaerobic, lactate is produced locally, and this has been used, for example, as an indication of ischemia during cardiac catheterization. Normally, uptake of lactate from the arterial blood by the normal myocardium is greater than 10 per cent. With the onset of ischemia, however, tissue lactate is formed as the end-product of glycolysis and cannot be metabolized further because of ischemic depression of the citric acid cycle. This results in a level of coronary venous lactate higher than in arterial blood; that is, lactate is produced by the myocardium. Lactate production demonstrated by arteriovenous measurements across the heart is typical of the regional ischemia associated with coronary artery disease.

Hypertrophy

Hypertrophy may be physiologic, and is seen in patients with congenital malformations of the heart which result in volume or pressure overload. In acquired heart disease, hypertrophy is seldom physiologic, although the degree of intrinsic abnormality of hypertrophied muscle varies widely. For example, reduction in cardiac size with normal dynamics may occur in some patients with aortic stenosis without heart failure following valve replacement. In others, the enlarged heart remains unchanged with abnormal dynamics.

One of the compensatory mechanisms available to the heart as it begins to fail is the ability to hypertrophy. The increased mass of hypertrophied myocardium can produce greater pressure and restore the heart's function as a pump. Several studies of the mechanics of hypertrophied muscle have suggested, however, that this muscle is not normal and is functioning at a lower level of contractility than normal cardiac muscle. Similarly, failing myocardium in various experimen-

TABLE 10–4 THE FAILING MYOCARDIUM

A. Mechanical alterations
1. Decrease in force development/cross-sectional area
2. Decrease in maximum rate of force development
3. Decrease in velocity of shortening
B. Biochemical alterations
1. Catecholamines
   a. Reduced tissue content
   b. Reduced synthesis (tyrosine hydroxylase)
2. Biochemical
   a. Reduced actomyosin-ATPase
   b. Increased hydroxyproline (hypertrophy)
   c. No reduction in ATP
   d. Decreased calcium binding by sarcoplasmic reticulum
   e. Decreased adenyl cyclase activity
3. Exogenous
   a. Increased cortisol, catecholamines, and free fatty acids
   b. ? Myocardial depressant factor in shock

tal studies has been shown to have an apparent decrease in contractile state. Table 10–4 lists some of the factors that have been studied in hypertrophy and heart failure which bear a relationship to the depressed function of the myocardium.

Mechanical Factors

In several animal models it has been noted that failing heart muscle has a decreased ability to shorten with a normal velocity. Since the shortening velocity at zero load (Vmax) has been used as an index of contractile state (see Chapter 8), this decrease in velocity of shortening suggests a decrease in the contractile state of the failing muscle. Furthermore, the muscle is unable to develop the same force per unit mass as normal muscle and has a reduced maximum rate of force development.

Biochemical Factors

Numerous studies have been carried out to investigate the potential reasons for these findings. For example, tissue catecholamines are reduced in the failing myocardium, suggesting that there has been an increased excretion rate by augmented sympathetic tone in an attempt to maintain compensation. This is not responsible for the decrease in contractile state, however, since contractile state is not affected by depletion of catecholamines by either reserpinization or denervation. Additional studies in failing heart muscle have noted a reduction in activity of the enzyme tyrosine hydroxylase, which is in the synthetic pathway of norepinephrine in the myocardium. Thus, there may be not only an increased

excretion of norepinephrine but a decreased rate of synthesis to help account for the depletion of tissue catecholamines. It also has been noted that during the process of hypertrophy there is an increased collagen content of the myocardium, as manifested by an increased hydroxyproline concentration. Whether or not this collagen tissue interferes with the process of contraction is not clear. Even if one corrects contractile measurements for this dilution of normal cardiac tissue by connective tissue, the remaining myocardium still appears to be functioning at a reduced level of contractile state.

Actomyosin-ATPase

One biochemical alteration of considerable importance in the failing heart is a reduction in actomyosin-ATPase activity. This enzyme is intimately associated with the myosin filament and actin-myosin cross bridges and is responsible for splitting the ATP that provides the energy for contraction. Previous studies by Barany have demonstrated that actomyosin-ATPase activity in a wide variety of species is closely related to contractile state, as measured by Vmax, the maximal velocity of shortening at zero load. Thus, there is a mechanical-biochemical correlation in failing heart muscle in that both velocity of muscular contraction and baseline actomyosin-ATPase activity are reduced. ATP serves as the immediate source of high-energy phosphate bonds for the process of contraction, although creatinine phosphate also contains high-energy bonds. In order for this latter energy to be utilized, however, there must be an interchange between creatinine phosphate and ADP to form ATP, which is the final source of energy for cardiac contraction. Studies in failing heart muscle have suggested that the levels of ATP are not reduced in the failing myocardium, so that a reduction in energy supply does not appear to be the reason for a decrease in contractile state.

It has also been noted that there is decreased binding of calcium by the sarcoplasmic reticulum in the failing myocardium. Calcium is the initiator of cardiac contraction by binding with troponin and releasing troponin's inhibition of the interaction of actin and myosin. The reduced ability of the sarcoplasmic reticulum to bind calcium might lead to reduced stores of calcium in the myocardium. Theoretically, this might produce a decreased availability of calcium to the myoplasm and a consequent decrease to contractile state.

In guinea pigs with inherited cardiomyopathy, it has also been noted that adenyl cyclase activity is decreased. This enzyme is intimately associated with the actions of the catecholamines via the beta-adrenergic pathway. Catecholamines, such as norepinephrine, stimulate adenyl cyclase activity and convert ATP to cyclic AMP. Cyclic AMP in turn activates phosphorylase activity and promotes glycogenolysis, making more glucose available for the glycolytic cycle. In addition, cyclic AMP also enhances calcium availability to the myofilaments and produces an increase in contractile state. This reduction in adenyl cyclase activity, however, does not appear to be the mechanism responsible for the decrease in contractile state, since the level of this enzyme can vary considerably (depending on the catecholamine content of the myocardium) without affecting basal levels of contraction.

Exogenous Factors

Several exogenous factors have important effects on cardiac function during heart failure. For example, circulating myocardial depressant factor has been identified in animal models in shock, which is released or activated by substances released from the splanchnic circulation. Although this isolated factor has been demonstrated to produce depression of cardiac function in isolated tissue, its function in the intact circulation is uncertain, since there is a concomitant increase in circulating catecholamines, which increase the contractile state of the myocardium. This catecholamine response is apparently part of the over-all response of the body to the stress associated with heart failure and also includes elevations of cortisol and free fatty acids. Of some interest is the potential role of increased levels of catecholamines and free fatty acids in producing arrhythmias in the setting of acute heart failure, particularly acute myocardial infarction. Whether the elevation of these substances is responsible for the arrhythmias observed or merely reflects the serious nature of the underlying heart disease is not yet clear.

In summary, although there are several biochemical alterations of importance in the failing heart, it is not yet known whether these various abnormalities are merely associated with or in some way are responsible for the decreased contractility of the failing heart.

RENAL PHYSIOLOGY IN CONGESTIVE HEART FAILURE*

Renal mechanisms are intimately involved in the retention of fluid and electrolytes and thus the peripheral edema that follows congestive heart failure. The basic response of the kidney to a fall in cardiac output is retention of salt and water. This receptor response apparently has difficulty in discriminating between a true fall in plasma volume, such as might occur with blood loss or fluid depletion, and a fall in effective circulating volume caused by a depression of cardiac function. The stimulus for retention of salt and water, however, will persist until adequate cardiac output is restored. This results in an increase in extracellular fluid volume, in total body water, and in total exchangeable sodium and chloride. Aldosterone secretion and the concentration of antidiuretic hormone also are increased.

Normally, about 98 per cent of the sodium filtered by the glomeruli is reabsorbed by the tubular system. The great bulk of this is reabsorbed in the proximal tubules. A smaller amount is absorbed in the collecting duct and the ascending loop of Henle, while the remainder, which is not excreted in the urine, is reabsorbed in the distal tubule by ion exchange with hydrogen or potassium. This mechanism is the principal means for excretion of potassium ion. Under the influence of enhanced aldosterone, total exchangeable potassium in the body may actually be reduced owing to this reabsorption of sodium in the distal tubule.

The rate of sodium excretion is determined by the balance between glomerular filtration and tubular reabsorption. In congestive heart failure, the glomerular filtration rate is commonly reduced to at least one half the normal rate. However, there appears to be increased tubular reabsorption of sodium, suggesting that this latter factor is the most significant cause of sodium accumulation, whereas the fall in glomerular filtration rate is only a contributory factor. Although it is not the exclusive factor, the role of aldosterone in this regard appears to be of primary importance in producing the retention of sodium ions. The sequence of events in this series apparently includes the release of renin from the renal afferent arterioles and juxtaglomerular cells, which transforms angiotensin to a decapeptide, angiotensin I. A plasma-converting enzyme converts this material to an octapeptide, angiotensin II, which is the immediate factor stimulating the secretion of aldosterone by the zona glomerulosa of the adrenal cortex. Presumably, decreased pressure or volume in the afferent arterioles is the signal mechanism that activates this system. The retention of sodium, therefore, is accompanied by the retention of water and expansion of the circulating blood volume. This in turn leads to filtration of the retained fluid as edema into tissue spaces and occasionally as pleural or peritoneal effusions.

Associated with this retention of fluid is also a decrease in free water clearance. Therefore, patients who have a continued large intake of water will be unable to clear this water through their kidneys and may develop dilutional hyponatremia. Thus, in severe heart failure, it is clear that

---

*See also Chapter 14.

therapy must include not only a restriction of salt intake but also some limited restriction of fluid intake, together with appropriate diuretics. Because of the propensity for potassium loss with increased aldosterone secretion and the administration of certain diuretics such as the thiazides it is often important to provide oral potassium supplements, particularly in patients who are digitalized. Alternatively, the use of aldosterone antagonists in addition to other diuretics may maintain reasonable potassium balance.

CONTROL OF PERIPHERAL CIRCULATION

In the normal circulation at rest, the total blood flow is divided in a relatively constant proportion among the different organ systems of the body (Table 10–5). Skeletal muscle and the splanchnic and renal beds each receive approximately 20 per cent of the total cardiac output. The cerebral circulation and blood flow through the skin each account for a further 10 per cent of total blood flow. The coronary vascular system receives 4 per cent of the total cardiac output. During activity the cerebral blood flow remains relatively constant. Flow in other segments of the circulation alters in accord with metabolic demand. Thus, during exercise, skeletal muscle blood flow increases promptly and may account for more than 50 per cent of the total cardiac output. At the same time, there is a major increase in skin blood flow, presumably to facilitate the loss of metabolic heat from the body. While the proportion of blood flow passing to the other

TABLE 10–5 REGIONAL DISTRIBUTION OF CARDIAC OUTPUT

	Normal		Cardiac Failure	
	Rest	Exercise	Rest	Exercise
Cardiac Output (L./min./M.^{2})	3.0	6.0	1.5	2.3
Blood Flows (% of cardiac output)				
Muscle	20	50	36	60
Splanchnic	25	12	25	10
Renal	20	9	10	4
Cerebral	12	6	12	12
Coronary	4	4	9	10
Skin	9	15	3	1
Blood Flows (absolute values in ml./min./M.^{2})				
Muscle	600	3000	540	1380
Renal	600	540	150	92
Coronary	120	240	135	230

(From Mason, D. T.: Mod. Conc. Cardiovasc. Dis., *36*: 25, 1967. By permission of The American Heart Association, Inc.)

circulatory elements is decreased, the absolute level of blood flow is still maintained.

In skeletal muscle, the arterioles are under essentially local control. The local vascular resistance is determined by the relative degree of vasodilatation resulting from the production of metabolites in skeletal muscle. When the muscle is relatively inactive, the production of metabolites is low and the "net" vascular tone remains high. As metabolic products are formed and their concentration rises, vasodilatation occurs, which has the autoregulatory effect of enhancing the removal of these substances with a tendency to restore the previous level of vasomotor tone. In addition, skeletal muscle is under modest degrees of autonomic control. The circulation in the skin is principally regulated by the autonomic nervous system. Vasodilatation occurs by reason of release of constrictor tone centrally mediated. This appears to be predominantly a heat regulatory mechanism.

Heart Failure

In heart failure, however, there is a reduction in total cardiac output at rest, and there is a failure to increase cardiac output proportionate with activity. Hence, there is a redistribution of the absolute magnitude of organ blood flow in this state, which is further accentuated during exercise. In patients with borderline cardiac compensation of heart failure, the coronary blood flow is preserved. In fact, the coronary blood flow may be much greater proportionate to cardiac output in patients with heart failure than in patients with normally compensated circulations. Relatively speaking, there is a diminution in renal blood flow and, to a lesser extent, in splanchnic blood flow. The skeletal muscles retain their usual proportion of blood flow (Table 10–5).

During activity, there is a pronounced alteration in the distribution of blood flow. Cerebral blood flow is maintained, but there is a marked reduction in blood flow to the splanchnic and renal beds. Within the limits of total cardiac output, blood flow to actively exercising skeletal muscle increases. This, however, is strictly limited by the availability of blood flow. In contrast, normal skin blood flow is not increased in heart failure, owing to sustained vasoconstriction. Vascular reactivity is profoundly altered in heart failure. First, there is an increased resting peripheral resistance throughout the organ systems, both collectively and individually. Thus, the balance between the concentration of dilating metabolites and the vascular tone in skeletal muscle is substantially altered so that a greater concentration is necessary to sustain a given level of vasodilatation. This may also be seen in the responses of skeletal muscle and skin to reactive hyperemia. In such instances, the magnitude of dilatation is greatly reduced. In addition, there is an abnormal response to ordinary autonomic reflexes. The vasodilatation in the skin is significantly reduced following heating, and responses to such mechanisms as acute tilting or the Valsalva maneuver are altered. In a normal subject, there is a significant and transient overshoot in arterial blood pressure following the Valsalva maneuver. This overshoot is absent in patients with heart failure, suggesting that the peripheral vascular tone is already high and is not particularly modified during the Valsalva maneuver, nor is stroke volume substantially increased. Heart failure is characterized by an increase in sympathetic vascular tone, which is in direct proportion to the severity of the failure.

Shock. One particular syndrome characterizing the failing heart is worthy of note. In the shock state, peripheral vascular responses may be grossly abnormal. Initially there is a marked increase in peripheral vascular resistance in such patients, although occasionally reduced peripheral vascular resistance and reflex vasodilation due to stimulation of cardiac receptors have been described. However, in the presence of prolonged and severe hypoxia with resulting lactic acidemia and acidosis, a specific paralysis of peripheral vessels occurs. In the shock syndrome, the ability of skeletal muscle vessels to dilate is almost completely abolished. The reactive hyperemic response is negligible in spite of the fact that presumably high levels of vasodilating substances are present in both the resting as well as the exercising muscle.

HEART FAILURE IN ISCHEMIC HEART DISEASE AND ACUTE MYOCARDIAL INFARCTION

Occlusive coronary artery disease is a special disorder of cardiac function which warrants separate consideration from a practical as well as a pathophysiologic standpoint. The processes of atherosclerosis result in the formation of obstruc-

tive lesions in the coronary vascular tree which, because of either degree or location, may substantially interfere with the magnitude of coronary blood flow. When the myocardial oxygen demand of the tissue in the distribution of each vessel exceeds the capacity of the restricted arterial bed to supply it with oxygenated blood, ischemic changes result. These changes are usually characterized by the development of chest pain of cardiac origin — angina pectoris — but this is a variable symptom. It is now clear that patients with coronary artery disease and angina pectoris have significant but reversible ventricular dysfunction due to ischemia alone. When the degree of ischemia is extremely severe or the vessel is acutely and completely blocked, major changes occur, both in the structure of the myocardium and in ventricular function. The dynamic nature of this process is shown in Figure 10–6. Patients with acute myocardial infarction are usually classified as being (1) uncomplicated, (2) uncomplicated apart from transient cardiac arrhythmias, (3) exhibiting heart failure of mild degree, (4) exhibiting heart failure of moderate degree, and (5) exhibiting cardiogenic shock. This classification is not always entirely precise, since a true reduction of cardiac performance is not always coincidental with the signs and symptoms of pulmonary venous congestion, which are the usual clinical hallmarks of the diagnosis of heart failure (Fig. 10–7). Thus, the measured values for cardiac performance may show the cardiac output, stroke volume, and stroke work to be normal or even increased in a given patient; may be reduced moderately to levels consistent with normal cardiac performance; or may be reduced profoundly. Indices of ventricular contractile state (Vmax, max dp/dt) show the same variability. The disease dominantly affects the left ventricle; isolated disease of the right ventricle is rare.

Left ventricular filling pressure may be normal, but it is frequently increased. The level of left ventricular filling pressure or pulmonary venous and distending pressure correlates with the presence of increased vascular markings of the lungs on chest x-ray, clinical signs of pulmonary

MYOCARDIUM:	HEALTHY ⇄ ISCHEMIC → INFARCTED → HEALED (SCAR)

| METABOLISM | DECREASED: | ← | | |
| | INCREASED: | → | → | |

| CONTRACTILE STATE: | N | ↓ | O | O |

| COMPLIANCE: | N | ↓ (?) | N, ↑ | ↓ |

Figure 10–6 Dynamic representation of the changes in the function of myocardium in coronary heart disease. There is a reversible relation between healthy and ischemic myocardium determined by the level of cardiac metabolism. The reaction becomes irreversible when ischemic tissue passes into the infarcted state and undergoes necrosis and healing in the form of fibrosis or scar. The contractile state is reduced to a varying degree (frequently severely) in ischemia and of course is absent in infarcted or scarred myocardium. The compliant state of myocardium may be decreased during ischemia (ventricular stiffening) and may be normal or increased in infarcted myocardium. Following healing, myocardial scars are noncompliant and extremely stiff, with a minimal mechanical disadvantage.

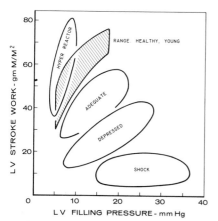

Figure 10–7 Relation of ventricular performance to filling pressure in patients with coronary heart disease and myocardial infarction. A wide spectrum of ventricular response exists. Certain patients may exhibit normal performance characteristics or performance characteristics that are inappropriately enhanced for the sedated, resting individual. Differing degrees of depression of ventricular performance exist that are related dominantly to the magnitude and location of the infarcted-ischemic tissue and the presence of additional mechanical lesions such as mitral valve incompetence. Patients with profound depression of ventricular function usually exhibit the shock state and experience a very high mortality.

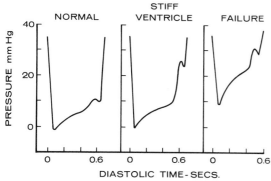

Figure 10–8 Left ventricular diastolic pressure pulses in patients with and without heart disease. In each instance ventricular systole is excluded and the tracing represents only the events in diastole. Note (left) the early diastolic pressure approaching zero with an "a" wave of approximately 10 mm. Hg in magnitude. In acute myocardial infarction the early diastolic contour of the pressure pulse remains unchanged, but there is an "a" wave of large magnitude, possibly owing to an increased ventricular stiffness and, therefore, a shift to the left of the diastolic pressure-volume relation. In the right panel is a tracing of a patient with chronic congestive heart failure and elevated early diastolic as well as late diastolic and "a" wave pressures.

venous congestion, and clinical signs of enhanced filling pressure—third and fourth heart sounds (Fig. 10–8). However, the relationship of cardiac performance to filling pressure is poor, in that patients may have normal cardiac performance with low or high ventricular filling pressures and reduced cardiac performance with low or high ventricular filling pressure.

The time course of changes in these hemodynamics is somewhat variable. Left ventricular filling pressure usually decreases in two to four days to normal levels, irrespective of whether the cardiac output has been normal or moderately decreased. Pulmonary congesting pressure — pulmonary venous pressure — falls spontaneously without any treatment or with diuretics, which initially act by enhancing venous capacitance and then have a later (½ hour) effect on salt and water excretion.

In myocardial infarction, agents such as digitalis or the catecholamines do not exhibit a powerful inotropic effect. In patients with normal or increased cardiac output there is a small increase in cardiac output or stroke work of approximately 10 to 15 per cent. On the contrary, in patients with severe depression of cardiac function, this does not take place. Hence, patients who are severely ill and who require the use of cardiac stimulators do not respond favorably to inotropic agents. This may be due to total failure of the infarcted or ischemic tissue to respond, while the normal myocardium is already maximally active. A wide variety of effects appear to result from myocardial infarction (Fig. 10–7). In a small infarct, there are few contractile elements that are rendered inactive. In addition, acute myocardial ischemia and/or infarction appears to mediate strong sympathetic activity. Therefore, certain patients in the ischemic-infarction syndrome exhibit tachycardia or hypertension in the presence of a normal or increased cardiac output. A second group of patients have an infarct of medium size. In this instance more contractile elements have been rendered ineffective and the cardiac output is usually more depressed. However, the diastolic compliant state of the ventricle is variable. In many patients there is good evidence that the ventricle is stiff and may be exhibiting ischemic contracture. This diastolic stiffness also appears to have a time course similar to that of the change in diastolic filling pressure, so that in two to five days diastolic pressure has declined and the characteristics of diastolic stiffness have disappeared. The presence of a loud fourth heart sound in the majority of patients with acute myocardial infarction and the typical configuration of the left ventricular pressure pulse renders an increased diastolic stiffness likely.

If the infarct is large, many contractile elements are rendered nonfunctional, and the ejec-

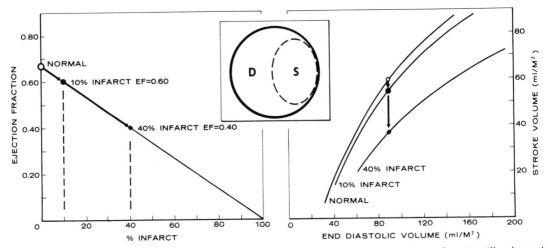

Figure 10–9 Diagrammatic representation of the effect of reduction in the number of contractile elements activated during ventricular systole. In myocardial ischemia or infarction, as the contractile units are rendered nonfunctional the overall performance of the ventricle falls. This is expressed in the left panel as the ejection fraction, or the portion of ventricular content expelled during systole, and on the right panel as isopleths of stroke volume as a function of end-diastolic volume. Note that obligatory reductions in stroke volume must occur as a function of the increasing magnitude of cardiac muscle involved. Further, the ventricle cannot dilate rapidly to compensate for this loss.

tion fraction (EF) is proportionately reduced (Fig. 10–9). Not infrequently, additional mechanical lesions are present. Of these, perhaps the most important is paradox of the area of the myocardial infarct. If the infarct does not stiffen (decreased ventricular compliance), it distends as intraventricular pressure rises (Fig. 10–10). The work performed by the normally contracting elements is therefore wasted in the distention of the infarct. In addition, mitral insufficiency due to chronic papillary muscle dysfunction or new and recent as a consequence of ventricular dilatation or papillary muscle abnormality can add to the burden of the already disordered ventricle. In the same way as ventricular paradox, mitral insufficiency or intraventricular flow can acutely and profoundly depress cardiac pump function. In this regard, a soft systolic murmur at the apex of the

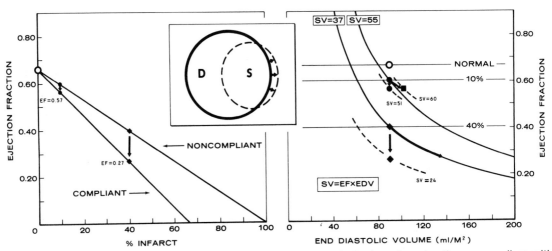

Figure 10–10 Ventricular performance as a consequence of substitution of contracting myocardium with noncontracting but compliant elements. In this instance the nonfunctional fibers elongate and the ventricle distends as a consequence of the rise in intraventricular pressure occasioned by contraction of the healthy elements. The mechanical disadvantage is evident (see Figure 10–9 for comparison).

heart in patients with acute myocardial infarction should never be regarded as an innocent, inconsequential sign. It may be evidence of mitral insufficiency of only moderate magnitude, but of a degree sufficient to account for a substantial proportion of the reduced cardiac output. In certain instances the mitral insufficiency may be completely silent, with the murmur returning only as cardiac compensation is partly restored.

The most profound form of depression of cardiac function results in a clinical syndrome known as *shock*. Shock may be associated with a number of causes, including acute infection, acute loss of blood volume, and acute profound destruction of myocardial elements. The reduction of approximately 40 per cent of the contractile elements in the myocardium causes a fall in cardiac performance to the order of magnitude seen in patients in or close to cardiogenic shock. If, however, additional mechanical lesions are present, these effects are additive to the factors depressing the circulatory state and result in a sufficient depression of cardiac function to cause shock in spite of the presence of an infarct of lesser size.

It has been found that patients exhibiting the shock state do indeed fall into appropriate pathophysiologic groupings. The younger patients with a first infarction who progress rapidly through their illness and die in cardiogenic shock have large myocardial infarcts, usually resulting from an acute anterolateral or anteroseptal infarction consequent on a major occlusion in the left coronary arterial system. This amounts to approximately 55 per cent of all patients. Another 15 to 20 per cent of patients have an additional definable mechanical lesion such as those indicated above, while the balance of approximately 30 per cent of cases have end-stage heart disease. In these latter cases, the imposition of new small myocardial infarction upon chronic heart disease is sufficient to depress function so that an adequate performance can no longer be maintained.

SYMPTOMS AND SIGNS OF HEART FAILURE

We shall relate the symptoms and signs of heart failure to the four subsystems previously introduced, that is, the left ventricle, the right ventricle, the pulmonary venous circulation, and the systemic venous circulation.

Left Ventricular Failure

The principal symptom associated with failure of the left ventricle as a pump consists of those complaints related to reduced organ perfusion (Table 10–6). Weakness, easy fatigability, and extreme weakness of the musculoskeletal system are characteristic. Dyspnea is principally due to the associated pulmonary venous congestion. The extremities are frequently cool and pale. At times there is mental forgetfulness, and if the condition is prolonged and severe, there is ultimately evidence of dysfunction in many organ systems, including the gut, kidney, and liver. Severe peripheral cyanosis and indeed gangrene may occur in profound chronic heart failure. The signs include tachycardia, with a heart rate exceeding 100 beats per min., and a slight reduction in blood pressure. The pulse pressure is usually narrowed. Cardiomegaly may be present, owing to the nature of the underlying disease, but the heart size may be normal. The first sound is usually muffled and less distinctive than normal. If diastolic blood pressure is diminished, the second heart sound at the pulmonary and aortic areas is reduced. Diagnostic physical findings in significant heart failure include the presence of third and fourth heart sounds (Fig. 10–8). These sounds

TABLE 10–6 PRINCIPAL CLINICAL SYMPTOMS AND PHYSICAL SIGNS OF RIGHT AND LEFT HEART FAILURE

	Left Heart Failure	*Right Heart Failure*
Symptoms	Fatigue, weakness	Weight gain
	Obtundation	Ankle swelling, pigmentation
	Cyanosis	Abdominal distention
	Exertion dyspnea	Subcostal pain
	Cough	Neck pulsations
	Orthopnea, paroxysmal nocturnal dyspnea	Jaundice
	Anorexia	
	Diaphoresis	
Signs	Tachycardia	Edema, ascites
	Apex diffuse	Increased 2nd sound (second component)
	First sound ↓	of pulmonary area
	Third and fourth sounds present	Left parasternal lift
	Moist rales, pleural effusion	Increased jugular venous pressure

relate to heightened filling pressure in the left ventricle: the former is associated with a rapid filling of an already partially filled ventricle at the beginning of atrial emptying; the latter is associated with an enhanced rate of pressure rise in the ventricle at end diastole. If a murmur is present, it usually is related to the underlying disease but is reduced in intensity. In heart failure, the diastolic murmur of mitral stenosis may be totally absent. In like manner, in acute myocardial infarction a systolic murmur associated with papillary muscle disease may not be apparent but will be detected as cardiac function improves. The apex beat is usually diffuse and rather weak, with or without associated abnormal pulsation. The carotid pulse may be slow in its upstroke, although this is not a consistent finding.

Right Ventricular Failure

Right ventricular dysfunction may be associated with dyspnea, as in patients with acute pulmonary embolization. More importantly, there is moderate fatigue, which is not so severe as that associated with comparable degrees of left heart failure. Frequently, a right ventricular lift and an accentuated second heart sound at the pulmonary area may be evidence of the presence of concomitant pulmonary hypertension. Occasionally, a pulmonary diastolic murmur is heard, owing to the presence of extremely severe pulmonary hypertension. The second sound of the pulmonary area may also be widely split (Table 10–6).

Pulmonary Venous Congestion

The principal symptom of pulmonary venous congestion is dyspnea, as occurs following exertion in patients with a serious degree of heart failure. If the precipitating cause is acute, as with rupture of a cardiac valve, sudden severe shortness of breath may rapidly disable the patient. Orthopnea exists when the patient is unable to lie flat and is due to a high level of pulmonary venous pressure. Paroxysmal nocturnal dyspnea usually is not associated with severe elevation of pulmonary venous pressure but occurs when a patient with more moderate elevations sleeps flat, allowing a slow accumulation of fluid throughout the interstitial spaces of the lungs. When this reaches a critical value, it is necessary for the patient to assume the upright posture, so that redistribution of interstitial and alveolar fluid can allow effective respiration to be restored. Acute pulmonary edema is associated with a very rapid development of severe dyspnea, even with the patient in the upright position. It may be associated with the producion of frothy bright red sputum. The patient will (naturally) be extremely apprehensive. On examination, patients with overt heart failure will be found to exhibit an increase in the frequency and depth of breathing. On auscultation of the chest, the findings are dependent on the degree of pulmonary venous hypertension. Patients with mild heart failure may have relatively few rales at both bases. In patients with acute pulmonary edema, it is possible to identify rales up to the thoracic apex. Unequal distribution of rales in the right and left chest is a frequent finding. Pleural effusion is often an accompaniment and may be so small as to be detectable only by chest x-ray, usually involving the right thoracic cavity. Radiographs of the chest reveal several changes that relate to the severity of the heart failure. In the mildest examples, there are increased vascular markings in the lower lobe pulmonary veins. As the pulmonary congestion becomes more severe, the upper pulmonary veins become more prominent, while the lower lobe veins actually appear to become smaller. Hilar congestion and interstitial edema are followed by generalized edema, with a ground-glass appearance across the thorax. Pleural effusions may be noted as indicated above, in the right or left chest cavities or bilaterally.

Systemic Venous Congestion

The principal symptoms relate to swelling of the ankles and dependent parts, abdominal swelling, and subcostal pain. The neck veins may be distended and pulsatile. On examination, edema may be identified and abdominal swelling found associated with ascites or a large and tender liver. The liver may pulsate in the presence of tricuspid incompetence. Neck veins are frequently distended with a high venous pressure, so that even with the patient sitting at 45 to 60 degrees from the horizontal, the neck veins remain filled. In the presence of tricuspid incompetence, venous pulsation characterized by "a" and "v" waves may be identified.

PHYSIOLOGIC PRINCIPLES IN THE THERAPY OF HEART FAILURE

Effective therapy requires an adjustment of the environment or creation of a milieu that will favorably influence the cardiac state. Hence, rational treatment depends on effective measures to reverse altered physiology.

The principles in the management of heart failure are to reduce cardiac demand, improve cardiac performance, maximize the rate and completeness of healing, and reverse associated disorders of organ function and fluid balance. It is not our purpose to discuss the mode of action or practical uses of inotropic or diuretic drugs or other conventional therapeutic modalities, or the mechanical benefits consequent on successful surgical treatment of congenital or valvar disease.

Alterations of Preload, Afterload, and Contractile State

It is convenient to think of the mechanical function of the heart in terms of its three principal determinants: preload, afterload, and contractile state (Table 10–7). *Preload* refers to initial and diastolic fiber length. Thus, changes in preload describe the Starling function curve. In the intact heart, preload is often considered in terms of either end-diastolic pressure or end-diastolic volume.

Since patients with power failure may have either high or low filling pressure, it is important to optimize the filling pressure to the most beneficial place on the Starling curve. Studies in patients with acute myocardial infarction, for example, have shown that a pulmonary capillary wedge pressure of approximately 15 to 18 mm. Hg provides the optimum cardiac performance, as measured by stroke volume or stroke work. Higher values of left ventricular filling pressure do not augment stroke volume any further, and lower values of filling pressure may reduce stroke volume by the Starling mechanism. Furthermore, high levels of filling pressure may lead to pulmonary congestion, increased work of breathing, and increased myocardial oxygen consumption due to cardiac dilatation and the Laplace relation. These factors emphasize the importance of optimizing the left ventricular filling pressure in patients with cardiac failure.

Afterload refers to the load against which the heart must work. It is convenient to think of afterload as aortic pressure, although in reality the afterload corresponds to wall stress, which is related to pressure by the Laplace relationship. Of importance is the fact that changes in afterload may affect cardiac performance at a given preload. For example, if afterload is abruptly increased, there will be a corresponding reduction in stroke volume, with subsequent compensatory mechanisms tending to return toward normal. Similarly, if there is a corresponding reduction in afterload, there is an initial increase in stroke volume. This latter fact is receiving considerable attention recently in patients with severe heart failure and elevated filling pressure. Such patients are being treated with such drugs as Regitine, nitroprusside, or nitroglycerin to reduce arterial pressure and systemic vascular resistance. This therapy is very beneficial in many patients in that it produces an increase in cardiac output and a reduction in left ventricular filling pressure in association with a fall in systemic vascular resistance and arterial pressure. The fall in left ventricular filling pressure is probably due to both venodilation, with a reduction in venous return, and more complete systolic emptying as a result of a reduction in afterload.

Among patients who might especially benefit from a reduction of afterload are those with acute myocardial infarction and a hypertensive reaction. Reduction of blood pressure would markedly reduce oxygen needs of the heart and might limit the size of the infarct by reducing the surrounding ischemic zone. Reduction of the afterload has also been shown to be effective in patients with heart failure associated with severe mitral regurgitation. A fall in afterload reduces the regurgitant fraction and increases forward flow and cardiac output. It should be noted, however, that reduction of afterload also reduces diastolic filling pressure, which is the coronary perfusing pressure. Too great a reduction of arterial pressure, therefore, may be deleterious by reason of a concomitant reduction of coronary blood flow.

The third determinant of mechanical performance, *contractile state*, refers to the ability of the heart to alter its contractile force at a given preload and afterload in response to such factors as intrinsic catecholamine stimulation; circulating catecholamines; or exogenous interventions such as digitalis, norepinephrine, isoproterenol, paired electrical stimulation, and so on. In chronic heart failure, the use of digitalis to increase contractile force, improve systolic emptying, and reduce heart size is accepted as having beneficial effects on the circulation. In the case of acute power failure due to acute myocardial infarction, however, the potential role of these positive inotropic agents is unclear. The effects of drugs such as digitalis, isoproterenol, and norepinephrine are relatively slight in this setting and may even be deleterious, owing to their propensity to produce arrhythmias and the obligatory increase in myocardial oxygen needs because of the increase in contractile state. The general lack of response to positive inotropic agents in acute power failure following infarction may be related to the fact that much of the myocardium is nonresponsive

TABLE 10–7 EFFECTS OF ALTERATIONS IN PRELOAD, AFTERLOAD, AND CONTRACTILE STATE ON STROKE VOLUME

	Preload (LVEDP)	Afterload (Arterial Pressure)	Contractile State
Increase in S.V.	↑	↓	↑
Decrease in S.V.	↓	↑	↓

(infarcted) and therefore unable to increase its contractile state. In addition, the normally responsive myocardium is already maximally stimulated by intrinsic sympathetic tone or circulating catecholamines. Studies of myocardial mechanics have shown that there is a ceiling of contractility; if reached by using one agent, this ceiling cannot be exceeded, even though another potent inotropic agent is added. Therefore, the relative lack of response of patients with power failure following myocardial infarction to all inotropic agents may be due to these factors and suggests that these agents may have limited value in this particular setting. Of equal or greater importance may be the correction of such factors as anoxia, arrhythmias, acidosis, and relative hypovolemia.

A knowledge of the factors that determine myocardial oxygen consumption is of importance in several clinical settings. For example, in coronary artery disease with a fixed proximal stenosis of a major vessel it would appear that a potent inotropic agent might be deleterious, since it would increase oxygen consumption by increasing contractile state, while the coronary circulation would be unable concomitantly to increase coronary flow because of the fixed proximal obstruction. This imbalance between oxygen supply and demand might produce or worsen ischemia and angina pectoris. In certain circumstances, however, it has been noted that digitalis will alleviate angina pectoris when given to some patients with ventricular failure. The reason for this observation apparently relates to the fact that when heart size is decreased by digitalis the decrease in myocardial oxygen consumption then offsets the increase in oxygen consumption associated with the increase in contractility produced by digitalis. Since digitalis has only modest inotropic effects, however, this beneficial effect on angina is not observed with other more potent inotropic agents such as isoproterenol.

A further point of clinical importance relates to the use of beta-adrenergic blockers such as propranolol in the treatment of angina pectoris. Such drugs may improve angina by decreasing oxygen consumption. For example, propranolol blocks neural sympathetic tone to the heart and, in addition, blocks the effects of circulating catecholamines, thus reducing oxygen consumption by preventing the increase in contractile state produced by these interventions. Furthermore, propranolol also has a direct depressive effect on the contractile state of the myocardium, which may further decrease oxygen needs. Because of these combined effects, propranolol and similar drugs may improve the relationship between oxygen supply and demand and decrease the frequency and severity of angina pectoris. It should also be noted, however, that when propranolol is given to patients with heart failure, it may worsen the congestive failure. This occurs because propranolol blocks sympathetic tone and the influence of circulating catecholamines, which may be needed to support the cardiovascular system. If propranolol increases congestive heart failure and produces further cardiac dilatation, myocardial wall tension will be increased by the Laplace relation, with a possible increase in myocardial oxygen consumption. Thus, although propranolol may favorably influence the relationship of oxygen supply and demand in a patient with angina pectoris and a small heart, it may actually aggravate angina pectoris in a patient in whom further cardiac dilatation occurs. Thus, the effects of any particular drug on angina pectoris must be evaluated in terms of its effects on heart rate, arterial pressure, contractile state, and cardiac size.

The concept of angina pectoris reflecting an imbalance between oxygen supply and demand has additional clinical implications. For example, in patients with aortic stenosis, large pressure gradients across the aortic valve, and a thick-walled ventricle, the symptoms of angina pectoris can occur, despite normal coronary arteries. This is not surprising when we consider the tremendous increase in oxygen cost produced by the level of systolic pressure in the ventricle and the hypertrophied myocardium. In a similar way, the relief of angina pectoris by nitroglycerin reflects a better balance between oxygen supply and demand, which is unrelated to any direct effect on the coronary arteries. Thus, the reduction in venous return by peripheral venodilation reduces end-diastolic volume and wall stress by the Laplace relation. Similarly, a reduction in arterial pressure by arterial vasodilation reduces the tension-time index. Both effects, therefore, reduce myocardial wall stress and oxygen consumption and are beneficial in relieving angina pectoris.

The importance of myocardial oxygen consumption has also recently been emphasized in the setting of acute myocardial infarction. In established infarction, there is a central zone of dead tissue surrounded by a zone of ischemic muscle with a marginal blood supply and oxygen delivery. The potential viability of this area, therefore, is critically dependent on the balance between oxygen supply and demand. Thus, the importance of maintaining coronary perfusion pressure has been emphasized in that it tends to reduce the surrounding area of ischemia as monitored by direct ST segment mapping of the ventricular epicardium in dogs. On the other hand, the use of inotropic agents which increase contractile state tends to enlarge the surrounding area of ischemia by increasing the need for oxygen. The desire to minimize the area of infarction by protecting this zone of ischemic muscle is receiving increasing attention in consideration of various modes of therapy for acue myocardial infarction.

MECHANICAL CIRCULATORY ASSIST

When one considers the management of cardiac decompensation, it is logical to examine the possibility of adding to the circulating bloodstream energy other than that provided by the contracting left ventricle. With this objective in mind, recent attention has been paid to the possibility of total or partial circulatory support by artificial mechanical devices.

Total cardiac replacement by an auxiliary heart has been attempted in a few patients. In most of these endeavors, the cardiac chambers themselves have not been removed but have been used in a nonfunctional manner as part of the conduit traversed by blood to an auxiliary ventricle, either in a portion of the arterial system or between the apex of the left ventricle and the aorta. These devices have sustained the circulation for short periods of time. They require the provision of an external power source with an appropriate transcutaneous connection to the working pump. In addition, the technical problems associated with insertion and vascular connections and the formation of thrombi on the surfaces in contact with flowing blood have not yet been satisfactorily resolved. In the relatively short duration of total cardiac function thus far attempted in man, no limitation seems to be imposed by the strength-durability characteristics of the materials utilized.

An artificial heart powered by an atomic energy source appears to be feasible in the future. Prototype heart pumps have been used for relatively long periods in calves. An atomic power source would allow total implantation, probably within the abdomen, and the problems of radiation shielding and heat dissipation are solvable. It is predicted that such devices will be developed within the next decade with approximately a 10-year life, determined by the stress-strain characteristics of the pump materials. There is no foreseeable limitation imposed by the energy source.

Temporary circulatory assist implies that fundamental abnormal processes may be reversible if the cardiovascular system is supported for a finite period of time, or until more definitive forms of therapy can be undertaken. Circulatory support for hours, or even several days, is now feasible and has been utilized in human patients. However, it has been found that in many instances the degree of myocardial damage which has caused the need for circulatory support is so great as to preclude long-term survival. Hence, many patients must be subjected subsequently to procedures to correct mechanically disadvantageous cardiac lesions or to provide cardiac revascularization by means of aorta-coronary artery anastomosis.

The use of the heart-lung bypass machine conventionally employed in cardiovascular surgery has been suggested for the temporary support of the circulation. Although this is feasible for periods of approximately three hours, the oxygenators do not allow prolonged total support of the circulation. Newly developed membrane oxygenators apparently more adequately preserve the structure of the formed elements in the blood and do not lead to thrombus formation. With these devices, total circulatory support has been undertaken for 24 to 60 hours in a small number of patients. As an extension of this principle, total support of the circulation utilizing the patient's lung as the oxygenator has been proposed. However, there are significant technical difficulties in recovering the oxygenated blood effectively from the left atrium or in the procedures necessary to totally empty the ventricle.

Mechanical counterpulsation refers to a form of partial mechanical support of the circulation. It is well known that when the heart exhibits failure, it is an extremely poor pressure pump, but it is less disabled than a volume pump. Therefore, reduction of the opening pressure at the aortic valve and a reducion of blood pressure during ventricular systole favor the more complete emptying of the left ventricle. Although this can be accomplished by the reduction of peripheral vascular resistance by spinal anesthesia or dilating drugs, it is done so at the expense of coronary perfusion, since a sustained pressure greater than 60 mm. Hg is probably needed during diastole to maintain coronary perfusion. Hence, the most favorable circumstance would be a fundamental reversal of the normal sequence of the cardiac cycle, that is, a fall in aortic pressure during ventricular systole and a rise in pressure during ventricular diastole. A number of procedures have been employed to accomplish these ends. Of these, the best known is accomplished by insertion into the descending thoracic aorta of a sausage-shaped 30-ml. balloon, supported by a rigid catheter. The balloon is connected to a source of compressed helium, which is allowed access to the balloon via a control valve synchronized with the cardiac cycle. Thus, just before or at the time of ventricular systole, the balloon is evacuated of gas and hence the volume in the aorta is acutely reduced by approximately 30 ml. Consequently, there is a brisk fall in aortic pressure, so that ventricular ejection occurs at a point earlier in the cardiac cycle and at a much lower pressure level. When cardiac ejection is complete

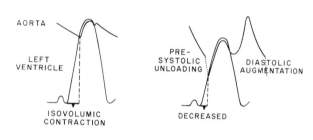

Figure 10–11 The mechanical consequences of counterpulsation. This diagram represents aortic and left ventricular pressure pulses *(left panel)* and the changes consequent upon counterpulsation *(right panel)*. During counterpulsation the pressure in the aorta during the isometric phase of ventricular contraction suddenly falls. Hence, the aortic valve can open at a lower pressure and early in the cardiac cycle. This may favorably influence the level of myocardial oxygen consumption. Since the aortic capacitance has been increased (see text), the absolute magnitude of pressure generated during ventricular systole is reduced. When the aortic valve closes, aortic pressure is artificially increased by the counterpulsation device, thus providing a higher head of pressure for the maintenance of coronary arterial blood flow.

and the aortic valve closes, the balloon is reinflated, adding a volume equivalent to 30 ml. to the aortic content, thus raising the intra-aortic pressure. These events are indicated diagrammatically in Figure 10–11. Coronary perfusion pressure is increased during ventricular diastole, while the stimulus to myocardial oxygen consumption is diminished because isometric contraction is shortened and maximal left ventricular wall tension is decreased.

Usually within 10 to 15 minutes after its initiation, this form of circulatory support can reverse profound depression of cardiovascular pump function. There is a prompt improvement in cardiac output, reduction in filling pressure, improved organ perfusion, and reversal of metabolic alterations. However, this technique necessitates surgical insertion of the balloon into the vascular system, a precise synchronization of the electrical action of the heart with the inflation and deflation sequences, and an experienced team of investigators and clinicians to manage other aspects of patient care.

REFERENCES

Braunwald, E.: The determinants of myocardial oxygen consumption. Thirteenth Bowditch Lecture. The Physiologist, *12*:65, 1969.

Braunwald, E., Chidsey, C. A., Pool, P. E., et al.: Clinical Staff Conference. Congestive heart failure: Biochemical and physiological considerations. Ann. Intern. Med., *64*:904, 1966.

Braunwald, E., Ross, J., and Sonnenblick, E. H.: Mechanisms of contraction of the normal and failing heart. Little, Brown and Co., Boston, 1968.

Chatterjee, K., and Parmley, W. W.: The role of vasodilator therapy in heart failure. Prog. Cardiovasc. Dis., *19*:301, 1977.

Dodge, H. T., and Baxley, W. A.: Hemodynamic aspects of heart failure. Am. J. Cardiol., *22*:24, 1968.

Ford, L. E.: Heart size. Circ. Res., *39*:297, 1976.

Friedberg, C. K. (Ed.): Congestive Heart Failure. Grune & Stratton, New York, 1970, pp. 1–70, 97–171, 195–288.

Ganz, W., Tamura, K., Marcus, H. S., et al.: Measurement of coronary sinus blood flow by continuous thermodilution in man. Circulation, *44*:181, 1971.

Herman, M. V., and Gorlin, R.: Implications of left ventricular asynergy. Am. J. Cardiol., *23*:538, 1969.

Katz, A. M., and Brady, A. J.: Mechanical and biochemical correlates of cardiac contraction (I and II). Modern Conc. Cardiovasc. Dis., *40*:39 and *40*:45, 1971.

Maroko, P. R., Kjekshus, J. K., Sobel, B. E., et al.: Factors influencing infarct size following experimental coronary artery occlusions. Circulation, *43*:67, 1971.

Mason, D. T.: Control of peripheral circulation in health and disease. Modern Conc. Cardiovasc. Dis., *36*:25, 1967.

Parmley, W. W., Tyberg, J. V., and Glantz, S.: Cardiac Dynamics. Ann. Rev. Physiol., *39*:277, 1977.

Spann, J. F., Jr., Mason, D. T., and Zelis, R.: Recent advances in the understanding of congestive heart failure. Modern Conc. Cardiovasc. Dis., *39*:73, 1970.

Swan, H. J. C., Forrester, J. S., Diamond, G., et al.: The hemodynamic basis of shock and acute myocardial infarction: a conceptual model. Circulation, *45*:1097, 1972.

11

Heart Sounds, Murmurs, and Precordial Movements*†

JOHN F. STAPLETON AND W. PROCTOR HARVEY

During each cardiac cycle the heart generates many vibrations which are transmitted through surrounding tissues to the chest wall. These arise from the contractile and expansile movements of the cardiac chambers, from valvular opening and closure, from tissue motion caused by blood flow, and from the bloodstream itself.

Vibrations having low frequency (0 to 30 cycles per second) cause subaudible chest wall pulsations which can be palpated when sufficiently forceful. Vibrations having higher frequency (30 to 500 cycles per second) enter the range of human audibility and can be heard at the chest surface when sufficiently loud. Such audible vibrations are called heart sounds when brief and murmurs when sustained. Figure 11–1 illustrates the sensitivity of the human ear to cardiovascular sound.

HEART SOUNDS AND MURMURS

The first heart sound (S_1) begins as the ventricles start to contract. Minor vibrations coinciding with the earliest contractile movement may initiate S_1, occurring as early as 0.02 to 0.03 sec. after electrocardiographic QRS begins. The first major vibrations then commence 0.06 sec. after the onset of QRS (Fig. 11–2), 0.02 to 0.04 sec. after rising left ventricular pressure exceeds left atrial pressure. These vibrations begin when flow ceases across the mitral valve, coinciding with the peak of the left atrial C wave caused by the suddenly arrested bulge into the left atrium of the closed mitral leaflets. Since this sound relates to mitral valve closure, it is called M_1.

A second set of vibrations, beginning about 0.03 sec. after the onset of M_1, coincides with the peak of the right atrial C wave. Since it relates to tricuspid valve closure, it is called T_1 (Figs. 11–3, 11–4). A few minor vibrations may follow T_1, completing the first heart sound. These final vibrations coincide with beginning movement of the aortic valve cusps and could derive from this structure. The total first sound lasts 0.04 to 0.10 sec., including the small initial and final oscillations.

The first sound is usually loudest over the cardiac apex, where M_1 predominates and T_1 is normally absent or faint. At the lower left sternal border, T_1 is often well heard following M_1. Many normal individuals have distinct splitting of S_1 at this area (Fig. 11–3). When T_1 is accentuated, it may be louder than M_1 at the apex. When this occurs, abnormally forceful tricuspid closure is present, as commonly occurs with atrial septal defect. Ebstein's anomaly often causes a singularly loud and late T_1.

At the cardiac base, the normal S_1 consists solely of M_1 unless T_1 is exaggerated.

The electrocardiographic PR interval influences the intensity of S_1. Short intervals intensify S_1; long intervals diminish it. When PR is less than 0.20, the intervals relate inversely to

*Supported in part by U.S. Public Health grants, The Benjamin May Memorial Fund, and Metropolitan Heart Guild.

†We wish to express our appreciation to Mr. Bernard Salb for his assistance in preparing this chapter.

335

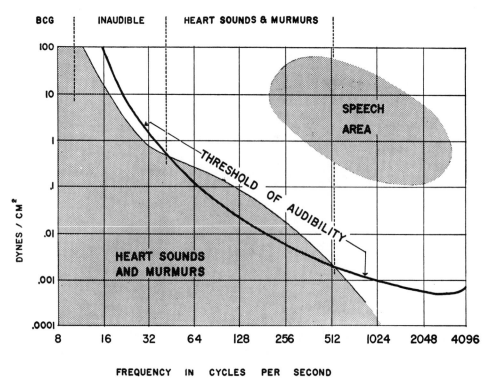

Figure 11-1   The graph illustrates the frequency spectrum of human hearing. Note that only a small component of total cardiac sound can be detected by the human ear. (By permission from Butterworth, J. S., Chassin, M. R., and McGrath, R.: Cardiac Auscultation including Audiovisual Principles, 2nd ed. Grune and Stratton, New York, 1960.)

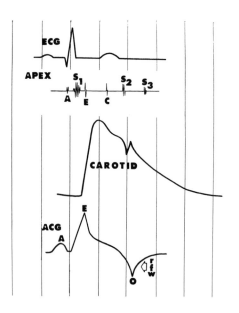

Figure 11-2   Heart sounds heard at the apex correlated with the electrocardiogram *(ECG)*, carotid artery pulse tracing *(CAROTID)*, and apex cardiogram *(ACG)*.

Sound tracing: *A,* atrial sound or S_4 (left atrial); S_1, first heart sound; *E,* aortic ejection sound; *C,* systolic click; S_2, second heart sound; S_3, ventricular filling sound.

Apex cardiogram *(ACG): E,* Peak of apical impulse; *O,* beginning of ventricular rapid filling *(rfw)*.

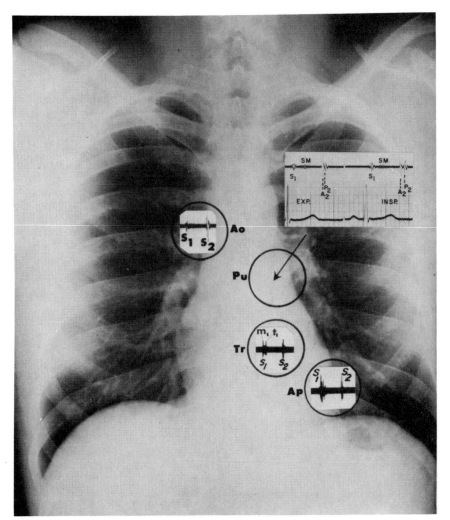

Figure 11–3   Heart sounds as heard over different valve areas. *Ao*, aortic area: Here the first sound *(S₁)* is faint and the second sound *(S₂)* is loud and single. *Pu*, pulmonary area: Here S₁ is reduced and S₂ is loud and split into two components, *A₂* (aortic closure) and *P₂* (pulmonary closure). The split S₂ widens with inspiration and narrows with expiration. *Tr*, tricuspid area: S₁ splits into two components, *M1* (mitral closure) and *T1* (tricuspid closure). *Ap*, apex: S₁ is loud with faint before and after vibrations. S₂ is single and less intense than S₁, at the apex. *SM*, systolic murmur; *INSP*, inspiration; *EXP*, expiration.

the loudness of S₁. Intervals longer than 0.20 are associated with faint first sounds. When PR exceeds 0.50 sec., the first sound may recover normal intensity.

The first sound–PR relationship is explained by the proximity of ventricular systole to atrial systole. The mitral and tricuspid leaflets are opened wide by atrial contraction. When ventricular systole occurs promptly there is greater leaflet excursion than when ventricular contraction is delayed, allowing the leaflets to float passively together before systole begins. The loudness of S₁ varies directly with the magnitude of leaflet excursion.

Conditions that increase the force of ventricular contractions usually increase the intensity of the first sound. Such conditions include thyrotoxicosis, severe anemia, exercise, excitement, and stimulatory drugs such as epinephrine. Mitral stenosis, by stiffening the mitral leaflets, causes a loud and often high-pitched first sound. Conditions that diminish cardiac function, such as myocardial infarction or myxedema, tend to soften the first sound, irrespective of the P-R interval.

Delayed onset of the first sound characterizes mitral stenosis, which impairs leaflet mobility and elevates left atrial pressure. The delay can be

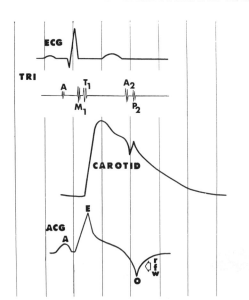

Figure 11–4 Heart sounds heard over the tricuspid region *(TRI)* correlated with the electrocardiogram *(ECG)*, carotid artery pulse tracing *(CAROTID)*, and apex cardiogram *(ACG)*.

Sound tracing: A, atrial sound or S_4 (right atrial); M_1, mitral valve closure sound; T_1, tricuspid valve closure sound; A_2, aortic valve closure sound; P_2, Pulmonary valve closure sound.

Apex cardiogram *(ACG): E*, peak of apical impulse; *O,* beginning of ventricular rapid filling *(rfw).*

heard over the pulmonary area and along the mid-left sternal border (Figs. 11–4 and 11–5). Aortic closure usually causes a louder sound than pulmonary closure, even in the pulmonary region; however, in some young individuals P_2 may normally exceed A_2 in the pulmonary region.

The interval between aortic valve closure and A_2 averages 0.01 to 0.015 sec., whereas the interval between pulmonic valve closure and P_2 is longer, ranging from 0.03 to 0.09 sec. The greater distensibility of the pulmonary vascular bed probably accounts for this longer interval. When pulmonary capacitance is further increased by inspiration, P_2 occurs even later. At the same time, inspiratory venous inflow lengthens right ventricular systole, delaying pulmonic valve closure, while inspiratory increase in pulmonary vascular capacity reduces flow into the left heart, thereby shortening left ventricular systole and causing slightly earlier aortic valve closure. These inspiratory events, leading to earlier A_2 and later P_2, cause audibly widened splitting of the second heart sound in many normal people. Usually expiration fuses the two components of S_2 (Fig. 11–3).

Inspiratory splitting of the second sound, described by Potain in 1866, has been reemphasized by Leatham. Complete right bundle branch block, by retarding right ventricular depolariza-

detected by measuring the interval between the onset of QRS on the electrocardiogram and the onset of the first major vibrations of the first sound as recorded on a phonocardiogram. This measurement correlates with the severity of mitral obstruction. Systemic hypertension may also delay the onset of the first heart sound.

When systolic ejection ends, aortic and pulmonic pressures exceed the declining pressures of the relaxing ventricles, causing the aortic and pulmonic valves to shut. The second heart sound (S_2) arises from this process. Echocardiographic tracking of semilunar valve closure reveals that this event slightly precedes S_2, which actually coincides with the arrest of the closed valve leaflets as they bulge into the ventricles, abruptly halting reverse blood flow. Normally the second sound splits into two distinct components, the first relating to aortic valve closure, followed by the second relating to pulmonary valve closure. The aortic component (A_2) normally can be heard all over the precordium, being maximal in the aortic area. The pulmonary component (P_2) is usually loudest in the pulmonary area (Fig. 11–5) but often extends to the tricuspid region (Fig. 11–4). Hence, splitting of the second sound is best

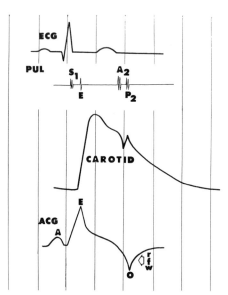

Figure 11–5 Heart sounds heard over the pulmonary area *(PUL)* correlated with the electrocardiogram *(ECG)*, carotid artery pulse tracing *(CAROTID)*, and apex cardiogram *(ACG)*.

Sound tracing: S_1, first heart sound; *E*, pulmonary ejection sound; A_2, aortic valve closure sound; P_2, pulmonary valve closure sound.

Apex cardiogram *(ACG): E,* Peak of apical impulse; *O,* beginning of ventricular rapid filling *(rfw).*

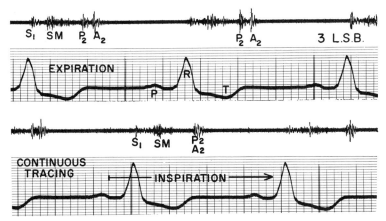

Figure 11–6   Paradoxical splitting of the second sound. The aortic valve closure sound *(A₂)* follows the pulmonary valve closure sound *(P₂)*. Inspiration delays P₂, narrowing the split. Compare with Figure 11–3, which illustrates normal inspiratory separation of A₂ and P₂. S₁, first heart sound. *SM,* systolic murmur. (Reproduced from Levine, S. A., and Harvey, W. P.: Clinical Auscultation of the Heart, 2d ed. W. B. Saunders Co., Philadelphia, 1959.)

tion, delays pulmonary valve closure, resulting in wide splitting of the second sound even during expiration; inspiration further widens the split. Conversely, conditions which prolong or delay left ventricular systole may cause A₂ to follow P₂. When this occurs, splitting increases with expiration and narrows with inspiration, a finding called paradoxic or reversed splitting of the second sound (Fig. 11–6). Complete left bundle branch block commonly causes this phenomenon by impeding left ventricular depolarization and so delaying aortic closure. Severe aortic stenosis occasionally prolongs left ventricular ejection sufficiently to cause paradoxic splitting. Right ventricular pacing and right ventricular extrasystoles simulate left bundle branch block by depolarizing the right ventricle before the left, causing reversed splitting of S₂. Other infrequent causes of reversed splitting include patent ductus arteriosus, angina pectoris, myocardial infarction, and, rarely, systemic hypertension.

In uncomplicated atrial septal defect with significant left-to-right shunt, the right and left ventricles share a functionally common atrium and have similar duration of systole. A₂ and P₂ remain clearly separate during both inspiration and expiration, exhibiting little or no respiratory variation (Fig. 11–7). This phenomenon, known as fixed splitting, characterizes left-to-right shunting of blood at the atrial level and is a valuable diagnostic sign, although occasional patients with atrial septal defects may present normal splitting of S₂.

Splitting of S₂ is "fixed" and widened in atrial septal defect because P₂ is unduly delayed. Although left and right ventricular systole end together, the copious pulmonary vascular bed takes longer than usual to reverse pulmonary flow and distend the pulmonic cusps. This mechanism explains persistence of "fixed" splitting of S₂ after surgical closure of atrial defects, since large pulmonary vascular capacitance persists.

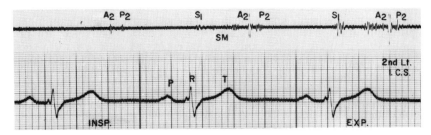

Figure 11–7   Fixed splitting of the second sound. Widely split second sound without significant respiratory variation of the interval between aortic closure *(A₂)* and pulmonary closure *(P₂)*. This finding characterizes most individuals with atrial septal defect. S₁, first heart sound; *SM,* systolic murmur.

Pulmonary or systemic hypertension produces forceful closure of the pulmonary or aortic valve. Loud A_2 or P_2 often accompanies aortic or pulmonary hypertension. The accentuated P_2 of pulmonary hypertension is sometimes palpable, if sought. It often occurs early, close to, or fused with A_2, causing a resounding single S_2 over the pulmonic area. This results from the quick reversal of pulmonary blood flow upon valve closure, owing to the high resistance–low capacitance vascular bed of severe pulmonary hypertension. Cor pulmonale due either to acute massive pulmonary embolism or chronic lung disease may lengthen right ventricular systole. In these cases, P_2 is both loud and late; the second sound becomes widely split with accentuation of the delayed pulmonic component. The hyperactive circulation of thyrotoxicosis or severe anemia also intensifies the second sound; however, these disorders increase the first heart sound, unlike hypertension, which selectively augments the second sound.

Impaired mobility of a semilunar valve will diminish its closure sound. The aortic second sound of calcific aortic stenosis is sometimes faint or even absent, whereas congenital aortic stenosis with its supple valve structure usually gives rise to a normal or increased closure sound. Severe pulmonary stenosis greatly diminishes (and delays) P_2 (Fig. 11–10), whereas mild pulmonary stenosis does so only slightly.

Posterior location of the pulmonary valve, as in certain congenital defects such as transposition of the great vessels, may also diminish or even abolish P_2.

Most children and many young adults have a normal third heart sound (S_3) in early diastole. This sound coincides with the rapid filling phase of left ventricular diastole and is variously known as a physiologic third sound, a ventricular filling sound, or simply S_3. Its genesis is unclear; it probably derives from vibrations of the ventricular wall and/or the mitral valve structure resulting from the sudden ventricular dilatation of rapid filling. The third heart sound is low pitched, best heard at the apex, and usually faint, although occasionally this sound is prominent and may have after-vibrations which extend its duration. Although a third sound during left ventricular rapid filling is physiologic during childhood and youth, this sound in middle life and beyond denotes cardiac dysfunction, usually myocardial failure. It is an early and subtle sign of cardiac decompensation, having great diagnostic and prognostic value. Its detection often requires deliberate listening in a quiet room. Occasionally, regurgitant disease of the aortic or mitral valve exaggerates ventricular filling enough to produce a third sound.

Another extra heart sound may occur during atrial systole. This sound, known as the atrial or fourth heart sound (S_4), probably arises from movement of the ventricular wall and/or the atrioventricular valve structure caused by sudden ventricular distention induced by atrial contraction. Atrial sounds may be heard in apparently healthy individuals, particularly in the older age groups. When atrioventricular block separates atrial from ventricular contraction, atrial sounds frequently become audible.

Left atrial sounds begin about 0.17 second (range: 0.14 to 0.24) after the onset of the electrocardiographic P, coinciding with the peak of the precordial atrial movement. The sound is low-pitched, apical, and usually faint. Its closeness to the first sound at times may simulate wide splitting of the first sound. Firm stethoscope pressure will frequently eliminate the low frequency atrial sound, but will not abolish M_1 or T_1. When prominent, the sound can be heard medial to the apex, sometimes extending to the sternal border. Right atrial sounds begin about 0.12 second (range: 0.09 to 0.16) after the onset of P and are low pitched, usually faint, and best heard over the tricuspid area. Right atrial sounds may increase during inspiration. Faint vibrations often can be recorded preceding an audible atrial sound; these vibrations, usually inaudible, probably arise from myocardial contraction.

Atrial sounds are likely to appear whenever there is increased resistance to ventricular filling. Various myocardial diseases increase resistance to ventricular filling by reducing myocardial compliance and thereby cause atrial sounds. Cardiomyopathies frequently cause atrial sounds; the concentric hypertrophy of aortic stenosis and systemic hypertension also stiffens the ventricular wall, leading to vigorous atrial contraction. Atrial sounds regularly accompany these diseases. Acute myocardial infarction often causes high diastolic ventricular filling pressure, low ventricular compliance, and atrioventricular block; hence, atrial sounds appear in most patients with acute myocardial infarction and usually persist after the acute stage.

When atrial and ventricular diastolic sounds result from heart disease, the term "gallop rhythm" is often applied, because these extra sounds impart the cadence of a cantering horse to the heart rhythm — particularly when the ventricular rate is rapid. Thus, the atrial and ventricular sounds of heart disease are usually called gallop sounds. A patient with cardiac failure may have a ventricular (or third sound) gallop, an atrial (or fourth sound) gallop, or both. When tachycardia is present, a diastolic gallop sound may be difficult to classify. When slowing occurs, identification can be made by noting a constant relationship of the ventricular gallop to the second sound and a constant relationship of the atrial gallop to the electrocardiographic P and, usually, to the first sound (Fig. 11–8).

Atrial and ventricular sounds frequently coex-

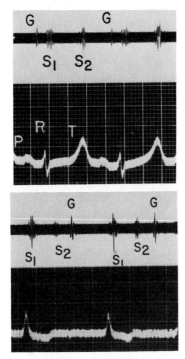

Figure 11–8 Upper panel displays a gallop sound (G) related to atrial systole. This sound is known as an atrial gallop or as an atrial sound or as a fourth heart sound (S_4). S_1, first heart sound; S_2, second heart sound.

Lower panel displays a gallop sound (G) related to ventricular rapid filling. This sound is known as a ventricular filling sound or as a ventricular gallop or as a third heart sound (S_3). S_1, first heart sound; S_2, second heart sound.

ist. When close together, this combination of sounds may resemble a short, low-pitched rumbling murmur. At times, as in an occasional patient with cardiomyopathy, the rumble is erroneously diagnosed as mitral stenosis. When diastole so shortens that these sounds fuse, a single sound may result, known as a summation gallop sound.

Patients with constrictive pericarditis often present an extra sound in early diastole which coincides with the sudden arrest of the expanding ventricle as the constricting pericardium abruptly halts diastolic filling.

A third sound often follows closely upon the second sound in mitral stenosis. Known as the "opening snap," it probably derives from the suddenly arrested descent (or "checking") of the stiffened mitral valve that occurs as the valve opens in early diastole. This sound signifies the end of isovolumetric relaxation; it is usually high pitched and is best heard at the apex but can transmit widely. It follows the aortic closure sound by 0.06 to 0.12 second. This measurement, which can readily be made with a phonocardiogram and approximated by careful auscultation, correlates with the severity of mitral obstruction, the shorter A_2-opening snap periods corresponding to higher grades of stenosis. This interval varies with heart rate, since shorter cycle lengths are associated with higher left atrial pressure and earlier mitral valve opening. When mitral stenosis greatly reduces valve mobility, as with dense calcification, the mitral opening snap may become fainter and occasionally disappears. Valve rigidity also can, occasionally, diminish the intensity of the first sound.

An opening snap may also occur without valvular stenosis when vigorous blood flow causes brisk opening and forceful arrest of the descending leaflets. Atrial septal defect, mitral regurgitation, thyrotoxicosis and other high-flow conditions occasionally cause opening snaps.

Extra heart sounds also occur during systole. Patients with congenital aortic or pulmonary stenosis often have an early systolic sound which closely follows the first sound. Known as an aortic or pulmonary ejection sound, it signifies the end of isovolumetric contraction, coinciding with the maximum excursion of the deformed semilunar valve and the beginning of ejection. Loudness of ejection sounds correlates with the magnitude of valve cusp movement. Aortic ejection sounds are best heard in the aortic area (Fig. 11–10) and at the apex (Fig. 11–2). Pulmonary ejection sounds are best heard in the pulmonary area (Fig. 11–4) and characteristically diminish with inspiration; they are generally faint or absent at the apex. Ejection sounds often occur with pulmonary or systemic hypertension or with abnormal dilatation of the ascending aorta or pulmonary artery; these ejection sounds arise from vigorous cusp distention with abrupt halt of reversed flow. An aortic ejection sound may be heard over the aortic and apical areas with coarctation of the aorta, and a pulmonic ejection sound is common with idiopathic dilatation of the pulmonary artery. Aortic ejection sounds can occur with thyrotoxicosis and other high-output states.

Other sounds may also occur during systolic ejection; such sounds are frequently brief, high pitched, and therefore called "clicks." The "midsystolic click" is a commonly used expression denoting the usual timing of such sounds (Figs. 11–2 and 11–9). A systolic murmur, usually in late systole, is often also present. This is known as the "systolic click–murmur" syndrome, prolapsing mitral valve leaflet syndrome, floppy valve syndrome, Barlow's syndrome, etc. Angiograms of patients with this finding commonly demonstrate one or both mitral leaflets to be so copious as to prolapse into the left atrium during late systole, permitting regurgitation; the posterior leaflet is most commonly involved. The click coincides with maximum leaflet excursion and probably arises from the suddenly arrested motion of the affected leaflet(s) and chordae tendineae. Clicks may be single or multiple. The standing position may intensify clicks, cause them to occur earlier in systole or produce clicks not audible during recumbency.

Audible vibrations that persist beyond the brief acoustic impact of a discrete heart sound constitute a heart *murmur*; a murmur is a rapid succession of heart sounds. Most investigators have attributed murmurs to blood flow through irregular or narrowed orifices or through dilated segments of major arteries, through abnormal intracardiac and arteriovenous communications, or backward through incompetent valves. Murmurs also can arise from rapid blood flow through normal structures. The actual genesis of murmur vibrations has not been established with certainty. There are two sources of sound which account for the many varieties of murmurs: the bloodstream itself and solid structures which are caused to vibrate by flowing blood. Murmurs arising from the blood itself are thought to derive from vortex (eddy) formation or from turbulence created as blood flows through varying orifices, chambers, and tubes at varying rates. Murmurs arising from solid structures usually represent the vibrations of heart valves or other cardiac or vascular tissue set into motion by the bloodstream.

Murmurs are classified according to timing, location, and loudness. Most murmurs are either systolic or diastolic; occasional murmurs that continue throughout systole and diastole are called continuous murmurs. The examiner may categorize loudness according to six grades of intensity. Grade I describes a murmur so soft that intent listening is required over several cardiac cycles. A Grade II murmur is also faint but audible immediately upon listening. Grades III and IV represent increasing loudness. Grade VI murmurs are so loud as to be audible through the stethoscope head held just off the chest wall. A Grade V murmur is very loud but cannot be heard off the chest. Grade IV, V, and VI murmurs cause palpable chest wall vibrations, felt by the hand as a gentle, throbbing sensation resembling the purr of a cat. This finding, known as a *thrill*, occurs where the murmur is loudest and represents the tactile counterpart of a loud murmur. The significance of a thrill is that of the underlying murmur.

The examiner localizes the murmur according to the area of maximal intensity. Thus, he may record a Grade III apical systolic murmur or a Grade II pulmonary diastolic murmur or a Grade VI aortic systolic murmur. Many murmurs have special pitch characteristics which merit description. Thus, diastolic flow across a stenotic mitral valve causes low-pitched vibrations usually described as a "rumble." A high-pitched murmur is often called a "blow" or "blowing murmur." Another category, the musical murmur, includes many curious harmonic patterns colorfully labeled as "sea gull," "cooing dove," "twanging string," and other epithets. The musical tonality derives from a single predominating frequency which usually arises from a vibrating structure within the heart, such as a perforated valve cusp or ruptured chordae tendineae.

Expert auscultation refines timing beyond the simple designation of systolic, diastolic, or continuous. A murmur may extend throughout systole or may be limited to early or late systole. A murmur may steadily intensify (crescendo), may steadily decline (decrescendo), or may have a midway loudness peak. Such variations often have meaning and should be noted. The term holosystolic (or pansystolic) signifies vibrations that commence with the first heart sound and cease at the second heart sound. A holosystolic murmur invariably indicates systolic regurgitation through the mitral or tricuspid valve or through a ventricular septal defect. Holosystolic murmurs are often called regurgitant murmurs. These murmurs are holosystolic because left ventricular pressure exceeds left atrial pressure throughout systole (mitral regurgitation) or because right ventricular pressure exceeds right atrial pressure throughout systole (tricuspid regurgitation) or because left ventricular pressure exceeds right ventricular pressure throughout systole (ventricular septal defect).

The systolic murmur of significant mitral regurgitation is typically a holosystolic murmur heard best at the cardiac apex (Fig. 11–9). Mitral regurgitation commonly results from the leaflet distortion caused by rheumatic fever. Fusion of the cusps and shortening and fusion of the chordae tendineae prevent normal valve closure and permit leakage into the atrium. Left ventricular dilatation of any cause may displace the papillary muscles and dilate the mitral annulus, disrupting normal valve closure. Left atrial enlargement itself may further impede closure by exerting traction on the mitral annulus. Other causes of mitral regurgitation recognized with increasing frequency are papillary muscle dysfunction, ruptured chordae tendineae, calcified mitral annulus fibrosus, myxomatous mitral cusps, bacterial endocarditis, endocardial fibroelastosis, and various congenital anomalies.

Mitral regurgitation does not always lead to a holosystolic murmur. Acute mitral regurgitation often causes a murmur which is loud in early and midsystole but subsides before the second sound. The tense left atrial wall of sudden mitral incompetence does not dilate in response to overfilling; instead, mounting left atrial pressure develops during ventricular systole until atrial pressure exceeds the declining pressure of late ventricular

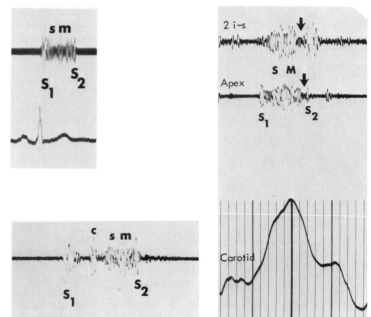

Figure 11–9 Upper left panel displays the holosystolic murmur of severe mitral regurgitation. The murmur *(sm)* extends from the first sound *(S₁)* to the second sound *(S₂)*.

Lower left panel displays the late systolic murmur *(sm)* of mitral regurgitation due to prolapse of posterior mitral leaflet. S_1, first sound; S_2, second sound; C, systolic click; *sm*, systolic murmur.

Vertical panel on right displays the systolic murmur *(SM)* of acute mitral regurgitation due to rupture of chordae tendineae. Note rapid decline of systolic vibrations in late systole (arrows). Upper sound tracing recorded in aortic area *(2 i-s);* lower sound tracing recorded over the cardiac apex. S_1, first heart sound; S_2, second heart sound.

systole, thereby reducing regurgitation and its resultant murmur in late systole (Fig. 11–9). This murmur often transmits well to the cardiac base.

A systolic murmur confined to late systole characterizes mitral incompetence caused by leaflet prolapse. This has been termed the late apical systolic murmur. It is frequently preceded by one or more systolic clicks as described previously (Fig. 11–9). It may be produced or lengthened and intensified by the standing posture.

The systolic murmur of tricuspid regurgitation is maximal in the fourth left interspace at the lower sternal edge. It may be holosystolic but sometimes fades out in the latter half of systole. It is often faint and easily overlooked. The murmur usually becomes louder during inspiration. This important characteristic results from the increased right ventricular filling caused by inspiration. Respiratory change can be subtle, requiring careful listening. Tricuspid regurgitation may result from leaflet deformity due to rheumatic fever. It is peculiarly common in heroin addicts, resulting from tricuspid bacterial endocarditis in these individuals. Tricuspid regurgitation frequently accompanies severe right ventricular hypertension of any cause, since dilatation of the right ventricle may displace the papillary muscles and dilate the tricuspid ring to such an extent that normal valve closure is not possible.

Blood flow across an irregular or stenotic semilunar valve causes a systolic murmur which commences after the first sound, increases to a peak in the middle third of systole, and then declines

in late systole, ceasing before closure of the affected pulmonary or aortic valve. Sound tracings reveal a diamond shape; this acoustic pattern has been termed an ejection murmur. Such murmurs are often harsh and loud, radiate widely, and may be associated with decreased intensity of A_2 or P_2 when valvular stenosis reduces leaflet mobility (Fig. 11–10).

Murmurs of aortic and pulmonary stenosis are generally loudest at the aortic or pulmonary areas of the chest wall, respectively. Good transmission to the clavicles and neck characterizes the murmurs of semilunar valve stenosis, although in older patients with aortic stenosis, particularly those with increased anteroposterior chest diameter, the aortic murmur may be loudest at the apex, and sometimes has a high frequency musical quality.

Some ejection murmurs relate to high velocity of blood flow through a normal semilunar valve. Such murmurs are common in conditions such as thyrotoxicosis, pregnancy, fever, excitement, and other states which increase stroke volume. Murmurs like these, which do not arise from structural alteration within the heart, are called functional murmurs in contrast to those arising from anatomic defects, which are called organic or significant murmurs.

Innocent murmurs are those which arise in healthy individuals who have no evidence of increased cardiac output or other circulatory alteration. They are most common in children but are also frequently encountered in the adult. The usual murmur is early to midsystolic, of Grade I

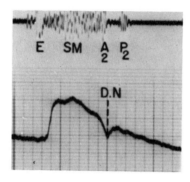

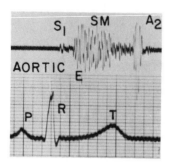

Figure 11–10 Upper panel displays the ejection systolic murmur of pulmonary valve stenosis. Note the pulmonary ejection sound *(E)* which initiates the diamond-contoured murmur which subsides before a late and softened pulmonary closure sound *(P₂)*. A₂, aortic closure sound; *SM,* systolic murmur; *DN,* dicrotic incisura.

Lower panel displays the systolic ejection murmur of aortic stenosis. This murmur begins after S₁, has midsystolic peak, and then declines before aortic closure *(A₂)*. *E,* aortic ejection sound; *SM,* systolic murmur; *S₁,* first heart sound.

or II intensity, occasionally Grade III. It is most common in the lower, left parasternal region or in the pulmonary area, although also frequently heard over the aortic and apical areas. Innocent murmurs are seldom loudest at the apex. The genesis of these murmurs is not known, though some appear to arise from high-velocity blood flow through the aortic or pulmonic valves.

Most systolic murmurs are innocent; most diastolic murmurs are organic. Abnormal vibrations during diastole usually result from regurgitation through an incompetent aortic or pulmonary valve or from stenosis of the mitral or tricuspid valve. Incompetence of a semilunar valve leads to a high-pitched decrescendo murmur, commencing with A₂ or P₂ and subsiding in mid- or late diastole (Fig. 11–11). Incompetence of the aortic valve results from the leaflet thickening and fusion of rheumatic fever; from dilatation of the aortic valve ring and separation of cusps

associated with syphilis or ankylosing (rheumatoid) spondylitis; from cusp perforation or laceration due to bacterial endocarditis or injury; from cusp prolapse due to dissecting aneurysm or due to loss of supporting septal tissue with certain ventricular septal defects; or from poor apposition of congenital bicuspid leaflets. All these anatomic deformities permit regurgitation when aortic pressure exceeds ventricular pressure during diastole. This pressure differential is highest in early diastole and declines as aortic pressure declines, hence the decrescendo pattern of murmur intensity.

Pulmonary valve insufficiency most commonly results from marked pulmonary arterial hypertension. Elevated pulmonary artery diastolic pressure may dilate the pulmonary valve ring sufficiently to prevent complete cusp apposition. A high-pitched, usually soft, decrescendo murmur is heard in the pulmonary region. Rarely, congenital deformity of the pulmonary leaflets permits regurgitation. Here the pulmonary artery pressure is normal, and the diastolic pressure gradient across the valve is small. The murmur may be similar to that caused by pulmonary hypertension but in some patients it is short, is medium- to low-pitched, and does not commence promptly with P₂ but develops in early diastole, separated from P₂ by a brief pause (Fig. 11–11). It also may increase coincident with inspiration.

The low-pitched apical diastolic murmur or rumble of mitral stenosis is separated from the second sound by a brief interval (0.06 to 0.12 second) which corresponds to left ventricular isovolumetric relaxation period. The rumble begins when the mitral valve opens and blood flows through the obstructed orifice at greater than normal velocity. The murmur usually commences with the mitral opening snap sound. As the pressure gradient between atrium and ventricle subsides in mid and late diastole, the rumble diminishes. If atrial systole, by raising left atrial pressure and/or by constricting the mitral orifice, increases the gradient, the murmur will accentuate just before the first sound, creating a crescendo rumble terminating in the exaggerated first sound of mitral stenosis (Fig. 11–11). This atrial systolic component of the murmur disappears when atrial fibrillation develops, although low-frequency antecedent vibrations may still initiate the first sound in atrial fibrillation, owing to ventricular contractions that precede valve closure.

Tricuspid stenosis causes a diastolic murmur that is similar to the rumble of mitral stenosis but usually subsides earlier in diastole, probably because the gradient across the stenotic tricuspid valve is generally smaller than that across the stenotic mitral valve. This murmur is maximal along the lower, left parasternal region. It characteristically accentuates with inspiration.

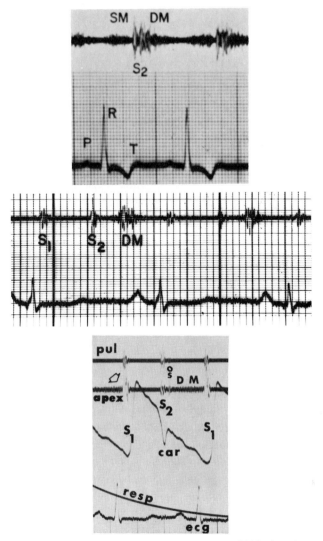

Figure 11–11 Upper panel displays the decrescendo diastolic murmur *(DM)* of aortic regurgitation which begins at aortic closure *(S₂)* and fades out in late diastole. Most patients with significant aortic regurgitation have a systolic ejection murmur in the aòrtic region as shown here *(SM)*.

Middle panel displays the short, early diastolic murmur *(DM)* of congenital pulmonary regurgitation. Note the brief pause between the second heart sound *(S₂)* and the onset of this diamond-contoured murmur which subsides quickly as pulmonary artery and right ventricular pressure equalize in mid-diastole. S_1, first heart sound. (By permission from Collins, N., Braunwald, E., and Morrow, A.: Am. J. Med., *28*:159, 1960).

Lower panel depicts the rumbling diastolic murmur *(DM)* of mitral stenosis which begins after opening snap *(OS)* which is present in the pulmonary area *(pul)* as well as at the apex. The murmur accentuates with atrial systole (arrow). *Car,* carotid pulse; *resp,* respiration; *ecg,* electrocardiogram.

This interesting diagnostic feature relates to increased venous return to the right atrium and greater flow through the tricuspid valve as inspiration lowers intrathoracic pressure, thereby facilitating venous flow into the chest.

One of the most striking cardiac murmurs is that caused by patent ductus arteriosus and other arteriovenous communications. Since arterial pressure exceeds venous pressure throughout the cardiac cycle, such murmurs are continuous, waxing and waning as pressure gradients and flow velocity wax and wane. The murmur may be high pitched but often contains loud vibrations of medium and low frequency. When this is so, the

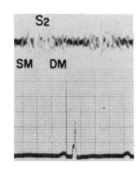

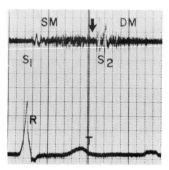

Figure 11–12   Upper panel displays the continuous murmur of patent ductus arteriosus which persists throughout the cardiac cycle, reaching its peak in late systole and early diastole, forming an envelope about the second sound *(S₂)*. *SM,* systolic component of murmur; *DM,* diastolic component of murmur. Contrast this murmur with the to-and-fro systolic *(SM)* and diastolic *(DM)* murmurs of ventricular septal defect and aortic regurgitation seen in the lower panel. Note declining late systolic vibrations *(arrow)* in contrast to the late systolic crescendo of the continuous murmur.

larger pressure gradient at this time between upper descending aorta and main pulmonary trunk. These murmurs must be distinguished from "to-and-fro" systolic and diastolic murmur of aortic stenosis and regurgitation or of ventricular septal defect and aortic regurgitation which do not envelop S_2 as does the continuous murmur of patent ductus arteriosus (Fig. 11–12).

Pericarditis causes a characteristic rough, scraping sound called a pericardial friction rub. The inflamed pericardial and epicardial surfaces move against each other to create this sound. Since the rub relates to movement, it occurs with three major movements of the cardiac cycle — atrial systole, early ventricular systole, and rapid ventricular diastolic filling. Therefore, the typical friction rub will often have three discrete, high-pitched grating noises corresponding to the cardiac movements described (Fig. 11–13). Frequently, only two components can be heard, as when atrial fibrillation eliminates atrial systole; rarely, only a single rub is present.

The sounds are usually maximal over the lower left parasternal area and often have to be sought intently, with the stethoscope diaphragm pressed firmly against the skin. A typical three-component pericardial friction rub is a highly specific and therefore valuable finding which indicates the presence of some form of pericarditis. A two component rub is also important evidence of pericardial disease but a single rubbing sound does not reliably implicate the pericardium, since an occasional cardiac murmur has a similar scratchy or grating quality. The pericarditis is nearly always acute, although chronic pericardial disease, such as a calcified plaque, may rarely account for a pericardial rub.

murmur has a characteristic musical cadence which has earned the descriptive label of "machinery murmur." The murmur of patent ductus arteriosus peaks in late systole and early diastole, *enveloping* S_2. This contour relates to the

PRECORDIAL MOVEMENTS

Four major pulsations dominate the precordial movement pattern. These are (1) a brief, small outward thrust coinciding with atrial contrac-

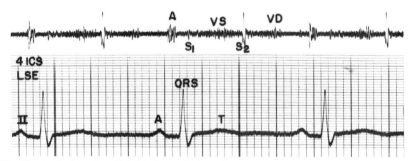

Figure 11–13   The typical pericardial friction rub has three components corresponding to the three major movements of the cardiac cycle: atrial systole *(A)*, ventricular systole *(VS)*, and early diastolic filling *(VD)*, *4ICS/LSE,* fourth intercostal space, left sternal edge. S_1, First heart sound; S_2, second heart sound.

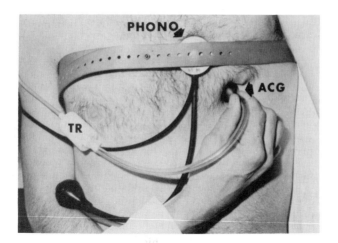

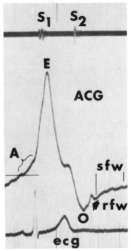

Figure 11–14 The upper panel depicts the recording of an apex cardiogram by means of a funnel which is handheld over the apex and which transmits the increased air pressure caused by displacement to a transducer and graphic recorder. *Phono,* phonocardiographic microphone; *ACG*, apex cardiographic funnel pickup; *TR*, transducer.

The lower panel displays the apex cardiogram *(ACG)* of a healthy young male adult. Note the four major precordial movements: (1) Atrial contraction *(A);* (2) early systolic outward thrust peaking at E; (3) steep downward deflection following *E*, representing systolic retraction. The nadir of the systolic inward movement, labeled O, approximates atrioventricular valve opening. (4) Outward diastolic movement to the presystolic baseline, commencing at O, with the brisk upward deflection of rapid ventricular filling *(rfw)* followed by the more gradual ascending deflection of slow ventricular filling *(sfw).*

tion; (2) a larger, brisk outward movement which starts during isovolumetric contraction and is followed quickly by (3) a steep, inward movement as systolic ejection begins; and (4) an outward movement then develops in early diastole which corresponds to ventricular filling. This last movement ascends at first rapidly, then more slowly, to a diastolic plateau which precedes the next atrial systole.

Improved recording techniques and hemodynamic correlation have led to better understanding of chest wall motion. The most prevalent method

of recording these movements is apex cardiography. According to this technique, a funnel or cup pickup is held to the precordium over the cardiac apex; chest wall displacement causes this device to transmit impulses to a transducer recording system (Fig. 11–14). The pulsations are so inscribed that upward deflections indicate outward movements and downward deflections represent inward movements. The apex cardiograph best records localized impulses, since diffuse pulsations which move the pickup device as a whole do not adequately register. For this reason, recordings usually are made with the patient turned on his left side so as to exaggerate the cardiac apex impulse.

Figure 11–14 depicts a normal apex cardiogram. Note the four major movements just described: a small atrial thrust, labeled A, is followed by a steep upward deflection corresponding to beginning ventricular contraction. Systolic ejection starts at E, whereupon the tracing descends, at first steeply but then more slowly, leveling off in late systole. The curve descends abruptly again in early diastole to a nadir labeled 0. At this point, the mitral valve opens and rapid diastolic filling begins, causing a steeply ascending deflection followed by a more gradual ascent during slow ventricular filling until atrial systole starts another cardiac cycle.

Another recording system less commonly used, but more precise, is kinetocardiography. This technique differs from apex cardiography in that the pickup device is held to the chest wall by an external supporting clamp (Fig. 11–15). This instrument can detect displacement, whether diffuse or localized, small or large. Tracings are obtained from many different precordial sites. The standard kinetocardiogram (KCG) contains leads from all the precordial electrocardiographic positions, each lead being labeled K instead of the electrocardiographic V. Figure 11–15 displays a kinetocardiogram recorded from the apex (K₄). The four major movements are again readily seen, the contour differing somewhat from the apex cardiogram.

Displacement cardiography (DCG) is another recording system that produces curves similar to kinetocardiograms. This method records the changing electromagnetic field of the moving heart by means of an oscillator suspended above the precordium.

Aside from these recording methods, there are other techniques, such as impulse cardiography and precordial accelerocardiography, which yield useful information when properly interpreted.

Numerous physiologic studies of intracardiac pressure and flow as well as bidimensional angiocardiography have clarified the cardiac events which cause precordial pulsations. Normally only the ventricles contact the chest wall, the right ventricle underlying the lower, left parasternal area while the left ventricle relates to the lateral precordium at the cardiac apex. The right ventricle, therefore, is the anterior ventricle which accounts for most of the anterior surface of the heart.

During atrial systole the ventricles move slightly forward, causing a diffuse outward precordial movement, which is not normally palpable but is readily recorded. As systolic contraction begins, a brief outward thrust occurs which can be recorded across the precordium and which is often palpable in the fourth or fifth left intercos-

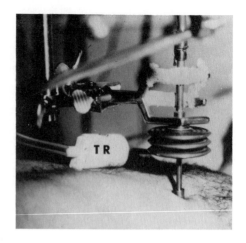

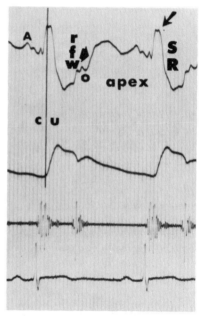

Figure 11–15 The upper panel depicts the recording of a kinetocardiogram with a flexible metal bellows probe held to the chest wall by external support. Air pressure changes within the bellows — as caused by chest wall displacement — are transmitted to a transducer *(TR)* and graphic recorder.

The lower panel displays a normal apex kinetocardiogram recorded with carotid pulse, heart sound, and electrocardiographic tracings. Note the four major movements: Atrial *(A)*, apical impulse *(arrow)*, systolic retraction *(SR)*, and early diastolic filling *(rfw)*. CU, carotid upstroke; O, beginning of ventricular filling.

tal space within 10 cm. of the midsternal line. This movement represents the apical impulse or point of maximal impulse (PMI). It corresponds anatomically to the anteroseptal region of the left ventricle above the actual apex. The apex impulse begins during isovolumetric contraction. When the left ventricular base begins to descend, the heart rotates slightly counterclockwise, and the apex thrusts against the chest wall. The impulse rises briskly to a peak which coincides with the onset of left ventricular ejection. At this instant the outward thrust quickly retracts; during the remainder of systole the apex tracing registers sustained retraction. This inward component of the systolic precordial movement sequence is larger and more prolonged than the apical impulse, yet is less easily appreciated. Systolic retraction is diffuse; it can be detected sometimes by observing the motion of an unheld stethoscope head resting on the left parasternal precordium during held expiration. As ventricular contraction ceases, the atrioventricular valves open, ventricular rapid filling begins, and the retracted precordium returns to its pre-atrial systolic baseline — at first swiftly, then more slowly. This movement can usually be recorded but is not normally seen or felt.

Increased left ventricular volume due to hypertrophy and/or dilatation affects the location, amplitude, duration, and area of the apical impulse. Normally, in the supine posture, this impulse occupies an area less than 3 cm. in diameter and is confined to one interspace. Increased area often indicates underlying cardiac disease but may represent normal heart action in young, slender individuals, particularly when the anteroposterior chest diameter is narrowed by sternal depression, by straightening of the thoracic spine, or by simple disproportion between the lateral and anteroposterior chest dimensions which places the heart closer than usual to the anterior chest wall.

It is difficult to establish normal values for amplitude of chest wall pulsations. Most recording techniques do not accurately quantitate movements, though some investigators have developed measurable values which are useful when properly interpreted. Every physician must determine for himself what constitutes normal amplitude by palpating many normal patients and developing a "feel" for the average apical

impulse. Abnormal amplitude often indicates underlying heart disease but may occur in patients with normal hearts and overactive circulation due to thyrotoxicosis, severe anemia, or other extracardiac causes of high cardiac output. Increased outward excursion of the apical impulse also may occur in young patients with slender chest configuration, especially if anteroposterior diameter is narrow.

Left ventricular hypertrophy and dilatation of any cause can heighten the amplitude and extend the area of apical impulse and may also displace it leftward. Conditions which greatly increase left ventricular diastolic volume such as severe aortic or mitral regurgitation cause the most marked displacement of the apical impulse. Conditions which elevate left ventricular systolic pressure such as aortic stenosis or hypertension do not increase total left ventricular volume as much as the regurgitant disorders just cited. Hence, leftward displacement of the apical impulse is found later in pressure overloading than in volume overloading conditions.

The normal apex impulse is a quick, early systolic thrust. Prolongation of this movement is an important and sensitive indication of abnormality. Impulse duration is easily measured on recordings and readily appreciated on palpation, especially if the examiner auscultates at the same time. Abnormally sustained outward movement correlates better with early left ventricular hypertrophy than does any other impulse characteristic and sometimes better than does the electrocardiogram or x-ray. Prolongation of the apical impulse is a more specific abnormality than increased amplitude or area, since there is little overlap with the normal brief impulse. Moreover, the patient with sustained systolic outward movement often has reduced stroke volume and ejection fraction as compared to the patient with abnormally heightened but unsustained apical impulse who usually has normal stroke volume and ejection fraction. Thus, the prolonged apical impulse is not only a more specific but often a more serious finding. Figure 11–16 displays the sustained outward apex movement of a patient

Figure 11–16 Apex impulse tracing (kinetocardiogram) of a patient with severe aortic regurgitation and congestive heart failure. Note the pronounced, sustained outward systolic movement, preceded by a smaller outward thrust corresponding to atrial systole *(A)*.

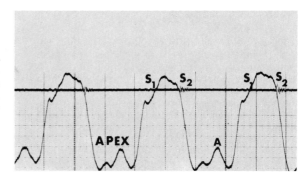

with advanced left ventricular hypertrophy and dilatation (cf. Figure 11–15).

Mitral regurgitation may cause a characteristic precordial movement pattern. Initially this lesion can cause leftward displacement of a localized pulsation which may evolve, with increasing duration and severity of disease, into a diffuse, systolic impulse, extending from apex to sternum owing to medial rotation of the anterior left ventricular wall. A prominent late systolic outward movement especially characterizes mitral regurgitation. This pulsation is maximal over the lower sternum and left parasternal region and peaks just after the second heart sound (Fig. 11–17). It relates to forward thrust of the ventricles

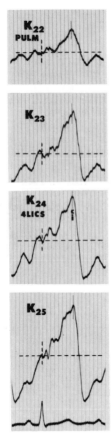

Figure 11–17 Movement tracings (kinetocardiogram) recorded along the left sternal border of a patient with severe mitral regurgitation. A prominent late systolic outward thrust is present from the pulmonary area (K_{22}) to the fifth left interspace (K_{25}). This results from forward displacement of the ventricles owing to late systolic distention of the dilated left atrium. CI, carotid incisura. Vertical dotted line represents peak of R of electrocardiogram. Horizontal dotted line represents baseline of kinetocardiogram. (By permission from Stapleton, J., and Groves, B.: Amer. Heart J., 81:409, 1971.)

caused by filling of the distended left atrium, which probably impinges on the vertebral column, thereby moving the heart forward. When this movement coexists with the apical impulse of left ventricular hypertrophy, the asynchronous timing of the two movements can be readily appreciated by simultaneous palpation with both hands.

Since the right ventricle underlies the midprecordium, conditions enlarging this ventricle affect chest wall pulsation in this area. Volume overloading conditions such as atrial septal defect cause brisk diffuse early systolic outward movement of the lower left parasternal area, with rapid decline in late systole. Pressure overloading disorders such as pulmonary stenosis give rise to more sustained, diffuse systolic outward movement, often extending from sternum to apex. Mitral stenosis with pulmonary hypertension causes a more medial systolic movement; the maximal thrust is often sternal.

Transmural myocardial infarction frequently causes abnormally sustained systolic outward movement, usually of the midprecordium or apex but occasionally of the sternal or even epigastric areas. This impulse, commonly called a systolic "bulge," relates to the failure of infarcted myocardium to contract normally. Sometimes this expansile movement derives from an anatomic ventricular aneurysm; more often the bulge correlates with contraction failure of infarcted tissue in the absence of true aneurysm. This movement pattern may characterize old or recent myocardial infarction and may occur transiently during angina pectoris.

Cardiomyopathies can also lead to precordial movement abnormalities that typify enlargement of either ventricle or both. Combined hypertrophy can be suspected when abnormal apical and lower left parasternal systolic outward movements are separated by a zone of quiescence or even systolic retraction.

Atrial systole, when exaggerated, may sufficiently amplify atrial chest wall pulsations so as to render them palpable. This occurs when resistance to ventricular filling is high, as with the concentric hypertrophy of aortic or pulmonary stenosis or of systemic or pulmonary hyertension. The altered myocardial compliance of cardiomyopathies or myocardial infarction also may lead to palpable presystolic impulses. Atrial sounds usually accompany atrial movements. Since atrial hypertrophy often coexists with ventricular hypertrophy, palpable atrial movement is frequently associated with the lifting thrust of ventricular enlargement. The examiner then feels a double or bifid impulse. Such double pulsations are common in clinical practice.

Important pulsations may also occur during diastolic filling. A loud ventricular gallop sound may be associated with a simultaneous brief precordial thrust which corresponds to an exaggerated diastolic rapid filling wave. Thus, the examiner may see, feel, and hear the vibrations of the ventricular gallop phenomenon. Atrial and ventricular rapid filling movements are exaggerated in the left lateral recumbent posture. Palpation in this posture will sometimes detect pulsations not felt with the patient supine.

Constrictive pericarditis and restrictive cardiomyopathy may cause a vigorous, outward impulse in early diastole which is easily mistaken for the movement of ventricular hypertrophy unless the physician carefully times his palpation.

This movement corresponds to the sudden arrest of rapid early diastolic filling by restricting pericardium or myocardium.

Careful auscultation and palpation of cardiac vibrations will yield many valuable diagnostic and prognostic clues without patient discomfort and at minimal cost. The examination requires only a few moments of intent observation and knowledge of fundamental normal and abnormal findings. As with other sources of evaluative information, the physician must fit auscultatory and palpatory findings into the total clinical context.

REFERENCES

Adolph, R. J., and Fowler, N. O.: The second heart sound: a screening test for heart disease. Mod. Concepts Cardiovasc. Dis., 39:91–95, 1970.

Conn, R. D., and Cole, J. S.: The cardiac apex impulse. Ann. Intern. Med., 75:185, 1971.

Craige, E., and Millward, D. K.: Diastolic and continuous murmurs. Progr. Cardiovasc. Dis., 14:38, 1971.

Davie, J. C., Langley, J. O., Dodson, W. H., and Eddleman, E. E.: Clinical and kinetocardiographic studies of paradoxical precordial motion. Am. Heart J., 63:775, 1962.

Deliyannis, A. A., Gillam, P. M. S., Mounsey, J. P. D., and Steiner, R. E.: The cardiac impulse and the motion of the heart. Br. Heart J., 26:396, 1964.

Eddleman, E. E., and Thomas, H. D.: The recognition and differentiation of right ventricular pressure and flow loads. Am. J. Cardiol., 4:652, 1959.

Fortuin, N. J., and Craige, E.: Echocardiographic studies of genesis of mitral diastolic murmurs. Br. Heart J., 35:75-81, 1973.

Harvey, W. P., and Stapleton, J. F.: Clinical aspects of gallop rhythm with particular reference to diastolic gallops. Circulation, 18:1017, 1958.

Heintzen, P.: The genesis of the normally split first heart sound. Am. Heart J., 62:332, 1961.

Leatham, A.: Systolic murmurs. Circulation, 17:601, 1958.

Leatham, A., and Towers, M.: Splitting of the second heart sound. Br. Heart J., 12:575, 1951.

Levine, S. A., and Harvey, W. P.: Clinical Auscultation of the Heart, 2nd ed. W. B. Saunders Co., Philadelphia 1958.

McCall, B. W., and Price, J. L.: Movement of the mitral valve cusps in relation to first heart sound and opening snap in patients with mitral stenosis. Br. Heart J., 29:417, 1967.

McDonald, I. G.: The shape and movements of the human left ventricle during systole. Am. J. Cardiol., 26:221, 1970.

McKusick, V. A. (Ed.): Symposium on Cardiovascular Sound. Circulation, 16:270, 1957.

Reddy, P. S., Shaver, J. A., and Leonard, J. J.: Cardiac systolic murmurs: Pathophysiology and differential diagnosis. Progr. Cardiovasc. Dis., 14:1, 1971.

Ronan, J. A., Steelman, R. B., DeLeon, A. C., Waters, T. J., Perloff, J. K., and Harvey, W. P.: The clinical diagnosis of acute severe mitral insufficiency. Am. J. Cardiol., 27:284, 1971.

Stapleton, J. F., and Harvey, W. P.: Systolic Sounds. Am. Heart J., 91:383-392, 1976.

Sutton, G. C., and Craige, E.: Quantitation of precordial movement. Circulation, 35:476, 1967.

Sutton, G. C., Taylor, A. P., and Craige, E.: Relationship between quantitated precordial movement and left ventricular function. Circulation, 61:179, 1970.

Tantouzas, P., and Shillingford, J.: Impulse cardiogram in early diagnosis of left ventricular dysfunction in hypertension. Br. Heart J., 31:97, 1969.

Weitzman, D.: The mechanism and significance of the auricular sound. Br. Heart J., 17:70, 1955.

12

The Electrocardiogram

J. A. ABILDSKOV

INTRODUCTION

The electrocardiogram is a record of electrical phenomena which occur in the heart and result in an electrical field distributed throughout the body. The usual electrocardiographic examination for medical diagnostic purposes is carried out with electrodes located at multiple sites on the body surface. When two electrodes are connected by a conductor, current flows in the conductor, and a suitable instrument placed in this current path records evidence of the potential difference between the electrode sites. Such instruments are designated electrocardiographs and the electrode arrangement constitutes an electrocardiographic lead. The electrocardiograph furnishes records in which deflections are calibrated in terms of voltage on the vertical axis and time is represented on the horizontal axis. The conventional electrocardiogram is thus a Cartesian coordinate graph in which voltage variations are plotted against time, as illustrated in Figure 12–1. Many other displays of the same data are possible, one of which has been designated the vectorcardiogram, also illustrated in Figure 12–1. In that display, voltage variations from one set of electrodes are plotted against those from another electrode combination rather than against time as in the electrocardiogram. It should be recognized that different displays of data from particular electrode combinations involve the same information from the body surface, but the accessibility of particular items of this information varies with the display. Thus, the relation of voltage to time is clearly evident in the electrocardiogram but not in the vectorcardiogram. In the vectorcardiogram, however, the relation of voltage variations from one set of electrodes to those in another electrode set is precisely indicated. The precision of this relation in the vectorcardiogram when it is recorded from a cathode ray oscilloscope is difficult to achieve even with simultaneously recorded electrocardiographic leads and is impossible to establish with non-simultaneous leads.

The time-based electrocardiogram is the most widely used and widely useful examination of cardiac electrical activity for medical diagnostic purposes. The vectorcardiogram has more limited diagnostic utility and is less often employed, while the many other possible displays of electrical events in the heart are still less frequently used. The discussion to follow will concern the time-based electrocardiogram unless otherwise specified.

As it is used at present, electrocardiographic examination is a major diagnostic method. Certain abnormalities of waveform are the best available clinical evidence of myocardial infarction. Other abnormalities, although often less specific, are useful evidence of a variety of cardiac and extracardiac states ranging from cardiac enlargement and myocardial ischemia to electrolyte and neurologic disorders. The electrocardiogram is the most certain means of identifying the cardiac rhythm at the time of examination and of detecting changes of rhythm when the record is continuously monitored. The ease and almost risk-free nature of electrocardiographic examination enhance its medical usefulness.

The present role of the electrocardiogram in medical diagnosis has been achieved in two ways. One of these has been the empiric correlation of electrocardiographic findings with particular states, the nature of which has been established by other clinical or by pathologic observations. This is the most certain means of establishing the

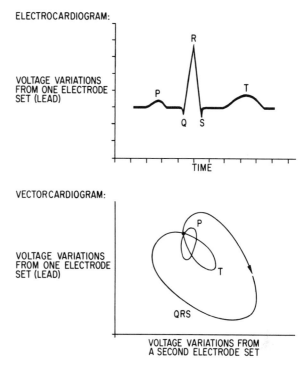

ELECTROCARDIOGRAM:

VOLTAGE VARIATIONS
FROM ONE ELECTRODE
SET (LEAD)

TIME

VECTORCARDIOGRAM:

VOLTAGE VARIATIONS
FROM ONE ELECTRODE
SET (LEAD)

VOLTAGE VARIATIONS FROM
A SECOND ELECTRODE SET

Figure 12–1 The electrocardiogram and vector-cardiogram. Both records reflect potential differences between electrode combinations. In the electrocardiogram these potential differences are recorded as voltage vs. time. The vectorcardiogram presents voltage variations from one electrode set, constituting a lead, vs. voltage variations from another lead.

diagnostic utility of particular electrocardiographic findings, and findings for which the diagnostic significance is suspected on other grounds must still be subjected to the actual test of diagnostic success or failure in patients.

The other means by which the diagnostic role of the electrocardiogram has been established is that of defining the physiologic basis of the record in normal and abnormal states. Increasing knowledge of the pertinent physiologic mechanisms has increased the degree to which electrocardiographic findings can be explained in these terms. Such explanation of electrocardiographic findings on the basis of their physiologic mechanism is unquestionably desirable for teaching purposes and is the appropriate subject for this text on pathologic physiology. This approach is also likely to be the major means by which further improvements in electrocardiographic diagnoses are achieved, and understanding of the physiologic mechanisms will be the best preparation for the utilization of these improvements.

The material to follow has been organized into seven sections. The first of these describes the *total system* involved in electrocardiography. The various components of the electrocardiographic system are not equally well understood nor are they equally important to diagnostic electrocardiography. This section will therefore specify those components of the total system for which the roles are most fully defined and application of

which to diagnostic electrocardiography is most important.

The second section presents a brief description of *electrocardiographic leads,* including those which constitute the present routine electrocardiographic examination. This is an extremely complex subject and detailed consideration is not appropriate in this text. The section will be largely limited to those items which must be appreciated in order for subsequent sections of this text to be understood. These items include description of the electrocardiogram in terms of the electrical axis.

The third section will consider the cardiac basis of the electrocardiogram in general terms applicable to both atrial and ventricular muscle and to the specialized conduction system. The description in this section of the relation between cardiac events and the waveform of the body surface electrocardiogram is, in the author's opinion, the most useful approach to employing the electrocardiogram in medical diagnosis available at present.

In the fourth and fifth sections, the relation of cardiac events during *excitation* to electrocardiographic waveform will be specifically applied to *atria* and *ventricles,* and the process of *atrial recovery* will be considered briefly.

Ventricular recovery and its electrocardiographic expressions in the ST-T deflection will be considered in the sixth section. The discussion will emphasize similarities between the cardiac state during recovery and that during excitation and will attempt to elucidate the physiologic basis of the ST-T deflection and QRS complex in the same terms.

The seventh and last section will concern *pathologic states* and their electrocardiographic manifestations using the same terms employed in previous sections to explain the normal electrocardiogram. The pathologic states considered in this section have been chosen as examples and are only a few of those in which the electrocardiogram has diagnostic utility. Texts of medicine, cardiology, and clinical electrocardiography which describe the diagnostic range of the electrocardiogram are available. The purpose of this text is to describe physiologic mechanisms and this is done through the use of selected examples of pathologic states.

THE ELECTROCARDIOGRAPHIC SYSTEM

The total system involved in electrocardiography is illustrated in diagrammatic form in Figure 12–2. The major component of the system is the heart, which is the site of origin of events reflected in the electrocardiogram. As the generator of the electrocardiogram, the heart can be considered at the level of intra- and extracellular ion relations in the resting and excited states. The generator can also be considered at the level of the cell membrane across which ion concentration gradients exist and ion movements occur. At still another level, the generator can be considered at the cellular level in terms of the transmembrane action potential. Finally, the generator can be considered at the organ level, at which the gross sequence of electrical events during excitation and recovery can be described.

At present, the most useful level at which to consider the physiologic basis of the body surface electrocardiogram is the gross sequence of electrical events together with certain information from the transmembrane action potential. It is at these levels that the cardiac basis of the electrocardiogram will be described in the next section.

Extracardiac components of the electrocardiographic system include a complex, three-dimensional conductive medium. This medium consists of tissues with different conductive properties and the geometrically complex and variable boundaries of the body. These portions of the electrocardiographic system undoubtedly influence the body surface electrocardiogram, and the degree and nature of their influence has been and continues to be the subject of intensive study. At present, however, the role of these factors has not been sufficiently well defined that they can be usefully considered in routine diagnostic electrocardiography. Further definition of the role of non-uniform conductive properties and complex boundary conditions can be expected to refine electrocardiographic diagnosis in the future, however.

The remaining portions of the electrocardiographic system are the electrodes with which potentials on the body surface are sampled, the combinations of electrodes which constitute "leads," and the instruments with which potentials are displayed and/or recorded.

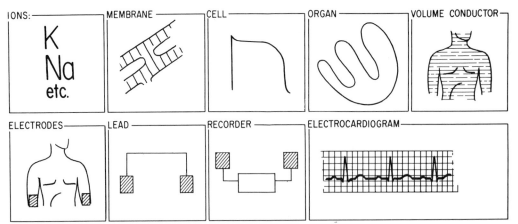

Figure 12–2 The total electrocardiographic system, consisting of ionic gradients across cell membranes, cellular events reflected by the transmembrane action potential, the sequence of electrical events at the organ level, and extracardiac portions of the system, including the conducting medium, recorder, and records.

ELECTROCARDIOGRAPHIC LEADS

The combination of a minimum of two electrodes in contact with the body and connected to provide a path for current flow between them constitutes an electrocardiographic lead. The term "lead" is also generally used to refer to the actual electrocardiogram recorded from an electrode combination. The waveform in the electrocardiogram is a description of potential differences at the electrodes constituting the lead as they vary with time. Electrocardiographic examination usually consists of obtaining electrocardiograms from multiple electrode sites. The examination considered to be routine at present includes nine electrode sites with 12 leads consisting of various combinations of these electrodes. Electrodes on the right and left arms and left leg and at six specified sites on the precordium are employed. Leads are designated as standard, precordial, and unipolar limb leads.

The standard lead designated as I consists of right and left arm electrodes, with the polarity of the recording system so arranged that an upright deflection in the recording occurs when the left arm potential is positive with respect to the right arm. Standard leads II and III consist of electrodes on the right arm and left leg and on the left arm and left leg, respectively, both arranged to yield an upright deflection when the left leg potential is positive with respect to the arm.

Precordial leads consist of six electrodes at specified sites on the anterior and left lateral thorax, and a central terminal to which right and left arm and left leg electrodes are all connected. These leads are designated V_1 through V_6 and each consists of a precordial electrode and the central terminal, with the polarity arranged to result in an upward deflection when the precordial electrode is positive with respect to the central terminal.

The remaining three "unipolar" limb leads consist of electrodes on the arms and the left leg, each of which is combined with a modified central terminal to which the other two limb electrodes are connected. The polarity of these leads is so arranged that an upward deflection results when the single limb electrode is positive with respect to the modified central terminal. Leads recorded with the modified central terminal yield larger deflections than would occur with a terminal to which all three limb electrodes were connected and are designated as augmented leads and by the symbols aV_L, aV_R, and aV_F for the three unipolar limb leads. It should be noted that the term "unipolar" lead is a misnomer, since a complete circuit is required to record an electrocardiogram. The term is applied to leads in which one side of the circuit is connected to all three limb electrodes in the case of precordial leads, or to two of these in the case of augmented limb leads. It is applied because potential variations at the central terminal, although neither zero nor negligible, are small, and potential variations at the precordial or limb location of the other electrode are chiefly responsible for the electrocardiographic waveform. Examples of standard, precordial, and unipolar limb leads are shown in Figure 12–3.

The electrode sites used in the routine 12-lead electrocardiographic examination have been selected according to a combination of technical considerations such as ease and reproducibility of electrode placement; theoretic considerations, including design of the central terminal; empiric evidence of their diagnostic merit; and informed intuition. It is unlikely that they constitute the optimum possible electrocardiographic examination. They do, however, furnish a large amount of diagnostically useful information, and this is the standard by which possible future modifications must be evaluated.

One of the fundamental problems of diagnostic electrocardiography can be appreciated by realizing that a pattern of potential variation due to cardiac electrical events exists at all points on the body surface. This pattern can be defined by recording from extremely large numbers of electrode sites and determining the potential distribution at multiple moments during the cardiac cycle. These patterns constitute virtually all the electrocardiographic information present on the

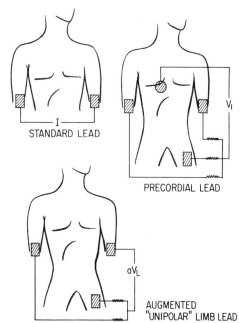

Figure 12–3 Examples of the three varieties of leads employed in the usual 12-lead electrocardiographic examination.

body surface, but sampling from such large numbers of electrodes presents major technical problems. Research is in progress in this area using computer techniques to display the data as isopotential maps at frequent intervals during the cardiac cycle. These studies have definitely demonstrated diagnostically useful information beyond that furnished by the present routine electrocardiographic examination, and this is an extremely promising area for improved electrocardiographic diagnosis in the future. Improved automated methods may make examinations with large numbers of electrodes practical, or it may be possible to identify limited numbers of electrode sites which furnish all or most of the diagnostic information possible from body surface electrocardiograms. This information will include that provided by leads with selective sensitivity to particular cardiac areas and may make regional cardiac examination by electrocardiography possible. Such examination may permit the identification and quantification of localized hypertrophy; measurement of myocardial infarct and other localized lesion size; and the recognition, localization, and estimation of size and severity of local abnormalities of ventricular repolarization.

Electrode arrangements or systems designated as vectorcardiographic or orthogonal lead systems are in actual clinical use, usually for the purpose of recording vectorcardiograms with the cathode ray oscilloscope or collecting electrocardiographic data for programs of computer analysis. These systems consist of multiple electrodes which in various combinations and with the contribution of individual electrodes weighted by resistor networks yield effects of cardiac electrical activity on three mutually perpendicular axes, namely, horizontal (X), vertical (Y), and anteroposterior (Z) axes. These systems have been designed on the basis of the dimensions and geometry of the human thorax and position of the heart within the thorax. Some of the systems also include qualitative consideration of the nonuniform conductive properties of the body. Evidence has been obtained that the three leads from such electrode systems contain most of the information furnished by the routine 12-lead examination. In addition, there is evidence that the range of normal variability of such leads is less than that of the 12-lead examination. Despite such findings, which suggest that a simpler examination may provide an equal, or nearly equal, amount of diagnostic information with less normal variability and may be more sensitive to abnormalities, these leads are not extensively employed. The major deterrents to their widespread use have probably been the extensive experience and familiarity with 12-lead examination, the relative lack of standards for interpretation of orthogonal leads, and particularly the lack of convincing evidence that their actual diagnostic merit is substantially greater than the 12-lead examination now in use.

Electrical Axis

Certain features of the electrocardiogram can be conveniently described as the "electrical axis." This description is usually applied to the QRS complex, but there is no inherent reason why it cannot be used to describe other electrocardiographic deflections. In essence, the description consists of relating features in one electrocardio-

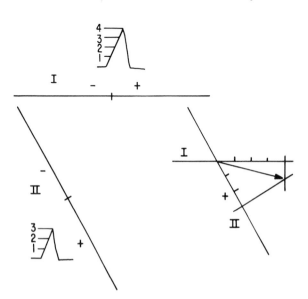

Figure 12–4 The electrical axis. In this description of electrocardiographic features, the geometric relation of the leads must be known or assumed. Here, leads I and II are assumed to form sides of an equilateral triangle. The peak QRS deflection in each is indicated, and these values have been employed to plot a vector. In the portion of the illustration showing this vector, the midpoint of the leads has been superimposed.

graphic lead to those in one or more additional leads. A deflection in one lead can be specified as having a particular amplitude and a positive or negative polarity. As one which can be specified by two terms, this is a scalar quantity, and individual ECG leads are often referred to as "scalar leads." If the relation of one lead to another is known, the magnitude and polarity of electrocardiographic deflections in both may be specified by a single vector quantity which has the additional feature of a specific direction. An example is shown in Figure 12–4. The peak deflection in two leads is illustrated, together with the geometric relation assumed to exist between these levels. The vector shown identifies the deflection in lead I as positive and having an amplitude of four units, while that in lead II is also positive and has a magnitude of three units. The term for this vector as usually employed in diagnostic electrocardiography is "electrical axis."

This description of electrocardiographic deflections may be applied to the instantaneous deflection in two simultaneous leads and then constitutes the "instantaneous axis." A number of successive instantaneous axes during the QRS complex would have their termini located on the QRS loop of the vectorcardiogram. An axis can also be plotted using the area of deflections. The axis plotted from QRS area in two leads is properly referred to as the mean electrical axis of the QRS. In actual routine interpretation of electrocardiograms an approximation of the mean axis is usually employed. The algebraic sum of peak deflections in a lead is determined and used with a similar sum from another lead to determine the vector which identifies these quantities in the leads being considered.

THE CARDIAC BASIS OF THE ELECTROCARDIOGRAM

As stated earlier, the most useful level at which to consider the physiologic basis of the electrocardiogram is the gross sequence of electrical events on the organ level together with certain information provided by the cellular transmembrane action potential. At the gross level, the cardiac state reflected by an electrocardiographic deflection at a given moment is that of a boundary between areas in different electrical states. When the heart is uniformly in the resting state, no such boundaries exist and the isoelectric reference line of the electrocardiogram is established. When excitation is in progress, one or more boundaries exist between excited muscle and that still in the resting state. The varying size and geometry of boundaries during atrial excitation determine the form of the P wave and those during ventricular excitation determine

the QRS complex waveform. After excitation in ventricular muscle there is a period during which the electrical state changes slowly, as reflected by the plateau of the transmembrane action potential. During this period all ventricular muscle is in the same or near-same electrical state, and the isoelectric or nearly isoelectric ST segment of the electrocardiogram reflects this condition. As more rapid changes in electrical state occur during the downstroke of the transmembrane action potential, boundaries of potential difference appear between areas in which the stage of recovery differs from that in an adjacent area.

One of the fundamental and most useful relations in electrocardiography is that between a boundary of potential difference in the heart and the potential at recording electrodes on the body surface. Potential at a recording electrode is influenced by the distance of the recording electrode from the boundary, the magnitude of potential difference across the boundary, and the geometry of the boundary. Figure 12–5 diagrams a closed boundary of potential difference in excitable tissue. If the boundary illustrated is considered to be an excitation front, the magnitude of potential difference across the boundary will be that between excited and resting tissue and will be related to the height of the transmembrane action potential upstroke. Tissue on the excited side of the boundary will have a potential related to the end of the upstroke of the transmembrane action potential, while tissue not yet excited will be at resting membrane potential level. The polarity of potential difference will be negative in

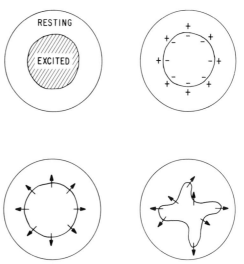

Figure 12–5 Diagrammatic representation of boundaries of potential difference. As described in the text, closed boundaries will not be expressed as electrocardiographic deflections.

excited tissue and positive in resting tissue. When the boundary is closed as illustrated, potential differences in all directions are present and the electrocardiographic effects of one segment of the boundary are canceled by effects of an opposing portion of the boundary. A closed boundary of potential difference will not be expressed by an electrocardiographic deflection, regardless of the dimensions of the boundary and regardless of the magnitude of potential difference across the boundary. The foregoing is true of closed boundaries, regardless of their shape, and is true of three-dimensional boundaries as well as those located in a single plane.

It is extremely important that the implications of this relation for diagnostic electrocardiography be appreciated. It should be evident, for example, that the size of electrocardiographic deflections is unlikely to have a simple and direct relation to heart size. It should also be evident that the size of a myocardial infarct or other destructive lesion will not necessarily be proportional to the magnitude of electrocardiographic alterations produced by the lesion. It should further be evident from the relation described that the electrocardiographic effect of a given unclosed boundary will be related to the degree by which it fails to be a closed boundary. A boundary with uncanceled portions is shown in Figure 12–6. The boundary

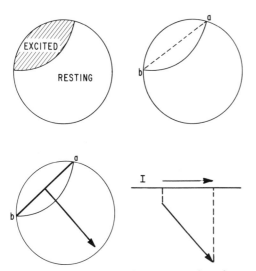

Figure 12–6 Diagrammatic representation of an unclosed boundary of potential difference. The electrocardiographic expression of such a boundary will be related to the quantity necessary to close the boundary. This quantity is the line a–b in the example shown. The electrocardiographic effect of such a boundary is conveniently obtained by constructing a vector perpendicular to the closing line, with a magnitude equal or proportional to the line and projecting the vector on lead axes.

shown can be closed by the line ab and the length of this line will be related to uncanceled portions of the boundary and to the magnitude of electrocardiographic effects of the boundary. In relating boundaries of potential difference to the electrocardiogram it is convenient to employ vectors as shown in the figure. A vector directed toward the positive side of the boundary, perpendicular to the line closing the boundary and having a magnitude equal or proportional to the closing line, indicates the polarity and magnitude of the electrocardiographic deflection in a particular lead by its projection on the lead axis. If the boundary has spatial form it cannot be closed by a line, and the electrocardiographic effect will be related to the area of the surface necessary to close the boundary.

Although the cardiac events responsible for electrocardiographic deflections during excitation and recovery are similar in that both consist of boundaries of potential difference between areas in different electrical states, they differ in significant ways. These differences in the cardiac states of activation and recovery will be introduced here and further explained in a subsequent section. One of the differences between excitation and recovery is the greater time required for the latter process. In individual cells, excitation occurs during the upstroke of the transmembrane action potential and requires only 1 or 2 milliseconds for completion. Recovery as reflected by the transmembrane action potential downstroke begins immediately after excitation but, because of the special features of cardiac recovery reflected by the plateau of the action potential, excited tissue remains at a potential level near that of the peak upstroke during the normal propagation of excitation. These events make it possible to regard excitation as a moving boundary of potential difference. If sequential boundaries are considered, the electrocardiographic effects of later boundaries can be considered without reference to those of earlier boundaries.

Because of the substantially longer time required for recovery, the potential difference boundaries which exist during that process cannot be related to the electrocardiogram in the same manner as excitation. When potential differences arise between two areas which have reached different stages of recovery, the resulting boundary continues to exist until recovery is complete in both areas. During this time, additional boundaries between other areas which reach different stages of recovery are established and also remain present until recovery is complete in the areas involved. The cardiac state responsible for the ST-T deflection of the electrocardiogram cannot therefore be considered as a moving boundary of potential difference, but must be considered as one in which multiple boundaries coexist. Potential differences across these boundaries vary according to the stage of recovery reached on the two sides of each boundary. The relations between each boundary of potential difference during recovery and an electrocardiographic lead are similar to those during excitation. The electrocardiographic expressions of both are related to the magnitude of potential difference across the boundary, polarity of this difference, and the quantity necessary to close the boundary which defines the uncanceled portion of the boundary.

ATRIAL EXCITATION AND THE P WAVE

Normal cardiac excitation begins in the right atrium, specifically in the specialized tissue constituting the sino-atrial node. This structure is located near the junction of atrium and superior vena cava. According to James, the human sino-atrial node is approximately $2 \times 5 \times 15$ mm. in size and is pierced by a central artery which provides the arterial supply of the node and a large area of surrounding atrial myocardium.

On the cellular level, excitation consists of a sudden increase in membrane permeability to sodium, probably due to inactivation of mechanisms which normally extrude sodium from cells during the resting state. The property of automaticity or pacemaker activity normally exhibited by the sino-atrial node consists of slow diastolic depolarization in which the potential difference between interior and exterior of the pacemaking cell declines to a critical point. At the threshold value of membrane potential, the rapid changes of membrane potential characteristic of excitation occur in the pacemaker cell. Propagation of excitation to surrounding cells occurs as a result of local current flow between excited and nonexcited cells. This acts as a depolarizing current in the same manner as current supplied from an external stimulus source.

The property of automaticity is not restricted to the sino-atrial node, and other portions of the specialized conduction system are also capable of pacemaker activity. Normally, however, slow diastolic depolarization occurs at a higher rate in the sino-atrial node than in other sites also capable of pacemaker activity. The normal sequence of atrial excitation during sinus rhythm is determined by the exact pacemaker site within the sino-atrial node and by the atrial properties which determine the velocity of propagation.

In addition to the sino-atrial node, other sites in both right and left atria have been demonstrated to be capable of pacemaker function. It is not yet clear how frequently or under what conditions these areas are likely to initiate the cardiac rhythm, but the wide variability of P waveform may be partially due to such extra sinus node origins of supraventricular rhythm.

In the thin-walled atria, activation sequence in the endocardial epicardial dimension is not a significant factor in determining P waveform, and atrial activation can be considered a surface phenomenon. It has usually been considered an atrial property that activation spreads with uniform velocity from the pacemaker site. There is, however, both anatomic and functional evidence of specialized preferential conduction paths. Anatomic evidence of three paths containing specialized fibers in direct continuity and extending from the sino-atrial to atrioventricular node and to the left atrium has been reported. Physiologic evidence of such paths, including the effect of localized lesions on P waveform, has also been reported. Conflicting physiologic findings have also been reported, however, ranging from evidence of simple radial spread of excitation with uniform velocity to evidence that excitation spreads in broad areas corresponding to gross anatomic landmarks. These areas are reported to form separate inputs to the AV node but without evidence of narrow specialized internodal tracts.

Whether atrial excitation is propagated uniformly or via specialized tracts, the physiologic basis of many features of normal and abnormal P waves can be reasonably well explained. Even uniform propagation of excitation would result in geometrically complex boundaries of potential difference in the anatomically complex atria. The location of the sino-atrial node determines some of the major features of atrial excitation sequence and P waveform. The normal pacemaker has a superior and slightly posterior location within the right atrium; thus, the over-all direction of atrial excitation is obliged to be leftward, downward, and slightly anteriorly. This results in

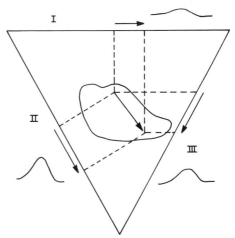

Figure 12–7 Diagrammatic representation of the atria and standard electrocardiographic leads. The average direction of spread of atrial excitation is indicated by the vector and the usual normal relation of P wave amplitude in the standard leads is shown.

upright P waves in leads I, II, and aV$_F$ and usually in all precordial leads. The relation of the overall direction of atrial excitation to the standard leads is illustrated diagrammatically in Figure 12–7. As shown in that figure, the normal P wave amplitude in lead II is likely to be larger than that in lead I, while lead III may show isoelectric P waves or waves of either polarity with only minor differences in the geometric relation of atrial excitation to that lead axis.

The relation of sequential boundaries of potential difference during atrial excitation to electrocardiographic leads I and II is illustrated in Figure 12–8. It should be noted that the time of onset of the P deflection differs in this example. The first boundary is so located that it produces no effect in lead I but results in a deflection in lead II. This illustrates that the duration of the P wave in any one lead is not necessarily indicative of the total time required for atrial excitation. Similar considerations apply to other electrocardiographic deflections and the actual duration of the cardiac process which they reflect.

Atrial repolarization results in an electrocardiographic deflection, usually designated the Ta wave, whose peak amplitude is smaller and duration is longer than the P wave. The Ta wave is responsible for the level of the P-R segment in relation to the isoelectric interval of the electrocardiogram. The wave also extends into and modifies the form of the QRS complex and the level of the ST segment. Although the Ta deflection has not been extensively studied, it is usually of opposite polarity to the P wave it follows and its area is approximately equal to that of the P wave. At present, the major diagnostic significance of the Ta wave concerns its influence on ST segment level. When large upright P waves are present in a given lead, the Ta deflection can be expected to be proportional and may result in ST segment depression in that lead. Such ST segment depression is not the result of ventricular abnormalities but may be erroneously attributed to these if the effects of atrial repolarization on ST segment level are not appreciated. The Ta wave and its effect on ST segment level is illustrated diagrammatically in Figure 12–9. P wave amplitude and area are often increased with increases in heart rate, and the resulting increase in amplitude and area of the Ta deflection may result in ST segment displacement. Diagnostic errors are therefore especially likely in postexercise electrocardiograms in which ST segment displacement is a frequent manifestation of ischemic heart disease. The tachycardia produced by exercise may result in increased amplitude of the P waves, which are then followed by larger Ta waves superimposed on and displacing the ST segment.

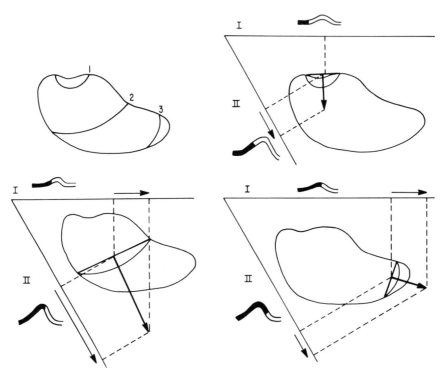

Figure 12–8 Diagrammatic representation of the atria and three sequential excitation boundaries. The electrocardiographic expressions of these boundaries on leads I and II are illustrated.

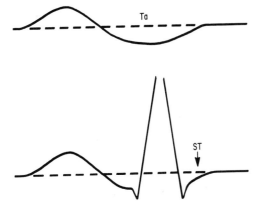

Figure 12–9 Diagrammatic representation of the P and Ta wave and the influence of the latter on ST segment level.

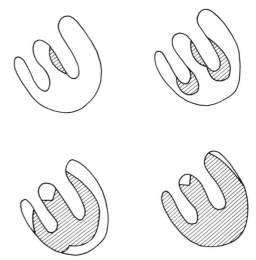

Figure 12–10 Representation of some of the major features of the normal ventricular activation sequence.

VENTRICULAR EXCITATION AND THE QRS COMPLEX

Normal cardiac excitation originating in the sino-atrial node and spreading through the atria is delivered to the atrioventricular junctional tissues and via these to the specialized intraventricular conduction system. Major components of the junctional and intraventricular conduction system are the atrioventricular node, bundle of His, right and left bundle branches, and the subendocardial Purkinje network. Activation of junctional and intraventricular conduction systems is not expressed as a distinct deflection in the body surface electrocardiogram and normally occurs during the P-R segment of that record. Catheter-mounted intracardiac electrodes positioned near portions of the junctional and specialized intraventricular conduction system show evidence of excitation in these structures and are providing valuable data concerning normal cardiac physiology, drug effects, and, in some cases, diagnostically useful information concerning cardiac rhythm.

The QRS complex reflects excitation in ventricular muscle after the process has reached that level via the Purkinje network. The pattern or sequence of ventricular activation has been defined in considerable detail in the hearts of several species, including man. The time of activation of multiple small areas has been determined, and the major features of the activation sequence so demonstrated account for the principal features of the QRS complex.

Figure 12–10 illustrates diagrammatically some of the major features of ventricular activation order. Excitation of ventricular muscle occurs first on the left side of the interventricular septum in approximately its midportion. The process continues to spread in this area and next appears on the endocardial surfaces of both right and left ventricles near their apices. Excitation then spreads from these three zones from endocardium toward epicardium and from apex toward base in the free ventricular walls and from both right and left, although chiefly from the left, in the interventricular septum. Activation of the thick basal portion of the left ventricular wall and activation of the superior portion of the interventricular septum are the latest events during ventricular excitation.

The relation of boundaries representative of the normal ventricular activation sequence to some leads of the routine electrocardiogram is illustrated diagrammatically in Figure 12–11. As described in previous sections, the electrocardiographic effects of each boundary are related to the quantity necessary to close the boundary and the magnitude of potential difference across the boundary. It is probable that the latter quantity is equal, or nearly so, for all normal activation boundaries, so that the relative size of closing boundaries is directly related to electrocardiographic effects. Early activation in the left side of the interventricular septum results in a boundary of potential difference with the negative side on the left. This is reasonably consistently expressed in the normal electrocardiogram by negative deflections in leads having one electrode on the left (I, aV_L, V_5 and V_6) and polarity so arranged that an upward deflection occurs when the left electrode is positive with respect to the other electrode involved in each lead. Since the negative deflection in these leads is the initial portion of

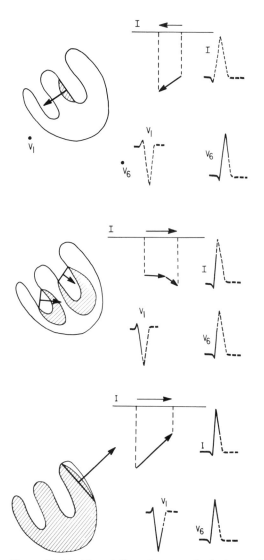

Figure 12–11 The relation of some major features of ventricular activation sequence to electrocardiographic deflections in leads I, V_1, and V_6.

the QRS complex, it constitutes a Q wave. In contrast, precordial lead V_1, in which one electrode is located to the right of the chest midline and has a polarity such that an upward deflection occurs when that electrode is positive with respect to the central terminal which is the other connection of that lead, reflects early septal activation as an R wave. In a similar fashion the other boundaries illustrated in Figure 12–11 account for R waves in leads I and V_6 and S waves in V_1 as well as major features of the QRS complex in other leads not illustrated.

 Cardiac events responsible for late portions of

the QRS complex include activation of the basal portion of the left ventricular wall and of the upper portion of the interventricular septum. The latter event is variable and sometimes occurs in a rightward direction, resulting in a late negative deflection or S wave in lead I and other leads with an electrode on the left side. Absence of S waves in these leads is a normal variant, however.

 One of the informative relations between cardiac events during ventricular excitation and the electrocardiogram is the degree to which the events cancel their electrocardiographic expression. The normal magnitude of this effect provides a useful insight into the diagnostic limits of electrocardiography. A totally closed boundary, as previously described, has no expression in the electrocardiogram and can be said to be 100 per cent canceled. Actual boundaries during ventricular excitation are not usually completely closed but during much of the normal process the quantity necessary to close boundaries is small in comparison to the boundaries themselves. Theoretic, experimental, and clinical estimates of the degree to which events during normal ventricular excitation cancel their electrocardiographic effects suggest that 70 to 90 per cent of the ventricular mass is excited without contributing to the body surface electrocardiogram. This is illustrated in Figure 12–12 with a boundary characteristic of left ventricular activation during the midportion of the QRS complex. Such considerations indicate that large destructive lesions may have only minor electrocardiographic effects when they involve areas whose excitation is not normally expressed in the electrocardiogram. They further suggest that small lesions appropriately located in areas whose normal excitation is expressed in the QRS waveform with only a small degree of cancellation may have marked effects on that form.

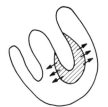 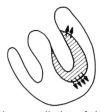

Figure 12–12 Illustration of the cancellation of electrocardiographic effects of portions of a representative boundary during ventricular activation. As shown in the diagram on the left, some portions of the boundary constitute equal and oppositely directed potential differences and cancel each other's electrocardiographic expression. Only those portions of the boundary indicated in the diagram on the right which do not have opposing portions result in electrocardiographic deflections.

VENTRICULAR REPOLARIZATION AND THE ST-T DEFLECTION

The cardiac state responsible for the ST-T deflection is similar to that responsible for the QRS complex in certain respects, but there are also important differences. Both excitation and recovery result in states in which boundaries of potential difference exist between cardiac areas in different physiologic states. In the case of excitation these boundaries are located between areas of excited and resting muscle. During recovery, boundaries are located between areas which have reached different stages of repolarization. If particular excitation and recovery boundaries are considered, their electrocardiographic effects are determined by the same factors. In both cases, the geometry of the boundary and its relation to the electrocardiographic lead under consideration are determinants of the electrocardiographic effect. A closed boundary between areas in different stages of recovery is similar to a closed excitation boundary in having no electrocardiographic expression. The effect of both excitation and recovery boundaries is related to the degree to which they fail to be closed and thereby fail to cancel their electrocardiographic effects.

Both excitation and recovery boundaries produce electrocardiographic effects related to the magnitude of potential difference across the boundary. In the case of excitation boundaries, this value is the potential difference between excited and resting muscle and is related to the height of the transmembrane action potential upstroke. During recovery, the potential difference across a particular boundary is determined by the stage of recovery present on the two sides of the boundary as reflected by the relative height of action potential downstrokes and is always a fraction of the potential difference between excited and resting tissue. Potential differences at any one time during recovery are therefore smaller than the potential difference across activation boundaries. The difference across activation boundaries represents the maximal difference in potential between fully excited and resting muscle, whereas the potential difference at a given moment during recovery is some portion of that between fully excited and resting levels. Another difference in the cardiac states of excitation and recovery is that potential difference across recovery boundaries varies with time in relation to variations in the relative height of transmembrane action potential downstrokes on the two sides of the boundary. In addition, there is a marked difference in the length of time during which activation and recovery boundaries persist. Activation of individual cells is accomplished during 1 or 2 milliseconds as the action potential upstroke occurs, and individual activa-

tion boundaries persist only that length of time. Successive activation boundaries separated by more than that amount of time can be considered individually. The first produces an electrocardiographic effect and then disappears by the time the second boundary comes into existence and produces its electrocardiographic result. This is equivalent to considering activation as a process in which boundaries of potential difference move within cardiac muscle. In contrast, recovery in individual cells requires a considerably longer time, and a given boundary between areas recovering at different rates continues to exist until the repolarization process is complete on both sides of the boundary. During this time, additional boundaries between other cardiac areas with different recovery rates are established. At a given moment during repolarization, the cardiac source of the ST-T deflection may thus be multiple boundaries of potential difference which are widely distributed in ventricular muscle.

To illustrate some of the relations between the cardiac state of recovery and the ST-T deflection it is helpful to consider a simplified activation sequence and organization of recovery properties. As illustrated in Figure 12–13, consider ventricular muscle as two groups of fibers, with all those in each group activated simultaneously and having particular recovery properties. The activation sequence can then be described as excitation of area A, followed by excitation of area B. This sequence of activation is illustrated in the figure by the upstrokes of action potentials designated A and B. In the interval between upstrokes A and B, a boundary of potential difference between car-

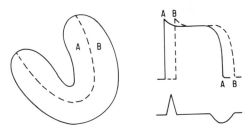

Figure 12–13 Relations between the cardiac state of recovery and the ST-T deflection. In this figure, ventricular muscle is illustrated as two groups of fibers with an excitation sequence such that fiber group A is excited first. The transmembrane action potentials for fiber groups A and B are shown, and the interval between upstrokes A and B represents the QRS interval. The interval in which action potentials A and B are both at the plateau level represents the ST segment portion of the electrocardiogram, and the onset to completion of rapid downstrokes corresponds to the T wave. Action potentials of the same form and duration for the two fiber groups are shown and, as illustrated, result in QRS and T deflections of opposite polarity.

diac areas A and B exists, and the magnitude of potential difference across this boundary is related to the height of the action potential upstroke in area A. After area B has also been excited and during the action potential plateau in both areas there is no potential difference between them. During the downstroke of the action potential, however, potential differences again exist between cardiac areas A and B. At any moment the magnitude of this difference is a fraction of that between fully excited and resting muscle.

Figure 12–13 can also be used to illustrate the relation of QRS and T wave polarity. An electrocardiographic lead has been arranged so that the potential difference between cardiac areas A and B results in an upward deflection when A is in the excited and B in the resting state. As shown in the figure, that polarity of potential difference is represented by the action potential from area A being located above that from area B. If action potentials are of equal duration, as shown in the figure, the action potential from area A will be completed before that from area B. During the downstroke of these action potentials the polarity of potential differences between cardiac areas A and B will be opposite that which existed during excitation. This state will result in a T wave of opposite polarity to the QRS deflection.

One of the major features of the normal electrocardiogram is a T wave with the same polarity as the major QRS deflection in most leads and under most circumstances. This suggests action potentials are of non-uniform duration and is, in fact, compatible with an inverse sequence of activation and of recovery. Actual physiologic data concerning the normal recovery sequence is difficult to obtain and is limited, but that which is available is compatible with such an inverse excitation and recovery sequence in ventricular muscle. Subendocardial muscle is excited early during ventricular excitation but has been demonstrated to have a longer refractory period and longer action potential downstroke than subepicardial muscle. Limited data suggest that an apex to base gradient of recovery properties also exists and apical muscle which is normally excited earlier than that at the ventricular base has the longer recovery time. The physiologic mechanism or mechanisms responsible for these normal variations in recovery properties have not been established. Variations in tension to which fibers are subjected, temperature differences, and other mechanisms have been suspected. Whatever the responsible mechanisms are, the normal recovery properties are such that they tend to equalize actual recovery times following a normal sequence of ventricular excitation. This probably has protective functions in that inequalities of recovery time have been strongly implicated in the mechanism of cardiac arrhythmias.

PATHOLOGIC STATES

The physiologic basis of electrocardiographic abnormalities in certain pathologic states will be considered in this section. The pathologic states to be considered have been selected on the basis of their diagnostic importance and because understanding of the mechanisms by which they modify the electrocardiogram is sufficiently complete to make these mechanisms diagnostically useful.

Atrial Enlargement

The physiologic basis of electrocardiographic features associated with atrial enlargement can

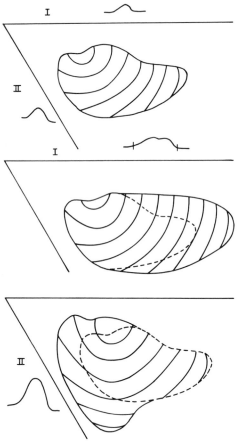

Figure 12–14   Diagrammatic representation of excitation in normal atria and in the states of left and right atrial enlargement. As illustrated, left atrial enlargement results in several successive fronts that are of similar geometry and are so oriented that a flat-topped or notched P wave in lead I results. Right atrial enlargement results in excitation boundaries directed roughly parallel to the axis of standard lead II and results in high P waves in that lead.

be qualitatively appreciated even with simplifying assumptions concerning atrial anatomy and activation order. A diagrammatic representation of the atria and a simple radial excitation spread is illustrated in Figure 12–14, together with P waves in the standard electrocardiographic leads. A representation of left atrial enlargement is also shown and, as illustrated, results in several successive excitation boundaries of nearly equal length and approximately the same relation to standard electrocardiographic leads. Potential differences across these boundaries are oriented roughly parallel to the left-right axis of the body so that the most characteristic evidences of left atrial enlargement are likely to occur in lead I. In that lead the greater time necessary for completion of excitation is evidenced by prolongation of the P wave, and the nearly identical successive boundaries characteristically result in a flat-topped or notched P wave.

Right atrial enlargement is also diagrammatically illustrated in Figure 12–14. As illustrated, activation boundaries extended into the enlarged atrium result in greater potential differences in the vertical axis of the body which are reflected by abnormally high and often peaked P waves in lead II and lead aV_F. Larger than normal P waves often occur in lead I as well but are less characteristic of right atrial enlargement than those in leads II and aV_F.

Myocardial Infarction

Recognition of this frequent and significant lesion is one of the major areas of clinical utility of the electrocardiogram. Positive electrocardiographic findings are the best available evidence of this lesion and the physiologic mechanisms of these are sufficiently well defined to explain the findings in a useful fashion. Alterations of the waveform of the ventricular complex are the major electrocardiographic manifestations of myocardial infarction; and all portions of this complex, including QRS, ST, and T deflections, may be changed.

The QRS alterations are most specific and provide evidence of the location as well as the presence of infarction. Two major mechanisms operate to alter the QRS complex. One of these is the simple loss of excitable tissue which during its activation contributed to QRS complex waveform prior to infarction. The second mechanism is alteration of the excitation sequence in ventricular muscle not actually involved by the infarct.

The loss of ventricular muscle which during its excitation previously contributed to the form of the QRS complex is the mechanism responsible for the most characteristic and diagnostically useful evidence of the presence and location of myocardial infarction. This mechanism is illus-

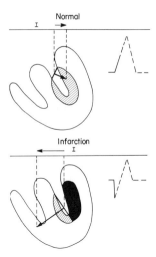

Figure 12–15 The mechanism of alteration of the QRS complex by loss of excitable tissue in myocardial infarction. In the upper diagram a representative excitation boundary in the left ventricle is shown and, as illustrated, is responsible for an upward deflection in lead I. The lower diagram shows part of the same boundary remaining after tissue loss indicated by the solid area. As shown, the remaining portion of the boundary results in a Q wave in lead I.

trated in Figure 12–15. Under the heading of "normal" in that figure, an activation boundary is shown on a diagrammatic ventricular section. As illustrated, the uncanceled portion of the boundary results in a positive deflection in lead I. In the diagram headed "infarction," loss of excitable tissue in the lateral left ventricular wall is illustrated, together with the remaining portion of the excitation boundary previously illustrated. The uncanceled portion of the remaining boundary now results in a negative deflection in lead I. This is the general mechanism by which myocardial infarction results in Q waves in leads in which normal ventricular activation is represented by upward deflections. The leads in which Q deflections occur are dependent on the location of infarction. As illustrated, lateral wall infarction may result in Q waves in lead I which are actually the result of activation in ventricular muscle not involved in the infarct. Similarly, lateral wall lesions may produce Q waves in lead aV_L and precordial leads V_5 and V_6. A similar mechanism accounts for Q waves in leads II, III, and aV_F with inferior wall location of infarction and leads V_1 through V_4 with anterior wall infarcts. Posterior wall infarcts are also reflected by QRS alterations in precordial leads V_1 through V_4, but the changes consist of increased amplitude of R waves, since normal activation in the posterior wall is reflected by downward deflections in these leads and destruction of part of that wall leaves anteriorly directed activation unopposed.

The portion of the QRS complex in which changes due to the loss of excitable tissue occur depends on the location of the infarct with respect to the normal ventricular activation sequence. Abnormally deep or wide Q waves in leads normally containing an R wave reflect an infarct or portion of an infarct involving areas normally activated during early portions of the QRS complex. Subendocardial and intramural lesions or the subendocardial and intramural portions of transmural lesions are thus most likely to produce pathologic Q waves, which are the most definitive electrocardiographic evidence of infarction. Destructive lesions in this location are also more likely to produce marked QRS alterations than similar lesions located in subepicardial areas. Early activation boundaries in subendocardial and intramural regions surround the ventricular cavities and include portions with potential differences oriented in multiple directions. When tissue loss removes a portion of such a boundary having a particular potential difference direction, portions of the boundary with potential differences in other directions determine QRS form which is often markedly different after infarction. Subepicardial lesions alter activation fronts in which potential differences are largely present in a particular direction. Removal of part of such a boundary can be expected to alter late portions of the QRS complex, but the direction of the boundary before and after such a destructive lesion is likely to be similar. The presence of subepicardial destructive lesions is thus likely to alter the detailed form of the QRS complex, but changes will be small compared to those associated with lesions in other locations. Actual myocardial infarcts are often transmural, or nearly so, but transmural involvement is not a necessity for diagnostically significant alterations of the QRS complex.

It should be clearly recognized that pathologic Q waves do not occur with all infarcts or with all infarct locations. These waves have special diagnostic significance because they represent a marked deviation from normal QRS waveform and do not overlap the range of normal variation of that waveform. Less marked QRS waveform changes may be expected with infarcts of particular size and in particular locations. For example, a lateral wall infarct may reduce the amplitude of R waves in leads I, aV_L, V_5, and V_6 but fail to produce Q waves if the size or location of the lesion is appropriate. Such a QRS waveform may not lie outside the range of normal variation and is less useful diagnostically than the more marked change to a pathologic Q wave.

The second factor which may alter QRS waveform with myocardial infarction is altered excitation sequence in ventricular muscle other than that destroyed by infarction. This mechanism is sometimes titled peri-infarction block and that term will be employed in this text, although the term has also been used with a more limited meaning. Whatever terminology is employed, a destructive myocardial lesion may alter activation sequence in remaining excitable muscle by affecting the spread of excitation in that muscle. Specialized conduction fibers may be interrupted by the lesion, so that areas normally excited via these fibers must be activated by other routes. Even without interruption of specialized fibers, the route of normal activation to a particular area through ventricular muscle may include the area of the destructive lesion, and other paths bypassing the lesion are then taken by the excitation process.

Alterations of the QRS complex by the mechanism of peri-infarction block mainly occur in mid and terminal portions of the complex. In actual diagnostic use it is difficult to distinguish such alterations from ones due to tissue loss in areas normally excited during these portions of the QRS complex. Only if the destructive lesion is known to be restricted to areas normally activated during early portions of the QRS complex can alterations of later QRS deflections be attributed to peri-infarction block with certainty. Since this information is not available ante mortem, the QRS alterations due to peri-infarction block are considerably less helpful diagnostically than those due to tissue loss. In addition, QRS alterations by the mechanism of peri-infarction block of necessity involve later portions of the QRS complex, which has a wider range of normal variability than initial deflections, so that changes in the late QRS may not be recognizable unless a preinfarction electrocardiogram is available.

QRS changes due to loss of excitable tissue are likely to be systematic, particularly when areas normally excited during early portions of the ventricular activation process are involved. At this time during the activation process, excitation is spreading in multiple directions and the localized loss of excitable tissue is likely to leave excitation fronts directed away from the area of lesion. In a similar manner, there is at least a tendency for QRS alterations due to peri-infarction block to be systematic. In this case, however, the muscle near the destructive lesion is likely to be the area in which activation sequence is most markedly altered and the spread of excitation into this region is thus directed toward the lesion. These systematic features of QRS alteration by tissue loss and peri-infarction block may be visualized by an electrocardiographic lead containing an R and S wave during normal excitation. Destruction of excitable tissue during early portions of ventricular activation may alter the initial QRS deflection by changing it from an R to a Q deflection, while the mechanism of peri-infarction

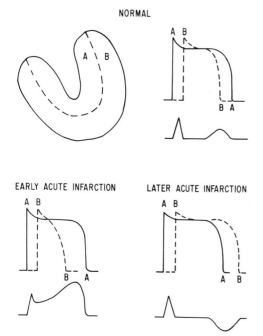

NORMAL

Figure 12–16 The relation of transmembrane action potential alterations by myocardial infarction to ST-T abnormalities. The normal state in which ventricular areas activated early have shorter action potentials and in which QRS and T deflections have the same polarity is illustrated in the upper portion of the figure. Early acute infarction results in reduced action potential duration, and ST displacement due to loss of the action potential plateau and increased T wave amplitude due to shorter action potential duration result. In later stages of infarction, action potential duration in ischemic tissue is prolonged and T wave inversion occurs, as illustrated in the lower right portion of the figure.

block may alter the terminal QRS in an opposite direction, changing the S wave to an R deflection.

ST segments and T waves are also likely to be altered by acute infarction and to change serially over a period of weeks or months. In old infarction, T wave abnormalities often persist, and ST segment displacement may persist in instances of ventricular aneurysm. The physiologic mechanism of both ST segment displacement and T wave abnormalities includes alteration of the duration and form of intracellular action potentials. An additional mechanism, namely reduced resting membrane potential, is also involved in ST segment displacement during acute infarction. Figure 12–16 illustrates the relation of action potential form to the electrocardiogram at various stages of myocardial infarction. For the purposes of this text, the heart may again be considered as consisting of two populations of cells with different intrinsic recovery properties. The normal

state in which the area activated earliest is represented by the action potential of longest duration is illustrated. The area represented by action potential B is excited at a later time but completes the recovery process first. As illustrated, potential differences between these areas during the plateau characteristic of cardiac muscle are small and the ST segment is near isoelectric. The polarity of potential differences between the two areas is the same during excitation and recovery, so that a lead reflecting an upright QRS complex also reflects an upright T wave.

Acute ischemia shortens the duration of the transmembrane action potential and increases the slope of that portion of the record normally represented by a plateau. The mechanism of these action potential changes is not certain, but it is most likely that they are the result of local hyperkalemia due to potassium release from injured cells. As illustrated under the heading of "early acute infarction," such alterations are associated with ST segment displacement and increased amplitude of the T waves but with normal polarity of the latter deflection.

Later in the course of acute infarction, ischemic cells exhibit prolonged recovery time. As illustrated, this produces a state in which the polarities of potential differences during excitation and recovery differ from each other and the polarities of QRS and T deflections therefore differ, the latter being abnormal. ST segment displacement decreases as cells recover and action potentials exhibit a more nearly normal plateau, or as injured cells become inexcitable.

Intraventricular Conduction Disorders

Abnormalities in the delivery of excitation to ventricular muscle by the intraventricular portion of the specialized conduction system result in abnormal atrioventricular relations or abnormalities of the QRS complex waveform. Abnormal atrioventricular relations occur with conduction disorders in the junctional tissues, including atrioventricular node and bundle of His, or bilaterally in more distal portions of the intraventricular conduction system and range from prolonged conduction time, resulting in a prolonged P-R interval in the electrocardiogram, to total failure of conduction, resulting in independent cardiac rhythms in the atria and ventricles, with the electrocardiogram showing unrelated P waves and QRST complexes.

Abnormalities of conduction in the specialized conduction system below the level of bifurcation of the bundle of His into right and left bundle branches result in abnormalities of QRS waveform. Some of these abnormalities have considerable diagnostic utility and they can only be recognized by electrocardiographic examination.

The physiologic basis of the distinctive QRS

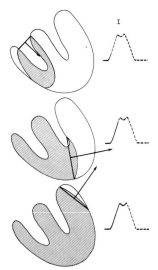

Figure 12–17 Ventricular activation sequence and QRS waveform in lead I in complete left bundle branch block.

waveform associated with complete failure of conduction through the left bundle branch is shown in Figure 12–17. Ventricular excitation reaches ventricular muscle exclusively via the right bundle branch, and its spread through ventricular muscle necessarily occurs in a right-to-left direction. Leads in which one of the electrodes is located on the left side of the body and which result in an upward deflection when that electrode is positive with respect to the other electrode involved in the lead thus show exclusively positive QRS deflections. Leads I, aV_L, V_5, and V_6 of the 12-lead electrocardiogram have this characteristic in left bundle branch block. In addition, most leads will reflect the abnormally long time required for the completion of ventricular activation by prolongation of the QRS complex. Normal ventricular activation delivered via both right and left bundle branches spreads simultaneously in right and left ventricles and determines the normal QRS duration. When bundle branch block is present and activation is delivered only via the functioning branch, an abnormally long time is required for completion of activation in the contralateral ventricle. A QRS duration of 0.12 second or more is usually considered the most useful index of complete bundle branch block.

The physiologic basis of QRS form in right bundle branch block is illustrated in Figure 12–18. As with left bundle branch block, the QRS duration is prolonged. In right bundle branch block, however, excitation occurs normally in the left ventricle. Early left septal activation may therefore give rise to a small Q wave in leads I, aV_L, V_5,

and V_6 as in the normal state. This is followed by normal left ventricular activation proceeding leftward in the free left ventricular wall and rightward in the interventricular septum. As illustrated, this combination of events gives rise to an R wave in lead I and similarly oriented leads. After completion of left ventricular activation including activation of the interventricular septum, activation of the free right ventricular wall takes place and results in an S wave in leads I, aV_L, V_5, and V_6. This deflection together with the prolonged QRS duration constitute characteristic electrocardiographic features of right bundle branch block. In addition, the anterior location of the free right ventricular wall results in additional major electrocardiographic evidence of right bundle branch block. The late activation of this structure is proceeding anteriorly as well as to the right and results in prominent late R waves in one or more of the precordial leads V_1 through V_3. These deflections are preceded by normal R and S waves in these leads and are therefore designated as R prime waves.

The T waves associated with bundle branch block are influenced by the abnormal ventricular activation sequence as well as by the intrinsic recovery characteristics of ventricular muscle. The gross abnormalities of activation sequence and QRS form in these states also result in gross alterations of T waveform, even if ventricular recovery characteristics are normal. In general, the recovery sequence alterations secondary to activation sequence abnormalities in bundle branch block tend to produce QRS and T com-

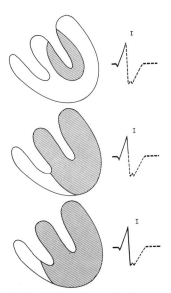

Figure 12–18 Ventricular activation sequence and QRS waveform in lead I in complete right bundle branch block.

plexes of opposite polarity, even if intrinsic recovery properties remain the same. The clinical significance of bundle branch blocks is an appropriate subject for texts of diagnostic electrocardiography and cardiology. As previously mentioned, however, the recognition of these states can only be accomplished by electrocardiographic means.

In addition to block at the level of major right and left bundle branches, other abnormalities of intraventricular conduction occur. Slower than normal conduction can occur under appropriate circumstances at any level in the heart, and in the case of the intraventricular conduction system distal to bifurcation of the bundle of His such conduction can alter QRS form in fashions which resemble bundle branch block but are less marked.

Furthermore, conduction defects may occur at sites more distal than the major bundle branches. Evidence has been reported that the left bundle branch consists of two major subdivisions, one of which is distributed to anterosuperior and the other to posteroinferior left ventricular muscle. Classification of electrocardiograms on the basis of findings to be expected with block of each of these has been proposed under the titles of anterosuperior and posteroinferior left fascicular block. Anatomic evidence for distinct subdivisions of the left bundle is conflicting, but classification of electrocardiograms as evidencing fascicular block is being widely employed. The major criterion proposed for recognition of these entities is the electrical axis of the QRS with anterosuperior fascicular block resulting in left axis deviation and posteroinferior block resulting in right axis deviation. Axis deviation compatible with these entities is often associated with right bundle branch block, and the presence of this conduction defect is compatible with the view that the axis deviation is also the result of a conduction disorder.

13

Arrhythmias — Mechanisms and Pathogenesis

Yoshio Watanabe, and Leonard S. Dreifus

A cardiac arrhythmia is any deviation from the normal rhythm of the heart beat, the requirements for "normal" being as follows: (1) The rhythm originates in the sinus (sino-atrial) node. In other words, the sinus node assumes the role of pacemaker of the heart. (2) The frequency of sino-atrial impulse formation is within an optimal range — usually between 60 and 100 per minute in adults. (3) Within this range, the rate must be reasonably regular. (4) Every sinus impulse is transmitted to the ventricles through the normal atrioventricular (AV) conducting system, and with a normal, constant conduction time. (5) Intraventricular conduction is also normal, with the impulse traveling through the His bundle, bundle branches or fascicles, and the peripheral Purkinje network. From this definition, it becomes readily apparent that cardiac arrhythmias include alterations in the site, frequency, or regularity of impulse formation, as well as abnormalities in the order, velocity, or regularity of conduction of excitation. Thus, disorders such as first-degree AV block and bundle branch block are included among the cardiac arrhythmias, even though the rhythm is of sinus origin and quite regular.

For clinical purposes, classification of cardiac arrhythmias is usually based on the origin of impulses (supraventricular or ventricular) and their mode of appearance (premature systole, tachycardia, flutter, fibrillation, and so on). From the electrophysiologic standpoint, on the other hand, genesis of cardiac arrhythmias is often divided into three categories: (1) disturbances of

impulse formation; (2) disturbances of conduction; and (3) a combination of both (Table 13–1).

ABNORMALITIES OF IMPULSE FORMATION

Alterations in Physiologic Automaticity

Physiologic automaticity is a property of the fibers of the specialized conducting system to generate their own impulses under physiologic conditions. Transmembrane potentials, as recorded with the use of glass microelectrode techniques, usually remain at a constant level (which is negative intracellularly) in the working muscle fibers of the atria and the ventricles when the fibers are not excited. In the fibers of the sinus node, in contrast, the membrane potential becomes gradually less negative during the electrical diastole (phase 4), a phenomenon called diastolic depolarization. When the loss of membrane potential reaches a critical level called the threshold potential, a rapid reversal of the membrane potential (phase 0 depolarization) ensues, generating a new action potential. These relationships are illustrated in Figures 13–1 and 13–2.

It is apparent from Figure 13–2 that the frequency of impulse formation due to automaticity is determined by the time required for the membrane potential to reach the threshold potential. More specifically, the cycle length is increased and the frequency of discharge decreased when either (1) the distance between the maximal dias-

TABLE 13–1 ELECTROPHYSIOLOGIC MECHANISMS OF CARDIAC ARRHYTHMIAS

I. Abnormalities of Impulse Formation:
  A. Alterations of physiologic automaticity in the specialized conducting fibers.
    1. Enhanced automaticity
    2. Depressed automaticity
  B. Development of abnormal automaticity in the atrial and ventricular muscle fibers.
  C. Other mechanisms of impulse formation
    1. Oscillations of membrane potential
    2. Delayed afterdepolarization (transient depolarization)
    3. Early afterdepolarization
    4. Local potential differences causing re-excitation of certain fibers, either due to asynchronous repolarization or partial depolarization

II. Disturbances of Conduction of Excitation:
  A. Decremental conduction
  B. Inhomogeneous conduction
  C. Conduction delay and block
  D. Unidirectional block
  E. Re-entry

III. Combined Disturbances of Impulse Formation and Conduction:
  A. Parasystole
  B. Ectopic rhythms with exit block
  C. Fibrillation

---

vous system. For instance, an increase in the vagal tone would make the maximal diastolic potential more negative and farther away from the threshold potential (hyperpolarization) and also decrease the velocity of diastolic depolarization, thus resulting in prolongation of the sinus cycle length (sinus bradycardia). Contrariwise, an increased sympathetic tone will increase the slope of diastolic depolarization and accelerate the sinus mechanism (sinus tachycardia). The respiratory sinus arrhythmia results from phasic alterations in the automaticity of the sinus node due to variations in the autonomic nervous tone associated with respiratory movement. Maneuvers stimulating the vagus nerve, such as carotid sinus massage, will release acetylcholine in the sinus node region, and a marked suppression of the sinus automaticity may result in sinus arrest. Marked sinus bradycardia, often seen in athletes during rest, is ascribed to the dominance of vagal over sympathetic tone. The frequency of impulse formation in the sinus node is higher in infants and children, often exceeding 100 beats per minute, whereas 60 to 100 beats per minute is considered the normal range for adults. Furthermore, the sinus rate tends to be lower in the aged.

Automatic fibers outside the sinus node are found in the so-called intra-atrial conducting system including the bundles of Bachmann, Wenckebach, and Thorel, the AN and NH regions of the AV node, His bundle, the right and left bundle branches, and the more peripheral Purkinje fibers. Hence, impulse formation can arise from various portions of the AV conducting system. However, the slope of phase 4 depolarization usually is steepest in the fibers of the sinus node, and the loss of membrane potential reaches the threshold level there earlier than in other automatic fibers. This is the reason why the sinus node becomes the pacemaker of the entire heart under normal conditions. Figure 13–2 shows that the transmembrane potential of the His-Purkinje

tolic potential (the deepest membrane potential attained at the end of an action potential) and the threshold potential is greater, or (2) the slope of the diastolic depolarization is less steep. This second factor is especially important, and the enhancement and depression of automaticity usually are associated with an increase and decrease in the slope of phase 4 depolarization, respectively. The automaticity in the sinus node is significantly affected by alterations in the autonomic ner-

Figure 13–1 Transmembrane action potentials from the sinus node (*left*) and a ventricular muscle fiber (*right*). The sinus nodal action potential is characterized by a gradual decrease in the resting membrane potential during phase 4 (DD, diastolic depolarization), a less negative membrane potential, small action potential amplitude (APa), slower rate of depolarization during phase 0 (RD), and the lack of phase 2 (plateau) in its repolarization phase. Other abbreviations are RP, membrane resting potential; APd, action potential duration, the time relationships between the ventricular complexes in the electrocardiogram and ventricular action potential as shown with ECG. (Reproduced from Watanabe, Y.: Electrophysiology of Cardiac Arrhythmias. Clin. Res., *51*: 607, 1974, in Japanese).

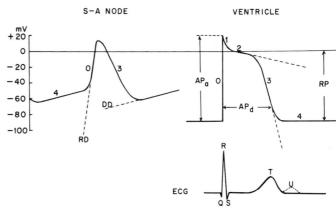

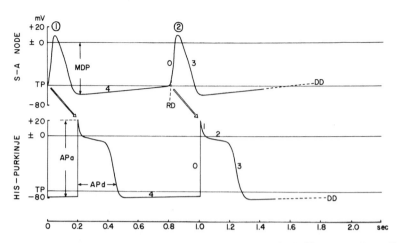

Figure 13–2 Transmembrane potentials of the SA nodal and the His-Purkinje fibers are schematically shown. The slope of diastolic depolarization (Dd) is steeper, and the threshold potential (TP) is attained earlier in the SA nodal fiber than in the His-Purkinje fiber. Thus, the His-Purkinje system is discharged by propagated sinus impulses (*arrows*). Note the differences in the action potential amplitude (APa), the action potential duration (APd), the rate of phase 0 depolarization (RD), and the time course of repolarization (phases 1, 2 and 3) between the two fiber types. MDP, maximal diastolic potential. (Reproduced with permission from Watanabe, Y., and Dreifus, L. S.: Am. Heart J., 76:114, 1968.)

fibers (bottom diagram) has a slower rate of phase 4 depolarization than that of the sinus node (top diagram); hence, the next sinus impulse will be transmitted to these His-Purkinje fibers and will produce phase 0 depolarization before their own threshold potential is reached. The fibers of the specialized conducting system, rather than the sinus node, thus remain as a latent pacemaker. Recently, one reason for the lower automatic activity of these subsidiary pacemakers has been attributed to the mechanism of so-called "overdrive suppression." For instance, when the sinus nodal fibers are excited by extrinsic electrical stimuli at a higher frequency, the rate of diastolic depolarization is temporarily decreased, resulting in a decrease in the frequency of impulse formation. The higher the frequency of stimulation and the longer its duration, the more marked the depression of automaticity. Thus it is possible that other fibers of the specialized conducting system would sustain certain degrees of suppression of their automaticity because of their repetitive depolarization by the sinus impulses.

Several mechanisms related to the genesis of cardiac arrhythmias will be readily apparent from the diagrams in Figure 13–2. First, if the arrival of the sinus impulses to the automatic fibers in other portions of the specialized conducting system is delayed for any reason, the diastolic depolarization in those fibers will proceed uninterrupted, eventually reaching their threshold potential and generating a new impulse. An impulse thus generated usually causes ventricular excitation and prevents a prolonged period of ventricular asystole. This is a physiologic safety mechanism that manifests itself on the electrocardiogram as an escape beat. A series of these escape beats will constitute an escape rhythm. Major causes for such an escape impulse formation include sinus arrhythmia, sinus arrest, and non-conducted atrial premature systoles (which delay the sinus impulse formation), and sinoatrial (SA) block or AV block (which prevents the transmission of normally formed sinus impulses to the downstream fibers). It is also readily understood that escape beats appear after an interval longer than the cycle length of the basic rhythm. The AV junction usually possesses the next highest order of automatic activity, and escape beats most commonly arise in this area. Less frequently, escape beats may originate from the Purkinje fibers below the bifurcation of the His bundle or within the atrial tissue. When the level of the AV conduction block is located below the bifurcation of the His bundle, the escape impulse formation should naturally arise below the site of block and take the form of idioventricular beats. A rare example of sinus escape beats has previously been observed when a slowing of the basic AV junctional rhythm permitted impulse formation in the sinus node, which had a lower intrinsic automaticity than the AV junctional pacemaker.

In the so-called "sick sinus syndrome," the presence of lesions in the AV junctional area is often suggested when failure of escape impulse formation in the AV junction produces long periods of asystole. This indicates depression of subsidiary automatic foci, an insufficient physiologic safety mechanism. There are occasions where automaticity is depressed in the sinus node and in most portions of the AV conducting system. In these instances, the site of impulse formation may gradually shift from the sinus node to the AV junction and further down to the intraventricular conducting system, eventually leading to ventricular standstill. Such "downward displacement of the pacemaker" is often seen immediately prior to death in a patient with acute myocardial infarction or other types of organic heart disease. It constitutes the most serious type of arrhythmia caused by depression of physiologic automaticity (Fig. 13–3).

In contrast to the rhythm disorders resulting from decreased automaticity, enhanced automaticity in the fibers of the specialized conducting system other than the sinus node may cause a higher rate of impulse formation in these fibers compared with the sinus rhythm. Then, such ectopic impulses (impulses originating outside the sinus node) could control the atria, the ventricles, or both. Ectopic tachycardias resulting from this mechanism would not show sudden onset and offset, and probably take the form of non-paroxysmal tachycardia. A diagram illustrating the relationship of enhanced ectopic automaticity and the sinus node and an electrocardiographic example of non-paroxysmal AV junctional tachycardia are shown in Figure 13–4. Depending on the site of enhanced ectopic automaticity, an atrial, AV junctional, or ventricular variety of non-paroxysmal tachycardia will be identified.

It is apparent from the above discussion that changes in the physiologic automaticity in fibers of the AV conducting system can produce various types of cardiac arrhythmia. The automaticity of the His-Purkinje system is enhanced by excessive administration of cardiac glycosides, catecholamines, and hypokalemia, whereas their automaticity can be depressed by hyperkalemia and various antiarrhythmic agents.

Development of Abnormal Automaticity

Under certain abnormal conditions, diastolic (phase 4) depolarization and resultant spontaneous impulse formation may be observed in the working muscle fibers of the atria and the ventricles. These ordinarily possess no such ability. Such phenomena can be termed abnormal automaticity. A report by Müller in 1965 showed that when the atrial or ventricular muscle fibers were perfused by a solution containing neither potassium nor calcium, these fibers developed a prominent diastolic depolarization, leading to regular impulse formation. A decrease in the resting membrane potential, or a partial depolarization of the cell membrane, was observed before the development of such automatic impulse formation. Particularly in the atrial muscle fibers, the reduction of the membrane potential reached about −45 millivolts. Müller explained these findings as a combination of the following two events:

(1) loss of membrane potential due to decreased potassium permeability brought about by the

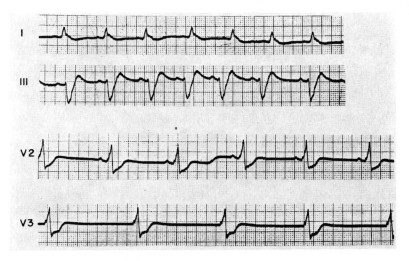

Figure 13–3 An example of so-called "downward displacement of the pacemaker." In leads 1 and 3, sinus rhythm at the rate of 70 per minute with a marked intraventricular conduction disturbance is seen. The sinus rate is decreased to approximately 45 per minute in lead V2, whereas a slow AV junctional or idioventricular rhythm at the rate of 33 per minute without any discernible P waves is noted in V3. Ventricular stand-still soon supervened. (Reproduced from Watanabe, Y.: Genesis of Cardiac Arrhythmias. Intensivmedizin, *10*:109, 1973).

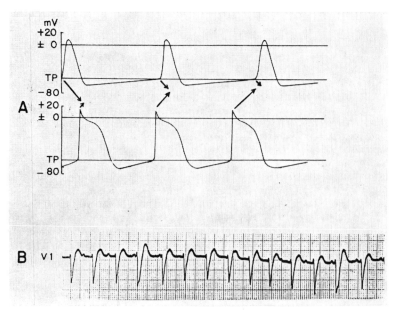

Figure 13–4 A, Diagram similar to Figure 13–2 illustrates an accelerated impulse formation in the His-Purkinje system. The sinus node is discharging at a normal rate. However, the His-Purkinje fiber generates its own impulses before a propagated sinus impulse arrives at this region because of an enhanced automaticity (increased phase 4 depolarization). Interference (or collision) of the two independently formed impulses may occur at different levels within the AV transmission system (*arrows*).

B, A clinical example of AV junctional tachycardia. The RR intervals are shorter than the PP intervals, and AV dissociation is present. (Reproduced with permission from Watanabe, Y.: Genesis of Cardiac Arrhythmias. Intensivmedizin, *10*:109, 1973).

lack of potassium ions; (2) an increased sodium permeability caused by the absence of calcium. Although the above results show clearly that even the working myocardial fibers outside the specialized conducting system can develop typical phase 4 depolarization and automatic impulse formation, perfusion of these tissues with potassium- and calcium-free solution is highly unphysiologic and incompatible with life. Therefore it was considered at that time that the development of such abnormal automaticity could not play a major role in the genesis of clinical cardiac arrhythmias.

It has also been shown that local application of barium chloride ($BaCl_2$) to the working myocardial fibers can produce regular impulse formation due to diastolic depolarization. Partial depolarization of the cell membrane again preceded this type of impulse formation, suggesting the importance of decreased membrane potential levels in the production of abnormal automaticity. However, the presence of barium ions at the high concentrations used in these experiments cannot be expected in the clinical setting.

More recently, partial depolarization of myocardial fibers due to the passage of a depolarizing current to the cell membrane has been shown to produce abnormal automaticity. This indicates that, under certain pathophysiologic conditions in the presence of organic heart diseases, ectopic impulse formation due to such an abnormal automaticity may indeed produce various arrhythmias. For instance, in the presence of myocardial infarction, ischemic ventricular fibers with a reduced membrane potential may develop diastolic depolarization and acquire abnormal automaticity. It is therefore evident that the role of this mechanism in the genesis of clinical arrhythmias requires more extensive studies.

Oscillations of Membrane Potential and Afterdepolarizations

Oscillations of the membrane potential, or socalled "oscillatory afterpotentials," have been observed in several different fiber types under various conditions. In 1959, Matsuda observed in ventricular muscle fibers after the application of aconitine that the completion of repolarization was followed by a decrease in the membrane potential which produced several small oscillations of the membrane potential not reaching the threshold level. The first of these oscillatory afterpotentials was the largest, and a gradual decrease in their amplitude was followed by their disappearance. When the drug effects were exaggerated, the first afterpotential became greater, reached the threshold potential, and generated a new action potential. The second action potential was again followed by a similar afterpotential, finally resulting in a repetitive discharge at frequencies of 150 to 450 per minute. One criticism of this report noted that such repetitive discharges were produced in Purkinje fibers contained in the preparation.

In any event, it is apparent that abnormal impulse formation at high frequencies may arise in some portions of the ventricle in the presence of this alkaloid. As indicated by the term "afterpotential," such alterations of the membrane potential are predicated on the presence of an initial action potential. This is the major difference between this mechanism and physiologic or abnormal automaticity, as the latter does not require an initiating beat.

West observed oscillations of the membrane potential in the sinus node of the rabbit heart. When the sinus node preparation was perfused with a solution containing 30 per cent of the normal sodium concentration and 20 μg. per liter of isoproterenol, an action potential produced by electrical stimulation was followed by a series of spontaneous discharges of progressively decreasing amplitude leading to subthreshold oscillations. After several (up to ten) small oscillations of 2 to 3 millivolts, the amplitudes again gradually increased until, on reaching the threshold potential, a series of spontaneous impulses occurred. The frequency of such subthreshold oscillations of the membrane potential was 200 to 250 per minute, similar to that of the action potentials.

Oscillations of the membrane potential also have been observed in Purkinje fibers under various experimental conditions. For example, Cranefield and others have observed that canine Purkinje fibers superfused with a sodium-free perfusate or with $BaCl_2$ develop phasic variations of the resting membrane potential. A gradual increase in their amplitudes to the threshold potential resulted in the generation of an action potential. This action potential was followed by hyperpolarization of the cell membrane, which, in turn, was followed by depolarization and a spontaneous discharge. Since this type of potential change precedes the development of a spontaneous rhythm, these authors termed it "oscillatory prepotential" in contradistinction to oscillatory afterpotentials. The frequency of these oscillations was about 10 to 20 beats per minute, as was the resultant spontaneous rhythm. In some of the perfused Purkinje fibers, the spontaneous rhythm was terminated by a premature response due to a single electrical stimulus. Sub-

sequent development of subthreshold oscillations was associated with a phenomenon similar to that observed in the sinus node, with initial waning and subsequent waxing until repetitive action potentials were formed. This mechanism of sustained rhythmic activity resulting from a progressive increase in amplitude of the oscillatory potentials may superficially appear similar to the diastolic depolarization in physiologic automaticity. In this experimentally induced mechanism, however, it is said that a rather rapid transition from hyperpolarization to partial depolarization brings about a loss of membrane potential to the threshold level; hence, it requires a preceding action potential.

Although these oscillations of the membrane potential may appear quite important as a mechanism of impulse formation in the myocardium, most of the experimental conditions producing the phenomena are unphysiologic and are not expected to occur clinically. One exception, reported by Vassalle, showed the development of oscillatory prepotentials with subsequent periods of spontaneous impulse formation in Purkinje fibers when the extracellular potassium concentration was lowered from 5.4 to 2.7 millimoles. Since this degree of hypokalemia can be observed in patients, ectopic impulse formation in the ventricles due to this mechanism may not definitely be ruled out.

Two types of afterdepolarization have been noted. (1) When Purkinje fibers are electrically stimulated in the presence of rather high concentrations of cardiac glycosides, the termination of an action potential is often followed by a transient loss of membrane potential. This is termed either "delayed afterdepolarization" or "transient depolarization." When the frequency of electrical stimulation is relatively low, the degree of depolarization is small and the membrane potential returns to a more negative level. In contrast, stimulation at higher frequencies causes an increase in depolarization sufficient to attain the threshold potential and to generate a new action potential. Usually, only one action potential is formed, and it is followed by a subthreshold transient depolarization. The amplitude of such afterdepolarizations increases when the extracellular calcium concentration is high or the potassium concentration is low. These observations led Ferrier and Moe to suggest that coupled ventricular premature systoles in the form of ventricular bigeminy as an expression of so-called "digitalis arrhythmia" probably result from this mechanism. Clinical observations of aggravation of digitalis arrhythmias by hypercalcemia or hypokalemia may support this contention. It has also been shown that the ionic mechanism producing this delayed afterdepolarization is what is now known as slow inward currents carried mainly by calcium ions. Indeed, this transient depolarization is abolished by manganese ions, which inhibit such slow inward currents.

(2) The second variety, called "early afterdepolarization" represents the following events: When ventricular muscle fibers are perfused with aconitine, the repolarization process is often brought to a halt at a membrane potential level of about -70 millivolts, at which point partial depolarization resumes. This depolarization may reach the threshold potential and produce several short action potentials in the form of spike discharges. These are finally followed by the completion of phase 3 repolarization and a return to the resting membrane potential level. Rather like the oscillatory afterpotentials described earlier, generation of these abnormal impulses under the influence of aconitine is observed only when the myocardial preparations are electrically stimulated. In other words, aconitine arrhythmias appear to require a preceding beat. Other reports have shown that aconitine produces similar phenomena in Purkinje fibers, whereas veratrine causes an extreme prolongation of phase 2 of repolarization (plateau) from which repetitive spike discharges may arise. These observations suggest the possible role of early afterdepolarizations in the genesis of arrhythmias, although questions can be raised about their clinical significance.

On the other hand, the following mechanism might possibly occur in the clinical setting. In a patient given a moderate amount of ouabain, when the membrane potential in the Purkinje fibers is reduced to -40 to -60 millivolts by the passage of a depolarizing current, repetitive impulse formation could develop at a frequency higher than that of the original spontaneous rhythm due to physiologic automaticity. The changes in the transmembrane potential during such sustained rhythmic activity appear similar to enhanced diastolic depolarization. However, this particular type of repetitive discharge occurred at a membrane potential level of -40 to -60 millivolts, whereas diastolic depolarization in the presence of physiologic automaticity starts at a level of -85 to -90 millivolts. Furthermore, the maximal rate of depolarization during phase 0, or the upstroke velocity of the action potential, is quite rapid in the latter, whereas it is extremely slow in the former. These two modes of impulse formation thus appear to show qualitative rather than quantitative differences. Transition between the two mechanisms is easily produced by applying either depolarizing or hyperpolarizing currents to the cell membrane. The possibility that this form of abnormal impulse formation may occur in injured Purkinje fibers, especially in the presence of excessive cardiac glycosides, cannot be ruled out.

It must be re-emphasized here that these abnormal mechanisms of impulse formation—abnormal automaticity, oscillations of the membrane potential, and afterdepolarizations — occur in Purkinje fibers as well as ventricular muscle when their transmembrane potential is reduced to a level similar to that found in a normally automatic sinus node. Furthermore, it is now widely accepted that both the sinus nodal action potentials and these abnormal modes of impulse formation depend on ionic currents through the so-called "slow channels" (slow inward currents). Certain investigators have therefore suggested two classifications of mechanisms of impulse formation: (1) those occurring at a membrane potential level of -90 to -70 millivolts and (2) those occurring at -60 to -40 millivolts.

Still another method of classification is to group the physiologic automaticity of the specialized conducting system with abnormal automaticity of the working myocardial fibers and then to contrast them with oscillatory potentials and afterdepolarizations. The former varieties represent true spontaneous impulse formation; the latter are triggered by a preceding action potential.

The classification we have adopted in this chapter is based more on clinical considerations, as automatic activity under physiologic conditions is seen only in the sinus node and other fibers of the specialized conducting system. Other mechanisms of impulse formation appear to occur only under abnormal conditions.

Re-excitation of certain fibers due to local potential differences, as listed in Table 13–1, probably plays a role in the genesis of rhythm disorders, particularly in the initiation as well as maintenance of fibrillation. A new term, "reflection," has been given to this phenomenon by certain investigators, although its differentiation from the so-called "microreentries" and other mechanisms of abnormal impulse formation in partially depolarized fibers may be rather difficult.

Possible clinical implications of these abnormal mechanisms of impulse formation can be suggested. If the rate of impulse formation caused by abnormal automaticity in the working myocardial fibers exceeds that of the sinus rhythm, non-paroxysmal ectopic tachycardias may be produced, whereas oscillatory afterpotentials and the various afterdepolarizations may result in coupled premature systoles. It has further been suggested that paroxysmal ectopic tachycardias, usually ascribed to re-entry movements, could be caused by these oscillatory events. The role of these mechanisms in the genesis of digitalis arrhythmias and of either unifocal or multifocal impulse formation in the initiation of cardiac fibrillation perhaps cannot be ruled out.

TABLE 13–2 FACTORS CONTROLLING
IMPULSE TRANSMISSION

I. Primary determinants of conductivity:
A. Physiologic factors:
  1. Effectiveness of stimuli produced by depolarization of upstream fibers
  2. Excitability of responding downstream fibers
  3. Temporal fluctuation of 1 or 2
B. Anatomic factors:
  1. Fiber diameter
  2. Geometric arrangement of fibers

II. Abnormal conduction phenomena resulting from alterations in the primary determinants of conductivity:
A. Decremental conduction
B. Inhomogeneous conduction
C. Conduction delay and block
D. Unidirectional block
E. Re-entry

III. Abnormal conduction phenomena secondarily affecting conductivity:
A. Conduction delay and block:
  1. Effects of conduction delay on the action potential duration (prolongation)
  2. Effects of conduction block on the action potential duration of fibers proximal to the site of propagation failure (shortening)
  3. Effects of conduction block on the action potential duration of fibers distal to the site of propagation failure (prolongation)
  4. Effects of conduction delay or block on excitability of the downstream fibers
  5. Conduction delay or block causing impulse formation in the downstream fibers
B. Re-entry:
  1. Collision of re-entrant impulse with the more slowly advancing, antegrade wave of excitation resulting in cancellation of both wave fronts
  2. Further disorganization of the excitation front (increased inhomogeneity) in subsequent impulse transmission
  3. Reorganization of the excitation front (decreased inhomogeneity) in subsequent impulse transmission

DISTURBANCES OF CONDUCTION OF EXCITATION

Factors Controlling Impulse Transmission

The various factors that control impulse transmission in the myocardium are listed in Table 13–2. Since an extensive review of these problems has previously been published elsewhere, only some of the more important factors will be discussed in this chapter.

The primary determinants of conductivity include: (1) effectiveness of impulses produced by depolarization of the upstream fibers; and (2) the excitability of downstream fibers responding to such impulses. With respect to the first factor, it can be generalized that the greater the amplitude and the upstroke velocity of phase 0 of an action potential, the higher its effectiveness as an impulse and the greater its conduction velocity. Smaller action potential amplitudes and decreased rates of phase 0 depolarization will be associated with depressed conductivity. Under physiologic conditions, Purkinje fibers have the most rapid rate of phase 0 depolarization (several hundred volts per second) of all fiber types and also show the highest conduction velocity (3.0 to 3.5 m. per second).

In fibers of the atria, ventricles, and the Purkinje system, whose phase 0 depolarization depends on a rapid inflow of sodium ions across the cell membrane (fast sodium channel), a greater (more negative) membrane potential immediately prior to excitation will be associated with both a greater amplitude and a greater rate of rise of the action potential. This is explained by more complete activation of the so-called "sodium carriers" as a function of the transmembrane potential, and this relationship is expressed by membane responsiveness curves (Figure 13–5).

The membrane responsiveness curve in a given myocardial fiber should remain constant as long as its physiologic environment is stable, but can vary with changing conditions. Quinidine, for instance, is known to shift the membrane responsiveness curve downward and to the right. The

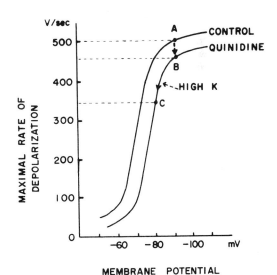

Figure 13–5 Membrane responsiveness curves correlating the level of membrane potential and the maximal rate of depolarization. The shift of the curve downward and to the right by quinidine (A → B) and the effect of a decrease in the membrane potential due to high potassium (B → C) are illustrated.

upstroke velocity of an action potential would then be decreased, even though the level of membrane potential remains unchanged (Fig. 13–5). A shift of this curve upward and to the left will increase the rate of phase 0 depolarization and improve conductivity without any changes in the transmembrane potential. On the other hand, various factors that reduce the membrane potential will consequently decrease the rate of depolarization and conduction velocity. Increased extracellular potassium concentrations, myocardial ischemia (hypoxia), and excessive administration of certain antiarrhythmic agents will produce partial depolarization of the cell membrane and depress conduction. Contrariwise, an increase in the resting membrane potential (hyperpolarization) tends to improve conductivity. Certain degrees of hypokalemia (for example, 1.5 millimolar) may exert such effects on atrial and ventricular muscle fibers.

In fibers of the AV conducting system showing automatic activity, the transmembrane potential will be progressively decreased during electrical diastole because of phase 4 depolarization. Then, action potentials produced by impulses arriving at these fibers later in diastole will show a slower rate of rise and a smaller amplitude of phase 0, and the conduction velocity is decreased. Depression of conductivity due to this mechanism becomes more marked in the presence of a longer electrical diastole or a greater rate of phase 4 depolarization. Conduction disturbances resulting from this mechanism are often called phase 4 block (Fig. 13–6, bottom).

The interval between two impulses may affect conductivity through the change in the membrane potential in a way different from that seen in phase 4 block. This is a sudden shortening of the cycle length of stimulation. In this instance, the wave of excitation arrives at the downstream fibers before the repolarization from a previous excitation is complete. Then, even when these fibers respond with a second action potential, its phase 0 will start from a reduced membrane potential level and show a much slower upstroke velocity. Since this type of conduction disturbance results from encroachment of the phase 3 repolarization by an excitation front, it is often called phase 3 block in contrast to the phase 4 block described above (Figure 13–6, top).

In addition to the levels of membrane potential at the onset of excitation (so-called "take-off potential"), the level of threshold potential also may affect the rate of rise of an action potential. It has been shown that a more marked diastolic depolarization is associated with a less negative threshold potential, and hence with a slower rate of phase 0 depolarization. Conductivity will thus be depressed in those fibers showing distinct phase 4 depolarization. Exit block from an ectopic pacemaker and the so-called "protection block" around a parasystolic focus could possibly be explained by this mechanism, since impulse formation in these ectopic sites results from automatic activity in a group of fibers. The role of slow channels may deserve special attention with reference to these phenomena.

Ever since the ionic theory was developed in

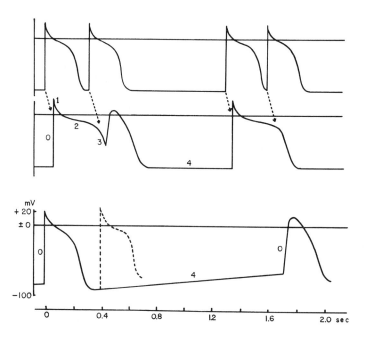

Figure 13–6 Schematic diagrams illustrating the mechanisms of phase 3 block (*top*) and phase 4 block (*bottom*). In phase 3 block, a premature impulse may arrive at certain downstream fibers during their phase 3 of repolarization because of their longer action potential duration compared with the upstream fibers. This will result in a premature action potential with a reduced amplitude and slower upstroke velocity and conduction may become decremental (*left*). Still earlier arrival of an impulse may find the downstream fibers refractory, resulting in a complete block (*right*). In phase 4 block (*bottom diagram*) impulses arriving later in electrical diastole (phase 4) cause an action potential with decreased amplitude and rate of rise of phase 0 because of the loss of membrane potential due to phase 4 depolarization. Note that depolarization of this fiber immediately after a preceding action potential produces an action potential with a better conductivity (*broken lines*).

TABLE 13–3 COMPARISON OF FAST CHANNEL AND SLOW CHANNELS

	Fast Channel	*Slow Channel*
Activation and inactivation	Proceed rapidly; inactivated upon loss of membrane potential	Proceed slowly; activated at lower (less negative) membrane potential levels
Maximal rate of phase 0 depolarization	Usually several hundred volts per second	Usually in the order of 1–10 V/sec
Propagation of excitation	Rapid, with high safety factor	Slow, with low safety factor
Ions carrying the current	Sodium	Mainly calcium; partly sodium (and certain other ions?)
Factors which inhibit the channel(s)	Tetrodotoxin	Manganese, lanthanum, verapamil, D 600, etc.; insensitive to tetrodotoxin

neurophysiology by Hodgkin and others, it has been postulated that ionic currents similar to those observed in nerve fibers are responsible for the generation of myocardial action potential. However, various experimental data gradually accumulated in the last decade have forced a major revision of that concept. It has been demonstrated that the slow channels, in addition to the fast sodium channel, play a major role in the production of cardiac action potentials. This important development in cardiac electrophysiology has been extensively reviewed by several investigators, and a brief discussion here appears in order.

It is now widely accepted that the initial rapid depolarization (phase 0) of the myocardial action potential is produced by a rapid inflow of sodium ions across the cell membrane, exactly as in nerve fibers (fast channel or fast sodium current). The prolonged action potential characteristically seen in myocardial fibers, on the other hand, appears to depend on a much slower influx of ions, and these slow inward currents are thought to be carried mainly by calcium and in part by sodium. The electrophysiologic characteristics of these two channels are compared in Table 13–3, which indicates their qualitative rather than quantitative differences. When the membrane potential is significantly decreased, e.g., by partial depolarization, the fast sodium channel is partially inactivated and the phase 0 depolarization becomes mostly dependent on slow inward currents. Slower rate of rise of the action potential and the depression of conduction in these circumstances (so-called "slow responses") are thus explained by a change in the ionic mechanism. This further illustrates the importance of the level of membrane potential in determining conduction of excitation.

It has been pointed out in the previous section that the development of abnormal automaticity or afterdepolarizations in the atrial, ventricular, or Purkinje fibers is observed when these fibers are partially depolarized to a membrane potential level similar to that of sinus nodal fibers. Also with reference to conduction of excitation, the fibers of the sinus node as well as the AV node appear to act like partially depolarized fibers of the working myocardium and the Purkinje system. In other words, the slowly rising action potentials seen in the sinus node and the N region of the AV node, under physiological conditions, are now considered to depend on slow inward currents, whereas the role of the fast sodium channel in these fibers is minimal, if any. The ions carrying these slow inward currents in sinus and AV nodal fibers again appear to be mainly calcium, but several experimental studies have shown that the presence of slow sodium current cannot be ruled out.

The various mechanisms that cause alterations of conductivity, as described above, depend mostly on the changes in the membrane potential. They are said to be *voltage-dependent*, except in the case of a shift of membrane responsiveness curve. In contrast, the possibility of *time-dependent* changes in conductivity has recently been suggested. For instance, in ventricular muscle fibers under the influence of certain drugs, including quinidine and chlorpromazine, partial refractoriness may continue beyond the completion of repolarization. Then, action potentials generated immediately after the end of phase 3 repolarization will show a slower upstroke velocity than those occurring later in electrical diastole, even though the same level of resting membrane potential has been attained. This phenomenon is different from a rightward shift of the membrane responsiveness curve. The rate of phase 0 depolarization varies as a function of time during phase 4 in the former, whereas the rate of rise of action potentials may remain steady at a new lower level throughout electrical diastole in the latter. These time-dependent disturbances in conduction are explained by delayed recovery of the fast sodium channel from its inactivation, compared with the restoration of the resting membrane potential. Nevertheless, it will be understood that the effectiveness of an impulse produced by depolarization of upstream fibers is affected by various factors in a complex manner.

The excitability of downstream fibers is the second primary determinant of conductivity. The diastolic threshold of excitation is determined by the minimal strength of stimulus (or the minimal amount of current) required to produce full depolarization of fibers during their phase 4. When this current requirement is greater, the excitability of the fibers is lower, and vice versa. One mechanism for an increased threshold of excitation is increased distance between the membrane resting potential and the threshold potential. If for some reason, the diastolic threshold of excitation in a given myocardial tissue is elevated, the strength of stimulus originally sufficient to excite this tissue may now become ineffective (subthreshold stimulation), causing a conduction block.

Generally speaking, the excitability of the myocardium tends to remain constant during electrical diastole, but undergoes a significant change with the onset of electrical systole (action potential). These fibers usually do not respond to a second stimulus from the beginning of phase 0 through phase 2 (plateau), until a certain point in phase 3 of repolarization is reached, regardless of the strength of the currents applied. This is called the effective refractory period, and it is followed by a relative refractory period. During the latter phase, cellular excitability is less than that during electrical diastole, and fibers respond only to stronger stimuli producing an action potential with a slower upstroke velocity and a reduced amplitude.

With reference to the excitability of downstream fibers, brief comments are in order on the phenomena of supernormal excitability and the Wedensky effect. Principally in fibers of the specialized conducting system, excitability toward the end of the relative refractory period may transiently become higher than during electrical diastole. This is termed the supernormal period of excitability and its mechanism is as follows. When repolarization has proceeded just beyond the level of the threshold potential but has not reached the resting potential, a small amount of current, or a weaker stimulus, could possibly decrease the membrane potential to the threshold level and excite these fibers. When the strength of impulses transmitted to a group of myocardial fibers is only slightly below the diastolic threshold, those fibers may respond only during the supernormal period of excitability and produce an action potential. Such phenomena are often observed clinically when the batteries of an electronic pacemaker are depleted.

The Wedensky effect, on the other hand, represents a transient increase in tissue excitability after a supramaximal impulse. One major difference between the Wedensky effect and supernormal excitability is that the latter has a very brief duration (i.e., less than 50 milliseconds), whereas the Wedensky effect lasts much longer and may affect excitability in several subsequent depolarizations. These two phenomena have often been invoked to explain the genesis of coupled premature systoles. For instance, an abnormal source of current (such as an injury current between ischemic and nonischemic myocardial fibers) may produce a propagated response only during the supernormal period of excitability and, hence, a premature beat with a fixed time interval from the preceding excitation. If impulses arriving from upstream fibers are barely sufficient to excite an area of conduction disturbance with a lower excitability, propagation of an excitation front may occur only during this period of supernormality, not during electrical diastole. This mechanism may possibly explain one type of supernormal AV conduction. On the other hand, the Wedensky effect may explain the observation that, in the presence of high grades of AV block, one successfully conducted beat sometimes is followed by conduction of several subsequent supraventricular impulses. Here, propagation of one excitation front may have increased the excitability of the depressed fibers at the site of the conduction failure.

These two physiologic factors which primarily determine the conductivity in the myocardium may not always remain stable in a given cardiac tissue and could vary depending on conditions. Fluctuations in cardiac hemodynamics, oxygen supply to the myocardium, autonomic nerve tone, or heart rate may cause slight variations in conductivity. Although these subtle changes probably do not have a significant effect on cardiac fibers under the normal physiologic conditions, they may well determine the success or failure of propagation in fibers with reduced conductivity. Certain cases of so-called "Mobitz Type II AV block" could possibly be explained by this mechanism.

In addition to these physiologic determinants of conductivity, several anatomic factors also must be considered. It is known that conductivity usually is better in fibers with larger diameters, and the high conduction velocity seen in Purkinje fibers can be ascribed in part to their larger diameter. Geometric arrangement of the fibers also appears to play a role in impulse transmission. When a larger fiber strand divides into several smaller ones, conductivity may be decreased because of the division of the wavefront of excitation and a decreased current density. On the other hand, summation of several different wavefronts, with appropriate timing, may improve the conductivity in more distal tissue. Indeed, increased amplitude and upstroke velocity of an action potential due to summation have often been demonstrated in the AV node as well as Purkinje fibers. In a preparation where two larger pieces of atrial tissue were connected by a small strand of fibers, conduction block tended to develop when the excitation front attempted to invade the larger tissue through the isthmus, whereas propagation from the larger tissue to the smaller strand was well maintained. These observations are in keeping with the concepts discussed above and have been used to explain the intermittency of conduction through accessory pathways that occurs in the WPW syndrome. It must be pointed out that summation of excitation fronts is more easily demonstrated in the presence of slow responses.

Abnormal Conduction Phenomena Caused by Alterations in the Primary Determinants of Conductivity

Changes in the various determinants of conductivity, whether alone or in combination, may produce several abnormal conduction phenomena. These are listed in Table 13–2. (1) Decremental conduction can be defined as a gradual decrease in the effectiveness of stimulus and in the magnitude of response along a pathway of conduction that is anatomically uniform but functionally depressed. Such decremental conduction will develop more easily in the presence of reduced membrane potentials. In a group of partially depolarized fibers, for example, the rate of rise of an action potential will be lower than in more normal cardiac tissue, and its effectiveness as a stimulus will be decreased. When the downstream fibers also have a lower transmembrane potential, their response may be progressively reduced, even to the point of propagation failure. Small action potentials due to slow inward currents may again be important in the development of this phenomenon. In fibers having lower membrane potentials and slower upstroke velocity of the action potential under physiologic conditions (e.g., the N region of the AV node), decremental conduction due to various pathophysiologic factors can be expected more frequently. (2) The next variety of abnormal conduction phenomena, which we have termed inhomogeneous conduction, is explained as follows. When depression of conductivity results in a nonuniform decrement at a given portion of the conducting system, the wavefront of excitation becomes fractionated. This fractionation will be associated with a decreased effectiveness of the stimulus compared with the smoother and more organized wavefront that produces synchronous

depolarization in adjacent fibers. It can then be suggested that decremental conduction is unlikely to develop in a tissue where fibers run parallel to one another, forming a compact strand. In sharp contrast, fractionation of the excitation front could be observed more frequently in the AV node, where frequent ramifications and anastomoses of small fibers form a complex network.

This concept of inhomogeneous conduction presupposes that a smooth excitation front with synchronous depolarization of a group of fibers is accompanied by better conductivity and the opposite also holds true. When impulses from atrial and ventricular tissues attempt to invade the AV node, their synchronous arrival at the fibers of the N region produce an action potential with greater amplitude and upstroke velocity. It has also been demonstrated that synchronization of two excitation fronts invading AV nodal tissue from two atrial sites causes a successful transmission of the impulse across the AV node, whereas the arrival of only one of the wavefronts or their asynchronous arrival is associated with an intranodal conduction block. The significance of inhomogeneous conduction in determining AV nodal conductivity has thus been established. When this inhomogeneity is markedly exaggerated, transmission of an impulse may be blocked on one side of the AV node while slow but successful conduction occurs on the other side. This phenomenon is called functional longitudinal dissociation and is considered to be responsible for reciprocal beating and reciprocal tachycardia (paroxysmal AV junctional tachycardia). The distinction between this mechanism and the more recently advocated mechanism of so-called "dual AV nodal pathways" probably requires more extensive study. Functional longitudinal dissociation has been shown to occur in myocardial tissues other than the AV node (e.g., in the His bundle or peripheral Purkinje fibers). Nevertheless, it may be said that inhomogeneous conduction is a transverse or parallel expression of depressed conductivity, whereas decremental conduction is a longitudinal or series expression of depressed conduction. (3) The third variety of abnormal conduction phenomena, conduction delay and block, can result from any of the mechanisms described above. However, the most common causes of conduction block, at least in tissues other than the AV node, are probably: (1) loss of the membrane potential due either to partial depolarization or diastolic depolarization) and the resultant appearance of slow responses; (2) the presence of a refractory tissue (or a tissue with lowered excitability) in the pathway of conduction. The role of conduction delay and block in the genesis of various arrhythmias will be discussed in the next section. (4) Unidirectional block or unidirectional con-

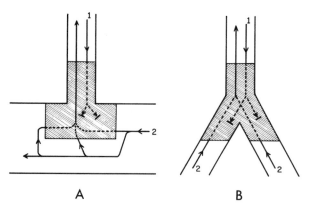

A   B

Figure 13–7 Schematic diagrams illustrating possible mechanisms of unidirectional conduction. In *A*, conductivity is depressed at the junction of a small fiber strand and a larger myocardial tissue (*shaded area*). Excitation front invading this area from above (*arrow 1*) is blocked as the action current is "diluted" at this junction, whereas retrograde wave front of excitation (*arrow 2*) successfully traverses this area because of summation of impulses. Similar relationship exists at the branching portion of a fiber strand (*B*).

duction is a special type of conduction block. It was first demonstrated experimentally by Schmitt and Erlanger and is considered responsible for re-entry movements. The genesis of this phenomenon is usually attributed to different degrees of decrement, depending on the direction of conduction. We believe that anatomic structures, as illustrated in Figure 13–7, may facilitate the production of unidirectional block. The wavefront of excitation could become irregular and fractionated in one direction while merging and summation of excitation fronts may occur in an opposite direction. We have previously demonstrated unidirectional block within the AV node, and similar phenomena also appear to occur in the Purkinje fibers.

(5) Re-entry is one of the mechanisms most frequently invoked in various cardiac arrhythmias. The requirements for the production of re-entry movement include: (1) either the presence of two anatomically separated pathways or functional longitudinal dissociation in the conducting tissue with different degrees of depression of conductivity in those two pathways; (2) the development of unidirectional block in one of the pathways (Fig. 13–8). One additional factor is a shortened refractory period in those fibers which are to be invaded by the re-entrant impulse that allows them to be re-excited after an initial depolarization. Although re-entry movement is often classified into macrore-entries and microreentries (depending on the size of the re-entry circuit), the distinction between these two varieties is far from clear. However, WPW tachycardias, most instances of atrial flutter, and reciprocal movements within the AV junction probably represent macrore-entry, whereas microre-entry movements may develop in any portion of the myocardium, causing various premature systoles, paroxysmal ectopic tachycardias, and fibrillation. As has been shown in Table 13–2, these several abnormal conduction phenomena will secondarily affect transmission of subsequent impulses in a complex manner. Readers are referred to the original articles for more detailed discussion.

The Role of Conduction Delay and Block in the Genesis of Arrhythmias

Conduction delay and block (failure of propagation) can cause numerous varieties of arrhythmia. Their direct expressions in the clinical setting are usually called some kind of "block," e.g., sinoatrial (SA) block, atrioventricular (AV) block, exit block from the pacemaker site in the presence of an ectopic rhythm, and intraventricular conduction disturbances (bundle branch block and fascicular block). In these arrhythmias, disturbances of conduction will produce irregularities in the PP, PR, or RR intervals or an abnormal prolongation of the PR or QRS interval. These usually are identified in electrocardiographic records.

SA block generally becomes of clinical significance only when some of the impulses regularly formed in the sinus node fail to excite the atrial tissue (second degree block). Resultant longer PP intervals then correspond to simple multiples of a basic sinus cycle length. Two different mechanisms for SA block appear to exist. When a P wave drops out in the presence of high extracellular potassium concentrations or certain types of drugs, the atrial tissue is not depolarized in its entirety because of decrements in atrial conduction. Thus, this condition may be considered intra-atrial block (Fig. 13–9). It has been suggested that, under these conditions, sinus impulses may be successfully transmitted to the ventricles without being accompanied by identifiable P waves, a phenomenon termed "sinoventricular conduction." An increased resistance of the fibers of the intra-atrial conducting system (or internodal tracts) greater than that of the working atrial muscle fibers against elevated potassium concentrations or depressant drugs probably

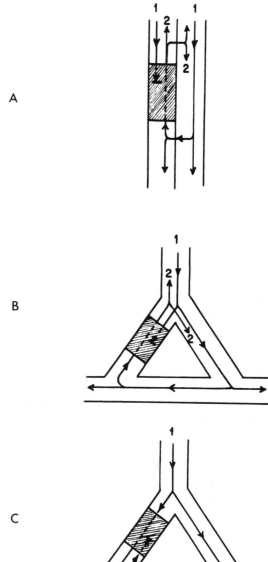

Figure 13–8 Diagrammatic explanation of re-entry mechanism. Localized areas of depressed conductivity with the property of unidirectional block (*shaded areas*), in the presence of either functional longitudinal dissociation (*A*) or two anatomically separate pathways (*B*), cause reexcitation of the initially depolarized tissue by the impulse traversing these depressed areas in a retrograde fashion (*arrow 2*). In *C*, an excitation wave traversing the depressed area at a reduced speed may finally emerge from this area (*arrow 2*) to reexcite the distal tissue, which once was depolarized by the same impulse rapidly traveling down a second pathway with a better conductivity (*arrow 1*). Presence of unidirectional conduction is required also in this model. (Reproduced from Watanabe, Y.: Electrophysiologic knowledge necessary for the understanding of cardiac arrhythmias. Medicina, *13*:17, 1976, in Japanese).

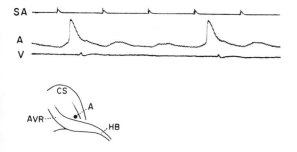

Figure 13–9 An experimental record showing SA or intra-atrial block observed in an isolated, perfused rabbit heart. Note a decreased rate of phase 0 depolarization in propagated response in this atrial fiber (*A*) adjacent to the AV node and two successive local responses upon failure of AV transmission. SA, electrogram from the SA nodal region; V, ventricular electrogram. Bottom diagram shows the AV junctional region. CS, ostium of coronary sinus; AVR, fibrous atrioventricular ring; HB, His bundle. (Reproduced from Watanabe, Y., and Dreifus, L. S.: Cardiac Arrhythmias: Electrophysiologic Basis for Clinical Interpretation. Grune & Stratton, New York, 1977.)

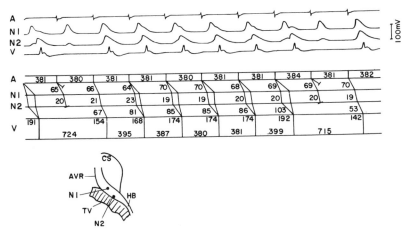

Figure 13–10 Mobitz type 1 block with higher (7:6) conduction ratio. Fibers N1 and N2 are located in the NH region. Note progressive step formation in downstream fiber (N2) and concomitant development of hump in repolarization phase of upstream fiber (N1).

could explain such a mechanism. On the other hand, transmission of sinus impulses to the surrounding atrial muscle or to the internodal tract may fail at the atrial junction when an organic lesion involves the so-called "perinodal fibers." This second mechanism was simulated by Sano when small incisions were made adjacent to the sinus nodal tissue. Until recently, first degree SA block (or simple prolongation of the SA conduction time) was considered only a theoretic entity. However, diagnosis of this condition now appears to be possible by measuring the SA conduction time from the difference between the return cycle after an atrial premature systole and the basic sinus cycle.

AV block usually is classified as first, second, and third degree block depending on the severity of the conduction disturbance. Second degree AV block has been further classified into Type 1 (Wenckebach periodicity) and Type 2 (Mobitz Type II). Precise electrophysiologic mechanisms underlying these two types have not been fully illustrated, although it has been shown that the former is caused mainly by conduction disturbances within the AV node, whereas the latter in most instances is produced by disorders of His-Purkinje conduction. These observations suggest a propensity toward the development of Wenckebach type block in the presence of slow responses. Indeed, this type of conduction phenomenon also has been demonstrated in Purkinje fibers or ventricular muscle when their membrane potential was significantly reduced and their conductivity markedly depressed. The possible role of inhomogeneous conduction in the production of Wenckebach phenomenon has been suggested experimentally (Fig. 13–10). On the other hand, certain instances of Mobitz Type II

block have been shown to result from an abnormal premature depolarization of certain portions of the conducting system, which creates a refractory tissue and prevents the transmission of an impulse arriving from the upstream fibers. Such a premature depolarization may be produced by various mechanisms of impulse formation, as discussed earlier, or it possibly may result from reentry movement caused by conduction disturbance. An example of the latter mechanism is shown in Figure 13–11. Disturbances of impulse

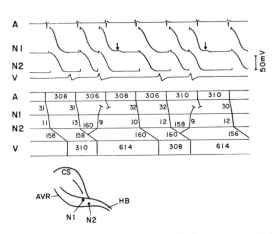

Figure 13–11 Mobitz type 2 block due to concealed re-excitation in AV junction. Fibers N1 and N2 are located in NH region. The third group of action potentials is premature. The action potentials show reversed order of excitation (depolarization of fiber N1 follows that of N2), suggesting retrograde activation of NH fibers. The third atrial impulse is blocked in NH region. (Reproduced from Watanabe, Y., and Dreifus, L. S.: Am. Heart J., 70:505, 1965).

transmission due to such premature depolarizations constitute one variety of concealed conduction, and are considered a direct expression of conduction delay and block.

In the case of so-called "protection block" around a parasystolic pacemaker, the presence of a conduction disturbance is not immediately apparent on the electrocardiogram. This is often called entrance block as compared to exit block; it prevents the invasion of a parasystolic pacemaker by other impulses, enabling the pacemaker to maintain its regular impulse formation. Protection block around the parasystolic focus and exit block from the site of ectopic impulse formation will be discussed in greater detail in the following section on the combination of abnormal impulse formation and disturbances of conduction.

Various intraventricular conduction disturbances as another direct expression of abnormal impulse transmission do not reveal themselves as irregularities of the heart beat. However, they may indirectly facilitate the production of various ventricular arrhythmias. In contrast to the cases with normal ventricular conduction, those cases with bundle branch or fascicular blocks show a higher incidence of ventricular premature systoles, which tend to originate from the regions of blocked bundles or fascicles. Ventricular tachycardias also appear to arise in areas of conduction disturbance. Although certain reservations must be made before accepting these observations as evidence for re-entry movements, the role of conduction disturbances in the genesis of abnormal impulse formation appears to be well established.

Supernormal Conduction

Supernormal AV conduction has been the focus of great clinical interest, although similar supernormal conduction in the intra-atrial conducting system has also been suggested. Supernormal AV conduction is defined as an apparently paradoxic improvement in the conduction of an impulse when its conductivity is expected to be further depressed from the previous sequence of AV conduction. Several varieties of supernormal AV conduction have been identified in clinical electrocardiograms and their electrophysiologic mechanisms may well differ from one patient to the next.

In this chapter, three varieties will be briefly discussed. In the first, in a second degree AV block showing the Wenckebach phenomenon, one conducted beat is associated with a shorter PR interval after the PR intervals of preceding beats had shown a progressive increase. The second variety of supernormal AV conduction is diagnosed when P waves occurring later in the electrical diastole of the ventricles are not conducted because of a high degree of AV block, whereas the P waves

occurring immediately after a QRS complex produced by a subsidiary pacemaker (either AV junctional or idioventricular) are conducted successfully to the ventricles. Alternation of short and long PR intervals, in the presence of regular sinus rhythm and 1:1 AV conduction, has been considered yet another type of supernormal AV conduction.

When a phenomenon similar to the first variety of supernormal AV conduction was observed in an experiment on an isolated perfused rabbit heart, transmission of the first several atrial impulses to the ventricles was accompanied by changes in the AV nodal action potentials, suggesting a progressive increase in inhomogeneous conduction in this tissue. The following AV nodal action potential showed a much smoother upstroke, suggesting reorganization of the excitation front, and the AV conduction time was shortened. Although the reason for the recovery of homogeneity of intranodal conduction is still unknown, several mechanisms, such as slight variations in atrial cycle length, different modes of invasion of the AV node by atrial impulses resulting from alterations in the atrial excitation process, and temporal fluctuations of conductivity within the AV node may be postulated.

In contrast, the second variety of supernormal AV conduction has been explained by several investigators through the concept of a "peeling back" of the refractory barrier. These investigators have demonstrated that a premature atrial impulse which ordinarily is blocked within the AV junction can be transmitted successfully to the ventricles when the AV junctional tissue is depolarized by a retrograde impulse that originates in the ventricles just before the supraventricular impulse arrives in this region.

A possible explanation for these findings is that, since the fibers in the region of propagation failure are prematurely depolarized by the retrograde impulse, both their repolarization process and their refractoriness will be terminated earlier, allowing these fibers to recover their excitability before the atrial impulse arrives. Blockage of premature atrial impulses in these instances is predicated on the presence of markedly prolonged refractoriness in the AV junction. It is, however, still questionable whether the same mechanism can be invoked in the presence of a regular sinus rhythm with high grades of AV block.

The concept of inhomogeneous conduction may provide us with an alternative explanation. When high grade AV block in the orthograde direction is caused by a marked inhomogeneity of intranodal conduction, invasion of this region by a retrograde impulse may cause more homogeneous depression of conductivity in this area; therefore, the next atrial impulse is associated with a better organized wavefront of excitation and a successful impulse transmission.

Still another explanation for this type of supernormal AV conduction invokes the mechanism of so-called "phase 4 block." When certain fibers of the AV conducting system show marked diastolic depolarization, their transmembrane potential will be progressively decreased later in electrical diastole and their conductivity depressed. When the sinus cycle is relatively long, most of the sinus impulses may arrive at these fibers when their membrane potential is sufficiently reduced to cause orthograde conduction block. Contrariwise, a sinus impulse arriving immediately after the completion of the action potential produced by the impulse from a subsidiary pacemaker may depolarize these fibers at the time their membrane potential is most negative (the maximal diastolic potential), generate an action potential with a greater upstroke velocity and amplitude, and sustain a lesser degree of decrement. Further studies are clearly needed to elucidate the two mechanisms of this interesting conduction phenomenon.

On the other hand, the following considerations lead us to believe that the third variety, as described above, may not satisfy the criteria for supernormal AV conduction. It has been argued that in the presence of regular sinus rhythm with alternation of short and long PR intervals, the P wave following a beat conducted with a prolonged PR interval would appear closer to the preceding QRS and have a shorter RP interval. This suggests the invasion of an atrial impulse into the AV conducting system after a shorter interval and at a time when the conducting fibers are less fully recovered. Since this should be accompanied by a further prolongation of the AV conduction time, the paradoxic shortening of the PR interval in the following beat has been considered an expression of supernormal AV conduction. It must be pointed out, however, that the shorter RP interval may not necessarily indicate an early arrival of an impulse in the AV conducting system. If the preceding QRS complex has been produced by an impulse from a subsidiary pacemaker, a shorter RP interval definitely indicates an earlier arrival of the impulse with reference to the preceding depolarization of the AV junctional fibers. Under a regular sinus mechanism, on the other hand, all the atrial impulses will attempt to invade the AV junction with a constant PP interval; the RP interval would have no significance in determining the subsequent conduction phenomena. It is known that a slow propagation of excitation is accompanied by a prolonged action potential in fibers in such regions. If the subsequent atrial impulse arrives immediately after the repolarization of these fibers, and if a diastolic depolarization is present, the concept of "phase 4 block" may again be invoked, as in the previous variety, to explain the shorter PR interval or a

paradoxic improvement in AV conduction. Inhomogeneous conduction again may be offered as an alternative mechanism. If, in the presence of functional longitudinal dissociation of the AV junction, one portion of the AV junctional tissue maintains a 1:1 conduction while the other portion shows a 2:1 block, a better organized excitation front with a higher conduction velocity will alternate with a poorly organized and slowly conducting wavefront. The concept of so-called "dual AV nodal pathways" may have the same significance as long as the term does not necessarily imply two anatomically separated pathways. Admittedly, all these mechanisms are still hypothetical, and the phenomena of supernormal AV conduction require more extensive experimental study.

COMBINED DISTURBANCES OF IMPULSE FORMATION AND CONDUCTION

The close association between abnormal impulse formation and disturbances of conduction in the genesis of cardiac arrhythmias can be readily understood by recognizing the fact that a localized conduction disorder with re-entry movements will produce a premature systole or an ectopic tachycardia, and that premature depolarization of the AV junction by an ectopic impulse can make the AV junction refractory and block a subsequent atrial impulse. Furthermore, abnormal impulse formation in one portion of the myocardium (atria) may accompany a conduction disturbance in another portion (AV conducting system), as is the case in atrial tachycardia with AV block. In this section, however, the term "combined disturbances of impulse formation and conduction" will be used in the narrower sense in that an arrhythmia is generated by the combination of these two mechanisms in a rather localized area of myocardium.

Two major types of arrhythmia included in this category are ectopic rhythms with exit block, and parasystole. Atrial fibrillation and ventricular fibrillation also will be discussed in this section, although their classification within this category may be subject to controversy.

Exit block from an ectopic pacemaker is seen most frequently in the presence of either AV junctional rhythm or non-paroxysmal AV junctional tachycardia, but also is often seen in idioventricular rhythm in cases of third degree AV block, Type B. We have previously demonstrated the actual occurrence of exit block from an AV junctional pacemaker with microelectrode techniques in isolated perfused rabbit hearts (Fig. 13–12). The difficulty in the exit of impulses from an automatic focus may be explained by the con-

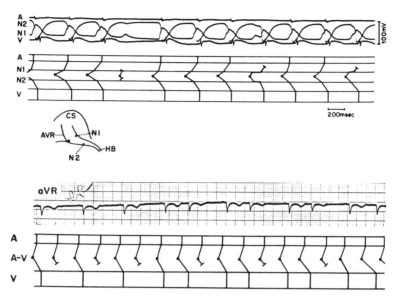

Figure 13–12 An experimental record showing exit block from an AV nodal pacemaker (*top*) and an equivalent clinical electrocardiogram (*bottom*). Transmembrane potential N1 was recorded from the N region of the AV node, and N2 (with reversed polarity) from the NH region. Site of impulse formation in this AV junctional rhythm (X mark) is shown in the inset. Either conduction delay or block in the exit of impulses from this pacemaker produces notched upstroke of phase 0 or incomplete depolarization in these fibers and dropping out of atrial (A) or ventricular excitation (V). In the bottom record, AV junctional rhythm with exit block in forward direction is diagnosed from regular appearance of positive P waves (this suggests retrograde conduction in lead AVR) and irregular R-R intervals (see attached diagram).

cept of phase 4 block, as diastolic depolarization in fibers within and around the pacemaker will cause a gradual loss of membrane potential, thus decreasing the rate of rise and amplitude of the action potential. This will cause decremental conduction. Indeed, phase 4 depolarization was observed in several recording sites adjacent to the point of earliest depolarization or the origin of ectopic impulses. In other words, automaticity in the localized area of the myocardium in this type of arrhythmia produces an ectopic rhythm on the one hand and, on the other, facilitates the development of exit block.

Regarding parasystole, disturbance of impulse transmission is considered to play a role in the form of so-called "protection block" around the site of impulse formation. The electrophysiologic mechanisms of such protection of the parasystolic pacemaker are still subject to controversy. Certain investigators postulate extremely rapid impulse formation in the parasystolic focus so that the region of the pacemaker remains almost always in the state of refractoriness, thereby preventing depolarization by extrinsic stimuli. Although cases of parasystole with such a high frequency discharge may indeed exist, the rather slow parasystolic rhythms most commonly seen clinically are not easily explained by this mechanism unless a rather high degree of exit block is postulated.

A second explanation proposes that, since the fibers within the parasystolic focus have a higher stimulation threshold than the surrounding tissue, impulses of the basic rhythm fail to excite the pacemaking fibers, whereas the impulses formed within this focus can depolarize the surrounding fibers with a relatively low threshold of stimulation and can make an exit. Since the difference of excitability between fiber groups is causing a conduction disturbance, this mechanism may be considered one type of protection block. Still another possibility is that the tissue around the site of parasystolic impulse formation has an abnormally prolonged refractory period, which prevents the invasion of extrinsic stimuli into the area. Distinguishing this mechanism from protection block due to conduction disturbance again may be rather difficult.

These three theories invoke either refractoriness or lowered excitability in or around the parasystolic pacemaker; however, phase 4 block in surrounding fibers also may explain such a protection mechanism. In this instance, diastolic depolarization in certain fibers of the specialized conducting system produces regular automatic impulse formation and, at the same time, prevents their discharge by extraneous impulses. Then the electrophysiologic mechanism of parasystole becomes quite similar to that of ectopic rhythms with exit block. If the site of phase 4 block-induced unidirectional conduction acts mainly to protect this focus from invading sinus impulses, parasystolic rhythm will be produced. Conversely, if the mechanism of unidirectional conduction due to phase 4 block mainly inhibits 1:1 outward spread of automatic impulses, an ectopic rhythm with exit block may ensue. It must be pointed out that parasystole occasionally is associated with exit block, suggesting the development of bidirectional block. We have previously demonstrated that impulse formation in ventricular parasystole in cases with intraventricular conduction disturbances tends to develop in the regions of the bundles or fascicles in which conduction is disturbed. Such observations may indirectly suggest the interrelationships between automaticity (diastolic depolarization), intraventricular conduction disorder due to phase 4 block, and the protection block. It may be speculated further that, if a region of unidirectional conduction is indeed playing a major role in protecting a parasystolic pacemaker, transition between simple, coupled premature systoles and parasystolic impulse formation may possibly be observed, as re-entry movement also is predicated on the presence of unidirectional block. Reports showing the occurrence of coupled premature systoles, which were considered re-entrant in nature, near the site of parasystolic impulse formation appear to support the above concept.

Regarding the phenomenon of cardiac fibrillation, theories of unifocal impulse formation, multifocal impulse formation, and re-entry have been advocated by different investigators. In the first two theories, abnormal impulse formation is considered to play a major role in the genesis of this arrhythmia, whereas the re-entry theory invokes mainly disturbances of conduction. Since it is our current feeling that cardiac fibrillation probably is explained either by re-entry alone or by the combination of unifocal impulse formation and re-entry, this arrhythmia has been included in this section.

In the theory of multifocal impulse formation, an entire disorganization of the atrial or ventricular excitation process results from the coexistence of numerous foci of impulse formation that cause independent and random depolarization of multiple points. In contrast, the unifocal impulse formation theory postulates a single site of impulse formation at an extremely high frequency through which some fibers cannot respond in a 1:1 fashion. Then, islands of conduction block will result in irregular spread of ventricular excitation. In this instance, however, the development of multiple areas of localized conduction block would most likely generate numerous microre-entry circuits, and resort to a combination with the re-entry theory may become mandatory.

The genesis of fibrillation triggered by a single premature impulse occurring in the so-called "vulnerable period" is explained by the theory of re-entry in the following manner. Because of the non-uniformity of the action potential duration, as well as the refractory period between fiber groups, a premature stimulus may produce different degrees of response in individual fibers. Thus, the wavefront of excitation will become grossly irregular, leading to multiple areas of microre-entry.

Findings that apparently support this concept have been observed experimentally, an example being shown in Fig. 13–13 (part A, lower record). When ventricular fibrillation was initiated in isolated perfused rabbit hearts with a premature systole, the two adjacent epicardial fibers showed markedly different responses to this premature impulse, with increased asynchrony of depolarization and dissimilar upstroke velocity and amplitude of the action potentials. A rapid transition to ventricular fibrillation is clearly noted in the electrocardiogram. Disorganized spread of ventricular excitation caused by premature stimulation is thus evident, and the development of microore-entry circuits may readily be anticipated. Such a rapid development of fibrillatory movement during the vulnerable period (termed Type A by us) appears to be explained by the re-entry theory.

Part B of Figure 13–13 illustrates another mode of onset of fibrillation observed both clinically and experimentally. In this instance, abnormal spread of ventricular excitation is gradually exaggerated after a more prolonged period of ectopic tachycardia, finally deteriorating into fibrillation. The experimental findings shown in the bottom record revealed that the transmembrane potentials recorded in one of the two adjacent ventricular muscle fibers develop an alternation of action potential amplitude, and asynchrony of depolarization in these two fibers not only becomes greater but also fluctuates from beat to beat. These findings will suggest the development of localized conduction block and marked variations of the excitation process from one beat to the next. Again, formation of numerous microre-entry circuits will be easily envisioned. Hence, also in this concept of onset of fibrillation (termed Type B), the role of conduction disturbance cannot be disregarded.

In view of experimental observations, as discussed, as well as numerous reports in the literature, it appears that the role of the re-entry mechanism is now widely accepted, at least in the maintenance of fibrillation. On the other hand, we have often observed in our experimental studies on the antifibrillatory actions of antiarrhythmic agents that a transition from ventricular fi-

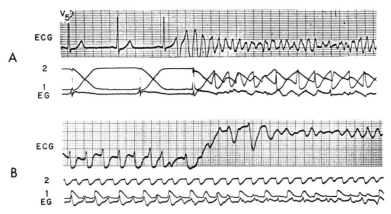

Figure 13–13 Two mechanisms of ventricular fibrillation.
A, Sudden onset of ventricular fibrillation (V₅) after a ventricular premature complex occurring at the apex of the T wave. Lower strip, experimental record showing premature action potentials (3rd beat). Note slight delay in the inscription of the inverted action potential followed by marked disorganization of excitation and abnormal action potentials.
B, Gradual onset of ventricular fibrillation following continued disorganization of excitation process (lower strip). Clinical record shown above.

brillation to what appears to be a ventricular tachycardia occurred after the administration of various antiarrhythmic agents. This either was sustained for a prolonged period or eventually returned to a normal sinus rhythm, which may suggest the possible role of unifocal impulse formation in the initiation of fibrillation. Demonstration of the localized area of high frequency discharge at the beginning of experimental atrial fibrillation produced by premature electrical stimulation, as reported by Sano and Scher, is of great interest in this regard. Furthermore, since

the various mechanisms of abnormal impulse formation dependent on slow inward currents are activated when the cell membrane is partially depolarized, and since this latter condition facilitates marked conduction disturbances through the production of so-called "slow responses," increased attention will be directed to the significance of slow channels in the genesis of cardiac fibrillation. A more detailed discussion on the mechanisms of cardiac fibrillation has been published elsewhere.

REFERENCES

Antoni, H., and Oberdisse, E.: Elektrophysiologische Untersuchungen über die Barium-induzierte Schrittmacher Aktivität in der Arbeitsmuskulatur des Säugetierherzens. Arch. Exp. Pathol. Pharmakol., *247*:329, 1964.

Arita, M., Nagamoto, Y., and Saikawa, T.: Automaticity and time-dependent conduction disturbance produced in canine ventricular myocardium. New aspects for initiation of ventricular arrhythmias. Jap. Circ. J., *40*:1401, 1976.

Aronson, R. S., and Cranefield, P. F.: The effect of resting potential on the electrical activity of canine cardiac Purkinje fibers exposed to Na-free solution or to ouabain. Pfluegers Arch., *347*:101, 1974.

Beeler, G. W., Jr., and Reuter, H.: Membrane calcium current in ventricular myocardial fibers. J. Physiol., *207*:191, 1970.

Bellet, S.: Clinical Disorders of the Heart Beat, 3rd ed. Lea & Febiger, Philadelphia, 1971.

Bigger, J. T., Jr., Bassett, A. L., and Hoffman, B. F.: Electrophysiological effects of diphenylhydantoin on canine Purkinje fibers. Circ. Res., *22*:221, 1968.

Bigger, J .T., Jr.: Electrical Properties of Cardiac Muscle and Possible Causes of Cardiac Arrhythmias. *In* Dreifus, L. S., and Likoff, W., (eds.): Cardiac Arrhythmias. Grune & Stratton, New York, 1973, p. 13.

Brooks, C. McC., Hoffman, B. F., Suckling, E. E., and Orias, O.: The Excitability of the Heart. Grune & Stratton, New York, 1955.

Brooks, C. McC., and Lu, H. H.: Sinoatrial Pacemaker of the Heart. Charles C Thomas, Springfield, Ill., 1972.

Castellanos, A. Jr., Lemberg, L., Johnson, D., and Berkovits, B. V.: The Wedensky effect in the human heart. Br. Heart J., *28*:276, 1966.

Cranefield, P. F., Klein, H. O., and Hoffman, B. F.: Conduction of the cardiac impulse. I. Delay, block and one-way block in depressed Purkinje fibers. Circ. Res., *28*:199, 1971.

Cranefield, P. F., and Hoffman, B. F.: Conduction of the cardiac impulse. II. Summation and inhibition. Circ. Res., *28*:220, 1971.

Cranefield, P. F.: The Conduction of the Cardiac Impulse. Futura Publishing Co., Inc., Mount Kisco, New York, 1975.

delaFuente, D., Sasyniuk, B., and Moe, G. K.: Conduction through a narrow isthmus in isolated canine atrial tissue. A model of the W-P-W syndrome. Circulation, *44*:803, 1971.

Dreifus, L. S., Watanabe, Y., Haiat, R., and Kimbiris, D.: Atrioventricular block. Am. J. Cardiol., *28*:371, 1971.

Elizari, M .V., Lazzari, J. O., and Rosenbaum, M. B.: Phase-3 and phase-4 intermittent left anterior hemiblock. Report of 1st case in the literature. Chest, *63*:673, 1972.

Ferrer, M. I.: The sick sinus syndrome in atrial disease. J.A.M.A., *206*:645, 1968.

Ferrer, M. I.: The sick sinus syndrome. Circulation, *47*:635, 1973.

Ferrier, G. R., and Moe, G. K.: Effect of calcium on

acetylstrophanthidin-induced transient depolarizations in canine-Purkinje tissue. Circ. Res., 33:508, 1973.

Gettes, L. S., and Surawicz, B.: Effects of low and high concentrations of potassium on the simultaneously recorded Purkinje and ventricular action potentials of the perfused pig moderator band. Circ. Res., 23:717, 1968.

Goto, M.: Physiology of Circulation — Heart and Systemic Circulation. Asakura Book Co., Tokyo, 1971.

Hellerstein, H. K., and Turell, D. J.: The Mode of Death in Coronary Artery Disease. An Electrocardiographic and Clinicopathological Correlation. In Surawicz, B., and Pellegrino, E. D. (eds.): Sudden Cardiac Death. Grune & Stratton, New York, 1964, p. 17.

Hoffman, B. F., and Cranefield, P. F.: Electrophysiology of the Heart. McGraw-Hill Book Co., New York, 1960.

Hoffman, B. F.: The Pathophysiology of Failure of Impulse Transmission to the Ventricles. In Surawicz, B., and Pellegrino, E. D. (eds.): Sudden Cardiac Death. Grune & Stratton, New York, 1964, p. 78.

Hoffman, B. F.: The Electrophysiology of Heart Muscle and the Genesis of Arrhythmias. In Dreifus, L. S., and Likoff, W. (eds.): Mechanisms and Therapy of Cardiac Arrhythmias. Grune & Stratton, New York, 1966, p. 27.

James, T. N.: The connecting pathways between the sinus node and A-V node and between the right and left atrium in the human heart. Am Heart J., 66:498, 1963.

Katz, B.: Electrical properties of the muscle fiber membrane. Proc. Roy. Soc., 135:506, 1948.

Katz, L. N., and Pick, A.: Clinical Electrocardiography. Part I: The Arrhythmias. Lea & Febiger, Philadelphia, 1956.

Kimura, E.: Paroxysmal tachycardias. Heart, 3:1395, 1971 (in Japanese).

Konishi, T., and Matsuyama, E.: Effect of changes in inputs to atrioventricular node on AV conduction. Jap. Circ. J., 40:1392, 1976.

Matsuda, K., Hoshi, T., and Kameyama, S.: Effects of aconitine on the cardiac membrane potential of the dog. Jap. J. Physiol., 9:419, 1959.

Matsuda, K.: Function of the node of Tawara. Clin. Res., 50:3514, 1973 (in Japenese).

Matsuda, K.: Significance of slow inward current in the myocardium. Heart, 7:617, 1975 (in Japanese).

Miller, H. C., and Strauss, H. C.: Measurement of sinoatrial conduction time by premature atrial stimulation in the rabbit. Circ. Res., 35:935, 1974.

Moe, G. K., and Abildskov, J. A.: Atrial fibrillation as a self-sustaining arrhythmia independent of focal discharge. Am. Heart J., 58:59, 1959.

Moe, G. K., Childers, R. W., and Merideth, J.: An appraisal of "supernormal" A-V conduction. Circulation, 38:5, 1968.

Moore, E. N., and Spear, J. F.: Experimental studies on the facilitation of A-V conduction by ectopic beats in dogs and rabbits. Circ. Res., 29:29, 1971.

Muller, P.: Ca- and K-free solution and pacemaker activity in mammalian myocardium. Helv. Physiol. Acta, 23:C38, 1965.

Noble, D.: A modification of the Hodgkin-Huxley equations applicable to Purkinje fiber action and pacemaker potentials. J. Physiol., 160:317, 1962.

Ogawa, S., Watanabe, Y., and Dreifus, L. S.: Double ventricular parasystole. Am. Heart J., 93:767, 1977.

Pamintuan, J. C., Dreifus, L. S., and Watanabe, Y.: Comparative mechanisms of antiarrhythmic agents. Am. J. Cardiol., 26:512, 1970.

Pick, A., Langendorf, R., and Katz, L. N.: The supernormal phase of atrioventricular conduction. I. Fundamental mechanisms. Circulation, 26:388, 1962.

Reuter, H.: Divalent cations as charge carriers in excitable membranes. Prog. Biophys. Mol. Biol., 26:1, 1973.

Rosen, K. M., Rahimtoola, S. H., and Gunnar, R. M.: Pseudo A-V block secondary to premature nonpropagated His bundle depolarizations: Documentation by His bundle electrocardiography. Circulation, 42:367, 1970.

Rougier, O., Vassort, G., Garnier, D., Gargouil, Y. M., and Coraboeuf, E.: Existence and role of a slow inward current during the frog atrial action potential. Pfluegers Arch., 308:91, 1969.

Ruiz-Ceretti, E., and Ponce-Zumino, A.: Action potential changes under varied Na+ and Ca2+ indicating the existence of two inward currents in cells of the rabbit atrioventricular node. Circ. Res., 39:326, 1976.

Sano, T., and Scher, A. M.: Multiple recording during electrically induced atrial fibrillation. Circ. Res., 14:117, 1964.

Sano, T., Iida, Y., and Yamagishi, S.: Changes in the Spread of Excitation from the Sinus Node Induced by Alterations in Extracellular Potassium. In Sano, T., Mizuhira, V., and Matsuda, K. (eds.): Electrophysiology and Ultrastructure of the Heart. Bunkodo, Tokyo, 1967, p. 127.

Sano, T., and Hiraoka, M.: Studies on the site and mechanism of sinoatrial block. J. Jap. Med. Assoc., 63:866, 1974.

Scherf, D., and Schott, A.: Extrasystoles and Allied Arrhythmias. William Heinemann, Ltd., London, 1953.

Scherf, D., and Bornemann, C.: Parasystole with a rapid ventricular center. Am. Heart J., 62:320, 1961.

Scherf, D., and Cohen, J.: The Atrioventricular Node and Selected Cardiac Arrhythmias. Grune & Stratton, New York, 1964.

Schmidt, R. F.: Versuche mit Aconitin zum Problem der spontanen Erregungsbildung im Herzen. Pfluegers Arch., 271:526, 1960.

Schmitt, F. O., and Erlanger, J.: Directional differences in the conduction of the impulse through heart muscle and their possible relation to extrasystolic and fibrillary contractions. Am. J. Physiol., 87:326, 1928.

Singer, D. H., Lazzara, R., and Hoffman, B. F.: Interrelationships between automaticity and conduction in Purkinje fibers. Circ. Res., 21:537, 1967.

Singer, D. H., Parameswaran, R., Drake, F. T., et al.: Ventricular parasystole and reentry: Clinical-electrophysiological correlations. Am. Heart J., 88:79, 1974.

Vassalle, M.: Cardiac pacemaker potentials at different extra- and intracellular K concentrations. Am. J. Physiol., 208:770, 1965.

Vitek, M., and Trautwein, W.: Slow inward current and action potential in cardiac Purkinje fibers. Pfluegers Arch., 323:204, 1971.

Watanabe, Y., Dreifus, L. S., and Likoff, W.: Electrophysiologic antagonism and synergism of potassium and antiarrhythmic agents. Am. J. Cardiol., 12:702, 1963.

Watanabe, Y., and Dreifus, L. S.: Inhomogeneous conduction in the A-V node. A model for re-entry. Am. Heart J., 70:505, 1965.

Watanabe, Y.: Antagonism and Synergism of Potassium and Anti-arrhythmic Agents. In Bajusz, E. (ed.): Electrolytes and Cardiovascular Disease. S. Karger AG Medical Publishers, Basel, 1965, p. 86.

Watanabe, Y., and Dreifus, L. S.: Mechanisms of ventricular fibrillation. Jap. Heart J., 7:110, 1966.

Watanabe, Y., and Dreifus, L. S.: Second degree atrioventricular block. Cardiovas. Res., 1:150, 1967.

Watanabe, Y., and Dreifus, L. S.: Sites of impulse formation within the atrioventricular junction of the rabbit. Circ. Res., 22:717, 1968.

Watanabe, Y., and Dreifus, L. S.: Newer concepts in the genesis of cardiac arrhythmias. Am. Heart J., 76:114, 1968.

Watanabe, Y.: Effects of Electrolytes and Antiarrhythmic Agents on Atrioventricular Conduction. In Sandøe, E., Flensted-Jensen, E., and Oleson, K. H. (eds.): Symposium on Cardiac Arrhythmias. A B Astra, Södertälje, Sweden, 1970, p. 535.

Watanabe, Y.: Reassessment of parasystole. Am. Heart J., 81:451, 1971.

Watanabe, Y., and Dreifus, L. S.: Antifibrillatory action of antiarrhythmic agents. Fed. Proc., 30:554 (Abs), 1971.

Watanabe, Y., and Dreifus, L. S.: Levels of concealment in second degree and advanced second degree A-V block. Am. Heart J., 84:330, 1972.

Watanabe, Y.: Cardiac Arrhythmias. Electrophysiologic and Clinical Aspects. Bunkodo, Tokyo, 1973 (in Japanese).

Watanabe, Y.: Genesis of cardiac arrhythmias. Intensivmedizin, 10:109, 1973.

Watanabe, Y.: Extrasystoles and parasystole: mechanisms involved. Triangle, 12:69, 1973.

Watanabe, Y.: Conduction disturbances in cardiac arrhythmias from the electrophysiological standpoints. Clin. Physiol., 3:575, 1973 (in Japanese).

Watanabe, Y., Pamintuan, J. C., and Dreifus, L. S.: Role of intraventricular conduction disturbances in ventricular premature systoles. Am. J. Cardiol., 32:188, 1973.

Watanabe, Y.: Mechanisms of A-V conduction. Heart, 6:604, 1974 (in Japanese).

Watanabe, Y.: Electrophysiology of cardiac arrhythmias. Clin. Res., 51:607, 1974 (in Japanese).

Watanabe, Y.: How to read electrocardiograms: Arrhythmias (7):High grade A-V block and unidirectional A-V conduction. Clin. All-round, 24:492, 1975 (in Japanese).

Watanabe, Y., and Dreifus, L. S.: Factors controlling impulse transmission with special reference to A-V conduction. Am. Heart J., 89:790, 1975.

Watanabe, Y.: The role of conduction disturbances in cardiac arrhythmias (Editorial). Indian Heart J., 28:3, 1976.

Watanabe, Y.: Clinical Pharmacology of Circulatory Diseases. 6. Antiarrhythmic Drugs. In I to Y (ed.): Handbook of Clinical Cardiology, Vol I: Diagnosis and Treatment in General. Kanehara Publishing Co., Tokyo, 1976, p. 276.

Watanabe, Y., and Dreifus, L. S.: Cardiac Arrhythmias. Electrophysiologic Basis for Clinical Interpretation. Grune & Stratton, New York, 1977.

Weidmann, S.: The effect of the cardiac membrane potential on the rapid availability of the sodium-carrying system. J. Physiol., 127:213, 1955.

Weidmann, S.: Effects of calcium and local anesthetics on electrical properties of Purkinje fibers. J. Physiol., 129:568, 1955.

West, T. C.: Effects of Chronotropic Influences on Subthreshold Oscillations in the Sino-Atrial Node. In Paes de Carvalho, A., de Mello, W. C., and Hoffman, B. F. (eds.): The Specialized Tissues of the Heart. Elsevier Press, Inc. Amsterdam, 1962.

Zipes, D. P., and Fischer, J. C.: Effects of agents which inhibit the slow channel on sinus node automaticity and atrioventricular conduction in the dog. Circ. Res., 34:184, 1974.

14

Renal Disease:
Water and Electrolyte Balance

Dana L. Shires, Jr.

INTRODUCTION

The opportunity to review, condense, and present information currently pertaining to the pathophysiologic status of the human kidney is at the same time an awesome and exciting undertaking. That only the high points can be brushed upon in the space allotted is a statement that needs no further elaboration. As a student of Nephrology during the past fifteen years, I have never been disappointed by the continuing amassment of useful information relating to this truly remarkable organ and the role it plays in the regulation of our internal milieu in both health and disease.

The kidneys represent only 0.04 per cent of total body weight. Despite this relatively insignificant mass, they receive, on an average, 20 per cent of the total cardiac output. They play an intricate if not dominant role in the regulation of total body volume, composition of electrolytes and acid-base balance, mineral metabolism, amino acid metabolism, erythropoiesis, blood pressure control, and no doubt many additional undefined metabolic and endocrine functions yet to be described.

THE RENAL CIRCULATION

The kidneys in man compositely receive 20 per cent of the cardiac output, or roughly 500 ml./min. of blood. This circulation gives the kidney the highest per-gram blood flow of any organ. Under usual circumstances, each kidney is supplied by a single artery from the aorta which

divides into a dorsal and a ventral branch within the hilus. These vessels in turn divide into several interlobar arteries that ascend into the cortical-medullary area. At this point the arcuate arteries are formed, from which arise the majority of the interlobular vessels. As the interlobular vessels pass through the cortex they give off the afferent arterioles. These, in turn, supply blood to the functioning filter of the kidney, the glomerulus (see Fig. 14–1).

The afferent arteriole contains smooth muscle as well as myoepithelial cells. These cells occur in the distal portion of the afferent arteriole in continuity with the macula densa. This composite structure has been termed the juxtaglomerular apparatus. Within the glomerulus the afferent arteriole gives off five to eight branches which further subdivide into 20 to 40 capillary loops. These capillary loops coalesce to form the efferent arteriole through which the circulation exits the glomerulus. In the superficial cortex the efferent arteriole from a given glomerulus may exclusively supply the tubule of the parent glomerulus. In the deeper subcortical glomeruli, the efferent arterioles run toward the superficial or deep regions of the cortex and may surround tubules quite distant from their point of origin. In juxtamedullary nephrons, there are two main types of efferent arterioles. The cortical-medullary efferent arteriole is a thin-walled vessel which divides into a capillary network in the area of the cortical-medullary junction and the outer medulla. The medullary efferent arteriole is a larger vessel which contains smooth muscle and divides into multiple vasa recta. The cortical-medullary efferent arterioles are present in 25 to 40 per cent

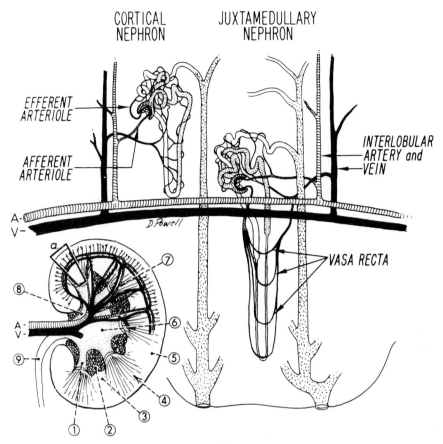

Figure 14–1 The sagittal surface of a bisected kidney is illustrated diagrammatically (lower left). Numbers (1) through (9) indicate the following: (1) minor calix; (2) fat in sinus; (3) renal column of Bertin; (4) medullary ray; (5) cortex; (6) pelvis; (7) interlobar artery; (8) major calix; and (9) ureter. The letter A indicates the renal artery; the letter V indicates the renal vein. Insert (a) from the upper pole is enlarged to illustrate the relationships between the juxtamedullary and the cortical nephrons and the renal vasculature. (From: Brenner, B. M., and Rector, F. C., Jr. (eds.): The Kidney. W. B. Saunders Company, Philadelphia, 1976.)

of the juxtamedullary nephrons and are the major vascular supply to the outer medulla. As the vessels descend into the medulla, most of these arteriolar vasa recta end in the capillary plexus, leaving only two to four branches which enter the inner medulla. These do not branch until they reach the tip of the papillae; they then empty into the ascending venous vasa recta.

Anatomically speaking, the venous circulation generally parallels the course of the arterial system.

Mass blood flow through the renal tissue is not evenly distributed. A number of methods for evaluation of blood flow distribution have been devised and applied. They include both direct and indirect methods — each having built-in discrepancies to make them less than perfect. This subject has been extensively reviewed in recent publications from which several important conclusions can be drawn. Under normal physio-

logic circumstances, the greater circulation is to the cortical areas of the kidney, representing roughly 85 per cent of the total blood flow to the kidney. No more than 15 per cent of blood flow enters the juxtamedullar nephrons. Most, if not all, of blood flow destined for the medulla traverses the juxtaglomerular nephrons. The osmolar concentration at the papillary tip is inversely related to blood flow to that area. Changes in medullary blood flow are an important determinant in the regulation of water balance. There is evidence that alteration in urinary sodium excretion is due, at least in part, to preferential redistribution of renal cortical blood flow to the juxtamedullary nephrons, which have a greater capacity for sodium reabsorption. Conversely, redistribution of blood flow to the outer cortical nephrons results in natriuresis. There are two types of juxtamedullary nephrons: those with a postglomerular circulation which is distributed only in the outer medulla; and those with the larger vasa recta which enter the inner medulla. Nephrons with the larger vasa recta make up 60 to 75 per cent of the glomeruli in the juxtamedullary cortex. There is a direct relationship between renal oxygen consumption and absolute sodium resorption or total renal blood flow. Over a wide range of sodium resorption, the ratio of sodium transport to oxygen utilization remains constant.

The kidney has a remarkable ability to maintain a constant blood flow, regardless of arterial pressure. This capability is independent of renal innervation and has been termed *autoregulation.* Under usual circumstances, autoregulation can be maintained with alterations of mean perfusion pressure from 60 to 180 mm. Hg. Mechanisms intrinsic to the kidney for autoregulation are exceedingly complex. Despite the fact that the kidneys receive a rich supply of both adrenergic and cholinergic nerve fibers, complete denervation of a kidney fails to alter the autoregulatory mechanisms materially. This leads to one of two conclusions: the kidney maintains an intrinsic neural distribution independent of extrinsic neural supply; or, intrinsic humoral factors are primarily responsible for autoregulation. There is no doubt that certain humoral mechanisms play an important role in the distribution of renal blood flow. Angiotensin II, generated by the release of renin from the juxtaglomerular apparatus, is the most potent vasoconstrictor known to man. Prostaglandins have been shown to be powerful renal vasodilators. It seems appropriate to conclude, at this stage of the art, that an intrinsic balance of these two humoral factors and possibly as yet undetermined additional humoral factors play a paramount role in this autoregulatory mechanism so crucial to renal homeostasis.

THE GLOMERULUS

The glomerulus is the primary filtering unit of the kidney. The highest concentration of glomeruli appears in the outer cortex; a lesser concentration in the juxtaglomerular area. The outer cortical glomerulus, although more frequent, is somewhat smaller in size than the juxtamedullary glomerulus. The juxtamedullary glomerulus has been shown to have a higher filtration rate per glomerular unit than does the cortical glomerulus. Each glomerulus receives its individual blood supply from an afferent arteriole. That arteriole, shortly after entering Bowman's capsule, divides into several branches. These, in turn, produce 20 to 40 capillaries per glomerulus. These capillaries then coalesce to form the efferent arteriole, which exits from Bowman's capsule in close proximity to the afferent arteriole. There

are roughly two million glomeruli in each individual. These glomeruli are permanently formed shortly after birth, and, although they may enlarge as the individual matures, no new glomeruli are formed.

The total filtering surface has been calculated for both kidneys to represent roughly one square meter. The thickness of the basement membrane in man has been established by electron microscopy as being roughly 3,500 Å. The membrane itself can be divided into at least three anatomic divisions. The first is the endothelial component of the capillary wall; the second is a continuous basement membrane; the third is the epithelial portion of the basement membrane. The structure and function of these component parts have been studied extensively. Each component plays an integral role in establishing permeability of the membrane to the various solute components of the plasma. Suffice it for this discussion to say that the membrane is freely permeable to solutes with a molecular weight equal to or less than inulin — inulin having a molecular weight of 5200 and an effective radius of 14 Å. Stated another way, molecules of this size and smaller will occur in concentrations when measured in Bowman's capsule equivalent to their concentration in the plasma. Larger molecules will be progressively restricted in their ability to pass this capillary membrane, depending on size and molecular shape.

The glomerulus is composed of three separate cellular elements; (1) the mesangial cell which constitutes the cellular matrix and supporting structures of the glomerulus; (2) the endothelial cell which forms and contributes to the endothelial lining of the basement membrane; (3) the epithelial cell which forms the external component of the capillary loop as well as the lining of Bowman's capsule.

Under usual circumstances in a 70-kilogram man, 180 liters of glomerular ultrafiltrate will be formed daily, of which less than 1 per cent is normally excreted in the form of urine. This ultrafiltrate, as noted above, contains small solute particles in roughly the same concentration as they are measured in plasma. It is almost totally free of larger molecular weight substances. It might be noted that the concentration of albumin with a molecular weight of 68,000 is less than 1 per cent of the concentration of inulin in the ultrafiltrate as measured in Bowman's capsule.

THE TUBULES

The human kidney has at least two populations of nephrons. Those nephrons derived from cortical glomeruli are composed of a proximal convoluted segment, a straight descending segment

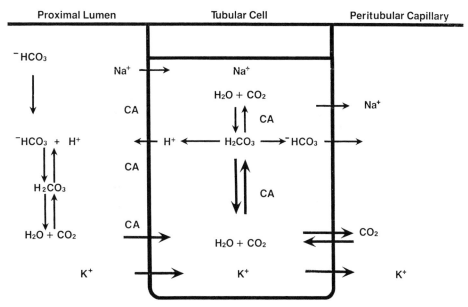

Figure 14-2 Luminal bicarbonate (HCO_3^-) combines with hydrogen (H^+) ion to form carbonic acid (H_2CO_3). In the presence of abundant carbonic anhydrase (CA), H_2CO_3 rapidly dissociates to carbon dioxide (CO_2) and water (H_2O). CO_2 diffuses back into the cells of the proximal tubule, where it is available for conversion to H^+ and HCO_3^-. The result is the generation of HCO_3^- and the excretion of H^+.

(pars rectus), a short diluting segment (short loop of Henle), and a thick ascending segment terminating at the macula densa where it becomes the distal convoluted tubule. For the purpose of conceptualizing various physiologic events as they relate to tubule function, renal physiologists have assigned functions to specific anatomic areas on the basis of in-vivo and in-vitro studies. It is worthy of mention that nature may not be as anatomically precise as the scientific community would choose; however, for the sake of simplicity, I shall observe the more precise assignments of function and duty.

In addition to the anatomic structures described for nephrons derived from cortical glomeruli, nephrons from the juxtamedullary glomeruli have a long descending and ascending medullary thin segment, some of which extend to the very tip of the renal papillae.

The proximal convoluted tubule is lined by thick cuboidal cells with a prominent brush border along the luminal surface. The ultrafiltrate of plasma is delivered in toto to this segment from Bowman's space, where roughly 60 per cent of the transluminal volume is reabsorbed by both active and passive mechanisms. Luminal fluid remains isosmotic to plasma as it transcends this tubule segment.

Within this segment active transport mechanisms have been demonstrated for sodium, potassium, glucose, amino acids, phosphate, and other less prominent cations and anions. The transport

of sodium appears to be of major importance in total volume removal, with a lesser role assigned to bicarbonate and potassium. Although a number of investigators have strongly suggested a direct transport mechanism for bicarbonate, the consensus of opinion at this writing favors the more classic description of hydrogen ion diffusion from the transluminal cells, formation of carbonic acid, rapid dissociation to $CO_2 + H_2O$ in the presence of abundant carbonic anhydrase, and diffusion of CO_2 intracellularly where it again becomes available for formation of the bicarbonate ion (see Fig. 14-2.)

Water passively follows the active transport of solute. The cells of the proximal tubules are aligned with their luminal membranes joined by so-called "tight junctions" (see Fig. 14-3). Between these tight junctions and the contraluminal membrane is an intercellular compartment, a site at which active transport of sodium ion is thought to occur. As sodium enters this paracellular channel, it increases the tonicity of the fluid, and water then moves toward the osmotic gradient thus created. These low resistant paracellular channels may play a major role in passive transfer of water and solute in the proximal tubule.

The nephrons of the juxtamedullary glomeruli have a long descending and ascending thin segment (see Fig. 14-4) which descends for a variable distance into the inner medulla. It is this highly specialized segment of tubule which in

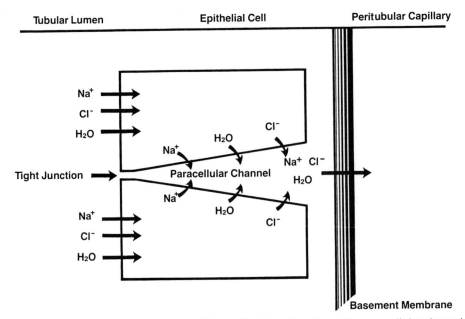

Figure 14–3 The cells of the proximal tubule with the "tight junctions" and the paracellular channel, a site at which active transport of sodium ion (Na^+) is thought to occur, creating an osmotic gradient for water (H_2O) and solute removal.

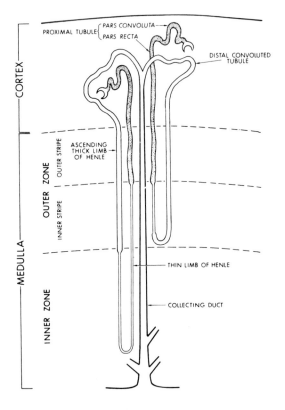

Figure 14–4 Diagram of the structural organization of the mammalian kidney to demonstrate the relationships between the various segments of the nephron and the zones of the kidney, especially the medulla. (From: Brenner, B. M. and Rector, F. C., Jr. (eds.): The Kidney. W. B. Saunders Comnpany, Philadelphia, 1976.)

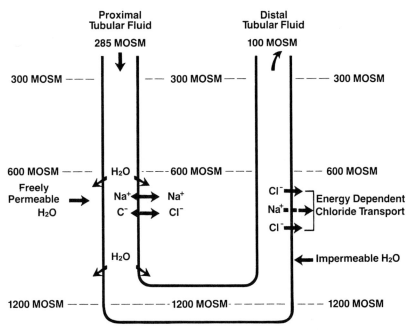

Figure 14–5 The descending limb is freely permeable to water (H_2O) and less so to solute. The ascending limb is impermeable to H_2O, coupled with an energy-dependent mechanism for the active transport of chloride.

conjunction with its closely associated vasa recta and collecting ducts provides the concentrating mechanism so critical to the mammalian kidney. Many models have been proposed to explain the complexities of this countercurrent system. Most have in common two major factors: (1) selective segmental permeability or impermeability to solute and water; (2) an energy-dependent active transport mechanism (see Fig. 14–5).

A simplified explanation of this countercurrent mechanism follows. Tubule fluid enters the descending thin segment of the loop of Henle from the pars rectus of the juxtamedullary nephron. At the point of entry it is isotonic to plasma. The descending thin segment is freely permeable to water and, to a lesser extent, solute. As the intraluminal fluid proceeds toward the inner medulla it is exposed to increasingly higher osmolalities and, because of the permeability factors noted, becomes progressively more hypertonic.

The ascending limb is highly impermeable to water; however, the active transport of chloride ion allows for the production of an increasingly dilute luminal fluid to a point where fluid is hypotonic to plasma as it enters the distal convoluted tubule. It is estimated that 25 per cent of the filtered load of sodium is absorbed by this chloride transport mechanism in the ascending thick segment and represents the primary source of energy expenditure for both concentration and dilution of urine.

The anatomic segment of the nephron extend-ing from the macula densa to the point of junction with other tubules to form the collecting duct is designated *the distal convoluted tubule*. The urine at its point of delivery to this tubule segment is hypotonic to plasma. Depending on the state of hydration, urine may be maintained in this hypotonic state or returned toward isotonicity — antidiuretic hormone (ADH) directly affects tubule permeability to water in the distal portions of this nephron segment. In addition to its role in concentration and dilution, the distal nephron plays a major role in the regulation of potassium and hydrogen excretion by the kidney. Renal handling of potassium and hydrogen will be discussed in greater detail in a later section of this chapter.

The collecting ducts are formed by the coalescence of several distal convoluted tubules and terminate in the ducts of Bellini. The epithelial cells lining this duct are selectively impermeable to the flux of water in the absence of ADH, resulting in the excretion of a highly dilute urine. In the presence of ADH, membrane permeability is enhanced many fold, allowing water to diffuse down a concentration gradient into the hypertonic interstitium of the medulla, resulting in final concentration of the urine. ADH has been shown to enhance selectively the diffusion of urea in segments of the collecting duct, further enhancing the establishment and maintenance of medullary hypertonicity. The collecting duct is capable of maintaining hydrogen ion gradients and plays an important role in the active transport of sodium from the tubule fluid. Although the absolute amount of sodium is small when compared to total filtered sodium, the collecting duct may serve as the ultimate fine tuning for sodium excretion.

SUMMARY

Roughly 25,000 mEq. of sodium ion are filtered by the normal glomerular mass in 24 hours. Approximately 65 per cent of the filtered sodium ion is absorbed in the proximal tubule by a process of active transfer. Twenty-five per cent is absorbed in the loop of Henle secondary to active transport of chloride ion in the ascending thick segment. Less than 10 per cent is absorbed by an active process in the distal convoluted tubule; approximately 1 per cent is absorbed in the collecting duct; and less than 1 per cent is finally excreted in the urine.

The renal handling of water is entirely passive — movement of water throughout the kidney is dependent on solute concentration. Bulk water movement is dependent on the active transport of sodium ion. The kidney is unique as far as we know in that the ascending loop of Henle and the collecting duct have the capability of remaining impermeable to water despite continued solute transport. It is this property which allows the kidney to form a dilute urine and at the same time to establish osmotic gradients necessary for final urinary concentration.

Potassium is filtered at the glomerulus, with 85 to 90 per cent active reabsorption occurring in the proximal tubule. Some additional absorption occurs in the ascending limb of Henle's loop secondary to chloride transport. Intraluminal fluid reaching the distal tubule is almost potassium-free. In this tubule segment there is a bidirectional flux of potassium ion. The intracellular potassium ion of tubule cells is high and enters tubule fluid probably by passive flux from the higher concentration in the cell to the lower concentration in the tubule fluid. Final concentration may be determined by the rate at which potassium ion is actively pumped against the gradient back into the cell.

Potassium transport in the distal segment is under partial control of aldosterone. Although there is a loose relationship between potassium ion concentration, sodium, and hydrogen ion, there is not a tightly coupled exchange mechanism as was previously thought to exist.

The kidneys are responsible for the removal of roughly 75 mEq. of hydrogen ion per 24 hours under usual conditions of intermediary metabolism. Metabolic derangements associated with various pathologic states may produce a many

fold increase in hydrogen ion excretion. At least three physiologic mechanisms exist within the kidney to meet this need. There may be more.

Bicarbonate, because of its small molecular size, is freely filterable at the glomerulus and reaches the proximal convoluted tubule in concentration equivalent to that found in plasma (24 to 26 mM. per liter). Transcending the early portion of this tubule segment it is rapidly removed from the tubule fluid as it combines with hydrogen ion entering the lumen from the paratubular cells ($H^+ + HCO_3^- \rightarrow H_2CO_3 \rightarrow H_2O + CO_2$). The CO_2 and H_2O are free to diffuse across the peritubular membrane (see Fig. 14–2). By this process one hydrogen ion molecule has been effectively eliminated and a bicarbonate radical returned to the general circulation to sustain the intact bicarbonate buffering system. As the luminal fluid proceeds down the tubule, there is a slight rise in hydrogen ion concentration as bulk bicarbonate is removed and is no longer available for combination with hydrogen ion. There is little reason to believe that the loop of Henle plays a major role in renal acidification mechanisms.

Tubule fluid reaching the distal segment of the nephron under normal circumstances contains little or no bicarbonate. In certain pathologic or drug-induced states, bicarbonate may be delivered to this segment, and under these circumstances regeneration of bicarbonate takes place in the distal nephron. Under more usual physiologic conditions, hydrogen ion is secreted into tubule fluid against a concentration gradient, allowing the hydrogen ion concentration to rise selectively. Tubule cells here are relatively impermeable to the back diffusion of hydrogen ion, a property also inherent to the cells of the collecting duct.

Ammonia production plays a major role in the kidney's ability to excrete an excess hydrogen ion load. The ability to produce ammonia by the selective degradation of the amino acid glutamine is a property inherent in all tubule cells. Ammonia thus formed is free to diffuse into the luminal fluid, where it binds with accessible hydrogen ion forming the ammonium radical, NH_4^+. The peritubular cell membranes are much less permeable to this radical. In essence it is now trapped in the tubular lumen, has buffered a hydrogen ion, and is excreted in the final urine. Under conditions of excessive hydrogen ion load, this accounts for the major route of hydrogen ion removal.

CLINICAL EVALUATION OF RENAL FUNCTION

The problem facing the physician in diagnosing renal disease is the relatively long asymptomatic period found in almost all types of kidney disorders. When the patient finally seeks attention, it is frequently too late to alter the course of his basic disease process. The importance of finding early disease cannot be overstressed. Only through a complete history and physical examination and the proper use of laboratory procedures does a physician have a chance to offer his patient help before it is too late.

The *urinalysis* is the most helpful and frequently the most overlooked renal function study in clinical medicine. It is often relegated to the least skilled member of the laboratory staff, who does it without interest or skill. In addition, the importance of collection and rapid evaluation after collection is overlooked. The best specimens are collected by the "clean-catch" method and examined promptly. Allowing urine to sit for any amount of time leads to destruction of the formed elements through changes in pH and osmotic pressures. I strongly recommend that in any patient suspected of having renal disease the physician examine each urine specimen under the microscope.

The finding of *protein* in the urine — by any method and in any amount — is reason for further evaluation. Proteinuria is the hallmark of renal disease. The lack of protein in the urine suggests that renal disease is not present; however, even this is not conclusive. A number of disease processes may present with minimal or no proteinuria. Examples are obstruction, hypercalcemia, hypokalemia, chronic pyelonephritis, arterio- and nephrosclerosis, polycystic disease, congenital diseases of the tubule, analgesic abuse nephritis, neoplasms, stones, and congenital malformations. The amount of protein found in 24 hours is of prime importance, both diagnostically and prognostically. Persistent proteinuria inevitably indicates renal disease. Even amounts only minimally in excess of normal may be of significance. Under normal circumstances, very little albumin is filtered at the glomerulus. Various investigators have estimated the rate of albumin filtration at 12 mg. per kg. per 24-hour period: a normal excretion rate at 2 mg. per kg. per 24-hour period. The 10-mg. per kg. per 24-hours represents proximal tubule transport of albumin by an energy-dependent process of pinocytosis. This means that a 70-kg. man would be expected to excrete no more than 140 mg. of albumin in any 24-hour period. The kidney normally secretes, probably by tubule cells, a globulin (Tamm-Horsfall protein) which occurs naturally in the urine in very minute quantities. The amount of protein excreted in any 24-hour period is useful in making a clinical assessment of the area of the kidney involved in the disease process. Patients with primary tubule disease usually will excrete less than 3 g. per day. Patients with disease processes related to glomerular basement membrane damage may be expected to excrete protein in excess of 3 g. per day and can reach values of 30 to 40 g. per day.

Normally a small amount of *glucose* appears in the urine in the range of 100 to 200 mg. per 24 hours. The appearance of glucose in excess of this amount is indication that the tubule process for glucose transport has been exceeded. This may indicate that plasma glucose is high or that tubule defects exist which have lowered the renal threshold for glucose. Renal glycosuria is frequently found in association with other proximal tubule transport defects, such as aminoaciduria, uric acid, and phosphate wasting.

The *pH* of the urine is routinely tested in the standard urinalysis. The kidney is capable of excreting urine over a wide range of pH's from 4.5 to 8.5. Man normally excretes the hydrogen ion produced from the metabolism of carbohydrate, lipids, and sulfa-containing amino acids in two forms. Thirty to 50 mEq. of hydrogen ion per 24 hours are excreted in combination with ammonia. Ten to 30 mEq. per 24 hours of hydrogen ion are excreted as so-called titratable acidity. Hydrogen ion in this form is, for the most part, buffered by either phosphate or creatinine. The finding of a pH of 5.5 or below in a urinalysis signifies that tubule mechanisms of acidification are intact. The finding of a value above this in a routine urinalysis does not imply that these mechanisms are defective. This can only be evaluated by stressing the patient with a hydrogen ion load. Failure to acidify may suggest such diseases as renal tubule acidosis, early pyelonephritis, primary aldosterone secreting tumor, or hypokalemia. The failure of the kidney to excrete hydrogen ion in renal disease results in its retention and leads to chronic metabolic acidosis, which is always seen with severe azotemia. In certain types of renal disease systemic acidosis may develop even though the glomerular filtration rate is well preserved. Renal tubule acidosis and analgesic-abuse nephritis are two examples of disease processes in which a relatively alkaline urine may be excreted in the face of metabolic acidosis.

Specific gravity is an indirect measurement of urine osmolality and thus of the kidney's ability to concentrate or dilute urine. Because specific gravity depends on the density and number of particles of solute rather than their absolute concentration, at times it may be misleading. Large amounts of protein or glucose in the urine may give the false impression of an ability to concentrate when that ability no longer exists. A direct measurement of urine osmolality is much more specific in establishing concentration or dilution abilities. This is done on as little as 2 ml. of urine by freezing point determination: osmolalities may range from as low as 40 to as high as 1400 mOsm. per kg. water. The finding of a fixed urine osmolality indicates a significant loss of functional renal mass. Tests of concentrating ability are frequently used to determine early damage to the kidney, especially in pyelonephritis or other forms of interstitial nephritis. Ability to form a highly concentrated urine indicates a relative intact medulla, ascending and descending loop of Henle, collecting duct and posterior pituitary. In the oliguric patient a specific gravity of 1.020 or an osmolality of 600 or above is considered indication of prerenal etiology for oliguria.

The *microscopic examination* of the urinary sediment is the most important part of the study to be done by the physician. This should be done only on a fresh specimen of urine. First, an unspun specimen should be searched for bacteria and cells. If bacteria are present, the assumption can be made that their numbers in the urine exceed 100,000 per ml. The urine should then be spun for five minutes at 2000 rpm. Staining is used in some laboratories for cell differentiation; however, in general it is not necessary. The quantitative evaluation of cells and types and number of casts produced by the kidney can be done with a 12- or 24-hour Addis count. In the 12-hour Addis count one normally expects to see 2000 hyaline casts, 130,000 to 300,000 red cells, and 650,000 to 1,000,000 white cells. In the normal urinalysis a small number of cells can often be seen: 2 to 3 red cells; 4 to 5 white cells per high powered field on a spun specimen, and an occasional hyaline cast are accepted as normal. The finding of red blood cells in the urine is indicative only of blood loss. The origin of these red cells cannot be localized to bladder, prostate, urethra, ureter, or kidneys. The finding of red blood cell casts indicates primary renal parenchymal involvement. Red cell casts do not persist in alkaline or hypotonic urine, and, therefore, repeated examinations may be necessary to rule out the presence of casts when one is searching for a primary glomerular lesion. Red cell casts are strongly suggestive of primary glomerular involvement, whether it be glomerulonephritis, angiitis, lupus, or periarteritis. They may also be found in malignant hypertension, acute tubular necrosis, and following trauma to the kidney. White blood cells and white blood cell casts may be found in increased numbers in any type of renal parenchymal lesion. White cells may be excreted at any point along the urinary tract, and their origin cannot be determined specifically by examination of the urine. The occurrence of large numbers of white cell casts is a strong indication that the renal parenchyma itself is involved in the disease process.

Routine biochemical evaluation of most patients entering the hospital includes a blood urea nitrogen (BUN) as an indicator of renal dysfunc-

tion. Unfortunately, as a screening test the BUN lacks sensitivity, as significant rises occur only after substantial loss of renal function. Changes in BUN are also dependent on the state of protein catabolism and may be found artificially low or high on that basis, independent of normal renal function.

A more informative clinical study is a direct or indirect measurement of *glomerular filtration rate*. In order to determine glomerular filtration rate, a substance must have the following characteristics: (1) It should neither be absorbed nor secreted by the renal tubule. (2) It must not be protein bound. (3) It must be easily measured in the serum and urine and be non-toxic. (4) It must have a molecular weight compatible with unimpeded filtration at the glomerulus.

The reference standard for measuring glomerular filtration rate in humans is inulin. Unfortunately, the performance of a clearance evaluation using inulin is cumbersome and necessitates a constant intravenous infusion and catheterization of the bladder. Urea, which is the end-product of protein metabolism, does not come close to fulfilling any of the prerequisites of a substance for measuring glomerular filtration rate. Urea is not only filtered — it is absorbed in significant quantities along the tubule and the collecting duct. Its clearance depends to a large extent on the rate of urine formation. As urine flow decreases, larger amounts of urea are resorbed, leading to significant decreases in clearance rate in the face of a normal glomerular filtration. At high urine flow rates, the clearance of urea is roughly 70 per cent of the clearance of inulin.

A more reliable marker of clinical renal function is creatinine. Creatinine is a normal end-product of muscle metabolism. Its plasma concentration and 24-hour urinary excretion are relatively constant. They are not influenced by diet, metabolic rate, exercise, or urine flow. It is these several advantages over urea that have made it acceptable as a routine measurement of glomerular filtration rate. The usual formula for calculating the glomerular filtration rate is: GFR is equal to the urinary concentration (U) of creatinine times the volume (V) divided by the plasma concentration (P) of creatinine: $GFR = U V/P$. Unfortunately, in man creatinine is not only filtered, but small quantities are also secreted by the renal tubule. Fortuitously, the Jaffe chemical determination of plasma creatinine measures not only true creatinine, but also a group of substances known as creatinine chromogens. These substances are not secreted and do not appear in the urine. This results in a falsely high plasma creatinine value which is balanced by the increase in creatinine excretion secondary to tubule secretion. As renal function fails, the serum creatinine rises, but the chromogens remain relatively unchanged. The result is that creatinine clearance in patients with renal disease reflects a certain amount of secretion, producing an artificially high creatinine clearance in patients with far advanced renal failure. Serial determinations and observations are therefore superior to any single observation, and the use of multiple determinations allows for a check on accuracy and the rate of progression of the disease. The following substances may interfere with the Jaffe reaction for creatinine: acetone, aceto-acetic acid, ascorbic acid, barbiturates, BSP, and PSP. The normal creatinine clearance values are as follows: men, creatinine clearance of 120 ± 25 ml./min.; women, creatinine clearance of 96 ± 13 ml./min. When corrected for body surface area, the values are: men, 103 ± 15 ml./min. per 1.7M.^{2}; women, 97 ± 9 ml./min. per 1.73M.^{2}

The creatinine clearance is by far the most sensitive regular clinical test of renal function available today. It is necessary to reemphasize the importance of obtaining serial values rather than trusting a single determination. The use of serum creatinine as an estimate of renal function is not as accurate as a clearance value, but it is a much more sensitive reflection of early changes of renal function than is the BUN. Normal values of creatinine vary depending on the method and specimen used. When plasma and the Jaffe method are used, the upper limits of normal values are as follows: men, creatinine 0.8–1.2; women, 0.6–1.1 mg./100 ml. A rough estimate of renal function ability can be made using the following schedule: serum creatinine of 1 mg. = 100 per cent normal function; serum creatinine of 2 mg. = 50 per cent or less of normal renal function; serum creatinine of 4 mg. = 25 per cent or less of normal renal function.

The BUN/creatinine ratio is a commonly derived function in many automated clinical laboratories and, under certain circumstances, can be used to draw additional clinical data about the status of renal function. This comparison takes advantage of the two different patterns of excretion of these compounds. Normal individuals are expected to maintain a BUN/creatinine ratio of approximately 10. The following is a list of reasons for this ratio exceeding 10:

1. Excessive ingestion of protein in a patient with depressed renal function.
2. Blood in the small intestine.
3. Excessive protein catabolism. This may be due to a variety of reasons, such as burns, fever, steroids, wasting, or trauma.
4. Marked glomerular-tubule imbalance — a finding most often related to underperfusion of the kidney. The glomerular filtration is relatively maintained, but absorption of urea becomes more complete. Dehydration and congestive heart failure are common examples of this phenomenon.

In certain circumstances the BUN/creatinine ratio may be less than 10, e.g., a patient with very low protein intake in renal disease. Low protein diets are frequently used in the treatment of renal failure, and the BUN in these patients no longer reflects the reduced functional capacity of the kidney. In these incidences, BUN's falling within the normal range may occur in patients with creatinine clearances of less than 20. Other examples can relate to excessive vomiting, diarrhea, or hepatic insufficiency.

The laboratory functions and studies which we have discussed are those commonly available to any physician from a routine reference laboratory. It is beyond the scope of this discussion to evaluate the application of more sophisticated radiologic, immunologic, and isotope studies in evaluation of renal function. It is pertinent to know that they exist and that their application is often indicated to delineate further the extent of renal embarrassment. The importance of serial testing should always be kept in mind. The use of multiple tests on individual patients will give a better evaluation than any single determination. The rate of change of functional testing is more important than the information gained from a single battery of tests.

DISORDERS OF SODIUM METABOLISM

Sodium is the major extracellular cation. The normal plasma sodium is 142 mEq. per liter. The intracellular sodium is less than 10 mEq. per liter of cell water (normal muscle cell). The total body sodium of a normal adult male averages 60 mEq. per kg. of body weight. A 70-kg. man contains some 4200 mEq. of sodium. Bone contains between 40 and 45 per cent of the total body stores of sodium. Accordingly, about 50 per cent of total sodium is extracellular, 40 per cent is associated with bone, and 10 per cent is intracellular. Exchangeable sodium amounts to 42 mEq. per kg. of body weight. This fraction includes all extracellular and intracellular sodium and slightly less than half of the bone sodium. If sodium is lost in sweat, urine or diarrheal fluid, that present in the exchangeable reservoir, including the exchangeable sodium of the cancellous bone is available to mitigate the decrease in concentration which would otherwise occur when body water is restored. When sodium is retained it is distributed into the subject's exchangeable reservoir.

The average American diet contains sodium far in excess of usual body requirements calculated at roughly 50 mEq. per day. The normal gastrointestinal tract has an almost unlimited capacity for sodium absorption. There is little net transport of sodium in the stomach. The bulk of ingested sodium absorption occurs in the small bowel (both jejunum and ileum), with final conservation occurring in the colon, leaving a residual stool sodium for excretion of between 5 and 10 mEq. per 24 hours. It must be recalled that sodium is also a major ionic constituent of gastrointestinal secretions, and the net absorption of sodium by the bowel may, under normal conditions, exceed 1500 mEq. per 24 hours. Sodium transport, at least in the colon, is facilitated by the presence of aldosterone.

Under normal physiologic circumstances, the kidney is the major route for excretion of excess body sodium. Under conditions of stress, such as continued vomiting or prolonged diarrhea, the gastrointestinal tract can make a major contribution to the depletion of total body sodium. Cutaneous losses of sodium vary widely with the individual, his activity and conditioning, and with environmental factors. Sweat sodium varies directly with the rate of sweat formation. An individual in a resting state may have less than 30 mEq. of sodium per liter in his sweat. As the ambient temperature rises, or his endogenous production of heat increases, his rate of sweating increases as does the concentration of sodium in the sweat. At high rates of sweating (as much as 700 ml./hr. under maximal stimulation), sodium losses increase dramatically, sometimes in excess of 100 mEq. per liter of sweat. It is apparent that prolonged exposure to conditions associated with sweating at a maximal rate can lead rapidly to severe body depletion of both salt and water. It is important to note that sweat is always hypotonic to plasma, and thus profuse sweating without access to water replacement can lead to a clinical state of hypernatremia. Sodiums of 165 to 170 mEq. per liter have been reported in otherwise healthy athletes undergoing vigorous exercise and denied free access to fluid replacement.

The normal functioning kidney is the ultimate regulatory organ for total body sodium. A 70-kg. man will form roughly 180 liters of plasma ultrafiltrate per day at the glomerulus. This means that in excess of 25,000 mEq. of sodium are presented to the renal tubule each 24 hours, where more than 99 per cent is selectively reabsorbed. Under conditions of maximum stress and salt loading, individual cases have been reported where 65 per cent of the filtered load of sodium can be excreted by the appropriately functioning kidney. I have previously discussed the more intricate details of tubule handling of sodium, and the reader is referred back to that section of this chapter for review.

Hypernatremia can be divided into two major classifications: (1) that associated with dehydration; or (2) the inappropriate conservation of water. Dehydration occurs when excessive body water is lost in comparison to total body sodium. This state of affairs is most commonly associated with disease processes which either limit the access of the individual to water, or associated with excessive losses of water, most commonly through the gastrointestinal tract. Increased insensible water losses may also lead to a state of hypernatremia and dehydration. Common causes for this pathologic state to develop are associated with hyperventilation or fever. Inappropriate conservation of water is usually divided into central and nephrogenic *diabetes insipidus.*

Central diabetes insipidus is always associated with the absence or less than normal release of antidiuretic hormone (ADH) secondary to appropriate stimuli. Central diabetes insipidus is associated with some form of central nervous system disease, although the idiopathic variety has been recognized with no demonstrable central nervous system pathology. Nephrogenic diabetes insipidus is either an acquired or hereditary disorder. The hereditary disorder is characterized by insensitivity of the collecting duct to antidiuretic hormone. The disorder usually presents in childhood with recurrent dehydration, a dilute urine and failure to thrive. In this disorder ADH has no effect on renal concentration. There is no other demonstrable renal lesion. Proximal tubule anatomic anomalies have been described, but their significance is uncertain. Inheritance is sex-linked dominant, and most cases occur in males; heterologous females may have some limitation of concentrating ability.

A more common form of nephrogenic diabetes insipidus is the acquired variety. This may be related to metabolic anomalies, certain disease processes or the administration of a variety of drugs. Examples of nephrogenic diabetes insipidus in which the distal nephron and collecting duct have become insensitive to the action of antidiuretic hormone include: hypokalemia, hypercalcemia, sickle cell disease, amyloidosis, Sjogren's syndrome, de-Toni-Fanconi syndrome, post-urinary tract obstruction, acute tubule necrosis, radiation nephritis, the administration of methoxyflurane, lithium, colchicine, vincristine, and demeclocycline. In the syndrome secondary to drug administration the process is usually a reversible one and the sensitivity to the actions of ADH returns with the removal of the drug.

Hyponatremia is one of the more common fluid and electrolyte anomalies seen in the practice of clinical medicine (Table 14–1). Dilutional hyponatremia is the most commonly occurring disorder of sodium metabolism. With dilutional hyponatremia, the total body sodium in relation to ideal body weight is normal, but the patient is incapable of excreting a water load. Frequently sodium has been restricted while free access to water continues and the patient becomes volume-

TABLE 14–1 HYPONATREMIA

1. Dilutional
2. Depletion
3. Factitious
   a. Hyperglycemia
   b. Hyperlipemia
   c. Hyperproteinemia
4. Diuretic-Induced
   a. Dilutional
   b. Depletion
   c. Hypokalemia
5. Hypothyroidism
6. Adrenal Insufficiency
7. Inappropriate Secretion Antidiuretic Hormone
   a. Malignant tumors
   b. Central nervous system disease
   c. Pulmonary disease
   d. Drugs

thought to relate to the activation of compensatory mechanisms to maintain volume. The continued and inappropriate elaboration of antidiuretic hormone results in expansion of total body fluid volume. Proximal tubule transport of sodium is depressed in an attempt to correct volume expansion, and significant sodium losses result. A number of drugs have been implicated in the production of this syndrome. The drug actions may be one of two varieties. The drug may act at the central nervous system level to stimulate excessive elaboration of pitressin or facilitate its action at the distal nephron and collecting duct. Examples of drugs which have been implicated in the production of inappropriate antidiuretic hormone syndrome are: barbiturates; morphine; nicotine; chlorpropamide; cytoxin; vincristine; clofibrate; norepinephrine; and prostaglandins.

expanded relative to the total body sodium. Classic examples include congestive heart failure and liver disease. This form of hyponatremia is simply corrected by restricting the patient's free access to water in conjunction with sodium restriction. Hyponatremia on the basis of total body sodium depletion is commonly associated with the administration of various diuretics and, again, the continued access to unlimited intake of volume. In this case, as opposed to the dilutional process, the total body sodium is depleted over a period of time, volume is replaced and hyponatremia is the end result. Factitious hyponatremia may be seen as the direct result of at least three common alterations of internal metabolism. In patients with severe hyperglycemia, the osmotic gradients produced in the interstitial space and plasma volume by excess glucose result in an influx of water in an attempt to maintain osmotic neutrality, and the serum sodium is artificially depressed. Total body sodium is normal and correction of hyperglycemia results in the correction of hyponatremia.

A second cause of hyponatremia on a factitious basis is hyperlipemia. In this case the distribution of sodium within the water component of the vascular space is entirely normal. That component has been significantly reduced by the high circulating concentrations of lipids. A syndrome similar to this has been described with hyperproteinemia exemplified by multiple myeloma and other disproteinemic syndromes. Hyponatremia may develop in cases of severe hypothyroidism and has long been recognized as a potential component of adrenal insufficiency.

The syndrome of *inappropriate ADH secretion* occurs secondary to a variety of clinical diseases. These include various malignant tumors, central nervous system disorders, and pulmonary disease. The pathophysiology which develops is

DISORDERS OF POTASSIUM METABOLISM

Potassium is the major intracellular cation. An average man has a total body potassium of 40 mEq. per kilogram and a woman slightly less. Ninety-eight per cent of the potassium pool is concentrated within the cells. Direct measurements of potassium within muscle intracellular water record values of 160 mEq. per liter. Normal concentration of extracellular potassium are recorded between 3.5 and 5.5 mEq. per liter of plasma. These transmembrane gradients for potassium are maintained within narrow limits by active transport of sodium from the cell and active transport of potassium into the cell.

The human diet is high in potassium and greatly exceeds daily body requirements. The kidney is the primary organ of excretion, gastrointestinal losses accounting for less than 10 mEq. per day. With prolonged nausea and/or diarrhea, gastrointestinal losses of potassium may be enhanced to the point of producing a clinical state of hypokalemia.

A number of mechanisms contribute to the regulation of total body potassium and its distribution within the body. The status of hydrogen ion concentration has a major impact on distribution and excretion of potassium. With hydrogen ion in excess, there is an increased flux of potassium from the cells as hydrogen ion enters. A direct result is a rise in serum potassium. At the same time, intracellular potassium is lowered, becoming less readily available for secretion by the distal tubule segment and/or the collecting duct, impairing renal mechanisms for potassium excretion.

Bicarbonate has an action on transmembrane potassium transport independent of hydrogen ion concentration. When pH is maintained by elevating the CO_2 and bicarbonate is increased, there is a significant shift of potassium intracellularly. This has been suspected by clinicians for many years, but only recently confirmed in experimental animals.

The mineralocorticoid, aldosterone, plays a major role in the internal regulation of potassium. In all probability, aldosterone promotes the intracellular flux of potassium of all cells. This may assume particular significance in the renal handling of potassium. In the presence of aldosterone, cells of the distal nephron and collecting duct are able to concentrate potassium, allowing for its increased flux into the tubule fluid and ultimate excretion. The ability of the distal nephron and collecting duct to secrete potassium is dependent upon the rate of flow of tubule fluid. When the flow rate is diminished, the secretion of potassium also diminishes. In states of potassium depletion the distal nephron and collecting duct have the ability to further the conservation of potassium by selectively removing it from the tubule fluid. In states of chronic potassium overload and perhaps uremia, the ability of these segments to secrete potassium is enhanced. The action of aldosterone on sodium transport mechanisms in these tubule segments is thought to be independent of this effect on potassium.

Insulin has been shown to promote cellular uptake of potassium independent of its action on glucose. Epinephrine infusion is followed by an initial rise in plasma potassium, followed shortly thereafter by a prolonged period of hypokalemia. This action is explained by an initial release of potassium from cells followed by an increase in potassium uptake by the liver.

It is beyond the limited scope of this discussion to review all known clinical disorders with which

TABLE 14–2   CLINICAL STATES ASSOCIATED WITH HYPOKALEMIA

1. Inappropriate Intake
2. Disorders Internal Distribution
   a. Metabolic alkalosis
   b. Hyperinsulinism
   c. Periodic paralysis
3. Inappropriate Excretion
   a. Renal tubule acidosis
   b. Mineralocorticoid excess
   c. Licorice abuse
   d. Salt-losing nephropathies
   e. Bartter's syndrome
   f. Interstitial nephritis
   g. Diuretic therapy
4. Inappropriate Gastrointestinal Losses
   a. Vomiting
   b. Nasogastric suction
   c. Diarrhea
   d. Laxative abuse
   e. Villous adenoma

hypokalemia may be associated (Table 14–2). Rather, I shall concentrate on broad categories based on the mechanisms of potassium regulation.

Hypokalemia.   Maintaining a normal potassium balance requires: (1) *adequate intake*; (2) *appropriate internal distribution* between intra- and extracellular fluid compartments, and appropriate control and function of (3) *mechanisms of excretion*. A state of clinical hypokalemia can result from alteration in any of these integrated functions. Hypokalemia may result following upper gastrointestinal disease with associated vomiting or nasogastric suction. Depending on its level of secretion, GI contents may contain potassium concentrations in excess of 20 MEq. per liter. Over a prolonged period, losses of this nature can result in serious depletion. With loss of accompanying hydrogen ion, the situation may be complicated by metabolic alkalosis with further depression of serum potassium.

Disease processes associated with alterations of internal mechanisms of control are exemplified by primary hyperaldosteronism, where hypokalemia results from a combination of inappropriate distribution, excessive excretion, and metabolic alkalosis.

Disease processes associated with alteration in the mechanisms of potassium excretion may result in hypokalemia. A classic example is renal tubule acidosis, Type I, where failure of appropriate hydrogen ion excretion results in excessive losses of potassium. A more complete list of known causes of hypokalemia appears in Table 14–2.

The clinical manifestations associated with hypokalemia relate to the skeletal muscle, smooth muscle, kidneys, and the cardiac conducting system. Reduction in plasma potassium concentration leads to an increase in resting membrane potential by altering the ratio of the concentration of intracellular potassium to extracellular potassium. Membrane excitability is reduced, and muscle weakness, or even paralysis, is the result. Signs and symptoms of muscle weakness do not commonly occur until plasma potassium values drop below 2.5 mEq. per liter; however, many factors such as plasma calcium, hydrogen ion concentration, and the state of intracellular potassium stores may modify response. The distribution of muscular weakness is characteristic, with early involvement of the lower extremities, followed by muscles of the trunk, upper extremities, and ultimate involvement of the muscles of respiration. In severe cases, rhabdomyolysis and myoglobinuria may occur. Smooth muscle involvement can lead to paralytic ileus.

In the human kidney potassium deficiency after a period of time leads to a characteristic vacuolar lesion in the tubule cells of the proximal nephron, which rarely may occur in the distal nephron as well. A common clinical manifestation is impairment in the ability to excrete a concentrated urine. This inability to concentrate is secondary to a decreased sensitivity to antidiuretic hormone. The degree of polyuria is less than that described with diabetes insipidus of a central origin.

Metabolic alkalosis is a commonly associated phenomenon in states of hypokalemia. With reduction in intracellular potassium, the hydrogen ion concentration rises. Hydrogen ion is then more available for resorption, thus sustaining the continuing metabolic alkalosis. Hypokalemia reduces the ability of the kidney to excrete or conserve a sodium or water load appropriately. In the face of a high sodium diet, this can lead to fluid retention and the formation of edema.

The electrocardiogram reflects the electrical events of the heart. The P wave represents atrial depolarization, the QRS complex ventricular depolarization, and the ST segment, T, and U waves ventricular repolarization. Hypokalemia produces characteristic changes in the electrocardiogram that are primarily due to delayed ventricular repolarization. The result is ST segment depression, decreased amplitude or inversion of the T wave, and increased height of the U wave with prolongation of the Q-U interval. With more severe hypokalemia, increased amplitude of the P wave, prolongation of the P-R interval, and widening of the QRS complex may occur. There may be a variety of associated cardiac arrhythmias, including premature atrial or ventricular beats, sinus bradycardia, paroxysmal atrial tachycardia, Wenckebach block, atrioventricular dissociation, nodal tachycardia, or ventricular fibrillation. The frequency and severity of arrhythmias are increased in the presence of digitalis preparations.

Hyperkalemia. In clinical medicine hyperkalemia can be divided into but two categories. The first is inappropriate internal distribution between the intracellular and extracellular fluid compartments. A classic example is untreated diabetic ketoacidosis, where total body potassium is oftentimes reduced despite significant elevations in serum potassium.

The second category includes the pathologic states associated with the inability of the kidney to excrete potassium appropriately. Whether as the result of reduction in functioning renal mass or the absence of aldosterone, the end result is the same — inadequate excretion of potassium with all the hazards pursuant thereto. A list of common causes of hyperkalemia is presented in Table 14–3.

Clinical signs and symptoms of hyperkalemia relate to the skeletal muscles and conducting system of the myocardium. Muscle weakness is the most common finding. It characteristically begins in the lower extremities. This muscle weakness or

TABLE 14–3 CLINICAL STATES ASSOCIATED WITH HYPERKALEMIA

1. Disorders of Internal Distribution
   a. Acidosis
   b. Insulin deficiency
   c. Tissue catabolism
   d. Periodic paralysis—hyperkalemic
   e. Succinylcholine
2. Disorders of Urinary Excretion
   a. Renal failure
   b. Adrenal insufficiency
   c. Administration of potassium-sparing diuretics
      1. Triamterine
      2. Spironolactone
   d. Volume depletion

paralysis is a result of a reduction in resting membrane potential as the ratio of intracellular potassium to extracellular potassium shifts toward unity. The cell membrane is unable to repolarize after a single depolarization stimulus. Elevations in serum potassium lead to a number of characteristic changes in the electrocardiogram, which may be progressive to the point of ventricular stand-still or fibrillation as potassium continues to rise. Although observations of changing electrocardiographic signs are helpful, it is critical to note that there is no clear-cut correlation with serum potassium. Any electrocardiographic changes of hyperkalemia are considered signs of serious intoxication and a need for prompt institution of corrective measures. The earliest changes in the cardiogram are peaking of T waves with shortening of the Q-T segment, reflecting rapid repolarization. More advanced changes include widening of the QRS complex, widening of the PR interval, diminished amplitude, and widening of P waves with eventual disappearance. The QRS complex will finally widen out to blend with the T wave in the so-called "sine-wave."

DISORDERS OF HYDROGEN ION CONCENTRATION

Disorders of acid-base balance are, by today's standards, entirely too commonplace in the practice of clinical medicine. No doubt they have always been present; however, with the advent of arterial blood gases and pH as common laboratory determinants, they are more readily recognized, requiring an appropriate understanding and response on the part of the physician. Understanding is critical if response is to be appropriate.

pH is a physical-chemical term with which we physicians have been saddled and befuddled since our thought processes turned toward an under-

TABLE 14–4 COMPARISON OF HYDROGEN ION [H⁺] TO pH

pH	[H⁺] nanomoles/L.
7.8	16
7.7	20
7.6	26
7.5	32
7.4	40
7.3	50
7.2	63
7.1	80
7.0	100
6.9	125
6.8	160

standing of internal metabolism, and, like so many anachronisms of medicine, would best be discarded. Unfortunately — I am afraid for the foreseeable future — we will continue to suffer with this term, but may still overcome if we learn automatically to convert our thinking from pH to hydrogen ion concentration [H⁺]. [H⁺] is a reciprocal function of pH, therefore, as [H⁺] rises, pH drops, and vice versa. [H⁺] can be considered in exactly the same fashion we consider Na^+, K^+, CO_2^-, HCO_3^-, Cl^-, recognizing that [H⁺] is found in the plasma in concentrations at roughly one-millionth the concentration of the other commonly measured cations and anions. [H⁺] can be expressed concurrently as nanomoles or nanoequivalents, which is 10^{-6} millimoles. A value of 40 nanomoles of [H⁺] per liter equals a pH value of 7.40. The entire range of [H⁺] compatible with life covers only a tenfold range, from a low of 16 nanomoles per liter to a high of 160 nanomoles per liter (see Table 14–4).

With this simple understanding we have taken a giant step forward. When a patient is acidotic, [H⁺] is high; when a patient is alkalotic, [H⁺] is low. This is an absolute and never changes. We now have only to establish the cause and we are well on our way to appropriate correction.

The concentration of hydrogen ion in the body is interrelated with the concentrations of the major extracellular cation, sodium, and the major intracellular cation, potassium. The absolute status of hydrogen ion concentration is controlled by but three known mechanisms. These mechanisms are: (1) Buffering, which takes place both intra- and extracellularly — in simple terms, this is any molecule which can readily give up or receive a hydrogen ion in response to minor changes in concentration. (2) The ability of the lung to remove CO_2, raising or reducing the alveolar partial pressure of CO_2 and, thus, plasma CO_2. (3) The ability of the kidney to increase or decrease plasma bicarbonate by hydrogen ion secretion in response to changes in [H⁺]. A brief discussion of each of these mechanisms is in order.

Extracellular Buffers. In the extracellular fluid bicarbonate is the most important buffer due to its relatively high concentration and the ability to vary the P_{CO_2} through changes in alveolar ventilation. An appropriate formulation of this reaction is: $CO_2 + H_2O \rightleftarrows H_2CO_3 \rightleftarrows H^+ + HCO_3^-$. All gases dissolve in water to a greater or lesser extent, the degree to which this occurs is proportional to the partial pressure of the gas in the solution. In the human, the partial pressure of CO_2 in arterial blood is in equilibrium with that in the alveolar space and normally approximates 40 mm. Hg. At 37° C. the amount of CO_2 dissolved in the plasma is: dissolved $CO_2 = 0.03\ P_{CO_2} = 0.03 \times 40 - 1.2$ mM./L., where 0.03 is the solubility constant for CO_2. The equilibrium of the reaction, dissolved $CO_2 + H_2O = H_2CO_3$, under normal physiologic circumstances, favors the reaction to the left. Approximately 500 molecules of CO_2 are in solution for each molecule of H_2CO_3. The degree to which H_2CO_3 dissolves into $H^+ + HCO_3^-$ can be appreciated from the law of mass action for this reaction:

$$K\alpha = \frac{[H^+]\ (HCO_3^-)}{(H_2CO_3)}$$

$K\alpha = 2 \times 10^{-4}$ and the normal [H⁺] –
$$40 \times 10^{-9}\ mol./L.$$

thus, $2 \times 10^{-4} = \dfrac{40 \times 10^{-9}\ (HCO_3^-)}{(H_2CO_3)}$

$$\frac{(HCO_3^-)}{(H_2CO_3)} = 5 \times 10^3$$

Thus, there are approximately 5000 molecules of bicarbonate for each molecule of H_2CO_3. From the preceding equation it is obvious that, for all practical purposes, H_2CO_3 does not exist in a physiologic state within the body; therefore we can concentrate our thinking on the partial pressure of CO_2 and the concentration of bicarbonate. There are other quantitatively less important buffers in the extracellular space — plasma proteins and inorganic phosphate representing two of these — however, their importance is not so critical as the bicarbonate buffering system because of the ability of the lung to vary the concentration of dissolved CO_2 in the plasma.

Intracellular Buffers. The intracellular buffers of importance are proteins, organic and inorganic phosphates, and, within the red cell, hemoglobin. The buffering of hydrogen ion in the cells has an important effect on plasma K^+ concentration. To maintain electroneutrality, the movement of hydrogen ion into the cells is associated with the movement of sodium and potassium out of the cells. The result may be a potentially serious increase in the plasma potassium concentration from the normal plasma concentration of 4 mEq./L. to 7 or 8 mEq./L. If, conversely, the extracellular hydrogen concentration is reduced, hydrogen ions are released from the intracellular buffers and enter the extracellular fluid space. In this setting, sodium and potassium enter the cells, resulting in a fall in the concentration of potassium in the plasma. Similar changes may occur in the concentration of plasma sodium, however, since the normal plasma sodium concentration is 140 mEq./L., small variations in the plasma sodium of several milliequivalents are not of physiologic importance.

Bone Buffers. Bone carbonate represents a large store of buffer which contributes to the buffering of hydrogen ion. For example, after an acid load, bone carbonate is released into the extracellular space. This is accompanied by the uptake of extracellular phosphate or by the release of calcium and sodium from the bone. It is difficult to measure the exact contribution of bone bicarbonate. It has been suggested, however, that as much as 40 per cent of the buffering of an acute acid load takes place in this fashion.

Ventilatory Responses to Changes in Hydrogen Ion Concentration. The main physiologic stimulus to respiration is a change in hydrogen ion concentration in arterial blood. This response is mediated by chemoreceptors sensitive to hydrogen ion concentration located in the medulla of the brain and chemoreceptors in the carotid bodies and in the aortic arch. As hydrogen ion concentration rises, respiration is stimulated, there is a concomitant drop in arterial CO_2, shifting the reaction: dissolved $CO_2 + H_2O \leftrightarrows H^+ + HCO_3^-$ to the left, effectively reducing the hydrogen ion concentration within the arterial circulation. This response occurs within a matter of minutes following a rise in the effective concentration of hydrogen ion in the arterial circulation.

Renal Response to a Change in Hydrogen Ion Concentration. I have previously discussed the handling of hydrogen ion by the kidney. It is important to recognize that the kidney's response to a sudden shift in hydrogen ion concentration within the arterial circulation occurs over a prolonged period of time and is not complete until probably three to five days after the initial change in hydrogen ion concentration occurred. The kidney responds in a number of interrelated fashions, i.e., by the conservation of bicarbonate, by the rise in absolute excretion of hydrogen ion as measured by titratable acidity, and by the production and excretion of increased concentrations of ammonia.

Clinical Disorders of Hydrogen Ion Concentration

There are four clearly defined metabolic states associated with anomolies of hydrogen ion concentration. They are: metabolic acidosis; metabolic alkalosis; respiratory acidosis; and respiratory alkalosis. It is important to remember that the hy-drogen ion concentration as determined in the laboratory may be the end result of altered physiologic mechanisms in more than one system of control, and we therefore oftentimes see a state of mixed metabolic acidosis-alkalosis or any other combination one chooses to put together.

Metabolic Acidosis. A state of metabolic acidosis exists when the ingestion of hydrogen ion or endogenous production of hydrogen ion exceeds the body's capabilities for elimination. This presumes that the respiratory mechanisms for alveolar ventilation are intact. Under these circumstances we would expect to see an absolute rise in the concentration of hydrogen ion in the general circulation where excess hydrogen ion would combine with the readily available bicarbonate in the reaction $H^+ + HCO_3^-$. Following the law of mass action, this would lead to an increased formation of CO_2 and H_2O. At the same time, the chemoreceptor centers described previously would stimulate respiration and the increased removal of CO_2 by the alveolar mechanism. Thus, we would find that hydrogen ion concentration is reduced, Pco_2 is reduced, and the hydrogen ion concentration returned toward the normal concentration of 40 nanomol./L. It is important to note that the respiratory compensation for metabolic acidosis is never complete and that plasma concentration of hydrogen ion will remain elevated. The respiratory response is prompt, occurring within minutes of the initial rise in hydrogen ion concentration. As the intracellular concentration of hydrogen ion rises, the kidney is stimulated to reabsorb more

TABLE 14–5 CAUSES OF METABOLIC ACIDOSIS

I. Inability to excrete the dietary hydrogen load
  a. Diminished ammonia production
    1. Renal failure
  b. Diminished hydrogen ion secretion
    1. Distal renal tubule acidosis
    2. Hypoaldosteronism
II. Increased hydrogen ion load or bicarbonate loss
  a. Ketoacidosis
  b. Lactic acidosis
  c. Ingestions
    1. Salicylates
    2. Ethylene glycol
    3. Methanol
    4. Paraldehyde
    5. Ammonium chloride
    6. Hyperalimentation fluids
  d. Gastrointestinal bicarbonate loss
    1. Diarrhea or fistula
    2. Cholestyramine
    3. Ureterosigmoidostomy
  e. Renal bicarbonate loss
    1. Renal failure
    2. Proximal renal tubule acidosis

bicarbonate and excrete more hydrogen ion, thus returning the hydrogen ion concentration of the body toward normal. The major causes of metabolic acidosis are listed in Table 14–5.

ANION GAP. The calculation of anion gap is a simple clinical tool and can be calculated from the readily available blood electrolytes as determined in any clinical laboratory. The causes of metabolic acidosis can be divided into those which elevate the anion gap and those which do not. Determining the anion gap is then very helpful in the beginning differential diagnosis of a patient with metabolic acidosis. The anion gap is simply determined by adding the chloride and bicarbonate and subtracting the total from the serum sodium. The anion gap normally should measure 10 to 14 mEq. per liter. As hydrogen ion accumulates in the body, there is rapid extracellular buffering by HCO_3^-. If the acid is HCl, then that effect is the mEq.-for-mEq. replacement of extracellular bicarbonate by chloride. Since the sum of chloride and bicarbonate concentrations remains constant, the anion gap is unchanged. Because of the increase in the plasma chloride concentration, this is referred to as a "hyperchloremic acidosis." Gastrointestinal or renal loss of sodium bicarbonate produces the same result, i.e., the exchange of bicarbonate for chloride, since the kidney retains sodium chloride in an effort to preserve the volume of the extracellular fluid. Conversely, if hydrogen ion accumulates with any ion other than chloride, extracellular bicarbonate is replaced by an unmeasured anion. As a result, there is a decrease in the sum of chloride and bicarbonate concentration and an increase in the anion gap. In disorders of this form, identification of the specific disease process can be obtained by measuring the serum concentrations of BUN, lactate, glucose, and pyruvate and by checking for the presence of ketones or exogenous intoxicants (see Table 14–6).

Metabolic Alkalosis. Metabolic alkalosis is characterized by a disorder of hydrogen ion in which there is an absolute decrease in hydrogen ion concentration, an increase in plasma bicarbonate concentration, and a compensatory rise in PCO_2 produced by depressed alveolar ventilation. A state of metabolic alkalosis is produced by either the excessive loss of hydrogen ion or the excessive retention of bicarbonate. It should be pointed out that the retention of bicarbonate will ultimately result in the excessive loss of hydrogen ion and that alkalosis can only exist when total hydrogen ion concentration is depressed, whatever the mechanism of that depression may be. Metabolic alkalosis is most commonly associated with gastrointestinal losses of hydrogen ion. This is usually accomplished by prolonged nasogastric suction. For every hydrogen ion that is secreted by the gastric mucosa, there is generated a bicarbonate ion which is returned to the extracellular space. If we return to our old friend, the formula, $CO_2 + H_2O \rightarrow H_2CO_3 \rightleftharpoons H^+ + HCO_3^-$, it is apparent that we are overloading the right-hand side of this reaction and driving the reaction to the left, with an over-all reduction of circulating hydrogen ion.

Excessive renal retention of bicarbonate may be stimulated by mineralocorticoid excess, volume contraction, or hypokalemia. Again, for every hydrogen ion loss, we are generating bicarbonate at the renal tubule and effectively decreasing circulating concentration of hydrogen ion. Additional unusual causes of metabolic alkalosis are the chronic ingestion of bicarbonate or milk-alkali syndrome.

In considering metabolic alkalosis, it usually is not difficult to establish the initial cause; however, recognizing the sustaining events which surround metabolic alkalosis may be more difficult. Two conditions play a major role in sustaining metabolic alkalosis once it has been established. A state of chronic volume contraction will consistently stimulate the tubule cells of the proximal nephron to reabsorb bicarbonate, despite existing alkalosis. The state of volume deficiency overrides the need for bicarbonate excretion and correction of alkalosis. This results in the facilitation of salt and water conservation despite the persisting state of alkalosis.

With potassium deficiency we see a similar process. As hydrogen ion moves into cells to replace

TABLE 14–6 ANION GAP IN METABOLIC ACIDOSIS

Normal Anion Gap
  a. Gastrointestinal loss of bicarbonate
    1. Diarrhea and fistulas
    2. Cholestyramine
    3. Ureterosigmoidostomy
  b. Renal bicarbonate loss
    1. Proximal RTA
    2. Renal insufficiency
  c. Ingestions
    1. Ammonium chloride
    2. Hyperalimentation fluids
  d. Renal dysfunction
    1. Pyelonephritis and obstructive uropathy
    2. Hypoaldosteronism
    3. Distal RTA
High Anion Gap
  a. Ketoacidosis
  b. Lactic acidosis
  c. Renal insufficiency
  d. Ingestions
    1. Salicylate
    2. Ethylene glycol
    3. Methanol
    4. Paraldehyde

potassium ions that have been lost, there is a facilitation of bicarbonate resorption in the proximal tubule produced by the presence of the additional hydrogen ion within these tubule cells. Persistent bicarbonate resorption occurs despite a continuing state of alkalosis. The point to be gained by all this is, if metabolic alkalosis is to be effectively corrected, any existing volume depletion or potassium depletion must be recognized and corrected.

Respiratory Acidosis. Respiratory acidosis is a metabolic state of increased hydrogen ion concentration secondary to CO_2 retention. It may be either acute or chronic. In acute respiratory acidosis, a minimum amount of buffering can occur from the shifts of intracellular bicarbonate, and there will be a small but significant rise in plasma bicarbonate levels, rarely exceeding 3 or 4 mEq. This is extremely helpful in determining whether the respiratory acidosis is of sudden onset or has been a long-standing process. With long-standing respiratory acidosis, renal compensation begins to play a major role with increased resorption of bicarbonate, and the bicarbonate levels may become significantly elevated.

Respiratory Alkalosis. A reduction in alveolar P_{CO_2} secondary to hyperventilation leads to respiratory alkalosis as plasma P_{CO_2} falls concomitantly. Hyperventilation can result from primary central nervous system pathology, primary lung disease, anxiety, various intoxications, or overvigorous artificial ventilation. This metabolic state is characteristically acute in nature and of a readily recognizable etiology. Therapy revolves around treatment of the underlying pathology. Hydrogen ion concentrations are lowered with reduction of P_{CO_2} as follows: $\downarrow P_{CO_2} \leftrightarrows HCO_3^- + H^+$.

DIURETICS

Diuretics as a group are one of the most widely used categories of drugs in modern medicine. By the very nature of their function, diuretics must alter the physiologic functions of the kidney, and any discussion of basic pathophysiologic mechanisms of acid base balance and fluid and electrolyte disturbances must include at least a brief look at this broad category of drugs. The diuretics currently employed in clinical medicine can be divided into seven general categories. Although diuretics in each class do not necessarily have a similar formula, their clinical activity can be grouped conceptually into one of these categories, and this provides a reasonable way to remember their clinical application. The seven categories are: (1) xanthine compounds; (2) carbonic anhydrase inhibitors; (3) osmotic diuretics; (4) organomercurials; (5) thiazides; (6) spironolactone–triamterene; and (7) ethacrynic acid–furosemide.

1. Xanthine Compounds. Xanthine compounds in themselves are very weak diuretic agents that have been available to clinicians for many years. They are rarely, if ever, used alone as a diuretic agent, but may have a significant potentiating effect when used in association with the more potent diuretic agents commonly in clinical use. Their action appears to be threefold. There is an inotropic effect on the myocardium which increases cardiac output and secondarily increases renal plasma flow. There is a suggested mechanism directly affecting renal hemodynamics with increased filtration fraction, and a third possible role in inhibition of active sodium transport in the proximal tubule.

2. Carbonic Anhydrase Inhibitors. Approximately 90 per cent of the filtered load of bicarbonate is reabsorbed in the proximal tubule. Bicarbonate is absorbed as a direct result of hydrogen ion secretion in the following formulation: $HCO_3^- + H^+ \rightarrow H_2CO_3 \rightarrow CO_2 + H_2O$. The CO_2 diffuses into the paratubular cell, where it is used to reconstitute bicarbonate. These reactions are greatly facilitated by the presence of the enzyme, carbonic anhydrase, which is abundantly present in the proximal tubule cells and in high concentration in the brush border of the paraluminal surface of the proximal nephron. Inhibitors of carbonic anhydrase exert a diuretic effect by reducing the efficient reabsorption of bicarbonate and thus sodium. The diuresis induced is characterized by high content of bicarbonate in the urine and the tendency, after prolonged administration, to the development of metabolic acidosis. Diuresis is self-limited in that a new bicarbonate steady state will shortly be reestablished and no further diuretic action will occur.

3. Mannitol. The mechanisms of mannitol diuresis include: (a) osmotic retention of water in the proximal tubule, which; (b) decreases sodium concentration in the lumen, thus creating a sodium gradient between the lumen and blood sufficiently large to reduce proximal sodium transport; (c) increased renal blood flow and reduced medullary hypertonicity; (d) reduced movement of sodium and water from Henle's loop into the medullary interstitial spaces; (e) reduced medullary hypertonicity due to osmotic retention of water in medullary tissues. Mannitol enhances excretion of calcium, phosphorus, magnesium, potassium, uric acid, and urea. These effects are brought about by producing osmotic dilution of these substances in the lumen, creating a gradient unfavorable for their transport and favorable for secretion.

4. Organomercurials. The organomercurials were for many years the most potent diuretics available and the mainstay of diuretic therapy. Because, for effective clinical application, they must be given intramuscularly or intravenously, the advent of the potent oral loop diuretics, exemplified by ethacrynic acid and furosemide, has significantly reduced their clinical application. Recent experimental data based primarily on the findings at micropuncture presents a persuasive argument that this class of drugs acts by the inhibition of active transport of chloride and that the natriuresis is secondary to the chloruresis. The mode of action of the mercurials at the cellular level has not yet been defined. Available evidence strongly suggests that this diuretic has its main site of action on the ascending thick segment of the loop of Henle.

5. Thiazide Diuretics. The thiazides are the most prescribed group of diuretics in clinical medicine. Micropuncture data suggests that their site of action is in the thick segment of the ascending loop of Henle at some point distal to the site of action of mercurials, ethacrynic acid, and furosemide. They apparently have no effect on proximal tubule transport of sodium and no distal action in terms of sodium or water resorption. Independent of their diuretic effect is an effect on glomerular filtration rate, which in animal experimentation has been shown to produce a reduction in effective glomerular filtration rate by as much as 25 per cent. They exert a primary effect on free water clearance, i.e., the ability of the kidney to form a dilute urine, but do not interfere with the ability of the kidney to achieve maximal water resorption from the collecting duct.

6. Spironolactone–Triamterene. Spironolactone and triamterene have different sites of action at the cellular level but can be lumped together in terms of their clinical action as diuretic agents. Spironolactone acts by blocking the effect of aldosterone in the distal tubule and possibly the collecting duct, while the action of triamterene is independent of the presence of aldosterone, although its site of action is similar to that of spironolactone. The major action is to block the distal tubule transport of sodium. At the same time, there is interference with the secretion of potassium at the distal tubule nephron. This group of diuretics is relatively ineffective when used alone, but becomes of clinical significance when used in conjunction with one or more of the other available diuretic agents or when a potassium-sparing effect is desired.

7. Ethacrynic Acid–Furosemide. The loop diuretics, exemplified by ethacrynic acid and furosemide, are the most recent group of diuretic agents introduced into clinical practice and the most potent currently available. Their site of action is thought to be in the medullary and cortical segment of the ascending loop of Henle. Like the mercurial diuretics, evidence suggests that their major pharmacologic effect inhibits the active transport of chloride in this tubule segment, producing a chloruresis and a natriuresis. Because the site of action is both medullary and cortical in the ascending loop, they interfere with both free water clearance and the ability of the kidney to maximally concentrate. They have not been demonstrated to have a clinical effect on glomerular filtration rate when volume is maintained. In large doses — doses usually in excess of those applied in clinical practice — a proximal tubule effect has been demonstrated in some animal species. This proximal tubule effect appears to be a direct inhibition of active sodium transport, but plays little or no role in production of diuresis in current clinical practice.

Complications of Diuretic Therapy

The most important complication of diuretic therapy is excessive and unwarranted depletion of extracellular volume. This may lead to hypotension and various complications of organ hypoperfusion, including syncope, confusion, transient ischemic attacks, oliguria, azotemia, and angina. In the cirrhotic patient, hepatorenal syndrome and hepatic coma may be induced by excessive volume reduction. In some cases, particularly in the patient with advanced cirrhosis, elimination of ascites and edema cannot be achieved without an unacceptable reduction of effective plasma volume.

None of the available diuretics is known to enhance potassium secretion directly. The potassium losses and the resulting hypokalemia seen as the direct result of diuretic therapy are secondary to increased delivery of volume to the distal nephron. Increased volume enhances the secretion of potassium at these sites with excessive potassium losses occurring in the final urine. There may exist slight differences in potassium-losing effect among the various thiazide diuretics, but none are of practical importance. It is suggested that, in addition to potassium loss, a redistribution of potassium from the extracellular to the intracellular space may result from thiazide administration. Whether potassium supplement is a necessity with thiazide or other diuretic therapy has been brought into serious dispute by recent studies which tend to show that total body potassium depletion is minimal and the administration of exogenous potassium salts does little to correct this deficiency.

The risk of hyperkalemia must always be considered in patients with compromised renal function placed on spironolactone or triamterene. These drugs interfere with the secretion of potassium into the distal tubule segments, where the bulk of potassium excretion must occur.

Hyperuricemia has been shown to be associated with the administration of thiazide diuretics, furosemide, ethacrynic acid, and acetazolamide. The effect of mercurials is much less clear. Thiazide diuretics and ethacrynic acid become uricosuric when given in larger doses or after intravenous administration.

Instantaneous sudden deafness may occur with rapid intravenous administration of furosemide or ethacrynic acid. In rare cases deafness has been reported after the oral administration of these drugs as well. This effect usually lasts for no more than a few hours and seems related to the action of the diuretics on the electrolyte composition of the endolymph. It has been shown that ethacrynic acid can cause a complete reversal of the sodium/potassium ratio in the endolymph ten minutes after administration.

The occurrence of transient and sometimes fatal arrhythmias has been reported after rapid administration of large doses of furosemide. This is probably due to alterations of sodium/potassium ratios within the heart itself. A number of other complications have been described, including idiosyncratic or hypersensitive reactions, but these are not directly related to the biochemical effects of the diuretic agents themselves.

Additional Clinical Application of Diuretic Agents

1. Hypertension. Thiazides, chlorthalidone, ethacrynic acid, and furosemide have been used in the management of hypertension. While it has been definitely established that one effect of diuretic therapy resulting in lower blood pressure is produced by contraction of extracellular volume, additional mechanisms have been suggested. At equipotent diuretic doses, thiazides seem to be somewhat better antihypertensive agents than do the other diuretics available. Their postulated action on arteriolar smooth muscle has not been definitely established.

2. Acute Pulmonary Edema. Rapid reduction of extracellular volume by furosemide or ethacrynic acid is a frequently used therapy in the emergency treatment of acute pulmonary edema. The major effect is the reduction of pre-load and after-load on the myocardium in addition to the clearing of the pulmonary transudate.

3. Acute Renal Failure. Mannitol, furosemide, and ethacrynic acid have been used to induce diuresis during the early phases of acute tubule necrosis in hopes of reversing the underlying process. The effectiveness of this procedure remains in doubt and there is clinical evidence to suggest that, although volume may be increased acutely by this approach, the long-term effect on the underlying disease process is not a clinically significant one.

4. Diabetes Insipidus. Diuretics reduce the volume and increase the osmolality of the urine in diabetes insipidus, whether the diabetes insipidus is central or nephrogenic in origin. The urine becomes less hypotonic, but never hypertonic. The effect is not due to any ADH-like activity. One explanation given is enhanced proximal tubule resorption secondary to volume depletion. This results in a reduction in the volume delivered to the distal tubule and the collecting duct. The diuretics most frequently used for this purpose are thiazides, although other diuretics are effective as well. The therapeutic benefit is potentiated by salt restriction and neutralized by high salt intake.

Under conditions of hyponatremia and inappropriately low free water clearance, furosemide and ethacrynic acid can enhance free water clearance. This is particularly true in the presence of a high glomerular filtration rate. This property has been used to induce diuresis of a dilute urine, which together with the administration of salt corrects the hyponatremia in the syndrome of inappropriate secretion of antidiuretic hormone.

5. Renal Tubule Acidosis. Hypovolemia produces metabolic alkalosis by enhancing proximal tubule transport of bicarbonate. Diuretic-induced volume contraction can help improve the acidosis of renal tubule acidosis. The action is particularly effective with the administration of thiazide diuretics.

6. Hypercalcemia. Diuresis induced by furosemide or ethacrynic acid produces calcium loss and a correction of hypercalcemia. It is important to note that thiazides are contraindicated in hypercalcemia and, under certain circumstances, can produce a hypercalcemic state. A possible explanation for the difference lies in the fact that most of the non-proximal calcium resorption takes place in the medullary segment and very little in the cortical segment of the ascending limb of Henle's loop.

CONGENITAL ABNORMALITIES OF THE KIDNEY

Congenital Malformations

Normal Embryology. During embryologic development of the human, three distinct excretory organs are formed. The first is the *pronephros*, the remnants of which rarely persist. The second is the *mesonephros*, parts of which persist in the adult male as epididymis and vas deferens and as vestigial appendages in the female. The *metanephros*, which forms the adult kidney, derives from two sources: (1) the ureteric bud, a diverticulum from the mesonephric duct, which forms the ureter, pelvis of the kidney, and collecting ducts; (2) mesoderm from the nephrogenic cord, which invests the distal end of the ureteric bud and forms the convoluted tubules and loops of Henle. The glomeruli develop within the mesodermal tissue and obtain arterial supply.

The kidneys are first formed at the fourth lumbar segment and ascend cephalad to the level of T12 or L1, their final position. During ascent they are squeezed together as they arise from the pelvis and rotate a quarter turn so that the pelves are medial and the convex borders are lateral. Arterial supply for the developing kidneys arises from vessels supplying the segments through which they ascend.

Congenital abnormalities of the adult kidney can be ascribed to errors or abnormalities of development at specific stages.

Bilateral agenesis, which is of course incompatible with life, is rare. The true incidence is difficult to ascertain. It apparently affects males more frequently than females. In true agenesis one would expect to find no ureter. However, in a large reported series, ureters were absent in only about one half. This suggests either that some cases of agenesis were actually extreme hypoplasia or that there was specific failure of the metanephric part of the holonephros. Agenesis of both kidneys is associated with oligophydramnios, fetal malformations of ears, eyes, and legs, and pulmonary hypoplasia.

Unilateral agenesis is not extremely rare and is compatible with normal development. Associated malformations apparently are not common. There may be absence of the fallopian tube or nondescent of the testis on the same side. The single kidney is hypertrophic and prone to infection. Recognition of a single kidney in cases of infection, stones, or tumor is, of course, important.

Supernumerary kidneys occur rarely. These by definition should have their own blood supply and own ureter. The supernumerary kidney is usually smaller than normal.

Hypoplastic kidneys are small kidneys with smaller than normal cells and a reduced number of nephrons. The arteries and ureters are likewise hypoplastic. Bilateral hypoplasia usually is incompatible with life. The hypoplastic kidney is prone to infection. The *Ask-Upmark kidney* is one in which there is hypoplasia of a single renal lobule and its calyx.

Fetal lobulation of the adult kidney is a retention of the surface marking of individual lobules. It is of no significance.

The *dysplastic kidney* represents a disturbed differentiation of nephrogenic tissue and consists of nonfunctional cystic structures and may contain cartilage. It may be associated with other organ defects but, if unilateral, has the same significance as unilateral agenesis. A unilateral dysplastic kidney is the most common palpable abdominal mass in the newborn, exceeding Wilms' tumor.

Ectopic kidneys may be located from pelvis to thorax. They may be retained in the pelvis by persistence of vascular attachments or allowed to migrate to the thorax through diaphragmatic defects. They are prone to infection, may cause compression of adjacent structures, and may be mistaken for a tumor.

Fused kidneys occur in two forms: the horseshoe kidney and the cake kidney. The *horseshoe* kidney is the more common, with an incidence of 1:300 to 1:800. The two kidneys are fused at the lower poles in 90 per cent of cases. While horseshoe kidney is not incompatible with a normal life-span, it may be associated with symptoms of abdominal pain and vasomotor disturbances. They are susceptible to trauma, infection, and ureteral obstruction and are associated with other urogenital tract abnormalities and defects of the gastrointestinal and cardiovascular systems. *Cake, lump,* or *shield* kidney is quite rare. Symptoms and complications are similar to horseshoe kidney. It may be palpable and mistaken for a neoplasm.

Malrotation of the kidney may occur to any degree, i.e., pelvis of kidney facing anteriorly, laterally, or dorsally. It is of no clinical significance other than its appearance on an IVP.

Otherwise normal kidneys may be supplied with more than the usual one renal artery. They may enter from above or below to supply the upper or lower pole of the kidney. They may cause complications if they pass ventral to the ureter and cause obstruction. There are a large number of anomalies of the ureters. There may be two separate ureters supplying two separate pelves of the same kidney and emptying into the bladder at separate locations. The ureter may divide anywhere along its length from bladder to hilus. There may be an anomaly involving stenosis of a valve or megaloureter. These are of concern as they predispose to infections and can then require urologic evaluation.

Several congenital abnormalities of the kidney have been reported to be hereditary, e.g., hydronephrosis and megaloureter. Available data does not give conclusive evidence of the mechanism of inheritance. Renal tumors have been observed to appear in families.

Hereditary Renal Diseases

Hereditary renal diseases may be divided into two major classifications, cystic and non-cystic. The most common cystic disease affecting the kidney is the so-called classic polycystic kidney disease of the adult. It is first recognized in adult life, usually in the fourth or fifth decade. In the typical patient, cystic changes are grossly apparent throughout the renal parenchyma, with a wide variation in size. Microscopically, cystic ectasia of all tubule elements abounds. In most instances adult polycystic disease is inherited as an autosomal dominant trait, but the disorder may also occur without clear-cut evidence of genetic transmission. Polycystic kidney disease is one of the more important causes of recurrent painful hematuria unassociated with nephrolithiasis. Polycystic disease of the liver, a cystic ectasia of the bile duct radicals, frequently attends this syndrome and can result in hepatomegaly as striking as the renomegaly. The common symptom of abdominal fullness in these patients is often a consequence of enlargement of both liver and kidneys. Only rarely does the liver involvement lead to portal hypertension. Progressive azotemia and uremia are characteristic of patients with polycystic disease. Hypertension is a usual and often fatal complication in these patients, and intracranial aneurysm is frequently found in association. The characteristic intravenous pyelogram reveals an over-all increase in size of both kidneys. The width of the renal parenchyma is characteristically increased, the pelvocaliceal system is frequently elongated, and the caliceal stalks can be so narrowed by impinging cysts that the pelvocaliceal pattern appears to be stretched out. The prognosis is one of progressive uremia and death unless intervention by dialysis or transplantation occurs.

Infantile polycystic disease refers to a variety of hepato-renal polycystic disorders that occurs in infancy and early childhood and is genetically transmitted as an autosomal recessive trait. Throughout both kidneys there is a uniform distribution of fusiform cysts. The glomeruli, intratubular tissue, calices, pelves, ureters, and lower urinary tract are normal. In the liver there is a bizarre infolding proliferation and dilatation of well-differentiated portal bile ducts and ductules associated with a variable degree of periportal fibrosis. Various investigators have attempted to sub-categorize infantile polycystic disease on the basis of onset and pathology. Unfortunately, regardless of categorization, prognosis appears to be uniformly poor.

Medullary Cystic Disease

Medullary cystic disease is another form of microcystic involvement of the renal medulla, and usually manifests itself by the insidious onset of uremia leading to death, frequently in the second or third decade of life. This disease should not be confused with medullary sponge kidney, another form of microcystic disease of the renal medulla, which is compatible with a normal life span and, in most cases, is asymptomatic. Medullary cystic disease is predominantly one of youth: the average age at death has been reported to be 27 years, with no predilection for sex. The disease seems to have an autosomal recessive inheritance pattern. Cysts appear to be derived from distal tubules or collecting ducts. They vary in size from 100 μ to 1 cm. or more in diameter and are restricted to the corticomedullary junction. The cortex is usually thin and poorly demarcated, with the majority of the glomeruli partially or completely hyalinized. The interstitial tissue shows diffuse fibrosis and round cell infiltration. Blood pressure is characteristically normal at the beginning of the disease, but may become moderately elevated later in the clinical course as uremia develops. The urinary sediment may be normal, and daily excretion of protein rarely exceeds 150 mg. per 24 hours. The prognosis is poor, with uniform progression to renal insufficiency as the rule.

Medullary Sponge Kidney

Medullary sponge kidney designates a rather benign renal disorder oftentimes diagnosed by intravenous pyelogram. It is quite unlike classic polycystic kidney disease. The intravenous pyelogram is characterized by multiple discrete urographic opacifications clustered around the caliceal cups of the pelvocaliceal system. In most cases there appears to be no evidence of genetic transmission. Nephrocalcinosis, indistinguishable from that seen with renal tubule acidosis can occur in these patients. An increased incidence of hypercalciuria has been described. The most common symptoms of patients with medullary sponge kidney relate to urinary tract infection, hematuria, and renal colic, which have been ascribed to their increased propensity for infection and stone formation. In contrast to patients with classic polycystic kidney disease, there is no associated hypertension or liver disease.

Hereditary Chronic Nephritis

A second major classification of hereditary renal disorders can be grouped under *hereditary chronic nephritis*. An hereditary form of renal disease, often clinically indistinguishable from chronic glomerulonephritis or pyelonephritis, has been recognized for many years; however, it was not until 1927 that its association with nerve deafness was first noted by Alport. Males are more severely affected than females and affected males appear to have a deficiency of affected sons. Affected females often have an excess of both affected sons and daughters. The hereditary complexities of this syndrome have not been firmly established. The syndrome is best regarded, at this point, as being inherited in an autosomal dominant manner. Many females with hereditary nephritis remain asymptomatic for most, if not all, of their lives, but some females and most males develop the progressive symptoms of chronic glomerulonephritis or pyelonephritis. The earliest manifestations of the disease are albuminuria and hematuria. In affected males, death generally occurs in the second or third decade of life, either from renal failure or from the vascular and cardiac complications of hypertension. Death of females usually occurs much later. The basic renal lesion has been variously described as chronic glomerulonephritis, chronic pyelonephritis, interstitial nephritis, or a combination of all these. The principal glomerular abnormalities include cellular proliferation and swelling, capsular adhesions, and thickened basement membranes with periglomerular fibrosis. The characteristic abnormality of the tubules is atrophy, alternating with discrete areas of tubule dilatation, hypertrophy, and regeneration. The prominence of lipid-laden "foam cells" is a characteristic feature of hereditary nephritis. The recognition of foam cells is not limited to this form of renal disease, and to date what role, if any, these cells may play in the pathogenesis of this syndrome has not been defined. The incidence and severity of deafness in this disease appears to be greater in males than in females, and audiometry may be necessary to detect a hearing loss in the latter. The hearing loss is bilateral and usually symmetrical. Loss of high frequency perception is the earliest lesion, and this may progress to profound deafness. Although various eye anomalies including myopia and macular lesions have been described in association with hereditary nephritis, the most characteristic lesions are associated with lens defects. There is no specific treatment and management other than that associated with the care of any patient suffering from advancing renal failure.

A third category of hereditary kidney diseases relates to *primary tubular disorders*. The discussion may be divided into disorders of proximal tubule and disorders of distal tubule. The proximal tubule is concerned with resorption of amino acids, glucose, phosphate, uric acid, and other substances filtered at the glomerulus. Proximal tubule syndromes are characterized by various combinations of glycosuria, aminoaciduria, increased clearance of phosphate, and high uric acid clearance. Distal tubule syndromes more classically relate to abnormalities in the final adjustment of urinary pH, salt, and water balance.

Hereditary Proximal Tubule Defects

Cystinuria. In cystinuria there is a defect in a single amino acid transport system in the proximal tubule resulting in excessive excretion of cystine, lysine, arginine, and ornithine. Until recently these amino acids were thought to be reabsorbed by the same transport system. There is now good evidence that lysine, arginine, and ornithine are reabsorbed by the same transport system, but the abnormal excretion of cystine conforms more closely to a pattern of tubule secretion rather than defective reabsorption, the theory being that lysine and cystine interact by sharing an efflux mechanism and that cysteine is the intracellular form of cystine. Thus a defect in lysine transport inhibits efflux of cysteine into capillaries, causing a build-up of cysteine in cells and inhibiting luminal uptake of cystine. All other renal functions are normal early in life. Cystine is one of the least soluble of the amino acids. Between pH 5 and 7 it is soluble to the extent of only 300 to 400 mg./L. Cystinuric patients excrete on the average of 0.73 gm. of cystine per day. The problem occurs when urine is saturated with cystine and calculi form. The other amino acids excreted are freely soluble.

Calculi predispose to obstruction and infection. They may begin to form early and cause symptoms even in infancy. Most commonly symptoms of nephrolithiasis occur between the ages of 20 and 25. Cystinuria accounts for a large proportion of stones in infancy. In adults it may account for as much as 1 per cent of renal calculi. The stones are radiopaque but less dense than calcium stones. They can contain calcium in their matrix or may be pure cystine. Symptoms are those ascribed to any type of calculi. Diagnosis is made by stone analysis and the finding of increased amounts of cystine, lysine, arginine, and ornithine in the urine. Cystine may be excreted in large amounts in other disorders which produce broad tubule damage and generalized aminoaciduria. Cystinuria must also be distinguished from cystinosis. Cystinosis is a defect in protein metabolism resulting in the deposition of cystine in many organs including the kidney. Cystinosis of the kidney results in proximal tubule damage with generalized aminoaciduria. Cystinosis is one of the known causes of Fanconi syndrome in children.

Cystinuric families can be divided into two distinct groups. In the first group there are two classes of individuals, affected and non-affected. The hereditary pattern in this group is typical mendelian recessive. The second group, less common than the first, has three types of individuals: (1) severe cystinurics; (2) mild cystinurics who have increased excretion of cystine and lysine, but normal amounts of arginine and ornithine; and (3) the unaffected individuals. The disease can be passed from generation to generation in this group, and the hereditary pattern is termed incomplete recessive.

Hartnup's Disease is a rare congenital defect of recessive inheritance. The clinical manifestations are a pellegra-like rash with variable attacks of cerebellar ataxia and other neurologic abnormalities. The biochemical abnormality is a specific aminoaciduria involving glutamine, asparagine, histidine, serine, threonine, phenylalanine, tyrosine, and tryptophan. The four amino acids found in the urine in cystinuria, i.e., cystine, arginine, ornithine, and lysine, are not found in greater than normal amounts. There is a specific defect in renal tubule absorption of the above amino acids. There is also a defect in jejunal absorption of tryptophan, which results in increased gastrointestinal formation of indoles by bacteria and increased absorption and urinary excretion of these substances.

The pellegra-like rash results from tryptophan deficiency secondary to defective jejunal absorption and increased urinary excretion. The attacks of cerebellar ataxia are due to intoxication of the central nervous system, probably secondary to action of bacteria on intestinal amino acids. The disease is not serious unless the patient develops central nervous system involvement. It shows a tendency to remit with increasing age, especially after adolescence. During attacks, treatment is directed toward reducing bacterial degradation of amino acids by measures similar to those used in hepatic coma, i.e., reduction in dietary protein intake and an attempt to sterilize the intestinal tract with neomycin.

The Fanconi syndrome is characterized by multiple proximal tubule defects. Typically, these defects involve the tubule's handling of phosphate, glucose, and amino acids. There is usually proteinuria with a high concentration of globulins, reflecting tubule cell damage rather than increased glomerular permeability to albumin. On occasion tubule damage is more widespread and associated with difficulties in water absorption, bicarbonate absorption, and absorption of potassium. Children with Fanconi syndrome develop rickets, fail to thrive, and suffer dehydration. In adults, osteomalacia and weakness associated with acidosis may occur. Symptoms are a result of bone anomalies, acidosis, and potassium depletion. The glycosuria and aminoaciduria produce no symptoms. There appear to be several forms of Fanconi syndrome. An idiopathic congenital type of uncertain inheritance occurs in childhood, with the child developing progressive renal failure terminating in death.

Lowe's syndrome is a rare hereditary renal disorder with diffuse and variable abnormalities. These are similar to the Fanconi syndrome, with diffuse renal aminoaciduria, proteinuria of the tubule type, systemic acidosis, increased phosphate clearance, and defects in concentration and acidification of the urine. With Lowe's syndrome, there is also mental retardation and severe congenital anomalies of the eyes. Tubule atrophy is a pathologic finding frequently associated with thickening of the basement membrane of the tubules. Transmission is sex-linked. The full syndrome occurs only in males.

Hypophosphatemia and rickets resistent to vitamin D is characterized by rickets in children and osteomalacia in adults. It is unresponsive to physiologic doses of vitamin D. There is a failure of reabsorption of phosphate in the proximal tubules and, therefore, high phosphate clearance. Kidney function is otherwise normal. Intestinal absorption of calcium and phosphate may be concomitantly affected. It is transmitted by the unusual mode of a sex-linked dominant. Heterozygous females are affected much less severely than homozygous males. Homozygous females are unknown.

Renal glycosuria is a benign congenital condition which requires no treatment. It does not cause polyuria, polydipsia, or ketoacidosis. The main problem is to differentiate it from diabetes mellitus, avoiding inappropriate treatment. It occurs in two types. The most common is due to an unusual heterogenicity of proximal tubule function regarding glucose resorption. The transport maximum for glucose is normal, but the titration curve exhibits an abnormally marked splay so that glucose is spilled at low serum levels. This appears to be transmitted as a mendelian recessive and is due to a single defect in transport. In the second type, there is a reduction in transport maximum for glucose throughout the kidney. Most cases of the later type are associated with other generalized proximal tubule defects.

Distal Tubular Syndromes

Nephrogenic diabetes insipidus is an hereditary disorder characterized by an insensitivity of distal tubule and collecting duct epithelium to antidiuretic hormone. This disorder presents in childhood with recurrent dehydration, hypernatremia, a dilute urine, and failure to thrive. Mental and physical retardation and death may occur. With early therapy a normal life span may be possible. Vasopressin has no effect on renal concentration in these individuals. There appears to be no other renal defect. Proximal tubule anatomic anomalies have been described, but their significance is not clear. Inheritance is sex-linked; most cases occur in males. Heterozygous females may have some limitation in concentrating ability.

Renal Tubule Acidosis. The renal acidification process contributes to acid-base balance by regulating the concentration of plasma bicarbonate. In normal man this process operates to maintain plasma bicarbonate at physiologic concentrations. Bicarbonate that is filtered by the glomerulus is reabsorbed and hydrogen ion is excreted in an amount equal to the bicarbonate thus generated. The bulk of bicarbonate resorption occurs in the proximal tubule, and the final regulation of hydrogen ion concentration in the urine occurs in the distal tubule and collecting duct. Metabolic acidosis can occur with defects at either level.

Proximal renal tubule acidosis results from an incomplete reabsorption of bicarbonate in the proximal tubule. The distal tubule cannot absorb the excess bicarbonate, and bicarbonate is lost until the patient becomes acidotic. Distal renal tubule acidosis is the result of an inability to establish or maintain a hydrogen ion gradient at the distal tubule and collecting duct epithelium. Complications of acidosis such as bone disease, nephrocalcinosis, and renal calculi are more com-

mon in distal tubule acidosis. In distal renal tubule acidosis the kidney is unable to form an acid
urine with a pH below 6. In proximal renal tubule
acidosis, an acid urine of pH 5 or less may be
formed once severe acidosis has developed and the
filtered load of bicarbonate is reduced. Both forms
of renal tubule acidosis occur as a primary disorder. Familial distal renal tubule acidosis occurs
as an autosomal dominant with variable penetrance with greater expressivity in females. Familial proximal renal tubule acidosis occurs more
commonly in males. Secondary causes of proximal
renal tubule acidosis are cystinosis, Wilson's disease, Lowe's syndrome, multiple myeloma, heavy
metal poisonings, and galactosemia. Secondary
causes of distal renal tubule acidosis include vitamin D excess or deficiency, analgesic-abuse
nephritis, and pyelonephritis.

PATHOPHYSIOLOGY OF GLOMERULAR DAMAGE

It is now generally accepted that immunologic
mechanisms normally concerned with host protection play a major role in the pathogenesis of most,
if not all, forms of glomerulonephritis. This appreciation of the role played by the immunologic
system is due in large part to studies conducted in
experimental animal models. The resemblance of
these diseases in the models to those in man is
particularly striking.

Two general mechanisms have been implicated
in the genesis of these diseases. The first involves
antibodies with a specificity for antigenic components of the glomerular basement membrane
(GBM). The second is dependent on the formation
of immune complexes, i.e., circulating antibody-
antigen complexes, in which the antigen is not
necessarily of glomerular origin. The focusing of
antibodies or immune complexes within glomeruli
is not of itself pathogenic. Tissue damage results
from the inflammatory response which these components trigger via the activation of the complement system. This in turn may trigger the coagulation system, resulting in additional glomerular
damage. Glomeruli destruction then is the end
result of a vicious cycle of a number of interacting
components. The development and severity of glomerulonephritis is dependent on these various
factors and the delicate balance between them.
Consideration of only one of these components, for
example that of the antibody involved, indicates
that the immunoglobulin class, kinetics of appearance, amount, specificity, and avidity may all influence the development and/or severity of the disease.

A third immunologic mechanism has been implicated more recently in the triggering of the

disease process. Antibody may be involved in the
activation of the complement cascade by the alternate pathway of the properdin system. Although
the triggering event may be different, the end
result is the same.

A fourth mechanism, that of cellular mediated
immunity, may also be involved in these disease
processes. Although patients with glomerulonephritis possess lymphocytes which are specifically
sensitized to glomerular or cross-reactive antigens, their possible role in the pathogenesis is not
yet clear. It seems quite likely, however, that all
these aforementioned mechanisms may contribute at some point to the disease process. The
following outline is neither intended to be all-
inclusive nor a complete summary of the role of
immunologic reactions in renal disease. Rather it
is but one of many possible ways to organize our
thoughts concerning the triggering events, the
role immunologic mechanisms may play, and the
points in these sequences that we may logically
attack with methods for therapy or possible prevention.

Several types of bacterial infections in man
have been treated by passive immunization with
xenogeneic serum, such as horse anti-tetanus
toxin. This particular form of therapy has been
largely discontinued. However, use of xenogeneic
serum or globulin therapy such as horse antilymphocyte serum is expected to increase. Recipients of such treatment often develop the serum
sickness syndrome characterized by fever, enlarged lymph nodes and spleen, erythematous and
urticarial rashes, painful joints, and renal involvement. The acute form (or "one-shot") may
result in a renal lesion at 10 to 14 days, which
usually heals spontaneously. In contrast, a chronic form of the disease may result from continued or
repetitive treatment, in which a severe and progressive glomerular lesion with resultant structural damage is evident. Investigations of the
serum sickness syndrome have been the spring-
board for our understanding of the pathologic immunogenic mechanisms involved in renal disease.
These mechanisms have been more carefully delineated in the experimental models discussed
below. Their human disease correlates have been
well documented.

Experimental Models

Heterologous Anti-GBM. This model, first provided by Masugi, involves the injection of heterologous antibody of anti-host kidney specificity
into recipient animals, (such as rabbit anti-rat
kidney serum injected into rats). These immunoglobulins combine with the glomerular basement
membrane or with other vascular tissues which
are antigenically similar to GBM, such as in the

lung. There they trigger a sequence of pathologic events by the activation and fixation of complement, the infiltration of polymorphonuclear (PMN) leukocytes, and destruction of basement membrane. A second round of immunologic insult results when the host makes antibody to the foreign immunoglobulins which are bound to its own basement membrane. This antibody-antigen complex may again trigger an inflammatory response, leading to additional membrane destruction.

Autologous Anti-GBM.   In this model the experimental animal is immunized with homologous or heterologous GBM. His immunologic response results in a clinical picture very similar to the Masugi type of nephritis, except in this case the triggering antibody is of host origin, i.e., an autoimmune phenomenon. That such antibody is pathogenic is demonstrated by the fact that transfer to normal animals of such antibody isolated from the serum of immunized animals (or eluted from their affected kidneys) may result in severe glomerular damage.

Immune Complex.   The classic model has involved the single injection of a rather large dose of radio-labeled bovine serum albumin as antigen into the rabbit. Analysis of the immunologic events that followed has been a significant contribution in our understanding of the pathogenesis of glomerulonephritis. The antigen is seen to disappear from the circulation in three phases: equilibration; metabolic decay; and immune elimination. During the latter phase, antibody forms complexes with the antigen. These may be deposited in tissues including heart, joints, and kidneys. Renal involvement occurs during the time interval when immune complexes are in slight antigen excess. The presence of such complexes within the glomeruli has been documented. When free noncomplexed antibody makes its appearance in the circulation, the complexes disappear along with the manifestations of renal disease. Coincident with the complex formation and renal disease there is a decrease in the serum complement level.

A different course of events is noted if the antigen is given in smaller repeated doses over a prolonged period. This form of chronic stimulation produces a severe and progressive glomerular lesion causing structural damage. Rabbits undergoing such experimentation fell into three groups according to their antibody response. The first group did not produce antibody and did not have any renal lesions despite the presence of foreign antigen in the circulation and tissues for prolonged periods of time. A second group of animals synthesized very large amounts of antibody which efficiently cleared the reinjected antigen from the circulation. Some of these Group Two animals developed an acute glomerulonephritis within the first two weeks, which usually resolved quickly with no further lesions observed. The third group produced an intermediate amount of antibody such that the repeatedly introduced antigen was cleared in a delayed fashion. Most of these animals developed chronic glomerular lesions. Thus it is apparent that soluble immune complexes must be present in the circulation for some period of time to cause glomerular injury. In addition, only complexes of the appropriate size of lattice formation (those in slight to moderate antigen excess) are potentially pathogenic. The fact that not all rabbits developed glomerular lesions indicates that the character of the animal's antibody response also influences the development of such lesions. Quantitative relationships between antigen and antibody appear crucial in determining the eventual response we may expect to see.

Spontaneous Glomerulonephritis in Animals.   A particularly interesting animal model which has been useful in unraveling the mechanisms inherent in the development of glomerulonephritis is the New Zealand mouse. F1 hybrids of the black and white strains (NZB/W F1) spontaneously develop a disease process which closely resembles systemic lupus erythematosus (SLE) in man. Females are more susceptible, beginning to die at six months of age. Mortality increases with advancing age, and 98 per cent are dead at one year. This fatal autoimmune glomerulonephritis is characterized by the presence of immune complexes within renal tissues. Approximately 50 per cent of the antibody eluted from these immune complexes reacts specifically with host deoxyribonucleic acid (DNA). Another 15 to 20 per cent react with "C" type oncogenic virus endogenous to these animals. Experimentally-induced infection — with lymphocytic choriomeningitis (LCM) virus, for example — markedly enhances or accelerates the immune response to DNA and the resultant nephritis. In contrast, rendering these animals tolerant to DNA prevents the disease. Although of the immune complex type (DNA-anti DNA), this model provides an example of spontaneous development of this disease triggered by endogenous materials.

Mechanisms of Immune Injury

As I have indicated, the trigger to the sequence of events that terminates in irreversible kidney damage — that of antibody or immune complex deposition within glomeruli — is not pathogenic of or in itself. The destruction is the result of the inflammatory response that follows, which in turn triggers the clotting, fibrinolytic, and kinin-generating systems.

Antibody Specificity. Antibody with GBM specificity produced either endogenously or exogenously reacts directly with these structures. A smooth continuous ribbon-like deposition of antibody along the basement membrane can be visualized by immunofluorescent techniques. The kidney, and occasionally the lung, are specific target tissues for antibodies of anti-GBM specificity. In contrast, the discontinuous granular immunoglobulin deposits of immune complex disease consist of antibodies of varied and widely ranging specificities together with their respective antigens. The complexes visualized in SLE consist of DNA and antibodies to nuclear factors. These tissues are innocent bystanders when immune complexes containing antibody and antigen of non-glomerular origin are deposited within them. Both forms of antibody-antigen interaction are capable of triggering the complement cascade.

Quantity and Quality. The formation of pathogenic immune complexes is dependent on the immune response of the individual to a given antigenic challenge. Those individuals producing minimal or no antibody will have either none or very small non-pathogenic immune complexes formed. Those individuals responding vigorously with large amounts of antibody will form very large complexes in antibody excess which are rapidly cleared by the reticuloendothelial system. Individuals intermediate in their response, i.e., barely keeping up with the job of clearing antigen, will form immune complexes in slight to moderate antigen excess. Such complexes are of sufficient size to be deposited within glomeruli, are most efficient at triggering the complement cascade, and are thus potentially pathogenic. Recent studies in the NZB/W F1 model suggest that antibody affinity may be of critical importance. The time of onset, time course, and severity of the murine lupus syndrome, are associated with the presence of increasing levels of low avidity anti-DNA antibody. Likewise, avidity of anti-DNA antibody in the serum of SLE patients with renal disease is lower than that in the SLE patient without renal involvement. Low affinity antibody is less efficient at antigen clearing and allows for the production and persistence in the circulation of potentially pathogenic immune complexes. In this sense the development of immune complex nephritis can be considered a consequence of a relative immunodeficiency, that of making poor quality (low affinity) antibody.

Immunoglobulin Class. IgM and IgG are capable of triggering the classic pathway of the complement system. IgA, in contrast, employs the alternative or properdin pathway, in addition to the other properdin-triggering materials such as aggregated immunoglobulins and endotoxins. Involvement of IgE antibody is suggested by some investigators. They suggest that antigen induces the release of platelet-activating factors and histamine from basophils sensitized with specific IgE antibody. The clumping of platelets releases vasoactive amines which along with histamine increase vascular permeability, allowing for the entry and deposition of immune complexes along the glomerular basement membrane.

Complex Size. Very large complexes (relative antibody excess) are inefficient at triggering complement. Although they may remain in the circulation for extended periods, they apparently do not have a propensity for accumulation within the glomeruli. Intermediate complexes (slight to moderate antigen excess with molecular weights $>10^6$) are soluble, very efficient at fixing complement, and show a propensity for accumulation within tissues.

The Inflammatory and Coagulation Response

The Complement (C′) System. Several lines of evidence implicate the involvement of the complement system in the pathogenesis of nephritis. These include: depression of total serum complement levels during immune complex deposition; identification of complement components (usually C′3) within glomeruli in a pattern similar to antibody deposition, either ribbon-like or lumpy-bumpy; prevention of arteritis and glomerulitis by depleting or inhibiting complement components (i.e., the use of cobra venom factor). Activation of the complement system by the classic or alternative pathway results in the liberation of anaphylatoxins, which increase vascular permeability and facilitate deposition of immune complexes. Chemotactic factors attract leukocytes which release their enzymes, causing degradation of the basement membrane and exposing collagen structures. In addition, stimulation of platelet aggregation and the amplification loop of the complement system ensues. The complement system in turn triggers and/or is triggered by the coagulation systems.

Clotting and Coagulation Systems. The ability to prevent glomerulitis by depleting or inhibiting components of this system points a finger of blame at these processes. Hageman factor is activated by the exposed collagen of damaged basement membrane, which in turn leads to the coagulation mechanism. Plasminogen is converted to plasmin, which in turn activates C′1 and C′3. Hageman factor converts prekallikrein to kalligrein, which is chemotactic for leukocytes, as well as activating the complement system. The cleavage of kininogen to bradykinin, a vasoactive amine, results in further reinforcement of this vicious cycle. A protease released by the leukocyte is also capable of activating C′3. Activated C′3 in turn promotes platelet clumping, fibrin deposition, and so the cycle continues.

CLINICAL EXAMPLES OF COMMONLY OCCURRING GLOMERULAR LESIONS IN MAN

We have enjoyed a brief look at immune mechanisms recognized as contributing factors in the development of certain glomerular lesions. The basic research is related to experiments performed primarily in animals. There are comparable examples well recognized in man and a brief examination of some of those examples is in order. It is beyond the scope of this text to examine the broad spectrum of recognized glomerular syndromes in their entirety and we must therefore limit our discussion to classically-described examples of disease.

Acute proliferative glomerulonephritis has long been recognized as a syndrome closely associated with streptococcal infections. That this syndrome may be temporally related to infections with many other organisms is well-recognized, and documentation exists for bacterial, viral and fungal infections as an antecedent event leading to the development of acute glomerulonephritis. There are, in addition, many cases for which no antecedent infectious agents can be recognized and these, for lack of better definition, have been lumped into an idiopathic variety. For the sake of this discussion I will reserve my remarks to the well-recognized poststreptococcal glomerulonephritis.

This disease entity occurs with the highest frequency in children, although it may occur at any age. There is a latent period between the recognition of streptococcal infection and the onset of the renal lesion. The classic clinical presentation includes hematuria, proteinuria, a rapidly rising BUN and creatinine, diminution in urinary output, fluid retention, and elevation in blood pressure. The presence of any or all of these clinical findings is highly variable, and in all probability, many cases are never clinically recognized. These clinical findings are associated with well-documented pathologic changes within the glomerular tufts. The glomeruli are bloodless, hypercellular, enlarged, and fill Bowman's space; there is marked proliferation of mesangial and endothelial cells with a variable degree of infiltration with polymorphonuclear leukocytes in the capillary lumina and the mesangial space. All glomeruli are affected and involvement is relatively uniform. Capillary walls are thin and delicate, except for occasional irregularities which, by light microscopy, can be recognized as discrete deposits on the epithelial surface of the basement membrane. Changes in the parietal epithelial cells are inconspicuous, although a few segmental epithelial

crescents may be seen. Necrosis of the tufts and hilus thrombi are unusual. Interstitial edema, focal tubule degeneration, and scattered collections of mononuclear cells may be seen. Blood vessels are usually normal.

By electron microscopy, the most consistent finding is the presence of discrete electron-dense nodular deposits on the epithelial surface of the basement membrane. The overlying epithelial cell cytoplasm is condensed adjacent to the hump, and the deposits are most often located at the site of the epithelial cell slit pore. Leukocytes may be seen impinging upon basement membrane denuded of endothelial cell cytoplasm. Epithelial cell foot processes show coalescence with obliteration of the slit pore complex. Mesangial cells are notably increased in number. Examination by immunofluorescent staining may reveal irregular deposits of immunoglobulin-G, immunoglobulin-M and, less commonly, immunoglobulin-A. Components of the complement system are found in frequent association with the immunoprotein deposits. Deposits of fibrin may be found distributed in a segmental fashion within the mesangium or in association with epithelial crescent formation.

These clinical, morphologic, and serologic features suggest that classic acute post-streptococcal glomerulonephritis is an immune complex disease. Repeated attempts have been made to localize soluble streptococcal products in association with the immune complex deposits, but results have either been negative, inconclusive, or difficult to repeat.

The immediate prognosis for post-streptococcal glomerulonephritis is favorable. With modern management, less than 1 per cent of pediatric patients can be expected to die in the acute stages of the illness. Long-term prognosis, however, remains controversial. Available evidence suggests that in the majority of pediatric patients the prognosis is excellent. The complete disappearance of urinary abnormalities may be delayed for several years; serial biopsies may display focal glomerular abnormalities and persistent deposits within the mesangium of immune globulins and/or complement. The situation in adults is quite different. Collective evidence available would suggest that the older the patient at the onset of disease, the less likely the individual to enjoy a total and complete recovery.

The treatment of acute post-streptococcal glomerulonephritis is entirely symptomatic until all clinical signs of disease have abated. Most patients can be expected to undergo a diuresis within one to three weeks of the onset of illness. Prolonged oliguria and persistent massive proteinuria are indications for serious concern, and under these conditions, a renal biopsy should be performed to assess prognosis and confirmation of the original diagnosis. The administration of cytotoxic agents such as cyclophosphamide or Imuran has not been demonstrated to alter the course of acute post-streptococcal glomerulonephritis, and to date there is no evidence to recommend the use of steroid preparations.

Rapidly Progressive Glomerulonephritis. This disorder is relatively uncommon and, in one recently reported series, accounted for less than 2 per cent of cases presenting with glomerulonephritis. The patients are usually young to middle-aged males, with a male-to-female predominance of roughly two to one. The onset of the disease may be abrupt and resemble acute post-streptococcal glomerulonephritis, except severe oliguria occurs much more commonly. An antecedent history of streptococcal infection does not exist, more commonly a history will be elicited of a recent upper respiratory tract or flu-like syndrome. In most cases, there is an insidious onset of disease with presenting complaints referable to the development of uremia or fluid retention. The absence of pulmonary hemorrhage distinguishes this syndrome from that of Goodpasture's disease. Examination of the urine classically reveals red blood cells and red blood cell casts in association with a varying degree of proteinuria. Circulating antiglomerular basement membrane antibody may be demonstrated early in the course of the disease. Fibrin degradation products are frequently elevated in plasma and urine; serum levels of complement are usually normal, although C'3 may be depressed in some cases. Examination of renal tissue by light microscopy reveals extensive extracapillary proliferation of the parietal epithelial cells which line Bowman's capsules into *epithelial crescents*. In usual cases, more than 50 per cent of glomeruli will evidence crescent formation. The glomerular tufts may be compressed by this proliferation of epithelial cells. Extensive necrosis of glomerular tufts can be seen in association with leukocyte infiltration and collapse of capillary loops. Over a period of days or weeks, progressive sclerosis and fibrosis of glomeruli occur.

Immunofluorescent studies are highly variable, and at least three patterns have been described. The linear deposit of IgG, diffuse granular IgG, or, less commonly, IgM deposits accompanied by complement, specifically C'3, deposits in both the peripheral capillary loops and the mesangial interstitium. Fibrin-related deposits are also found, frequently in the crescents and in Bowman's space, or, less commonly, the lumina of involved tubules. Electron microscopy may reveal subendothelial deposits of electron-dense material indicative of immune complex disease. Biopsies may fail to reveal any deposits, with the principal pathologic alteration that of increasing mesangial matrix, collapse of denuded capillary walls, and fibrin thrombi. The crescents, by electron microscopy, demonstrate proliferation of parietal epithelial cells.

The diffuse IgG pattern in rapidly progressive glomerulonephritis with or without pulmonary hemorrhage is indicative of an antiglomerular basement membrane pathogenesis. The presence of diffuse granular deposits of IgG is more indicative of an immune complex pathogenesis. The third pattern consisting of scanty or irregular deposits of IgG with extensive fibrin deposition is relatively uncommon. It seems possible that each of the described patterns are compatible with a common pathologic basis, i.e., immune complexes leading to initial damage, subsequent exposure of basement membrane antigen, an endogenous immune response to the antigen thus exposed, and a cascading of the complement system in association with fibrin deposits leading to the various described pathologic entities, depending on timing of the tissue taken for examination.

The outlook for recovery in rapidly progressive glomerulonephritis is extremely poor. Recently, several authors have reported favorably on a combination therapy of cytotoxic agents, steroids, and repeated plasmapheresis. At the time of this writing, long-term results are not available.

Membranous Glomerulonephritis. Membranous glomerulonephritis may result from a number of known causes; the majority of cases, however, will fall under the catch-all term of "idiopathic membranous glomerulonephritis" (see Table 14–7). This disease process can occur at any age. The majority of patients are over the age of 40 at the time of diagnosis. The onset is insidious, without antecedent upper respiratory tract infection or history of streptococcal or other known infection. Hypertension and azotemia occur late in the course of the disease. Proteinuria is commonly non-selective. Microscopic hematuria is common; complement levels in the plasma are usually normal. Patients classically present with asymptomatic proteinuria or frank nephrotic syndrome. The rate at which the disease progresses to renal failure is highly unpredictable. Examination of tissue by light microscopy reveals the characteris-

TABLE 14–7 CLINICAL CONDITIONS COMMONLY ASSOCIATED WITH MEMBRANOUS GLOMERULONEPHRITIS

1. Idiopathic
2. Systemic lupus erythematosus
3. Heavy metals
4. Syphilis (congenital and secondary)
5. Malaria
6. Chronic active hepatitis
7. Sarcoidosis
8. Sjogren's syndrome
9. Sickle cell disease
10. Neoplasia
11. Renal vein thrombosis
12. Diabetes mellitus

tic feature of diffuse and uniform thickening of the capillary walls without significant proliferation of endothelial, mesangial, or epithelial cells. With progression, capillary walls become increasingly thickened; even with advanced progression of the capillary lesion, tubule alterations are minimal. Crescents, if present at all, are focal and are considered a late manifestation of the disease. Electron microscopy reveals small, discrete subepithelial deposits of electron-dense material producing some distortion of the foot processes. As the disease progresses, the electron-dense deposits enlarge, and projections of basement membrane-like material develop, giving the characteristic positive spikes seen by silver staining in light microscopy. This gives an irregular contour to the epithelial side of the basement membrane. With time the deposits become larger and more heterogeneous in size and distribution, and may vary in their degree of electron density. Foot processes demonstrate progressive distortion and disruption. By immunofluorescence, IgG is nearly always present in a granular distribution corresponding to the capillary loops sparing the mesangium. In advanced cases, IgG deposits may be weak and irregular, or even negative, corresponding to the decreased electron-density seen by electron microscopy. IgM and IgA deposits are scanty; complement is usually found in a pattern similar to that of IgG. The natural history and course of this disease is a highly irregular progression, punctuated by clinical remissions, which may be spontaneous. There is no clear-cut evidence that any form of therapy currently available has played a significant role in either retardation of the progression of this disease process or in the clinical remissions that have been noted.

Minimal Change Disease, known by several other synonyms such as lipoid nephrosis, or nochange by light microscopy, has no clear-cut or documented association with an alteration in immune mechanisms. It is commonly seen in younger age groups, occurring less and less frequently with advancing age. Usually there is a sudden onset of edema associated with massive proteinuria. Males predominate by a ratio of 1.5:1 in most series. Hypoalbuminemia and hyperlipemia are commonly demonstrated in association with the onset of edema. Hypertension is uncommon, and azotemia occurs rarely, unless hypovolemia is severe. Microscopic hematuria may be seen in a minority of cases; C'3 and C'4 levels are usually normal; C'1q levels may occasionally be decreased. The proteinuria is most often selective in nature, particularly in children. In adults, however, poorly selective proteinuria may be seen in a substantial number of cases. Examination by light microscopy reveals a paucity of pathologic findings. Electron microscopy detects abnormalities of epithelial cells of the glomerular capillaries

which are typical but not specific. Juxtaposition of the foot processes of epithelial cells and the obliteration of the slit pore membrane is noted in all glomeruli and glomerular capillaries. There is an associated vacuolation of cell cytoplasm. The glomerular basement membrane is normal in thickness. Examination by immunofluorescence fails to reveal significant deposits of IgG, IgM, or complement. The pathogenesis of this clinical entity remains to be delineated. Spontaneous remissions apparently occur frequently and a high percentage of cases respond dramatically following the initiation of steroid therapy. In patients who fail to respond to steroids, or relapse following their withdrawal, the administration of cyclophosphamide may be therapeutic. The mechanism of action of steroids and alkylating agents in lipoid nephrosis is unknown.

Nephrotic Syndrome. Nephrotic syndrome is a flexible term that is difficult to define with any degree of accuracy. It has been defined in the past as the association of edema, proteinuria, hypoalbuminemia, and hyperlipemia with renal disease. The presence of all these findings is considered necessary for its diagnosis, but, if these criteria are too rigidly enforced, several forms of the disease may be overlooked. It is true that most patients will exhibit all these manifestations at one time or another during the course of their illness, but it is also true that all manifestations may not be present at the same time, especially at an early stage. A better definition for the nephrotic syndrome is the one offered by Kark, in which he defines it as the metabolic, nutritional, and clinical consequences of massive proteinuria. Its presence does not imply a single disease entity. It can be observed in various forms of primary renal disease, as well as in association with certain generalized systemic diseases.

The nephrotic syndrome may be found at any age, occurring more commonly in children and young adults, but it is still observed frequently in the middle and older age groups. Edema is usually the first clinical manifestation noted and frequently brings the patient to the attention of the physician. It may appear gradually in the course of weeks, or may be of rapid and sudden onset. The edema is usually pitting in nature and is influenced by gravity. As a consequence, it varies with position, noticed in the face in the morning and in lower extremities in the evening. It may be minimal or extensive, involving the various serous cavities producing hydrocele, ascites, and pleural effusion. Visceral edema can occur in the more advanced cases of anasarca. Cases of acute edema of the larynx have been reported. Retinal sheen and skin pallor are manifestations of local edema. The presence of edema is not necessary for the definition of nephrotic syndrome and in early stages a moderate proteinuria may be the only clinical manifestation. Weakness, anorexia, and headaches are common complaints. Changes in the fingernails are observed consisting of paired horizontal white lines on the nail bed and pinking of the normally white semilune. These changes are secondary to hypoproteinemia.

The most important change in the urine is proteinuria. Its intensity varies greatly from 2.5 gm. to as high as 70 gm. per 24 hours. It is usually found in excess of 3.5 gm. per 24 hours. Proteinuria is related to an increased permeability of the glomerular basement membrane to plasma proteins. Albumin constitutes the bulk of protein present. Protein losses may be highly specific for albumin or relatively non-specific, with the presence of Alpha-1 globulin, Alpha-2 globulin, and lipoproteins, depending on the basic underlying pathology. The degree of selectivity may have a prognostic value, those with the non-selective type having the worst prognosis. Examination of the urinary sediment will reveal the presence of casts, birefractile bodies, and oftentimes minimal concentrations of red and white blood cells. The lowering of the plasma protein level, particularly of albumin, is another characteristic feature of the nephrotic syndrome. Increased lipemia and hypercholesterolemia are consistently present in association with minimal change disease. Hypercholesterolemia may be absent in other forms of the syndrome. The evolution of the nephrotic syndrome will depend on the nature of the underlying renal disease. It may present a wide spectrum of clinical disease, from the benign course associated with minimal change commonly seen in children, to the picture of progressive renal failure and uremia observed in older adults. Infection is a common complication, and before the advent of antibiotics it was the major cause of death. It has been proposed that the propensity for infection is associated with the demonstrated low levels of circulating IgG commonly associated with relapse.

The major pathophysiologic event in the nephrotic syndrome is the increase of the permeability of the glomerular basement membrane to protein. The mechanism of this increased permeability is not well understood, but it would appear that the increased filtration of plasma proteins is due to a diffuse change in the basement membrane at the micromolecular level.

TUBULO-INTERSTITIAL DISEASES (INTERSTITIAL NEPHRITIS)

Pathologists have long recognized a disease syndrome characterized by renal failure in association with bilaterally small kidneys and a normal caliceal system by gross examination. Microscopic examination reveals relative glomerular sparing,

TABLE 14–8 COMMON CAUSES: TUBULO-INTERSTITIAL DISEASE

1. Antibiotics: e.g., Methicillin
2. Analgesics: Phenacetin, Acetaminophen, ASA
3. Diuretics: Lasix, Hydrodiuril
4. Heavy Metals: Gold, lead, etc.
5. Metabolic Disorders: Hypercalcemia, hypocalcemia, hyperuricemia
6. Hyperproteinemia: Multiple myeloma
7. Anesthetics: Methoxyflurane
8. Infections

periglomerular fibrosis, a remarkable amount of interstitial fibrosis with or without round cell infiltration, marked flattening of tubule epithelial cells with dilatation of tubule lumina which are filled with a pink proteinaceous material on H & E staining. Distribution of these changes is not uniform and they occur in varying degrees of severity. It has been common practice to lump all disease patterns which approximated these findings into a single disease process believed to be caused by infection. Although apparent that infection may lead to this clinical-pathologic state, many other etiologies are now recognized and most probably account for the majority of cases described (see Table 14–8).

The onset and progression of interstitial nephritis may be acute and fulminating, with accompanying oliguria and rapidly progressive renal failure. A more common presentation is that of slowly progressive and often unrecognized renal failure with clear-cut clinical symptomatology developing only after the renal damage has become far advanced. Many of the recognized and, to some extent, previously discussed physiologic functions of the kidneys predispose them to injuries of the type described in tubulo-interstitial diseases. In all probability as yet undefined functions may make additional contributions to the initiation and progression of disease. Specific factors related to the kidney include the following:

1. The kidneys receive a remarkably high blood flow calculated at 20 per cent of cardiac output. This fluid flow perfuses tissue representing only 0.4 per cent of total body weight. Ninety per cent of that blood flow is directed to the renal cortex. Despite small differences in arterial-venous oxygen, renal oxygen consumption is high. This makes renal tissue susceptible to any factor that interferes with oxygen availability, transport, or utilization.

2. Cells of the renal tubule epithelium have the ability selectively to uncouple protein binding. Many potential cellular toxins are effectively inactivated while circulating bound to plasma proteins. Unbound by the uncoupling mechanism of

the kidney, they may become toxic to the cells in which the uncoupling has taken place. At the same time, concentration and acidification of urine is taking place, adding a further burden of susceptibility.

3. Compounds which may be relatively nontoxic at a pH of 6.8 to 7.4 may become highly toxic when hydrogen ion concentration increases and pH values fall to the range of 4.5 to 6.5.

4. Phagocytosis by white blood cells is impeded by rising osmolality and ceases altogether when values exceed 600 milliosmoles.

5. Ammonia production is a usual and important function of normal kidney tissue and rises rapidly in the face of an increased hydrogen ion load. High concentrations of ammonia interfere with complement activation and may interfere with the usual immunologic response to potential injury.

6. The vascular bed of the kidney is extensive per gram of tissue and may in itself predispose to injury beyond that seen in other organs.

The clinical presentation is remarkably variable. In the acute fulminating form, the patient experiences oliguria associated with a rapid rise in BUN and serum creatinine. He may have a concomitant cutaneous rash and peripheral eosinophilia in association with eosinophils in the urine. Protein, WBC's, RBC's, and a variety of urinary casts are present in the urine but are in no way diagnostic.

Chronic forms are insidious in onset and, under most circumstances, have no antecedent history of an acute episode. As opposed to the usual finding of normal size or enlarged kidney by x-ray in the acute form, kidneys are classically small and scarred. The caliceal system is normal unless papillary necrosis or obstruction is present or has occurred in the past. In many cases anemia may be out of proportion to the degree of uremia. Proteinuria is present, but rarely exceeds 2 gm. per 24 hours. White blood cells and, to a lesser extent, red blood cells may be present in the urine.

While it is beyond the scope of this discussion to consider in detail all of the known causes of tubulo-interstitial disease, several of the more common categories can be reviewed.

Disorders Due to Hypersensitivity. Agents included in this grouping are methicillin, ampicillin, penicillin, sulfonamides, diuretics, anticonvulsants, and antituberculin drugs. The lesion is not dose-related and oftentimes follows the second exposure to the drug. Antibodies to specific agents (e.g., methicillin) have been demonstrated. With appropriate recognition of the inciting agent and its prompt removal, recovery is the rule, although cases have been reported with chronic renal failure as the end result.

Toxic Factors. Agents falling into this category have a direct toxic effect on tissues, either alone or in combination. Examples include: phenacetin, acetaminophen, and acetylsalicylic acid (oftentimes referred to as analgesic-abuse nephritis). The usual course is one of injury occurring with prolonged exposure. Apparently an individual susceptibility exists and injury does not occur in every individual so exposed. A wide variety of antibiotics have been implicated. Diuretics have been implicated on occasion.

Metabolic Factors. Hypercalcemia can lead, either abruptly or gradually, to renal failure. Crystallization may occur in the interstitial area with or without intraluminal crystallization. Calcium ion in high concentrations may have a direct toxic effect on tubule cells without any demonstrable crystal formation and produce a concomitant drop in renal blood flow leading to a rapid fall in glomerular filtration rate. An associated nephrogenic diabetes insipidus syndrome may occur.

Other examples of metabolic factors which may lead to interstitial nephritis include hypokalemia and hyperuricemia. Renal changes usually occur only after prolonged states of potassium deficiency and appear to be largely reversible. Cases of persistent changes have been reported but are difficult to document.

Pyelonephritis. The role of urinary tract infection in the pathogenesis of acute or chronic renal disease has undergone major reassessment in recent years. Data currently available suggest that primary infection of the kidney in the absence of other renal pathology is an unusual cause of extensive renal parenchymal damage in the adult.

The bacteria commonly responsible for infections in the urinary system are: *Escherichia coli, Proteus* species, *Klebsiella, Enterobacter* and *Pseudomonas.* Various species of enterococci have been implicated. All these agents are usual and common constituents of bowel flora. The majority of uncomplicated infections are *E. coli.* If the patient has undergone prior antibiotic therapy, instrumentation, or has an associated urinary tract anomaly, the prevalence of infection with organisms other than *E. coli* rises sharply.

Infection may occur in any segment of the urinary tract without necessary involvement of other segments. The mere presence of bacteria in the urine cannot directly implicate the area primarily involved.

Spread of infection to involve the renal parenchyma may occur in one of three ways: (1) direct invasion by ascending the urethra, bladder, and ureter; (2) lymphatic invasion; (3) hematogenous spread. Evidence suggests that lymphatic spread is a rare event. The most common route of infection occurs by direct ascent. Hematogenous infection is much less common and when it does occur is related to specific organisms such as tuberculosis, staphylococcus, and pseudomonas.

The usual site of infection is the medulla, with

direct extension into the cortex in a segmental fashion. The susceptibility of the medulla to small numbers of organisms of relatively low virulence can be explained by a number of factors unique to that renal segment. Among those are: (1) high ammonia level; (2) hypertonicity; (3) relatively low blood flow; (4) depressed leukocyte immigration.

Renal parenchymal infection without associated pathology is self-limited and can be expected to resolve spontaneously in a period of six weeks to six months with or without therapy. Underlying pathology such as stones, reflex, obstruction, or scarring can contribute to sustained and widespread infection, resulting in significant and permanent loss of parenchyma.

In our discussion of tubulo-interstitial diseases, I have touched on only a small number of known causes of this type of renal damage. No doubt a wide variety of as yet unidentified compounds exist with the potential for producing nephrotoxicity in addition to those already identified. This is particularly disturbing in a society where new chemical agents in a variety of forms and exposure reach the environment each day. Only after long exposure, as in the case of analgesic-abuse nephritis, will many of these agents be documented as potential toxins to renal tissue. It behooves us all as physicians to keep this point in mind when searching for a potential cause of renal failure and, more importantly, in doing our part to see that exposure is limited to an absolute necessity in an area over which we have control — that is, exposure to prescription drugs.

REFERENCES

REVIEW OF NORMAL RENAL PHYSIOLOGY

Neutze, J. M., Wyler, F., and Rudolph, A. M.: Use of radioactive microspheres to assess distribution of cardiac output of microspheres. Am. J. Physiol., 215:496, 1968.

Kaihara, S., Rutherford, R. B., Schwenker, E. P., and Wagner, H. N.: Distribution of cardiac output in experimental hemorrhagic shock in dogs. J. Appl. Physiol., 27:218, 1969.

Boyer, C. C.: The vascular pattern of the renal glomerulus as revealed by plastic reconstruction from serial sections. Anat. Rec., 125:435, 1956.

Elias, H., Hosman, A., Barth, I. B., and Solmon, A.: Blood flow in the renal glomerulus. J. Urol., 83:790, 1960.

Edwards, J. G.: Efferent arterioles of glomeruli in the juxtamedullary zone of human kidney. Anat. Rec., 123:521, 1956.

Smith, J. P.: Anatomical features of the human renal glomerular efferent vessel. J. Anat., 90:290, 1956.

Trueta, J., Barclay, A. E., Daniel, P. M., Franklin, K. J., and Prichard, M. M. L.: Studies of the renal circulation. Blackwell Scientific Publications Oxford, 1948.

Horster, M., and Thurau, K.: Micropuncture studies on filtration rates of single superficial and juxtamedullary glomeruli in rat. Arch. Ges. Physiol., 301:162, 1968.

Brenner, B. M., Troy, J. L., and Daugharty, T. M.: The dynamics of glomerular ultrafiltration in the rat. J. Clin. Invest., 50:1776, 1971.

Brenner, B. M., and Galla, J. H.: Influence of postglomerular hematocrit and protein concentration on rat nephron fluid transfer. Am. J. Physiol., 220:148, 1971.

Stein, J. H., Congbalay, R. C., Karsh, D. L., Osgood, R. W., and Ferris, T. F.: Effect of bradykinin on proximal tubular sodium resorption in the dog: evidence for functional nephron heterogeneity. J. Clin. Invest., 51:1709, 1972.

Forster, R. P., and Maes, J. P.: Effect of experimental neurogenic hypertention on renal blood flow and glomerular filtration rates in intact denervated kidneys of unanesthetized rabbits with adrenal glands demedullated. Am. J. Physiol., 150:534, 1947.

Mitchell, G. D. G.: The nerve supply of the kidneys. Acta Anat. (Basel), 10:1, 1950.

Hollenberg, N. K., Solomon, H. S., Adams, D. F., Abrams, H. L., and Merrill, J. P.: Renal vascular responses to angiotensin and norepinephrine in normal man. Circ. Res., 31:750, 1972.

Hardaker, W. T., Jr., and Wechsler, A. S.: Redistribution of renal intracortical blood flow during dopamine infusion in dogs. Circ. Res., 33:437, 1973.

Johnson, H. H., Herzog, J. P., and Lauler, D. P.: Effect of prostaglandin E_1 on renal hemodynamics, sodium and water excretion. Am. J. Physiol., 213:936, 1967.

Zins, G. R.: Renal prostaglandins. Am. J. Med., 58:14, 1975.

Kirschenbaum, M. A., and Stein, J. H.: The effect of inhibition of prostaglandin synthesis on urinary sodium excretion in conscious dogs. J. Clin. Invest., 57:517, 1976.

Swain, J. A., Heynkricky, G. R., Boettcher, D. H., and Vatner, S. F.: Prostaglandin control of renal circulation in unanesthetized dog and baboon. Am. J. Physiol., 229:826, 1975.

Hardwicke, J., Hulme, B., Jones, J. H., and Ricketts, C. R.: Measurement of glomerular permeability to polydisperse radioactively labeled macromolecules in normal rabbits. Clin. Sci., 34:505, 1968.

Maddox, D. A., Bennett, C. M., Deen, W. M., Glassock, R. J., Knudson, D., Daugharty, T. M., and Brenner, B. M.: Determinants of glomerular filtration in experimental glomerulonephritis in the rat. J. Clin. Invest., 55:305, 1975.

Jamison, R. L.: Intrarenal heterogeneity. The case for two functionally dissimilar populations of nephrons in the mammalian kidney. Am. J. Med., 54:281, 1973.

Maddox, D. A., Deen, W. M., and Brenner, B. M.: Dynamics of glomerular ultrafiltration. VI. Studies in the primate. Kidney International, 5:271, 1974.

Windhager, E., and Giebisch, G.: Proximal sodium in fluid transport. Kidney International, 9:121, 1976.

Maude, D. L.: The role of bicarbonate in proximal tubular sodium chloride transport. Kidney International, 5:253, 1974.

Maren, T. H.: Chemistry of the renal absorption of bicarbonate. Canad. J. Physiol. Pharmacol., 52:1041, 1974.

Malnic, G., and Steinmetz, P. R.: Transport processes in urinary acidification. Kidney International, 9:172, 1976.

CLINICAL EVALUATION OF RENAL FUNCTION

Doolan, P. D., Alpen, E. L., and Theil, G. B.: A clinical appraisal of the plasma concentration and endogenous clearance of creatinine. Am. J. Med., 32:65, 1962.

Healy, J. K.: Clinical assessment of glomerular filtration rate by different forms of creatinine clearance and a modified urinary phenolsulphonphthalun excretion test. Am. J. Med., 44:348, 1968.

Wesson, L. G.: Physiology of the human kidney. Grune & Stratton, New York, 1969.

Jelliffe, R. W.: Creatinine clearance: bedside estimate. Ann. Int. Med., 79:604, 1973.

Spinel, C. H.: The Fe Na test used in the differential diagnosis of acute renal failure. J.A.M.A., 236 (6):579, 1976.

Anderson, R. J., Linas, S. T., Berns, A. S., Henrich, W. L., Miller, T. R., Gabow, P. A., and Schrier, R. W.: Non oliguric acute renal failure. N. Engl. J. Med., 269:1134, 1977.

Jones, L. W., and Weil, M. H.: Water creatinine and sodium excretion following circulatory shock with renal failure. Am. J. Med., 51:314, 1971.

DISORDERS OF SODIUM METABOLISM

Albrink, M. J., Hald, P. M., Mann, E. B., and Peters, J. P.: The displacement of serum water by the lipids of hyperlipemic serum: A new method for the rapid determination of serum water. J. Clin. Invest., 31:1483, 1955.

Bartter, F. C., and Schwartz, W. B.: The syndrome of inappropriate secretion of antidiuretic hormone. Am. J. Med., 42:790, 1967.

Brenner, B. M., Falchuk, K. H., Keimowitz, R. I., and Berliner, R. W.: The relationship between peritubular capillary protein concentration and fluid resorption by the renal proximal tubule. J. Clin. Invest., 48:1519, 1969.

Carter, N. W., Rector, F. C., and Seldin, D. W.: Hyponatremia in cerebral disease resulting from the inappropriate secretion of antidiuretic hormone. N. Engl. J. Med., 264:67, 1961.

DeRivera, J. L.: Inappropriate secretion of antidiuretic hormone from fluphenazine. Ann. Int. Med., 82:811, 1975.

DiScala, V. A., and Kinney, M. J.: Effects of myxedema on the renal diluting and concentrating mechanisms. Am. J. Med., 50:325, 1971.

Earley, L. E., and Friedler, R. M.: The effects of the combined renal vasodilatation and pressor agents on renal hemodynamics and the tubular resorption of sodium. J. Clin. Invest., 45:542, 1966.

Moses, A. M., and Miller, M.: Drug induced dilutional hyponatremia. N. Engl. J. Med., 291:1234, 1974.

Klahr, S., and Slatopolsky, E.: Renal regulation of sodium excretion. Arch. Int. Med., 131:780, 1973.

Pitts, R. F.: Physiology of the kidney and body fluids. Yearbook Medical Publishers, Chicago, 1974.

Arieff, A., and Guisado, R.: Effects on the central nervous system of hypernatremia and hyponatremic states. Kidney International, 10:104, 1976.

DISORDERS OF POTASSIUM METABOLISM

Flear, C. T. G., Cook, W. T., and Quentin, A.: Serum potassium levels as an index of body content. Lancet, 1:458, 1957.

Simmons, D. H., and Avedon, M.: Acid-base alterations in plasma potassium concentration. Am. J. Physiol., 197:319, 1959.

Gennari, F. J., and Cohen, J. J.: Role of the kidney in potassium homeostasis: Lesson from acid-base disturbances. Kidney International, 8:1, 1975.

Fordtran, J. S., and Dietschy, J. M.: Water and electrolyte movement in the intestine. Gastroenterology, 50:263, 1966.

Schwartz, W. B., and Relman, A. F.: Metabolic and renal studies in chronic potassium depletion resulting from overuse of laxatives. J. Clin. Invest., 32:258, 1953.

Knochel, J. P., Dotin, L. N., and Hamburger, R. J.: The pathophysiology of intense physical conditioning in a hot climate. Mechanisms of potassium depletion. J. Clin. Invest., 51:242, 1972.

Schwartz, W. B., and Relman, A. S.: Effects of electrolyte disorders on renal structure and function. N. Engl. J. Med., 276:383, 1967.

Beck, N., and Webster, S. K.: Impaired urinary concentrating ability and cyclic AMP in potassium depleted rat kidney. Am. J. Physiol., 231:1204, 1976.

Davidson, S., and Surawicz, B.: Incidence of superventricular and ventricular ectopic beats and rhythms of atrioventricular conduction disturbances in patients with hypopotassemia. Circulation, 34, Suppl 3: 85, 1966.

Tannen, R. L., Wedell, E., and Moore, R.: Renal adaptation to a high potassium intake. The role of hydrogen ion. J. Clin. Invest., 52:2089, 1973.

Goldfarb, S., Cox, M., Singer, I., and Goldberg, M.: Acute hyperkalemia induced by hyperglysemia: Hormonal mechanisms. Ann. Int. Med., 84:426, 1976.

Khuri, R. M., Wiederholt, M., Strieder, N., and Giebisch, G.: Effects of flow rate and potassium intake on distal tubular potassium transfer. Am. J. Physiol., 228:1249, 1975.

Giebisch, G.: Some reflections on the mechanism of renal tubular potassium transport. Yale J. Biol. Med., 48:315, 1975.

Wright, F.: Sites and mechanisms of potassium transport along the renal tubule. Kidney International, 11:415, 1977.

Brautbar, N., Levi, J., Rosler, A., Leitsdorf, E., Epstein, M., and Kleeman, C. R.: Familial hyperkalemia, a probable defect in potassium secretion. Clin. Res., Feb., 1976, p. 125A.

ACID-BASE DISTURBANCES

Brackett, N. C., Cohen, J. J., and Schwartz, W. B.: Carbondioxide titration curve of normal man. Effect of increasing degrees of acute hypercapnia on acid-base equilibrium. N. Engl. J. Med., 272:6, 1965.

Schwartz, W. B., Orning, K. J., and Porter, R.: The internal distribution of hydrogen ion with varying degrees of metabolic acidosis. J. Clin. Invest., 36:373, 1957.

Kurtzman, N. A., White, M. G., and Rogers, P. W.: Pathophysiology of metabolic alkalosis. Arch. Int. Med., 131:702, 1973.

Lemmon, E. J., and Lemann, J., Jr.: Defense of hydrogen ion concentration in chronic metabolic acidosis. Ann. Int. Med., 65:265, 1966.

Morris, R. C., Jr.: Renal tubular acidosis: mechanisms, classification and implications. N. Engl. J. Med., 281:1405, 1969.

Morris, R. C., Jr., Sebastian, A., and McSherry, E.: Renal acidosis. Kidney International, 1:322, 1972.

Oliva, P. B.: Lactic acidosis. Am. J. Med., 48:209, 1970.

Rector, F. C., Jr., Blommer, H. A., and Seldin, D. W.: Effect of potassium deficiency on the resorption of bicarbonate in the proximal tubule of the rat kidney. J. Clin. Invest., 43:1976, 1964.

Rector, F. C., Jr., Carter, N. W., and Seldin, D. W.: The mechanism of bicarbonate resorption of proximal distal tubules of the kidney. J. Clin. Invest., 44:278, 1965.

Seldin, D. W., and Rector, F. C., Jr.: Symposium on acid-base homeostasis. The generation and maintenance of metabolic alkalosis. Kidney International, 1:306, 1972.

ACTION OF DIURETIC DRUGS

Kessler, R. H., Lozano, R., and Pitts, R.: Studies on structure-diuretic activity relationships of organic compounds of mercury. J. Clin. Invest., 36:656, 1957.

Clapp, J. R., and Robinson, R. R.: Distal sites of action of diuretic drugs in the dog nephron. Am. J. Physiol., 215:228, 1968.

Seeley, J. F., and Dirks, J. H.: Micropuncture study of hypertonic mannitol diuresis in the proximal and distal tubule of the dog kidney. J. Clin. Invest., 48:2330, 1969.

Suki, W., Rector, F. C., Jr., and Seldin, D. W.: The site of action of furosemide and other sulphonamide diuretics in the dog. J. Clin. Invest., 44:1458, 1965.

Burg, M. B.: Tubular chloride transport in the mode of action of some diuretics. Kidney International, 9:189, 1976.

Clapp, J. R., and Robinson, R. R.: Distal sites of action of diuretic drugs in the dog nephron. Am. J. Physiol., 215:228, 1968.

Seeley, J. F., and Dirks, J. H.: Micropuncture studies of hypertonic mannitol diuresis in the proximal and distal tubule of the dog kidney. J. Clin. Invest., 48:2330, 1969.

Maren, T. H.: Carbonic anhydrase: chemistry, physiology and inhibition. Physiol. Rev., 47:595, 1967.

Burg, M., and Green, N.: Effect of ethacrynic acid on the thick ascending limb of Henle's loop. Kidney International, 4:301, 1973.

Burg, M.: The mechanism of action of diuretics in renal tubules. In Wessen, L., and Fanelli, G. (eds.): Recent Advances in Renal Physiology and Pharmacology. University Park Press, Baltimore, 1974.

Suki, W., Rector, F. C., Jr., and Seldin, D. W.: The site of action of furosemide and other sulphonamide diuretics in the dog. J. Clin. Invest., 44:1458, 1965.

Muth, R. G.: Diuretic properties of furosemide in renal disease. Ann. Int. Med., 69:249, 1968.

Cannon, P. J., Heinemann, H. O., Albert, M. S., Laragh, J. H., and Winters, R. W.: "Contraction" alkalosis after diuresis of edematous patients with ethacrynic acid. Ann. Int. Med., 62:979, 1965.

Burg, M. B.: Tubular chloride transport and the mode of action of some diuretics. Kidney International, 9:189, 1976.

Kunau, R. T., Jr., Weller, D. R., and Webb, H. L.: Clarification of the site of action of chlorothiazide in the rat nephron. J. Clin. Invest., 56:401, 1975.

CONGENITAL ANOMALIES OF THE KIDNEY

Hayman, J. M., Jr.: Congenital Malformations of the Kidney. *In* Strauss, M. B. and Welt, L. G. (eds.): Diseases of the Kidney, 2nd ed. Little, Brown & Co., Boston, 1971.

Morris, R. C., Jr., McInnes, R. R., Epstein, C. J., Sebastian, A., and Scriver, C. R.: Genetic and Metabolic Injury of the Kidney. *In* Brenner, B. M., and Rector, F. C., Jr. (eds.): The Kidney, Volume II. W. B. Saunders Co., Philadelphia, 1976.

Perkoff, G. G.: The Hereditary Renal Diseases. N. Engl. J. Med., 277:79, 1967.

Purriel, P., Drets, M., Pascal, E. E., Cestaur, S., Borras, A., Ferreira, W. A., Deluca, A., and Fernandes, L.: Familial hereditary nephropathy (Alport's Syndrome). Am. J. Med., 49:753, 1970.

Segal, S.: Disorders of renal amino acid transport. N. Engl. J. Med., 294:1044, 1976.

Bigelow, N. H.: The association of polycystic kidneys with intracranial aneurysms and other dilated disorders. Am. J. Med. Sci., 225:485, 1953.

Bricker, N. S., and Patten, J. F.: Cystic disease of the kidneys. A study of dynamics and chemical composition of cyst fluid. Am. J. Med., 18:207, 1955.

Bricker, N. S., and Patten, J. F.: Renal function studies in polycystic disease of the kidneys with observation on the effect of surgical decompression. N. Engl. J. Med., 256:212, 1957.

Dalgaard, O. Z.: Bilateral polycystic disease of the kidneys: Follow-up of 284 patients and their families. Acta. Scand., 328:1, 1957.

Morris, R. C., Yamauchi, H., and Palubinskas, A. J.: Medullary sponge kidney. Am. J. Med., 38:883, 1965.

Osath, A., Nondh, V., and Patter, E. L.: Pathogenesis of polycystic kidneys. Arch. Pathol., 77:466, 1964.

Stella, F. J., Massry, S. G., and Kleeman, C. R.: Medullary sponge kidney associated with parathyroid adenoma. Nephron, 10:332, 1973.

PATHOPHYSIOLOGY OF GLOMERULAR DAMAGE

McCluskey, R. T., and Classen, J.: Immunologically mediated glomerular tubular and interstitial renal disease. N. Engl. J. Med., 288:564, 1973.

Dickson, F. J., Feldman, J. D., and Vasquez, J. J.: Experimental glomerulonephritis. The pathogenesis of a laboratory model resembling the spectrum of human glomerulonephritis. J. Exp. Med., 113:899, 1961.

MacIntosh, R. M., Tinglof, B., Kaufman, D., Dornfeld, L., Gon-

ick, H., Smith, F. G., and Vernier, R. L.: Immunohistology in renal disease: diagnostic, prognostic, therapeutic and etiology value and limitations. Q. J. Med., 40:385, 1971.

Wilson, C. B., and Dixon, F. J.: Antiglomerular basement membrane antibody induced glomerulonephritis. Kidney International, 3:74, 1973.

Cochrane, C. G.: Immunologic tissue injury mediated by neutrophilic leukocytes. Adv. Immunol., 9:97, 1968.

Lambert, P. H., Perin, L. H., Mahieu, P., Nydigger, U. E., and Miescher, P. A.: Activation of complement in human nephritis. Adv. Nephrol., 4:79, 1974.

Peters, D. K., and Williams, D. G.: Complement and mesangial capillary glomerulonephritis: Role of complement deficiency in pathogenesis of nephritis. Nephron, 13:189, 1974.

di Belgiojoso, G. B., Tarantino, A., Bazzi, C., et al: Immunofluorescence patterns in chronic membranoproliferative glomerulonephritis. Clin. Nephrol., 6:303, 1976.

Wilson, C. B., and Dickson, F. J.: Immunopathology and glomerulonephritis. Ann. Rev. Med., 25:83, 1974.

Lange, K., and Treser, G.: Acute poststreptococcal glomerulonephritis. Clin. Nephrol., 1:55, 1973.

Baldwin, D. S., and Gluck, M. C.: The long term course of poststreptococcal glomerulonephritis. Ann. Int. Med., 80:342, 1974.

Hinglais, N., Garcia-Torras, R., Kleinknecht, D.: Long term prognosis in acute glomerulonephritis. Am. J. Med., 52:56, 1974.

Merrill, J. P.: Glomerulonephritis. N. Engl. J. Med., 290:257, 1974.

Baldwin, D. S., and Schact, R. G.: Late sequelae of poststreptococcal glomerulonephritis. Ann. Rev. Med., 27:49, 1976.

Lockwood, C. M., Rees, A. J., and Pearson, T. A.: Immunosuppression and plasma-exchange in the treatment of Goodpasture's Syndrome. Lancet, 1:711, 1976.

Kluthe, R., Vogt, A., and Batsford, S. R. (eds.): Glomerulonephritis: International Conference on Pathogenesis, Pathology and Treatment. John Wiley & Sons, New York, 1977.

TUBULO-INTERSTITIAL DISEASES (INTERSTITIAL NEPHRITIS)

Suki, W. N., and Eknoyan, G.: Tubulo-Interstitial diseases. *In* Brenner, B. M., and Rector, F. C., Jr. (eds.), The Kidney. W. B. Saunders Co., Philadelphia, 1976, pp. 1113–1137.

Drago, J. R., Rohner, T. J., Sanford, E. J., Engle, J., and Schoolwerth, A.: Acute interstitial nephritis. J. Urol., 115:105, 1976.

Andres, G. A., and McClusky, R. T.: Tubular and interstitial disease due to immunological mechanisms. Kidney International, 7:271, 1975.

Fuller, T. J., Barcenas, C. G., and White, M. G.: Diuretic induced interstitial nephritis. J.A.M.A., 235:1998, 1976.

15

Pulmonary Ventilation and Blood Gas Exchange*

W. Keith C. Morgan
and Douglas Seaton

The primary purpose of the lungs is to maintain the oxygen and carbon dioxide content of the arterial blood within a relatively narrow range. This range must be maintained even though both oxygen need and carbon dioxide production are constantly changing with the degree of activity and metabolic rate of the subject. The lungs achieve this homeostasis by allowing venous blood to come into contact with the alveolar gases; such contact taking place over an enormous surface area, the alveolo-capillary bed. Three basic mechanisms are involved in gas exchange: (1) *ventilation* or, as it is often known, the "bellows" function of the lungs; (2) *diffusion* or the transfer of gas from the alveolus to the capillary; and (3) *perfusion* or pulmonary blood flow.

VENTILATION

The ventilatory capacity of the lungs depends first on their size (lung volumes), second on the resistance to flow present in the airways, and third on the elastic properties or compliance of the lungs and the chest wall. Movement of air in and out of the lungs can be compared to the action of a pair of bellows, and is dependent on the pressure difference between the mouth and the

alveoli at various phases of breathing. At times of no flow, alveolar and mouth pressures are equal. During *inspiration,* the thorax enlarges, the diaphragm descends, and, as a result, the chest cage increases in volume as do the lungs. In contrast, *expiration* is largely passive and depends on the elastic recoil of the chest wall and lungs. The pressure that acts upon the lungs and causes them to expand during inspiration is that which exists in the pleural cavity. Intrapleural pressure is negative as compared to the atmospheric pressure, and during normal breathing varies between −5 and −9 cm. of water. Much larger pressure changes occur during forced expiratory and inspiratory maneuvers; for example, at total lung capacity, the intrapleural pressure is −35 to 40 cm. of water, whereas at residual volume the pressure may become slightly positive, especially at the lung bases. A detailed description of the mechanical events involved in inspiration is beyond the scope of this chapter but can be found in *The Respiratory Muscles* (Campbell, et al., 1970).

At this stage it is necessary to point out there is a gradient in pleural pressure from the top to the bottom of the lung. This gradient is largely gravity dependent and is thought to be related to the weight of the lung. Pleural pressure increases from the apex to the base; there being a gradient of around 7 to 8 cm. of water from top to bottom of the lung. This gradient has profound effects on regional ventilation and perfusion and will be discussed in more detail later in this chapter.

---

*Much of this chapter has previously been published in *Occupational Lung Disease* by W. K. C. Morgan, M.D. and A. Seaton, M.D., W. B. Saunders Company, Philadelphia, 1975.

Static Lung Volumes

Certain lung volumes can be measured with a spirometer; however, others require more complicated apparatus. The volume of each breath exhaled during quiet respiration is known as the tidal volume (V_T). The total volume of air that the lungs and bronchial tree contain after maximal inspiration is known as the total lung capacity (TLC). If the subject then exhales as much air as he can, the volume of air remaining in the lungs after the expiration is known as the residual volume (RV); that which has been expelled is known as the vital capacity (VC). It must be stressed that during the measurement of VC, the patient is permitted to take as long as he likes to complete the maneuver. If after maximal inspiration, he exhales as rapidly and as forcibly as possible, then the measurement obtained is known as the forced vital capacity (FVC). In normal persons the FVC and the VC are not significantly different; however, in certain types of airway obstruction (e.g., emphysema), the FVC may be considerably less than the vital capacity as a result of collapse of the smaller airways during forced expiration — a phenomenon known as air trapping. The volume of air remaining in the lung at the end of a normal expiration is known as the functional residual capacity (FRC), whereas the volume that can be exhaled from FRC is known as the expiratory reserve volume (ERV). Similarly the volume of air that can be taken in from FRC is known as the inspiratory capacity (IC); needless to say, the sum of the ERV and IC equals the VC (Fig. 15–1). The VC, ERV, and IC can be measured with a spirometer; TLC and its derivatives, FRC and RV, require other means, namely, closed circuit helium equilibration, the nitrogen washout, a radiographic method, or plethysmography.

The helium equilibration method requires that the subject rebreathe a known volume of helium in a closed circuit until equilibration is reached. The carbon dioxide produced during the rebreathing is absorbed. If the volume of helium reservoir is known, and if the initial and final concentrations of helium in the system are known, it is therefore possible to calculate the FRC. The nitrogen washout depends on giving the subject 100 per cent oxygen and collecting all the expired air in a large spirometer. When the nitrogen has been completely washed out from the lungs and collected along with the expired air in a Tissot spirometer, the volume of the expirate and the nitrogen concentration are measured. Since the concentration of nitrogen in the lungs at the start of the maneuver is known, it is therefore possible to calculate the volume of nitrogen present in the lungs and hence the FRC.

The plethysmographic method is probably the best and most accurate way of determining lung volumes, since it measures all the gas in the thoracic cage. In contrast, the helium equilibration and nitrogen washout methods do not include regions of poorly ventilated lung that contain trapped gas — e.g., bullae are not included — and thus falsely low estimates are obtained. A body plethysmograph consists of an airtight box in which the subject sits. As the subject breathes in and out, the pressure inside the box changes and is recorded by sensitive transducers. If the change in lung volume with each breath is also known, then by simple application of Boyle's Law it is possible to calculate the intrathoracic gas volume.

Total lung capacity can also be accurately determined from the chest film. Barnhard and his colleagues have described a method which utilizes anteroposterior and lateral films. The method depends on treating the lungs as a series of elliptical cylindroids and calculating the area of each. Allowance is made for heart size, pulmonary blood volume, the spine, and the domes of the diaphragm. The method has been simplified by Reger and his co-workers, is accurate, and has application to epidemiologic surveys. If the VC is determined by spirometry, it then becomes possible to measure the RV and hence the RV/TLC.

In a healthy young adult, the residual volume (RV) is around 20 per cent of the total lung capacity (TLC). As the subject grows older, the RV slowly increases so that by age 60 it may constitute up to 40 per cent of the TLC. The increase in RV is related to the fact that with increasing age the lung loses some of its elasticity. The decreased elastic recoil of the older person is opposed by an unchanged but relatively greater intrapleural pressure which maintains the lungs at a higher level of inflation than that present when the subject was younger. The increased lung volumes and associated increased radiographic translucency that occur with age used to be known as "senile emphysema;" however, since there is neither airways obstruction nor disrup-

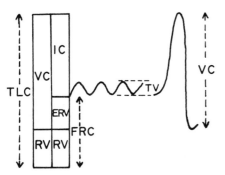

Figure 15–1 Lung volumes and spirometric tracing of a slow vital capacity maneuver in a normal subject.

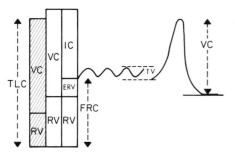

Figure 15–2 Lung volumes and spirometric tracing of a slow vital capacity maneuver in a subject with airways obstruction. The hatched area represents predicted values.

tion of the alveolo-capillary surface, that term is a misnomer.

In obstructive airways disease and emphysema, the RV/TLC is increased, and in many instances the RV may be well over 50 per cent of the TLC (Fig. 15–2). An increased RV/TLC is an almost invariable finding in air flow obstruction, but lesser increases in the ratio are sometimes seen in diffuse fibrosis such as fibrosing alveolitis or asbestosis. Such increases often are more apparent than real for the most part, and often are related either to inadequacies in the predicted values for RV and TLC or sometimes to an appreciable decrease in TLC, with the RV being less affected. In most subjects with emphysema, the TLC is increased above the predicted figure owing to a decrease in the elastic recoil of the lungs; however, the increase in TLC is not as dramatic as is the increase in RV. In the diffuse fibroses all the lung volumes tend to be smaller than the predicted figure, and this is particularly true of the VC and TLC (Fig. 15–3). In contrast, and for the reasons mentioned above, changes in RV are sometimes less spectacular in pulmonary fibrosis. Thus in an individual subject small increases in the RV/TLC are not necessarily diagnostic of any particular type of physiologic im-

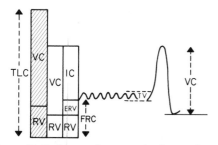

Figure 15–3 Lung volumes and spirometric tracing of a slow vital capacity in a subject with diffuse fibrosis. The hatched area represents predicted values.

pairment. In many subjects there is a mixed effect, the subject having some degree of airways obstruction and subsequently contracting another disease that produces stiff and smaller lungs. In epidemiologic studies a knowledge of the RV/TLC in large groups of persons is much more useful than it is in the individual. Thus the demonstration of an increased RV/TLC in a particular group of subjects as compared to a comparable control group indicates a higher prevalence of airways obstruction.

Dynamic Lung Volumes

Ventilatory capacity also depends to a large extent on the resistance to airflow in the bronchial tree. If a normal subject is asked to breathe in as far as possible and then to breathe out as rapidly and as forcibly as possible, he should be able to get out 80 per cent of his FVC in one second ($FEV_{1.0}$) and 95 per cent in 3 seconds. Although this is true in the young subject, there is a fall in the $FEV_{1.0}$/FVC ratio with age. By the time the subject is 55 or over, the ratio will often be around 65 to 70 per cent. Expiratory flows are most rapid early in the forced expiratory volume maneuver, but as the subject begins to approach RV there is a marked slowing. This is most evident once the subject gets below his FRC; when RV is reached, flow ceases entirely (Fig. 15–4). Subjects with airway obstruction, that is to say, those who have an increased resistance to flow of air in and out of their lungs (e.g., asthmatics, chronic bronchitics, and those with emphysema), all show a flatter curve with decreased flow rates. In some instances, there is also a loss of VC. In asthma, but not in the other two conditions, the use of bronchodilators such as isoproterenol or ephinephrine by nebulization will appreciably lessen the obstruction so that the forced expiratory volume curve becomes steeper and more closely resembles that of a normal person. As indices of obstruction, both the one-second and three-seconds timed vital capacity tests (percentage of FVC exhaled in one and three seconds respectively) are frequently used. Some workers, on the other hand, prefer to measure the actual volume of air exhaled in the first 0.75 second ($FEV_{0.75}$). A less popular but still commonly used measurement is the maximal expiratory flow rate (MEFR), this being the rate of flow between 200 and 1200 ml. on a forced expiratory volume tracing. Another index that has its advocates is the MMF (FEF 0.25–0.75) or the maximal expiratory flow over the mid-half of a forced expiratory spirogram. The latter measurement is more sensitive but it is also more variable, and if the forced expiratory volume maneuver is not recorded for an adequate period, spurious results are frequently obtained. All these indices have

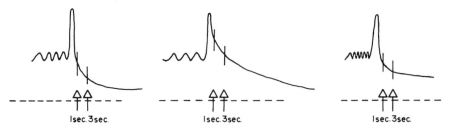

Figure 15–4 Forced expiratory volume maneuvers in a normal subject (left) and in subjects with obstructive (center) and restrictive (right) impairment.

their proponents, but there are valid reasons for preferring the $FEV_{1.0}$ and the MMF.

An additional method by which the ventilatory capacity can be assessed is the maximal breathing capacity (MBC). This should preferably be known as the maximal voluntary ventilation (MVV) and is the maximal volume of air breathed over one minute. As the test is very tiring to subjects with airways obstruction, the volume is usually measured over a period of 15 to 20 seconds and the result multiplied by the necessary factor. This test is effort-dependent and has little advantage over the single breath tests. The simple expedient of multiplying the FEV_1 by 35 yields an excellent approximation to the measured MVV.

The normal respiratory rate (f) of a young adult is around 12 per minute. With increasing age there is an increase to 14 or 16. Since the tidal volume is normally around 500 ml., the minute ventilation is 12 × 500 ml. = 6 L. ($V_T \times f$). Not all of every breath reaches the alveoli; some air remains in the nose, nasopharynx, and bronchi and therefore does not come into contact with the alveolo-capillary surface. The non-gas-exchanging part of the respiratory system is known as the anatomic dead space (V_{D_A}) and is normally around 150 ml. In a normal subject the volume of gas reaching the alveoli with each breath is 500 − 150 ml. = 350 ml. ($V_T - V_{D_A}$). Alveolar ventilation per minute therefore equals 350 ml. × 12 = 4.2 L. The anatomic dead space has to be distinguished from the physiologic dead space (V_{D_P}) which consists of the anatomic dead space plus the fraction of each breath wasted, either to ventilate underperfused alveolar units or to overventilate alveolar units relative to perfusion. In a normal subject the anatomic and physiologic dead spaces are approximately the same, but with mismatching of ventilation and perfusion, the V_{D_P} increases. Lung volumes are generally expressed at the subject's body temperature saturated with water vapor and at the atmospheric pressure (BTPS). When expressed at BTPS, the various indices represent the actual volume in the lungs.

Airflow Resistance

During quiet breathing, most of the respiratory effort goes toward overcoming the compliance of the lungs and chest wall. By comparison, the work necessary to overcome airflow resistance is small, but when breathing becomes deeper and more rapid, the work expended overcoming airways resistance increases rapidly. When the airways are narrowed or obstructed by mucus, there is a huge increase in airways resistance and the work of breathing, especially at lower lung volumes where the lumina of the airways normally are narrower.

Gas flow in the airways is governed by the same factors that regulate the flow of fluid in tubes or, if it comes to that, the flow of the electricity in a conductor. Ohm's Law (C = E/R, where C is the current or flow, E the voltage or pressure gradient, and R the resistance) applies equally well to the flow of gas in the airways. Airflow may be either turbulent or laminar. When flow is turbulent, the pressure gradient necessary to produce a certain flow rate is appreciably higher. With laminar flow, the pressure gradient necessary to produce a certain flow is directly proportional to the viscosity of the gas. In contrast, for turbulent flow, the viscosity of the gas becomes less important and the density more important. Under normal circumstances, flow in the larger airways tends to be turbulent and, in addition, eddy currents are set up at the bifurcation of the airways. In contrast in the smaller airways, that is to say from the 12th generation and down, flow is mainly laminar. Thus, flow in the central airways is mainly density-dependent, while in the smaller airways it is related more to the viscosity of the gases present. Poiseuille's Law ($P = K_1 V$, where P is driving pressure, V is flow, and K_1 is a constant that depends on the viscosity of the gas) applies only to laminar flow in a straight line in a tube whose cross-sectional diameter does not change. Clearly this situation does not apply in lungs, where the cross-sectional diameter is constantly changing, where the airways are repeatedly dividing, and where, owing

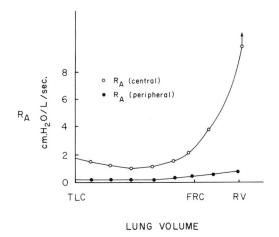

Figure 15–5 Relationship of central and peripheral airways resistance to lung volumes.

to disease, the diameter of the airways may be either narrowed and distorted or occasionally dilated. Nonetheless, despite all these variables, it is useful to apply to clinical situations the concept of airways resistance and the basic physical laws.

Airways resistance depends not only on the number of patent airways but on the total cross-sectional area of the airways. The intrathoracic resistance of the airways may be partitioned into central and peripheral components. The central component includes the resistance from the trachea to roughly the 11th generation of bronchi. The peripheral component is made up of the resistance from the 12th generation to the alveoli. Central resistance in normal subjects makes up 85 to 90 per cent of the total airway resistance (R_A). Thus the peripheral resistance constitutes only 10 to 15 per cent of the total resistance and, moreover, at high lung volumes is negligible (Fig. 15–5). It is therefore possible for a subject to have diffuse disease of the small airways and yet have a normal airway resistance and normal spirometry. When the resistance in the peripheral airways is increased, the lungs become less distensible, although total resistance may still be within normal limits. The peripheral airways usually are not uniformly and diffusely affected; rather the pathologic processes producing small airways disease tend to lead to patchy or regional involvement.

Airways resistance is normally expressed at FRC. This is related to the fact that the cross-sectional diameter of the airways varies greatly with lung volume. Thus at TLC the airways are widely patent and with expiration there is a fairly minor change in a cross-sectional diameter until FRC is approached, at which time the air-

ways start to narrow rapidly. For this reason, R_A remains relatively unchanged until FRC, at which time it starts to rise geometrically. It is also important to remember that in airways obstruction both the R_A and the FRC are likely to increase, although not always to the same extent.

Airways resistance can be measured directly in several ways. These include the body plethysmograph, the simultaneous recording of alveolar pressure and flow using an esophageal balloon, the interrupter technique, and also the oscillator method. A description of these various techniques is beyond the scope of the present chapter; however, suffice it to say that the plethysmographic method is to be preferred since it is most accurate in the clinical situation. There is little doubt that measurement of R_A in many instances adds little, and is not as useful as is spirometry in most clinical situations. However, determination of R_A can be most useful in challenge tests and in the assessment of various bronchodilator drugs. Under the latter circumstances, objective measurements of resistance may be preferable to spirometry.

The normal airways resistance is around 1.5 $H_2O/L./Sec$. In comparison, the nasal airflow resistance is two to three times as high. In bronchitis and emphysema the airways are irreversibly obstructed, and R_A may be increased four- to six-fold, under which circumstances most of the increased resistance is located in the respiratory bronchioles and smaller airways. In asthma, even greater increases in R_A occur, but here the obstructions usually are located in both smaller and large airways.

Compliance of the Lungs

Ventilation also depends on the compliance of the lungs. This is a measurement of the distensibility of the lungs, and is expressed as the change in lung volume that occurs when the pressure gradient between the pleura and the alveoli is changed by 1 cm. of water. It may be measured during breathholding (static compliance) or during regular breathing (dynamic compliance). If the increase in volume were directly proportional to the pressure change through the range of inflation and deflation, then a single value for static compliance would describe the elastic properties of the lungs. In reality this is not the case; the lungs becoming less compliant at high lung volumes; only in the tidal volume range is the relationship approximately linear. Lung compliance also depends on lung size, and the larger the lungs the more compliant they are. Thus an infant's lung is less compliant than is an adult's; likewise, there is disparity in the compliance of the lungs of large and small men. The reason for

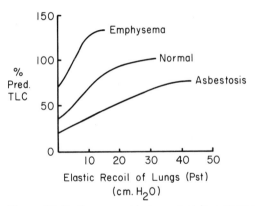

Figure 15–6 Pressure volume curves in a normal subject, and in subjects with emphysema and diffuse fibrosis (i.e. asbestosis).

this can be clearly seen if one considers the hypothetical case of a man whose vital capacity is 5 L. and whose static compliance is 0.2 L./cm. H_2O. Under such circumstances increasing his negative intrapleural pressure by 1 cm. H_2O increases the volume of his lungs by 200 ml. Were he then to have one lung removed, this would reduce his vital capacity to 2.5 L., and a pressure change of 1 cm. would then increase his lung volume by only 100 ml. In short, his compliance would be halved although the elastic properties of his lung would be unchanged. This is an oversimplification of the problem, since following pneumonectomy some compensatory overdistention of the remaining lung occurs. The latter phenomenon, nonetheless, is responsible for only a marginal increase in the volume of the remaining lung.

To get around the problem of lung size, a measurement known as specific compliance has been introduced. This relates compliance to lung volume and is obtained by dividing the static compliance by the FRC. If the lungs become stiff and fibrotic, as frequently occurs in asbestosis, sarcoidosis, berylliosis, and certain other diffuse fibroses, the compliance is markedly reduced and values of 0.04 L./cm. H_2O and less may be found. In subjects who have a marked reduction of compliance the vital capacity usually is concomitantly decreased. In conditions in which the lung has lost elasticity, a small change of pressure may produce a large increase in lung volume (Fig. 15–6). Under such circumstances, the lungs are said to be more compliant than normal. This is the usual state of affairs in emphysema and status asthmaticus. Measurement of compliance usually is carried out by relating intrapleural pressure changes as reflected by changes in esophageal pressure to volume change in the lungs. Esophageal pressure is recorded by placing a cylindrical balloon attached to a fine plastic tube in the lower third of the esophagus. The measurement of compliance is objective, but care must be taken to see that the balloon is situated correctly.

Dynamic compliance may be defined as the ratio of tidal volume to the difference between pressure at end-inspiration and end-expiration at points of no flow during breathing. In normal subjects measurement of dynamic compliance gives similar values to the static compliance; however, when airway resistance is increased an appreciable difference is often present. This is best explained by considering a state of affairs in which there is partial obstruction of a lobe or lung. In the unobstructed region, flow is maximal and there is an appropriate increase in flow volume for this area. In contrast the flow of gases into the region with increased airways resistance takes place more slowly, thereby causing smaller increase in volume per head of pressure.

Surfactant

The compliance of the lungs is also dependent on the presence of surfactant. The latter is a substance that lines the alveoli and respiratory bronchioles and tends to prevent their collapse. Radford first demonstrated that the lungs of an animal that had been filled with saline distend more easily than they did with air. This phenomenon suggests that saline either removed or rendered ineffective a substance that regulates the surface tension of the gas-tissue interface. Pattle subsequently showed that pulmonary edema fluid has a much lower surface tension than does plasma, an observation that suggests there is a substance lining the alveoli and influencing surface tension. Subsequently, Clements and his colleagues demonstrated that the surface retractive forces are appreciable during lung expansion; however, during deflation of the lungs and as the surface area contracts these forces decrease.

In normal subjects, there is a difference between the inspiratory and expiratory limbs of a pressure volume curve: a phenomenon usually referred to as *hysteresis*. By way of contrast, the saline-filled lung fails to show hysteresis, which suggests that the difference in the inspiratory and expiratory limbs in the normal subject is a consequence of a substance that regulates surface tension at the air-liquid interface. This substance has been shown to be surfactant, a complex of dipalmitoyl-lecithin with protein. It can be extracted from minced lungs or by washing out the lungs with saline. It appears to be secreted by the alveolar cells and has been shown to be present in decreased amounts in hyaline membrane disease, in conditions in which the blood flow to the lungs is decreased, and in sundry other conditions including the prolonged inhalation of 100 per cent oxygen.

IMPAIRMENT OF THE SMALL AIRWAYS FUNCTION

The detection of changes in air flow resistance and function in the small airways is a challenge to the ingenuity of the physiologist, but several techniques have been devised that can be used to this end. Moreover, in many subjects such changes have been shown to be reversible and it has therefore been suggested that if the abnormalities are detected early before there are accompanying spirometric abnormalities, and if further exposure to the responsible agent is avoided, irreversible disease may be avoided. Whether such tests will prove useful in prognosticating whether a particular subject is going to develop irreversible airways obstruction remains undecided. Three approaches are at present in vogue:

1. **Flow Volume Loop.** The standard method of recording a forced expiratory volume maneuver plots volume against time. In contrast, the flow volume loop, as the name suggests, plots flow against volume. There are several types of flow volume curves and each needs a definition. The maximal expiratory flow volume curve (MEFV) is a plot of maximal expiratory flow (Vmax) against volume during a forced expiratory maneuver. The term flow volume loop refers to a loop obtained when a maximal forced expiration is followed immediately by forced maximal inspiration, both being presented on the same tracing.

The typical flow loops are shown in Figure 15–7. Peak flow is largely effort-dependent and is mainly a reflection of the state of the large airways. Flow at 50 per cent of vital capacity (FEF_{50}) reflects both large and small airways function, with the former probably predominating. The latter part of the curve is felt to represent flow in the smaller airways. Also shown in Figure 15–7 is the curve of a subject with airways obstruction.

Figure 15–8 shows a series of curves with dif-

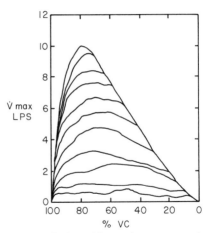

Figure 15–8 Series of flow volume curves showing graded respiratory efforts and different inspiratory volumes.

ferent efforts. Although the peak flow varies, it can be seen that eventually the latter part of the curve blends with that of the MEFV; in short, there is a final common pathway. These phenomena stimulated Hyatt to construct iso-volume pressure flow curves (IPPV), in which he measured transpulmonary pressure. These showed that as driving pressure increased, flow concomitantly increased until a maximum value was attained, after which further increases in pressure produced no further increase in flow (Fig. 15–9). Although flow usually is expressed as a percentage of vital capacity, it is preferable to relate it to total lung capacity (TLC) for the following reasons. When the MEFV is being used to evaluate bronchodilator drugs or to assess changes in air flow resistance over a relatively short period, e.g., during challenge tests or when subjects may have been exposed to cotton dust or agents likely to produce an acute change in the airways, in some

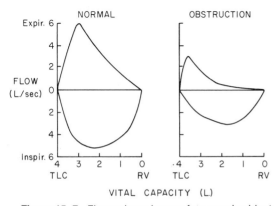

Figure 15–7 Flow volume loops of a normal subject and of a subject with airways obstruction.

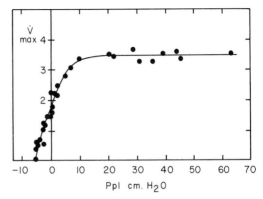

Figure 15–9 Iso-volume pressure flow showing limitation of flow at pressure of 15 cm./H_2O.

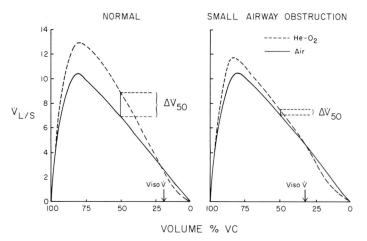

Figure 15–10 Helium oxygen and air flow volume curves in a normal subject and a subject with small airways obstruction. Note the point of identical flow (V_{iso} V) is farther from RV in the subject with small airways obstruction.

instances not only do the flow rates decrease but in addition lung volumes and VC may likewise show a decrease. Thus it is possible for a "before and after" challenge FEF_{50} when expressed as a percentage of VC to remain relatively unchanged; however, were the FEF_{50} related to TLC, a marked difference would become apparent.

In large airways, because flow is partly turbulent the pressure necessary to produce a particular flow rate increases with gas density. In contrast, flow in the peripheral airways is for the most part laminar and therefore independent of gas density. If one measures airways resistance (R_A) when the subject is breathing a 4:1 helium and oxygen mixture (HeO_2) it is found that the R_A is substantially decreased. If a subject with peripheral airways obstruction alone breathes a helium-oxygen mixture, there is little change in

R_A since flow in small airways is mainly laminar. Since the effective pressure necessary to produce maximal flow is independent of the gas mixture breathed, and since the difference in flow between breathing air and helium oxygen mixture is determined by how much the peripheral airways contribute to the total resistance, the higher the resistance to flow in the peripheral airways, the less will be the helium responses (Fig. 15–10).

At a particular lung volume, the flows on HeO_2 and air coincide. This is known as the point of identical flow (PIF). It is usually expressed as a percentage of vital capacity. In normal subjects it varies from 0 to 6 per cent and is rarely elevated above 10 per cent. In small airways obstruction it may be elevated to around 30 per cent (Fig. 15–10).

The flow volume curve is also useful in detect-

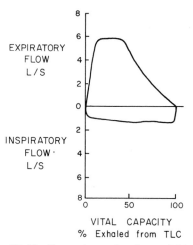

Figure 15–11 Flow volume showing variable extrathoracic obstruction.

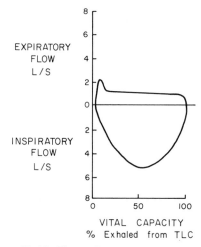

Figure 15–12 Flow volume curve showing variable intrathoracic obstruction.

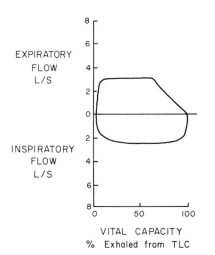

Figure 15–13 Flow volume curve showing fixed extrathoracic obstruction.

ing obstructing lesions of the right and left main bronchi, the trachea, and larynx. Figures 15–11, 15–12 and 15–13 show typical examples of the major airways obstruction. Figure 15–11 is a tracing from a subject with a variable extrathoracic obstruction, namely, bilateral vocal cord paralysis. It is apparent that inspiratory flows are more affected than are expiratory flows. A variable intrathoracic obstruction, e.g., a tracheal cylindroma, is represented in the tracing shown in Figure 15–12. Expiratory flows are more affected since the trachea collapses during exhalation. Figure 15–13 shows a fixed extrathoracic obstructive lesion in which inspiration and expiration are both affected, e.g., stenosis of the larynx following surgery or injury.

2. Closing Volume. It has been shown that small airways start to close somewhat between functional residual capacity (FRC) and residual volume (RV). Closure depends on the pressure difference acting on the wall of the airway and on the elastic properties of the small airways. If the lumina of peripheral airways are narrowed by mucus or some pathologic process, or if the concentration of surfactant is reduced, the surface forces acting on the airways become greater and a tendency to collapse occurs.

Fowler originally observed that when a person exhaled to residual volume and then took a breath of oxygen and achieved total lung capacity (TLC), during a subsequent slow expiratory maneuver, a tracing of the percentage of nitrogen exhaled showed four distinct phases (Fig. 15–14). In phase 1 there is an absence of nitrogen owing to the fact that the dead space contains pure oxygen. Phase 2 begins as the subject starts to exhale a mixture of gas from the dead space and alveoli; it is characterized by a sharp increase in the concentration of expired nitrogen. Phase 2 is followed by an alveolar plateau known as phase 3. Finally there is an abupt increase in the concentration of nitrogen (phase 4). The junction of phases 3 and 4 is thought to be the volume at which the basal airways close, and the volume between the junction of phases 3 and 4 and RV is known as closing volume (CV). CV plus RV is known as closing capacity (CC). The upward inflection at the end of phase 3 is best explained by the effects of gravity on the distribution of inspired gas. In a normal subject there is a gradient of transpulmonary pressure from the top to the bottom of the lung. When a sitting or standing subject takes a breath from RV, the first portion of the breath is distributed to the apices, while the latter portions are distributed to the lower lobes. During a subsequent exhalation, the

Figure 15–14 Single breath oxygen test showing the four phases.

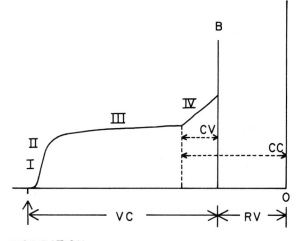

FULL INSPIRATION

air that is exhaled first comes from both the upper and lower zones, but toward the end of the breath small airways in the lower zones close and the upper zones make a relatively greater contribution. This principle has been aptly named "First In–Last Out."

Measurement of closing volume can be carried out in several ways. The most simple is the resident nitrogen method, in which the subject takes a breath of 100 per cent oxygen. The nitrogen remaining in the airways forms a bolus of tracer gas. Other methods involve labeling the inspired air with a foreign gas such as argon, xenon, or helium. Differences in measurement of closing volume in the same subject have been noted according to the method used. A normal closing volume implies that the distribution of inspired gases is mainly dependent on gravity, and that the lungs empty relatively homogeneously. When filling and emptying become discordant, the principle of "First In–Last Out" is broken and a closing volume may not be apparent on the tracing. Phase 3 represents gas coming from alveoli, and as such the alveoli must contain different concentrations of nitrogen in order to account for the slope. The steepness of the slope is therefore an indication of abnormal distribution, since the concentration of nitrogen in each alveolus after a breath of oxygen depends on how much oxygen enters each alveolus.

Measurement of CV is influenced by the rate at which the inspired breath is taken, by expiratory flow, and by prolonged breath-holding, which leads to a greater percentage of oxygen being absorbed. Expiratory flow should be regulated to between 0.4 and 0.5 L./sec. CV, (CV/VC%) (CC/TLC%) all have higher coefficients of variation than do the FEV_1 and FVC. In this regard, CV and CV/VC% are the most variable, viz., 20 to 25 per cent. Moreover, while intelligent subjects have no difficulty in carrying out the CV maneuver, its applicability in field studies is severely limited by the inability of a substantial proportion of the less well educated population to carry out the respiratory maneuvers in a satisfactory fashion. Abnormalities of CV, in the presence of normal spirometry have been reported in obesity, cigarette smokers, asthmatics in remission, coal miners, and in patients with skeletal deformities such as kyphosis. As such, an elevated CV is thought to indicate early disease; nonetheless, the prognostic significance of CV remains a topic of controversy.

3. Frequency Dependence of Dynamic Compliance.
The history of the development of this technique begins with the mechanical time constant theory elaborated by Otis, et al., and used to explain the relationship between mechanical factors and the intrapulmonary distribution of inspired gas. Theory suggests that differences in time constants (resistance × compliance) between parallel lung units would be associated with a decrease in dynamic compliance as breathing frequency increased. This would mean that a progressively smaller portion of the lung would be ventilated as breathing frequency increased.

Macklem and Mead reported that the time constants of the distal lung units (airways smaller than about 2 mm.) were in the order of 0.01 second. They concluded that a fourfold difference in these time constants would cause dynamic compliance to fall with any increase in respiratory frequency because there would be less time for air to enter and leave the affected regions. Thus an increased resistance to flow in the smaller airways should lead to a fall in dynamic compliance at faster rates of breathing. This raised the possibility that the frequency dependence of dynamic compliance could be used as a test of obstruction in peripheral airways.

For widespread time constant discrepancies to occur, the obstruction must be unevenly distributed; that is, some airways must remain patent while others are narrowed. Other criteria must be met before it can be assumed that frequency-dependent dynamic compliance is a consequence of peripheral airway narrowing rather than of lesions in large airways or other parts of the lung. If the static pressure/volume (compliance) curve of the lung is normal, then it is not likely that frequency-dependent dynamic compliance is due to abnormal elastic properties of the lung. It has been assumed that regional differences in elastic properties sufficient to cause a detectable fall in dynamic compliance at rapid respiratory rates should result in an abnormal static compliance curve. Thus, if a patient has normal pulmonary resistance, spirometry, and static pressure/volume curve, any fall in dynamic compliance with increased frequency of respiration (frequency-dependent compliance) is assumed to be due to peripheral airways obstruction. The time constants and ventilation of peripheral gas-exchanging units of the lung will be affected by:

1. Regional obstruction due to bronchiolar narrowing or obstruction by mucus.
2. Regional increases in elastic recoil produced by the interstitial fibroses; for example, in asbestosis and berylliosis.
3. Regional loss of elastic recoil with airways collapse; for example, in centrilobular emphysema and the focal emphysema of coalworkers' pneumoconiosis (CWP).

All three of these pathologic processes may lead to unequal time constants in the lung and hence to an uneven distribution of ventilation that is more pronounced at faster rates of ventilation. All should produce a fall in dynamic compliance at higher respiratory rates.

The detection of frequency-dependent dynamic compliance involves measuring dynamic compliance at various rates of respiration, e.g., 20, 40, 60, and 80 breaths/minute. The dynamic changes in volume are obtained using a pneumotachograph; the intrapleural pressure changes are measured with an esophageal balloon.

WORK OF BREATHING

A certain amount of energy is expended with each breath we take. Part of the energy expenditure is related to moving air in and out of the lungs, and part to moving the thoracic cage and diaphragm. Normal values for the work of breathing are 0.5 kg./min at rest and up to 250 kg./min. with a maximal voluntary ventilation maneuver. In asthma and emphysema, the main increase in the work of breathing is related to overcoming the increased airflow resistance; in pulmonary fibrosis the additional work is necessary to overcome the stiffness of the lungs. The respiratory muscles under normal circumstances use about 2 to 4 per cent of the energy requirements at rest.

REGIONAL DISTRIBUTION OF VENTILATION AND PERFUSION

Ventilation

Quantitative studies of the regional distribution of gas over large zones of excised lung using radioactive xenon have shown relatively even distribution of inspired gas per unit lung volume. The situation in life, with the lungs suspended within the chest wall, is very different in that the intrapleural pressure is no longer uniform as in the isolated preparation. Instead, in the erect posture there is a vertical gradient of intrapleural pressure, with a progressive reduction in pressure from the base to the apex of the lung. As the static transpleural pressure (i.e., pressure difference between pleural surface and atmosphere, during breath-holding with the glottis open) is more negative at the apex, the upper zone alveoli tend to be more expanded than those in the lower zones. An analogy is a loosely-coiled spring which, when suspended by its uppermost coil, becomes progressively more expanded by its own weight from bottom to top (Fig. 15–15). The pleural pressure gradient in the chest always occurs in the direction of gravitational pull; thus in a supine subject the differences in alveolar expansion occur dorso-ventrally. Because of these regional differences in alveolar expansion, the static lung compliance of the more stretched upper zones is less than that of the lower zones in the erect posture, and therefore during tidal

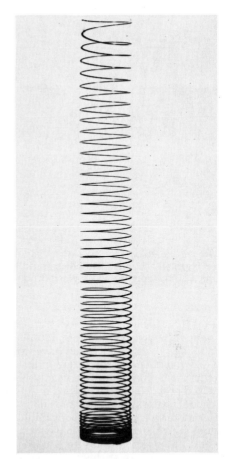

Figure 15–15 A spring suspended by the uppermost coil showing the relative separation of the coils at the top and bottom.

breathing at low flow rates basal ventilation tends to exceed that of the apices. As inspiratory flow rate increases, regional airways resistance is thought to become more influential than compliance in determining regional ventilation, which is then more evenly distributed. It is of note that in elderly normal subjects, particularly in the supine posture, regional ventilation may be altered by small airways closure occurring in dependent lung zones during tidal breathing, and that this may result in a reduction in arterial oxygen tension.

Perfusion

Studies using a variety of different radioactive tracer techniques have also demonstrated that pulmonary perfusion is not uniformly distributed, and that there is a vertical gradient of increasing pulmonary perfusion per unit lung vol-

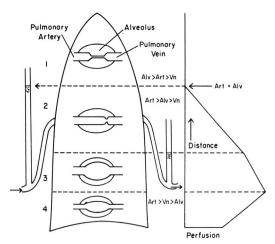

Figure 15–16 Relationship of pulmonary arterial, venous, alveolar, and interstitial pressures in the various zones of the lung (Based on West).

ume from apex to base in the erect posture, apart from some reduction over the most dependent 6 to 10 cm. of lung. West and Hughes have explained these regional differences in terms of the interaction of pulmonary arterial, venous, alveolar, and interstitial pressures in the lungs (Fig. 15–16). In zone one of the upright lung there is no pulmonary arterial perfusion because pericapillary lung pressure, which under static conditions can be thought of as "alveolar" pressure, exceeds pulmonary arterial pressure at this level, and alveolar vessels therefore collapse. The junction of zones one and two, at which pulmonary arterial perfusion commences, is represented by the height of a column of blood in an open manometer tube connected to the pulmonary artery. Below this level, pulmonary arterial pressure exceeds atmospheric pressure and can therefore open the vessels, perfusion increasing down this zone as the hydrostatic pressure of the column of pulmonary arterial blood rises. The amount of perfusion at any level in this zone is determined by the difference between the pulmonary arterial and alveolar pressure which still exceeds pulmonary venous pressure. In the third zone, pulmonary venous pressure now also exceeds alveolar pressure. Here there is a continued slower increase in perfusion probably due to distention of intra-alveolar vessels as a result of a continued increase in the hydrostatic pressure in both pulmonary artery and pulmonary vein, whereas alveolar pressure remains atmospheric. A fourth zone was added to this scheme when it was observed that there was some fall-off of basal blood flow, particularly at lung volumes below functional residual capacity. This is attributed to a lung volume-related change in the resistance of extra-alveolar pulmonary vessels, whose caliber

is related to changes in surrounding interstitial pressure rather than alveolar pressure.

Regional Variation in the Matching of Ventilation and Perfusion

Although in the normal lung both alveolar ventilation (V_A) and perfusion (Q) vary regionally in the same direction, according to vertical gravity-dependent gradients, the rate of increase of perfusion from apex to base is steeper than that for ventilation. Consequently the regional matching of V_A to Q, which may be conveniently expressed as V_A/Q ratios, is not uniform, but decreases down the length of the lung. The total V_A/Q ratio for a normal upright lung with cardiac output of approximately 6 L. per minute and alveolar ventilation of 5 L. per minute lies between 0.8 and 0.9; however, regional V_A/Q ratios vary considerably from about 3.3 at the apex to 0.6 at the lung base. The predilection of post-primary pulmonary tuberculosis for the lung apices has been attributed to the high apical V_A/Q ratio, which results in an alveolar oxygen tension and hence tissue tension over 40 mm. Hg higher than that at the lung base. This idea is supported by observations of a higher incidence of this disease in patients with pulmonary stenosis whose apical perfusion is still further reduced. Conversely, tuberculosis usually affects the lung bases in bats since they hang upside down. Regional alterations in the normal pattern of V_A/Q matching are important as they determine the overall efficiency of the lung in its principal function as a gas-exchanger. Exercise and the assumption of the supine position even out the regional differences. In disease, most abnormalities of gas exchange result from mismatching of ventilation and perfusion and these inequalities may be expressed in terms of wasted blood flow or ventilation.

(a) Wasted Perfusion. If an alveolus is totally unventilated but remains perfused ($V_A/Q = 0$), then the arterial end of the capillary supplying it will still contain blood of venous composition, and perfusion will have been useless and is often referred to as a "true shunt." Suppose that the supply of fresh air to the alveolus is not completely interrupted, but merely reduced disproportionately to its blood supply. It may be felt intuitively that some of the perfusion is still surplus to the requirements of that alveolus. We can imagine that the reduced amount of inspired gas will be totally accommodated by some fraction of the same volume of perfusing blood, and the rest will remain venous. In both these situations "venous" blood will mix with arterialized blood, reducing its oxygen content and increasing its carbon dioxide content. This process, which is called "shunting" or "venous admixture," may, if sufficient alveoli are involved, produce measurable changes

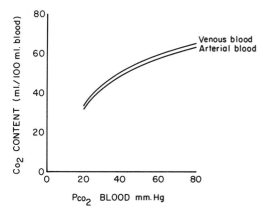

Figure 15–17 Carbon dioxide dissociation curve.

in the gas tensions of arterial blood. It should be noted that both oxygen and carbon dioxide transfer are impaired in shunting; however, usually the respiratory center responds to hypercarbia by increasing ventilation, which lowers the pco_2 of ventilated alveoli. Since the carbon dioxide dissociation curve is nearly linear (Fig. 15–17), this will be accompanied by an approximately equal fall in CO_2 content for a given fall in pco_2 over the physiologic range, and, as a result, in shunts a normal arterial pco_2 can usually be maintained. In the absence of a hyperventilatory response carbon dioxide retention would occur. Arterial oxygen content is less easily maintained because increasing the po_2 of relatively well ventilated alveoli on the flat part of the non-linear oxyhemoglobin dissociation curve (Fig. 15–18)

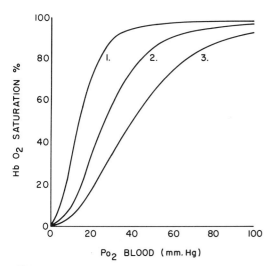

Figure 15–18 Oxygen dissociation curves showing right and left shifts. (See text for explanation.)

will produce only minimal improvement in the oxygen saturation of the blood perfusing these units, which cannot therefore compensate for unventilated units. The arterial blood gas abnormality most commonly found in significant shunts is a lowered arterial po_2 in the presence of a normal or low arterial pco_2.

The direct passage of blood from the arterial to the venous side of the pulmonary circulation without any contact with ventilated alveoli is called true shunting, and is physiologically indistinguishable from the small amount of anatomic shunting that occurs in normal individuals through the bronchial circulation and Thebesian veins of the heart. Any remaining shunt is due to alveoli with low V_A/Q ratios and is really a shunt-like effect or physiologic shunt. Total shunt in a resting normal individual does not usually exceed 5 per cent of the cardiac output, of which true shunt comprises about 2 per cent.

(b) Wasted Ventilation. Now consider the opposite situation of a normally ventilated alveolus receiving no perfusion (V_A/Q ratio = infinity). This alveolus will act as an extra space in which air is moved to and fro without participating in gas exchange, and is therefore dead space or wasted ventilation. In terms of function, this dead space produces the same effect as an enlargement of the anatomic dead space, which comprises the whole of the non-alveolated respiratory tract from the mouth and nose to the respiratory bronchioles. If the perfusion of the alveolus is not completely interrupted but only reduced disproportionately to its ventilation, then a fraction of that ventilation will now be sufficient to meet the gas-exchanging potential of the reduced blood flow, and the remaining ventilation is therefore useless. This process will also contribute to alveolar dead space. Alveolar dead space is therefore the volume of inspired gas entering alveoli but not taking part in gas exchange due to local V_A/Q imbalance. It is more conceptual and less tangible than anatomic dead space, which, as it is a volume contained within a physical structure, is easier to picture. Alveolar and anatomic dead space together are conventionally referred to as physiologic dead space. The measured physiologic dead space in health is usually not more than 30 per cent of the tidal volume.

If anatomic dead space is increased artificially, for example by mouth breathing through a length of tube, and if the rate and depth of breathing are unaltered, then less fresh air will reach the alveoli with each inspiration. It follows that alveolar po_2 will fall and alveolar pco_2 rise, with consequent hypoxemia and hypercapnia. Suppose now that alveolar dead space is increased by relative underperfusion of a group of normally ventilated alveoli, and that the rate and depth of breathing and over-all pulmonary perfusion remain unaltered. Although the oxygen tension of the reduced volume of blood perfusing these alveoli will be increased, it will be insufficient to compensate for a greater reduction of oxygen tension in blood coming from other normally ventilated alveoli, which are now overperfused as they receive additional blood that normally would have been directed to the first group of alveoli. The result will be a reduction in arterial oxygen tension. Even though over-all alveolar ventilation may remain normal, wasted regional ventilation will also reduce carbon dioxide exchange, tending to produce a raised arterial carbon dioxide tension. In disease this tendency is often corrected by compensatory hyperventilation, although hypoxemia often persists.

Alveolo-arterial Oxygen Gradient [(A − a) DO₂]

Were the matching of ventilation and perfusion perfect, with the assumption that gas diffusion occurred across the alveolo-capillary membrane to equilibrium, then arterial and alveolar oxygen tensions would be equal. When mismatching occurs, an alveolo-arterial oxygen tension difference $(A-a)DO_2$ will develop. The measurement of arterial oxygen tension is easy, but that of average alveolar oxygen tension presents problems. Although end-expiratory samples of alveolar gas may not be contaminated by dead space air in normal subjects, in pulmonary disease some lung units may take much longer to empty than others, so that end-expiratory po_2 measured at the mouth changes continually, and spot sampling introduces error. Consequently for clinical purposes "ideal" alveolar po_2 is estimated indirectly. This is the alveolar po_2 that would be found in a given subject if, for the same over-all rate of consumption of oxygen and production of carbon dioxide, ventilation and perfusion were to become perfectly matched throughout the lung. The calculation requires the analysis of an expired air and arterial blood sample. A simplified version of the ideal alveolar gas equation is:

$$\text{ideal } pAo_2 = PIo_2 - \frac{Paco_2}{R}$$

where PIo_2 is the inspired oxygen tension, $Paco_2$ is the arterial carbon dioxide tension, and R is the respiratory quotient (rate of production of carbon dioxide divided by the rate of uptake of oxygen, which usually is 0.8). The ideal $(A-a)DO_2$ underestimates true $(A-a)DO_2$ because it fails to account for alveoli with a raised po_2 due to high $\dot{V}_A/\dot{Q}$ ratios. It is used as a non-specific indicator of impaired gas exchange due to diffusion or distribution abnormalities. It remains normal (4 to 15 mm. Hg) in patients with over-all alveolar hypoventilation, and is increased by hyperven-

TABLE 15–1 CHANGES IN ARTERIAL BLOOD GASES AND (A–a)O₂ GRADIENT IN VARIOUS PHYSIOLOGIC IMPAIRMENTS

	Po₂	Pco₂	(A–a) Do₂
Regional V̇/Q̇ mismatching	↓	↑ or N or ↓	↑
"Pure" diffusion block	↓	N or↓	↑
Overall Alveolar Hypoventilation	↓	↑	N
Overall Alveolar Hyperventilation	N or ↑	↓	↑

tilation, whether voluntary or induced by anxiety (Table 15–1).

Estimation of Shunt

Physiologic shunt (anatomic plus alveolar shunt) may be estimated using the following equation:

$$\frac{\dot{Q}s}{\dot{Q}} = \frac{Cio_2 - Cao_2}{Cio_2 - C\bar{v}o_2}$$

where $\dot{Q}s/\dot{Q}$ is the proportion of total pulmonary flow taking part in the shunt, Cao_2 and $C\bar{v}o_2$ are the arterial and mixed venous oxygen contents, and Cio_2 is the ideal arterial oxygen content (that which would result from an arterial po_2 equal to the ideal alveolar po_2) which can be obtained from a knowledge of the ideal alveolar po_2, by use of the oxyhemoglobin dissociation curve. True shunt (anatomic shunt plus shunt through totally ventilated alveoli) may be separated from shunt-like effects (alveoli with low $\dot{V}_A/\dot{Q}$ ratios) by the administration of 100 per cent oxygen for 20 minutes. This washes out all alveolar nitrogen and fully oxygenates even poorly ventilated alveoli (alveolar po_2 approximately 670 mm. Hg), thereby abolishing shuntlike effects. The only possible cause for persisting hypoxemia in this situation is a true shunt, where venous blood unexposed to ventilated alveoli continues to dilute oxygenated blood. It should be noted that the arterial po_2 will rise to some extent in true shunts due to the increased alveolar po_2, and only in large shunts (greater than 25 per cent of the cardiac output) will the blood remain desaturated. A widened $(A-a)DO_2$ will persist in true shunts but not in shuntlike effects.

Estimation of Physiologic Dead Space and Effective Alveolar Ventilation

Physiologic dead space (anatomic dead space plus alveolar dead space) may be estimated using Bohr's equation in terms of alveolar and mixed expired pco_2:

$$V_{D_P} = V_T \frac{(P_A CO_2 - P_{\bar{E}} CO_2)}{P_A CO_2}$$

The difficulties inherent in measuring average alveolar pCO_2 are avoided by equating it to arterial pCO_2 (equals ideal alveolar pCO_2). The proportion of the tidal volume (V_T) made up by the physiologic dead space V_{D_P} may now be given by:

$$\frac{V_{D_P}}{V_T} = \frac{P_a CO_2 - P_{\bar{E}} CO_2}{P_a CO_2}$$

Alveolar ventilation has already been defined in terms of anatomic dead space and minute ventilation. If the physiologic dead space is known, it is possible to estimate the effective alveolar ventilation, this being the proportion of total ventilation being used effectively in carbon dioxide exchange according to the equation:

$$\begin{array}{ccc} V_A \text{ (eff)} = & f & \times (V_T - V_{D_A}) \\ \text{ml./min.} & \text{Breaths/min.} & \text{ml.} \end{array}$$

In clinical practice, however, arterial pCO_2 alone is generally taken as a reliable and readily available indicator of the level of effective alveolar ventilation. Hypoventilation, by reducing the delivery of fresh air to gas exchanging areas, inevitably reduces arterial pO_2 and increases arterial pCO_2. The resultant hypoxemia may be eliminated by the administration of a high concentration of oxygen, but the raised arterial pCO_2 cannot be corrected unless the level of alveolar ventilation is increased. Conversely, conditions that result in effective alveolar hyperventilation are associated with a lowered arterial pCO_2. This may be seen in hysterical overbreathing, and occasionally following the hyperventilatory response to hypoxemia found in diffusion impairment or ventilation-perfusion mismatching in which sufficient normal lung tissue remains to eliminate carbon dioxide.

THE TRANSPORT OF GASES BY THE BLOOD

In a mixture of different gases, the pressure exerted by each of the constituents (commonly referred to as the partial pressure (p)) is the product of its fractional concentration by volume and the total pressure of the mixture. For inspired air containing 20.93 per cent oxygen, 0.03 per cent carbon dioxide, and 79 per cent nitrogen and other inert gases, whose total pressure is 760 mm. Hg (barometric pressure at sea level) and whose water vapor pressure is 10 mm. Hg, the pO_2 will be:

$$\frac{20.93}{100} \times (760 - 10) = 157 \text{ mm. Hg}$$

Water vapor pressure is subtracted because volumes of gases are conventionally estimated dry.

Similarly the atmospheric pCO_2 will be 0.2 mm. Hg and the P_{N_2} 592 mm. Hg. If a mixture of gases is brought into contact with a fluid, then the constituent gases will continue to diffuse into it until their partial pressures in solution are equal to those of the gas phase. At this point equilibration is said to have occurred. The partial pressure of a gas in fluid is often referred to as its *tension*.

The content of a gas in a fluid is derived from the product of the gas's solubility coefficient (α) and its partial pressure, and is expressed in ml. gas measured at standard temperature and pressure dry (STPD) per 100 ml. of liquid or in volumes percent. The solubility coefficient of oxygen is 0.003 ml./dl./mg. Hg and its average partial pressure in the alveoli is approximately 100 mm. Hg. This is less than that of atmospheric air because of mixing with oxygen-depleted and carbon dioxide-rich gas already present in the lung, and since it also becomes saturated with water vapor during its passage to the gas exchanging surfaces; the saturated water vapor pressure at 37° C being 47 mm. Hg. The average content of dissolved oxygen in pulmonary capillary plasma at equilibrium with alveolar air will therefore be 0.003 × 100 = 0.3 ml./dl.

A normal resting subject's oxygen requirement is around 300 ml./min., and were all dissolved oxygen in the plasma removed by the tissues on each complete circuit, the minimum cardiac output necessary to support life would be 60 L./min., a level impossible to sustain. This difficulty is overcome by the reversible binding of most oxygen to hemoglobin, of which whole blood contains approximately 15 gm./dl. Hemoglobin is a tetramer formed by a globulin molecule bound to four heme molecules, each of which may react with a single oxygen molecule. This complex structure is capable of binding 1.34 ml. of oxygen/gm. and the hemoglobin capacity is therefore 1.34 × 15 = 20.1 ml./dl. Percentage saturation is the oxygen content, which may be measured by Van Slyke's method, expressed as a percentage of the blood oxygen hemoglobin capacity.

Oxyhemoglobin Dissociation Curve

The content of a gas dissolved in fluid, expressed in volumes percent, is related to its partial pressure in a linear fashion (Henry's Law). This contrasts markedly with the S-shaped relationship of blood oxygen tension to saturation that results from the presence of hemoglobin (Fig. 15–19). The curve owes its distinctive shape to the so-called heme-heme reaction, in which the oxygenation of each heme molecule in the tetramer in turn affects the oxygen affinity of the other subunits, so that the molecule as a whole has four successive equilibrium constants. Notice

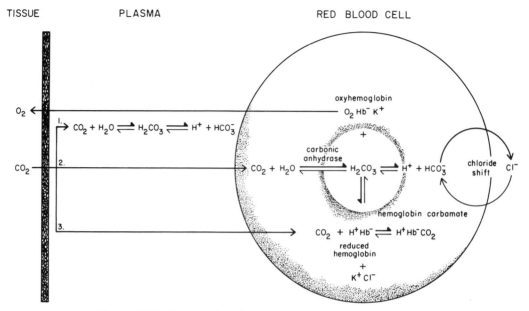

Figure 15–19 Modes of carriage of carbon dioxide in the blood.

that the upper part of the curve is relatively flat, so that a drop in oxygen tension from 100 to 60 mm. Hg is associated with a relatively small fall in oxygen saturation. As a result persons who live at an altitude of 10,000 feet, at which the alveolar po_2 is about 60 mm. Hg, still maintain an oxygen saturation of about 90 per cent, which is clearly to their advantage. Conversely, a rise in the po_2 of arterial blood in this range produces only a minimal increase in oxygen saturation. Consequently hyperventilation of normal lung tissue may be unable to compensate for hypoxemia resulting from areas of impaired gas exchange elsewhere. The lower, steeper part of the curve is also physiologically important, as a small fall in the po_2 of blood is associated with a relatively large change in its oxygen content. Thus the transfer of oxygen from blood to metabolically active tissues is facilitated.

Factors Affecting the Oxyhemoglobin Dissociation Curve

The relation of the po_2 of blood to hemoglobin saturation may be altered by a number of factors which are capable of causing a "shift" of the oxyhemoglobin dissociation curve to either the right or the left, so that the flat part of the curve corresponding to high hemoglobin saturations is either expanded or contracted (Fig. 15–18). The most important of these factors are: pH, pco_2, 2,3-diphosphoglycerate level (2,3, DPG), and temperature. These shifts may be defined in terms of the po_2 of blood at which hemoglobin is half satu-

rated (P_{50}). If the oxyhemoglobin dissociation curve shifts to the right, the P_{50} rises, and with a shift to the left, it falls. Although it might at first seem that a raised P_{50} would be disadvantageous, since a smaller amount of oxygen is being transported for a given po_2, careful examination of the diagram shows that as a result of the shape of curve 3, a raised P_{50} implies that for a given reduction in arterial po_2 in the physiologic range, a greater amount of oxygen becomes available to the tissues. If on passing through the systemic capillaries the po_2 of arterial blood falls from 90 to 40 mm. Hg (arteriovenous O_2 difference), then according to curve 2 the oxygen saturation would fall by only 20 per cent, whereas if curve 3 is applied, the fall would be 40 per cent.

When hemoglobin is oxygenated, hydrogen ions are released from the molecule. If the pH of the red cell, which is linearly related to that of the plasma, is reduced by the addition of hydrogen ions, then by the principle of mass action, this process tends to reverse, hemoglobin reverting to its deoxygenated state with the release of oxygen. In practice metabolically active tissues constitute a more acid environment for the blood perfusing them as a result of the local production of CO_2 and lactic acid, and this low pH therefore assists the transfer of more oxygen to the tissues for the same arteriovenous fall in po_2. In other words, a fall in pH results in an increase in P_{50}, or shift of the oxyhemoglobin dissociation curve to the right. This is known as the Bohr effect. It might be thought that the reduced oxygen affinity of venous blood which is more acid would be detrimental to the uptake of oxygen in the lungs; however, at a higher po_2, the dissociation curves come closer together and oxygen uptake is little affected. P_{50} may be altered by a change of both pH and pco_2, for the shift to the right will still occur if pH is kept constant and pco_2 increased, showing the latter has an effect independent of pH.

The organic phosphate 2,3 DPG is an intermediate in erythrocyte carbohydrate metabolism, and constitutes most of the phosphate in red cells. If the concentration of 2,3 DPG is increased, it competes with oxygen for binding sites on deoxygenated hemoglobin, thereby reducing its oxygen affinity, shifting the oxyhemoglobin dissociation curve to the right. The level of 2,3 DPG is regulated by erythrocyte enzyme systems which are pH dependent, so that acidity or alkalinity tend to suppress or stimulate its production, respectively. We have seen that a fall in plasma pH causes an immediate shift of the curve to the right, thereby reducing the affinity of hemoglobin for oxygen. If this fall in pH persists for several hours, 2,3 DPG production is reduced, exerting a counterbalancing effect on the pH-mediated right shift. Consequently, when long-standing acidosis is quickly corrected with bicarbonate, a persisting low 2,3 DPG level may have a deleterious "overshoot effect" by increasing the oxygen affinity of hemoglobin and reducing its supply to the tissues. Deoxygenated hemoglobin, which is a weaker acid and therefore relatively alkaline, stimulates 2,3 DPG production, reducing the affinity of hemoglobin for oxygen and causing the shift to the right that is associated with long-standing hypoxemic conditions such as cyanotic heart disease or chronic bronchitis. Similarly, the rise in plasma alkalinity that occurs at high altitudes causes a shift to the left with increased hemoglobin-oxygen affinity, and also stimulates 2,3 DPG production which has a counteraction. Other situations in which 2,3 DPG may be depleted with a reduction in blood oxygen transferring efficiency, include the storage of transfusable blood, hypophosphatemia, certain congenital hemoglobinopathies, and the raised blood levels of carboxyhemoglobin associated with cigarette smoking.

A rise in the temperature of blood reduces the oxygen affinity of hemoglobin and facilitates its removal by metabolizing tissues, the temperature of which is slightly higher than that of the lungs.

Carbon Dioxide Transport

The partial pressure gradient between metabolizing tissues and the capillaries perfusing them results in the diffusion of carbon dioxide into the blood, in which it is carried in three forms: (1) in solution in plasma; (2) combined with hemoglo-

bin; and (3) as bicarbonate (Fig. 15–19). Plasma alone is an inefficient carrier of carbon dioxide, and only 5 per cent of total carbon dioxide is carried in this way. Although the volume of dissolved carbon dioxide is linearly related to the pco_2 of blood, the slope of this relationship is not steep enough to enable the elimination of sufficient carbon dioxide by the lungs to keep pace with its production by the tissues. A small proportion of dissolved carbon dioxide in the plasma reacts with water to form carbonic acid which then ionizes according to the equation:

$$CO_2 + H_2O \rightleftharpoons H_2CO_3 \rightleftharpoons H^+ + HCO_3^- \text{ (Equation 1)}$$

Carbon dioxide also diffuses into red blood cells, and here the above reaction proceeds rapidly as a result of the action of the enzyme, carbonic anhydrase. This results in a concentration gradient of bicarbonate between the erythrocyte and the plasma, so that bicarbonate diffuses out of the cell in exchange for chloride which passes in to maintain electrical neutrality, a process known as the *chloride shift*. The hydrogen ions are largely buffered by hemoglobin, although venous blood is rendered slightly more acid than arterial blood. Ninety per cent of total blood carbon dioxide is carried as bicarbonate in this way. The remaining 5 per cent combines reversibly with NH_2 on deoxygenated hemoglobin to form hemoglobin carbamate:

$$HbNH_2 + CO_2 \rightleftharpoons HbNHCOOH \rightleftharpoons HbNHCOO^- + H^+$$

When venous blood in the lungs comes into contact with alveolar gas, carbon dioxide in the plasma diffuses into the air spaces, causing the equations illustrated in Figure 15–19 to proceed in the opposite direction. It is clear that the red blood cell is essential not only for oxygen, but also for carbon dioxide transport.

ACID–BASE BALANCE

The acidity or alkalinity of blood is expressed as pH, which is the negative logarithm of the hydrogen ion concentration, $[H^+]$. If an acid is added to water (pH 7) it dissociates and the hydrogen ion concentration increases, producing a fall in pH:

$$HCl \rightleftharpoons H^+ + Cl^-$$

The addition of a base has the opposite effect, reducing hydrogen ion concentration and therefore increasing pH:

$$NaOH + H^+ \rightleftharpoons Na^+ + H_2O$$

There is a constant tendency for the body to increase its acidity by the production of both gaseous and non-gaseous acid metabolites. This tendency is controlled by the excretion of hydrogen ions indirectly by the lungs and by the kidneys, and involves a number of chemical buffering systems. These mechanisms are normally able to maintain the pH in a narrow range between 7.36 and 7.44; a departure above or below these limits being referred to as alkalosis or acidosis, respectively.

A *buffer solution* is one whose pH is relatively unchanged following the addition of an acid or alkali. In general buffers are effective only over a certain range of pH. An example of such a buffer system is a solution containing a weak acid (by which is meant one that does not completely dissociate in solution) and a salt of that acid. A buffer system substitutes the stronger, more dissociable acid with one that is weaker and less dissociable, therefore reducing the hydrogen ion concentration. In man there are a number of buffers, the most important of which is the carbonic acid/bicarbonate system which buffers non-gaseous acidic metabolites such as lactic and pyruvic acids. Thus, sodium bicarbonate reacts with lactic acid to produce carbonic acid and sodium lactate:

$$NaHCO_3 + HLac \rightleftharpoons NaLac + H_2CO_3$$

Since carbonic acid is a weaker acid, it is less dissociated than lactic acid and fewer hydrogen ions are released into solution. The buffer system has therefore "mopped up" a number of hydrogen ions that otherwise would have been released were lactic acid alone dissociated in solution.

In addition to non-gaseous tissue metabolites, it can be seen from Equation (1) that the continual production of carbon dioxide also has an extremely important influence on pH in that each molecule of carbon dioxide produced releases one hydrogen ion. We have seen (Fig. 15–19) how this is buffered by reduced hemoglobin and its neutral salt:

$$H_2CO_3 + KHb \rightleftharpoons HHb + KHCO_3 \xrightarrow{\text{chloride shift } Cl^-}$$

Reduced hemoglobin is an even weaker, less dissociable acid than carbonic acid, and necessarily reduces hydrogen ion concentration, thereby preventing acidemia. Although the role of hemoglobin in buffering tissue carbon dioxide is important, the over-all level of carbon dioxide retained in the body depends on the rate at which it can be eliminated from the blood; this in turn is dependent on the level of alveolar ventilation. If alveolar ventilation is reduced disproportionately to the rate of carbon dioxide production, then Equation (1) moves to the right, with a consequent fall in pH.

The ability of these buffer systems to maintain pH within a given range is related to the readiness or otherwise with which the weak acid dissociates. This may be expressed mathematically:

$$K' = \frac{[H^+] \times [A^-]}{[HA]} \qquad \text{(Equation 2)}$$

where K' is the dissociation constant of HA which is a weak acid, the brackets denoting concentration. The higher the value of the dissociation constant, the more readily the acid dissociates. Just as hydrogen ion concentration is for convenience expressed as the logarithm of its reciprocal: $-\log_{10}[H^+]$ or pH, so the dissociation constant is conventionally written as: $-\log_{10}K'$ or pK'. Equation (2) may therefore be rewritten:

$$-\log K' = -\log[H^+] - \log\frac{[A^-]}{[HA]}$$

$$pK' = pH - \log\frac{[A^-]}{[HA]}$$

By adding the last term to both sides of this equation we obtain:

$$pH = pK' + \log\frac{[A^-]}{[HA]} \qquad \text{(Equation 3)}$$

The relationship of the pH of blood to its carbon dioxide content and tension may be derived by substituting carbonic acid from Equation (1) as the weak acid in equation (3):

$$pH = pK' + \log\frac{[HCO_3^-]}{[H_2CO_3]} \qquad \text{(Equation 4)}$$

This is the Henderson-Hasselbalch equation. The dissociation constant of carbonic acid at 37° C. is 6.10, and measurement of the remaining two factors will allow the pH to be calculated. In practice the concentration of carbonic acid in plasma is about 700 times lower than that of dissolved CO_2, as the reaction in Equation (1) is driven to the left by HCO_3^- ions derived from sodium and potassium salts:

$$NaHCO_3 \rightleftharpoons Na^+ + HCO_3^- \qquad \text{(Equation 5)}$$

Dissolved CO_2 also bears a constant relationship to carbonic acid concentration; it can therefore be substituted for it in Equation (4):

$$pH = pK' + \log\frac{[HCO_3^-]}{[CO_2]} \qquad \text{(Equation 6)}$$

The quantity of CO_2 in solution is the product of its solubility coefficient ($\alpha = 0.03$) and partial pressure and the latter can be measured directly with a CO_2 electrode. Carbonic acid contributes insignificantly to the plasma concentration of HCO_3^- ions which are largely accounted by the reaction shown in Equation (5). The plasma bicarbonate of arterial blood may be derived by subtracting dissolved from total carbon dioxide content and is normally 24 mM./L. With substitution of these values in Equation (6) we find:

$$pH = 6.10 + \log \frac{24}{40 \times 0.03}$$
$$= 7.4$$

The practical importance of the Henderson-Hasselbalch equation is that in order for pH to remain constant, any change in bicarbonate (the numerator) has to be matched by a proportional change in CO_2 (the denominator). If this ratio, which is normally 20:1, is altered, a change in pH is inevitable. Disturbances of pH primarily due to alteration in CO_2 are referred to as respiratory; those primarily due to alteration in HCO_3^- are called metabolic. Any primary change in one component of the HCO_3^-/CO_2 ratio leads to a similar change in the other component in an attempt to maintain normal pH. If for some reason the lungs are unable to remove CO_2 as fast as it is produced, arterial pCO_2 will rise and pH will fall. In order to correct this respiratory acidosis, the kidneys act by conserving HCO_3^- and excreting H^+ ions, leading to a compensatory rise in HCO_3^-. In disturbances of acid-base balance the compensatory change in HCO_3^- or CO_2 is less than the primary change and is also usually insufficient to return the pH to the normal range. The following analyses of arterial blood samples will illustrate this.

Example One: $pCO_2 = 60$ mm. Hg, plasma bicarbonate = 26 mM./L.

Here the rise in pCO_2 is greater than that of bicarbonate and is therefore likely to reflect respiratory acidosis rather than a metabolic alkalosis. The pH of 7.29 confirms this. Normally a rise in pCO_2 leads to an increase in output of the medullary respiratory center, resulting in increased ventilation which "blows off" CO_2. A failure of this homeostatic mechanism to compensate can uncommonly occur with widespread airway obstruction, producing ventilation-perfusion mismatching as seen in chronic bronchitis, or with failure of the bellows function due to muscle weakness as in myasthenia gravis or depression of the respiratory center by drugs.

Example Two: $pCO_2 = 50$ mm. Hg, plasma bicarbonate = 40 mM./L.

Here the greatest rise has occurred in bicarbonate with a smaller compensatory rise in pCO_2 and is therefore likely to result from a metabolic alkalosis rather than a respiratory acidosis. This is confirmed by the pH of 7.53. This situation might follow the excessive ingestion of alkali or after repeated vomiting, and may also occur in hypokalemia in which depleted intracellular potassium is replaced by hydrogen ions, resulting in extracellular alkalosis.

Example Three: $pCO_2 = 30$ mm. Hg, plasma bicarbonate = 12 mM./L.

Here the major fall is in bicarbonate with a smaller compensatory fall in pCO_2. This is therefore likely to be a non-respiratory or metabolic acidosis rather than a respiratory alkalosis. This is confirmed by the pH of 7.24. This situation is commonly seen in renal failure and in diabetic ketoacidosis, in which the excretion of hydrogen ions fails to keep pace with the production of non-gaseous acid metabolites.

Example Four: $pCO_2 = 25$ mm. Hg, plasma bicarbonate = 20 mM./L.

Here the major change is in pCO_2, with only a small fall in bicarbonate. The fact that this is a respiratory alkalosis is confirmed by the pH of 7.53. This picture may be seen in hysterical hyperventilation or with overbreathing due to other causes such as salicylate poisoning or diffusion defects.

GAS TRANSFER

Diffusing Capacity

The rate of diffusion of a gas in a gaseous medium is inversely proportional to the square root of its density (Graham's Law). Thus in such a medium CO_2 diffuses less easily than does oxygen, however, diffusion in the lungs involves a gaseous phase and a liquid phase. For this reason the solubility of the gas in the liquid is an important factor and is governed in this instance by Henry's Law. This law states that the volume of the gas that dissolves in a given volume of a liquid is directly proportional to the partial pressure of that gas. Since CO_2 is 24 times more soluble than oxygen, it has a greater rate of diffusion.

Factors Influencing the Diffusing Capacity of the Lungs (Table 15–2)

1. The Pressure Gradient Between the Alveoli and the Capillary Blood. Under normal circumstances blood remains in the pulmonary capillaries for 0.75 seconds. Even this short time is more than enough to allow equilibrium to take place; the latter being reached in 0.3 seconds in a normal subject breathing ambient air at sea level. Under these conditions the alveolar pO_2 is around 100 mm. Hg. With moderate impairment of diffusion, equilibration takes longer to occur;

TABLE 15–2 PHYSIOLOGIC FACTORS AND DISEASE PROCESSES AFFECTING THE DIFFUSING CAPACITY

	$D_{L_{CO}}$	Principal Determinants
Loss of lung tissue		
e.g., emphysema, lung resection	↓ ⎫	
Diffuse infiltrations	⎬	Dm
e.g., asbestosis, sarcoid, scleroderma	↓ ⎭	
Altered pulmonary blood volume		
e.g., mitral stenosis	↑ or ↓	Vc/Dm
left to right cardiac shunt	↑ ⎫	
exercise	↑ ⎬	Vc
supine posture	↑ ⎪	
Valsalva maneuver	↓ ⎭	
Altered Hb binding capacity		
e.g., anemia	↓ ⎫	
polycythemia	↑ ⎬	θ
reduced PaO_2	↑ ⎪	
increased PaO_2	↓ ⎭	

but, even so, it is still achieved in less than 0.75 seconds. Only when alveolo-capillary block is severe does anoxemia result. During exercise, however, the time the blood remains in the capillaries is shortened, so although the subject may not be anoxemic at rest, he may become so with exercise. The pressure difference responsible for the diffusion of oxygen is not as might be expected the initial alveolo-arterial gradient (100 − 40 = 60 mm.) nor the end capillary gradient (100 − 99.9 = 0.01 mm.), but is an integrated mean value that depends on a variety of complex factors including the time oxygen takes to traverse the membrane and combine with hemoglobin.

2. The Length of the Pathway of Diffusion. Before an oxygen molecule can combine with hemoglobin it must traverse the following:

a. Surfactant lining of alveoli;
b. The alveolar membrane;
c. The capillary endothelium;
d. The plasma in the capillary;
e. The RBC membrane;
f. The intracellular RBC fluid.

The distance across the membrane is usually about 0.2μ. In certain disease states this distance may be increased by edema fluid, fibrous tissue, or the presence of additional alveolar cells.

3. The Surface Area Available for Diffusion. The area available for diffusion depends on the number of functioning alveoli rather than the total number of alveoli present in the lungs. In man, it is approximately 70 square meters. Thus, loss of diffusing surface occurs in emphysema,

following resection, and in a fibrothorax with compression of the adjacent lung. Owing to the fact that in exercise many non-functioning alveoli open up, the diffusing capacity increases with exercise.

4. The Number and Character of the Red Blood Cells Available to Accept Diffused Oxygen. Anemia reduces the diffusing capacity since there are less red blood cells to take up the diffused gas. In addition, were the red cells affected in some anatomic or physiologic way which impaired the acceptance of diffused oxygen, then the diffusing capacity would likewise be reduced. The latter is mainly a theoretic concept.

Measurement of Diffusing Capacity

To measure the capacity it is necessary that the gas used be more soluble in blood than in the alveolo-capillary membrane and in the tissue fluid. Both oxygen and carbon monoxide fulfill this criterion because they combine with hemoglobin. Other gases such as N_2O are equally soluble in tissues and blood and therefore can be used to measure pulmonary capillary blood flow. They are not, however, suitable for the measurement of the diffusing capacity.

The equation for measurement of the diffusing capacity for oxygen is expressed thus:

$$D_{O_2} = \frac{ml./O_2 \text{ taken up by capillaries/min.}}{\text{Alveolar } po_2 - \text{Pulmonary capillary } po_2}$$

$$= ml.O_2/min./mm. \ Hg$$

To measure D_{O_2} necessitates a knowledge of the po_2 of mixed venous blood since this datum is necessary in order to calculate the alveolo-capillary gradient. In addition, since the capillary po_2 rises as the blood traverses the capillary, the gradient and hence the rate of diffusion falls. To calculate the D_{O_2} requires that a knowledge of the Pao_2 is available at every moment as the blood traverses to the capillary. Although these data can be derived mathematically, the calculations are tedious and many assumptions are made. Thus for the most part, persons seldom measure the diffusing capacity of the lungs for oxygen. In this regard CO is far more convenient and is used almost exclusively now. The advantages of the use of CO are that the pco in the mixed venous blood is zero except in the case of heavy smokers and hence need not be measured. In addition, CO has 210 times the affinity for hemoglobin and consequently only very low concentrations of inhaled CO (0.3) are necessary to measure the D_{LCO}.

There are a number of methods for obtaining D_{LCO} of which the most commonly used is the single breath technique. This requires the subject to make a vital capacity inspiration of a mixture containing 0.3 per cent carbon monoxide, 10 per cent helium, and 21 per cent oxygen, and to breath-hold at total lung capacity for 10 seconds, so that some of the carbon monoxide diffuses into the blood. A forced expiratory volume maneuver is then made, and once dead space gas has been displaced, an "alveolar" sample is taken and is analyzed for the final carbon monoxide concentration (F_ECO). The carbon monoxide concentration that was present in the alveolar gas before transfer had taken place is estimated from the dilution of inspired helium (He) according to the equation:

$$F_{INCO} = \frac{F_E He}{FiHe \times FiCo}$$

(initial CO concentration
in alveolar gas)

where:

$F_E He$ = He concentration in expired alveolar sample
$FiHe$ = Inspired He concentration
$FiCO$ = Inspired CO concentration

The change in carbon monoxide concentration during breath holding is now known and so D_{LCO} can be calculated according to Krogh's equation:

$$D_{LCO}(ml./min./mm.\ Hg) = \frac{Alveolar\ Volume\ (L.) \times 60}{Time\ (secs) \times (BaPr - 47)}$$

$$\times \log_N \frac{F_{INCO}}{F_{ECO}}$$

Alveolar volume in this equation may be taken either as the sum of the inspired volume and the residual volume (measured separately), or the "effective" alveolar volume (V_{Aeff}) may be calculated from the dilution of helium contained in the mixture according to the equation:

$$V_{Aeff} = \frac{FiHe}{F_E He} \times (Vi - V_{D_A})$$

where:

Vi = inspired volume
V_{D_A} = anatomic dead space

The effective alveolar volume tends to give a lower value for D_{LCO} in obstructive lung disease than does the former method.

D_{LCO} may also be measured by a steady state technique in which the subject rebreathes a mixture containing a small concentration of carbon monoxide in air, during which the rate of removal of the gas is measured. This method has the advantage that it may be used during exercise; however, errors may occur in the estimation of al-

veolar pco, particularly at rest when the tidal volume is small and dead space gas may not be entirely flushed out when sampling is made.

D_L is analogous to an electrical conductance and its reciprocal is therefore comparable to a resistance. Resistances arranged in series may be added to give the over-all resistance; and so in the lungs:

$$\frac{1}{D_L} = \frac{1}{D\ alveolar\ walls} + \frac{1}{D\ capillary\ walls}$$
$$+ \frac{1}{D\ plasma} + \frac{1}{D\ red\ cells}$$

Although it is not possible to estimate each of these smaller values separately, they may be incorporated into two measurable terms to give:

$$\frac{1}{D_L} = \frac{1}{D_m} + \frac{1}{\Theta V_c}$$

where D_m is the diffusing capacity of the alveolo-capillary membrane and ΘV_c is the diffusing capacity of the blood (V_c being the volume of alveolo-capillary blood to which the gas is exposed in the lungs, and Θ being the rate of reaction of the gas with hemoglobin in ml./min.). D_{LCO} falls following oxygen breathing because the value of Θ, which can be determined in vitro, depends on the degree of saturation of hemoglobin, which in turn determines the number of binding sites available for carbon monoxide. If two measurements of D_{LCO} are made after breathing first room air and then oxygen, and Θ is known for each level, then simultaneous equations may be solved for the two unknowns D_m and V_c. The membrane component (D_m) falls in diseases in which the surface area available for diffusion is reduced, i.e., emphysema or following lung resection. It is also reduced in conditions causing abnormal thickening of the alveolo-capillary membrane, such as fibrosing alveolitis or sarcoidosis. The alveolo-capillary blood volume (V_c) is labile because the pulmonary circulation has a large reserve capacity, and it may not fall until pulmonary disease is advanced. It tends to increase in normal subjects when they exercise or lie flat. It is also increased in patients with left-to-right cardiac shunts. In mitral stenosis D_{LCO} may be initially raised due to an elevation of V_c (Table 15–2). This may later fall due to "pruning" of the lungs' vasculature as a result of pulmonary hypertension. The picture may be further complicated by pulmonary edema which leads to a reduction of D_m. Θ is lowered in anemia and raised in polycythemia and D_{LCO} may be corrected for hemoglobin concentration by the equation:

$$D_{L.C} = D_{L.O} (14.6a + Hb) \div (1+a)Hb$$

where $D_{L,C}$ and $D_{L,O}$ are corrected and observed D_{LCO} respectively, Hb is the hemoglobin concentration and a is the D_m/V_c ratio which is assumed to be 0.7.

In bronchial asthma the D_{LCO} is normal, which is a useful point in distinguishing this condition from irreversible airflow obstruction due to emphysema. The measurements of D_m, V_c and Θ are laborious and, for clinical purposes, the simpler measurement of D_{LCO} usually suffices. It should be clear that this is influenced by a variety of factors other than thickening of the alveolo-capillary membrane as was once thought, and it is therefore sometimes called the transfer factor (T_{LCO}).

Carbon Dioxide

Because of its solubility, carbon dioxide diffuses from the pulmonary capillaries to the alveoli about 20 times more rapidly than does oxygen. For this reason diffuse pulmonary fibrotic or granulomatous diseases, such as asbestosis or sarcoidosis which are associated with impaired diffusion of oxygen, do not affect the diffusion of carbon dioxide sufficiently to cause a rise in arterial pCO_2. By the time this stage is reached, the arterial pO_2 is too low to support life. A raised arterial pCO_2 usually indicates alveolar hypoventilation.

Control of Respiration

The regulation of ventilation, by which the arterial pO_2 and pCO_2 are maintained within a fairly narrow range, is complex and incompletely understood. The involuntary rhythmic nature of breathing depends primarily on the integrity of collections of interrelated, reciprocally-acting inspiratory and expiratory neuronal pathways contained in the reticular formation of the medulla oblongata. These are known as the medullary respiratory centers, although they have no distinct anatomic boundaries. Their output to the respiratory neurones in the spinal cord is modified by cortical and pontine activity, by the aortic and carotid body chemoreceptors, and by vagus-mediated signals from the lungs and chest wall. They are extremely sensitive to the arterial pCO_2 level, and a 5 per cent increase causes the minute ventilation to double. Carbon dioxide will cross the blood-brain barrier more readily than will bicarbonate, and the subsequent dissociation of carbonic acid releases hydrogen ions into the cerebrospinal fluid (CSF), which is less able to buffer them than is blood. The medulla possesses receptors on its ventral surface which, when bathed with acid CSF, respond by increasing first tidal volume and later respiratory rate. If the acidity of the CSF is prolonged, as may occur in respiratory acidosis due to chronic obstructive airways disease, a compensatory change occurs in which CSF bicarbonate is increased, raising the pH again. As a result, a patient with an elevated arterial pCO_2 due to chronic bronchitis may have a diminished hyperventilatory response to carbon dioxide, and depends instead on hypoxic drive. Uncontrolled oxygen therapy in such a patient may produce apnea by raising arterial pO_2 above the normal level, thereby leading to secondary hypoventilation and a further rise in pCO_2 which raises the intracranial pressure and acts as a respiratory depressant. Depression of the respiratory center also occurs physiologically during sleep, and may be deepened by hypnotic drugs or anesthetics.

The carotid body and aortic arch chemoreceptors are stimulated mainly by hypoxia and to a lesser extent by hypercarbia. The carotid bodies are also sensitive to a fall in pH. These peripheral chemoreceptors are highly active metabolically, and it has been suggested that they are stimulated by the local accumulation of products of anaerobic metabolism occurring either as a consequence of a reduction in arterial pO_2 or from diminished perfusion in the presence of normoxemia as may occur in hemorrhagic shock. Their afferent signals are carried to the medulla by the glossopharyngeal and vagus nerves. The peripheral chemoreceptor response to hypoxia is not as sensitive as the medullary carbon dioxide response and the alveolar pO_2 is usually reduced to about 50 mm. Hg before the chemoreceptors take over. Variation in the intensity of hypoxic drive between normal individuals has been reported, and it is possible that this might explain the differing clinical presentations of chronic obstructive airways disease, in which the "blue bloater" with a poor hypoxic response may be found at one end of the scale, and the "pink puffer" with a normal response at the other.

A number of vagally mediated afferent stimuli pass to the respiratory centers from the lungs and chest wall. The Hering-Breuer reflex is initiated by receptors in the bronchial and bronchiolar walls. Inhibitory signals are generated when these are stretched on inspiration. These do not affect central respiratory drive, but modify tidal volume and breathing rate during exercise and hypoxic or hypercarbic stimulation. Their role during quiet breathing is minimal. In addition to brain-stem and cortical controls, the diaphragm, intercostal, and abdominal muscles, which drive the "respiratory pump," are also subject to reflex influences at the spinal level. Like other voluntary muscles, they contain length-sensitive spindle fibers, which when stretched produce signals which are transmitted to the spinal cord by α-afferent fibers. Here these synapse with α-motor neurons supplying the corresponding muscle fibers. It is thought that the α-afferent system may have a coordinative function, providing proprioceptive information about the respiratory muscles, so that motor output may be modified accordingly.

In *metabolic acidosis,* as occurs in renal failure or diabetic ketosis, non-gaseous acid metabolites which do not cross the blood-brain barrier may stimulate respiration by acting on the peripheral carotid body chemoreceptors, leading to Kussmaul breathing. Cheyne-Stokes breathing is characterized by a cyclical waxing and waning of tidal volume and respiratory frequency, and is commonly seen in severe cardiac failure associated with hypotension and following cerebrovascular accidents. This instability of the ventilatory control system may result from a variety of causes, such as prolonged circulation time resulting in delayed feed-back signals to the respiratory centers, or from increased sensitivity of the CO_2 control system as a consequence of damage to higher centers, or paradoxically from depression of CO_2 responsiveness due to brain-stem disease, enabling the less stable O_2 control system to take over.

PARTICLE DEPOSITION AND CLEARANCE

Tyndall first made the observation that inspired air contains numerous bacteria and other particles, whereas in contrast expired air is sterile, provided one does not sample the air that has come from the dead space. Both inorganic and organic particles are inhaled with each breath. Included among the latter are bacteria, fungi, and viruses. The vast majority of larger particles (5 to 10 μ) and a varying proportion of smaller particles (1 to 5 μ) are deposited in the nose. Of those particles that pass through the nose, a small but significant number are deposited in the trachea and bronchi, with the majority of such particles being in the range of 5 to 10 μ. Those that are not deposited in the nose or in the trachea and bronchi reach the gas-exchanging portions of the lung and are likely to be deposited there. A few of the smaller particles are breathed out again.

Deposition depends on three physical processes: sedimentation; inertial impaction; and diffusion or Brownian movement. Sedimentation is the main cause of deposition of particles of 3 μ or over in size; however, some particles of between 0.5 and 3 μ also settle due to this process. In contrast, most small particles between 0.1 and 1.5 μ come into contact with the alveolar walls through Brownian movement. A smaller proportion of the larger particles are deposited through inertial impaction. This process comes into play when a particle is being carried along by an air current and when at a bifurcation of an airway the momentum of the particle is such that it will carry along its original path so that it comes in contact with the wall of the airway and hence is deposited.

Over 99 per cent of deposited particles are removed by the lung clearing mechanisms. Those that are deposited in the dead space are cleared by the mucociliary escalator; those that are deposited in the parenchyma are taken up by the alveolar macrophage and either transported to the terminal bronchiole and hence to the mucociliary escalator or else they migrate into the interstitium of the lung and hence into the lymphatics to be carried to the regional nodes.

REFERENCES

Bake, B., Wood, L., Murphy, B., Macklem, P. T., and Milic-Emili, J.: The effect of inspiratory flow rate on the regional distribution of inspired gas. J. Appl. Physiol., 37:8, 1974.

Barnhard, H. J., Pierce, J. A., Joyce, J. W., and Bates, J. H.: Roentgenographic determination of total lung capacity. Am. J. Med., 28:51, 1966.

Campbell, E. J. M., et al.: The Respiratory Muscles. Philadelphia, W. B. Saunders Co., 1970.

Clements, J. A.: Surface phenomena in relation to pulmonary function. Physiologist, 5:11, 1962.

Comroe, J. H.: The Lung, 2nd ed. Chicago, Year Book Medical Publishers, 1962.

Evans, J. W., Wagner, P. D., and West, J. B.: Conditions for reduction of pulmonary gas transfer by ventilation — perfusion inequality. J. Appl. Physiol., 36:533, 1974.

Fahri, L. E., and Rahn, H.: A theoretical analysis of the alveolar oxygen difference with special reference to the distribution effect. J. Appl. Physiol., 7:699, 1955.

Filley, G. F., MacIntosh, D. J., and Wright, G.: Carbon monoxide uptake and pulmonary diffusing capacity in normal subjects at rest and during exercise. J. Clin. Invest., 33:530, 1954.

"First In-Last Out." Editorial, Br. Med. J., 3:119, 1973.

Fowler, W. S.: Lung function studies, III. Uneven pulmonary ventilation in normal subjects and in subjects with pulmonary disease. J. Appl. Physiol., 2:283, 1949.

Glazier, J. B., Hughes, J. M. B., Maloney, J. E., and West, J. B.: Vertical gradient of alveolar size in lungs of dogs frozen intact. J. Appl. Physiol., 23:694, 1967.

Hughes, J. M. B., Glazier, J. B., Maloney, J. E., and West, J. B.: Effect of lung volume on the distribution of pulmonary blood flow in man. Resp. Physiol., 4:58, 1968.

Hyatt, R. E., Schilder, D. P., and Fry, D. L.: Relationship between maximum expiratory flow to degree of lung inflation. J. Appl. Physiol., 13:331, 1950.

Lenfant, C., Wayes, P., Aucutt, C., and Couz, J.: Effect of chronic hypoxic hypoxia on the O_2-Hb dissociation curve and respiratory gas transport in man. Resp. Physiol., 7:7, 1969.

Macklem, I. T., and Mead, J.: Resistance of central and peripheral airways measured by retrograde catheter. J. Appl. Physiol., 22:395, 1967.

Milic-Emili, J., Henderson, J. E. M., Dolovich, M. B., Trop, D., and Kaneko, K.: Regional distribution of inspired gas in the lung. J. Appl. Physiol., 21:749, 1966.

Ogilvie, C. M., Forster, R. E., Blakemore, W. S., and Morton, J. W.: A standardized breath holding technique for the clinical measurement of the diffusing capacity of the lungs for carbon monoxide. J. Clin. Invest., 36:1, 1957.

Otis, A. B., McKerrow, C. B., Bartlett, R. A., Mead, J., McIlroy, M. B., Selverstone, N. J., and Radford, E. P.: Mechanical factors in the distribution of pulmonary ventilation. J. Appl. Physiol., *26*:732, 1969.

Pattle, R. E.: Lining layer of the lung. Br. Med. Bull., *19*:41, 1963.

Perutz, M. F.: Stereochemistry of cooperative effects of haemoglobin. Nature, *228*:726, 1970.

Radford, E. P.: Recent Studies of the Mechanical Properties of Mammalian Lungs. *In* Remington, J. W. (ed.): *Tissue Elasticity*. Washington, D.C., American Physiological Society, 1957.

Reger, R. B., Young, A., and Morgan, W. K. C.: An accurate and rapid radiographic method of determining total lung capacity. Thorax, *27*:163, 1972.

Riley, R. L., and Cournand, A.: "Ideal" alveolar air and the analysis of ventilation — perfusion relationships in the lungs. J. Appl. Physiol., *1*:825, 1949.

Roughton, F. J. W., and Forster, R. E.: Relative importance of diffusion and chemical reaction rates in determining rate of exchange of gases in the human lung, with special reference to true diffusing capacity of pulmonary membrane and volume of blood in the lung capillaries. J. Appl. Physiol., *11*:277, 1957.

West, J. B.: Regional differences in gas exchange in the lung of erect man. J. Appl. Physiol., *17*:893, 1962.

16

Protective Mechanisms of The Lungs; Pulmonary Disease; Pleural Disease

JOHN H. KILLOUGH

INTRODUCTION

For the lungs to perform their basic function as a membrane for two-way gaseous exchange between the external and internal environments, it is necessary that they be in constant contact with air. Thus, the lungs are exposed to air which may contain dust, bacteria, fungi, viruses, and various other noxious agents. For defense against these potentially harmful materials the lungs possess a complex of protective mechanisms. Disruption of these mechanisms by internal changes or overwhelming onslaught from without accounts for many pulmonary diseases. To understand these disease processes, some knowledge of the structure and function of the various elements of the respiratory system is necessary.

Although the respiratory tract may be divided arbitrarily into upper and lower portions, it functions as a physiologic unit directed toward the cleansing, warming, and humidification of ventilated air and the exchange of gases. From the nasopharynx to the alveoli there are many gross and microscopic changes in structure which reflect these different physiologic functions.

Nasopharynx

Air entering the upper passage is grossly filtered by hairs in the nose and further filtered, warmed, and humidified as it comes in contact with the moist mucous membranes of the turbin-

ates. At sites where air currents strike the membrane, cilia are present which beat in a coordinated fashion, so that particles are swept toward areas where they can be expectorated, swallowed, or expelled by nose blowing. Absorption from the olfactory area occurs rather freely; thus, various allergens and infectious agents as well as medications may enter at this level.

Trachea and Bronchi

The trachea branches into the right and left bronchi, and this pattern of dichotomous division is repeated with decreasing cross-sectional diameters to the level of the respiratory bronchioles. Here the branching becomes much more extensive and gives rise to alveolar ducts, alveolar sacs, and alveoli.

Structurally, the trachea and bronchi contain more or less the same elements, although there are important quantitative variations. They have been divided into layers on cross section: the epithelial, the subepithelial, the muscular, and the adventitial layers. The first three layers are most important in terms of protective mechanisms and diseases and will be briefly described.

The *epithelial layer* consists of ciliated columnar cells, among which are interspersed goblet cells. This pattern persists throughout the trachea and bronchi until bronchioles are reached which are 0.4 mm. in diameter. Here the goblet cells disappear and the cilia-bearing cells become

451

cuboidal and interspersed with non-ciliated cuboidal cells. Finally, in smaller bronchioles the ciliated cells disappear altogether.

Sensory fibers of the trigeminal, glossopharyngeal, and vagal nerves are present at various levels in the mucous membranes of the pharynx, larynx, trachea, and bronchi. Stimulation of these fibers by irritating substances results in cough. At present it is not known whether ciliary action is under nervous control; however, it is quite evident that the activity of the cilia is coordinated by some means.

The *subepithelial layer* lies between the basement membrane upon which the epithelial cells rest and the muscular layer. It is composed largely of connective tissue elements, arterioles, venules, and capillaries of the bronchial vasculature. There are also fibers of the vagi and sympathetics distributed to the blood vessels. The lymphatic vascular system is found in this layer and it should be appreciated that it represents one of the most extensive in the body. The lymphatic capillaries do not extend to the alveoli but appear at the level of the alveolar ducts. From Miller's diagrams it is evident that the lymphatics form a plexus about the arteries and the airways and anastomose at the level of the alveolar ducts, with a somewhat separate system about the pulmonary veins. Lymph flow in the periarterial and peribronchial vessels is believed to be centrifugal, whereas the flow in the perivenous vessels is centripetal and into the hilar lymph glands. Peripheral connections are made with the lymphatic plexus in the pleura. The pleural lymphatics form a set which unites into a variable number of trunks and drains into lymph nodes at the hilum. One of the peculiarities of the pulmonary lymphatic system is that nearly all the lymph from both lungs drains into the right lymphatic duct. Only lymph from the left upper lobe drains into the thoracic duct. There are, however, frequent connections between the two sides, so that this separation is not entirely complete. These patterns are of importance in the understanding of metastatic spread of infection and malignant disease. As in other parts of the body, lymph flow is dependent on the movement of tissues. In the central portions of the lung, movement is restricted by large vascular and bronchial structures, with resultant sluggish lymph flow. As a consequence, in certain disease states accompanied by pulmonary edema, the edema, as revealed radiographically, may be more marked centrally and in a "butterfly" arrangement.

The *muscular layer*, composed entirely of smooth muscle, is so extensive that it is said to be impossible to cut through a cubic millimeter of lung without encountering muscle. It extends from the trachea to the alveoli, where occasional delicate muscle fibers have been identified in the walls. The helical turns of crisscrossing muscle fibers are almost circular in the larger bronchi, but the turns become steeper peripherally. This more or less circular arrangement of the muscle fibers provides efficiency in constriction as well as strength against high intraluminal pressures. Innervation of the musculature is via the vagi and sympathetics, which, by their activity, may produce constriction and relaxation, respectively. However, it is most likely that the changes in bronchial diameter during normal respiration are a passive phenomenon without an element of alternating vagal and sympathetic activity. Beneath the smooth muscle are the longitudinal elastic fibers which passively resist the expansion of inspiration and by elasticity alone bring the airways back to their resting length on expiration.

The submucosal glands which extend throughout the three outer layers produce a mucoprotein secretion of varying viscosity. Secretion occurs on vagal stimulation, but the effect is largely a quantitative rather than a qualitative one.

Cartilage, which at first is regularly disposed and almost surrounds the trachea and large bronchi, eventually becomes fragmented into irregular plaques, and in bronchioles disappears altogether. Where cartilaginous support is absent, the encircling muscle fibers can produce maximal constriction.

Alveoli

The respiratory bronchiole divides twice, giving rise to three orders of respiratory bronchioles. The third order then divides into two alveolar ducts, which in turn divide five to eight times and terminate as alveolar sacs. There are occasional small projecting spaces, the alveoli, on the walls of the first-order respiratory bronchioles. With continued branching, the frequency of these alveoli increases markedly until at the level of the alveolar sacs the walls are beset solidly with alveoli. The walls of the alveoli consist of a moist surface (see Surfactant, p. 432), a thin alveolar epithelium which is one cell thick, a narrow "basement membrane," and the underlying capillary membrane. Through these tissues, gaseous diffusion occurs between the air and the blood. Various mononuclear cells are found on and within these thin structures. Lymphocytes which become sensitized to antigen interact with the bone marrow–derived alveolar macrophages, and the macrophages become activated. Activated macrophages are more phagocytic, possess more bactericidal activity and have a higher lysosomal enzyme level. These activated cells remove offensive matter which, by damaging the alveolar epithelium, would interfere with the essential process of gaseous diffusion.

Minute openings called alveolar pores exist between adjacent alveoli, and considerably larger epithelium-lined communications exist between bronchioles and alveolar sacs. These two types of communications are of importance, for they permit the direct passage of air from alveolus to alveolus and bronchioles to alveolar sac. This situation is referred to as collateral ventilation, since alveoli may continue to be ventilated in the presence of obstruction of their normal ventilatory pathways.

PROTECTIVE MECHANISMS

The protective mechanisms of the lung are directed toward maintaining the integrity of the alveoli, their blood supply, and ventilation. This requires the cleansing, humidification, and temperature regulation of relatively large volumes of air. The size of the task is impressive when one realizes that air contains bacteria, fungi, viruses, and many other forms of particulate matter which are potentially damaging to the 70 or 80 sq. m. of alveolar surface area. Air that seems clean may contain as many as 3 million particles per cubic foot, whereas visibly dusty air may contain over 100 million particles per cubic foot. The efficiency of these protective mechanisms is evident from the fact that the alveoli are maintained essentially sterile and free of foreign matter in the presence of these agents and a necessary basal alveolar ventilation of approximately 4 liters each minute.

A large portion of the cleansing of air, humidification, and temperature adjustment occurs in the nose. From the moment air enters the nose, the processes for removing particulate matter are at work. Larger material is immediately trapped by hairs in the nose, and those particles getting past this gross filter still may be removed in the nose by coming in contact with the moist turbinates. If this happens, the particles are swept away by cilia for elimination by swallowing or nose blowing.

In the trachea and bronchi the process becomes somewhat more elaborate. Mucus, produced by the goblet cells and mucous glands, enters the lumen of the bronchi and forms a continuous, moist, sticky surface. Beneath the surface lies the ciliated epithelium. The wavelike movements of the cilia are coordinated in such a way as to move the mucus sheet upward at a rate which increases from less than 1 mm./minute in small airways to as much as 2 cm./minute in the main bronchi and trachea. Thus, a tubular "conveyer belt" is provided which continuously moves upward in the normal individual and is being replenished continuously throughout the airways from the level of the alveolar ducts on up. The ciliated epithelium is interrupted only by stratified squamous epithelium over the vocal cords, but recurs again above them. It is believed that the mucus sheet is drawn uninterrupted over the vocal cords through its cohesive and elastic properties. Airways are somewhat tortuous, and where particles impinge upon the walls, they adhere and are swept out of the respiratory tract. As will be noted in the subsequent discussion of lung disorders, there are many factors which alter the efficiency of this self-cleansing mechanism. For example, cold air, sedatives, anesthetics, tobacco smoke, systemic alcohol, sulfur dioxide, and possibly high concentrations of oxygen may depress ciliary action; ciliary efficiency may be disrupted seriously by dry air and various drugs which render the mucus sheet too viscous for efficient ciliary action. Even here there is considerable latitude, for as much as 50 per cent of the water may be removed from mucus before there is a great increase in its consistency.

The movement of the mucus sheet and the expelling of foreign matter are assisted to some extent by changes in the diameter of airways on inspiration and expiration. Bronchi have been observed to widen and elongate on inspiration and narrow and shorten on expiration. The narrowing on expiration increases the rate of air flow considerably and therefore has a tendency to blow out mucus and other intraluminal matter.

Normally, the cleansing secretions of the lung are handled entirely by ciliary action with some assistance from the expulsive forces of quiet respiration. However, when bronchial or tracheal secretions become slightly excessive, acceleration of the expiratory air flow by clearing of the throat may be necessary to clear the nonciliated vocal cords. If this is ineffective, a more forceful mechanism, the cough, may be called forth to blast the secretions upward. The cough reflex is initiated by stimulation of afferent nerve endings in the laryngeal, tracheal, or bronchial mucosa. The act itself can be divided into three parts. First, there is a deep inspiration, followed immediately by closure of the glottis. Second, with the glottis still closed, positive pressure develops in the thorax by contraction of muscles of the chest and the abdominal wall. Lastly, the glottis is suddenly opened and the air under pressure is rapidly expelled. If the offending substance is eliminated, or if it is moved upward to an insensitive area, coughing ceases. There may, however, be continuous paroxysms of coughing which move the offensive matter little by little until it is eliminated or until the cough reflex is suppressed by medication.

In addition to the cleansing action of the mucus sheet and the expulsive forces of normal respiration and coughing, peristaltic movements in the finer bronchi probably assist in eliminating secretions. Jarre and Di Rienzo, in separate studies using radiopaque material, have demonstrated peristalsis in the bronchi of man. It is believed that the peristaltic waves assist in moving foreign material to larger airways where coughing may be more effective.

Up to this point the mechanisms of defense that have been described are the ones which are at work in the airways lined with a ciliated epithelium and coated with a moving mucus sheet. However, some respired matter may penetrate beyond these barriers. Very small particles, 10 μ or less in diameter, are respirable, and after inhalation can be found rather uniformly deposited over the alveolar walls. Heppleston has observed this in coal miners who have died very shortly after exposure to such particles in dusty mines. Disposal of foreign material at this level of the respiratory tree is quite different from what has been described thus far. It depends upon phagocytosis and, from the observations of Heppleston, must occur rapidly. If the ingested material is bacterial, it may be destroyed within the macrophage. If, as in the case of various dusts, it is resistant to digestion, the phagocyte moves upward to an alveolar duct. This is the level of termination of both the ciliated epithelium and the lymphatic system. Disposition may then be accomplished by ciliary action sweeping the phagocyte upward, or the cell may enter the lymphatic vessels and arrive in nearby lymphoid collections or hilar lymph nodes. Some of the variations in this process of removing dust particles are discussed in the section on Pneumoconiosis.

The mechanisms which trap inspired dry material are not as successful against liquids or even insoluble material suspended in a liquid. For example, Barclay found in his experimental studies that finely powdered lead-glass insufflated into lungs did not reach the alveoli and frequently was eliminated from the larger airways within a matter of hours. Yet, the same material suspended in a liquid reached the alveoli and might still be visible on roentgenography for weeks. The significance of this observation to patients with sinusitis, bronchitis, and other morbid conditions characterized by excessive pulmonary secretions is quite obvious.

The inhalation of irritating fumes may elicit reflex constriction of the bronchioles. This is similar to the response in asthma, and although it may be looked upon as a mechanism for protecting the alveoli, it is a two-edged sword. If the irritation is long maintained, as in the case of industrial fumes, it can produce bronchitis and asthmatic symptoms. Voluntary breath-holding or limitation of ventilation as an obvious defense against inhalation of noxious material can be effective for only short periods of time.

Defensive mechanisms can be active to extremes which are disadvantageous. The dry cough which does not become productive even when expectorants are employed may be exhausting to the patient and accomplish nothing toward removing the irritative focus. Occasionally, the cough reflex has been incriminated in the spread of infection from one area of the lung to another. The risk of spreading infection which is inherent in excessive liquid secretions has been alluded to above. In general, however, the effectiveness of the self-cleansing mechanisms of the lungs is quite impressive when one considers how much extraneous material must be removed even from air that seems to be clean.

Although self-cleansing mechanisms are impressive, potential pathogens and allergens are deposited in the lung. Immunologic defenses are then activated to protect the person from microbial invasion. IgA is the primary mechanism in the lung, and the quantity of this antibody in the pulmonary secretions correlates better with resistance to infection than the quantity of any serum antibody. Immunofluorescent studies of bronchial and nasal mucosa have shown a predominance of cells containing IgA and relatively few containing IgM, IgG, or IgE. There is evidence suggesting that IgE may be antiviral. Thus there is a local humoral mucosal immunity. Several studies suggest that the IgA-producing cells predominate in the upper and middle portions of the respiratory tract but diminish considerably at the level of the bronchioles. In fact, studies of alveolar washings reveal IgG:IgA ratios resembling serum at this lowest level of the respiratory tract. Several recent reports have described a local cell-mediated immune response.

For many years it has been known that the alpha-1-globulin fraction of serum contains a factor which inhibits the activity of proteolytic enzymes. This factor has been designated alpha-1-antitrypsin and recognized as the chief biologic substance responsible for the alpha-1-globulin band on electrophoresis. The biologic function of this antitrypsin is not well understood at the present, but it probably has a role in protecting the lungs.

The lysis of inflammatory exudate by the proteolytic enzymes of macrophages and granulocytes is an important supplement to cough and mucociliary action in clearing the lungs of inflammatory products. However, it is postulated that the released leukocytic enzymes, if uncontrolled, could lead to the excessive destruction of pulmonary tissue. The role, then, of alpha-1-antitrypsin is thought to be the inhibition of excessive proteases and thus protection of the lung. Whether this is the biologic function of antitrypsin is not proved, but it is recognized that abnormally low concentrations of antitrypsin are associated with "hereditary" emphysema.

Maintenance of the integrity of alveoli depends on defense mechanisms not only against foreign matter but also against the tendency of surface tension of the moist lining to collapse the alveoli. Patency of alveoli is accomplished in part by negative intrathoracic pressure and supporting tissues; however, these alone do not prevent collapse under certain pathologic conditions. The relationship between pressure (P) within a sphere, tension (T) in the wall, and the radius (r) of the sphere is expressed in the Laplace equation, $P = \frac{2T}{r}$. A moist sphere such as an alveolus with airway connections to the atmosphere would tend increasingly to collapse as the radius diminished were it not for the presence of a "surfactant system" which adjusts surface tension in relation to radius. Normally there is believed to be a complex mixture of lipids, protein, and carbohydrates — the surface-active system — lining the alveolus. This surface-active material, or surfactant, reduces surface tension as the surface area of alveoli decreases. By thus varying the surface tension of the alveolar wall (in relation to radius), the right side of the equation $\frac{2T}{r}$ is maintained relatively constant, so that an antiatelectatic effect is produced. The exact site of surfactant production is unresolved; however, the larger cells of the alveolar epithelium are suspect.

Additional physiologic functions of surfactant are postulated as protecting the integrity of the alveolus. By maintaining a lower surface tension, and thus a lower tension on the alveolar wall, the capillary hydrostatic pressure is augmented to a lesser degree than would otherwise be the case. This diminishes the tendency of hydrostatic pressure to move fluid into the alveoli. Another characteristic of surface-active agents, the spreading tendency, may be important in moving bacteria, cellular debris, and foreign particles to phagocytic alveolar macrophages. This is a physical phenomenon in which a surfactant tends to move from areas of high concentration and a low surface tension to areas of low concentration and a high surface tension.

PULMONARY DISEASE

A virulent infectious organism introduced into the respiratory tract in one individual may result in progressive disease. In another, the organism may obtain a temporary foothold only to be eliminated later or held in a quiescent state, though still alive. In still another, the infectious agent may be eliminated promptly without any measurable effect on the host. Thus, there are varying degrees of effectiveness of the protective mechanisms. Pulmonary disease, whether infectious or not, may be looked upon as the result of the disruption or undesirable response of one or more of these mechanisms. The pulmonary protective mechanisms probably are modified by many factors, including heredity, age, sex, nutritional status, environment, and ill-defined fluctuations in individual resistance to disease. It must be remembered that very little information is available concerning the physiologic effects of these

factors. The body's defenses are many and varied so that the failure of one mechanism is generally compensated for by other processes. As a consequence, many pulmonary disorders are reversible, and on recovery the functional status of the lungs is little or none the worse for the experience.

In the consideration of pulmonary disorders, it is desirable to interpret the pathologic alterations in terms of effects on physiologic processes. Thus, pulmonary disease should be considered in the light of the various components of pulmonary function that are discussed in the preceding chapter. When doing this, however, it must be remembered that a patient may have pulmonary disease without significant deviation from normal in functional studies. This may be due to the statistical range of normal values, limited extent of the pathologic process, or the inherent limitations of testing techniques.

Asthma

Bronchial asthma is characterized by diffuse airway obstruction which is largely at the bronchiolar level (see p. 430). Hypersensitivity to inhaled extrinsic allergens or to intrinsic infectious agents of the respiratory tract are believed, in the majority of patients, to initiate the pathophysiologic changes. However, once the asthmatic reaction pattern is established, psychophysiologic reactions, smoke, fumes, physical exertion, and changes in the temperature or humidity of the air may precipitate attacks. Whether or not there is a single common abnormality for these various triggers is unknown.

The obstructive characteristics of asthma arise mainly from two physical changes in the airways which increase the resistance of gas flow: irregularities of the walls and narrowing of the lumina by spasm of smooth muscle. Slight irregularities in larger airways such as the bronchi increase the resistance to flow by producing turbulence. The physical accompaniment of this is audible wheezing. In smaller airways, turbulence, if it occurs at all, is less important, and viscosity of the air becomes dominant because of the extreme degrees of bronchiolar narrowing.

The narrowing is brought on by at least three factors. One is the inflammatory reaction with its accompanying vascular engorgement, edema, leukocytic infiltration, and eventual fibroblastic proliferation. Another is the excessive, tenacious secretions produced by the hyperactive mucous glands. This sticky material adheres, narrows, blocks, and produces irregularities and increased thickness in the walls of the bronchi and bronchioles. Lastly, there is constriction of smooth muscle in the bronchial walls.

Various bronchoconstrictors initiate these narrowing processes. The induction of asthma by allergens occurs in the presence of IgE antibodies fixed to basophils and mast cells. The interaction of allergens and these antibodies results in the release of histamine and the slow-reacting substance of anaphylaxis, thus causing edema of mucous membranes and smooth muscle spasm.

The ventilatory alterations of bronchial asthma are those of bronchiolar obstruction and as such are not diagnostic for asthma alone, but occur with any process obstructing small airways. Diffusing capacity, however, remains relatively normal in uncomplicated asthma. Hypercarbia may occur with marked airway obstruction or diminished sensitivity of the respiratory center and hypoxemia from an inhomogeneity of ventilation/perfusion ratios. The primary value of function tests is that they are objective and allow better evaluation of the disability as well as the results of therapy. In the early stages there is a high degree of reversibility of the changes in bronchial asthma, and the lungs may be normal between paroxysms. This is the chief point of functional differentiation from emphysema, which is characterized by relative irreversibility. As paroxysms of asthma are repeated over and over again, the narrowing of airways may become persistent as a consequence of smooth muscle hypertrophy, thickening of the basement membrane and mucous plugs. There is disruption of alveolar walls, and the pulmonary-cardiac abnormalities become indistinguishable from those of obstructive emphysema. Thus, the pathophysiologic changes described in the section on emphysema are applicable in various degree to bronchial asthma.

Emphysema

Obstructive pulmonary emphysema is a pathologic entity characterized by obstructive phenomena at the level of the smaller bronchioles. As such it is clearly distinguished from compensatory emphysema and the normal aging lung, conditions which lack the obstructive element. Etiologic factors are not sharply defined. In more than 60 per cent of patients, obstructive emphysema is accompanied or preceded by chronic bronchitis. The etiology of that disease is unclear, but the continued accumulation of data incriminates irritants such as cigarette smoke and air pollutants as well as repeated bouts of respiratory tract infection. An interesting fact is that cigarette smoke lowers the surface tension of lung extracts. This might contribute, if true in vivo, to the pathogenesis of emphysema by promoting the hyperinflation of alveoli. Cigarette smoke, which is ciliatoxic and inhibits the phagocytic activities of macrophages, may also contribute by diminishing the protection from foreign matter. Other factors cited are pneumoconiosis, sarcoidosis, bronchiectasis, mucoviscidosis, and tuberculosis. An etiologic role for bronchial asthma is highly questionable. Since 1963, when a deficiency of alpha-1-antitrypsin in the serum was first noted to be associated with obstructive pulmonary emphysema in certain patients, there have been many reports of "familial" or "hereditary" emphysema. Phenotyping has demonstrated that approximately 0.1 per cent of the population have the homozygous antitrypsin deficiency (ZZ). There are, however, multiple alleles that occur at the autosomal locus, hence varying degrees of the deficiency.

The initial pathophysiologic lesion in obstructive emphysema is unknown. An interesting speculation is based on the fact that an appropriate stress from continuing irritants or infections leads to an outpouring of leukocytes and macrophages. This might in turn lead to increased amounts of protease released by these cells which would more easily overcome the reduced concentration of alpha-1-antitrypsin in the person with the hereditary antitrypsin deficiency but also might overcome normal levels of the antienzyme. The excess concentrations of enzyme would in turn lead to tissue damage.

Concomitants of tissue damage are edema, exudate, hyperactivity of the muscular layers and, in time, fibrosis. Each of these by narrowing pulmonary airways, particularly at the bronchiolar level, may cause air trapping in the alveoli. There are several factors which facilitate the passage of air beyond the partial obstruction in inspiration yet do not assist in its egress on expiration. One of these is the fact that airways are wider on inspiration than on expiration. Thus, an obstruction which is of minor significance on inspiration may increase to a serious degree on expiration. If the narrowing is further increased, the discrepancy between the forces of inspiration and those of expiration comes into play. Air is taken into the lungs by the powerful contraction of the diaphragm supplemented by the levator muscles of the ribs which enlarge the diameter of the thorax. Forces of expiration consist of fibroelastic recoil of the lungs, the use of depressor muscles of the ribs, relaxation of the diaphragm, and contraction of the abdominal muscles so as to force the diaphragm up. From the studies of von Neergaard, it is clear that the surface tension of the air-liquid interface of the approximately 300 million alveoli is also a significant contributory factor in expiration. These combined forces do not approximate those of inspiration; thus, with airway narrowing, air can be forcibly pulled into the alveoli but expiration is less effective in discharging it. Even with complete obstruction, the alveoli distal to the obstruction may receive air via collateral pathways from alveoli which are normally aerated. These pathways also narrow on expiration, and, in addition, this collateral ventilation is tortuous, so that air trapping is continued. On expiration, and particularly when expiration is forced, there is a sharp, abnormal rise in pressure in the areas of trapped air, leading to compression and further narrowing of adjacent bronchi and bronchioles. All these processes lead to an increasing accumulation of air and a rising pressure beyond the obstruction. Eventually, distention becomes so great that there is disruption of alveolar walls and the encircling mesh of musculoelastic tissue about the smaller airways. Paroxysms of coughing increase the intrapulmonary pressures still further and contribute to the hyperinflation.

With repetition of acute exacerbations of the underlying disease there may be excessive amounts of tenacious mucus, mucopurulent secretion, hypertrophy and spasm of bronchial muscle, and permanent thickening of the mucosa. Each of these, by interfering with mechanisms such as ciliary action, cough, and collateral ventilation, serves to increase the obstructive process and trapping of air. When the lungs enlarge, their bases push the diaphragm downward toward its position of maximal inspiration so that its excursion becomes less and less. As distention continues, the intrapleural pressure becomes less negative and, during expiration, actually may be 1 or 2 cm. of water pressure above atmospheric, so that when the sternum is removed at autopsy, the lungs balloon out of the thoracic cavity. With increasing intrapleural pressure, the ribs elevate, the chest becomes barrel-shaped, and the diaphragm flattens. This is the position of full inspiration; hence, the ability to inspire additional air and maintain effective ventilation is markedly impaired. An improvement in ventilation might be anticipated if the diaphragm could be returned to a more normal position on expiration — the rationale behind the use of emphysema belts, breathing exercises, and pneumoperitoneum.

In obstructive emphysema, as during acute attacks of asthma, the timed vital capacity is reduced and the total lung volume is increased. This is the result of expiratory air trapping beyond narrow airways, producing an increase in the residual volume. As noted previously, rapid expiration increases the obstructive element and augments air trapping still further. Under these circumstances, therefore, the vital capacity varies with the speed of expiration — hence, the importance of the timed vital capacity as a measure of obstruction. The midexpiratory flow rate and maximal breathing capacity are reduced and the work of breathing is increased.

The physiologic and pathologic changes are not uniform throughout the lungs; some areas are better ventilated than others. The effect of this variation is that inspiratory and expiratory gaseous mixing is poor or absent in some regions and relatively better in others. Venous blood passing through poorly ventilated regions with impaired mixing of gases is exposed to a low pressure of oxygen and a high pressure of carbon dioxide. If this defect is pronounced, there will be a fall in the oxygen saturation of arterial blood and a rise in the partial pressure of carbon dioxide. Contributing to the fall in oxygen saturation is a reduction of diffusing capacity. This reduction is due to a disruption of normal alveolar architecture and a decrease in the functioning capillary bed, both of which decrease the effective surface area for diffusion.

In advanced obstructive emphysema, cyanosis and respiratory acidosis develop, and the same may occur in acute asthmatic attacks if the attack continues long enough. With severe respiratory acidosis the medullary respiratory centers lose their sensitivity to the normal carbon dioxide stimulus for respiration. In this circumstance, hypoxia provides the respiratory drive. If this is not recognized and high concentrations of oxygen are given to relieve cyanosis without mechanical aids to respiration, the result may be fatal.

Several factors operate to produce pulmonary hypertension: destruction of interalveolar septa, which diminishes the area of the capillary bed; vasoconstriction due to hypoxia; increased viscosity of blood due to secondary polycythemia; and hypervolemia and high intra-alveolar pressure coincident to air trapping which squeezes small pulmonary vessels. With hypoxia the cardiac output is normal or somewhat elevated. The combination of relatively normal cardiac output and increased pulmonary vascular resistance increases right heart work and leads to the development of cor pulmonale. If the process continues, cardiac failure follows. Elevated intrapleural pressure and prolonged expiration add to the elevation of systemic venous pressure by impeding venous return to the heart.

The *aged lung* is characterized by minimal functional changes which have sometimes been referred to as senile emphysema. This term has been used in the past to describe a form of nonobstructive pulmonary overdistention secondary to kyphotic distortion. In the absence of complicating pulmonary disease, vital capacity is slightly reduced, residual lung volume is increased, maximal breathing capacity may be reduced by half, and there is a mild increase in airway resistance. These changes are related to a reduction of pulmonary elasticity, dilatation of alveolar ducts, and weakening of alveolar septal membranes with confluence of adjacent alveoli. There is frequently some reduction of PaO_2 but carbon dioxide values remain within the limits of normal.

Compensatory emphysema is a nonobstructive panacinar dilatation called forth by a decrease in volume of lung parenchyma, most commonly from atelectasis, surgical resection, or fibrosis. The remaining pulmonary tissues overdistend to fill the available space and, to this extent, compensate for the loss. If the diseased pulmonary segment becomes functional again, the emphysema may disappear. But, if the emphysema persists, as after pneumonectomy, there is a gradual loss of pulmonary elasticity with some associated functional impairment.

Interstitial emphysema occurs when air from ruptured alveoli or bronchi enters the interstitial tissues of the lung and dissects along the peribronchial and perivascular sheaths into the mediastinum. From here it may enter the pleural space or travel to the subcutaneous tissues of the suprasternal notch and extend over the neck, face, arms, and trunk. Pain which may simulate angina pectoris often heralds the onset of interstitial emphysema. If the volume of air is large and if it is under pressure, it may interfere with venous return to the heart and be associated with dyspnea and cyanosis. Most commonly interstitial emphysema occurs in association with trauma, surgery, asthma, obstructive pulmonary processes, and pulmonary infections.

Hypersensitivity Pneumonitis

There are several clinical entities of interstitial pneumonitis which are recognized as hypersensitivity reactions to protein dusts inhaled during certain activities of man. Pigeon-breeder's disease, farmer's lung, bagassosis, sequoiosis, maple-bark disease and mushroom worker's lung are examples. The hypersensitivity reaction results in a sarcoid-like granulomatous reaction with associated interstitial plasma cells, lymphocytes, areas of focal histiocytosis, and multinucleated giant cells. Alveolar walls and bronchioles are involved in the process. Precipitating antibodies to the appropriate inciting antigen generally are demonstrable. The chief pulmonary functional defect is a low diffusing capacity which correlates with the alveolar and bronchiolar involvement. However, low compliance and a disturbed ventilation-perfusion relationship are also noted in some patients. Studies suggest that prolonged exposure to the offending antigen in some patients leads to airway obstruction, although in most patients there is no obstructive element. On removal of the offending agent, there is in the majority an impressive abatement of the various symptoms and laboratory abnormalities, but with chronic exposure there may be irreversible damage.

Eosinophilic Pulmonary Infiltration (Loeffler's Syndrome)

Eosinophilia associated with transient, migratory, and symptomless roentgenographic shadows was described first by Loeffler in 1932. Subsequently, he suggested that an allergic mechanism might be responsible, and this seems compatible with later opinions. The meager amount of autopsy material indicates that the lesion is a pneumonitis composed largely of aggregates of eosinophils together with macrophages and giant cells in a background of edema fluid. Eosinophils are predominant both in the interstitial and alveolar exudates and in the sputum. The size of the lesions is such that significant alterations in pulmonary function have not been described. Similar areas of eosinophilic pulmonary infiltrates with systemic eosinophilia have been reported in bronchial asthma, helminthiasis, chronic brucellosis, tuberculosis, tropical eosinophilia, coccidioidomycosis, aspergillosis, drug sensitivities, chemical sensitivities, and polyarteritis nodosa.

Pulmonary Alveolar Proteinosis

This chronic disease of the lungs, characterized by the accumulation of eosinophilic material in alveoli, was described first by Rosen, Castleman, and Liebow in 1958. To date, the etiology remains unknown. Certain histologic similarities to pneumocystis infection have led to intensive but unsuccessful searches for this parasite. Efforts to isolate other infectious agents or to identify an inhalant or aspirant common to all cases have also been unsuccessful. The material has the chemical composition of pulmonary surfactant but has decreased surface-active properties. At present the disease is believed to be a consequence of decreased clearance of surfactant rather than overproduction.

In the early stages of pulmonary alveolar proteinosis, septal cells in the walls of alveoli increase in both size and number. Increasing further, they may line the alveoli, project into the lumina, slough, disintegrate, and give rise to PAS-positive granular and floccular material with numerous small acicular spaces. Continuation of this sequence leads to the filling of the alveoli and distal air spaces, including respiratory bronchioles. In these areas of consolidation there is a striking absence of cellular infiltration into the interalveolar septa and there is no evidence of vascular congestion. The ultimate histologic fate is not clearly defined, although it is known from clinical studies that regression may occur. Biopsy studies of areas believed to have been involved previously have shown slight interstitial fibrosis of questionable significance and some residual granularity of the alveolar lining cells.

In this disease, although the distal parenchyma is not normal and air-containing, there is no primary involvement of the airways. Hence, spirographic studies show no evidence of obstruction to air flow. There is, however, filling of alveoli by "proteinaceous" material and replacement of functioning lung volume by consolidation. As a consequence of this, there is a restrictive pattern of ventilation with a decrease in vital capacity. The patient may complain of dyspnea and there may even be objective hyperventilation at rest. Inspiration of high concentrations of oxygen does not relieve the hyperventilation, although it does decrease any arterial unsaturation which may be present. As in many other forms of diffuse lung disease, the hyperventilation is believed to be due to an alteration in the proprioceptive reflex mechanism within the diseased lung.

The increase in size and number of alveolar septal cells and the early partial coating of alveoli with eosinophilic material interferes with the diffusion of oxygen across the alveolar-capillary membrane. This does not permit full saturation of hemoglobin passing such alveoli and results in various degrees of arterial unsaturation and its clinical manifestation, cyanosis. Further arterial oxygen unsaturation is caused by venous blood passing through the intact vasculature of consolidated alveoli which contain no air at all. Thus, the pathophysiology of pulmonary alveolar proteinosis is a consequence of a ventilation-perfusion imbalance. There is no evidence of impaired carbon dioxide excretion. If clinical improvement occurs, the oxygenation of blood may return to normal.

From clinical studies thus far published, patients with pulmonary alveolar proteinosis seem unusually susceptible to superimposed infections. In the presence of pulmonary insufficiency, such infections, even though minor in extent, may lead to death. Those who have died without recognized infection showed progressive respiratory failure in the form of dyspnea and cyanosis.

Hyaline Membrane Disease

One of the causes of the respiratory distress syndrome of infancy is hyaline membrane disease, a diagnosis that can be established with certainty only on necropsy. The characteristic findings are dilation of respiratory bronchioles and of alveolar ducts as well as extensive alveolar collapse and hyaline membranes. Functionally, there is diminished lung volume, reduced compliance, arterial oxygen desaturation, right-to-left vascular shunts, increased physiologic dead space, respiratory and metabolic acidosis, decreased cardiac output, and decreased effective pulmonary blood flow. Although the pathophysiology of hyaline membrane disease is not established in each patient as attributable to a deficiency or absence of surfactant, it is evident that in most such patients there is an absence of the material. However, surfactant has been found in certain infants who had hyaline membrane disease. It is postulated that infants may be born

with an immature mechanism for producing surfactant and, although they have a hyaline membrane and the associated symptoms, the mechanism may mature so that surfactant is produced five to 15 days after birth. Thus, at death both the hyaline membrane and surfactant may be present. As for the hyaline membrane itself, it appears to consist of plasma from alveolar capillaries and possibly fibrin. The absence of the action of surfactant in reducing surface tension would result in transmitting the surface tension of the alveoli to the alveolar walls and thus would augment the capillary hydrostatic pressure and in this manner move fluid into the alveoli. The tissue asphyxia would add to the tendency to plasma loss and the membrane would be created. The collapse of the alveoli themselves would be governed by the theorem of Laplace, as discussed in the section on Protective Mechanisms.

Congenital Cystic Disease

Although it is difficult in a given case to be certain that a cystic pulmonary lesion did not develop after birth, there is little doubt as to the existence of true congenital cysts. It is believed that if intrauterine lung development is arrested at an early stage, a large solitary cyst may be formed; whereas, if the arrest occurs later, multiple cysts may result. The cysts, as observed in the patient, may be walled off and filled with serous fluid or they may be partly or entirely air-containing if there are communications to functioning bronchi. The lining epithelium of the cyst may be invested partially with cartilage and smooth muscle. Other cysts may be thin-walled and lined by a flattened epithelium.

There is a great tendency for these lesions to become infected, because bacteria gaining access to cysts cannot be removed by normal mechanisms. The absence of any connections to an airway or the inadequate size where a connection does exist prevents drainage of infected material and elimination by ciliary action and coughing. In those cysts connected to airways, infection, mucus accumulation, and the valvelike mechanism from changes in duct sizes on inspiration and expiration cause air trapping.

Pulmonary Embolism

The pulmonary vascular tree is an efficient filter which can remove emboli of neoplastic cells, bacteria, blood clots, fat globules, air, and the debris of amniotic fluid. Frequently overlooked is the fact that pulmonary infarction is not an invariable accompaniment of embolism. Pulmonary embolism alone is much more common than pulmonary infarction. The collateral bronchial circulation is, in many cases, adequate to maintain viability of the area involved. In the presence of conditions such as diminished ventilation, pulmonary infection, or cardiac disease which tend to produce vascular stasis, an embolus is much more likely to produce frank infarction.

Embolic obstruction leads to hyperemia and edema, which, if some of the above conditions are present, will progress in about 24 hours to infarction with alveolar wall necrosis and hemorrhage into the alveoli and associated bronchi. This gives rise to the so-called "meaty sputum" which contains dark red clots. Within two weeks, fibroblastic proliferation is in progress and the end result is a contracted scar which may not be visible on roentgenographic examination.

The severity of response to embolism is a function of the previous cardiovascular status and the subsequent degree of blood pressure elevation in the pulmonary arterial tree. In general terms, the obstruction of a small pulmonary artery may be silent, whereas occlusion of the main trunk of the pulmonary artery is followed by cessation of cardiac output, gasping respirations, and death. Between these extremes is a spectrum of variations in the pathophysiologic response.

If the vascular bed obstructed is of intermediate size, the systemic blood pressure falls suddenly and there is a concomitant rise in the pulmonary artery pressure, the right ventricular end-diastolic pressure, and the venous pressure. The mechanism or mechanisms producing the pulmonary hypertension continue to be a source of considerable controversy. Experimental studies in animals indicate that embolus-particle size is important. Emboli lodging at the precapillary level elicit hypertension by vasoconstriction, whereas emboli trapped in muscular and larger elastic arteries produce hypertension by mechanical blockage. Clinical data seem to be compatible with this concept of particle size. Pulmonary hypertension in some patients is demonstrated as being based on mechanical obstruction; in others, the hypertension is secondary to vasoconstriction; and in a third group there is a combination of obstruction and vasoconstriction.

With embolism there is a sudden onset of dyspnea which has been explained variously as a consequence of anoxia and reflexes from stimulation of receptors in the pulmonary artery. Tachycardia occurs as a response to the fall in systemic blood pressures, anoxia, and apprehension. Cyanosis is a manifestation of arterial unsaturation rather than the stasis cyanosis seen after myocardial infarction. This unsaturation may be the result of shunting through normal arteriovenous anastomoses and a decreased area of functional pulmonary capillaries, as with atelectasis and alveolar duct constriction. Pulmonary embolism *per se* is generally not accompanied by fever and leukocytosis; however, both may occur as a consequence of an underlying infection or pulmonary infarction with the embolism. When cough

occurs, it is probably in response to the inflammation of bronchial mucosa within the area of infarction. With involvement of the visceral pleura by infarction there is frequently pleuritic pain, but there may also be substernal discomfort reminiscent of myocardial ischemia. This discomfort may be attributable to the mechanical block of pulmonary arteries reducing, in turn, the cardiac output and coronary blood flow. Distention of the right cardiac chambers may also impede coronary flow by interfering with coronary venous return. Since pulmonary hypertension of other types has been noted to produce similar pain, it is also possible that some of the pain may result directly from distention of the pulmonary arteries.

One consequence of pulmonary embolism is that alveoli may continue to be ventilated although there is no capillary circulation. In the absence of effective circulation, the CO_2 tension in these alveoli will fall to very low levels instead of remaining approximately equal to the CO_2 tension of arterial blood, as in the normal state. On the basis of this, it was thought that a pulmonary embolus could be detected and quantitated on the basis of a comparison of arterial CO_2 and mixed expired alveolar CO_2. In practice this has not been too successful for three reasons: first, any pulmonary disease such as obstructive emphysema which alters ventilation-perfusion relationships may give similar results; second, when an area of lung loses its circulation, there is, in fact, reduction of ventilation of the area; and third, the effects of smaller emboli are not detected. Although the theory has had some practical application, the identification of embolization by perfusion lung scan or angiography is much more sensitive.

Pneumoconiosis

If large airborne particles are inhaled, they impinge upon the walls of the tortuous airways and are either swept out in the mucus sheet by ciliary action or expelled by the cough mechanism. However, if the particles are small, less than 10 μ in diameter, they are respirable and, as such, a portion of them will reach the alveoli and become scattered evenly over the walls. With surprising rapidity these particles are engulfed by phagocytes and transported toward the respiratory bronchioles. Even in normal lungs this is a relatively inefficient process, and silting up of these dust cells occurs in the respiratory bronchioles. Thus, not all the material reaches the continuous layer of ciliated epithelium which could expel the dust from the lung. Those cells which do not progress up the bronchial tree enter the interstitial tissues. Furthermore, some of the dust cells take a short cut via interstitial routes, arriving in the walls of other alveoli, or they aggregate about venules. The possibility that some dust particles enter the interstitial tissues without previous phagocytosis is not ruled out.

Once within the interstitial tissues, the dust particles may remain in situ or enter the lymphatics lying in relation to the airways, arteries, and veins. Much of this dust is arrested in foci of lymphoid collections at the divisions of the airways or vessels, while the remainder is carried to the tracheobronchial and hilar lymph nodes. In many instances, more distant lymph nodes such as those in the supraclavicular area also contain the inspired particles. There is no clear-cut evidence that phagocytes have any destructive action on the contained inorganic particles. Apparently, they act merely as vehicles to free the alveoli from foreign matter.

As dust particles arrive within the pulmonary tissues, a foreign-body type of response is elicited. Reticulum cells are transformed into fibroblasts and there is a deposition of fibrous tissue. When this reaction occurs about small bronchioles, there is impairment of air flow at the site, distortion and disruption of alveoli, the development of focal emphysema, and a sequence of events similar to that in obstructive emphysema. In advanced pneumoconiosis in which conglomerate lesions appear, there will be a decrease in lung volume in such areas from scarring and a compensatory emphysema in other areas. If the process is extensive, not only is the ventilatory function affected but there is disruption of the pulmonary capillary bed. Fibrosis occurring within the lymphatics impedes lymph flow, so that the irritating dust and phagocytes escape into the areolar tissue about the blood vessels. In this position, further fibrosis, with the added element of decreased capillary bed, contributes to the development of pulmonary arterial hypertension. In time this may eventuate in cor pulmonale and right heart failure. The obstruction of the lymphatics is possibly related to the known susceptibility of these patients to superimposed pulmonary infections. The severe ventilatory disturbances are those found in emphysema and fibrosis. In a given patient the changes may be predominantly those of emphysema or fibrosis, or a combination of the two. The decreases in arterial blood oxygen saturation are due primarily to poorly ventilated or non-ventilated alveoli which are perfused with blood. This, in effect, is a right-to-left shunt of blood and, if severe, will be attended by cyanosis, secondary polycythemia, and clubbing of the fingers.

Each type of dust invokes a particular response, and there is considerable variation in the pathologic characteristics and the attendant physiologic alterations. In general, carbon particles cause only mild changes in the lymphatic vessels and nodes with which they come in contact; silica produces intense fibrosis; and asbestos, diffuse fibrosis. The sputum produced in pneumoconiosis can be revealing. With anthracosis it may be black with carbon. In asbestosis, asbestos bodies may be found. Chronic infection is a common complication of the pneumoconioses, and the mucopurulent sputum produced is suggestive of tuberculosis. The possibility of superimposed tuberculosis always must be considered, for it is a frequent secondary invader, particularly in silicosis and anthracosilicosis. In asbestosis, bronchogenic carcinoma and, less frequently, mesothelioma must be considered as possible complications.

Pulmonary Fibrosis

Pulmonary fibrosis is not an etiologic entity, but it may occur as a consequence of tuberculosis, scleroderma, sarcoidosis, roentgen irradiation of the lungs, the inhalation of various noxious dusts and fumes, the Hamman-Rich syndrome, the administration of a number of drugs, various degrees of pulmonary venous obstruction, aspiration pneumonia, the organization of inflammatory exudates of pneumonia, as well as a familial variety which is hereditary. Systemic symptoms in this group of diseases vary widely and are generally characteristic of the particular clinical entity, but the pulmonary manifestations may be strikingly similar. The spectrum of pulmonary signs and symptoms varies from none at all in the earlier stages to cough, mucopurulent sputum, chest pain, cyanosis, clubbing of the digits, severe dyspnea, weight loss, and fatigue. As fibrosis progresses, pulmonary hypertension, cor pulmonale, and cardiac failure ensue. The common denominator pathologically is interstitial fibrosis, which may be localized, as in the case of irradiation pneumonitis following therapy for cancer of the breast, or diffuse, as in many of the other diseases. When the lesions are small, there may be no detectable alteration of pulmonary function. However, if the lesions become diffuse and the fibrosis becomes extensive, the lung will lose its elastic distensibility and there will be a decrease in total lung capacity, vital capacity, and residual volume. The dyspnea reflects the poor compliance and results in a concomitant increase in the work of breathing. If the fibrosis is not evenly distributed throughout the lungs, compensatory emphysema develops in the uninvolved tissue. An element of airway obstruction may also be present from fibrosis about bronchioles. Frequently, the fibrosis disturbs the relationship between the air-containing alveoli and the alveolar capillaries so as to impair gaseous diffusion. If extensive, this results in chronic hypoxemia, hyperventilation, and lowered Pco_2. These may be the predominant aberrations of pulmonary physiology in the Hamman-Rich syndrome, miliary tuberculosis, sarcoidosis, scleroderma, beryllium granulomatosis, and certain neoplasms with lymphangitic spread in the lungs.

Atelectasis

A bronchus may become obstructed either by an intraluminal mass or by external pressure so that the passage of air beyond is prevented. When obstruction occurs and is complete, gas in the segment supplied by the bronchus is absorbed into the bloodstream, leaving the lung airless and collapsed. Secondary to the collapse, there is a decrease of surfactant activity in the affected area of the lung. Although not known with certainty, the decrease of surfactant in atelectasis may be related to its short half-life (14 hours) and the fact that normal ventilation is required for its constant replenishment. Adjacent normal lung retains normal activity of the antiatelectatic surfactant.

Depending on the size of the atelectatic area, various aberrations in pulmonary function may be observed. The vital capacity is reduced through the absolute reduction in functioning lung tissue. Arterial oxygen saturation is reduced owing to the passage of desaturated venous blood through alveolar capillaries which are no longer in contact with air. Pulmonary elasticity is reduced. If the collapsed volume of lung is large, these physiologic changes are manifested as dyspnea and cyanosis. Fever is usual and is due either to the process initiating the atelectasis or to bacteria already present in the bronchi or introduced from aspiration, bloodstream, or lymphatics. In most cases, antibody and leukocytic activity controls the infective agents, but at times pulmonary abscess or chronic bronchiectasis may develop in the affected area. If infection does not intervene, restoration of normal function may occur after removal of the obstruction, even though atelectasis has been long persistent.

A type of atelectasis which is not obstructive may occur in the presence of processes which decrease the effective intrathoracic space. This is commonly observed in patients with sizable pleural effusions or pneumothorax and may also be noted with the high diaphragm and retracted intercostal spaces of patients with respiratory paralysis. The atelectasis is a consequence of compression from outside the lung and represents an adjustment to a new intrathoracic volume. Among the terms used for this entity are adjustment atelectasis, compression atelectasis, and disc, or platelike, atelectasis.

Atelectasis in association with pneumonia may occur as a consequence of obstruction of airways by viscid bronchial secretions, inflammatory exudate, or edema. It also may occur in the absence of obstruction and in any stage of the disease, including even convalescence. The mechanism is not entirely clarified. There is evidence that smooth muscle elements extend as far distal as alveolar walls. It is postulated that these muscular elements are under autonomic control and might under certain circumstances give rise to "contraction atelectasis." There is also a decrease in surfactant activity in infected portions of lungs and contiguous areas which might contribute to pulmonary collapse.

At birth, various degrees of atelectasis might well be anticipated, since intrauterine life is essentially aquatic. A certain amount of physiologic atelectasis exists in the normal full-term infant but generally disappears during his first week of life (see Hyaline Membrane Disease, p. 459).

In children, atelectasis has no predilection for a particular area, presumably because all the bronchi are narrow. Adults, however, are particularly vulnerable to obstruction of the right middle lobe. This fact led E. A. Graham to coin the term "middle lobe syndrome." Since the etiologic factors are many, this unusual susceptibility would seem to be on an anatomic basis. The middle lobe bronchus is not only relatively narrow but also more compressible by virtue of the acute angle that informs with the main bronchus. Brock has emphasized that this situation is made more precarious by the fact that the bronchus is surrounded closely by lymph nodes draining not only the middle lobe but also the lower lobe. Thus, infection in any part of these two lobes may produce sufficient lymphadenopathy to be obstructive.

Atelectasis as a postoperative complication is attributed to bronchial obstruction from retained secretions. Many of the processes which normally protect the bronchi from occlusion by secretions are rendered ineffective by surgery. Anesthesia, narcotics, pain, and fear of damage to the wound interfere with the expulsion of secretions by eliminating or making ineffective the cough reflex and by diminishing the tidal volume and associated bronchial movements. Also, as shown by Brock, lying on one side for long periods of time allows secretions to gravitate to the dependent lung segments. Aggravating each of these deficiencies is the increased viscosity of the sputum as a consequence of drugs administered for premedication, anesthesia, and postoperative pain. Not only is the sputum so sticky that it is difficult to move by coughing, but this same viscid characteristic impairs the movement of the cilia. Consideration of these various surgical effects on the pulmonary protective mechanisms provides the rationale for effective therapy of atelectasis — thinning of the sputum, restoration of the cough, changing body positions, alleviation of pain on respiration, and increasing the depth of respiration.

Tumor of the Lung

The respiratory symptoms of tumor of the lung are largely manifestations of partial or complete mechanical obstruction of an airway. Intraluminal tumors obstruct by direct growth into a bronchus, whereas parenchymal tumors produce similar effects through external pressure on the airways. As the tumor enlarges, asthmatic type breathing or stridor may be observed over the area of one lung or lobe in approximately 10 per cent of the cases. Since bronchi enlarge on inspiration and narrow on expiration, there may be localized emphysema beyond the tumor. This can be demonstrated often if roentgenograms are taken in both full inspiration and full expiration. Cough is an early symptom which is difficult to evaluate, since most of these patients are heavy smokers and chronic cough is such a prevalent symptom in this group. However, as ulceration occurs the sputum changes and there may be blood streaking or frank hemoptysis. Drainage from the bronchus is impaired and secondary infection appears. The sputum becomes more abundant and is mucoid or mucopurulent. Pneumonia may develop and respond to antibiotics, only to recur. Lung abscess, either distal to the obstructing lesion or within the necrotic tumor, is relatively common. With complete obstruction there is atelectasis. All these symptoms are predominantly attributable to mechanical effects of the tumor and are not indicative of its origin or cell type, benign or malignant.

As the malignant tumor spreads to the pleura, or as a consequence of pneumonia, there is pleuritis with pain and effusion. Extension to the mediastinum may produce back pain and obstruction to the superior vena cava. Rarely, a primary or metastatic carcinoma in the lungs may have a lymphangitic spread throughout the lungs. Pulmonary hypertrophic osteoarthropathy, which may resemble rheumatoid arthritis, is said to occur in approximately 10 per cent of malignant lung tumors.

Pulmonary Infections

The remarkable effectiveness of protective mechanisms of the lung maintains the alveoli essentially free of particulate matter such as dust and bacteria. This is in striking contrast to the upper respiratory tract, where there is a wide variety of bacteria which, if permitted to travel downward into the alveoli, would produce serious disease. However, like all defensive mechanisms, those of the lung are not perfect, and infectious disease of the lung still ranks high among infections as a cause of death.

Consideration of the fact that mechanisms are in action to remove particles from the air from the moment it enters the nares until the time it reaches the alveoli would suggest that the major onslaught would be in the trachea and bronchi. Experimentally, this theory is supported by the radiologic studies of Jarre, in which opaque dusts insufflated into lungs did not appear to enter the alveoli, although bronchi were rendered opaque. Clinically, it is supported by the fact that the majority of respiratory tract infections actually are limited to the trachea and bronchi. Ordinarily, the mucus lining of the bronchi and trachea is being constantly swept upward for elimination of foreign material deposited on it from ventilation. When the foreign material is irritating and produces inflammation of the larger airways, the cough mechanism and orally directed peristaltic waves help to move the mucus sheet more rapidly. Yet this constant cleansing action is not impregnable. During sleep, for example, defenses are lowered and septic material from the nose and pharynx, particularly if it is abundant, gravitates readily into the lungs. Other factors which must be taken into consideration when there is a breakdown of protective mechanisms are the virulence of organisms inhaled, the dosage of the infectious material, and variation in the patient's native resistance to pathogenic organisms. Once an organism invades and produces an inflammatory reaction, secondary defenses involving phagocytes and antibodies, still assisted by the expulsive mechanisms, are manifested.

Acute Tracheitis and Bronchitis

The inflammatory reaction may be a consequence of infectious diseases such as influenza or pertussis, drainage from suppurative sinusitis, allergies, dust, or chemical irritants. Among the latter, excessive cigarette smoking and atmospheric pollution are relatively common. Treatment is directed toward assisting the normal protective mechanisms. Termination of exposure to dust or chemical irritants; thinning of secretions with expectorants, steam, or aerosols; antihistaminics for allergy; and correctly directed antibiotic or chemotherapeutic agents for infections are used as indicated in a given situation. Occasionally, bronchodilators are useful when there is a bronchospastic element. If the cough is excessive or non-productive, it may be desirable to suppress this reflex to avoid undue exhaustion of the patient.

Chronic Bronchitis

When the etiologic factors considered in the section on acute tracheitis and bronchitis are constant or frequently repeated, so that the bronchial inflammation cannot be completely eliminated, chronic bronchitis is said to exist. In the

British Isles, chronic bronchitis as a reported cause of death is exceeded only by heart disease, cerebrovascular accidents, and carcinoma. By contrast, chronic bronchitis does not appear frequently as a diagnosis on death certificates in the United States. The difference in incidence may be in part real, but it is certainly in part a matter of definition. Gaensler and Lindgren in the United States reinvestigated the medical histories of their patients who had been given a diagnosis of chronic obstructive emphysema on the basis of pulmonary function tests. They found that 68 per cent of their patients with the physiologic alterations of obstructive emphysema met the British criteria for chronic bronchitis. Patients with chronic bronchitis had a progressive increase of a productive cough, worse in the mornings and in cold or inclement weather, and, ultimately, dyspnea. In patients who had a productive cough with chronic obstructive emphysema, the dyspnea antedated the cough. This study suggests that chronic bronchitis is an important etiologic factor in most of the patients presenting with obstructive emphysema.

The etiologic relationship of chronic bronchitis to obstructive emphysema emphasizes the need for more serious regard of "bronchial troubles." Chronic bronchitis may lead to rigidity and thickening of the bronchial mucosa from vasodilatation, congestion, and edema. There is infiltration of the mucosa by lymphocytes and polymorphonuclear cells and there may be an increase in the tonicity of the bronchial musculature. Mucous glands are enlarged and the excessive secretion interferes with ciliary activity, as does tobacco smoke, so that the cough mechanism must assist in the expulsion of mucus. The pathologic changes also involve the smaller bronchi and bronchioles. It is not clear why the "antiseptic mucosal paint" of immunoglobulins is ineffective in eliminating bacterial pathogens that are present.

Thickening of the bronchial mucosa, excessive mucus secretion, and increased tone of the bronchial musculature first slow the rate of maximal expiratory air flow and subsequently that of maximal inspiratory flow. Initially there is a normal total lung capacity, normal vasculature by x-ray examination, and a normal diffusing capacity. However, as the disorder continues, the results of functional pulmonary tests may become those of obstructive emphysema.

Treatment is directed along physiologic lines of assisting the normal pulmonary defenses: antibiotics for infectious elements; removal from exposure to airborne irritants; thinning of secretions with expectorants and aerosols; and treatment for allergy, if such is present. Histologic examination of the secretion is of considerable value in establishing the type of bronchitis.

Lung Abscess

Aspiration of infectious material from the upper air passages is probably the most common cause of lung abscess. When dental or surgical procedures on the mouth or surgical procedures on the paranasal sinuses are performed under general anesthesia, the incidence of acute pulmonary abscess is relatively high. Blood clots and other material, along with organisms from the mouth, are inhaled into the lungs at a time when the cough reflex is depressed by general anesthetics and sedatives. Simultaneously, viscosity of the bronchial secretions is increased, as a consequence of premedication, anesthesia, and dehydration, rendering ciliary action ineffective. With the inactivation of these mechanisms for clearing foreign material and the presence of a culture medium in the form of blood, the groundwork is laid for bacterial multiplication and abscess formation. The anatomic distribution of these bronchogenic abscesses has been presented admirably by Brock.

All pulmonary abscesses, however, are not sequels to *aspiration* of infectious material. Bronchogenic mechanisms such as strictures and tumors may disrupt the processes which normally remove foreign material from the lower respiratory tract. Necrotizing vasculitis of Wegener's granulomatosis and polyarteritis nodosa may also result in abscess. Occasionally abscesses arise from hematogenous spread of organisms in septicemias and in septic pulmonary infarcts, as from right-sided endocarditis. Even aseptic infarcts, by devitalizing pulmonary parenchyma, may precipitate abscess formation. Necrotizing pneumonitis caused by Friedländer's bacillus, staphylococci, streptococci, mixed flora, and poorly drained bronchogenic cysts may also overwhelm local defenses. It is rare for a simple pneumococcal pneumonia to progress to abscess formation. Infrequently, pulmonary abscess may result from transdiaphragmatic spread of infectious material. Amebic hepatic abscess is generally considered in this situation if the abscess is in the base of the right lung, but this same route may be taken by any subdiaphragmatic abscess. Progress of the infection is usually slow enough to allow symphysis of the pleura, so that the lung is invaded without empyema occurring first.

In most cases of simple abscess the defense mechanisms discussed in the section of Pneumonia, when aided by antibacterial agents, bronchoscopy, and postural drainage, will be adequate. The abscess wall collapses, fibrosis occurs, and the end result may be a scar which is invisible on roentgenography. The chronic abscess with a thick fibrous wall which will not collapse even on adequate bronchial drainage is seen less frequently than in the past — even in tuberculosis — because of earlier diagnosis and effective antibiotic agents.

Bronchiectasis

Prolonged bronchial obstruction, whether by tumor, foreign body, viscid mucous, scar, or lymphadenopathy, and parenchymal disease with infection are the two chief pathogenic factors in bronchiectasis. Among the most frequently cited parenchymal diseases are pulmonary atelectasis, chronic bronchial infection with parenchymal scarring, pneumonitis, and pulmonary fibrosis. Although the pathogenesis varies somewhat, each of these is characterized by some reduction in air-containing lung and concomitant traction on bronchial walls. This traction combined with weakening of the bronchial walls by infection results in dilatation or bronchiectasis. When the parenchymal infection is reversible and of short duration, so is the bronchiectasis. Pneumonia and atelectasis are notable examples of this type of clinically reversible bronchiectasis. However, when the bronchial obstruction is prolonged and complicated by infection, bronchiectasis results. Thus, infection complicating obstruction from tenacious mucus in mucoviscidosis, lymphadenopathy in the middle lobe syndrome, or healing with fibrosis in tuberculosis may progress to bronchiectasis. There is also a congenital form in which embryologic development is arrested after the outgrowth of bronchial buds but before there is differentiation into alveolar tissue. This is more frequently referred to as congenital cystic disease. Another congenital defect, intralobar bronchopulmonary sequestration with aberrant systemic arterial supply, is also generally complicated by persistent infection and bronchiectasis.

In the diseases mentioned there is a relative lack of aerated alveoli distal to the bronchiectasis. As a consequence, the current of air generated in coughing is inadequate to expel secretions from the bronchi. Thus, secretions tend to stagnate and become secondarily infected because the weakened cough mechanism cannot eliminate completely the dependent secretions. The accumulated secretions destroy much of the bronchial wall, including cilia and muscle, if the disease is long continued. Large anastomotic communications develop between the bronchial and pulmonary vasculature and may give rise to hemoptysis. Since the bronchiectatic lung is often functionless in terms of gaseous exchange, these segments may constitute a considerable area of arteriovenous shunting. It is therefore not surprising that pulmonary osteoarthropathy is a frequent finding. So-called "dry bronchiectasis" does exist as a clinical entity, but it is confined most commonly to the upper lobes where gravitational drainage exists.

Pneumonia

When an acute infectious process involves the alveoli, pneumonia results. The route of transport of the infectious agent to the alveoli varies somewhat with the organism, being via the airways, blood vessels, or lymphatics.

The pattern of response to a particular organism has a tendency to be characteristic. For example, the pneumococcus (*Streptococcus pneumoniae*) and Friedländer's bacillus tend to elicit a lobar type of consolidation, whereas the streptococcus is more apt to lead to bronchopneumonia and the staphylococcus to abscess formation. With earlier etiologic diagnosis and specific treatment this anatomic differentiation has lost much of its diagnostic significance, and infections are frequently arrested at the stage of scattered consolidation, resulting in bronchopneumonia.

Among the bacterial pneumonias, the pathogenesis of pneumococcal pneumonia has been the most extensively studied. The current concept is that the pneumococci reach the alveoli via the airway in droplets of mucus or saliva. Because of gravity and the absence of acute angles of the bronchi leading to the right lower and left lower lobes, these areas are the most frequently involved. Once established in the alveolus, the pneumococcus elicits an acute outpouring of edema fluid with neutrophilic leukocytes and small numbers of erythrocytes. This fluid constitutes not only a favorable culture medium for the organisms but also the vehicle for spread. With respiration and coughing this watery exudate laden with bacteria is carried via the smaller air passages and collateral pathways to adjacent areas. As the lesion enlarges it may be divided into three zones. The peripheral zone consists largely of bacteria floating in edema fluid and represents the advancing wave of infection. Beneath this there is an area of leukocytes, fibrin, and bacteria where phagocytosis is occurring. In the central zone the infection is under control and advanced consolidation is present. The alveoli contain many leukocytes, but there is a relative absence of bacteria. It is in this inner zone that resolution first appears.

With increasing numbers of leukocytes and the appearance of macrophages, the outer zone is invaded by the phagocytes and the lesion ceases to progress in size. When, or whether, this occurs is a function of many factors, including the dose, virulence, and rate of multiplication of the infecting bacteria, antibody formation, and the general health of the patient.

In the early stages, when the infection is spreading rapidly, bacteremia is commonly observed in patients with underlying disease but infrequently in the otherwise healthy. However, it may occur at any stage should the defense mechanisms of the host be overwhelmed. When bacteremia occurs it is believed that the organisms gain access to the bloodstream via the lymphatics. The consequence of bacteremia may be metastatic lesions such as meningitis, bacterial endocarditis, peritonitis, and arthritis.

The development of antibodies such as precipitins, lysins, and opsonins constitutes an important aspect of host defense. Before the development of chemotherapeutic and antibiotic agents, type-specific antipneumococcus serum was an important agent in therapy. This serum is thought to be effective largely by its enhancement of phagocytosis. Pneumococci in the presence of opsonins tend to agglutinate, presumably through altered surface tension, and agglutinated organisms are more readily ingested by phagocytes.

By the time of crisis, living bacteria have been disposed of and the temperature falls to normal. Consolidation is still present but liquefaction sets in rapidly and the debris is removed largely via the lymphatics but in part by coughing and ciliary activity. Complete resolution may be delayed for several weeks, particularly in older individuals, but in the absence of complications proceeds in most patients with striking rapidity. Rarely, the process is not completely resolved and the involved area is replaced by fibrous tissue. Lung abscess is an extremely rare complication of pneumococcal pneumonia, apparently because there is little or no necrosis of lung tissue. The pleura is involved in most instances and small pleural effusions occur. If there is delay in the initiation of specific therapy, an empyema may develop.

Systemic manifestations depend upon the characteristics of the organism, the host, and the degree of impairment of lung function. Fever and cyanosis, if the process is extensive, are constant. At the outset of lobar pneumonia and throughout bronchopneumonia, cyanosis is due to imperfect oxygenation of the blood which passes through the affected lobes. As a consequence of consolidation of alveoli and obstruction of airways, the venous blood is not exposed to high levels of oxygen and, in effect, venous blood is shunted through these areas into the pulmonary veins and systemic circulation. When consolidation of one lobe is complete, cyanosis improves somewhat, since all the alveoli have lost their function and there is a decrease in pulmonary blood flow to the lobe.

When pain occurs in pneumonia, it is indicative of involvement of the parietal pleura. The localization of pain by the patient is generally accurate because the impulse travels over fibers of the corresponding spinal nerves. The pulmonary parenchyma and the visceral pleura are themselves devoid of pain fibers. When the diaphragmatic pleura is involved, pain may be referred less accurately to the abdomen and simulate acute disorders for which surgery is indicated.

Similarly, as a consequence of the cervical origin of the phrenic nerves, pain of diaphragmatic pleuritis may be experienced in the shoulder region.

Pneumonia also is associated with many viral and rickettsial infections, such as influenza, parainfluenza, measles, mumps, chickenpox, respiratory syncytial virus, adenovirus and several related viruses, psittacosis, and *Coxiella burnetti* (Q fever). *Mycoplasma pneumoniae* (Eaton agent), which is a pleuropneumonia-like organism (PPLO), has been identified as the cause of 30 or 40 per cent of adult pneumonias. Adenovirus and Mycoplasma frequently have been identified in civilian and military populations as an agent in primary atypical pneumonia (PAP). The term "primary atypical pneumonia" was coined to describe a clinical syndrome, not an etiologic entity. Now that approximately 50 per cent of acute viral lower respiratory tract infections can be identified etiologically, the term is of less value clinically.

Lipoid Pneumonia

Certain oils, particularly mineral oil and vitamin oils, when introduced into the lungs, produce an acute pneumonitis which may progress to fibrosis. Access to the airways is through the use of oily nasal drops or sprays, forceful administration of oily preparations to crying infants, defective swallowing mechanisms, or the aspiration of oily laxatives taken at bedtime.

The lesion produced is an organizing bronchopneumonia with an abundance of macrophages with large lipid-containing vacuoles. There are also giant cells and desquamated alveolar lining cells. In time the lesion may progress to fibrosis with obliteration of the pulmonary vasculature and contraction of the area, producing bronchial distortion and even bronchiectasis. If the involvement is extensive, there may be some reduction in the vital capacity. Oil is partly ingested by macrophages and carried off into the lymphatics and partly eliminated in sputum. When the latter occurs, the etiology of the pneumonitis may be established by cytologic and histochemical studies of 24-hour sputum specimens. The clinical spectrum varies from asymptomatic to simulation of most of the usual pulmonary diseases, including carcinoma.

There is also an endogenous variety of lipoid pneumonia commonly secondary to abscesses, non-resolving pneumonia and carcinoma. The main differences from the exogenous type is the lack of a gravitational distribution and fine, dispersed lipid droplets in the macrophages.

Aspiration Pneumonia

Although not invariably true, aspiration generally occurs when the patient's state of consciousness is depressed. The more commonly associated conditions are the administration of an anesthetic agent or debilitation, stroke, brain tumor, drugs, and alcoholic intoxication. Each of these conditions may either depress or eliminate the normal protective mechanism of reflex glottic closure associated with vomiting and swallowing. When large solids are aspirated, bronchi may be occluded, with consequent distal pulmonary collapse, mediastinal shift, cyanosis, dyspnea, tachypnea, and tachycardia. The pathophysiologic mechanisms are those discussed in the section on Atelectasis.

The most virulent form of aspiration pneumonia results from the aspiration of acidic gastric fluid. When the pH of the aspirate is below 2.5 and the volume is sufficiently large, the mortality is high — over 70 per cent in some reports. The pathologic manifestations vary from acute inflammatory reaction, with the destruction of epithelium, hemorrhage, and an outpouring of plasma-like fluid, to near complete pulmonary parenchymal destruction. Data on the pathophysiology of the acute process in man are not available and must be inferred from animal studies. Initially, there is acute intense bronchospasm, a brief period of apnea, followed by shallow tachypnea, a prompt rise in pulmonary artery pressure, and a fall to shock levels of the systemic blood pressure. The pressures return to normal levels within an hour, but later may fall again until death occurs. Bloody froth appears as a consequence of hemorrhage and the outpouring of plasma-like fluid. The net result is an increasing hematocrit and a fall in plasma volume. There is a fall in blood pH and evidence of significant right-to-left shunting of blood in the lungs. With severe injury the arterial blood pH falls and there is an increase in Pco_2. With minimal injury, the blood gas changes are those of hyperventilation, i.e., a rise in pH and a fall in Pco_2. With survival, the sequelae may be those of interstitial pulmonary fibrosis.

Tuberculosis

In primary pulmonary tuberculosis, the bacilli are inhaled and arrive at the alveoli in the same manner as other small particulate matter. Because ventilation is greater in the lower two thirds of the lungs, most bacilli and consequent primary lesions occur in this area, where, depending on the number of organisms, their virulence, and the native resistance of the host, there may be little prompt reaction or the formation of a relatively acute inflammatory exudate. The latter develops into a patch of bronchopneumonia with bacillary proliferation, neutrophils, and other inflammatory changes which are not unique to tuberculosis. However, whatever the initial reaction, tuberculous necrosis occurs with a surrounding zone of tuberculous granulation tissue consisting of blood vessels, lymphocytes, epithelioid and Langhans' cells, and collagen fibrils. Bacilli become scarce in the areas of necrosis for reasons that are not understood, although it has been suggested that caseation itself may be the defense mechanism. With the development of adequate acquired resistance the lesions become quiescent with the formation of a hyalinized connective tissue capsule from the zone of granulation and a consequent reduction in the size of the lesion. The caseous material may be resorbed, inspissated, calcified, or subsequently liquefied. Bacilli in such a primary lesion may be completely eliminated or they may remain quiescent but virulent for years.

Simultaneous with the development of the pulmonary lesion, bacilli appear in the hilar lymph nodes. Although these areas of involvement are larger than those in the pulmonary parenchyma, the progressive anatomic changes are similar. If the hilar lesion and the pulmonary parenchymal lesion both become calcified, a Ghon complex is formed.

It is believed that, in the evolution of the primary lesion, bacilli reach the blood stream either directly from the parenchyma or via the hilar lymph nodes and thoracic duct into the subclavian vein. Generally, the seeding is slight, the lesion is minute, and the end result is encapsulation, calcification, or complete absorption. Infrequently, persistent, viable bacilli in these extrapulmonary sites later may give rise to progressive disease in the organ in which they are situated. Tissues with a high oxygen tension constitute a preferential site for the bacilli to proliferate, hence the prime frequency of pulmonary infections with a lesser tendency to metastatic lesions of the kidney, brain, and the epiphyses of bones before maturation.

Postprimary adult tuberculosis occurs in many patients despite the defense mechanisms of specific immunity and the walling-off of necrotic lesions. In the past this has been called reinfection tuberculosis, largely because it may become evident many years after the primary infection; however, from epidemiologic data it is now evident that the "reinfection" is largely endogenous in origin. This is true in nations such as the United States where the annual tuberculin-reaction conversion is low, but it is not necessarily true in developing nations where the high endemnicity of tuberculosis suggests that reinfection from exogenous sources is still the predominant process.

For reasons that are not understood, softening and liquefaction occurs in the necrotic foci of some patients. As noted previously, bacilli are scarce in areas of necrosis, but concomitant with liquefaction they multiply and may reach large numbers. With rupture of the softened lesion into a bronchus, discharged infectious material is washed through previously uninfected airways establishing a mechanism for further spread and repetition of the sequence of caseation and cavitation. The cavitary lesions are prolific sources of bacilli, since the establishment of an airway connection makes growth-promoting oxygen available.

The gross mechanisms of defense are evident from the preceding accounts of primary and postprimary tuberculosis. As in other infectious processes, it is an inflammatory reaction with exudation, phagocytosis, fibrosis, and walling-off of the involved area. There are, however, unique characteristics of tuberculosis and the host response which make it inadvisable, if not impossible, to make dogmatic statements regarding other protective mechanisms. The mechanism of variation of racial resistance, for example, is not understood, although it is an evident fact. White adults respond to the presence of tubercle bacilli by inhibiting their multiplication and spread by marked reparative fibrosis. Blacks of all age groups and white children are deficient in these responses and, hence, less well protected. Hereditary constitutional characteristics, age, and sex are factors influencing the course of tuberculosis in the individual; yet the role of these parameters in causing fluctuations in the level of resistance to infection is not understood. Although antibodies develop in response to the tuberculous focus, their role in acquired resistance is not yet clear. Still, acquired resistance can be demonstrated in experimental animals and there is indirect evidence for its occurrence in man. In 1886, Marfan observed that individuals who had healed cervical adenitis before puberty subsequently did not develop pulmonary tuberculosis as frequently as others. This "Law of Marfan" has been held to be true even in African natives who are highly susceptible to tuberculosis. Rich has indicated the important role of mononuclear phagocytes in ingesting free bacilli as well as dead polymorphonuclear cells with their contained bacilli. In the susceptible host, bacilli may not only survive but also multiply within the monocytes. Yet, once resistance is acquired through infection, not only do these mononuclear phagocytes continue to ingest bacilli but in addition they then inhibit multiplication and increase the rate of destruction of bacilli.

When tuberculin is injected into a person who has never had a tuberculous infection, the material is harmless and no significant reaction occurs. When injected into the skin of a person who has or has had a tuberculous infection, the tuberculin causes a sterile inflammatory reaction. Using a pure culture of tubercle bacilli rather than tuberculin, Koch observed this altered reactivity in infected guinea pigs, and subsequently the altered reaction to reinfection has been referred to as the "Koch phenomenon." This hypersensitiveness has been a source of considerable controversy. Some investigators have considered it an important protective mechanism, since acceleration and augmentation of the inflammatory response occur in response to tubercle bacilli in the hypersensitive organism. This response and the concomitantly accelerated tubercle formation are believed to represent an acceleration of the normal body defense. Others have regarded hypersensitivity as undesirable because of the associated necrosis of connective tissue, epithelium, blood vessels, and even the inflammatory cells themselves. In considering this problem, Rich comes to the conclusion that acquired resistance and hypersensitivity are separate phenomena and that hypersensitivity is at times decidedly deleterious and at other times is neither deleterious nor beneficial. This role of hypersensitivity as an advantageous defense mechanism remains an unsettled question and it is even doubted by many that it in any way participates in the development of acquired immunity.

From the standpoint of systemic symptoms the presence or absence of hypersensitivity is important. The very hypersensitive patient with a focus producing tuberculoprotein may have malaise, fever, headache, anorexia, and the other constitutional symptoms of tuberculosis. But another individual who is anergic may have a more extensive process with active bacilli and yet fail to develop any appreciable systemic response. The experimental counterpart of this is the desensitized tuberculous animal that will tolerate enormous doses of tuberculin which would be fatal to a hypersensitive but similarly infected animal.

The tendency of postprimary adult tuberculosis to localize in the posterior portions of the upper lobes is well recognized, but the mechanism of the localization has not been defined clearly. Various theories have been proposed based upon diminished respiratory movement in the apices, direct retrograde spread from cervical lymphatics, streaming of blood flow to the lungs so that blood from the superior vena cava flows preferentially to the apices, and relative anemia of the apices due to man's erect posture. There is now increasing evidence that the hydrostatic effect of gravity diminishes circulation to the apical areas of the lung. It is postulated that there is also a decreased transport of humoral factors and possibly a decrease in lymph flow. All these factors might contribute to increased susceptibility to infection in the apices.

The functional alterations in advanced pulmonary tuberculosis are secondary to parenchymal infiltration, loss of lung substance, fibrosis and pleural disease. Infiltrations result in destruction of alveoli and localized stiffening of the lung. The loss of lung substance in itself is infrequently serious owing to the large pulmonary reserve. The normal minute ventilation is of the order of 5 liters and this can be increased, on demand, to as much as 150 liters. However, the loss may be critical when combined with extensive fibrosis of the lung parenchyma and pleura, resulting in increased lung stiffness (loss of compliance) and slowing of both inspiration and expiration, defects in gas mixing, and compensatory emphysema. Pulmonary function tests reveal these pathologic changes as decreases in vital capacity, an increase in dead space, an increase in the ratio of the residual air to total lung capacity, and a decrease in arterial oxygen saturation on exercise. Although cor pulmonale is less common in tuberculosis than in chronic bronchitis and emphysema, it does occur in long-standing cases as a consequence of extensive vascular destruction from inflammation and fibrosis and increased shunting of blood from the bronchial arteries into the pulmonary veins.

In recent years it has become evident that mycobacteria other than *M. tuberculosis* and *M. bovis* may produce human pulmonary disease. These strains, such as *M. kansasii* and *M. intracellularis* (Battey mycobacteria), are generally referred to as "atypical" mycobacteria. Early skepticism as to their pathogenicity was based on the lack of virulence for guinea pigs. Repeated recovery in culture from sputa and tissue specimens in the absence of other organisms has been convincing evidence of their primary role in certain cases. Although pulmonary disease caused by these unclassified mycobacteria is uncommon, it is now evident that the disease produced is indistinguishable from tuberculosis, both clinically and pathologically. Although not yet demonstrated, it is supposed that the pathologic physiology will closely resemble that of tuberculosis.

Fungus Infections

There are many systemic mycoses which at times involve pulmonary tissues. Among the more important are histoplasmosis and coccidioidomycosis. Others, less frequently encountered, are actinomycosis, nocardiosis, cryptococcosis, candidiasis, blastomycosis, aspergillosis, geotrichosis, and mucormycosis. These various mycoses may occur as independent infections, but it is not unusual for them to appear as complications in the terminal stages of diseases such as the lymphomas, leukemia, and cancer. Candidiasis is often reported as a complication of broad-spectrum antibiotic therapy and mucormycosis as a complication of uncontrolled diabetes mellitus. The use of corticosteroids and immunosuppressive agents is a contributing factor to the increased incidence of fungal diseases.

As a group, the fungi are poor antigens, and they do little to stimulate resistance mechanisms. In some, the response is more reminiscent of that to a foreign body than to a living infectious agent. Like the tubercle bacillus, fungi have a tendency to elicit hypersensitivity in the patient, and it is believed that the necrosis of tissue and abscess formation are consequences of this.

Clubbing of Fingers and Toes

The bizarre phenomenon of clubbing is associated with pulmonary neoplasms and various chronic disorders of the lung, as well as chronic disorders of the heart, gastrointestinal tract, liver, thyroid, and parathyroids and subacute bacterial endocarditis. In its more advanced stages, clubbing may be associated with periostitis and synovitis in the triad referred to as hypertrophic osteoarthropathy. The sequence, however, may be reversed so that the osteoarthropathy precedes the clubbing, and at times the manifestations may be unilateral or unidigital. There are also two hereditary-familial conditions, congenital clubbing and idiopathic hypertrophic osteoarthropathy, which are of little clinical significance except that their presence may be interpreted incorrectly.

Clubbing is a process of soft tissue proliferation at the base of the nail which elevates the nail root. The bony aspect is a proliferative periostitis which most commonly involves the distal portion of long bones of the forearms and legs and metacarpals and metatarsals. When joints are involved, there are osteoporosis, chronic synovitis, and non-specific changes in the cartilage.

The pathogenesis is not clearly understood. Increased peripheral blood flow is a constant feature in the acquired form, but the flow is believed to be largely through dilated arteriovenous anastomoses. Limitation to fingers, toes, and occasionally the nose is attributed to the fact that these areas are endowed richly with arteriovenous anastomoses. Various hypotheses as to how clubbing is brought about have included endocrine imbalance, reduced oxygen tension of the blood, and reflex circulatory changes mediated through efferent nerves of the lung. Hall has postulated that digital clubbing may be the result of long-term action of a vasoactive substance on the arteriovenous anastomoses. On the basis of experimental studies he suggests the substance to be reduced ferritin which has not been oxidized by circulation through normal lung tissue. At present, however, one need not assume that there is a single cause of clubbing.

PLEURAL DISORDERS

The pleura is a thin, serous membrane. It is composed of an outer mesothelial layer, which rests on an avascular elastic layer and an areolar layer, consisting of elastic and collagenous fibers, blood vessels, lymph vessels, and nerves. The blood vessels of the visceral pleura are derived from the bronchial artery and, after breaking up into capillaries, reunite into branches of the pulmonary vein. The lymphatics drain into the hilar lymph nodes.

Since the relationship of the pleura to the subpleural alveoli is an intimate one, disorders involving these alveoli are readily reflected in pleural disease. This is well illustrated by the pleurisy and serous exudate that occur as a result of a small tuberculous focus in the lung. Cardiac decompensation, trauma to the thoracic duct, or any generalized disease affecting blood vessels or lymphatics also may lead to the appearance of fluid in the pleural space. Pleural effusion associated with the ascites of hepatic cirrhosis or solid ovarian tumors is occasionally observed. Examination of such fluid for its physical, chemical, and cellular characteristics is a useful clinical procedure.

Although there are various means of driving fluid into the pleural space, there are probably only two defense mechanisms for its subsequent removal. In those circumstances in which the protein concentration of the fluid is low, the resorption is probably at the venous end of the pleural blood capillaries. This is a consequence of the colloidal osmotic pressure of the blood plasma. However, in the presence of fluid of high protein content, the hydrostatic effect is nullified and the absorption of fluid, as well as of any particulate matter, is through pleural lymphatics.

Tumors of the Pleura

The true, primary pleural origin of tumors which are found in the pleura is under considerable question. In a given case it is extremely difficult to rule out the possibility of a primary pulmonary origin with growth of secondary lesions in the pleura. The localized tumors have the characteristics of lipomas, fibromas, fibrosarcomas, and differentiated neural tissue. As a group, they are slow-growing and may reach huge size without evidence of metastases. The only diffuse tumor is the mesothelioma, and it may involve the entire pleural surface. Whether metastases of this neoplasm ever extend beyond mediastinal lymph nodes is open to question, but the clinical course may nevertheless be rapidly downhill. The symptoms of pain, dyspnea, and cyanosis associated with pleural tumors are due to the interference with ventilation from the space occupied by the tumor, stiffening of the lung, and the accompanying effusion. Clubbing of the fingers may occur. Cytologic examination of the massive serous or serosanguineous fluid may be diagnostic.

Pleuritis

Inflammatory reaction of the pleura is almost always a consequence of spread of infection from contiguous structures. Thus, the primary site may be within the lungs, mediastinum, chest wall, diaphragm, or subdiaphragmatic area. Pulmonary infarctions, neoplasms, and systemic diseases such as the so-called "collagen diseases" are at times the causes of pleurisy. The early reaction to insult is erythema and edema of the pleura, followed promptly by the exudation of cellular elements and fibrin deposition. As the inflammatory reaction involves the parietal pleura and as the rough fibrinous surface stimulates parietal pain receptors during respiration, the symptoms and signs of pleurisy are evident. The pain of diaphragmatic pleuritis may be referred to the abdomen or the shoulder area, whereas involvement of the parietal pleura of the chest wall is rather accurately localized by the patient. Partial relief is obtained by voluntary and involuntary splinting which, by decreasing the amplitude of pleural excursions, reduces the stimulation of parietal pleural nerves. This limitation of tidal ventilation is partially compensated for by an increase in the rate of respiration. The clinical manifestation is tachypnea and the patient may complain of dyspnea if he resorts to any exertion. A friction rub may be audible over the area of disease. Pleural pain is absent in interlobar pleurisy, and any symptoms produced are those of the primary lesion or those of decreased lung volume should the effusion be very large.

If the disease progresses from the stage of dry pleurisy, an exudate which is usually serofibrinous is produced and this may become frankly purulent. As fluid separates the inflamed pleural surfaces, there will be alleviation of the acute pleuritic pain and the appearance of a more generalized chest pain. With large effusions, dyspnea is largely a consequence of volume displacement and reduced vital capacity.

Protective mechanisms brought into play are those that deal with the pulmonary problem precipitating the pleuritis, as well as absorption of fluid through the pleural capillaries and lymphatics and formation of adhesions that tend to seal the pleural surfaces together and wall off the process. The latter is readily induced, particularly when pulmonary movement is retarded, as it normally is at the apices.

At times the needle aspiration of pleural fluids is attended by symptoms of dizziness and faintness, even in the absence of pain. This is attributable to a fall in blood pressure, and its degree is a rough function of the volume aspirated and the rate of removal. Infrequently, the reaction to thoracentesis may be more serious and has even been reported to be a cause of death. Capps and

Lewis studied this phenomenon in dogs and demonstrated that the aspiration of fluid with stimulation of the visceral pleura in the presence of inflammation is attended by a much greater risk than in the absence of inflammation. Their studies indicated that two different reflex mechanisms are involved. One is cardio-inhibitory, with slowing of the cardiac rate and usually slowing of respiration. This type of reflex is infrequently fatal. The other reflex is of the vasomotor type and is characterized by a rapid fall in blood pressure and more frequent termination in death unless therapy is directed toward the restoration of arteriolar tone.

Empyema

In thoracic empyema the pleural surfaces are abscess walls which are thickened, inflamed, and granular. Initially, there is an acute pleuritis which may be a consequence of pulmonary infection, surgery, trauma, or extension of an infection from the subdiaphragmatic area, mediastinum, or esophagus. When the origin is neither traumatic nor iatrogenic, the infectious agent most generally reaches the pleural space by direct extension from the lung, by rupture of a subpleural abscess, by lymphatic drainage into an effusion, or by septic embolization. Once the organism is established, an inflammatory exudate appears, and the previously glistening pleural surface becomes a dull, thickened, granulating surface and pyogenic membrane. Further progress results in fibrous bands crisscrossing the empyema space and loculation of the exudate so that complete removal by thoracentesis is not possible. The wall of the empyema becomes organized into elastic fibrous tissue which may, as in tuberculous empyema, effectively limit the infection and lead to quiescence for years.

If the empyema is small, the only alteration in pulmonary function may be a decrease in the excursions of the diaphragm and ribs. This is secondary to pain and reduces the vital capacity and maximal breathing capacity. If the empyema is large, the lung is compressed and the mediastinum is shifted toward the opposite lung, decreasing its volume also. The total pulmonary volume is reduced, vital capacity decreases, and pulmonary blood flow diminishes. Reduced oxygenation of the blood is generally evident. Although the loss of volume may not be great, the development of a non-elastic fibrous peel over the pleurae will reduce ventilatory function by mechanically limiting changes in volume. With maturation of the fibrous tissue, contraction occurs, which may reduce the lung volume severely by pulling the mediastinum toward the affected side and elevating and fixing the diaphragm. Particularly when this develops in early life, there may be a deforming scoliosis. With the

decrease in volume on the side of disease, there is an absolute increase in volume in the normal hemithorax which results in compensatory emphysema.

The principles of management are directed toward the elimination of the infection by use of appropriate antibiotics, aspiration of the exudate, and enzymatic debridement if the purulent exudate is thick. If this is delayed or unsuccessful, surgical drainage of the abscess or decortication of the fibrous peel will be required to restore more normal pulmonary function. It has been observed repeatedly that bacteria may occur in pleural effusions and be eliminated by host defenses so that empyema does not develop. This situation, however, is a risky one, because if empyema does develop, the defense mechanisms walling off the empyema may in themselves result in crippling pulmonary disease.

Epidemic Pleurodynia

Epidemic pleurodynia, or Bornholm disease, is an acute febrile illness due to Coxsackie virus, Group B. In experimental animals the typical lesion in striated muscle resembles Zenker's hyaline degeneration. In man, the histologic changes are unknown because the illness is self-limited and followed by complete recovery. There may be severe pain and tenderness of muscles in the trunk and extremities, suggesting that the basic lesion is perhaps a myositis which also involves the diaphragm. Pleuritis, pleural effusion, exanthems, orchitis, diarrhea, hepatitis, meningitis, and pulmonary infiltrations have been noted. There are no significant alterations in pulmonary function. Recovery is characterized by a rise in specific neutralizing antibodies.

Pneumothorax

Pneumothorax occurs when air enters the pleural space. If entry of the air is via the bronchial tree, the condition is termed closed pneumothorax, and if via the thoracic wall, open pneumothorax. The latter is a consequence of trauma, whereas the causes of closed pneumothorax are many. Most commonly, closed pneumothorax is a consequence of the rupture of emphysematous blebs, but there are other entities occasionally incriminated: abscess, staphylococcal infections, tuberculosis, various forms of pulmonary fibrosis, and, rarely, malignant disease.

The physiologic complications are related to the loss of or, at least, decrease in normal intrapleural negative pressure, which in turn interferes with the return of venous blood to the heart. If there is a valvelike mechanism at the site of the tear in the visceral pleura, a tension pneumothorax with pressures many times atmospheric may be obtained. Valsalva maneuvers associated with sneezing or coughing continue to force air into the pleural space. The lung first collapses with the loss of negative pressure and eventually is compressed toward the mediastinum. This structure may be forced toward the opposite side, resulting in partial compression of the intact lung, and the diaphragm may be forced downward. Dyspnea and cyanosis may occur as a consequence of pain, impairment of the volume of ventilation, and the passage of blood through non-aerated lung.

The vast majority of pneumothoraces are simple in that the pressures developed are not strikingly elevated and the process does not proceed beyond partial collapse. The pleural opening closes spontaneously and the healthy pleura absorbs the air within a matter of a few weeks. Complications such as tension pneumothorax, hemopneumothorax, bilateral spontaneous pneumothorax, and infectious processes require intervention to remove air, halt bleeding, and eradicate infection.

REFERENCES

Altschule, M. D.: Physiology in Diseases of the Heart and Lungs. Harvard University Press, Cambridge, 1949.

Barclay, A. E., Franklin, K. J., and Macbeth, R. G.: Roentgenographic studies of the excretion of dusts from the lungs. Am. J. Roentgenol., 39:673, 1938.

Basch, F. P., Holinger, P., and Poncher, H. G.: Physical and chemical properties of sputum. II. Influence of drugs, steam, carbon dioxide and oxygen. Am. J. Dis. Child., 62:1149, 1941.

Bates, D. V.: Chronic bronchitis and emphysema. N. Engl. J. Med., 278:546, 600; 1968.

Bates, D. V.: The fate of the chronic bronchitic: A report of the 10 year follow-up in the Canadian Department of Veterans' Affairs coordinated study of chronic bronchitis. Am. Rev. Respir. Dis., 108:1043–1065, 1973.

Blanshard, G.: Sputum viscosity and postoperative pulmonary atelectasis. Dis. Chest, 37:75, 1960.

Brock, R. C.: The Anatomy of the Bronchial Tree with Special Reference to the Surgery of Lung Abscess. Oxford University Press, London, 1954.

Cameron, J. L., Anderson, R. P., and Zuidema, G. D.: Aspiration pneumonia, A clinical and experimental review. J. Surg. Res., 7:44, 1967.

Canetti, G.: Pathogenesis of tuberculosis in man. Ann. N. Y. Acad. Sci., 154:13, 1968.

Capps, J. A., and Lewis, D. D.: Observations upon certain blood-pressure-lowering reflexes that arise from irritation of the inflamed pleura. Am. J. Med. Sci., 134:868, 1907.

Cherniack, N. S., and Carton, R. W.: Factors associated with respiratory insufficiency in bronchiectasis. Am. J. Med., 41:562, 1966.

Comroe, J. H., Jr.: Physiology of Respiration. Year Book Medical Publishers, Inc., Chicago, 1974.

Corssen, G.: Changing concepts of the mechanism of pulmonary atelectasis. J.A.M.A., 183:314, 1963.

Cudkowicz, L., and Armstrong, J. B.: The bronchial arteries in pulmonary emphysema. Thorax, 8:46, 1953.

Dalen, J. E., and Alpert, J. S.: Natural history of pulmonary embolism. Prog. Cardiovasc. Dis., 16:257–270, 1975.

Dickson, J. A., Clagett, O. T., and McDonald, J. R.: Cystic disease of the lungs and its relationship to bronchiectatic cavities. J. Thoracic Surg., 15:196, 1946.

Di Rienzo, S.: Radiologic Exploration of the Bronchus. Charles C Thomas, Springfield, Illinois, 1949.

Ellis, F. H., Jr., and Carr, D. T.: The problem of spontaneous pneumothorax. Med. Clin. North Am., 38:1065, 1954.

Fraimow, W., Cathcart, R. T., and Taylor R. C.: Physiologic and clinical aspects of pulmonary alveolar proteinosis. Ann. Intern. Med., 52:1177, 1960.

Gordon, R. B., Lennette, E. H., and Sandrock, R. S.: The varied clinical manifestations of Coxsackie virus infections. Arch. Intern. Med., 103:63, 1959.

Hall, G. H.: The cause of digital clubbing. Testing a new hypothesis. Lancet, 1:750, 1959.

Hamman, L., and Rich, A. R.: Acute diffuse interstitial fibrosis of the lungs. Bull. Johns Hopkins Hosp., 74:117, 1944.

Head, J. R.: Cystic disease of the lung with emphasis on emphysematous blebs and bullae. Am. J. Surg., 89:1019, 1955.

Heppleston, A. G.: The pathogenesis of simple pneumoconiosis in coal workers. J. Path. Bact., 67:51, 1954.

Ishizaka, K.: Immunoglobulin E and reaginic hypersensitivity. Johns Hopkins Med. J., 135:67–90, 1974.

Jarre, H. A.: Roentgenologic studies on physiologic motor phenomena. Radiology, 15:377, 1930.

Krahl, V. E.: Anatomy of the mammalian lung. In Fenn, W., and Rahn, H. (eds.): Handbook of Physiology, Vol. I. American Physiological Society, Washington, D.C., 1964, p. 213.

Kueppers, F., and Black, L. F.: Alpha-1 antitrypsin and its deficiency. Am. Rev. Resp. Dis., 110:176–194, 1974.

Lewis, P. A., and Sanderson, E. S.: The histological expression of the natural resistance of rabbits to infection with human type tubercle bacilli. J. Exper. Med., 45:291, 1947.

Liebow, A. A.: Atlas of Tumor Pathology. Tumors of the lower respiratory tract. Armed Forces Institute of Pathology, Washington, D.C., 1952.

Loeffler, W.: Zur Differential-Diagnosis der Lungeninfiltrierungen. II. Über flüchtige Succendan-Infiltrate (mit Eosinophilie). Beitr. Klin. Erforsch. Tuberk., 79:368, 1932.

Macklin, C. C.: The dynamic bronchial tree. Am. Rev. Tuberc., 25:393, 1932.

Mallory, T. B.: The pathogenesis of bronchiectasis. N. Engl. J. Med., 237:795, 1947.

Mayer, E., and Rappaport, I.: Developmental origin of cystic, bronchiectatic and emphysematous changes in the lungs. A new concept. Dis. Chest, 21:146, 1952.

McIntyre, K. M., and Sasahara, A. A.: The hemodynamic response to pulmonary embolism in patients with prior cardiopulmonary disease. Am. J. Cardiol., 28:288, 1971.

McLaughlin, R. F., and Tueller, E. E.: Anatomic and histologic changes of early emphysema. Chest, 59:592, 1971.

Miller, W. S.: The Lung. Charles C Thomas, Springfield, Illinois, 1947.

Mittman, C., Lieberman, J., Marasso, F., and Miranda, A.: Smoking and chronic obstructive lung disease in alpha-1-antitrypsin deficiency. Chest, 60:214, 1971.

Morgan, T. E.: Pulmonary surfactant. N. Engl. J. Med., 284:1185, 1971.

Morrow, P. E., Gibb, F. R., and Gozioglu, K. M.: A study of particulate clearance from the lung. Am. Rev. Resp. Dis., 96:1209, 1967.

Motley, H. L.: Pulmonary function impairment in pneumoconioses. J.A.M.A., 172:1591, 1960.

Newhouse, M., Sanchis, J., and Bienenstock, J.: Lung defense mechanisms. N. Engl. J. Med., 295:990–1052, 1045–1052, 1976.

Nicholson, D. P.: Extrinsic allergic pneumonias. Am. J. Med., 53:131–136, 1972.

Norris, R. F., and Tyson, R. M.: The pathogenesis of congenital polycystic lung and its correlation with polycystic disease of other epithelial organs. Am. J. Path., 23:1075, 1947.

Reynolds, E. O. R., Robertson, N. R. C., and Wigglesworth, J. S.: Hyaline membrane disease, respiratory distress, and surfactant deficiency. Pediatrics, 42:758, 1968.

Rich, A. R.: The Pathogenesis of Tuberculosis. Charles C Thomas, Springfield, Illinois, 1951.

Rococeanu, S. F., Mendlowitz, M., Suck, A. F., Wolf, R. L., and

Naftchi, N. E.: Digital capillary blood flow in clubbing. Ann. Intern. Med., 75:933, 1971.

Sasahara, A. A.: Pulmonary vascular responses to thromboembolism. Mod. Conc. Cardiovasc. Dis., 36:55, 1967.

Sladen, A., Zanca, P., and Hadnott, W. H.: Aspiration pneumonitis — The sequelae. Chest, 59:448, 1971.

Sodeman, W. A., and Stuart, B. M.: Lipoid pneumonia in adults. Ann. Intern. Med., 24:241, 1946.

Steinberg, I.: Lipoid pneumonia associated with paresophageal hernia. Angiocardiographic study of a case. Dis. Chest, 37:157, 1960.

Stevens, P. M., Hnilica, V. S., Johnson, P. C., and Bell, R. L.: Pathophysiology of hereditary emphysema. Ann. Intern. Med., 74:672, 1971.

Stewart, P. B.: The rate of formation and lymphatic removal of fluid in pleural effusions. J. Clin. Invest., 42:258, 1963.

Sturm, A.: Der Lungenkrampf (Kontraktionsatelektase durch Pulmonalen Spasmus). Deutsch. Med. Wschr., 71:201, 1946.

Sutnick, A. I., and Soloff, L. A.: Atelectasis with pneumonia. A pathophysiologic study. Ann. Intern. Med., 60:39, 1964.

Vogl, A., Blumenfeld, S., and Gutner, L. B.: Diagnostic significance of pulmonary hypertropic osteoarthropathy. Am. J. Med., 18:51, 1955.

von Meyenburg, H.: Eosinophilic pulmonary infiltration: Pathologic anatomy and pathogenesis. Schweiz. Med. Wochenschr. 72:809, 1942.

von Neergaard, K.: Neue Auffassungen über einen Grundbegriff der Atemmechanik, abhängig von der Oberflächenspannung in den Alveolen. Z. Ges. Exp. Med., 66:373, 1929.

West, J. B., Holland, R. A. B., Dollery, C. T., and Mathews, C. M. E.: Interpretation of radioactive gas clearance rates in the lung. J. Appl. Physiol., 17:14, 1962.

Wood, W. B., Jr.: Studies on the mechanism of recovery in pneumococcal pneumonia. I. The action of type specific antibody upon the pulmonary lesion of experimental pneumonia. J. Exp. Med., 73:201, 1941.

Woods, W. B., Jr., Smith, M. R., and Watson, B.: Studies on the mechanism of recovery from pneumonia. The mechanism of phagocytosis in the absence of antibody. J. Exp. Med., 84:355, 1946.

Yoo, O. H., and Ting, E. Y.: The effects of pleural effusion on pulmonary function. Am. Rev. Resp. Dis., 89:55, 1964.

Zimmerman, L. E.: Fatal fungus infections complicating other diseases. Amer. J. Clin. Path., 25:46, 1955.

Zohman, L. R., and Williams, M. H., Jr.: Cardiopulmonary function in pulmonary fibrosis. Am. Rev. Resp. Dis., 80:700, 1959.

RHEUMATOLOGY, ALLERGY, INFECTIOUS DISEASE, AND HEMATOLOGY

17

Rheumatic Diseases

GILES G. BOLE, JR.

The rheumatic diseases are grouped together because they produce symptoms in and impairment of function of the musculoskeletal system as well as other body systems. The musculoskeletal system can be visualized as a highly integrated apparatus consisting of (1) the bones which provide the skeletal supports of the body, (2) the joints between the osseous structures which permit mobility while maintaining the capacity for stability, and (3) the neuromuscular apparatus for moving or stabilizing the supporting structures as needed. This chapter will be concerned primarily with the articulations and with the disturbances in function of the musculoskeletal system produced by diseases of the joints and closely related structures. It will also deal with other closely related diseases of connective tissue.

The joints and the tendinous structures which transmit the motivating forces to permit smooth and efficient motion represent specialized forms of connective tissue. Basic information regarding the structure and function of connective tissues is needed for an understanding of normal function of these structures and the alteration produced by disease.

STRUCTURE AND FUNCTION OF CONNECTIVE TISSUES

It is no longer possible to regard connective tissue as an inert stuffing material, supporting and binding together the parenchymatous, neural, and vascular structures of multicellular organisms. As a result of numerous investigations, there has emerged a concept emphasizing the complex and dynamic state of these tissues,

their importance in maintaining the physiologic integrity of the musculoskeletal system, and the significance of pathologic alterations in diseases of the connective tissues. The several types of connective tissues which differentiate from the mesenchyme include loose (areolar) connective tissue, dense fibroelastic connective tissue, reticular, adipose and elastic connective tissue, as well as bone, cartilage, and synovium.

Connective tissue can be regarded as composed of *cellular* and intercellular elements, with the intercellular components consisting of an *amorphous ground substance* interlaced with extracellular *fibrillar* materials. The proportion of these three constituents varies greatly with anatomic location and functional requirements: tendons and fascia are largely fibrillar, Wharton's jelly of the umbilical cord is predominantly ground substance, and cartilage and synovium are relatively rich in cells.

Connective tissue has the obvious important function of mechanical support and protection. In addition, it is essential for the smooth transmission of mechanical energy derived from muscle contraction to move the organism or its parts, facilitated by lubrication from ground substance components located in the gliding planes of joints, bursae, and tendon sheaths. Since connective tissue is everywhere interposed between capillaries and cellular structure, it has an important transport function, influencing the passage of essential nutrients to the cells and the return of metabolic wastes to the circulation. Particularly noteworthy is the remarkable potential of connective tissue in the process of anatomic repair. Following tissue injury, cellular components usually neutralize or destroy noxious agents, remove debris,

476

and produce a framework of fibers and ground substance which bridges the anatomic defect and frequently restores functional capacity.

Connective Tissue Cells

The cellular elements of connective tissue control the formation, maintenance, and breakdown of the extracellular components. Primordial mesenchymal cells may differentiate to become macrophages, mast cells, plasma cells, lymphocytes, and fibroblasts. Fibroblasts are capable of mitotic division and are not dependent on a "stem cell" for their perpetuation. Tissue macrophages, widely distributed throughout the connective tissue, arise from hematogenous precursors and serve a scavenger role, ingesting foreign substances and removing debris. These cells form an important part of the mononuclear phagocytic system, which also includes the Kupffer cells of the liver, alveolar macrophages of the lung, and splenic and bone marrow mononuclear phagocytes. Tissue mast cells, also diffusely distributed, may be present in significant numbers in certain tissues. They represent 3 per cent of the cells in the superficial aspect of the synovial membrane. Their role in the physiology of connective tissue is not clear; they contain heparin, histamine, and 5-hydroxytryptamine. Plasma cells, lymphocytes, and eosinophils, derived from the bloodstream, are sparsely and irregularly distributed throughout connective tissue.

Fibroblasts are responsible for the formation and maintenance of fibrous and fibroelastic connective tissues. Specialized variants of fibroblasts — the chondrocytes, osteocytes, and synoviocytes — are credited with the formation of cartilage, bone, and the synovial fluid, respectively. The fibroblast appears as a stellate or spindle-shaped cell with a large pale nucleus and faintly staining cytoplasm under conventional light microscopy. Ultrastructural studies demonstrate that these cells are equipped for complex biosynthetic activities. By tissue culture it has been convincingly demonstrated that the fibroblast synthesizes the glycosaminoglycans (acid mucopolysaccharides) of the ground substance. In addition, the fibroblast produces collagen and elastic fibers, which are first detectable in aggregated form outside of, but close to, the cell periphery.

Fibrillar Components

Three types of intercellular fibers can be distinguished by staining techniques and light microscopy. The most abundant is collagen, composing one third of total body protein. With conventional histologic techniques this appears as wavy bundles of fibers with the smallest units appearing to be non-branching fibers with a uniform diameter of 0.3 to 0.5 μ. Under the electron microscope these fibers appear to be made up of submicroscopic fibrils with a characteristic periodic banding measuring 68 nm.

The formation of collagen and its molecular characteristics have been intensively investigated. The fundamental unit is referred to as tropocollagen which is rod shaped (1.5 × 300 nm.) and consists of three α (alpha) chains in triple helical configuration. Five different α chains with distinctive amino acid sequences are recognized: $\alpha 1$ (I), $\alpha 2$, $\alpha 1$ (II), $\alpha 1$ (III), $\alpha 1$ (IV). Each chain has a molecular weight of 95,000 to 100,000 daltons and contains high concentrations of the unique amino acids hydroxyproline and hydroxylysine, as well as glycine, alanine, lysine, and proline. Four types of tropocollagen can be identified by their α chain content: Type I contains $[\alpha 1(I)]_2 \alpha 2$; Type II $[\alpha 1(II)]_3$; Type III $[\alpha 1(III)]_3$; and Type IV $[\alpha 1(IV)]_3$. These collagens demonstrate differences in carbohydrate content, number of cross-links, and the degree of hydroxylation of prolyl and lysyl residues. Tissue distribution of the four major types of collagen can be related to these structural differences and the functional requirements within each tissue. Type I collagen contains fibrils of high tensile strength and occurs in tissues which contain sparse amounts of ground substance materials. It is the most common type of collagen, and is found in large amounts in bone, skin, and tendons. In cartilage the collagen is Type II, contains a high concentration of carbohydrate, does not form prominent fibrils, and is complexed with large amounts of proteoglycan. Chondroblasts are the only cells known to synthesize this form of collagen. Type III collagen is found in fetal tissues, occurs in association with Type I collagen, and contains the amino acid cysteine and a high content of hydroxyproline. Basement membranes contain Type IV collagen, which is rich in carbohydrates including mannose and hexosamines. In addition, this form of collagen contains 3-hydroxyproline and large amounts of cysteine, plus hydroxylysine.

The biosynthesis of collagen molecules follows the general process established for proteins that are to be secreted from the cell. Collagen messenger RNA (mRNA) is transcribed from structural genes specific for each α chain. The precursor of α chains is a larger molecule (pro α chain, 150,000 daltons) which contains noncollagenous sequences at the N- and C-terminals of the molecule. These parts of the molecule are cleaved after secretion and are thought to maintain solubility, to facilitate orientation of troprocollagen, and to inhibit cross-link formation. Within the endoplasmic reticulum each pro α chain is synthesized; then three chains form triple helix protropocollagen, lysyl and prolyl residues are

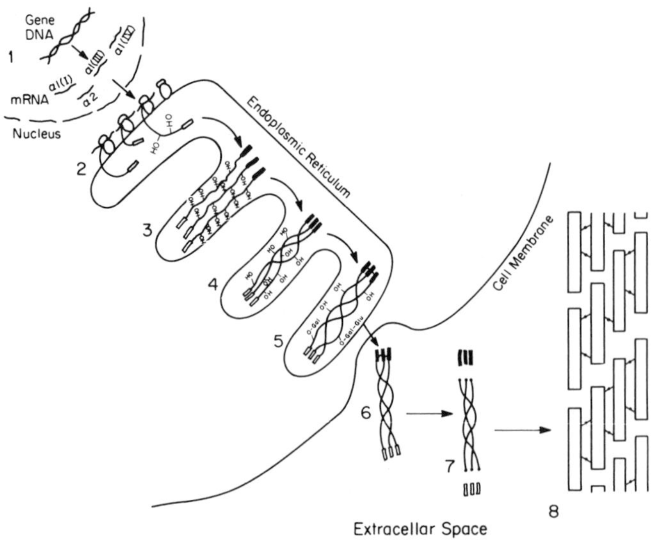

Figure 17–1 Diagrammatic representation of collagen biosynthesis, and extracellular formation of collagen fibrils. The major steps in the process are outlined:

1. *Transcription* of structural genes produces messenger ribonucleic acid (mRNA) specific for each α chain type.

2. *Translation:* The mRNA molecules are transported to ribosomes lining the rough endoplasmic reticulum. Pro α chain synthesis includes N-terminal ☐, and C-terminal ■ non-collagen peptides.

3. *Hydroxylation:* The middle collagen pro α chains are enzymatically hydroxylated at certain prolyl and lysyl residues.

4. *Triple helix formation:* Three pro α chains are aligned and form protocollagen.

5. *Glycosylation* involves addition of galactose (Gal) and the disaccharide glucosylgalactose (Glu-Gal).

6. *Secretion:* The completed molecule is transported to the Golgi apparatus (not shown) and secreted from the cell.

7. *Propeptide cleavage:* Extracellular protolytic enzymes remove the N- and C-terminal non-collagen peptides.

8. *Collagen fibril* polymerization and cross-link formation. Interchain cross-links (—•—) are initiated by the enzyme lysyl oxidase. The degree of cross-linking depends on the collagen type.

hydroxylated, glycosylation occurs, and the molecule is secreted from the cell. This process is schematically outlined in Figure 17–1.

After secretion of protropocollagen, proteolysis of the noncollagen N-terminus peptides occurs first (procollagen peptidase), followed by cleavage of the C-terminus peptides, leaving helical tropocollagen. The latter polymerizes into fibrils in a highly specific fashion in Type I and II collagen, with each tropocollagen molecule overlapping its neighbor by 68 nm. or a multiple of this length. Cross-linking occurs through action of lysyl oxidase on lysine to form an aldehyde (allysine) which interacts with a hydroxylysine residue on an adjacent chain. These steps can be inhibited by copper deficiency, β-aminoproprionitrile, or penicillamine. Other cross-linking reactions also occur, and their number determines the tensile strength of the collagen fibrils in different connective tissues.

Collagen in triple helical configuration resists degradation by most proteases. Bacterial and vertebrate collagenases, as well as cathepsin B1, found in lysosomes, act upon the intact collagen molecule. The latter acts only at acid pH's, whereas cathepsin D, also active at acid pH, will not cleave helical collagen. The vertebrate collagenases are found in several tissues (skin, bone, rheumatoid synovium, tadpole tail, in-vitro cultures of granulocytes, macrophages, fibroblasts). They are less active against denatured collagen, inhibited by serum alpha globulins (except granulocyte-derived collagenase), and cleave tropocollagen between glycine-isoleucine three fourths of the distance from the N-terminus of the molecule. Both fragments of the molecule are then susceptible to denaturation at 37°C., and in non-helical form can be degraded by a broad spectrum of extracellular proteases active at neutral pH or in phagolysosomes at acid pH. These mechanisms are visualized as responsible for collagen turnover and tissue destruction within an inflammatory focus.

The second type of intercellular fiber, reticulin, defined by its intense black appearance after reaction with silver methionine stain using light microscopy, has no certain counterpart identifiable by electron microscopy. These fibers are found around blood and lymph vessels, nerves, and muscle fibers; in basement membranes; and in the lymphoid organs. The exact composition of reticulin has not been determined, but it appears to consist of collagen, non-collagen proteins, lipid, and proteoglycans. The fibers are labile to collagenases, but resist proteolytic digestion by trypsin.

Elastic fibers, the third type of intercellular fibers, quite clearly differ from collagen. They have less tensile strength than collagen fibers, but have a much greater tendency to return to their previous fiber length after removal of a distorting force. The elastic fiber viewed by electron microscopy consists of a fibrillar and an amorphous component. Most of the classic efforts to characterize elastic fibers have utilized bovine ligamentum nuchae, although large blood vessels, lung, and most tissues also contain this fibrillar protein. The extreme insolubility of elastic fibers has made their biochemical characterization difficult. The two components of the elastic fiber differ in chemical composition. The microfibrils are rich in polar and sulfur-containing amino acids, but no hydroxyproline or cross-links are present. In the amorphous component the amino acid composition conforms to that of "elastin." It contains non-polar amino acids, no cysteine or methionine; while cross-links and hydroxyproline have been detected. The precursor to elastin is tropoelastin which is synthesized by fibroblasts and smooth muscle cells. A high content of lysine in tropoelastin is critical to the development of the three major cross-links in elastin (desmosine, isodesmosine, lysinonorleucine). The enzyme lysyl oxidase is responsible for aldehyde formation (as in collagen) which leads to the development of cross-links between tropoelastin chains. In copper deficiency or osteolathyrism the cross-linking is impaired and elastic fiber tensile strength reduced. Cross-linked elastin invests the microfibrils to form mature elastic fibers. The microfibrils contain cystine disulfide bonds, and as noted above differ in chemical composition from elastin. They are glycoproteins that contain hexose and hexosamines which are labile to a fairly broad spectrum of proteases. Turnover of elastin and presumably elastic fibers occurs slowly (as studied in aortic tissue). The enzyme elastase is thought to be involved in the degradation process; it is susceptible to inhibition by naturally-occurring substances in phagocytic cells.

Ground Substance

The cellular and fibrillar components of connective tissue are embedded in an amorphous sol-gel continuum known as ground substance. In routine histologic preparations much of the ground substance is leached out, leaving empty spaces between cells and fibers. By special fixation and appropriate histochemical procedures a dramatic staining of ground substance is produced. Although these methods are not specific for glycosaminoglycans, they identify the acidic nature of the extracellular materials. Information concerning its chemical composition has increased considerably in recent years, but much remains to be learned about variations with anatomic location and alterations with aging and in disease states. It is clear that this optically structureless sol-gel is an aqueous solution of electrolytes, proteins, highly polymerized carbohydrate-containing substances known as glycosaminoglycans which (except perhaps for hyaluronic acid) are covalently linked to protein and called proteoglycans, combinations of amino acids and carbohydrate substances known as glycoproteins, and lipoproteins.

By extraction procedures the proteins of ground substance have been characterized as quite distinct in amino acid content from the fibrillar proteins, and as closely resembling certain of the plasma proteins in electrophoretic properties. The glycoprotein content of connective tissue is somewhat higher than in plasma, and there is evidence that at least some of these glycoproteins are synthesized by connective tissue cells.

The best characterized constituents of ground substance are the proteoglycans, which contain protein covalently linked to glycosaminoglycans (GAG). The detailed structure of the protein portion is not well defined, but the ester linkage to GAG is through the amino acid serine or threonine. The GAG chains are arranged perpendicular to the protein "core" and are visualized as bristles on a test tube brush. In most instances 30 to 100 GAG chains are attached to the protein molecule. Within the GAG chain a repeating disaccharide unit consists of specific monosaccharides: glucosamine or galactosamine (with acetyl and sulfate substituents), plus glucuronic or iduronic acid. In keratan sulfate the simple sugar galactose replaces the uronic acid. In the hyaluronic acid polymer the presence of protein is disputed; however, the number of disaccharide units may approximate 2500. Currently, seven different GAG have been recognized: hyaluronic acid, chondroitin-4-sulfate, chondroitin-6-sulfate, dermatan sulfate, heparin, heparan sulfate, and keratan sulfate. The proteoglycans are named for the GAG contained in the molecule; their structure is outlined in Table 17–1.

The initiation of biosynthesis of the protein core of proteoglycans is believed to follow the mechanisms responsible for development of a protein destined for secretion. Attachment of individual sugars is initiated at the serine or threonine residue of the core protein through the action of specific transferases which utilize nucleotide sugars as precursor molecules. Before development of the repeating disaccharide portion of the GAG chain a "linkage region" of monosaccharides is attached to the protein core through action of individual enzymes. All the enzymes responsible for growth of the carbohydrate chains, including the addition of sulfate groups, are found in the endoplasmic reticulum and the Golgi apparatus. It has been shown that fibroblasts, synoviocytes, chondrocytes, and endothelial cells synthesize certain of the GAG or proteoglycans. Heparin is synthesized by mast cells. Degradation of GAG has been shown to occur in several of the heritable diseases of connective tissue (mucopolysaccharidoses) through action of specific lysosomal enzymes. In these situations GAG are degraded in phagolysosomes. Phagocy-

TABLE 17–1 COMPOSITION OF GLYCOSAMINOGLYCANS AND THE CARBOHYDRATE PORTION OF CERTAIN PROTEOGLYCANS

Glycosaminoglycan	Hexosamine	Hexuronic Acid	Hexose	Disaccharide Units
Hyaluronic acid	N-acetyl-D-glucosamine	D-Glucuronic	—	500–2500
Chondroitin-4-sulfate	N-acetyl-D galactosamine 4- or 6-sulfate	D-Glucuronic	—	60
Dermatan sulfate	N-acetyl-D galactosamine 4-sulfate	L-Iduronic + D-Glucuronic 5–15%	—	40–60
Heparin*	N-sulfamido-glucosamine 6-sulfate	D-Glucuronic + L-Iduronic trace	—	10–20
Heparan sulfate*	N-sulfamido-glucosamine or N-acetylglucosamine 6-sulfate	D-Glucuronic	—	10–20
Keratan sulfate	N-acetyl-D-glucosamine	—	D-Galactose	10–20

*The degree of sulfation of heparin and heparan sulfate varies in the disaccharide units. For heparin SO_3^- radical can occur at the 2-position of the uronic acid and/or 2- and 6-position of the hexosamine. For heparan sulfate SO_3^- radical can occur at the 2- and/or 6-position of the hexosamine.

tic cells such as macrophages are probably responsible for the intracellular breakdown of GAG and/or proteoglycans.

Tissue culture and isotope studies indicate that connective tissue cells from many sources synthesize glycosaminoglycans locally from simple precursors, including glucose. Cultures of human synovial tissue synthesize hyaluronic acid from the components of a chemically defined medium. Turnover rates determined with isotopes indicate that the GAG and/or proteoglycans of connective tissue are continuously in active flux, in contrast to the relatively static collagen. The half-life of hyaluronic acid is two to four days, and that of chondroitin sulfate(s), seven to ten days.

The anatomic distribution of GAG and proteoglycans has considerable functional significance. Synovial fluid and vitreous humor contain only hyaluronic acid. Cartilage ground substance contains chondroitin-4 and 6-sulfate, and keratan sulfate. The major mucopolysaccharide in adult bone is chondroitin-4-sulfate. Mixtures of the chondroitin sulfates and hyaluronic acid occur in diverse tissues such as umbilical cord, skin, tendon, heart valve, and aorta. Heparan sulfate, a family of compounds with variable acetyl and

sulfate ratios, has been isolated from aorta, lung, liver, and amyloid tissue. Certain of these substances are excreted in large amounts in the urine by some patients with a hereditary disease of connective tissue. Heparin can be isolated from lung and aorta as well as liver. Keratan sulfate I or II has been identified in cornea, nucleus pulposus, aging cartilage, and growing bone. Chondroitin has been found only in the cornea.

Formation of Connective Tissue

An orderly sequence of connective tissue formation has been demonstrated in the healing wound and in a variety of experimental granulomas. Such studies frequently combine histochemical and analytical chemical techniques. The connective tissue defect is promptly flooded with plasma proteins and leukocytes from the circulatory system. Early in the reparative phase there is an impressive increase in the number of cells. This active proliferation of connective tissue cells is accompanied by a striking change in the tinctorial properties of the ground substance, characterized by prominent metachromatic staining that indicates high local concentrations of acidic substances, including glycosaminoglycans. Soon fine intercellular collagen fibers can be detected. As the repair continues, the fibers become more numerous and individually larger, the cellular elements decrease in size and number, and the metachromatic hue of the ground substance subsides. Chemical analyses along the time course of this process show the hexosamine content (from glycoproteins and glycosaminoglycans) to peak in the first few days and then fall steadily, while hydroxyproline (an index of collagen content) rises steadily.

Information concerning factors which regulate the formation and maintenance of connective tissue in health and disease may be of fundamental importance; as yet, such information is fragmentary. There is evidence that aging, nutritional factors, and hormonal influences may be significant.

Protein depletion prior to wounding is known to retard healing and decrease wound tensile strength. The granulation tissue in healing wounds of protein-depleted animals contains decreased amounts of hexosamine and hydroxyproline, suggesting that fibroblastic synthesis of both ground substance and collagen has been retarded. Ascorbic acid deficiency in guinea pigs and in man results in the failure to form collagen fibers, probably owing to the inability to hydroxylate proline to hydroproline. Correction of the vitamin C deficiency is followed within hours by the appearance of collagen fibers.

The effect of adrenal glucocorticoids on connective tissue has been extensively studied. An excess of hydrocortisone (in many studies doses exceed maximum pharmacologic doses in humans) will interfere with wound healing and the forma-tion of granulation tissue. It will also reduce the cellularity and thickness of skin following local application, reduce the ratio of hexosamine to collagen in rat connective tissue, suppress the uptake of labeled sulfate into the sulfated glycosaminoglycan of rodents, and suppress both oxidative and glycolytic metabolism of rheumatoid synovium in vitro. Cell culture studies show that near-physiologic concentrations of hydrocortisone induce multiple effects on human fibroblasts, including accelerated mitosis, suppression of collagen deposition, and depression of the specific rate of hyaluronate synthesis.

Recently, "connective tissue activating peptide(s)," which markedly stimulates the glycolysis of synovial cells in culture and increases the formation of hyaluronic acid by 10 to 40 times over the basal rate, has been demonstrated in a variety of mammalian cells, including leukocytes and platelets. These substances have been proposed as mediators that bridge the gap between the exudative and reparative phase of inflammation. In pathologic states of inflammation they might play a critical role in perpetuating the inflammatory response along with immune mediators that amplify the inflammatory reaction.

STRUCTURE AND FUNCTION OF JOINTS

Simple gliding joints (diarthroses) consist of two bone ends covered by articular hyaline cartilage and held together by a sleeve of white fibrous connective tissue — the joint capsule. The inner layers of this capsule consist of specialized connective tissue cells — the synovium or syn-

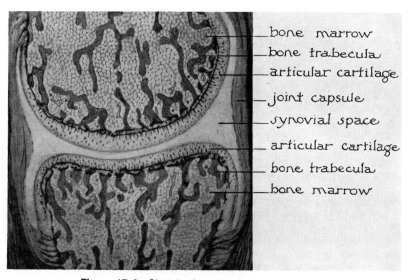

bone marrow
bone trabecula
articular cartilage
joint capsule
synovial space
articular cartilage
bone trabecula
bone marrow

Figure 17–2 Sketch of a normal diarthrodial joint.

ovialis. Within the joint space is a small amount of synovial fluid. In the human embryo, the future joint can be identified by the fifth to seventh week as a remnant of mesenchyme interposed between two chondrogenous zones. Later, the center of this zone appears to liquefy, owing to elaboration of soluble ground substance, and the mesenchyme appears to retract peripherally and to produce large numbers of closely packed fibrils. This is the future joint cavity, and its lining is the embryonic equivalent of the synovium.

Joint Capsule

The joint capsule consists largely of fibrous collagenous tissue with few elastic fibers. It is reinforced in areas by ligaments. It blends with periosteum of the bone shaft above and below the joint, and with tendinous and ligamentous periarticular structures. Stability and normal movement of the joints require that the relationships of the articulating bones maintain a normal alignment. This is accomplished to some extent by the anatomic configuration of the articulating surfaces ("congruity"), by the slight negative pressure in the joint cavity (−2 to −12 cm. water), and by the molecular cohesive properties of the synovial fluid. But the most important stabilization is provided by the strong fibrous outer part of the joint capsule and its reinforcing ligaments. When the joint capsule is weakened, joint stability and function are threatened or destroyed. The collagenous layers determine the mechanical properties of the joint capsule. It has very little elasticity, but its resistance to a stretching force is 30 times that of a sheet of pure rubber of equal thickness. Like tendinous connective tissue it has a high resistance to tear. The pliability of the synovium helps it to withstand the stresses of joint motion.

The blood vessels which supply the joint usually arise in common with those supplying adjacent bone and form a prominent arterial circle around the joint. Those that supply the joint ultimately pass into a rich capillary network which is prominent in the cellular and areolar areas of the synovium.

Articular nerves carry fibers from several spinal nerves and may supply more than one joint. They contain sensory fibers and autonomic fibers. The branches are widely distributed to joint capsule, ligaments, and synovium. The larger sensory fibers form proprioceptive endings in the capsule and ligaments which are very sensitive to position and motion. They play an important role in reflex control of posture, locomotion, and kinesthetic sensation. The smaller sensory fibers form pain endings in the capsule and ligaments and along the blood vessels. Twisting and stretching are the most effective pain stimuli to the joint

capsule. Joint pain is perceived as diffuse and poorly localized; when severe, it may be felt distally over most of the extremity. Like visceral pain, it may be referred to another anatomic location. Joint pain not uncommonly leads to reflex contraction of adjacent muscles, which may take the form of a protective spasm.

Articular Cartilage

Cartilage is tough, resilient connective tissue consisting of cells embedded in a firm extracellular matrix which is made up of a spongelike network of Type II collagen fibers into which proteoglycans are tightly packed. The proteoglycans exist in large aggregates of molecular weight of a million or more, which consist of a highly polymerized chain of hyaluronate and tissue glycoproteins which stabilize the interaction of 30 to 40 proteoglycan molecules with the hyaluronate chain (Fig. 17–3). Since the collagen fibers have nearly the same refractive index as the matrix, they are not visualized by conventional light microscopy. With polarized light the fibers are seen to be arranged so as to provide optimal resilience (Fig. 17–4). They extend as a looping curve resembling a croquet wicket with the ends anchored in the deeper calcium-rich zone of cartilage adjacent to the underlying bone. In relation to the cartilage surface this provides a surface zone of closely packed fibers parallel to the surface, an intermediate zone where the fibers are tangential, and a deeper zone where the direction is perpendicular to the surface. The proteoglycan aggregates can bind large amounts of water, but are constrained by the collagen mesh from binding excess amounts of water. This arrangement restricts access of molecules larger than 70,000 daltons, such as proteolytic enzymes. This capacity of the cartilage mass to change in

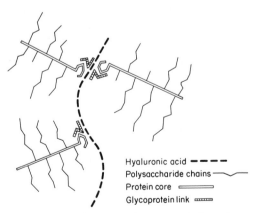

Hyaluronic acid
Polysaccharide chains
Protein core
Glycoprotein link

Figure 17–3 Diagrammatic representation of a proteoglycan aggregate.

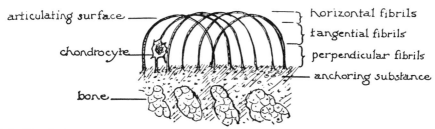

Figure 17–4 Sketch showing arrangement of collagen fibrils in articular cartilage as seen with polarized light. Note the three zones of fibrils aligned in horizontal, tangential, and radial positions.

shape and "weep water" under pressure provides a cushioning effect protecting the subchondral bone and is the major method of buffering the blows and jolts received by the skeleton. The surface arrangement of the fibers assists the cartilage in providing a smooth gliding surface for the opposing bone ends. Under frequent intermittent pressures cartilage continues to be elastic. But with continuous compression its expansile power is decreased and the time for recovery becomes longer. Elasticity is also reduced as water content decreases.

Articular cartilage has no blood supply. It receives most of its nourishment from the synovial fluid, probably augmented by the pumping action of intermittent compression and decompression. Some nutrition may be derived from diffusion from vessels in the underlying subchondral bone or subsynovial vessels located at the junction of the capsule and cartilage at the periphery of the joint.

Articular cartilage contains relatively few cells; therefore, the rate of respiration is relatively low. However, the rate of metabolism per cartilage cell is in the range exhibited by other connective tissues. New cartilage is formed interstitially by chondrocytes which are most numerous in the deeper layers of the cartilage. The cells of adult articular cartilage have restricted mitotic ability. Consequently, the capacity of this tissue to repair itself or to regenerate after injury is distinctly limited. Nevertheless, there is evidence that in normal use some replacement of articular cartilage may occur, and that opposition of articular surfaces is necessary for maintenance of cartilage integrity. Reaction to injury depends on the depth of the damage to the cartilage. Superficial cuts show little or no reaction. Peripheral lesions reaching the joint capsule or central lesions extending to the subchondral bone are promptly filled with fibrous tissue. Sclerosis of the subchondral bone may also lead to microfractures with alteration in the structure and function of the overlying cartilage.

The Synovium

Synovial tissue, a vascular connective tissue basically similar to connective tissue elsewhere in the body, lines the inner surface of the joint capsule but does not cover the articular cartilage. It consists of cells, fibers, and ground substance. The cells near the surface have long cytoplasmic processes which overlap and intertwine. They may be one to several layers thick, forming a relatively smooth surface from which villi, folds, and fat pads may project into the joint cavity. Tissue deep to the surface may be fibrous, fatty, or areolar. The surface cells do not form a complete lining, so that intercellular material may be directly adjacent to the synovial space. Thus, the joint cavity is not a body cavity like the pleura, pericardium, and peritoneum. It is a specialized connective tissue space.

The synovium is richly supplied with blood vessels, lymph vessels, and some nerve fibers. The capillary network and lymphatic network are adjacent to the joint cavity, and diffusion takes place readily between these vessels and the joint cavity. Most substances in the bloodstream enter the joint cavity easily, and many substances injected into the joint cavity readily enter the blood. The size and configuration of large molecules appear to influence the ease with which they may pass. Colloidal solutions, fine suspensions, and proteins, when injected into the joint cavity, enter into the subsynovial tissue and are removed chiefly by the lymphatics. Large particles are removed with difficulty and leave the joint by way of the lymphatics after phagocytosis. Motion of the joint definitely facilitates removal of materials injected into the joint cavity by both vascular and lymphatic routes.

Since the synovium is quite cellular and has an excellent blood supply, it is not surprising that it has a very good capacity for regeneration. After surgical removal, it will be formed again either from remnants of synovial tissue or from the joint capsule.

Synovial Fluid

The fluid within the joint cavity is highly viscous and sticky, resembling egg white in consistency. It is slightly alkaline and ranges from colorless to pale yellow. It contains relatively few cells (see Table 17–2), predominantly mononuclear cells derived from the synovium. Normal fluid

TABLE 17–2   CHARACTERISTICS OF SYNOVIAL FLUID IN NORMAL JOINTS AND IN COMMON FORMS OF ARTHRITIS

		Appearance	Viscosity	Mucin Clot	Cell Count (per mm.³)	Crystals	"R.A." Cells*	Bacteria (on stain or culture)
Group I Noninflammatory	Normal	Straw colored, clear	High	Good	±200 WBC 20% PMN	0	0	0
	Traumatic Arthritis	Yellow to bloody, often turbid	High	Good	±2000 WBC 30% PMN Many RBC	0	0	0
	Osteoarthritis	Yellow, clear	High	Good	±1000 WBC 15–25% PMN	0	0	0
Group II Inflammatory	Rheumatoid Arthritis	Yellow to greenish, cloudy	Low	Fair to poor	15,000 to 40,000 WBC 60–90% PMN	Occasionally cholesterol	+	0
	Rheumatic Fever	Yellow, slightly cloudy	Low	Good	10,000 to 12,000 WBC ±50% PMN	0	0 or +	0
	Systemic Lupus Erythematosus	Straw colored, slightly cloudy	High	Good	±5000 WBC 10–15% PMN	0	0 or +	0
	Gout	Yellow to milky, cloudy	Low	Fair to poor	10,000 to 30,000 WBC 60–80% PMN	Urate +	0	0
	Pseudogout	Yellow, clear to slightly cloudy	Low	Fair to poor	1000 to 10,000 WBC 25–50% PMN	Calcium pyrophosphate +	0	0
Group III Septic	Tuberculous Arthritis	Yellow, cloudy	Low.	Poor	±25,000 WBC 50–60% PMN	0	0	+
	Septic Arthritis	Grayish or bloody, turbid to purulent	Low	Poor	80,000 to 200,000 WBC 75–90% PMN	0	0	+

*"R.A." cells—Inclusion-bearing cells, not morphologically specific, but most frequently found in large numbers in rheumatoid arthritis.

is 95 per cent water and has a specific gravity around 1.010. In normal joints the amount of synovial fluid present is small; one can expect to aspirate only 1 to 2 ml. of fluid from a normal knee.

The relative viscosity of normal joint fluid ranges from 50 to 200 or more times that of water. This viscosity is due to the hyaluronic acid content which averages 3.5 mg. per gram of fluid. The viscosity increases exponentially with increases in concentration of hyaluronic acid and is also clearly related to the degree of polymerization of this polysaccharide. The viscosity of hyaluronic acid is due to the complex, highly asymmetric long-chain structure of the high molecular weight polymer. This structure confers the property of binding large amounts of water to form a viscous sol. Thus, the joint fluid is provided with high viscosity with negligible osmotic properties. A protein solution with comparable viscosity would produce an osmotic pressure far beyond the physiologic range.

In joint fluid, the hyaluronic acid is conjugated with but easily separated from a protein compo-

nent; the protein content is less than 2 per cent of the total complex. This protein-polysaccharide forms a clotted precipitate when treated with dilute acids, forming *mucin*. The characteristics of the mucin clot formed on addition of dilute acetic acid provide a crude index of the degree of polymerization of the hyaluronic acid. In normal joint fluids, a tight adherent clot is formed. Such good mucin clot formation is also seen in fluids from traumatized joints, in degenerative joint disease, and in most types of acute inflammatory arthritis. In more chronic types of inflammatory joint disease this "mucin clot test" produces a flocculent, loosely adherent precipitate or even a powdery precipitate (Table 17–2).

The electrolyte content of joint fluid is comparable to that of the blood plasma. The amount of non-protein nitrogenous substances and uric acid is lower than in plasma. The glucose content varies with the level in the plasma, with changes in joint fluid sugar lagging behind fluctuations in blood sugar. The total protein content is lower than plasma, ranging from 1 to 2 grams per 100 ml. In normal joint fluids the protein is largely albumin, with albumin-to-globulin ratios as high as 20:1. This is attributed to the smaller size of the albumin molecule.

Thus, synovial fluid, aside from its hyaluronic acid content, can be considered as a dialysate of plasma. Just as the joint cavity can be considered a specialized connective tissue space structurally and functionally, the synovial fluid can be visualized as a specialized type of ground substance, composed of a dialysate of plasma to which the synovial cells have added a characteristic polysaccharide.

Joints as Functional Units

The structure of joints appears to be well adapted to serve the primary purposes of bearing weight and providing motion. Stability with motion is afforded by the fibrous joint capsule, ligaments and tendons, and muscle tone. The elasticity of articular cartilage permits adaptation to changing pressures and buffers impacts to which the skeleton is subjected. Viscous synovial fluid forms a strong fluid interface with the cartilage surface, so that motion can occur with negligible friction.

Joint lubrication is so extremely efficient that the coefficient of friction is less than that of ice sliding on ice. The rheologic properties of synovial fluid contribute to this end. Since the viscosity of synovial fluid is non-Newtonian in character, it offers high resistance to static pressures, while at the same time providing lowered resistance to the increasing rates of shear encountered in joint motion. Joint lubrication is usually considered to be an example of fluid film or "floating" lubrication. Since the articular surfaces do not fit perfectly throughout the whole range of motion, this incongruity permits the development of wedge-shaped spaces filled with synovial fluid. The intra-articular pressure increases during motion, and it is greatest where the articular cartilages are closest together. Since this pressure is great enough to keep the articular surfaces apart, the intervening film of synovial fluid, rather than the bearing surfaces, takes up the effects of friction. In many joints, intra-articular fibrous and fibrocartilaginous structures such as menisci and discs, as well as fat pads and synovial folds, aid in distributing the synovial fluid. In the joints, this classic concept of hydrodynamic lubrication must be modified to take into consideration the fact that synovial fluid is absorbed by articular cartilage and oozes from the cartilaginous surfaces under pressure. This provides an element of boundary lubrication where the moving surfaces are separated by a layer of lubricant which is adherent to or incorporated into the surface and need be only a few molecules thick.

Like all moving mechnical systems, the human joint wears with time. Some wear and tear is inevitable with normal activity. The most evident result is wearing away of the articular cartilage to some degree. Articular cartilage is subjected to wear and tear unequaled by any other tissue except the skin. Since articular cartilage has no blood supply and since adult cartilage cells have largely lost the power of mitosis, the potential for regeneration of cartilage is limited.

In contrast, the highly vascular and cell-rich synovium has great capacity for regeneration. But alterations in the synovium can result in modifications in exchange equilibria between plasma and synovial fluid and changes in the characteristics of the protein-polysaccharide of synovial fluid. Since the articular cartilage is dependent primarily on the synovial fluid for its nutrients, sooner or later the cartilage can be expected to reflect the results of functional aberrations of the synovialis.

FUNDAMENTAL PATHOLOGIC CHANGES OF JOINT DISEASE

Virtually all forms of joint disease can be understood in terms of two pathologic processes — degeneration and inflammation. Degenerative changes are dependent primarily on the limited capacity of articular cartilage to repair itself. Inflammation may be predominantly exudative or predominantly proliferative, or a combination of the two. It is not surprising that both degenerative and inflammatory changes can often be seen in the same joint. Cartilage which has been damaged as a result of inflammation is rendered more vulnerable to subsequent degenerative changes. In older persons, degenerative changes which have developed over the years do not render the joint immune to superimposed inflammation.

Degenerative Joint Changes

Much of the knowledge of the sequence of degenerative changes has been obtained from studies of the normal aging process in the joints. Bennett, Waine, and Bauer reported the gross and microscopic appearance of 63 knee joints obtained postmortem or following amputation and covering a wide age span. Abnormality of articular structure was first seen in the second decade and increased with advancing age. The first changes appear in the articular cartilage and show a predilection for those areas which are subjected to weight-bearing or shearing pressures. These are seen as localized areas of softening of the cartilage associated with a fine velvety disruption of the surface. In these areas, dehiscence of the cartilage occurs along the planes of the collagen fibers. The most superficial dehiscences are oriented parallel to the surface and, when confined to the tangential layers at the surface, produce "flaking." As the dehiscences proceed to the deeper layers they arch downward in a more vertical direction, producing "fibrillation" of the cartilage. An early change in the ground substance in these areas of cartilage is indicated by decrease in proteoglycan content in perichondrocyte regions and more conspicuous fibrillar elements— the "unmasking" of the collagen fibrils. Chemical studies show a decrease in the proteoglycan content and size of aggregates relative to the collagen in such areas.

With abrasion of the fibrillated cartilage, clefts and fissures develop, followed by erosion and progressive denudation of the underlying bony cortex. Associated with this progressive wearing away of the cartilage is new bone formation in two separate locations relative to the joint surface: (1) exophytic growth at the margins of the articular cartilage and (2) in the marrow and cortex of the subchondral bone immediately underlying the articular cartilage. The latter has been proposed as a primary event which leads to microfractures in the subchondral bone and disruption of the integrity of overlying cartilage. The marginal osteophytes develop at the periphery of the articular cartilage where the joint capsule blends with the periosteum covering the shaft of the bone. They may extend into the joint cavity and tend to develop within capsular and ligamentous attachments to the joint margins, generally growing in a direction governed by the lines of mechanical forces exerted on the area. Such marginal bony lipping may be seen in the knee joint as early as the fourth decade of life. The osteophyte consists largely of bone which merges imperceptibly with the cortical and cancellous structure of subchondral bone. Proliferation of bone in the subchondral area results in increased density of the bony structure underlying the cartilage. It is most marked in areas that have been denuded of their covering of cartilage. Here the exposed bone becomes dense and hardened and takes on a highly eburnated appearance.

The synovial tissue itself is largely unaffected in degenerative joint disease. Some thickening and hypertrophy of the villous processes may occur. Synovitis occurs rarely and is usually due to mechanical irritation. The joint cavity is not obliterated and ankylosis does not develop.

Because of the development of marginal osteophytes and sclerosis of subchondral bone, degenerative joint disease is called *osteoarthritis* or *osteoarthrosis*. There is difference of opinion as to whether the disease represents an exaggeration of the normal process of aging, or whether other additional pathologic processes are operating. Predisposing factors may be grouped as (1) those which influence the integrity of the articular cartilage and (2) those which accentuate or acceler-

ate normal wear and tear. One hypothesis suggests that abnormal stress stimulates increased formation and release of hydrolytic enzymes from chondrocytes. This leads to degradation of matrix proteoglycans with concomitant proliferation of chondrocytes and synthesis of proteoglycan. When reparative processes fail to keep pace with cartilage breakdown, the manifestations of osteoarthritis appear (Fig. 17–5).

Genetic influences may be important determinants of the resistance of cartilage to wear and tear. Stecher demonstrated a hereditary pattern in the occurrence of *Heberden's nodes*, osteophytes which form at the base of the distal phalanges of the fingers and which are more common in women than in men. *Acromegaly,* in which there is excessive proliferation of cartilage, is associated with osteoarthritis with an unusual degree of bony overgrowth. In ochronosis which complicates alkaptonuria an abnormal pigment discolors articular cartilage and intervertebral discs, with gross alterations of their physical properties; this is often associated with unusually severe osteoarthritis. A disease of growing children characterized by defective growth and maturation of the epiphyses results, despite the age of the patient, in joint changes indistinguishable from osteoarthritis. This disorder, known as Kaschin-Beck disease, is seen in Manchuria and eastern Siberia and is clearly of nutritional origin. In *hemophilia,* repeated hemorrhage into the joint leads to deposition of hemosiderin in the articular cartilage and eventually results in severe osteoarthritis. These rare forms of degenerative joint disease suggest that extreme endocrine, metabolic, and dietary influences may alter the integrity of articular cartilage and predispose to the development of osteoarthritis. Whether more subtle influences of the same nature are operative in the more common types of degenerative joint disease is as yet in the realm of speculation.

It is much easier to document the role of predisposing factors which accentuate or accelerate the wear and tear on the joints. *Secondary osteoarthritis* can result from excessive or abnormal stresses and strains related to postural or orthopedic abnormalities. A variety of structural abnormalities of the hip joint in childhood such as congenital dysplasia, Legg-Perthes disease, slipped femoral epiphysis, and congenital coxa vara lead to premature osteoarthritic degeneration. It may be a late result of trauma to the joint structures or of chronic irritation produced by derangement of internal joint structures — for example, a torn semilunar cartilage in the knee. It may appear in joints previously damaged by other types of inflammatory arthritis.

The clinical features of osteoarthritis are readily explained by the underlying pathologic

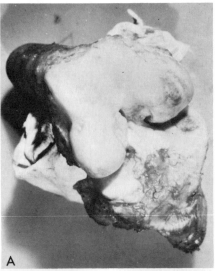

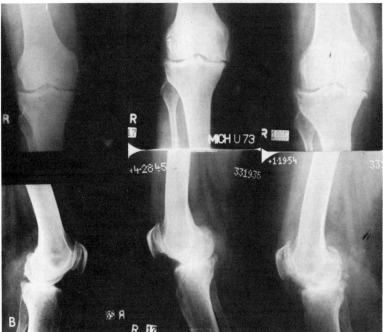

Figure 17–5 Osteoarthritic erosions on the medial and lateral femoral condyles and tibial plateau of the knee (*A*). Roentgenograms of the knee joint of a patient at ages 45, 52, and 61 years demonstrating progressive changes due to osteoarthritis. Over this 16-year interval there is loss of joint space due to cartilage degeneration, development of marginal osteophytes, and irregularity and eburnation of subchondral bone (*B*).

changes in the joint. It affects chiefly older individuals and characteristically involves weight-bearing joints. It is a localized disease of the joints and is not accompanied by systemic symptoms. The most common complaint is an aching pain which occurs on use, is rarely intense, and is relieved by rest. Stiffness after sitting is noted, particularly with the first few motions involving use of the part. Such stiffness is dissipated rapidly and rarely persists more than a few minutes. Objectively, the joints may appear normal, but bony enlargements may be felt around the joint margins. Occasionally these are tender. Crepitus, creaking, or grating on motion can usually be detected. Increase in synovial fluid is uncommon; when it does occur — usually in the knees — it subsides within a day or two after elimination of weight bearing. The range of motion is usually only slightly impaired except in osteoarthritis of the hip. The roentgenographic features of osteoarthritis are decrease in thickness of articular cartilage (erroneously termed "loss of joint space"), formation of intra-articular and marginal osteophytes ("lipping"), and increased density of the subchondral bone. In advanced disease there may be crumbling and remodeling of the subchondral bone.

Neurologic disorders which result in loss of proprioceptive and pain sensation may be complicated by *neuropathic joint disease,* which has many features of osteoarthritis. Deprived of its protective reflexes the joint is subject to severe and cumulative injury. There is relaxation of supporting structures with chronic instability of the joint. The degenerative changes progress rapidly and cartilage damage is extensive. With relative absence of pain, continued use results in extensive damage to cartilage and subchondral bone. These structures fragment, leaving loose bodies of cartilage and bone free in the joint cavity. These loose bodies and the extensive erosion of bone stimulate the synovium, with a resulting proliferative synovitis and persistent joint effusion. Subluxations and dislocations are common, as are intra-articular and juxta-articular fractures. The degenerative changes are accompanied by exuberant overgrowth of bone. The characteristic clinical features are the relative absence of pain and remarkable hypermotility of the affected joint. Radiographic features are the combination of extensive destructive and hypertrophic changes.

Classically, neuropathic joints occur as a complication of tabes dorsalis ("Charcot's joints"). Syringomyelia and spinal cord degeneration accompanying diabetes and pernicious anemia may also be the basis. Usually one joint only is affected — most often the hip, knee, ankle, midtarsal joints, and the lumbar and the lower spine. In syringomyelia, joints in the upper extremity may be involved.

Effects of Trauma

The simplest type of joint abnormality is that which results from injury. The trauma may be slight and cause only a strain on the fibrous capsule or ligaments. The response of edema and congestion produces swelling around the joint, with pain and stiffness from stimulation of the nerve endings which are abundant in the periarticular tissues. Since the tissues affected have a good blood supply, healing is usually rapid and complete. With more severe trauma, the synovium may be injured, followed by traumatic synovitis and effusion within the joint cavity. In the

absence of repeated trauma, such sterile inflammation persists for a relatively short time and recovery is usually complete. More severe trauma can damage the cartilage and, at times, the underlying bone and may provoke changes in the dynamics of the joint which, after a period of time, result in post-traumatic degenerative changes. If the injury is to the cartilage located centrally in the joint, little regeneration takes place and the irregularity of the joint surface places a strain on the periarticular structures at the joint margins, stimulating proliferation of bone. If the injury is at the articular margin of the cartilage, abnormal bone formation may develop rapidly. The late changes resulting from severe joint trauma are those of osteoarthritis, with rapidity of development determined by severity and location of the damage to joint structures.

Joint Inflammation — Synovitis

The vascular phase of inflammation can be visualized as a progressive impairment of the microcirculation of a tissue, initiated by a variety of agents and mediated by mechanisms that are incompletely characterized. The classic manifestations of heat, redness, swelling, pain, and impaired function correlate with alterations in the microcirculation, dominantly increased local blood flow, and increased vascular permeability ("leaks"). Since the vascular and lymphatic supply to the joint is predominantly in and just beneath the synovium, it is this tissue which is initially and principally involved in joint inflammation.

In acute synovitis, exudative inflammation predominates. The joint is swollen, warm, tender to touch, and painful to move. Redness and heat over the joint vary with the type and severity of inflammation. The joint capsule is distended by an outpouring of synovial fluid with an increased content of inflammatory cells, nearly always polymorphonuclear neutrophils. Microscopically, the venules and capillaries of the synovium are dilated; the synovium and subsynovial tissues are edematous and infiltrated to a varying degree with inflammatory cells. Some types of arthritis such as the synovitis of serum sickness and acute rheumatic fever, which are self-limited and subside without residual joint damage, can be regarded as examples of purely exudative inflammation of the synovium.

However, in the more chronic forms of arthritis, the proliferative phase of inflammation develops and may dominate the pathologic and clinical features of the disease. Rheumatoid arthritis is the prototype of such combined exudative and proliferative inflammation, with extensive formation of granulation tissue accounting for the

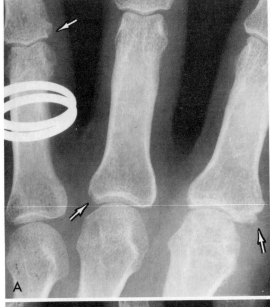
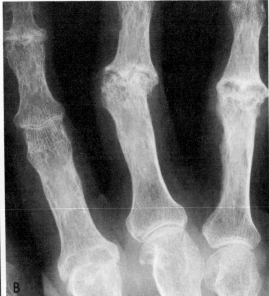
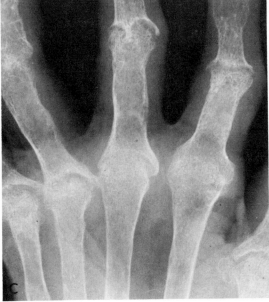

Figure 17–6 Progressive changes in the proximal interphangeal (PIP) and metacarpophangeal (MCP) joints of patients with rheumatoid arthritis. In panel *A* early marginal inflammatory erosions are identified by the arrows. In panels *B* and *C* progressive destructive changes due to rheumatoid pannus are shown. In addition, secondary osteoarthritic alterations and bony ankylosis of PIP and MCP joints have developed as sequelae of the rheumatoid process.

joint destruction and disability (Fig. 17–6). The synovium is swollen and deep red in color and there is hypertrophy of the villous processes. There is reduplication of the synovial lining cells and proliferation of fibroblasts. The inflammatory cells are chiefly lymphocytes (T cells predominating), plasma cells, and macrophages, and may appear in a follicle-like arrangement. Many of the cells found in the tissue lesions are designated as immunocompetent. The fibroblastic and angioblastic proliferation forms granulation tissue which replaces the synovium and invades the joint capsule and periarticular structures. Particularly significant is the invasion of the interior of the joint by a reddish, roughened, tongue-like protrusion of granulation tissue, growing over the articular cartilage from the joint margins (pannus formation).

By lysis of cartilage ground substance and fibers, interference with nutrition of the cartilage, and actual invasion, this inflammatory tissue slowly destroys the articular cartilage. It may join with similar granulation tissue arising from subchondral marrow. The capsular inflammation and proliferative granulation tissue tend to persist and to progress slowly, with remissions and exacerbations leading to cumulative damage to cartilage and subchondral bone. This damage, consequences of the original inflammation, accounts for the deformities and crippling that characterize the later stages of rheumatoid arthritis. In these later stages the evidences of exudative inflammation usually lessen and may appear to subside completely. The granulation tissue becomes primary fibrous and is converted to a dense scar. This tough fibrous scar limits or prevents joint motion (fibrous ankylosis). On occasions, this scar becomes calcified and is converted to osseous tissue (bony ankylosis).

Alterations in Joint Fluid Produced by Disease

It is to be expected that changes in the permeability of the synovial tissues and vessels will be reflected by changes in the joint fluid. The increased permeability accompanying inflammation permits more ready passage into the joint cavity of water, electrolytes, and easily diffusible colloids. The passage of protein molecules is enhanced, and the increase in total protein content of the joint fluid is proportional to the intensity of the inflammation. The proportion of globulin increases with lowering of the ratio of albumin to globulin. This increased permeability also accounts for the presence of fibrinogen, immune globulins, leukocytes, and proteins with enzymatic activity in the joint fluid during inflammation. The glucose content tends to decrease as the leukocyte content increases, and is characteristically low or absent in septic joints. This is attributed to the increased glycolytic activity of the leukocytes and synovial cells.

The viscosity of joint fluid is reduced in inflammatory disease, particularly in rheumatoid arthritis. This is explained in part by a decrease in concentration of hyaluronate; however, since the volume of joint fluid is increased severalfold, the total amount of hyaluronate is considerably greater than in the normal joint. Some of the decrease in viscosity is also due to the presence of less highly polymerized molecules of hyaluronate, which is also evidenced by deterioration of the mucin clot produced by the addition of dilute acetic acid. These changes are usually considered to reflect alterations in metabolic activity of synovial cells during inflammation, a concept supported by the observation that rheumatoid synovial cells in culture produce larger amounts of less highly polymerized hyaluronate as compared with synovial cell cultures from noninflamed joints. The possibility of degradation in vivo by enzymes released from leukocytes and synovial lining cells into the synovial fluid cannot be ruled out.

The characteristic changes in the synovial fluid in the more common forms of arthritis are listed in Table 17–2. As an aid in differential diagnosis, examination of the synovial fluid by simple methods is of greatest help in differentiating noninflammatory from inflammatory synovial effusions, in the detection of septic arthritis, and in the demonstrations of characteristic crystals in gout and pseudogout. Effusions in traumatic and degenerative joint disease are relatively clear, do not clot, and characteristically show only a modest increase in number of white blood cells but may contain increased numbers of red blood cells. Viscosity is well maintained and the mucin clot is firm, ropy, and non-friable. Inflammatory fluids are more turbid, may clot on standing owing to the presence of fibrinogen, and usually contain more than 5,000 leukocytes per mm.[3] and may range as high as 60,000 to 80,000 in chronic inflammation. The leukocytes are predominantly polymorphonuclear neutrophils. Varying degrees of deterioration in viscosity and characteristics of the mucin clot reflect alterations in the hyaluronate. In septic joints the fluid is turbid to frankly purulent, the leukocyte count is 80,000 to 200,000 per mm.[3], almost all of which are polymorphonuclear leukocytes, and the responsible microorganism may be demonstrated by direct staining or by culture.

PATHOGENESIS OF JOINT INFLAMMATION

Extensive investigation is beginning to elucidate the physiologic, immunologic, and biochemical mechanisms by which inflammation is produced. Since the joint in an extremity is a well-demarcated tissue space which can be sampled easily and repeatedly by needle aspiration or biopsy, studies of joint inflammation have contributed significantly to concepts relating inflammatory mechanisms to human disease. Present knowledge permits what must be regarded as an evolving concept of the mechanisms and mediators of the changes in the microcirculation which is the "final common pathway" of inflammatory damage. Factors which have been considered mediators of the microcirculatory effects can be conveniently grouped under headings of small molecular mediators, plasma factors, leukocyte factors, immune mechanisms, and tissue necrosis, with full appreciation of the interplay between such factors and others yet to be identified.

The role of *immune mechanisms* in producing tissue damage and inflammation is covered in Chapter 4. The biologic activities of immune complexes, lymphokines, immunocompetent cells, phagocytic cells, complement components, and lysosomal enzymes, have been shown to be of importance in the pathogenesis of rheumatic disease.

Plasma factors implicated in inflammatory reactions include Hageman factor, the kininogen system, and the fibrinogen and plasminogen systems. Each of the systems involves specific substrates, enzyme activators, cofactors, and inhibitors.

Small molecular mediators include histamine, the kinin peptides, serotonin, slow reactive substance, cyclic nucleotides, and prostaglandins. Several of these chemicals, produced by body cells, have profound effects on the microcirculation in extremely small concentrations. In model systems, injections of histamines, bradykinin, and serotonin produce only an immediate and transient effect on the microcirculation. Whether such substances serve only to initiate the inflammatory response or whether continued production of them may sustain the inflammation is not clear. Kinin peptides in synovial fluids from inflamed knees have been demonstrated by bioassay. High concentrations of prostaglandin E have been identified in rheumatoid synovium and may subvert immune defenses in this tissue. It is noteworthy that several of the anti-inflammatory drugs are potent inhibitors of prostaglandin synthetase activity.

Among leukocyte factors, the concept of *lysosomes* has attracted much attention in recent years. This concept, originated by DeDuve, visualizes many types of cells to contain small subcellular aggregates (granules) of hydrolytic enzymes active against a variety of substrates. These enzymes are active only when leaks develop in the wall of the lysosomal structure that contains them. Once released, the enzymes all have optimal activity at an acid pH. The key to the lysosome is its lipoprotein membrane, which can be either stabilized or weakened by a number of exogenous factors. The lysosomal membrane can be disrupted by mechanical means, by chemical means, and by enzymes. It may be stabilized by compounds such as corticosteroids, cholesterol, and chloroquine.

It is convenient to measure the activity of one or more of these enzymes as an index of lysosomal disruption; acid phosphatase and beta glucuronidase are most often measured. It is of interest that lysosomal hydrolyases have been demonstrated in the cytoplasm of proliferating fibroblasts. Several lysosomal hydrolyases have been found in the synovial fluid from inflamed joints, with levels paralleling the number of polymorphonuclear leukocytes.

While lysosomes are found in many types of cells, the polymorphonuclear leukocytes are particularly rich in them, and they constitute the familiar neutrophilic granules seen with the Wright's stain. Three mechanisms of disruption of the lysosomes of these cells have been described. (1) During phagocytosis of particulate matter the cell membrane invaginates to surround the ingested particle, forming an autophagic vacuole; the lipid wall of the lysosome fuses with the vacuole and discharges the hydrolytic enzymes into the vacuole as well as to the extracellular environment. Leukocytes exuding in response to particulate matter such as bacteria and crystals die in a few hours. (2) Certain bacterial exotoxins, such as streptolysin O and S, can rupture lysosomes within the cytoplasm of the leukocyte, resulting in rapid death of the cell. This phenomenon has led some workers to refer to lysosomes as "suicide bags." (3) A staphylococcal exotoxin, "leukocidin," causes the granules to swell into vesicles, some of which fuse with the cell membrane and rupture to the outside. The end-result in each case is a degranulated leukocyte showing the nuclear and cytoplasmic changes of cell death, and nearly every exudate rich in polymorphonuclear leukocytes has shown elevation of the activity of those enzymes which serve as an index of lysosomal disruption.

The interrelations among these various factors and their relative importance in producing the microcirculatory alterations and tissue changes characteristic of inflammation are not completely understood at the present time. Nevertheless, it is possible to examine these mechanisms as they apply to the various types of inflammatory joint disease. Much of the remainder of this chapter represents an attempt to do this.

SPECIFIC INFECTIOUS ARTHRITIS

Almost every type of microorganism can infect joint tissues and cause inflammation. Rarely, the entry to the joint is directly by laceration or by extension of infection from contiguous bone. Usually the infection is carried by the bloodstream, with initial localization of the microorganism in the synovial and subsynovial tissues. The inflammatory reaction in the joint has the same characteristics as that provoked by the particular microorganism in other body tissues.

Bacteria most commonly responsible for purulent inflammation of the joint are staphylococcus, streptococcus, gonococcus, meningococcus, and pneumococcus. Infection by these organisms in their more usual habitat may be evident but at times must be searched for carefully. The large joints, such as the hip, knee, or wrist are most commonly affected, although any articulation, either spinal or peripheral, can be involved. The process usually involves only one or a few joints, although with gonococcal or meningococcal infection there may be an early migratory phase with pain in several joints before the bacteria settle down to provoke a true septic arthritis. The inflammation is dominated by the purulent exudate, and the "leukocyte factors" are undoubtedly principally responsible for the intensity of the inflammatory reaction. These factors also account for the rapid destruction of articular cartilage which accompanies the presence of pus in the joint cavity. Proteolytic and other hydrolytic enzyme activity can be demonstrated in leukocyte autolysates, and purulent synovial fluids. Fluids containing 110,000 or more leukocytes per mm.[3] are capable of digesting small pieces of cartilage, whereas synovial fluid with leukocyte counts of 6,000 to 20,000 are not. If septic arthritis is not recognized promptly and treated with appropriate antibiotics, extensive joint destruction may occur. Also, the natural repair of joint tissue which has harbored prolonged purulent inflammation results in granulation tissue with ensuing scar formation, and fibrous ankylosis may result.

Tuberculous infection usually involves only one joint, provoking a slowly progressive low-grade synovitis dominated by the granuloma formation and proliferative inflammation characteristic of the response to the tubercle bacillus. Doughy swelling of the joint with slight to imperceptible increase in local heat may be present, owing to the thickened synovium rather than increase in synovial fluid. The tuberculous synovitis forms a pannus of granulation tissue which tends to spread over and destroy the cartilage and also infiltrates under the cartilage, resorbing the bony articular cortex and the lower layers of the cartilage. In some cases this results in detachment of the articular cartilage. Since the synovial fluid in tuberculous arthritis is not rich in proteolytic and other hydrolytic enzymes, such loosened cartilage may persist for months but is eventually destroyed. Early destruction of periarticular bone is one of the roentgenographic features of tuberculous arthritis. An exception is the knee joint, where tuberculous synovitis of low grade may persist for months or years with little discomfort and little bone destruction. However, in almost all cases the joint tuberculosis should be regarded as involving synovium, cartilage, and bone. The tuberculous process may extend into periarticular tissues, producing a "cold abscess" about the joint, or it may travel between muscle and fascial planes and drain to the exterior through sinus tracts.

Mycotic infections of the joint, which develop in the disseminated granulomatous phase of coccidioidomycosis, histoplasmosis, blastomycosis, cryptococcosis, and actinomycosis, provoke an inflammatory reaction which has many of the clinical, radiographic, and pathologic features of tuberculous arthritis.

CRYSTAL-INDUCED SYNOVITIS

Acute Gouty Arthritis

The rediscovery in 1960 of the vital role of urate crystals in the acute gouty attack has stimulated extensive studies of mechanisms involved in acute joint inflammation. Crystals of sodium urate were demonstrated to be a constant finding in synovial fluid of patients with gout and to be uniformly absent from non-gouty fluids. The presence of such crystals within leukocytes is characteristic of acute gouty inflammation. The crystals are seen in wet preparations as short rod shapes with rounded ends, or as needle-like. Under polarized light they show a strong negative birefringence, which is definitive. Injection of urate crystals ($0.5-8\mu$ in length) into the joints or subcutaneously into experimental animals or human subjects (both normal and gouty) produces an acute inflammatory response, whereas amorphous urates produce only a mild response, and urates in solution produce no response. Other crystalline substances of similar configuration produce a similar inflammatory reaction, indicating that the phenomenon is dependent on the physical rather than the chemical nature of the crystal. In man the inflammatory response strikingly resembles the acute gouty attack.

It has been convincingly demonstrated that this inflammatory response requires leukocytes. Dogs rendered profoundly leukopenic by prior administration of vinblastin or by the use of specific antileukocyte serum displayed suppression of the inflammatory response to intra-articular injection of urate crystals. The ability to respond was restored when the injected joint was perfused by blood from a normal animal. Following intra-articular injection of microcrystalline urate, the joint pressure increases and the pH of the synovial fluid falls, owing to a rise in the concentration of lactic acid resulting from increased metabolic activity of the leukocytes. The crystals are phagocytized and either destroyed or released if the leukocyte ruptures and may be reingested by others. After entry into a phagosome the plasma-derived protein coating of the crystal may be digested away by lysosomal enzymes, leading to crystal perforation of the lysosomal membrane with escape of hydrolytic enzymes into the cell sap, which is responsible for death of the cell and extracellular escape of hydrolytic enzymes.

Such observations support the concept of the pathogenesis of acute gouty arthritis as originally proposed by Seegmiller and associates. This is illustrated in Figure 17–7. The initial event is precipitation or release of urate crystals locally. The presence of even a few crystals in supersaturated body fluids promotes further crystallization. The crystals provoke a polymorphonuclear

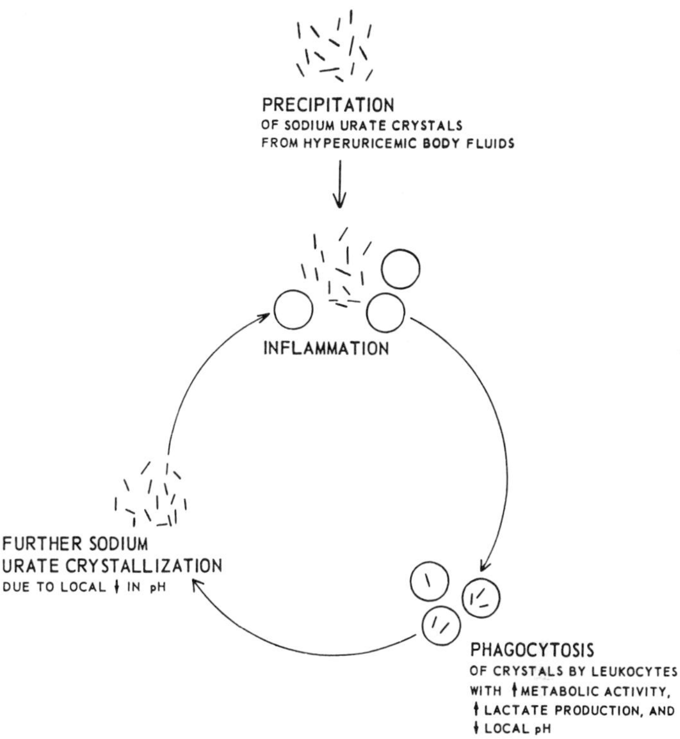

Figure 17–7 Concept of pathogenesis of acute gouty arthritis as a self-propagating inflammatory reaction. (From Seegmiller, J. E., and Howell, R. R.: Arthritis Rheum., 5:616, 1962.)

leukocyte response. These leukocytes phagocytose the urate crystals; accompanying phagocytosis, leukocyte metabolic activity increases, and lactic acid production increases, producing a lowering of local pH. Because urate solubility decreases at a more acid pH, this change tends to promote further precipitation of urate crystals and a self-perpetuating cycle is produced. Colchicine, the drug which for centuries has been the classic and highly specific treatment for the acute gouty attack, appears to interrupt this cycle by a direct effect upon the leukocyte, with inhibition of its metabolic and biological activity. One specific action has been shown to be related to inhibition of organization of microtubules within the cell. These subcellular constituents are essential to the structure and mobility of cells.

This system has also permitted study of possible mediators of the inflammatory response. Considerable evidence has accumulated to support the role of kinin polypeptides in this response. It has been demonstrated that urate crystals are capable of activating Hageman factor (factor XII). In addition to its role in initiating coagulation, Hageman factor has the ability to activate kallikrein, the enzyme regulating the formation of bradykinin from kininogen. It has been established that Hageman factor is present in normal synovial fluid and that kinins are present in the synovial fluid in acute gout (and in other inflammatory joint diseases), decreasing in con-

centration as the inflammation subsides. There is evidence that Hageman factor (and urate crystals without the intervention of Hageman factor) can activate C1-esterase; this in turn promotes activation of complement components which produce increased vascular permeability, phagocytosis, and chemotaxis. The leukocytes may also significantly contribute to the production of kinins. It has also been demonstrated that phagocytosis of crystals leads to rapid release of a chemotactic protein from the leukocyte. Alternatively, or in addition, they contribute to the inflammatory process by release of lysosomal enzymes.

Gout is fundamentally a disorder of purine metabolism, usually genetically determined but sometimes acquired, characterized by persistent elevation of urate in the plasma.

A detailed description of the mechanisms responsible for hyperuricemia will not be attempted; however, a brief review of major advances in our understanding of human purine metabolism will be undertaken. The reader is referred to recent reviews for more detailed discussion. It is now evident that hyperuricemia occurs as a result of excessive production of uric acid, reduced renal excretion, or a combination of these two events. Identification of specific enzyme defects leading to both uric acid over- and underproduction have helped to clarify the regulatory mechanism that operates in the purine pathway. Al-

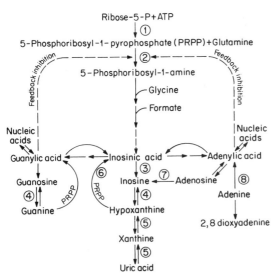

Figure 17–8 The purine pathway in man. The following enzymes are identified: (1) PRPP synthetase; (2) amidophosphoribosyltransferase; (3) 5'-nucleotidase; (4) purine nucleoside phosphorylase; (5) xanthine oxidase; (6) hypoxanthine-guanine phosphoribosyltransferase; (7) adenosine deaminase; (8) adenine phosphoribosyltransferase.

though these enzymatic defects account for only a small fraction (1–5 per cent) of gouty overproducers (20–25 per cent) within the total population of patients with primary gout, their recognition is important. Key reactions relevant to this discussion are outlined in Figure 17–8. The synthesis of purine nucleotides (adenylic, guanylic, inosinic acid) occurs directly from purine bases (adenine, guanine, hypoxanthine) or de novo from precursors which lead to the formation of inosinic acid (IMP). The latter is a common intermediate for the other purine nucleotides used in the formation of nucleic acids and critical nucleotide intermediates. Degradation of purine nucleotides leads to the formation of xanthine and, finally, uric acid. The enzyme amidophosphoribosyltransferase is the rate limiting step in de novo purine synthesis, which is itself regulated by the intracellular concentration of PRPP (Fig. 17–8). When PRPP levels in the cell are increased, the rate of uric acid synthesis is increased, and vice versa.

Clinical disorders leading to overproduction of uric acid and gout include the Lesch-Nyhan syndrome, which is due to complete deficiency of hypoxanthine-guanine phosphoribosyltransferase (HGPRT). This X-linked disorder afflicts children and is further characterized by self-mutilation, spasticity, choreoathetosis, and mental retardation. Partial deficiency of HGPRT leads to onset of acute gout and renal stone formation in patients 15 to 25 years of age who are

neurologically normal. Another enzyme abnormality leading to gout has been shown to be due to overactivity of PRPP synthetase in a small number of patients. Deficiency of this enzyme has been identified in one Japanese child who had hypouricemia, orotic acidemia, and mental retardation. The first two manifestations can be traced to the deficiency of intracellular levels of PRPP. Xanthine oxidase deficiency leads to increased urinary excretion of oxypurines and reduced plasma levels and urinary excretion of uric acid. Three patients with a homozygous deficiency of adenine phosphoribosyltransferase were found to have renal calculi composed of the compound 2,8-dioxyadenine. Recently adenosine deaminase deficiency has been identified in patients with severe combined immunodeficiency (severe T-cell and mild B-cell dysfunction). Other patients with immune deficiency disease have defects in the enzyme purine nucleoside phosphorylase. These abnormalities unrelated to aberrations in uric acid metabolism have linked purine metabolism with regulation of the immune system. Elucidation of other genetic defects relevant to gouty arthritis and their relation to the larger population of patients with primary gout are to be anticipated. The renal mechanisms of handling uric acid also require further investigation.

Clinically gout is manifested by recurrent attacks of a characteristic type of acute arthritis, by depositions of sodium urate monohydrate in and around joints of the extremities and by renal disease which may include deposits of urate crystals in the kidney and formation of urate calculi. The clinical manifestations are ultimately dependent on the fact that, even in normal humans, uric acid is present in concentrations near the limit of its solubility in body fluids.

Acute attacks of gout are characterized by abrupt onset and extremely severe inflammation which may easily be mistaken for a septic joint. Although the victim of this disease may be totally incapacitated, the synovitis subsides in several days to a week or two, with complete resolution of the inflammation and restoration of normal joint function. The concepts outlined above provide an explanation for many features of the acute episodes, including the abruptness of onset, the severity of the synovitis, and the intermittent pattern of attacks. However, the events leading to the initial crystallization of sodium urate from the supersaturated fluid are incompletely defined. Furthermore, these concepts do not clarify how and why the untreated attack resolves spontaneously.

Chronic Gouty Arthritis

In gout, urates tend to deposit in cartilage, epiphyseal bone, periarticular structures, and the kidneys. Such deposits may form visible tophi and may be responsible for permanent joint damage or chronicity of symptoms. Such urate deposition is dependent on the height of the serum uric acid concentration, the severity of the renal involvement, and the duration of the disease. Tophi are seen most often in patients who have had gout for six to ten years or more. Lowering of the serum urate concentration with appropriate medication can prevent urate deposition and can actually lead to disappearance of tophi that have previously developed.

Deposition of urates produces a local necrosis and (unless the tissue is avascular) an ensuing foreign-body reaction with proliferation of granulation tissue. In the joint, synovial proliferation with pannus formation may develop, producing chronic synovitis with capsular fibrous thickening. Deposits of urate on the surface of the articular cartilage are often present with associated cartilaginous degeneration and accelerated appearance of degerative joint changes. Destruction of subchondral bone with depositions of urate in the marrow results in the punched-out lesions of bone commonly seen in roentgenograms of gouty patients. These marrow tophi often communicate with the urate crust on the articular surface through erosions and defects in the articular cartilage.

Pseudogout

When, stimulated by the findings in gout, microscopic examination of wet preparations of synovial fluid by compensated polarized light was applied to examination of many synovial fluids, non-urate crystals were discovered in the joint fluids of patients whose clinical diseases had many features of gout. The crystals appear as rodlike or rhomboid forms with sharp corners, and under polarized light they demonstrate weakly positive birefringence. By x-ray diffraction these crystals were identified as calcium pyrophosphate dihydrate. Fluids removed from acutely inflamed joints with pseudogout invariably showed such crystals within polymorphonuclear leukocytes, indicating that they had been phagocytosed. Crystals with morphologic features identical to the natural crystals were synthesized. Injection of synthetic or natural crystals into human and canine joints was followed by acute inflammation associated with phagocytosis of the crystals by polymorphonuclear and mononuclear leukocytes. The inflammation was related in severity to the dose of crystals injected and was completely reversible. Although the details of mediation of the inflammation in this condition have not been studied as completely as in gout, it is clear that this condition is another example of crystal-induced synovitis.

As this disease was recognized, it soon became apparent that it was associated with miliary calcium deposits in fibrocartilaginous structures, articular cartilage, ligaments, and joint capsule which can be seen on roentgenograms (chondrocalcinosis). These punctate and linear densities are seen most frequently in the menisci of the knee; other fibrocartilaginous structures calcified in this fashion are the articular disks of the distal radio-ulnar articulation, the symphysis pubis, the glenoid and acetabular labra, and the annulus fibrosus of the intervertebral disks. Calcification in the hyaline articular cartilage appears as a midzonal radiopaque line paralleling the contour of the underlying bone. Calcification may also be seen in the articular capsules of the larger joints. The deposits visualized radiographically have been studied at necropsy and have been convincingly demonstrated to be calcium pyrophosphate dihydrate crystals.

The clinical pattern of the arthritis ranges from intermittent acute attacks with complete remission between attacks, to clusters of almost continuous acute episodes in a number of joints, to a chronic progressive arthritis with superimposed acute episodes. Synovial biopsy shows inflammatory and reparative changes consistent with the clinical appearance of the joint. Some patients show only a chronic progressive arthritis without acute episodes; in such patients often the crystals cannot be demonstrated in the synovial fluid. Some patients with chondrocalcinosis are completely asymptomatic, and many patients will show calcific deposits in the tissues of joints which have never been the site of acute or chronic inflammation.

The mechanism for deposition of the calcium pyrophosphate crystals in cartilage and periarticular structures is unknown. Undoubtedly, local tissue changes must be favorable for the physical-chemical formation of the crystals. Aside from the occasional patient with hyperparathyroidism, serum values for calcium and phosphorus are normal. Diseases associated with calcium pyrophosphate crystal deposition disease include hemochromatosis, hyperparathyroidism, degenerative and destructive joint disease, and possibly hypophosphatasia and neuropathic joints.

Calcareous Tendinitis (with Subacromial Bursitis)

Inflammatory involvement of tendons and contiguous bursae associated with deposition of calcium in and about the tendon is presumably another example of crystal-induced inflammation. This occurs commonly around the shoulder, with calcium deposition in one or more of the tendons in the rotator cuff, notably the supraspinatus tendon. Such deposits, visualized radiographically, are the most frequent abnormality encountered in acutely and subacutely painful shoulder. However, similar calcifications are found in many asymptomatic patients. The deposition of calcium is believed to be associated with degenerative changes in the tendon, perhaps related to wear and tear. As long as the calcium is confined to the relatively avascular fibrous tendon, it excites little or no reaction. But with encroachment into more vascular areas, a severe acute inflammatory reaction with hyperemia and edema is aroused. In the shoulder, the floor of the subacromial bursa forms part of the sheath for the supraspinatus tendon. Fluid collects within the tendon sheath and bursa and produces pressure, pain, and muscle spasm.

The calcium deposits in calcareous tendinitis have been found to resemble hydroxyapatite, although the characteristics of the inflammatory response have not been well studied. Most recently apatite crystals have been found by electron microscopic study in synovial effusion cells in acute undiagnosed arthritis and exacerbation of synovitis in patients with osteoarthritis. This suggests that apatite found as the principal normal mineral of bone can under certain circumstances induce an acute inflammatory reaction. The inflammation in calcareous tendinitis is self-limited, and subsidence may be accelerated by removal of the calcium by needle aspiration or by the injection of anti-inflammatory agents. Often, as a result of the hyperemia of the inflammation, the calcium densities seen radiographically may appear to be resorbed.

IMMUNOLOGICALLY MEDIATED INFLAMMATION

As experimental immunologic observations have been correlated with clinical experience, a workable system of general classification of the immunologic reactions producing tissue injury has emerged. As proposed by Gell and Coombs, the system is based on four general types of reactions. Those of principal interest in rheumatic diseases are types II, III, and IV, or a combination thereof. Humoral antibody responses are mediated by B lymphocytes, and cellular immune responses by T lymphocytes and their influence on mononuclear phagocytes (macrophages). Type II reactions (complement-dependent cytotoxic reactions) are dependent on the interaction of antibody with cell-bound antigen, with consequent activation of the complement system to produce cell damage or lysis. Type III reactions (immune-complex reactions) are mediated by the deposition of soluble antigen-antibody complex at a reaction site. Following complex formation, complement fixation occurs, with sequential activation of the complement system accounting for the biologic alterations of the reaction. Among the diverse biologic consequences of the interaction of antigen, antibody, and the complement system are activation of the kallikrein-kinin system, the attraction of polymorphonuclear leukocytes, and increase in capillary permeability. The kinin peptides induce vasodilatation, pain, and increased vascular permeability. The infiltrating leukocytes have been shown to ingest complexes, then to degranulate and release their lysosomal enzymes, which in turn act as even more powerful chemotactic agents and mediators of the inflammatory response.

Type IV reactions (delayed or cellular reactions) depend on the interaction of specifically sensitized small lymphocytes (T cells) with the antigen. Developmentally, these small lymphocytes with the capacity for immunologic memory are thymus-dependent. A brief and undoubtedly oversimplified summary of the mechanism of this type of delayed reaction is as follows. Contact of these small lymphocytes with antigen leads to blast transformation and biosynthetic events producing a "sensitized lymphocyte." Cell-free extracts of disrupted leukocytes from individuals displaying delayed hypersensitivity are capable of transferring this capacity to sensitize the small lymphocyte (transfer factor). Upon recurrent contact with the antigen, these sensitized lymphocytes can recruit other mononuclear cells to the reaction site by the elaboration of effector substances called lymphokines. The lymphokines can be subdivided into groups according to their biologic activity. They include cytotoxic factors, chemotactic substances, inhibitory factors, and a group of substances that activate or alter the function of macrophages. Cytolysis of antigen-bearing cells may then result from adherence of sensitized cells and elaboration of lytic substances. Under the microscope the delayed or cellular reaction may show variable accumulation of fluid and polymorphonuclear leukocytes for the first 24 hours but thereafter is dominated by mononuclear cells, predominantly macrophages and monocytes with occasional small lymphocytes. The macrophages may coalesce to form giant cells. In severe reactions, necrosis in the central portion of the lesion may develop. More detailed analysis of immune mechanisms operative in several of the rheumatic diseases can be found in Chapters 4 and 5.

Serum Sickness

The basic mechanism of serum sickness is a type III antigen-antibody interaction. In studies with suitably tagged foreign protein, the concentration of circulating antigen shows a gradual decrease for 10 to 14 days. This corresponds to the latent period between introduction of the foreign protein and the appearance of symptoms, a period of development of the immune response. Circulating antibody is not easily detected at this time because of the formation of soluble complexes with the circulating antigen. This is indicated by a sudden drop in the level of circulating antigen, and onset of the inflammatory lesions corresponds to the appearance of circulating soluble immune complexes. The disease continues until complexes are entirely removed from the circulation. Antibodies to the foreign protein are easily demonstrated in the patient's serum during convalescence and for long periods of time thereafter. Readministration of the foreign antigen leads to prompt formation of antibodies and immune complexes and recurrence of the clinical disorder.

In experimental animals, localization of immune complexes containing antigen, antibody, and complement has been demonstrated in the endothelium of vessels of several organs. In synovial tissue this immune complex deposition leads to inflammatory infiltration, edema, and tissue necrosis.

Clinically, serum sickness is characterized by fever, arthralgia, skin eruptions, and edema. Objective evidence of synovitis may be present. It is a self-limited disease, the manifestations usually subsiding in 1 to 3 weeks. With the advent of antimicrobial therapy the use of serum for the treatment of bacterial infection has declined markedly. At the present time the most common cause of serum sickness is an administered drug, most often an antibiotic.

Rheumatic Fever

Rheumatic fever is an uncommon but by no means rare sequela to an upper respiratory tract infection caused by Group A hemolytic streptococci. Although most, if not all, serologic M types of Group A streptococcal infections of the pharynx can lead to rheumatic fever, only 3 per cent or less of all patients who do not receive adequate antimicrobial treatment for streptococcal infection will develop subsequent rheumatic fever. There is a latent period of two to four weeks between the streptococcal infection and the appearance of signs and symptoms. Multiple focal aseptic inflammatory lesions are the basis of the acute manifestations. These include migratory arthritis, carditis, chorea, skin lesions, and subcutaneous nodules. The acute disease is of limited duration, but the carditis can lead to permanent valvular damage.

The arthritis in rheumatic fever is characterized by an inflammation which develops and subsides in the joints first affected, only to occur in other joints which were initially spared ("migratory polyarthritis"). The inflammation can be mild, with only vague discomfort in the region, but is often severe, with acutely inflamed red swollen joints which are very painful to touch or on attempted motion. The fluid in such joints is turbid and contains inflammatory leukocytes (Table 17–2) but is sterile on bacteriologic culture.

An immunologic mechanism in the production of at least the acute inflammatory lesions in rheumatic fever is inferred rather than established. Such a mechanism is strongly suggested in the production of the synovitis by the intriguing parallelism between the latent period of serum sickness and rheumatic fever and by the fact that the inflammation in both conditions is self-limited, subsiding completely and without residual joint damage. Antibodies to numerous components of the streptococcus appear in the circulation of patients during pharyngeal infection by this organism, regardless of whether they subsequently develop rheumatic fever. Therefore, an increase in the titer of antistreptococcal antibodies is evidence of a recent streptococcal infection and is not diagnostic of rheumatic fever. Most but not all of those who develop rheumatic fever have a higher antibody response which may persist longer than in those who do not develop this complication after streptococcal pharyngitis.

The mechanism for production of the carditis and the late valvular lesions is not clear. Autologous antibodies that react with mammalian muscle including myocardial elements occur in the sera of patients with rheumatic fever in concentrations greater than those in the sera of patients who do not develop this complication. This autologous antibody cross-reacts with a streptococcal antigen. The source of the antigenic stimulus for this antibody and the role which it plays in the pathogenesis of the disease remain to be determined.

Rheumatoid Arthritis

Much evidence has accumulated in recent years implicating immunologic mechanisms in the pathogenesis of rheumatoid arthritis. This dates from the identification over 20 years ago of the presence of autologous immune globulins ("rheumatoid factors") in the serum of most patients with rheumatoid arthritis. This immune globulin has the characteristics of an antibody to normal human gamma globulin. Later, the presence of complexes of this antigen and antibody in the leukocytes of rheumatoid synovial fluid was demonstrated. In the past few years, impressive evidence for activation of the complement system by way of both the classic and alternate pathways in rheumatoid synovial fluid has emerged. These findings correlate with the presence of immune complexes in the synovial fluid.

It has long been recognized that the sera of some patients with rheumatoid arthritis could cause the agglutination of a number of different particles. These included certain strains of streptococci and staphylococci, collodion particles, and various erythrocytes, such as those of sheep coated with subagglutinating quantities of rabbit antiserum. It was then found that the particle involved was nonspecific, and that the essential reaction was between the gamma globulin coating the particle and a factor in rheumatoid serum. It was shown that tanned sheep erythrocytes and inert particles such as latex or bentonite, when coated with gamma globulin, are agglutinated by rheumatoid sera.

The factor responsible for these reactions was identified as gamma globulin with a sedimentation constant in the ultracentrifuge of a macroglobulin (19S). It is frequently found in serum in a complex with 7S gamma globulin. Thus, classic rheumatoid factor was defined as IgM with antibody binding sites directed toward determinants of IgG. Later, globulins of the IgG (and possibly IgA) classes were found to have anti-IgG activity, and polymorphism among the rheumatoid factors is well established. Rheumatoid factors react most avidly with IgG that has been partly denatured or aggregated, presumably owing to exposure of additional binding sites by the alteration in molecular configuration. Immunofluorescent studies indicate that rheumatoid factor is produced by lymphoid tissues in the "large pale cells" in the germinal centers of lymph nodes and in plasma cells surrounding the germinal centers. The same distribution of staining is seen in the lymphoid nodules within the synovial membrane of rheumatoid joints.

As this information developed there was difficulty in visualizing the way in which rheumatoid factor was involved in producing the pathologic lesions and clinical manifestations of rheumatoid arthritis. Rheumatoid factor cannot be detected in some 30 per cent of patients who meet the criteria for the diagnosis of rheumatoid arthritis ("seronegative" rheumatoid arthritis). It has been found in high titers in other disorders without arthritis and in some normal subjects. In short-term studies, infusion of serum containing high titers of rheumatoid factor did not induce the disease in normal recipients.

By 1965, several observers using phase contrast microscopy for examination of wet film preparations of synovial fluid had demonstrated the presence of particulate inclusions in the cytoplasm of leukocytes in a high proportion of rheumatoid synovial fluids. Rheumatoid factor was released when these leukocytes were disrupted. Determinants of both IgG and rheumatoid factor were identified in these cytoplasmic particles by immunofluorescent techniques. This finding was not restricted to rheumatoid arthritis, being seen at times in other forms of inflammatory synovitis. IgM globulins were more frequently found in seropositive patients with rheumatoid arthritis, and some of these inclusion bodies were shown to contain certain components of complement. Rheumatoid synovial fluid was found to contain both kinin polypeptides and lysosomal enzymes. Reaction of rheumatoid factor with IgG complexes produced larger complexes that were phagocytosed by synovial cells and by leukocytes with release of lysosomal enzymes. Injection of autologous IgG into inactive or clinically uninvolved joints of patients with rheumatoid arthritis produced inflammation in some, but not all, patients studied.

Immunofluorescence studies demonstrated certain components of complement in tissue sections of rheumatoid synovium along with deposits of immunoglobulins. Although the serum level of complement in patients with rheumatoid arthritis is in the normal range, the complement activity of the synovial fluid usually is definitely lower in rheumatoid fluids as compared with other joint effusions. This lowered complement activity is most consistently found in the fluids from seropositive patients. Such determinations first were done in terms of total hemolytic complement activities (CH50). As the 12 serum proteins constituting the complement system (nine "components" and three "inhibitors" or "inactivators") were identified, methods became available for quantitative studies of the sequential activation of this complicated system. Several investigators have applied such methods to measure the activities of components of the complement sequence involved in both the classic and alternate (properdin) pathways in synovial fluids from patients with seropositive or seronegative rheumatoid arthritis or osteoarthritis. Certain of the fluids from seropositive patients demonstrated marked reduction in activity of the first component (C1). Although depressed activities of C1 were not uniformly found, there was ample evidence of activation of this component in the striking reduction in the second (C2) and fourth (C4) components. These two components are the natural substrates for activated C1 ($C\bar{1}$). There was also reduction of for third component (C3), indicating generation of C3 convertase by the action of $C\bar{1}$ on C4 and C2. Additional products of complement activation — namely, C3a, which increases vascular permeability, and chemotactic fragments C5a and the trimolecular complex $C\overline{567}$ — have been found in synovial fluid. Taken together, these alterations in complement component activities are consistent with the intrasynovial activation of the complement system in rheumatoid synovial fluids by an immune complex or its equivalent. Although such evidence for complement activation was most impressive in fluids from seropositive patients, borderline reductions in activities

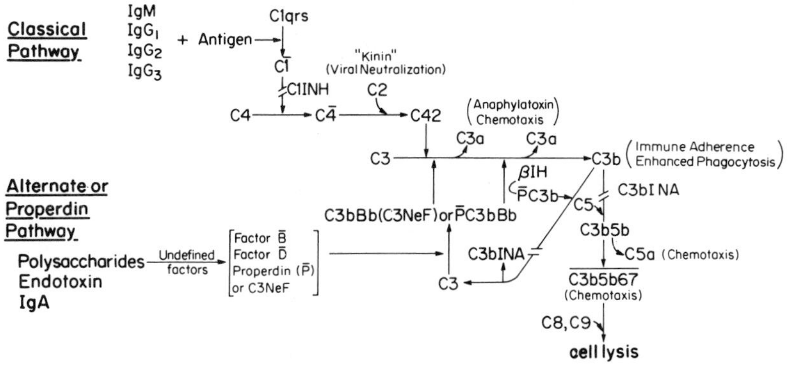

Classical Pathway

IgM
IgG$_1$
IgG$_2$ + Antigen
IgG$_3$

C1qrs

C1̄

"Kinin" (Viral Neutralization)

↓C1INH   C2

C4 ——→ C4̄ ——→ C42
Anaphylatoxin Chemotaxis

C3a   C3a

C3 ——→ ———→ C3b   Immune Adherence Enhanced Phagocytosis

βIH
P̄C3b   C5   C3bI NA

Alternate or Properdin Pathway

C3bBb(C3NeF)or P̄C3bBb   C5   C3bINA   C3b5b

Polysaccharides ——Undefined factors——→   Factor B̄ / Factor D̄ / Properdin (P̄) or C3NeF ———→   C3bINA   C5b   C5a (Chemotaxis)

Endotoxin
IgA

C3 ←———   C3b5b67 (Chemotaxis)

C8, C9

cell lysis

Figure 17–9 Pathways of complement activation and some of the biologic factors generated during the process of activation.

of the C2 and C4 components suggest that activation of C1 also occurs in fluids from seronegative patients. The reaction sequences and some of the biologic activities of complement by-products generated by activation of the complement system are outlined in Figure 17–9.

Such observations have led to the concept that immune complexes activate the complement system within the joint, with diverse biologic consequences which lead to the inflammatory response. The role of rheumatoid factor of the 7S class (7S-anti-IgG) may be particularly important in activating the complement system. Complexes of IgG–7S-anti-IgG are demonstrable in rheumatoid synovial fluid, and the extent of complement depletion can be correlated with the quantities of these complexes contained in the fluid. There is evidence that the presence of 19S (IgM) rheumatoid factor may greatly augment the activating effects of these complexes. This would account for the fact that the most profound alterations in the complement system are observed in synovial fluids from seropositive patients.

It is clear that several steps remain obscure in the elucidation of a completely satisfactory immunologic explanation of rheumatoid arthritis. The nature of the original antigenic stimulus remains unknown. The question remains whether it is an exogenous foreign antigen or an autoantigen. If the rheumatoid factors are antibodies, presumably IgG should be the antigen. Several observations suggest that some alteration in the molecular configuration of IgG is required to provide such antigenic properties. There is ultrastructural evidence that mononuclear cells within the rheumatoid synovium are undergoing blast cell transformation. There is also evidence that the synovium is heavily infiltrated with T-lymphocytes which generate immune mediators (lymphokines). Several of the latter act upon polymorphonuclear and mononuclear phagocytic cells. These cells can release lysosomal enzymes (collagenases, elastase, cathepsins, other glycosidases, proteases) which could mediate the damage to articular cartilage, soft tissues, and bone. These responses encompass almost every immune reaction found in the several forms of chronic immunologic disease.

One of the most exciting findings related to rheumatoid arthritis has been the discovery that the genes of the major histocompatibility complex (HLA system of man), specifically at the HLA-D region, show strong correlation with this disease. This association is with immune response genes (Ir genes) which exercise control over the entire immune system. It has been shown that HHL-A-Dw4 identified by mixed lymphocyte culture reaction occurs in up to 40 per cent of patients with classic rheumatoid arthritis. It is presumed that through further study a locus with even higher association will be found. It is assumed that the frequent association of ankylosing spondylitis and Reiter's disease (not discussed in the chapter) with the HLA-B27 antigen (>90 per cent) is a similar marker for a yet unidentified Ir gene abnormality. Further details regarding the HLA system and disease can be found in other recent publications on this topic.

In contrast to some of the other immunologically mediated forms of arthritis, rheumatoid synovitis is characterized by fluctuating but continuing inflammatory activity with predominance of the proliferative and granulomatous reaction. The basis for this chronicity is not easily explained. There may well be continuing release of biologically active substances by the mechanisms outlined above, but the process may also be perpetuated by other means. Several differences in the biologic activity of fibroblasts from rheumatoid synovium as compared to normals have been reported. These "abnormalities" are reproducible on successive subculture. Comparable "abnormalities" in the biologic activity of normal

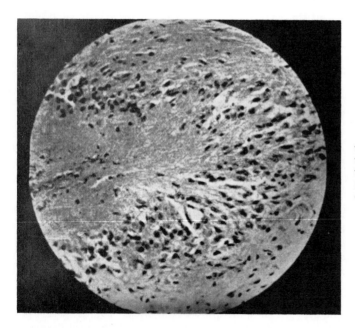

Figure 17–10 Extra-articular inflammatory lesions in rheumatoid arthritis. Subcutaneous rheumatoid nodule. Note the central zone of fibrinoid necrosis, the middle palisading zone of epithelioid cells, and the outer fibrous zone.

fibroblasts in culture result from the addition of small amounts of "connective tissue activating peptide," which is widely distributed in mammalian cells (including lymphocytes and platelets). Substantial amounts of these peptides can be extracted from leukocytes and from the granulation tissue of rheumatoid joints.

Rheumatoid arthritis, however, is not just a localized disease of the joints. It is a systemic disease, and constitutional manifestations such as ease of fatigue, weight loss, weakness, and at times fever and anemia are common. The outstanding characteristic is a chronic proliferative synovitis in multiple joints with a predilection for smaller joints such as the proximal interphalangeal, the metacarpal-phalangeal, and the metatarsal-phalangeal and a tendency for symmetrical distribution of the joint involvement once the disease has become established. Yet inflammatory lesions are seen throughout the connective tissues of the body. Both the constitutional symptoms and the inflammatory activity are subject to fluctuations in severity, with a strong tendency to remission and exacerbations without apparent reason.

Prominent among the extra-articular manifestations is the rheumatoid nodule. These nodules occur in 20 to 30 per cent of patients at some time during the course of their disease. They arise as a microvascular lesion and are found most frequently in patients positive for rheumatoid factors. These are granulomas with a characteristic microscopic appearance (Fig. 17–10). They are most common over bony prominences and often are attached to the articular capsule or to bursae, but they may be attached to the periosteum, lie loose in the subcutaneous tissue, or involve the deeper layers of the skin. They may persist for months or years. Such nodules are occasionally seen in pleura and pulmonary tissue, and actually have been found in virtually every connective tissue structure throughout the body. Other systemic manifestations include pericarditis, pleuritis with or without effusion, rheumatoid pneumoconiosis, scleritis, uveitis, peripheral neuropathy, and vasculitis. Vasculitis may be found in about 15 per cent of patients with rheumatoid arthritis, and an arteritis, at times difficult to distinguish from polyarteritis nodosa, is occasionally encountered in severe cases. The occurrence of these extra-articular lesions can be correlated in many instances with the presence of serum antinuclear antibodies, and deposition of immunoglobulins and complement in vessel walls in affected tissues. It may also be significant that more than 95 per cent of patients with nodules are seropositive for rheumatoid factor, and that patients with the severe complications of rheumatoid arthritis usually have uncommonly high titers for rheumatoid factor in their circulating blood.

Systemic Lupus Erythematosus

Systemic lupus erythematosus (SLE) is a chronic autoimmune disease affecting connective tissue, cells, and many organ systems, either individually or in various combinations. The clinical course may be fulminating or indolent but usually is characterized by periods of remission and exacerbations. Typically, patients with this disease manifest a host of immune phenomena, with circulating antibodies to their own cells, cell constituents, and proteins. Among these, particular significance is usually attributed to antibodies to nuclear materials. One of these antinuclear antibodies (deoxyribonucleoprotein, anti-DNP) is responsible for the LE cell phenomenon — an in-vitro "happening" dependent on the traumatization of some leukocytes with release of nuclear material, then the binding of the antibodies to nuclear material, and the subsequent phagocytosis of this complex by white blood cells, usually polymorphonuclear neutrophils. In the sera of patients with SLE there are multiple antinuclear antibodies with specificities to various nuclear constituents. These include double stranded DNA, (ds DNA); single stranded DNA (ss DNA); histones; non-histone acidic nuclear proteins (Sm, RNP, others). Antibodies to ds DNA are felt to be almost specific for SLE; however, antibodies to ss DNA and denatured DNA may react with incompletely purified test antigen. Detection of antibodies to Sm antigen have been found to be highly diagnostic of SLE. Identification of antinuclear antibodies using cell or tissue section substrates and indirect immunofluorescent techniques is positive in 95 to 100 per cent of patients with SLE.

Clinically, SLE has a bewildering array of acute and chronic manifestations. Nearly all patients have constitutional symptoms, ranging from malaise and weight loss to high fever and prostration in fulminating cases. Ninety per cent will have joint and muscle pain, and of these about 70 per cent will have objective evidence of synovitis. Most characteristic is episodic inflammatory arthritis, especially of joints around the hands and feet, which develops rapidly and persists for only a few days. Although more persistent synovitis can occur, major joint swelling, capsular thickening, development of deformities, and ankylosis are uncommon. A variety of skin and mucous membrane lesions occur, especially in skin areas exposed to the sun. The identification of immunoglobulin deposits in the basement membrane of biopsies of normal and involved skin ("Band Test") by direct immunofluorescence is a useful diagnostic procedure. The classic erythematous "butterfly rash" on both cheeks and over the bridge of the nose is seen in less than half the patients. Involvement of serosal surfaces with pleuritis, pericarditis, or, less often, peritonitis may dominate the clinical picture. There may be pulmonary infiltrates. The myocardium and endocardium can be involved as well as the pericardium. Depression of one or more of the formed elements in the blood with anemia, neutropenia, or thrombocytopenia is common. The Coombs' antiglobulin test is frequently positive. Involvement of the central nervous system may be reflected in organic neurologic disturbances or psychiatric syndromes, and peripheral neuropathy is not uncommon. Elevations of spinal fluid gamma globulin levels occur during CNS involvement; however, detection of depressed C4 complement content is unreliable as an index of cerebritis owing to technical problems. Renal involvement occurs in about half of patients with SLE, presenting as either nephritis or the nephrotic syndrome. SLE is frequently the explanation for false positive serologic reactions for syphilis. Rarely do all these manifestations occur at the same time in any one patient, but they may present simultaneously in various combinations. When it is possible to follow patients with SLE over long periods of time the sequential development of these varied manifestations is impressive. Such acute episodes, dominated at one time by one manifestation and later by another, are often separated by months or years of apparent good health.

The pathologic changes of SLE, even in organs and tissues known to be clinically involved, are often minor when examined by usual histologic techniques. Vasculitis and fibrinoid deposition produced by immunologic mechanisms are the most common findings in inflammatory sites such as pleura, pericardium, synovium, skin lesions, and in Libman-Sacks non-bacterial verrucous endocarditis. Vasculitis can involve venules, capillaries and arterioles, and occasionally arteries. Fibrinoid is an amorphous eosinophilic material deposited along tissue fibers and in blood vessels. By immunofluorescent methods fibrin and serum proteins, including immunoglobulins, complement, and DNA, have been detected in fibrinoid. Deposits of immune complexes have been eluted from glomeruli taken from patients with SLE. The only in-vivo analogue of the LE cell is the "hematoxylin body," a rounded hematoxylin-stained mass, roughly the size of nuclei, occasionally seen in areas of inflammation.

Renal involvement in SLE is of special interest. From a practical point of view, progressive impairment of renal function terminating in uremia is still a common cause of death in this disease. The renal involvement also provides the best insight into immunologic mechanisms which are important in the pathogenesis of SLE. The renal lesions may vary from mild to severe. The mildest form consists of deposits of immunoglobulins (chiefly IgG) and complement (especially C3) in the mesangium and along the glomerular basement membrane, without any other apparent abnormality. The most common renal lesion is focal glomerulitis with fibrinoid change, focal thickening of basement membrane, and slight increase in cellularity. These changes have been found in patients in the absence of clinical evidence of nephritis. In SLE glomerulonephritis these lesions are more generalized and severe, with a mixture of proliferative and membranous changes and hypercellularity leading to crescent formation. Some kidneys show only a diffuse membranous glomerulonephritis with considerable thickening of the glomerular basement but little hypercellularity.

It is in SLE nephritis that the most definite changes in the immune mechanisms have been noted. The LE cell phenomenon and the titer of antibody to nucleoprotein do not correlate closely with clinical activity of the disease or with the presence or absence of renal involvement. However, the titers of antibodies to DNA are characteristically higher during periods of clinical activity, especially nephritis, than during remissions. Minute amounts of DNA have been demonstrated in serum at the same time that anti-DNA antibodies are present. Markedly decreased levels of circulating complement are seen primarily in active lupus glomerulitis. This can be measured as whole complement (CH50) or complement components (C3 and C4). Less impressive decreases in complement levels occur at some time during the course of SLE in 95 per cent of patients. These low levels are evidence of in-vivo activation of the complement system and fixation of complement components by circulating immune complexes.

The demonstration of these immunologic phenomena has led to the concept that these antibodies with determinants directed against the patient's own cells, cell constituents, and proteins are "autoantibodies," and that SLE, rheumatoid arthritis, and related diseases are "autoimmune" diseases. The nature of the antigenic stimulus in SLE remains a mystery. A viral etiology for SLE has long been suspected. This possibility has received added impetus by the study of animal models of SLE (NZB/NZW mouse) where type-C virus is present, and by detection, under the electron microscope, of cytoplasmic microtubules in the glomerular endothelium of patients with this disease. Although not specific or pathognomonic for SLE, such virus-like particles are demonstrable very frequently in the kidneys and other tissues of patients with the disease, and their recognition has some diagnostic value. However, these particles may represent ultrastructural manifestations of endothelial cell injury due either to secondary imposition of a viral infection in a more vulnerable host or tissue or to some other deleterious mechanism. The pathogenic significance of virus infection in the initiation of SLE may be clarified by further studies of excellent animal models (mouse, dog) that simulate human SLE.

OTHER CONNECTIVE TISSUE DISEASES

Other diseases often grouped together with rheumatoid arthritis, rheumatic fever, and SLE under the heading of connective tissue diseases ("collagen diseases") are progressive systemic sclerosis, polymyositis, and polyarteritis nodosa. Recently, an additional disorder referred to as "mixed connective tissue disease" has been described. These diseases of unknown etiology are grouped together because of common or overlapping clinical and histopathologic features. An estimate of prevalence of these diseases per 1.0 million population per year compared to rheumatoid arthritis (500) and SLE (30) is 12 cases of progressive systemic sclerosis, 10 cases of polymyositis, and is undetermined for polyarteritis nodosa. The common histologic features are widespread inflammatory damage to connective tissues and blood vessels, often associated with deposition of immune material. Clinical findings which justify a common grouping include the occurrence of major features of more than one entity in the same patient; sequential transitions between one entity and another in the same patient; suggestions of familial aggregation of more than one disease; and serologic abnormalities which predominate in one entity but have an appreciable incidence in others. For example, approximately 15 per cent of patients with rheumatoid arthritis have positive tests for antinuclear antibodies, while 15 to 20 per cent of patients with SLE have positive serologic reactions for rheumatoid factor.

Progressive systemic sclerosis (scleroderma) was first recognized as a disease of the skin characterized by dermal fibrosis and fixation of the skin to underlying structures. Later, involvement of visceral organs (notably gastrointestinal tract, lungs, kidney, and heart) were recognized as part of the same process. The pathologic lesions are essentially those of mild to moderate vascular inflammation followed by excessive laying down of collagen in both appropriate and inappropriate sites, with ensuing fibrosis. There is limited evidence of a qualitative abnormality in this excessive collagen. In vitro cultures of scleroderma fibroblasts show augmented synthesis of collagen which is sensitive to serum supplementation. About 70 per cent of patients with progressive systemic sclerosis have circulating antinuclear antibodies, usually of the type directed against various components of the nuclear material rather than against nucleoprotein. Also in contrast to patients with SLE, immunochemical analysis of the vascular lesions in systemic sclerosis has not demonstrated deposition of immunoglobulins or complement. Rheumatoid factor is present in 20 to 40 per cent of patients with systemic sclerosis. Recently a late cell mediated immune abnormality has been ascribed to a subclass of T cells in some patients. Perhaps a cell-mediated immune reaction may prove to be involved in the pathogenesis of this disease.

Polymyositis (also termed dermatomyositis if

there is an associated dermatitis) is a less common disease in which weakness of skeletal muscle is the outstanding clinical feature. Although inflammatory degenerative and regenerative changes are seen in the muscle, inflammation and pain are rarely prominent among the clinical manifestations. Aside from dysphagia due to involvement of muscle in the pharynx and upper third of the esophagus, visceral involvement is rare. Occasionally, patients show features of both polymyositis and systemic sclerosis. Overlapping with features of rheumatoid arthritis and SLE also occurs at times. The muscle biopsy may show edema and inflammatory cells, particularly around blood vessels in the connective tissue between muscle fibers, with degeneration of muscle fibers and phagocytosis of remnants of muscle necrosis. Other features include evidence of efforts at muscle regeneration, non-necrotizing perivasculitis, and interstitial fibrosis.

Evidence of muscle involvement can be documented by electromyographic abnormalities and by characteristic biochemical changes. Release of several enzymes normally found in muscle is reflected by elevated serum levels of creatinine phosphokinase, aldolases, transaminases, and lactic dehydrogenases. There is usually creatinuria. Measurement of serum myoglobin levels provides a new approach to evaluation of disease activity. An immunologic mechanism has been suggested by the association of malignant disease in 15 to 20 per cent of adults with polymyositis, but attempts to demonstrate antibodies to the patient's own tumor have rarely been successful. About 5 per cent of patients with polymyositis exhibit the LE cell phenomenon; frequency of positive tests for rheumatoid factor has ranged from 10 to 50 per cent in various series. In vitro studies indicate that lymphocytes from polymyositis patients are cytotoxic for skeletal muscle cells, suggesting that a cell-mediated abnormality is present in this disease.

Mixed Connective Tissue Disease (MCTD) is defined as a disorder characterized by overlapping features of systemic lupus erythematosus, progressive systemic sclerosis, and polymyositis. Serologically, these patients have been shown to have antibody to ribonucleoprotein (RNP), a ribonuclease-sensitive antigenic component of extractable nuclear antigen (ENA) in high titer. ENA, isolated chemically from calf thymus, has been reported to be a loose molecular complex with several antigenic sites. Two major antigenic components are RNP and a ribonuclease-resistant non-nucleoprotein fraction termed Sm. Besides Sm, other minor antigenic components have been found in the ribonuclease-insensitive ENA fraction. The antibody to RNP, although found in high titer in MCTD, has been found in patients with SLE, progressive systemic sclerosis, and in some series in patients with polymyositis or cases with "undifferentiated connective tissue disease." A recent multicenter study of MCTD demonstrated that the most common clinical features of this disorder include Raynaud's phenomenon, polyarthralgia and arthritis, swollen hands, esophageal hypomobility, abnormal pulmonary diffusion capacity, inflammatory myositis, speckled nuclear fluorescent antinuclear antibodies, and high titers of RNP antibodies. In contrast to those with SLE, these patients appear to have a low incidence of nephritis, and are said to demonstrate a good response to corticosteroid therapy. Long-term follow-up of these patients is required before their ultimate prognosis can be established. It is clear that not all patients with overlapping features of the several major forms of connective tissue disease can be accounted for as cases of MCTD. It is worth noting that MCTD is the first connective tissue disease originally identified by an antibody reaction to a nuclear antigen followed by correlation of this response (anti-RNP antibody) with clinical symptomatology.

Polyarteritis Nodosa (Periarteritis Nodosa)

The term polyarteritis is applied to a disease characterized pathologically by inflammation and fibrinoid necrosis of medium-sized or small arteries. The widespread distribution of these arterial lesions produces a diversity of clinical manifestations which depend on the particular organ system which has suffered impairment of its arterial supply. Common presentations include renal disease, hypertension, abdominal symptoms which may simulate conditions requiring emergency surgery, coronary artery disease, cerebrovascular disease, peripheral neuritis, and fever of unknown origin with weight loss. A majority of patients complain of migratory muscle and joint aching, but true synovitis is uncommon.

The pathologic lesions typically involve one or more segments of small or medium-sized arteries with necrosis, fibrinoid change, and infiltration with polymorphonuclear neutrophils and varying numbers of eosinophils. The media is involved with extension to the intima and adventitia. Weakening of the arterial wall may lead to dissection or aneurysmal dilatation with rupture and hemorrhage. As the areas of fibrinoid necrosis are replaced by cellular granulation tissue, proliferation of the intima may lead to thrombosis with arterial occlusion and infarction. As the involved segment is finally replaced by scar tissue the periarterial fibrosis may be sufficient in rare instances to produce gross nodules and partial vascular occlusion. Characteristically, both fresh and healing inflammatory lesions are found together in an individual case.

No clear line of demarcation can be drawn between the pathologic lesions of polyarteritis and other types of systemic necrotizing angiitis, including those which may be associated with any of the other connective tissue diseases. Necrotizing vascular lesions resembling those of human polyarteritis can be produced in rabbits by repeated injections of foreign protein. Indeed, it was from such studies that the current understanding of the mechanism of serum sickness and the concept of the type III immunologic reaction developed. Recent evidence that some patients with polyarteritis have chronic hepatitis B (HBs) antigenemia has led to the demonstration that vascular lesions result from deposition of immune complexes containing HBs antigen. The circulating immune complexes form in the presence of excess viral antigen. The clinical findings in these cases compared to patients who were HBs antigen negative were quite comparable. The extent to which this important finding can be correlated with all cases of "classic form" polyarteritis remains undetermined. In recent series HBs positive cases have accounted for as few as 10 per cent to as many as 41 per cent of patients with polyarteritis. Some of the HBs-positive patients were found to have chronic active hepatitis. Response to treatment did not differ in HBs-positive or negative cases. There is a very low incidence of positive tests for either rheumatoid factor or antinuclear antibodies in patients with polyarteritis. Some pathologists distinguish the angiitis (hypersensitivity angiitis) related to hypersensitivity to serum and drugs from classic polyarteritis on the basis of inflammatory and necrotic changes in arterioles and venules (which are characteristically spared in classic polyarteritis); the development of changes first in the intima and then by extension involving the entire vessel wall; the relatively uniform character of the lesions at any particular evolutionary stage; and the frequent involvement of pulmonary vessels. It seems reasonable to conclude that several syndromes associated with necrosis and inflammation of arteries cannot yet be clearly distinguished, and that they may well be produced by diverse mechanisms.

NONARTICULAR RHEUMATISM

In addition to the diseases which affect the joints themselves, discomfort and dysfunction of the musculoskeletal system can be caused by disorders of the muscles which move the joints, by neurologic diseases, and by circulatory disturbances. Pain and interference with joint function can also be produced by disorders in periarticular connective tissue structures such as tendons, tendon sheaths, bursae, and fascia; these are termed non-articular rheumatism.

Inflammation of tendon sheaths (tenosynovitis) and bursae can result from specific infections, with or without accompanying joint involvement. Sterile inflammation of these structures occurs in rheumatoid arthritis, gout, and systemic lupus erythematosus; it may also develop as a local disturbance without other disease. Bursitis around the shoulder has been discussed under the heading of calcareous tendinitis. Inflammation of tendons and bursae located around the elbows, knees, ischial tuberosities, hips, and Achilles' tendons can cause similar pain and interference with function of the adjacent joint, although seldom as troublesome as that produced by bursitis around the shoulder. Tenosynovitis may interfere with free motion of the enclosed tendon, impairing motion of the joint moved by the tendon. The sheaths of the flexor tendons of the fingers are common sites of such inflmmation, with fibrous tissue reaction leading to adhesive tenosynovitis, so that if the finger is flexed, it cannot be extended without assistance ("trigger finger"). In some cases, inflammation of the flexor tendon sheaths and palmar fascia may result in adhesions so strong that the fingers become fixed in a partially flexed position. A fibroblastic reaction in the palmar fascia may cause adhesions with contractures resulting in flexion deformities of the fourth and fifth fingers (Dupuytren's contracture).

Primary fibrositis is the term applied to a symptom complex characterized by generalized or localized muscle stiffness and discomfort, particularly after rest, made worse by cold and usually alleviated by heat, massage, and exercise. It is also called "muscular rheumatism." It may occur in acute attacks, accounting for the "stiff neck" or low back pain of "lumbago," which nearly everyone experiences at some time in life. It may also occur in more chronic forms, involving many structures at one time, or it may migrate from one part to another. Although the name fibrositis implies an inflammation of fibrous tissue, biopsies have failed to show histologic abnormalities in either connective tissue or muscle. The symptom complex is presumed to be an expression of localized biochemical disturbances in the muscle or connective tissue. Sleep disturbances have been demonstrated in some patients with fibrositis syndrome; however, the exact significance of this finding remains obscure.

Like any other system in the body, the musculoskeletal system may serve as the means of somatic expression of psychiatric disorders. Such expression is more common in psychoneurosis than in psychosis, although complaints referred to the musculoskeletal system are not uncommon in depression. Such manifestations are sometimes termed "psychogenic rheumatism."

REFERENCES

Structure and Function of Connective Tissue

Castor, C. W.: Synovial cell activation induced by a polypeptide mediator. Ann. N.Y. Acad. Sci., *256*:304, 1975.

Copenhaver, W. M., Bunge, R. P., and Bunge, M. B. (eds.): Bailey's Textbook of Histology, 16th ed. Williams & Wilkins Co. Baltimore, 1971.

Gallop, P. M., Blumenfeld, O. O., and Seifter, S.: Structure and metabolism of connective tissue proteins. Annu. Rev. Biochem., *41*:617, 1972.

Grant, M. E., and Prockop, D. J.: The biosynthesis of collagen. N. Engl. J. Med., *286*:194, *242*, 291, 1972.

Gross, J.: Collagen biology: structure, degradation, and disease. Harvey Lect., *68*:351, 1973.

Harris, E. D., and Krane, S. M.: Collagenases. N. Engl. J. Med., *291*:557, *605*, 652, 1974.

Pras, M., and Glynn, L. E.: Isolation of a noncollagenous reticulin component and its primary characterization. Br. J. Exp. Pathol., *54*:449, 1973.

Rosenberg, L., Margolis, R., Wolfenstein-Todel, C., Pal, S., and Strider, W.: Organization of extracellular matrix in bovine articular cartilage. *In* Slavkin, H. C., and Greulich, R. C. (eds.): Extracellular Matrix Influences on Gene Expression. Academic Press, New York, 1975.

Ross, R.: The elastic fiber: A review. J. Histochem. Cytochem., *21*:199, 1973.

Schubert, M., and Hamerman, D. (eds.): A Primer on Connective Tissue Biochemistry. Lea & Fibeger, Philadelphia, 1968.

Silbert, J. E.: Biosynthesis of mucopolysaccharides and protein-polysaccharides. *In* Perez-Tamayo, R., and Rojkind, M. (eds.): Molecular Pathology of Connective Tissues. Marcel Dekker, New York, 1973.

Wahl, L. M., Wahl, S. M., Mergenhagen, S. E., and Martin, G. R.: Collagenase production by lymphokine-activated macrophages. Science, *187*:261, 1975.

Structure and Function of Joints

Castor, C. W.: Microscopic structure of human synovial tissue. Arthritis Rheum., *3*:140, 1960.

Engin, A. E., and Korde, M. S.: Biomechanics of normal and abnormal knee joint. J. Biomechanics, 7:325, 1974.

Gardner, E.: Structure and function of joints. *In* Hollander, J. L. (ed.): Arthritis and Allied Conditions. Lea & Febiger, Philadelphia, 1972.

Hascall, V. C., and Heinegård, D.: Aggregation of cartilage proteoglycans. I. The role of hyaluronic acid. J. Biol. Chem., *249*:4232, 1974.

Kempson, G. E., Muir, H., and Pollard, C.: The tensile properties of the cartilage of human femoral condyles related to the content of collagen and glycosaminoglycans. Biochim. Biophys. Acta, *292*:456, 1973.

Kremer, D., Deodhar, S. D., and Dick, W. C.: A function of synovial membrane of normal and diseased humans in relation to movement of small-molecular-weight ions. Clin. Sci., *44*:611, 1973.

Radin, E. L.: The physiology and degeneration of joints. Semin. Arthritis Rheum., *2*:245, 1973.

Woodburne, R. T. (ed.): Essentials of Human Anatomy. Oxford University Press, New York, 1973.

Pathologic Changes of Joint Disease

Bennett, G. A., Waine, H., and Bauer, W.: Changes in the Knee Joint at Various Ages, with Particular Reference to the Development of Degenerative Joint Disease. Commonwealth Fund, New York, 1942.

Howell, D. S., and Moskowitz, R. W.: Symposium on osteoarthritis. Arthritis Rheum., *20*:S96, 1977 (Suppl.).

Jessar, R. A.: The Synovial Fluid. *In* Hollander, J. L. (ed.): Arthritis and Allied Conditions. Lea & Febiger, Philadelphia, 1972.

Lichtenstein, L.: Diseases of Bone and Joints. C. V. Mosby Co., St. Louis, 1975.

Muir, H.: Molecular approach to the understanding of osteoarthrosis. (Heberden Oration, 1976). Ann. Rheum. Dis., *36*:199, 1977.

Pinals, R. S.: Traumatic arthritis and allied conditions. *In* Hollander, J. L. (ed.): Arthritis and Allied Conditions. Lea & Febiger, Philadelphia, 1972.

Ropes, M. W., and Bauer, W.: Synovial Fluid Changes in Joint Disease. Harvard University Press, Cambridge, 1953.

Serafini-Fracassini, A., and Smith, J. W.: The Structure and Biochemistry of Cartilage. Churchill, Livingston (Longman Inc.), Edinburgh, 1974.

Ziff, M.: Symposium on rheumatoid arthritis. Arthritis Rheum., *20*:S31, 1977 (Suppl.).

Pathogenesis of Joint Inflammation

Coleman, R. W., Mason, J. W., and Sherry, S.: The kallikreinogen-kallikreinin enzyme systems of human plasma. Assay of components and observations in disease states. Ann. Intern. Med., *71*:763, 1969.

DeDuve, C.: The lysosome. Sci. Am., *208*:64, 1963.

Mannik, M., and Haakenstad, A. O.: Circulation and glomerular deposition of immune complexes. Arthritis Rheum., *20*:S148, 1977 (Suppl.).

Robinson, D. R., McGuire, M. B., and Levene, L.: Prostaglandins in the rheumatic diseases. Ann. N. Y. Acad. Sci., *256*:318, 1975.

Stossel, T. P.: Phagocytosis. N. Engl. J. Med., *290*:717, 774, 833, 1974.

Ward, P. A.: Part V. Acute and chronic inflammation. The inflammatory mediators. Ann. N.Y. Acad. Sci., *221*:290, 1974.

Weissmann, G.: Lysosomes and rheumatoid joint inflammation. Arthritis Rheum., *20*:S193, 1977 (Suppl.).

Wihelm, D. L.: Mechanism responsible for increased vascular permeability in acute inflammation. Agents Actions, *3*:297, 1973.

Willoughby, D. A., Coot, A., and Turk, J. L.: Complement in acute inflammation. J. Pathol., *97*:295, 1969.

Specific Infectious Arthritis

Berney, S., Goldstein, M., and Bishko, F.: Clinical and diagnostic features of tuberculous arthritis. Am. J. Med., *53*:36, 1972.

Brandt, K. D., Cathcart, E. S., and Cohen, A. S.: Gonococcal arthritis: clinical features correlated with blood, synovial fluid, and genitourinary cultures. Arthritis Rheum., *17*:503, 1974.

Goldenberg, D., and Cohen, A. S.: Acute infectious arthritis. A review of patients with nongonococcal joint infections. Am. J. Med., *60*:369, 1976.

Handsfield, H. H., Wiesner, P. J., and Holmes, K. K.: Treatment of the gonococcal arthritis-dermatitis syndrome. Ann. Intern. Med., *84*:661, 1976.

Karten, I.: Septic arthritis complicating rheumatoid arthritis. Ann. Intern. Med., *70*:1147, 1969.

Lightfoot, R. W., and Gotschlich, E. C.: Gonococcal disease. Am. J. Med., *56*:347, 1974.

Crystal-Induced Synovitis

Kellermeyer, R. W., and Breckenridge, R. T.: The inflammatory process in acute gouty arthritis. I. Activation of Hageman factor by sodium urate crystals. J. Lab. Clin. Med., *65*:307, 1965.

Kelley, W. N.: Symposium on gout and other disorders of purine metabolism. Arthritis Rheum. *20*:S219, 1977.

Klineberg, A. R. (ed.): Proceedings of the second conference on gout and purine metabolism. Arthritis Rheum., *18*:659, 1975 (Suppl.).

McCarty, D. J. (ed.): Proceedings of the conference on pseudogout and pyrophosphate metabolism. Arthritis Rheum., *19*:275, 1976 (Suppl.).

McCarty, D. J., Jr., and Hollander, J. L.: Identification of urate crystals in gouty synovial fluid. Ann. Intern. Med., *54*:452, 1961.

McCarty, D. J., Kohn, N. N., and Faires, J. S.: The significance of calcium phosphate crystals in the synovial fluid of arthritis patients: The "pseudogout syndrome." I. Clinical aspects. Ann. Intern. Med., 56:711, 1962.

Phelps, P., and McCarty, D. J., Jr.: Crystal induced inflammation in canine joints. II. Importance of polymorphonuclear leukocytes. J. Exp. Med., 124:115, 1966.

Seegmiller, J. E., and Howell, R. R.: the old and new concepts of acute gouty arthritis. Arthritis Rheum., 5:616, 1962.

Shumacher, H. R., Somlyo, A. P., Tse, R. L., and Mauer, K.: Arthritis associated with apatite crystals. Ann. Intern. Med., 87:411, 1977.

Thompson, G. R., Ting, Y. M., Riggs, G. A., Fenn, M. E., and Denning, R. M.: Calcific tendinitis and soft tissue calcification resembling gout. J.A.M.A., 203:464, 1968.

Wyngaarden, J. B.: Gout and Hyperuricemia. Grune & Stratton, New York, 1976.

IMMUNOLOGICALLY MEDIATED INFLAMMATION

Austen, K. F.: Inborn and acquired abnormalities of the complement system of man. Trans. Assoc. Am. Physicians, 83:49, 1970.

Castor, C. W.: Connective tissue activation. II. Abnormalities of cultured rheumatoid cells. Arthritis Rheum., 14:55, 1971.

Dixon, F. J.: Experimental Serum Sickness. In Samter, M. (ed.): Immunologic Diseases. Little, Brown & Co., Boston, 1965.

Dubois, E. L. (ed.): Lupus Erythematosus. A Review of The Current Status of Discoid and Systemic Lupus Erythematosus and Their Variants. University of Southern California Press, Los Angeles, 1974.

Evans, R. L., Beard, J. M., Lazarus, H., Schlossman, S. F., and Chess, L.: Detection, isolation, and functional characterization of two human T-cell subclasses being unique differentiation antigens. J. Exp. Med., 145:221, 1977.

Gell, P. G. H., and Coombs, R. R. A. (eds.): Clinical Aspects of Immunology, 2nd ed. F. A. Davis Co., Philadelphia, 1969.

Glynn, L. E., and Schlumberger, H. D. (eds.): Experimental Models of Chronic Inflammatory Diseases. Springer-Verlag, Berlin, 1977.

Hargraves, M. M.: The L.E. cell phenomenon. Adv. Intern. Med., 6:133, 1954.

Hollander, J. L., McCarty, D. J., Jr., Astorga, G., and Castro-Murrilo, E.: Studies on the pathogenesis of rheumatoid inflammation. I. The "R.A." cell and a working hypothesis. Ann. Intern. Med., 62:271, 1965.

Kunkel, H. G.: The immunologic approach to SLE. Arthritis Rheum., 20:s139, 1977 (Suppl.).

Lawrence, H. S.: Transfer factor. Adv. Immunol., 11:195, 1969.

McCluskey, R. T., and Cohen, S. (Eds.): Mechanisms of Cell Mediated Immunity. John Wiley & Sons, New York, 1974.

Mellors, R. C., Heimer, R., Corcos, J., and Korngold, L.: Cellular origin of rheumatoid factor. J. Exp. Med., 110:875, 1959.

Miescher, P. A., and Müller-Eberhard, H. J. (eds.): Textbook of Immunopathology, 2nd ed. (Vols. I and II). Grune & Stratton, New York, 1976.

Pekin, T. J., and Zvaifler, N. J.: Hemolytic complement in synovial fluid. J. Clin. Invest., 43:1372, 1964.

Pollack, V. E., and Pirani, C. L.: Renal histologic findings in SLE. Mayo Clin. Proc., 46:630, 1969.

Ruddy, S., and Austen, K. F.: The complement system in rheumatoid arthritis. Arthritis Rheum., 13:713, 1970.

Ruddy, S., Gigli, I., and Austen, K. F.: The complement system in man. N. Engl. J. Med., 287:489, 545, 592, 642, 1972.

Sasazuki, T., McDevitt, H. O., and Grumet, F. C.: The association between genes in the major histocompatibility complex and disease susceptibility. Ann. Rev. Med., 28:425, 1977.

Stastny, P.: HLA-D typing in rheumatoid arthritis. Arthritis Rheum., 20:S45, 1977 (Suppl.).

Stollerman, G. H.: Rheumatic Fever and Streptococcal Infection. Grune & Stratton, New York, 1975.

Tisher, C. C., Kelso, H. B., Robinson, R. R., Gunnels, J. C., and Burkholder, P. M.: Intraendothelial inclusions in kidneys of patients with systemic lupus erythematosus. Ann. Intern. Med., 75:537, 1971.

Williams, R. C.: Lymphocyte abnormalities in rheumatoid arthritis. Arthritis Rheum., 20:s35, 1977 (Suppl.).

Williams, R. C.: Rheumatoid Arthritis as a Systemic Disease (Major Problems in Internal Medicine, Volume IV). W. B. Saunders Co., Philadelphia, 1974.

Yoshiki, T., Mellors, R. C., and Strand, M.: The viral envelope glycoprotein of murine leukemia virus and the pathogenesis of immune complex glomerulonephritis of New Zealand mice. J. Exp. Med., 140:1011, 1974.

Zwaifler, N. J.: The immunopathology of joint inflammation in rheumatoid arthritis. Adv. Immunol., 16:265, 1973.

OTHER CONNECTIVE TISSUE DISEASES

Adams, R. D. (ed.): Diseases of Muscle, 3rd Ed. Harper & Row, New York, 1975.

Barnes, B. E.: Dermatomyositis and malignancy: a review of the literature. Ann. Intern. Med., 84:68, 1976.

Campbell, P. M., and LeRoy, E. C.: Pathogenosis of systemic sclerosis: a vascular hypothesis. Semin. Arthritis Rheum., 4:351, 1975.

Christian, C. L., and Sergent, J. S.: Vasculitis syndromes: clinical and experimental models. Am. J. Med., 61:385, 1976.

D'Angelo, W. A., Fries, J. F., Masi, A. T., and Shulman, L. E.: Pathologic observations in systemic sclerosis (scleroderma). Am. J. Med., 46:428, 1969.

Farber, S. J., and Bole, G. E.: Antibodies to components of extractable nuclear antigen. Arch. Intern. Med., 136:425, 1976.

Gocke, D. J., Hsu, K., Morgan, G., and Christian, C. L.: Association between polyarteritis and Australia antigen. Lancet, 2:1149, 1970.

Rodnan, G. P.: Progressive Systemic Sclerosis, (Scleroderma) In Hollander, J. L., and McCarty, D. J. (eds.): Arthritis and Allied Conditons. Lea & Febiger, Philadelphia, 1972.

Rodnan, G. P., et al: Primer on the rheumatic diseases. J.A.M.A., 224: No. 5, 1973 (Suppl.), 7th ed.

Sack, M., Cassidy, J. T., and Bole, G. G.: Prognostic factors in polyarteritis. J. Rheumat., 2:411, 1975.

Sharp, G. C.: Mixed connective tissue disease, current concepts. Arthritis Rheumat., 20:S181, 1977 (Suppl.).

NON-ARTICULAR RHEUMATISM

Berges, P. U.: Myofascial pain syndromes. Postgrad. Med., 53:161, 1973.

Clark, D. D., Ricker, J. H., and MaCollum, M. S.: The efficacy of local steroid injection in the treatment of stenosing tenovaginitis. Plast. Reconstr. Surg., 51:179, 1973.

Smythe, H. A., and Moldofsky, H.: Two contributions to understanding the "fibrositis" syndrome. Bull. Rheum. Dis., 28:928, 1977–78.

Weiss, E.: Psychogenic rheumatism. Med. Clin. North Am., 39:601, 1955.

18

Allergy and Asthma

RICHARD F. LOCKEY, AND SAMUEL C. BUKANTZ

INTRODUCTION

Advances in biochemistry and immunology have yielded information which better explains the pathophysiologic differences of the allergic diseases. This chapter will elaborate upon pathophysiologic mechanisms in which an allergic etiology is present. It will also describe those pathologic entities which mimic diseases of allergic etiology through similar clinical manifestations or diseases previously thought to be purely allergic in etiology but which now are known to have a different pathophysiologic mechanism.

Although there is general agreement that a genetic basis for asthma, allergic rhinitis, and atopic eczema exists, there is considerable disagreement about the exact mode of inheritance. The family tendency to develop these diseases does not depend on a single dominant or recessive gene with variable penetrance, but, like diabetes, hypertension, and other familial diseases, probably results from polygenic inheritance dependent on the interaction of several genes at more than one locus. The only satisfactory explanation of why monozygotic twins have only a slightly higher coincidence of the atopic diseases than do dizygotic twins is that appropriate exposure to environmental influences is also necessary to induce these disorders. For similar reasons, individuals with familial but not identical genetic predisposition and comparable environmental exposure may develop symptoms at different periods of life and of differing severity, or may not develop them at all.

Those persons with a genetic predisposition to develop extrinsic asthma, allergic rhinitis and conjunctivitis, and atopic eczema are referred to as atopic individuals. Atopy, therefore, is the genetic capacity to develop IgE-mediated disease secondary to exposure to normally innocuous substances commonly found in the environment. Other allergic states in which an IgE mechanism is operative include anaphylaxis secondary to an insect sting or an ingested food. According to one part of the definition of atopy, these diseases are atopic; however, evidence supporting a genetic predisposition to develop IgE-mediated insect, drug, and food allergy remains contradictory and inconclusive. There is also a genetic predilection to develop asthma, although often not mediated by IgE. Accordingly, separate genes or combinations of genes predispose individuals to develop atopy and/or asthma. Depending on the constellation of genes acquired and the existence of proper environmental influences, asthma may assume various forms with or without atopy.

Allergy is defined as increased reactivity (hypersensitivity) to normally innocuous substances, the reaction being mediated by an immunopathologic mechanism. All atopic diseases are allergic, but not all allergic diseases are atopic, since many are not mediated by IgE and do not have a familial tendency. All persons have the capacity to develop an allergic disease: for example, serum sickness, which can be induced by the injection of horse serum. Patients with serum sickness secondary to horse serum are not genetically predisposed to it but develop the disease because of a characteristic response of the normal immune system to the parenteral introduction of a foreign substance. This consists of the production of antihorse serum antibodies, immune complex formation, and activation of the complement cascade that causes the disease.

IMMUNOPATHOLOGIC CLASSIFICATIONS OF ALLERGIC DISEASES

The most commonly accepted classification of immunopathologic or allergic reactions is that suggested by Gell and Coombs, who assigned numerical designations to refer to four different mechanisms. These have been labeled Type I, the immediate hypersensitivity or anaphylactic reaction; Type II, the cytotoxic reaction; Type III, the immune complex or Arthus reaction; and Type IV, the cell-mediated or delayed hypersensitivity reaction. There are other immunopathologic reactions which do not fit into these four groups. These include cutaneous basophil hypersensitivity (CBH or Jones-Mote hypersensitivity reaction) and the granulomatous reaction, which is most likely an extension of the Type IV reaction.

This section will discuss these reactions as they relate to various disease states.

Type I: Immediate Hypersensitivity or Anaphylactic Reaction

The Type I reaction partially or completely explains the pathophysiology of allergic rhinitis, allergic conjunctivitis, extrinsic asthma, insect hypersensitivity, most cases of anaphylactic shock, and some cases of urticaria and angioedema. The reaction appears to be involved in allergic bronchopulmonary aspergillosis (ABPA) and atopic eczema. The Type I reaction has been clearly defined over the past decade following the Ishizakas' identification of IgE as a separate immunoglobulin class. Prior to the identification of IgE, it was known that a wheal and flare reaction developed within 20 minutes following a cutaneous or intracutaneous test with ragweed antigen in the skin of an atopic individual with allergic rhinitis due to ragweed pollen. Inhalation of the ragweed pollen or an aqueous extract of that pollen reproduces the disease. Immunoglobulin E, previously referred to as reagin or skin-sensitizing antibody, is one of five immunoglobulins. It can be inactivated by heating at 56° C. for two to four hours. It is homocytotropic in that it fixes to the surface of tissue mast cells and circulating basophils. It can be transferred to the skin of a normal individual, and, when that same area of skin is subsequently challenged with ragweed antigen, an identical wheal and flare reaction is produced in the normal recipient. This transfer of skin reactivity is referred to as the passive transfer or Prausnitz-Kustner reaction. Another class of antibody, IgG homocytotropic antibody, which is thermostable, may also exist in man and may be responsible for similar types of slightly delayed immediate hypersensitivity reactions, especially in certain asthmatic patients.

The bridging of at least two antigenically specific IgE antibody molecules by one molecule of antigen takes place on the mast cell surface with the subsequent release of various chemical mediators. The IgE molecules attached to the mast cell surface are in dynamic equilibrium with serum IgE. Chemicals such as histamine, slow-reacting substance of anaphylaxis (SRS-A), eosinophilic chemotactic factor (ECF-A), platelet-activating factor (PAF), and other mediators such as the prostaglandins are released from the mast cell, causing the secondary physiologic effect. The occurrence of this reaction on mucosal surfaces where mast cells are numerous — for example, in the nose — induces edema, vascular engorgement, leaking of intravascular fluids onto the mucosal surface, and attraction of eosinophils. These are the pathologic changes of allergic rhinitis, and affected patients present with the symptoms of nasal pruritus, sneezing, clear rhinorrhea, and nasal stuffiness. The nasal mucosa becomes pale and edematous, and clear mucus can readily be visualized. If the reaction occurs in the intravascular compartment secondary to injection of penicillin or from a honey bee sting in an allergic individual, the immediate release of chemical mediators into the intravascular system may cause urticaria, angioedema, wheezing, and nausea and vomiting. In severe cases, massive vasodilatation and cardiovascular collapse or anaphylactic shock can occur. If the reaction occurs in the bronchopulmonary tree secondary to inhalation of an allergen to which the person is allergic, it causes bronchial constriction or extrinsic asthma. Apparently, the biochemical defect in the effector cells or in the autonomic regulation may also be inherited along with the atopic tendency to develop IgE-mediated disease. This defect may augment the immunologic reaction in individuals who develop these diseases (see Chapters 4 and 5).

The exact mode by which sensitization takes place in atopic individuals is unknown. These individuals may have a mucosal surface abnormality that enables sensitization to take place. Individuals may develop penicillin hypersensitivity, insect hypersensitivity, or other hypersensitivity reactions mediated by IgE and other immunoglobulins without mucosal contact. These individuals may also have cells that are genetically programmed to manufacture IgE but do not require mucosal contact and absorption.

Type II or Cytotoxic Reaction

The Type II or cytotoxic reaction involves cell surface antigens, immunoglobulin G or M, and, at times, complement. An example of a disease mediated by this reaction is an acute hemolytic crisis caused by an immunologic reaction of erythrocyte surface antigens with isoagglutinins.

which are naturally occurring IgM antibodies. Anti-A and Anti-B are the major isoagglutinins. These naturally occurring antibodies react with the red blood cell surface antigens and agglutinate them. Many are sequestered in the liver, some are phagocytized, and others are lysed. In some cases the combination of antibody with the red blood cell surface antigen causes complement to be fixed, beginning with protein fraction C1, followed by activation of C4, C2, and C3. Activation of C3 and C5 results in formation of C3a and C5a (anaphylatoxins) which trigger histamine release from mast cells, followed by anaphylaxis and/or anaphylactic shock. The activation of the complement cascade proceeds from C3 through C9 and results in lysis and phagocytosis of red blood cells.

The Type II reaction or a modification of the Type II reaction is also involved in the pathogenesis of Goodpasture's disease, hemolytic disease of the newborn, isoallergic neonatal thrombocytopenia, complement-dependent autoimmune hemolytic anemia, Coombs' positive hemolytic anemia secondary to alpha methyldopa, and possibly lupus erythematosus and various vascular diseases. Complement is involved in some of these reactions and not in others.

In Goodpasture's syndrome, anti-glomerular basement membrane antibodies (anti-GBM antibodies) for unknown reasons are produced by the host with specificity to react with antigens of the basement membrane of the renal glomeruli. When the antibody attaches to the basement membrane antigens, the complement cascade is activated, forming chemotactic factor which attracts polymorphonuclear cells to the area. The lysosomes from the polymorphonuclear cells release enzymes, leading to enzymatic destruction of the basement membrane, liberating more antigen into the circulation, and thus causing further antibody formation. The antigenic similarity between lung basement membrane and glomerular basement membrane may result in cross reactivity of the antibody with lung tissue, causing pulmonary disease in some of these patients. This immunologic reaction triggers the pathophysiologic process, leading to an acute or chronic life-threatening disease, manifested clinically by pneumonia, fever, hemoptysis, general toxicity, and the signs and symptoms of glomerulonephritis.

Myasthenia gravis is a neurologic disease manifested by muscle weakness and fatigability in which both IgG antibodies and C3 have been localized to the postsynaptic region of the motor end-plate. It has been proposed that they enhance the defect of the already deficient neuromuscular acetylcholine receptor. If this hypothesis proves correct, it will be yet another example of cytotoxic-induced disease.

Type III or Immune Complex Disease or Arthus Reaction

Type III or immune complex disease involves complement fixing antibodies (IgG or IgM). In this immunopathologic reaction, a soluble immune complex composed of an aggregate of antibody in antigen excess is the basic molecular unit responsible for initiating the disease. The soluble antigen-antibody complexes, because of their molecular weight and characteristics, impinge on certain endothelial membranes throughout the body, including synovial tissue, the basement membranes of kidneys, and blood vessel walls.

The antigen-antibody complex activates complement, which produces anaphylatoxin, enhancing vascular permeability through the release of histamine and other chemical mediators from mast cells. This enables more antigen-antibody complex to be deposited on the endothelial surface. C567, C3a, and C5a are chemotactic and attract polymorphonuclear cells into the area. The release of lysosomal enzymes from polymorphonuclear cells in vessel walls in various tissues of the host causes focal vascular lesions.

Serum sickness is an example of an immune complex disease. The illness usually begins seven to 14 days after the initial injection of foreign protein. If prior sensitization has occurred, the time interval between the injection and the onset of symptoms is shortened. As long as immune complexes are formed, the immunopathologic reaction continues and may be the pathogenic pathway for some forms of chronic vasculitis. The vasculitis can affect various organ systems, including the skin, heart, liver, muscles, pancreas, and testes. Laboratory abnormalities include mild leukocytosis, an increased sedimentation rate, eosinophilia, albuminuria, and decreased serum complement levels.

Other diseases in which immune complexes play a role include several forms of chronic glomerulonephritis. Antistreptococcal antibodies may be produced in response to streptococcal pharyngitis or an antiplasmodial antibody in response to infection with *Plasmodium falciparum*, which causes quartan malaria. Subsequently, each antigen-antibody system may combine to form immune complexes which circulate and, when in appropriate antigen excess, diffuse onto the epithelial surface of the basement membrane. As immune complex is deposited, complement is activated with subsequent migration of polymorphonuclear leukocytes to the glomeruli. Lysosomal enzymes are released from the polymorphonuclear cells and destroy additional basement membrane. This releases basement membrane protein fractions, including antigen for additional immune complex formation, causing an autoimmune or autoallergic disease. Only a small proportion of persons with chronic glomerulonephritis have had previous acute poststreptococcal nephritis. Other antigens such as drugs, foreign proteins, and viruses may also initiate this series of events. In lupus erythematosus, immune complexes of DNA-anti-DNA are continuously formed, accounting for the chronicity of the disease.

The pathogenesis of hypersensitivity pneumonitis, an example of which is farmer's lung, probably involves Type III and/or Type IV reactions. Precipitin antibodies are formed to an organic dust which are the antigens of thermophilic actinomycetes found in moldy hay. When the farmer is continually exposed to inhalation of this antigen, immune complexes may form, with subsequent complement fixation and the inflammatory reaction characteristic of this disease. This process does not explain the entire pathophysiology, since precipitins can be demonstrated in a large percentage of asymptomatic patients. The Type IV reaction appears to be responsible for the experimental pneumonitis induced in rats and rabbits by inhalation of *Micropolyspora faeni* and may play a major role in human disease.

Immune complexes are found in many diseases of unknown etiology, including multiple sclerosis, chronic active hepatitis, primary biliary cirrhosis, idiopathic interstitial pneumonia, hepatitis associated arthritis, rheumatoid arthritis, bacterial endocarditis, and others. The implications of these findings remain unknown, but they may prove to be important in the pathophysiology of many of these diseases.

Type IV or Delayed Hypersensitivity Reactions

The fourth immunopathologic process is the Type IV cell-mediated or delayed hypersensitivity reaction. This immunopathologic reaction is operative in tuberculin hypersensitivity, tissue transplant rejection, and diseases such as allergic contact dermatitis, hypersensitivity pneumonitis (also involving a Type III reaction), and allergic encephalomyelitis. The latter is an experimental disease which appears to have human counterparts in such diseases as postvaccinial encephalitis secondary to immunization with rabies vaccine containing myelin and in multiple sclerosis.

The most common contact dermatitis in the United States results from sensitization to poison ivy, poison oak, or poison sumac. The simple plant catechol antigen penetrates the superficial layer of the skin and attaches to a "carrier protein" in the area of the dermal-epidermal junction. The catechol, a hapten, combines with the tissue protein, forming an antigen to which the previously unsensitized small T-lymphocyte reacts. Sensitization requires the period of time it takes for the T-cell to acquire specific activity, i.e., seven to 14 days. Rechallenge with that chemical after sensitization has occurred results in an eczematous eruption. This second antigenic challenge releases various effector molecules, lymphokines, from the sensitized lymphocyte. Lymphokines have specific biologic activities which amplify the immunologic response and cause the pathologic reaction and attract other lymphocytes and macrophages to the reaction site.

Other Immunopathologic Reactions

Evidence exists which indicates that the contact dermatitis reaction may be more appropriately included under cutaneous basophil hypersensitivity (CBH), separate from the classic delayed hypersensitivity reaction. This is a reaction in which the skin develops a lymphocyte-mediated delayed hypersensitivity reaction that differs both clinically and histologically from classic tuberculin hypersensitivity or Type IV reaction. The main difference is that basophils appear upon antigenic challenge, and the reaction in the skin causes erythema, but without induration, both of which are seen in the Type IV reaction. At this point, this reaction appears to have experimental importance, and it also may be important in allergic contact dermatitis.

Another reaction which appears to have unique characteristics separate from the major four classes is neutralization or inactivation of antigen by antibody, such as occurs in neutralization of insulin in insulin-resistant patients with diabetes mellitus. Molecular inactivation of insulin takes place when it interacts with its specific antibody, preventing the insulin from acting on the target cell.

The granulomatous reactions are differentiated from delayed hypersensitivity reactions by some investigators. This differentiation may be an arbitrary one based more on morphologic observations than on biologic responses to various foreign substances. Delayed hypersensitivity reactions (Type IV) occur more rapidly than do the granulomatous hypersensitivity reactions, which require weeks or months to develop. These granulomatous reactions may be identified morphologically by the appearance of reticuloendothelial cells, including histiocytes, epitheloid cells, giant cells, and, in some instances, mononuclear cells arranged in a characteristic round or oval laminated structure called a granuloma. This granuloma can be seen in tuberculosis, zirconium and beryllium exposure, sarcoidosis, leprosy, and in certain parasitic diseases.

ASTHMA

Definition

The definition which best characterizes asthma was suggested by the Committee on Diagnostic Standards of the American Thoracic Society in 1962: "Asthma is a disease characterized by an increased responsiveness of the trachea and bronchi to various stimuli and manifested by widespread narrowing of the airways that changes in severity either spontaneously or as a result of therapy." This statement was qualified by the Committee with the following: "The term asthma is not appropriate for bronchial narrowing which results solely from widespread bronchial infection, e.g., acute or chronic bronchitis; from destructive disease of the lung, e.g., pulmonary emphysema; or from cardiovascular disorders. Asthma, as here defined, may occur in subjects with other bronchopulmonary or cardiovascular diseases, but in these instances, the airway obstruction is not causally related to these diseases."

The diagnostic term, "asthma," is used in the same way as are many other diagnostic terms in medicine, for example, arthritis, hypertension, diabetes, urticaria and glaucoma, to describe clinical entities that require additional clarification before the nature of the disease may be defined more completely. Examples of further subclassification of asthma include extrinsic asthma, intrinsic asthma, and mixed asthma. These forms of asthma can be subclassified as intrinsic exercise-induced asthma, intrinsic aspirin-intolerant asthma, and extrinsic pharmacologic asthma.

Many persons with bronchitis and/or emphysema have significant reversible obstructive airways disease (ROAD, a term synonymous with asthma) which responds to stimuli, resolves either spontaneously or as a result of therapy and is a significant part of the disease. Persons with these diseases are most often referred to as having either emphysema, bronchitis, or chronic obstructive lung disease (COLD), when, in fact, they have two or three diseases simultaneously, one of which is asthma (Fig. 18–1).

To simplify these obvious differences, one can classify these combinations of several diseases as bronchitic intrinsic asthma, emphysematous intrinsic asthma, and bronchitic emphysematous intrinsic asthma — listed in order of clinical importance. Pulmonary function studies may help to characterize the disease in numerical terms, i.e., FeV_1 of 500 cc., 1000 cc., 1500 cc., or in relative percentages of predicted normals, which are terms universally employed for these clinical entities. Measurements can be made of other ventilatory functions. Both bronchitis and emphysema are described in Chapter 16; however, they will be discussed here to some extent when they co-exist with asthma.

Types of Asthma

Asthma can be classified clinically as outlined in Table 18–1. Pathophysiologically, there may be similarities in various clinical states, and there may even be different pathophysiologic mechanisms operative in the same clinical state. The severity of the asthma should also be included as part of the formal clinical diagnosis, i.e., mild, moderate, or severe. The latter would be reserved primarily for those in whom systemic glucocorticosteroids are necessary for adequate treatment. By so classifying asthma, not only is communication among physicians, insurance carriers, and statisticians possible, but a general idea as to the type, severity, prognosis, and treatment of the individual is possible. Few patients have the pure form of any of these clinical types; however, most can be categorized into one of the following clinical classes: extrinsic, intrinsic, or mixed. Further subclassifications is possible in most cases.

Extrinsic Asthma (Asthma Triggered by Environmental Substances). EXTRINSIC IMMEDIATE ATOPIC ASTHMA. Extrinsic immediate atopic asthma is explained primarily by the Type I immunopathologic reaction, although an underlying defect in autonomic regulation also may be present, and, indeed, may be present in one way or another in all forms of asthma. Chemical mediators such as histamine, slow-reacting substance of anaphylaxis (SRS-A), eosinophilic chemotactic factor (ECF), platelet activating factor (PAF), and prostaglandins are released secondary to allergenic exposure. Aeroallergens that may provoke this type of asthma include tree, weed, and grass pollens, animal epithelials, dust, and mold particles. An example is the patient who develops

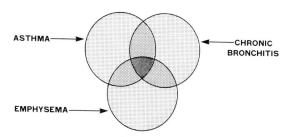

Figure 18–1 Nonproportional Venn diagram indicating the overlapping relationships of asthma, chronic bronchitis and emphysema. Each entity occurs alone; many patients present features of two entities; occasional patients combine features of all three disorders. (With permission from Snyder, G. L.: Interrelationships of Asthma, Chronic Bronchitis and Emphysema. *In* Weiss, E. B., and Segal, M. S. (Eds.): Bronchial Asthma, Mechanisms and Therapeutics. Little, Brown & Co., Boston, 1976, p. 32.)

TABLE 18–1   CLASSIFICATIONS OF ASTHMA

Types of Asthma	Mechanism(s)	Examples	Synonymous Terms	Comments
A. Extrinsic asthma	One or more of several mechanisms including immunopathologic plus altered autonomic regulation of bronchopulmonary tree	Immediate atopic asthma; late non-atopic allergic asthma; irritant and pharmacologic asthma	When the term extrinsic asthma is used, it most often refers to extrinsic atopic asthma	Extrinsic implies that the primary cause is external
1. Extrinsic immediate atopic asthma	Type I with IgE; ? modified Type I with homocytotropic IgG	Ragweed pollen-induced asthma. Grass pollen-induced asthma. Allergic bronchopulmonary aspergillosis.* Occupational asthma implies it is associated with work. This is rarely a pure form of the disease. Examples include castor bean dust exposure; enzymes from *Bacillus subtilis* (detergent industry); trimellite anhydride used in plastic industry**	Allergic asthma; Type I asthma; immediate hypersensitivity asthma; reaginmediated asthma; early-onset asthma; extrinsic asthma	Common form of asthma which begins immediately after allergenic exposure. It may occur in combination with extrinsic immediate or late non-atopic allergic asthma (cytotropic IgG)
2. Extrinsic late non-atopic allergic asthma	IgE plays role in some ?IgE in TMA; ? Type III and/or Type IV	Trimellitic anhydride** (plastics) "TMA flu syndrome;" any form of late-onset asthma, which is asthma denoting bronchial airway obstruction beginning at least one hour after exposure to allergen	The term "late-onset asthma" can also refer to asthma beginning late in life	Some individuals have both the characteristic atopic asthma with the immediate phase and the non-atopic with the late-onset phase. May begin one hour, last 2-3 hours; may begin 3-4 hours, last 24-36 hours
3. Extrinsic irritant asthma	Irritant; ? pharmacologic in some	Sulfur dioxide, nitrogen dioxide, chlorine, trimellitic anhydride** (plastics). If associated with occupation, it can be referred to as extrinsic occupational irritant asthma	Chemical asthma, occupational asthma	Many forms of asthma may be exacerbated by numerous chemicals. Some chemicals appear to cause asthma by their direct irritant effect. Others have an effect through an immunologic (possibly IgE as in TMA) or pharmacologic mechanism

4. Extrinsic pharmacologic asthma	Pharmacologic; i.e., direct release of mediators or direct effect on pharmacologic receptors	Toluene diisocyanate (TDI); complex salts of platinum in metal refining; nickel salts; organic phosphorus insecticides; byssinosis. If associated with occupation, can be referred to as extrinsic occupational asthma, such as meat wrappers' asthma	Pharmacologic asthma, occupational asthma	If removal from the irritant or chemical causes resolution of the disease, the definition of irritant or pharmacologic asthma applies. If asthma persists, the chemical in question is an irritant in one of the forms of extrinsic or intrinsic asthma
B. Intrinsic	All forms have altered autonomic regulation of bronchopulmonary tree (possibly beta receptor blockade)	Intrinsic asthma is a common form of asthma. Various types have specific characteristics	Asthma associated with viral respiratory tract infections	Immunologic mechanisms have not been demonstrable
1. Intrinsic aspirin intolerant asthma	Aspirin and other nonsteroidal anti-inflammatory agents may alter prostaglandin synthesis and cause severe asthma. Possible altered chemoreceptor response to these chemicals	Asthma exacerbated by ingestion of aspirin. Also may be exacerbated by indomethacin, mefanamic acid, naproxen, ibuprofen, fenoprofen, phenylbutazone, dipyrone, diclofenac, tartrazine (FD&C yellow #5 dye)	ASA triad; aspirin asthma; aspirin triad; aspirin-induced asthma	Can have associated extrinsic atopic asthma. Onset usually in middle-age, but can be seen in children. ? familial incidence. Nasal polyps and/or chronic sinusitis common
2. Intrinsic infectious asthma	The infectious agent may exacerbate underlying autonomic defect (increase beta receptor blockade)	Asthma exacerbated by certain viral respiratory tract infections	Intrinsic asthma; asthmatic bronchitis (during flare)	Children primarily affected. Patients completely well between infections. Many viruses implicated, including respiratory syncytial and parainfluenza. Bacterial infections uncommon triggers. Patients immunologically appear to be normal
3. Intrinsic asthmatic bronchitis	Autonomic dysfunction	Asthma with cough and sputum production	Infectious asthma; intrinsic asthma; reversible obstructive airway disease (ROAD) with bronchitis	Viruses most commonly exacerbate asthma causing severe flare and production of copious amounts of sputum

TABLE 18–1   CLASSIFICATIONS OF ASTHMA *(Continued)*

Types of Asthma	Mechanism(s)	Examples	Synonymous Terms	Comments
4. Intrinsic exercise-induced asthma	Hyperexcitable airway due to autonomic imbalance	Asthma with onset usually after exercise	Exercise-induced asthma	Very common in children. Exercise-induced broncho-spasm occurs commonly in many forms of asthma
5. Intrinsic asthma associated with various degrees of irreversible obstructive lung disease. Listed in order of severity:				
a. Bronchitic intrinsic asthma	Damage to the broncho-pulmonary tree with im-paired autonomic regulation	Chronic sputum production with asthma. Significant smoking history usually present	Asthma and bronchitis; ROAD with bronchitis; asthmatic bronchitis; chronic obstructive pul-monary disease (COPD); chronic obstructive lung disease (COLD)	The diseases are listed in order of importance. This is primarily a clinical im-pression. It can be supported with pulmonary function data. Exacerbated by viral and bacterial infection
b. Emphysematous intrin-sic asthma	Damage to alveoli with impaired autonomic regulation	Combination of emphysema with asthma. Significant smoking history usually present	Emphysema with asthma; emphysema with ROAD; COPD; COLD	
c. Bronchitic emphysema-tous intrinsic asthma (emphysematous bronchitic intrinsic asthma, intrinsic asthmatic bronchitic emphysema)	Autonomic dysfunction with damage to broncho-pulmonary tree and alveoli	Combination of asthma with emphysema and bronchitis. Significant smoking history usually present	ROAD with emphysema and bronchitis; COPD; COLD	
C. Mixed asthma (individual types which predominate listed in order of impor-tance), i.e., mixed, primarily extrinsic atopic with intrin-sic asthma or vice versa, etc.	Combination of any form of extrinsic and intrinsic asthma	The patient could have seasonal asthma secondary to weed aeroallergens and severe asthma associated with viral respiratory tract infections	None	Any combination of the above types of asthma or the above clinical profiles could be included in mixed asthma

*The asthma in this form of disease is primarily IgE-mediated, although it appears that the type III and IV reactions are also pathogenetically important.
**TMA may cause different forms of asthma in various individuals.

asthma upon exposure to cats or dogs. If he is a veterinarian, extrinsic immediate atopic occupational asthma may best describe his disease.

EXTRINSIC LATE NONATOPIC ALLERGIC ASTHMA. Asthma in certain individuals begins at least one hour following exposure to airborne allergens. This is in contrast to extrinsic immediate atopic asthma, which begins shortly after exposure. This may be secondary to a modified Type I reaction or to an immunoglobulin other than IgE, i.e., an IgG homocytotropic antibody. Some individuals with hypersensitivity pneumonitis wheeze following antigenic exposure. This has led to speculation that this asthma may be secondary to the Type III and/or Type IV immunopathologic reaction.

EXTRINSIC IRRITANT AND PHARMACOLOGIC ASTHMA. An immunologic basis for these diseases has not been established; however, the asthma is precipitated by extrinsic factors. Most asthmatics are exacerbated by chemical exposure. Some chemicals appear to cause asthma by their direct irritant effect on the bronchial mucosa. Others appear to have an effect through some unexplained pharmacologic mechanism. The definition of irritant or pharmacologic asthma applies if removing the patient from the chemical triggering this form of asthma causes resolution of the disease and reexposure exacerbates it. If the asthma persists in spite of removal, but to a lesser degree, the inciting agent becomes an irritant in another form of asthma. Sulfur dioxide, nitrous oxide, and chlorine are examples of chemicals capable of inducing extrinsic irritant asthma. Toluene diisocynate (TDI), which is a polymerizing agent used in manufacturing polyurethanes, is an example of a chemical that will cause pharmacologic asthma on continuous exposure to minute concentrations. Other chemicals such as salts of platinum and soldering fluxes appear capable of causing a similar type of asthma, which has also been referred to as chemical asthma. The mechanism for this form of extrinsic asthma remains unknown. Finally, it has been demonstrated that in certain individuals, such as those working with trimellitic anhydrides used in the plastics industry, immunologic as well as irritant and/or pharmacologic mechanisms are operative in this extrinsic form of asthma.

Intrinsic Asthma. Intrinsic asthma was originally conceived as that form of reversible obstructive airway disease, the cause of which "lies within the patient." It is now suspected that a primary defect exists in autonomic regulation of the bronchial tree, since immunologic abnormalities previously thought to exist have not been demonstrable in this form of asthma. Viral respiratory tract infections are common precipitators of asthmatic paroxysms, as are many other non-specific factors. These include meteorologic changes; physical factors such as exercise, coughing, laughing; exposure to chemical substances; and various irritants. Sub-groups of intrinsic asthma have distinct characteristics.

INTRINSIC ASPIRIN-INTOLERANT ASTHMA. These asthmatics often have associated chronic sinusitis and nasal polyposis. They usually have asthma which can be severely exacerbated by the ingestion of aspirin (acetylsalicylic acid), or, in certain individuals, by the ingestion of indomethacin, mefenamic acid, naproxen, ibuprofen, fenoprofen, phenylbutazone, dipyrone, diclofenac, and tartrazine (FD & C yellow #5 dye). This reaction does not appear to be immunologic in etiology. Theories have been proposed, but the mechanism remains unknown.

INTRINSIC INFECTIOUS ASTHMA. This is a common form of asthma in children. These asthmatics are susceptible to recurrent viral upper respiratory tract infections which cause asthma. Bacterial infections rarely cause asthmatic exacerbations. The patients are usually well between infections, and they generally become less symptomatic with age. This clinical profile of asthma also occurs in adults.

INTRINSIC ASTHMATIC BRONCHITIS. This is a combination of asthma and chronic bronchitis. The patients may or may not have been smokers; however, both asthma and bronchitis play an important role in the clinical presentation.

INTRINSIC EXERCISE-INDUCED ASTHMA. It is primarily seen in children who wheeze only after vigorous exercise. Exercise-induced bronchospasm is commonly seen in association with many forms of asthma.

INTRINSIC ASTHMA WITH IRREVERSIBLE AS WELL AS REVERSIBLE OBSTRUCTIVE AIRWAYS DISEASE (FIG. 18–1). These patients almost always have a smoking history. The most treatable element of their disease is usually the reversible obstructive airways disease (ROAD).

Bronchitic Intrinsic Asthma. These patients have bronchitis, i.e., chronic cough with sputum production associated with reversible airways disease. They develop recurrent viral and bacterial respiratory tract infections and have a high susceptibility to pneumonia.

Emphysematous Intrinsic Asthma. These patients have emphysema with intrinsic asthma. They are also susceptible to bacterial and viral respiratory tract infections.

Bronchitic Emphysematous Intrinsic Asthma, Emphysematous Bronchitic Intrinsic Asthma, Intrinsic Asthmatic Bronchitic Emphysema. This is the combination of three diseases. They are exacerbated by similar factors. The most severe of the three diseases should be listed first and the others in order of importance.

Mixed Asthma. Both extrinsic and intrinsic factors are operative in this form of asthma. The patient may have certain seasons of the year during which allergenic exposure will exacerbate his asthma. The disease can also be triggered by many non-specific factors, such as exercise, weather changes, viral infections, and irritants. In order to emphasize the predominant forms, for example, a patient can be classified as a mixed asthmatic, primarily intrinsic, with extrinsic atopic asthma. Although somewhat elaborate, this description is more precise than the term "mixed asthma" used alone.

There are inadequacies in this classification of asthma; however, it is workable and useful in caring for patients. If several forms of asthma co-exist with or without other diseases such as emphysema or bronchitis, they can be included in order of clinical importance. The severity of the affliction should also be included. By using this classification, the physician has a definition of the patient's disease in reasonable pathophysiologic and clinical terms, and appropriate treatment can be initiated.

The Autonomic Nervous System in Asthma

An immunologic etiology partially explains the pathophysiology of extrinsic asthma. Inhalant allergens such as pollens, dust, cat dander, and molds trigger a Type I immunopathologic response with subsequent release of chemical mediators.

These mediators cause asthma by their secondary effects on the effector cells (smooth muscle and exocrine cells) of the bronchopulmonary tree. Intracellular levels of cAMP and cGMP have a notable effect on the release or formation of these mediators. However, because allergic mechanisms cannot explain all asthma, other equally important abnormalities are now thought to exist in the asthmatic lung. An imbalance in effector cell response to sympathetic and parasympathetic activity may be the common denominator for all asthma. Allergic reactions play a role in only certain forms of asthma, such as extrinsic imme-

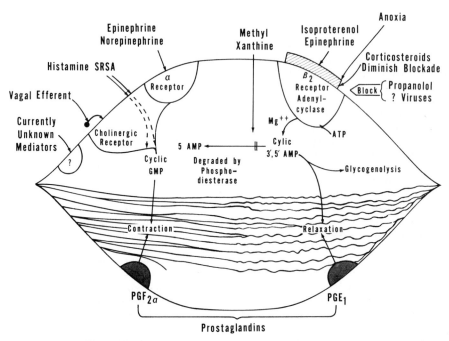

Figure 18–2 Schematic presentation of the pharmacologic and biochemical forces which modulate bronchial smooth muscle contraction and relaxation. Known pharmacologic receptor sites are depicted. Propranolol, a beta receptor blocking agent, augments the suspected blockade at this receptor site. Viruses, which commonly flare asthma and anoxia, may also act by increasing the blockade at the beta receptor. Drugs used to treat asthma pharmacologically influence the effector cell. Isoproterenol and epinephrine stimulate the beta receptor and cause bronchial relaxation. Glucocorticosteroids may diminish the beta blockade. Methylxanthines block the degradation of cAMP and cause smooth muscle relaxation. (With permission from Stevenson, D. D.: Bronchial asthma. *In* Lockey, R. F. (Ed.): Clinical Immunology and Allergy for Students and Practicing Physicians. Medical Examination Publishing, Inc., New York, in press.)

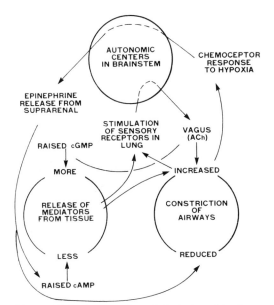

Figure 18–3 Autonomic activity induced by the release of pharmacologic activity in lung during an asthmatic attack. (With permission from Brocklehurst, W. E.: Richet Lecture, 1977. The role of mediators and homeostatic processes in asthma. Ann. Allergy, *40*:1, 1978.)

diate atopic asthma or mixed asthma (Fig. 18–2). Figures 18–2 and 18–3 schematically illustrate how autonomic activity is induced by the release of pharmacologic activity in the lung during an asthmatic attack.

A genetically predisposed derangement in the effector cell as regulated by the autonomic nervous control of the lung theoretically could be secondary to: (1) an excessive cholinergic response, since cholinergic stimulation causes bronchial smooth muscle contraction and increased mucous gland secretion; (2) an inadequate beta adrenergic response, since beta adrenergic stimulation relaxes smooth muscle in the airways; (3) increased alpha receptor effect, since alpha stimulation causes bronchial smooth muscle contraction. This abnormal autonomic response could also co-exist in mucous membranes and other tissues in atopic diseases such as atopic eczema, allergic rhinitis, and allergic conjunctivitis and in patients who have a history of nasal polyps and chronic sinusitis associated with their asthma. If atopy exists, IgE disease occurs. However, if atopy is absent, the inherent mucosal defect leads to intrinsic rhinitis quite often associated with nasal polyps and chronic sinusitis. These persons are exacerbated by non-specific stimuli similar to those which precipitate bronchospasm in intrinsic asthmatics.

At least two intracellular cyclic nucleotides, cGMP and cAMP, are important secondary messengers which, through their action within cells,

regulate smooth muscle tone in the bronchopulmonary tree. Theories have been proposed to explain the apparent functional imbalance in asthma. These include postulates that there may be an excessive cholinergic influence mediated directly or indirectly by cGMP, the cyclic nucleotide regulator which is increased by vagal stimulation. There may also be a suboptimal beta adrenergic response mediated through a relative deficiency of cAMP, the cyclic nucleotide of the beta adrenergic receptor. In-vitro, cGMP facilitates allergic mediator release and smooth muscle contraction, whereas cAMP facilitates mediator release and muscle relaxation.

Evidence that excessive vagal response is present is supported by the fact that atropine sulfate and vagotomy abolish bronchoconstriction in certain animals induced by mechanical factors, chemicals, and chemically inert dust. These same stimuli trigger asthma in humans. Antigen-induced bronchoconstriction in monkeys is not prevented by atropine, although low doses of cholinergic agonists increase the response to subsequent exposure to antigens. Gold has also demonstrated in animals that reflex activity through the vagus is important, since unilateral bronchopulmonary challenge causes bilateral bronchoconstriction. Other evidence exists which may indicate the presence of an abnormality in vagal regulation. Increased cGMP activity in lungs of experimental animals occurs during anaphylaxis-induced bronchospasm. Similarly, an increase in venous cGMP/cAMP ratio occurs in asthmatics following inhalation challenge with acetylcholine. In addition, an imbalance of the cGMP/cAMP ratio in leukocytes apparently is present in asthmatics; however, it remains unknown whether this imbalance also exists in airway smooth muscle.

The sympathetic influence in the lung is secondary to circulating catecholamines since minimal direct sympathetic innervation is present. The majority of the receptors on smooth muscle in the lung appear to be adrenergic. Beta stimulation causes bronchial dilation and alpha stimulation bronchial constriction; however, beta influence predominates. Szentivanyi in 1968 proposed that a partial beta blockade would physiologically explain the pathophysiology of asthma. He had observed that *Bordetella pertussis*-vaccinated mice behaved as did mice given a beta adrenergic blocking agent. They demonstrated markedly enhanced reactivity to histamine and other smooth muscle spasmogens. Rats treated similarly produced more homocytotropic antibody (rat reagin) than did controls. Other animals behaved in a similar fashion. Several lines of evidence lend support to this theory. First, asthmatics generally respond poorly to epinephrine in comparison to normals. When given epinephrine, there is a lessened reduction in the number of eosinophils and in peripheral arterial resistance. Mobilization of blood glucose, fatty acids, pyruvate, and lactic acid is also impaired. Second, leukocytes from asthmatics show less increase in intracellular levels of cAMP in response to beta stimulators. Third, drugs such as propranolol (a beta blocker) increase airway resistance and increase the response to methacholine and aeroallergenic challenge. A similar response may be seen in persons with allergic rhinitis who have no history of asthma. Fourth, many of the drugs that benefit asthmatics, such as the glucocorticosteroids, sympathomimetics, and methylxanthines appear to benefit the patient by enhancing the effectiveness of the cAMP system.

Evidence that the alpha receptor is overactive is lacking; however, some evidence supporting the partial beta blockade theory could likewise be applied to alpha overactivity. Alpha blockers have been used successfully to block histamine-induced bronchospasm. They also have been used with some benefit in treating isolated cases of asthma.

Evidence to support any unifying concept explaining the underlying abnormality in all asthma is based more on theory than fact. It is most probable that more than one pathophysiologic mechanism will explain various forms of asthma — just as multiple etiologic explanations explain various forms of arthritis, glaucoma, diabetes, and hypertension.

Pathophysiology of Asthma

Most asthmatics have periodic symptoms manifested by wheezing, cough, and shortness of breath. These can interfere with normal activity, but rarely threaten life or require emergency care. Intrinsic asthmatics and persons with irreversible lung changes and asthma are the patients who most commonly develop life-threatening disease. Most of this discussion will deal with extrinsic, intrinsic, and mixed asthma, since there are major differences in respiratory failure in those persons who have emphysema and/or chronic bronchitis with asthma.

A ventilation-perfusion abnormality is the primary defect in progressively severe asthma. It ultimately can and does lead to death. Obstruction of the bronchopulmonary tree initially causes impaired ventilation of obstructed segments of the lung and hyperventilation in those units which are not obstructed. Pulmonary blood flow continues to both aerated and poorly ventilated units, the former saturated and the latter unsaturated with oxygen. As the total population of alveolar ventilation units with low ventilation and high perfusion increases, arterial hypoxemia increases. This occurs because blood O_2 content increases only slightly with O_2 tension above 60

mm. Hg — thus, hyperventilation of well-ventilated units cannot compensate to any extent for the low O_2 content of underventilated alveoli. Hyperventilation of functional segments will prevent carbon dioxide retention early in the disease because of a more linear relationship between CO_2 content and tension. Because of these relationships early in the disease, arterial blood gases are normal or low in pCO_2 with alkaline pH. As more units become impaired, CO_2 retention occurs, resulting in respiratory acidosis. This becomes a life-threatening situation that requires medical intervention for survival. Status asthmaticus is severe asthma which has become refractory to treatment with standard pharmacologic agents such as epinephrine and aminophylline. These patients may go on to respiratory failure.

Measuring reversible airways obstruction by pulmonary function studies can assess the degree of reversible obstructive airways disease. Early in the course of an asthmatic exacerbation, the peripheral airways constrict, and, as the disease progresses, the central and larger airways obstruct. The last pulmonary units to revert to normal after treatment and remission are the smaller airways.

Descriptions of the pathology of asthma are based largely on studies of patients who have died with severe asthma. As far as can be determined, anatomic changes in various forms of asthma without bronchitis and/or emphysema are similar: hyperinflated alveoli; widespread mucous plugging of bronchi; loss of ciliated and globular cell layers of mucosal epithelium; cellular infiltrates with large numbers of eosinophils together with lymphocytes, histiocytes, and plasma cells; and hypertrophy of the basement membrane and smooth muscles surrounding the bronchioles are present in varying degrees. Effects on the heart, liver, and other organs are unusual, of little consequence, and, if present, likely occur very late in the disease.

ALLERGIC EMERGENCIES

Allergic emergencies result from the release of chemical mediators triggered by an immunologic reaction. The clinical conditions so mediated and threatening life are anaphylaxis and laryngeal edema. Anaphylactoid reactions mimic the clinical presentations of anaphylaxis but are not caused by an immunologic reaction. Certain definitions are necessary to discuss the events which cause allergic emergencies:

Anaphylaxis. Any or all of the acute symptom complex mediated by an immunologic reaction which includes generalized erythema and pruritus, urticaria, angioedema, nausea, vomiting, crampy abdominal pain, diarrhea, asthma, with or without collapse or hypotension.

Anaphylactic shock. Anaphylaxis associated with hypotension.

Anaphylactic. Refers to the Type I allergic reaction.

Anaphylactoid. The symptom complex of anaphylaxis induced by a foreign substance but not caused by an immunologic mechanism.

Susceptibility

The mechanism by which certain individuals become susceptible to these types of reaction is unknown. The existence of atopy as a predisposing factor to the development of anaphylaxis has not been established.

Pathogenesis

Penicillin, pollens, insect venoms, certain foods, horse serum, and other substances normally tolerated by man induce the synthesis of specific IgE immunoglobulin in certain individuals. This homocytotropic antibody attaches to the surfaces of the human mast cell and basophil. Upon rechallenge with the sensitizing antigen, the antigen-antibody interaction on the mast cell surface initiates a Type I reaction, causing mediator release and the clinical syndrome of anaphylaxis.

The target organ systems involved in anaphylaxis in experimental animals and man determine what subsequently occurs. The guinea pig target organ is the smooth muscle of the bronchi. This leads to a respiratory death. The rabbit develops severe pulmonary arterial constriction and subsequent right heart failure. The dog's shock tissue is the venous system of the liver, which contracts, causing hepatic congestion. The lung and cardiovascular system are primarily affected in man.

Histamine, which is found in greatest concentrations in mast cell granules, increases capillary permeability, contracts bronchiolar smooth muscle, and stimulates exocrine gland secretion in humans. SRS-A, an acidic lipid, may also play a role in human anaphylaxis. ECF-A attracts eosinophils to the site of the reaction. Human lung tissue passively sensitized with serum containing IgE releases SRS-A upon specific antigenic challenge. Isolated human smooth muscle preparation from lung is also contracted by SRS-A. Despite these persuasive in-vitro experiments, more conclusive evidence is needed before stating unequivocally that SRS-A plays a role in human anaphylaxis. Both kinins and serotonins have been implicated in animal anaphylaxis. Experimental evidence for their role in human anaphylaxis remains inconclusive.

A second immunopathologic reaction that can cause anaphylaxis is the Type II or cytotoxic reaction. The antigen is located on cell surfaces with which the antibody reacts. Complement may or may not be required, the primary example of which would be an acute hemolytic transfusion reaction.

A third reaction, aggregate anaphylaxis, results from the direct release of chemical mediators. It does not involve a latent period of sensitization. Human gamma globulin in-vitro tends to aggregate, and, when administered in-vivo, can cause complement activation and subsequent anaphylaxis. It may also cause the direct release of mediators from target cells. In a similar fashion, rabbit anti-rat gamma globulin injected intravenously into rats will react with rat gamma globulin and produce anaphylaxis. Patients with IgA deficiency who have received human gamma globulin or whole blood may develop an anti-IgA gamma globulin, which subsequently aggregates with IgA molecules on administration of gamma globulin or whole blood. This causes complement activation and formation of anaphylatoxins, followed by release of chemical mediators by mast cells and basophils. The pathogenesis of this phenomenon fits the Type III or immune complex immunopathologic or allergic reaction.

Mechanisms not yet defined are involved in various anaphylactoid reactions. These reactions follow the ingestion or injection of a foreign substance to which an immunologic reaction cannot be demonstrated. These foreign substances may cause a direct release of chemical mediators in certain individuals and precipitate the clinical syndrome. Complement activation may also play a role, particularly in iodinated contrast dye reactions.

Pathology

James and Austen summarized numerous reports of the pathologic findings in deaths secondary to anaphylaxis. The descriptions include acute pulmonary emphysema, laryngeal edema, and, in fatal cases without significant respiratory difficulty, either visceral congestion or no significant postmortem findings. They studied six fatal cases: five of these patients developed angioedema of the larynx or pulmonary emphysema or both; neither was present in the sixth case. The interval between parenteral antigen administration and death ranged from 16 to 120 minutes (penicillin in three patients and, in one patient each, skin tests with bee venom, ragweed extract, or guinea pig hemoglobin).

Predominant pathologic abnormalities were seen in the respiratory tract, including the hypopharynx, epiglottis, larynx, and trachea. Two patients with laryngeal edema and the fifth patient with respiratory symptoms had acute pulmonary hyperinflation which was felt to be secondary to outflow obstruction in the upper respiratory tract. The sixth patient suffered pain and shock without respiratory distress, and the postmortem examination did not reveal the cause of death. Increased numbers of eosinophils were seen in the sinusoids of the spleen, liver, lamina propria of the upper respiratory tract, and the pulmonary vessels in several patients.

Specific Causes

Agents that can precipitate anaphylaxis include drugs, particularly penicillin; allergy extracts; other therapeutic agents; insects, specifically of the order Hymenoptera (bees, wasps, yellow jackets, hornets, ants); certain foods, such as peanuts, nuts, fish, and shellfish; blood group substances; and gamma globulin. Substances such as iodinated contrast material, aspirin, and other agents cause anaphylactoid reactions through a non-immunologic mechanism.

ALLERGIC RHINITIS AND CONJUNCTIVITIS

The physiologic response of the nasal mucosa to various environmental stimuli is regulated by the autonomic nervous system. Alteration of these normal physiologic processes can be secondary to anatomic, physiologic, or allergic abnormalities. Proper humidification, temperature regulation, filtration of air, and smell and taste depend on normal upper airway function.

Hay fever refers to a constellation of symptoms experienced by various atopic individuals in the fall of the year. Weeds, including ragweed, pollinate at this time of year and are responsible for this disease, which is more properly referred to as seasonal allergic rhinitis. If the conjunctiva is affected, the patient has concomitant allergic conjunctivitis. Seasonal allergic rhinitis can occur in allergic individuals at those times of the year when sufficient numbers of tree, grass, weed, or mold aeroallergens to which they are specifically sensitive are in the atmosphere. The aeroallergens precipitate nasal symptoms, which may include nasal stuffiness, pruritus, rhinorrhea, decreased smell and taste, itching of the palate and ears, and mild facial pain.

Inhaled aeroallergens contact mucosal surfaces and release antigenic fractions which react with specific IgE attached to mast cell surfaces. Chemical mediators such as histamine, eosinophilic chemotactic factor of anaphylaxis (ECF-A), slow-reacting substance of anaphylaxis (SRS-A), and others are released and cause mucosal surface changes, which include edema and clear mucus discharge.

Allergic rhinitis that occurs throughout the year is referred to as perennial allergic rhinitis. The most common allergens which cause perennial rhinitis are usually located in the immediate environment and include dust, animal epithelial debris from cats or other household pets, and household mold particles. Pollen aeroallergens can also be important in perennial allergic rhinitis and/or conjunctivitis.

Differential Diagnosis

Several diseases of the upper airway can mimic the clinical manifestations of seasonal and perennial allergic rhinitis. Vasomotor rhinitis (intrinsic rhinitis) is a disease in which the autonomic regulatory system of the upper airway appears to be impaired. Its etiology remains unknown. Symptoms similar to those seen with seasonal or perennial allergic rhinitis occur. Sudden changes in ambient temperature or humidity, postural changes, emotional changes, and exposure to airborne irritants cause nasal stuffiness, sneezing, clear rhinorrhea, and upper airway discomfort. These same physical stimuli can trigger increased symptoms in allergic rhinitis patients.

Rhinitis medicamentosa results from the chronic use of sympathomimetic nasal sprays. When these drugs are repeatedly insufflated into the nose to relieve upper airway congestion, they may worsen rather than alleviate nasal congestion. This results from a mucosal rebound phenomenon. Certain antihypertensive agents such as alpha methyldopa, reserpine, and propranolol can also cause similar nasal obstruction by interfering with normal autonomic regulation of the nose.

Chronic infectious sinusitis or infectious rhinitis occurs secondary to various microbes that infect the upper airway. These infections may begin secondarily to a viral infection of the upper respiratory tract, an anatomic abnormality that interferes with proper airways function, or they may accompany the chronic use of nasal sprays. Microbes most responsible for the infectious process include various anaerobes and aerobes.

Nasal polyps are grapelike cystic masses which arise from the nasal mucosa. They are commonly associated with infectious sinusitis and/or rhinitis but can also occur with allergic rhinitis. The etiology is often undetermined, but they occur with increased frequency in persons with intrinsic asthma, particularly those who have severe bronchospasm after ingesting acetysalicylic acid and other non-steroidal anti-inflammatory agents. Histopathology reveals scanty cellular infiltration. The surface epithelium demonstrates squamous metaplasia, the stroma has a fibromyxomatous appearance, with stellate and spindle-shaped cells, and a large number of eosinophils may be present.

Allergic Conjunctivitis

It is uncommon to have allergic conjunctivitis in the absence of significant allergic rhinitis. Conjunctival tearing, erythema, and pruritus are commonly seen. Acute viral conjunctivitis can mimic allergic rhinitis, but this disease is self-limiting and usually does not occur seasonally.

Vernal Conjunctivitis

Vernal conjunctivitis is a disease of the conjunctival mucosal membranes. It occurs primarily in young people and is of an undetermined etiology. The conjunctiva have a "cobblestone" type of appearance. There is usually a thick, ropy, white discharge over these papillae. Although an allergic cause has been suspected, it remains a disease of unknown etiology.

ATOPIC DERMATITIS (ATOPIC ECZEMA)

Atopic dermatitis (atopic eczema) is a chronic eczematoid skin disease of unknown etiology and pathogenesis associated with high IgE levels and a high incidence of atopic disease. The exact mode of genetic inheritance of atopic eczema remains unknown. The majority of affected individuals also develop allergic rhinitis and/or asthma. Histologically, the skin lesions resemble other chronic dermatoses: cellular and intercellular edema and non-specific cellular infiltrates with a predominance of lymphocytes and eosinophils. In the chronic form there is a thickening of the cellular epidermis (acanthosis) and stratum corneum (hyperkeratosis) and retention of the nuclei in the stratum corneum (parakeratosis).

The exact role of allergy in the pathogenesis of the disease remains uncertain. High IgE levels are characteristically found associated with a peripheral blood eosinophilia. The ingestion of certain foods and inhalation of certain aeroallergens may exacerbate the disease in individual cases. However, in most individuals, allergic exposure does not correlate with the severity of the disease.

The skin of the person with atopic dermatitis differs in many ways from normal skin. Normal skin responds to stroking with the triple response of Lewis, i.e., red line followed by erythema (flare) and a central wheal. The atopic dermatitic skin responds initially with an erythema which is rapidly replaced by a white line that disappears rather rapidly. Pharmacologic abnormalities also exist. Agents such as acetylcholine, various catecholamines, histamine, kallikrein, and nicotinic acid have different effects on the normal versus the affected individual's skin. It also appears that some individuals with the more severe form of atopic dermatitis have impaired cellular immunity.

Infants present with a severe, weeping, erythematous eruption on the face, scalp, and other areas of the body. With increasing age, the rash typically affects popliteal and antecubital areas, face, neck, hands and chest. Lichenification becomes the predominant feature of the disease. The patient complains of severe pruritus which is difficult to relieve. Some patients become secondarily infected with skin pathogens which can lead to sepsis. Persons with atopic eczema are also susceptible to disseminated vaccinia because of secondary innoculation from the primary site and an apparent defect in cellular immunity. Disseminated herpes simplex and herpes zoster are other viral complications. These patients also have a higher incidence of cataract formation than does the normal population. Most patients with eczema improve as they age; however, some continue to have problems throughout life.

URTICARIA AND ANGIOEDEMA

Urticaria and/or angioedema is a common clinical problem. Although most cases of acute urticaria and angioedema are of an allergic etiology, previously held theories that most chronic problems were allergic or psychic have not been scientifically validated. Even though the clinical manifestations are similar, the pathophysiology is complex and differs in the various forms of the disease.

The histopathology is unimpressive: there is dermal edema, dilatation and engorgement of cutaneous blood vessels and lymphatics, and little or no perivascular eosinophilic infiltration. Angioedema affects the deeper dermal or connective tissues of certain organ systems, whereas urticaria affects the upper corium of the skin.

Urticaria secondary to Type I, II, and III allergic mechanisms usually is readily identified. However, the pathophysiologic mechanisms that cause many forms of urticaria and angioedema are poorly understood. Although histamine appears to be the most important mediator of the disease, other biologic products such as bradykinin, acetylcholine, and complement are important in individual forms of the disease (Fig. 18–4).

Many associated or etiologic factors may cause urticaria and angioedema. Some of these include drugs; infections such as hepatitis, infectious mononucleosis, and Coxsackie viral infections; inhalant allergens; physical stimuli, i.e., mechanical pressure, thermal, and solar; insect bites and stings; connective tissue disorders; and neoplasms. A few types of urticaria are of genetic origin: a heredofamilial syndrome of urticaria, deafness, and amyloidosis; familial cold urticaria;

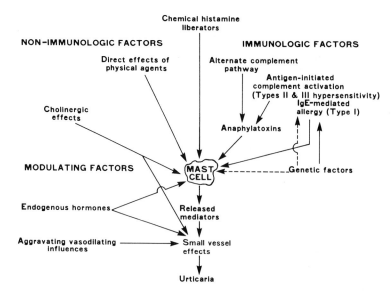

Figure 18–4 Schematic representation of various factors which can produce urticaria and angioedema. (With permission from Mathews, K. P.: A current view of urticaria. Med. Clin. North Am., *58*:188, 1974.)

familial localized urticaria; a familial vibratory urticaria; and erythropoietic protoporphyria with solar urticaria. Hereditary angioedema is a genetically-determined disease not associated with urticaria in which there is a deficiency or lack of function of the inhibitor (C$\bar{1}$ INH) of the first component of complement, Cl$_r$. C$\bar{1}$ INH also inhibits kallikrein, activated Hageman factor, plasmin, and activated thromboplastin antecedent. Thus, it is also an important modulator of bradykinin generation. Life-threatening angioedema of the larynx occurs and is the major cause of death in this disease. These patients also experience one- to two-day episodes of vomiting, severe abdominal pain, abdominal rigidity, and leukocytosis in the absence of fever. The clinical signs and symptoms are secondary to edema of the bowel wall. Trauma to skin can also precipitate angioedema. The method by which this deficiency leads to angioedema is unknown, but it is thought to be secondary to activation of the complement system with some suggestion the activation is Hageman factor-dependent.

Clinically, acute urticaria and angioedema can be defined as of less than six weeks' duration, whereas chronic urticaria and angioedema are of greater than six weeks' duration. The etiology for most cases of chronic urticaria and angioedema remains unknown. It is therefore referred to as idiopathic urticaria and angioedema. It may persist for months or years.

CONTACT DERMATITIS

Allergic contact dermatitis refers to a type of contact dermatitis caused by the Type IV immunopathologic reaction. The term "contact dermatitis" is often used to refer to other forms of dermatitis, which include photoallergic contact dermatitis, phototoxic contact dermatitis, irritant dermatitis, and contact urticaria.

The contact allergen (for example, pentadecyl catechols in the plants of the genus *Rhus*, which include poison ivy, oak, and sumac) penetrates and attaches to tissue proteins (carrier protein) in the skin, causing lymphocytic cellular sensitization. On subsequent exposure, lymphokines are released by the sensitized T-cells and cause the pathophysiologic changes of allergic contact dermatitis.

The dermopathology is characterized by the appearance of vasodilatation, edema, and perivascular infiltration with mononuclear and polymorphonuclear cells. In certain forms of the disease, basophils are also a prominent finding. Clinically, edema and vesicular eruptions apppear on the skin where contact with the allergen has occurred. Chronic exposure causes thickening of the skin, fissure formation, and hyperpigmentation.

Chemicals producing phototoxic or photoallergic contact allergic dermatitis require light to activate the chemical by absorption in certain wavelengths, usually between 2800 and 4300 angstroms. The activated chemical sensitizes in a fashion similar to that of those chemicals which cause allergic contact dermatitis. Phototoxic contact dermatitis refers to a non-immunologic exaggeration of the normal response of the skin to sunlight. Irritant dermatitis is induced by various irritants which may come in contact with the skin. The pathologic changes in all forms of contact dermatitis are not unlike those changes seen with allergic contact dermatitis.

EXTRINSIC ALLERGIC ALVEOLITIS (HYPERSENSITIVITY PNEUMONITIS)

The lung and bronchopulmonary structures are accessible to many airborne allergens. Extrinsic asthma and its immunobiochemical mechanisms have already been described. During the past several decades, other immunologically-mediated diseases of the lung have been studied and characterized. The first is farmer's lung, a disease induced by exposure to antigens in moldy hay. The same disease may be induced by other organic antigens under varying exposure circumstances. Microbiologic and immunologic techniques have identified the most common antigens responsible for this entity and the diseases they induce (Table 18–2).

A major contribution to understanding Farmer's lung resulted from Pepys' discovery of IgG precipitins against antigen derived from moldy hay. Antigen-specific IgG alone is produced in non-atopic persons in contrast to IgG and IgE antibody which atopic individuals make when exposed to these same antigens.

There is overwhelming evidence that extrinsic allergic alveolitis results from a hypersensitivity reaction, although the exact mechanism or mechanisms are not certain. Most of the patients are non-atopic, have normal serum concentrations of IgE, and have an absence of eosinophilia and significant bronchoconstriction. This suggests that the Type I mechanism is not involved.

Arguments in favor of a Type III immune complex-mediated disease are persuasive. There are serum-precipitating antibodies against the suspected organic antigens in most patients. The titers of these antibodies increase with the severity and, conversely, decrease with remission. Furthermore, there is a 4- to 6-hour time interval between exposure and the onset of symptoms. Antigen, immunoglobulin, and complement are demonstrable in the lung lesions characteristic of immune complex disease.

TABLE 18–2

Antigen (Organic Dusts)	Disease
Actinomycetes (Thermophilic) Microspolyspora faeni, Thermoactinomycetes vulgaris and Thermomycetes sacchari	Farmer's lung, mushroom worker's lung, humidifier lung, bagassosis
Antigen (Mold) Cryptostroma corticale, Aspergillus species, Penicillium, others	Maple bark disease, malt worker's lung, sequoiosis, suberosis
Antigen (Animal) Pigeon, dove, parrot, parakeet, gerbil	Pigeon-breeder's disease, bird-fancier's lung, gerbil-keeper's lung

Disturbing to this explanation alone are the virtual absence of vascular lesions of the lung, the detection of precipitating antibody to the organic antigen in a large proportion of asymptomatic but exposed persons, and the inability to transfer the disease passively to nonhuman primates with antibody-containing serum.

The Type IV mechanism may also play a role in the pathogenesis of this disease. Granuloma formation may occur, which is consistent with this mechanism. There are also in-vitro correlates (MIF production and lymphocyte transformation) in symptomatic persons, but not among the asymptomatic exposed subjects. Skin tests, however, do not result in the typical 48-hour delayed hypersensitivity reaction.

Animal models of allergic alveolitis have been developed by immunization in the guinea pig, mouse, rat, rabbit, and monkey. These animals will react with a pathologic process resembling hypersensitivity pneumonitis only when both precipitating antibody is formed and delayed hypersensitivity develops.

It therefore seems probable that Type III and IV mechanisms are contributors to the development of allergic alveolitis.

Allergic Bronchopulmonary Aspergillosis (ABPA)

The *Aspergillus* mold is hearty, ubiquitous, lives on substrates with low moisture, and has been demonstrated in diverse sources. It is one of the most commonly cultured molds in houses, and is found in basements, among bedding, and in house dusts and crawl spaces. Although classic extrinsic allergic alveolitis (malt worker's lung) may be induced by a species of the *Aspergillus*, there are at least four other types of disease which may be caused by the species or some member of the genus. These include invasive or septic aspergillosis, aspergilloma, bronchial asthma, or ABPA.

The latter condition was first described in 1952 and is characterized by pulmonary eosinophilia, infiltrates of the lung, and both blood and sputum eosinophilia. The disease occurs in atopic individuals who have had a history of bronchial asthma. Inhaled *Aspergillus fumigatus* spores grow in the bronchial secretions and form mycelia. Thus, a cardinal feature of ABPA is the capacity of the fungus to grow in the bronchial lumen and continue to shed its antigen. These antigens are capable of combining with both IgG and IgE and initiate immunologic reactions which result in bronchial wall damage and pulmonary eosinophilic consolidation.

A significant laboratory finding in ABPA is the marked elevation of serum IgE, in some cases as high as 78,000 ng./ml. Total IgE and IgE specific for *Aspergillus* species have been found highest during symptomatic episodes associated with pulmonary infiltrates and eosinophilia.

Pathogenetically, both IgE skin-sensitizing antibody and IgG precipitating antibody may be required to develop the dual skin test reaction that characterizes this condition. The same antibodies may be responsible for the pathogenesis of the disease. Although serum of patients with ABPA may contain only small amounts of precipitating antibody, their skin tests demonstrate a vigorous late reaction when challenged with the appropriate antigen. The low titer of precipitins provides a condition of moderate antigen excess which is conducive to the formation of toxic immune complexes. In experimental animals, an IgE-mediated reaction enhances the toxic effect of immune complexes. The dual role of IgE and IgG antibodies has also been demonstrated in passive transfer and aerosol challenge experiments in monkeys.

Other immunologic reactions that affect the lung include those mediated by cytotoxic antibodies. These Type II reactions are relatively rare in the lung. They are mediated by an antibody cytotoxic for target cells in the basement membrane of the lung and cross-reactive with the basement membrane of the kidney. The reactions are cytolytic, involve the activation of the complement system, and result in destructive lesions in the lung and kidney (Goodpasture's disease).

DRUG ALLERGY

This discussion considers hypersensitivity to drugs to be a synonym for drug allergy and excludes those adverse drug reactions not mediated by immunologic processes. Antigens capable of inducing allergic responses are large molecules which are foreign to the host. Most drugs, however, are simple chemicals of molecular weights under 1000. They must conjugate with macromolecules, usually proteins, which act as carriers. These complete antigens stimulate either specific humoral or cellular hypersensitivity. Under these circumstances, the small drug acts as a hapten, conferring specificity on the conjugated molecule.

The precise mechanisms by which drugs or their metabolic products become conjugated is unknown. Little is known also about genetic influences on the development of drug allergy. There is scanty evidence to support the predisposition of atopic patients to develop drug allergy, but some evidence exists for a genetic influence on drug metabolism which may affect the incidence of drug allergy. In at least one study of drug-induced systemic lupus erythematosus (SLE) with hydralazine, those who developed the SLE syndrome

were found to possess slow activity of the enzyme acetyl transferase. However, with rare exceptions, genetic influences of this type are more apt to affect the incidence of non-allergic drug reactions.

Drug allergic reactions may manifest any of the four immunopathologic mechanisms classified by Gell and Coombs. Type I reactions associated with IgE antibodies include anaphylaxis, urticaria, asthma, and allergic rhinitis. Serum from such patients usually contain specific IgE antibodies to large molecular weight substances. When simple chemical drugs are involved, such as with penicillin, specific serum IgE antibodies to the stable penicilloyl conjugate have been found with some regularity. The penicilloyl forms spontaneously from penicillin in solution and has been conjugated for use in skin testing.

Type II reactions due to cytotoxic antibodies are most frequent when mismatched blood is transferred. Under these conditions, transfused red cells, platelets, or leukocytes are readily destroyed by IgG or IgM antibodies in the presence of complement. A similar phenomenon may occur by a hapten cell mechanism which, for example, is present in penicillin-induced hemolytic anemia. IgG penicillin-specific antibodies react with red cells to which stable derivatives of penicillin have become attached. Red cell destruction may then occur primarily extravascularly.

Type III reactions due to drug antibody immune complexes are probably responsible for most allergic drug reactions involving formed blood elements. As an example, complexes may bind and activate complement near the cell surface. The cells, which are damaged, are designated as "innocent bystanders," since the action of antibody is not specifically directed at their surface.

Type IV reactions due to drugs are best exemplified by allergic eczematous contact dermatitis. These lesions are characterized by lymphocytic and mononuclear infiltration. Sensitized lymphocytes release lymphokines and cause tissue injury. The drug causing the reaction can be identified by a patch test in which a positive delayed response, as in the tuberculin test, is elicited at the application site by the drug interaction with specifically sensitized cells.

IMMUNOTHERAPY FOR ALLERGIC DISEASE

Immunotherapy for allergic disease consists of periodic injections of increasing amounts of allergens to which the patient has demonstrated Type I hypersensitivity, such as allergic rhinitis and extrinsic asthma. The patient, successfully treated, demonstrates a progressive capacity to accept increasing quantities of the injected allergen to a defined maximum level or maintenance dose. Immunologic changes which occur include the appearance of blocking antibody, an IgG immunoglobulin which is specific for the allergen being administered. The proposed mechanism by which blocking antibody induces improvement is that it competes for allergen with mast cell and basophil-bound IgE. Thus, less allergen reaches the sensitized mast cell and basophil, resulting in decreased mediator release. Blocking antibody may also bind allergen, thereby preventing it from reaching immunocompetent cells involved in IgE production. This would result in a reduced production of IgE antibody.

An effect of long-term immunotherapy is to diminish IgE titers specific for allergen, including the usual postallergic seasonal increase in IgE production. This normal increase is diminished in some treated patients. An additional immunologic change is the diminished histamine release by sensitized basophils in response to allergenic challenge. The possibility that increased suppressor T-cell activity may decrease IgE production secondary to immunotherapy has also been suggested.

CELL-MEDIATED IMMUNITY; TRANSFER FACTOR; ANERGY

Cell-Mediated Immunity

Cell-mediated immunity (CMI) consists of those immune reactions mediated by sensitized cells, not by antibodies. Initially, CMI was considered primarily as a diagnostic tool for evidence of prior contact or infection with certain microbes. It is now realized that CMI is vital in immunoprotection of the host and immunologic surveillance in neoplasia.

The nature of the antigen, the route of administration, and the functional integrity of the thymus-derived lymphocyte (T-cell) all influence the induction phase of CMI. The development of adequate populations of T-cells depends on several factors: (1) presence of a stem cell derived from the fetal yolk sac, liver and bone marrow; (2) differentiation of these cells in the thymus, probably triggered by an intracellular thymic epithelial factor called thymosin or thymopoietin; (3) migration of these modified immunocompetent T-cells to the deep cortical areas of lymph nodes, periarteriolar sheaths of the spleen, and peripherally in the blood and thoracic duct lymph.

Induction of CMI results from the interaction of antigen, either exogenous or endogenous, with T-lymphocytes having specific affinity for the antigen. This interaction may be facilitated by or dependent on participation by the macrophage.

The effector phase of CMI can be measured by delayed hypersensitivity (DH) skin testing with appropriate soluble antigens, which results in erythema and induration at the test site. The reaction peaks at 48 hours and resolves after several days.

The effector phase response of CMI results from the release from sensitized lymphocytes of one or more non-antibody humoral substances called lymphokines or products of activated lymphocytes (PALs). These include migration inhibition factor (MIF) and a variety of aggregation, activation, blastogenic, chemotactic, and skin-reactive factors affecting macrophages, non-sensitive lymphocytes, granulocytes, eosinophil, and other cells.

Transfer Factor

A notable property of CMI is its transferability to naive recipients by infusing sensitized lymphocytes. CMI manifested by DH has also been transferred with a subcellular dialyzable material of low molecular weight derived from disrupted lymphocytes. This low molecular weight material (less than 10,000 daltons) known as transfer factor has not been completely characterized and is still under intensive study. It may exert specific as well as non-specific adjuvant action and, since it is not antigenic, is a substance of considerable therapeutic potential. It may be of benefit to anergic patients whose CMI capacity is lost or severely diminished.

Anergy

This term was originally applied to the transient loss of tuberculin hypersensitivity following measles. The term has since been expanded to include patients who have lost the capacity, either completely or relatively, to express DH when tested with ubiquitous microbial antigens. The occurrence of either partial or complete anergy is affected by many factors. Transient DH depression, which occurs in pregnancy, malnutrition, and acute illness, is of less importance than the prolonged depression, which may occur in Hodgkin's disease, rheumatic disorders, non-lymphomatous malignancies, and chronic infections, such as TBC, coccidiomycosis, chronic mucocutaneous candidiasis and leprosy. Although common in occurrence, the underlying mechanism responsible for anergy is often ill-defined. Anergy is also manifest by in-vitro abnormalities such as diminished responsiveness of T-lymphocytes to stimulation by either phytohemagglutinin (PHA) or specific antigens. Another significant finding in anergic patients is their incapacity to become sensitized by dinitrochlorbenzene (DNCB), which is a universal sensitizer of contact dermatitis.

REFERENCES

BASIC MECHANISMS IN ALLERGY

Dixon, F. J., Vazquez, J. J., Weigle, W. O., et al.: Pathogenesis of serum sickness. Arch. Pathol., 65:18, 1958.

Gell, P. G., and Coombs, R. R. (Eds.): Clinical Aspects of Immunology, 2nd ed. F. A. Davis Co., Philadelphia, 1969.

Hunsicker, L. G.: Immunology of Renal Disease. In Lockey, R. F. (Ed.): Clinical Immunology and Allergy for Students and Practicing Physicians. Medical Examination Publishing Company, Inc., New York, 1978, pp. 287–311.

Ishizaka, K., and Ishizaka, T.: Immunology of IgE-Mediated Hypersensitivity. In Middleton, E., Reed, C. E., and Ellis, E. F. (Eds.): Allergy, Principles and Practice. C. V. Mosby Co., St. Louis, 1978, pp. 52-78.

Ishizaka, K., Ishizaka, T., and Hornbrook, M. M.: Physiochemical properties of human reaginic antibody. IV. Presence of a unique immunoglobulin as a carrier of reaginic activity. J. Immunol., 97:75, 1966.

Johansson, S. G. D., and Bennich, H.: Immunological studies of an atypical (myeloma) immunoglobulin. Immunology, 13:381, 1967.

Kohler, P. F.: Immune Complexes and Allergic Disease. In Middleton, E., Reed, C. E., and Ellis, E. F. (Eds.): Allergy, Principles and Practice. C. V. Mosby Co., St. Louis, 1978, pp. 155–176.

Lockey, R. F.: Immunopathologic (Allergic) Mechanisms. In Lockey, R. F. (Ed.): Clinical Immunology and Allergy for Students and Practicing Physicians. New York Medical Examination Inc., New York, 1978, pp. 121–140.

Plaut, M., and Lichtenstein, L. M.: Cellular and Chemical Basis of the Allergic Inflammatory Response. In Middleton, E., Reed, C. E., and Ellis, E. F. (Eds.): Allergy, Principles and Practice. C. V. Mosby Co., St. Louis, 1978, pp. 115–138.

Richerson, H. B., Dvorak, H. F., and Leskowitz, S.: Cutaneous basophil hypersensitivity. I. A new look at the Jones-Mote reaction, general characteristics. J. Exp. Med., 132:546, 1970.

Sell, S.: Immunology, Immunopathology, and Immunity, 2nd ed. Harper and Row, Hagerstown, Maryland, 1975.

Stanworth, D. R.: Immediate hypersensitivity. American Elsevier Publishing Co., Inc., New York, 1973.

ASTHMA

Aldolphson, R. L., Abern, S. B., and Townley, R. G.: Demonstration of alpha adrenergic receptors in human respiratory smooth muscles. Clin. Res., 18:629, 1970.

Austen, K. F., and Orange, R. P.: Bronchial asthma: the possible role of the chemical mediators of immediate hypersensitivity in pathogenesis of subacute chronic disease. Am. Rev. Resp. Dis., 112:423–436, 1975.

Brockelhurst, W. E.: Many facts, but insufficient knowledge: the story of asthma. J. Pharm. Pharmacol., 28:(4 Suppl.) 361–368, 1976.

Brockelhurst, W. E.: Pharmacodynamics and Mechanisms of Asthma. In Weiss, E. B., and Segal, M. D. (Eds.): Bronchial Asthma, Mechanisms and Therapeutics. Little, Brown and Co., Boston, 1976, pp. 117–136.

Gold, W. M.: Cholinergic Pharmacology in Asthma. In Austen, K. F., and Lichtenstein, L. M. (Eds.): Asthma: Physiology, Immunopharmacology and Treatment. Academic Press, New York, 1973, pp. 169–182.

Kaliner, M. A., Orange, R. P., and Austen, K. F.: Immunological release of histamine and slow reacting substance of anaphylaxis from human lung. J. Exp. Med., 136:556, 1972.

Lichstenstein, L. M., and Margolis, S.: Histamine release in vitro: inhibition by catecholamines and methylxanthines. Science, 161:902, 1968.

Nadel, J. A.: The parasympathetic system and its role in asthma. Adv. Asthma, Allerg. Pul. Dis., 4:15–21, 1977.

Stevenson, D. D.: Bronchial Asthma. In Lockey, R. F. (Ed.): Clinical Immunology and Allergy for Students and Practicing Physicians. Medical Examination Publishing Company, New York, 1978, pp. 712–761.

Szentivanyi, A.: The beta adrenergic theory of the atopic abnormality in bronchial asthma. J. Allergy, 42:203, 1968.

Szentivanyi, A., Krzanowski, J. J., and Polson, J. B.: The Autonomic Nervous System; Structure, Function, and Altered Effector Responses. In Middleton, E., Reed, E. E., and Ellis, E. F. (Eds.): Allergy, Principles and Practice. C. V. Mosby Co., St. Louis, 1978, pp. 265–300.

Weiss, E. B., and Segal, M. S.: Bronchial Asthma, Mechanisms and Therapeutics. Little, Brown and Co., Boston, 1976.

ALLERGIC EMERGENCIES

Austen, K. F.: Histamine and Other Mediators of Allergic Reactions. In Samter, M. (Ed.): Immunologic Diseases, 2nd ed. Little, Brown and Co., Boston, 1971, pp. 332–355.

Austen, K. F., and Orange, R. P.: Bronchial asthma: the possible role of the chemical mediators of immediate hypersensitivity in the pathogenesis of sub-acute chronic disease. Am. Rev. Resp. Dis., 112:423, 1975.

Austen, K. F.: Systemic anaphylaxis in man. J.A.M.A., 192:108, 1965.

Becker, F. L., and Austen, K. F.: Anaphylaxis. In Miescher, P. A., and Muller-Eberhard, H. J. (Eds.): Textbook of Immunopathology, Vol. I. Grune and Stratton, New York, 1968, pp. 76–93.

Idsoe, O., Gruthe, T., Willcox, R. R., and DeWeck, A. L.: Nature and the extent of penicillin side reactions, with particular reference to fatalities from anaphylactic shock. Bull. WHO, 38:159, 1968.

James, L. P., and Austen, K. F.: Fatal systemic anaphylaxis in man. N. Engl. J. Med., 270:597, 1964.

Lockey, R. F.: Allergic Emergencies. In Lockey, R. F. (Ed.): Clinical Immunology and Allergy for Students and Practicing Physicians. Medical Examination Publishing Company, Inc., New York, 1978, pp. 906–918.

Lockey, R. F., and Bukantz, S. C.: Allergic emergencies. Med. Clin. North Am., 58:147–156, 1974.

Parker, C. W., and Snider, D. E.: Prostaglandins and asthma. Ann. Intern. Med., 78:963, 1973.

Stember, R. H., and Levine, B. B.: Prevalence of allergic diseases, penicillin hypersensitivity, and aeroallergen hypersensitivity in various populations. Abstract. J. Allerg. Clin. Immunol., 51:100, 1973.

Van Arsdel, P. P.: Risk of penicillin reactions. Ann. Intern. Med., 69:1071, 1968.

ALLERGY: NOSE, EYES, AND SKIN

Brestel, E. P.: Contact Dermatitis. In Lockey, R. F. (Ed.): Clinical Immunology and Allergy for Students and Practicing Physicians. Medical Examination Publishing Company, Inc., New York, 1978, pp. 848–860.

Brestel, E. P.: Atopic Dermatitis. In Lockey, R. F. (Ed.): Clinical Immunology and Allergy for Students and Practicing Physicians. Medical Examination Publishing Company, Inc., New York, 1978, pp. 835–846.

Connell, J. T.: Non-Infectious and Non-Surgical Nasal Diseases. In Lockey, R. F. (Ed.): Clinical Immunology and Allergy for Students and Practicing Physicians. Medical Examination Publishing Company, Inc., New York, 1978, pp. 691–711.

Connell, J. T.: Quantitative intranasal pollen challenge. II. Effect of daily pollen challenge, environmental pollen exposure and placebo challenge on the nasal membrane. J. Allergy, 41:123–139, 1968.

English, G. M.: Nasal Polyps and Sinusitis. In Middleton, E., Reed, C. E., and Ellis, E. F. (Eds.): Allergy, Principles and Practice. C. V. Mosby Co., St. Louis, pp. 977–1001, 1978.

Lieberman, P. L., and Wood, T. O.: Allergy and immunology of eye disease. In Lockey, R. F. (Ed.): Clinical Immunology and Allergy for Students and Practicing Physicians. Medical Examination Publishing Company, Inc., 1978, pp. 457–471.

Mathews, K. P.: A current view of urticaria. Med. Clin. North Am., 58:185–205, 1974.

Mathews, K. P.: Chronic urticaria revisited. J. Allerg. Clin. Immunol., *61*:347–349, 1978.

Patterson, R.: IgE mediated rhinitis. Med. Clin. North Am., *58*:43–54, 1974.

Patten, J. T., and Allansmith, M. R.: Ocular Allergy. In Middleton, E., Reed, C. E., and Ellis, E. F. (Eds.): Allergy, Principles and Practice. C. V. Mosby Co., St. Louis, pp. 1116–1132, 1978.

DRUG ALLERGY

Agrup, G.: Patch Testing in Drug Allergy. *In* Dash, C. H., and Jones, H. E. H. (Eds.): Mechanisms in Drug Allergy. The Williams and Wilkins Co., Baltimore, 1972.

The Boston Collaborative Drug Surveillance Program. Excess of ampicillin rashes associated with allopurinol or hyperuricemia. N. Engl. J. Med., *286*:505, 1972.

The Boston Collaborative Drug Surveillance Program. Drug induced anaphylaxis: a cooperative study. J.A.M.A., *224*:613, 1973.

Juhlin, L., and Wide, L.: IgE Antibodies and Penicillin Allergy. *In* Dash, C. H., and Jones, H. E. H. (Eds.): Mechanisms in Drug Allergy. The Williams and Wilkins Co., Baltimore, 1972.

Levine, B. B., and Zolov, D. M.: Prediction of penicillin allergy by immunological tests. J. Allergy, *43*:231, 1969.

Parker, C. W.: Drug allergy. N. Engl. J. Med., *292*:732, 1975.

Reisman, R. E., Rose, N. R., Witebsky, E., et al.: Serum sickness. II. Demonstration and characteristics of antibody. J. Allergy, *32*:531, 1961.

Samter, M., and Parker, C. W.: Hypersensitivity to Drugs, Vol. I. Pergamon Press, Elmsford, N. Y., 1972.

VanArsdel, P. P., Jr.:Serum Antibodies to Red Cell Conjugates. *In* Stewart, G. T., and McGovern, J. P. (Eds.): Penicillin Allergy. Charles C Thomas, Springfield, 1970.

VanArsdel, P. P., Jr.: Adverse Drug Reactions. *In* Middleton, E., Reed, C. E., and Ellis, E. F. (Eds.): Allergy: Principles and Practice. C. V. Mosby Co., St. Louis, 1978, p. 1133.

EXTRINSIC ALLERGIC ALVEOLITIS AND ALLERGIC BRONCHOPULMONARY ASPERGILLOSIS

Banaszak, E. F., Thiede, W. H., and Fink, J. N.: Hypersensitivity pneumonitis due to contamination of an air conditioner. N. Engl. J. Med., *283*:271, 1970.

Buechner, H.A., Prevatt, A. L., Thompson, J., et al.: Bagassosis — a review. Am. J. Med., *25*:234, 1958.

Campbell, J. M.: Acute symptoms following work with hay. Br. Med. J., *2*:1143, 1932.

Dickie, H. A., and Rankin, J.: Farmer's lung: an acute granulomatous interstitial pneumonitis occurring in agricultural workers. J.A.M.A., *167*:1069, 1958.

Fink, J. N., Sosman, A. J., Barboriak, J. J., et al.: Pigeon breeder's disease — a clinical study of a hypersensitivity pneumonitis. Ann. Intern. Med., *68*:1205, 1968.

Fink, J. N.: Hypersensitivity pneumonitis: a case of mistaken identity. Hosp. Practice, *9*:119, March, 1974.

Hargreave, F. E., Pepys, J., Longbottom, J. L., et al.: Bird breeder's (fancier's) lung. Lancet, *1*:44, 1966.

Hinson, K. F. W., Moon, A. J., and Plummer, N. S.: Bronchopul-

monary aspergillosis: a review and a report of eight new cases. Thorax, *73*:317, 1952.

Lopez, M., and Salvaggio, J.: Hypersensitivity pneumonitis: current concepts of etiology and pathogenesis. Ann. Rev. Med., *27*:453, 1976.

McCarthy, D. S., and Pepys, J.: Cryptogenic pulmonary eosinophilia. Clin. Allerg., *3*:339, 1973.

Patterson, R., et al.: Serum immunoglobulin levels in pulmonary allergic aspergillosis and certain other lung diseases, with special reference to immunoglobulin E. Am. J. Med., *54*:16, 1973.

Pepys, J.: Hypersensitivity diseases of the lungs due to fungi and organic dusts. Monogr. Allerg., *4*:69, 1969.

Pepys, J., and Jenkins, P. A.: Precipitin (FLH) tests in farmers lung. Thorax, *20*:21, 1965.

Roberts, R. C., and Moore, V. L.: Immunopathogenesis of hypersensitivity pneumonitis. Am. Rev. Resp. Dis., *116*:1075, 1977.

Salvaggio, J. E., Buechner, H. A., Seabury, J. H., et al.: Bagassosis. I. Precipitins against extracts of crude bagasse in the serum of patients with bagassosis. Ann. Intern. Med., *64*:748, 1966.

Slavin, R. G.: Hypersensitivity diseases of the lung. Adv. Asthma Allerg., *5*:25, 1978.

Slavin, R. G.: Allergic Bronchopulmonary Aspergillosis. *In* Middleton, E., Reed, C. E., and Ellis, E. F. (Eds.): Allergy: Principles and Practice. C. V. Mosby Co., St. Louis, 1978, p. 843.

CELL-MEDIATED IMMUNITY, ANERGY AND TRANSFER FACTOR

Bloom, V. R., and Chase, M. W.: Transfer of delayed-type hypersensitivity: a critical review and experimental study in the guinea pig. Progr. Allerg., *10*:151, 1967.

Burnet, F. M.: Immunological surveillance in neoplasia. Transplant Rev., 7:3, 1971.

Chase, M. W.: Persistence of tuberculin hypersensitivity following the cellular transfer between genetically similar guinea pigs. Fed. Proc., *22*:617, 1963.

David, J. R., and David, R. R.: Cellular hypersensitivity and immunity: inhibition of macrophage migration and lymphocyte mediators. Prog. Allerg., *16*:300, 1972.

Eltringham, J. R., and Kaplan, H. S.: Impaired delayed hypersensitivity response in 154 patients with untreated Hodgkin's disease. Nat. Cancer Inst. Monogr., *36*:107, 1973.

Grossman, J., Baum, J., Gluckman, J., et al.: The effect of aging and acute illness on delayed hypersensitivity. J. Allerg. Clin. Immunol., *55*:268, 1975.

James, D. G., Neville, E., and Walker, A.: Immunology of sarcoidosis. Am. J. Med., *59*:388, 1975.

Kantor, F. S.: Infection, anergy and cell mediated immunity. N. Engl. J. Med., *292*:629, 1975.

Lawrence, H. S.: Transfer factor and cellular immunity. Harvey Lecture Series 63, Academic Press, New York, 1974.

Schwartz, R. S.: Current concepts: another look at immunological surveillance. N. Engl. J. Med., *290*:181, 1974.

Zweiman, B., and Levinson, A. I.: Cell-Mediated Immunity. *In* Middleton, E., Reed, C. E., and Ellis, E. F. (Eds.): Allergy: Principles and Practice. C. V. Mosby Co., St. Louis, 1978, p. 79.

19

Pathogenic Properties of Invading Microorganisms

LOUIS WEINSTEIN,
AND MORTON N. SWARTZ

INTRODUCTION

Although the terms "health" and "disease" are mutually exclusive, "health" and "infection" are not. For example, within a few days of birth an infant is "infected" with a variety of bacteria and remains so infected throughout his lifetime. Thus, bacterial (and viral) colonization of body surfaces and the intestinal tract is the early and inevitable consequence of the ubiquitous distribution of microorganisms in man's surroundings. A delicate but peaceful balance is ordinarily maintained between the host and his normal flora through the operation of a variety of natural antibacterial defenses. These serve to limit the flora to areas where it may be tolerated safely such as the surfaces of the upper respiratory tract, the skin, and the intestinal tract. However, there are two ways in which microorganisms may gain access to tissues not normally colonized: (1) The intrinsic pathogenicity of the organism may be such that it is capable of breaching the natural protective physical or biochemical barriers. *Streptococcus pyogenes* (Group A streptococcus) is an example of a bacterial species with such potential. (2) Natural defenses may be sufficiently compromised (trauma, immunosuppression, phagocytic malfunction, etc.) to allow commensal organisms to enter tissues not normally infected and to produce disease. This situation has become increasingly familiar during the past several decades as advances in the treatment of a variety of diseases have been won at the price of decreasing the host's natural resistance to invasive infection

by elements of his own flora. Such infections have been designated "opportunistic." In this setting, ordinarily bland organisms such as *Staphylococcus epidermidis. Serratia,* and *Herellea* may produce life-threatening invasive infection.

Whatever the mechanism of microbial invasion, once invasion has taken place the clinical manifestations of the infection are the result of the interaction of several major factors: (1) the intrinsic virulence of the microorganisms, (2) the nature of the host response to infection, and (3) specific anatomic features at the site of infection. The role of these factors in the pathophysiology of the infectious process and thus in the development of characteristic signs and symptoms will be the theme of this and the succeeding chapters in this section. An attempt will be made not to be encyclopedic but rather to examine some of the important examples of the aforementioned interactions. Since the presentation of most infections is that of involvement of a specific organ, and since this is necessarily the focus of the clinician's initial attention, considerable emphasis will be given to the particular pathophysiologic features of infection at specific sites such as the heart, central nervous system, skeletal system, and so on.

BASIC MECHANISMS OF PATHOGENICITY

Bacteria produce disease by either (1) the elaboration of toxins or (2) the invasion of tissues. The

528

pathogenicity of certain bacterial species appears to reside exclusively in their ability to elaborate a potent toxin (e.g., *Clostridium tetani,* the causative organism in tetanus), while that of other species appears to be due to bacterial multiplication and invasiveness alone (e.g., *Streptococcus pneumoniae*). However, the combination of invasive and toxigenic potential accounts for the pathogenicity of many other species (e.g., *Streptococcus pyogenes*).

TOXIN PRODUCTION

There are two major types of bacterial toxins: *exotoxins* and *endotoxins.* The former are produced within the interior of the cell and appear in filtrates of growing cultures and in infected tissues. Some exotoxins diffuse readily through the bacterial cell wall and appear in greatest concentration in culture filtrates toward the end of the logarithmic phase of growth (e.g., alpha toxin of *Clostridium perfringens*). Others, sometimes designated "protoplasmic toxins," do not diffuse through the cell wall as easily and do not appear in appreciable amounts in culture fluid until the cells have autolyzed (e.g., tetanus and botulinum toxins). Those toxins that have been purified thus far appear to be proteins. In contrast, endotoxins are lipopolysaccharides of the cell wall of many gram-negative bacteria and are released into culture media only on autolysis or disruption of the organisms. In the case of several of the potent bacterial exotoxins, rather specific mechanisms

of action have been elucidated at both the gross physiologic and subcellular levels. Although endotoxins have been studied extensively and although a variety of consequences of their administration have been demonstrated, their exact role in human disease is less specific and remains unclear.

EXOTOXINS

The number of bacterial exotoxins that have been reasonably well characterized is now rather extensive. Most of these, but not all, are produced by gram-positive bacteria, and they are listed in Table 19–1. No attempt is made here to provide a complete catalogue. In several instances, a given organism produces a variety of toxic products but only an illustrative example of clear clinical import is listed. Thus, *Clostridium perfringens* produces, in addition to the α toxin (lecithinase), κ toxin (collagenase) and λ toxin (protease), and so on. A variety of exotoxins similar to those produced by *Cl. perfringens* are produced by other clostridial species. Very recent additions to the list of toxigenic bacteria include enteropathic strains of *E. coli* and certain enteropathic strains of Shigella. In the case of certain exotoxins, the altered physiology they produce is now understandable at a subcellular or molecular level (diphtheria toxin, α toxin of *Clostridium perfringens, Vibrio cholerae* enterotoxin); in other instances, the biochemical lesion is not as clearly understood but the cellular localization of the toxin and the ensuing functional alterations have

TABLE 19–1 SOME TOXIGENIC BACTERIA AND THEIR EXOTOXINS

Bacterial Species	Disease	Toxin	Mechanism of Action
Corynebacterium diphtheriae	Diphtheria	Diphtheria toxin	Neurotoxic; generally cytotoxic
Clostridium tetani	Tetanus	Tetanus toxin	Neurotoxic (spastic)
Clostridium botulinum	Botulism	Botulinum toxin (5 immunologic types)	Neurotoxic (paralytic)
Clostridium perfringens	Gas gangrene; bacteremia	Alpha toxin	Lecithinase (necrotizing, leukotoxic, hemolytic)
Streptococcus pyogenes (Group A streptococcus)	Pyogenic infections; scarlet fever	Streptolysin 0 and DPNase	Leukotoxic (?)
		Erythrogenic toxin	Vascular dilatation and injury
Staphylococcus aureus	Pyogenic infections; food poisoning	Alpha toxin	Necrotizing
		Leukocidin	Leukotoxic (?)
		Enterotoxin	Enterotoxic (vomiting; diarrhea)
		"Exfoliatin"	Exfoliation
Bacillus anthracis	Anthrax	Lethal toxin	Lethal; edema production
Pasteurella pestis	Plague	Plague toxin	Necrotizing (?); vascular injury causing shock
Vibrio cholerae	Cholera	Cholera enterotoxin	Intestinal loss of water and electrolytes
E. coli (enterotoxigenic strains)	Gastroenteritis	*E. coli* enterotoxin	Intestinal loss of water and electrolytes
Shigella	Gastroenteritis	Shigella enterotoxin	Intestinal loss of water and electrolytes
Pseudomonas aeruginosa	Pyogenic infections	Exotoxin A	Lethal; necrotizing

been reasonably well characterized (botulinum and tetanus toxins). On the basis of their mechanisms of action, certain of the exotoxins can be characterized as *general cytotoxins, neurotoxins,* or *enterotoxins.*

General Cytotoxins

Diphtheria Toxin. The variety of clinical manifestations which may develop in the course of diphtheria are directly due to the production of toxin at the site of the pharyngeal (or rarely cutaneous) infection. The hallmark of the disease, the gray faucial membrane, is due to the local effect of the potent necrotizing exotoxin and the inflammatory response of the body. This membrane may progress downward and involve the larynx and trachea, causing airway obstruction. Absorption of exotoxin into the general circulation may lead to abnormalities in many distant organ systems.

Cardiac involvement (in the second week or later) occurs in about two thirds of patients with diphtheria, as judged by electrocardiographic observations. Frank myocarditis is seen in 10 to 25 per cent of patients. Conduction abnormalities are prominent features: bundle branch block (commonly), complete heart block, sinus tachycardia, atrial fibrillation, increased ventricular irritability or ventricular tachycardia and fibrillation. Congestive heart failure and cardiogenic shock may occur owing to the toxic myocarditis and are ominous developments. Diffuse involvement of the myocardium with granular and hyaline myofiber degeneration, mononuclear cell infiltration, and scarring has been found on pathologic examination of the heart in fatal cases. These findings are consistent with the expected effects of a potent cytotoxin (see below).

Nervous system complications occur in about 10 per cent of patients with diphtheria. Postdiphtheritic paralysis affects cranial and peripheral nerves. In severe cases, paralysis of the soft palate may appear early (first one to two weeks) and is probably due to the direct action of the toxin on the pharyngeal motor nerve endings. More commonly, neuritis involving cranial nerves III, VI, VII, IX, and XI, or peripheral nerves occurs in the second to sixth week. Motor loss is the predominant feature. A late (two to three months) form of peripheral neuritis, initially characterized by symmetrically distributed sensory loss and identical to the Guillain-Barré syndrome, also may occur. Very rarely diphtheria is associated with encephalitis.

Hepatitis and nephritis are occasionally seen in diphtheria and are probably due to effects of the toxin. Necrosis, fatty infiltration, and cellular degeneration are demonstrable histologically in the liver, kidney, and adrenal glands.

Diphtheria toxin is highly toxic for many species (man, guinea pig, rabbit); but a few (rat, mouse) are notably resistant. As little as 50 to 100 nanograms per kg. is lethal in a sensitive species. Diphtheria toxin is a single polypeptide chain of 62,000 daltons, which on cleavage of a single peptide bond and a disulfide linkage, is split into two fragments. Fragment A (21,000 daltons) is the toxic moiety; fragment B (40,000 daltons) is non-toxic by itself but is required for recognition of specific surface receptors in susceptible cell membranes. In the absence of the B portion of the molecule (or of fragment B), fragment A is not toxic because it cannot cross the plasma membrane and gain entry into the cell. A number of other toxins (cholera, *E. coli* enterotoxin) consist, similarly, of A and B polypeptide chains where the latter interacts with membrane receptors and the former is the "toxic" fragment.

Clinical evidence suggests that a variety of types of body cells are injured by diphtheria toxin. The work of Pappenheimer and his colleagues on the molecular basis of the action of diphtheria toxin is in keeping with these observations. The toxin interferes with mammalian cell protein synthesis, a process common to all cells of the body. Diphtheria toxin at a concentration of approximately 1 μg per ml. completely suppresses protein synthesis when added to HeLa cells or to cell cultures derived from animal species that are sensitive in vivo to the toxin. In cell-free systems from mammalian sources, the toxin (or fragment A) promptly inhibits the incorporation of amino acids into protein in the presence of the cofactor nicotinamide adenine dinucleotide (NAD). Transfer of amino acids from aminoacyl-tRNA to the growing polypeptide chains on the polyribosomes is blocked. This inhibition of polypeptide chain elongation is the result of the specific inactivation of the eukaryotic translocating enzyme (elongation factor-2 [EF-2], also known as transferase II), a soluble protein required for the guanosine triphosphate (GTP)-dependent translocation of peptidyl transfer RNA from the aminoacyl ("A") site to the peptidyl ("P") site on the ribosome (Figs. 19–1 and 19–2). An inactive adenine diphosphate ribosyl (ADPR) derivative of EF-2 is formed in a reaction catalyzed by diphtheria toxin:

$$NAD^+ + EF\text{-}2 \underset{\text{(active)}}{\overset{\overset{\text{Diphtheria}}{\text{toxin}}}{\rightleftharpoons}} \underset{\text{(inactive)}}{ADP\text{-ribosyl } EF\text{-}2} +$$

$$nicotinamide + H^+$$

The effect of toxin can also be demonstrated in cell-free extracts prepared from a diphtheria-toxin-susceptible species such as the guinea pig.

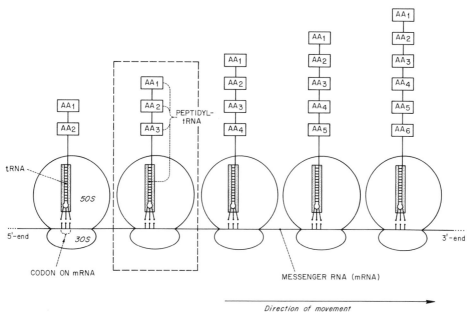

Figure 19–1 Polypeptide synthesis on polyribosome. Schematic representation showing polypeptide chain elongation during movement of the ribosomes (made up of 30S and 50S subunits) along the messenger RNA (mRNA) molecule. Five ribosomes are shown bound to the mRNA. Initiation of protein synthesis begins at the 5' end of the mRNA and polypeptide chain elongation proceeds on each ribosome as it moves toward the 3' end of the mRNA. The ribosomes shown on the right of the diagram (toward the 3' end of the mRNA) bear the longer polypeptide chains. The tRNA molecule is shown in a specific site (darkened area) on each ribosome, positioned in relation to the codon on the mRNA by its complementary codon (anticodon). The tRNA serves as an "adapter" to which an amino acid is attached, so that the latter can be adapted to the triplet-based (nucleotide) genetic code. When an incoming amino acid is added to the initiating aminoacyl-tRNA, the latter is converted to a peptidyl tRNA. The initial amino acid is designated as AA_1. Subsequent amino acids added to the nascent polypeptide chains are designated AA_2, AA_3, and so on. Because each of the five ribosomes above are traveling down the same mRNA molecule, the same five polypeptide chains will ultimately be made. The detailed steps involved in the addition of a single amino acid to form the peptidyl-tRNA shown in the boxed area in the figure are illustrated in Figure 19–2. The molecular site of action of diphtheria toxin is located there.

Relatively small amounts of toxin (less than 25 M.L.D.) administered parenterally render inactive the "soluble enzyme fraction" (EF-2), prepared from heart and skeletal muscle, that is an essential component of the in-vitro protein synthesizing system. Polyribosomes prepared from intoxicated guinea pigs function normally in in-vitro protein synthesis, provided that the "soluble enzyme fraction" is obtained from animals that have not been treated with toxin.

The toxin is extremely potent. Only a few molecules located in the cell membrane of a HeLa cell in the presence of the internal NAD concentration are capable of converting the entire cell content of free EF-2 to its inactive ADP-ribosyl derivative. In vivo, certain tissues, such as the heart and skeletal muscle, are particularly sensitive to small amounts of toxin. The inhibition of protein synthesis in subcellular components is consistent with the clinical and pathologic findings. Since the turnover rate of protein in muscle is slow, the toxin may inhibit synthesis at a functionally critical site (the S-A node or conduction

system) or of specific enzymes involved in maintaining normal cardiac function. In vitro, the direct addition of diphtheria toxin to brain and liver tissue extracts of the susceptible guinea pig inhibits polypeptide synthesis. However, the protein-synthesizing ability of the in-vitro system prepared from brain tissues of intoxicated guinea pigs is not significantly impaired. This is in contrast to the aforementioned results with heart and skeletal muscle. The reason for this apparent difference is obscure. A possible explanation may lie in the number of surface receptors for the toxin on brain cells. It would be informative to study the protein-synthesizing system in peripheral nerves, since the major impact of diphtheria toxin is registered there rather than in the brain. Nonetheless, the available body of evidence is sufficient to strongly suggest that diphtheria toxin acts in the susceptible animal in a manner analogous to its action in cell cultures and in cell-free systems, namely, by inactivation of EF-2.

Clostridium Perfringens Toxins. *Clostridium*

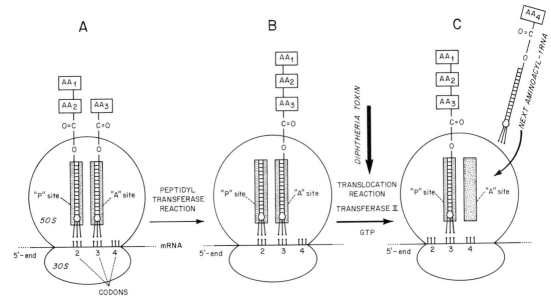

Figure 19–2 Schematic view of the individual steps involved in polypeptide chain elongation on an individual ribosome.

A, A ribosome (made up of its 50S and 30S subunits) is shown bound to a segment of mRNA. Two sites (aminoacyl or "A"; peptidyl or "P") are shown on the ribosome. The incoming aminoacyl-tRNA (bearing AA_3) is bound to the "A" site, positioned in accordance with the complementary nucleotide sequence it bears to the next codon (codon 3) of the mRNA. The "P" site is occupied by a peptidyl-tRNA (in this case bearing the two amino acids, AA_1 and AA_2).

B, The addition of AA_3 to the growing polypeptide chain involves peptide bond formation between the amino group of AA_3 and the esterified carboxyl group of AA_2 of the peptidyl-tRNA. This reaction is catalyzed by the enzyme peptidyl transferase, a part of the 50S subunit of the ribosome. As a result of this reaction, AA_1 and AA_2 are displaced from their tRNA in the "P" site to the tRNA in the "A" site, forming a new, elongated peptidyl-tRNA. The tRNA portion of the peptidyl-tRNA formerly in the "P" site (tRNA-AA_2-AA_1) remains (without its amino acid charge) bound to the "P" site.

C, The next step in polypeptide chain elongation is the translocation reaction, a complex step involving a specific protein (elongation factor-2 in mammalian cell systems; also designated "transferase II") and the ribonucleoside triphosphate GTP. This reaction involves the physical movement of peptidyl-tRNA (tRNA-AA_3-AA_2-AA_1) from the "A" site to the "P" site, with resulting displacement of the empty (uncharged) tRNA from the latter site. This is shown in Section C of the figure. As a result of this movement, the "A" site is now open and available to receive a new incoming aminoacyl-tRNA coded for by codon 4. The cycle can then be repeated. Diphtheria toxin acts to inhibit the transferase II-requiring translocation reaction by causing the adenosine diphosphate ribosylation of the protein (see text).

perfringens is an obligate anaerobe normally inhabiting the lower gastrointestinal tract of man. Wound contamination with this organism is very common; however, significant infection is rare. Clostridial infections are not due to uniquely pathogenic strains but rather to local circumstances such as low oxidation-reduction potential, ischemia, and necrosis that are favorable for multiplication. The critical pathogenetic step which transforms the relatively mild gas-forming infection (anaerobic cellulitis) into the devastating, rapidly advancing anaerobic myositis ("gas gangrene") capable of involving healthy muscle is as yet unknown. Several of the exotoxins, such as κ toxin and λ toxin, produced by the organisms may contribute to the rapid advance of the highly lethal infection through their collagenolytic and proteolytic activities respectively. However, it is important to recognize that the mere fact of production of these toxins is not sufficient evidence to establish their role in the pathogenesis of the infection. The alpha toxin, or lecithinase (phospholipase-C), of *Cl. perfringens* has been implicated in both the local tissue necrosis and toxemic features of gas gangrene. However, it should be noted that some strains of *Cl. perfringens* isolated from severe gas gangrene have been poor producers of alpha toxin. Furthermore, specific antitoxin to the lecithinase will not protect against the development of gas gangrene, not stop its spread, and not alleviate the toxemia and shock which are features of this disease. The interaction of alpha toxin or other extracellular enzymes with injured muscle is thought by some to be the source of the as yet unidentified toxic factor in gas gangrene. Although the direct role of alpha toxin has been somewhat de-emphasized in the foregoing discussion, it should be appreciated that it is nonetheless an extremely potent and lethal product. Intravenous administration in experimental animals produces fever, hypotension, intravascular hemolysis, jaundice, hemoglobinuria, renal shutdown, and death. The clinical counterpart with the identical constellation of findings develops in the course of high-grade *Cl. perfringens* bacteremia. This does not occur ordinarily in gas gangrene but is a fairly common complication of clostridial infection of the uterus following a septic abortion. The lethal effects of the lecithinase are due to splitting of lecithin (Fig. 19–3) which is present in the membranes of a variety of cells in the body. These cells include erythrocytes, which are hemolyzed by this enzyme; leukocytes are probably similarly injured, accounting for the paucity of these cells in the exudate of gas gangrene. Recent studies indicate that purified phospholipase-C does not have primary hemolytic activity; rather it acts in concert with the theta toxin (an hemolysin) of *Cl. perfringens*. The initial action of the theta toxin on erythrocyte membranes exposes buried phospholipid groups to subsequent phospholipase-C action; the latter in turn renders the red blood cell more susceptible to hemolysis.

Pseudomonas Aeruginosa Exotoxin A. This protein exotoxin can be demonstrated in the blood of experimental animals moribund with systemic infection due to *P. aeruginosa*. Injection of purified toxin intraperitoneally in mice produces leukopenia, hepatic necrosis, renal tubular necrosis and death. This toxin is more than 20,000 times as toxic (on a weight basis) as Pseudomonas endotoxin. The role of the toxin in the clinical manifestations of localized (pneumonia, pyelonephritis, etc.) and systemic (bacteremia) Pseudomonas infection in man is as yet unclear. It is tempting to relate the hemorrhagic, necrotizing features of these infections to this exotoxin. However, in view of the prominent bacterial arteritis (prominent growth of bacilli in arterial walls) seen with Pseudomonas infections, another explanation can be offered. This toxin appears to act at a molecular level like diphtheria toxin: it interferes with

protein synthesis by effecting ADP-ribosylation of eukaryotic elongation factor-2 (EF-2). However, clinically these two toxins appear to have different cellular specificities. Whether these variations stem from differences in cell membrane receptors remains to be elucidated.

Tetanus Toxin. Tetanus is an intoxication with the exotoxin of *Clostridium tetani* and is characterized by intense, severe muscle spasms. The toxin, known as tetanospasmin, is one of the most potent bacterial toxins known. Spores of the etiologic agent, *Clostridium tetani*, are introduced by contamination of a wound. The wound may be an extensive laceration, gun shot or puncture wound, or a very trivial lesion into which spores of the organism have been introduced. The mere presence of *Cl. tetani* in a wound does not mean that tetanus will develop. Transformation of the spores into toxin-producing vegetative forms requires a lower oxidation-reduction potential than is present in normal tissues. Necrotic tissue produced by the trauma or by invasion by pyogenic bacteria simultaneously present and the introduction of foreign material can lower the reduction-oxidation potential sufficiently to allow this to occur. There is little or no capacity of the organism to invade tissues, and often the wound hardly appears to be infected. All the clinical manifestations of the disease are due to the physiologic changes produced by the toxin in the nervous system — spinal cord, brain stem, and sympathetic nervous system. Toxin introduced into muscle spreads centrally along motor nerves and up the spinal cord. Toxin may also be spread via the bloodstream, and this route may be the more important one in generalized tetanus. Despite the violent and widely distributed symptoms of the disease, no lesions are detectable in the nervous system (or other tissues), even with the electron microscope.

The major clinical manifestation of tetanus is muscular rigidity. This may be mild in "local tetanus," in which rigidity affects only one limb or one group of muscles (the site of injury) and usually occurs in patients with a limited degree of immunity. More often, the initiating injury is followed within a matter of days by local muscu-

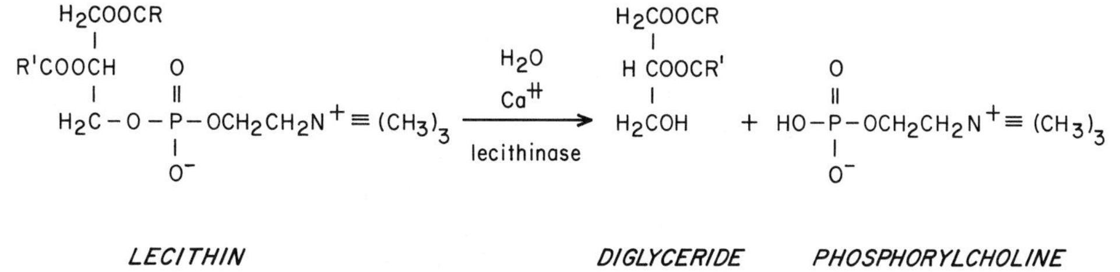

Figure 19–3 Action of *Cl. perfringens* lecithinase (α toxin) on lecithin. Cleavage of the bond between the phosphoric acid and glycerol moieties yields a diglyceride and phosphorylcholine. R and R′ represent fatty acids esterified with glycerol.

lar spasm about the wound and then trismus. Stiffness of the facial muscles may produce a bizarre sneering expression (*risus sardonicus*). Stiffness of the back, neck, and abdomen may become marked enough to produce pain as a prominent symptom. Dysphagia and hydrophobia are due to spasm of the pharyngeal and glottal muscles. With the progression of generalized tetanus, opisthotonos and violent spasmodic contractions of the neck, trunk, and limb muscles occur. Despite the severity of such manifestations the sensorium is still clear. Sudden stimuli (noise, bright light, an injection) may precipitate a generalized tonic convulsion, with accompanying spasm of the larynx and respiratory muscles, resulting in respiratory arrest. Thus, afferent stimuli appear to produce an exaggerated effect. This suggests that the toxin produces its characteristic effects by disturbing the normal regulation of the reflex arc. Reciprocal innervation is abolished and as a result both the stimulated muscle groups and the opposing groups contract simultaneously. This produces the characteristic muscular spasm. The particular features of this spasm are determined in each area by the relative bulk (strength) of the opposing muscle groups. Thus, since the masseters are stronger than the opposing mylohyoid and digastricus muscles, trismus results. The masseters generally show greater sensitivity to tetanus toxin than the muscles of the extremities. It has been suggested that this is because the masseters are normally maintained in a state of partial contraction when man is awake. In the lower extremities the strength of the extensor groups exceeds that of the flexors, and the predominant posture in tetanus is that of extension at the hips and knees.

The neurophysiology of the action of tetanus toxin now seems reasonably clear, particularly as a result of the studies of Sir John Eccles. The main impact of the toxin is on the spinal cord. Grossly, the effects of the toxin are very similar to those of strychnine. The toxin does not act on reflex arcs which include only sensory and motor neurons (two-neuron or monosynaptic reflexes). It profoundly affects the more complex reflexes (polysynaptic reflexes that involve interneurons), blocking the normal postsynaptic inhibition of spinal motorneurons that results from afferent impulses. This action of the toxin in selectively blocking inhibitory synapses in the central nervous system results in multiplication of excitatory impulses which run in unchecked fashion and are not coordinated by inhibitory mechanisms. This produces the muscular spasms (tetanic seizures) characteristic of tetanus.

In the normal resting state, muscle tone is maintained by the constant mild tension of opposing muscle groups. Thus, motion at the elbow is controlled by two sets of muscles — the extensor (triceps) and the flexor (biceps). When the biceps contracts slightly, the triceps is stretched, activating stretch-sensitive receptors. These, in turn, send afferent impulses to the spinal cord, where they stimulate the motor neurons and cause contraction of the triceps opposing the stretch. The stretch reflex thus plays an important role in maintaining postural tone. However, for proper functioning of the elbow joint, for example, it is essential that the biceps not be opposed too vigorously by the triceps. Otherwise, the forearm would be locked into spasm by the action of the opposing muscles, and voluntary movement would be impossible. Therefore, the afferent impulse that causes the activation of the biceps must facilitate relaxation of the triceps. This inhibition is effected in the spinal cord by branching of the axon carrying the afferent impulse. One branch excites the biceps and the other excites the internuncial neuron ("inhibitory cell") to release an inhibitory transmitter (Fig. 19–4). This inhibitory transmitter in turn acts on the anterior horn cells innervating the triceps, thus opposing the action of the excitatory transmitter released there from the stretch-sensitive afferent nerve. The net result is that triceps motor neurons are not excited and the triceps does not contract; the biceps is then able to flex the forearm unhindered. Tetanus toxin acts in the spinal cord to disrupt this balanced reciprocity by suppressing the normal inhibition through the internuncial connections. The toxin appears either to reduce the amount of inhibitory transmitter (glycine) available for release or to block its release. As a result, in the absence of inhibition the normal stretch reflex of the triceps is unopposed, and when the biceps contracts, the antagonist muscle, the triceps, does likewise, locking the forearm in spasm.

An unusual form of tetanus results from action of the toxin primarily on the motor innervation (in the brain stem) of the facial, glossal, pharyngeal, jaw, and ocular muscles. Whether the toxin reaches these areas by the neural or hematogenous route is not clear. This form of tetanus is known as "cephalic tetanus." It occurs when the spores of *Cl. tetani* are introduced into wounds involving the eye, during tonsilloadenoidectomy, during the course of chronic otitis media, or following trauma to the head or neck. In this form of tetanus the affected muscles appear to be paralyzed, especially those involving facial and ocular movements. The apparent facial palsy in reality is a pseudoparalysis. Hypertonia involves all the muscles supplied by the facial motor neurons, and voluntary movements are prevented. Although "cephalic tetanus" may be the only clinical presentation, it is important to emphasize the fact that generalized disease may develop subsequently.

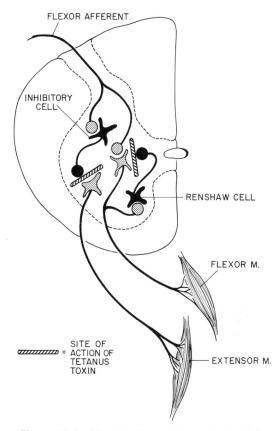

FLEXOR AFFERENT

INHIBITORY CELL

RENSHAW CELL

FLEXOR M.

SITE OF
= ACTION OF
TETANUS
TOXIN

EXTENSOR M.

Figure 19-4 Site of action of tetanus toxin. Schematically shown are neural connections involved in controlling the action of opposing flexor and extensor muscle groups such as the biceps and triceps. Contraction of the biceps normally stretches the triceps, activating receptors which pass to the spinal cord (this afferent is not shown on the illustration) and stimulating the motor innervation of the triceps. Another afferent to the biceps is shown which synapses with an inhibitory cell ("interneuron"). The latter releases an inhibitory transmitter, preventing the stretch-induced excitation of the triceps. Also shown is a second inhibitory pathway, involving an axon collateral from the flexor motor neuron extending to a Renshaw cell. This cell, in turn, synapses with the flexor motor neuron, producing postsynaptic inhibition, controlling the stimulation of flexor contraction. Tetanus toxin appears to act by blocking both of the above inhibitory pathways in the spinal cord.

Overactivity of the sympathetic nervous system has been observed in patients with severe tetanus, suggesting that tetanus toxin may also directly affect this portion of the nervous system. Among the manifestations that may develop, in any combination, are labile hypertension, tachycardia, peripheral vasoconstriction, irregularities of cardiac rhythm, profuse sweating, increased respiratory rate, increase in the urinary excretion of catecholamines, and, in some instances, during the late stage of the disease, hypotension. These manifestations do not appear to be related to hypoxia secondary to involvement of the innervation of the muscles of respiration or to pulmonary infection. Such evidences of sympathetic overactivity are not generally observed in other paralyzed patients treated in identical fashions to support respiration and maintain adequate oxygenation.

"Localized tetanus" is an unusual clinical form of tetanus in which intermittent twitching and spasm of muscles occur in a circumscribed area of the body, with or without a known wound or injury in that area. Stiffness of the muscles in the involved area, usually a limb, may be the initial symptom. The manifestations may persist over several weeks or months restricted to the initial area of involvement, or the process may progress to generalized tetanus within a few days. Although it was originally believed that this form of tetanus was due to the local action of the toxin on muscle near the site of injury, it is now thought that the manifestations of this form of tetanus are also due to suppression of spinal inhibitory mechanisms. Toxin reaching the spinal cord either by passage along regional nerves or by hematogenous spread (as seems more likely) produces an increased central excitatory state. This, however, is so slight in localized tetanus as to be inapparent if it were not for the increased afferent inflow from the periphery provided by the local skin and muscular lesion at the site of trauma.

The pathophysiology of the action of tetanus toxin at the molecular level is unknown. However, Van Heyningen has demonstrated that the site of toxin binding in nervous tissue is the synaptic membrane of the nerve endings. The chemical substance binding the toxin is a ganglioside, a compound containing fatty acid, sphingosine, sialic acid, and several sugars. The role of toxin binding in clinical tetanus is not clear; there is no detectable change in the ganglioside molecule where the toxin is bound. Binding may not be an essential feature of the action of toxin but may simply be a means of channeling this toxin to the central nervous system. Like diphtheria toxin, tetanus toxin can be dissociated by proteolytic cleavage and thiol reducing agents into two polypeptide chains (α and β). The ganglioside-binding site of the intact toxin molecule resides in its β chain.

Botulinum Toxin. Botulism is an intoxication with the exotoxin of *Clostridium botulinum* and is characterized by profound weakness of both skeletal and smooth muscle. The disease results from the ingestion of food (canned meats and vegetables, packaged fish, sausages) in which the organism has grown under anaerobic conditions and elaborated its potent exotoxin. There is absolutely no invasive potential to the organism itself and all the clinical manifestations are due solely to the toxin. The toxin is heat labile; cooking at boiling temperature for a few minutes destroys it. Clinical symptoms usually develop 18 to 36 hours after ingestion of contaminated food. The cranial nerves are involved earliest, resulting in paresis of accommodation, diplopia due to weakness of the external ocular muscles, dysphagia, difficulty talking, and weakness of the jaw muscles. Subsequently, the muscles of the trunk and limbs become weak. The deep tendon reflexes remain normal; sensory abnormalities are absent. A curious neurophysiologic response, a facilitated muscle-action potential after repetitive nerve stimulation, is typical of botulism.

Like tetanus toxin, botulinum toxin is extremely potent yet produces no apparent structural damage. There is no evidence of involvement of the central nervous system. In contrast to the diffuse muscular overactivity of tetanus, the characteristic feature of botulism is a flaccid weakness; this is not due to any loss of contractile power of the muscles themselves, since they respond normally to direct electrical stimulation.

After absorption from the gastrointestinal tract, toxin reaches susceptible neurons via the circulation and there becomes bound to presynaptic terminals. The molecular nature of the toxin receptor in the presynaptic membrane is not certain but is suggested by the finding that certain gangliosides bind botulinum toxin. Burgen, Dickens, and Zatman have reported that the toxin acts at the neuromuscular junctions, preventing release of acetylcholine, the excitatory transmitter. They noted that the quantity of acetylcholine liberated by stimulation of phrenic nerve-diaphragm preparations of rats was very much smaller in the presence of botulinum toxin than in control preparations. Thus, excitatory impulses are blocked between the efferent nerve endings and the muscle; this leads to flaccid weakness. Electron microscopic studies indicate that the toxin blocks exocytosis of acetylcholine-containing vesicles at presynaptic release sites.

Enterotoxins

Cholera Enterotoxin. Cholera, an infection due to *Vibrio cholerae,* is characterized by dramatic and devastating diarrhea, resulting in enormous fluid and electrolyte losses. It occurs endemically and epidemically in Asia but recently has spread to Africa and southern Europe. The disease is usually transmitted by contaminated water but occasionally by fruits or vegetables contaminated with human feces. Its onset is sudden and the course is, as a rule, fulminant. Chills and fever are not prominent features; the body temperature may, in fact, be depressed. Abdominal pain and vomiting may accompany the initial diarrhea.

Later, however, the striking feature of the disease is the prodigious fluid loss from the intestine. This may exceed one liter of fluid per hour. The "rice water" stool is watery, odorless, and mucoid. The various clinical manifestations that develop later are secondary to the severe degree of dehydration and the loss of electrolytes. These include hypotension and shock, metabolic acidosis, muscle cramps, stupor and coma, hypokalemic flaccid paralysis, acute tubular necrosis, and, occasionally, myocardial infarction.

The primary pathophysiologic disturbance in cholera is severe loss of fluid and electrolytes from the small intestine. These changes occur in the absence of any invasion of the intestinal mucosa by the organisms or a significant inflammatory response. The initial outpouring of large volumes of fluid into the lumen of the intestine occurs at a time when there is no disruption of the intestinal mucosa. Denudation of the mucosa is a late phenomenon and is secondary to severe hypovolemia in the end stages of cholera. The only histologic changes noted consistently in early human cases and in the experimental animal (rabbit) are mild hyperemia of the mucosal capillaries and edema of the tunica propria of the small intestine.

The fluid lost from the intestine is isotonic and has a low protein content similar to that found in the intestinal fluid of normal persons. The bicarbonate concentration of this fluid is about twice and the potassium concentration about four times that of normal plasma. All the clinical manifestations of the disease can be corrected by prompt intravenous administration of appropriate fluid and electrolytes.

Recent studies of the effects of cholera enterotoxin indicate that it produces increased fluid and electrolyte movement across the small intestine from plasma to the gut lumen. This could be due to either increased filtration of electrolytes from intestinal capillaries across the mucosal cells, or to active secretion of one or more electrolytes by the epithelial lining cells. Present evidence suggests that the former is not the case. For example, decreasing the mesenteric blood flow in the dog by as much as 70 per cent does not reduce the rate of fluid production by intestinal loops treated with cholera enterotoxin. Even more telling evidence against the filtration hypothesis is provided by the examination of the intestinal clearance of mannitol and sodium in patients with acute cholera. Gordon has demonstrated that the clearance of intravenously administered ^{14}C mannitol is only 25 per cent of the clearance of sodium, indicating less resistance to the flow of sodium than of mannitol.

Considerable insight into electrolyte movement across the normal and cholera enterotoxin-treated intestine has been provided by study of the isolated rabbit ileal mucosa. Normally, the net secretory flux of HCO_3^- balances the net absorptive flux of Cl^-. There is also a net absorptive flux of Na^+, and this can be increased by the addition of glucose to the solution on the luminal side of the isolated ileum. (This experimental observation has a very important therapeutic implication. Indeed, orally administered glucose-containing solutions can reduce considerably the electrolyte loss of patients with the disease.) The addition of cholera enterotoxin to the mucosal side of such an in-vitro preparation produces distinct changes after a latent period of about an hour. These consist of (1) complete disappearance of the net absorptive flux of Na^+ and (2) reversal of the direction of chloride transport, the net absorptive flux being replaced by a net secretory flux. The HCO_3^- net secretory flux remains unchanged. *Thus, the effect of enterotoxin on solute transport consists of stimulation of chloride secretion and inhibition of sodium absorption.* The toxin-induced secretion of anion would then cause isosmotic accumulation of water. Fluid pouring into the intestine in the cholera patient, or in the rabbit ileal loop, is indeed isotonic. Large losses of HCO_3^- occur when the reabsorptive capacity of the colon for diarrheal fluid is exceeded. The same mechanism may be responsible for substantial losses of potassium.

Cyclic AMP (3',5'-AMP), when applied to the isolated rabbit ileal mucosa preparation, produces changes in ion flux similar to those produced by cholera enterotoxin. This suggests that the cholera enterotoxin-induced fluid and electrolyte loss may be mediated by cyclic 3',5'-AMP. There is a large body of evidence in support of this concept: (1) Adenylate cyclase, the enzyme involved in the synthesis of 3',5'-AMP from ATP, is demonstrable in the mucosa at all levels of the small intestine but is present in highest concentration in the duodenum. Outpouring of fluid and solute in response to cholera enterotoxin occurs at all levels of the small bowel; the highest rate of secretion is in the duodenum. (2) Theophylline, an inhibitor of the phosphodiesterase that normally breaks down 3',5'-AMP to 5'-AMP, produces effects similar to those of cholera enterotoxin: infusion of theophylline into the superior mesenteric artery of dogs produces fluid and solute secretion into the small intestine comparable to that produced by cholera enterotoxin, and theophylline produces alterations of ion flux similar to those produced by cholera enterotoxin on the isolated rabbit ileal mucosa. (3) Cholera enterotoxin increases the adenylate cyclase activity of membranes prepared from rabbit small intestine. (4) 3',5'-AMP levels in intestinal mucosa are increased several fold after preincubation with the toxin either in vitro (membrane preparations) or in vivo (intact mucosal cell in the experimental animal).

The detailed molecular events in the action of cholera toxin are currently in the process of being defined in many laboratories. Cholera toxin, molecular weight 84,000, consists of two subunits (or protomers): A and B. The entire toxin molecule is necessary for intoxication of intact cells through activation of adenylate cyclase. The first step in the activation process appears to be the binding of the B protomer of the toxin to cell surface receptors containing the monosialoganglioside G_{M1}. The A protomer then appears to penetrate the cell membrane at least as far as the inner surface, where it activates the adenylate cyclase. The lag between exposure of intact cells to toxin and the first rise in adenylate cyclase activity probably represents the time needed for the A protomer to cross the membrane and reach its site of action. In disrupted cell preparations the initial B protomer binding step is unnecessary, and the A protomer alone can activate adenylate cyclase. Cholera toxin and its A protomer catalyze the hydrolysis of nicotinamide adenine dinucleotide (NAD) to ADP-ribose and nicotinamide. It can also catalyze the ADP-ribosylation of the amino acid L-arginine. It has, therefore, been proposed that activation of adenylate cyclase by cholera toxin involves ADP-ribosylation of an arginine or similar amino acid residue in some acceptor protein (even adenylate cyclase itself). This would be analogous to the mechanism of action of diphtheria toxin (or its active fragment A) which catalyzes the ADP-ribosylation of a protein, elongation factor-2.

Several other acute infectious diarrheal diseases of man may be produced by a mechanism identical to that operative in cholera. These are disorders in which bacterial invasion of the bowel wall does not take place, but in which exotoxins may have a major pathogenetic role. These include the gastroenteritides due to enterotoxin-producing strains of *E. coli,* *Shigella,* and *Clostridium perfringens.* Extracellular products of these organisms have been shown experimentally to stimulate small intestinal fluid secretion. *E. coli* enterotoxin has been shown to cause diarrhea by increasing adenylate cyclase levels in intestinal mucosa. A peptide released from enterotoxic *E. coli* appears very similar to the A protomer of cholera toxin, and like the latter is able to activate adenylate cyclase in vitro.

ENDOTOXINS

Bacterial endotoxins are integral parts of the bacterial cell wall and are released only upon disruption of the bacterial cell. Endotoxins differ in a variety of ways from bacterial exotoxins: (1) Endotoxins are particulate macromolecules. Although originally isolated as phospholipid-polysaccharide-protein complexes, their biological activity resides in an extractable lipopolysaccharide fraction. Their toxicity appears to reside predominantly in the phospholipid component; the major antigenic determinants are in the polysaccharide fraction. On the other hand, bacterial exotoxins are proteins, usually of relatively small size (M.W. 50,000 to 100,000, occasionally as large as 1,000,000). (2) True endotoxins are found predominantly, if not exclusively, in gram-negative bacteria. In contrast, exotoxins are produced by many types of bacteria, most frequently by gram-positive bacilli. (3) Endotoxins are less potent by at least several orders of magnitude than most exotoxins. (4) Endotoxins from a variety of bacterial species elicit the same responses after parenteral administration, even though the intrinsic pathogenicity of the organism from which they were derived shows considerable differences. (5) Endotoxins are relatively heat-stable, unlike bacterial protein exotoxins (with the exception of the enterotoxin of *Staphylococcus aureus*). (6) Bacterial endotoxins are much more varied in their activity and less specific in their cytotoxic actions. Thus, no effects of endotoxin can compare with the exquisite selective neuro-tropism of the toxins of *Cl. tetani* and *Cl. botulinum*.

Endotoxins have been identified in *E. coli*, Salmonella, Shigella, *Vibrio cholerae,* Brucella, *Neisseria gonorrhoeae, Neisseria meningitidis,* and other gram-negative organisms. When injected intravenously in experimental animals, they produce a variety of biologic effects. These include fever, diarrhea, hypotension, shock, transient leukopenia followed by leukocytosis, hyperglycemia, abortion, capillary hemorrhages, diffuse intravascular coagulation, altered resistance to bacterial infections, and the Shwartzman phenomenon. Despite this large number of physiologic derangements produced by endotoxins, their role in the clinical features of illnesses due to gram-negative bacteria remains speculative. Tolerance, or refractoriness to the pyrogenic and other biologic effects of endotoxin, develops on repeated injection. The state appears to be independent of the development of demonstrable circulating antibody, since it subsides after one to two weeks following a course of repeated injections, whereas active immunity persists much longer. Tolerance results from an increased clearance of injected endotoxin by cells of the reticuloendothelial system (RES); it can be prevented by prior injection of particulate material (Thorotrast, India ink) which is readily taken up by the RES, resulting in "blockade" of its ability to clear subsequently injected endotoxin. It has been suggested that circulating endotoxin plays an important role in sustained gram-negative infection and that the development of tolerance is an important aspect of recovery from the illness. Tolerance to endotoxin is not a feature of infections of man produced by gram-negative bacteria (brucellosis, typhoid, tularemia). There is, in fact, an

enhanced reactivity to its effects. Indeed, in experimental typhoid fever an enhanced pyrogenic response to injected endotoxin can be elicited from late in the incubation period through the early phase of convalescence. As the convalescent phase progresses, tolerance to the pyrogenic effects of endotoxin develops. Tolerance to endotoxin, induced in man by daily injections, disappears during the active stage of typhoid fever and reappears when chemotherapy has produced a favorable response.

Biologic Effects

1. *Fever* is produced by the intravenous injection of endotoxin in most laboratory animals and man. The febrile response occurs in humans after a lag period which may be as long as 90 minutes. Clearer understanding of the febrile response to endotoxin has come from the animal studies of Atkins and Wood. Immediately following the injection of endotoxin, blood was found to contain a weak pyrogen which had all the properties of the originally injected material. This then disappeared from the blood, which became non-pyrogenic; 90 to 120 minutes after the endotoxin injection a second pyrogen appeared in the circulation. The properties of this substance differed in many ways from those of endotoxin and appeared to be identical with those of pyrogenic material ("endogenous pyrogen") isolated from polymorphonuclear leukocytes (see Chapter 20). The marked neutropenia produced by the injection of endotoxin has been presumed to be evidence of direct damage to leukocytes by this macromolecule. Release of the leukocytic pyrogen from the injured neutrophils is the most likely cause of the later fever. The non-identity of leukocytic pyrogen and endotoxin has been demonstrated in several ways. Leukocytic pyrogen is active in animals previously rendered tolerant to the pyrogenic effects of bacterial endotoxin. Unlike endotoxin, leukocytic pyrogen produces a single febrile peak after a very brief lag period when injected into animals.

2. *Granulocytopenia* appears promptly after intravenous injection of endotoxin, persists for three to six hours, and is followed by a marked leukocytosis. The short period of granulocytopenia is associated with impairment of leukocytic migration into areas of active inflammation. Granulocytopenia develops as neutrophils shift from the circulating pool to the marginal one, as a result of increased adherence of leukocytes to the vascular endothelium, particularly in the lung.

3. *Hypotension and shock* are produced in animals by the injection of large doses of endotoxin. Species difference among animals with regard to the pattern of vascular response to this substance has been a source of confusion in attempts to

understand the pathophysiology of endotoxic shock and to relate the circulatory changes in bacteremia due to gram-negative organisms in man to "endotoxic shock." For example, in the dog the early systemic hypotension that develops after injection of endotoxin stems from a decreased cardiac output. This follows a marked decrease in venous return that is due primarily to pooling in the portal system secondary to constriction of hepatic veins produced by release of histamine. Recovery from the initial hypotension occurs within a few minutes. A second fall in blood pressure occurs in one to two hours; this is more gradual, and spontaneous recovery is not usual. There is gradual slowing of blood flow in the microcirculation and vasospasm of arterioles and venules. Decreased perfusion of many organs ensues, with the greatest effects occurring in the renal and splanchnic circulation. Catecholamines are released and produce an increase in total peripheral arterial resistance. When endotoxin shock has gone on for several hours in the dog the process becomes irreversible. This stage is featured by arteriolar and capillary dilatation, venular contraction, stasis, and morphologic evidences of damage to capillaries and veins (hemorrhage and edema, especially of the intestine). In contrast to the response to endotoxin in the dog, the circulatory changes in man are less clear and well-defined. The cause of the circulatory changes occurring in patients with sepsis due to gram-negative bacteria is uncertain. Many of the features may be attributed to the bacteremia itself or to endotoxemia alone.

4. *Coagulation* may be profoundly altered following injection of endotoxin into experimental animals. The changes in hemostasis are biphasic. After a lag period there is a hypercoagulable state (associated with an increased amount of circulatory fibrinogen), followed in a matter of hours by a prolonged hypocoagulable period. The latter is characterized by depletion of plasma fibrinogen, thrombocytopenia, and other changes associated with intravascular clotting. In-vitro studies of human and animal plasma suggest that endotoxin initiates intravascular clotting by activating Factor XII (Hageman factor) which appears to be capable of activating plasma prekallikrein to the active protease kallikrein. This in turn releases bradykinin (an extremely powerful vasodepressor) from its inactive plasma precursor kininogen. Bradykinin, with its ability to increase vascular permeability and its vasodepressor effects, may be responsible for many of the circulatory effects of septic shock. Thus, it is likely that the same site of endotoxin action (activation of Factor XII) may initiate both the coagulation and hemodynamic alterations associated in some instances with shock.

5. The *Shwartzman phenomenon* is a peculiar toxic reaction observed in rabbits following two injections of endotoxin. Two types of this phenomenon have been described. The *local Shwartzman reaction* consists of gross hemorrhage and necrosis in the skin. It occurs after an initial *cutaneous* injection of endotoxin (or endotoxin-containing bacteria), which is then followed in some hours by an *intravenous* injection of endotoxin. The initial ("preparatory") and second ("eliciting") injections may utilize endotoxin from different bacterial species. Non-bacterial materials such as washed antigen-antibody precipitates may be employed for the "eliciting" reaction. Polymorphonuclear leukocyte "cuffing" develops about the small veins at the skin site following the "preparatory" injection. Peripheral vasoconstriction, particularly at the prepared skin site, is produced by the intravenous injection. Leukocyte-platelet thrombi develop and occlude capillaries and small veins, resulting in necrosis of vessel walls and secondary hemorrhage.

The *generalized Shwartzman reaction* develops when both the "preparatory" and "eliciting" injections of endotoxin are given intravenously approximately 24 hours apart. The typical histologic lesion that develops is characterized by deposition of fibrinoid material within capillaries. This occurs most dramatically in the kidney and produces bilateral renal cortical necrosis. The histologic findings appear to be the result of disseminated intravascular coagulation. Polymorphonuclear leukocytes are essential to the development of the Shwartzman phenomenon; the prior induction of leukopenia will prevent both the localized and generalized forms of the reaction.

The striking incidence of purpuric skin lesions in meningococcemia, in comparison with the incidence in bacteremias due to gram-negative bacilli, appears to be related to the properties of meningococcal endotoxin (lipopolysaccharide). Whereas the lipopolysaccharides (LPS) from the meningococcus and from enteric gram-negative bacilli (*E. coli, S. typhimurium*) are of comparable potency for the general Shwartzman reaction and for mouse lethality, the meningococcal LPS is five to ten times more potent in inducing the localized (dermal) Shwartzman reaction. Histologic examination of purpuric skin lesions of patients with acute meningococcemia reveal large numbers of meningococci in endothelial cells and neutrophils, endothelial necrosis, and thromboses. Immunoglobulins and complement are present in the vascular walls, suggesting possible immunologic factors in the genesis of the skin lesions. Although it is tempting to ascribe the characteristic hemorrhagic necrotic skin lesions of meningococcemia to the Shwartzman reaction, convincing proof that this reaction occurs during disease in man is still lacking.

INVASION OF TISSUES

Local Effects

Most infectious agents produce demonstrable damage to host cells in the area immediately surrounding their site of invasion. In many instances, this is due primarily to multiplication of the infecting agent (usually bacteria or fungi) or to its growth (parasites). Among the invasive bacteria, *S. pneumoniae* (pneumococcus) is an example of an agent the pathogenicity of which appears to be solely related to its capacity to multiply rapidly and successfully in the susceptible host. No toxins capable of producing local or distant effects have been demonstrated in infections produced by this organism. The essential ingredient in its pathogenicity is the antiphagocytic activity of its capsular polysaccharide. Thus, smooth encapsulated strains are capable of resisting surface phagocytosis, the first line of host defense, prior to the appearance of specific antibody. Pneumococci invading the lung are thus capable of extensive multiplication and of eliciting marked edema and an acute inflammatory response in the alveoli. The extensive lobar involvement that occurs is responsible for the characteristic dyspnea and tachypnea due to both arterial oxygen undersaturation (secondary to continued perfusion of the poorly ventilated area of lung) and splinting of the chest (secondary to spread of the bacterial inflammation to the pleural surface with its attendant pain). Rarely, the unrestrained growth of pneumococci may be so extensive that frank tissue destruction and abscess formation occur. This is almost invariably due, when present, to type 3 pneumococci, strains which, because they produce unusually abundant capsular material, are almost totally insulated from surface phagocytosis.

Localized pyogenic foci (abscesses) due to a large variety of bacteria may develop almost anywhere in the body and increase in size sufficiently to produce obstructive or pressure phenomena. However, when they occur in the central nervous system their effects may be most dramatic because of their anatomic location and the lack of elasticity of the surrounding structures. Thus, an abscess in the cerebrum or cerebellum can produce marked neurologic deficit by two mechanisms: neuronal destruction by the invading microorganisms, and swelling of surrounding brain tissue due to edema and the inflammatory response. The abscess may be well walled-off by a thick capsule, and there may be little or no fever or other manifestations of infection. The clinical picture may then mimic that of an enlarging cerebral mass lesion such as a brain tumor. Manifestations of increased intracranial pressure such as headache, papilledema, and sixth and third cranial nerve palsies may dominate the clinical picture. If untreated, the lesion may go on to cause herniation of the temporal lobe and midbrain compression, or it may rupture into the ventricular system and cause fulminating meningitis. A temporal lobe lesion that may present in a similar way may occasionally be seen in viral infection of the central nervous system, especially encephalitis due to *Herpes hominis*.

The dramatic mass effects of infection are particularly prominent in certain parasitic infestations. Heavy loads of adult Ascaris may produce abdominal pain and even intestinal obstruction. Migration of these worms into the biliary tree may produce obstruction and ascending cholangitis. Cysticercosis represents the invasion of various tissues by the larval form of the pork tapeworm, *Cysticercus cellulosae*. The brain is most commonly involved. The parasitic cyst surrounded by a thick capsule can mimic a neoplasm and cause seizures, personality changes, long tract signs, or increased intracranial pressure. The larvae of *Toxocara canis* may migrate in man to a variety of organs such as liver, lung, or eye. In the ocular form, a space-occupying granulomatous mass resembling a retinoblastoma may develop and distort the retina.

Effects of Widespread Dissemination of Infection

Bacteremia may result when initial host defenses are insufficient to contain the invading microorganism locally. Thus, *Staphylococcus aureus* bacteremia following an initial skin or other focus of infection may produce abscess formation in distant organs such as kidney, bone, and brain. The symptoms and signs of the infection that develops in this situation are related to dysfunction of the particular organ involved. A transient bacteremia may become high grade and continuous when staphylococcal infection is superimposed on a previously damaged (or entirely normal) heart valve to produce acute bacterial endocarditis (see Chapter 21). Rarely, the density of staphylococci in the blood may be sufficiently high as to be visible in Gram-stained smears of a "buffy-coat" preparation of venous blood. The nature of the factors that contribute to staphylococcal pathogenicity is unclear. Clinical isolates do not appear to contain an antiphagocytic capsule component.

Another organism that, in the setting of nosocomial infection, is notoriously capable of producing abscesses in multiple organs following bacteremia is *Pseudomonas aeruginosa*. It is an aggressive secondary invader in open wounds, in decubiti, at the sites of foreign bodies (e.g., indwelling venous catheters), and particularly in extensive third-degree thermal burns. It is an opportunist par excellence in patients suffering from complicated, debilitating illness, in premature or malnourished infants, in individuals whose normal bacterial flora has been altered by prior antibiotic therapy, and in persons with neoplastic disease (especially leukemia) whose antibacterial defenses are compromised by deficiencies of circulating and/or cellular immunity or by defective circulating granulocytes. Invasion of the bloodstream by *P. aeruginosa,* unlike that due to *S. aureus,* is frequently followed by the development of widespread bacterial vasculitis. Growth of the organism in the walls of small and medium-sized arteries leads to thrombosis and septic infarction in many organs. Nodular, necrotic septic lesions occur, particularly in lung, kidney, heart, and brain. Unusual but characteristic bullous, hemorrhagic, and necrotic lesions of a similar pathogenesis may develop in the skin. Involvement of the lung results in pneumonia characterized by multiple nodular areas of consolidation which may rapidly undergo abscess formation. Dyspnea, pleuritic pain, and hemoptysis are prominent clinical manifestations. Involvement of the heart may lead to endocarditis, myocardial infarction secondary to coronary artery occlusion by the arteritis, or pericarditis, as a result of spread of infection to the pericardial sac by the bacteremic route or by contiguity from a septic myocardial infarct. The cellular or extracellular factors involved in the invasive propensity of *P. aeruginosa* in the compromised host have not been characterized. The very recent isolation and characterization of *P. aeruginosa* exotoxin A (see earlier section on General Cytotoxins) as a lethal toxin may provide valuable insights into the pathogenicity of this highly invasive organism. The role of exotoxin A in the production of the striking bacterial arteritis that occurs in *P. aeruginosa* is not known at present. In view of the extensive bacterial proliferation in and about blood vessels in such infections, direct bacterial invasiveness must be an important, if not the only, determinant of pathogenicity.

Widespread dissemination of infection leading to involvement of multiple organs is not restricted exclusively to bacterial disease. Although viral infections often demonstrate rather remarkable tropism for specific organs (poliomyelitis for anterior horn cells, infectious hepatitis for the hepatocytes, influenza for respiratory epithelial cells), certain viruses may, under special circumstances, proliferate in many organs and produce tissue damage. Thus, *Herpes hominis* infection in the neonate may eventuate in viremia which is followed by invasion of multiple sites. Destruction of cells of the skin, brain, liver, lung, and adrenal glands may occur as a result and contribute to the usually lethal outcome. Overt, clinically evident pneumonia, encephalitis, and hepatitis may dominate the picture.

Widespread involvement of organs may also occur in protozoan disease such as malaria. In infection due to *Plasmodium vivax,* up to 2 per cent of erythrocytes may be parasitized; in disease produced by *P. malariae,* such involvement usually does not exceed 1 per cent. *P. falciparum* has the greatest invasive propensity of the three major species of malarial parasites and may parasitize as many as 10 per cent of the red blood cells of a patient. The consequences of such marked multiplication may be extensive and produce a variety of organ dysfunctions secondary to circulatory changes. Hemolysis produced by red cell rupture at the time of schizogony leads to the rapid development of severe anemia. Evidence suggests that the hemolysis in malaria is related to the loss of erythrocyte membrane function. This appears to be the consequence of the usurpation by the parasite of the metabolic machinery of the red cell needed for the maintenance of the membrane. Further, hemolysis may be related to splenic removal of parasitic inclusions from the erythrocytes ("pitting") as they pass between the walls of splenic sinusoids. The red cells that survive this procedure re-enter the circulation as spherocytes. Some of these spherocytes are damaged in the process and subsequently exhibit a shortened survival in the circulation. Capillary distention and blockage by parasitized red cells result in anoxia that may produce irreversible damage in brain, liver, and kidneys. Pulmonary edema may develop as a consequence of cerebral, pulmonary, and cardiovascular injury in patients with acute falciparum malaria.

COMBINATION OF TOXIN PRODUCTION AND INVASIVENESS AS BASIS OF PATHOGENICITY

The clinical manifestations of certain infections are due exclusively to the effects of potent exotoxins in the absence of bacterial invasion (tetanus, botulism). The primary features of other infectious processes, on the basis of current evidence, appear to be related almost exclusively to the local or disseminated proliferation of the invading microorganism itself. A third class of infectious diseases is one in which clinical manifestations appear to be related both to the activity of exotoxin and to the multiplication of and invasion by bacteria. Three different diseases produced by three distinct bacterial species serve as examples of this type of infection.

Scarlet fever is a syndrome characterized by a localized infection, usually of the pharynx but occurring anywhere in the body, accompanied by a toxic rash. The eruption is produced by an erythrogenic toxin elaborated by the organisms at their site of multiplication and absorbed into the bloodstream. This toxin is produced by the majority of strains of Group A and by occasional strains of Group C and G streptococci. Its production is related to the presence of a temperate bacteriophage in the streptococcus, a phenomenon very similar to that involving diphtheria toxin elaboration by lysogenic strains of *Corynebacterium diphtheriae*.

The signs and symptoms of scarlet fever consist of two groups: (1) The *local manifestations of infection* in the pharynx are the result of the inflammatory reaction and response of the lymphoid tissues to bacterial invasion. These account for the redness of the pharyngeal mucosa, the development of soft, yellow exudate that fills the crypts of the tonsils and may overflow onto the pharynx and over the uvula, the edema and enlargement of lymphoid tissues including those of the posterior pharynx. In an occasional patient with streptococcal tonsillitis, bacteremia may develop as a complication. Although an abundance of extracellular products are produced by Group A streptococci and although it is tempting to assign them a role in the invasiveness of the organism (e.g., streptolysin 0 and DPNase are leukotoxic; hyaluronidase may assist in breaking down tissue barriers; streptokinase is fibrinolytic and might account for lack of localization of many streptococcal infections), there is no clear evidence to establish such a role. (2) *The manifestations of scarlet fever due to the erythrogenic toxin* are a characteristic skin eruption and various peripheral signs. This agent acts primarily on the capillary bed to produce dilatation, congestion, and increased fragility.

The typical scarlatiniform eruption, a punctate rash superimposed on an erythematous base, the bleeding lines (Pastia's lines), the suggestive early "strawberry" and later "raspberry" tongue, the increased excretion of red blood cells in the urine, and the swelling of the hands and feet that may be present at the onset of the disease are all due to activity of erythrogenic toxin in the vascular bed. The generalized abdominal pain, nausea, and vomiting that may be early features have a similar pathogenesis. The diffuse erythema of the skin is related to the dilatation of the capillaries; the punctate erythematous lesions are manifestations of the same effect on the tufts of blood vessels in the dermal papillae, causing them to be raised and somewhat darker than the surrounding skin. Histologic study reveals dilatation of small blood vessels which are surrounded by an accumulation of neutrophilic exudate. When injected into the skin of normal non-immune subjects, purified erythrogenic toxin produces a localized area of erythema (Dick test). The action of the toxin on the capillary tuft in the papillae may be sufficiently intense to cause increased fragility and the appearance of petechiae. The effect of the toxin on the integrity of the capillary vasculature is readily shown by the occurrence of "bleeding lines" and hematuria. Because of increased fragility, vessels in skin folds (e.g., inguinal, axillary, and antebrachial areas), which are subjected to considerable movement and minor trauma, rupture and produce linear extravasations of blood (Pastia's lines). The renal glomerular capillaries are also injured by the toxin and leak small numbers of red cells in the urine early in the disease and for as long as a week.

The changes in the tongue characteristic of scarlet fever are also due to the effects of the erythrogenic toxin on the capillary bed of this organ. The "strawberry" tongue, present at the onset of the disease, is not pathognomonic of scarlet fever. It represents the early effect of toxin on the capillaries in the lingual papillae, which become enlarged, reddened, and protrude through the white coat on the surface of the tongue, giving the appearance of an unripe strawberry. The "raspberry" tongue appears after three to four days and is much more characteristic of the disease. It is the result of continued activity of the toxin on the blood vessels, which are now diffusely dilated, accounting for the deep red color of the tongue after the coat has been shed. Because of the greater number of capillaries in the lingual papillae, these become large and deeper in color than the surrounding tissue, standing out as strikingly elevated structures.

Within a week or so, desquamation of the skin and tongue begins. This represents shedding of superficial dermal and lingual layers of these organs that have borne the brunt of the activity of the erythrogenic toxin and have eventually been destroyed. This leads to separation of large patches of skin from the hands and feet, "brawny" desquamation on the trunk, and loss of lingual papillae (to such an extent that the surface of the tongue becomes quite smooth).

The diffuse abdominal pain, nausea, and vomiting that often characterize severe scarlet fever are probably the result of the effects of erythrogenic toxin on the capillary vasculature of the intestinal tract as well as on the lymphoid tissues in the intestinal wall and mesenteric nodes. The fact that lymph nodes may be affected by erythrogenic toxin in the absence of bacteremia is strongly suggested by the presence of generalized lymphadenopathy in most cases and splenomegaly in about 10 per cent of patients.

Jaundice, accompanied by evidence of dysfunction of the liver, may be a feature of severe scarlet fever and is probably due to a toxic hepatitis produced by the erythrogenic toxin.

When scarlet fever is severe, it is not uncommon for patients to complain of arthralgia and to exhibit a considerable degree of swelling of the hands and feet. Since these findings appear during the first one or two days of the disease, it is clear that they are not manifestations of rheumatic fever but are manifestations of the activity of erythrogenic toxin on blood vessels, resulting in the development of edema. An unusual feature of the early stage of scarlet fever is the presence of meningeal irritation, with stiff neck and back and positive Kernig and Brudzinski signs. Examination of the cerebrospinal fluid discloses a pleocytosis (up to 1000 cells per mm.[3], practically all of which are lymphocytes), a moderate increase in the concentration of protein, and a normal content of sugar. This is the "serous meningitis" of scarlet fever and has been considered to be due to the effect of the erythrogenic toxin or other extracellular products of *Streptococcus pyogenes*.

Toxic epidermal necrolysis (Lyell's disease or "scalded-skin" syndrome) is a dramatic and serious skin disease, usually occurring in infancy. It is characterized by tenderness of the skin and striking erythema, followed by desquamation in sheets over most of the body. Because of the extensive exfoliation, temperature regulation and fluid balance are particular problems in the newborn. The characteristic histologic changes are the formation of a cleavage plane high in the epidermis, in the granular cell layer, and separation of the epidermal layer by edema fluid producing typical bullae. This disorder has been associated with the presence on the epidermis or at other sites of infection of large numbers of *S. aureus* of phage group II. Such strains produce an extracellular toxic protein ("exfoliatin") capable of causing exfoliation in neonatal mice following subcutaneous or intraperitoneal administration; this is presumed to be the agent responsible for the scalded-skin syndrome in infants. This toxin is separate and distinct from the alpha and delta toxins of the organism. It has been proposed that the rare case of scarlatiniform eruption associated with some infections due to *S. aureus* is a forme fruste of the scalded-skin syndrome in which systemic spread of the toxin has occurred without the full picture of exfoliation, due to less toxin production or to undefined host factors.

Anthrax is a disease in which bacterial multiplication and dissemination and toxin production in vivo proceed pari passu. Recent evidence has suggested a predominant role for a toxin in the pathophysiologic changes that occur in the lethal form of the disease. Anthrax is an infection, primarily of animals, caused by *Bacillus anthracis*. It is occasionally transmitted to man by exposure to animal products (wool, bone, etc.). The commonest manifestation of the disease in man is a necrotic skin or mucous membrane ulcer ("malignant pustule") surrounded by a wide zone of gelatinous edema. Dissemination of infection from the original focus may occur via the bloodstream and may lead to the development of a hemorrhagic mediastinitis or hemorrhagic meningitis. Following inhalation of anthrax spores, a fulminant form of the disease may occur, characterized by a hemorrhagic mediastinitis and meningitis. When dissemination of the infection occurs, blood cultures are usually positive. The bacteremia is often high grade and it may be possible to identify the bacilli on stained smears of centrifuged sediment of blood. No quantitative data are available on the number of organisms per milliliter of blood in man. However, in the experimental animal, 10^8 to 10^9 organisms per ml. of blood may be found terminally. Although it was originally thought that death was due to widespread capillary blockage produced by the large number of bacilli in the circulation, this hypothesis is no longer accepted.

A toxin has recently been demonstrated in the edema fluid of the anthrax lesion and in the plasma of animals dying of anthrax. This substance appears to be made up of a complex of three serologically distinct components: an *edema-producing factor*, a *protective antigen*, and a *lethal factor*. The level of the toxin in the blood roughly parallels the degree of bacteremia. The most recent experimental evidence strongly suggests that the exotoxin contributes significantly to the pathophysiology of the infection. Purified anthrax toxin complex is lethal for several animal species. Its main effect is to increase vascular permeability; this may account for the gelatinous edema about the local lesion and the terminal pulmonary edema in fatal disease in experimental animals. The molecular mechanism of action of the toxic moiety is unknown. It is now generally believed that death from anthrax is due to the effects of this toxin.

REFERENCES

GENERAL CYTOTOXINS

Bornstein, D. L., Weinberg, A. N., Swartz, M. N., and Kunz, L. J.: Anaerobic Infections: Review of current experience. Medicine, *43*:207, 1964.

Bowman, C. G., and Bonventre, P. F.: Studies on the mode of action of diphtheria toxin III. Effect on subcellular components of protein synthesis from the tissues of intoxicated guinea pigs and rats. J. Exp. Med., *131*:659, 1970.

Collier, R. J.: Effect of diphtheria toxin on protein synthesis: Inactivation of one of the transfer factors. J. Molec. Biol., *25*:83, 1967.

Collier, R. J., and Pappenheimer, A. M.: Studies on the mode of action of diphtheria toxin II. Effect of toxin on amino acid incorporation in cell-free systems. J. Exp. Med., *120*:1019, 1964.

Davis, B. D., et al.: Anaerobic spore-forming bacilli. *In:* Microbiology. 2nd ed. Hoeber Medical Division of Harper and Row, New York, 1973.

Gill, D. M., Pappenheimer, A. M., Brown, R., and Kurnick, J. T.: Studies on the mode of action of diphtheria toxin. J. Exp. Med., *129*:1, 1969.

Honjo, T., Nishizuka, Y., Kato, I., and Hayaishi, O.: Adenosine diphosphate ribosylation of aminoacyl transferase II and inhibition of protein synthesis by diphtheria toxin. J. Biol. Chem., *246*:4251, 1971.

Iglewski, B. H., and Kabat, D.: NAD-dependent inhibition of protein synthesis by *Pseudomonas aeruginosa* toxin. Proc. Nat. Acad. Sci., 72:2284, 1975.

Lehninger, A. L.: Ribosomes and protein synthesis. *In:* Biochemistry — The Molecular Basis of Cell Structure and Function. Worth Publishers, Inc., New York, 1970.

Liu, P. V.: Extracellular toxins of Pseudomonas aeruginosa. J. Infect. Dis., *120*(S):594, 1974.

MacLennan, J. D.: The histotoxic clostridial infections of man. Bact. Rev., *26*:177, 1962.

Pappenheimer, A. M., and Brown, R.: Studies on the mode of action of diphtheria toxin VI. Site of the action of toxin in living cells. J. Exp. Med., *127*:1073, 1968.

Pappenheimer, A. M., Jr.: Diphtheria toxin. Ann. Rev. Biochem., *46*:69, 1977.

NEUROTOXINS

Burgen, A. S. V., Dickens, F., and Zatman, L. J.: The action of botulinum toxin on the neuromuscular junction. J. Physiol., *109*:10, 1948.

Eccles, J. C.: The Physiology of Synapses. Springer-Verlag Publishers, Berlin, 1964.

Koenig, M. G., Spickard, A., Cardella, M. A., and Rogers, D. E.: Clinical and Laboratory Observations of Type E Botulism in Man. Medicine, *43*:517, 1964.

Prys-Roberts, C., Kerr, J. H., Corbett, J. L., Crampton Smith, A., and Spalding, J. M. K.: Treatment of sympathetic overactivity in tetanus. Lancet, *1*:542, 1969.

Struppler, A., Struppler, E., and Adams, R. D.: Local tetanus in man. Arch. Neurol., 8:162, 1963.

Wright, G. P.: The Neurotoxins of *Clostridium botulinum* and *Clostridium tetani*. Pharmacol. Rev., 7:413, 1955.

Zacks, S. I., and Sheff, M. F.: Tetanism: Pathobiological aspects of the action of tetanal toxin in the nervous system and skeletal muscle. Neurosciences Res., 3:209, 1970.

ENTEROTOXINS

Field, M.: Intestinal secretion: Effect of cyclic AMP and its role in cholera. N. Engl. J. Med., *284*:1137, 1971.

Gill, D. M.: Involvement of nicotinamide adenine dinucleotide in the action of cholera toxin *in vitro*. Proc. Nat. Acad. Sci., 72:2064, 1975.

Gill, D. M., Evans, D. J., Jr., and Evans, D. G.: Mechanism of activation of adenylate cyclase *in vitro* by polymyxin-released, heat-labile enterotoxin of *Escherichia coli*. J. Infect. Dis., *133* (S): S103, 1976.

Gordon, R. S.: Moderator-Combined Clinical Staff Conference at the National Institutes of Health. Ann. Intern. Med., *64*:1328, 1966.

Keusch, G. T., Grady, G. F., Mata, L. J., and McIver, J.: The pathogenesis of Shigella diarrhea I. Enterotoxin production by *Shigella dysenteriae*. J. Clin. Invest., *51*:1212, 1972.

Kimberg, D. V., Field, M., Johnson, J., Henderson, A., and Gershon, E.: Stimulation of intestinal mucosal adenyl cyclase by cholera enterotoxin and prostaglandins. J. Clin. Invest., *50*:1218, 1971.

Moss, J., and Vaughan, M.: Mechanism of action of choleragen. J. Biol. Chem., *252*:2455, 1977.

Moss, J., Manganiello, V. C., and Vaughan, M.: Hydrolysis of nicotinamide adenine dinucleotide by choleragen and its A protomer: possible role in the activation of adenylate cyclase. Proc. Nat. Acad. Sci., *73*:4424, 1976.

Pierce, N. F., Greenough, W. B., III, and Carpenter, C. C. J.: *Vibrio cholerae* enterotoxin and its mode of action. Bact. Rev., 35:1, 1971.

ENDOTOXINS

Cluff, L. E.: Effects of endotoxins on susceptibility to infections. J. Infect. Dis., *122*:205, 1970.

Davis, C. E., and Arnold, K.: Role of meningococcal endotoxin in meningococcal purpura. J. Exp. Med., *140*:159, 1974.

Elin, R. J., and Wolff, S. M.: Biology of endotoxin. Ann. Rev. Med., *27*:127, 1976.

Greisman, S. E., Hornick, R. B., Carozza, F. A., and Woodward, T. E.: The role of endotoxin during typhoid fever and tularemia in man. I. Acquisition of tolerance to endotoxin. II. Altered cardiovascular responses to catecholamines. III. Hyperreactivity to endotoxin during infection. J. Clin. Invest., *42*:1064, 1963, and *43*:986, 1774, 1964.

Landy, M., and Braun, W. (Eds.): Bacterial Endotoxins. Institute of Microbiology, Rutgers University, New Brunswick, 1964.

Nowatny, A. (Ed.): Symposium on Molecular Biology of Gram-Negative Bacterial Lipopolysaccharides. Ann. N.Y. Acad. Sci., *133*:277, 1966.

Sotto, M. N., Langer, B., Hoshino-Shimizu, S., and deBrito, T.: Pathogenesis of cutaneous lesions in acute meningococcemia in humans: light, immunofluorescent, and electron microscopic studies of skin biopsy specimens. J. Infect. Dis., *133*:506, 1976.

Thomas, L.: The physiologic disturbances produced by endotoxins. Ann. Rev. Physiol., *16*:467, 1954.

Zweifach, B. W., and Janoff, A.: Bacterial endotoxemia. Ann. Rev. Med., *16*:201, 1965.

INVASIVE INFECTIONS

Brooks, M. H., Malloy, J. P., Bartelloni, P. J., Tigertt, W. D., Sheehy, T. W., and Barry, K. G.: Pathophysiology of acute falciparum malaria. I. Correlation of clinical and biochemical abnormalities, Am. J. Med., *43*:735, 1967.

Conrad, M. E.: Pathophysiology of malaria. Ann. Intern. Med., *70*:134, 1969.

Lincoln, R. E., and Fish, D. C.: Anthrax toxin. *In:* Montie, T. C., Kadis, S., and Ajl, S. J. (Eds.): Microbial Toxins. Vol. III. Academic Press, New York, 1970.

Melish, M. E., Glasgow, L. A., and Turner, M. D.: The staphylococcal scalded-skin syndrome: Isolation and partial purification of the new exfoliative toxin. J. Infect. Dis., *125*:129, 1972.

Melish, M. E., Glascow, L. A., Turner, M. D., and Lillibridge, C. B.: The staphylococcal epidermolytic toxin: its isolation, characterization, and site of action. Ann. N.Y. Acad. Sci., *236*:317, 1974.

Neva, F. A., Sheagren, J. N., Shulman, N. R., and Canfield, C. J.: Malaria: Host defense mechanisms and complications. Combined Clinical Staff Conference of the National Institutes of Health. Ann. Intern. Med., *73*:295, 1970.

Nungester, W. J.: Proceedings of the Conference on Progress in the Understanding of Anthrax. Fed. Proc., *26*:1491, 1967.

Rabin, E. R., Graver, C. D., Vogel, E. H., Finkelstein, R. A., and Tumbusch, W. A.: Fatal Pseudomonas infection in burned patients: A clinical, bacteriologic, and anatomic study. N. Engl. J. Med., *265*:1225, 1961.

Rogers, D. E.: The current problem of staphylococcal infections. Ann. Intern. Med., *45*:748, 1956.

Wood, W. B., Jr.: Studies on the cellular immunology of acute bacterial infections. The Harvey Lectures, *Series XLVII*:72, 1951–52.

20

Host Responses to Infection

Louis Weinstein,
and Morton N. Swartz

INTRODUCTION

The host response to an invading microorganism may be varied in nature, in extent, and in pathophysiologic consequences.

1. *In some circumstances the response may be minimal.* The majority of individuals exposed to *Mycobacterium tuberculosis* do not develop symptomatic pulmonary involvement or manifestations of disseminated infection. The host response is sufficient to contain the infectious process without progression to overt clinical disease. The only evidence that infection has taken place is the development of delayed hypersensitivity to antigens of *M. tuberculosis* as indicated by positive skin tests. A similar situation prevails in certain areas of the western United States where a fungus, *Coccidioides immitis,* is present in the soil; the majority of the population in such areas are infected with the organism (positive skin reactions) but do not develop an identifiable illness.

2. *In other circumstances the response of the host may be significant but the major impact of the infection is the result of the invasive properties and/or toxigenicity of the organism.* Examples of such infections (anthrax, cholera, streptococcal and staphylococcal sepsis) have been discussed in Chapter 19.

3. *In another group of infectious processes, the host response may be so exaggerated and troublesome, or so specific in nature, that it alone induces pathophysiologic consequences of considerable magnitude.* These responses may then account for various disorders that dominate the clinical picture. The invasive or toxin-producing phase of the infection may never develop, or if it does, it is concluded by the time symptoms become manifest. The signs and symptoms due to the host response become paramount or, in effect, constitute the entire clinical illness itself. It is this third category of infection that is the focus for discussion in this chapter. A variety of general responses may be elicited by most infections. Some, such as fever, are so common as to be considered a hallmark of this kind of disease. Others, such as disseminated intravascular clotting, are relatively uncommon but are being recognized more and more frequently as the laboratory criteria for their diagnosis have been clarified.

GENERAL HOST RESPONSES

Fever

Fever is an almost universal response of warm-blooded animals to infection. The normal oral body temperature is 98.6° F. (37° C.). However, this represents a mean value derived from studies of large numbers of normal people, and the "normal" for occasional individuals may deviate from this value by as much as 0.5 to 1.0° F. During the course of the day body temperature varies over a range of 0.5 to 2.0° F., the low point occurring in the early morning hours during sleep and the peak being reached late in the afternoon. In addition to disease, a variety of physiologic and environmental factors may transiently elevate the temperature by temporarily overwhelming the mechanism available for heat loss. For example, in very warm weather body temperature may rise 0.5° to 1.0° F. Similarly, after vigorous exercise or a hot shower even greater increases may occur. Commencing at the time of ovulation and persisting during the second half of the menstrual cycle, a more prolonged physiologic rise in morning temperature (0.50 to 0.75° F.) occurs and continues until the onset of menstruation. Such elevations are minor and, in most instances, only transitory. The term fever is commonly reserved for more sustained elevations of greater magnitude occurring in the course of disease.

The role of fever as a potential defense mechanism is obscure. There is as yet no clear evidence that a rise in body temperature confers a selective advantage to the host over the invading microorganism. However, this may be the case in a few infections. The optimal temperature for the retention of the infectivity of *Treponema pallidum* in vitro is 34° to 35° C. Higher temperatures are progressively more unfavorable for the spirochete. It is not unreasonable to suggest that this sensitivity to temperature is involved in the predilection of this organism for the skin. In addition, the occasional favorable response of certain forms of syphilis subjected to fever therapy in the pre-antibiotic era may be accounted for on this basis. It is very difficult to design an experiment with ordinary laboratory animals to determine whether the febrile response of the host augments resistance to infection, because the measures required to suppress fever are themselves capable of producing complicating side-effects. However, an interesting study of the role of fever in survival from bacterial infection has been carried out in lizards, reptiles whose body temperature can be kept constant over a wide range by simply controlling the ambient temperature. In lizards inoculated with the pathogenic bacteria *Aeromonas hydrophila,* an elevation of body temperature from 34° to 40° C. increased survival from 0 to about 70 per cent, suggesting enhanced host defenses at the elevated temperature. (The in-vitro bacterial growth rate was stable between these two temperatures.) If fever evolved in reptiles as a protective response to infection, a similar role might be anticipated in mammals. If the febrile response to infection *is* beneficial, then the common use of antipyretic agents in the treatment of mild infectious fevers might be ill-advised.

Although fever is usually associated with infection, this is by no means an exclusive relationship. Thus, it may be a manifestation of neoplastic disease (e.g., lymphoma), non-infectious inflammatory disorders (e.g., vasculitis, rheumatoid arthritis, ulcerative colitis, regional enteritis), or excess catabolism in certain metabolic states (e.g., pheochromocytoma, thyrotoxicosis). On the other hand, severe infection may exist without eliciting hyperpyrexia. Hypothermia (accompanying hypotension) may be present in the course of overwhelming infections. The presence of certain metabolic abnormalities (myxedema, uremia) may completely quench the usual febrile response to infection.

Normal Thermoregulation.   Normal body temperature is the result of a delicately maintained balance between heat production and heat loss. In the resting state, the major sites of heat production, under normal circumstances, are the liver and skeletal muscles; during exercise or in disease-associated febrile states the latter is the major site. Loss of heat takes place at the surface of the body (skin and lungs) through radiation, convection, and vaporization. The primary mechanisms by which control of temperature is maintained involve the nervous system. Generation of heat is produced through the somatic motor efferents (shivering); conservation or loss of heat is achieved through the control, by the autonomic nervous system, of cutaneous blood supply (loss of heat) and sudomotor activity (sweating). The central guidance for these efferent connections is the thermoregulatory center in the anterior hypothalamus. It responds to stimuli from two sources: (a) the superficial thermoreceptors of the skin that respond to changes in surface temperature and (b) the deep thermoreceptors located in or near the hypothalamus that respond to slight changes in the temperature of the blood perfusing this part of the central nervous system. The thermoregulatory center in the hypothalamus operates as a thermostat, with a "set point" at 98.6° F., and responds to superficial and deep stimuli from external heat load (e.g., high environmental temperature) by initiating loss of heat via sweating and vasodilatation.

Thermoregulation in Febrile Disease States.   An endogenous febrile reaction consists of four phases which are fairly sharply defined and which follow in regular sequence; these are (1) prodrome, (2) chill, (3) flush, and (4) defervescence. During the prodrome, there are only nonspecific complaints such as fleeting aches and pains, mild headache, nausea, and malaise; the circulation through the skin is normal. The initial discernible event in the chill phase is cutaneous vasoconstriction — the patient complains of being cold, and often covers up with more bedclothes. He becomes increasingly pale and the extremities appear somewhat cyanotic. The skin is cool and dry, except perhaps for a little perspiration of the forehead or upper lip. This phase lasts approximately 1½ hours. These changes suggest that during the early phases of a febrile illness the hypothalamic thermostat responds as though its "set point" had been raised to a new higher maintenance level. If the decrease in surface temperature due to reduced blood flow is of sufficient magnitude, the superficial cutaneous thermoreceptors are triggered. Feedback from the latter to the hypothalamus reflexly produces increased muscular activity in the form of shivering or, when this is maximal, a shaking chill. Production of heat is markedly increased by this muscular activity. During the chill phase the low skin temperature makes the patient feel cold even though the rectal temperature is rising. In fact, since the most severe chills are associated with the most marked rises in rectal temperature, patients feel coldest when they are storing the most heat. The patient continues to feel cold; a disproportion between internal and cutaneous temperatures may be responsible in part for the sensation of cold. The clinical and physiologic manifestations of chills may be precipitated or aggravated by exposure to cold when the subject is in the chill phase of a febrile reaction.

The effectiveness of shivering as a means of increasing heat production for the maintenance of the body heat balance can be gauged in a quantitative way. Thus, in an experiment in a calorimeter at 23° C. reported by Hardy, production of heat prior to a chill was 63 kcal. over an hour, and heat loss was 87 kcal. In the next half hour, during a chill, the rate of heat production was 164 kcal. per hour and heat loss was 116 kcal. per hour. Shivering is a more efficient means of increasing body temperature than exercise because loss of heat can be minimized by reducing the body surface area (site of convection loss) by curling up and by maintaining some degree of insulation by simultaneous vasoconstriction.

As the temperature of the skin rises with prolonged shivering, a sensation of warmth develops, and the shivering ceases. Cutaneous vasodilatation proceeds rapidly and the flush phase begins. The increased flow of blood in the skin causes an increase in the rate of heat loss, balancing the abnormally high level of heat production. As a result, body temperature remains poised at the newly established higher level. When the skin temperature reaches about 34° C., sweating occurs and marks the defervescent phase of the febrile response. Stimulation of the sweat glands is produced by efferent impulses from the hypothalamus, stimulated itself both by afferent impulses from the skin and by the elevated temperature of the blood flowing through the brain.

As already suggested, deviations of body temperature from the "set point" initiate mechanisms that tend to restore body temperature to the programmed level. Fever appears to represent, in essence, a rise in the "set point." In keeping with this is the observation of Cooper and coworkers that in man, when body temperature is elevated but stable, the skin vasomotor responses to a heat load are normal. In a normal subject infused with endogenous pyrogen (see below), prepared by preincubation of the subject's blood with bacterial endotoxin, an abrupt rise in temperature ensues and reaches its peak in about an hour. This is associated with marked cutaneous vasoconstriction, myalgias, and chills. Following this, there is a stable period (several hours) in which the peak temperature level is maintained. An additional heat load (generated by immersion of an arm in warm water) during the phase of rising temperature causes no cutaneous vasodilatation measured in the other hand. In contrast, immersion during the stable phase at the peak temperature produces a transient rise in oral temperature with increased elimination of heat on the other hand. The elevation of temperature required to induce vasodilatation is very small (0.10 to 0.15° C.) in contrast to the increase (1.70° C.) induced by the administration of pyrogen. These observations are compatible with the view that fever represents an alteration in the level at which the thermostat is set, and that, at this new setting, thermostatic control is as well exercised as at the former lower setting.

A variety of pathophysiologic changes involving the cardiorespiratory system accompany the febrile state. Changes in respiration may be prominent. In the chill phase, respiratory rate and minute volume increase and the tidal volume decreases. There may be a small decrease in arterial Po_2 due to rapid shallow breathing, but respiratory alkalosis is the more common finding. The increased respiratory activity during fever serves to eliminate some of the heat. The stimulus for this is thought to be the increased temperature of the blood supplying the respiratory center; accumulation of carbon dioxide in the respiratory center as a result of decreased cerebral blood flow during the chill phase may also play a role.

Cardiac output differs in the various phases of the febrile state. With severe chills a considerable decrease in cardiac output may occur, resulting in hypotension. During the flush phase, the cardiac output is increased in excess of the rise in oxygen consumption. During defervescence, cardiac output and oxygen consumption return toward normal. During the febrile period, the pulse rate in man roughly parallels the temperature; a rise of nine beats per minute occurs for each degree Fahrenheit increase in rectal temperature. However, the pulse rate is a poor indicator of changes in cardiac output during fever, since it often increases disproportionately and may rise when the cardiac output falls.

Mediators of Fever. The well-known clinical association of fever with inflammatory processes led to an early examination of purulent exudates for materials capable of evoking a febrile response in experimental animals. The results of such studies were obscured by the probable presence, in the soluble fractions of the exudates, of endotoxin, a pyrogenic lipopolysaccharide from the cell envelopes of contaminating gram-negative bacilli. In 1948, Beeson, employing procedures to exclude endotoxins, was able to extract from granulocytes a fever-producing material that he termed *endogenous pyrogen* (E.P.). Since then this substance has been the subject of considerable interest and study by many investigators. Most of the current knowledge concerning E.P. has been derived from investigations of experimental fever in animal models. When rabbits are given injections of endotoxin (typhoid vaccine) intravenously, fever develops and lasts for five to eight hours. Serum obtained at intervals during the febrile period elicits a febrile response when injected into normal animals. Except for the serum obtained early in the experiment, the development of fever in the recipient animal is not due to carry-over of endotoxin, since elevation of temperature is produced in endotoxin-refractory (tolerant) animals as well. Thus, the febrile response is induced by another pyrogenic material which appears to have properties indistinguishable from the pyrogen obtained from granulocytes.

The granulocyte pyrogen (E.P.) is released from exudate neutrophils incubated in isotonic saline. This in-vitro system has been the major source for isolation and purification of the pyrogen. Leukocytes from circulating blood rather than exudates are less capable of releasing E.P. when incubated with 0.15 M NaCl. However, leukocytes from blood are better producers of E.P. than those from exudates, when exposed to endotoxin in vitro. Little if any active E.P. is present in exudate or blood granulocytes. Incubation of the former with saline or of the latter with endotoxin causes apparent conversion of an inactive precursor molecule to an active pyrogen during its release from the cell. Conversion to active pyrogen in blood granulocytes (but not exudate cells) is blocked by inhibitors of protein synthesis. It appears that exudate cells have already passed the preliminary activation step which requires protein synthesis. Purification of pyrogen from rabbit exudate has reached the stage at which injection of as little as 30 to 50 nanograms produces fever in a rabbit. It has been characterized as a heat-labile (56° C.) protein with a molecular weight of 10,000 to 20,000 (small amounts of carbohydrate or lipid may be present also).

Sources of Endogenous Pyrogen. The prominent role of granulocytes in the production of E.P. is suggested by the association of an initial leukopenia (mainly granulocytic) with the experimental fever induced by endotoxin. (Margination of polymorphonuclear leukocytes along blood vessel walls occurs at the same time.) Animals in which leukopenia has been induced by nitrogen mustard respond to endotoxin with less fever and less circulating E.P. than normal ones.

The stimulus for the release of E.P. from circulating granulocytes in vivo or in vitro is not restricted to endotoxin. Intravenous injection of various bacteria or viruses in normal or specifically sensitized rabbits has been followed by fever and the appearance of demonstrable E.P. in the circulation. Release of E.P. from suspensions of rabbit granulocytes occurs when they have been incubated in vitro with bacteria, viruses, tuberculin, or antigen-antibody complexes. Successful phagocytosis appears to be an important feature of the bacteria-induced E.P. release.

Granulocytes are not the only cells capable of releasing E.P. That there are other sources of endogenous pyrogen has been suggested by the common occurrence of fever in patients with marked and prolonged agranulocytosis. Monocytes and macrophages have recently been shown to be sources of E.P. Alveolar macrophages obtained from the lungs of rabbits sensitized to tuberculin by intravenous injection of BCG release abundant E.P. when incubated with tuberculin in vitro. This finding may provide an explanation for the fever occurring in diseases like tuberculosis in which mononuclear cells are histologically the major element. Kupffer's cells of the liver, but not hepatocytes, produce E.P. in vitro when activated by endotoxin, bacterial phagocytosis, or tuberculin. The common functional characteristic of all cell types capable of E.P. production is their ability to phagocytose. Lymphocytes from human blood, in contrast to monocytes and macrophages, do not release pyrogen in vitro when subjected to a variety of stimuli. Nonetheless, lymphocytes may have a somewhat indirect role as activators of the febrile state in diseases in which delayed hypersensitivity is a prominent feature. Lymphocytes of rabbits sensitized to a foreign protein, when exposed to that specific antigen in vitro release a nonpyrogenic substance that stimulates blood leukocytes to release E.P.

Site of Action of Endogenous Pyrogen. The introduction of endotoxin or any of many other activators of E.P. in a susceptible animal or man appears to set off the following sequence of events in which E.P. is the final common pathway (see formula below). The central site of action of E.P. has been demonstrated in rabbits. When this substance is infused slowly into the carotid artery to perfuse the brain directly, a more rapid and greater febrile response is generated than when it is given intravenously. In contrast, the degree

Endotoxin (or similar activator)		Cell Injury (granulocytes, monocytes, macrophages)		Endogenous Pyrogen Activation and Release		Stimulation of Hypothalamic Thermoregulatory Centers		Fever

of fever produced by endotoxin is the same when given by either route. These observations are consistent with the concept that E.P. acts directly on the hypothalamus, and that endotoxin activates circulating leukocytes to release E.P. Direct perfusion of the anterior hypothalamus of rabbits with extremely small amounts of E.P. via microcannulas causes an immediate rise in body temperature.

Mechanism of Fever Production During Overt Infections. Crucial to the definition of the role of E.P. in fever production is the demonstration of its presence in some common infectious processes. In experimental pneumococcal peritonitis produced in rabbits, the substance is present in the peritoneal cavity in the early stages of infection; it is detectable in thoracic-duct lymph and in blood later in the course of the fever. When the infection is controlled by therapy with penicillin, fever subsides and E.P. can no longer be demonstrated.

The possible role of continuing endotoxemia from *Salmonella typhosa* in typhoid fever has been studied by Greisman, et al. in human volunteers. Endotoxin tolerance, induced immediately before or during experimental typhoid fever, did not inhibit the febrile course or toxemia characteristic of the disease. This appeared to eliminate continuing circulation of endotoxin as responsible for the sustained fever in this infection. Thus, it seems likely that in this disease persistence of fever is due to the production of E.P. by phagocytes in areas of inflammation.

Headache

Headache is a common symptom of systemic infection and is usually associated with fever. We are concerned here only with elevations of temperature unrelated to specific infections of the central nervous system such as meningitis or brain abscess. The febrile headache is usually throbbing in character at the onset of the febrile reaction and then becomes a deep dull ache of varying severity. It is usually generalized but may be predominantly in the frontotemporal, occipital, or suboccipital areas. It is aggravated by bodily movement. Several mechanisms may be active in the pathogenesis of headache occurring in the course of fever related to infection. First, there may be microscopic evidence of central nervous system inflammation without obvious meningeal signs. Thus, an occasional patient with mumps and a more severe than usual headache will have a small (but abnormal) number of lymphocytes in the cerebrospinal fluid. In most other infections in which febrile headaches occur, however, there is no evidence of active infection of the central nervous system or its linings. Such headaches may be a particularly prominent feature of

influenza, typhoid fever, typhus and other rickettsial diseases, mycoplasma pneumonia, and infectious mononucleosis. It usually parallels the fever but may precede or outlast it.

The pain-sensitive structures in the central nervous system are the dural sinuses and their principal branches, the arteries in the dura and the areas immediately surrounding them, and the large intracranial arteries. It seems reasonable to suggest that disturbance of one or more of these structures during infection is responsible for febrile headaches.

Present evidence strongly suggests that pyrexial headaches result from stretching of sensitive structures about the intracranial arteries due to dilatation of these vessels. Sutherland and Wolff have reported that after intravenous administration of typhoid vaccine an increased amplitude of pulsations of the cerebrospinal fluid preceded the onset of headache, the severity of which closely paralleled the magnitude of the oscillations which occurred synchronously with the pulse. In addition, a direct relation was noted between the intensity of the headache and the amplitude of pulsations in the temporal artery. Direct visualization of pial vessels through skull windows in experimental animals has shown that intravenous administration of typhoid vaccine is followed by cerebral vasodilatation. The immediate factor(s) directly responsible for the cerebral vasodilatation is unknown at present. It is of interest that the headache following injection of histamine is similar in character, and that dilatation of intracranial arteries is the basis of the pain.

It appears reasonable to consider the following sequence of events in the development of the headache produced by infections in which direct invasion of the central nervous system is not a feature: Phagocytosis of the infecting agent → Activation of granulocyte or mononuclear pyrogen (E.P.) → Action of E.P. on the thermoregulatory center, generating a febrile response → Cerebral vasodilatation mediated in some way directly by E.P. or through alterations secondary to the E.P.-induced fever.

Hypotension and Shock

Shock associated with bacteremia is the major cause of mortality in infections otherwise amenable to antibiotic therapy. Although gram-negative bacteria are the most frequent offending organisms, the syndrome may develop in the course of disease produced by viruses, fungi, and rickettsiae. Shock in bacteremia is not due simply to endotoxin; studies with the Limulus amebocyte gelation assay for circulating endotoxin have revealed no correlation between positive assays and the number of circulating gram-negative bacilli or the occurrence of shock or death. The pathophysiology of the changes observed in bacteremia and septic shock in man are still incompletely understood. It was formerly believed that the fundamental problem was a low pressure state due to loss or paralysis of vasomotor tone. Thus, treatment in the past was directed at restoration of circulating blood volume and correction of defective vasomotor tone by administration of vasopressor agents. The more recent concept of the mechanism of septic shock is that it is due to redistribution of blood within the vascular bed in a manner precluding maintenance of an adequate circulating blood volume. Tissue ischemia and anoxia are a consequence of this pooling and lead to decreased renal function, myocardial failure, lactic acidemia, and ultimately to cell death.

Commonly, when hypotension develops during the course of bacteremia due to gram-negative bacilli, the patient is febrile and the extremities are warm. During this early pyrogenic phase of acute circulatory failure cardiac output, stroke volume, and pulse pressure are increased, and arterial vasodilatation predominates. This is the syndrome that has been labeled "warm shock." Adrenergic effects are not prominent at this stage. There is an increased circulatory demand which cannot be met. As a result hypoxia, oliguria, and alterations in the sensorium begin to occur. With progression of shock, cardiac output is decreased secondary to a reduction in effective blood volume due to what appears to be pooling of blood in the venous capacitance bed. At this stage (so-called "cold shock") the more typical clinical changes of shock (pallor; cold, clammy extremities; peripheral cyanosis) are observed and adrenergic response dominates the picture. This stage of shock is characterized by reduced cardiac output, increased peripheral arterial resistance, decreased central venous pressure, and decreased tissue perfusion and oxygenation. Decline in renal perfusion results in reduction of urine output. As tissue hypoxia increases, serum lactic acid levels rise, and blood pH and bicarbonate fall. If the shock is of severe degree and persists for a protracted period, the picture of "shock lung" develops. The accompanying elevation of pulmonary vascular resistance increases the work load on the right ventricle and raises the right ventricular end-diastolic volume. Patients in whom prolonged septic shock has been reversed may nevertheless die from acute respiratory insufficiency as a result of this type of pulmonary difficulty. Persistence of shock leads to intense vasoconstriction of both the arterial and venous sides of the microcirculation. Eventually the precapillary arterial vasoconstriction diminishes without a concomitant decrease on the venous side. A consequence of this is a high degree of congestion in the pulmonary capillary bed. Hypoxia and lactic acidosis intensify. Congestion and edema, hemorrhage, and capillary thrombi are the characteristic changes in the lung.

Other Circulatory Changes

The elevation of body temperature accompanying infection is usually associated with a proportional increase in heart rate. Relative bradycardia is seen during infections due to gram-negative bacilli (e.g., typhoid fever, tularemia). Endotoxin has been suggested as the element inducing this peculiar response. The definition of the actual microbial component inducing the response seems more complex than this, however, since relative bradycardia is also observed in viral diseases (dengue, yellow fever), mycoplasma infections (primary atypical pneumonia), and during illness due to Bedsoniae (psittacosis). Bradycardia (accompanied by hypertension) may be present in infections of the central nervous system (meningitis, subdural empyema, brain abscess, and encephalitis) as a consequence of increased intracranial pressure.

Reversible Alterations of Sensorium — Confusion, Delirium, Stupor, and Coma

Alterations of sensorium occur in many infectious diseases in the absence of cerebral invasion by the attacking microorganism or of histologic evidence of inflammatory brain disease. Stupor and coma are usually more evident and more severe in systemic infections in which high fever and hypotension are prominent features. However, such changes may occur in the absence of hypotension or extreme hyperthermia. They are usually reversible and disappear when the infection is brought under control. The usual sequence involves a progressive change from a state of drowsiness and confusion to stupor and finally coma. The pathophysiologic alterations producing these changes are not well understood.

In the presence of severe hypotension (systolic level below 70 to 75 mm. Hg), the cerebral metabolic rate is reduced as a result of decreased blood flow to the brain. This may account for the stupor or coma often seen in septic shock. Extremes of hyperthermia (106° F. or higher) or hypothermia (below 97° F.) may develop during bacteremia or septic shock and are thought to induce coma by altering neuronal metabolism nonspecifically. Hyperthermia due to any cause may initiate a convulsion (febrile seizure) in infants and young children presumably through temporary alterations in cerebral cortical function. Alterations in sensorium that occur in some bacterial infections are thought to be due to "toxins" elaborated by the organisms. However, such toxins have not been isolated and their role remains hypothetical. Cerebral metabolic rate is reduced while blood flow remains normal in the course of coma associated with some systemic infections.

A severe and extreme example of alteration of cerebral function during the course of infection is *acute toxic encephalopathy*. This syndrome occurs during or following bacterial or viral disease. It is characterized by fever, confusion, stupor, and coma. Generalized convulsive seizures are prominent and, unlike simple febrile convulsions, are recurrent. Focal disease of the cerebrum or brain stem is absent. Although bacterial "toxins" have been proposed as the cause of the cerebral changes, no clear-cut substantiating evidence is available. There does not appear to be a close correlation between the severity of the initiating infection and the degree of neurologic dysfunction. Contributing factors initiating the process may be fever, hypoxia, and cerebral edema secondary to water intoxication.

Skin Reactions in Disseminated Infection

Skin eruptions of differing morphology are frequently associated with systemic bacterial or viral infections. The cutaneous changes may be produced in several different ways: (1) Bacteremic or viremic spread to the skin, with local proliferation of the organism (subcutaneous abscesses in *S. aureus* bacteremia, cutaneous vesicles in disseminated *Herpes simplex* infection of infants). (2) Development of a cutaneous vasculitis. The etiologic agent (bacteria or virus) may or may not be found in the vessel wall or surrounding dermis. (3) The damaging effect of antigen-antibody complexes on the skin, or possibly by the development of delayed hypersensitivity to the infecting agent. Staphylococcal infections are an example of bacteremic skin lesions due to direct invasion of bacteremic skin. Frank, fluctuant subcutaneous abscesses, nodular subcutaneous lesions, pustules, and purulent purpura (a small area of hemorrhage with a white purulent center) may be present. *S. aureus* can be demonstrated without any difficulty in any of these lesions. Vasculitis involving small blood vessels of the skin may occur in the absence of demonstrable localization of bacteria. The macular, papular, nodular, and petechial lesions of chronic meningococcemia are examples of this phenomenon. The painful, nodular pretibial lesions of erythema nodosum exhibit a prominent element of vasculitis, but the instigating organism in certain cases is located at a distance from the subcutaneous lesions (e.g., streptococcal pharyngitis). Vasculitis of the skin may also be associated with direct invasion of the vessel wall by bacteria. A characteristic example of this is the widespread involvement of blood vessels that occurs in the course of Pseudomonas bacteremia. Bullous, hemorrhagic, and necrotic skin lesions develop as a result of intramural bacterial proliferation which leads to occlusion of vessels by fibrin thrombi.

Immunologic factors may play a role in the production of the skin lesions in certain systemic infections, particularly in the case of some viral exanthems. Measles is a good example of this. The pathogenesis of the rash in this disease is not clearly established. It could be produced by direct viral invasion of the epidermal and vascular endothelial cells or the result of damage induced locally by a virus-antibody complex. There is some evidence in support of the latter concept. The time of appearance of the rash coincides with the appearance of circulating antibody. Another intriguing bit of evidence is the absence of rash in some children, usually those with leukemia, who develop chronic measles with giant cell pneumonia but do not produce specific antibody. The use of inactivated measles virus vaccine has suggested an altered cutaneous reactivity in the host. Individuals previously immunized with this agent develop an atypical measles syndrome characterized by unusual skin lesions (petechiae, purpura, urticaria, or vesicles superimposed on a maculopapular rash) following exposure several years later to the natural disease. Local reactions, consisting of erythema and vesicle formation, have developed at the site of live measles vaccine injection in patients who had previously received inactivated measles vaccine. Little is known of the exact basis of these reactions. It is of interest in this regard, however, that a high incidence of delayed hypersensitivity to antigens in inactivated measles vaccine has been demonstrated in recipients of the killed vaccine.

Hematologic Changes

A variety of alterations of blood elements occur during the course of human infectious diseases. They are common; the magnitude of the changes is usually minor and contributes little to the over-all symptomatology or clinical findings. On occasion, however, they may be so profound as to completely dominate the clinical picture or to influence significantly the host response to the infection. The roles of the neutrophil in phagocytosis and bacterial killing as well as in producing leukocytic pyrogen establish its importance in the initial host response to infection.

Changes in Circulating Neutrophils. Most infections due to pyogenic bacteria are accompanied by a polymorphonuclear leukocytosis. A relation between this response and the inflammatory reaction at the site of the infectious process has been inferred from the known phagocytic function of these cells and their presence in abundance in the early stages of inflammation. The best insights into the dynamics of the neutrophil response to infection have evolved from studies of neutrophil kinetics employing radioactive isotopic techniques.

Polymorphonuclear leukocytes are produced continuously in the bone marrow through the differentiation of precursor myeloid cells. Upon maturation, the granulocytes enter the marrow storage pool, one of several "pools" in the body. From the *marrow pool* they are discharged into the circulation, where they enter either the *circulating granulocyte pool* (CGP) or the *marginal granulocyte pool* (MGP). The former is made up of actively circulating cells, whereas the latter consists of granulocytes which are sequestered or "marginated" in various capillary beds. Prompt increases in numbers of circulating granulocytes that result from exercise or injection of catecholamines involve movement of the marginated leukocytes into the circulating pool. The size of the CGP depends on three concurrent processes: (1) rate of release from marrow, (2) proportion of granulocytes held in MGP, and (3) rate of loss of granulocytes into tissues.

It has been difficult to study leukokinetics in acute infections of man because patients are not seen until disease is well established and treatment initiated. However, acute infections have been studied in experimental animals (pneumococcal pneumonia in the dog) and have provided valuable insights into the kinetics of the response. The sequence of events that takes place is as follows: (1) Infection produces an increased demand for migration of granulocytes from the CGP. (2) Egress from the blood is via diapedesis from the MGP; an increase in the size of this pool is required for this. However, migration from the MGP to the tissues is a one-way street; there is no evidence that the granulocytes re-enter the circulation from infected areas. (3) The marrow responds to the foregoing with acceleration of the rate of release of cells from the marrow storage pool. This might involve a feedback loop mediated by a serum factor. Also contributing to the marrow response is a subsequent wave of differentiation down the myeloid pathway to the granulocyte level. (4) Enlargement of the CGP occurs only after the acceleration of release from the marrow storage pool has exceeded the enhanced rate of movement from the blood into the tissues. Within four hours of inoculation of pneumococci, an accelerated rate of release of neutrophils from bone marrow to blood, as indicated by an increase in the ratio of band forms to segmented forms, can be observed. This can sometimes be detected before there is an increase in the numbers of circulating neutrophils in venous blood. This lag period before the rise in neutrophil count appears to be the result of restoration of the MGP before the CGP.

An occasional patient with severe pneumococcal pneumonia will develop severe neutropenia. When this same response occurs in the experimental animal, it is associated with an acceleration of marrow neutrophil release and a marked increase in the ratio of band to segmented forms. Neutropenia in this situation stems from inability of the marrow to replenish the accelerated cell loss to the sites of tissue inflammation. Data from kinetic studies with labeled cells as well as examination of marrow (loss of mature neutrophils) suggest exhaustion of the marrow granulocyte pool. There is no evidence that infection blocks release of neutrophils from the marrow. The well-known poor prognosis of such severe pneumococcal (and other bacterial) infections is more readily understandable if the mechanism of the neutropenia is depletion of the marrow granulocyte reserve.

In certain bacterial infections, particularly typhoid fever, leukopenia is a common finding. The basis for this phenomenon is not known. However, it is of interest that a similar blood picture features the initial response in rabbits and man to the injection of gram-negative bacilli or of bacterial endotoxin. This occurs at the time of the chill and is followed by leukocytosis in 1/2 to 4 hours. The initial leukopenia is due to enlargement of the MGP before that of the CGP. The subsequent leukocytosis is secondary to release of cells from both the MGP and the marrow storage pool.

Anemia of Infection. Anemia is a common feature of chronic infections but may occasionally complicate acute ones. In the latter case, the anemia is usually hemolytic. High-grade bacteremia with *Clostridium perfringens* may produce massive intravascular destruction of erythrocytes, with shock and anuria. The production by this organism of a lecithinase (α toxin) and hemolysins (e.g., θ toxin) which act on the membranes of red cells and cause their lysis is the basis for the hemolytic anemia of clostridial bacteremia (see Chapter 19). Primary atypical pneumonia due to *Mycoplasma pneumoniae* is, on rare occasions, complicated by severe hemolysis related to the development of autoantibodies, the cold agglutinins. These are IgM antibodies, most often directed against the I antigen on red blood cells. There is some evidence that certain infectious agents like *M. pneumoniae* may interact with the red blood cell, thus altering the I antigen and making it immunogenic. In patients with congenital deficiency of the erythrocyte enzyme glucose-6-phosphate dehydrogenase (G6PD), episodes of hemolysis may be precipitated by a variety of infections. Bacterial infections (pneumonia) and viral infections (infectious hepatitis) have been associated with hemolytic episodes. Accumulation of metabolites capable of oxidizing glutathione, and thus decreasing the concentration of the reduced form of this compound, has been suggested as the basis for the hemolysis. However, direct exposure of G6PD-deficient erythrocytes to influenza virus produces increased hemolysis; this suggests a direct effect on the red cell rather than an indirect one due to toxic metabolites produced in the host.

The anemia associated with chronic infections is usually normocytic and normochromic but may be normocytic and hypochromic. The infectious process is usually of many weeks' duration, since the life span of the normal erythrocyte is 120 days. Anemia is common in cases of subacute bacterial endocarditis, tuberculosis, brucellosis, and chronic pulmonary infections such as lung abscess and empyema. A decrease in serum iron, serum iron-binding capacity, and saturation of transferrin with iron are the biochemical changes characteristic of this type of anemia. Ferrokinetic and erythrokinetic studies have revealed the following: (1) A rapid rate of clearance of injected iron from the plasma. (2) Normal or only moderately increased erythropoiesis. (3) Mildly shortened erythrocyte survival. The latter finding suggests a *hemolytic process,* yet the usual evidences of increased blood destruction (increased serum bilirubin and urobilinogen excretion) are not present. (4) Increased iron stores in bone marrow and reticuloendothelial system (RES). The reason for this avidity of the RES for iron is unclear. The serum transferrin levels are low and its turnover rate is increased, findings thought to be due to increased catabolism and decreased synthesis of transferrin.

The pathophysiologic basis for the anemia of infection is not clear. The defect may be in erythropoietin production (the bone marrow has more than enough potential for the replacement of the red cells lost as a result of the shortened red cell survival), RES function, transferrin metabolism, or a combination of these factors. The manner in which bacterial products or the inflammatory response affects any or all of these targets remains a mystery.

Coagulation Defects.   Isolated thrombocytopenia may develop during the course of some acute gram-positive and gram-negative bacterial infections. It may also appear immediately before, during, or after some systemic viral diseases such as measles. During bacteremia and viremia, platelets tend to adhere to each other and the vascular endothelium; this probably accounts for their depletion. This adherence may be due to the action of bacterial toxins or other products on the platelet. For example, staphylococcal alpha toxin causes agglutination and lysis of rabbit platelets in vitro. The extent of thrombocytopenia may be sufficient to cause bleeding, usually in the form of petechiae and purpura. Bone marrow depression secondary to the infection may also contribute to the thrombocytopenia in a lesser degree.

A more profound coagulation defect, *disseminated intravascular coagulation* (DIC), may occur as a complication of infections with a variety of agents: gram-positive organisms (Group A and Group B streptococci, Pneumococcus, *S. aureus, Clostridium perfringens*); gram-negative bacteria (Meningococcus, *E. coli,* Proteus, Pseudomonas, etc.); viruses (varicella, variola, rubella, rubeola, hemorrhagic fevers, etc.); rickettsiae (*Rickettsia rickettsii* of Rocky Mountain Spotted Fever); protozoa (malaria, *Leishmania donovani* of kala-azar). DIC is a distinct clinical entity in which the clinical manifestations are fever, petechial or purpuric eruption, hypotension, and a widespread hemorrhagic diathesis. Renal failure is usually evident secondary to hypotension or, occasionally, to renal cortical necrosis. Histologically, there is evidence of fibrin deposition in blood vessels of various organs, particularly in the capillaries and venules of the skin. The basic pathophysiology of DIC involves a host response to an underlying illness (many processes other than infection may also trigger this response) that sets off a generalized activation of the normal clotting mechanism. As a result of systemic infection, endothelial damage and inflammation of blood vessel walls occur. The subsequent depletion of fibrinogen and other clotting components and the ensuing clinical bleeding diathesis are the results of two fundamental processes: (1) activation, by endothelial damage, of the coagulation sequence, leading to the generation of thrombin; and (2) activation of the natural defense of the body (fibrinolytic system) against widespread clotting initiated by uncontrolled thrombin production.

The current state of knowledge suggests that the following sequence of events is involved in the coagulation aspect of DIC. The initiating event is a vascular injury such as occurs in meningococcemia, Rocky Mountain Spotted Fever, and so on. This can activate the clotting mechanism in three ways:

1. *Activation of the Intrinsic Clotting System:* Loss of integrity of the vascular endothelium exposes the circulating blood to collagen, which converts Factor XII (Hageman factor) from an inert precursor to its enzymatically active form, which then initiates the intrinsic clotting cascade (Fig. 20–1) by converting Factor XI, plasma thromboplastin antecedent (PTA), from the precursor to the active form. Activated Factor XI then activates Factor IX [Christmas factor or plasma thromboplastin component (PTC)]. Activated Factor IX forms a complex with Factor VIII (antihemophilic factor) and with platelet phospholipids (platelet Factor III). This complex then activates Factor X (Stuart factor). Activated Factor X, in the presence of platelet phospholipids and Factor V (proaccelerin), forms a complex which converts prothrombin (Factor II) into thrombin. Thrombin then transforms soluble fibrinogen (Factor I) to the still soluble fibrin monomer. The latter than polymerizes and is converted to the stable insoluble fibrin polymer by the action of

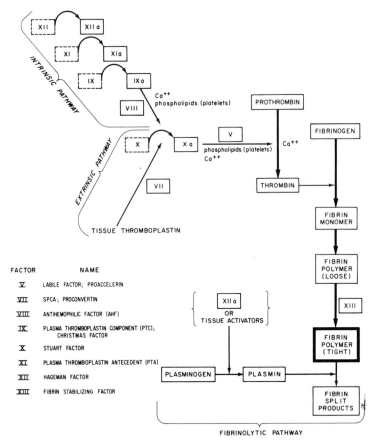

Figure 20–1   Coagulation cascade and fibrinolytic pathway. Clotting factors in ⌐⌐⌐⌐⌐ represent inert precursor forms of the factors. Clotting factors with subscript a in ▭ represent activated forms of the factors. *Intrinsic pathway* for prothrombin conversion to thrombin is initiated by conversion of Hageman factor to its activated form. Cascade follows, in which various clotting factors are sequentially converted from their precursor form to their active form. Activated Factor X with Factor V, platelet phospholipids, and Ca^{++} forms a *prothrombin converting principle,* which liberates thrombin from its precursor, prothrombin. Once thrombin forms, it converts fibrinogen to the fibrin monomer, which after several steps becomes a tight fibrin polymer (clot). *Extrinsic pathway* is initiated by tissue thromboplastins (present in many tissues, particularly blood vessel walls, lung, and brain) which interact with Factor VII, calcium ions, Factor X, and Factor V to form the prothrombin converting principle. This then converts prothrombin to thrombin.

The *fibrinolytic pathway* is initiated by the conversion of the inactive proteolytic enzyme plasminogen, present in all body fluids, to its active form, plasmin. This conversion is activated either by Factor XIIa or by activators present in tissues and vascular endothelium. Plasmin then cleaves fibrin, releasing fibrin split products.

Factor XIII (fibrin stabilizing factor). Factor XIII exists as an inert precursor and must be activated by thrombin before it can act on the fibrin polymer. In addition to converting fibrinogen to fibrin and to activating Factor XIII, thrombin also enhances the activities of both the activated Factor IX-Factor VIII-phospholipid complex and the activated Factor X-Factor V-phospholipid complex, thus accelerating its own formation.

2. *Activation of the Extrinsic Clotting System:* Vascular injury secondary to infection releases tissue thromboplastin (probably from the walls of blood vessels) which interacts with calcium and Factor VII (serum prothrombin conversion accel-

erator) to form a complex capable of activating Factor X. At this point the extrinsic clotting system joins the intrinsic system, and the steps leading to the formation of fibrin are identical.

3. *Activation of the Plasma Kallikrein System:* Shock may occur during the course of infections with a wide variety of organisms. However, shock per se, regardless of its cause, can induce intravascular coagulation. Endothelial damage due to infection or due to endotoxin is capable of activating Factor XII (Fig. 20–2). Activated Factor XII or its derivatives are able to activate plasma prekallikrein to the active enzyme kallikrein. This results in elaboration of bradykinin, a highly po-

tent vasodepressor, from its precursor plasma kininogen. Thus,the same trigger point, Factor XII activation, appears capable of initiating both activation of the coagulation pathway directly and bacteremic shock via the kallikrein-kinin system. Once developed, shock itself may elicit further intravascular coagulation. In keeping with this interrelation is the clinical observation that DIC commonly occurs in patients with bacteremia and hypotension, but does not develop when infection is unaccompanied by hypotension. However, it is still not clear whether the intravascular coagulation appears first and causes shock and hypoxia, or vice versa.

Once thrombin has been generated in the circulation during the coagulation process, several mechanisms come into play to limit its unimpeded action. One is its rapid removal by adsorption to the newly formed fibrin gel and another is its slow inactivation by a serum factor, antithrombin III. The most important mechanism for interfering with the action of thrombin involves plasmin

(fibrinolysin), which destroys fibrinogen, the substrate for thrombin. Plasmin is a potent but relatively non-specific proteolytic enzyme which degrades many proteins, including fibrinogen. Activation of the plasmin system involves cleavage of an inert circulating protein, plasminogen, by activated Factor XII. This results in the conversion of plasminogen to the active enzyme plasmin, which then acts on fibrinogen to degrade it into a series of large and small fragments. It also digests fibrin; this results in the production of polypeptides (fibrin split products). A potent anticoagulant activity is produced when fibrinogen is cleaved by plasmin. The anticoagulants are two large fragments of fibrinogen which act as (1) competitive inhibitors of fibrinogen for thrombin and (2) blockers of the formation of a tight fibrin gel by interposing between fibrin polymers as they are forming.

The inappropriate and extensive clotting process proceeds at an accelerated rate in DIC. Fibrin deposition extends throughout the vascular tree

Figure 20–2 Pathogenesis of disseminated intravascular coagulation (DIC). The chain of events initiated by bacteremia is shown schematically. Vascular injury has a central role. It causes activation of Factor XII, release of tissue thromboplastins (TPL), and aggregation of platelets. All three then initiate activation of clotting factors, XIIa by the intrinsic pathway and TPL and platelet aggregation by the extrinsic pathway. Thrombin generation and fibrinogen conversion to fibrin occur intravascularly.

Activation of Factor XII contributes to intravascular coagulation by another mechanism as well. Factor XIIa (activated factor XII) interacts with the kallikrein-kinin system, converting prekallikrein (kallikreinogen) to its active form kallikrein. Plasma kallikrein, in turn, acts on its major substrate, bradykininogen, releasing the nonapeptide bradykinin, a powerful vasodilator. Hypotension and shock develop as a result of the activity of bradykinin. The effect of these circulatory changes is to decrease the hepatic clearance rate of activated clotting factors and to induce additional intravascular clotting. Hypotension induced directly as a result of bacteremia by mechanisms other than the kinin pathway similarly decreases hepatic processing of clotting factors and enhances intravascular coagulation.

Activation of Factor XII has a third major effect, one related to its role in the activation of plasminogen to plasmin. Plasmin furthers the incoagulability of blood in DIC by attacking fibrinogen and fibrin to produce split products which inhibit thrombin and fibrin polymerization.

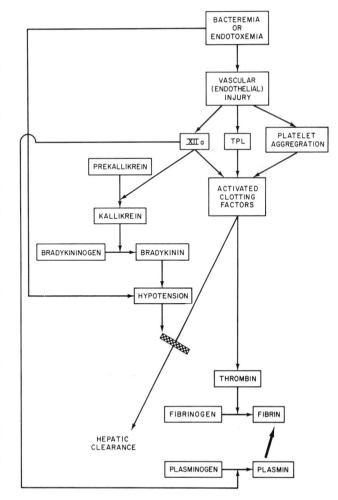

causing local tissue necrosis and more extensive organ damage. Soon, hemorrhage becomes a major clinical feature as blood coagulation factors are depleted (V, VIII, prothrombin, fibrinogen) and fibrin can no longer be formed. Aggravating the coagulation picture is the activation of the fibrinolytic system. Five major events are involved to produce the net result — incoagulable blood: (1) Depletion, during coagulation, of blood clotting components; (2) depletion of fibrinogen by the intravascular clotting; (3) plasmin-mediated digestion of fibrinogen and possibly Factors V and VIII; (4) suppression of thrombin action by the split products of fibrinogen and fibrin; and (5) inhibition of fibrin polymerization by the split products of fibrinogen and fibrin.

Treatment of DIC is aimed at control of the underlying infection with the appropriate antibiotic and management of any accompanying shock. The potent anticoagulant heparin has been used in the treatment of DIC accompanying septicemia when there have been evidences of bleeding, but it appears to have been effective in only a minority of patients.

SPECIAL HOST RESPONSES

Eosinophilia and Eosinopenia

Eosinophils are present in all species above the most primitive vertebrates, and their appearance in evolution roughly parallels that of complex lymphocyte-mediated immune systems. Although eosinophils do not seem important in defense against most invading microorganisms, they do appear to confer some protection against certain helminthic parasites. In addition, eosinophils serve to modulate tissue reactions in which mast cells or basophils degranulate and release potent mediators of inflammation (histamine, slow-reacting substance of anaphylaxis). Previously it was thought that phagocytosis of immune complexes was a unique function of the eosinophil, but it is now clear that such complexes are readily phagocytosed by polymorphonuclear neutrophils and mononuclear cells as well. The fact that eosinophils are not commonly present in tissues in immune-complex diseases (glomerulonephritis, lupus nephritis) further indicates that the eosinophil does not have a special role in the removal of such complexes. Infection can profoundly affect the number of circulating eosinophils: a striking eosinophilia develops in the course of infection with certain metazoan helminths, and a marked diminution occurs during acute bacterial infections.

The circulating eosinophil is believed to be an end-cell. Its maturation takes place in the bone marrow, where it enters a reserve pool several orders of magnitude larger than the total of circulating eosinophils. Upon release from the marrow it circulates for only a few hours in the blood before migrating into tissue sites where it dies or is extruded from a mucosal surface.

Much of current knowledge of the eosinophilic response has developed from the studies of Beeson and his co-workers on parasitic infection of the rat with the nematode *Trichinella spiralis*. Following intravenous injection larvae are trapped (and die) in the lungs, where they elicit a granulomatous response. Eosinophilia develops in about three days and appears to be the result of interaction between intact parasites and host cells, since it does not occur if homogenized larvae (fragments small enough to pass through the pulmonary vessels) are infused intravenously.

Production of eosinophils by the bone marrow consists of an inductive and a proliferative stage analogous to the phases of antibody production to a specific antigen. A role for the lymphocyte in the inductive phase is suggested by the fact that depletion of the pool of recirculating lymphocytes (antilymphocyte serum, cortisone) a few hours before (but not 24 hours after) the intravenous injection of *T. spiralis* blocks the development of eosinophilia. More direct evidence of a role for the lymphocyte in inducing an eosinophilic response is provided by lymphocyte transfer studies: injection of thoracic duct lymphocytes from animals in the early (intestinal) phase of the natural form of trichinosis into recipients causes an eosinophilia three or four days later. Also, a role for the lymphocyte can be shown in the test model employing intravenous injection of *T. spiralis* larvae. Whole body irradiation blocks development of the eosinophilic response, which can be restored by infusion of bone marrow cells and lymphocytes from normal syngeneic donors. An enhanced response occurs in irradiated animals reconstituted with normal bone marrow and lymphocytes from animals with trichinosis, suggesting a cooperative interaction between lymphocytes (exhibiting "memory" from prior contact with *T. spiralis*) and eosinophil precursors in the marrow. Analogous to the secondary antibody response, a second intravenous challenge with *T. spiralis* larvae produces an enhanced eosinophil response, as an indication also of immunologic memory. The stimulation of eosinopoiesis by lymphocytes appears to be mediated by a diffusible product: thoracic-duct lymphocytes from rats with naturally acquired trichinosis evoke eosinophilia in syngeneic recipients when placed into the peritoneal cavity with a millipore diffusion chamber.

The T lymphocytes (thymus-processed) appear to be the ones involved in inducing the eosinophilic response. Thymectomized mice fail to develop an eosinophilic reaction to trichinosis, but do respond to acute bacterial infections with an increase in neutrophils. Reconstitution of these animals with graft of thymus tissue permits a normal eosinophil response to trichinosis. The use of antisera to effect selective removal of B or T lymphocytes further supports the role of the T cell.

Following the induction phase, the proliferative phase of the eosinophilic response occurs, characterized by a 16- to 64-fold increase in formation of eosinophils. This phase cannot be blocked by antilymphocyte serum, but it is inhibited by immunosuppressive drugs, such as methotrexate and cyclophosphamide, administered 24 hours after the antigen. A role for "eosinophilopoietin," a small polypeptide recently described by Mahmoud, et al., in the proliferative phase has been suggested. This material is found in the serum of mice rendered eosinopenic by repeated administration of rabbit anti-mouse eosinophil serum. Injection of serum from such eosinopenic mice into normal mice produces an increased production of marrow eosinophils. It is not yet known whether "eosinophilopoietin" is a product of T lymphocytes.

Eosinopenia is a characteristic feature of the host response to acute bacterial infections. A similar response occurs in experimental animals with pneumococcal, E. coli, and Coxsackie virus infections and with sterile inflammation due to turpentine. This suggests that the effect is not due to a specific pathogen or toxin but rather to an acute inflammation but this can be reversed by elimination of the inflammatory (infectious) stimulus. Such inflammation can markedly suppress the eosinophilia of trichinosis. Eosinopenia is part of the normal response to stress. Since administration of glucocorticosteroids causes eosinopenia, it had been assumed that the eosinopenia of acute infection is a non-specific aspect of the hormonal response to the stress of acute infection. However, recent studies indicate that the eosinopenia of acute infection is independent of the adrenal response to non-specific stress: the eosinopenic response to acute inflammation occurs prior to the rise in serum corticosterone level and occurs normally in adrenalectomized animals. The marked decrease in circulating eosinophils during acute inflammation is due to both a rapid accumulation of eosinophils at the periphery of the inflammatory lesion and a suppression of the discharge of eosinophils from bone marrow. Prolongation of the inflammation causes suppression of eosinopoiesis as well. A protein (molecular weight of greater than 30,000 daltons) capable of producing an eosinopenic response when injected into mice with trichinosis has been found in inflammatory exudates. The response it induces is so rapid as to suggest a direct effect on eosinophils; e.g., by inducing intravascular margination.

The best evidence for the possible role of the eosinophil in defense against multicellular parasitic invaders comes from recent studies of schistosomiasis and trichinosis. Resistance to reinfection with *Schistosoma mansoni* develops in mice and rats after primary infection, and it can be passively transferred with serum (but not cells). This immune response is directed mainly at the migration of young worms (schistosomules) following cercarial penetration of the skin. Such penetration elicits a prompt eosinophilic inflammatory response in the immune animal. Within 12 hours degenerating schistosomules can be observed in the dermis surrounded by masses of eosinophils. Pretreatment of immune mice with non-specific anti-eosinophil serum (but not antilymphocyte, antimacrophage, or antineutrophil serum) abrogates the immunity, and the numbers of schistosomules and adult worms increase to the levels found in non-immune animals. Sera from partially immune mice, passively transferred to uninfected mice, confer marked resistance to infection as measured by decreased recovery of schistosomules. Anti-eosinophil serum administered to the recipient also blocks this passively transferred immunity. Thus, it appears that antibody-dependent cell-mediated immunity to schistosomiasis occurs in vivo and involves the eosinophil. A similar role for the eosinophil in defense against *T. spiralis* is suggested by the markedly increased number of viable encysted larvae found in muscles of animals depleted of eosinophils by treatment with anti-eosinophil serum.

Lymphocytosis

An absolute lymphocytosis of great magnitude and consisting of mature lymphocytes is characteristic of two infectious diseases: pertussis and infectious lymphocytosis (an unusual viral disease of children). The parenteral injection of killed virulent *B. pertussis* organisms produces a marked lymphocytosis in a variety of vertebrate species. Lymphocytosis-promoting factor (LPF), a polypeptide of molecular weight approximately 70,000 released into the supernatant of cultures of *B. pertussis*, evokes a lymphocytosis on intravenous injection. Morse and his co-workers have elucidated the mechanism of this lymphocytosis by demonstrating that the peripheral lymphocytosis is accompanied by depletion of small lymphocytes in thymus, spleen, and lymph nodes. The lymphocyte content of thoracic duct lymph is markedly reduced, indicating that the cells enter the circulation from lymphoid organs by a more direct route. Once in the circulation, lymphocytes no longer migrate back to lymph nodes, etc., across postcapillary venules. It appears that migration is impaired due to changes on the lymphocyte surface, possibly produced by adsorption of LPF onto the cell membrane. Lymphocytosis featured primarily by atypical lymphocytes ("viral cells") develops in other diseases such as infectious mononucleosis and infectious hepatitis. The Epstein-Barr virus, the etiology of infectious mononucleosis, infects only B lymphocytes. The atypical lymphocytes that are so prominent in this disease are T cells, suggesting that these uninfected cells play an important role in the immune response to this viral agent.

Alterations Due to the Immune Response of the Host

One of the major defenses of the host against bacterial and viral disease is the mounting of an antibody response. This may be of great importance in the complement-dependent bactericidal reaction against gram-negative bacilli and in the phagocytosis and intracellular killing, by polymorphonuclear leukocytes, of various species of bacteria and viruses. The presence of specific circulating antibody also provides protection against reinfection on re-exposure to the same microorganism. The role of type-specific antibody to the pneumococcal capsular polysaccharide in the response of the host to pneumococcal infection (pneumonia) was manifest, during the pre-antibiotic era, in the dramatic clinical improvement that occurred coincident with the appearance of circulating antibody. The development of an immune response against an invading organism is, however, not invariably a salutary event. Occasionally, this may result in injury to the host and the appearance of overt clinical disease. Several examples will be cited here to illustrate this phenomenon, but no attempt will be made to be encyclopedic.

Immune Complex Disease. Circulating antigen-antibody complexes contribute to the pathophysiology and pathology of at least several human diseases such as acute poststreptococcal glomerulonephritis and viral hepatitis.

Poststreptococcal glomerulonephritis appears to be primarily an immunologic disorder in which antigen-antibody complexes are produced and subsequently trapped in or adjacent to the glomerular capillary walls. Evidence for this is the following: (1) The appearance of the disease after a latent period following streptococcal infection. (2) The high titers of antibodies to streptococcal products present in the sera of patients. (3) The involvement of only certain type-specific strains of Group A streptococci in outbreaks of acute glomerulonephritis. (4) The reduction of complement levels in the sera of patients. (5) The presence of granular and lumpy deposits of complement and bound gamma globulin in the glomerular capillary walls and near the renal basement membrane. These deposits are similar to those observed on electron microscopy and by immunofluorescence in experimentally induced immune complex glomerulonephritis. (6) Demonstration of streptococcal antigen (cell wall rather than cell membrane in origin) in the glomeruli. However, the presence of streptococcal antigen in the nodular, gamma globulin and complement-containing deposits in the kidney must be proved by elution techniques. (7) Development of a possible laboratory model in the rat of experimental poststreptococcal glomerulonephritis. This involves intraperitoneal implantation of millipore chambers containing Group A streptococci. Proteinuria develops a short time after the appearance of type-specific antibodies in the serum and simultaneous with the demonstration of bound gamma globulin, complement, and streptococcal M-protein in the region of the glomerular basement membrane.

The circulating soluble immune complexes appear capable of mediating immunologic injury following deposition on the glomerular basement membrane through activation of complement and stimulation of an inflammatory response consisting of polymorphonuclear leukocytes. This glomerular inflammation accounts for many of the clinical manifestations of acute glomerulonephritis such as hematuria, proteinuria, edema, hypertension, and azotemia.

Immunopathologic mechanisms appear to be involved also in the development of glomerulonephritis following pneumococcal infection. Glomerular bound C3, pneumococcal polysaccharide, and properdin are observed as well as subepithelial and intramembranous electron-dense deposits, suggesting that activation of the alternate complement pathway by the pneumococcal capsular antigen has occurred.

Circulating immune complexes appear to be involved in the pathogenesis of the glomerulonephritis that occurs in other infections such as bacterial endocarditis, quartan malaria, infected ventriculo-atrial shunt pathways, and possibly secondary syphilis. With the exception of secondary syphilis, the feature common to these disorders is a chronic relapsing course. Instances of diffuse glomerulonephritis as a complication of bacterial endocarditis due to a variety of organisms have been reported. These include *Streptococcus viridans, Staphylococcus aureus, Staphylococcus epidermidis,* and Group G streptococcus.

Antibody-Induced Agglutination and Hemolysis of Erythrocytes. Cold agglutinins develop in 50 per cent or more of individuals with primary atypical pneumonia due to *Mycoplasma pneumoniae.* They may also appear in high titer in patients with the protozoan disease trypanosomiasis. Although the incidence of these antibodies in mycoplasma pneumonia is high, acute hemolytic anemia develops only rarely, most often toward the end of the second week of illness and is featured by fever, prostration, and hypotension. The latter, or less commonly hemoglobinemia and hemoglobinuria, may lead to renal failure.

Amyloid Disease. A variety of chronic infectious diseases may be complicated by the development of amyloidosis. These include tuberculosis, leprosy, chronic osteomyelitis, and chronic bronchiectasis. The clinical manifestations and pathophysiologic consequences depend on the major sites of deposition of the amyloid. The kidneys, spleen, liver, and adrenal glands are most commonly affected, but the nervous system, gastrointestinal tract, blood vessels, and heart may be damaged as well. Deposition in the kidney is usually manifest by proteinuria and the nephrotic syndrome and may lead to progressive renal insufficiency. Nervous system amyloidosis is characterized by a peripheral combined sensory-motor polyneuropathy involving the distal extremities initially. Involvement of the heart usually occurs in the older age group and its clinical correlates include myocardial failure, conduction disturbances, coronary artery insufficiency, and restrictive cardiomyopathy presenting a clinical picture of chronic constrictive pericarditis.

Recent studies have established that in many, if not all instances, amyloidosis consists of the deposition in various organs of specific fragments of immunoglobulins. The insolubility of partially purified amyloid fibrils had raised some question as to the relation of amyloid to the immunoglobulins and presented problems in its further purification. However, it has recently been possible to solubilize these fibrils and to analyze their composition. Most amyloid fibrils are made up of the amino-terminal variable portion of the kappa or lambda light chain of immunoglobulin molecules as determined by amino acid sequencing studies. Further support for the immunoglobulin origin of amyloid fibrils is derived from the in-vitro conversion, by proteolytic digestion, of a soluble light chain (Bence Jones protein), with production of insoluble fibrils having the staining properties of amyloid and a partial amino acid sequence derived from the amino-terminal variable region of the Bence Jones protein.

The mechanism of formation and the specific localizations in tissues of amyloid are not clearly understood. It has been reported that Bence Jones proteins from patients with amyloidosis have a greater tendency to bind to kidney, liver, and heart muscle than those from individuals with myeloma uncomplicated by amyloidosis. The possible route for generation of the amyloid fibril is unclear. It has been suggested that antigen-antibody complexes may be processed by macrophages and the immunoglobulin degraded in such a manner as to produce fibrils which are then deposited in the macrophage-rich organs such as liver and spleen. It has also been postulated that free whole immunoglobulins (as in chronic infections) or free light chains (as in myeloma) circulating in increased concentrations may be the immediate source of the fibrils in the vascular system.

Unusual Responses of the Host to Viral Disease

Hypersensitivity Induced by Viral Agents—Postinfectious Encephalomyelitides. Demyelinating encephalitis occasionally follows some viral infections, particularly measles, vaccinia, rubella, and varicella. The disorder occurs most commonly on the fourth or fifth day after the rash, but may develop earlier or later. The histologic pattern is that of a lymphoplasmacytic infiltration of the adventitia of cerebral blood vessels with microglial proliferation in the perivascular spaces. Distinctive perivenous demyelinization is a prominent feature. The infecting virus has not been isolated from the brain or spinal cord of patients with this disease. However, it is important to note that in a few cases of measles encephalitis, cytoplasmic and nuclear inclusion bodies as well as small multinuclear giant cells have been found, suggesting direct viral invasion of brain tissue.

Similar histologic lesions are observed in the brain and spinal cord of laboratory animals in which experimental allergic encephalomyelitis has been produced by a single injection of brain or spinal cord tissue suspended in Freund's adjuvant. The immunologic basis of this disease is suggested by several features: (1) It occurs nine days or more following the injection; there is a shorter latent period when animals that have recovered are re-injected, as would be expected in a secondary response. (2) The inciting ingredient is specific, namely, myelin-containing tissues. (3) The pathologic changes are distinctive and are limited, for the most part, to the white matter. (4) Brain-reactive antibodies are demonstrable in serum, and lymphoid cells cause cytopathic effects on myelinated brain tissue and glial cells in tissue culture. Although antibodies are present in serum the lesions appear to be due to the cellular type of immunity as judged by (a) a delayed type skin response to intradermal injection of myelinated tissue in affected animals and (b) transfer of the disease from affected animals by lymphocytes but not by serum. The neurologic signs are extremely varied, reflecting the patchy distribution of the lesions; they may include pyramidal tract involvement, akinetic mutism, cortical blindness, cerebellar ataxia, choreiform movements, and so on.

It is tempting to relate the experimental disease to the naturally occurring encephalomyelitis that develops following viral infections. However, this is still hypothetical; the lesions of the experimental and natural disease are not absolutely identical.

Chronic Viral Infections of the Central Nervous System. There are four known chronic viral infections ("slow virus" diseases) of man: subacute sclerosing panencephalitis (SSPE), kuru,

Creutzfeldt-Jakob disease, and progressive multifocal leukoencephalopathy. Common to all these are an incubation period of many months to years and a clinical course of prolonged motor and mental deterioration. The unusual features may be related primarily either to unique properties of the virus or to an unusual host response to a typical viral agent. The agents of kuru and Creutzfeldt-Jakob disease have been transmitted to chimpanzees but have not been cultivated in tissue culture, and thus are not yet well characterized. However, the agent of SSPE has been identified as the measles virus in tissue culture. (Recently a syndrome of progressive rubella panencephalitis with insidious deterioration of mental and motor function in the second decade of life also has been described.) This disease is uncommon (1 case per million population in the United States), with the onset in childhood. Clinically, it is characterized by progressive motor and mental dysfunction with myoclonic movements. Extremely high levels of measles antibody are present in the spinal fluid and blood. SSPE (measles) viruses have been isolated from lymph nodes as well as from the brains of patients with the disease, suggesting that the infection may be a disseminated one. These viruses have biologic properties that are more characteristic of the laboratory-adapted vaccine strains of measles than of isolates of the wild virus. It has been suggested that these features may be the result of defective viral replication in nondividing neurons. Another, perhaps more appealing, suggestion is that the disease represents an unusual host response to the virus, one characterized by a specific defect in cellular immunity to the agent of measles.

Metabolic Alterations in Infection

A variety of metabolic changes accompany systemic infection. Some may be the direct result of the activity of the infecting agent, some may represent the consequences of epiphenomena such as fever and infection-induced glucocorticoid and aldosterone excess, and others may be related to specific organ dysfunction due to localization of the infectious process (e.g., hepatitis or pyelonephritis). The sorting out of the contributions to the over-all picture by each of these elements has not thus far been achieved.

Changes in electrolyte metabolism have been described in a variety of infectious diseases due to extracellular and intracellular agents. Increased urinary losses of sodium and chloride occur in the immediately prefebrile and early symptomatic periods. This may be due to increased renal perfusion and sodium delivery to renal tubules secondary to increased cardiac output early in the febrile phase. Poor dietary intake, vomiting, diarrhea, and sweating may contribute to electrolyte loss. In sum, these factors probably account for the hyponatremia and hypochloridemia observed at the height of symptoms. The initial heightened urinary sodium and chloride loss is followed by renal retention of sodium coincident with increasing compensatory aldosterone excretion.

In chronic infections involving the lung (slowly resolving pneumonias, pulmonary tuberculosis) and central nervous system infections (tuberculous meningitis), water retention and hyponatremia may develop secondary to inappropriate antidiuretic hormone activity (ADH). The role of hyponatremia in the symptoms of acute infections is not established but it may contribute to the asthenia and malaise that commonly occur.

The most obvious metabolic consequences of acute infection are catabolic. A negative nitrogen balance occurs regularly during infections but does not begin until after the onset of symptoms. It is usually paralleled by potassium losses. The role of these catabolic changes in the not infrequent occurrence of the troublesome and prolonged postinfectious asthenia is still speculative.

Alterations in whole blood amino acid concentrations have been observed during the course of a variety of experimentally-induced infections in man. An increase in the total amino acid concentration occurs during the incubation period of typhoid fever. This is followed by a decrease in amino acid concentrations, accompanying the development of overt clinical illness. It is not clear whether these alterations are the direct effect of the infectious agent on host amino acid metabolism, or the consequence of a non-specific host response to stress mediated by adrenocorticosteroids. No clinical manifestations have been directly attributable to these biochemical changes.

Marked elevations in the concentrations of total serum lipids have occurred in patients with severe infections, particularly bacteremia, due to gram-negative bacilli. The lipid pattern consists of a predominant increase in free fatty acids, accompanied by lesser increases in triglycerides and phospholipids. In contrast, similar changes in serum lipids have not been observed in severe infections caused by gram-positive cocci. In experimental animals injection of endotoxin has produced hyperlipidemia, and this component of gram-negative bacilli may be responsible for the changes in lipids during bacterial infections.

REFERENCES

FEVER

Altschule, M. D., and Freedberg, A. S.: Circulation and respiration in fever. Medicine, 24:403, 1945.

Atkins, E.: Pathogenesis of fever. Physiol. Rev., 40:580, 1960.

Atkins, E., and Bodel, P.: Fever. N. Engl. J. Med., 286:27, 1972.

Bennett, I. L., Jr., and Beeson, P. B.: The properties and biological effects of bacterial pyrogens. Medicine, 29:365, 1950.

Cooper, K. E.: Temperature regulation and the hypothalamus. Br. Med. Bull., 22:238, 1966.

Cooper, K. E., Cranston, W. I., and Snell, E. S.: Temperature regulation during fever in man. Clin. Sci., 27:345, 1964.

Greisman, S. E., Hornick, R. B., Carozza, F. A., and Woodward, T. E.: The role of endotoxin during typhoid fever and tularemia in man. I. Acquisition of tolerance to endotoxin. II. Altered cardiovascular responses to catecholamines. III. Hyperreactivity to endotoxin during infection. J. Clin. Invest., 42:1064, 1963; 43:986, 1774, 1964.

Hardy, J. D.: Physiology of temperature regulation. Physiol. Rev., 41:521, 1961.

Hornick, R. B., Greisman, S. E., Woodward, T. E., et al.: Typhoid fever: Pathogenesis and immunologic control. N. Engl. J. Med., 283:686, 739; 1970.

Kluger, M. J., Ringler, D. H., and Anver, M. R.: Fever and survival. Science, 188:166, 1975.

Wood, W. B., Jr.: Studies on the cause of fever. N. Engl. J. Med., 258:1023, 1958.

Wood, W. B., Jr.: The pathogenesis of fever. In Mudd, S. (Ed.): Infectious Agents and Host Reactions. W. B. Saunders Co., Philadelphia, 1970.

HEADACHE ASSOCIATED WITH FEVER

Scott, R. B., and Warin, R. P.: Observations on the headache accompanying fever. Clin. Sci., 6:51, 1948.

Sutherland, A. M., and Wolff, H. G.: Experimental studies on headache: Further analysis of the mechanism of headache in migraine, hypertension, and fever therapy. Arch. Neurol. Psychiat., 44:929, 1940.

Wolff, H. G.: Headache and Other Head Pain. Oxford University Press, New York, 1963.

SEPTIC SHOCK

Blain, C. M., Anderson, T. O., Pietras, R. J., and Gunnar, R. M.: Immediate hemodynamic effects of gram-negative vs. gram-positive bacteremia in man. Arch. Intern. Med., 126:260, 1970.

Christy, J. H.: Pathophysiology of Gram-negative shock. Am. Heart J., 81:694, 1971.

Gilbert, R. P.: Mechanisms of the hemodynamic effects of endotoxin. Physiol. Rev., 40:245, 1960.

Mills, L. C., and Moyer, J. H. (Eds.): Shock and Hypotension: Pathogenesis and Treatment (The 12th Hahnemann Symposium). Grune and Stratton, New York, 1965.

Nishijima, H., Weil, M. H., Shubin, H., and Cavanilles, J.: Hemodynamic and metabolic studies on shock associated with gram-negative bacteremia. Medicine, 52:287, 1973.

ALTERATIONS OF SENSORIUM

Lyon, G. Dodge, P. R., and Adams, R. D.: The Acute Encephalopathies of Obscure Origin in Infants and Children. Brain, 84:680, 1961.

HEMATOLOGIC CHANGES

Bass, D. A.: Behavior of eosinophil leukocytes in acute inflammation. II. Eosinophil dynamics during acute inflammation. J. Clin. Invest., 56:870, 1975.

Bass, D. A.: Reproduction of the eosinopenia of acute infection by passive transfer of a material obtained from inflammatory exudate. Infect. Immunol., 15:410, 1977.

Basten, A., and Beeson, P. B.: Mechanism of eosinophilia. II. Role of the lymphocyte. J. Exp. Med., 131:1288, 1970.

Basten, A., Boyer, M. H., and Beeson, P. B.: Mechanism of eosinophilia. I. Factors affecting the eosinophil response of rats to Trichinella spiralis. J. Exp. Med., 131:1271, 1970.

Beeson, P. B., and Bass, D. A.: The Eosinophil. Vol XIV: Major Problems in Internal Medicine. W. B. Saunders Co., Philadelphia, 1977.

Cartwright, G. E., and Wintrobe, M. M.: The anemia of infection XVII. A review. In Dock, W., and Snapper, I.: Advances in Internal Medicine. Vol. V. Year Book Medical Publishers, Inc., Chicago, 1952, p. 165.

Coleman, R. W., Girey, G. J. D., Zacest, R., and Talamo, R. C.: The human plasma kallikrein-kinin system. Progr. Hematol., VII:255, 1971.

Corrigan, J. J., Ray, W. L., and May, N.: Changes in the blood coagulation system associated with septicemia. N. Engl. J. Med., 279:851, 1968.

Deykin, D.: Thrombogenesis. N. Engl. J. Med., 276:622, 1967.

Marsh, J. C., Boggs, D. R., Cartwright, G. E., and Wintrobe, M. M.: Neutrophile kinetics in acute infection. J. Clin. Invest., 46:1943, 1967.

Mahmoud, A. A. F., Warren, K. S., and Peters, P. A.: A role for the eosinophil in acquired resistance to Schistosoma mansoni infection as determined by anti-eosinophil serum. J. Exp. Med., 142:805, 1975.

Mahmoud, A. A. F., Stone, M. K., Kellermeyer, R. W.: Eosinophilopoietin: a circulating low-molecular-weight peptide-like substance which stimulates production of eosinophils in mice. J. Clin. Invest., 60:675, 1977.

Minna, J. D., Robboy, S. J., and Coleman, R. W.: Disseminated Intravascular Coagulation in Man. Charles C Thomas Co., Springfield, Ill., 1974.

Morse, S. I., and Riester, S. K.: Studies on the leukocytosis and lymphocytosis induced by Bordetella pertussis. II. The effect of pertussis vaccine on the thoracic duct lymph and lymphocytes of mice. J. Exp. Med., 125:619, 1967.

Rodriguez-Erdmann, F.: Bleeding due to increased intravascular blood coagulation. N. Engl. J. Med., 273:1370, 1965.

Taub, R. N., Rosett, W., Adler, A., and Morse, S. I.: Distribution of labeled lymph node cells in mice during the lymphocytosis induced by Bordetella pertussis. J. Exp. Med., 136:1581, 1972.

Wilhelm, D. L.: Kinins in human disease. Ann. Rev. Med., 22:63, 1971.

MISCELLANEOUS

Beisel, W. R., Sawyer, W. D., Ryll, E. D., and Crozier, D.: Metabolic effects of intracellular infections in man. Ann. Int. Med., 67:744, 1967.

Feigin, R. D., Klainer, A. S., Beisel, W. R., and Hornick, R. B.: Blood amino acids in experimentally induced typhoid fever. N. Engl. J. Med., 278:293, 1968.

Gallin, J. I., Kaye, D., and O'Leary, W. M.: Serum lipids in infection. N. Engl. J. Med., 281:1081, 1969.

Glenner, G. G., Ein, D., and Terry, W. D.: The immunoglobulin origin of amyloid. Am. J. Med., 52:141, 1972.

Gutman, R. A., Striker, G. E., Gilliland, B. C., and Cutler, R. E.: The immune complex glomerulonephritis of bacterial endocarditis. Medicine, 51:1, 1972.

Lennette, E. H., Magoffin, R. L., and Freeman, J. M.: Immunologic evidence of measles virus as an etiologic agent in subacute sclerosing panencephalitis. Neurology, 18:21, 1968.

Miller, H. G., Stanton, J. B., and Gibbons, J. L.: Parainfectious encephalomyelitis and related syndromes. Q. J. Med., 25:427, 1956.

Payne, F. E., Baublis, J. V., and Itabashi, H. H.: Isolation of measles virus from cell cultures of brain from a patient with subacute sclerosing panencephalitis. N. Engl. J. Med., 28:585, 1969.

Swartz, M. N., and Weinberg, A. N.: Infections due to gram-positive bacteria. Gram-negative coccal and bacillary infections. In Fitzgerald, T. B.: Dermatology in General Medicine. McGraw-Hill Book Co., New York, 1971.

Zabriskie, J. B.: The role of streptococci in human glomerulonephritis. J. Exp. Med., 134:180, 1971.

21

Pathophysiologic Changes Due to Localization of Infections in Specific Organs

LOUIS WEINSTEIN,
AND MORTON N. SWARTZ

The major impact of a number of human infections is directly related to the specific anatomic site of disease, and the pathophysiologic abnormalities that develop are due primarily to dysfunction of the single or principal organ involved. In some instances, a wide variety of organisms are capable of localizing at the same site, where they produce roughly similar pathophysiologic changes (e.g., infective endocarditis due to any of a number of bacterial and mycotic species). In others, a specific discrete site may be involved by only a very limited group of infectious agents (e.g., involvement of the motor neurons of the spinal cord in disease due to poliomyelitis or Coxsackie viruses).

The pathophysiology of many of the common infectious diseases represents, in effect, the changes due to dysfunction of a particular organ. These are little different from those that might be induced in the same area by non-infectious processes. Thus, the abnormalities that develop in viral hepatitis have much in common with those that appear in acute alcoholic hepatitis. This is also true for chronic pyelonephritis and chronic renal disease due to other causes such as hypertension and chronic glomerulonephritis. The cardiovascular alterations associated with myocarditis are much the same whether it is due to viral infection or alcoholic cardiomyopathy. Likewise, the dramatic circulatory consequences of cardiac tamponade are similar whether this is the result

of viral or tuberculous pericarditis on the one hand, or pericardial invasion by a neoplastic process on the other. The pathophysiology of these and many other infectious diseases is considered in sections devoted to organ-system physiology elsewhere in this book. The focus in this chapter is on selected organ involvement in which the pathophysiologic changes, although reflecting primarily organ dysfunction, are quite uniquely produced by infectious agents. Emphasis is put on a limited number of illustrative examples rather than on a comprehensive listing of infectious diseases appropriate to this category.

The characteristic pathophysiologic changes to be considered may be centered about one organ primarily (e.g., osteomyelitis) or the ramifications may be broad, involving many other organs in a specific fashion (e.g., infective endocarditis, syphilis with its multiple stages).

INFECTIONS WITH PATHOPHYSIOLOGIC CONSEQUENCES IN MULTIPLE ORGAN SYSTEMS

Infective Endocarditis

Although this infection involves primarily the heart valves or mural endocardium, the peripheral changes secondary to bland (or septic) emboli,

562

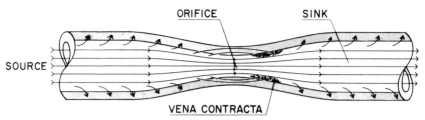

Figure 21-1 Venturi model of high-pressure source driving a bacterial aerosol into a low-pressure sink. Typical location of bacterial colonies is noted at the vena contracta. (Reproduced from Rodbard with permission of the publisher. Circulation 27, 18, 1963.)

associated vasculitis, or antigen-antibody complexes may be so striking as to become pre-eminent. Thus, neurologic dysfunction, skin and joint changes, or renal failure may dominate the picture and draw attention to organs other than the heart.

Pathogenesis of Endocarditis. The pathophysiologic processes involved in the development of subacute bacterial endocarditis are strikingly different from those operative in the development of the acute form of the disease. Four mechanisms are responsible for the initiation of the subacute infection: (1) a previously damaged cardiac valve, or a hemodynamic situation in which a "jet effect" is produced by blood flowing from an area of high pressure to one of relatively low pressure; (2) a sterile platelet-fibrin thrombus; (3) bacteremia (often transient); and (4) a high titer of agglutinating antibody for the infecting organism.

By the introduction of a bacterial aerosol into an air stream moving through an agar Venturi tube, Rodbard has shown clearly how high pressure drives an infected fluid into a low pressure sink and produces a characteristic pattern of colony distribution, concentrating in the low pressure region just distal to the orifice (Fig. 21-1). This model helps to account for the distribution of lesions observed in endocarditis complicating various cardiac valvular and septal defects (Fig. 21-2). In mitral insufficiency a "jet effect" is produced when blood is driven from a high-pressure site (left ventricle) into a low-pressure area (left atrium); vegetations of endocarditis are typically located on the atrial (low-pressure) side of the valve and on the adjacent atrial endocardium where the impacting regurgitant stream produces a fibrous area, MacCallum's patch. In aortic insufficiency the aorta is a high-pressure area and the left ventricle is a low-pressure zone; vegetations of endocarditis characteristically are located on the ventricular (low-pressure) surface of the aortic cusps. In addition, in the presence of active infection on the aortic valve, a regurgitant "jet" of blood can inoculate bacteria onto the adjacent anterior leaflet of the mitral valve, where a secondary infection can result in mitral insufficiency and further compromise left ventricular function. In a small ventricular septal defect with

a left-to-right shunt, a Venturi effect can result in the development of vegetations around the orifice on the right ventricular side or on the right ventricular wall opposite the defect at the site of jet impact.

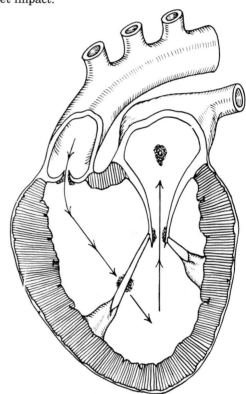

Figure 21-2 High-velocity streams in mitral and aortic insufficiency and locations of endocarditic lesions. Arrows at the left indicate regurgitant flow from aortic high-pressure area into left ventricle. Endocarditic lesions appear at the ventricular surface of the aortic valve. The "jet" stream through the incompetent aortic valve may produce secondary lesions on the chordae tendineae of the anterior leaflet of the mitral valve. In the presence of mitral insufficiency, the regurgitant "jet" stream (arrow at right) will enter the sink of the left atrium during ventricular systole, and bacterial vegetations will tend to develop on the atrial surface of the mitral valve and on the site of impact on the atrial endocardium. (Adapted from Rodbard with permission of the publisher.)

As blood flows over a valve leaflet that has been distorted by acquired heart disease such as acute rheumatic fever, or malformed because of a congenital defect, a "whipping" effect is produced, inducing platelet deposition. Platelet aggregation occurs, initiating coagulation factor activation and local fibrin formation. A platelet-fibrin thrombus is thus deposited at the site of the deformity on the valvular surface. The valvular defect responsible for this phenomenon is occasionally of insufficient magnitude to cause enough turbulence of flow to produce a murmur. Although transient bacteremias probably occur very frequently in man, they are usually without clinical significance, even in the individual with abnormal cardiac valves on which sterile platelet-fibrin thrombi may be situated. In most instances, the failure of implantation of organisms on such a valve is related to the small number of bacteria in the circulation at any given time. A factor that possibly plays an important role in the development of valvular infection is the level of circulating antibody, especially agglutinins. These may result in conglutination of a sufficiently large number of bacterial cells to allow their successful multiplication, and the establishment of infection within the platelet-fibrin thrombus. This phenomenon may be of particular importance in the pathogenesis of subacute endocarditis because of the relatively low invasive capacity of the bacterial species usually involved.

The pathophysiologic changes involved in the development of acute bacterial endocarditis are, in most respects, quite different. In at least 50 to 60 per cent of cases of acute endocarditis, previously normal valves are the site of infection. It appears, therefore, that the presence of a sterile platelet-fibrin thrombus is unnecessary in the pathogenesis of this form of the disease. Because the organisms responsible for this type of infection (Staphylococcus aureus, pneumococci, meningococci, gonococci, Streptococcus pyogenes, and Haemophilus influenzae) are highly invasive, only small numbers are required to establish infection. Thus, the only requirement for the establishment of acute endocarditis is bacteremia due to an invasive organism. It should be pointed out, however, that in the instances in which underlying valvular damage, either acquired or congenital, is present, sterile platelet-fibrin thrombi may develop and facilitate the initiation of this type of infection. The exact mechanism by which "pathogenic" bacteria invade normal valve leaflets is unknown. Although small blood vessels have been suggested as the route by which organisms reach and invade a normal valve in the course of bacteremia, there is little or no anatomic evidence to support this hypothesis. In fact, most observers have failed to demonstrate a distinct blood supply in the leaflets of undamaged valves.

In a great many cases of subacute bacterial endocarditis, the bacteremia responsible for the infection originates not from an infectious process, but from trauma to an area where the causative organisms normally reside as components of the indigenous flora (e.g., the teeth, urinary tract, and intestine). This is in sharp contrast to acute infective endocarditides, in which the inducing bacteremia has its origin in an active infection at a site remote from the heart.

Support for the concept that non-bacterial thrombotic endocarditis is the initial lesion that is converted to subacute bacterial endocarditis comes from studies of an experimental model of this disease by Durack and Beeson. In this model, non-bacterial thrombotic endocarditis is produced by insertion of a polyethylene catheter into the right side of the heart of a rabbit. Subsequent intravenous injection of Streptococcus viridans results in adherence of the bacteria to the vegetation, where they multiply rapidly and serve as a source of continuing bacteremia. Microcolonies appear beneath and within a superficial layer of material that appears to be fibrin.

Selective bacterial adherence to valvular endothelium has been suggested as an important characteristic of bacteria capable of causing endocarditis in man. On incubation in vitro with excised valve leaflets, strains of enterococci, viridans streptococci, and S. aureus adhere more readily than E. coli and Klebsiella. These gram-positive organisms are the commonest causes of endocarditis, whereas E. coli and Klebsiella are rarely implicated despite their frequency as causes of bacteremia. Although these findings are suggestive, adherence is not the sole determinant of bacterial pathogenicity in endocarditis, as is indicated by the fact that P. aeruginosa, a rare cause of endocarditis, exhibits marked adherence.

Pathophysiology of the Clinical Features of Endocarditis. Four mechanisms are responsible for the clinical features of infective endocarditis: (1) the infectious process on the involved valve; (2) the occurrence of emboli; (3) metastatic infection; and (4) the deposition of immune complexes and clinical manifestations of immunologic injury, including vasculitis. All these are not found in every patient. There are also striking qualitative and quantitative differences in their roles in the acute and subacute forms of the disease.

THE INFECTIOUS PROCESS ON THE INVOLVED HEART VALVE. The striking differences in the clinical course of subacute and acute endocarditis can be related almost entirely to the patho-anatomic and pathophysiologic changes induced at the primary site of infection, the heart valve. Microscopic study of the lesions in subacute bacterial endocarditis reveals evidence of both slowly progressive activity and early or complete healing. Neutrophils, lymphocytes, plasma cells, and Anitschkow cells compose the cellular infiltrate. The impression is one of simultaneous slow destruction and healing, with the latter not quite "catching up" with the former. In contrast to this are the anatomic changes characteristic of acute endocarditis. Grossly, the vegetations on the involved valve surface are often larger, softer, and more friable than the smaller, harder thrombi observed in the subacute infection. In the more fulminant forms or when the lesion has been present for some time, a variety of destructive changes may occur in proximity to the valvular vegetation (Table 21–1). Tears, aneurysms, and/or perforation of one or several cusps of the aortic valve may take place during the course of active infective endocarditis. Eversion or extreme distortion of the aortic valve cusps may occur in some instances after bacteriologic cure has been achieved. Free aortic regurgitation is produced, and marked acute left ventricular failure ensues.

A mycotic aneurysm of the sinus of Valsalva may develop in the course of acute or subacute bacterial endocarditis involving the aortic valve. The aneurysm occasionally enlarges by burrowing through the commissure into the wall of the ventricle and there forms an abscess, destroying myocardial fibers. The aneurysmal sac may even dissect into the septum and rupture into the right atrium. This occurrence is characterized by the sudden development of a roaring continuous thrill and murmur over the upper left sternal border along with peripheral signs of aortic and tricuspid regurgitation, the sudden onset of con-

TABLE 21–1 INTRACARDIAC COMPLICATIONS OF INFECTIVE ENDOCARDITIS

AORTIC VALVE
1. Eversion or distortion of a cusp
2. Fenestration, rupture, or avulsion of a cusp
3. Erosion of aortic annulus; aortic ring abscess
    a. Rupture into pericardium → tamponade
4. Mycotic aneurysm of sinus of Valsalva or of the mitral-aortic intervalvular fibrosa
5. Dissection of a valve ring abscess or of a mycotic aneurysm into the upper (membranous) interventricular septum
    a. Perforation of the septum producing a shunt between left ventricle and right atrium
    b. Perforation of the septum producing a shunt between left ventricle and right ventricle
6. Occlusion of the valve orifice by vegetations (fungal endocarditis; prosthetic valve endocarditis)

MITRAL VALVE
1. Distortion of leaflet
2. Mycotic aneurysm of mitral valve
3. Rupture of chordae tendineae
4. Papillary muscle dysfunction
5. Dissecting infection involving mitral annulus
6. Occlusion of valve orifice by vegetation (fungal endocarditis; prosthetic valve endocarditis)

TRICUSPID VALVE
1. An uncommon site of endocarditis; distortion, etc., of leaflets producing valvular insufficiency

PULMONIC VALVE
1. A rare site of endocarditis; distortion, etc., of leaflets producing valvular insufficiency

MYOCARDIUM
1. Abscess (wall or septum)
2. Diffuse myocarditis
3. False aneurysm
4. Rupture of abscess → cardiac tamponade

PERICARDIUM
1. Pericarditis
    a. Fibrinous or hemorrhagic pericarditis secondary to aortic annulus erosion or to burrowing of aortic root abscess into the epicardium

SEPTAL ABSCESS
1. Dissection of infection from aortic ring abscess or from infection involving mitral annulus
2. Bacteremic or embolic infection of septum

CORONARY ARTERIES
1. Embolus → myocardial infarction
2. Mycotic aneurysm

gestive failure, and the absence of radiologic findings of marked pulmonary edema. Infection of the aortic valve may also burrow into the root of the aorta (erosion of aortic annulus; aortic ring abscess), and the inflammation may extend posteriorly to the pericardial wedge between the aorta and pulmonary artery, producing fibrinous or hemorrhagic pericarditis. A ring abscess may secondarily involve the mitral-aortic intervalvular fibrosa (the junctional zone between the aortic and mitral valves) and form an expanding false aneurysm, ultimately rupturing with hemorrhage into the pericardial cavity and causing death from cardiac tamponade.

Similarly destructive changes may involve the mitral valve and produce rupture of the chordae tendinae or of a head of a papillary muscle. Catastrophic mitral regurgitation with a loud pansystolic murmur then develops, accompanied by sudden dyspnea and attacks of acute pulmonary edema. Infection involving the mitral valve may burrow into the mitral annulus and even become superimposed on degenerative calcification of the mitral annulus.

Myocardial abscesses may develop not only by extension from valvular vegetations but also as a result of seeding of the coronary circulation with organisms from the vegetations on the aortic valve, or as a consequence of septic embolization. Hectic fevers with or without positive blood cultures (while the patient is receiving antibiotic therapy) and rapidly progressive left-sided heart failure are prominent features. Myocardial abscesses in a strategic location in the septum may cause striking changes in conduction. Infection that involves this area may have (1) spread down the septum from the aortic valve to the A-V bundle, causing disruption of A-V conduction; (2) spread from the mitral valve through the annulus to the region of the A-V bundle or node; or (3) reached the septum by embolization through the coronary circulation. The proximity of the aortic valve (right and non-coronary cusps) to the conduction system and of the mitral annulus to the atrioventricular node and the common bundle of His accounts for the development of conduction defects when infection has extended beyond the valve annulus (Fig. 21–3). Prolongation of the PR interval, a new left bundle branch block, or a new right bundle branch block with left anterior hemiblock could indicate extension of infection from the aortic valve into the interventricular septum. Extension of infection from the mitral annulus into the atrioventricular node or proximal bundle of His might be indicated by the onset of nonparoxysmal junctional tachycardia, second degree A-V (Wenckebach) block, or complete heart block with a narrow QRS on the electrocardiogram. Rupture of the interventricular septum secondary to a septal abscess occurs very rarely and is characterized by the abrupt appearance of a pansystolic murmur and thrill, as well as rapidly developing cardiac failure.

The constitutional reaction to the valvular infection is manifested by elevated temperature, rigors and generalized malaise; it is, in general, less intense in subacute than in acute endocarditis. Although the level of fever may be the same in either type of disease, it is lower, as a rule, in the chronic form and may never exceed 100 to 101° F.; in about 5 per cent of cases, particularly in patients with azotemia, it may be absent en-

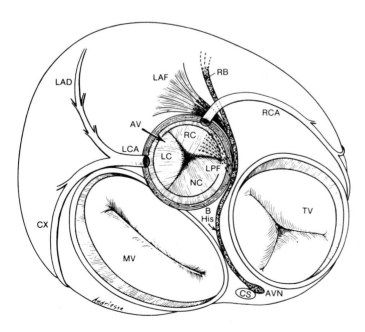

Figure 21–3 Anatomic relationships between cardiac valves and conduction system as viewed from above (superiorly). MV indicates mitral valve; TV, tricuspid valve; AV, aortic valve; LC, left coronary cusp; RC, right coronary cusp; NC, non-coronary cusp; LCA, left coronary artery; LAD, left anterior descending artery; CX, circumflex artery; RCA, right coronary artery; CS, coronary sinus; AVN, atrioventricular node; B His, common bundle of His; LPF, left posterior fascicle of left bundle branch; LAF, left anterior fascicle of left bundle branch; and RB, right bundle branch. (Adapted from Hutter and Moellering with permission of publisher.)

tirely. In contrast, the temperature is very often high in the acute disease and commonly reaches 103 to 104° F. or more. Although rigors may occur at the beginning or during the course of untreated subacute bacterial endocarditis, they are more frequently present in acute endocarditis. Anemia is usually present in both types of disease and may develop quite rapidly in the absence of overt intravascular hemolysis; it is usually the anemia of infection (see Chapter 20).

A changing murmur has been considered a common and characteristic feature of subacute endocarditis. However, broad experience has made it clear that this is rarely the case when *Streptococcus viridans,* the usual cause of this disease, is involved. In contrast, murmurs often undergo rapid and striking changes in intensity and quality in patients with acute valvular infections. This is due to several factors: (1) decrease or increase in size of the relatively soft valvular thrombi, (2) tears or fenestration of valve leaflets, (3) rupture of chordae tendineae or papillary muscles, (4) perforation of the ventricular septum, or (5) development of an aneurysm in an aortic cusp or in the sinus of Valsalva. Of great importance is the fact that murmurs may be absent in patients with subacute bacterial endocarditis, even when the disease has been present for some weeks. Also, about one third of patients with *acute* valvular infections involving the left side of the heart, or patients with right-sided endocarditis (commonly acute) may have no detectable murmurs early in the course of the disease.

Valvular infection due to enterococcus occupies a clinical position between that produced by *S. aureus* (acute) and *S. viridans* (subacute). Distant septic complications may develop but are most uncommon in endocarditis due to *S. viridans.*

Although the white blood count may be elevated (10,000 to 20,000 per mm.³), it is commonly not increased in patients with subacute bacterial endocarditis. Indeed, the presence of a leukocytosis usually suggests the occurrence of embolic complications or an infecting organism other than *S. viridans* (e.g., enterococcus). Leukocytosis is common in the acute type of disease; however, the number of white cells in the peripheral blood may be normal or even strikingly decreased.

The interval between the onset of infection and the establishment of the diagnosis, as well as the duration of disease in untreated patients with endocarditis is directly related to the character of the valvular lesion. The progression of the infectious process in the acute form is so rapid that severe constitutional manifestations force the patient to seek early medical attention. If undetected, and therefore untreated, death may occur in one or two weeks as the result of marked destruction of the involved valve, multiple metastatic infections, or embolization to a vital area. The course of subacute endocarditis is strikingly different. In this, the symptoms of infection are often very insidious in onset, mainly low-grade fever and slowly developing anemia. The patient's only complaints may be loss of appetite, increasing fatigue, weight loss or night sweats. The interval between the onset of symptoms and definitive diagnosis in 100 cases of subacute bacterial endocarditis was about 3.5 months. Life expectancy after development of this disease is usually rather long, even in the absence of antimicrobial therapy, unless rupture of a mycotic aneurysm or lethal embolization occurs. The chronicity of the disease reflects the slow progress of the pathologic process on the infected valve. Survival for three to six months is common. It may be even longer (over one year) when *Staphylococcus epidermidis* is the responsible organism.

EMBOLIC PHENOMENA. Embolic episodes are common in both acute and subacute bacterial endocarditis. Although they occur most often when infection is still present, they may supervene at any time in the course of the disease, even well into convalescence when the active process has been eliminated. Almost any organ may be the site for embolic deposition. However, the kidneys, heart, brain, spleen, and eyes are more frequently involved than other organs. The areas of resulting infarction may be solitary and large, or multiple and quite small; the clinical manifestations that develop as well as the risk of death depend on the organ involved and the extent of damage. Cerebral embolism is the most common of the neurologic complications of bacterial endocarditis and occurs in 15 to 20 per cent of patients with this disease; it is particularly common in patients with mitral valve involvement and in those with infection due to pyogenic organisms such as *S. aureus* and enteric gram-negative bacilli. Although emboli in both acute and subacute endocarditis usually contain organisms early in the course of infection, there is a striking difference in the changes that develop at the sites of deposition. The areas of infarction that occur in the subacute disease are, as a rule, sterile. Thus, in subacute endocarditis one observes the paradox of an infected embolus producing a bland infarct. In contrast, infarcts that develop in the course of acute valvular infections, especially those caused by *S. aureus,* rapidly suppurate. Emboli that occur in patients with mycotic endocarditis or atrial myxoma tend to be large. Occlusion of major vessels should, therefore, suggest the presence of these diseases rather than the commoner bacterial infections of valves.

Myocardial infarction secondary to coronary embolization may occur in the course of bacterial endocarditis. Pericarditis may result from extension of the area of infarction to the pericardial surface. Although this is the basis of the pericardial involvement in some patients with endocarditis it is not the only cause for pericardial inflammation in this setting. Other causes include myocardial abscess, erosion of a mycotic aneurysm of the sinus of Valsalva, extension of aortic valve infection into the pericardial wedge between the root of the aorta and the pulmonary artery, uremia, bacteremic spread of infection to the pericardium, and reactivation of acute rheumatic fever.

METASTATIC INFECTIONS. One of the most striking differences between subacute and acute bacterial endocarditis is the high frequency with which metastatic infection occurs in the latter. Infarcts in subacute infection usually do not become infected. This may be attributed to several factors: (1) the invasive capacity of the organisms involved is relatively low, (2) the number of organisms present in the embolus is insufficient to establish metastatic infection, and (3) a high titer of specific antibody results in killing of the few bacteria that are deposited at the local site. Thus, while infarction of the kidneys, heart, and brain occurs in patients with subacute bacterial endocarditis, abscesses in these organs, meningitis, pyelonephritis, or suppurative myocarditis develop only very rarely. However, a sterile meningitis, with the biochemical and cellular characteristics of "aseptic" meningitis, is not an uncommon occurrence in the subacute form of the disease. Mycotic aneurysms of the aorta and its branches that may develop in the course of subacute valvular infection are usually not due to suppuration in and about the vessel walls. In most instances, the vascular necrosis, mural weakening, and aneurysmal dilatation result from sterile occlusion of the vasa vasorum; histologic study of such lesions rarely reveals evidence of active inflammation. Mycotic aneurysms may occur intracranially, particularly in the distribution of the middle cerebral artery. Leakage or rupture of such aneurysms may produce neurologic dysfunction secondary to intracerebral or subarachnoid bleeding. Cerebral mycotic aneurysms now tend to occur more frequently in the course of acute than subacute endocarditis; when they occur in the latter it is late in the course of the disease. Healing of mycotic aneurysms, as shown on sequential angiography, can occur during the course of effective antimicrobial therapy. Mycotic aneurysms may also develop in a coronary artery, in the mesenteric arterial tree, or in arteries of the extremities. Because the organisms contained in emboli in acute infective endocarditis are usually highly invasive, they are able to successfully multiply and establish infection in the infarcted areas. Thus, when valvular disease is due to *S. aureus,* multiple abscesses are often detectable, particularly in the kidney and myocardium.

Brain abscesses, often small and multiple, may complicate acute endocarditis, particularly when *S. aureus* is the cause. Purulent meningitis may occur also owing to seeding during bacteremia. It is important to recognize that the symptoms of headache, nuchal rigidity, and a mild cerebrospinal fluid pleocytosis during endocarditis do not necessarily represent pyogenic meningitis; they may result from cerebral emboli. Such emboli may involve relatively silent areas of the cortex and produce few if any localizing neurologic findings.

IMMUNOLOGIC ASPECTS AND HYPERSENSITIVITY PHENOMENA. Agglutinating, complement-fixing, and opsonizing antibodies specific for the infecting bacteria in subacute bacterial endocarditis are regularly present. There is an increased level in the serum of both IgG and IgM. Over 50 per cent of patients develop some type of antiglobulin factor. The latex fixation test for rheumatoid factor is positive in about 50 per cent of cases when the disease has been present for 6 weeks or longer. Large amounts of cryoglobulins and macroglobulins may be present. About one third of patients with endocarditis have high levels (above 100 μg. per ml) of circulating immune complexes; high levels are much more frequent in patients with extravalvular manifestations of endocarditis (arthralgias, sterile arthritis, splenomegaly, Roth spots in the retina, glomerulonephritis) than in those without such signs. This suggests, but does not prove, that immune complexes may be important in the pathogenesis of all these features of endocarditis. It has been suggested that the articular symptoms, a prominent feature in some patients with subacute endocarditis, are related to the presence of the rheumatoid factor. Arthralgia or florid arthritis may occur early or late in the course of subacute endocarditis. The synovial fluid is usually sterile. Changes in serum globulins are much less marked and less frequently present in the acute endocarditis, because death occurs early if the disease is untreated.

Renal lesions often develop in the course of bacterial endocarditis, particularly the subacute variety. These are of several types: (1) diffuse membranous glomerulonephritis, both acute and subacute, in which immune complexes consisting of antigen, antibody, and complement are deposited as "lumpy-bumpy" aggregates on the glomerular basement membrane (see Chapter 20); (2) renal infarcts, both large and small; and (3) so-called "focal embolic glomerulonephritis," an entity presumed in the past to be the result of multiple small emboli, but now also considered to be due to an immune complex mechanism. The renal lesions appear to play an important role in death from prolonged and untreated endocarditis. Disease that has persisted for protracted periods may no longer require the active participation of viable bacteria. A "bacteria-free stage" of chronic bacterial endocarditis has been described, the predominant features of which are those of chronic renal failure.

The classic peripheral signs of subacute bacterial endocarditis, originally considered to be of embolic origin, have been thought more recently to represent lesions of allergic vasculitis involving small arteries. Among such signs are *Osler's nodes* (painful and tender bluish-red lesions in the pulp spaces over the terminal phalanges of the fingers or toes); *Janeway's lesions* (nontender, irregular, erythematous or hemorrhagic lesions situated most often in the skin over the thenar and hypothenar eminences of the hands or on the soles of the feet); *Roth's spots* (boat-shaped exudates with a surrounding zone of hemorrhage in the retina); *subungual* or *"splinter"* hemorrhages in the nail beds; and *petechial skin lesions.* Histologic and bacteriologic study of Osler's nodes has been performed in only a few patients with endocarditis. Pathogenic organisms have been isolated from aspirates of Osler's nodes in four patients (*S. aureus* in three patients and *Candida albicans* in one); histologic examination of the skin lesion from one of these patients with *S. aureus* endocarditis revealed a microabscess in the dermis and microemboli in adjacent arterioles. These four patients had acute bacterial endocarditis due to virulent organisms. Thus, in acute bacterial endocarditis Osler's nodes may be due to septic microemboli. In contrast, in subacute bacterial endocarditis due to viridans streptococci and other microorganisms of limited pathogenicity, convincing proof of an embolic origin for Osler's nodes is lacking. It is thought that Osler's nodes are painful because of the location of the lesion in the densely-packed, extensively-innervated tissues of the digital pulp space.

Salmonella Infections (Salmonellosis)

Infections caused by different species of salmonella have in common a number of clinical features such as fever, chills, and diarrhea. However, careful consideration of the pathophysiologic processes involved in the syndromes of "acute gastroenteritis," "enteric fever," and isolated "bacteremia" produced by this group of organisms clearly indicates striking differences that sharply distinguish one disease pattern from another. In fact, these are distinct disorders in most respects, the only common denominator being invasion by salmonella, some species of which are more commonly responsible for certain clinical pictures.

Salmonella Gastroenteritis. A very large number of species of salmonella are capable of producing acute gastroenteritis. This form of infection is usually limited to the intestine. Unlike cholera, this enteritis appears to be related to bacterial invasion of the intestinal mucosa and not to elaboration of a specific enterotoxin. The presence of polymorphonuclear leukocytes in the feces is consistent with an inflammatory reaction in the bowel. Only salmonella strains capable of penetrating the intestinal mucosa induce the appearance of inflammatory cells or of enhanced fluid electrolyte loss; non-invasive strains that merely proliferate in the bowel lumen do not produce these changes. Not all invasive strains induce fluid secretion. Evidence suggests that some strains of salmonella which cause fluid secretion may induce intestinal prostaglandin secretion which in turn stimulates adenylate cyclase, resulting in fluid and electrolyte loss. Bloodstream invasion is very uncommon except in young infants and elderly individuals. Metastatic infections of the hepatobiliary and other organ systems is also very infrequent. Several abnormal states appear to be of importance in increasing susceptibility to this type of intestinal infection. Among these are *subtotal gastrectomy* (probably related to a decrease in gastric acid production which permits viable organisms to pass through the stomach), *neoplastic diseases, hemoglobinopathies,* the *administration of antimicrobial agents* (related to suppression of competing components of the normal intestinal flora), and the *use of corticosteroids* (possibly due to alteration in immune mechanisms).

Enteric Fever. The enteric fevers include typhoid *(S. typhi)* and the paratyphoid *(S. paratyphi, S. schottmülleri,* and *S. hirschfeldii)* fevers. A similar clinical picture may be produced occasionally by others of the approximately 1500 salmonella species. The pathogenesis and pathophysiologic phenomena involved in this group of infections are quite distinct and different from those that characterize salmonella gastroenteritis. The enteric fevers are not primary diseases of the intestinal mucosa but rather affect principally the lymphoid tissues in certain areas of the small intestine. The clinical manifestations of dysfunction of the intestine that occur are secondary to this anatomic localization of the infection. The following sequence takes place after ingestion of an inoculum of one of the salmonella species causing enteric fever. Organisms in contaminated water or food pass through the stomach into the small intestines, where they enter the smaller lymphatic channels and are deposited in the lymphoid tissues within the bowel wall. The organisms multiply in the lymph follicles and are often found intracellularly within plasma cells. This intracellular location may be responsible for persistence of infection in the presence of circulating antibodies. A marked macrophage response is induced locally, and a varying degree of necrosis of the nodes occurs. At the end of about two weeks, the average length of the incubation period for the enteric fevers, the organisms invade the bloodstream from the lymphatics. At this point clinical manifestations of disease (fever, chills, and other constitutional reactions to infection) appear. The bacteremic phase may, in fact, be made up of two periods, as suggested by studies of experimental typhoid fever in the mouse. The initial bacteremia is a transitory one, rapidly brought to an end by the removal of the bacilli by the reticuloendothelial system, particularly in the liver and spleen. This is followed by a period of very active bacterial proliferation in the reticuloendothelial cells of these organs. A secondary and more intense bacteremia then ensues, resulting in widespread dissemination of the bacteria. The bacteremia usually persists for several days but may last as long as ten days; during this time salmonella ordinarily cannot be recovered from the feces. However, after this they are demonstrable in fecal cultures. During the bacteremic phase, salmonella reinvade the intestine via the gallbladder and bile ducts. Ulcerations occur in Peyer's patches in the ileum, and salmonella appear in the feces. Because of the location of the collections of lymphoid tissue in the intestinal wall, the ulcerations are not linear but encircle the bowel. The fact that intestinal involvement is secondary to disease in the lymphoid structures is supported by the absence of diarrhea in over half the patients with enteric fevers. The two commonest complications of this type of salmonella infection, intestinal hemorrhage and perforation, are directly related to the active inflammatory and destructive process in the submucosal aggregations of lymphoid cells. Despite the prominent bacteremia, it is uncommon for metastatic infections of various organs to occur in the course of typhoid and paratyphoid fever.

Salmonella Bacteremia. A number of unrelated factors play important roles in the pathogenesis of salmonella bacteremia. Although not known for some, the pathophysiology of others has been partly defined. *Advancing age* appears to predispose to this type of disease. Individuals with *hepatic cirrhosis* are also more prone to develop this syndrome. This may be related to their greater susceptibility to bacteremia in general because of the decreased effectiveness of the liver in removing members of the intestinal microflora from the portal circulation. *Various types of neoplastic disease* predispose to this type of salmonellosis; although not proved, it is likely that this is related to the immunosuppressive effects of certain malignant diseases. The *administration of antimicrobial agents and corticosteroids* may play a role in the pathogenesis of salmonella bacteremia; the former by eradicating competing elements of the normal flora, and the latter by decreasing immunocompetence. A group of disorders characterized by *chronic or acute episodes of hemolysis —* malaria, sickle cell anemia (or other hemoglobinopathies), louse-borne relapsing fever *(Borrelia recurrentis),* and Oroya fever *(Bartonella bacilli-*

formis) — are associated with a markedly increased risk of intestinal infection and bacteremia due to salmonella. The loading of macrophages with large quantities of hemoglobin breakdown products may make it possible for these cells, the major defense against salmonella, to ingest and kill the organisms. It has also been suggested that hyperferremia, consequent on acute hemolysis, is responsible for the increased susceptibility to invasion by salmonella. There is some evidence, from animal studies, that hypoferremia may be associated with some increase in resistance to certain infections, whereas excessive levels of iron in the serum may be associated with a decrease in resistance. The association of salmonella osteomyelitis with hemoglobinopathies is well recognized. The microscopic areas of bone infarction that commonly occur in sickle cell anemia appear to serve as a nidus for the engraftment and multiplication of salmonellae that have previously entered the circulation. An increased susceptibility to invasion by salmonella occurs in patients with schistosomiasis. Chronic salmonella urinary tract infection can complicate *S. hematobium* infection in this area. Salmonella are able to penetrate and multiply within schistosomes *(S. mansoni),* protected from the effects of antibody and antimicrobial agents. From this sanctuary they may be the source for persisting or recurrent bacteremias.

One of the most interesting pathophysiologic phenomena that may play a very important role in the pathogenesis of continuing salmonella bacteremia is an *arteriosclerotic aneurysm of the aorta,* or one of its major branches. The aneurysmal sac or the clot may become infected during a transient salmonella bacteremia. This then becomes the site of a bacterial endarteritis, which thereafter is a source for a continuous intense bacteremia. However, in some patients with this syndrome, neither clot nor infection of the aneurysmal wall can be demonstrated. An aortic aneurysm in a rare patient with salmonella infection of a vertebral body may become infected as the result of direct spread of infection to its outer wall from the adjacent area of osteomyelitis. The pathophysiologic changes in salmonella bacteremia consist of three groups of phenomena: (1) those due to the presence of viable gram-negative bacilli in the circulation; (2) those related to circulating endotoxin (myalgias, fever, and even disseminated intravascular coagulation in an occasional patient); and (3) the tendency for metastatic infections to develop. The lungs, meninges, synovial membranes, bones, and endocardium (valvular) are most often involved.

Syphilis

Syphilis may involve any part of the body, particularly in its late stages, and may produce profound functional changes in many organs. The pathophysiologic phenomena in this disease are the result of inflammatory and vascular changes in organs where *Treponema pallidum*, the etiologic agent, has been deposited during the early phase of invasion of the bloodstream. The changes are conveniently considered under three major groupings: *early, late, and congenital* syphilis. The relative impact of the disease on various organ systems depends on the stage of the process; the latter is determined to a large measure by the effectiveness of the immunologic response to the invading spirochete. Certain organs such as the heart and aorta, the central nervous system, and the eye are prominently involved; important functional derangements occur as a result. The natural history of untreated early syphilis, as observed at the turn of this century, suggested that in about two thirds of individuals the disease became latent and produced no major manifestations. However, it was found, 50 to 60 years later, that 10 per cent of these patients had syphilitic cardiovascular disease and another 6.5 per cent had neurosyphilis.

Early Syphilis. The usual portal of entry for *T. pallidum* is skin or mucous membrane. Symptomatic early syphilis is made up of two stages. The initial lesion of *primary syphilis* is a papule which evolves into a painless, eroded or crusted lesion (chancre), usually located on the genitals but occasionally at extragenital sites. The chancre develops two to six weeks after inoculation of the organism. Painless regional lymphadenopathy appears shortly thereafter. Pathologically, the primary lesion shows a dermal infiltrate (lymphocytes and plasma cells), a proliferation of capillaries, and endarteritis. *T. pallidum* is present in the lesion and in the regional nodes. The chancre, even if untreated, slowly heals over the next two to six weeks. During the evolution of the primary lesion and extension of infection to regional lymph nodes, the treponemes enter the circulation and are widely disseminated. Metastatic foci develop, particularly in the skin, the mucous membranes, and the nervous system.

Secondary syphilis occurs five to six weeks after the appearance of the chancre and is a manifestation of treponemal multiplication in metastatic foci. The principal features are a generalized measles-like rash (often accompanied by erosive superficial lesions in the oral, genital, or anal mucous membranes) and generalized lymph node enlargement. The *secondary eruption,* even if untreated, disappears within several weeks; and the treponemes in other foci appear to die out, presumably as a result of the immunologic response of the host. Occasionally, sufficient numbers of the organisms survive to initiate another round of treponemia. This is responsible for one or more recurrent episodes of secondary syph-

ilis (mucocutaneous relapse). Meningitis due to invasion by treponemes is not uncommon in secondary syphilis. In addition to the usual findings common to many types of aseptic meningitis, delirium and seizures occasionally occur. Damage to the third, sixth, seventh, and eighth cranial nerves may develop as a result of reactive fibrosis of the leptomeninges about the base of the brain. Acute hydrocephalus with papilledema may rarely complicate the process. The cerebrospinal fluid shows a pleocytosis of up to 500 cells, predominantly lymphocytes. The duration of the meningitis is usually less than a month. Other areas that may be involved in secondary syphilis are the *eye* (visual loss due to iritis or optic perineuritis secondary to meningitis); *kidney* (interstitial nephritis; nephrotic syndrome due to membranous glomerulonephritis, with proteinuria and edema); *liver* (hepatitis mimicking viral hepatitis in its manifestations); and *bones* (pain and tenderness of long bones due to periostitis).

Late Syphilis. In about one third of patients with untreated early syphilis sufficient immunity does not develop to render the disease asymptomatic (latent) for the remainder of the patient's life. Instead, chronic destructive inflammatory and vascular changes slowly progress over many years and produce late manifestations. These occur principally in the skin and mucous membranes, bones, joints, central nervous system, and heart and great vessels.

The characteristic lesion in late syphilis is the gumma, a granulomatous lesion in which there is coagulation necrosis due to obstructive inflammation of small arteries; treponemes are usually absent.

SKIN AND MUCOUS MEMBRANES. The changes of late syphilis in the skin consist of gross, nodular, ulcerating lesions. Gummas also may occur in the oral mucosa and cause perforation of the palate and destruction of the nasal septum.

SKELETAL SYSTEM. Gummatous periosteal involvement of bones produces pain and swelling, particularly of the tibia and clavicle. Destructive involvement of weight-bearing joints ("Charcot's joints") is not due to invasion of the synovia by treponemes, but rather to the effects of constant trauma on joints lacking pain sensation because of the neurologic changes of syphilis (tabes dorsalis).

CENTRAL NERVOUS SYSTEM. There are five definable patterns of late syphilis of the central nervous system. (1) *Meningovascular syphilis:* This develops a few years after the primary lesion and lacks the usual features of acute bacterial meningitis. The fundamental lesion is an arteritis. The clinical features result from arterial thromboses and fibrosis. A variety of neurologic syndromes may develop, depending on the site of vascular occlusion. These may be located in the cerebral cortex and produce hemiplegia, aphasia, homonymous hemianopia, or seizures. Occlusions of the anterior spinal artery may lead to paraplegia. Other vascular lesions may produce sensory loss and impairment of bowel and bladder function. A mild lymphocytic pleocytosis (up to 100 cells) of the cerebrospinal fluid is common. (2) *Tabes dorsalis:* This occurs 10 to 30 years after the initial infection. Atrophy of the dorsal roots and demyelinization of the sensory fibers that ascend in the posterior columns of the spinal cord are the characteristic pathologic changes. These are produced by the inflammatory arteritis in the meninges, and not by direct invasion of the cord substance by treponemes. As a result of posterior column involvement, position sense is grossly impaired. Patients have difficulty walking, particularly in the dark. Sharp stabbing pain over the extremities or trunk occurs episodically and is due to the changes in the dorsal roots. Involvement of the sacral nerve roots causes impotence, incontinence, and constipation. Atrophy of the optic nerve and changes in function of the pupil (poor responsiveness to light but normal reaction to accommodation — Argyll Robertson pupil) is common. (3) *Primary optic atrophy:* This may occur in the absence of tabes dorsalis. Damage to the optic fibers results from continuous leptomeningitis. This is confirmed by the observation that the outer portions of the optic nerve are first affected, causing impairment of peripheral vision. Subsequent decrease in central visual acuity develops, owing to involvement of the deeper placed fibers in the optic nerve. (4) *General paresis:* This is a very serious form of central nervous system syphilis, involving primarily the cerebral cortex, meninges, and cerebral arteries. Large numbers of *T. pallidum* are found in the cortex, and diffuse neuronal destruction with reactive gliosis is prominent. Atrophy of the frontal and temporal lobes and dilatation of the ventricles are marked. As a result of these extensive pathologic changes in the cerebral cortex, evidence of a wide range of mental and neurologic dysfunction is present. Delusions, hallucinations, hypomania, and paranoia may be prominent. As in tabes dorsalis, patients with paresis may have the Argyll Robertson pupil (irregular miotic pupil responsive to accommodation but not to light). Seizures and strokes secondary to the syphilitic endarteritis are not uncommon. Once developed, general paresis progresses rapidly, with profound mental deterioration followed by physical incapacitation. If untreated, the disease is uniformly fatal. (5) *Gummas of the central nervous system (intracranial or intraspinal):* These are rare and present with manifestations consistent with an expanding lesion, such as a tumor.

Very rarely, *T. pallidum* appears to persist (as evidenced by dark-field microscopy and immunofluorescent antibody techniques) in cerebrospinal fluid or aqueous humor of the eye (or even lymph nodes) following heretofore-considered adequate penicillin treatment of latent or late syphilis. Progression of central nervous system syphilis in an occasional patient after conventional penicillin therapy may be related to persistence of the spirochete in areas where antibiotic penetrance is poor. Higher penicillin dosage to provide maximal treponemicidal concentrations in the cerebrospinal fluid is now recommended for such patients.

CARDIOVASCULAR SYSTEM. Cardiovascular syphilis takes the form of either an aortitis of the ascending aorta, producing the clinical features of aortic insufficiency with left ventricular strain, or an aneurysm of the ascending aorta. Involvement of the coronary ostia in the aortitis may lead to coronary insufficiency. Syphilitic aortic aneurysms cause hoarseness (impingement on the recurrent laryngeal nerve); cough and dyspnea (pressure on the trachea and bronchi); dysphagia (compression of the esophagus); and pain (erosion of ribs, sternum, or vertebrae).

Congenital Syphilis. As a result of treponemia occurring after the fourth month of pregnancy, the fetus becomes extensively infected. The placenta is enlarged and there is extensive proliferation of fibrous connective tissue. Similar fibrotic lesions with mononuclear cell infiltrations are present in many viscera. The most characteristic findings are in the lungs ("pneumonia alba"), which show a marked increase in fibrous tissue and poorly developed alveoli filled with macrophages. Periostitis and osteochondritis are also common.

Late congenital syphilis is a prenatally acquired infection that has been less acute and the clinical manifestations are not evident until the child is over two years of age. Osseous changes (saddle nose, saber-shaped tibia from periostitis), synovitis of the knees, dental deformities (upper central incisors), and eighth nerve deafness are usually present. The most common manifestation is interstitial keratitis, an inflammatory process of the cornea complicated by neovascularization, which may progress to blindness. Central nervous system involvement may occur, as in the acquired disease, and result in meningitis, meningovascular disease, juvenile paresis, and, rarely, tabes dorsalis.

INFECTIONS WITH PATHOPHYSIOLOGIC CONSEQUENCES IN A SINGLE ORGAN OR ORGAN SYSTEM

Lobar Pneumonia

The pneumococcus is the commonest cause of lobar pneumonia, but other organisms such as *Klebsiella pneumoniae* may produce a similar lesion. The onset of pneumococcal infection of the lung is usually preceded by a viral upper respiratory tract infection of several days' duration. Aspiration of the infected mucus from the nasopharynx into the distal ramifications of the bronchial tree, usually in the lower lobes, sets up the initial focus of pulmonary infection. The occurrence of such an aspirational event is enhanced by alcoholic intoxication, anesthesia, or depressant drugs, all of which are known to diminish the epiglottal reflex.

Following establishment of infection in the alveoli a characteristic sequence takes place in the evolution of pneumococcal pneumonia. First, bacterial invasion by the encapsulated diplococci evokes an outpouring of edema fluid. This thin fluid serves as a vehicle for carrying the organisms into terminal bronchioles and through the alveolar pores of Kohn into adjoining alveoli. Inspiratory movements aid the rapid spread of infection toward the lung periphery. Polymorphonuclear leukocytes quickly enter the infected area and soon reach sufficient numbers to completely fill the alveoli and produce frank consolidation. At this stage phagocytosis by leukocytes begins to take place even though type-specific opsonizing capsular antibodies have not yet appeared. Such early phagocytosis ("surface phagocytosis") follows the trapping by the leukocytes of pneumococci against alveolar walls or against the surface of other leukocytes. Unspecific heat-labile opsonins (capable of acting on bacteria in general) contribute to the effectiveness of this early phagocytic process and the subsequent destruction of the organisms. After the untreated patient has been ill for some days, monospecific anticapsular antibody appears. By neutralizing the antiphagocytic properties of the capsular polysaccharide, this antibody considerably enhances phagocytosis and intracellular killing. Once most of the organisms have been ingested, macrophages derived from the monocytes of the blood and the lining cells of the alveoli enter the lesion to clear away the bacterial and leukocytic debris.

Although the events described above occur sequentially in a given area of involvement, all are going on simultaneously when the entire spreading lobar process is considered. Three areas of activity are discernible. The peripheral portion of the lesion, the edema zone, is composed of alveoli filled with bacteria and serous fluid containing few if any cells. Inside this is a second zone characterized by the presence of leukocytes and red blood cells which have entered through injured alveolar walls. These two peripheral areas, exhibiting edema and hemorrhage together, present the gross appearance of "red hepatization." The third or central zone is one in which the alveoli are crowded with polymorphonuclear leukocytes and in which the appearance of macrophages may herald early resolution. This dense consolidation, when viewed in the gross, is the area of "gray hepatization."

The spreading pneumonic process may rapidly involve a whole lobe, extending as far as the pleural surface. Aspiration of infected edema fluid into the bronchial tree may spread the infection to several lobes. The infection may not be contained by the pleural boundaries but may enter the pleural space and produce empyema.

Clinical Manifestations of Pneumonia. A variety of clinical manifestations develop in association with the progression of the histologic changes in the lung. The pathophysiologic basis of the signs and symptoms that characterize this kind of pneumonia is understood to a varying degree.

COUGH. This is usually an important feature of the disease. The cough reflex is stimulated by irritation of the lower respiratory tract and by the accumulation of purulent exudate in the bronchial tree. Pink, bloody, or "rusty" sputum is produced by the majority of patients and is the result of the bleeding into alveoli that characterizes the early inflammatory process.

CHILL AND FEVER. The first major symptom of lobar pneumonia is frequently a single shaking chill which is temporally related to the stage of bacterial invasion of the lung. Whether a specific pyrogenic component of the pneumococcus analogous to the endotoxin of gram-negative bacilli is involved in stimulating endogenous leukocytic pyrogen (EP) is not known. Phagocytosis stimulates the production and release of EP and thus may be the responsible mechanism. Bacteremia is present in approximately one third of cases of pneumococcal lobar pneumonia and is usually detectable when patients enter the hospital some time after the chill has occurred.

PLEURITIC PAIN. Severe chest pain occurs in the majority of patients with pneumococcal pneumonia. It often occurs at the onset of the disease and is the result of inflammation of the pleural surface following peripheral extension of the pneumonia. The pain is usually referred directly to the overlying chest wall. However, when the diaphragmatic pleura is involved, it is referred to the shoulder. The discomfort is strikingly accentuated by inspiratory movement; this leads to splinting of the affected side of the chest and rapid, shallow, and grunting respiration.

CYANOSIS. Cyanosis of the lips and nail beds is commonly present, in the absence of shock, in pneumococcal lobar pneumonia. This indicates a significant degree of arterial hypoxemia. Several mechanisms may be involved in the pathogenesis of this phenomenon: (1) *Shunting of blood through consolidated lung tissue.* The extensive exudate that completely fills the alveoli in much of the involved lobe decreases or abolishes effective gas exchange in this area. However, blood flow to the consolidated, poorly aerated lobe continues. Thus, venous blood perfusing the area is not exposed to high oxygen tensions and is, in effect, physiologically shunted into the pulmonary veins, and then to the systemic circulation. (2) *Postpulmonary shunting.* This results from admixture of unsaturated blood that occurs distal to the pulmonary capillaries from such venous channels as thebesian vessels, bronchial veins, and anastomoses between portal vein collaterals and the pulmonary circulation (portopulmonary shunt). (3) *Ventilation-perfusion disturbances in unconsolidated areas of the lung.*

Most of the hypoxia in patients with lobar pneumonia is accounted for by a right-to-left shunt. When the disease is moderately severe, essentially all of the shunt is pulmonary. When it is severe, both pulmonary and postpulmonary shunting is markedly accentuated. The increase in the postpulmonary shunt in severe pneumonia has been attributed to an increase in bronchial circulation. However, a more likely explanation is that the heightened tissue metabolism in the area of infection causes an increase in the observed total shunt (without affecting the pulmonary shunt) by decreasing the oxygen content of pulmonary venous blood. Later in the course of pneumonia (after four days) the magnitude of the shunt declines. After four days of illness, ventilation-perfusion disturbances begin to contribute relatively more to the observed hypoxia in some instances. This may be due to altered lung mechanics known to be present in acute pneumonia (decrease in lung compliance out of proportion to the amount of lung tissue involved as observed in roentgenograms of the chest). The reason for this increased rigidity of apparently normal parts of the lung may be the reduction of surface activity that has been noted in grossly normal areas from lungs containing lobar consolidations. The causes of hypoxemia in lobar pneumonia clearly appear to depend to some extent on both the severity and the duration of the pulmonary infection.

CIRCULATORY CHANGES. Cardiovascular function may be taxed heavily by the stress of pneumonia. The impact on the heart may be so severe that death results. The adequacy of the circulation and tissue perfusion can be appraised by measurement of the arteriovenous (A-V) oxygen difference. A normal (not exceeding 5.5 vol. %) or narrowed A-V difference is an indication of a physiologically adequate circulation. In the presence of fever, the cardiac output is normally increased in parallel or in excess of the increase in oxygen consumption. The net effect is that the A-V O_2 difference remains normal or is narrowed. In two thirds of patients with pneumonia, tissue perfusion is adequate as judged by evidence of an appropriate circulatory response — an increased cardiac output associated with increased oxygen consumption, and an A-V O_2 difference not in excess of 5.5 vol. %. In the other one third of patients there is an inadequate hemodynamic response, consisting of a relatively low cardiac output that results in a widened A-V O_2 difference. This occurs in patients who have no apparent evidence of pre-existing heart disease and whose venous pressure is normal. These individuals also have an abnormally high total peripheral resistance and an increased hematocrit. The hypodynamic state in this group appears to be due principally to depressed myocardial function which returns to normal during convalescence. Relative hypovolemia due to decreased fluid intake, fluid losses secondary to fever, and shifts out of the vascular compartment may also contribute to the lowered cardiac output. The underlying nature of the myocardial dysfunction is unknown. T-wave changes have been reported in the ECG during pneumonia; infiltration of the myocardium with inflammatory cells has been noted in some fatal cases. Whether these represent direct effects of a bacterial product or of hypoxia is not known.

ILEUS. Adynamic ileus and gastric dilatation may be prominent features in pneumococcal pneumonia. They may be of sufficient magnitude to add to the patient's discomfort and interfere with respiration. The cause of the ileus is not established, but it may result from the low O_2 saturation of the blood supplying the bowel.

HERPES LABIALIS. Pneumococcal pneumonia is frequently accompanied by an attack of herpes labialis. By means not yet understood, this pulmonary infection (as well as a variety of other events) can stimulate herpes simplex virus release from trigeminal ganglia in which it resides quiescently. After passage of the virus down the nerve fibers to the skin, infection of epidermal cells occurs, with development of characteristic vesicles on the lips.

Complications of Pneumococcal Pneumonia. A variety of complications may occur and produce pathophysiologic consequences depending on their location.

PULMONARY AND PLEURAL INVOLVEMENT. Lung abscess is a rare complication of pneumococcal pneumonia and is almost always due to infection with type III strains. These organisms possess an abundant "slime layer" of antiphagocytic capsular polysaccharide. This interferes with initial surface phagocytosis as a result of which the density of bacteria in the pneumonic focus may reach an extremely high level and produce local necrosis of the lung. Pleural involvement may lead to the development of an effusion or a frank empyema. Fever and evidence of infection will persist if the latter is not properly drained. Compression of the lung may become chronic owing to fibrosis and produce restrictive changes in pulmonary function.

CARDIAC INVOLVEMENT. Purulent pericarditis and acute bacterial endocarditis are the serious cardiac complications of pneumococcal pneumonia and are due to direct bacterial invasion. Pericarditis may produce cardiac tamponade with limitation of venous return and cardiac output as the physiologic consequences of this constrictive process.

MENINGITIS. This complication is the result of bacteremic spread of infection.

ARTHRITIS. This is a suppurative process due to growth of pneumococci in the synovia and extension into the joint space.

PERITONITIS. Although pneumococcal peritonitis may occur in the course of pulmonary infection due to this organism, it is rare. Patients with either postnecrotic hepatic cirrhosis or the nephrotic syndrome are particularly susceptible to the development of peritoneal involvement. The clinical picture is that of a septic process complicated by adynamic ileus.

FULMINANT PNEUMOCOCCAL BACTEREMIA. Splenectomized patients, particularly children whose spleens have been removed because of thalassemia or other hemolytic anemia, are particularly susceptible to severe pneumococcal infections with intense bacteremia complicated by shock and disseminated intravascular coagulation.

Interstitial Pneumonia

Interstitial pneumonia is a diffuse inflammatory process of the lung in which the pathologic changes are located mainly in the alveolar walls and, to a varying degree, within the alveoli. There is involvement of the alveolar ducts and bronchioles to a lesser extent. Histologically, there is an extensive interstitial inflammatory infiltration, usually consisting of mononuclear cells, in the walls of alveoli and in the connective tissue septa about the small pulmonary vessels. This process usually accompanies or immediately follows an initial intra-alveolar inflammatory reaction. It may be manifest clinically as an acute process and resolve completely or occasionally lead to severe interstitial fibrosis and run a subacute or chronic course.

A wide range of infectious agents may be involved in the pathogenesis of interstitial pneumonia: (1) viruses, such as influenza, varicella, adenovirus, and Herpes hominis; (2) Mycoplasma pneumoniae (the cause of the common type of "atypical pneumonia"); (3) Chlamydia (psittacosis or ornithosis); (4) Rickettsia, principally Coxiella burnetii (Q fever); (5) bacteria, primarily Haemophilus influenzae; (6) fungi such as Histoplasma capsulatum; and (7) protozoa (Pneumocystis carinii). However, a somewhat similar clinical and pathophysiologic picture can also be produced by a variety of non-infectious processes. These include (1) infiltrative disorders (sarcoidosis, histiocytosis); (2) pneumoconioses; (3) collagen vascular diseases; (4) radiation pneumonitis; (5) drug sensitivity (busulfan, methotrexate); and (6) unusual pathologic process of unknown etiology ("desquamative interstitial pneumonia," "lymphocytic interstitial pneumonia").

Non-productive cough, fever, and slight shortness of breath are the principal symptoms in mild cases of interstitial pneumonia. Breathing is rapid and shallow, even at rest, in more severe cases. Roentgenographic changes are usually minimal and consist of fine mottling and a reticular pattern. The oxygen saturation of arterial blood may be markedly reduced, and cyanosis, incompletely relieved by oxygen administration,

may be present. The P_{CO_2} of arterial blood is normal or decreased (owing to hyperventilation). The low arterial oxygen tension (P_{O_2}) was originally interpreted to be the result of impairment of diffusion of oxygen through a thickened alveolar membrane ("alveolar-capillary block" syndrome). However, physiologic studies have indicated that it is unlikely that this can account for the observed arterial oxygen unsaturation. A more likely explanation stems from the finding that there are irregularly distributed areas of lung with altered mechanical properties in this disease. Alveoli in such areas of reduced compliance have somewhat decreased ventilation but are still normally perfused. Thus, abnormalities of ventilation-perfusion and ventilation-diffusion ratios result in inadequate oxygenation of blood leaving certain areas of the lung (venous admixture).

Physiologic studies of patients with acute interstitial pneumonias have been very limited. Varicella pneumonia, a disease seen almost exclusively in adults, has been examined more extensively than others. Dyspnea, non-productive cough, and cyanosis are common features due to pulmonary involvement in patients with extensive and severe chickenpox. Death may occur from respiratory failure. X-ray examination discloses prominent bronchovascular markings and diffuse nodular densities. There is no evidence of obstructive ventilatory difficulty. Increased venous admixture has been found during the acute phase of illness. There may be chronic impairment of gas transfer after resolution of the pneumonia. Scattered, small nodular pulmonary calcifications may develop some time after recovery.

Bacterial Meningitis

The syndrome of uncomplicated bacterial meningitis represents a combination of the nonspecific manifestations of infection (fever, malaise, headache), the signs of meningeal irritation (stiff neck and back, positive Kernig's and Brudzinski's signs), and abnormalities of the spinal fluid (variable numbers and types of cells, and changes in content of sugar and protein). These alterations are induced by pathophysiologic processes which are, for the most part, reasonably well understood.

Manifestations of Infection. As with infections of most types, fever is an almost universal accompaniment of meningitis; chills are often, but not invariably, present. Generalized malaise, often with pain in the muscles and joints, is common. Myalgia appears to be a more prominent feature during the prodromal stages of meningococcal meningitis than during other bacterial meningitides. This may be a manifestation of the accompanying meningococcemia or of endotoxemia.

Manifestations of Meningeal Irritation and Intra-

cranial Infection. The signs of meningeal irritation are produced by the inflammatory reaction about the pain-sensitive spinal roots and nerves. As attempts are made to flex the neck or back or to extend the lower legs on the flexed thighs, traction occurs on the spinal roots and nerves; this produces pain and results in involuntary spasm of the muscles innervated by these nerves. The inability to flex or extend respective muscle groups is responsible for the stiffness of the neck and back and the positive Kernig's and Brudzinski's signs.

Headache, often extremely severe and "pounding" in character, is the most common symptom of meningitis. Although an increase in intracranial pressure is relatively frequent, the pain in the head is usually not due to this, but appears to be related to distortion of the meningeal vessels which are usually encased in the inflammatory exudate.

A common occurrence in the course of the bacterial meningitides is the development of *cerebral edema.* This may be of a degree severe enough to produce changes in the state of consciousness, confusion, or even localizing neurologic signs. It may develop early during meningitis and may be accentuated by excessive administration of parenteral fluids in the course of treatment. The primary danger is herniation of the temporal lobe or cerebellum with compression of the midbrain at the tentorium, producing respiratory arrest. Removal of cerebrospinal fluid in the presence of heightened intracranial pressure may precipitate herniation. Marked brain swelling is usually reflected clinically by coma, by signs of third nerve dysfunction (irregularity of the size or fixation of the pupils), or by respiratory arrest. Papilledema may occur in various types of meningitis. However, the majority of patients with meningitis and increased CSF pressure do not have papilledema. Elevated CSF pressure in the early stages of bacterial meningitis is, in most instances, due to brain swelling and not to obstructive hydrocephalus or intraspinal block. It is important to remember, however, that meningeal infection may be the consequence of intraventricular leakage of a cerebral abscess, or may be accompanied or complicated by subdural empyema. Both cerebral abscess and subdural empyema are space-occupying lesions which can produce increased intracranial pressure and papilledema. Since their treatment is different from that of meningitis, early diagnosis is essential.

Seizures frequently complicate bacterial meningitis. The incidence is higher in infants. However, convulsions are known to be frequent in young children with fever due to a variety of causes. The seizures associated with meningeal infection may be focal or generalized. A common type of focal episode consists of rhythmic jerkings of the eyes conjugately to one side. Seizures may occur during the peak of the meningitis or may appear for the first time during the second or third week of the disease when evidence of active meningeal infection has all but disappeared. Delayed thrombosis of cortical veins is responsible for late seizure activity; it can also account for seizure activity which develops earlier in the disease. Brain swelling may be responsible for seizures during the course of meningitis. Seizures during treatment of meningitis may be a manifestation of penicillin neurotoxicity if this antibiotic is being administered in high dosage to a patient with reduced renal function.

Focal cerebral signs, aside from seizures and alterations of consciousness, occur in meningitis infrequently. Focal cerebral signs that appear early are commonly due to cortical necrosis or occlusive vasculitis (usually venous). Among these are hemiparesis, quadriparesis, visual field defects, disorders of conjugate gaze, and dysphasia. Temporary hemiparesis (persisting up to several hours or longer) can occur as a postictal phenomenon, and its significance can be considerably different from that of a true dense hemiplegia. Prominent and persisting focal cerebral signs always raise the spectre of an associated pyogenic process such as brain abscess, subdural empyema, or possible cerebral embolism from bacterial endocarditis.

Cranial nerve dysfunction is not uncommon in bacterial meningitis. Impaired ocular movement (paresis of third or sixth cranial nerve) is the most frequently encountered evidence of such dysfunction. Facial weakness (seventh nerve) and deafness (eighth nerve) are the other principal signs of cranial nerve involvement. In general, dysfunction of the cranial nerves is transient and disappears shortly after recovery from the meningitis. It is generally assumed, but not yet proved, that damage to these nerves results from their entrapment by the meningeal exudate. Deafness and labyrinthine deficits tend to persist, in contrast to the transient character of the disturbance of other cranial nerve functions. This suggests the possibility that damage to the inner ear is the result of the activity of bacteria or their products. Deafness is not correlated with the presence of otitis media. In fact, deafness is observed more frequently after meningococcal than after other types of meningitis; yet otitis media is much less common in meningococcal meningitis than in meningitis due to *S. pneumoniae* or *H. influenzae.*

Sterile subdural effusions occur in about 10 per cent of patients under the age of two years with bacterial meningitis. They are only rarely reported in children older than this. However, this is misleading, since the usual techniques for diagnosis (transillumination of the skull and subdural taps) cannot be employed in older children or adults. Repeated vomiting, persistence or recurrence of fever, increasing irritability, seizures, fullness of the fontanelle, or increasing cranial circumference have been attributed to subdural effusion when they occur later in the course of meningitis. Transillumination has proved to be a useful means of making the diagnosis. In many infants with meningitis such sterile subdural effusions disappear without the need for subdural tap. Indeed, they may be found (on routine transillumination of infants with meningitis) in the absence of any clinical manifestations attributable to the process. Rarely, subdural effusions are invaded by bacteria as a result of penetration of the arachnoid by the infectious process. The resulting subdural empyema is characterized by high fever, considerable toxicity, and a variety of cortical signs (seizures, hemiplegias, visual field defects). The latter signs are due to (1) inflammation and thrombosis of the cortical veins that run through the subdural space and (2) pressure phenomena secondary to the often large accumulation of pus over one or both cerebral hemispheres.

Abnormalities of Cerebrospinal Fluid. An increase in the number of cells is demonstrable, with very rare exceptions, in patients with bacterial meningitis. Almost without exception, the predominant cell in the early stages of the disease is the neutrophil. In rare instances, mobilization of inflammatory cells into the spinal fluid may not occur, and culture of the spinal fluid may yield organisms that are too few in number to be detectable in stained preparations. Although not frequent, this phenomenon appears to be most common in the early stage of meningococcal infection. This may be due to the fact that insufficient time had elapsed for the developing inflammatory exudate in the meninges to extend into the spinal fluid. Rarely, the cerebrospinal fluid may be strikingly turbid in the absence of cells; the turbidity then is due entirely to large numbers of organisms. The pneumococcus is the usual etiologic agent in these circumstances. In such cases, studies of bone marrow and peripheral blood have revealed no abnormalities; in fact, a leukocytosis with a shift to the left is commonly present. Patients with leukemia may develop meningitis with similar findings; in this instance, the lack of cerebrospinal fluid pleocytosis is attributable to the marked reduction in circulating neutrophils.

The increased content of protein in the spinal fluid in cases of meningitis is the result of leakage of serum proteins, the release from the meninges of the products of inflammation, and the breakdown of leukocytes introduced during the infectious process. The pathophysiologic basis of very high levels of protein (up to 1 gram or more per 100 ml.) in fluid removed from the lumbar sac is intraspinal block, usually complicating more chronic forms of meningitis such as that due to *Mycobacterium tuberculosis;* excessive concentrations in ventricular fluid are suggestive of block in the internal circulation of spinal fluid, most commonly due to obstruction of the sylvian aqueduct.

Reduction of the concentration of glucose in the spinal fluid is usually, but not always, observed in the active, untreated phase of bacterial meningitis. Although levels may be normal in the very early stage of the disease, these decrease, as a rule, as the infection progresses. It must be stressed that the content of glucose in the cerebrospinal fluid in healthy individuals is directly related, except in uncommon instances, to the concentration of glucose in the blood. High blood sugar levels in a patient with diabetes may be accompanied by a normal or elevated concentration in the spinal fluid. In contrast, quite low levels of glucose in the spinal fluid of young infants do not necessarily indicate infection but may reflect hypoglycemia due to vomiting or poor food intake.

Although extensive bacterial multiplication may play some role in the fall in cerebrospinal fluid glucose concentration in certain types of experimentally produced meningitis (pneumococcal) in animals, it is clear that the metabolic demands of the bacteria or of the leukocytes alone do not account for the lowered levels of glucose. The limited surface phagocytosis that occurs in early bacterial meningitis may contribute in a small measure to lowering CSF glucose through augmented glucose utilization, a characteristic of the phagocytic event. However, interference with the transport of glucose from blood to cerebrospinal fluid appears to be the major factor contributing to the lowering of the concentration of glucose in the spinal fluid. Under physiologic conditions the transfer of glucose from blood to spinal fluid is mediated by two processes: simple diffusion and carrier-facilitated diffusion. The facilitated diffusion of glucose from blood to the cerebrospinal fluid and outward diffusion of glucose from spinal fluid to blood are impaired in bacterial meningitis. This may be secondary to alterations in the blood-CSF barrier due to increased metabolism of the cells involved, or due to structural changes produced by the inflammatory process. In addition there may be greater utilization of glucose by the brain in the course of meningeal infection.

An increase in the concentration of cerebrospinal fluid hydrogen ion has been reported in some patients with bacterial meningitis or subarachnoid hemorrhage. The decrease in pH is associated with a rise in the level of lactic acid in the CSF. It has been suggested that some of the changes in respiration and sensorium that occur in the course of bacterial infection of the meninges may result from this. The decreased pH of CSF may stimulate medullary chemoreceptors and induce hyperventilation, an event that occurs occasionally, in severe meningitis. The respiratory alkalosis produced by hyperventilation may then reduce cerebral perfusion, and, in this way, exacerbate the CSF acidosis.

The pathophysiologic processes described above are common to practically all the bacterial meningitides. However, each etiologic type of meningeal infection has individual physiologic and anatomic features which may account for some of their special clinical characteristics.

Meningococcal Meningitis. Meningococcal infection may have its sole impact as a meningeal disease. However, there may also be widespread effects on other organ systems. Infection of the upper respiratory tract is the most common form of meningococcal disease in man, but produces few if any symptoms. In a small percentage of these patients, there is a sequential development of clinical manifestations: bacteremia, meningitis, and/or other metastatic localizations. The presence of circulating antibodies specific for the various serologic groups of meningococci affords protection against bloodstream invasion.

The occurrence of meningococcal bacteremia (meningococcemia) precedes the development of meningococcal meningitis. The pathophysiologic consequences of meningococcemia vary.

MILD MENINGOCOCCEMIA. The onset is usually acute, with fever, chilliness, myalgias, arthralgias, nausea, and vomiting. Macular skin lesions, particularly on the extremities, are replaced by petechiae and, at times, purpuric lesions. The petechiae that are so common in this disease often contain a necrotic center surrounded by a small zone of hemorrhage. Meningococci may sometimes be demonstrated in Gram stains or culture of material obtained by needle from the pale center of such lesions. The pathophysiologic basis of the lesions in the skin may be a bacterial vasculitis, an endotoxin-induced Shwartzman-like reaction, or thrombocytopenia secondary to the bacteremia. Meningitis quickly follows the bacteremia in some cases; in others, meningeal infection never develops. Some patients develop meningitis without even exhibiting any manifestations in the skin, despite the presence of organisms in the circulation.

ACUTE FULMINATING MENINGOCOCCEMIA (WATERHOUSE-FRIDERICHSEN SYNDROME). The striking feature of this process is the abruptness of its onset and the rapidity with which it inexorably progresses. Shock, extensive purpura, and rapid death (within 24 hours of the intrusion of meningococci into the bloodstream) are attributable to the overwhelming bacteremia and the effects of endotoxin. Circulatory collapse, coma, and disseminated intravascular coagulation (see Chapter 20) may occur within a few hours of onset of the disease. The coagulopathy is responsible for widespread but patchy gangrene of the skin, digits, ears, and nose that may lead to spontaneous amputation of the involved areas. Gastrointestinal bleeding may occur secondary to mucosal lesions of the bowel. Bilateral hemorrhages of the adrenal glands are often present in fatal cases. Levels of corticosteroids in the circulation are usually normal or elevated in fulminant meningococcemia. Thus, acute adrenal insufficiency is probably not the major pathophysiologic basis of the shock occurring in this form of disease.

METASTATIC INFECTIONS SECONDARY TO MENINGOCOCCEMIA. The meninges are the commonest sites of metastatic infection in the course of meningococcemia. However, the organisms may be deposited at many other sites. This usually occurs early in the disease and most often coincides with the meningitis. Metastatic infections of joints, endocardium, myocardium, pericardium, eye, testes, and lungs have been recorded.

CHRONIC MENINGOCOCCEMIA. This is a rare syndrome characterized by recurrent episodes of fever, chills, arthralgias (or arthritis), and an erythematous papular rash. These tend to occur at intervals of 48 to 72 hours and last for one to two days. Blood cultures usually yield meningococci early in the febrile stage. The source of the organisms cannot be defined in every case; in some instances, however, they may be recovered from the upper respiratory tract. Recurrent attacks may go on for weeks to months if treatment is not instituted; meningitis or endocarditis may develop in patients who are not treated.

The clinical characteristics of the meningitis due to *N. meningitidis* are, in general, similar to those present in other types of pyogenic meningeal infections. However, several features are more often associated with disease caused by the meningococcus than with that in which the pneumococcus or *H. influenzae* is involved. Among these are severe agitation, delirium, and maniacal behavior in the early stages of the meningitis; acute brain swelling also appears to be more common and, indeed, may be the pathophysiologic basis of the cerebral signs.

An interesting group of late complications may appear in a small percentage of patients in the course of meningococcal bacteremia or meningitis. Among these are marked arthralgia or frank arthritis, pericarditis (usually with effusion), and myocarditis (primarily electrocardiographic abnormalities). These usually develop during convalescence and are not prevented or abolished by effective antimicrobial therapy. The synovial or pericardial fluids contain a moderate number of polymorphonuclear leukocytes but are sterile. This process is distinct from the septic arthritis or pericarditis that accompanies or complicates the acute phase of meningococcemia or meningitis. It has been suggested that these manifestations represent immunologic reactions, involving complexes of meningococcal polysaccharide antigens and antibody deposited in various tissues. In several patients who developed sterile arthritis during recovery from meningococcal meningitis, circulating immune complexes have been demonstrated in sera and synovial fluid. Deposits of meningococcal antigen, immunoglobulin, and complement (C_3) have been detected in leukocytes in synovial fluid and in skin lesions. Host responses to the antigen-antibody complexes are thought to produce the ensuing sterile inflammation in the involved areas.

Haemophilus influenzae Meningitis. The age

distribution of *H. influenzae* meningitis is striking, the vast majority of cases occurring between the ages of six months and three years. The presence of bactericidal antibody appears to be a crucial determinant in this predilection of the young for this disease. Antibody to type B *H. influenzae,* the strain principally responsible for human infection, is transferred across the placenta to the fetus and persists at effective levels until somewhere between the ages of three and six months. Thereafter, infants are without this protective antibody until they are three years of age, when they begin to acquire it as a result of contact or of relatively minor infections. By the time most individuals are 12 to 15 years old they are immune to invasion by the type B organism. This accounts for the relative infrequency of this type of meningitis in otherwise normal adults. However, recent studies indicate an increasing incidence of this infection in the latter age group. This has been associated with an increase in the number of older individuals lacking specific bactericidal antibody, owing to lack of contact with the organism or to very prompt treatment of respiratory infections in the past.

The pathophysiology of meningitis due to *H. influenzae* is, for the most part, similar to that produced by the meningococcus. Bacteremia originating from the respiratory tract occurs frequently in this type of infection but is not necessary for initiation of meningeal infection. Suppurative arthritis is a rare complication. Petechial rashes may develop rarely in patients in whom the organisms have invaded the bloodstream.

Seizures and sterile subdural effusions occur more commonly with meningitis due to *H. influenzae* than with that caused by the meningococcus. This does not stem from a difference in the invasive properties of the organisms but rather from the age distribution of the two types of meningitis. *H. influenzae* meningitis commonly occurs in infants or young children, whereas the peak age incidence of meningococcal meningitis is in older children and young adults. The prominence of seizures in *H. influenzae* meningitis may reflect merely the frequency of "febrile convulsions" in young infants prone to develop this disease. The higher incidence of subdural effusions with *H. influenzae* meningitis may similarly reflect the age distribution of this type of meningitis, and the availability of easy methods of detecting the presence of subdural fluid (transillumination or subdural tap) in children less than two years of age.

Pneumococcal Meningitis.   Many, but not all, instances of pneumococcal meningitis are secondary to bacteremia. This is particularly so when the source of the organisms is pneumonia. In about 25 per cent of patients, the primary infection involves the middle ear or paranasal sinuses from which it extends to the lining of the central nervous system along venous channels that drain these areas, or the disease reaches the meninges by direct invasion of bone (e.g., the mastoid).

Most instances of recurrent bacterial meningitis are caused by the pneumococcus; as many as 20 episodes have occurred in the same patient. The anatomic basis for this disease is the presence of a cranial lesion that permits communication between the external environment and the meninges. Organisms then can pass directly from the upper respiratory tract, most commonly the nose and its accessory structures, to the central nervous system. The predisposing conditions are usually tears in the dura, fractures of the cribriform plate, nasal meningoceles, and osteomyelitis of the floor of the anterior fossa of the skull.

Meningitis due to the pneumococcus tends to be a more severe disease with a significantly higher mortality than that due to the meningococcus or *H. influenzae.* The exudate tends to be thicker, particularly over the convexity of the brain, in pneumococcal meningitis. Cerebral venous and arterial occlusions leading to hemiplegia or other syndromes appear to be more common in this type of meningeal infection than in the other two types, probably reflecting the effect of the markedly purulent exudate that is often present.

Tuberculous Meningitis.   Bacteremia is probably not the immediate predisposing event in tuberculous meningitis. The most likely focus from which *Mycobacterium tuberculosis* reaches the meninges is a pre-existing small tuberculoma within the cerebral substance or abutting on the meninges. These lesions usually develop during the course of a transient postprimary tubercle bacillemia. The tuberculoma is quickly walled off by host defenses and then remains quiescent for many years or for the lifetime of the patient; however, in a rare instance, breakdown of the lesion occurs later and leads to spread of organisms to the meninges. Meningitis may develop occasionally as a complication of disseminated (miliary) tuberculosis, particularly in children. Even under these circumstances it is probable that the meningeal infection is not the result of direct implantation of organisms, but is secondary to the development of microscopic tuberculomas within the central nervous system. In support of this is the observation that injection of tubercle bacilli into the carotid arteries of dogs produces tuberculomas of the brain and meninges but not tuberculous meningitis. Overt pulmonary tuberculosis is not a prerequisite for the development of meningitis; infection of the lung is not apparent in about one third of instances of central nervous system disease. Two pathophysiologic features of tuberculous meningitis account for several characteristic aspects of this form of meningitis. These are the basilar location of the inflammatory exudate and the common involvement of blood vessels, particularly in the form of an occlusive arteritis. These are responsible for the frequent development of cranial nerve dysfunction, especially bilateral paralysis of the sixth nerve, and the sudden appearance of signs of vascular thrombosis, including hemiplegia and other manifestations of localized brain or spinal cord damage. Ventricular block or spinal block may occur secondary to the chronic inflammatory process and may lead to obstructive hydrocephalus.

The abnormalities in the spinal fluid in tuberculous meningitis differ from those found in meningitis due to pyogenic bacteria. The cellular response consists predominantly of lymphocytes, whereas in untreated pyogenic meningitis over 80 per cent of the cells are polymorphonuclear leukocytes. While the cell count in meningitis caused by other bacteria is usually between 1000 and 10,000 per mm.^{3}, it rarely exceeds 500 per mm.^{3} in tuberculous meningitis. The other changes in the spinal fluid in this disease are qualitatively the same as those in the other bacterial meningitides; they are, however, quantitatively different. In contrast to other infections of the meninges, the sugar content of spinal fluid falls much more slowly and the quantity of protein usually increases to appreciably higher levels. Although it was formerly thought that a reduced concentration of chloride in the cerebrospinal fluid was characteristic and even diagnostic of tuberculous meningitis, this is now known not to be the case. Decreased levels of chloride may occur in other types of meningeal infection and are directly related to hypochloremia, a not uncommon phenomenon in this disease due to the loss of chloride from the profuse sweating and vomiting that frequently occur in the early stages of infection. The syndrome of inappropriate antidiuretic hormone secretion, though not common, occurs more frequently in tuberculous than in other types of meningitis, perhaps related to its longer course and the accompanying chronic pulmonary tuberculosis. It may contribute significantly to the low levels of chloride in the serum and spinal fluid.

Serous tuberculous meningitis is an unusual clinical entity that occasionally develops in children with tuberculosis. The clinical features associated with this syndrome are similar to those characteristic of the early stage of infection of the meninges by the tubercle bacillus — fever, apathy, irritability, headache, vomiting, and stiff neck. Cranial nerve abnormalities do not occur. Serous meningitis differs from caseous tuberculous infection in several ways: (1) It may resolve spontaneously in several weeks or less, whereas true tuberculous meningitis is almost invariably fatal without antimicrobial therapy. (2) Tubercle bacilli are not found in the cerebrospinal fluid. (3) Chemical alterations are generally not observed in the CSF: the glucose concentration is normal and the protein level is, at most, only slightly increased. (4) The number of cells, usually predominantly lymphocytes, is sometimes normal, but is frequently increased to as high as 300 per mm.^{3}

Serous meningitis is thought to be an inflammatory response of the meninges to the presence of localized adjacent (parameningeal) caseous foci, the result of hematogenous infection. These foci induce a "sympathetic" response in the meninges that is similar to that which occurs in pyogenic intracranial infections (brain abscess, subdural empyema), without creating a diffuse meningitis due to seeding with tubercle bacilli. Another interesting, but unproved, hypothesis for the mechanism of serous meningitis is based on the concept of a tuberculin reaction restricted to the meninges. The setting for this process is thought to be an individual with an "inactive" pulmonary lesion and a quiescent tuberculoma of the meninges. Release of tuberculoprotein into the circulation when the pulmonary process becomes active may initiate a response of delayed hypersensitivity (tuberculin reaction) in the meningeal focus. This results in development of fever, signs of meningeal irritation, and CSF pleocytosis.

Since the introduction of effective antituberculous drugs, calcification of intracranial tuberculous lesions (located in the basal meninges and in the brain itself) has been observed more frequently. In occasional patients the late onset (several years after recovery from tuberculous meningitis) of dysfunction of the hypothalamic-pituitary axis (diabetes insipidus, hypopituitarism, precocious puberty) has become evident, apparently related to chronic scarring or necrosis secondary to the meningeal inflammation.

Poliomyelitis

Poliomyelitis virus, acquired by a non-immune person from a patient with active disease or from a healthy carrier, enters the body by the oral route. It multiplies in the oropharynx for a short period, then disappears from this site. At the same time that the virus becomes established in the upper respiratory tract, it also is implanted in the intestine. There it continues to replicate throughout the incubation period and active stage of the disease, and for some time during and after convalescence. From the intestine, the infectious agent invades the regional lymphatic channels; from there, it reaches the bloodstream. The virus enters the central nervous system at many points by direct passage from capillaries to the motor neurons.

A number of physiologic processes play important roles in determining susceptibility and response to infection by poliomyelitis virus. The mechanism by which these processes operate is obscure in most instances. (1) Age is an important determinant of severity of the disease. Young children with spinal involvement usually have paralysis of one extremity, most commonly a leg. In contrast, a quadriplegia is the most frequent consequence of involvement of the spinal cord in adults. Paralysis of the bladder is about 10 times more common in older individuals than in youngsters. (2) Pregnancy increases the risk of developing poliomyelitis. Women who come in contact with the virus at about the time of ovulation are more prone to infection than if they are exposed at other times in the menstrual cycle. (3) Muscles that have been subjected to trauma or intense exercise may be particularly vulnerable. Muscles that are sites of injection of vaccines, particularly those containing *B. pertussis*, are prone to becoming paralyzed, if immunization is carried out during a period of endemicity of poliomyelitis. (4) Patients who have undergone tonsilloadenoidectomy are much more susceptible to the development of the bulbar form of the disease than those not subjected to this procedure, regardless of when the operation had been performed.

The clinical pictures that characterize poliomyelitis are primarily the direct result of pathophysiologic phenomena involving areas of the nervous system invaded and injured by the virus. The sore throat, often present as a prodromal manifestation of the disease, is due to the growth of and accompanying local inflammatory reaction initiated by the virus. The gastrointestinal manifestations (nausea, vomiting, diarrhea) are related to multiplication of the agent in this area and to its effect on the function of the plexuses of Meissner and Auerbach. The anterior horn cells of the spinal cord are the site of predilection for viral invasion; but this occurs in a scattered ("skip") fashion, with variation in the degree and distribution of neuronal involvement. This is manifested by varying degrees of asymmetrical paresis or paralysis of extremities and of weakness of the muscles of respiration. The neurologic findings are characteristic of a lower motor neuron lesion: flaccid weakness, loss of reflexes, and fasciculation of muscles. Sensory modalities are unimpaired. Alterations in blood pressure, irregularity of cardiac rhythm, variation in skin and muscle temperature, and a variety of skin rashes may be related to invasion of autonomic ganglia by the virus.

When neurons in the medulla are involved, two pathophysiologic consequences are observed. Striking irregularity in the rate and depth of breathing (Biot respiration) is the result of involvement of the respiratory center. As the disease progresses, there are longer periods of apnea until breathing ceases completely. Hiccupping, probably related to irritation of the respiratory center, is often present in the early phase of involvement of this area. Hypoxia, without visible cyanosis, is common and may produce transient elevations of blood pressure. Viral injury to the neurons in the vasomotor center in the medulla is manifested by hypertension initially, followed by fluctuations in the level of blood pressure, and

finally by severe hypotension together with the clinical manifestations of shock. Myocarditis is not uncommon in poliomyelitis; it is probably due to direct invasion by the virus. Electrocardiographic abnormalities, mainly T and ST and P-R alterations, are present in from 10 to 20 per cent of cases. Irregularities in cardiac rhythm, including sinus tachycardia or bradycardia, atrial fibrillation, premature ventricular contractions, and ventricular fibrillation, may supervene. Hyperpyrexia, with temperatures of 106° or higher, often develops in the late stages of the type of disease in which the medulla is involved.

The brain may be affected, to a varying degree, by poliomyelitis. Encephalitic manifestations occur as isolated syndromes, or together with bulbar or spinal disease. The diffuse form of encephalitis is featured by confusion, agitation, anxiety, or somnolence. Quivering and jerking of the facial muscles and extremities, flushing of the face, tremor of the hands, and restless movements occur. In focal polioencephalitis, there may be clinical evidence of dysfunction, or the lesions may be silent and demonstrable only at necropsy. Visual-verbal agnosia, myoclonic jerks, grand mal seizures which occasionally persist long after recovery, spastic hemiparesis, ataxia of one arm or leg, and hydrocephalus have been described.

Dysfunction of the peripheral vascular tree may accompany severe poliomyelitis in some cases. This is probably related to invasion of the sympathetic ganglia by the virus. A variety of skin eruptions including miliaria, morbilliform rashes and scarlatiniform eruptions may develop in the severely paralyzed patient; these are usually transient but tend to recur. Abnormalities of sweating are quite common. Autonomic disturbances may be reflected in coldness, pallor, and even cyanosis of the paralyzed limbs. These have been attributed to persisting spasm of the peripheral blood vessels. However, it has been suggested that, while peripheral vasoconstriction is probably a very common phenomenon in chronically paralyzed muscles, angiospasm may not be a feature of the early phase of poliomyelitis. The exact mechanism involved in this phase is not clear.

There is considerable evidence that artificial respiration effected in a tank respirator under negative pressure is physiologically the same as that produced by application of positive pressure to the upper airway. Positive airway and negative intratank pressures produce identical changes in intrapulmonary, intrapleural, intracardiac, and systemic arterial and venous pressures. These result in (1) impairment of the circulation and decrease in cardiac output, (2) increase in cerebral venous and spinal fluid pressures, (3) rise in central venous pressure, (4) loss of blood volume, and (5) increased filling of the venous bed and arteriolar constriction. In the individual who has normal hemodynamics at the time of institution of artificial respiration, compensatory mechanisms tend to counteract these deleterious circulatory effects. Positive pressure applied to the airway results in transmission of a large fraction of the increase to the pleural space, great veins, and right atrium. The elevated pressure in the right atrium produces a momentary decrease in the venous gradient. Although venous return and cardiac output are momentarily decreased, they return to normal rapidly because there is a rise in peripheral venous pressure which reconstitutes the venous gradient and re-establishes venous return. The reconstitution of the venous gradient is dependent upon the existing vascular tone, the capacity for reflex vasoconstriction, and the presence of a normal circulating blood volume. The increase in peripheral venous pressure required to establish the venous gradient causes a rise in capillary filtration pressure; this results in a reduction of the circulating blood volume. When the sympathetic pathways are affected in severe poliomyelitis, re-establishment of the venous gradient after the application of positive pressure to the airway is greatly hindered. Because of this, venous return, cardiac output, and blood pressure fall in direct proportion to the degree of pressure applied. When intense generalized vasoconstriction is present in poliomyelitis because of diffuse involvement of the autonomic nervous system, positive pressure breathing produces a decline in arterial pressure, because the mechanisms responsible for re-establishing the venous gradient are already maximally active. Although this discussion has been limited to the pathophysiologic changes in the circulation that develop when respiratory assistance is required during poliomyelitis, it must be pointed out that similar phenomena are present in other situations which require the use of artificial respiration.

Life-threatening pulmonary edema develops in some individuals with poliomyelitis, especially those who are severely ill because of medullary involvement or because of difficulty in respiration as a result of paralysis of the diaphragm and intercostal muscles. Although the exact mechanisms involved in the pathogenesis of this phenomenon are unknown, several factors that may contribute to its development have been suggested. Among these are hypoxia, oxygen toxicity (overuse of 100 per cent oxygen), constriction of the pulmonary vessels, pulmonary infection, circulatory changes produced by artificial respiration, and myocardial dysfunction.

An interesting and clinically important pathophysiologic phenomenon that develops in practically all patients severely paralyzed by poliomyelitis is mobilization of calcium from the bones. This is responsible for the nephrolithiasis that commonly complicates the prolonged course of illness in these cases. The presence of stones is often the factor responsible for infection of the urinary tract which leads, if untreated, to chronic pyelonephritis and subsequent renal failure. The stones that are formed may be so large as to produce sufficient obstruction to require nephrostomy.

Some of the clinical features of poliomyelitis may have as their basis direct viral involvement of extraneural tissues. Thus, some of the cardiovascular abnormalities are unquestionably related to invasion of the myocardium resulting in interstitial lymphocytic infiltration in most instances or in severe necrosis in others. Generalized lymphadenopathy, a common feature of the disease, is probably due to multiplication of the virus in lymph nodes.

Herpes Zoster

Herpes zoster and varicella are produced by the same virus, and the initial event in the natural history of the herpetic syndrome is an episode of chickenpox at any age, but usually in childhood. It has been proposed (but not proved) that recovery from varicella is sometimes accompanied by passage of the virus from the lesions in the skin and mucous membranes into the sensory nerve endings of these tissues. From here, it is thought, the agent is transported up the sensory fibers to the sensory ganglia, where it may become established in the nuclei of the ganglion cells and remain quiescent for varying periods, often for many years. During this latent period, small quantities of virus might possibly enter the circulation from the ganglia but would be quickly and effectively neutralized by specific antibody. Such periodic intrusions of the virus into the circulation, when they occurred, would be expected to stimulate production of neutralizing antibody.

It appears most likely that activation of the latent varicella-zoster agent is responsible for clinical herpes zoster. In most instances, provoking factors are not readily apparent. However, a variety of disorders which lead to generalized immunosuppression (or drugs such as corticosteroids and cytotoxic agents that produce the same effect) seem to predispose to the development of clinical herpes zoster, presumably by activating the latent virus. Among such diseases are the lymphomas, leukemia (usually lymphatic), and multiple myeloma.

It has been postulated (but not proved) that when antibody levels are reduced, the virus, which has remained latent in the nucleus of sensory ganglia, emerges and travels antidromically down the sensory nerve. In its passage from the ganglia along the sensory nerve it may produce a severe neuritis; this is thought to account for the severe pain commonly present in the pre-eruptive stage (before skin lesions are apparent) of herpes zoster. The virus may travel over only a portion of the length of the nerve and may not reach the skin; the only manifestation in this situation is severe root pain without dermal lesions, so-called *herpes zoster sine eruptione* or *zoster sine herpete*.

If, as is the case in most patients, the virus reaches the dermal sensory nerve endings, the typical vesicular eruption develops; the lesions are always in the most precise anatomic relation to the neurons of the sensory ganglia that have been involved or destroyed. Virus is shed from the vesicles and may lead to the development of characteristic varicella if acquired by non-immune individuals.

Although the spinal ganglia are most frequently involved, others may be the site for presumed long-term residence of the virus. Activation of the virus may produce a variety of syndromes characterized by neurologic dysfunction related to the area affected. The fifth cranial nerve is the apparent pathway for transport of the virus from its ganglion (gasserian). When virus in this location is activated, any one of the three main branches of the fifth nerve may be involved; pain and skin lesions are distributed along the course of the mandibular, maxillary, or ophthalmic divisions. Involvement of the latter (herpes zoster ophthalmicus) produces lesions of the cornea; the earliest sign is loss of the corneal reflex. Enlargement of the ipsilateral preauricular lymph nodes and conjunctivitis (Parinaud's syndrome) are common. When the nasociliary branch of the ophthalmic division is affected, the skin lesions usually appear at the end of the nose; other manifestations of this syndrome include conjunctivitis, keratitis, retinopathy, and retrobulbar neuritis which may lead to blindness. The necrotizing retinopathy is presumed to be the result of migration of virus along the ophthalmic branch of the fifth cranial nerve, along the nasociliary branch, and ultimately to the long ciliary nerve extending to the retina. Typical intranuclear inclusions have been identified in the involved sensory retina. The geniculate ganglion may be involved (Ramsay Hunt syndrome). In this situation, the skin lesions are present on the pinna, tympanic membrane, or external ear canal. The accompanying neurologic abnormalities are facial palsy alone or together with diminished hearing and tinnitus. If the chorda tympani is involved, there is loss of the sensation of taste over the anterior two thirds of the tongue.

In rare instances, paralysis of the muscles of the arms, legs, abdomen, and diaphragm has been described. This suggests involvement by the virus of anterior horn cells, but proof is lacking as yet. An unusual syndrome of ophthalmic herpes zoster followed in a few weeks by an acute contralateral hemiparesis or aphasia has occurred in rare patients. An unusual segmental granulomatous arteritis (possibly due to varicella-zoster virus) confined to the central nervous system is believed to be responsible for the contralateral neurologic findings. Bladder hypertonia results from mild inflammation in dorsal root ganglia; urinary retention may develop with more extensive involvement of parasympathetic fibers innervating the bladder (second, third, and fourth

sacral segments) as well as meninges and possibly anterior-horn cells. Vesicles and hemorrhagic cystitis may be observed on the bladder mucosal surface. Transient ileus may rarely occur in herpes zoster. On occasion, the lesions of herpes zoster may be diffusely distributed in the skin in a centripetal fashion similar to that of initial episodes of varicella. "Cropping," that is, the continuing appearance of new lesions of varying structure in the same area of skin, as is the case in varicella, does not occur in the disseminated form of herpes zoster. These lesions are practically always painless. This is probably so because only latent virus in the skin (not that in the ganglia) is activated. The appearance of this form of the infection, especially in patients with Hodgkin's disease, is an ominous prognostic sign.

Osteomyelitis

Osteomyelitis may take the form of either an acute or a chronic infection. However, there is no abrupt shift from acute to chronic disease but rather a gradual blending of one into the other. On the basis of the pathogenesis of the lesion, cases of osteomyelitis fall into one or another of three categories: (1) hematogenous osteomyelitis; (2) osteomyelitis secondary to a contiguous focus of infection (including postoperative wound infections, osteomyelitis in which bacteria have been introduced following a puncture wound, and bone involvement from an adjoining soft tissue focus of infection); and (3) osteomyelitis associated with peripheral vascular disease.

Hematogenous Osteomyelitis. Acute hematogenous osteomyelitis most frequently involves rapidly growing bone, as evidenced by the fact that over 85 per cent of cases occur in children. There is often a history of antecedent trauma to the area subsequently involved in the septic process. The disease characteristically affects the metaphysis of long bones. The anatomic features of the microvasculature adjacent to the metaphyseal side of the growth plate provide the most satisfactory explanation for the localization of blood-borne bacteria and initiation of infection. The capillary ramifications of the nutrient arteries supplying bone loop sharply just below the epiphyseal growth plates and then enter large sinusoidal veins, where the flow of blood is sluggish (Fig. 21–4). These sinusoidal vessels connect with the venous channels of the medullary cavity. In the experimental animal (and probably also in man) the inability of the metaphysis to handle infection is related to several factors: (1) The afferent loop of the metaphyseal capillary lacks phagocytic lining cells, and the phagocytic cells present in the efferent loop (a sinusoidal structure) are functionally inactive; (2) flow in the descending loops of the metaphyseal capillaries is slower and more turbulent because the descending loops are often multiple and have a diameter two to seven times as great as that of the ascend-

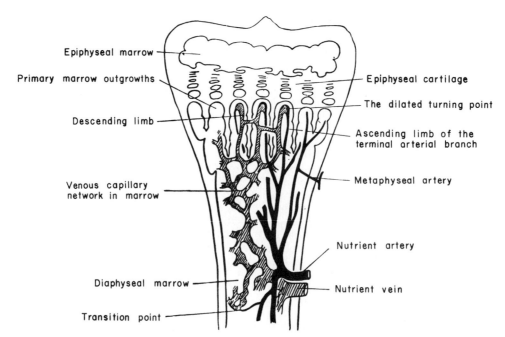

Figure 21–4 Schematic representation of the blood supply of a long bone in the region of the metaphyseal growth plate (epiphyseal cartilage). (From Waldvogel, F. A., Medoff, G., and Swartz, M. N., Osteomyelitis: A Review of Clinical Features, Therapeutic Considerations and Unusual Aspects, 1971. Courtesy of Charles C Thomas, Publisher, Springfield, Illinois.)

ing loops; (3) the capillary loops adjacent to the epiphyseal growth plates are non-anastomosing branches of the nutrient artery, and obstruction (by bacterial growth or microthrombi) would be expected to result in small areas of avascular necrosis, a mechanism conducive to progressive infection.

Once infection has started, the local decrease in pH, the edema, and the accumulation of leukocytes (and possibly their collagenase) all contribute to tissue necrosis and breakdown of bone trabeculae. The infection extends to the neighboring bone through the haversian and Volkmann canals, occludes vascular channels, and causes the death of more osteocytes in the process. Larger segments of bone, deprived of blood supply by this process of vascular compromise, may become separated and form sequestra. These act as foreign bodies, converting the infection into a chronic one and rendering eradication by antibiotic therapy impossible until the devitalized bone is removed. Osteoblastic apposition can take place on smaller pieces of already dead bone, further compounding the problem by burying the infection behind a rampart within which bacteria can multiply uninhibited by circulating bactericidal factors and phagocytic cells. The suppurative process may also produce a septic thrombophlebitis of the diaphyseal vessels, impairing venous return and increasing the high pressure created within bone. Upon reaching the outer part of the cortex the infection causes an inversion of the slow periosteal blood flow and enters the subperiosteal space. This then may progress to formation of a

subperiosteal abscess which is associated with considerable local pain, tenderness, and swelling because of accumulation of pus under pressure. The local presence of heat, pain, and erythema may be so prominent that a subcutaneous abscess is erroneously suspected. Incision and drainage may be carried out in the mistaken belief that the process is a soft tissue infection, when, in fact, the process merely represents extension from a focus of acute osteomyelitis. Subperiosteal infection may induce exuberant circumferential growth of the periosteum (involucrum). Progressive chronic destruction of the cortex is followed by spontaneous pathologic fracture in some instances.

MANIFESTATIONS IN DIFFERENT AGE GROUPS. The clinical course of hematogenous osteomyelitis may vary somewhat, depending on the age of the patient. These differences are related to certain anatomic features and their changes during growth. In the infant below the age of one, infection begins in the metaphyseal sinusoidal veins. However, at this age some patent capillaries still perforate the epiphyseal growth plate, and infection can spread rapidly via this route to the epiphysis. This results in septic arthritis, thrombosis of nutrient vessels, and possible destruction of the epiphyseal growth anlage. Such destruction may result in loss of hip joint function and eventual shortening of the involved leg. *Between the age of one and puberty,* the initial metaphyseal infection is contained by the epiphyseal growth plate and spreads laterally through the paths of least resistance. It commonly perforates the cortex, lifting off the periosteum which is loosely adherent, and produces a subperiosteal collection of pus. The epiphysis in this age group is protected from the spread of infection by the epiphyseal plate, and normal growth is usually not impaired. *In the adult,* because resorption of the growth cartilage has occurred, anastomoses between metaphyseal and epiphyseal blood vessels are reestablished and make spread of the infection to the subarticular space a distinct possibility. Subperiosteal abscess formation and extensive periosteal proliferation are unusual in this age group, since the periosteum is firmly attached to the underlying bone.

About one third of patients with acute hematogenous osteomyelitis have demonstrable bacteremia and exhibit a toxic, febrile course. *Staphylococcus aureus* is the most common etiologic agent but other pyogenic gram-positive cocci (pneumococcus, Group A streptococcus) are occasionally implicated. Salmonella infections are a relatively common complication of sickle cell anemia. If salmonella bacteremia occurs in patients with this disease, it is almost always associated with subsequent localization in bone. It has been suggested that the small "bone infarcts" that occur in sickle cell anemia secondary to occlusion of small blood vessels by the deformed red cells are favorable sites for the initiation of infection.

FEATURES DUE TO SPECIFIC SITES OF INVOLVEMENT. Vertebral body involvement in hematogenous osteomyelitis has been seen with increasing frequency in recent years, usually in adults, and often complicating pelvic surgery and urinary tract infections. Infection of the vertebral body spreads readily to adjacent ligaments and adjoining vertebral bodies by anastomosing venous channels. Thus, this type of osteomyelitis frequently involves two adjacent vertebral bodies and the intervening intervertebral disk. Special problems may arise with this type of osteomyelitis because of proximity to the spinal cord. Infection may extend through the thin vertebral periosteum, and pus may accumulate between the periosteum and the dura mater (spinal epidural abscess). Further extension of infection through the dura, either directly or through venous channels, into the subarachnoid space may lead to acute bacterial meningitis. The initial site of bone infection may, not infrequently, fail to produce prominent manifestations. In this situation, the illness is heralded by the sudden onset of the complicating spinal epidural abscess (compressing the spinal cord) or bacterial meningitis. Compression of the cord with concomitant paraplegia may result from the epidural extension of the infectious process itself, from secondary vascular impairment with infarction of the cord, or from

compression fractures of the involved vertebrae.

The particular anatomic features of the hip and shoulder joints account for the common occurrence of septic arthritis secondary to osteomyelitis of the femur and humerus in children. Although the epiphyseal plate serves as an effective barrier to the direct extension of infection from the metaphysis to epiphysis (and thence to the joint space) in this age group, an alternative route is available. The synovial capsules in these joints reach beyond the epiphyseal growth plate; thus, infection can rupture through the cortex and spread directly from the metaphyseal focus into the joint.

Osteomyelitis Secondary to a Contiguous Focus of Infection. This type of disease is at present most common after surgical procedures such as open reduction of fractures, craniotomy, and reconstruction of joints severely affected by degenerative arthritis. However, it may follow burns, infection of the ears or paranasal sinuses, animal bites, and infection of soft tissue produced by trauma. Because the route of infection is different than in hematogenous osteomyelitis, metaphyseal localization of the process is much less frequent. In contrast to hematogenous osteomyelitis, which is predominantly a disease of the young, most patients with this form of bone disease are over 50 years old. These infections tend to be chronic, recurrent, and difficult, if not impossible, to eradicate until all foreign bodies (plates, screws, and other orthopedic appliances) have been removed. The most frequent clinical manifestations are local pain and drainage from a sinus tract. *S. aureus* is the organism most commonly involved. However, less invasive bacteria can produce this syndrome when infection of an orthopedic prosthesis takes place. The usual manifestations of acute infection are often absent in this setting. There may be only minimal local erythema and only low-grade fever. Pain and limitation of motion secondary to spasm of muscle due to inflammation in and around bone may be important features.

Osteomyelitis Associated With Vascular Insufficiency. The pathogenesis of the process in this situation involves extension of infection to bone secondary to ischemic ulceration of the skin. The toes or the small bones of the feet are almost invariably involved. This is a problem almost always in patients with long-standing diabetes mellitus, occasionally in individuals with severe atherosclerosis, and rarely in persons with vasculitis secondary to a connective tissue disorder. Local symptoms (pain, swelling, erythema) dominate the clinical picture. There are few systemic manifestations of infection.

REFERENCES

INFECTIVE ENDOCARDITIS

Alpert, J. S., Krous, H. F., Dalen, J. E., O'Rourke, R. A., and Bloor, C. M.: Pathogenesis of Osler's nodes. Ann. Intern. Med., 85:471, 1976.

Angrist, A. A.: Pathogenesis of bacterial endocarditis. J.A.M.A., 183:249, 1963.

Arnett, E. N., and Roberts, W. C.: Valve ring abscess in active infective endocarditis. Circulation, 54:140, 1976.

Bayer, A. S., Theofilopoulos, A. N., Eisenberg, R., Dixon, F. J., and Guze, L. B.: Circulating immune complexes in infective endocarditis. N. Engl. J. Med., *295*:1500, 1976.

Durack, D. T., and Beeson, P. B.: Experimental bacterial endocarditis. I. Colonization of a sterile vegetation. Br. J. Exp. Path., *53*:44, 1972.

Gould, K., Ramirez-Ronda, C. H., Holmes, R. K., and Sanford, J. P.: Adherence of bacteria to heart valves *in vitro.* J. Clin Invest., *56*:1364, 1975.

Hutter, A. M., and Moellering, R. C.: Assessment of the patient with suspected endocarditis. J.A.M.A., *235*:1603, 1976.

Kaye, D. (Ed.): Infective Endocarditis. University Park Press, Baltimore, 1976.

Lerner, P. I., and Weinstein, L.: Infective endocarditis in the antibiotic era. N. Engl. J. Med., *276*:199, 323, 388, 1966.

Pruitt, A. A., Rubin, R. H., Karchmer, A. W., and Duncan, G. W.: Neurologic complications of bacterial endocarditis. Medicine, *57*:453, 1978.

Rodbard, S.: Blood velocity and endocarditis. Circulation, *27*:18, 1963.

Weinstein, L., and Schlesinger, J. J.: Pathoanatomic, pathophysiologic and clinical correlations in endocarditis. N. Engl. J. Med., *291*:832 and 1122, 1974.

Ziment, I.: Nervous system complications in bacterial endocarditis. Am. J. Med., *47*:593, 1969.

SALMONELLA INFECTIONS

Bennett, I. L., Jr., and Hook, E. W.: Infectious diseases (some aspects of salmonellosis). Ann. Rev. Med., *10*:1, 1959.

Black, P. H., Kunz, L. J., and Swartz, M. N.: Salmonellosis — a review of some unusual aspects. N. Engl. J. Med., *262*:811, 864, 921; 1960.

Giannella, R. A., Gots, R. E., Charney, A. N., Greenough, W. B., III, Formal, S. B.: Pathogenesis of salmonella-mediated intestinal fluid secretion: activation of adenylate cyclase and inhibition by indomethacin. Gastroenterology, *69*:1238, 1975.

Gill, F., Kaye, D., and Hook, W.: The influence of erythrophagocytosis on the interaction of macrophages and salmonella *in vitro.* J. Exp. Med., *124*:173, 1966.

Greisman, S., Hornick, R. B., Carozza, F. A., Jr., and Woodward, T. E.: The role of endotoxin during typhoid fever and tularemia in man. I. Acquisition of tolerance to endotoxin. J. Clin. Invest., *42*:1064, 1963.

Hook, E. W.: Salmonellosis: Certain factors influencing the interaction of salmonella and the host. Bull. N. Y. Acad. Med., *37*:499, 1961.

Kaye, D., and Hook, E. W.: The influence of hemolysis on susceptibility to salmonella infections: Additional observations. J. Immunol., *91*:518, 1963.

Rubin, R. H., and Weinstein, L.: Salmonellosis — Microbiologic, Pathologic, and Clinical Features. Stratton Intercontinental Medical Book Corporation, New York, 1977.

SYPHILIS

Clark, E. G., and Danbolt, N.: The Oslo study of the natural history of untreated syphilis. J. Chronic Dis., *2*:311, 1955.

Merritt, H. H., Adams, R. D., and Solomon, H.: Neurosyphilis. Oxford University Press, New York, 1946.

Sparling, P. F.: Diagnosis and treatment of syphilis. N. Engl. J. Med., *284*:642, 1971.

Turner, T. B.: Syphilis and the treponematoses. *In:* Mudd, S. (Ed.): Infectious Agents and Host Reactions. W. B. Saunders Co., Philadelphia, 1970.

Yobs, A., Clark, J. W., Jr., Mothershed, S. E., Bullard, J. C., and Artley, C. W.: Further observations on the persistence of *Treponema pallidum* after treatment in rabbits and humans. Br. J. Vener. Dis., *44*:116, 1968.

PNEUMONIA

Benson, H., Akbarian, M., Adler, L. A., and Abelmann, W. H.: Hemodynamic effects of pneumonia. I. Normal and hypodynamic responses. J. Clin. Invest., *49*:791, 1970.

Bocles, J. S., Ehrenkranz, N. J., and Marks, A.: Abnormalities of respiratory function in varicella pneumonia. Ann. Intern. Med., *60*:183, 1964.

Davidson, F. F., Glazier, J. B., and Murray, J. F.: The components of the alveolar-arterial oxygen tension difference in normal subjects and in patients with pneumonia and obstructive lung disease. Am. J. Med., *52*:754, 1972.

Herzog, H., Staub, H., and Richterich, R.: Gas-analytical studies in severe pneumonia. Observations during the 1957 influenza epidemic, Lancet, *1*:593, 1959.

Marshall, R., and Christie, R. V.: The visco-elastic properties of the lungs in acute pneumonia. Clin. Sci., *13*:403, 1954.

Mellemgaard, K.: The mechanism of hypoxemia in lobar pneumonia. Scand. J. Resp. Dis., *48*:109, 1967.

Triebwasser, J. H., Harris, R. E., Bryant, R. E., and Rhoades, E. R.: Varicella Pneumonia in Adults. Report of seven cases and review of the literature. Medicine, *46*:409, 1967.

Wood, W. B., Jr.: Studies on the cellular immunology of acute bacterial infections. The Harvey Lectures, *Series XLVII*:72, 1951–52.

INFECTIONS OF THE CENTRAL NERVOUS SYSTEM

Bodian, D.: Histopathologic basis of clinical findings in poliomyelitis. Am. J. Med., *6*:563, 1949.

Controni, G., Rodriguez, W. J., Hicks, J. M., Ficke, M., Ross, S., Friedman, G., and Khan, W.: Cerebrospinal fluid lactic acid levels in meningitis. J. Pediatr., *91*:379, 1977.

Denny-Brown, D., Adams, R. D., and Fitzgerald, P. J.: Pathologic features of *Herpes zoster.* Arch. Neurol. Psychiat., *51*:216, 1944.

Dodge, P. R., and Swartz, M. N.: Bacterial meningitis. II. Special neurological problems, post meningitic complications and clinicopathological correlations. N. Engl. J. Med., *272*:954, 1003; 1965.

Feigin, R. D., and Dodge, P. R.: Bacterial meningitis: newer concepts of pathophysiology and neurologic sequelae. Ped. Clin. North Am., *23*:541, 1976.

Fishman, R. A.: Carrier transport of glucose between blood and cerebrospinal fluid. Am. J. Physiol., *206*:836, 1964.

Greenwood, B. M., Whittle, H. C., and Brynceson, A. D. M.: Allergic complications of meningococcal disease. II. Immunological investigations. Br. Med. J., *2*:737, 1973.

Harter, D. H., and Petersdorf, R. G.: A consideration of the pathogenesis of bacterial meningitis: Review of experimental and clinical studies. Yale J. Biol. Med., *32*:280, 1960.

Hope-Simpson, R. E.: The nature of *Herpes zoster.* A long-term study and a new hypothesis. Proc. Roy. Soc. Med., *58*:9, 1965.

Horstmann, D. M., McCollum, R. W., and Mascola, A. D.: Viremia in human poliomyelitis. J. Exp. Med., *99*:355, 1954.

Lincoln, E. M., and Sewell, E. M.: Tuberculosis of the meninges and central nervous system. *In:* Tuberculosis in Children. McGraw-Hill Book Co., New York, 1963.

Miller, L. H., and Brunnel, P. A.: Zoster, reinfection or activation of latent virus? Observations on the antibody response. Am. J. Med., *49*:480, 1970.

Petersdorf, R., and Harter, D.: The fall in cerebrospinal fluid sugar in meningitis. Arch. Neurol., *4*:21, 1961.

Swartz, M. N., and Dodge, P. R.: Bacterial meningitis — a review of selected aspects. I. General clinical features, special problems, and unusual meningeal reactions mimicking bacterial meningitis. N. Engl. J. Med., *272*:725, 779, 842, 898; 1965.

Weinstein, L.: Cardiovascular disturbances in poliomyelitis. Circulation, *15*:735, 1957.

Weinstein, L.: Influence of age and sex on susceptibility and clinical manifestations in poliomyelitis. N. Engl. J. Med., *257*:47, 1957.

Weller, T. H., Witton, H. M., and Bell, E. J.: The etiologic agents of varicella and *Herpes zoster.* Isolation, propagation, and cultural characteristics *in vitro.* J. Exp. Med., *108*:843, 1958.

OSTEOMYELITIS

Collins, D. H.: *In* Dodge, O. G. (Ed.): Pathology of Bone. Butterworth, London, 1966.

Diggs, L. W.: Bone and joint lesions in sickle cell disease. Clin. Orthop., *52*:119, 1967.

Trueta, J.: The three types of acute hematogenous osteomyelitis: a clinical and vascular study. J. Bone Joint Surg., *41B*:671, 1959.

Waldvogel, F. A., Medoff, G., and Swartz, M. N.: Osteomyelitis — clinical features, therapeutic considerations, and unusual aspects. N. Engl. J. Med., *282*:198, 260, 316; 1970.

22

Pathophysiology of Hematologic Disorders

ALLAN J. ERSLEV AND THOMAS G. GABUZDA

BONE MARROW

With the exception of lymphocytes, blood cell formation in the normal adult is the exclusive prerogative of bone marrow. Even lymphocytes, however, both T and B cells, are bone marrow derived, and multipotential stem cells in the bone marrow cavities are probably directly or indirectly responsible for all blood cell formation. Other areas can support hematopoiesis, but the bones appear to provide an optimal environment for differentiation and multiplication of blood cells. Before bone cavities form during the fifth fetal month, blood cell formation takes place first in the yolk sac and then in the liver and spleen (Fig. 22–1). During the brief yolk-sac phase the erythrocytes produced are nucleated and contain an embryonic hemoglobin but the subsequent crops of fetal erythrocytes produced by the liver, spleen, and bone marrow are non-nucleated and contain fetal hemoglobin with $\alpha_2\gamma_2$ polypeptide chains. Although the spleen in the human fetus plays only a brief role in hematopoiesis between the third and the seventh months, the splenic microcirculation appears to be well suited for blood cell formation, and the spleen serves as the principal back-up organ for the bone marrow. At time of birth the splenic and hepatic phases have ceased, the slow transformation from fetal to adult hemoglobin production is under way, and all bone cavities are actively involved in blood cell formation.

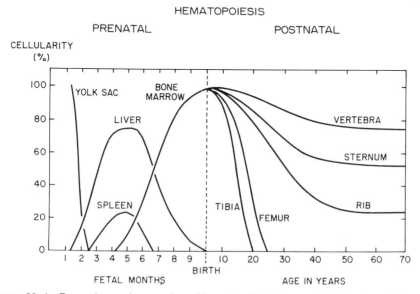

Figure 22–1 Expansion and regression of hematopoietic tissue during fetal and adult life.

For the first few years of life there is a precarious balance between the need for blood cells of a rapidly growing infant and the available bone marrow space, and reactivation of hepatic and splenic hematopoiesis takes place whenever there is an increased demand for blood cell formation. At about the age of 4 the growth of bone cavities has outstripped the growth of the circulating blood cell mass, and fatty reserve bone marrow becomes noticeable. Fatty replacement occurs first in the diaphysis of the peripheral long bones, then slowly creeps centripetally until at the age of about 18 hematopoietically active bone marrow is found only in the vertebrae, ribs, sternum, skull, and proximal epiphyses of the long bones. This obviously must mean that the available bone marrow space has continued to grow faster than the circulating blood cell mass, since the ratio between progenitor cells in the marrow and mature cells in the circulation is the same at all ages. In support of this assumption are measurements by Hudson which indicate that the volume of bone marrow cavities increases from about 1.5 per cent of body weight at birth to about 4.5 per cent of body weight in the adult, while the blood volume actually decreases from about 8 per cent of body weight at birth to about 7 per cent of body weight in the adult. During adult life the expansion of bone cavities continues, owing to bone resorption, and there is a gradual increase in the amount of fatty tissue present in all bone marrow areas. Because of the abundant bone marrow space, compensatory reactivation of extramedullary sites rarely takes place in later life, even during periods of accelerated hematopoietic activity. When present, extramedullary hematopoiesis often indicates inappropriate rather than compensatory blood formation.

Measurements of blood flow and hematopoietic activity have shown a close relationship between cellular production and blood supply, and some interesting experiments by Huggins suggest that this relationship goes in both directions and that induced vascularization is followed by increased hematopoietic activity. Huggins and co-workers implanted the tip of a rat's tail into the abdominal cavity or enclosed it in a heating chamber and found after some weeks that the inactive fatty marrow had become red and hematopoietically active. The conclusion from these experiments was initially that the low peripheral temperature in the long bones impairs blood cell formation and is responsible for the centripetal regression of active marrow in the adult. However, fatty marrow appears in the fingers even before birth and active marrow is found in peripheral epiphyses when more proximal diaphyses are completely inactive. It seems more likely that temperature is merely one of many variables which control vascularization and that it is the vascular density of the bone marrow which determines hematopoietic activity. Recent studies by Crosby suggest that this vascular density is inherently

lower in the peripheral areas of the body rendering them particularly vulnerable to decreased temperature.

Structurally, the bone marrow is highly organized with a spokelike pattern of venous sinuses and cords of hematopoietic tissue (Fig. 22–2). The cords are percolated by arterial blood draining into the central venous sinuses through a fenestrated basement membrane (Fig. 22–3) partly covered on the inside by endothelial cells and on the outside by reticular cells. Projections from the reticular cells subdivide the cords and provide support for hematopoietic cells (Fig. 22–4). They also control available hematopoietic space by gaining or losing lipid globules. Within the cords, the megakaryocytes lie close to the outside of the sinus wall and appear to reel off strings of cytoplasmic platelets directly into the sinus. The erythroblasts also lie close to the venous sinuses in distinctive clusters or islands. Each island consists of a central macrophage, or nurse cell, with maturing and dividing erythroblasts nestled in cytoplasmic pockets (Fig. 22–5). When mature enough for independent existence, the erythroblasts squeeze through the sinus apertures usually losing their pyknotic and non-deformable nuclei (Fig. 22–6). The maturing and dividing granulocytic precursors are situated deep in the hematopoietic cords and do not move toward the sinus wall until they reach a motile metamyelocytic stage.

The nervous supply to the bone marrow is quite extensive, as everyone having experienced a bone marrow aspiration can attest. Some of the nerves are in close contact with the hematopoietic islands and may sense pressure changes caused by cellular proliferation. If such signals are transmitted to the nerves attached to the vessel walls, an autoregulatory system may well exist, adjusting the flood flow to permit undisturbed proliferation and maturation before the cells are released into the circulation.

The fatty tissue which in the adult fills about 50 per cent of the bone cavities probably serves merely as a space-occupying material. Attempts have been made to assign primary regulatory functions to it, but the evidence presented so far has been unimpressive.

As described in the section on the spleen, the bone marrow is one of the major lymphomacrophage organs and is involved in antigen processing, cellular and humoral immunity, and the recognition and removal of senescent cells. Its main mission is, however, the production of differentiated blood cells (Fig. 22–7). These cells are derived from pools of self-perpetuating stem cells — a multi- or pluripotential pool capable of differentiation in several directions and unipotential pools committed to erythropoiesis, granulopoiesis, or thrombopoiesis (Boggs and Chervenick, 1970). The multipotential stem cells are believed to provide a dormant bone marrow reserve. They are not destroyed by tritiated thymi-

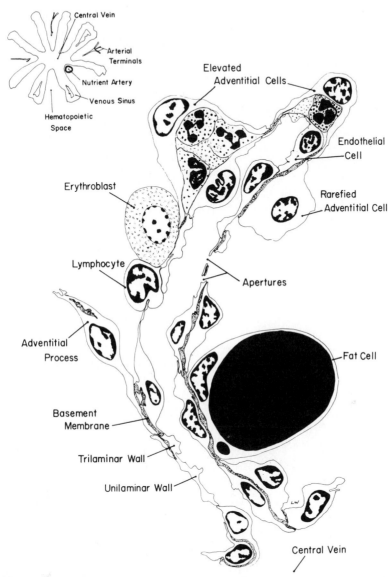

Figure 22–2 Sketch in upper left depicts cross section of bone marrow with spokelike sinusoids draining into a central longitudinal vein. Larger sketch depicts sinusoidal basement membrane covered on the outside by adventitial reticular cells guarding the fenestrations in the basement membrane and providing structural support for hematopoietic cells. (From Weiss, L.: *In* Gordon, A. S. (Ed.): Regulation of Hematopoiesis. Vol. 1. New York, Appleton-Century-Crofts, 1970.)

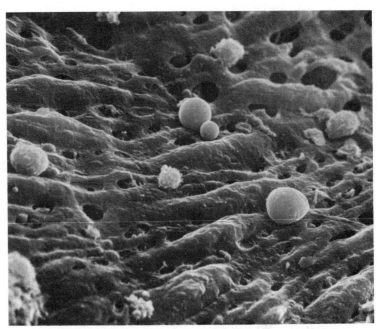

Figure 22–3 Fenestrated basement membrane of venous sinus in rat bone marrow (Courtesy of LeBlond, P.-F., Nouv. Rev. Franc. d'Hemat., *13*:771, 1973).

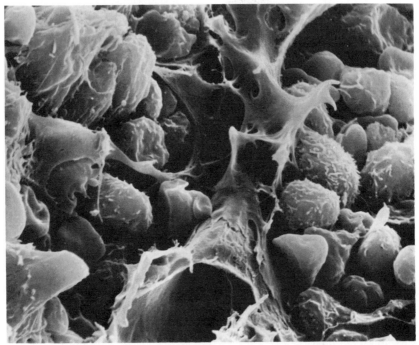

Figure 22–4 A venous sinus crossing the field with luminal endothelium exposed to the right but otherwise covered by adventitial reticular cells. The cytoplasm of these cells extends far into the hematopoietic compartment and provides structure and support for hematopoietic cells. (Courtesy of Weiss L.: Anat. Rev., *186*:161, 1976.)

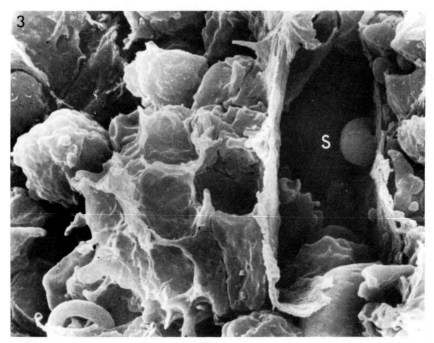

Figure 22-5 An erythropoietic island lying on the wall of a sinusoid (s) in rat bone marrow. The erythroblasts, nestled in the pockets of the island, were removed during the preparation of this scanning electron microscopic picture. (Courtesy of Weiss, L. Anat. Rev., *186*:161, 1976.)

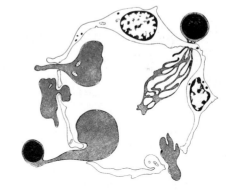

Figure 22-6 Nucleated and non-nucleated red blood cells squeezing through basement pores into a venous sinusoid. The nucleus is incapable of the necessary deformation and is snared off. (Courtesy of Bessis M. Life Cycle of the Erythrocyte. Sandoz Pharm., 1966.)

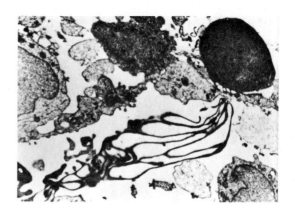

HEMATOPOIESIS

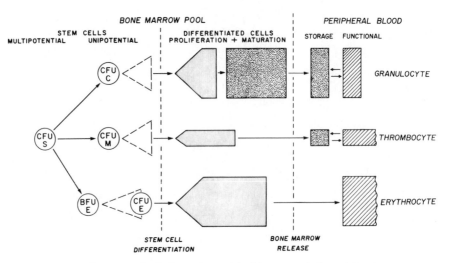

Figure 22-7   A dynamic model of hematopoietic activity.

dine when given in doses which will cause radiation-induced "suicide" of all cells using thymidine in the synthesis of DNA, unless they first have become activated by bone marrow depletion or injury. Such activation into a regenerative and differentiating cell cycle was first described by Till and McCulloch in their classic observations of the spleens of irradiated mice in which surviving or transplanted marrow attempts to replenish the hematopoietic tissues. Initially, the few available stem cells enter into intense proliferative activity and produce minute clonal colonies of undifferentiated stem cells. After the fifth day, specific differentiation takes place and discrete bone marrow colonies can be observed macroscopically on the surface of the spleen and microscopically in the parenchyma of the spleen and the bone marrow (Fig. 22-8). Since chromosomal studies have shown conclusively that each colony is derived from a single stem cell, it is possible to quantitate the number of multipotential stem cells [CFU — S (colony forming units — spleen)] present initially. In the mouse, it has been estimated that there are about 1 to 3 multipotential stem cells per 1000 nucleated bone marrow cells, or about 1 per 100 nucleated red blood cells.

In the human, CFU — S have been isolated by Barr and Wang-Peng in the lymphocyte fraction when peripheral blood cells were separated by velocity sedimentation. In this fraction they could be separated from B and T lymphocytes by their failure to form rosettes with sheep red cells, but otherwise they were found to be morphologically identical with small lymphocytes.

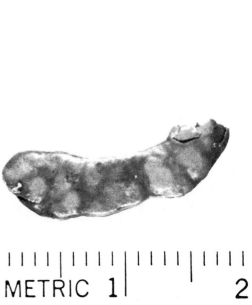

Figure 22-8   Each white raised plaque on the surface of the lower mouse spleen contains a colony of bone marrow cells. These colonies were found 7 days after total body radiation immediately followed by a transfusion of bone marrow cells obtained from an isogeneic donor. Each colony is derived from a single sequestered multipotential stem cell. The upper spleen is a normal control.

Studies on the distribution and composition of bone marrow colonies in the spleen have provided valuable information about the interrelationship between parenchymal structure and cellular differentiation. Each colony is made up of a mixture of hematopoietic cellular elements, usually with one cell type dominating. Although the specific differentiation probably is determined by humoral stimuli, it has been demonstrated by Trentin that the immediate cellular environment or HIM (hematopoietic inductive microenvironment) modifies the effectiveness of the stimuli. Colonies derived from stem cells lodged on the surface of the spleen are primarily erythroid, while colonies from cells lodged in the center of the spleen or in the bone marrow are primarily granulocytic and megakaryocytic. This effect of the microenvironment on cellular differentiation is undoubtedly of major importance for normal hematopoiesis but it is not known whether it is caused by a modification of the activities of stem cells or of differentiated cells.

The unipotential stem cells have been shown, by the use of "suicide" techniques, to be in active cell cycle and capable of self-renewal for a considerable period of time. However, they need the stimulus of a humoral "poietin" in order to undergo blast transformation and further differentiation. Erythropoietin is known to be the specific "poietin" for stem cells committed to erythropoiesis but there is also mounting evidence for the existence of a leukopoietin and a thrombopoietin responsible for the differentiation of stem cells committed to granulocytopoiesis and thrombopoiesis.

In the presence of even small amounts of erythropoietin, bone marrow suspensions plated on fibrin clots or on methyl cellulose plates will form tiny erythroid colonies consisting of from 8 to 64 hemoglobin-containing erythroblasts (Fig.

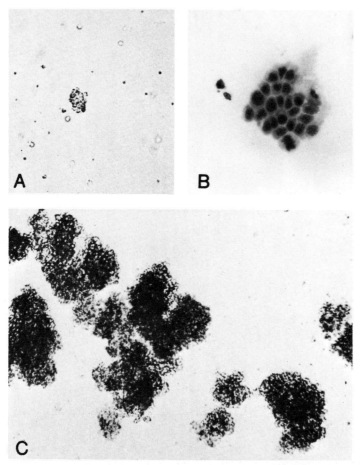

Figure 22–9   The appearance of a single CFU-E (*A*) and a single BFU-E (*C*) grown on a methyl cellulose medium (× 120) (courtesy of Gregory C. J. and Eaves A. C.: Blood, *49*:855, 1977) and of a single CFU-E (*B*) × 1,000.

22–9). The responsible cell has been identified by Clarke and Housman as a small mononuclear "lymphocyte." It has been designated as a CFU-E (colony forming unit-erythroid) and it is probably identical with the unipotential, erythropoietin-responsive stem cell. In addition to these early occurring CFU-E, a second kind of colony begins to appear after eight to ten days of culture if the medium contains large amounts of erythropoietin. These colonies grow to macroscopic size and may contain thousands of erythroblasts. Because of their irregular outline with many CFU-E sub-colonies they are called "bursts," and the responsible cell is called a "burst forming unit-erythroid" or BFU-E. BFU-E have been demonstrated both in peripheral blood and bone marrow while CFU-E have been found only in the bone marrow (Fig. 22–10).

Apparently, erythropoietin promotes both stem cell proliferation and blast transformation. Whether this dual effect is accomplished by a single effect of erythropoietin on stem cells or by multiple sequential actions (or multiple erythropoietin species) is not known. A current hypothesis envisions BFU-E as early descendants of CFU-S (Fig. 22–7). They contain a few erythropoietin receptors enabling them to respond to large concentrations of erythropoietin with proliferation and maturation. According to Gregory and Eaves, the progeny will contain an increasing number of erythropoietin receptors until at a certain point of maturation the stem cells acquire the properties of CFU-E and undergo blast transformation to hemoglobin-producing erythroblasts. A problem with this hypothesis is that erythropoietin-responsive stem cells appear to be in

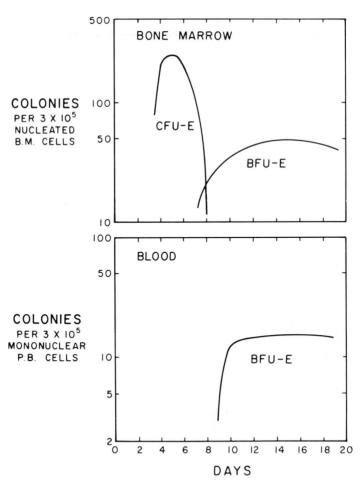

Figure 22–10 The sequential appearance and disappearance of erythroid colonies in bone marrow and peripheral blood suspensions plated on a methyl cellulose medium. (Slightly modified from Ogawa M. et al., Blood, *50*:1081, 1977.)

TABLE 22-1 NORMAL BLOOD CELL KINETICS

Cell Type	Marrow			Blood		
	Number (cells/kg)	Transit time (days)	Production (cells/kg/day)	Number (cells/kg)	Transit time (days)	Production (cells/kg/day)
I. Red cells						
Normoblasts	5.3×10^9	≈ 5.0	3.0×10^9	—	—	—
Reticulocytes	8.2×10^9	2.8	3.0×10^9	3.1×10^9	1.0	2.56×10^9
Erythrocytes	—	—	—	3.07×10^{11}	120.0	2.56×10^0
II. Megakaryocytes	15×10^6	≈ 7	2.0×10^6	—	—	—
Platelets	—	—	—	2.5×10^{10}	9.5	2.5×10^9
III. Granulocytes						
Proliferation pool	2.1×10^9	≈ 5.0	0.85×10^9	—	—	—
Postmitotic pool	5.6×10^9	6.6	0.85×10^9	—	—	—
Circulating	—	—	—	0.4×10^9	0.3	0.85×10^9

(Courtesy of Finch C. A., et al., Blood, *50*:699, 1977.)

active cell cycle even in the absence of erythropoietin. An explanation may be that these stem cells have a certain slow base line rate of proliferation with wastage and death of cells not exposed to erythropoietin. Studies, summarized by Craddock and co-workers, provide some support for this explanation by demonstrating the presence of short-lived "lymphocytes" in the bone marrow.

Bone marrow plated on agar plates has also been shown to grow large granulocytic colonies when exposed to a "colony stimulating factor, CSF." These colonies have been designated CFU — C (C for culture). The CSF originates from monocytes or macrophages and apparently is capable of transforming granulocyte-committed unipotential stem cells to myeloblasts. Although it acts as a leukopoietin in vitro, its physiologic significance, if any, for in vivo granulopoiesis has not been resolved. Megakaryocytic colonies (CFU-M) originating from bone marrow plated on fibrin plates have been described by Nakeff and Daniels-McQueen, but their relationship to physiologic thrombopoiesis is also unknown.

The newly formed proerythroblasts and myeloblasts will subsequently undergo three to five mitotic divisions, resulting in an eight to 32-fold multiplication (Fig. 22–7). The nucleus of the megakaryoblast will undergo the same number of endomitotic divisions, resulting in the formation of a few huge cells with multilobed nuclei. Concomitant with nuclear proliferation the cytoplasm will undergo specific maturation and three to five days after the initial differentiation the cells are almost completely mature and functional.

The maturing reticulocytes and the maturing granulocytes remain in the bone marrow for some days before they are released into the circulation. The length of this delay appears to be responsive to the immediate needs for circulating blood cells. However, because the circulating granulocyte mass is much smaller than the circulating red cell mass, a premature release of the marrow reserve of maturing cells is of importance only for the functional adjustment of the peripheral granulocyte count. After the release from the bone marrow, the erythrocytes are all in active use in circulating blood, while about 50 per cent of the granulocytes and 30 per cent of the thrombocytes are sequestered in the microvasculature or in the spleen as functional reserves. Figure 22–11 and Table 22–1 give a summary of the cellular morphology and composition of the hematopoietic tissue. The apparent discrepancy between the 2:1 ratio between erythroid and granulocytic cells and the 1:3 ratio found in bone marrow smears is caused by the fact that the bone marrow reticulocytes are included in Table 22–1 but usually not in bone marrow differential counts.

Figure 22-11 The normal morphology of the hematopoietic cells.

(See illustration on following pages)

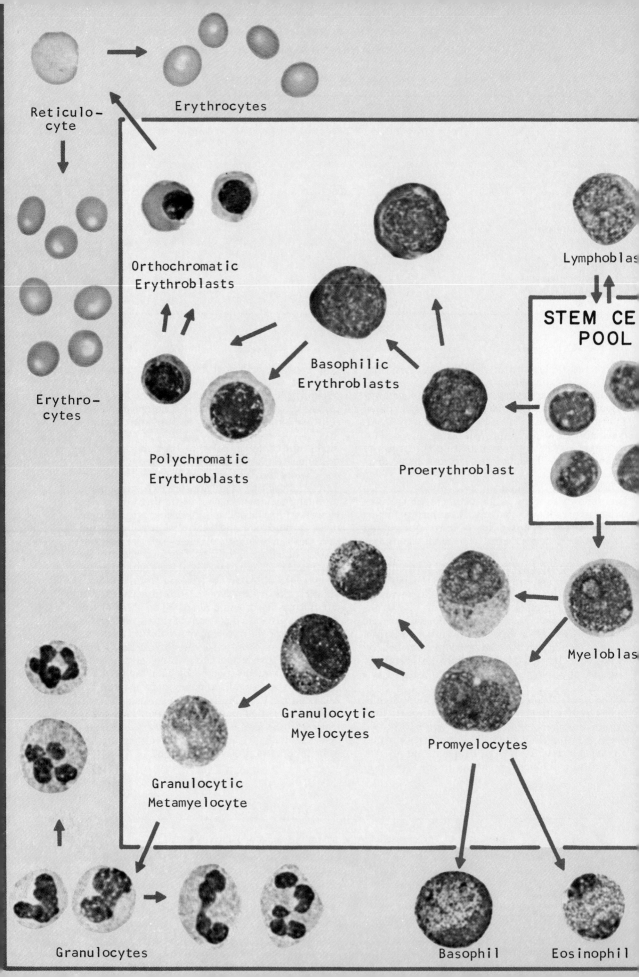

Erythrocytes

Reticulo-
cyte

Orthochromatic
Erythroblasts

Lymphoblas

STEM CE
POOL

Erythro-
cytes

Basophilic
Erythroblasts

Polychromatic
Erythroblasts

Proerythroblast

Myeloblas

Granulocytic
Myelocytes

Promyelocytes

Granulocytic
Metamyelocyte

Granulocytes

Basophil

Eosinophil

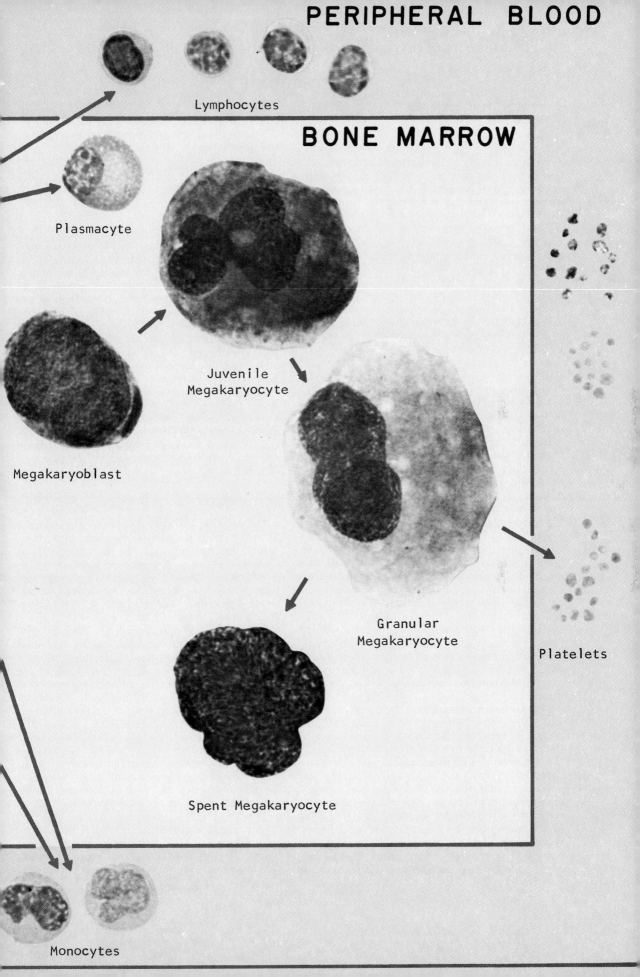

PERIPHERAL BLOOD

Lymphocytes

Plasmacyte

BONE MARROW

Megakaryoblast

Juvenile
Megakaryocyte

Granular
Megakaryocyte

Platelets

Spent Megakaryocyte

Monocytes

ERYTHROCYTES

STRUCTURE

The ultrastructure of the erythroid cells has by now been so closely correlated with metabolic activities that structure and function cannot be separated and will be dealt with together in this section. However, the morphology of blood cells stained with the Romanovsky dyes deserves some separate remarks, since stained blood and bone marrow smears are cornerstones in the clinical management of patients with hematologic disorders.

The earliest nucleated red blood cell, the proerythroblast is a large cell with a diameter of about 20 to 25 μ and a nucleus occupying about three fourths of the cell (Fig. 22–11). The nuclear chromatin, stained dark violet with the usual Wright or Giemsa stain, is finely dispersed, and the nucleus with its one or several nucleoli is clearly separated from the deep-blue cytoplasm by a distinct membrane. The nucleus is usually perfectly round and the cytoplasm devoid of granules. The subsequent proliferation and maturation through the stages of basophilic, polychromatophilic, and orthochromatic erythroblasts are characterized by a stepwise reduction in cellular and nuclear size, by a condensation of the nuclear chromatin into well-defined chunks, and by a dilution of the blue staining cytoplasmic ribosomes with newly synthesized hemoglobin. At the orthochromatic stage, the nucleus has become condensed into a small pyknotic mass and is extruded. Hemoglobin synthesis continues for a few more days until the nucleus-dependent synthetic machinery is exhausted. During this period precipitation and condensation of the remaining basophilic ribosomes with oxidant dyes such as brilliant cresyl blue and methylene blue will result in the characteristic appearance of the reticulocyte on a blood smear. The final transformation of reticulocytes to mature cells is associated with a considerable loss in volume due to cytoplasmic dehydration and loss of cellular membrane.

The mature erythrocyte is a biconcave disk with an average diameter of about 8 μ and a central pallor occupying the middle third of the cell. Owing to a relative excess of surface over volume, the cell is soft and pliable, accounting for the ease with which it can pass through tissue capillaries and splenic fenestrations with diameters considerably less than its own. Its membrane has a remarkable self-healing capacity, and red cell injury may cause the production of viable fragments rather than intravascular hemoglobin leakage. As the cell grows older it becomes slightly more dense, but it maintains its normal pliable biconcave appearance until enzymatic failure leads to rigidity, macrophage trapping, and destruction.

FUNCTION

ERYTHROBLASTS

Erythroblastic function is exclusively inner-directed. Each proerythroblast is programmed to undergo three to four mitotic divisions and to synthesize hemoglobin until its eight to 16 daughter cells contain about 300 million hemoglobin molecules each. This program has general and special metabolic requirements. The general requirements are common to all actively proliferating cells and include the building blocks and coenzymes needed for cellular construction. The special requirements are those needed for the synthesis of hemoglobin molecules and of enzymes designed to protect the integrity and function of these molecules. The various synthetic functions and their influence on red cell production have been reviewed by Marks and Rifkind and by Nienhuis and Benz and will be described later.

ERYTHROCYTES

The red blood cells are usually considered to be functionally quite unsophisticated, since their only obligations appear to be the transport and protection of the oxygen-carrying pigment, hemoglobin. Nevertheless, the survival of cells containing neither nuclei nor mitochrondria for about 4 months in a high oxygen and sodium environment demands the presence of efficient metabolic defenses and long-lived enzymes. The cargo of enzymes provided during the nucleated phase of development has to provide sufficient energy to maintain hemoglobin iron in its active ferrous state; to power the cation pump needed to maintain intracellular sodium and potassium concentrations despite the presence of unfavorable concentration gradients; to keep the sulfhydryl groups of globins, enzymes, and membranes in an active reduced state; and to preserve the integrity of the membrane. The metabolic pathways responsible for maintaining structure and function of the red cells will be described in the section dealing with the pathophysiology of red cell survival.

As mentioned earlier, the raison d'être for the existence of erythroid tissue and circulating red blood cells is the synthesis, transport, and protection of hemoglobin molecules. The importance of these molecules for oxygen transport has been known since 1862, when Hoppe-Seyler first isolated hemoglobin and demonstrated its affinity for oxygen. However, the molecular structure making a reversible oxygen binding possible has been clarified only recently.

The hemoglobin molecule is a tetramer consisting of two α and two β polypeptide chains, each with an attached heme group. The sequential mapping of the 141 amino acids of the α chain and 146 amino acids of the β chain has been of great importance for our identification of abnormal hemoglobins with specific amino acid substitutions. However, normal function of the hemoglobin molecules and the functional impact of such amino acid substitutions was not comprehended until the spatial positioning of the chains and of the individual amino acids had been established. Recent studies initiated by the classic x-ray crystallographic observations by Perutz and co-workers have shown that each of the four chains coils into eight helices (Fig. 22–12), forming an eggshaped molecule with a central cavity (Fig. 22–13). The polar, hydrophilic amino acid residues cover the surfaces while hydrophobic residues line four superficial pockets, each containing a heme group with its iron positioned between two histidine radicals. The proximal histidine is firmly bound to the ferrous atom while the distal histidine provides a protective and reversible link for deoxygenated iron. In our sequential nomenclature these histidine radicals are far apart (histidine 58 and 87 for α chains and histidine 63

and 92 for β chains) (Fig. 22–12), but spatially they are close together in the wells of the heme pockets.

The uptake and delivery of oxygen by the hemoglobin molecules are associated with considerable spatial rearrangement of the hemoglobin molecule, and as Perutz has pointed out, the well-known oxygen dissociation curve can best be explained on the basis of such rearrangement (Fig. 22–14). The oxygen affinity of deoxygenated hemoglobin is low, and it takes a relatively large increase in oxygen tension to attach an oxygen molecule to the first heme group. However, the oxygenation of this heme group causes a widespread molecular displacement, presumably initiated by changes in the distal histidine radical which formerly was linked to the ferrous atom (Fig. 22–13). A sliding motion in the α-β contact area reduces the size of the central cavity and makes the other heme pockets more available, so that two more oxygen molecules can be attached with only slight additional increases in the oxygen tension. Further molecular rearrangement is finally responsible for the fact that the last heme group has a low oxygen affinity and demands a considerable oxygen pressure to be oxygenated.

The sequential changes in oxygen affinity are reflected in the sigmoid shape of the oxygen dissociation curve and are responsible for the ease with which hemoglobin can be loaded with oxygen in the lungs and unloaded in the tissues. Hemoglobin variants with amino acid substitution in a heme pocket or in the α-β contact area

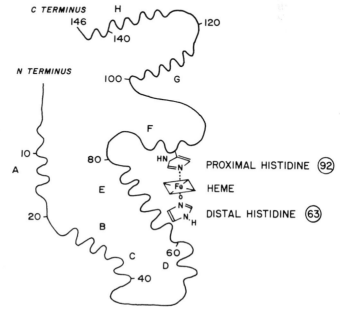

Figure 22–12 Diagram of the β polypeptide chain of hemoglobin with its eight helices (A to H) and the histidine enclosed heme group. (Adapted from Giblett, E. R.: Genetic Markers in Human Blood. Oxford, Blackwell Scientific Publications, 1969, p. 349.)

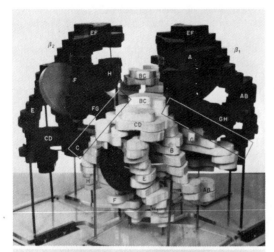

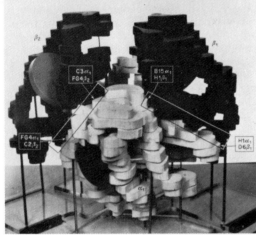

Figure 22-13 Model of the hemoglobin molecule depicting the α-β contact areas and the sliding motions which occur in the transformation from a deoxygenated form with a large central cavity (*top*) to an oxygenated form with a small cavity (*bottom*). (From Muirhead, H., et al.: J. Molec. Biol., *13*:646, 1965.)

often have altered oxygen dissociation curves. If these substitutions cause a shift to the left in the curve, the oxygen affinity is increased, the tissues become hypoxic, and a compensatory polycythemia ensues (Fig. 22–14). If the substitution causes a shift to the right, the oxygen affinity is decreased and the tissues can be provided with adequate amounts of oxygen at low hemoglobin concentrations. Obviously, if the amino acid substitutions involve the proximal or distal histidine in the heme pockets, much more severe changes will occur, with loss of the oxygen-carrying capacity of the heme pockets involved. The oxygen dissociation curve for hemoglobins made up by like

chains such as β^4 in hemoglobin H or γ^4 in hemoglobin Bart are not sigmoid but are shifted far to the left, making these hemoglobin variants useless as oxygen carriers.

It has been known for many years that the shape of the oxygen dissociation curve is dependent on the pH (Fig. 22–14). This so-called Bohr effect is responsible for the fact that the curve is shifted to the right in the acid microenvironment of hypoxic tissues, causing an enhanced capacity to release oxygen where it is not needed. The reason for this favorable shift in the oxygen affinity of hemoglobin is related to the oxygen-dependent acidity of the hemoglobin molecule. Oxyhemoglobin is a stronger acid than deoxyhemoglobin, and an acid environment will consequently facilitate deoxygenation.

In addition to the Bohr effect, the oxygen dissociation curve is also responsive to the intracellular concentration of certain organic phosphates. This recent discovery has explained the fact that oxygen affinity can be adapted to compensate for a decreased oxygen supply, such as at high altitudes, or an impaired oxygen supply system, such as in anemia. In both these conditions there is an alkalosis, respiratory hyperventilation alkalosis at high altitude and intracellular alkalosis due to accumulation of the more alkaline reduced hemoglobin in anemia. Since alkalosis stimulates glycolysis, there is an increase in the intracellular concentration of 2,3-diphosphoglycerate (2,3-

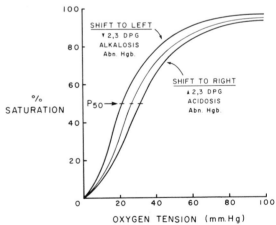

Figure 22-14 Oxygen dissociation curve of normal human blood showing that a shift to the right with an increase in P_{50} (the oxygen tension at which 50% of hemoglobin is deoxygenated) is found under conditions of acidosis or increased 2,3 DPG or with certain abnormal hemoglobins, whereas a shift to the left with a decrease in P_{50} is found under conditions of alkalosis or decreased 2,3 DPG or within other abnormal hemoglobins.

DPG). Furthermore, the binding of increased quantities of 2,3 DPG to deoxyhemoglobin depletes the unbound pool and thus also stimulates the increased synthesis of the low molecular weight phosphate. This phosphate fits into the expanded central cavity of deoxygenated hemoglobin and impedes the transformation of deoxyhemoglobin with a low oxygen affinity to oxyhemoglobin with a high oxygen affinity. The result is that the oxygen dissociation curve shifts to the right, permitting more oxygen to be released at a given tissue tension of oxygen. The opposite of such a facilitated oxygen unloading occurs in conditions in which the 2,3-DPG concentration is decreased, such as in stored bank blood. Here the shift of the curve is to the left, and the tissues may become hypoxic despite a normal oxygen carrying capacity of the perfusing blood.

The respiratory function of hemoglobin also includes support for carbon dioxide transport from the tissues to the lungs. Carbon dioxide will diffuse into the red cells and catalyzed by carbonic anhydrase becomes transformed into carbonic acid. The hydrogen ions of carbonic acid will be buffered by the relatively alkaline deoxyhemoglobin and the bicarbonate ion diffuses back into plasma. In the pulmonary capillary the same process in reverse will liberate carbon dioxide for pulmonary elimination. In addition to this so-called Bohr effect on carbon dioxide transport, the amino groups of globin form reversible carbamino groups with carbon dioxide and are responsible for about 10 per cent of carbon dioxide transport and excretion.

KINETICS

SELF-RENEWAL AND DIFFERENTIATION

The earliest recognizable erythroid cell is the proerythroblast. However, since it is synthesizing and accumulating hemoglobin from the time of its appearance, it cannot renew itself merely through mitotic division but must be replenished from an earlier undifferentiated stem cell (Fig. 22–15). The existence of such a precursor cell is supported by the fact that nonerythroid cells in an erythropoietically inactive mouse spleen are capable of being transformed into proerythroblasts (Fig. 22–16). The morphologic identity of this precursor cell has not as yet been firmly established, but it probably is a mononuclear lymphoid cell called BFU — E or CFU — E in accord with its cultural characteristics. As described in the bone marrow section, it is replenished from an earlier multipotential stem cell pool (CFU — S) but it is in active cell cycle and capable of some degree of self-renewal. It is solely committed to the erythroid series, and it is generally accepted that the hormone erythropoietin will induce proliferation, activate its potential as a hemoglobin synthesizing cell and transform it into a proerythroblast.

The mechanism by which erythropoietin induces proliferation and blast transformation is still obscure as noted in a 1978 report by Nienhuis and co-workers. It may directly cause a derepression of the production of a messenger RNA

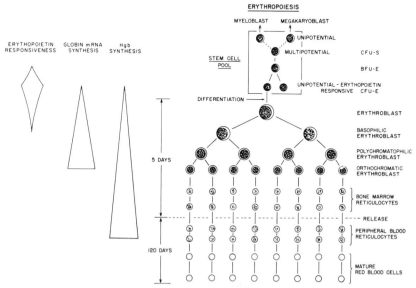

Figure 22–15 A pictorial model of the stem cell compartment and its differentiation by the action of erythropoietin to proliferating, maturing and hemoglobin producing erythroid cells.

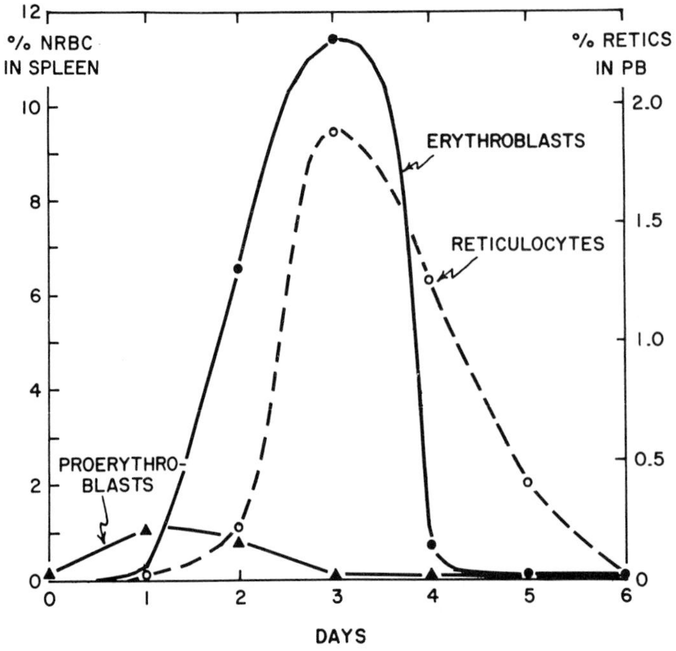

Figure 22–16 Erythropoietic effect of a single injection of erythropoietin at day 0 on a mouse spleen rendered erythropoietically inactive by prior hypertransfusion. (Redrawn from Filmanowicz, E., and Gurney, C. W.: J. Lab. Clin. Med., 57:65–72, 1961.)

coded for a key enzyme in the synthesis of hemoglobin such as ALA synthetase. It is also possible that it acts indirectly on DNA transcription by activating a membrane adenyl cyclase, which in turn increases the production of cyclic AMP, a common second messenger for hormonal action. In either case, the activated cell appears to differentiate and proliferate according to a preformed program with only little additional stimulation by erythropoietin (Fig. 22–16).

MULTIPLICATION AND MATURATION

Following erythropoietin-induced blast transformation of the unipotential erythropoietin-sensitive stem cells, the emerging proerythroblasts immediately begin an integrated and controlled process of protoporphyrin production, globin-chain synthesis, iron uptake, and hemoglobin assembly. In the mitochondria the newly formed ALA synthetase initiates synthesis of protoporphyrin by condensing activated glycine and succinic acid to ALA. The final step in this synthetic chain occurs again in the mitochondria and consists of the formation of heme from protoporphyrin and iron. Simultaneously, alpha and beta globin chains are produced in ribosomes strung together by mRNA. The synthesis of heme and globins is closely coordinated and it appears that heme plays an essential role in this coordination. It not only exerts an end-product control on ALA

synthetase activity but also a control on the transcription or processing of alpha and beta m RNA. The synthesis of other red cell proteins, such as membrane receptors, antigens and glycolytic enzymes, are also closely integrated with the formation of heme and globins.

Iron necessary for the transformation of protoporphyrin to heme is provided from iron-charged transferrin which becomes attached to specific receptors on the immature red cell membrane. The iron passes through the membrane while the iron-free transferrin possibly after a brief sojourn inside the cell is released and reused for shuttling iron from the macrophage system to erythroid cells. The intracellular iron is transported to the mitochondria for heme production or temporarily deposited as ferritin complexes in the cytoplasm. The fate of these so-called siderotic granules is not known. They may provide storage iron for further heme production, or they may be extruded and returned to the circulating iron pool.

Although transferrin-mediated delivery presumably provides adequate amounts of iron to the maturing cell, a second supply exists with iron provided by macrophages through direct cell-to-cell delivery. Since such an intercellular transport system also could facilitate removal or pitting of intracellular iron by the macrophages, the exact role played by these cells in cellular maturation is not clear. Nevertheless, it is known that erythroid development occurs in close physical proximity with macrophages (Fig. 22–17). This

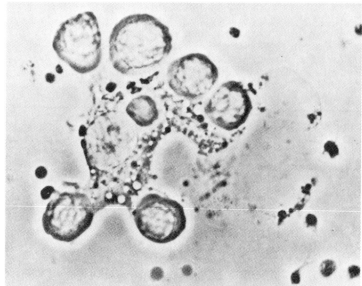

Figure 22–17 Phase contrast picture of a macrophage (nurse-cell) "servicing" attached erythroblasts. (From Lessin, L. S., and Bessis, M.: *In* Williams et al. (Eds.): Hematology. New York, McGraw-Hill Book Co., 1977, p. 105, by permission of Sandoz Ltd., Basel, Switzerland.)

proximity is not always apparent from observing regular bone marrow smears, since the cells are torn apart from each other and from the thin, wide-flung cytoplasmic veil of the macrophages. However, biopsy sections and in-vitro bone marrow cultures often show the presence of characteristic erythropoietic islands, each consisting of a macrophage and nucleated red cells at the same stage of maturation. As the cells mature and proliferate, the islands increase in size until they break up and release their finished cellular products.

Concurrently with the cytoplasmic maturation, the cell will undergo three to four mitotic divisions, causing a stepwise reduction in volume. Since all nucleated red cells are diploid, the reduction in nuclear size must be caused by a progressive condensation of nuclear protein, a condensation which eventually results in the appearance of a dense pyknotic nucleus incapable of further DNA synthesis. Occasionally in normal bone marrow and frequently in bone marrow from patients with accelerated red cell production the last division may be incomplete, with the production of a cloverleaf nucleus or satellite nuclear pieces, so-called Howell-Jolly bodies. In most non-mammalian species, the condensed nucleus is carried as an inert inclusion by the mature circulating red blood cells. In mammals, however, it is extruded by a process of intracellular demarcation and extracellular pressure. The cell is pitted either when it forces its way into the circulation through narrow endothelial openings in the bone marrow sinusoids or when it passes a similar sievelike hazard in the spleen. The extruded nucleus is surrounded by a thin layer of hemoglobin, and in patients with accelerated red cell formation the breakdown of this

hemoglobin may contribute significantly to the concentration of circulating bilirubin.

After the nucleus has been extruded, hemoglobin synthesis continues but at a gradually diminishing rate for another three to four days. The cells lose membrane receptors for transferrin-iron, the mitochondria diminish in number, and the polyribosomes disaggregate. When the ribosomes finally disappear, the cells no longer show the characteristic staining qualities of a reticulocyte and they have become mature red blood cells. The cells also diminish in size, and the stickiness which characterizes immature red cells is lost. This stickiness may be caused by a coating of transferrin, and the diminishing number of iron receptors could be responsible in part for the loss of cellular cohesion and adhesion and could promote the release of cells into the circulating blood.

According to nuclear size and degree of cytoplasmic maturation, the developing bone marrow cell goes through five stages designated respectively as proerythroblasts, basophilic erythroblasts, polychromatic erythroblasts, orthochromatic erythroblasts, and bone marrow reticulocytes. Since each of the first three stages appears to be separated from the next by a mitotic division, it is possible to estimate their duration or generation time by enumerating mitotic figures. The fraction of cells in mitosis (mitotic index) depends on the duration of the mitosis (about 30 to 60 minutes) and on the generation time:

$$\text{Mitotic Index} = \frac{\text{Number of cells in mitosis}}{\text{Total number of cells}}$$

$$= \frac{\text{Mitotic time}}{\text{Generation time}}$$

The mitotic index has been measured to be about 2.5 per cent for proerythroblasts, 5 per cent for basophilic erythroblasts, and 6 per cent for polychromatic erythroblasts, and the generation times are calculated to be 30 hours, 15 hours, and 13 hours, respectively. Unfortunately, when generation times are measured by other techniques, the results have been somewhat different. The most popular alternate method has been based on using tritiated thymidine to label cells during their synthetic phase (lasting about six hours) and employing radioautography to measure fraction of cells labeled, the so-called labeling index.

$$\text{Labeling Index} = \frac{\text{Number of cells in synthetic phase}}{\text{Total number of cells}}$$

$$= \frac{\text{Synthetic time}}{\text{Generation time}}$$

The generation times calculated from such studies by Skårberg are 11 hours for proerythroblasts, 16 hours for basophilic erythroblasts and 26 hours for polychromatic erythroblasts. In the absence of more consistent data, it seems permissible to use as a practical approximation 24 hours for each maturation phase. Since the orthochromatic erythroblasts and the bone marrow reticulocytes do not synthesize DNA or undergo mitotic divisions, the time spent in each of these stages is estimated from the turnover of appropriately labeled cells and is about 24 hours and 48 hours, respectively. Using a model based on these values (Fig. 22–15) one can estimate that the number of erythropoietic cells in the bone marrow is about 3 per cent of the circulating red cells, or, if the red cell mass is 30 ml. per kg. body weight and the mean red cell volume is $90\mu^3$, about 10×10^9 cells per kg body weight. More accurate methods for enumeration of erythropoietic bone marrow cells have disclosed somewhat higher values (Table 22–2), but a basic numerical agreement exists supporting the validity of the model presented in Figure 22–15.

TABLE 22–2 ERYTHROID POOLS

Cell Types	Number of Cells in 10⁹ per kg. Body Weight
Proerythroblast	0.10
Basophilic erythroblast	0.48
Polychromatophilic erythroblast	1.47
Orthochromatic erythroblast	2.95
Marrow reticulocytes	8.20
Blood reticulocytes	3.10
Mature red blood cells	307.00
Daily production and destruction	3.00

(Adapted from Donohue D. M., et al.: J. Clin. Invest., *37*:1571, 1958 and from Finch C. A., et al., Blood, *50*: 699, 1977.)

Part of the transformation of nucleated red cells to mature red cells takes place in circulating blood which contains about one third the reticulocyte pool. Under normal conditions, the reticulum persists for about one to two days, but in patients with accelerated red cell production, reticulocytes are released earlier and stay longer in the blood. As has been emphasized by Hillman and Finch, this has to be taken into account when reticulocytes are used to estimate the rate of red cell production. The earlier release of reticulocytes is also reflected by the fact that these so-called "stress reticulocytes" are larger and more immature than normal circulating reticulocytes and that the bone marrow transit time is shortened. It has been suggested by Leblond and coworkers that the early release is caused by a direct action of erythropoietin on the bone marrow release mechanism. However, it could also be due to ecologic crowding of the bone marrow by new erythroid cells derived from an overstimulated stem cell pool.

REGULATION

Maturation and proliferation of nucleated red cells proceed at an integrated speed and rate. Changes in the speed of cellular maturation or in the rate of cellular proliferation could influence the total output of red cells from the bone marrow but cannot be solely responsible for the remarkable range of erythropoietic activity. A shortened maturation time or an early release of cells will only augment the circulating red cell mass slightly, and several extra mitotic divisions are needed in order to provide the bone marrow with its capacity to increase its rate of red cell production five- to tenfold. Since most studies indicate that an accelerated rate of red cell production is associated with a shortened transit time, it seems most unlikely that added mitotic divisions can be squeezed in. Furthermore, direct measurements of cellular generation times have suggested that the maturation and proliferation of immature red cells proceed at fixed rates independent of the overall erythropoietic activity. Consequently, it seems more likely that the rate of red cell production depends on the number of operational erythropoietic units rather than on the activity within each unit. According to this widely accepted erythropoietic quantum theory, the rate of red cell production is controlled primarily, if not exclusively, by the rate at which stem cells differentiate to proerythroblasts and initiate the formation of an erythropoietic unit.

Under normal steady-state conditions the rate of differentiation provides just enough red cells to replace the daily loss of cells. Maintenance of such a homeostatic balance demands the existence of a feedback system responsive to red cell loss and capable of inducing the necessary adjustment in the production of red cells. Occasionally the reticulocyte count displays the oscillatory pattern which characterizes all feedback control systems (Fig. 22–18), but under normal conditions the system is usually too finely tuned to be visibly oscillatory. Under pathologic conditions with increased loss or destruction of red cells the compensatory adjustment in the rate of red cell production becomes evident. The triggering event in the activation of the adjustment must in some way be related to the physical or functional effect of red cell loss, and it has variously been suggested that red cell production is controlled by a device responsive to breakdown products of red cell destruction, to blood viscosity, to red cell volume, or to oxygen transport. Of these possibilities, a responsiveness to oxygen transport is by far the most likely, since oxygen transport is the main function of the red cell mass. Furthermore, numerous studies have shown that a decreased supply of oxygen to the tissues almost invariably is associated with an increased rate of red cell production.

The existence of an erythropoietic feedback system responsive to the tissue tension of oxygen was first suspected by Dennis Jourdanet, a French physician who in the 1860's practiced medicine in the highlands of Mexico. He observed that the dark blood of his surgical patients was thick and flowed slowly, and he suggested that there was a connection between a low arterial content of oxygen and thick blood. Subsequent studies by the famous Parisian physiologist, Paul Bert, on the physiologic effect of low barometric pressure led to the hypothesis that decreased arterial oxygen tension stimulates red cell production. Supporting evidence came from the fact that many patients with chronic pulmonary disorders or with right-to-left shunts were polycythemic. Since anemia, despite normal arterial oxygen tension, is also associated with increased red cell production, it was concluded that erythropoietic stimulation is caused by tissue hypoxia due to either a decreased oxygen tension or a decreased oxygen content of arterial blood.

Subsequent observations of the effect of an increased supply of oxygen to the tissues showed that the rate of red cell production is suppressed and that the tissue tension of oxygen apparently influences or controls the full range of red cell production. Direct confirmation of this hypothesis has been difficult to achieve because of our ignorance of the exact cellular location of the oxygen sensor. Measurements of the oxygen tension of subcutaneous tissue have disclosed an inverse relationship between oxygen tension and erythropoietic stimulation (Fig. 22–19). However, the oxygen sensor is probably not located in the subcutaneous tissue, and measurements of the oxygen tension in the kidney, a more likely site,

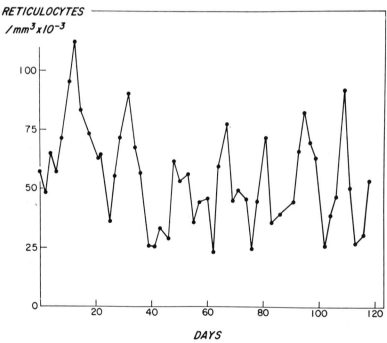

Figure 22–18   Absolute reticulocyte counts of a dog showing regularly spaced oscillations. The period is about 16 days, presumably twice the time from stem cell differentiation to reticulocyte maturation. (Redrawn from Morley, A., and Stohlman, F., Jr.: Science, *165*:1025, 1969. Copyright 1969 by the American Association for the Advancement of Science.)

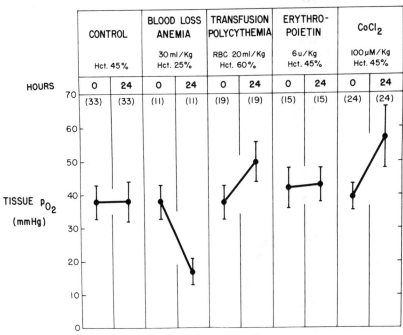

Figure 22–19 Oxygen tension of air pockets introduced subcutaneously in rats. The effects of bleeding, transfusion, erythropoietin, and cobalt on the oxygen tension are given. As expected, bleeding causes hypoxia, transfusion causes hyperoxia and erythropoietin has no immediate effect. Cobalt causes tissue hyperoxia, presumably reflecting reduced oxygen utilization because of inhibited cellular oxidative metabolism.

have not been too informative. This may be related to the fact that the oxygen sensor appears not to be responsive directly to the intercellular tissue tension of oxygen, but rather to a component of intracellular oxidative metabolism. Cobalt chloride administration, for example, causes an accelerated rate of red cell production despite an increase in the tissue tension of oxygen (Fig. 22–19), and the triggering event for the increase in both red cell production and tissue tension of oxygen appears to be impaired intracellular oxidative metabolism and oxygen utilization.

The mechanism which links the oxygen sensor to the bone marrow has recently been clarified and appears to consist of a feedback system mediated in one direction by red cell-bound oxygen and in the opposite direction by erythropoietin, a renal erythropoietic hormone (Fig. 22–20).

The suggestion that tissue hypoxia causes the release of a humoral mediator was given its first solid experimental support in 1950 when Reissmann demonstrated that hypoxia induced in one rat of a parabiotic pair caused increased red cell production in both partners. A few years later an erythropoietic factor was found in the serum of anemic rabbits (Fig. 22–21), and since then this factor, named erythropoietin, has been isolated and partially characterized.

Erythropoietin is a glycoprotein with a molecular weight of about 35,000 and a sialic acid content of about 13 per cent. It is present in both

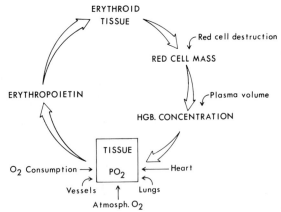

Figure 22–20 The feedback circuit that links red cell production to the tissue tension of oxygen. (From work reviewed by Erslev, A. J.: Medicine, *43*:661, 1964. © 1964. The Williams & Wilkins Company, Baltimore.)

plasma and urine of all mammals tested, and similar substances have been described in birds and fish. It man, it has a biologic half-life of about 4 to 6 hours, but its renal clearance is quite low (about 0.5 ml. per min.). Attempts to characterize and purify erythropoietin and to elucidate its site of production have been impeded by our crude and cumbersome assay technique. Agglutination inhibition tests and radioimmunoassays are being developed, but the only acceptable technique for measurement at present involves bioassay in mice. This assay utilizes mice in which endogenous erythropoietin production is first abolished by transfusion or by hypoxia-induced polycythemia. The technique is unfortunately not sensitive enough to detect erythropoietin in normal serum since its level of sensitivity is 50 mU/ml., and the normal level is about 5 to 20 mU/ml. (Fig. 22–22). Assay of urine, concentrated about 50 times, has shown that there is a linear relationship between the 24 hour erythropoietin excretion and the hemoglobin concentration and has also shown that the daily erythropoietin excretion in normal men is about 2 units and in normal women 3 units (Fig. 22–22).

Following the observations by Jacobson and co-workers that the production of erythropoietin ceases after bilateral nephrectomy, it has generally been accepted that erythropoietin has a renal origin. Support for this hypothesis has come from the observation that erythrocytosis occasionally occurs in patients with compromised renal blood supply or with renal ischemia due to space-occupying lesions. Although hypernephromas specifically have been reported to be a source of inappropriate production of erythropoietin, other tumors, as well as cysts or hydronephroses, have been associated with an increased rate of red cell production, and it seems more likely that erythropoietin is released by the compressed normal kidney tissues rather than by the pathologic lesion. Intrarenal injury due to experimental induction of microinfarcts or as a consequence of tissue rejection after kidney transplantation may also lead to overproduction of erythropoietin and erythrocytosis. However, the usual consequence of renal injury and renal failure is impaired erythropoietin production and anemia.

In order for the normal kidney to adjust erythropoietin production to the oxygen requirements of the body it appears that it, in addition to erythropoietin-producing tissue, also must contain an oxygen-sensitive device. The exact location of these two tissues is still unknown. The cortex appears most unsuited to act as an oxygen sensor since its large supply of blood with a high hematocrit (due to plasma skimming) should make it quite insensitive to small changes in the oxygen-carrying capacity of blood. The medulla, however, is relatively hypoxic owing to the shunting of oxygen between the descending and ascending capillaries at its base, and the apex of the medulla could serve as an oxygen-sensing apparatus. The fact that renal cysts made up of

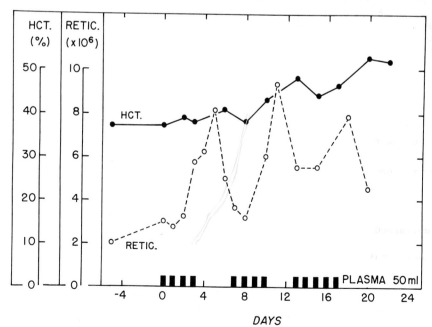

Figure 22–21 The erythropoietic effect of plasma from anemic donor rabbits when infused in large amounts to normal rabbits. (Redrawn from Erslev, A.J.: Blood, 8:349–357, 1953, by permission of Grune & Stratton Inc., New York.)

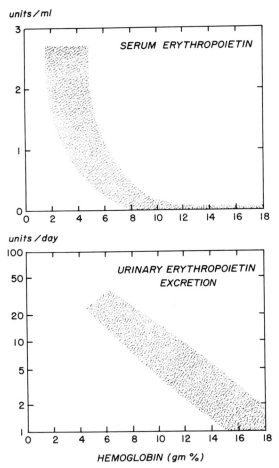

units / ml

units / day

HEMOGLOBIN (gm %)

Figure 22–22 The relationship between hemoglobin concentration and the content of erythropoietin in plasma (*upper panel*) and the 24 hour excretion of erythropoietin in urine (*lower panel*).

has been provided by Gordon and co-workers. They suggest that the kidney does not produce erythropoietin directly but rather produces an enzyme which is capable of transforming a circulating erythropoietin precursor into the active hormone. Considerable experimental support has been marshaled for the existence of such a renal erythropoietic enzyme, and the hypothesis has received wide acceptance because of its close analogy to the renin-angiotensinogen system and to many other cascade-activation schemes. Unfortunately, only trace amounts of erythropoietin can be generated by mixing the renal erythropoietic enzyme with normal plasma. Furthermore, in a 1975 study Erslev has shown that the isolated kidney perfused with a plasma-free amino acid mixture can synthesize erythropoietin almost as well as a kidney perfused with plasma. Consequently it appears that the kidney is the source of erythropoietin and that alternate explanations for the erythropoietic inactivity of renal homogenate must exist. One of these proposed by Erslev and co-workers is that erythropoietin is inactivated by an erythropoietin inhibitor during the processing of the kidney extract. Such an inhibitor has been demonstrated in crude renal homogenate and in its lipid component. This inhibitor is extremely powerful and could completely conceal the presence of many thousands of units of erythropoietin in kidney tissue. Whether or not this lipid inhibitor plays a physiologic role in the storage and release of erythropoietin is not known, but if erythropoietin is present in the kidneys, in an inactive lipid-bound form, practical recovery will have to await methods for inactivating the inhibitor or breaking the erythropoietin-inhibitor bond.

Recent studies of anephric animals and humans have disclosed that extrarenal erythropoietin production occurs. It amounts to a fraction of what is normally produced but the erythropoietic material produced is immunologically similar to renal erythropoietin. The site of production appears to be the liver and/or the mononuclear macrophage system. Since the production here is enhanced by severe anemia and hypoxia, the extrarenal site, like the kidney, must be linked to local or distant oxygen sensors. Extrarenal erythropoietin production has been described in association with various neoplasms, particularly cerebellar hemangiomas and hepatomas, but the relationship between this inappropriate secretion by neoplastic cells and the slight but appropriate secretion found in anephric mammals is completely unknown.

The action of erythropoietin on red cell precursors is better understood, although the exact target cells have not been morphologically identified or isolated. As outlined in Figure 22–15, the target cells are undoubtedly the unipotential stem cells committed to erythroid development. Stimulat-

dilated tubules occasionally contain erythropoietin would also suggest that the site of the erythropoietin-producing tissue may reside in the medulla. On the other hand, studies of the juxtaglomerular apparatus in anemia have suggested that this may be the site of erythropoietin production, a suggestion supported by the fact that fluorescent-tagged antibodies to erythropoietin are attracted to the glomerular tuft. In order to correlate some of these observations, it has been proposed that an oxygen sensor in the medulla controls erythropoietin production in the cortex by means of a short-range releasing hormone, but so far such a hormone has not been demonstrated.

The validity of many of these observations and speculations has recently been questioned because studies of renal extracts have disclosed that kidney tissue is not erythropoietically active. A possible explanation for this surprising finding

ing effects on other cell types have been de-scribed, but at present such effects appear to be related to increased stem cell activity rather than to a direct action of erythropoietin. Changes in granulocyte and thrombocyte counts are fre-quently observed under conditions of increased erythropoietin release. However, these changes are temporary and may depend on a secondary activation of multipotential cells with either an increased rate of differentiation in all directions or a possible competition by the unipotential stem cell pools for the attention of the multipo-tent cell compartment. Since an erythropoietin-stimulated bone marrow regularly displays a shortened erythroid transit time with an early release of large immature reticulocytes, a direct effect of erythropoietin on red cell maturation and release has been postulated. However, this effect could also be caused by the rapid growth of the early erythroid cells stressing the physical capacity of bone marrow to provide room for ma-turing erythroid cells.

Although the capacity of renal hypoxia to gen-erate erythropoietin and in turn to accelerate red cell production explains most clinical and experi-mental observations on the control of red cell production, the existence of additional regulatory mechanisms has been proposed. The pituitary, hypothalamus, and carotid bodies have all been claimed to be involved in the physiologic regula-tion of red cell production, but the experimental support for such neuroendocrine control is not convincing. More impressive are reports suggest-ing that hemolyzed red cells may exert an end product feedback stimulation on red cell produc-tion. Because of the high reticulocyte count in hemolytic anemias, it has usually been assumed that these anemias exert a more powerful stimu-lation on red cell production than similar ane-mias caused by blood loss. However, the differ-ence in the rate of red cell production between the two kinds of anemia may actually not be as pro-nounced as suggested by the reticulocyte counts, since hemolysis often causes a selective destruc-tion of old red cells, leaving relatively more reti-culocytes in the circulation. Nevertheless, hemo-lyzed red cells do appear to have some effect on red cell production, mediated either by their iron content or by a "stimulatory" effect on the erythropoietin-producing cells in the kidney or elsewhere.

In summary, it appears that the main, if not only, feedback system regulating red cell produc-tion is based on the capacity of the kidneys to sense tissue hypoxia and translate this informa-tion into production of erythropoietin. Figure 22–23 shows an updated feedback model which incorporates current concepts of erythropoietin production and action and more recent informa-tion about the compensatory adjustments of oxy-gen transport.

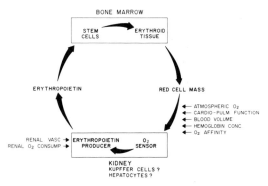

Figure 22–23 Current version of the feedback circuit.

PATHOPHYSIOLOGY

DEFINITION AND CLASSIFICATION OF POLYCYTHEMIAS AND ANEMIAS

The polycythemias and anemias are defined as hematologic disorders with either too many or too few red cells in the circulation. Functionally the polycythemias are better characterized by an in-creased hematocrit (more than 53 per cent) since their clinical manifestations are not caused by a change in oxygen delivery but rather by hyper-volemia and hyperviscosity, both consequences of a high hematocrit. The anemias on the other hand are functionally better characterized by a reduced hemoglobin concentration (less than 12 gm. per cent) since the clinical manifestations depend on the oxygen-carrying capacity of blood.

Based on the size of the red cell mass, both polycythemias and anemias can be classified as either relative, caused by changes in the plasma volume, or absolute, caused by changes in the red cell mass. Strictly speaking, the relative poly-cythemias or anemias are not primary hemato-logic disorders. However, from a differential diag-nostic point of view they play a considerable role in hematology.

The absolute polycythemias traditionally are subdivided into primary and secondary polycyth-emias, whereas the absolute anemias can be clas-sified further into anemias caused by decreased red cell production or decreased red cell survival (Table 22–3).

POLYCYTHEMIA

General Effects of Polycythemia

The pathophysiologic manifestations of poly-cythemia, or more correctly of erythrocytosis, are caused by hyperviscosity and hypervolemia asso-ciated with an increase in the red cell mass. Under normal conditions, the red cell mass is maintained carefully at about 30 ml. per kg. body

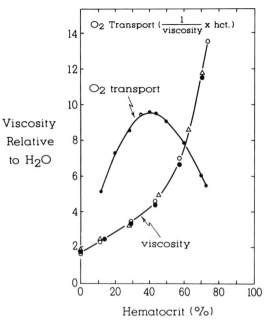

Figure 22-24 Oxygen transport as calculated from blood oxygen carrying capacity (hematocrit) and blood flow (reciprocal of viscosity).

weight, a value which presumably must be considered optimal. The reason for not maintaining a higher red cell mass does not reside in any bone marrow limitation, since a mere doubling of the rate of red cell production would sustain a red cell mass twice normal size. The reason seems to be that an increased red cell mass will be associated with a high viscosity and sluggish flow of circulating blood.

Such sluggish blood flow is responsible in part for the tendency to thrombosis found in patients with polycythemia and would, if not compensated for, result in decreased oxygen flow to the tissues (Fig. 22-24) and obviate any benefits derived from the development of secondary polycythemia. Fortunately, the high hematocrit and high viscosity are associated with an increase in blood volume (Fig. 22-25), and the resulting vasodilatation will enhance the tissue perfusion with blood and oxygen. Using measurement for cardiac output it can be shown directly that oxygen transport at a given hematocrit is greater in hypervolemic than in normovolemic dogs (Fig. 22-26). Furthermore, the optimal value for oxygen transport, which is about 45 per cent for normovolemic animals, is also increased, facilitating the mutual adjustment between hematocrit, red cell mass, and oxygen transport.

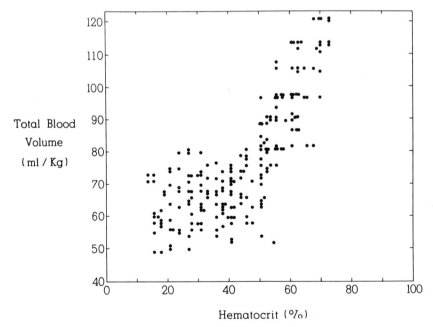

Figure 22-25 Relationship between blood volume and hematocrit. A reduction in hematocrit to about 15 per cent does not cause a significant change in blood volume, but an increase in hematocrit above 50 per cent appears to cause hypervolemia. (Data from Metcalfe, J., et al.: Circ. Res., *25*:47, 1969, by permission of The American Heart Association, Inc.)

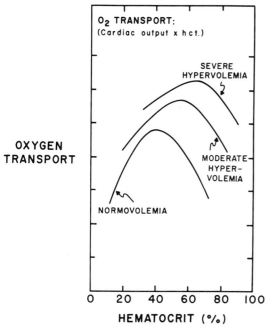

Figure 22-26 Calculated in vivo oxygen transport in normovolemic and hypervolemic conditions. As can be seen, the oxygen transport in hypervolemia is better than that in normovolemic states, even at higher hematocrits. The curves also indicate that the optimal value for oxygen transport is higher at higher blood volumes. (From Murray, J. F., et al.: J. Clin. Invest., *42*:1150, 1963, and Thorling, E. B., and Erslev, A.J.: Blood, *31*:332, 1968, by permission of Grune & Stratton, Inc., New York.)

The high blood volume in polycythemia is tolerated quite well, though symptoms such as headache, tinnitus, and dizziness and signs such as nose-bleeding and ruddy cyanosis probably are caused by the vascular dilatation needed to accommodate the blood volume. Since the increase in red cell production needed to sustain a polycythemia is quite moderate, clinical or laboratory signs of bone marrow hyperactivity are usually absent. However, a slight increase in uric acid, and lactic dehydrogenase levels may occur, reflecting an increase in the number of red cells destroyed daily.

Relative Polycythemia

A relative erythrocytosis with a hematocrit of more than 53 per cent can be found after severe fluid loss and the hematocrit may serve as a useful gauge of dehydration. A relative erythrocytosis has also been observed in otherwise healthy individuals with no apparent fluid volume deficit. Careful measurements by Brown and co-workers of red cell mass and fluid volume in such patients have suggested that the increase in hematocrit is

spurious and merely caused by the combination of a borderline high red cell mass and a borderline low plasma volume. Since many patients with such spurious polycythemia are tense, chain-smoking individuals, the condition has been called "stress polycythemia." However, tobacco by itself produces carbon monoxide hemoglobin leading to a compensatory increase in the red cell mass, and nicotine may have a diuretic, plasma volume lowering effect. Consequently "stress polycythemia," as pointed out by Smith and Landow, probably should be called "tobacco polycythemia" and designated as a secondary rather than a relative polycythemia.

Absolute Polycythemia

Primary. Polycythemia vera is a "myeloproliferative" disorder characterized by an uncontrolled proliferation of erythroid, myeloid, and megakaryocytic bone marrow elements. The proliferation is predominantly erythroid, and the circulating red cell mass is increased during the early part of the disease. The concomitant increase in granulocytes and platelets has led to the assumption that polycythemia vera is caused by an inappropriate activation of multipotential stem cells. However, the unipotential committed stem cells must also be involved in the disease process, since the erythropoietin-sensitive stem cells undergo differentiation despite the fact that the production of erythropoietin is almost completely suppressed.

Recent studies by Adamson, Prchal and co-workers have shown that polycythemia vera is a clonal disorder caused by autonomous overactivity of a single abnormal multipotential stem cell. These authors studied two polycythemic women who were heterozygous for the X-linked A and B glucose-6-phosphate dehydrogenase isoenzymes. As expected, their skin and bone marrow fibroblasts showed a mosaicism of cells with A and B isoenzymes, but all red cells, granulocytes, and platelets contained the same isoenzymes, type A, presumably derived from a single, type A, multipotential stem cell. Bone marrow from these patients cultured in the absence of erythropoietin grew out erythroid colonies, all with the same type A isoenzyme. When erythropoietin was added, the number of type A colonies increased but in addition, colonies with type B isoenzyme appeared. These findings suggest that the autonomous clones of polycythemia vera are responsive to the stimulating effect of erythropoietin and that the bone marrow from patients with polycythemia vera in addition contains a number of normal erythropoietin-dependent clones.

The cause for this autonomous overactivity of the stem cell pool is unknown, but the existence of a viral-induced polycythemia in mice has raised the possibility that the human disorder also is virus-related. However, as is the case for most neoplastic proliferative disorders, firm evidence for a viral etiology is not available.

The increased rate of red cell production causes a steady rise in red cell blood count and hematocrit. The plasma volume remains unchanged or increases slightly, and the erythrocytosis becomes characterized by an increase in both the red cell mass and the blood volume. This process may be quite slow and may be accomplished by a slight but sustained excess of red cell production over red cell destruction. For example, a mere doubling of the rate of red cell production for a period of four months will result in a doubling of the size of the red cell mass. Since the establishment of a clinically recognizable polycythemia may take much longer, it is not surprising that a routine bone marrow examination may not show evidence of much erythroid hyperactivity.

Ferrokinetic studies, measuring total bone marrow activity, are more apt to demonstrate the presence of a slight increase in erythroid bone marrow mass. Such studies also show that the red cell production in patients with polycythemia vera is effective with the release of normal, long-lived red blood cells. Because of the increase in the number of erythroid cells in the bone marrow and circulating blood, a greater than normal amount of iron is "trapped" in the hemoglobin of these cells, and the tissue iron stores may become depleted. This trend is aggravated by the frequent therapeutic use of phlebotomy, by spontaneous nose and gastric bleedings, and by the lack of an "anemic stimulus" to intestinal iron absorption, and leads to an iron-deficient erythropoiesis. Fortunately, the production of microcytic and hypochromic cells may be of considerable symptomatic benefit, since the hematocrit and in turn the viscosity will become disproportionately lower than the red cell count.

Most symptoms are related to hypervolemia and hyperviscosity and are alleviated by phlebotomy. They frequently consist merely of nonspecific headaches, dizziness, blurred vision, and a feeling of "fullness in the head." Engorgement of thin-walled vessels may cause nose and gastric bleedings, serving as convenient means for spontaneous bloodletting. However, more serious symptoms may occur if the hyperviscosity causes venous stagnation, thrombosis, and embolization. Such events can cause fatal vascular accidents when they occur in cerebral, coronary, hepatic or intestinal veins.

The characteristic splenomegaly found in polycythemia vera may be caused in part by vascular engorgement but is probably more closely related to the development of extramedullary hematopoiesis, especially extramedullary granulocytopoiesis. The granulocyte count in polycythemia vera is regularly increased, although it rarely exceeds 30,000 cells per cu. mm. The resulting increase in granulocyte turnover is often reflected by an increase in serum and urine muramidase levels and in the concentration of B_{12} and B_{12} binders in serum. The granulocytes are usually mature and normally functioning, but more immature granulocytic elements may be present. The leukocyte alkaline phosphatase is either normal or high, a finding of uncertain functional significance but of use in distinguishing the granulocytosis of polycythemia vera from the granulocytosis of chronic myeloid leukemia. The granulocytes of polycythemia vera reportedly contain an increased amount of histidine decarboxylase, an enzyme involved in the production of histamine from histidine. Excessive histamine may be responsible for the common complaint of itching, especially following warm baths or showers.

The platelet count is regularly increased, but frequently not as much as would be expected from examining bone marrow specimens. These often reveal sheets of megakaryocytes, a finding which may justify bone marrow aspiration as a differential diagnostic test in the polycythemias. The characteristic tendency of patients with polycythemia vera to develop thrombotic complications is frequently related to the increased platelet count. However, morphologic and functional studies of platelets indicate that their adhesiveness is reduced and that despite their increased numbers they may not be responsible for these complications. Actually, studies by Spaet and co-workers on the coagulation process in this disease suggest the presence of impaired hemostasis with poor clot formation rather than hypercoagulability. In evaluating the results from such studies, it is important to realize that the plasma volume is relatively decreased in polycythemic blood and that the amount of available coagulation factors may not be adequate for the establishment of a firm red cell clot.

It is usually not difficult to make a diagnosis of polycythemia vera in patients with full-blown pancytosis and splenomegaly. However, early in the course, polycythemia vera may be more difficult to recognize, and Table 22–4 gives some of the findings of value in the differential diagnosis of various polycythemias. As the disease progresses, patients with polycythemia vera develop specific and characteristic complications not seen in the other polycythemias. The paradoxic occurrence of both thromboses and hemorrhages occurs quite frequently, and cerebral, coronary, mesenteric, or portal thrombosis may cause life-threatening situations in a patient who displays nasal, gastric, or dermal hemorrhages. In a considerable number of patients the disease slowly changes in character, with myelofibrosis and myeloid metaplasia becoming predominant features. These features are the results of excessive fibroblastic activity, an integral part of the general myelo-

TABLE 22–3 CLASSIFICATION OF POLYCYTHEMIAS
AND ANEMIAS

                     Dehydration
                     "Stress", "Spurious", "Tobacco "
            Absolute
            Primary
                     Polycythemia Vera
            Secondary
                  Appropriate
                     Altitude
                     Cardio-pulmonary disease
                     Hemoglobin abnormality
                     Cobalt
                  Inappropriate
                     Renal cyst and tumor
                     Various neoplasms

Anemias
     Relative
                     Pregnancy
                     Macroglobulinemia
     Absolute
            Stem Cell Disorders
                  Multipotential
                     Aplastic Anemia
                  Unipotential
                     Anemia of renal disease
                     Anemia of chronic disease
                     Anemia of endocrine disorders
                     Pure red cell aplasia

     Multiplication Disorders
                     Vitamin B_{12} deficiency
                     Folate deficiency
                     Refractory megaloblastic anemias
                     Antimetabolite therapy (methotrexate, 6 mercaptopurine)

     Cytoplasmic Maturation Disorders
            Porphyrias
                     Hereditary porphyrias
                     Acquired porphyrias (lead poisoning)

Table continued on the following page

stimulatory disease process. The reduction in available bone marrow space and the increase in splenic size will lead first to anemia and eventually to pancytopenia.

Acute myelogenous leukemia develops ultimately in about 10 to 15 per cent of patients with polycythemia vera. The occurrence of this dreaded complication has been reviewed by Modan and Lilienfeld and it was believed initially to be related to the therapeutic use of radioactive phosphorus. Recent reports, however, suggest that the use of so-called radiomimetic agents such as busulfan also may be followed by the development of acute myelogenous leukemia. Polycythemia vera was the first "neoplastic" disease with a long enough survival to make possible prolonged follow-up studies after the use of myelosuppres-

sive agents. The more recent successes in the treatment of Hodgkin's disease, breast cancer, chronic lymphatic leukemia, and transplantation rejection have permitted similar prolonged follow-ups after the use of other forms of radiation or radiomimetic drugs, and it has become clear that the development of acute myelogenous leukemia is an appreciable therapeutic hazard. So far the therapeutic results have been well worth the risk, but obviously these agents should be used with reluctance and caution.

Secondary. Secondary polycythemia is a condition characterized by an enhanced, erythropoietin-mediated stimulation of red cell production and an increased red cell mass. In most cases the erythropoietin release is an appropriate response to tissue hypoxia, but in some the

TABLE 22–3 *Continued* CLASSIFICATION OF
POLYCYTHEMIAS AND ANEMIAS

Iron
Iron deficiency anemia
Iron loading anemias
Globin
Structural Abnormality
Hemoglobinopathies (Sickle Cell Anemia)
Quantitative Abnormality
Thalassemias

Survival Disorders
Intrinsic
Hereditary spherocytosis
Hereditary elliptocytosis
Paroxysmal nocturnal hemoglobinuria
Enzymopathies (G-6-PD, P.K.)
Hemoglobinopathies
Extrinsic
Toxic Factors
Thermal burn
Chemical damage
Infection (malaria)
Hyperoxia (hyperbaric conditions)
Oxidative hemolysis due to drugs (sulfonamides)
Hypersplenism
Mechanical Factors
March hemoglobinuria
Traumatic cardiac hemolysis
Microangiopathic hemolytic anemia
Plasma Lipid Abnormality
Spur cell anemia of cirrhosis
Hereditary acanthocytosis
Immune Hemolysis
Isoimmune
Transfusion reaction
Erythroblastosis fetalis
Autoimmune
Cold type
Warm type
Blood Loss
Acute blood loss anemia

release is inappropriate and the resulting erythrocytosis presumably serves no useful function.

APPROPRIATE SECONDARY POLYCYTHEMIA

High Altitude. The erythrocytosis experienced by high altitude dwellers is probably the most common of the secondary polycythemias and it must be considered an appropriate physiologic adaptation rather than a pathologic disorder. However, sustained physiologic adaptations are usually achieved at a certain biologic cost, and individuals at high altitudes pay for an enhanced oxygen transport by problems related to hypervolemia, hyperviscosity, and hyperventilation.

Most studies of high-altitude polycythemia have been carried out in the small town of Morococha at 15,000 feet in the Peruvian Andes. Only a few precarious settlements exist above this altitude, the highest permanent settlement probably being Aucanguilcha in the Chilean Andes at 17,500 feet. At this level the atmospheric oxygen pressure is not much higher than the mean capillary oxygen pressure at sea level, making it very difficult to provide a downhill gradient for oxygen from air to cells. Above 17,500 feet only short-term sojourns are possible and no one has yet managed to reach the top of the world, Mt Everest, at 29,000 feet without being sustained by supplemental oxygen (Fig. 22–27).

The ability of the inhabitants of the mining town of Morococha to live active, strenuous lives

TABLE 22–4 DIFFERENTIAL DIAGNOSIS
OF POLYCYTHEMIAS

	Relative Polycythemia	Polycythemia Vera	Secondary Polycythemia
Hematocrit	Increased	Increased	Increased
Red blood cell mass	Normal	Increased	Increased
Erythropoietin	Normal	Absent	Increased
White blood count	Normal	Increased	Normal
Platelet count	Normal	Increased	Normal
Bone marrow	Normal	Hyperplastic	Erythroid hyperplasia
Spleen	Normal	Enlarged	Normal
Arterial oxygen saturation	Normal	Normal	Decreased or normal
Serum iron	Normal	Decreased	Normal
Serum B$_{12}$	Normal	Increased	Normal
Leukocyte alkaline phosphatase	Normal	Increased	Normal
Muramidase	Normal	Increased	Normal

at 15,000 feet is directly related to their adaptable oxygen transport system. The tissue requirements for oxygen are the same as or higher than at sea level, but increased pulmonary function, increased oxygen carrying capacity of blood and increased blood volume succeed in reducing the oxygen gradient needed to bring oxygen from the air to the tissues (Fig. 22–28). Such a reduction will ensure that the oxygen molecules in the capillaries are under enough pressure for their subsequent diffusion into the tissues.

Sustained hyperventilation causes a reduction in the oxygen gradient between ambient and alveolar air. Because of the inherent effect of dead space and water vapors, this part of the gradient can only be moderately reduced. However, hyperventilation causes a pulmonary "stretch" with enlargement of the alveolar diffusing area and almost eliminates the alveolar-capillary gradient. The most important reduction occurs in the arterial-venous gradient, permitting unloading of oxygen throughout the length of the capillary at a relatively high pressure. Since the tissue demands for oxygen are not reduced, the maintenance of a shallow gradient demands an increased flow of oxygen-carrying red blood cells through the tissues. Although an increase in cardiac output would accomplish just this, the added workload on a vital organ is unacceptable for chronic adjustments. Of more importance for the maintenance of an increased oxygen flow to the tissues is an increase in the red blood cell count.

Tissue hypoxia will lead to the release of erythropoietin which in turn will increase the rate of red cell production and enhance the oxygen carrying capacity of blood. Furthermore, the increased rate of red cell production will cause an increase in blood volume, with dilatation and opening of vessels, and an increase in tissue perfusion. This dual effect on oxygen flow far outweighs the moderate disadvantages derived from the higher viscosity of circulating blood.

A shift in the oxygen dissociation curve to the right would also reduce the arteriovenous gradient and enhance the unloading of oxygen in the

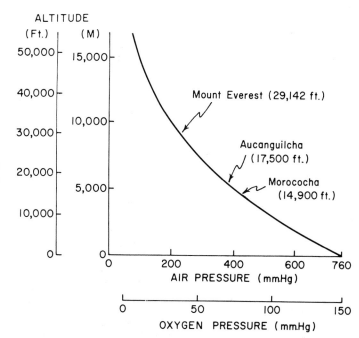

Figure 22–27 The oxygen pressure at altitudes inhabited or visited by man.

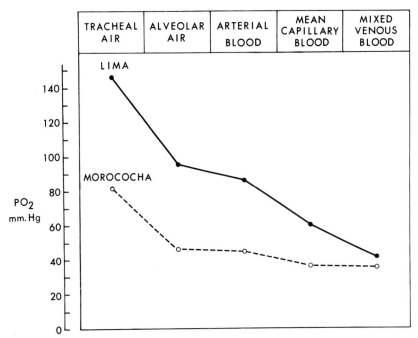

| TRACHEAL AIR | ALVEOLAR AIR | ARTERIAL BLOOD | MEAN CAPILLARY BLOOD | MIXED VENOUS BLOOD |

Figure 22-28 The oxygen gradient from lungs to tissues at sea level (Lima) or at 15,000 feet (Morococha). (Redrawn from Hurtado, A.: *In* Weihe, W. H. (ed.): Physiological Effects of High Altitude. New York, Pergamon Press, 1964, p.1.)

tissue capillaries (Fig. 22–29). Such a shift is undoubtedly of great importance in the initial adaptation to high altitudes, especially since it will tend to counteract the disadvantageous shift to the left induced by acute hyperventilation alkalosis. However, it is less certain whether it plays a significant role in chronic acclimatization. At that point the blood pH is usually normal and, as emphasized by Finch and Lenfant, an excessive shift to the right might significantly reduce the loading of hemoglobin in the lungs, an important consideration when the ambient oxygen pressure is about one half normal. It is of interest that the animals indigenous to high altitudes such as llamas and vicunas have oxygen dissociation curves positioned far to the left, suggesting that the adjustments of the shape of the curve in sustained acclimatization is aimed at improving the loading of oxygen in the lungs rather than at the unloading in the tissues.

The clinical manifestation of chronic high altitude acclimatization is dominated by ruddy cyanosis and physiologic emphysema. The vascular enlargement can be observed readily in the conjunctiva, mucous membrane, and skin and may contribute to the remarkable capacity of Sherpas to walk barefoot and sleep on ice and snow.

The blood studies reveal a normochromic and normocytic erythrocytosis, with increased red cell mass but only borderline increases in granulocyte or platelet counts. The plasma iron concentration is normal in contradistinction to polycythemia vera, in which it is usually low. This may

be due merely to blood loss and to therapeutic phlebotomies in polycythemia vera, but it has been suggested that tissue hypoxia as experienced at high altitudes enhances intestinal iron absorption. Erythropoietin titers in plasma and urine are increased, also in contradistinction to polycythemia vera, in which they are extremely low.

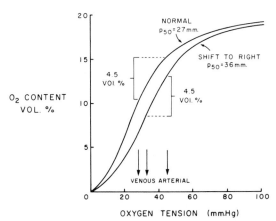

Figure 22-29 At low arterial oxygen tension (i.e., 45 mm.) the delivery of 4.5 vol % of oxygen from normal hemoglobin with a P_{50} of 27 mm. will reduce venous oxygen tension to 28 mm. A shift to the right, however, will permit the delivery of the same volume of oxygen with less reduction in venous oxygen tension (33 mm.).

It is difficult to evaluate the biologic cost of chronic acclimatization to high altitudes, since very few reliable data on the longevity and morbidity of high altitude dwellers exist. However, the compensatory reserves are undoubtedly decreased and the effect of cardiopulmonary disorders must be more serious than at sea level. So-called "chronic mountain sickness" (Monge's disease) is caused by an acquired refractoriness of the respiratory center leading to relative alveolar hypoventilation and excessive tissue hypoxia. Since this in turn will cause an increase in an already expanded red cell mass and higher blood viscosity, cardiovascular decompensation occurs. Therapeutic venesection provides symptomatic relief, but the individuals suffering from Monge's disease usually need to be brought down to sea level for permanent improvement.

Pulmonary Disease. Chronic pulmonary disease associated with cyanosis, clubbing, and arterial oxygen unsaturation is not always accompanied by an increase in hemoglobin concentration (Fig. 22–30). In some cases a concomitant increase in plasma volume may conceal the effect of an increased red cell mass, but in most cases true secondary polycythemia does not occur. The release of erythropoietin appears to be commensurate to the degree of tissue hypoxia, but for unknown reasons there is an unresponsiveness of the stem cells to this hormone or an impairment in the subsequent proliferation of nucleated red cells.

Cardiovascular Disease. Right-to-left shunt in congenital heart disease is characteristically associated with cyanosis, clubbing, and often extreme secondary appropriate polycythemia. Despite high hematocrit, hyperviscosity symptoms are rarely present, probably owing to the simultaneous increase in total blood volume. Whether or not to perform phlebotomy on blue babies prior to surgery is still an unanswered question, but most surgeons feel more comfortable if the hematocrit is brought down below 60 per cent by judicious phlebotomies. It certainly will provide a little more reserve if fluid intake becomes inadequate.

In acquired heart disease with chronic decompensation, erythrokinetic studies by Chodos and co-workers have shown that a mild increase in red cell production and red cell mass is usually present. However, the increased plasma volume prevents an accurate assessment of the size of the red cell mass from hematocrit determinations alone.

Alveolar Hypoventilation. Alveolar hypoventilation, whether related to central or peripheral impairment, causes arterial hypoxemia, cyanosis, and secondary polycythemia. Its two most colorful variants are Monge's chronic mountain sickness (see earlier) and the Pickwickian syndrome. In the latter syndrome, named by Ratto and co-workers, obesity, peripheral hypoventilation, hypercapnia, somnolence and central hypoventilation are involved in a vicious circle lead-

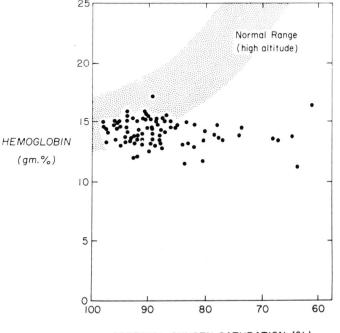

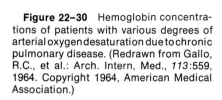

Figure 22–30 Hemoglobin concentrations of patients with various degrees of arterial oxygen desaturation due to chronic pulmonary disease. (Redrawn from Gallo, R.C., et al.: Arch. Intern, Med., *113*:559, 1964. Copyright 1964, American Medical Association.)

ing to the proverbial somnolent cyanosis of Mrs. Wardle's boy, Joe.

Defective Oxygen Transport. Secondary polycythemia is occasionally observed in patients with cyanosis due to acquired or congenital methemoglobinemia. However, the erythropoietic response in these patients is less than would be anticipated in cyanotic patients. Cyanosis may actually be present with as little as 1.5 grams of methemoglobin per 100 ml. in the circulation, an amount which in itself should not result in significant tissue hypoxia. An increase in oxygen affinity is also present in hemoglobin partially combined with carbon monoxide and is probably responsible for the polycythemia observed in heavy smokers.

Familial polycythemias have recently been described in a number of individuals with abnormal hemoglobins. In most of these, the amino acid substitution occurs in the contact area between the alpha and beta chains. Such substitutions interfere with the release of oxygen to the tissues, decrease the P_{50} and result in a compensatory erythrocytosis despite fully oxygenated arterial blood.

Drug-induced Tissue Hypoxia. Although a number of drugs and chemicals can induce histiotoxic anoxia, only cobalt has convincingly been associated with the development of a secondary appropriate polycythemia. Several recent studies have shown that cobalt administration causes the release of erythropoietin, and that this release presumably is related to its inhibitory effect on intracellular oxidative metabolism in the kidneys. Since histiotoxic anoxia is generalized (Fig. 22–19), the use of cobalt in the treatment of refractory anemias is of little benefit to the patient. His oxygen carrying capacity may increase, but merely enough to counteract the effect of the additional tissue hypoxia induced by cobalt.

INAPPROPRIATE SECONDARY POLYCYTHEMIA (TABLE 22–5)

Renal Disorders. A partial obstruction of the renal artery or its tributaries may cause localized renal hypoxia, the stimulus for erythropoietin production. However, an impaired blood supply to the kidneys usually causes structural damage and impaired erythropoietin production, and it is only the rare patient who responds with an increased release of erythropoietin and a secondary polycythemia. It is of potential importance that intrarenal vascular obstruction as observed in transplanted kidneys undergoing rejection will cause the release of erythropoietin. Unfortunately, the current assays are too laborious to permit the erythropoietin titer to be used to detect threatening rejection. However, the appearance of an increased number of nucleated red cells or reticulocytes in the circulating blood may be used as a warning signal.

TABLE 22–5   INAPPROPRIATE SECONDARY POLYCYTHEMIA

Location	Pathologic Condition	Number of Case Reports Until 1972
Kidney		
	Hypernephroma	118
	Other tumors	13
	Hydronephrosis	14
	Cystic disease	35
	Renal artery stenosis	2
	Transplantation rejection	7
	Bartter's syndrome	1
Liver		
	Hepatoma	64
Uterus		
	Leiomyoma	24
Cerebellum		
	Hemangioblastoma	50
Adrenal Gland		
	Pheochromocytoma	5

(Data from Thorling, E. B.: Scand. J. Haemat., Suppl. 17, 1972.)

A more common cause of secondary polycythemia is the presence of space-occupying renal lesions. These lesions can be cysts, either solitary or part of polycystic renal disease, hydronephrosis, or a variety of renal neoplasms. Erythropoietin assays of cyst fluid have disclosed the presence of erythropoietin, and it has been proposed that the tubular lining of cysts is capable of secreting erythropoietin. In regard to the neoplasms, assays of tumor extracts, especially extracts of hypernephromas, for erythropoietin have occasionally been positive. However, the fact that so many histologically different lesions can lead to an excessive production of erythropoietin has raised the suspicion that it is not the tumor cells which are engaged in inappropriate erythropoietin production, but it is the adjoining normal parenchyma which secretes this hormone in response to pressure-induced hypoxia.

Successful removal of renal tumors in patients with polycythemia has in many cases resulted in a normalization of the red blood cell count. Subsequent metastases in the opposite kidney have been associated with a recurrence of the polycythemia. However, the important question of whether or not extrarenal metastases can cause polycythemia has still not been answered.

Extrarenal Disorders. Cerebellar hemangiomas are an infrequent cause of secondary, inappropriate polycythemia. Cyst fluid from the tumor has, in a few cases, been shown to contain erythropoietic stimulatory material indistinguishable from erythropoietin. However, the proximity of the tumor to the respiratory center and to the hypothalamus has also suggested that central hypoventilation plays a role or that a hypothetical hypothalamic-renal connection is involved. In areas such as Hong Kong with a high incidence of hepatocarcinoma, 10 per cent of afflicted patients develop erythrocytosis. The most favored explanation is that the tumor is responsible for inappropriate secretion of erythropoietin, an explanation supported by direct assays of tumor extracts and by the finding that the liver normally produces small amounts of extrarenal erythropoietin. The rare polycythemia observed in patients with large uterine myomas may be caused by mechanical interference with renal blood supply. An inappropriate neoplastic production of erythropoietin by these fibrous, differentiated tumors seems unlikely in view of their histologic character. The occasional association with certain endocrine lesions such as Cushing's syndrome and pheochromocytomas is intriguing but has not been too informative. Steroid hormones appear to stimulate bone marrow activity mildly but the relationship between hypertension and erythropoietin is still quite tenuous. Although androgen-producing lesions have not been associated with polycythemia, androgens have empirically been found to be potent stimulators of erythropoiesis. This was first pointed out by Kennedy and co-workers, who 20 years ago observed the development of plethora and high hematocrits in women treated with androgens for breast cancer. The effect may be mediated via a release of renal erythropoietin, although some data suggest a direct action of androgens on the bone marrow stem cell pool.

ANEMIA

General Effects of Anemia

The pathophysiologic effects of a reduced oxygen carrying capacity of blood are all related to tissue hypoxia and to the compensatory mechanisms mobilized to alleviate this hypoxia. Tissue hypoxia occurs when the pressure head of oxygen in the capillaries is too low to provide distant cells with enough oxygen for their metabolic needs. This may happen despite the presence of several times the needed oxygen in the circulating blood. Using approximate figures for a normal adult, the red cell mass has to provide the tissues with about 250 ml. of oxygen per minute to support life. Since the oxygen-carrying capacity of normal blood is 1.34 ml. per gram hemoglobin or about 20 ml. per 100 ml. of normal blood and the cardiac output is about 5000 ml. per minute, 1000 ml. of oxygen per minute is made available at the tissue level. The extraction of one

fourth of this amount will reduce the oxygen tension of 100 mm. Hg in the arterial end of the capillary to 40 mm. Hg in the venous end. This partial extraction will maintain a diffusion pressure throughout the capillaries sufficient to provide all cells within a truncated cone segment with enough oxygen for their metabolism (Fig. 22–31). In anemia, the extraction of the same amount of oxygen would lead to greater hemoglobin desaturation and a lower oxygen tension at the venous end of the capillary. Since this would result in destructive cellular hypoxia or anoxia in the immediate vicinity, compensatory and frequently symptomatic adjustment in the supply of blood and oxygen must be mobilized in order to keep the oxygen gradient almost unchanged (see review by Finch and Lenfant in 1977).

Decreased Oxygen Affinity. One of the earliest and least traumatic adjustments is a shift in the oxygen dissociation curve to the right, permitting the extraction of increased amounts of oxygen without a decrease in oxygen pressure. As mentioned before, the position of the oxygen dissociation curve is in part dependent on the intracellular pH. At an acid pH, as experienced in tissues in which anemic hypoxia has led to anaerobic metabolism and lactic acid accumulation, the curve will be shifted to the right, the so-called Bohr effect (Fig. 22–14). More important, however, is a stimulation of the production of 2,3 diphosphoglycerate. The reason for this stimulation in anemia is not clear, but it has been suggested that the binding of free 2,3-DPG to deoxygenated hemoglobin, present in increased amounts in anemia, will result in a compensatory increase in glycolysis and 2,3-DPG production. Alternately, deoxygenated hemoglobin may cause enough intracellular alkalosis to stimulate glycosis and 2,3-DPG production. The binding of 2,3-DPG to reduced hemoglobin stabilizes the molecule in its low-affinity state and facilitates the unloading of oxygen in the tissues. According to Torrance et al., this change in oxygen affinity plays a substantial role in reducing the arteriovenous oxygen pressure gradient and in minimizing cellular hypoxia (Fig. 22–32).

Increased Tissue Perfusion. Redistribution of blood from tissues with fairly low oxygen requirements and high blood supply such as skin or kidneys to oxygen-dependent tissues such as brain and myocardium provides an early and efficient protection of these vital tissues. The metabolic price for maintaining a high oxygen tension in some selective organs or tissues appears reasonable. Subcutaneous vasoconstriction and oxygen deprivation are tolerated well, since dermal blood supply is geared more toward temperature regulation than toward oxygen delivery. The same is true for the kidney, in which the blood supply is far in excess of the oxygen requirement. The effect on renal excretory function is relatively minor, since

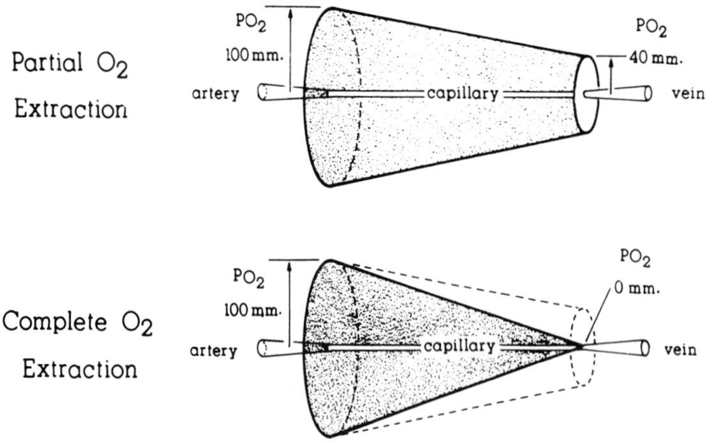

Partial O₂
Extraction

Complete O₂
Extraction

Figure 22–31   A hypothetical model of the tissue cone provided by oxygen when the blood is partially or completely extracted of oxygen.

the decrease in blood supply is offset by the increase in "plasma crit" of the perfusing anemic blood.

Increased Cardiac Output. In mild to moderate anemia, the combined effects of decreased oxygen affinity and selective redistribution of blood maintain oxygen pressure at close to normal levels, and these anemias are usually quite asymptomatic. However, with more severe anemias it becomes necessary to increase cardiac output in order to provide the tissues with enough oxygen. Although the low viscosity of anemic blood and the peripheral vasodilatation reduce the workload on the heart, the metabolic cost and the wear and tear on the moving part of the cardiac pump make an increase in cardiac output an undesirable device for long-term compensation.

The clinical manifestations of severe anemia are to a great extent caused by the compensatory cardiac overactivity. Pallor is due primarily to dermal vasoconstriction and blood redistribution, but tachycardia and symptoms of decreased cardiac reserve are related to cardiac stress. The characteristic shortness of breath of severe anemia may be a sign of incipient cardiopulmonary failure rather than a manifestation of ventilatory compensation to the anemia. Owing to the almost complete saturation of anemic blood with oxygen in the lungs, a pulmonary compensation would actually be of little practical importance.

Increased Red Cell Production. The most appropriate but also the slowest compensatory device in anemia is an increase in the rate of red cell production. Tissue hypoxia will lead to increased erythropoietin production within four to seven hours, but owing to the time lag from stem cell differentiation to the release of reticulocytes from the bone marrow, a compensatory increase in the number of circulating red cells does not begin until four to five days later. Increased erythropoietin titers in serum and urine (Fig. 22–22) causing increased bone marrow activity may be associated with sternal pain or tenderness and the presence of large immature reticulocytes on the blood smear.

These compensatory mechanisms are all designed to keep the capillary oxygen pressure up and the oxygen delivery adequate for the cellular needs. However, a complete rectification of tissue hypoxia cannot occur until the hemoglobin concentration has been restored to normal. Some degree of tissue hypoxia is needed in order to provide a driving force for the various compensatory devices. The symptomatology of such remaining hypoxia is difficult to separate from that of the compensatory mechanisms, but leg cramps, angina pectoris, and light-headedness appear to be caused directly by tissue hypoxia.

Stem Cell Disorders

Under physiologic conditions, the red cell mass is maintained at an optimal size by appropriate adjustments in the rate of transformation of stem cells to nucleated red blood cells. These adjustments are accomplished by feedback systems, and

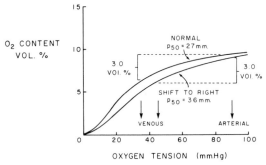

Figure 22–32 This figure depicts the effect on venous oxygen tension when 3.0 vol. % of oxygen is extracted from normal hemoglobin in an anemic individual. A shift to the right will permit this extraction of 3 vol. % with less reduction in venous oxygen tension and therefore an enhanced tissue oxygenation.

a disruption at any point in the circuits of these systems will lead to disordered stem cell function and anemia. A disordered function of the multipotential stem cells such as observed in patients with aplastic anemia is usually believed to be caused by an intrinsic defect of the stem cells themselves. However, very little is known of their regulation, and it is possible that cellular dysfunction is secondary to defective feedback signals from the immediate microenvironment.

The feedback system regulating the unipotential erythropoietin-sensitive stem cells is much better understood, and it is now possible to relate various aregenerative anemias to defects in specific key stations in this circuit. The major distinction between disorders of the multipotential and the unipotential stem cells is that multipotential stem cell disorders are characterized by pancytopenia and unipotential stem cell disorders by erythrocytopenia.

Disorders of Multipotential Stem Cells

APLASTIC ANEMIA. Aplastic anemia is a bone marrow disorder characterized by a reduction in the number and function of multipotential stem cells. This reduction leads in turn to a decrease in the volume of active blood-cell–producing bone marrow and to a pancytopenia. The remaining marrow becomes confined to small, often intensely active islands surrounded by fatty tissue. This fatty replacement is the sine qua non of true aplastic anemia.

The clinical manifestations are all directly related to the pancytopenia. The anemia may cause weakness, fatigue, and pallor; the granulocytopenia may cause fever and infections; and the thrombocytopenia may cause hemorrhages, hematomas, and petechiae. Hepatomegaly and splenomegaly are unusual findings in the early phase of the disease and their presence should lead to reevaluation of the diagnosis. However, after prolonged illness, recurrent infections may produce a reactive macrophage hyperplasia of the spleen, and transfusion hemosiderosis may lead to hepatomegaly and congestive splenomegaly.

The anemia is often macrocytic, and the reticulocytes are few in number but relatively immature. These findings reflect an accelerated bone marrow transit time and release, possibly caused by a high level of erythropoietin or by the crowded environment in the remaining bone marrow islands. Ferrokinetic studies reveal a reduced plasma iron turnover but this reduction may be difficult to appreciate, since the normal baseline value is quite low.

Of greater importance for the demonstration of a reduced rate of red cell production are the iron clearance time and the red cell utilization of iron. The reduced bone marrow mass can clear iron from plasma only slowly, giving extramedullary tissues such as liver or spleen extra time in which to compete with the marrow for circulating radio-

active iron. The result is a prolonged iron clearance time and a low red cell iron utilization. This combination is characteristic for all anemias caused by a reduction in erythropoietic tissue and distinguishes them from anemias caused by ineffective red cell production. In the latter anemias, intramedullary destruction of nucleated red cells will also cause a low utilization of radioactive iron, but the iron clearance is short because of an abundance of erythropoietic bone marrow (Fig. 22–33). This distinction is of particular importance in establishing whether pancytopenia is caused by bone marrow hypoplasia or by ineffective cellular production. This latter condition has been called "aplastic anemia with a hyperplastic bone marrow," a confusing term for a condition that often is preleukemic and may be pathogenetically quite different from aplastic anemia.

Both plasma iron and erythropoietin concentrations are high in aplastic anemia, probably reflecting decreased utilization by a reduced bone marrow mass. The high plasma iron concentration may cause excessive tissue incorporation of iron and eventually hemosiderosis. Bone marrow preparations disclose many siderotic granules in the reticulum cells, but since maturation of the individual nucleated red cells is normal, siderotic granules in these cells are seen only rarely. The high erythropoietin titer in plasma and urine has made patients with aplastic anemia useful sources for the preparation of erythropoietin concentrates.

In some patients with aplastic anemia, particularly in children, there may be a substantial increase in the production of fetal hemoglobin. This challenging but still unexplained finding is of great potential interest, since it may provide a clue for the mechanism by which gamma chain production can be activated, a mechanism of potential use for patients with sickle cell anemia or Cooley's anemia.

Absolute granulocytopenia is always present in aplastic anemia and its severity will determine to a great extent the immediate prognosis. As a rough guide, an absolute granulocyte count of less than 200 per cu. mm. suggests imminent danger of infectious complications and demands some kind of a sheltered environment. In addition to an absolute granulocytopenia, there is often a reduction in the total number of lymphocytes. The reason for this reduction is not known but the functional significance is apparently of little importance, since immunoglobulin synthesis and delayed sensitivity reactions are usually intact.

Thrombocytopenia with its dramatic and visible hemorrhagic manifestations is also always part of the clinical picture of advanced aplastic anemia. Because of the insidious onset of this disease, it is difficult to assess the sequence by which the various cytopenias appear. However, during the recovery phase, thrombocytopoiesis is often the last

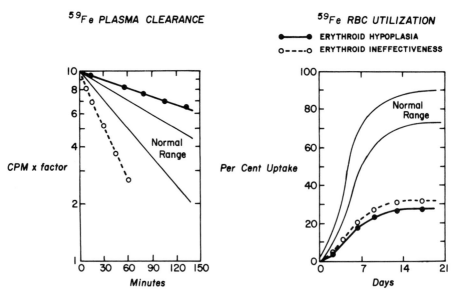

Figure 22–33 Plasma clearance and red cell utilization of radioactive iron in normals, patients with erythroid hypoplasia, and patients with ineffective red cell production. The clearance rate of ^{59}Fe injected intravenously at time 0 was determined by serial measurements of the radioactivity (C.P.M.) over a 3-hour period. The subsequent utilization of the ^{59}Fe for hemoglobin synthesis was estimated by measuring the total radioactivity in circulating red cells (Red cell mass × C.P.M.) and relating it in per cent to the total amount of ^{59}Fe injected. Although the utilization of ^{59}Fe is equally reduced in patients with erythroid hypoplasia or with erythroid ineffectiveness, the plasma clearance rate readily separates them from each other.

bone marrow function to recover and many patients may have thrombocytopenia for years after the other cytopenias have been corrected.

Etiology and Pathogenesis (Table 22-6). Numerous drugs, illnesses, and physical agents have the capacity to alter stem cell function presumably by interfering with intracellular metabolism.

TABLE 22-6 ETIOLOGIC CLASSIFICATION OF APLASTIC ANEMIA

I. Idiopathic
  A. *Constitutional* (Fanconi's anemia)
  B. *Acquired*

II. Secondary
  A. *Chemical and physical agents*
    Drugs
    Nonpharmacologic chemicals
    Radiation
  B. *Infectious*
    Viral (Hepatitis)
    Bacterial (Miliary TB)
  C. *Metabolic*
    Pancreatitis
    Pregnancy
  D. *Immunologic*
    Antibody
    Graft-vs.-host
  E. *Neoplastic*
    Myelophthisic anemia
  F. *Paroxysmal nocturnal hemoglobinuria*

However, these agents could also alter the stem cell microenvironment, and the relative importance of "seed" and "soil" in the pathogenesis of aplastic anemia is still not resolved. Although statistical and clinical cause-effect relationships between a specific agent or event and the development of aplastic anemia can be quite impressive, aplastic anemia is a disease in which the etiology can be only suspected, not established. No in-vitro test system is capable of duplicating the in-vivo events, and in-vivo tests in patients are too potentially dangerous to be justified. This makes the designation of an etiologic agent a question of judgment and clinical experience, hallowed but quite vulnerable criteria. In patients without exposure to a suggestive etiologic agent, the term "idiopathic" is used to conceal our ignorance. Obviously, even in these cases an etiologic agent must exist and may be present among the host of environmental toxins which have become part of our civilized existence.

Drugs and Chemicals. The drugs suspected of being potentially toxic for the hematopoietic stem cells have been listed in booklets published by the American Medical Association in 1965 and 1967 and include about 329 items. (See also review by Williams and co-workers, 1973). Table 22-7 lists those drugs with a strong etiologic relationship to aplastic anemia. It is a difficult list to interpret, since it does not give the actual incidence, the number of cases per number of patients receiving

TABLE 22-7 DRUGS LISTED BY A.M.A. AS BEING ASSOCIATED WITH THE DEVELOPMENT OF APLASTIC ANEMIA IN MORE THAN FIVE INSTANCES

	Number of Cases Receiving Drug Alone, or Drug in Combination with Nontoxic Drugs	Number of Cases Receiving Drug in Combination with Potentially Toxic Drug
Acetazolamide	3	7
Chloramphenicol	182	156
Chlordiazepoxide HCl	2	7
Chlorothiazide	2	13
Chlorpheniramine	2	15
Chlorpromazine	3	18
Chlorpropamide	4	2
Colchicine	2	3
Diphenylhydantoin sodium	3	21
Epinephrine	2	4
Gold salts	8	2
Mepazine	4	1
Meprobamate		15
Penicillin	4	91
Phenacetin	3	31
Phenantoin	9	14
Phenylbutazone	18	22
Potassium perchlorate	6	4
Primidone	2	6
Prochlorperazine	1	9
Pyrimethamine	2	3
Quinacrine HCl	3	2
Salicylamide	2	3
Streptomycin		31
Sulfadimethoxine	2	4
Sulfamethoxypyridazine	3	11
Sulfisoxazole	3	30
Sulfonamides	4	17
Tolbutamide	7	5
Trimethadione	2	4

the particular drug. However, it is possible to make a mental adjustment and realize that the incidence of aplastic anemia following treatment with aspirin or penicillin must be much lower than that following treatment with phenantoin, gold salts, or phenylbutazone. Furthermore, the incidence following treatment with the nitrobenzene compound chloramphenicol must be far higher than that following treatment with any other commonly used drug.

Many attempts have been made to relate potential toxicity to the presence of a benzene or nitrobenzene radical in the chemical structure of suspected drugs. Benzene itself is a major bone marrow toxin capable of inducing both aplastic anemia and leukemia, and in addition to chloramphenicol, many benzene-related chemicals such as trinitrotoluene, toluene, and the insecticides lindane and DDT have been strongly suspected of inducing aplastic anemia. However, many drugs without the benzene radical also appear to be toxic to stem cells, and the common denominator may reside in an intermediate metabolic product rather than in the parent molecule.

Because of the high incidence of aplastic anemia in patients receiving chloramphenicol special efforts have been made to clarify the mechanism of the toxic action of this drug on the bone marrow. Although we talk about "high" incidence, it has to be emphasized that only one out of 10,000 to 20,000 treated patients develops aplastic anemia and that prospective metabolic studies are almost impossible. However, mild, reversible bone marrow suppression is observed in most treated patients, a suppression related to drug dosage and length of treatment. Clinically it can easily be recognized by a decrease in reticulocyte counts and an increase in serum iron concentration. Bone marrow examination reveals vacuolization of erythroid cells. After prolonged treatment vacuolization can be observed in other cellular elements as well, and granulocytopenia and thrombocytopenia may ensue. These effects were initially thought to be related to a suppressive action on the ribosomal protein synthesis similar to the action of chloramphenicol on the bacterial cells. However, in-vitro studies of bone marrow suspensions by Yunis and co-workers have suggested that in the mammalian cell chloramphenicol inhibits mitochondrial protein synthesis. Since many consider the mitochondria to be intracellular inclusions of plant origin with independent mechanisms for replication and metabolism, this finding could provide a link between the bacteriostatic and the bone marrow suppressive actions of chloramphenicol.

It is tempting to consider the suppressive action of the bone marrow as an early, still reversible manifestation of a stem cell injury which eventually leads to irreversible aplastic anemia. However, it seems more likely that patients who develop aplastic anemia have an abnormal response to the bone marrow suppressive effect of chloramphenicol. Not only is the regularly occurring suppression readily reversible even after prolonged treatment with large amounts of chloramphenicol, but many patients who develop aplastic anemia do so weeks or months after exposure to relatively small amounts of this drug. It has been proposed that the few unfortunate victims have an underlying genetic or acquired hypersensitivity to chloramphenicol. This could reside in the rate or extent of detoxification of the drug or in a specific stem cell abnormality. In-vitro studies of bone marrow from patients who have recovered from aplastic anemia or from their immediate relatives have suggested a greater than normal susceptibility to the suppressive action of chloramphenicol. However, we are still far from having established the pathogenetic mode of action of chloramphenicol or from having learned how to predict individual hypersensitivity to this or to other potentially toxic drugs.

Radiation. Bone marrow suppression is a well-recognized side-effect of the diagnostic and therapeutic use of radiation. Radiation energy, whether mediated by a direct hit of waves or particles or by the production of highly reactive free radicals, is capable of breaking molecular bonds in critical intracellular macromolecules. Although all cells can be injured by radiation energy, organ systems dependent on a rapid cellular turnover of nucleic acids are particularly vulnerable. These systems can be ranked, according to Cronkite and Bond, with regard to radiosensitivity as follows: (1) germinal cells of the testes, (2) hematopoietic cells, (3) intestinal cells, and (4) epidermal basal cells.

Brief exposure to radiation of high energy as in reactor accidents leads to extensive destruction of the bone marrow and intestine, and death is usually caused by acute granulocytopenia and thrombocytopenia and by intestinal ulcerations. If the patient should survive the acute effects the recovery is usually almost complete, since the dormant multipotential stem cells will have sustained very little radiation injury and are capable of bone marrow repopulation. In the aftermath of the atomic attacks on Nagasaki, for example, Kirschbaum and his Japanese co-workers found that aplastic anemia was observed in only a very small number of survivors.

Prolonged exposure to more moderate doses of radiation, on the other hand, may cause chronic bone marrow failure and aplastic anemia. This has been described in patients vigorously treated with external or internal total body radiation and in Martland's famous report on watch-dial painters who accidentally ingested paint containing radium with a long biologic half-life. It has also been suspected as a pathogenetic mechanism in aplastic anemia occurring in physicians or radiologists exposed to minimal amounts of radiation for many years, but as is the case for exposure to drugs and chemicals a definite cause-effect relationship can never be firmly established. The reason for defective bone marrow repopulation after chronic radiation exposure may reside in the fact that multipotential stem cells are activated and then share in the radiation injury. An alternative explanation for the development of aplastic anemia after chronic radiation has been provided by Knospe and co-workers; namely, that radiation-induced damage to the "endothelial stem cells" will change the structural microenvironment of the bone marrow and prevent bone marrow regeneration.

Immunologic Rejection. Aplastic anemia has been associated with a variety of seemingly unrelated diseases. Miliary tuberculosis has always been listed prominently among such disorders, but a critical evaluation of reported cases indicates that this association is rare indeed. Hepatitis with its many immunologic manifestations looms much larger as a possible etiologic event, and aplastic anemia associated with complement-sensitive red cells and nocturnal hemoglobinuria has been described so frequently by Lewis and Dacie in England and Vincent and de Gruchy in Australia that this combination ought to contain some clue to etiology or pathogenesis.

The most reasonable explanation is that an immunologic mechanism underlies the development of aplastic anemia. Support for this hypothesis is that aplastic anemia has been described after the transfusion of whole blood or bone marrow into immunologically deficient children. Miller has suggested that the disease in these unfortunate patients reflects a graft-versus-host immunologic rejection of either hematopoietic or structural stem cells. The therapeutic implication of such a concept would be to use immunosuppressive drugs, a most difficult decision to make because of the inherent bone marrow suppressive effect of currently used drugs. The effect of prednisone in aplastic anemia has unfortunately been too erratic to be of use in pathogenetic considerations and at present the possibility that aplastic anemia is another "autoimmune" disorder is merely a hypothesis.

Constitutional. Fanconi's anemia is a form of aplastic anemia which occurs as an inborn defect associated with other congenital abnormalities such as skin pigmentations, renal hypoplasia, absent thumb or radius, and microcephaly. Multiple abnormalities of the chromosomal pattern of lymphocytes and bone marrow cells have been described, but whether or not the basic disorder resides in the hematopoietic or the structural stem cells is no better known here than in the acquired cases. Of great interest, however, has been the demonstration by Shahidi and Diamond that the hypoplastic bone marrow in Fanconi's anemia appears to be quite responsive to the myelostimulatory effect of androgens. Many patients have been kept alive and well on a maintenance regimen of androgens, and these results have led to a revival of the therapeutic use of androgens in all cases of aplastic anemia. Androgens do enhance erythropoietin release, but this cannot explain their occasional effect on granulocyte and thrombocyte production and, as emphasized by Gardner and co-workers, they must have some direct or indirect action on the hematopoietic or the structural bone marrow stem cells.

The pathogenesis of cellular aplasia in a bone marrow injured by various toxins or illnesses has been clarified by recent successes with bone marrow transplantation. Until then, it was argued vigorously whether aplastic anemia was a disease of the "seed" or of the "soil", of hematopoietic stem cells or of structural, supporting cells. However, as reported by Storb, Thomas, and co-workers, the clear-cut "takes" of transplanted bone marrow cells leading in some cases to cures of aplastic anemia have shown that aplastic anemia is a disease of the hematopoietic stem cells. Although these cells are present and may form small and even large foci of hematopoietic cells, they are not capable of normal renewal and growth and can not reseed the fatty bony marrow stroma, as emphasized by Kansu and Erslev, this defect in proliferation is associated with defects in differentiation leading to the production of macrocytic red cells containing excessive fetal hemoglobin and being abnormally sensitive to the action of complement. The therapeutic implication is obviously to attempt to replace these abnormal stem cells with transfused normal stem cells. This has been accomplished with identical twins and with bone marrow from well-matched siblings, but is still not feasible between unrelated donor-recipient pairs.

Disorders of Unipotential Stem Cells

RENAL DISEASE. Anemia is a hallmark of chronic renal disease and is roughly proportional to the degree of renal failure as measured by urea or creatinine retention. Since the pathogenesis of the anemia and the uremia is related to the failure of many independent functions, it is actually surprising that the proportionality is as good as depicted in Figure 22–34. The two major failing functions are the renal excretory function and the renal endocrine function.

Failure of Renal Excretory Function

HEMOLYSIS. The red cell of patients with uremia frequently shows multiple tiny spicles (Fig. 22–35). The presence of this so-called burring has been related to the accumulation of toxic end-products in the circulation and has been thought to be responsible for an impaired sodium-potassium pump activity and a shortened red cell life span. However, the correlation between azotemia and red cell life span is poor (Fig. 22–36), and when hemolysis occurs, it is often related more closely to changes in the microvasculature than to the degree of uremia. Indeed, extensive red cell fragmentation and hemolysis can be observed in patients with malignant vascular hypertension or with inflammatory vascular changes (hemolytic uremic syndrome) and with only mildly elevated BUN or creatinine concentrations. At present it seems most reasonable to relate the premature destruction of red cells in chronic renal disease to mechanical disruption of metabolically fragile red cells.

BLEEDING TENDENCY. As a manifestation of chronic renal disease, purpura is almost as characteristic as pallor. In addition to subcutaneous bleedings, gastrointestinal and uterine hemorrhage may cause a considerable loss of blood and increase the demands for an accelerated rate of red cell production. Iatrogenic blood loss should also not be forgotten. Patients with chronic renal disease are usually monitored by multiple laboratory tests and, if also hemodialyzed, may lose some blood in the dialysis coil. All in all, iron deficiency is one of the most common — but fortunately very treatable — problems in patients with chronic renal disease. The pathogenesis of the bleeding tendency is poorly understood, since thrombocytopenia and coagulation factor deficiency, when present, are rarely severe enough to be responsible for overt blood loss. Studies by Horowitz and co-workers, however, suggest that certain retention products may affect normal platelet function and cause an abnormal bleeding time, clot retraction, platelet adhesion, and platelet aggregation.

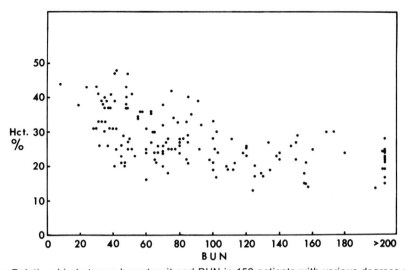

Figure 22–34 Relationship between hematocrit and BUN in 152 patients with various degrees of renal failure and uremia. (From Erslev, A. J.: Arch. Intern. Med., *126*:774–780, 1970. Reprinted from Wesson, L. G. (ed.): Physiology of the Human Kidney, 1969, by permission of Grune & Stratton, Inc., New York.)

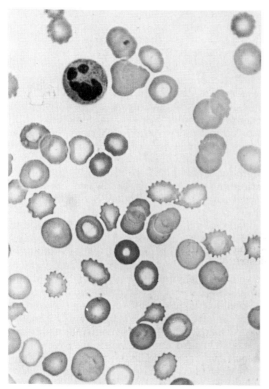

Figure 22–35 Burr cells in smear of blood from a patient with severe uremia.

The responsible toxic factor is believed to be a guanidino compound, and intensive dialysis has been found to reduce the bleeding tendency.

RESPONSIVENESS TO ERYTHROPOIETIN. In chronic renal failure there is both inadequate production of erythropoietin (see later) and decreased bone marrow response to erythropoietin (Fig. 22–37). The reason is not known, but the degree of responsiveness appears to be related to the severity of uremia. It seems probable that the improvement in erythropoietic function found after intensive dialysis is caused by an increased response to available erythropoietin rather than to an increased production of erythropoietin. Because of this refractory condition, it is anticipated that much more erythropoietin will be needed to abolish the anemia of chronic renal disease than is required for normal erythropoietic maintenance.

Failure of Renal Endocrine Function. The various effects of uremia on the rate of red cell destruction and production result in an increased demand for erythropoietin. This demand could easily be met by a normal but apparently not by an abnormal kidney. Impaired renal tissue is not capable of producing normal quantities of erythropoietin unless stimulated by intensive anemic hypoxia, and a balance between the rates of red cell destruction and red cell production is not achieved except at anemic levels. Under conditions of progressive kidney failure, the hypoxic stimulus needed to produce adequate amounts of renal erythropoietin becomes greater and the anemia more severe. However, even anephric individuals continue to manufacture red blood cells (Fig. 22–38). This residual erythropoietic activity appears to be generated by the release of extrarenal erythropoietin but the hemoglobin concentration which can be maintained in anephric patients is usually too low to be compatible with life and has to be augmented by transfusions.

CHRONIC DISORDERS. Although one of the most common of anemias, the anemia of chronic disorders is of relatively little clinical significance, since it is rarely severe enough to cause symptoms

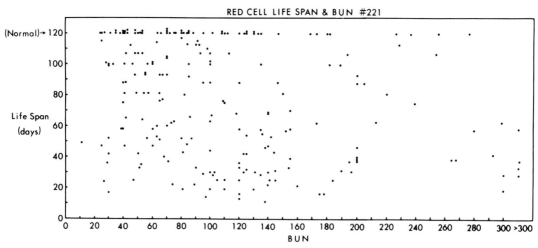

Figure 22–36 Relationship between red cell life span and BUN of 221 patients with various degrees of renal failure and uremia. (From Erslev, A. J.: Arch. Intern. Med., *126*:774, 1970. Copyright 1970, American Medical Association.)

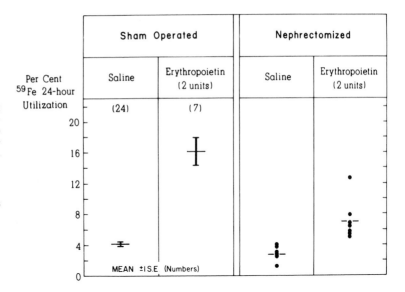

Figure 22–37 Erythropoietic response of normal and nephrectomized rats to the same amount of erythropoietin. On Day 0, the animals were transfused with 20 ml. per kg. of rat red cells. On Day 3, they were either nephrectomized or sham operated, and then given 2 units erythropoietin sc. On Day 4, ^{59}Fe was injected IV and its utilization determined 24 hours later.

or demand active transfusion therapy. On the other hand, it probably has been treated by more unneeded and ineffective hematinics than any other anemia, and the pathogenesis of this refractory anemia is still a fascinating enigma.

During the early part of this century, anemia was an invariable complication of many chronic debilitating infections, such as tuberculosis, osteomyelitis, or brucellosis, and it was known as anemia of chronic infection. With the change in the ecology of disease, it was realized that a similar anemia also occurred in patients with chronic, noninfectious diseases, such as rheumatoid arthritis, lymphomas, or disseminated carcinomas, and the anemia was given the noncommittal name of anemia of chronic disorders. It is characterized by a moderate reduction in hemoglobin concentra-

tion, a reduction in the level of both serum iron and iron-binding capacity, an increased amount of storage iron in the macrophages of the bone marrow, and a normal or elevated serum ferritin concentration.

The presence of decreased amounts of circulating iron, despite abundant iron stores, is probably caused by a defective iron release mechanism by the macrophages. The erythroid cells in the bone marrow apparently can handle available iron, and the utilization of radioactive iron is normal. However, the reutilization of iron is decreased (Fig. 22–39), indicating that hemoglobin iron, which normally is reutilized after being processed by the macrophages, is trapped in these cells and removed from the dynamic iron economy of the body. This relative iron deficiency is aggravated by a

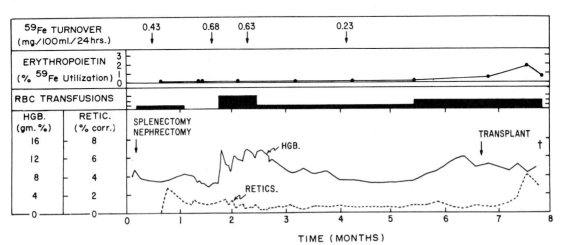

Figure 22–38 Erythropoietic status of a patient who underwent nephrectomy and splenectomy seven months before a successful kidney transplantation. Although erythropoietin levels were unmeasurable, reticulocytes were produced throughout the anephric period.

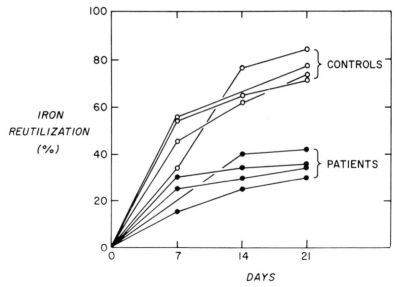

Figure 22–39 Reutilization of radioactive iron in normal individuals and in patients with anemia of chronic disease. Hemoglobin labeled with ^{59}Fe was injected intravenously and the combined process of hemoglobin sequestration, ^{59}Fe release and ^{59}Fe incorporation into new red cells (reutilization) was estimated by measuring the appearance of radioactivity in circulating red cells. (Redrawn from Haurani, F. I., Burke, W., and Martinez, E. J.: J. Lab. Clin. Med., *65*:560–570, 1965.)

moderate shortening of the red blood cell life span, resulting in a mild anemia. However, it has always been a puzzle why the anemia of chronic disorders does not display the morphologic characteristics of an iron deficiency anemia but is normocytic and normochromic, as if the basic defect resides in the stem cells. Recent studies by Ward and coworkers have suggested that there may indeed be an element of stem cell failure, since the serum level and the 24-hour excretion of erythropoietin are subnormal. No renal injury or abnormality can be held responsible for this defect, and studies so far have not shown any change in red cell oxygen affinity. Consequently, it is possible that the anemia of chronic disorders may reflect a primary defect in the oxygen sensing device or in the erythropoietin-producing cells. It is hoped that the unraveling of the pathogenesis of the anemia may provide us not only with means to correct the anemia but also with basic knowledge as to the relationship between erythropoietin production and iron metabolism.

ENDOCRINE DISORDERS

Pituitary and Thyroid Dysfunction. Pituitary and thyroid dysfunction or ablation are characteristically associated with a moderate normochromic, normocytic anemia. Although many attempts have been made to assign a specific erythropoietic effect to the thyroid, pituitary, or hypothalamic secretions, most current studies indicate that the anemia is an appropriate response to a decreased cellular demand for oxygen. The administration of thyroxin, triiodothyronine, or

desiccated thyroid will increase this demand, and the rate of red cell production will respond appropriately. It is questionable whether the administration of growth hormone, ACTH, or gonadal hormones are of additional benefit. In many cases of myxedema or other hypothyroid conditions, the anemia is somewhat atypical because of associated nutritional deficiencies. Malabsorption of B_{12} or folic acid may lead to a megaloblastic, macrocytic blood picture and the frequent uterine bleedings in hypothyroid females may lead to an iron-deficient, microcytic, hypochromic anemia. Even in hypothyroid men, the common achlorhydria may result in malabsorption of iron and an iron deficiency anemia.

Despite the erythropoietic effect of increased oxygen consumption induced by thyroid hormones, patients with hyperthyroidism or thyrotoxicosis are rarely polycythemic. This may be explained by the fact that thyroid hormones also increase cardiac output and tissue perfusion, making an increase in red cell mass less needed. Nevertheless, direct measurements by Muldowney and co-workers of red cell mass and plasma volume suggest that the absence of a high hematocrit in these conditions is caused by a concomitant increase in plasma volume, and that hyperthyroidism will cause true secondary polycythemia as defined by an increased red cell mass.

Gonadal Dysfunction. In normal mature men the hemoglobin concentration is about 1 to 2 grams higher than in normal females, whereas the male hemoglobin concentration in childhood, in advanced age, and in gonadal deficiency states is similar to that of females. This phenomenon has led to the assumption that physiologic excretions of androgens have an erythropoietic effect on the bone marrow. Conversely, it has been postulated that physiologic doses of estrogens cause a slight suppression of red cell production. Many experimental data on castrated animals have been marshaled to support these contentions, but unfortunately many studies were designed to prove rather than to test, and the erythropoietic effects of physiologic doses of gonadal hormones are still not quite clear. More impressive are the data indicating that androgens in pharmacologic doses can stimulate red cell production and even cause full-blown secondary polycythemia (Fig. 22–40). This effect may be mediated by a release of renal erythropoietin or by an enhanced effect of erythropoietin on the bone marrow or by both mechanisms as suggested by Shahidi.

Anemia of Pregnancy. Anemia of pregnancy is most often caused by an iron deficiency, and the routine use of iron in prenatal care is definitely in order. However, even under conditions of adequate iron intake, a mild anemia is present during the third trimester in almost all pregnant women. This anemia is normochromic and normocytic and unresponsive to any kind of treatment. Recent measurements of the red cell mass have shown it not to be caused by a lack of red cells but rather by

an increase in plasma, a so-called dilution anemia. The red cell mass actually increases about 20 per cent during pregnancy, but the plasma volume increases even more. The physiologic effect of such an increase in blood volume is very advantageous for oxygen transport (Fig. 22–26), and despite the moderate decrease in hemoglobin concentration, the pregnant woman and her fetus are undoubtedly well provided with oxygen for their metabolic demands.

IMMUNOLOGIC DYSFUNCTION. Pure red cell aplasia is an unusual but dramatic disease characterized by severe anemia due to the isolated depletion of the erythroid tissue and is believed to be related to an immunologic dysfunction. The production and turnover of erythropoietin appear to be normal but the bone marrow response to this hormone is inadequate, as evidenced by the absence of proerythroblasts and other nucleated red blood cells despite high plasma titers of erythropoietin.

An acute, self-limited form of pure red cell aplasia has been reported following "virus" infections in patients with hereditary spherocytosis or other congenital hemolytic disorders. The predominance of reports dealing with such patients may be due to the fact that a brief period of erythroid aplasia in a patient with a short red cell life span will have a much more noticeable effect on the hemoglobin concentration than the same period of

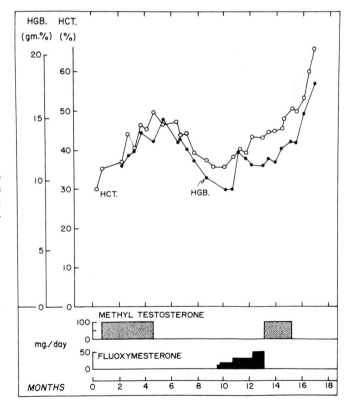

Figure 22–40 Erythropoietic response of a patient with myelofibrosis to various androgen preparations. (Redrawn from Gardner, F. H. and Pringle, J. C.: N. Engl. J. Med., *264*:103, 1961.)

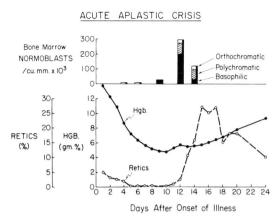

Figure 22–41 Acute aplastic crisis following a brief febrile illness in a patient with hereditary spherocytosis. (Redrawn from Owren, P. A.: Blood, *3*:231–248, 1948, by permission of Grune & Stratton, Inc., New York.)

aplasia would have if the red cell life span were normal (Fig. 22–41). Consequently, it is assumed that brief periods of asymptomatic erythroid aplasia may actually be quite common and if properly looked for found in many normals suffering from

upper respiratory infections or viral gastroenteritis. The exact pathogenetic mechanism is unknown but it has been proposed that the erythroid cells or their immediate erythropoietin-sensitive progenitors are affected by a viral-related antibody.

Chronic pure red cell aplasia is a far more unusual disorder, but its relationship to thymic tumors has recently caused a flurry of interest regarding its pathogenesis.

Thymomas are present in about 30 to 50 per cent of cases, and although thymectomy is rarely of dramatic benefit, "spontaneous" recoveries have been described in patients who have undergone thymectomy. Since so-called autoimmune disorders are frequently associated with thymus abnormalities, it is of additional pathogenetic importance that prednisone may occasionally cause a striking reticulocyte response (Fig. 22–42) and that remissions may be induced by the therapeutic use of immunosuppressive drugs. Studies by Krantz and co-workers have demonstrated antibodies directed against erythroid bone marrow cells in the serum of some patients. These antibodies presumably coat and possibly reject the erythroid cells or the erythropoietin-responsive stem cells, and their presence could explain

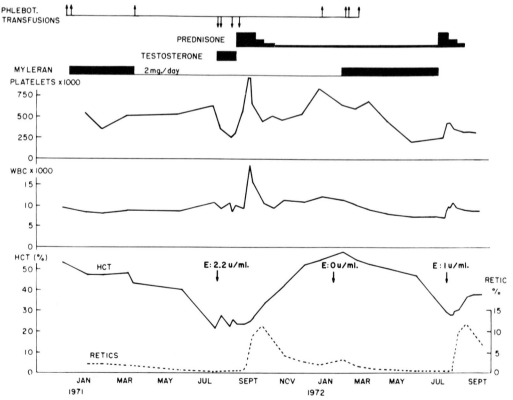

Figure 22–42 A patient with polycythemia vera, disseminated lupus erythematosus, and recurrent bouts of pure red cell aplasia. In each instance prednisone medication caused a striking increase in reticulocytes, followed by a return of the hematocrit to normal or even polycythemic values. (E = Erythropoietin).

the development of a pure red cell aplasia. The existence of antibodies directed against erythropoietin has also been reported, but since the erythropoietin titer is usually very high, these reports are difficult to accept. The cause-effect relationship of the autoantibodies to the thymic tumor is not clear, but it has been suggested that the tumor destroys normal thymic function and permits the survival of lymphocytic clones programmed to produce autoantibodies. Further studies of this fascinating disease may well lead to concepts of importance for the management not only of patients with pure red cell aplasia but also of patients with other autoimmune diseases.

Multiplication Disorders

Vitamin B$_{12}$ and Folic Acid. The identification of vitamin B$_{12}$ and folates as important anti-anemia principles ranks among modern medicine's greatest triumphs. The exemplary clinical investigations of Minot and Murphy and of Castle in the 1920s and 1930s were the first of a steady stream of basic and applied research accomplishments, the most recent of which has been the synthesis of vitamin B$_{12}$ in the laboratory. Kass has recently recounted with rich pictorial detail the history of this fascinating chain of discoveries extending for

more than a century after Addison's clinical description of pernicious anemia in 1849.

B$_{12}$ and folates participate as factors in a wide variety of biochemical reactions in the body. In some respects their biochemical reactions are interrelated. Their essential role in DNA synthesis explains why deficiencies of either or both lead to "megaloblastic anemia" and to disturbances in cell division not only in the marrow but in other proliferating cell populations, such as the gastrointestinal epithelium. Nervous tissue, which is not in a state of cellular proliferation, also has an important requirement for vitamin B$_{12}$.

Vitamin B$_{12}$ (molecular weight 1355) is built asymmetrically around cobalt much like heme is built around iron. Cobalt, like iron, has six coordinate positions four of which are bound to nitrogen atoms in a planar tetrapyrrole corrin ring (Fig. 22–43). Below and almost perpendicular to the plane of the corrin ring, a benzimidazole nucleotide occupies the fifth coordinate position, also in a nitrogen linkage. The sixth position is ionic, and in "cyanocobalamin," the parent compound of the family of vitamin B$_{12}$ relatives, it is occupied by cyanide. The presence of the cyanide ligand in this position, however, is an artifact of isolation. The physiologically active coenzyme forms of the vitamin contain either a methyl or a deoxyadenosyl

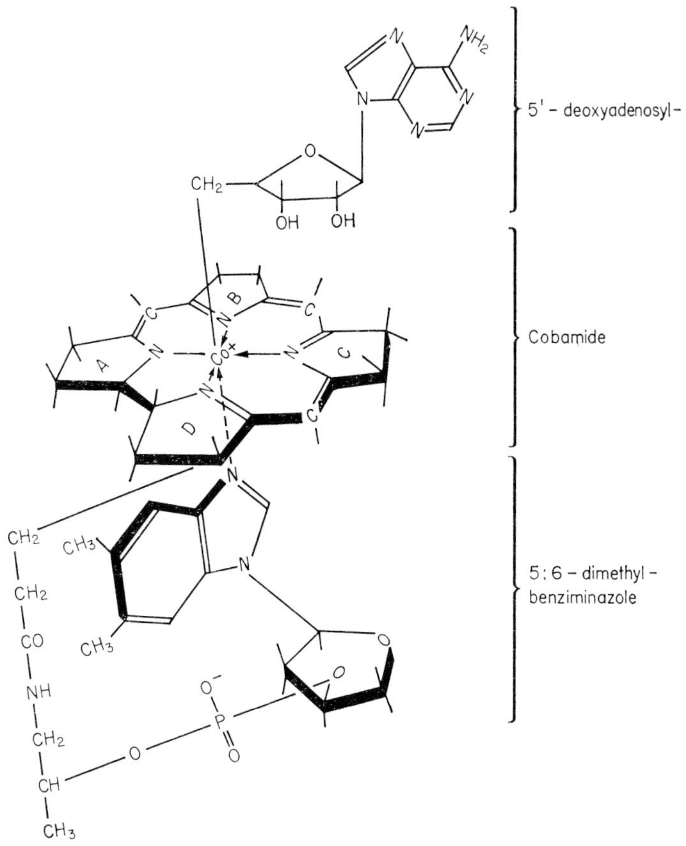

Figure 22–43 Structure of deoxyadenosyl cobalamin, a physiologically active form of vitamin B$_{12}$. (From Chanarin, I.: The Megaloblastic Anemias. F. A. Davis Co., Philadelphia, 1969, p. 16.)

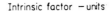

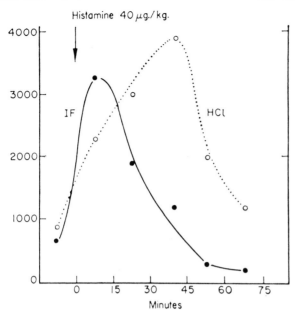

Figure 22–44 Stimulation of gastric secretion of intrinsic factor (IF) and hydrochloric acid by histamine. (Redrawn from Arderman, S., et al.: Br. Med. J., 2:600, 1964.)

group in this position. Cyanocobalamin, as well as its relative hydroxycobalamin, is readily converted to these active forms within the body.

The absorption of vitamin B_{12} is dependent upon a unique mechanism unshared by any other essential nutrient. The parietal cells of the stomach produce, along with hydrochloric acid, a glycoprotein known as "intrinsic factor" (IF), which tightly and specifically binds B_{12}, the "extrinsic factor," after it has been ingested and is released from complexes in foodstuffs (Fig. 22–44). IF has a molecular weight of 60,000 and binds B_{12} on a mole-for-mole basis. The binding occurs with the benzimidazole nucleotide moiety of B_{12} and is independent of the specific chemical form of the vitamin. Dimers are formed when the vitamin is bound. It then travels down the length of the intestinal tract, protected in the IF complex from the degradative activities of digestive enzymes. Specific receptors on the surface of the microvilli of the terminal ileum take up the IF-B_{12} complex in a process dependent upon a pH of above 6.5 as well as upon divalent cations (calcium and/or magnesium) (Fig. 22–45). It is still uncertain whether the entire complex enters the cell or whether IF is released back into the lumen after the vitamin is removed.

After a small dose of 1 μg of B_{12} about 60 to 80 per cent is absorbed. However, the proportion absorbed decreases as the amount of ingested B_{12} increases. About 1 to 5 μg. is absorbed from a dietary intake of 5 to 30 μg per day. A tiny amount of B_{12}, less than 1 per cent, is absorbed in an

IF-independent manner, but this is too small to be of physiologic significance. There is a substantial excretion of B_{12} from the biliary tract into the intestinal lumen, but this is efficiently reabsorbed in an IF-dependent enterohepatic circuit, and thus is not lost to the body economy.

In addition to IF, other specific vitamin B_{12} binding proteins are of importance to the body economy. A family of "R binders" (R for rapid electrophoretic mobility), found in plasma, saliva, milk, and other body fluids, share a common protein structure but differ in their carbohydrate content. Transcobalamin (TC) I and III are R-binders found in plasma. Most of the B_{12} present in plasma is attached to TC I and has a relatively slow rate of turnover according to Hall. TC III contains only a minor fraction of the plasma vitamin B_{12} and appears to arise from granulocytes largely as a result of in-vitro cell lysis. A third plasma binder, TC II, lacks carbohydrate and, like IF, differs in its protein make-up from the R-binders. TC II accounts for most of the unsaturated plasma vitamin B_{12} binding capacity and is responsible for binding newly absorbed vitamin B_{12} and rapidly transporting it to the tissues so its turnover rate is many times more rapid than that of TC I.

Much remains to be learned about the biologic roles of the vitamin B_{12} binding proteins. TC I seems to be dispensable since its congenital absence causes no clinically important abnormality. In contrast, congenital lack of TC II leads to megaloblastic anemia. Striking elevations of the plas-

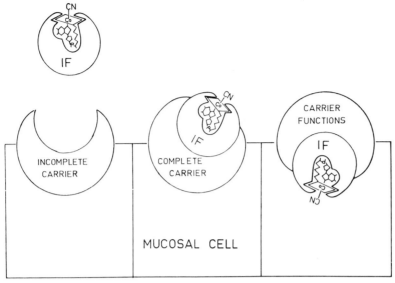

Figure 22-45   Mucosal absorption in the terminal ileum of vitamin B_{12} bound to intrinsic factor. (From Gräsbeck, R.: Scand. J. Clin. Lab. Invest., *19*:7 (Suppl. 95.), 1967. Universitetsforlaget, Oslo.)

ma R-binders and vitamin B_{12} levels are observed in patients with chronic myelogenous leukemia, other myeloproliferative syndromes, and in occasional patients with cancer.

Folic acid (pteroylmonoglutamic acid) consists of pteroic acid in combination with only one molecule of L-glutamic acid (Fig. 22-46). However, the term "folates" refers to a large family of related compounds containing as many as six or seven L-glutamic acid residues locked in gamma glutamyl polypeptide linkage. Most food folate is in the polyglutamate form and must be broken down in the intestine to the monoglutamate to permit efficient absorption. This is accomplished by the intestinal enzyme "conjugase" (Fig. 22-47).

Following its absorption, folic acid is reduced by the enzyme dihydrofolate reductase. The reduction is accomplished in two steps, each involving the addition of two hydrogen atoms to yield biologically active tetrahydrofolate (FH_4). Dihydrofolate reductase is inhibited by minute concentrations of the antifolate compound, methotrexate, an effective chemotherapeutic agent used in the treatment of neoplastic diseases.

Reduced folates, acting out their roles as agents of single carbon unit transfer, are methylated in a variety of ways. The active carbon may exist in one of several different chemical states (methyl, formyl, hydroxymethyl, methylene, methenyl, formimino), and it may be attached at several alternative sites on the parent FH_4 molecule (Fig. 22-46).

In addition to folic acid itself, the only other pharmacologically available folate is the N^5 formyl derivative, folinic acid (also called citrovorum factor, or Leucovorin). This agent is of use as an antidote for methotrexate toxicity, against which folic acid, the biologically inactive precursor of FH_4, is ineffective.

Plasma folate occurs almost entirely as the monoglutamate form of methyl FH_4, but following its uptake into cells the molecular size is once again increased by the enzymatic addition of multiple glutamic acid residues. This conversion (or reconversion) to the polyglutamate form markedly enhances coenzymatic activity. Thus, as reviewed by Hoffbrand, the intracellular pool of reduced and methylated polyglutamates is the principal source of folate biologic activity.

Although B_{12} and folates participate as cofactors in a number of biochemical reactions involving transfer of carbon or hydrogen atoms, their roles in DNA synthesis are of particular interest with respect to the pathogenesis of megaloblastic anemia. Patients with B_{12} deficiency show hematologic response to treatment with large doses of folic acid (although their neurologic symptoms may worsen). This clinical observation has for a long time aroused interest in the hypothesis that B_{12} and folates are interrelated in their roles as coenzymes in DNA synthesis. Several findings have shed some light on this interrelationship. Plasma levels of methyl FH_4 tend to be elevated in patients with B_{12} deficiency, while at the same time intracellular polyglutamate folates are decreased. This has suggested that B_{12} may play a role in cellular uptake of methyl FH_4 monoglutamate or in the conversion of monoglutamate to polyglutamate folate derivatives. However, the reciprocal changes in plasma and

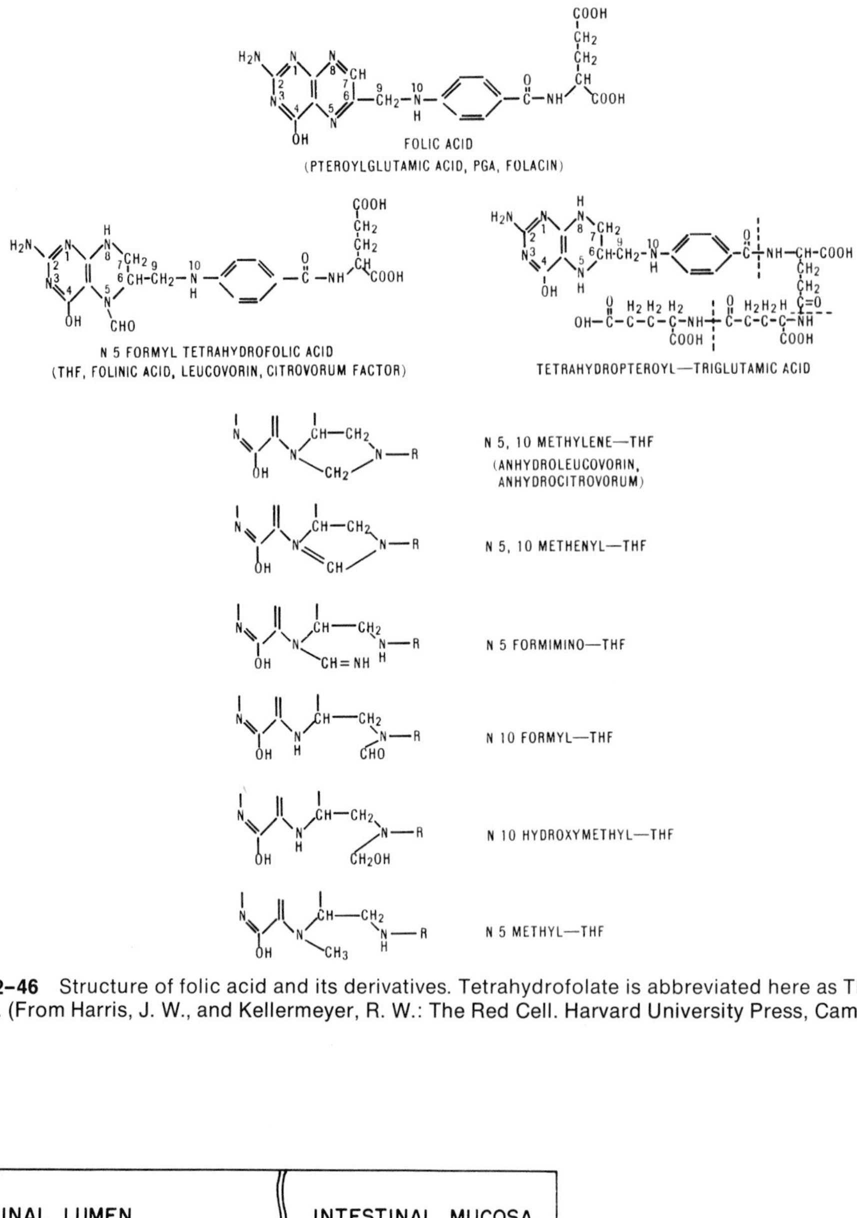

Figure 22–46 Structure of folic acid and its derivatives. Tetrahydrofolate is abbreviated here as THF and in the text as FH$_4$. (From Harris, J. W., and Kellermeyer, R. W.: The Red Cell. Harvard University Press, Cambridge, 1970, p. 395.)

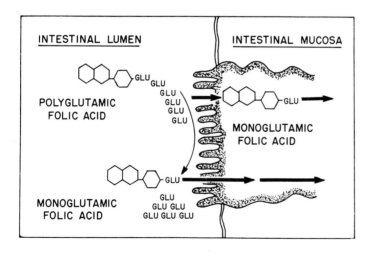

Figure 22–47 Intestinal absorption of the folate derivatives in food, present largely in polyglutamate form. The site of action of the enzyme conjugase, which degrades the polyglutamate to the monoglutamate, is not known, but may actually be within the mucosal cell rather than in the intestinal lumen. Folate appears in the plasma as the reduced monoglutamate N$_5$ methyl tetrahydrofolate. (From Streiff, R. R.: J.A.M.A., *214*, 105, 1970. Copyright 1970 by the American Medical Association.)

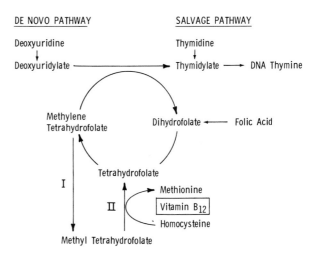

Figure 22–48 The methyl tetrahydrofolate "trap" hypothesis. Elevated plasma N_5 methyl tetrahydrofolate levels are observed in patients with vitamin B_{12} deficiency due to an inability to convert this, the major extracellular form, to tetrahydrofolate and other active coenzymic intracellular forms. Because of this lack of active intracellular folates (and specifically of $N_{5,10}$ methylene tetrahydrofolate) there is a deficient conversion of deoxyuridylate to thymidylate and consequently also of DNA synthesis. The unutilized folate is "trapped" as N_5 methyl tetrahydrofolate. (Redrawn from Waxman, S., et al.: J. Clin. Invest., *48*:284, 1969.)

intracellular folate levels may also be explained by the methyl FH_4 "trap" hypothesis, as explained in Figure 22–48.

The biochemical action of B_{12} in the nervous tissue is still controversial, but circumstantial evidence has pointed to its role in propionate metabolism (Fig. 22–49). Deoxyadenosyl cobalamin acts as co-factor in the rearrangement of active methylmalonate, formed as a result of carboxylation of propionate, to succinate. Indeed, increased urinary excretion of methylmalonate is a reliable indicator of B_{12} deficiency. An increase in the serum concentration as well as the urinary excretion is also seen in methylmalonic acidemia, a rare inherited defect of B_{12} conversion to its active deoxyadenosyl coenzyme form.

Although folate lack is not notable for the presence of neurologic sequelae, except inasmuch as other vitamin deficiencies may coexist, rare congenital deficiencies of the intermediary steps of folate metabolism may cause mental retardation and other neurologic problems early in infancy. This observation has stimulated interest in the possibility that folates are of importance in the normal development of the nervous tissue.

General Effects of Megaloblastic Anemia. The signs and symptoms are primarily related to the hematopoietic and gastrointestinal systems, although the neurologic system is also affected in B_{12} deficiency. The degree of anemia may be quite profound, but its onset is very slow and as a result it is amazingly well tolerated, unless congestive heart failure or angina pectoris supervenes. The sclerae are often slightly icteric, the tongue is usually atrophic and smooth, and splenomegaly may be present. There may be vague gastrointestinal complaints. The neurologic signs of B_{12} deficiencies include a spastic and incoordinate gait, paresthesias, and sometimes mental changes. Increased reflexes, Babinski signs, and loss of position and vibration sense are indicative of posterior

and lateral column demyelination (Fig. 22–50). Decreased reflexes and hypesthesia are signs of peripheral neuropathy, and altered behavior and impaired mentation may indicate cerebral involvement.

The deficiency affects all the proliferating hematopoietic elements, and therefore pancytopenia is commonly observed, but granulocytopenia and thrombocytopenia are usually not so severe that infectious susceptibility or hemorrhage results. The anemia is macrocytic, but wide variations of erythrocyte size on either side of the mean are characteristic, and indeed, some erythrocytes are microcytic. The presence of "macro-ovalocytes" is a particularly valuable morphologic sign. Mature segmented neutrophils have a greater than nor-

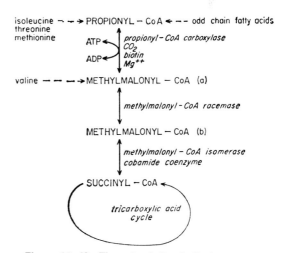

Figure 22–49 The role of vitamin B_{12} in propionate metabolism. The cobamide coenzyme is deoxyadenosyl cobalamin. (From Rosenberg, L. E., et al.: Science, *162*:805, 1968. Copyright 1968 by the American Association for the Advancement of Science.)

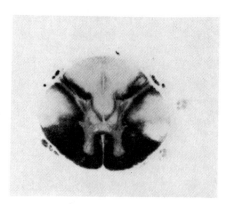

Figure 22–50 Degeneration of the posterior and lateral columns of the spinal cord in vitamin B$_{12}$ deficiency. (From Chanarin, I.: The Megaloblastic Anemias. Philadelphia, F. A. Davis Co., 1969, p. 576.)

mal mean number of lobes per nucleus; a few may contain as many as 7 or 8.

Not all macrocytic conditions are megaloblastic. An increase in mean corpuscular volume may be seen with reticulocytosis or if there is acquisition of excessive membrane surface area due to plasma lipid abnormalities (Table 22–8).

When the anemia is severe, megaloblastic erythroid precursors are found in the circulation, and a small proportion of mature erythrocytes contains nuclear remnants (Howell-Jolly bodies, Cabot's rings). The reticulocytes are not increased and polychromasia is not prominent. Distinctive morphologic changes are also seen in the gastrointestinal epithelial cells, but the diagnosis rests upon the finding of "megaloblastic" changes in the bone marrow. This term was originally applied to erythroid precursors only, but today it is used to refer to changes in all three cell lines — granulocytic and megakaryocytic as well as erythroid. The entire erythroid line of maturation is altered to form a "megaloblastic series." There is the appearance of a "maturation arrest" because of the marked shift to the left, with large numbers of early erythroid precursors having intensely basophilic cytoplasm. The arrest in nuclear development is reflected in an abnormally finely divided and open pattern of the nuclear chromatin. Hemoglobin formation proceeds in the cytoplasm, however, and "nuclear-cytoplasmic dissociation" is observed. The entire series of cells is larger than normal, and mature cells emerge as macrocytic erythrocytes. The marrow granulocytic precursors also show distinctive changes, in particular large horseshoe- and C-shaped nuclear forms at the band stage of maturation. The marrow shows a marked over-all increase in cellularity.

The deficient marrow, driven by the stimulus of "poietins," reacts with a hypercellular proliferative response. However, the defect in nuclear development leads to intramedullary destruction of the blood cell precursors. Heme catabolism from the breakdown of erythroid precursors in the marrow is the major factor contributing to the signs of hemolysis — the elevated serum indirect bilirubin, the absence of plasma haptoglobin, and the elevation of serum lactic dehydrogenase to levels rarely seen even in the hemolytic anemias. Megaloblastic anemia is a classic example of the pathophysiology of ineffective erythropoiesis. The number of reticulocytes in the peripheral blood is not elevated despite intense erythroid hyperplasia

TABLE 22–8 SOME CAUSES OF MACROCYTIC ERYTHROCYTES

Impairment of DNA synthesis
    Vitamin B$_{12}$ deficiency
    Folate deficiency
    Chemotherapy
        Antimetabolites (e.g., 6-mercaptopurine, methotrexate)
        Alkylating agents (e.g., cyclophosphamide)
    Primary refractory anemias
        Aplastic anemia
        Sideroblastic anemia
        Erythroleukemia and other myelogenous leukemia variants
        Refractory megaloblastic anemias (acquired)
    Rare hereditary blocks in DNA synthesis (e.g., orotic aciduria)

Reticulocytosis
    Hemolytic anemia
    Response to acute blood loss

Surface Membrane Excess
    Liver disease
    Obstructive jaundice
    Post-splenectomy
    Hereditary lecithin: cholesterol acyl transferase (LCAT) deficiency

---

in the marrow. The serum iron concentration is raised, and its rate of clearance from the circulation to the erythroid marrow is increased, with only small amounts appearing over subsequent days in the newly formed erythrocytes (Fig. 22–33). The amount of radioactive label appearing in the "early bilirubin" peak after administration of a tagged heme precursor is markedly increased (Fig. 22–8).

With treatment, the signs promptly revert to normal within several days: the serum iron concentration decreases and its utilization for the production of circulating erythrocytes becomes effective, the jaundice disappears, the elevated serum lactic dehydrogenase falls, and megaloblastic cells are no longer seen in the marrow. The reticulocyte count becomes elevated within three to four days, reaches a peak at 7 to 10 days, and then falls (Fig. 22–51). The reticulocyte response is the most reliable early sign of response, and in the more anemic individuals it may peak at 25 to 50 per cent. The neurologic symptoms of B_{12} lack are reversed, unless they have progressed to an advanced degree of severity. Pharmacologic doses of folic acid will produce a hematologic response in the B_{12}-deficient patient while worsening the neurologic complications. Presumably the folate causes a fall in serum B_{12} level, with a diversion of available B_{12} away from neural to hematopoietic tissue. Large doses of B_{12} will also give a hematologic response in the folate-deficient patient. Response to therapy is specific if the administered dose is limited to the range of the minimal daily requirement, about 1 μg. per day of B_{12} or 50 μg. per day of folate.

Vitamin B_{12} Deficiency

DIETARY LACK.   Inadequate intake is an exceptionally rare cause of B_{12} deficiency, since this vitamin is present in a wide variety of products of animal origin — meat, fish, eggs, butter, milk, and cheese — and the minimal daily requirement of 1 to 5 μg. is readily met unless a strict vegetarian diet is followed. Even then, the total body stores of 2000 to 5000 μg. are well conserved, with a loss of only 0.1 per cent per day of the total body pool, and the earliest signs of B_{12} deficiency are not seen until after 10 to 20 years on such a diet.

INTRINSIC FACTOR LACK.   The term "pernicious anemia" (PA) no longer seems appropriate, considering the fact that the condition can now be effectively cured. However, its historical roots are deep and it seems appropriate to continue to use this term but only for megaloblastic anemia caused by a lack of intrinsic factor.

Congenital PA is a rare autosomal recessive condition which is apparently clinically manifest only in the homozygous state. There is an isolated lack of IF without insufficiency of gastric acid or pepsin. Passively acquired B_{12} stores present at birth are exhausted in two or three years, and anemia then develops.

Adult PA is a disorder of mature and older adults. Genetic factors still not well defined play some role, since there is a significant intrafamilial occurrence as well as an ethnic predilection for individuals of northern and western European

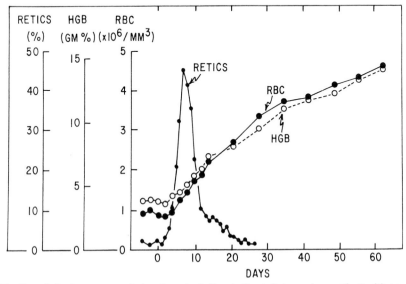

Figure 22–51   Hematologic response to treatment of vitamin B_{12} deficiency in a patient with pernicious anemia. (Redrawn from Castle, W. B. *In* Cecil and Loeb (eds.): A Textbook of Medicine. W. B. Saunders Co., Philadelphia, 1959, p. 1131.)

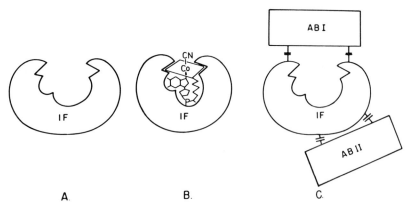

A.   B.   C.

Figure 22–52   Anti-intrinsic factor antibodies of the blocking (AB I) and binding (AB II) types. (From Gräsbeck, R.: Progr. Hemat., 6:233–260, 1969. By permission of Grune & Stratton, Inc., New York.)

background. The absence of IF in the gastric juice is always found in association with atrophic gastritis, and there is accordingly a lack of gastric acidity and pepsin, even after stimulation with histamine. Atrophic gastritis is not uncommon in the general population, and its incidence increases with age. Why certain affected persons develop pernicious anemia is still uncertain, but the following evidence supports an autoimmune theory of pathogenesis:

(1) The histologic appearance of lymphocytic infiltration of the gastric mucosa suggests a local immunologic process.

(2) Antibodies which react against the cytoplasm of the gastric parietal cell are present in the serum of 90 per cent of patients with adult PA. A significant incidence of such antibodies is present, however, in patients who do not have PA. These include 60 per cent of all individuals with atrophic gastritis, 30 per cent of blood relatives of PA patients, and slightly less than 10 per cent of a control population. PA patients frequently have serum antibodies directed against parenchymal endocrine glands, most notably the acinar cells of the thyroid. Conversely, patients with primary myxedema and Hashimoto's thyroiditis have a 30 per cent incidence of antiparietal cell serum antibodies and a 12 per cent incidence of coexisting PA.

(3) About three fourths of PA patients have anti-IF antibodies in serum, saliva, and gastric juice. These are much more specific for PA and are rarely found in its absence. These antibodies are polyclonal and may be either IgG or IgA. They apparently react at two different sites on the IF molecule (Fig. 22–52). "Blocking" antibodies prevent the binding of B_{12} to IF, presumably by obstructing the site of attachment. "Binding" antibodies do not interfere with the attachment of B_{12} to IF, but they do impede absorption in the ileum.

Whether these various autoimmune phenom-
ena associated with PA are cause or effect remains uncertain, but the properties of the anti-IF antibodies present in gastric secretions clearly suggest a role in its pathogenesis.

Total gastrectomy will predictably produce megaloblastic anemia after five or six years, but partial gastrectomy in most instances does not deplete IF sufficiently to lead to frank megaloblastosis. With the passage of years, however, an increasing proportion of partial gastrectomy patients develop low serum B_{12} levels, some of whom have mild megaloblastic changes in the marrow (Fig. 22–53). Iron deficiency is the commonest cause of postgastrectomy anemia, and its presence may mask concomitant megaloblastosis, the signs of which are brought out following iron repletion.

DECREASED ILEAL ABSORPTION.   Ablation of the specific site of B_{12} absorption in the terminal ileum by surgical resection or by such diseases as regional ileitis, lymphoma, or tuberculosis leads to B_{12} deficiency without an associated lack of IF or of gastric acid. Certain drugs (neomycin, colchicine, para-amino salicylate) reportedly interfere with B_{12} absorption by mechanisms which remain obscure. The gastrointestinal epithelial changes of tropical sprue are extensive and commonly cause B_{12} deficiency, especially in chronic cases. The megaloblastic alterations of B_{12} or folate deficiency themselves cause sufficient epithelial change to interfere with ileal absorption. Indeed, patients with folate deficiency tend to have lower than normal serum concentrations of B_{12}, with spontaneous correction after folate repletion (Fig. 22–54). Poor absorption may also occur consequent to pancreatic insufficiency primarily because pancreatic enzymes cleave R-binder B_{12} complexes and make the vitamin available for attachment to IF. *Imerslund's syndrome* is a rare congenital deficiency of the receptor site in the terminal ileum causing megaloblastic anemia in children. IF secretion is normal. Renal structural abnormalities and proteinuria are also commonly present.

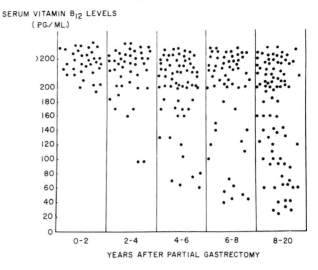

Figure 22–53 Serum vitamin B_{12} levels at various intervals after subtotal gastrectomy. Patients with B_{12} deficiency megaloblastic anemia have values in the range of 0 to 100 pg. per ml. (Redrawn from Hines, J. D., et al.: Am. J. Med., *43*:555, 1967.)

DECREASED AVAILABILITY. Decreased serum B_{12} levels and megaloblastic anemia are found in association with anatomic abnormalities of the gastrointestinal tract which lead to stasis and pooling of the luminal contents. Such "blind loop syndromes" — strictures, surgically created bypasses, fistulas, and large diverticula — have in common the presence of bacterial overgrowth along with steatorrhea. The anemia does not respond to orally administered B_{12}, but parenteral replacement is effective. Intrinsic factor is present in normal amounts, indicating that the IF-B_{12} complex is unavailable for absorption in the terminal ileum. The finding that therapy with broad-

spectrum antibiotics causes disappearance of the stigmata of B_{12} lack provides strong evidence that bacterial utilization is responsible for the deficiency. A similar mechanism explains the megaloblastic anemia associated with the fish tapeworm *(Diphyllobothrium latum)*. Infestation occurs because of eating improperly cooked fresh-water fish. The worms grow to great lengths in the intestinal tract and effectively compete with the host for available IF-B_{12} complex. The disorder is especially common in Finland.

Folate Deficiency

DIETARY LACK. Poor nutrition — an unusual cause of B_{12} deficiency — frequently gives rise to

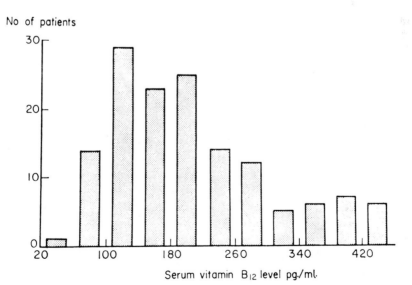

Figure 22–54 Serum vitamin B_{12} levels in patients with megaloblastic anemia due to folate deficiency. The normal range of values is 200 to 800 pg. per ml. (Redrawn from Mollin, D. L., Waters, A. H., and Harriss, E., *in* 2 Europaisches Symposium, Hamburg, 1961, (H. C. Heinrich, ed.), Stuttgart, Enke. Reprinted in Chanarin, I.: The Megaloblastic Anemias. F. A. Davis Co., Philadelphia, 1969.)

folate depletion. The elderly recluse, the "tea and toast" faddist, and the alcoholic are prototypes of deficiency in the United States. In other countries, excessive cooking of food, often limited in amount and diversity, destroys labile folates and causes leeching out of the soluble folates in the cooking water. Newborns procure sufficient amounts even from deficient mothers, but develop megaloblastic anemia when they reach the two-year stage of rapid growth if they are raised on low folate diets, such as goat's milk or boiled milk. Folates are present in many different foodstuffs — leafy green vegetables, fruits, meats, eggs — and food intake must be severely limited in diversity in order to fall short of the minimal daily requirement of 50 μg. Lack of ascorbate, thiamine, and other essential nutrients often coexists. In alcoholics, poor diet is not the only factor, since ethanol seems to interfere with folate absorption, its intermediary metabolism, and its hepatic storage. It also exerts a direct toxic suppression on the bone marrow elements.

The sequence of events after limitation of folate intake has been studied experimentally by Herbert (Fig. 22–55). The serum folate concentration is the most sensitive indicator of deficiency, falling within a month of deficient intake. Red cell folate concentration is more stubbornly defended, but it also falls as megaloblastic anemia appears after three to four months of deficiency. Folate stores are neither as ample, relative to daily requirement, nor as avidly guarded as B_{12} stores.

The minimal daily requirement of folate increases during pregnancy to about 400 μg. Serum folate levels tend to fall as pregnancy proceeds to term. A diet that maintains body folate in a marginal state of balance will prove inadequate in the face of such an increase in demands, and thus folate deficiency is the commonest cause of megaloblastic anemia of pregnancy. Conditions of increased cellular proliferation, such as hemolytic anemia, as well as thyrotoxicosis also raise the minimal requirement for folate.

MALABSORPTION. "Blind loop syndromes," which bring on B_{12} deficiency because of bacterial utilization, are not associated with folate lack. Possibly bacterial synthesis in the stagnant loop may actually add to the body's supply. On the other hand, gastrointestinal disorders affecting extensive areas of absorptive surface, with attendant malabsorption, frequently lead to folate deficiency. Gluten-sensitive enteropathy (nontropical sprue) most severely affects the upper reaches of the bowel — the duodenum and jejunum — where folate absorption normally is maximal, sparing the terminal ileum along with B_{12} absorption in many instances. In tropical sprue, the involvement extends throughout the gut, affecting B_{12} as well as folate absorption. Folic acid therapy often improves the malabsorption along with the megaloblastic anemia in tropical sprue, but in non-tropical sprue improvement in gastrointestinal function is achieved by eliminating gluten from the diet. Oral therapy with folic acid — the monoglutamate form — is effective, suggesting that the polyglutamates of food are not absorbed as well.

Other gastrointestinal disorders with malabsorption are lymphoma, scleroderma, amyloidosis, Whipple's disease, and extensive surgical resection. In addition to deficiencies of folate and/or B_{12}, iron lack is also commonly present in malab-

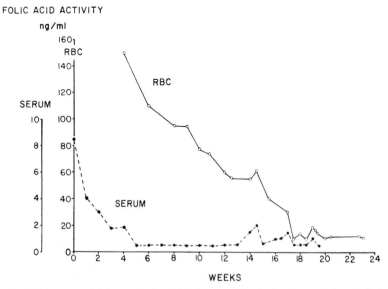

FOLIC ACID ACTIVITY

Figure 22–55 The fall in serum folate and red cell folate in a subject placed on a folate-deficient diet. (Redrawn from Herbert, V.: Trans. Am. Assoc. Physicians, 75:307, 1962.)

sorption syndromes, giving the picture of a combined deficiency anemia.

DRUGS. Patients on diphenylhydantoin therapy have a significant incidence of low serum folate levels and of megaloblastic anemia which responds readily to oral folic acid therapy. Estrogenic contraceptives occasionally have a similar side-effect. The notion that these agents interfere with the absorption of food folates by inhibiting intestinal conjugase activity has not yet withstood the test of scientific confirmation. Some evidence suggests that diphenylhydantoin may interfere with folate intermediary metabolism. The mechanism of megaloblastic anemia produced by the antimalarial pyrimethamine is more closely akin to that of methotrexate as a competitive inhibitor of folate metabolism.

Miscellaneous Megaloblastic Anemias. Therapy of neoplastic disease often leads to megaloblastic bone marrow and macrocytic red cells. Some of the cytotoxic agents in use which predictably inhibit nucleotide synthesis with secondary megaloblastic change are the antifolates (methotrexate), purine inhibitors (6-mercaptopurine, thioguanine, azathioprine), pyrimidine inhibitors (5-fluorouracil), and pentose analogues (cytosine arabinoside). *Primary refractory megaloblastic anemia* may represent a nuclear maturation defect of a myeloproliferative syndrome. When such a defect affects both the erythroid and granulocytic precursors with an increase in marrow myeloblasts it is known as *erythroleukemia (Di Guglielmo syndrome).* In some proliferative disorders of the bone marrow, local shortages are brought on by the increased requirements of the abnormal proliferation, causing morphologic signs of deficiency in neighboring cells. *Hereditary orotic aciduria* is a rare megaloblastic anemia of childhood caused by an inherited block in pyrimidine synthesis.

Maturation Disorders of the Erythrocyte Cytoplasm

Hemoglobin Synthesis. The circulating erythrocyte is the most specialized of the body's cells — 95 per cent of its cytoplasm consists of the respiratory pigment hemoglobin packed into the cell interior at a concentration almost five times that of the proteins of the exterior plasma. The formation of hemoglobin begins at the earliest precursor stage of the developing erythroid cell and is completed when the anucleate reticulocyte matures to an erythrocyte. No additional hemoglobin is produced during the 120-day period of the erythrocyte's life span in the circulation. The biosynthesis of hemoglobin is a complex series of distinct but delicately coordinated biochemical events, so well balanced that component parts are brought together assembly-line fashion, without significant shortages or surpluses, to form the completed molecule. Heme is formed in a sequential series of enzymatically controlled reactions. Dissimilar polypeptide globin subunits under separate genetic control are assembled on polyribosomes. The finished molecule has two pairs of such subunits, each linked with its own prosthetic heme group into a tetrameric macromolecule.

GENERAL EFFECTS OF DISORDERS OF HEMOGLOBIN SYNTHESIS. Deficiency in the quantity of hemoglobin leads to microcytic, hypochromic anemia. The hemoglobin lack comes either from a lack of heme, as in iron deficiency, or from insufficient globin, to which the designation "thalassemia" is given. Qualitative abnormalities of the hemoglobin may alter the internal consistency of the erythrocyte cytoplasm and cause increased cell rigidity which leads to premature destruction and hemolysis. Abnormal hemoglobin oxygen affinity or oxidation state gives rise to cyanosis or erythrocytosis. Many abnormal hemoglobins produce no pathophysiologic abnormality because they function quite normally.

Porphyrin. Of all the tissues in the body, the erythroid marrow and the liver are the preeminent porphyrin producers. The synthesis begins on the mitochondria and requires energy. The intermediate steps take place in the cytosol and the process is completed once again on the mitochondria with the insertion of iron into the completed porphyrin molecule to form heme. The brightly colored finished product contains four pyrrole rings connected into a larger cyclic tetrapyrrole structure by methene bridges. Side chains are attached to the ring structure: 4 methyl, 2 vinyl, and 2 propionyl. The structure of heme is shown in Figure 22-56.

The biochemical steps in heme synthesis are outlined in Figure 22-57. Active succinate is joined to glycine to form delta-amino levulinic acid (ALA). This enzymatic step, controlled by

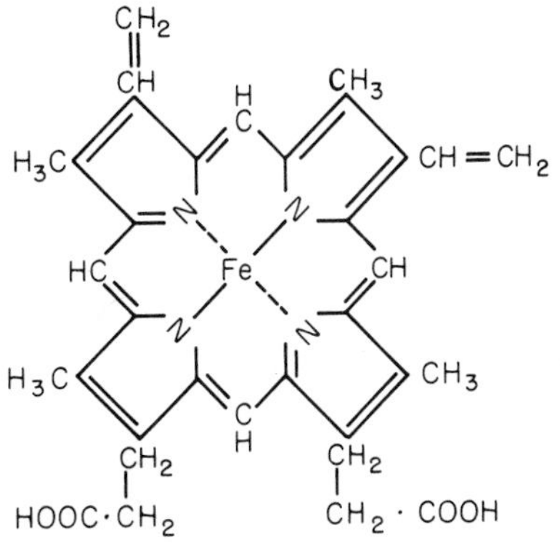

HEME (FERROPROTOPORHYRIN 9)

Figure 22-56 The structure of heme. (From Harris, J. W., and Kellermeyer, R. W.: The Red Cell. Harvard University Press, Cambridge, 1970, p. 3.)

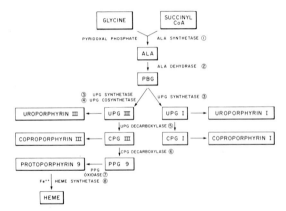

Figure 22–57 The synthesis of heme. Eight enzymatic steps are indicated. The initial step (1) is energy requiring, takes place on mitochondria, and uses pyridoxal phosphate as a co-factor. The final steps (6, 7, and 8) are also mitochondrial. The intermediate enzymes (2 through 5) are in the cytosol.

Demonstrated enzymatic deficiencies in hereditary porphyria are as follows: acute intermittent porphyria (3); erythropoietic porphyria (4); porphyria cutanea tarda (5); hereditary protoporphyria (8). Postulated defects, not proved, are: variegate porphyria (7 or 8); hereditary coproporphyria (6). In lead poisoning decreased activity of (2) and (8) are most pronounced, although (1) and (6) are also inhibited. As another example of "toxic" porphyria, the chemical compound hexachlorobenzene inhibits (5) and produces a clinical picture resembling porphyria cutanea tarda. The enzymatic lack in the various porphyria states is associated with induction of increased ALA synthetase activity due to the lack of feedback control and consequent overproduction of porphyrin precursors synthesized proximal to the site of the enzymatic block.

Abbreviations are as follows: ALA—δ amino levulinic acid; PBG—porphobilinogen; UPG—uroporphyrinogen; CPG—coproporphyrinogen; PPG—protoporphyrinogen.

ALA synthetase, is both rate limiting and regulatory. It is subject to negative feedback inhibition and, as will be subsequently explained, in a variety of deficiencies of enzymes in the porphyrin synthetic pathway, the lack of end product causes deficient inhibition along with marked overproduction of precursors synthesized at sites above the block. Pyridoxal phosphate, the active form of the vitamin pyridoxine, is also required for this initial synthetic step.

Monopyrrole porphobilinogen rings are then formed by head-to-tail linkages of two ALA molecules. Four porphobilinogens in turn condense into the cyclic tetrapyrrole structure, which then undergoes progressive decarboxylation from uroporphyrinogen (containing 8 carboxyl side chains) to coproporphyrinogen (containing 4 carboxyl side chains) to protoporphyrinogen (containing 2 carboxyl side chains). Progressive decarboxylation is associated with an increased degree of insolubility which determines fecal as opposed to urinary excretion, the less soluble being predominantly fecal and the more soluble urinary (Table 22–9). Oxidation converts these colorless heme precursors into the brightly colored uroporphyrins, coproporphyrins, and protoporphyrins.

The porphyrins may exist in a variety of isomeric states depending on the position of the side chains, but only a limited number of isomers are of biologic significance. The uro- and copro- derivatives are found biologically only as the I and III isomers. In the formation of uroporphyrinogen from porphobilinogen, a cosynthetase operating in conjunction with a synthetase directs the bulk of synthesis to the III isomer, which serves exclusively as heme precursor. In the absence of cosynthetase, uroporphyrinogen I is preferentially formed and this does not fulfill the requirements of heme synthesis. Following consecutive conversions from uroporphyrinogen III to coproporphyrinogen III to protoporphyrinogen 9 to protoporphyrin 9, four of the six coordinate positions of ferrous iron are chelated to the completed tetrapyrrole to form heme, ready for combination with globin or other apoproteins.

GENERAL EFFECTS OF DISORDERS OF PORPHYRIN SYNTHESIS. The porphyrias are caused by inherited or acquired blocks in the enzymatic steps governing heme synthesis, but the most pronounced consequence of the block is overproduction of the heme precursors above the site of the block. The liver is most commonly the major site of the defect with sparing of the erythroid cells ("hepatic porphyrias"), although in some conditions the erythroid tissue is affected. It is surprising that in those states affecting the erythroid cells heme synthesis is sufficient to meet almost completely the needs of hemoglobin synthesis, and hypochromia of the erythrocytes is either absent or minimal. Specific diagnosis is usually accomplished by quantification and characterization of the various heme precursors in the urine, feces, erythrocytes, and liver. The characteristics of the porphyrias are summarized in Table 22–10.

Pink or red urine may be observed if there is sufficient concentration of the colored derivatives uroporphyrin and/or coproporphyrin. The freshly passed urine is colorless, however, if the increase affects primarily colorless reduced precursors. In the case of protoporphyria the urine is normal; excretion is via the fecal route because of the insolubility of this derivative. Deposition of the colored derivatives in tissue slices is detected by observing the emission of red fluorescence upon exposure to ultraviolet light. Indeed cutaneous absorption of light in the 400 nm. wave length range produces photo-sensitive skin reactions with symptoms which range from mild itching and burning to erythema, edema, blistering, and even-

TABLE 22-9 NORMAL VALUES FOR PORPHYRINS AND PORPHYRIN PRECURSORS IN MAN

	Urine μg./24 hrs.	Stool μg./gm. dry wt.	Erythrocytes μg./100 ml. cells
ALA	trace–2000	—	—
PBG	trace–1500	—	—
uroporphyrin	10–40	trace	trace
coproporphyrin	100–250	trace–50	0.5–1.5
protoporphyrin	0	trace–120	25–75

(Abbreviations as in Figure 3–46; From Marver and Schmid, 1972.)

tually even scarring and disfigurement involving exposed areas, such as the face and the backs of the hands. Damage to other tissues may also occur, as will be subsequently discussed.

INHERITED DISORDERS OF PORPHYRIN SYNTHESIS. *Acute intermittent porphyria* is an autosomal dominant hepatic disorder with onset in young adult life. The overproduction of ALA and porphobilinogen in the liver is associated with acute attacks of abdominal pain, polyneuropathy, and neuropsychiatric disturbance, sometimes with a fatal outcome, but with relative freedom from symptoms between episodes. In some instances the attacks are provoked by any of a variety of medications, such as barbiturates, estrogens, or sulfa drugs, which further increase ALA synthetase activity. Fasting also provokes attacks, while a high carbohydrate diet appears to be of value in their prevention. There have been reports by Dhar and co-workers that intravenously administered heme derivatives successfully terminate attacks by means of end product inhibition of ALA synthetase activity. It has still not been established if the increased porphyrin precursors are the direct cause of the neuropathic symptoms of the disease. Freshly passed urine is colorless, but may darken after several hours' standing owing to spontaneous oxidation of porphobilinogen to porphobilin. In addition to the classic acute intermittent porphyria, there are two variants, also autosomal dominant with late onset, "variegate porphyria" and "hereditary coproporphyria." These variants are distinguished by light sensitive skin, with more marked lesions in the variegate variety, and by the increased excretion of porphyrin precursors further along the pathway of synthesis in addition to ALA and urobilinogen, as described in Table 22–10. The acute attacks resemble those of acute intermittent porphyria.

Congenital erythropoietic porphyria is a rare but dramatic autosomal recessive condition in which the increase of uroporphyrin and coproporphyrin I isomers affects primarily the erythroid cells, but red staining of all the tissues and of the urine is prominent. The onset is usually in childhood. Photosensitivity is especially severe and there are signs of hemolysis along with splenomegaly.

Porphyria cutanea tarda, also an hepatic porphyria, presumably originates from a combination of inherited enzyme deficiency in addition to acquired factors essential for the expression of the clinical signs and symptoms, which typically do not begin until middle age, as reported by Kushner and co-workers. Among the acquired factors, alcoholism and liver disease and exposure to certain medications, especially estrogen, are commonly observed, but increased liver iron is always present, often along with elevation of the plasma iron concentration and increased saturation of the plasma iron binding protein. The excess liver iron is of pathogenetic importance since its removal by a series of phlebotomies ameliorates both the clinical and biochemical manifestations of the disorder (Figure 22–58). Although the primary deficiency involves uroporphyrinogen decarboxylase, cosynthetase also appears to be in some manner affected, since urinary uroporphyrin I excretion exceeds that of uroporphyrin III. Urine urobilinogen excretion may be normal, or if elevated is commensurate with the degree of liver dysfunction. In addition to the symptoms of liver disease, photosensitivity and red urine are usually present.

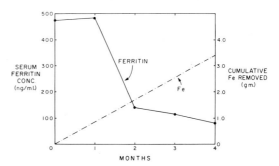

Figure 22-58 Decrease in serum ferritin concentration as iron stores were reduced by weekly phlebotomy in a patient with porphyria cutanea tarda. Initial liver biopsy documented markedly increased hepatocellular iron. The reduction in iron stores resulted in a marked decrease in the urinary porphyrin excretion (normal serum ferritin concentration 20 to 200 ng./ml.).

TABLE 22-10 CLASSIFICATION OF PORPHYRIAS

Condition	Photo Sensitivity	Tissue Primarily Involved Erythroid	Hepatic	Biochemical Abnormalities Useful in Diagnosis (Abbrevs. in Fig. 3-46)
Hereditary				
Acute intermittent porphyria	−	−	+	Increased urinary ALA and PBG.
Erythropoietic porphyria	+	+	−	Increased urinary and erythrocyte uroporphyrin I and coproporphyrin I.
Porphyria cutanea tarda	+	−	+	Increased urinary uroporphyrin I>III and coproporphyrin I and III. (Porphyrins also increased in liver, along with excess iron.)
Coproporphyria	+	−	+	Increased fecal and urinary coproporphyrin III. Increased urinary ALA and PBG during acute attacks.
Variegate porphyria	+	−	+	Increased fecal protoporphyrin 9 and coproporphyrin III. Increased urinary coproporphyrin III and, during acute attacks, ALA and PBG.
Protoporphyria	+	+	+	Increased erythrocyte and fecal protoporphyrin 9.
Acquired				
Lead poisoning	−	+	?	Increased urinary ALA and coproporphyrin III. Increased erythrocyte protoporphyrin 9.
Hexachlorobenzene toxicity	+	−	+	Increased urinary uroporphyrin I and III and coproporphyrin I and III.

Enzyme defects are listed in the legend to Figure 3-46. All inherited conditions are autosomal dominant, except erythropoietic porphyria which is autosomal recessive.

Hereditary protoporphyria is associated with high tissue concentrations of protoporphyrin 9 in both erythrocytes and liver. Symptoms may be entirely absent, but mild photosensitivity is often present from childhood. Cholelithiasis commonly occurs as a result of the high concentration of this relatively insoluble porphyrin in the bile. In some cases of long duration, chronic liver disease has developed. The excess porphyrin is excreted exclusively via the fecal route; the urine is normal. Mild anemia may be present, but there are no clinical signs of hemolysis, despite the fact that photohemolysis is demonstrable in vitro.

ACQUIRED DISORDERS OF PORPHYRIN SYNTHESIS. In *lead intoxication* several of the enzymes controlling heme synthesis are inhibited (Figure 22–57). Depression of ALA dehydrase activity is one of the earliest changes. Heme synthetase is also readily depressed as reviewed by Chisholm. Increases in urinary ALA and in erythrocyte protoporphyrin levels are accordingly observed early in the course of the disease. Urinary coproporphyrin III is also frequently increased, while urinary porphobilinogen is normal or only slightly increased. Photosensitivity is not a feature of lead toxicity because the increased intraerythrocytic protoporphyrin occurs as a zinc complex tightly bound to hemoglobin, in contrast to hereditary protoporphyria in which the protoporphyrin is loosely bound and passes out of the erythrocytes into the skin and other tissues, causing light sensitivity (Piomelli and co-workers). Increased amounts of ferritin and hemosiderin accumulate in the erythroid precursors because of the blocks in heme synthesis. The erythrocytes are slightly hypochromic and a significant proportion of them show punctate basophilic stippling due to the presence of aggregated incompletely degraded ribosomes. After having observed that hereditary deficiency of the red cell enzyme pyrimidine 5'-nucleotidase was associated with punctate basophilic stippling, Valentine and his co-workers found that this red cell enzyme was also low in patients with lead poisoning. Apparently this lack causes an impairment of ribosome ribonucleic acid degradation in reticulocytes. The anemia of lead toxicity is mild and the erythrocyte life span only slightly or moderately shortened. The neurologic symptoms are the most significant aspects of the disease — encephalopathy in the child and peripheral motor neuropathy in the adult. Abdominal pain as well as renal disease may also occur.

Toxic exposure to hexachlorobenzene mimics porphyria cutanea tarda. Affected individuals are photosensitive and have red urine. The resemblance is explained by the observation that the same enzyme, uroporphyrinogen decarboxylase, is depressed in both conditions. The original clinical observations, made following an outbreak in Turkey, have served to stimulate interest in experimental porphyria induced by this and other chemical agents.

Iron. NORMAL IRON METABOLISM. Iron, by far the most abundant heavy metal in the body is used chiefly for hemoglobin synthesis. About 1 mg. is required for each ml. of red cells produced, adding up to a daily need of 20 to 25 mg. for erythropoiesis. Almost all this iron is obtained through recycling and only about 5 per cent, or 1 mg. per day, is newly absorbed to balance losses incurred via fecal and urinary excretion and also in sweat and desquamated skin. The average menstruating female loses about twice this amount and so must absorb more to maintain balance. Menstrual loss of blood, however, is difficult to estimate and varies a great deal from woman to woman.

Absorption by the gastrointestinal epithelial cell is finely tuned to admit just enough iron to cover losses, without permitting either excess or deficiency of body iron to develop. Absorption normally admits about 5 to 10 per cent of a total dietary intake of 10 to 20 mg. per day. The physiologic signal between the size of the body iron

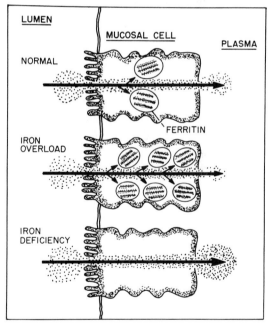

Figure 22–59 Regulation of iron absorption at the intestinal mucosa. Stippled dots represent iron molecules. Intracellular ferritin is symbolized by oval structures. The iron overloaded mucosal cell deposits more iron as ferritin, but admits relatively little into the plasma, while the iron deficient cell lowers its barrier to efficient transport of iron across into the plasma. Sloughing of mucosal cells into the intestinal lumen is a significant excretory route for iron, especially in states of iron overload. (Reprinted with permission of *Nutrition Today.* Copyright Summer, 1969, by Nutrition Today, Inc.)

Iron administered (mg)

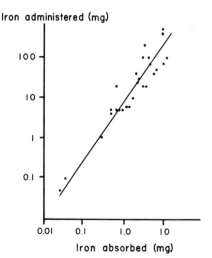

Figure 22–60 Augmentation of absolute amount of iron absorbed with increasing doses administered. (Redrawn from Bothwell, T. H., and Finch, C. A.: Iron Metabolism. Little, Brown & Co., Boston, 1962, p. 98.)

supply and the gastrointestinal mucosal cell is still only vaguely understood. The mucosal cell itself appears to act as a "ferrostat" by reflecting within its own cytoplasm the state of the body store of iron. A high concentration of cytoplasmic iron, present presumably almost entirely as ferritin, discourages further uptake, while an iron-poor intracellular environment encourages uptake into the cell and then on into the plasma for binding to transferrin (Fig. 22–59).

The absorption of iron is also increased in response to increased erythropoietic activity. The mucosal epithelial cells are in a constant state of renewal, proliferating from the crypts out toward the tips of the villi, where they are shed into the lumen. Such cellular loss is a significant source of iron excretion in the feces. The existence of a specialized iron transport protein within the mucosal cell remains open to question.

The barrier to excessive iron absorption set up by the mucosal cell is easily overcome, since increasing amounts of iron presented to the intestinal epithelial surface are met by additional increments of absorbed iron, although the proportion absorbed falls off (Fig. 22–60). The mucosal barrier is temporarily raised, however, by recently ingested iron, which decreases the absorption of a second dose given several hours later (Fig. 22–61).

The entire gastrointestinal tract has the capacity to absorb iron, but maximal activity is found in the duodenum and upper jejunum, probably because of the presence there of optimal conditions of pH and redox potential. Absorption occurs in the ferrous state, and ferric iron, which forms insoluble hydroxides at neutral and alkaline pH, must first be reduced before it is absorbed. For efficient reduction, an acid gastric juice is indispensable (Fig. 22–62). Chelation with low molecular weight compounds, such as fructose and amino acids, may also promote solubility preparatory to absorption. Whether the gastric juice itself contains special iron-chelating substances of either high or low molecular weight remains somewhat controversial. Dietary constituents such as phosphate and phytate render iron less soluble and thus less available for absorption. The concept that pancre-

RADIOIRON ABSORPTION
(% OF CONTROL)

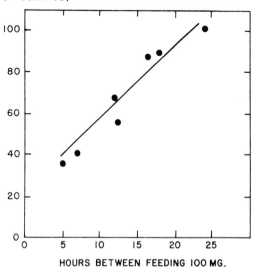

HOURS BETWEEN FEEDING 100 MG.
IRON AND RADIOIRON

Figure 22–61 The change in absorption of a test dose of radioactive iron at intervals after an initial loading dose of nonradioactive iron. (Redrawn from Stewart, W. B., et al.: J. Exper. Med., 92:375, 1950.)

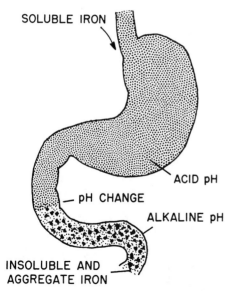

Figure 22–62 Relation of pH to the maximal site of iron absorption in the upper duodenum. (Reprinted with permission of *Nutrition Today.* Copyright Summer, 1969 by Nutrition Today, Inc.)

atic insufficiency, by reducing duodenal pH, causes increased iron absorption has been challenged. Food iron, in contrast to the inorganic ferrous form of medicinal iron, occurs as organic complexes, such as ferritin and myoglobin, much of it in the trivalent state. Some of the complexes are broken up and solubilized during acid digestion in the stomach, but the heme iron passes on and is readily absorbed intact into the mucosal epithelial cells, without dependence upon reducing systems and by a mechanism that is distinct from that for inorganic iron, as described by Weintraub and co-workers. The iron is stripped away from its complex with porphyrin only after cellular uptake. Myoglobin and hemoglobin are better nutritional sources of iron than ferritin and hemosiderin, which are not as well absorbed.

Effete red cells which have lived out their 120-day life span are taken up by the phagocytic macrophages, chiefly in the spleen, liver, and bone marrow. Inside these phagocytic cells the hemoglobin is broken down into its essential constituents, with an efficient salvage of the iron taken from degraded heme. This salvaged iron is packed in extremely high concentration inside apoferritin protein shells to form molecules of ferritin, each of which may contain up to 4000 atoms of iron (Fig. 22–63). Ferritin molecules, in turn, are com-

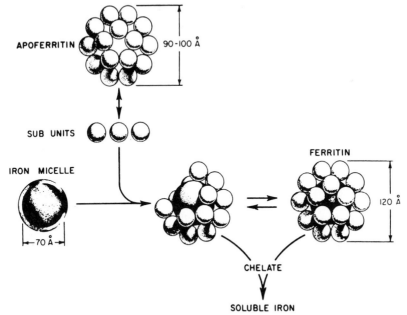

Figure 22–63 Structure of ferritin. A series of identical subunits is assembled to form a protein shell (apoferritin). An iron micelle, containing up to 4000 atoms of iron, is formed inside. Iron can be removed, leaving behind an intact apoferritin shell.

There are a series of isoferritins which differ depending on the tissue of origin. Thus, for example, ferritin extracted from macrophages differs from that found in erythroid cells or heart. Ferritin found in plasma also differs from that found in tissues, especially in its low iron content. It appears to originate predominantly from macrophages rather than parenchymal cells.

(Reprinted from Pape, L., et al.: Biochemistry, 7:606, 1968. Copyright 1968, American Chemical Society. Reprinted by permission of the copyright owner.)

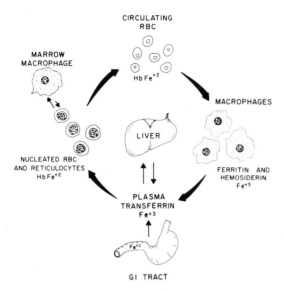

Figure 22–64 Metabolic pathways of iron. The bulk of body iron turnover goes to erythropoiesis in the marrow and is reutilized from hemoglobin degraded in macrophages located primarily in the liver, spleen, and marrow. Only a small proportion of the iron is newly absorbed from dietary sources to make up for excretory losses. Cell-to-cell interaction between erythroid precursors and macrophages takes place in the marrow with possible exchange of ferritin iron. The direction of this exchange is still uncertain, but most evidence suggests that marrow (and splenic) macrophages remove excess ferritin and hemosiderin iron from erythroid cells. Transferrin mediates iron transport from macrophages and the intestinal mucosa to immature erythroid cells. It also delivers iron to hepatic and other parenchymal cells, but at a much lesser rate.

pressed into still larger amorphous aggregates of insoluble material called hemosiderin, which form granules visible by light microscopy. Thus it is as ferritin and hemosiderin, chiefly in macrophages, that the bulk of the reserve iron is stored. It is from these depots that iron recycles, fulfilling the continuing need for iron in the production of red cells (Fig. 22–64).

The storage iron most recently obtained from degraded heme is the first to be reutilized for hemoglobin synthesis; the chronologically more archaic iron depots may remain untouched for very long periods of time. In a normal adult with 2500-ml. red cell mass, 2500 mg. of iron circulates as hemoglobin while another 500 to 1500 mg. is present as storage iron. Although the vast bulk of the storage iron is found in macrophages, ferritin is detectable in many of the tissues of the body, including erythroblasts and the intestinal epithelial cells. Other significant pools of body iron are in myoglobin (130 mg.) and a variety of enzymes, such as the cytochromes, catalase, peroxidase, and many others (8 mg.).

Iron is taken from storage depots and transported back to erythroid precursors by a highly specialized plasma protein, transferrin. Stored in ferritin in the trivalent state, the iron is first reduced to the ferrous form for removal from the apoferritin shell, and then it is carried in the ferric state, up to two atoms per molecule of transferrin. The normal concentration of iron in the plasma is about 100 μg. per 100 ml., one third the total binding capacity of available transferrin. The total amount of iron in the transferrin pool, assuming that approximately half of it is intravascular and half extravascular, is about 4 to 5 mg. Although this transferrin-bound iron is only 1 per cent of that in the body, its metabolic rate of turnover is extremely rapid — 50 per cent of it is cleared from the intravascular space every 60 to 120 minutes. Transferrin molecules deliver their iron at the surface of the erythroid precursors and return empty to the macrophages to pick up another load (Fig. 22–65).

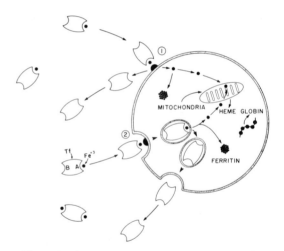

Figure 22–65 Schematic representation of the delivery of iron to erythroid precursors. *A* and *B* indicate the two iron-binding sites on the transferrin molecule. Transferrin preferentially delivers its iron to receptors present on the surface of nucleated erythroid cells and on reticulocytes, but absent from mature erythrocytes (Aisen and Brown, 1977). The presence of an anion, physiologically probably bicarbonate, is necessary to establish the extraordinarily high affinity between transferrin and Fe^{+3}; in its absence virtually no binding takes place. The cell frees iron from transferrin, possibly by removing the anion. Two mechanisms for delivery have been postulated. Pathway (1) envisions a receptor on the outer surface of the cell membrane. Pathway (2) pictures pinocytosis of the transferrin-iron complex, release of iron, and then ejection of the iron-free transferrin back to the plasma. Iron is transported within the cell to mitochondria for heme synthesis and is stored as ferritin and hemosiderin. Intracellular iron transport mechanisms have still not been elucidated.

Fletcher and Huehns have proposed a provocative, but still unproved, hypothesis stating that the two iron binding sites on the transferrin molecule, Site A and Site B, are unequal in their affinity for ferric iron and subserve different physiologic functions. Site A, they state, picks up iron at the intestinal mucosal cell and delivers it to receptors on immature erythroid cells (and the placenta). Site B preferentially gives up its iron to hepatocytes as well as to intestinal mucosal cells, the governors of the rate of iron absorption. The amount and distribution of iron on transferrin would then control its absorption as well as its distribution in the body. This remarkable hypothesis has had the merit of provoking a number of experimental tests, but the results so far have generally been at odds.

The rate of disappearance of radioactive iron from the plasma as well as its reappearance in the circulating red cells as newly produced labeled hemoglobin is a convenient method of measuring the functional state of erythropoiesis, as discussed by Ricketts and co-workers (Fig. 22–33). In hypoplastic conditions the utilization of iron is depressed, causing a rise in its plasma concentration along with a decrease in the rate at which it is cleared from the normal half-life of 1 to 2 hours to 3 to 4 hours or longer. In iron deficiency the clearance rate is more rapid than normal, as it is in conditions associated with increased proliferation of red cell precursors in the marrow, such as

hemolytic anemia. Normally about 70 to 80 per cent of the tracer iron reappears in circulating erythrocytes within 10 days of administration, but this figure may approach zero in the absence of red cell production. The red cell utilization of tracer iron is also depressed in conditions such as thalassemia or megaloblastic anemia, in which the marrow is rich in proliferating erythroid precursor cells and in their requirement for iron, but owing to extensive intramedullary destruction of these cells, little of the radioiron reappears in circulating erythrocytes despite its rapid clearance from the plasma. A labile pool of storage iron contributes a minor slow component to the plasma radioiron disappearance curve.

IRON LACK

General Effects. The first change in the development of iron deficiency is the loss of storage iron from the macrophages of the spleen, liver, and bone marrow. The evaluation of marrow iron stores is a convenient method of assessing the state of the body iron stores; if they are preserved, iron deficiency can be excluded as the primary cause of anemia. After the stores of iron are used up, the plasma iron concentration falls, at the same time stimulating an increase in the synthesis of transferrin. The saturation of transferrin with iron thus falls from 30 per cent to values often below 10 per cent (Fig. 22–66). Plasma ferritin concentration is always depressed and distinguishes the hypoferremia of iron deficiency from

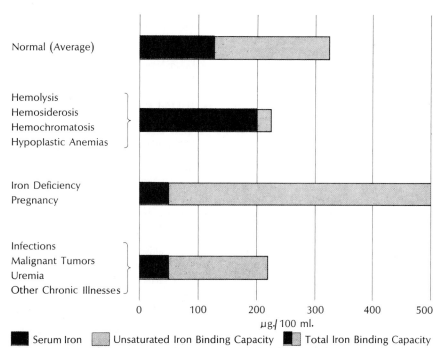

Normal (Average)

Hemolysis
Hemosiderosis
Hemochromatosis
Hypoplastic Anemias

Iron Deficiency
Pregnancy

Infections
Malignant Tumors
Uremia
Other Chronic Illnesses

0   100   200   300   400   500
μg./100 ml.

■ Serum Iron   ▨ Unsaturated Iron Binding Capacity   ▨ Total Iron Binding Capacity

Figure 22–66 The changes in serum iron and iron binding capacity in various disorders. (From McIntyre, P.: Hosp. Pract., March, 1972, p. 101.)

that seen in association with the anemia of chronic disease, in which plasma ferritin is normal or elevated. Erythrocyte protoporphyrin levels are increased secondary to the intracellular deficit of sufficient iron for heme synthesis. Anemia is the last change to be observed. At first, the erythrocytes may be normocytic and normochromic and show only a few shape changes, but microcytic, hypochromic, and misshapen erythrocytes emerge as significant anemia develops. Even with only a moderate degree of anemia, the deficit in body iron is thus already advanced.

Whether iron deficiency without anemia causes significant symptoms remains a controversial issue. The activities of certain iron-containing enzymes decrease, but this change may not be of pathophysiologic significance. When anemia develops it is often well tolerated, except when there is acute blood loss or cardiovascular limitation. Changes in epithelial tissues complicate more protracted deficiency. There is inversion of the normal curvature of the fingernails ("spooning"), which also become more brittle; hair splits and breaks off; and a smooth red tongue reflects glossitis. Dysphagia with web formation in the upper esophagus rarely complicates iron lack of many years' duration. Atrophic gastritis with anacidity is frequently associated with iron deficiency, whether primarily the result of it (through secondary epithelial changes) or the cause of it (through impaired absorption of food iron) or both is not clear. Infants with iron deficiency anemia frequently have detectable occult blood in the feces without demonstrable gastrointestinal disease, presumably because of mucosal friability secondary to the deficient state. Mucosal changes secondary to iron deficiency in infants reportedly may be of sufficient magnitude to cause malabsorption. A moderately elevated platelet count is often seen in infants with iron deficiency anemia. Thrombocytosis in iron-deficient adults seems to be less prominent and more often explainable on the basis of reactive changes to hemorrhage, tumor, or other underlying disorders.

Pathogenesis. Iron deficiency always arises because of the inability of diet and absorption to keep pace with the increased requirements imposed either by the expansion of the red cell mass or by blood loss. The efficiency of absorption depends not only on the total amount of food iron but also on its form as well as on the dietary content of phosphate and phytate. Habitual eating of laundry starch or clay is commonly seen among iron-deficient patients of certain population groups. Such materials may have an adverse effect upon iron absorption, but of even greater importance is the fact that among such patients the dietary intake of good sources of iron, such as meat, is also often severely limited. A peculiar craving for ice may develop. Iron deficient children with pica may develop lead poisoning because they eat lead-containing paint. These unusual eating patterns appear to respond to the treatment of the iron deficiency.

The growth spurt of the 2-year-old and of the adolescent are common times for iron deficiency to appear. The well-nourished milk-fed infant is particularly prone because such a diet, while adequate in calories, is sorely lacking in iron. Iron deficiency is very rare at the time of birth, even if the mother is deficient. However, the rapid growth which follows premature birth requires iron supplementation during the first weeks of life to prevent the development of anemia. During pregnancy, the red cell mass expands by 20 per cent, which may require about 400 mg. of additional iron. The fetus requires about 280 mg., which is lost to the mother along with blood loss at childbirth. The losses of lactation are about equal to those which would have occurred from menstruation (Fig. 22–67).

The proper absorption of food iron being dependent upon a normal gastric milieu, anacidity acquired from either atrophic gastritis or from partial or total gastrectomy very commonly leads to iron deficiency anemia. Billroth type II procedures, which bypass the duodenum, are more commonly associated than those procedures which leave this site of maximal iron absorption intact. Rapid intestinal transit time may limit the time available for absorption. Excessive gastrointestinal blood loss contributes to iron depletion in those clinical situations which require gastric surgery, such as peptic ulcer. Iron lack coexists with other multiple deficiencies in the intestinal malabsorption syndromes, but if the duodenal surface is well preserved, sufficient iron may be absorbed to meet requirements.

Blood loss is the most important factor in the development of iron deficiency. Identification of its origin may bring to light the presence of unsuspected but significant underlying disease, such as carcinoma of the colon. Hiatus hernia, hemorrhagic gastritis, and peptic ulcer disease are particularly frequent causes of upper gastrointestinal bleeding. Chronic aspirin users develop iron deficiency anemia because of increased gastrointestinal blood loss with or without demonstrable underlying disease. Menorrhagia, sometimes associated with such underlying disease as uterine fibroids, is the most frequent cause in premenopausal females. Sources of urinary blood loss include renal tumors as well as the chronic hemoglobinuria and hemosiderinuria associated with chronic intravascular hemolysis. Vasculitis of the pulmonary vessels with chronic hemorrhage into the lungs will cause pulmonary macrophages to become iron-laden in *Goodpasture's syndrome.* However, iron is not efficiently reutilized from these cells and an iron-deficient bone marrow with microcytic, hypochromic anemia ensues.

IRON
REQUIREMENT
MG / DAY

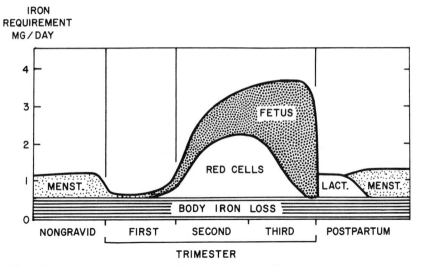

Figure 22–67 The change in iron requirement during pregnancy. (Redrawn from Bothwell, T.H., and Finch, C. A.: Iron Metabolism. Little, Brown & Co., Boston, 1962, p. 309.)

IRON EXCESS

General Effects. The accumulation of excessive quantities of iron in the body ultimately originates from increased absorption or from parenteral administration as transfusions or as pharmacologic iron complexes. The capacity of the macrophages to gather the extra iron within their protective confines is immense, but ultimately the degree of transferrin saturation rises, its synthesis is inhibited, and the plasma iron concentration approaches 200 µg. per 100 ml. with near 100 per cent saturation of the iron-binding capacity (Fig. 22–66). As the transferrin saturation rises above 50 per cent parenchymal cells are no longer protected from pathologic iron uptake and damage occurs over the years to various organs, especially the liver, heart, pancreas, pituitary, and synovial tissues. Signs of chronic liver disease appear, along with those of heart failure, diabetes mellitus, and endocrine insufficiency. A characteristic form of arthropathy may develop. The term *hemochromatosis* is used to describe the disease which thus arises from such chronic iron overexposure. Grayish pigmentation of the skin is caused by deposition of melanin in the deeper layers of the epidermis. Deposits of iron are seen in the glandular structures of the skin.

Acute iron poisoning occurs chiefly in children who accidentally swallow an overdose of iron pills. Nausea, vomiting, and intestinal bleeding are soon followed by vascular collapse and shock, with a high likelihood of a fatal outcome.

The detection of iron overload would be best accomplished by the direct measurement of total body iron stores, but no satisfactory technique is available for this. A rise in the plasma iron concentration and transferrin saturation is associated with increased iron stores, but similar changes are seen secondary to altered bone marrow function, such as hypoplastic and megaloblastic anemia. Furthermore, the hypoferremic response to inflammation may depress an elevated plasma iron level and mask a state of iron overload.

A time-honored but cumbersome method of measuring iron stores uses quantitative phlebotomy carried out over many months to the point of early iron deficiency anemia, a sign that the iron stores initially present have been depleted. The total amount of hemoglobin iron removed, assuming 1 mg. Fe per ml. erythrocytes, is roughly equivalent to the iron stores initially present.

A "labile" intracellular pool of iron may be assessed by measuring the urinary excretion of iron for 24 hours after a single injection of the chelating agent desferrioxamine (DFOM). The normal excretes about 0.5 mg., whereas the iron-loaded patient may excrete up to 10 to 20 mg. This labile pool is thought to be physiologically chelated within cells to low molecular weight substances, since the other biologic forms of iron (ferritin, transferrin, heme) are not significantly available for DFOM chelation.

The concentration of ferritin in plasma may be extraordinarily high in iron-overloaded states, but normal values also are observed. The plasma ferritin level usually reflects the iron pool of the macrophages rather than that of the parenchymal cells, and thus normal levels may be seen in the face of parenchymal iron excess. Breakdown of normal hepatic or neoplastic parenchymal cells, however, may cause release of ferritin into the plasma. Thus, elevated plasma ferritin levels also occur in patients with acute or chronic liver disease, leukemia, or cancer. Plasma ferritin measurements may be useful in the detection of iron deficiency, of iron excess, or in following changes on body iron status (Fig. 22–58), but caution must be exercised in correctly interpreting the value.

Perhaps the most sensitive method for the early detection of iron overload is direct measurement on samples obtained by liver biopsy. Estimation is made microscopically after suitable staining or by chemical measurement. Although bone marrow iron content is invaluable in the detection of iron deficiency, it is less helpful in hemochromatosis, as discussed below.

Pathogenesis. An increase in the body content of iron in *primary hemochromatosis* occurs because of an inappropriate and as yet unexplained increase in iron absorption by the intestinal mucosal cells as reviewed in 1977 by Jacobs. An increase in liver iron, predominantly in the hepatocytes, may be the sole manifestation early in the course of the disease, but elevation of the plasma iron and increased saturation of transferrin is also often present initially (Edwards and associates, 1977). Iron loading in macrophages and elevation of the plasma ferritin occur later. In advanced stages the body may contain 30 to 40 grams of iron. The fact that macrophage and intestinal mucosal cell iron content do not appear increased early in the disease has led to the postulate that the primary defect may be a deficient rate of ferritin synthesis in these sites, with breakdown of the mucosal barrier against increased absorption, reduction of the normal protective storage function of the macrophages, and consequent iron loading of transferrin and of parenchymal cells, especially hepatic. Erythrocyte morphology is normal, and erythropoiesis is unaffected. Indeed, anemia is noteworthy for its absence. Although the disorder runs in families, its hereditary nature has been disputed. Excess dietary iron — usually in the form of certain beers and wines with high iron content, food cooked in iron utensils, or medicinal iron — leads to a similar disorder. Instances of apparent primary hemochromatosis which develop in patients with alcoholic cirrhosis presumably are related to the fact that a small proportion of such patients develop increased iron absorption secondary to the liver disease. The pathogenesis of this increase is obscure.

Iron overload due to chronic transfusion (transfusion hemosiderosis) contrasts with primary hemochromatosis inasmuch as iron loading occurs first in the macrophages and only later in the parenchymal cells. Plasma ferritin is elevated early in the course of the iron overload, and a rise in the plasma iron and transferrin saturation occurs later. The iron overload may be readily detected in bone marrow macrophages or circulating blood monocytes, which are not reliable parameters of iron overload in early primary hemochromatosis, although their iron content increases as the disease progresses.

Hemochromatosis also complicates disorders of erythropoiesis in which iron is not properly utilized for hemoglobin formation. The increased iron absorption is apparently related to the hyperplastic, although ineffective, erythropoiesis which characterizes these conditions. Red cell morphology is abnormal. The anemia is of any degree from minimal to severe. An excessive number of hemosiderin granules accumulates in the cytoplasm of erythroid precursor cells as well as in mature erythrocytes, where their presence becomes much more obvious after splenectomy. The term "sideroblast" is applied to any nucleated erythroid precursor which contains stainable iron granules. In normal marrow about 25 per cent of erythroid precursors are sideroblasts containing two or three small cytoplasmic granules. The number and size of such iron granules as well as the proportion of erythroid cells containing them increase in a number of states of increased erythropoiesis, including hemolytic anemia and megaloblastic anemia. However, in the marrow of certain iron-loading anemias there are seen a large number of "ringed sideroblasts," erythroid cells in which a necklace of iron granules surrounds the nucleus. To these conditions the term "sideroblastic anemia" is applied. The ringed configuration is presumably related to the fact that the iron accumulation is concentrated on the mitochondria, which cling to the nuclear membranes in the fixed and stained preparations.

The *sideroblastic anemias* are classified as primary or secondary, hereditary or acquired (Kushner, et al., 1971). Hypochromic, small, misshapen erythrocytes are often seen in the midst of a population of normocytic or even macrocytic cells. Hereditary sex-linked hypochromic anemia is usually first detected in young adult or adolescent males, whereas primary acquired sideroblastic anemia is seen in patients of either sex over the age of 60. Occasionally, with observation the latter condition will ultimately prove to be a secondary variety associated with a myeloproliferative syndrome culminating in acute myelogenous leukemia. The condition can also occur secondary to certain drugs (isoniazid, cycloserine, chloramphenicol), to lead poisoning, or to alcoholic excess, but reversibility averts the development of hemochromatosis. Rare ringed sideroblasts are occasionally seen in the marrow of patients with certain chronic diseases, such as rheumatoid arthritis or carcinoma, but hyperferremia and iron-loading do not complicate the picture.

Some of the sideroblastic anemias are pyridoxine-responsive, as described by Harris. The doses required are pharmacologic, and signs of pyridoxine deficiency are absent. Anemia is improved and the serum iron decreases. The response is not complete, although it is generally more satisfactory in the hereditary than in the primary acquired cases. The explanation of responsiveness may reside in a defect in conversion of pyridoxine to its active form, pyridoxal phosphate, which is required for the first step in heme synthesis on the mitochondria, upon which iron accumulates. Recent studies have provided some evidence for superior therapeutic efficacy of pyridoxal phosphate, but it would appear that the entire group of disorders is at present too heterogeneous to be properly analyzed until a more precise biochemical classification is achieved. Indeed, megaloblastic erythropoiesis and macrocytic erythrocytes are also sometimes observed along with a degree of folic acid responsiveness.

Hemochromatosis is a major cause of morbidity and mortality in thalassemia, a primary deficiency of globin synthesis. Erythroid cells are iron-loaded, but ringed sideroblasts are not prominent. Transfusional hemosiderosis contributes to the iron-load in thalassemia major, as well as in any anemia of sufficient severity to require chronic transfusion therapy.

Primary hemochromatosis is treated with removal of iron by repeated phlebotomy over a long period of time, until iron stores become depleted and the serum iron falls. This approach has also been used in hemochromatosis secondary to iron-loading erythrocyte disorders in which the anemia is mild. Another approach has been the use of iron chelating agents such as desferrioxamine. Recent observations by Propper and co-workers have shown enhanced efficacy of desferrioxamine given by continuous infusion rather than bolus injection. Iron chelators may be life-saving in the treatment of acute iron poisoning.

Globin

NORMAL STRUCTURE AND SYNTHESIS. The primary structure of the globin molecule as well as its production rate is under genetic control. Its specific amino acid sequence is governed by the triplet code of DNA bases passed down in the chromosomes from generation to generation. The rate at which globin polypeptide chains are synthesized is a function of the rate at which the DNA code is transcribed into messenger RNA. The sequence of translational events which follow modifies the production rate of the completed chains. These include the initiation and assembly on, and the release of the polypeptide chains from, the messenger RNA-polyribosome complex upon which the amino acids are joined together in proper sequence.

At least six genetic loci direct globin synthesis. The α and β chains of normal adult hemoglobin (HbA) are produced in matched amounts, but under the control of separate genes located far apart from one another on different chromosomes. The δ chain closely resembles the β chain, to which it is genetically linked on the same chromosome, but it is synthesized at only 1/40 the rate of β chains. Thus the concentration of Hb A_2 ($\alpha_2\delta_2$) in the normal adult is only about 2.5 per cent of the total hemoglobin. Alpha chains are synthesized from early embryonic life on, but are combined

with different chains according to the stage of development (Table 22–11). The ζ and ϵ globin chains are embryonic products produced during the first trimester of intrauterine development. Beyond the first trimester α and γ chain synthesis predominates in the formation of fetal hemoglo-

TABLE 22–11 SELECTED HEMOGLOBINS— THEIR STRUCTURES AND STRUCTURAL MUTATIONS

Normal Amino Acid Sequence	
HbA	$\alpha_2\,\beta_2$
Hb A_2	$\alpha_2\,\delta_2$
Hb F	$\alpha_2\,\gamma_2$
Hb H	β_4
Hb Bart's	γ_4
Hb Portland	$\zeta_2\gamma_2$
Hb Gower-1	$\zeta_2\epsilon_2$
Hb Gower-2	$\alpha_2\epsilon_2$

Methemoglobinemia	
Hb M Boston	$\alpha^{58\ his} \rightarrow {}^{tyr}\,\beta_2$
Hb M Iwate	$\alpha^{87\ his} \rightarrow {}^{tyr}\,\beta_2$
Hb M Saskatoon	$\alpha_2\ \beta_2^{63\ his} \rightarrow {}^{tyr}$
Hb M Hyde Park	$\alpha_2\ \beta_2^{92\ his} \rightarrow {}^{tyr}$

Increased Oxygen Affinity with Erythrocytosis	
Hb Chesapeake	$\alpha_2^{92\ arg} \rightarrow {}^{leu}\,\beta_2$
Hb Rainier	$\alpha_2\ \beta_2^{145\ tyr} \rightarrow {}^{his}$
Hb Hiroshima	$\alpha_2\ \beta_2^{143\ his} \rightarrow {}^{asp}$

Decreased Oxygen Affinity with Cyanosis	
Hb Kansas	$\alpha_2\ \beta_2^{102\ asn} \rightarrow {}^{thr}$

Unstable Hemoglobin with Hemolytic Anemia	
Hb Torino	$\alpha_2^{43\ phe} \rightarrow {}^{val}\,\beta_2$
Hb Hammersmith	$\alpha_2\ \beta_2^{42\ phe} \rightarrow {}^{ser}$
Hb Zürich	$\alpha_2\ \beta_2^{63\ his} \rightarrow {}^{arg}$
Hb Tacoma	$\alpha_2\ \beta_2^{30\ arg} \rightarrow {}^{ser}$
Hb Philly	$\alpha_2\ \beta_2^{35\ tyr} \rightarrow {}^{phe}$
Hb Freiburg	$\alpha_2\ \beta_2^{23\ val} \rightarrow {}^{o}$
Hb Gun Hill	$\alpha_2\ \beta_2^{93-97} \rightarrow {}^{o}$
Hb Genova	$\alpha_2\ \beta_2^{28\ leu} \rightarrow {}^{pro}$
Hb Seattle	$\alpha_2\ \beta_2^{76\ ala} \rightarrow {}^{glu}$

"Exterior" Mutants	
Hb S	$\alpha_2\ \beta_2^{6\ glu} \rightarrow {}^{val}$
Hb C	$\alpha_2\ \beta_2^{6\ glu} \rightarrow {}^{lys}$
Hb E	$\alpha_2\ \beta^{26\ glu} \rightarrow {}^{lys}$
Hb C Harlem	$\alpha_2\ \beta_2^{6\ glu} \rightarrow {}^{val};$
	${}^{73\ asp} \rightarrow {}^{asn}$
Hb Korle-bu	$\alpha_2\ \beta_2^{73\ asp} \rightarrow {}^{asn}$
Hb G Accra	$\alpha_2\ \beta_2^{79\ asp} \rightarrow {}^{asn}$
Hb D Punjab	$\alpha_2\ \beta_2^{121\ glu} \rightarrow {}^{gln}$

Mutants with Low Synthetic Rate	
Hb Lepore	$\alpha_2\ \delta$-β_2 (fusion gene)
Hb Constant Spring	$\alpha_2^{141} \rightarrow {}^{172}\,\beta_2$

Globin polypeptide subunits, each under the control of separate genes, are designated alpha (α), beta (β), gamma (γ), delta (δ), epsilon (ϵ), or zeta (ζ). The subscript refers to the number of subunits. The superscript indicates the mutation site.

bin, Hb F ($\alpha_2\gamma_2$), which makes up 75 to 90 per cent of the total hemoglobin at birth. Schroeder and co-workers have shown that at least two genetic loci govern the production of different types of γ chains, one with glycine at the 136 position Gγ, the other with alanine Aγ. Although the synthesis of adult type β chains is begun early in intrauterine development, predominance is not established until its synthetic rate sharply rises in the weeks just preceding birth. Hb A then gradually replaces Hb F in the circulating erythrocytes until the normal adult level of Hb F (<2 per cent) is attained, usually at about 6 months of age, although slight elevations may persist for two years (Fig. 22–68).

Thanks largely to the work of Perutz, the three-dimensional fine structure of the hemoglobin molecule is rather well understood. The α and β subunits, similar but not identical in size and shape, possess a complementariness of structure which causes them to spontaneously associate with each other and form a dimer which constitutes the basis of both the function of the molecule as an oxygen transporter and its physicochemical stability. Unpaired, the subunits not only are incapable of oxygen transport but are also excessively unstable. The stability of the dimer ($\alpha_1\beta_1$) comes from the extensive area of surface contact between the two subunits, involving 34 amino acid residues in the contact site. When two dimers come together to form the complete tetrameric configuration, an "asymmetric" contact point forms between the α chain of one dimer and the β chain of the other (Fig. 22–69). This asymmetric ($\alpha_1\beta_2$) contact area is somewhat less extensive, involving only 19 amino acid sites, but this region is important in the regulation of the normal sigmoid shape of the hemoglobin oxygen dissociation curve. It is at this point that the allosteric properties of hemoglobin, as it combines with its substrate oxygen, are modulated. The initial attachment of oxygen to the α chain heme causes its iron to "snap back" as if released from a position under tension. This signal

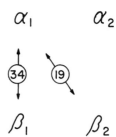

Figure 22–69   The α and β subunit contact regions in the hemoglobin molecule. The numbers of amino acids in the contact areas are indicated. (Redrawn from Weatherall, D. J., and Clegg, J. B.: the Thalassemia Syndromes. Blackwell Scientific Publications Ltd., Oxford, 1972, p. 17.)

then sends a "shock wave" through the molecule which increases the affinity of the β chain heme groups for oxygen atoms, producing the upward inflection of the oxygen dissociation curve and at the same time causing the β chains to move closer to another by 7 Å. The β chains shift back apart when oxygen is once again removed (Fig. 22–13). These intramolecular changes have led to the use of the terms "tense" (T) and "relaxed" (R) to describe the allosteric configurational states of deoxy- and oxyhemoglobin, respectively. The binding of low molecular weight phosphates, such as 2,3-diphosphoglycerate, takes place in the cleft between the two β chains when they are in the deoxy configuration, thus diminishing the oxygen affinity of the hemoglobin.

The globular subunit, which is divided into eight helical regions designated by the letters A through H, is physiologically submerged in an aqueous medium with which it blends because it carries all its hydrophilic groupings on its exterior surface. These include hydroxyl groups, such as those of serine and threonine, as well as polar carboxyl and amino groups. The molecular interior is arid and is lined with hydrophobic nonpolar groups. Each subunit has its heme group neatly tucked into a "heme pocket" which dips down from the molecular surface and is also completely lined with hydrophobic groups which exclude water from the region. The heme comes into contact at about 60 atomic sites with the surface of the pocket. The fifth coordinate position of the heme iron is bound to the "proximal histidine" residue (β^{92} and α^{87}). Molecular oxygen is carried between the sixth coordinate position of iron and the "distal histidine" (β^{63} and α^{58}) (Fig. 22–12).

Hemoglobinopathy Due to Structural Defects (Table 3–10)

Nomenclature. In the years that followed the first description of sickle hemoglobin (Hb S) in 1949 it became evident that the letters in the alphabet would not be sufficient to accommodate

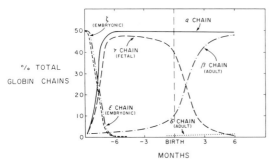

Figure 22–68   The change in globin chains during intrauterine development. (Redrawn from Bunn, H. F., Forget, B. G., and Ranney, H. M. Human Hemoglobins. W. B. Saunders Co., Philadelphia, 1977. p. 107.)

names for the large number of mutant hemoglobins being discovered. Family names and then place names were given as trivial expressions, to be followed by a specific designation of the amino acid substitution which characterized the abnormal hemoglobin. For example, "Hb Philly" was first observed in Philadelphia. It has normal α chains, but the β chains are affected by an inherited abnormality of the 35th amino acid from the N-terminal end of the β chains, at which phenylalanine is found in place of tyrosine (Fig. 22–70). This abnormal hemoglobin is thus designated $\alpha_2 \beta_2^{35tyr} \rightarrow {}^{phe}$. Mutations of the β chain outnumber those of the α chain. Abnormal δ and γ chains have also been discovered. Many abnormal hemoglobins produce no abnormality in erythrocyte appearance or function and are not pathogenetic. Some are harmful only in the homozygous state, while others are lethal in the homozygous state and thus are only observed in heterozygous carriers.

Methemoglobinemia. A substitution of tyrosine for histidine at either the proximal or distal histidine residues of either the α or the β chains locks the heme iron into a trivalent state resistant to the action of the enzyme methemoglobin reductase, which has the responsibility of maintaining the iron atoms of hemoglobin in the ferrous state. The affected heme groups in half the molecule are incapable of oxygen transport while the unaffected pair of hemes retains the ability to combine reversibly with oxygen. In the α chain methemo-

globinemias, the normal β partner has a somewhat decreased affinity for oxygen because of the absence of the "signal" which is normally sent across to the β chain from the α when it first combines with oxygen. In the β chain mutants, the oxygen affinity of the unaffected α submit is more nearly normal. Inheritance is autosomal dominant and homozygosity is apparently lethal, in contrast to inherited deficiency of methemoglobin reductase, which is an autosomal recessive state. The methemoglobinemia of mutant hemoglobins is resistant to therapy while that occurring as a result of deficiency of the enzyme responds to treatment with such reducing agents as methylene blue or ascorbic acid.

High Affinity Hemoglobin With Erythrocytosis. Mutant hemoglobins which raise the hemoglobin oxygen affinity shift the oxygen dissociation curve to the left, impeding oxygen unloading at the tissues (Fig. 22–71). The erythropoietin response evokes a secondary form of polycythemia which is familial and benign and is unassociated with increases in the platelet or leukocyte count. The mutation sites affect either the area of $\alpha_1\beta_2$ subunit contact or the C-terminal ends of the β chains close to the cove where low molecular weight phosphates are bound. Mutants such as Hb Chesapeake, which are located at the $\alpha_1\beta_2$ contact, have a raised oxygen affinity along with a loss in the normal sigmoid contour of the oxygen dissociation curve, but their Bohr effect is preserved. In Hb Hiroshima and Hb Rainier, which affect the C-terminal region of the β subunits, the Bohr effect is impaired. These substitutions presumably raise oxygen affinity by interfering with low molecular weight phosphate binding and allosteric movements.

Low Affinity Hemoglobin With Cyanosis. Hb Kansas is a mutation at the $\alpha_1\beta_2$ contact which causes a lowered oxygen affinity (Fig. 22–71). Cyanosis is reversed if the patient is placed in an atmosphere of sufficiently high partial pressure of oxygen. Oxygen unloading is facilitated in the tissues, with a decreased stimulus to erythropoietin secretion causing a mild but "physiologic" anemia.

Unstable Hemoglobin With Congenital Heinz Body Hemolytic Anemia. Amino acid replacements which loosen the attachment of heme in its pocket or the dimeric association of the subunits at the $\alpha_1\beta_1$ contact region cause the mutant hemoglobin to be inordinately susceptible to oxidation. Water entry into normally hydrophobic regions is followed by conversion to methemoglobin and oxidation of the hemoglobin into insoluble lumps. These impede erythrocyte pliability and cause hemolysis. The intact spleen plucks these precipitates from the erythrocytes. After splenectomy, a large proportion of the circulating erythrocytes contain Heinz bodies, the term which is used to describe these intracellular inclusions of precipi-

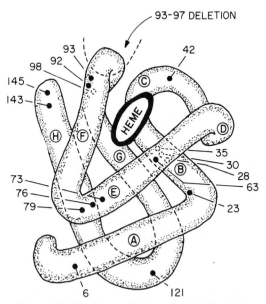

Figure 22–70 The β globin subunit. The letters *A* through *H* indicate the eight helical regions. The numbered positions indicate amino acid sites discussed in the text and in Table 22–11. (Redrawn from Giblett, E. R.: Genetic Markers in Human Blood. Blackwell Scientific Publications Ltd., Oxford, 1969.)

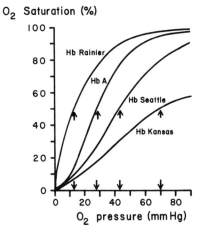

O₂ Saturation (%)

Figure 22–71 Examples of hemoglobins with abnormal oxygen affinity. Arrows indicate P_{50}. (Reproduced with permission from "Abnormal Hemoglobins with High and Low Oxygen Affinity" by G. Stamatoyannopoulos, A. J. Bellingham, C. Lenfant and C. A. Finch, Annual Review of Medicine, Volume 22. Copyright © 1971 by Annual Reviews Inc. All rights reserved.)

tated hemoglobin. The replacement of one hydrophobic amino acid for another inside the heme pocket, as in Hb Torino, causes only mild hemolysis, but when a hydrophilic group is placed into the heme pocket lining, as in the case of serine in Hb Hammersmith, heme loss is marked and hemolysis severe. A gross deletion of a block of five amino acids adjacent to the proximal histidine residue in Hb Gun Hill produces gross molecular distortion with heme-deficient globin subunits and marked hemoglobin instability. Hb Zürich affects the distal histidine residue of the β chain, which is replaced by arginine. The polar group of arginine lies poised just outside the heme pocket and leads to very mild hemolysis unless the patient is given certain "oxidant" drugs, such as sulfonamides, which explosively provoke episodes of severe hemolysis. Hb Philly and Hb Tacoma are unstable because they affect the $\alpha_1\beta_1$ contact area. The globin subunit also cannot bear disruption of its helical regions without suffering molecular instability. The insertion of the hydroxyl group of proline into the B helix of the β chain in Hb Genova breaks up the regular helical structure and causes a gross alteration in molecular configuration with hemolysis.

The oxygen affinity of the unstable hemoglobins may be raised or lowered, with an effect on the level of hemoglobin at which the patient compensates. When the affinity is high, the erythropoietin response is greater and the degree of anemia less than in those mutants with a lowered affinity, in which compensation is achieved at a lower concentration of circulating hemoglobin. The severity of the hemolytic process obviously also determines the severity of the anemia.

Exterior Mutants. Mutants placed on the hydrophilic exterior of the molecule do not alter either the oxygen affinity or the oxidative stability of the molecule. Relatively few of the more than 50 variants described in this class of abnormal hemoglobins cause any significant signs. Two major exceptions are the most common structural hemoglobinopathies, Hb S and Hb C. Both these hemoglobins are substituted at the 6 position from the N-terminal end of the β chain, where glutamic acid is replaced by valine in the case of Hb S and by lysine in the case of Hb C. Hb E, prevalent in Southeast Asia, also has a lysine in place of glutamic acid, but the affected site is 26 from the N-terminus of the β chain.

Erythrocytes which contain Hb S undergo jagged distortion of their membranes under reduced partial pressure of oxygen, a phenomenon known as sickling (Fig. 22–72). The sickling is visualized by electron microscopy as a linear molecular stacking of hemoglobin molecules, the filaments intertwining into cable-like structures illustrated in Figure 22–73. The process is reversible, and as the oxygen tension is raised, the semisolid gelled hemoglobin liquefies once again, and the cell reassumes its normal biconcave shape. The reversibility of the process is a function of the allosteric shift of the β chains, the deoxy T configuration causing a "fit" between the β chains of one molecule and the α chains of the next, on to a linear stacking of molecule upon molecule. With reoxygenation, the β chains relax and move closer together and the complementariness between adjacent molecules is broken. The erythrocyte membrane may undergo irreversible deformation. The cell will then remain irreversibly sickled, even

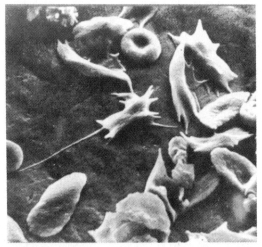

Figure 22–72 Sickled erythrocytes as demonstrated by scanning electron microscopy. (From Jensen, W. N., and Lessin, L. S.: Seminars Hematol., 7:409–426, 1970. By permission of Grune & Stratton, Inc., New York.)

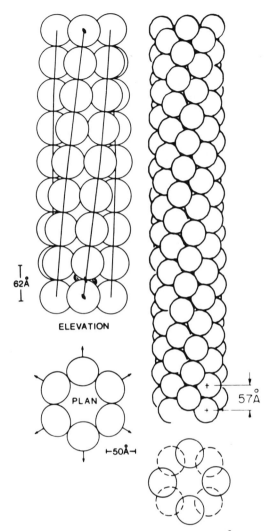

62Å

ELEVATION

PLAN

←50Å→

57Å

Figure 22–73 Two currently proposed models of the deoxy Hb S fiber. To the left is the six-stranded model of Finch and to the right the eight-stranded fiber of Josephs. Both models picture a helical structure. (With permission from Finch, J. T., et al.: Proc. N.A.S. U.S.A., 70:718, 1973, and Josephs, R., et al.: J. Mol. Biol., 102:409, 1976. Copyright by Academic Press Inc. (London) Ltd.)

though the interior structure of the oxyhemoglobin S is not in the gelled state. Sickled erythrocytes seen in routine blood films prepared from blood of sickle cell anemia patients are examples of irreversibly sickled cells, or, as designated by workers in the field, "ISC's."

Murayama proposed that the substitution of valine with its hydrophobic side chain in place of glutamic acid with its exterior polar carboxyl group causes, in a sense, an interiorization of a portion of the molecular exterior. He suggested that a cyclic hydrophobic valine-to-valine bond forms between the 1 and 6 amino acid residues of

the β chain of Hb S. This changes the exterior molecular configuration and causes a key and lock arrangement between molecules when the β chains are in the deoxy configuration.

Further considerations of the orientation of tetramers of deoxy Hb S within the multistranded sickle fiber lead to the conclusion that there are many contact sites between the entrapped molecules in both horizontal and vertical planes, not just the one area of contact envisioned by Murayama at the site of the amino acid substitution. Wishner and co-workers have drawn up a model depicting a multiplicity of contact sites with an asymmetric placement of the hemoglobin tetramers within the fibers such that only one of the two substituted valines of deoxy Hb S tetramer is situated at a contact point (Fig. 22–74).

Wishner's model is based on studies of hemoglobin crystals, but it correlates in many respects with clinical observations made in individuals who have inherited another abnormal hemoglobin present in the red cells along with Hb S. For example, Hb C Harlem has two amino acid substitutions in its beta chains, one identical to that of Hb S and the other at the 73 position, where asparagine replaces aspartic acid. Despite the fact that this molecule is more abnormal than Hb S, its presence in patients also heterozygous for Hb S inhibits the sickling process. Another mutant, Hb Korle-bu, has the same property of inhibiting sickle fiber formation. Hb Korle-bu is characterized by the same substitution at position 73 of the beta chain as that found in the Hb C Harlem, but otherwise its structure is normal. From this observation one is led to the conclusion that position 73 of the beta chain is an important site of contact between hemoglobin tetramers in the sickle fiber, as in fact shown in Wishner's model. Analogous observations have been made by Bookchin and co-workers with a number of other mutant hemoglobins that interact with deoxy Hb S to affect the sickling process.

The presence of fetal hemoglobin together with Hb S also inhibits gelation. Newborn infants do not suffer from sickle cell disease. Symptoms only become manifest as the fetal hemoglobin is replaced by the adult type. Hb F levels are commonly raised in sickle cell anemia to values from 5 to 15 per cent, but the fact that it is heterogenously distributed among the erythrocytes explains why its level is not generally related to disease severity. However, those erythrocytes with higher Hb F content do survive longer in the circulation. In the doubly heterozygous condition of hereditary persistence of fetal hemoglobin and sickle trait, erythrocytes uniformly have 20 to 30 per cent Hb F mixed together with Hb S and the result is a benign condition.

On the other hand, Hb C rather strongly interacts with Hb S in the gelation and its presence in erythrocytes together with Hb S in equal pro-

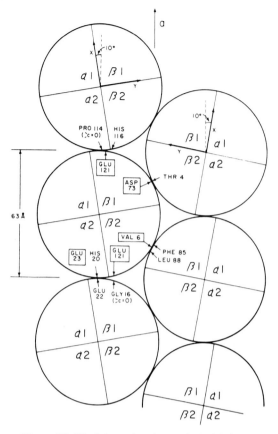

Figure 22-74   Intermolecular contact sites between deoxy Hb S molecules within fibers. The illustration is based on the results of x-ray crystallography of hemoglobin crystals and thus may not necessarily reflect physiologic conditions. (Wishner, B. C., et al.: J. Mol. Biol., 98:179, 1975. Copyright by Academic Press Inc. (London) Ltd.)

tion. Acidosis, by shifting the oxygen dissociation curve to the right, promotes sickling, while alkalosis inhibits it. The gelation of deoxy Hb S is also highly dependent upon the intracellular hemoglobin concentration, which is raised as water moves out of erythrocytes during their movement through a hyperosmolar environment. As a result individuals with sickle cell trait or other sickle hemoglobinopathies may incur episodes of sickling within the renal medulla leading to infarction and painless hematuria. Low molecular weight phosphates (inorganic phosphate as well as 2,3-DPG) also promote sickling by decreasing the oxygen affinity of the hemoglobin.

Sickle cell anemia is usually a severe disease in which erythrocytic sickling causes chronic hemolytic anemia in a setting of vaso-occlusive phenomena which may affect any organ of the body. Periodic bouts of occlusion of the microvasculature in one or several parts of the body cause "painful crises," which at their worst produce prolonged excruciating pain, sometimes associated with fever. Major arteries and veins may also suffer occlusion. There is a serious susceptibility to infection. Organ damage is cumulative over the years, and death, if not from infection, may come unannounced from a major occlusion affecting a vital function, or it may come in more chronic fashion from gradual failure of any one of several organs, such as liver, kidney, or heart. The sickle variants, Hb SC disease and Hb S thalassemia, also suffer vaso-occlusive phenomena, but symptoms are usually milder. Carriers of sickle cell trait are asymptomatic except for an incidence of hematuria due to renal infarction.

Vascular changes occur in reaction to erythrocytic sickling. These changes are demonstrable in the kidney and are presumably etiologically related to a renal concentrating defect which cannot be reversed in adults despite exchange transfusion of normal for sickle erythrocytes. Vascular changes are also present in the eye, and retinal aneurysms leading to vitreous hemorrhage cause blindness, a complication particularly associated with Hb SC disease, as described by Condon and Serjeant in 1972.

Therapy over the years has been essentially symptomatic. Acidosis is treated, hydration ensured, and occasionally the sickled erythrocytes replaced by normal transfused cells as a temporary expedient. The search for a pharmacologic agent which would prevent sickling has been elusive. Methemoglobin as well as such liganded states of hemoglobin as carboxyhemoglobin and cyanmethemoglobin all assume the oxy R configuration and therefore do not sickle, but these altered states of hemoglobin do not function in oxygen transport. More recently it was discovered that treatment of Hb S erythrocytes with cyanate results in a carbamylation of the hemoglobin molecules which not only inhibits sickling but also

portions causes significant in-vivo sickling in the disorder known as Hb SC disease. Normal Hb A, which is found in a proportion of about 60:40 relative to that of Hb S in individuals who are carriers of sickle cell trait, also interacts with Hb S in the gelation, but to a much lesser degree. How other hemoglobins become intertwined with Hb S during deoxygenation is still not understood in molecular terms. Bunn and McDonough have observed that dimers of $\alpha^A\beta^A$ and $\alpha^A\beta^S$ combine to form the hybrid $\alpha_2{}^A\beta^A\beta^S$. Thus, hybridization of different hemoglobin types within the same erythrocyte may be the explanation.

Heterozygous carriers of the sickle cell trait show no abnormality of erythrocyte morphology, life span, or function, except under certain extenuating circumstances, such as severe hypoxia. At the tips of the papillae in the renal medulla a number of factors combine to produce an optimal environment for erythrocyte sickling. The region is hypoxic and acidotic, with a high salt concentra-

results in a marked improvement in the life span of the treated erythrocytes. Cyanate is an example of a class of antisickling agents which inhibit sickling by raising the oxygen affinity of the chemically altered hemoglobin (Fig. 22–75). Carbamylation, alkylation, amidination, and other chemical modifications of hemoglobin may also introduce new configurations at critical contact sites on the molecular surface, causing steric hindrance to fiber formation, much in the same manner that the mutant hemoglobins Hb C Harlem and Hb Korle-bu inhibit sickling. Among the growing list of chemicals which are being found to have significant in vitro antisickling effects, none has yet reached the stage of clinical usefulness in the prevention or reversal of sickling in patients.

Individuals homozygous for Hb C have a mild chronic hemolytic anemia associated with splenomegaly. The pathogenesis of the hemolysis apparently lies in the fact that this abnormal hemoglobin spontaneously crystallizes at a slightly lower concentration than Hb A, as described by Charache and associates. As red cells age in the circulation they undergo a measure of water loss, with concomitant increase in the intracorpuscular concentration of hemoglobin to values approaching 36 grams per 100 ml. Hb A does not begin to crystallize into an insoluble state until its concentration is over 40 grams per 100 ml., but Hb C begins to develop this change in physical state at the values physiologically approached during red

cell aging in the circulation. At this point the cell becomes rigid and is subject to entrapment and destruction. The presence of this abnormal hemoglobin within erythrocytes causes a prominent tendency for the central deposition of a mass of hemoglobin into a "target cell" configuration. Intracellular crystals are readily demonstrable in vitro by suspending the erythrocytes in hypertonic saline, which raises intracorpuscular hemoglobin concentration, or in vivo after removal of the spleen. Heterozygotes have fewer target cells and do not show signs of significant hemolysis. The pathogenesis of Hb E disease presumably resembles that of Hb C.

Non-genetic Structural Alterations. As red cells age in the circulation glucose becomes attached to the N-terminal valines of one or both beta chains of hemoglobin in an irreversible ketoamine linkage. Older erythrocytes contain a higher level of glycosylated hemoglobin than young. The average value in normal individuals is about 7 per cent of the total hemoglobin. Several different glycosylated components are present, about one third hemoglobins A_{Ia} and A_{Ib}, and the remainder Hb A_{Ic}. The oxygen affinity of the modified hemoglobin is increased because of impaired binding of 2,3 DPG at the blocked N-terminus. The level of glycosylated hemoglobin is approximately doubled in patients with diabetes mellitus. Following its level in diabetics may provide a more valid index of the adequacy of treatment

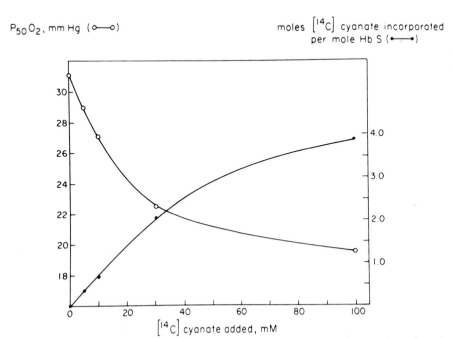

Figure 22–75 The increase in hemoglobin affinity after treatment of sickle cell anemia erythrocytes with cyanate, a possible mechanism for the inhibition of sickling. P_{50} is defined as the partial pressure of oxygen at which the hemoglobin is half saturated with oxygen. (Redrawn from deFuria, F. G., et al.: J. Clin. Invest., *51*:566, 1972.)

than serial blood sugar measurements according to Koenig and co-workers.

HEMOGLOBINOPATHY DUE TO QUANTITATIVE DEFECTS. The thalassemias are a heterogeneous group of disorders, usually inherited, characterized primarily by a deficiency in the rate of synthesis of specific globin chains. The deficit of one subunit may bring about an imbalance with surplus of another.

The structure-rate hypothesis as conceived by Itano in the 1950s postulated that the structure of an abnormal globin chain was an important factor which determined its synthetic rate. The fact that Hb S was synthesized at a slightly less efficient rate than Hb A provided support for this theory, but subsequent attempts to identify a mutant hemoglobin produced at a very low rate in thalassemic states were not successful, with the exception of two types of rare structural alterations which cause a marked slowing of their synthetic rate. One affects β chain production, and the other α. The first of these, Hb Lepore, is a globin chain which is a hybrid polypeptide consisting of a portion of the δ chain connected to a portion of the β chain to make a completed globin subunit of normal chain length which pairs with α chains in the completed tetrameric hemoglobin molecule. This hybrid globin subunit is the product of a fusion gene which presumably first originated in prior generations by a crossover occurring between homologous chromosomes slightly displaced during synapsis. Several different types of Lepore hemoglobins have been described, differing from one another in the proportion of the molecule which resembles the δ chain (Fig. 22–76). Protein synthesis is normally initiated at the N-terminal end of the molecule, which in the Lepore hemoglobins is always that of the δ portion of the chain, and thus its synthesis takes on the slow character of normal δ chain production. The deficit results in a β-thalassemia syndrome.

Hb Constant Spring, described by Milner and co-workers, is found in trace quantities in association with α-thalassemia states. In contrast to the normal α chain, which has 141 amino acids, this abnormal hemoglobin carries a defect in chain length which causes it to grow to an abnormal length of 172 amino acids, 31 too long. The pathogenetic basis of the defect appears to lie in the fact that at position 142 of the messenger RNA, where the triplet codon normally signals "terminate," a mutation signals instead for the insertion of a specific amino acid. Additional amino acids are then added until the next terminating codon is read from the messenger RNA strand at position 173. The defect in chain termination markedly slows its synthetic rate and causes an α-thalassemia syndrome.

However, these two examples notwithstanding, the basic pathogenesis of most of the thalassemia syndromes is not associated with the production of structural abnormalities of the globin chain. In some instances messenger RNA is absent due to deletion of the genetic locus responsible for its transcription. In other cases, messenger RNA is transcribed at an abnormally low rate. In still other cases messenger RNA is transcribed in sufficient quantity but it does not function properly in translation. These diverse results at the basic scientific level parallel the heterogeneity observed clinically and permit the conclusion that a variety of underlying mechanisms cause low synthetic rates of proteins. According to Nienhuis and Benz, the protein synthetic mechanism itself operates normally in most cases of thalassemia.

Any one or combination of the genes directing globin chain synthesis may hypothetically be affected by a thalassemic lesion causing depressed production rates, but only those affecting the α or the β loci are important. The degree of depression of globin chain formation may be minimal, moderate, or virtually complete, but it is relatively consistent within the affected members of the same family.

In the heterozygous carrier state one member of the chromosome pair produces globin chains at a normal rate and the clinical condition is asymptomatic. Anemia is minimal or mild, the erythrocytes are microcytic and are often present in greater than normal numbers, and the erythrocyte morphology is abnormal. Some thalassemic carrier states are so minimal that they are completely silent and exhibit no abnormalities whatsoever. The depressed β chain production in the carrier state of β-thalassemia is reflected in an increased proportion of Hb A_2 to approximately twice the normal value, the shortage of β chains altering the ratio of β to δ chain production. A few also have slight elevations of Hb F to about 2 to 6

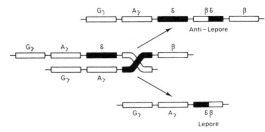

Figure 22–76 Hemoglobin Lepore, an example of a product of a fusion gene. Allelic chromosomes become misaligned. Crossover produces a fusion gene. Lepore hemoglobins resemble δ chain at their amino terminals and β chain at their C terminals. Anti-Lepore hemoglobins have the reciprocal structure, with β structure at their amino terminals. Several different Lepore hemoglobins have been described which differ from one another at the exact point of crossover. Also shown are the positions on the chromosome of the fetal globin genes Gγ and Aγ. (Wood, W. G., et al., 1977.)

per cent of the total hemoglobin. Hb F is more elevated and the Hb A$_2$ normal in a less common strain of β-thalassemia trait, designated δ-β thalassemia because the genetic lesion appears to affect the δ locus along with the adjacent β, thus, keeping the proportionality of β and δ globin subunits normal while evoking an especially strong stimulus for γ chain production. In carriers of α-thalassemia trait the proportions of Hb A$_2$ and Hb F are not altered, since these hemoglobins, in common with Hb A, are all affected by the shortage of α chains. Table 22–12 summarizes the heterozygous thalassemias.

Homozygosity for β-thalassemia (Cooley's anemia) is associated with little or no capacity to produce β chains (and thus Hb A), because both alleles responsible for β chain synthesis are affected. Hb F becomes the major hemoglobin type produced, usually exceeding 50 per cent and often approaching 95 per cent of the total. The Hb A and the Hb F are contained in variable mixtures in the erythrocyte population. The better filled cells containing more Hb F have a more prolonged survival time than the more empty Hb F-poor cells. The pathogenesis of the severe hemolysis is explained by imbalanced production of α as compared to β chains. The surplus unpaired α chains are exceedingly unstable and precipitate readily within nucleated erythroid precursor cells, causing marked intramedullary destruction, i.e., ineffective erythropoiesis. Those cell lines which retain a greater capacity for γ chain production not only are better filled with hemoglobin but also have fewer surplus unpaired α chains and thus are less rapidly hemolyzed. The patients are severely anemic, are transfusion dependent beginning in early childhood, develop massive enlargement of the spleen and of the liver, show prominent signs of extramedullary hematopoiesis, and suffer physical disfigurement because of the bone deformity brought on by the extreme erythroid hyperplasia in the marrow. Iron overload ultimately causes failure of the heart or liver, along with diabetes mellitus. Some apparently homozygous patients have a much milder anemia because one or both of their inherited thalassemic genes are mild or minimal. Patients in such a state, designated as "thalassemia intermedia," are not transfusion dependent but over the years are apt to develop hemochromatosis.

Homozygosity for α-thalassemia-1, so far observed only in Oriental newborns with an erythroblastosis fetalis-like picture, is a lethal condition. Severe anemia is associated with nearly 100 per cent Hb Bart's (γ_4) which lacks α chains and therefore does not function in oxygen transport, its affinity for oxygen being too great. Death thus occurs before or soon after birth. Hemoglobin H disease is a milder form of α-thalassemia in a subject who carries one mild and one severe gene. It is associated with about 20 per cent Hb Bart's at birth. This is subsequently replaced by its adult counterpart Hb H (β_4), which also cannot function in oxygen transport. Hb H is the product of surplus β chains in the face of a shortage of α chains. Its degree of instability is not as marked as that of unpaired α chains, and it precipitates in more mature circulating erythrocytes, causing hemolytic anemia without the same degree of intramedullary erythroid cell destruction seen in Cooley's anemia. Newborn heterozygous carriers of α-thalassemia trait have slight increases in Hb Bart's in the cord blood, but this disappears with development, leaving no disturbance in the proportions of Hb A or Hb F in the adult erythrocytes. Examples of combinations of thalassemia genes are contained in Table 22–13.

Sophisticated techniques have been developed to diagnose sickle hemoglobinopathy and thalassemia in the fetus during early intrauterine life. Minute samples of fetal blood are obtained by amniocentesis or by direct fetoscopy. The pattern of globin chain synthesis is then characterized from the pattern of incorporation of radioactive amino acids. Since adult type globin chains are synthesized as minor components along with the predominant fetal type chains early in gestation, accurate diagnosis of beta chain hemoglobinopathy is possible. Kan and co-workers have brought the full force of high technology to bear on the problem of early intrauterine diagnosis of α-thalassemia-1. They used purified α chain mes-

TABLE 22–12   HETEROZYGOUS THALASSEMIA

Type	Hemoglobin A$_2$	Hemoglobin F	Abnormal Hemoglobin
Beta	Increased	Normal or slightly increased	Absent
Delta-beta	Normal	Increased	Absent
Lepore	Normal or decreased	Slightly increased	6–15% Lepore
Alpha	Normal	Normal	Absent in adults; 1–6% Bart's in cord blood
Constant Spring	Normal	Normal	1–2% Constant Spring

Thalassemia is subclassified according to the degree of the genetic deficit of β or α chains. β° is used to designate a more severe defect with absent β chain production. β^+ is milder. In analogous fashion, α–1 is more severe and α–2 milder.

TABLE 22–13   SOME EXAMPLES OF COMBINATIONS OF THALASSEMIA GENES

Type	Hemoglobin A$_2$	Hemoglobin F	Abnormal Hemoglobin
Homozygous beta	Normal, decreased, or increased	10–90% (usually above 35%)	Free alpha chain
Homozygous alpha-1*	Absent	Absent	80–90% Bart's; remainder H and Portland
Alpha-1 alpha-2	Decreased	Normal	3–30% H; 0–5% Bart's
Homozygous delta-beta	Absent	100%	None reported

*These values relate to the newborn. All other values are beyond the newborn period.

senger RNA to prepare synthetic "DNA probes." Hybridization experiments demonstrated deletion of the α chain genetic locus in DNA extracted from fetal fibroblasts cultured from amniotic fluid. These approaches are still experimental, however, and not yet ready for widespread clinical use.

HEMOGLOBINOPATHY: POPULATION GENETICS. Inherited abnormalities of globin chain structure or production rate sporadically affect individuals from all population groups, but by far the most frequently affected are those originating from tropical or subtropical regions. Incidence figures are highest in Africa, the Mediterranean Basin, the Near and Middle East, and Southeast Asia. Hb S reaches its highest frequency in Africa, where it affects 20 to 30 per cent or more of the Negro population in regions of West, Central, and East Africa. There is also a significant incidence in the Mediterranean countries and in localized regions of Arabia and India. Hb C has a peak prevalence of 10 to 20 per cent among West African Negroes in the region of Ghana. Hb E attains a comparable frequency in areas of Southeast Asia. The α- and β-thalassemia genes are relatively frequent throughout the entire "hemoglobinopathy belt," but Southeast Asia and regions of Greece and Italy have an especially high incidence.

Red Cell Survival Disorders

General Signs of Hemolysis.   After a 4-month trip through the streams and bogs of the circulation, the normal erythrocyte ends its life span and is ingested by macrophages. Its death is heralded by cellular changes of aging: loss of surface membrane, decrease of cell water, and decline in activity of several enzyme systems. Premature disappearance of erythrocytes either by hemorrhagic loss from the circulatory compartment or by hemolysis may lead to anemia. Hemolysis occurs when the cell itself is intrinsically defective or when the milieu in which it is bathed contains noxious factors.

When the life span of the erythrocyte is only slightly shortened, the consequence may not be of significance. On the other hand, in severe hemolytic states a red cell life span of only 1/10 of 1/20 the normal period of 120 days severely strains the

capacity of the bone marrow to sustain erythroid cell production at a rate sufficient to maintain a circulating hemoglobin concentration compatible with health. The production of erythroid cells in the marrow is increased to meet the demands of increased erythrocyte turnover. This is reflected in hyperplasia of the erythroid precursor cells. Marrow normally occupied by fat is converted to hypercellular tissue. The proportion of erythroid to granulocytic precursors is increased. Young reticulocytes and sometimes nucleated erythroid cells are released into the circulation. The bone marrow is able to increase red cell production to a limited degree — about 6 to 8 times the normal rate. Therefore it is possible to compensate for shortened erythrocyte life spans that are 1/6 to 1/8 normal.

The hemolytic state is thus not necessarily associated with severe anemia. Indeed, the term "compensated hemolysis" is used to describe hemolytic states that are not associated with anemia at all. However, it is still not clear how the bone marrow, in the absence of the stimulus of anemic hypoxia, maintains a rate of red cell production high enough to compensate fully for the reduced erythrocyte life span.

Acute hemolysis causes a rapid reduction in red cell mass because the bone marrow is caught off guard; there is a four to five day delay before production is geared up in response to the anemia.

When chronic hemolysis is associated with anemia, the reduced red cell mass turning over at a faster rate represents the balance between production and destruction in a steady state condition. Limitations upon production may cause anemia even when the degree of erythrocyte hemolysis is moderate. Such limitation occurs secondary to other diseases, such as neoplastic or inflammatory states, or to deficiency of essential nutrients, especially iron and folate. The acute "aplastic crisis" is the most critical imbalance between production and destruction — erythroid precursors suddenly vanish from the marrow, the reticulocyte count drops, and soon after there is a rapid increase in the degree of anemia as the remaining short-lived erythrocytes, no longer being replenished from the marrow, disappear from the circulation. Fortunately, the period of aplasia of red cell formation, probably triggered by a minor infection, is usually short-lived, and recovery is the rule. Similar infections may well arrest erythropoiesis in normal individuals, but during the period of marrow arrest, the fall in blood count is imperceptible because of the longevity of normal erythrocytes.

In the Wright's stained peripheral blood film, reticulocytes are recognized as polychromatophilic macrocytes. Microspherocytes are small, round, densely stained erythrocytes seen in a variety of hemolytic states. Regular and irregular distortions of the erythrocyte membrane into spurs and burrs and the fracturing of erythrocytes into bits and pieces suggest metabolic or mechanical damage.

The biochemical signs of hemolysis are those of the release and breakdown of the pigment of the red cells. Erythrocyte destruction within the confines of the circulatory system ("intravascular hemolysis") causes leakage of hemoglobin directly into the plasma. Phagocytosis of intact erythrocytes or of erythrocyte fragments releases hemoglobin inside the phagocytic macrophages, where the heme is degraded to bilirubin ("extravascular hemolysis"). Hemolytic states are not exclusively intra- or extravascular, but when extensive cell damage causes the erythrocytes to "fall apart" in the circulation the signs of hemoglobin release into the plasma and urine are marked. Hemoglobin released from erythrocytes into the circulation is first bound to haptoglobin, a plasma protein with alpha-2 electrophoretic mobility (Fig. 22–77). The complex of hemoglobin with haptoglobin is then rapidly cleared from the plasma into the hepatocytes, promptly reducing the plasma concentration of haptoglobin to near absent levels.

Thus, a reduction of the plasma haptoglobin concentration (and of the alpha-2 fraction of the serum proteins) is often observed in hemolytic states, regardless of pathogenesis. Haptoglobin concentration, however, is subject to rather pronounced increases secondary to many inflammatory and neoplastic states, and its final level represents a balance between those factors promoting its synthesis and those producing its degradation, such as hemolysis. Haptoglobin normally is capable of binding hemoglobin to the extent of about 100 mg. per 100 ml. plasma. When the haptoglobin binding capacity is exceeded, hemoglobin is lost in the urine. Haptoglobin serves the purpose of conserving iron by preventing its loss in the urine as heme. Oxidized heme, split apart from its globin bond, may also be detected bound to hemopexin, a beta globulin of the plasma, as well as to albumin (as methemalbumin), giving the plasma a dirty brown color. Heme bound to hemopexin is also taken up into the hepatic parenchymal cells.

The detection of free hemoglobin in the plasma and urine indicates that the haptoglobin binding capacity has been exceeded and that the degree of intravascular hemolysis has been extensive. The free plasma hemoglobin, unattached to high molecular weight haptoglobin, is readily filtered through the glomerulus. Some passes through directly to produce urine benzidine positive for the presence of heme pigment. However, hemoglobin is also resorbed into the epithelial cells of the tubules, where its iron is removed and deposited within the cell as ferritin and hemosiderin. These iron-rich proteins are then sloughed with the normal loss of tubule epithelial cells into the urine, where they can be detected in the sediment by the Prussian blue reaction for iron (Fig. 22–78). Hemosiderinuria is a valuable sign that the patient either is suffering from intravascular hemolysis or has recently done so. After recovery from an acute intravascular hemolytic episode, the urine stain for hemosiderin will remain positive for some days after hemoglobinuria has stopped.

Jaundice is a common sign of hemolysis. Often the degree is subclinical and cannot be detected except by chemical measurement of the serum bilirubin concentration. The degree of jaundice is never intense; total serum bilirubin concentrations in excess of 6 mg. per 100 ml. suggest malfunction of the liver or of its biliary drainage system, since the capacity of the normal liver to process bilirubin is immense. Hemolytic jaundice involves primarily elevation of the unconjugated bilirubin (or indirect-reacting fraction). It circulates bound to plasma albumin and therefore is not lost in the urine. After its transport to the liver, bilirubin is processed by the hepatic cells and converted to the water-soluble diglucuronide derivative (direct-reacting, or conjugated), which is the major form excreted in the bile, as reviewed

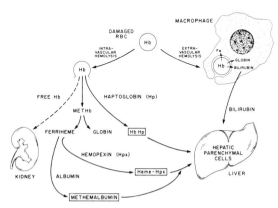

Figure 22–77 Extra- and intravascular disposal of erythrocytes. Intact erythrocytes and cell fragments are removed by extravascular uptake into phagocytic macrophages. Hemoglobin products leaked directly into the circulation are bound to several plasma proteins and redirected into hepatocytes. "Surplus" free hemoglobin is excreted in the urine.

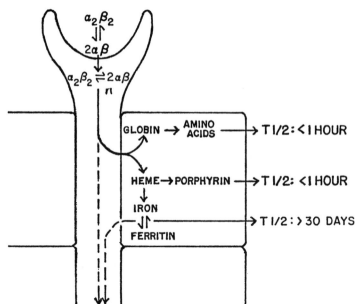

Figure 22–78 The renal handling of hemoglobin. Subunit dissociation into lower molecular weight components permits glomerular filtration. Some of the filtered hemoglobin is taken up into the epithelial cells of the tubules and degraded. The released iron is incorporated into ferritin and hemosiderin. Shedding of renal tubule cells causes persistence of hemosiderinuria for some time after hemoglobinuria has stopped. (From Bunn, H. F. and Jandl, J. H.: J. Exper. Med., *129*:925, 1969.)

by Schmid in 1972. A portion of this conjugated bilirubin is absorbed and undergoes enterohepatic circulation. Most of it is reduced by colonic bacteria to urobilinogen, which also has an enterohepatic circulation. In hemolysis the output of bile pigments into the intestinal tract is increased in direct proportion to the degree of heme degradation and thus to the extent of the hemolytic process. Measurement of the fecal urobilinogen excretion may be used to quantitate the extent of hemolysis as a function of heme degradation rate, but the procedure is too cumbersome for general use. Urine urobilinogen is likewise increased as a reflection of the increased enterohepatic circulation, but only a small proportion of the total is excreted by this route.

Bilirubin is produced in phagocytic cells throughout the body from degraded heme pigments of a variety of types, chief among which by far is hemoglobin. Phagocytes possess an efficient enzymatic mechanism which rapidly and voraciously strips away the iron for metabolic recycling, digests the globin into its constituent amino acids for re-entry into the body pool, and oxidizes the tetrapyrrole ringed structure of heme into biliverdin (Gemsa and co-workers, 1973). This conversion, mediated by heme oxidase, fractures open one of the four bridges (the alpha methene) that hold together the four pyrrole groups into a ringed tetrapyrrole structure. Carbon monoxide is produced in this reaction and is delivered to the lungs for respiratory excretion, one mole for each mole of heme degraded. Since there is almost no other source of endogenous carbon monoxide, measurement of its production rate accurately quantitates

the catabolism of heme compounds and thus also the rate of hemolysis (Fig. 22–79). Biliverdin, a green pigment, is reduced to bilirubin, which is then transferred from the phagocytic cells to the hepatic parenchymal cells for conjugation.

The load of heme pigments normally presented for degradation comes chiefly from dying senescent erythrocytes, but about 15 per cent is from other sources, some from the liver and some from the bone marrow (Fig. 22–80). The hepatic contribution may be increased in porphyria of hepatic origin or following the administration of certain drugs, as phenobarbital, which stimulate the endoplasmic reticulum along with heme synthesis. The bone marrow also produces heme which never reaches the safe haven of the circulating erythrocyte. This marrow heme, destined for early degradation, consists partly of hemoglobin shrouds which veil normoblast nuclei after their extrusion (Fig. 22–81), partly of defective normoblasts destroyed before they gain access to the circulation as mature erythrocytes, and possibly partly of heme which is never incorporated into hemoglobin but is "shunted" into an early catabolic demise. From the foregoing, it is apparent that hepatic or marrow defects can markedly affect the net pattern of heme degradation. The process of intramedullary hemolysis, i.e., ineffective erythropoiesis, so prominent in megaloblastic anemia and in homozygous β-thalassemia, may be the major contributor to heme catabolism and thus to the increased production of carbon monoxide and bilirubin associated with these disorders.

The measurement of red cell survival time would appear to be the most direct approach to the

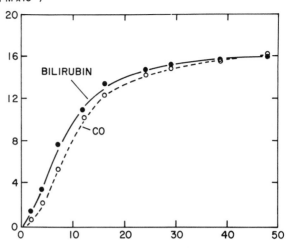

CUMULATIVE EXCRETION
($DPM \times 10^3$)

Figure 22–79 Parallel appearance of radioactivity into bilirubin and carbon monoxide after administration of radioactive hematin. (Redrawn from Landaw, S. A., et al.: J. Clin. Invest., *49*:914, 1970.)

HOURS AFTER HEMATIN-^{14}C INJECTION

diagnosis of hemolytic disorders, but this measurement presents a number of difficulties from practical as well as theoretical points of view. Not the least of these is the rather long time required, during which the patient should be in the steady state with regard to the maintenance of a constant red cell mass as well as to absence of significant loss of blood by hemorrhage. There are two basic approaches, both of which follow the behavior in the circulation of a tag on the erythrocytes. The first, called the cohort label, employs the use of a radioisotope which is administered and is then incorporated into a cohort of newly formed cells. Examples are isotopes of iron (e.g., ^{59}Fe) and of amino acids (e.g., glycine-2-^{14}C, ^{75}Se selenomethionine). Normally the cohort tag will appear in the peripheral blood erythrocytes and then rise to a plateau in about 10 days. This plateau is maintained until about 100 days, and at 120 days it reaches a maximum rate of decline as the cohort dies off. Mean erythrocyte survival time can be estimated from such curves, but this method is difficult to carry out and may be hampered by reutilization of these biologically active tags.

The second method, the population or random label, uses a nonphysiologic marker of a representative sample of the entire erythrocyte population. The sample should be uniformly tagged without difference or discrimination as to cell age, pathologic state, or any other cell variable, so that when it is reintroduced into the circulation, a clear picture is obtained of the rate of removal of the population of erythrocytes it represents. Normally a fixed number of erythrocytes reaches senescence and dies each day; the tag will represent this by a straight-line decline intercepting zero at 120 days, when the last of the tagged cells will have died off.

This is an age-dependent pattern of cell destruction. Many hemolytic states are characterized by random destruction of erythrocytes, without regard to their age. A fixed percentage of the remaining cells are destroyed per day; the tag disappears from the circulation at an exponential rate according to first order kinetics. The time required for disappearance of half the tag (the half-time or T/2) is the most conventional method of expressing erythrocyte survival time as measured with a population label.

No tags are ideal, but two of the best are diisopropylfluorophosphate (DF^{32}P) and sodium chromate (Na$_2$ ^{51}CrO$_4$). DF^{32}P attaches to red cell

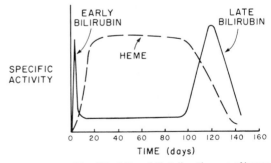

TIME (days)

Figure 22–80 "Early" and "late" pathways of heme degradation into bilirubin. The graph illustrates in a normal subject the incorporation of a radioactive precursor of heme into circulating red cells (interrupted line) and into "early" and "late" bilirubin, the latter corresponding to completion of the life span of the labeled erythrocytes. Early bilirubin originates from both bone marrow and hepatic heme. It is markedly increased in conditions associated with ineffective erythropoiesis.

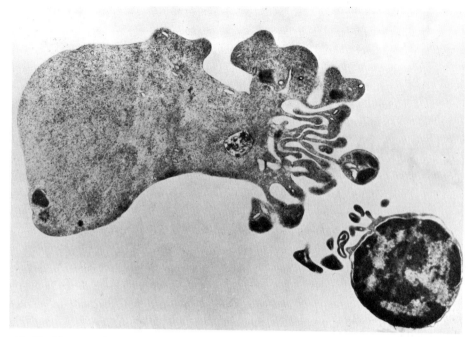

Figure 22–81   The extrusion from an erythyroid precursor of a nucleus covered with a shroud of hemoglobin, leaving behind a reticulocyte containing mitochondria and ribosomes. (Reproduced from the Sandoz-Monograph, The Life Cycle of the Erythrocyte. M. Bessis, Basel, Switzerland, 1966.)

cholinesterase to form a tight bond which lasts for the duration of the erthrocyte's life span; its disappearance rate from the circulation yields a value quite close to the true life span, but the method is inconvenient. $Na_2{}^{51}CrO_4$ penetrates the red cell membrane and is reduced to the chromic state, and then the chromium tag forms a chelate with the β chain of hemoglobin. Its bond to proteins is not nearly so tight and it elutes from red cells at a rate of about 1 per cent per day, with significant differences in various disease states. Consequently, its disappearance rate from the circulation does not give a true measure of erythrocyte survival but rather a composite of this function minus the elution rate of the chromium. The normal half-time of ^{51}Cr-labeled erythrocytes is 25 to 35 days, a value considerably shorter than the physiologic half disappearance time of 60 days. Despite these patent disadvantages, ^{51}Cr has practical virtues and has gained widespread acceptance as a convenient method for the clinical assessment of erythrokinetics. Since ^{51}Cr is a strong gamma emitter, the accumulation of chromium-labeled red cells can be detected by external probes, and body surface counting is used to determine the degree of splenic participation in excessive red cell destruction.

Membrane Function and Energy Metabolism.   The biochemistry of the erythrocyte has long been a subject of practical interest in the development of satisfactory methods of preserving shed blood in-

tended for transfusion therapy. This deceptively simple cell has also served as a model system in the basic investigation of glycolysis and of the structure and function of cell membranes. Along with the elucidation of the biochemical clock-works of the erythrocyte has come the definition in precise biochemical terms of a large number of different hemolytic states.

The red cell membrane consists of proteins embedded into lipids, chiefly phospholipids and cholesterol. The membrane proteins include the carbohydrate-rich blood group substances, a filamentous structural protein called spectrin, certain enzymes, and other proteins yet to be identified (Fig. 22–82). The membrane maintains a certain excess of surface area which, by dimpling into a biconcave shape, squeezes the hemoglobin into the peripheral ring of the doughnutlike cell. Weed and co-workers have shown that the preservation of this shape depends on energy expenditure. The extent of the surface area is subject to change; it normally decreases as the cell ages. However, mature erythrocytes, no longer able to synthesize lipid, may undergo volume changes through membrane interaction with the external environment. Rapid passive exchange of free cholesterol (but not esterified cholesterol) takes place between the membrane and the plasma. Phospholipid exchange also occurs, but at a much slower rate. The quantity of membrane free cholesterol can be manipulated by varying the free cholester-

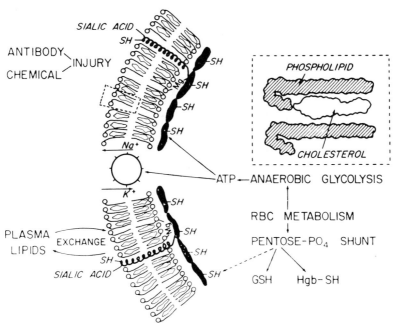

Figure 22–82 Diagrammatic representation of the erythrocyte membrane. (From Weed, R. I., and Reed, C. F.: Am. J. Med., *41*:681, 1966.)

ol content of the surrounding medium (Fig. 22–83). A high level will cause free cholesterol to accumulate in the membrane, thereby increasing its surface area. The increased surface-to-volume ratio confers upon the erythrocytes a greater distensibility in hypotonic media, i.e., their osmotic resistance is increased (Fig. 22–84). The redundant membrane of such cholesterol-replete cells produces a targeted appearance; the area of central pallor has a "bulls-eye" of hemoglobin deposited within. Conversely, suspension of erythrocytes in plasma or serum poor in free cholesterol will cause cholesterol loss from the membrane along with decreased osmotic resistance. Cooper has reported that other important factors such as the serum lipoproteins modify the plasma-membrane exchange.

A busy traffic hums through the pores of the erythrocyte membrane. Gas transport is high on the priority list in fulfillment of the cell's chief function. An active uptake of glucose is required to power the metabolic machinery. Of great interest — and still considerably a mystery — is the movement of electrolytes across the membrane. The pores, seemingly guarded by positively charged sentries (possibly calcium ions), freely allow anions to pass rapidly into the cell. Permeability to cations is quite another matter; cations diffuse across the membrane much more slowly. To oppose this slow, passive diffusion of cations, an active pumping mechanism in the membrane

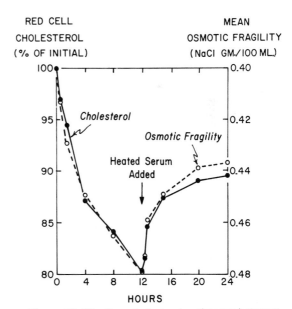

Figure 22–83 Free cholesterol exchanges between the serum and the erythrocyte membrane. After initial incubation with free cholesterol-poor serum, heated serum replete with free cholesterol was added. As the red cell cholesterol decreases, loss of membrane decreases the surface/volume ratio of the cell along with its osmotic resistance. Repletion of the red cell cholesterol reverses this change as the surface/volume ratio returns toward normal. (Redrawn from Cooper, R. A., and Jandl, J. H.: J. Clin. Invest., 48:906, 1969.)

HEMOLYSIS
(%)

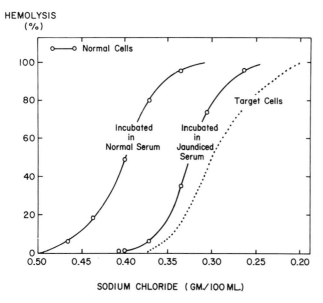

Figure 22–84 The erythrocyte membrane is affected by changes in its serum milieu. Osmotic resistance of normal erythrocytes increases when they are incubated in high free cholesterol serum from a patient with obstructive jaundice as compared to incubation in normal serum. The osmotic resistance of the patient's erythrocytes, which showed target cell formation, was likewise increased (dotted line). (Redrawn from Cooper, R. A., and Jandl, J. H.: J. Clin. Invest., 47:809, 1968.)

maintains concentration gradients of sodium and potassium. Sodium is actively extruded from the cell against a concentration gradient of 10 mEq. per liter inside the cell to 145 mEq. per liter in the extracellular plasma. Potassium is pumped into the cell against a concentration gradient from 4.5 mEq. per liter in the plasma to 100 mEq. per liter inside the cell. The active transport of cations requires ATP as an energy source; it consumes about 15 per cent of the erythrocyte ATP production. The membrane contains an ATPase to mediate its utilization there. Energy deprivation may therefore lead to a breakdown of the pumping mechanism, with serious consequences to the osmotic equilibrium of the cell.

The erythrocyte is the principal transporter of oxygen as fuel for the entire body. In addition to the high-energy phosphate bonds of ATP, it requires energy to perform biochemical reductions to protect its own parts from oxidative denaturation by this fuel. There are two major reducing systems. One, utilizing NADH, maintains the iron atoms of hemoglobin in the reduced state, a need imposed by the continuous slow conversion of hemoglobin to methemoglobin. The reduction is mediated by an enzyme, methemoglobin reductase (Jaffé and Hsieh, 1971). The other reducing system assumes responsibility for maintaining the cell's thiol groups — those of the membrane, the enzymes, and the hemoglobin — in the reduced state. This pathway is mediated through NADPH, which in turn ultimately works through maintaining glutathione in the reduced state.

Glucose is the sole source of energy. The mature erythrocyte consumes 90 per cent of its glucose through the anaerobic Embden-Meyerhof pathway, with conversion to lactate as the end-product and the net production of two moles of ATP and the

reduction of two moles of NAD to NADH per mole of glucose (Fig. 22–85). Normally about 10 per cent of the glucose is consumed through the pentose phosphate pathway with the reduction of two moles of NADP to NADPH per mole of glucose. Under the influence of certain redox compounds (for example, methylene blue) the amount of glucose processed through this route is markedly increased, a factor of considerable importance in the pathophysiology of hemolysis in patients lacking key enzymes in this pathway.

Reticulocytes possess mitochondria and therefore have an active Krebs cycle for the oxidative metabolism of glucose, but this apparatus is lost as the reticulocyte matures.

A third pathway of glucose metabolism in the erythrocyte does not participate in energy generation, but rather sacrifices energy production to the cause of an important adaptive mechanism for changing hemoglobin oxygen affinity. This pathway (the Rapoport-Luebering shunt), controlled by diphosphoglycerate mutase (DPGM), generates 2,3-DPG, which binds to deoxyhemoglobin and reduces its affinity for oxygen. As more 2,3-DPG becomes bound, the free unbound pool becomes depleted, thus coaxing DPGM into detouring triose intermediates to replenish the pool. This detour costs the cell a loss of 2 moles of ATP per mole of glucose, but this loss does not appear to have any significant effect on fulfilling total energy requirements.

Classification of Hemolytic States. The seeds of premature erythrocyte destruction may lie either within the erythrocyte or outside in a hostile environment. Hemolytic states are thus readily categorized as "intrinsic" or "extrinsic" disorders, although some represent combinations of both. Most intrinsic defects are inherited; most extrin-

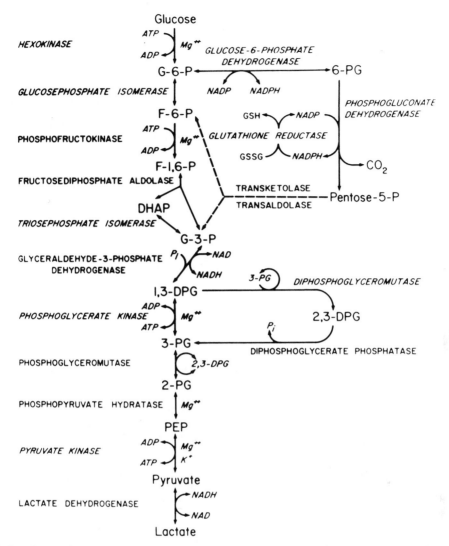

Figure 22–85 Glycolytic pathways in mature erythrocytes. (From Valentine, W. N.: Calif. Med., *108*:280, 1968.)

sic disorders are acquired. A classic experimental approach, no longer in common use, applied cross-transfusion techniques between the patient and a normal individual with compatible blood type. Erythrocytes from a patient with an intrinsic defect will exhibit a shortened survival time not only in the patient's own circulation but also in that of the normal recipient. Erythrocytes from a normal subject will survive as well in the patient's circulation as in his own. However, normal compatible erythrocytes will suffer a shortened survival time in the circulation of a patient with an extrinsic hemolytic disorder. Variations of this approach have also been applied to the study of combined disorders. Thus, tagged erythrocytes from a patient with glucose-6-phosphate dehydrogenase deficiency, an intrinsic drug-sensitive state, will survive quite normally in the circulation of a normal

compatible recipient until the offending drug is administered, which will cause hemolysis of the tagged abnormal erythrocytes but not of the normal person's own erythrocytes. The interaction of the intrinsically defective red cells of hereditary spherocytosis with the extrinsic splenic environment has been demonstrated by the observation that such erythrocytes, appropriately labeled, will exhibit a shortened survival in the bloodstream of a normal recipient with intact spleen (Fig. 22–86) but a normal survival time in a normal person lacking a spleen.

To establish that a hemolytic state exists, measurements of the reticulocyte count, the conjugated and unconjugated serum bilirubin, the serum haptoglobin, the plasma and urine hemoglobin, and the urine hemosiderin, along with careful morphologic examination of the peripheral blood and

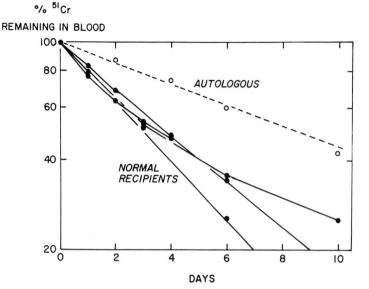

% ^{51}Cr

REMAINING IN BLOOD

DAYS

Figure 22–86 The survival of intrinsically defective ^{51}Cr-labeled erythrocytes from a patient with hereditary spherocytosis with intact spleen is even shorter in normal compatible recipients with intact spleen than in the patient. Survival time is normal in the absence of the spleen. (T/2 25–35 days.) (Redrawn from Wiley, J. S.: J. Clin. Invest., *49*:666, 1970.)

bone marrow should indicate its severity and point to the diagnosis. A second echelon of hemolytic tests may then pinpoint the precise cellular or extracellular pathophysiologic condition. These include osmotic fragility measured in a graded series of hypotonic NaCl solutions; the autohemolysis of erythrocytes incubated in vitro under sterile conditions; screening for enzyme defects; hemoglobin analysis; tests for immunologic factors, such as the Coombs antiglobulin, cold agglutinin, and cold hemolysin tests; and tests for the complement-sensitive erythrocytes of paroxysmal nocturnal hemoglobinuria (sucrose hemolysis and acid hemolysin tests). The morphology of the red cells or the clinical circumstances (such as the fact that the patient has cirrhosis or uremia) may alone readily yield the pathophysiologic classification.

Intrinsic Hemolytic Disorders. *Hereditary spherocytosis* (HS) is generally classified as a red cell membrane abnormality, but the molecular defect, inherited as an autosomal dominant trait, is not known (Weed, 1975). Its clinical expression is extraordinarily variable. At times it is first discovered incidentally in old age, but at the other extreme it may produce a severe hemolytic syndrome in the neonate or in early childhood. Many adults with HS maintain a state of completely compensated hemolysis. As with any chronic hemolytic disorder, there is a great likelihood that pigment gallstones will eventually develop. Spherocytosis is a prominent feature in the peripheral blood film along with polychromasia. Tests for autoimmune disorders are negative. The family study is typically positive. The autohemolysis and osmotic fragility tests, to be described, are abnormal. The enlarged spleen is the site of

the premature red cell destruction and its removal predictably restores the erythrocyte life span to almost normal, even though the intrinsic red cell defect remains.

Elegant investigations over the years have elucidated the cellular pathophysiology of HS. The membrane is leaky and allows sodium to enter the cells at a faster than normal rate. Osmotic balance is maintained at the cost of increased energy expenditure required to increase the pump rate of sodium out of the cell, a feat easily accomplished as long as an adequate supply of glucose is available to provide the necessary ATP. The circumstance, however, places the erythrocyte in a precarious state of dependence upon favorable surroundings; it is critically susceptible to glucose deprivation or other limitations on the availability of energy. If osmotic balance of the sodium ion cannot be maintained, water will enter the cell and cause it to swell and become a "macrospherocyte" and possibly eventually to rupture forth its contents.

This inability of the HS erythrocyte to withstand deprivation is demonstrated in the autohemolysis test. Whole blood is incubated at 37° C. under sterile conditions for 48 hours. The available glucose supply is sufficient to keep normal erythrocytes intact; less than 5 per cent will hemolyze. The HS erythrocyte consumes glucose at an increased rate. When the supply runs low, erythrocyte lysis is greatly increased, and 20 to 40 per cent autohemolysis is commonly observed. The addition of supplemental glucose prior to incubation has a salutary effect in reducing the degree of autohemolysis, sometimes to normal levels. Since lysis is produced by the osmotic imbalance between the cell interior and exterior, addition of impenetrable osmotically active agents, such as sucrose or ATP, to the plasma will also reduce autohemolysis.

In addition to increased cation permeability and glucose consumption, the cellular pathophysiology of HS is characterized by the loss of lipid materials from the membrane with a parallel loss of membrane surface area. The reduction in surface area without commensurate volume loss forces the biconcave erythrocytes to change into "microspherocytes" — small cells, densely stained, round, and lacking in central pallor. Since microspherocytes rather than macrospherocytes are the hallmarks of this and of other spherocytic hemolytic conditions, the loss of surface is probably the more important pathophysiologic event (Fig. 22–87). The microspherocyte contains its hemoglobin at a higher concentration than normal. Thus, the mean corpuscular hemoglobin concentration (MCHC) in HS frequently is elevated above 36 grams per 100 ml. Spherocytic erythrocytes (whether micro or macro) are exquisitely sensitive to osmotic lysis following suspension in hypotonic solutions of NaCl. Since as spheres they already have the minimum ratio of surface to volume, they can undergo no further volume expansion as water is taken into the cell. As the spherocyte attempts to swell further, the membrane pores distend and offer free permeability to cations soon to be followed by leakage of large molecules. The hemoglobin escapes from the cell interior into the surrounding medium, leaving behind the hollow "ghost."

The osmotic fragility test is always abnormal in HS, although at times it may be necessary to "bring out" the abnormality by first exposing the erythrocytes to glucose deprivation by a 24-hour in-vitro preincubation. The lipid-depleted microspherocytes represent a discrete subpopulation of especially osmotically fragile erythrocytes. These show up in the complete osmotic fragility test as a "fragile tail," some of them lysing even at a slight reduction of the NaCl concentration below 0.85

gram per 100 ml. The remaining nonspherocytic cells may exhibit normal osmotic fragility. But if the blood is incubated for 24 hours before being tested in graded concentrations of saline, the entire cell population will swell somewhat because of the cells' inability to maintain osmotic equilibrium. This limited degree of volume expansion produces spherodicity and increases osmotic susceptibility. Thus, the entire erythrocyte population in HS after 24 hours' incubation will show a marked shift toward increased fragility, much greater than that of normal red cells similarly treated.

Of crucial importance in the pathophysiology of hemolysis in HS is the unhappy interaction between the erythrocyte and the spleen. Removal of the spleen restores red cell life span to normal or near normal; all hemolytic manifestations are brought to a prompt halt, yet the cellular defect, along with the abnormal autohemolysis and osmotic fragility tests, remains. What is so unique about the splenic interior that these erythrocytes find so hostile to longevity? In many respects, the spleen subjects the red cells to the same stresses they undergo during sterile in-vitro incubation. The spleen is an organ of erythrostasis; erythrocytes linger in their passage through the splenic pulp. Plasma skimming concentrates erythrocytes to higher packed cell volumes. The splenic pulp has a lower glucose concentration and a more acid pH than the circulating blood. These factors place limitations upon glycolysis and cause lipid loss from the membrane surface. This damage may not be fatal to the erythrocyte during its first passage through the spleen, but with repeated passage the red cell becomes "conditioned," that is, it loses so much membrane surface area that it becomes a microspherocyte. This ball-like erythrocyte lacks the extreme pliability of the normal biconcave shape and it is finally retained in the splenic cords, unable to make the crossing through the finely fenestrated wall that separates the cords from the sinuses of the red pulp. The erythrocytes in the splenic cords must squeeze

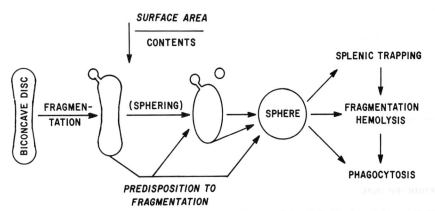

Figure 22–87 Microspherocyte formation. (From Weed, R. I., and Reed, C. F.: Am. J. Med., *41*:681, 1966.)

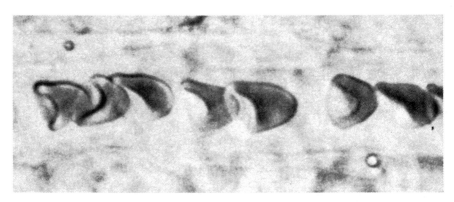

Figure 22–88 The pliability of normal erythrocytes as they move through small capillaries by assuming a parachute configuration. Rigid erythrocytes, such as microspherocytes, sickled erythrocytes, or erythrocytes containing Heinz bodies are subject to entrapment. (From Skalak, R., and Brånemark, P. I.: Science, *164*:717, 1969. Copyright 1969 by the American Association for the Advancement of Science.)

through this meshwork — past quality-conscious macrophages — to gain access into the splenic sinuses and on to drainage into the splenic vein. The small but plump spherocytes are detained, in the meantime suffering the ravages of the splenic environment to the point of outright cell destruction and phagocytosis. No other site in the body possesses such a finely tuned filtering mechanism as the spleen; it places the most stringent limitation upon rigid erythrocytes which cannot easily squeeze and twist through its small orifices (Fig. 22–88).

Hereditary elliptocytosis, an autosomal dominant condition about one fifth as common as HS, is just as obscure in terms of precise molecular genetics. The majority of erythrocytes have an elliptical shape. The diagnosis is clear from inspection of the peripheral blood film alone. Smaller numbers of elliptocytes are often present in the deficiency anemias, thalassemias, myeloproliferative syndromes, and other situations. The defect presumably resides in the membrane, but the pathogenesis of the shape change is not understood. About four fifths of cases exhibit little or no hemolysis. Those with clinical stigmata of hemolysis resemble HS in pathophysiology. Splenomegaly is also present and the hemolysis, as in HS, is corrected by splenectomy.

Paroxysmal nocturnal hemoglobinuria (PNH) is peculiar among the intrinsic red cell disorders in that it is acquired. Despite its rarity it has been intensively investigated, but a precise definition of its molecular basis is still lacking. At present PNH is considered to be an acquired defect of the red cell membrane that renders it pathologically sensitive to destruction by the complement system. This destruction is accomplished without the interposition of the antibodies which usually are required for the initiation of complement-related cell lysis. The onset may be at any age, and the disease usually has a chronic protracted course.

Its name is derived from the fact that intravascular hemolysis occurs at night, causing the first voided morning urine to be darkly colored by its hemoglobin content. In many cases, however, the nocturnal character is not prominent. Periods of exacerbation of the hemoglobinuria may follow infections, exercise, surgery, or other physical stresses. The most serious morbidity and mortality stem from a high incidence of intravascular thrombosis, chiefly venous and often involving the mesenteric and portal venous systems. Some patients become dependent on blood transfusion. Fortunately for them, normal compatible erythrocytes survive normally in their circulation.

The etiology of PNH is unknown. It bears an obscure relationship to aplastic anemia, both idiopathic and drug-induced. Interconversions from one syndrome to the other have been well documented. A few patients with PNH have developed acute leukemia, but this is decidedly a rare occurrence. Some exceptional cases of PNH have undergone complete and permanent remission. Along with the anemia and the elevated reticulocyte count and signs of intravascular hemolysis, the white cell and platelet counts are commonly reduced. Thus the disorder is "trilineage."

Although the red cell life span is shortened, the life span of the platelets is normal. Several odd cellular enzyme deficiencies are associated with PNH, including deficiency of granulocyte alkaline phosphatase and erythrocyte acetylcholinesterase, with unknown pathophysiologic significance.

The diagnosis usually is established by a positive stain of the urinary sediment for hemosiderin and a positive sucrose hemolysis test. The hemosiderinuria is a reflection of the predominantly intravascular nature of the hemolysis. Indeed urinary losses of iron, up to 20 mg. per day, frequently lead to iron deficiency, otherwise an uncommon complication of hemolytic anemia. The sucrose hemolysis test relies on the promotion of complement fixation to the PNH erythrocyte under the conditions of lowered ionic strength obtained when the cell-plasma suspension is diluted in an aqueous sucrose solution. The reason for using sucrose is to maintain osmotic balance, since the erythrocyte membrane is impermeable to it. Another simple screening test is the observation that gross hemolysis is present in the serum surrounding the retracted clot of freshly drawn PNH blood after 2 hours' incubation at 37° C.; autologous complement lyses the erythrocytes in vitro. The acid hemolysin (Ham) test utilizes still another property of complement activation, namely, its optimum at an acid pH of about 6.4. PNH erythrocytes suspended in fresh compatible complement-containing serum properly acidified will show lysis, absent when the serum is heated to 56° C. to inactivate complement. The hemolysis may be enhanced by the addition of crude bovine thrombin preparations (Crosby test), possibly because their heterophile antibody content promotes complement fixation.

The pathophysiologic basis of the disorder remains the subject of much speculation. There are two erythrocyte populations, one sensitive and the other insensitive (Fig. 22–89). The sensitive population, perhaps the offspring of stem cells with a somatic mutation or a self-perpetuating drug-induced change, undergoes hemolysis. The insensitive population has a more normal cell life span. Götze and Müller-Eberhard have reported that

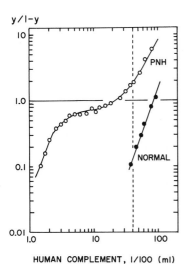

y/1-y

10

PNH

1.0

NORMAL

0.1

0.01

1.0   10   100

HUMAN COMPLEMENT, 1/100 (ml)

Figure 22–89 Complement sensitivity of normal and PNH erythrocytes. Two cell populations are evident in PNH. In some patients a third population of intermediate sensitivity can be demonstrated. Complement concentration is shown on the horizontal axis and the proportion of lysed to unlysed erythrocytes on the vertical. (Redrawn from Rosse, W. F., et al.: J. Exper. Med., *123*:969, 1966.)

properdin and the related serum proteins of the "alternate pathway" are able to fix C3 directly onto the PNH cell, without the usual prior attachment of C1, C4, and C2. The "membrane attack" unit, C5-9, then proceeds to pierce the erythrocyte membrane and bring on intravascular hemolysis.

Intrinsic enzyme deficiency of the erythrocytes may cause either overt hemolysis or hemolytic susceptibility under adverse environmental circumstances. Dacie recognized that a group of hereditary hemolytic disorders could be set apart from hereditary spherocytosis, which they otherwise resembled clinically. Their distinguishing features were the presence of few, if any, spherocytes in the peripheral blood and either a less favorable or no response to splenectomy. He also soon recognized that the "hereditary nonspherocytic hemolytic anemias" did not form a homogeneous group, and he classified them as Type I or Type II according to the results of the autohemolysis test. Type I showed a modestly positive test with correction by the addition of glucose. Type II showed marked autohemolysis without correction by the addition of glucose. The subsequent development of methods for the assay of red cell enzymes has led to the discovery of a large number of deficiencies which appear to explain the etiology of many of the hereditary nonspherocytic hemolytic anemias. Hemolysis has been attributed to deficiency of hexokinase, glucose phosphate isomerase, triose phosphate isomerase, diphosphoglyceromutase, phosphoglycerate kinase, glutathione reductase, pyruvate kinase, and glucose-6-phosphate dehydrogenase, among others. Only the two most common — pyruvate kinase and glucose-6-phosphate dehydrogenase deficiency — will be discussed here.

Pyruvate kinase deficiency, itself a rare disorder, ranks second only to G-6-PD deficiency in frequency among the red cell enzymopathies. The clinical severity is extremely variable, even within a given family. Inherited as an autosomal recessive, the disorder produces hemolysis only in the homozygous state. The heterozygote is hematologically normal, but demonstrates about half the normal enzyme activity. Most patients have splenomegaly. Splenectomy may produce some improvement if the anemia is severe, but the benefit is not nearly as predictable nor as great as it is in hereditary spherocytosis. The postsplenectomy changes in the peripheral blood also contrast with those in HS. In the latter the reticulocyte count promptly declines to near-normal levels within a week as the hemolysis is halted, while patients with PK deficiency often demonstrate a paradoxical rise in reticulocyte count along with the rise in hemoglobin concentration after splenectomy. This clinical observation has suggested that, as in paroxysmal nocturnal hemoglobinuria, the young erythrocyte population is particularly susceptible to hemolysis. In PK deficiency, the destruction of reticulocytes is in the spleen, whereas in PNH it is primarily intravascular.

Pyruvate kinase stands astride an important ATP generating step, the conversion of phosphoenol pyruvate to pyruvate. Deficiency thus leads to impairment of the erythrocyte's ability to provide an adequate supply of energy in the form of ATP necessary to power the membrane cation pump as well as other glycolytic reactions. PK-deficient erythrocytes exhibit a positive autohemolysis test of the Type II variety; adding glucose does not correct the positive test because of failure to utilize glucose. The reason for the inordinate susceptibility of reticulocytes to PK deficiency is not entirely clear, but their high energy requirement presumably narrows their margin for survival in the circulation of the spleen. Reticulocytes derive their energy primarily through the high ATP generating capacity of the oxidative Krebs cycle, which is lost as the reticulocyte matures. The conditions in the spleen — low glucose concentration, low pH, hemoconcentration, plus the delay of the passage of reticulocytes owing to their excessive stickiness in comparison with mature erythrocytes — all lead to a lower safety factor, especially when the mitochondria are in the process of being lost. Although, as with many enzymes, PK concentrations are higher in young than in old red cells, the activity is not high enough to prevent the cell damage which then subsequently leads to cell destruction in both the liver and spleen.

PK deficiency can be caused by a variety of different molecular defects, as is the rule in hereditary disorders. Some represent qualitative structural defects of the enzyme which lead to low activity; others presumably are a quantitative lack of a structurally normal enzyme. In either circumstance the result is a lack in enzyme function.

Glucose-6-phosphate dehydrogenase (G-6-PD) deficiency is by far the most common red cell enzyme abnormality, as discussed by Motulsky. A sex-linked condition, it affects 11 per cent of American black males. In Mediterranean regions it affects about 1 in 1000, but in certain isolated populations it has higher frequencies, affecting up to 50 per cent of male Kurdish Jews, for example. Over 100 genetic variants have already been discovered. From the clinical point of view, three major categories are recognized:

(1) Chronic hereditary non-spherocytic hemolytic anemia is a rare condition that occurs sporadically among various ethnic groups, including Northern European, and represents a variety of differing molecular genetic defects of the enzyme.

(2) The "Mediterranean" variety is one in which the loss of enzyme activity is profound (about 1 per cent of normal) but does not produce clinically significant hemolysis until the erythrocyte is exposed to an extrinsic stress, usually of an oxidative nature, to which the erythrocyte, unable to regenerate reduced glutathione, cannot respond in self defense. The extrinsic stresses include certain drugs as well as such acquired illness as hepatitis and other infections, acidosis, and uremia. Certain deficient individuals in this group are sensitive to fava beans, a sensitivity which may be so severe that it can lead to fatal hemolysis. Genetic factors apparently set these fava bean-susceptible patients apart from the others.

(3) The "Negro" variety resembles the Mediterranean variety but is less severe, deficient males having about 10 to 15 per cent of the normal G-6-PD activity. The affected individual also is hematologically normal until exposed to one of the extrinsic stresses mentioned previously (with the exception of fava beans).

Inheritance is sex-linked, and significant hemolytic episodes are thus observed among affected males and the relatively rare homozygous females. The identification of heterozygous females is not always possible because of the wide range of enzyme levels found in this group, many falling within the normal range, and hemolytic reactions are usually so mild that they pass unnoticed. Beutler and co-workers showed that random inactivation of the X chromosome in the female leads to a dual red cell population, some erythrocytes carrying the normal X chromosome and others in the affected heterozygote carrying the G-6-PD-deficient one. The mean enzyme level will depend upon the relative proportions of normal and deficient erythrocytes. Tests which utilize intact erythrocytes rather than cell lysates may thus be more successful in detecting female heterozygotes.

The two most common types — the "Mediterranean" and the "Negro" — form relatively homogeneous genetic groupings. In the normal black population there are two electrophoretic types of G-6-PD which differ in only one amino acid site on the molecule. The faster migrating type is designated A and the slower B. Thus, nondeficient normal black males possess either A or B (approximately 18 per cent carry A), while the female may be homozygous AA or BB or heterozygous AB. The deficient enzyme in the black has the same electrophoretic mobility as the A type and it is therefore called A⁻. Caucasians, including the Mediterraneans, have only the B type of G-6-PD, and the Mediterranean type of G-6-PD deficiency is called B⁻ (Fig. 22–90).

The clinical severity of the drug-induced hemolysis varies from a clinically inapparent episode to a life-threatening event in an individual who may experience flank and abdominal pains, faintness from shock, and dark-colored urine from massive intravascular hemolysis. The antimalarials such as primaquine, pamaquine, and quinine are the

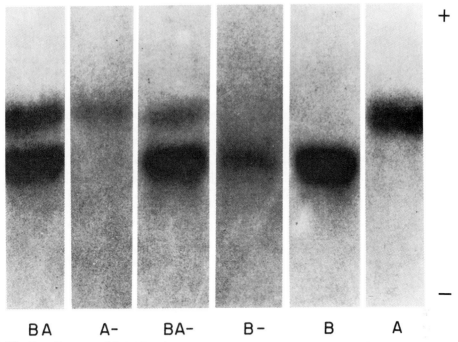

+

BA   A-   BA-   B-   B   A

−

Figure 22-90 Genetic types of G-6-PD deficiency identified by electrophoresis. BA is a normal Negro female heterozygote and BA− is a deficient Negro female heterozygote. The other patterns demonstrate normal and deficient male phenotypes. (From Giblett, E. R.: Genetic Markers in Human Blood. Blackwell Scientific Publications Ltd., Oxford, 1969.)

best known offenders, but sulfonamides, nitrofurans, analgesics, sulfones, and vitamin K derivatives are also frequently implicated. The hemolysis begins within 1 to 3 days of drug exposure, preferentially affecting the more aged erythrocytes because their level of enzyme is lower than that in the young cells. The initial change is a rapid drop in hemoglobin concentration in the peripheral blood. A reticulocyte elevation is observed 4 to 5 days later. After 7 to 10 days the patient enters into a phase of "drug resistance" during which the anemia becomes less pronounced and the patient appears to develop a tolerance to the drug (Fig. 22-91). The explanation for this apparent tolerance is that the younger erythrocytes have a higher enzyme level than the older ones and thus are somewhat better able to cope with the oxidative stress.

Some drugs act directly as oxidants, but most of the chemical agents which provoke oxidative hemolysis do so by interacting with oxyhemoglobin to cause the release of peroxide and other active states of oxygen. The normal erythrocyte meets this oxidative challenge by increasing the rate of glycolysis through the pentose phosphate pathway to maintain NADPH and glutathione in the reduced form. Reduced glutathione, through the good offices of glutathione peroxidase, rapidly detoxifies peroxide. The G-6-PD deficient erythrocyte cannot respond in this fashion. Its hemoglo-

bin is denatured into insoluble Heinz bodies attached to the inner membrane (Fig. 22-92). Between the increased rigidity caused by these inclusions and the direct oxidative damage wrought on the membrane and other cell constituents, hemolysis ensues. Some chemical agents, phenylhydrazine for example, are so potent they cause oxidative hemolysis in normal people. In addition to the potency of the agent and its dose, the genetic type of G-6-PD deficiency also determines the severity of the hemolysis. Pharmacogenetic differences in the population are sometimes important in determining whether or not oxidative hemolysis occurs. One person may metabolize a drug to a harmless intermediate, while another may convert the same agent to a by-product with toxic oxidative properties.

Direct enzyme assay is commonly used to establish the diagnosis of the G-6-PD–deficient state, but the result is affected by the average age of the red cell population. Thus, immediately following a hemolytic episode the levels may be nearly normal unless a correction is made for the mean cell age by the simultaneous measurement of another nonaffected enzyme such as hexokinase which also has a higher concentration in young than in old red cells. A number of simple screening tests have been devised, two of the more common in clinical use being the methemoglobin reduction test and the fluorescent spot test. The methemo-

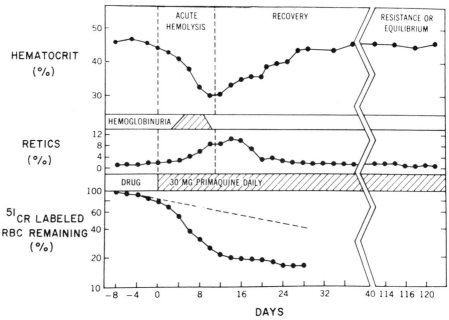

Figure 22–91 Drug-induced hemolysis in a male with G-6-PD deficiency. A period of hemolytic anemia is followed by compensation at higher hematocrit and relative drug resistance due to higher enzyme levels in the young population of erythrocytes. (Redrawn from Alving, A. S., et al.: Bull. WHO, 22:621, 1960.)

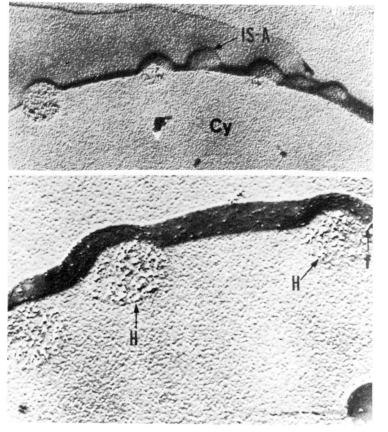

Figure 22–92 Heinz bodies (*H*) attached to the erythrocyte membrane demonstrated by freeze etching electron microscopy. *Cy* = cytoplasm; *IS-A* = intramembrane surface A. (From Lessin, L. S., et al.: Arch. Intern. Med., *129*:306, 1972. Copyright 1972 by the American Medical Association.)

globin reduction test takes advantage of the fact that methylene blue establishes a redox bridge between the pentose phosphate pathway and methemoglobin reduction with NADPH as hydrogen donor. Intracellular hemoglobin is first converted to methemoglobin by incubation with sodium nitrite. After addition of methylene blue, normal erythrocytes rapidly reduce the methemoglobin and change color from brown to red. G-6-PD–deficient erythrocytes, unable to increase glycolysis through the pentose phosphate pathway, remain the chocolate-brown color of methemoglobin. The fluorescent spot test is based on the reduction by lysate of NADP to NADPH, which fluoresces under ultraviolet light. G-6-PD–deficient erythrocytes, unable to accomplish this reduction, fail to produce fluorescence in the spot.

Intrinsic hemolysis may result from the presence of *abnormal hemoglobin*. As already discussed in detail, some abnormal hemoglobins are so unstable to oxidative stresses that they undergo spontaneous precipitation into insoluble deposits in the red cell, even in the presence of a normal enzymatic machinery. Some are drug sensitive, and in this respect resemble G-6-PD deficiency. The selective destruction of newly formed erythroid cells in homozygous β-thalassemia is reminiscent of a similar preferential susceptibility of young cells in paroxysmal nocturnal hemoglobinuria and in pyruvate kinase deficiency, but the pathogenetic mechanism is quite distinctive for each of these disorders. Sickle cell anemia, the most common of the hemoglobin diseases, results not from oxidative instability but from a physicochemical alteration of the hemoglobin which produces rigid erythrocytes. The final common pathway in the intrinsic hemoglobin disorders is membrane damage and reduction in cell pliability to the point of entrapment and destruction.

Extrinsic Hemolytic Disorders. Hemolytic conditions are caused by a wide variety of extrinsic physical and chemical factors. Extensive burns cause thermal damage to the erythrocyte membrane, with fragmentation, spherocytosis, and acute hemolysis. Acute poisoning with arsenate or copper or drowning (with hypotonic hemolysis) are other examples of acute hemolytic syndromes in patients suffering severe medical emergencies. Infections produce hemolysis indirectly, as in hypersplenism secondary to miliary tuberculosis or subacute bacterial endocarditis, or by direct invasion of the erythrocyte, as in the case of malaria or bartonellosis. In *Clostridium welchii* septicemia, the organism secretes a phospholipase which attacks the phospholipid backbone of the red cell membrane. The high oxygen tensions used in hyperbaric therapy cause hemolysis by peroxidation of membrane lipids. Chemical hemolysis by phenylhydrazine was once used therapeutically to reduce the red cell mass in patients with polycythemia. This agent, still commonly used to produce

hemolytic anemia experimentally in animals, causes a "Heinz body anemia" in normal erythrocytes quite similar to that observed in G-6-PD–deficient individuals given drugs to which they are sensitive.

The types of extrinsic hemolysis of greatest clinical interest from the pathogenetic point of view are those caused by mechanical damage and those which are the result of plasma factors.

Mechanical hemolysis is vividly illustrated by *march hemoglobinuria,* so called because it was observed in soldiers after the exertion of a long march (Davidson, 1969). The hemolysis is intravascular but benign and self-limited. The mechanical damage to the red cells occurs during the physical impact of the soles of the feet on hard surfaces. Ingeniously simple experiments have shown that it can be prevented among track athletes by placing shock absorbing material in the footwear or by running on soft grass instead of hard asphalt or concrete. The syndrome has even been seen in karate fighters, the damage in this instance coming from the palms of the hands as well as the soles of the feet.

Mechanical hemolysis also occurs because of damage to erythrocytes from physical impacts within the circulation. High pressure turbulence behind a stenotic aortic valve may cause mild cardiac hemolysis even in the unoperated patient. Modern cardiovascular surgery has contributed an important iatrogenic variety of *"traumatic" hemolysis* from red cell damage in the heart after insertion of prosthetic devices, as discussed by Marsh and Lewis. Its presence indicates an abnormal turbulence of blood or an exposed plastic surface not yet covered with endothelium. Examples of underlying causes are a loosened stitch at the base of a valve prosthesis through which a high-pressure jet of blood squirts; a bare Teflon patch used to close a septal defect upon which a regurgitant jet of blood strikes; and "ball variance," a late cause of postoperative hemolysis due to improper valve closure from slow swelling and distortion of the plastic ball. Technical improvements such as the use of a metal ball have reduced the frequency of postoperative traumatic hemolysis. Cardiac hemolysis is intravascular. When it is severe the loss of iron in the urine from the chronic hemoglobinuria and hemosiderinuria leads to iron deficiency and compromises the ability of the bone marrow to compensate for the reduced red cell life span.

Traumatic cardiac hemolysis has been aptly called the "Waring blender syndrome" because the morphologic alterations of the red cells suggest that they have been chopped by the whirling blades of this kitchen apparatus. They are sheared into bits and pieces, and display pointed and triangular forms, "helmet" shapes, and other distorted contours (Fig. 22–93). Microspherocytes and polychromasia are also present.

These morphologic changes are also a charac-

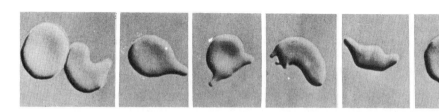

Figure 22–93   Irregular distortion of erythrocytes demonstrated by interference microscopy. (Reproduced from the Sandoz-Monograph, The Life Cycle of the Erythrocyte. Basel, Switzerland, Bessis, M., 1966.)

teristic feature of another group of hemolytic disorders which have in common an occlusive process of the microvasculature and hence have been called by Brain the *"microangiopathic hemolytic anemias."* The fragmentation has been reproduced experimentally in vitro by forcing red cells through a fibrin meshwork and in vivo by inducing intravascular coagulation in animals with injections of endotoxin or thrombin (Fig. 22–94). The clinical counterparts of these experiments are those conditions characterized by a thrombo-occlusive process in the small vessels, including the various disseminated intravascular coagulation syndromes, hemolytic uremic syndromes, and thrombotic thrombocytopenic purpura. Fragmentation hemolysis has also been encountered in patients with malignant hypertension or disseminated carcinoma.

Of the plasma factors that adversely effect erythrocyte survival time, antibodies against red cell antigens have received the most scrutiny. Much remains to be learned about the effects of non-immune plasma factors. The role of plasma lipids and lipoproteins in the hemolytic anemia of cirrhosis however warrants special consideration.

Anemia in cirrhosis is the result of a combination of factors — blood loss, iron and/or folate lack,

and hypersplenism. Even in the absence of these complicating factors, the erythrocyte life span is slightly to moderately reduced. Macrocytosis is a common feature of hepatocellular disease, often in association with target cells. The increased erythrocyte volume comes from accumulation of excessive lipid in the erythrocyte membrane, free cholesterol to a greater degree than phospholipid. The passive exchange between plasma and red cell membrane favors uptake into the latter because impairment of cholesterol esterification in liver disease leads to a relative increase in plasma free cholesterol at the expense of cholesterol esters. Indeed, inherited deficiency of the cholesterol esterifying enzyme, lecithyl cholesterol acyl transferase (LCAT), also causes macrocytosis with target cells. The increased levels of plasma free cholesterol secondary to obstruction of the biliary tract affect erythrocytes in a similar way. Marked hemolysis is not a feature of these forms of target cell anemia.

The *"spur cell"* anemia of cirrhosis is a more severe form of hemolysis. Its name is derived from the pointed thorny projections which protrude from the red cells (Fig. 22–95). This hemolytic disorder is seen in association with fulminating hepatocellular disease and is apparently a more extreme form of membrane accumulation of free

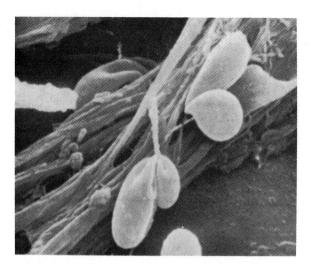

Figure 22–94   Erythrocyte fragmentation on fibrin strands. (From Bull, B. S., and Kuhn, I. N.: Blood, *35*:104–111, 1970, by permission of Grune & Stratton, Inc., New York.)

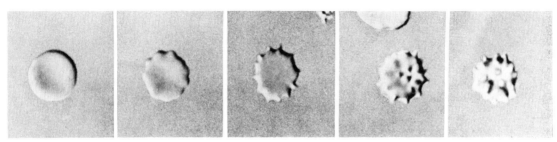

Figure 22–95 Regular distortion of an erythrocyte to form an acanthocyte. (Reproduced from the Sandoz-Monograph, The Life Cycle of the Erythrocyte. Basel, Switzerland, Bessis, M., 1966.)

cholesterol in excess of phospholipid. Plasma lipoproteins with abnormally high ratios of free cholesterol to phospholipid are important in its pathogenesis. The spur cells are susceptible to entrapment in the enlarged spleen commonly present in cirrhosis. Normal compatible erythrocytes transfused into affected patients soon acquire the membrane defect. Serum from patients with these disorders when added in vitro to normal compatible erythrocytes will produce macrocytosis and targeting or spur cell formation, as the case may be.

Hereditary acanthocytosis is characterized by absence of plasma beta-lipoproteins together with hypolipidemia and abnormal erythrocytes which closely resemble spur cells but are called "acanthocytes." The degree of hemolysis is mild. Acanthocytosis is occasionally seen in individuals after splenectomy who are otherwise hematologically normal. Spiculated erythrocytes are also seen. The pathogenesis of the erythrocyte shape change in these disorders remains unexplained.

Immune hemolysis may take place when antibodies present in the circulation react with antigens on the red cell surface. Hidden behind this deceptively simple theme lie the countless complexities of antigens, antibodies, and complement. *Isoimmune hemolysis* is the result of immunologic reactions between antibodies and antigens which reflect differences between individuals. Examples of isoimmune hemolysis include hemolytic transfusion reactions and immunohemolytic disease of the newborn, i.e., erythroblastosis fetalis. ABO incompatible erythrocytes are destroyed by "natural" isoantibodies normally present in the plasma. "Irregular" isoantibodies are produced only as a result of previous antigenic exposure, usually from transfusion or pregnancy. An autoantibody produced within a given individual with specificity directed against that individual's own autologous erythrocyte antigens brings on *autoimmune hemolytic anemia.*

The "natural" isoantibodies of the ABO system are predominantly IgM immunoglobulins with potent complement fixing ability. Isoimmune hemolytic reactions due to accidental transfusion of ABO incompatible erythrocytes are abrupt and life-threatening. The degree of complement fixation is extensive and provokes prompt intravascular hemolysis with hemoglobinemia and hemoglobinuria. Hypotension, disseminated intravascular coagulation, and acute renal failure are common complications.

"Irregular" antibodies directed against other red cell antigens, such as those of the Rh locus (CcDEe), are usually IgG immunoglobulins with a lesser propensity to fix complement. Their activity is maximal at 37°C. Demonstration of their presence requires the Coombs test. They are "warm" "incomplete" antibodies as distinct from the isoantibodies of the ABO system, which agglutinate erythrocytes in saline suspension at room temperature and therefore are "complete". Hemolysis secondary to irregular antibodies is less brisk and may be relatively more extravascular.

The Coombs test is central to the evaluation of immunohemolytic states. It is designed to detect either immunoglobulin or complement components coated on the erythrocyte surface. Coombs reagent, or "antiglobulin serum", is an antiserum raised in animals injected with these human plasma protein constituents. This antiserum when incubated with erythrocytes coated with immunoglobulin or with complement causes them to clump together. In general antiglobulin serum of broad specificity is used, sensitive to the presence either of immunoglobin or complement. Antiglobulin serum of more restricted specificity will distinguish immunoglobulin from complement on the erythrocyte surface. The term "gamma" Coombs refers to identification of immunoglobulin and "non-gamma" to the demonstration of complement. In experimental work, antiglobulin serum of even greater specificity permits identification of immunoglobulin subclasses. The "direct" Coombs test is performed on washed erythrocytes suspected of being coated in the circulation. The "indirect" test detects antibodies present in serum by first reacting the serum in vitro with erythrocytes and then testing these washed erythrocytes as described above.

Isoimmune hemolytic disease of the newborn is caused by the passage of 7S IgG antibodies across the placental barrier from the maternal into the fetal circulation, where they proceed to combine with antigens present on fetal erythrocytes. Although most of the natural isoantibodies of the ABO system are IgM antibodies too large to cross the placenta, some natural ABO isoantibodies are IgG and can cause erythroblastosis even during the first pregnancy. The usual incompatibility pairing is maternal type O and fetal type A or B. The hemolysis is generally mild and often requires no treatment. The antibody coating on the fetal erythrocyte may be so sparse that the Coombs test is negative.

Transplacental hemorrhage of fetal erythrocytes containing an antigen absent on the maternal red cell surface may raise the production of an irregular isoantibody in the maternal circulation, harmless to the mother but potentially detrimental to fetal erythrocytes once it crosses the placental barrier. Most significant is the D antigen of the Rh locus, although other antigens are occasionally responsible. ("Rh positive" indicates presence of the D antigen, "Rh negative" its absence.) Erythroblastosis fetalis due to Rh incompatibility causes severe hemolysis. The direct Coombs test on fetal erythrocytes is always positive. Hemorrhage of fetal erythrocytes into the maternal circulation is an event which most often occurs near term or at the time of labor and delivery. They can be demonstrated by a simple slide elution test which depends on the resistance of fetal hemoglobin to acid elution. Because of this requirement for prior immunization, first borns are usually spared, assuming that the mother has not been accidentally sensitized by previous transfusion of Rh incompatible cells.

A number of natural factors operate to reduce the incidence of Rh incompatibility neonatal he-

molytic disease. One of these is the dependence on prior occurrence of feto-maternal hemorrhage. Another is "ABO cancellation." If incompatibility within the ABO system coexists with Rh incompatibility, the rapid removal of the fetal erythrocytes by the natural isoantibodies anti A and/or anti B prevents active maternal immunization to the foreign Rh antigen on the fetal erythrocyte.

Following on this observation, it was reasoned that rapid removal of Rh incompatible fetal erythrocytes from the maternal circulation by the passive administration to the mother of a human gamma globulin preparation, hyperimmune with respect to its anti D titer, would prevent active maternal sensitization. This has indeed proved to be the case, and current practice calls for the routine prophylactic use of such gamma globulin preparations shortly after delivery in all Rh negative mothers at risk. Since this form of preventive therapy has been introduced, the incidence of Rh incompatibility neonatal hemolytic disease has decreased dramatically (Fig. 22–96). This remarkable reduction in cases deserves to rank among the major therapeutic achievements of recent years.

Kernicterus is the most dread complication of neonatal hemolytic disease, provided the infant survives the initial crisis. Lipid-soluble unconjugated bilirubin, present in excess of the plasma albumin binding capacity, is taken up into the nervous tissue, causing toxic damage. Therapeutic strategy is aimed at preventing the build-up of unconjugated bilirubin. This has traditionally been accomplished by exchange transfusion. More recent efforts have explored the use of albumin infusion, of pharmacologic agents such as phenobarbital to stimulate the hepatic enzymes to in-

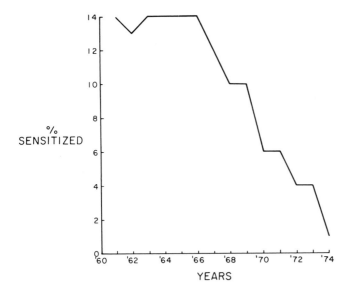

Figure 22–96 Following the routine prophylactic administration of anti Rh hyperimmune gamma globulin to mothers at risk, there has been a dramatic decrease in the incidence of erythroblastosis fetalis due to Rh incompatibility. The vertical axis represents the proportion of the Rh negative mothers sensitized to Rh. Clinical trials began in 1964 and routine use started in 1968. (Redrawn, by permission, from Freda, V. J., et al.: New England Journal of Medicine, 292:1014, 1975.)

crease the rate of bilirubin conjugation in the immature fetal liver, and exposure to light which appears to convert the bilirubin to less toxic derivatives.

The *autoimmune hemolytic anemias* are classified as "warm antibody" or "cold antibody" types. Warm antibody is an IgG immunoglobulin with maximal activity at 37°C. Its presence on the red cell is demonstrated by a positive Coombs test. It may or may not fix complement. Many of the warm antibodies have a specificity for the "core" antigen of the Rh locus. They react with all Rh phenotypes but not with the rare type Rh null, presumably a genetic deletion of the entire Rh locus.

Cold reactive autoantibody has increased activity as the temperature is reduced; the highest titer is at 4°C. It is demonstrated by the cold agglutinin test. In this simple procedure, dilutions of the patient's serum are mixed with normal type-compatible erythrocytes and incubated overnight at 4°C. The greatest dilution at which agglutination occurs is recorded. Titers greater than 1:64 are abnormal. Clinical hemolysis is associated with titers in excess of 1:1000, and they usually are considerably higher, some times as high as several million. The cold antibody, with one exception noted below, is an IgM immunoglobulin. It usually has specificity for the I antigen present on most adult erythrocytes, but absent on fetal erythrocytes which have the i antigen. Cord blood erythrocytes are thus usually not agglutinated by cold reactive antibody. A few cold antibodies have specificity for the i rather than the I antigen. Curiously, the reason for the cold reactivity of this class of antibodies does not appear to be a function of the antibody but rather of the Ii antigens. These presumably move to more accessible positions at the membrane surface as the temperature is reduced. Conversely, as the temperature is again increased the antigen sinks down into the more fluid lipid membrane, the immune complex is broken, and the antibody is released (Pruzanski and Shumak, 1977). However, the complement component, fixed by the cold antibodies to the membrane surface, remains and is responsible for the positive direct Coombs test usually observed in cold antibody hemolytic anemia (Table 22–14).

Warm antibody autoimmune hemolytic anemia is the most common of the immunohemolytic anemias. It affects all age groups. The onset may be insidious or acute, with fever, weakness, flank and abdominal pain. The spleen is commonly enlarged and the patient slightly jaundiced. The peripheral blood film shows microspherocytes mixed together with polychromatophilic macrocytes. It is distinguished from hereditary spherocytosis by the positive Coombs test. The autohemolysis test gives variable results. Osmotic fragility testing may show a "fragile tail" because of the population of osmotically susceptible microspherocytes.

Cold antibody autoimmune hemolytic anemia is almost always of the cold agglutinin type. It may occur in acute and self-limited form during the recovery phase of certain infections, most notably mycoplasma pneumonia and infectious mononucleosis. A chronic variety occurring usually in older patients is associated with a monoclonal autoantibody — and often with a monoclonal M-component on serum protein electrophoresis. This "idiopathic" condition is presumably "paraneoplastic" and closely related to the lymphoproliferative diseases. The degree of hemolysis is often mild in chronic cold agglutinin disease, even when the titer is very high. Exposed parts of the body — the fingers, toes, ears, and nose — may suffer the consequences of reduced temperatures with vaso-obstructive signs such as Raynaud-like symptoms or local tissue necrosis. The "thermal amplitude" refers to antibody activity as a function of temperature. The activity decreases as the temperature increases and usually no activity is present above 32°C. Spontaneous agglutination of anticoagulated blood at room temperature may cause technical errors in the laboratory unless precautions are taken to maintain the blood at temperatures above 32°C. Autoagglutination, along with spherocytosis, is a dominant feature of the peripheral blood film. The marrow is often infiltrated with lymphocytes in the idiopathic chronic variety.

Paroxysmal cold hemoglobinuria is a very rare acquired immunohemolytic anemia caused by an IgG cold reactive autoantibody demonstrated by the Donath-Landsteiner test. The antibody is bound at 4°C. and complement is fixed. Agglutination is not present, but as the sample is warmed complement induced hemolysis takes place. Acute hemolytic episodes are provoked by exposure to cold. Signs of intravascular hemolysis are marked. Some cases are idiopathic, while others are related to infections, especially syphilis.

The pathogenesis of the hemolysis in autoimmune hemolytic anemia has posed apparent paradoxes. For example, a strongly positive Coombs test may be associated with an absence of clinical

TABLE 22–14 LABORATORY DIAGNOSIS OF AUTOIMMUNE HEMOLYTIC ANEMIA

	Routine Coombs Test	"Gamma" Coombs Test	"Non-gamma" Coombs Test	Cold agglutinin Test
Warm type	+	+	+ or −	−
Cold agglutinin type	+	−	+	+

hemolysis on the one hand, while on the other an occasional case of acquired autoimmune hemolytic anemia may be discovered with a negative Coombs test. Some explanations for these apparent contradictions between laboratory tests and clinical events have in large measure been provided by new information about the subclasses of immunoglobulins and their relationships to complement fixation and to specific receptors on the surface of macrophages.

It stands to reason that the density of the antibody coating on the red cell is a major determinant of the severity of hemolysis, as Rosse and others have demonstrated (Fig. 22–97). About 500 IgG molecules per erythrocyte are necessary to produce a positive Coombs test. For a given antibody the greater this number the shorter the red cell life span. However, reduced erythrocyte life span may also be present at values less than 500.

The process of complement fixation is directly a function of the density of antibodies on the red cell surface. In order for the first component of complement to be fixed, two IgG molecules must achieve a certain critical distance apart from each other (250-400 Å). Low-density IgG coatings are thus not likely to fix complement. On the other hand, the pentameric IgM contains within its intrinsic structure five potential immunoglobulin binding sites. Since these five "feet" fall within the critical distance, IgM on the cell surface invariably fixes complement. If the antigenic sites on the red cell surface are spaced too far apart to permit the corresponding IgG antibodies to be placed within the critical distance, then complement fixation cannot take place. Such is the case with the Rh

antigens; immunohemolytic disease due to Rh antibodies lacks complement on the cell surface (Logue and Rosse, 1976).

The immunoglobulin subclasses do not fix complement equally well. In addition to IgM, IgG_3 and IgG_1 are active. IgG_2 has only weak activity. IgG_4, IgA, and IgE do not fix complement at all. Thus, the specific subclass to which the autoantibody belongs, along with its concentration, is important as a hemolytic determinant.

The specific details of the complement system have been clearly depicted by Müller-Eberhard. The "recognition unit" (C_1 qrs) is followed by "the activation unit" ($C_{4, 2, 3}$) which in turn may develop a "membrane attack unit" (C_{5-9}). An immense amount of C_1 must be fixed to bring on the membrane attack unit to punch holes through the cell surface and cause direct hemolysis. This usually does not occur in autoimmune hemolytic anemia. If complement fixation is achieved, it ordinarily is arrested at the level of the activation unit, which leaves C_3b on the cell surface. However, this component can also bring about cell damage by interaction with macrophages.

Macrophages have at least two specific receptors on their surfaces, one for the Fc fragment of IgG and the other for the C_3b component of complement. Once again the subclasses of IgG are important; receptor activity is greatest for IgG_3 and IgG_1 and absent for IgG_4 and IgA, in parallel to the complement fixing activity of these immunoglobulin types. Immunoglobulin and/or C_3b on the erythrocyte surface brings the coated erythrocyte into close juxtaposition to macrophages at these receptor sites. At the interface the macrophage proceeds about its work, gnawing bits and pieces

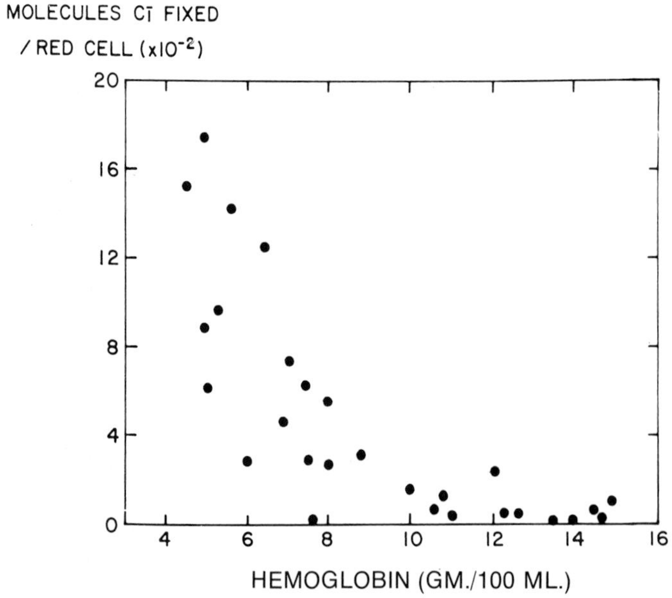

MOLECULES C̄1 FIXED

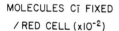

Figure 22–97 The relation between IgG density on the erythrocyte membrane and the degree of anemia in nonsplenectomized patients with warm antibody autoimmune hemolytic anemia. The measurement of membrane antibody density employs a sensitive technque of first reacting the coated erythrocytes with anti-human gamma globulin and then measuring complement fixation on the doubly coated cells. (Redrawn from Rosse, W. F.: J. Clin. Invest., 50:734, 1971.)

HEMOGLOBIN (GM./100 ML.)

away from the cell surface. Lost surface causes spherocytosis culminating in the eventual entrapment and engulfment of the entire erythrocyte. These events are depicted diagrammatically in Figure 22–98. Erythrocyte fragmentation at the cell-cell interface has been vividly documented by electron microscopy (Fig. 22–99).

Other variables also affect the severity of the hemolysis. One of these is the state of activation of macrophages. Another is C_3 inactivator. This ingredient of the complement system cleaves C_3b on the erythrocyte surface, leaving behind a fragment called C_3d. This is still detectable in the Coombs test, but its presence on the cell surface protects against further phagocytosis, thus limiting hemolysis (Jaffe and coworkers, 1976). In fact, C_3 inactivator appears to be able to release the C_3b coated erythrocyte from the grasp of the hepatic macrophage and allow it once again to circulate without further damage (Fig. 22–98).

Thus the lack of correlation between the results of routine clinical tests and clinical phenomena has become more understandable. The reason why IgG_4 or IgA do not produce hemolysis is clear; neither fix complement and neither bind to macrophages. Conversely an erythrocyte coated with both IgG_3 and C_3b is rapidly destroyed since both

moieties bring about lethal contacts with macrophage receptors.

What determines splenic as against hepatic hemolysis? In warm antibody hemolytic disease the IgG coating on the erythrocyte is often unaccompanied by complement and splenic macrophages are the preferred site of destruction. Hence splenectomy is often successful as a definitive means of therapy if glucocorticoids cannot adequately control the hemolysis. On the other hand, cold agglutinin hemolytic disease is predominantly hepatic, probably because C_3b on the erythrocyte surface favors interaction with the hepatic Kupfer cells. Splenectomy is usually unsuccessful and glucocorticoids of less benefit than in warm antibody hemolytic disease. By similar reasoning resistance of warm antibody hemolytic anemia to these therapeutic measures may be related to class and concentration of antibody and to complement fixation.

Glucocorticoids act primarily by blocking macrophage–erythrocyte interactions and inhibiting phagocytosis. Only later do they cause autoantibody concentrations to fall. Other immunosuppressive modalities have also been used in the treatment of resistant cases.

How does an autoantibody come to be produced

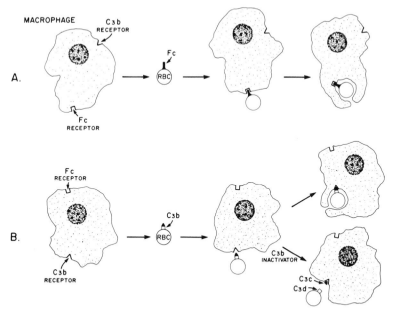

Figure 22–98 The role of macrophage surface receptors in immune hemolytic anemia, illustrated diagrammatically. Macrophages have separate receptors for immunoglobulins and for complement. The immunoglobulin receptors have a restricted specificity for the Fc fragment of the subclasses IgG_1 and IgG_3. The other immunoglobulins do not bind to macrophages. The complement receptor is specific for the C_3b component.

A. An IgG coated erythrocyte is attached to a macrophage. Erythrocyte fragmentation and/or outright engulfment follows.

B. A C_3b coated erythrocyte is attached to a macrophage. Phagocytosis may follow, as in A, or C_3b inactivator may cleave C_3b and cause release of the erythrocyte from the clutches of the macrophage. C_3d is left behind on the erythrocyte. This surface coating renders the erythrocyte resistant to further phagocytic damage.

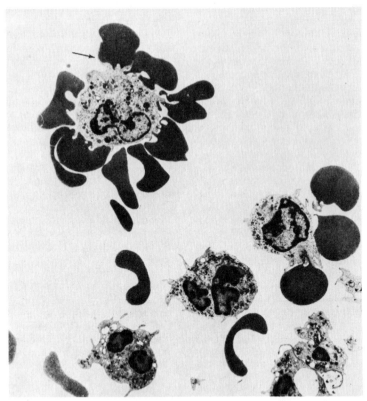

Figure 22–99 The adherence of IgG coated erythrocytes to macrophages, with fragmentation of small pieces of the erythrocyte membrane at the cell to cell interface. (From Abramson, N., et al.: J. Exper. Med., *132*:1191, 1970.)

in violation of the principle of immune self recognition and tolerance to autologous antigens? Hypotheses for this phenomenon as a pathogenetic factor in a variety of disease states have been put forth: (1) There is a shared antigenicity between an exogenous inciting antigen and an autologous antigen which brings on the immune attack upon the autologous tissue. (2) "Forbidden clones" of immunocytes emerge, perhaps due to lack of proper immunologic "suppressor" or "surveillance" activity, and these produce antibodies against autologous antigen. (3) A subtle change takes place in autologous antigen, rendering it immunogenic.

What is clear is that a large proportion of autoimmune hemolytic anemias occur in association with altered states of immunity. Acute self-limited syndromes appear in the recovery phase from certain infections while the immune response is taking place. Others occur in association with immune deficiency syndromes, such as agammaglobulinemia and a variety of chronic lymphoproliferative disorders, especially chronic lymphatic leukemia, lymphocytic lymphoma, and Hodgkin's disease. They also complicate the course of other autoimmune disorders, such as disseminated lupus erythematosus and ulcerative colitis. Many however remain unexplained and are designated "idiopathic."

Coombs-positive immunohemolytic anemias also occur as adverse reactions to certain medications, and a consideration of these may provide some further insight into pathogenetic mechanisms. They fall into three classes:

(1) The "haptene" (or penicillin) type. The serum of the patient contains antipenicillin antibodies of the 7S type. Penicillin, if given in very high doses, is soaked up into the erythrocyte membrane. The antipenicillin antibodies are not directed against red cell antigens but do bind to the penicillin in the membrane, giving rise to a positive "gamma" Coombs test and to hemolysis.

(2) The "immune complex" (or "innocent bystander") type. IgM antibody is formed to the drug (quinidine, quinine, stibophen) which is associated with an unidentified serum protein as carrier. The antibody then reacts with the antigen to form an immune complex, which attaches to the red cell membrane and fixes complement. The antibody

may then be detached, leaving complement behind. The "non-gamma" Coombs test is positive because of the complement coat. The red cell is considered the innocent bystander. The mechanism is the same as that of quinidine thrombocytopenia, except that the latter is characterized by the production of a 7S IgG antibody.

(3) The true autoimmune (or alphamethyldopa) type. In a time- and dose-dependent manner, the drug induces the formation of an antibody specifically directed against a normal red cell antigen, usually of the Rh complex. The autoimmune state persists for months after discontinuation of the drug, gradually subsiding without additional treatment. This drug-related form of autoimmunity suggests a possible pathogenesis of other types of autoimmune states by undefined exogenous agents.

PHAGOCYTES

STRUCTURE

A recent trend in dynamic morphology has been to separate the leukocytes into two major groups: the phagocytes and the immunocytes. This separation has taxonomic merits and will be followed in this book.

The phagocytes can be divided into the granulocytes and the monocyte-macrophages. Both types are bone marrow derived and it appears plausible that these cells have a common precursor, either a stem cell committed to the phagocytic cell lines or a blast cell designated as a myeloblast or a myelomonoblast. This blast cell is smaller, and both nucleus and cytoplasm are less basophilic than those of the proerythroblast. It is distinguished from the lymphoblast in that it has several visible nucleoli and a nucleus with an indistinct nuclear membrane and no perinuclear halo. The pale blue cytoplasm is scant and frequently present only as a faint outline on one side of the nucleus. The subsequent differentiation to granulocytes is heralded by the appearance of coarse granules made up of lysosomes staining blue or violet with Wright's stain. They contain large amounts of a myeloperoxidase as well as lysozymes and bactericidal cationic proteins. At this promyelocytic stage, the nucleus is still blastic with nucleoli, but at the next stage, the myelocytic stage, the nuclear chromatin becomes clumped and the capacity for mitotic division ceases. New species of lysosomal granules appear, giving the mature granulocytes their characteristic morphologic appearance. The neutrophilic granules are small and pink and contain a bactericidal lactoferrin and an alkaline phosphatase. The eosinophilic granules are large and round and contain red-staining, basic mucopolysaccharides. The basophilic granules are coarse, often concealing the nucleus, and contain histamine, heparin, and acid mucopolysaccharides. The background cytoplasm of all three cell types is pink, and the nucleus becomes lobulated with 2 to 5 distinct lobes connected by thin strands (Fig. 22–11).

The differentiation from myelomonoblast to mature monocytes is undoubtedly also a process of integrated proliferation and maturation, but distinct stages are difficult to recognize. The mature monocyte is a large cell with a diameter of about 20 to 30 microns and a prominent multishaped nucleus. The chromatin structure is less clumped than that of the mature granulocyte or lymphocyte and appears lace-like, with small chromatin particles tied together by fine strands. The cytoplasm is grayish-blue and contains many fine lysosomes stained pink with Wright's stain. Even on fixed smears, the cytoplasm gives an impression of being "free flowing," reflecting active ameboid motions right up to the time the cell becomes permanently fixed to the glass slide. The clear cytoplasmic vacuoles frequently observed may be artifactual and caused by the smearing technique. After the monocyte leaves the circulating blood it is transformed into a lysosome-filled macrophage. Cline and Golde have reviewed the sequence of this transformation which involves a sudden burst in metabolic activities (Fig. 22–100). Energy production is increased, synthesis of hydrolytic enzymes by the endoplasmic reticulum and their subsequent packing by the Golgi apparatus into lysosomes are enhanced, and the cell enlarges until it has taken on the appearance of the large mobile macrophage found in pulmonary alveoli, peritoneal cavities, and inflammatory exudate. These cells reach a diameter of 50μ or more and send out far-reaching cytoplasmic tentacles. The cytoplasm may contain lipid droplets and lysosomes with incompletely digested material such as carbon particles, and hemosiderin granules. The oval-shaped nucleus is off to one side, is relatively small in proportion to the cytoplasm and has an open lacy chromatin network (Fig. 22–101). Although the mobile macrophages retain common phagocytic properties, they develop characteristics of the or-

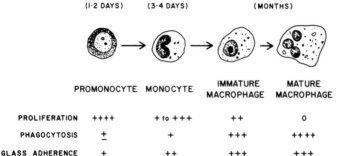

	MARROW (1-2 DAYS)	BLOOD (3-4 DAYS)	TISSUES (MONTHS)	
	PROMONOCYTE	MONOCYTE	IMMATURE MACROPHAGE	MATURE MACROPHAGE
PROLIFERATION	++++	+ to +++	++	0
PHAGOCYTOSIS	±	+	+++	++++
GLASS ADHERENCE	+	++	+++	+++
LYSOSOMES	+	++	++++	++++
IgG RECEPTORS	+	++	+++	+++
LYMPHOCYTE INTERACTION	?	++	++++	++++

Figure 22–100 Cellular kinetics and functional properties of the monocyte-macrophages. The mature macrophage is represented by a multinucleated epithelial giant cell, but other types include the alveolar macrophages, Kupffer cells, brain microglia, and the macrophages of the spleen, lymph nodes, marrow, and other tissues. (From Cline, M. J., and Golde, D. W.: Am. J. Med., 55:49, 1973.)

gan to which they belong. For example, alveolar macrophages depend on oxidative phosphorylation for their energy production, whereas other macrophages depend on glycolysis. The fixed macrophage in the liver, spleen, and bone marrow appears to exist in a dynamic equilibrium with the mobile macrophage, and the characteristic foreign body giant cell or Langhans cell may represent fusion of a number of mobile macrophages. The term "reticuloendothelial system" is traditionally used to describe this large system of mobile and fixed macrophages. Since neither reticular nor endothelial cells are phagocytic, a better, but still not widely used, term is "mononuclear phagocyte system," as suggested by Meuret in 1977.

FUNCTION

Although the functions of the granulocytes and the monocyte-macrophages overlap, it seems reasonable to suggest that granulocytes function primarily as the first line of defense against microbial organisms, whereas the monocyte-macro-

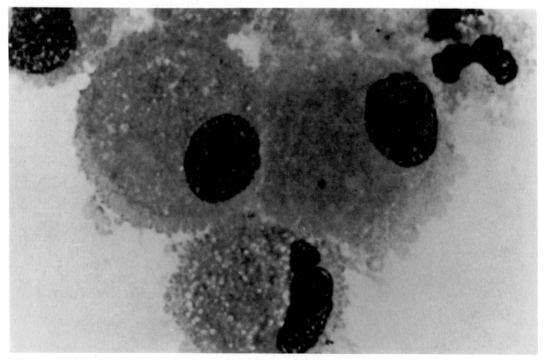

Figure 22–101 Alveolar macrophages. These macrophages live in aerobic circumstances and, in contrast to other phagocytic cells, they utilize aerobic metabolism for energy. (From Golde, D. W., Finley, T. N., and Cline, M. J.: N. Engl. J. Med., 290:875, 1974.)

phages provide final removal of such organisms and also clear the body of its own aged and damaged cells. In order to accomplish this, the phagocytes have to (1) accumulate in sufficient numbers at the right place, (2) become attached to the foreign or nonviable material, (3) engulf, (4) dissolve, and (5) dispose of this material (Stossel, 1974).

Granulocytes spend less than a day in the circulation before they migrate through the endothelial wall and are disposed of in various tissues. Inflammatory lesions will release specific leukotaxines which increase capillary permeability and induce local migration of the granulocytes. These leukotaxines are poorly defined but, as shown by Ward, Cochrane, and Müller-Eberhard, they may include fragments of the activated complement C3. In addition, transformed lymphocytes release both chemotactic lymphokines and a "migration inhibition factor" which acts by arresting macrophages at sites of antigen accumulation.

The process responsible for the attachment of granulocytes to antigens depends on the opsonization of the antigenic surface by activated complement C3. Antibodies will also cause opsonization, but primarily for monocytes and macrophages which have abundant binding sites for both the Fc region of IgG and for the C3 fragment. Consequently, cells coated with non-complement binding antibodies, as found, for example, in acquired hemolytic anemia or idiopathic thrombocytopenic purpura, are primarily phagocytized by the mononuclear phagocyte system. The mechanism responsible for the attachment of phagocytes to antigens prior to antibody formation and complement activation or to devitalized cells is still obscure.

After the attachment, the membrane responds by engulfing the material in toto (Fig. 22–102). Inside the cytoplasm the engulfed material is enveloped by internalized surface membrane and distinct phagosomes are formed. Lysosomal granules become attached and empty their cargo of hydrolytic enzymes into the phagosomes, killing and/or dissolving their content (Fig. 22–103) and morphologically degranulating the phagocytes. The process of killing involves peroxidation of H_2O_2, which in the presence of iodide derived from tyrosine will destroy microbial membranes. Subsequent dissolution involves the integrated action of numerous hydrolytic enzymes. The ingestion of foreign or devitalized material is associated with a rapid increase in energy production and the generation of H_2O_2. Since the granulocytes contain only a few mitochondria, the major energy-producing pathway is glycolysis, and phagocytosis appears to stimulate both the Embden-Meyerhof pathway and the hexose monophosphate shunt. It has been proposed that increased demands for ATP energy cause an accumulation of NADH, which in the presence of an oxidase

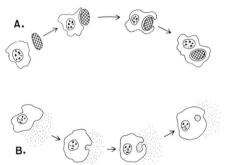

Figure 22–102 Endocytosis. The process of engulfing a portion of the cell's exterior into its interior. A. "Phagocytosis" refers to the inclusion of relatively large particles. The phagocyte membrane sends out pseudopodia to grasp the particle, utilizing a propulsive mechanism biochemically similar to that of muscle. B. "Pinocytosis" refers to the cellular interiorization of smaller particles included as a droplet of the fluid exterior into an interior membrane-lined vesicle.

generates H_2O_2. Excess H_2O_2 will in turn oxidize reduced glutathione and stimulate shunt activity (Fig. 22–104).

The final release of the degradation products tends to amplify the inflammatory response. Released lysosomal enzymes may cause injury to surrounding tissues, endogenous pyrogens cause fever, thromboplastic products may cause fibrin obstruction of vessels, and cationic proteins cause vasodilatation.

In addition to participating in the phagocytic inflammatory response to foreign antigens, the tissue macrophages play a key role in the important process of antigen-induced blast transformation of lymphocytes. This process may be dependent on a preliminary processing or digestion of the antigens by the macrophages. However, it is equally possible that the macrophage surface provides sites of attachment for both antigens and lymphocytes, permitting optimal interaction (Fig. 22–105).

The tissue macrophages are also responsible for the daily destruction of aged blood cells, denatured plasma proteins, and plasma lipids. This large and somewhat unappreciated function is accomplished through phagocytosis of whole cells and pinocytosis of small droplets containing plasma proteins and lipid microcolloids (Fig. 22–102). There still is no clear explanation of the process by which the macrophage recognizes non-viable blood cells or plasma constituents. Studies of red blood cells have revealed that aging is associated with a decreased membrane content of sialic acid resulting in a decreased negative change, but whether it be this or another subtle membrane change that is responsible for the fatal interaction with macrophages is unknown. The avidity of the tissue macrophage to slightly altered cells,

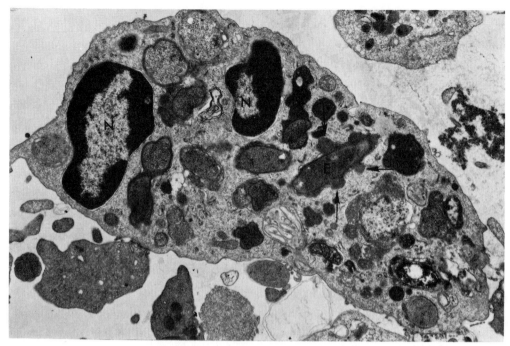

Figure 22–103   Electron microscopic picture of a human granulocyte after phagocytosis of *E. coli* (*E*). Coalescence of lysosomes with the phagocytic vacuoles is seen at arrows. *N* = nucleus. (From Zucker-Franklin, D., Elsbach, E., and Simon, P. J.: Lab. Invest., *25*:415, 1971. U.S.–Canadian Division of the International Academy of Pathology. The Williams and Wilkins Company [Agent].)

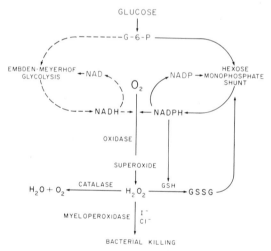

Figure 22–104   Generation of superoxide and hydrogen peroxide by an oxidase which transfers electrons from reduced pyridine nucleotides to molecular oxygen. The reduced pyridine nucleotides are primarily but not exclusively generated via the hexose monophosphate shunt. The H_2O_2 can be used for bacterial killing via a myeloperoxidase pathway utilizing the halides, iodide and chloride. Excess H_2O_2 is destroyed by catalase or by reduced glutathione (GSH), which in its oxidized state further activates the monophosphate shunt. (Adapted from Karnofsky, et al., 1970, and Stossel, 1977.)

to denatured proteins, or to macrocolloids has been used diagnostically to measure the size and blood flow of organs containing many macrophages — such as the liver, spleen, and bone marrow. The technique has been to label a cell or protein with a radioactive tracer, expose the labeled material to heat or chemicals, and use scanning techniques to determine the tissue transit or deposit of the isotopes. Similarly, certain isotopes of gold or technetium can be prepared in a colloidal form, and the clearance rate from blood and the uptake in the tissues can be used in the diagnostic evaluation of the size and function of mononuclear phagocyte organs (Fig. 22–106).

Macrophages are also placed in the mainstream of iron metabolism. A variety of tissue macrophages possess inducible heme oxidase activity, enabling them to break down red cell hemoglobin. The released iron is incorporated into ferritin and subsequently into insoluble hemosiderin. Macrophages of the liver, spleen, and bone marrow can again return iron to transferrin for transport back to the erythroid marrow. Alveolar macrophages are lacking in the ability to provide reutilization of iron, and indeed, in pulmonary hemosiderosis, abundant iron-laden alveolar macrophages are demonstrable even in the face of iron deficiency anemia and an absence of storage iron elsewhere.

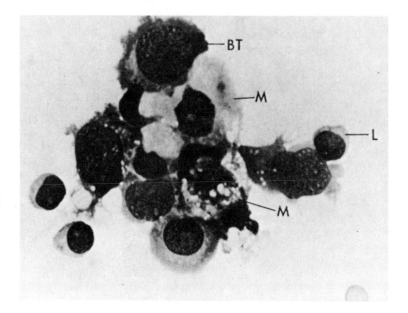

Figure 22–105 An "immunologic island" composed of central macrophages (*M*), surrounding lymphocytes undergoing blast transformation (*BT*) and untransformed lymphocytes (*L*). (From Cline, M. J.: *In* Williams et al. (Eds.): Hematology, 2nd Ed. McGraw-Hill Book Co., New York, 1977.)

Tissue macrophages presented with a phagocytic load may show a temporary decrease in efficiency, a phenomenon that Wagner and Iio called "blockade." There is a degree of specificity, however, since blockade induced by one injected material does not necessarily block the subsequent clearance of a different particle. Nevertheless, blockage produced by excessive hemolysis may cause impaired removal of foreign antigens. Fortunately, a chronic challenge to macrophage function causes "overwork hyperplasia" with an appropriate compensating increase in the mass of the mononuclear phagocyte system.

The pathophysiologic relationship of eosinophils and basophils to so-called "allergic reactions" is still unexplained. The basophils have been shown to contain sites of attachment for IgE antibody, and their degranulation is associated with the release of histamine. However, the eosinophils, which are much more closely identified

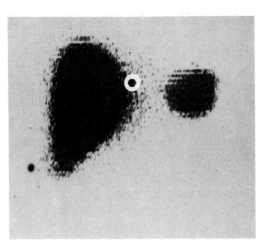
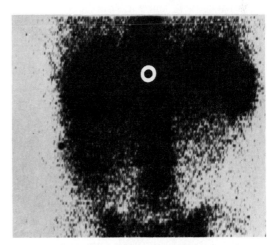

Figure 22–106 Body surface scans after intravenous injection of technetium (^{99m}Tc) sulfur colloid. Anterior views are shown. The position of the xiphoid is shown by the white circle. Left: In a normal individual 85–95% of the colloid is taken up by the macrophages of the liver because of the large hepatic blood flow, but the spleen is also well visualized. Right: In a patient with cirrhosis, hepatic uptake is reduced. The enlarged spleen is shown with increased colloid uptake, and the bone marrow macrophages now participate in the clearance, as shown by uptake over the vertebral column and pelvis. The clearance rate from the circulation is also slowed, leaving a heavy "background." (Kindly provided by Dr. M. Croll. Division of Nuclear Medicine, Lankenau Hospital, Philadelphia, PA.)

with allergy than the basophils, have not as yet been found to interact specifically with antigen-antibody complexes (Beeson and Bass, 1977).

KINETICS

Because of the relatively long tissue phase prior to and following the brief appearance of the granulocyte in the bloodstream, information about the rate and control of production and destruction has been difficult to obtain. However, reliable labeling techniques have been developed, both cohort labeling of DNA with ^{32}P or with tritiated thymidine and random labeling with radioactive diisopropyl fluorophosphate or with ^{51}Cr. Utilizing such techniques it has been possible to construct a model for granulocyte kinetics similar to models developed for erythrocytes and thrombocytes (Fig. 22–7).

In order to account for granulocyte renewal and control it is a necessity to accept the existence of a stem cell precursor pool. As described in the bone marrow section, this pool is probably divided morphologically or functionally into a multipotential stem cell pool and several unipotential stem cell pools committed to specific cell lines. The culturing of bone marrow on soft agar has disclosed the existence of a colony-forming cell, CFU-C, which, when stimulated by a colony-stimulating factor, CSF, will grow colonies containing thousands of granulocytes and monocytes. The CFU-C is believed to be the unipotential stem cell committed to the granulocyte-monocytic cell line. After blast transformation, the myeloblasts divide about three to five times and simultaneously mature into myelocytes. Warner and Athens have proposed that the number of divisions is not predetermined but actively regulated, and that skipped divisions or additional divisions may adjust the responsiveness of granulocytic production to peripheral demands. After the myelocytes have become mitotically inactive, maturing cells accumulate as a marrow granulocyte reserve. This reserve is under normal conditions made up by about five days' worth of granulocytes. Following their final release from the bone marrow, the granulocytes spend less than one day in the bloodstream, establishing two pools of about equal size — a circulating pool and a marginated pool. From the bloodstream they migrate into the tissues in which they will be destroyed either randomly in defense actions or by senescence about two to three days later (Boggs, 1967; Robinson and Mangalik, 1975).

Table 22–15 gives some approximations of the size of the various granulocytic pools. The combined size of the marrow pools is almost 1.5 times that calculated for the nucleated red blood cell pools, despite the fact that the daily production of

TABLE 22–15   GRANULOCYTIC POOLS

Cell Types	Number of Cells in 10^9 per kg. Body Weight
Proliferating Cells	2.1
Marrow Granulocytic Reserve	5.6
Circulating Granulocytes	0.3
Marginated Granulocytes	0.2
Daily Production and Destruction	0.9

red cells is about twice the daily production of granulocytes. This, of course, is due to the fact that the marrow contains a large reserve of maturing and mature granulocytes.

In peripheral blood, the normal granulocyte count should always be considered a range rather than a value. The fluctuating equilibrium between circulating and marginated cells precludes a completely stable granulocyte count and the existence of an extensive granulocyte reserve in the bone marrow permits the granulocyte count to adjust temporarily to the demands for phagocytic cells.

The exact mechanism regulating granulocyte production is still unknown, although it undoubtedly involves a feedback between circulating granulocytes and the bone marrow. In support of the existence of a feedback mechanism is the observation that the granulocyte count in some patients with depleted bone marrow reserves exhibits an oscillatory pattern and that each period in this pattern is about 11 to 15 days, about twice the length of time it takes for myeloblasts to become mature granulocytes (Fig. 22–107). The reason for not observing such oscillations more often probably is the fact that under normal conditions the large bone marrow reserve pool will dampen or obliterate the amplitude of oscillations.

Various factors have been claimed to be responsible for maintaining the feedback adjustment between the peripheral demands for granulocytes and the bone marrow supply of granulocytes. Several granulocyte-mobilizing factors have been described, including endotoxin, etiocholanolone, Menkin's tissue leukotaxines, and a leukocyte-mobilizing factor, but, as emphasized by Craddock and co-workers, it seems unlikely that any of these are involved in the physiologic regulation of granulocyte production. Other factors released by mature circulating granulocytes have been claimed to act as inhibitors or chalones of mitotic divisions within the myelocyte pool. Recent studies, summarized by Golde and Cline in 1974, have suggested that the true granulopoietin is a glycoprotein derived from monocytes and macrophages and named colony stimulating factor or CSF. This glycoprotein, which is present in both plasma and urine, is necessary for the

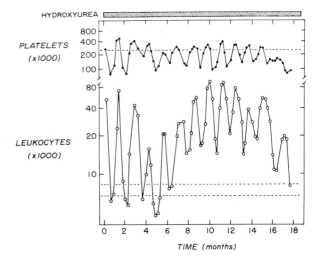

Figure 22–107 Regular oscillatory variations in the leukocyte and platelet count in a patient with chronic granulocytic leukemia receiving hydroxyurea therapy. (From Kennedy, B. J.: Blood, *35*:751, 1970, by permission of Grune & Stratton, Inc., New York.)

induction of clonal growth of granulocyte precursors in vitro (Stohlman and Quesenberry, 1972). Consequently it is tempting to construct a feedback model for the control of granulocyte production, as outlined in Figure 22–108. This model, however, is quite hypothetical since the existence of a granulopoietin and its identification with CSF are based primarily on in-vitro data. Nevertheless, Richard and co-workers have shown that CSF is present in higher concentrations in leukopenic individuals than in normals, and Metcalf and Stanley have shown that it may increase granulocyte production when injected into mice. Furthermore, the apparently well-established existence of a circulating eosinophilopoietin (Mahmond, et al., 1977) gives support to the operation of granulocytic feedback systems based on the release and action of specific poietins.

The kinetics and regulation of the monocyte-macrophage complex are even less understood than those of the granulocyte complex (van Furth, 1970). The monocytes appear to have a shorter intramedullary life span than the granulocytic precursors, since they tend to emerge earlier than the granulocytes after a temporary bone marrow suppression. The life span of the monocyte in the circulation is probably about 36 hours or three times longer than that of the granulocyte. The extravascular life span after it has been transformed to mobile of fixed macrophages is undoubtedly long and may be counted in months if not years.

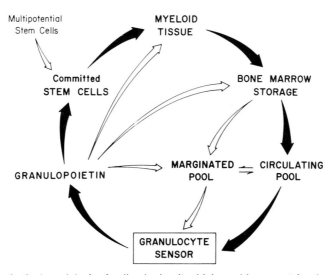

Figure 22–108 Hypothetical model of a feedback circuit which could account for the physiologic control of the granulocyte count.

PATHOPHYSIOLOGY

GRANULOCYTE DISORDERS

Classification and General Considerations

Disorders of the granulocytes are traditionally classified according to the number of circulating granulocytes into granulocytopenias and granulocytoses. However, a classification based on function and kinetics is of more contemporary importance. Using such criteria, the following classes of disorders can be recognized: quantitative abnormalities, qualitative abnormalities, and myeloproliferative disorders (Table 22–16). The pathophysiologic effect of quantitative disorders is determined by the size of the actual and potential granulocyte pools. In granulocytopenia the lack of defense against microorganisms and other foreign invaders dominates the clinical picture, whereas in granulocytosis the problems are more subtle. Although much larger and stickier than the red cells, the viscosity of blood with a high granulocyte count is about the same as for normal blood with the same total hematocrit (white cell crit plus red cell crit), and hyperviscosity due to granulocytosis is rare unless the white blood cell count measures in the hundreds of thousands. More common is bone tenderness caused by expansion of the bone marrow and uric acid arthropathy or nephropathy caused by destruction of granulocytes. The qualitative disorders are characterized by impaired granulocyte defense despite a normal number of circulating neutrophils. Finally, the clinical manifestations of myeloproliferative disorders are related to the extent and character of cellular proliferation and cellular replacement.

TABLE 22–16 CLASSIFICATION OF GRANULOCYTE DISORDERS

I. Quantitative Abnormalities
   Granulocytopenia
   Granulocytosis

II. Qualitative Abnormalities
   Defective delivery
   Defective phagocytic activity
   Defective bactericidal activity

III. Myeloproliferative Disorders
   Polycythemia vera
   Chronic granulocytic leukemia
   Myelofibrosis
   Thrombocythemia
   Erythroleukemia
   Acute granulocytic leukemia
   Acute myelomonocytic leukemia

Quantitative Abnormalities

Granulocytopenia. When the absolute granulocyte count is less than 3000 per cu. mm., the term granulocytopenia is used, but even at this level there are adequate numbers of granulocytes for normal defense activities. When the absolute number reaches 1000 per cu. mm., the patient becomes vulnerable to microbial attacks, but serious risk is usually first experienced at absolute counts of less than 500 per cu. mm. When playing this numbers game it is important to take into account the presence of monocytes which, although not as readily phagocytic as granulocytes, do contribute to the defense. The term *agranulocytosis* is usually reserved for the serious granulocytopenias in which both the marginated pool and the bone marrow reserve have been depleted. A depletion of the marrow reserve leaves the proliferating immature cells as the only myeloid cells present in the marrow and has given rise to the erroneous expression "maturation arrest." The immature cells are not arrested at all, but as soon as they reach maturity they are swept out of the marrow to shore up peripheral defenses.

The granulocytopenias may be caused by decreased production, ineffective production, or increased destruction. Decreased production is responsible for the granulocytopenia observed in patients with disorders causing bone marrow replacement or bone marrow aplasia. Most acutely it is seen after exposure to radiation or to radiomimetic drugs. The granulocytopenia here is part of a general suppression of cellular proliferation in the bone marrow, but because of the short granulocyte life span and the limited reserves, granulocytopenia is observed earlier than thrombocytopenia or anemia. Pisciotta has described a similar suppressive effect on the bone marrow of certain susceptible individuals by the use of phenothiazine-type drugs. These appear to have a predominant effect on the myeloid cells, with less suppression of the erythroid cells and almost complete sparing of the megakaryocytic elements. Underproduction of granulocytes has also been found to be responsible for a number of hereditary and acquired granulocytopenias. Of special interest is *cyclic neutropenia*, a disorder in which at regular intervals patients develop granulocytopenia, fever, mouth ulcerations, and infections. The pathogenesis has been linked to hormonal cycles, but recent studies indicated that the recurrent granulocytopenia may be caused by an undampened feedback between the peripheral granulocyte pool and granulocytic committed stem cells (Fig. 22–107).

Ineffective granulocytopoiesis is undoubtedly responsible for the granulocytopenia observed in *megaloblastic anemias* as well as in some of the *preleukemic syndromes.* Blume and co-workers have suggested that the granulocytopenia observed in *Chediak-Higashi's syndrome* may be caused by intramedullary autodestruction by the large abnormal lysosomes which characterize the cells in this interesting disease.

Increased peripheral destruction is caused by increased utilization, antibody-coating of the granulocytes or hypersplenism. As in patients with ineffective granulocytopoiesis the granulocytopenia is associated with a striking granulocytic hyperplasia in the bone marrow. Increased removal or destruction is an appropriate physiologic response to inflammation. An early transient granulocytopenia actually precedes the leukocytosis of bacterial infection. When the infection is particularly severe, as in septicemia, the marrow reserves of mature granulocytes may be used up, with granulocytopenia ensuing. Granulocytopenia is also commonly observed during and after viral infections, but here the mechanism is not known. Transient granulocytopenia is a feature of procedures involving exposure of large volumes of blood to foreign surfaces, such as hemodialysis coils and filtration leukopheresis columns. The surfaces presumably activate complement, which in turn causes the transient fall in granulocytes. Antibody destruction of circulating granulocytes is dramatic but rare. It is believed to involve the interaction of a drug hapten, such as aminopyrine, phenylbutazone or methyluracil, with a specific antibody and the subsequent attachment of the antigen-antibody complex to granulocytes, the so-called "innocent bystander" concept (Fig. 22–137). These coated granulocytes are then destroyed by the macrophages particularly in the spleen. Attempts to identify autoantibodies as a cause of *chronic idiopathic neutropenia* or of the granulocytopenia of collagen vascular diseases so far have not been successful. Hypersplenism or splenic neutropenia is observed in conditions without overt antibody production but with splenomegaly. Despite many studies of the pathogenesis of the hypersplenic syndrome we still do not understand why a large spleen should destroy otherwise healthy granulocytes. It may be a question of sequestration rather than destruction similar to hypersplenic thrombocytopenia or it may involve antibodies too few to be detected by current techniques.

Granulocytosis. Granulocytosis is present when the granulocyte count exceeds 10,000 per cu. mm. When it is over 30,000 per cu. mm. the term *"leukemoid reaction"* is often used. Although a nonleukemic granulocytosis may reach levels of 50,000 per cu. mm. or higher, counts in excess of 100,000 per cu. mm. are extremely rare.

An acute granulocytosis of moderate degree can be caused by a mere shift of granulocytes from the marginal pool and the bone marrow reserve pool into the circulation. It is frequently observed after exposure to acute infections, trauma, emotional or physical stress or after the administration of epinephrine, adrenal steroids and endotoxin. Chronic granulocytosis is observed under conditions of sustained overproduction of granulocytes. The most common causes are bacterial infections and tissue injury. Neoplasias presumably cause granulocytosis by inducing tissue necrosis with the release of hypothetical bone marrow-stimulating substances. Eosinophilic granulocytosis is observed primarily in conditions characterized by the sustained presence of antigen-antibody complexes such as in patients with chronic parasitic invasion or with dermatologic or allergic manifestations.

Qualitative Abnormalities

A decreased resistance to infection may occur despite normal granulocyte counts if the functional competence of the granulocytes is impaired. In the so-called *"lazy leukocyte syndrome"* described by Miller, Oski and Harris the granulocytes do not respond appropriately to chemotaxic factors, and the granulocytes fail to accumulate and produce an inflammatory focus. Similar dysfunction of chemotaxis and migration is also present if the classic or alternate activation of C3 is impaired. Defective attachment and phagocytosis of foreign bodies are usually caused by impaired antibody production and complement function. Impaired killing of ingested microorganisms causes recurrent and chronic infections and may lead to massive granuloma formation. Despite its rarity, this so-called *"chronic granulomatous disease,"* studied extensively by Holmes and coworkers and by Baehner and Nathan, has provided considerable insight into normal and abnormal bactericidal function. Morphologic and metabolic studies have shown that the granulocytes are capable of phagocytosis of microorganisms but incapable of their subsequent killing and disposal. The lysosomes, present in normal number, discharge their enzymatic cargo into the phagosomes, but the enzymes apparently are not bactericidal. The usual acceleration of glycolysis and hexose monophosphate shunt activity does not occur and the production of H_2O_2 is decreased. It has been proposed that in the absence of H_2O_2 the iodination of the microbial membrane cannot take place, and the organisms remain unharmed inside the phagosomes. Support for this hypothesis has been obtained from the fact that some hydrogen peroxide-producing organisms such as lactobacillus are killed by the granulocytes from patients with chronic granulomatous disease, and phagocytosis of latex particles coated with a hydrogen peroxide-producing oxidase will restore killing of simultaneously phagocytized bacteria. Chronic granulomatous disease encompasses both sex-linked and autosomal variants. Although an inherited deficiency of a NADH oxidase could explain both the lack of H_2O_2

production and hexose monophosphate shunt acceleration (Fig. 22–104), such deficiency has not been definitely established (Hohn and Lehrer, 1975).

A distinct disorder of lysosomal morphology is characteristic of the *Chediak-Higashi syndrome,* in which giant lysosomes can be observed in granulocytes, melanocytes, fibroblasts, and other cellular elements. As suggested by White, the granulocytic lysosome may be responsible for intramedullary autodestruction, ineffective granulopoiesis, and granulocytopenia. Whether phagocytosis and lysosomal killing also are abnormal is not known, since the decreased resistance to infection exhibited by these patients could easily be accounted for by their granulocytopenia. The abnormal melanocytic lysosomes may in some way be responsible for the hypopigmentation observed in patients with Chediak-Higashi syndrome and in the closely related lysosomal disorders of the Aleutian mink and the beige mouse.

Myeloproliferative Disorders

In 1951, Dameshek, with characteristic abandon, lumped all the disorders which involve uncontrolled proliferation of bone marrow cells into one syndrome, *the myeloproliferative syndrome.* Some investigators have objected to this blatant oversimplification of a difficult problem and marshalled impressive evidence for basic differences among the diseases included. However, so far the similarities are more numerous than the differences and the unified myeloproliferative concept has been useful in our pathophysiologic and clinical approach to these diseases.

The prototype for the myeloproliferative diseases is *polycythemia vera* (see page 35), with its uncontrolled proliferation of erythrocytic, granulocytic, and megakaryocytic elements and its frequent termination in myelofibrosis. The cellular proliferation characterizing the other members of the syndrome involves predominantly single cell lines.

Chronic Granulocytic Leukemia. This dramatic disease was undoubtedly the disorder observed by Rudolf Virchow in 1845 and reported under the catching title *"Weisses Blut"* or, in Greek terminology, *"leukemia."* Even today we occasionally see untreated patients in whom the white cell crit exceeds the red cell crit and the blood appears pale and the bone marrow whitish green as in Virchow's original case.

The characteristic of early chronic granulocytic leukemia is an expansion of all granulocytic pools overflowing into peripheral blood and spleen. Since the proportional sizes of the pools closely approximate those of normal bone marrow, it has been tempting to consider this disease as being caused by an impaired cellular control with autonomy of the granulocytic stem cells. However, the manifestations cannot be explained on the basis of uncontrolled normal stem cell function, but must include dysfunction of abnormal committed and multipotential stem cells.

In 1960, Nowell and Hungerford described a specific chromosomal abnormality in the myeloid cells of patients with chronic granulocytic leukemia, an abnormality which subsequently has been found to be present in about 90 per cent of cases. It consists of a deletion of part of the long arm of the number 22-G chromosome, leaving a tiny chromosome named the Philadelphia chromosome (Ph^1) (Fig. 22–109). A simultaneous lengthening of chromosome number 9 has suggested that the alteration is not a deletion but a translocation. This fortunate discovery has been of considerable diagnostic and biologic importance. It has separated the classic Ph^1 positive patients from a small subgroup of Ph^1 negative cases with similar physical and laboratory findings but apparently with a more aggressive course and poorer prognosis. It has also established that granulocytic, erythrocytic, and megakaryocytic cells are derived from the same stem cell, since all are Ph^1 positive in chronic granulocytic leukemia. Circulating lymphocytes and bone marrow fibroblasts are Ph^1 negative, suggesting that the mutagenic event which gave rise to Ph^1 positivity must involve a step in the stem cell hierarchy distal to the points at which the stem cells for the lymphocytes and fibroblasts branch off. Although the majority of marrow metaphases show the abnormal chromosome in patients with chronic granulocytic leukemia, normal stem cell lines must also be present since intensive chemotherapy may transform a Ph^1 positive marrow to a Ph^1 negative, as reported by Smalley and co-workers.

In most patients with chronic granulocytic leukemia there is no inkling as to the character of the insult which has caused such a somatic mutation. In a few cases, however, past exposure to radiation or to drugs suggests a cause-effect relationship. For many years radiation has been recognized to be leukemogenic in certain strains of mice, but its potential for inducing leukemia in humans was not appreciated until the early 1940s. At that time statistical studies of the incidence of leukemia in physicians showed an overall incidence of 1.7 times that in the general population, and more importantly the studies by March indicated that the incidence of leukemia in radiologists was nine times that of physicians with little personal radiation exposure. This startling finding was accentuated by the finding of a high incidence of leukemia among the Japanese survivors from the atomic bomb explosions in Hiroshima and Nagasaki. Here, as summarized by Bizzozero and co-workers, the incidence of

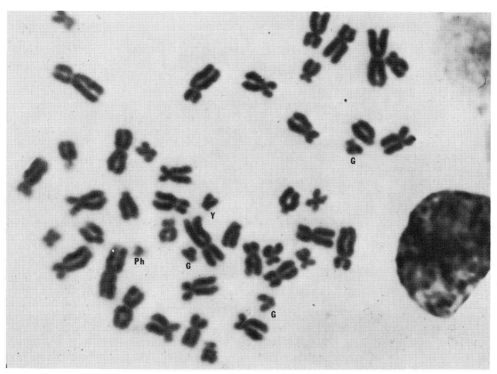

Figure 22–109 Chromosomal pattern of a male (Y chromosome) with chronic granulocytic leukemia (three normal G chromosomes and one tiny Ph[1] chromosome). (Courtesy of Dr. L. Jackson, The Thomas Jefferson University, Philadelphia.)

granulocytic leukemia, either acute or chronic, increased to about three times normal during the period from 1946 to 1955 and then slowly returned toward normal again. Studies of patients receiving therapeutic radiation have indicated that this form of radiation exposure also may be leukemogenic, but at present there are no convincing data showing that diagnostic radiation will cause leukemia. The obvious issue is whether or not the leukemogenic effect of radiation has a threshold. Some feel that any amount of radiation is potentially dangerous and should be avoided at all cost, whereas others feel that the leukemogenic risk of diagnostic radiation or radiation from natural sources or atomic bomb fallout is too small to be of public health concern.

The clinical and laboratory features of chronic granulocytic leukemia are predominantly caused by the increased body load of myeloid cells. This load may be increased up to 150 times normal and causes bone marrow expansion with sternal tenderness, anemia, splenomegaly, and granulocytosis. The nutritional demands made by the overproduction of myeloid cells may cause an increased metabolic rate, with fever and weight loss, and the final breakdown of these cells may cause uricemia, gouty arthritis, and renal stones. The red cell production is usually decreased in

unrestrained cases of chronic granulocytic leukemia, probably owing to decreased "Lebensraum" in the marrow. The same may be true for platelet production. When granulocyte production has become controlled by adequate therapy the red cell and platelet mass will return to normal. The differential count of the granulocytes of peripheral blood is similar to that of the myeloid cells in normal bone marrow and is distinctly different from that of patients with leukemoid reactions in whom the cells are predominantly mature. These cells also have a normal or high content of alkaline phosphatase, whereas the cells of chronic granulocytic leukemia characteristically have a reduced content. Despite this biochemical abnormality, the phagocytic and bactericidal functions of the leukemic granulocytes appear normal. The number of basophils is usually increased and may even dominate the granulocytic picture, an unexplained but prognostically ominous sign. Serum vitamin B_{12} levels are high as is the concentration of the main B_{12} binder, transcobalamin I. The latter appears to be derived from broken-down granulocytes, but its role in the symptomatology of chronic granulocytic leukemia is unknown.

Chronic granulocytic leukemia is usually successfully managed with the use of alkylating agents such as busulfan. Unmaintained remissions may last as long as several months to a year. Incipient relapses are readily recognized by the rising granulocyte count, often accompanied by a return of splenic enlargement. Radiation therapy delivered to the spleen also successfully produces hematologic and clinical remission, but currently is considered less satisfactory than chemotherapy.

After about two to five years the disease in most patients begins to take on a more aggressive character. Myeloblasts appear in the peripheral blood, anemia becomes more severe, and thrombocytopenia develops. The spleen increases in size and the response to treatment becomes increasingly unsatisfactory. Blast cells take over the marrow and the patient eventually succumbs to the metabolic and cellular effects of an acute refractory granulocytic leukemia, the so-called "blast crisis." Some patients enter the aggressive phase by developing rapidly progressive myelofibrosis. The blast cells in this leukemia are usually Ph[1] positive, but they also display the chromosomal breaks and duplications seen frequently in acute granulocytic leukemia (Pedersen, 1973). Recent observations by Rosenthal and co-workers suggest that some of these terminal blast cell leukemias are lymphatic rather than granulocytic — observations of potential biologic and therapeutic importance. As in patients with polycythemia vera, the question has been raised as to the pathogenetic role of treatment in the final development of acute leukemia. No definite answer can be given, since in the past patients with untreated chronic granulocytic leukemia usually died from the effects of their chronic leukemia and only a few lived long enough to reach the stage in which contemporary patients develop their blast crisis.

Myelofibrosis. Bone marrow fibrosis with distortion and obliteration of marrow cavities may occur as an independent disease or as a complication of polycythemia vera or chronic granulocytic leukemia. Because of this relationship, myelofibrosis is considered a member of the myeloproliferative family. However, it seems somewhat farfetched to give the proliferation of fibroblasts the same status as the uncontrolled proliferation of blood cell precursors. In the first place, fibroblasts and other bone marrow cells do not share the same stem cell as indicated by the fact that fibroblasts of patients with chronic granulocytic leukemia are Ph[1] negative. Secondly, similar fibrotic reactions have been observed in tuberculosis, Hodgkin's disease, and carcinomatosis involving the bone marrow and are presumably reactions to tissue destruction and necrosis.

The characteristic splenomegaly of this disorder is usually believed to be caused by compensatory extramedullary hematopoiesis. However, the adult spleen appears to have lost most of its fetal capacity as a primary hematopoietic organ,

and compensatory extramedullary hematopoiesis is rarely found in older people who develop an increased requirement for extra blood cell production. When foci of so-called extramedullary hematopoiesis in the spleen are found, they are probably made up of clones of bone marrow cells originating from immature cells prematurely released from the marrow and trapped in the sinusoids of the spleen. In myelofibrosis, the spleen is packed with hematopoietic tissue. Since this may occur at a time when the bone marrow is only minimally replaced by fibrous tissue and is in no need of supplementary extramedullary support, it seems more likely that the splenomegaly is caused by a pathologic myeloid metaplasia rather than by a physiologic extramedullary hematopoiesis. Foci of myeloid metaplasia are also observed in the liver but rarely elsewhere.

The most striking laboratory finding is an abnormal blood smear. The red blood cells show distorted and fragmented forms, and immature blood cells such as late erythroblasts, metamyelocytes, and myelocytes are present. It is usually assumed but has not been proved that such abnormalities are caused by cells being produced in and released from a microenvironment with less organized and regulated architecture than normal bone marrow. Progressive anemia is part of the disease, but the platelet count behaves erratically, and thrombocytosis may be as common as thrombocytopenia. It is of interest in this connection that biopsies of the fibrous marrow often reveal nests of megakaryocytes, as if these were the most hardy of the hematopoietic elements. When anemia or thrombocytopenia is severe, the question has to be raised whether the spleen destroys more cells than it produces. Erythrokinetic studies including organ scanning have been of only limited help in answering this question, and the decision to perform a splenectomy should be made only with great reluctance. The administration of androgens may cause striking improvement in the anemia in some cases (Fig. 22–40). Otherwise treatment does not appear to influence the slow but relentless progress of the disease.

Essential Thrombocythemia. Essential thrombocythemia is characterized by unrestrained proliferation of megakaryocytes. Large numbers of viable but ineffective platelets are produced causing a characteristic but unexplained mixture of bleeding and clotting problems. It is a chronic disorder, readily corrected by appropriate myelosuppressive therapy.

Chronic Erythroleukemia. Chronic erythroleukemia is a rare disorder characterized by the presence of macrocytosis, megaloblastic nucleated red cells in peripheral blood and bone marrow, ineffective erythropoiesis, and gradual progression into acute granulocytic leukemia. In the early stages it can be difficult to separate from chronic sideroblastic anemia since bone marrow examination may also disclose ringed sidero-blasts. However, granulocytopoiesis and thrombopoiesis in erythroleukemia are almost always abnormal and ineffective.

Acute Granulocytic Leukemia. Acute granulocytic leukemia is a rapidly progressive disease characterized by the replacement of the bone marrow with immature and undifferentiated granulocytic cells. At present we relate the acute granulocytic leukemia to the myeloproliferative syndrome on the one hand and to acute lymphocytic leukemia on the other, relationships which may be spurious but nevertheless are useful in the clinical approach to this frustrating and discouraging disorder.

About 50 per cent of all leukemias are of the acute variety. There appears to be a slow but definite increase in this percentage, possibly owing to better diagnostic skills, possibly to an increased exposure to leukemogenic agents.

The acute leukemias can be divided into two major groups: the acute granulocytic and the acute lymphocytic. This subdivision of a rapidly progressive and uniformly fatal disease was initially felt to be a wasteful exercise in morphologic hair-splitting. However, at the present we recognize a fundamental difference between these two groups with regard to incidence, etiology, course, and prognosis. Acute granulocytic leukemia is a disease of adulthood, occasionally related to past exposure to radiation or chemicals, frequently with a long preleukemic phase and discourag-

ingly resistant to chemotherapeutic agents. Acute lymphocytic leukemia is the predominant leukemia of childhood, rarely preceded by chemical exposure or preleukemic symptoms and highly responsive to chemotherapeutic agents. Acute granulocytic leukemia can further be subdivided into *acute granulocytic, acute promyelocytic, acute myelocytic, acute myelomonocytic,* and *acute erythroleukemia.* Acute promyelocytic leukemia is listed as a separate group because leukemias with a predominance of promyelocytes often display the characteristic syndrome of disseminated intravascular coagulation. However, owing to the high content of thromboplastic material in leukocytes, this syndrome has also been described in the other acute leukemias. The acute myelomonocytic designation is of considerable help in leukemias in which the immature cells have features of both myeloblasts and monoblasts, since it prevents the clinicians from getting into futile arguments about morphologic minutiae. The acute erythroleukemia, or so-called *Di Guglielmo's syndrome,* is a rare but dramatic acute granulocytic leukemia in which the bone marrow during the early stages is dominated by a profusion of abnormal, often multinucleated but always ineffective erythroblasts (Fig. 22–110).

The important separation of the acute leukemias into granulocytic and lymphocytic types is usually not too difficult for the experienced hematologist relying on blood and bone marrow smears stained by Wright's or Giemsa stain. Occasion-

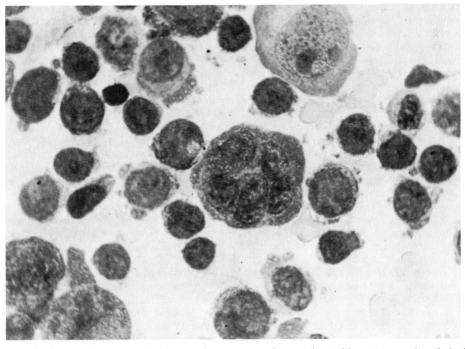

Figure 22–110 Multinucleated erythroblasts in bone marrow from patient with acute granulocytic leukemia of the Di Guglielmo variety.

ally, he is assisted by finding an eosinophilic rod in the cytoplasm of the leukemic blast cells. This so-called Auer rod is probably a giant lysosome and is never present in lymphoblasts, a useful diagnostic tidbit. Various cytochemical techniques also are being used in the differential diagnosis. The most important are the myeloperoxidase and Sudan black stains specific for the granules of acute granulocytic leukemia and tests for terminal deoxynucleotidyl transferase specific for acute lymphatic blast cells.

The etiology of acute leukemias is not known, but there is mounting evidence for the hypothesis that leukemia is caused by the action of a leukemogenic virus on stem cells rendered susceptible by genetic predisposition or chemical alteration. The presence of a genetic or chromosomal susceptibility is supported by statistical studies which indicate that the chance of developing acute leukemia is about 1 in 5 if one's identical twin has leukemia, 1 in 60 if one's nonidentical twin has leukemia, 1 in 700 if one's sibling has leukemia, and 1 in 3000 if no one else in the family has leukemia (Zuelzer and Cox, 1969). However, these data also tend to rule out an inborn mutation as the sole etiologic mechanism, since only 20 per cent of individuals with a leukemic identical twin develop the disease. Certain chromosomal defects, both congenital and acquired, appear to predispose to acute leukemia. Children with inborn chromosomal defects such as in *Down's syndrome, Fanconi's anemia,* and *Bloom's syndrome* all have an increased incidence of acute leukemia, and leukemogenic chemicals or radiation seems generally to have the capacity to cause chromosomal changes. However, the relationship between chromosomal defects and the development of acute leukemia cannot be too direct, since no single unifying chromosomal change has been found among patients with preleukemia or acute leukemia.

The potential leukemogenic effect of ionizing radiation has already been mentioned. Chemical leukemogens are playing an increasing role in the etiology of acute granulocytic leukemia. Any chemical interference with DNA replication must be considered potentially leukemogenic, and the widespread and successful use of cytotoxic and immunosuppressive agents will probably result in an increased incidence of leukemia in the future. Although these agents could cause a chromosomal mutation with the production of autonomous leukemic blast cells the possibility that they provide a latent leukemogenic virus with the opportunity for unchecked multiplication appears equally good. It has been known for about 65 years that avian leukemia is caused and transmitted by a virus, and studies by Gross 20 years ago provided strong evidence for the existence of a similar etiologic mechanism for murine leukemias. The murine leukemogenic viruses are RNA viruses and their mechanism of replication has recently been clarified by the discovery of a reverse transcriptase, an enzyme capable of incorporating the information coded in viral RNA into DNA of the host. Such an enzyme has been found in human leukemic cells but its presence there is of questionable significance, since it has also been found in human non-leukemic embryonic cells. Direct demonstration of viral particles in and around leukemic cells is difficult to achieve and, when found, their pathogenic importance is difficult to interpret (Jarrett, 1973).

Epidemiologic data suggesting direct transmission of leukemia are sparse, but strong indirect evidence for the presence of an infective agent has recently been provided by Fialkow and coworkers, who reported the course of leukemia in a girl who had received a bone marrow transplant from her brother. After some months the leukemia recurred, but this time the leukemic blast cells were cytogenetically XY cells. This unique case has generated considerable speculation and has even raised the possibility that leukemic relapses after prolonged remission are caused by reinfection rather than by the survival of a few leukemic cells, a most unorthodox view.

The orthodox view of cellular kinetics in acute leukemia is based on data obtained by Skipper and co-workers and suggests that the relapses and remissions of the disease are determined by the size of the leukemic mass. Manifest leukemia with the presence of leukemic cells in the bloodstream and with considerable leukemic bone marrow replacement is present when the leukemic mass is about 1 kg. in weight or 10^{12} cells in number. The reduction in mass to about 1 gram will cause a morphologic and symptomatic remission but will still leave about 10^9 leukemic cells at large. Further therapy will reduce the body load and prolong the remission but only total cell kill will provide a cure (Fig. 22–111). This latter assumption is derived from data in rodents in which the transplantation of a single leukemic cell into an inbred recipient will result in leukemia. However, immunologic assistance in an outbred species such as man may make it less mandatory to aim for total cell kill, a goal which probably could not be accomplished without irreparable damage to normal tissues.

By now, it has been shown convincingly that leukemic blast cells do not proliferate as actively as normal bone marrow cells (Killmann, 1968). The mitotic index and the tritiated thymidine labeling index are lower for leukemic blast cells than for normal blast cells. Even without the help of sophisticated quantitative techniques it is evident from looking at leukemic bone marrow smears that mitotic figures are relatively rare. This paradox that a rapidly growing tumor such as acute leukemia should consist of sluggishly proliferating cells has been difficult to accept.

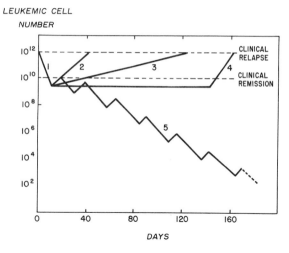

LEUKEMIC CELL
NUMBER

Figure 22-111 Hypothetical relationship between therapy of acute leukemia, leukemic cell number, and remission or relapse: (*1*) The effect of a successful induction therapy on cell count; (*2*) the immediate relapse which occurs after unmaintained therapy; (*3*) the slow relapse after partially effective maintenance therapy; (*4*) the prolonged remission on effective maintenance therapy; and (*5*) the hoped-for effect of repeated course of reinduction therapy on leukemic cell number. (Redrawn from Spiers, A. S. D.: Clin. Haematol., *1*:127, 1972.)

However, the therapeutic use of cytotoxic agents is based on the fact that normal bone marrow cells recover early, while there is a much more delayed recovery of leukemic blast cells; in other words, leukemic cells must have a longer generation time than normal cells. It is possible that the leukemic cell mass is made up of several cellular populations, with the majority of the cells being inert, long-lived, and slowly proliferating, while a minority have a rapid cellular turnover. It is the activity of this latter population which presumably accounts for the abrupt changes which occur in the bone marrow and peripheral blood during relapse.

In about 30 per cent of cases, the clinical and laboratory manifestations of acute granulocytic leukemia have been preceded for months or even for years by a prodromal phase which retrospectively can be designated *preleukemia*. Different degrees of neutropenia, thrombocytopenia, and anemia are present and associated with a cellular but ineffective bone marrow. Morphologic abnormalities, such as hyper- or hyposegmentation of granulocytes, megaloblastic changes, abnormal red cell morphology, ringed sideroblasts, and giant platelets, suggest defective cell development. Eventually myeloblasts appear in large enough numbers to establish a diagnosis of acute granulocytic leukemia.

The signs and symptoms of acute granulocytic leukemia usually can be attributed to mechanical or metabolic interference with the normal function of a number of organs. The leukemic cells will amass in great numbers in the bone marrow, spleen, liver, lymph nodes and blood. Bone marrow function is first and most seriously threatened, either because the finite marrow volume precludes compensatory expansion or because blast cells exert a suppressive effect on the remaining normal cells. The liver, spleen, and lymph nodes can expand considerably without

functional impairment, but a liver extensively infiltrated with leukemic cells may show signs of failure, an enlarged spleen may cause sequestration and injury to normal blood cells, and lymphatic tissue with architectural displacement may be immunologically less effective. Leukostasis in the lungs with pulmonary failure, or in the brain with cerebral hemorrhage, may occur if the white cell count is exceedingly high. The effect of leukemic cells on the function of blood is less clear Whole blood viscosity is probably not changed significantly, since an increase in the white blood cell mass usually is offset by a decrease in the red blood cell mass.

Anemia is almost invariably present at the time of diagnosis. Hypersplenic red cell destruction and ineffective erythropoiesis may contribute, but the cause is usually clear-cut — lack of space for the erythroid precursors. The anemia is best managed by judicious transfusions of packed red blood cells.

Hemorrhages and petechiae are most often the features which bring the patient to a physician. With few exceptions they are caused by thrombocytopenia and are ameliorated by transfusion of concentrated platelet preparations. The critical level of platelet count below which spontaneous bleeding occurs is hard to define, since the effect of thrombocytopenia may be aggravated by platelet dysfunction or even disseminated intravascular coagulation. In general, platelet counts below 30,000 per cu. mm. should cause concern, and platelet counts below 10,000 per cu. mm. are associated with spontaneous hemorrhages and petechiae.

Infections and fever are common and are most often caused by granulocytopenic impairment of host defenses. Although it has been claimed that an infection is always present when a leukemic patient develops fever, tissue necrosis and endogenous pyrogens undoubtedly contribute. Nevertheless, fever in a granulocytopenic patient in whom defenses often are reduced even further by steroids and immunosuppressive drugs should always be treated as if an infection were present. During the last decades important changes have occurred in the ecology of the infecting microorganisms. Bacteria and fungi of low virulence and high antibiotic resistance have emerged as major offenders and contribute to the chilling statistics which show that about 70 per cent of all leukemic patients die from infections. The preventive use of absorbable antibiotics has had little or no effect on infectious morbidity or mortality, but the use of careful reverse isolation techniques, laminar air flow chambers, and non-absorbable oral antibiotics has been of some help. Complete isolation in life islands tends to isolate

patients from good nursing care and compassionate personal attention. The transfusion of normal granulocytes harvested by centrifugation or filtration leukopheresis is coming of age, and Higby and Henderson have reported on its usefulness in the management of febrile leukemic patients during their leukopenic phases.

The triad of anemia, hemorrhage, and infection will respond to effective treatment of the leukemia. Unfortunately this treatment is not specific and normal hematopoietic elements are wiped out together with the leukemic cells. If the patient survives the initial weeks of severe bone marrow failure first brought on by the disease and then temporarily aggravated by the treatment, complete remission may be achieved with the restoration of a normal bone marrow picture

TABLE 22–17   CHEMOTHERAPEUTIC AGENTS CURRENTLY USED IN TREATMENT OF LEUKEMIA

Drug	Drug Category	Mechanisms of Action
Cytosine arabinoside	Pyrimidine antagonist	Inhibition of de-novo synthesis of deoxycytidine riboside and of DNA polymerase
6-Mercaptopurine 6-Thioguanine	Purine antagonists	Inhibitions of de-novo purine synthesis
Nitrogen mustard Cyclophosphamide Chlorambucil Busulfan Melphalan	Polyfunctional alkylating agents	Cross-linkage of DNA
Methotrexate	Folic acid antagonist	Inhibition of dihydrofolate reductase. Inhibition of DNA synthesis
Daunorubicin Doxorubicin	Anti-tumor antibiotics isolated from *Streptomyces peucetius*	Inhibition of DNA and RNA synthesis
Bleomycin	Anti-tumor antibiotics isolated from *Streptomyces verticillus*	Inhibition of DNA synthesis
Prednisone	Synthetic adrenocorticosteroid	Direct lysis of lymphocytes and lymphoblasts. Inhibition of cell cycle. Inhibition of DNA synthesis and/or DNA-directed RNA synthesis.
Vincristine	Alkaloid of periwinkle plant	Metaphase arrest resulting from inhibition of mitotic spindle (microtubule) formation
L-Asparaginase	Enzyme, catalyzing the hydrolysis of L-asparaginase	Depletion of exogenous L-asparagine needed for the metabolism of malignant cells incapable of synthesizing this amino acid

and peripheral blood counts. Without treatment, survival is about 3 to 6 months. Modern multiagent treatment induces a complete remission in about 40 to 50 per cent of patients, but the median survival is still only about one year. The selection of treatment programs remains quite empiric. Some drugs shown to be quite effective in animal studies, such as hydroxyurea, are relatively inactive. Other agents known to be very effective in acute lymphatic leukemia, such as vincristine and prednisone, are far less effective in acute granulocytic leukemia. Table 22–17 lists some of the agents used currently in the treatment of leukemia, along with their presumed modes of action.

MONOCYTE-MACROPHAGE DISORDERS

Disorders of the monocyte-macrophage complex can be classified as quantitative, qualitative and malignant cellular disorders (Table 22–18).

Quantitative Abnormalities

A monocytosis with an absolute increase in circulating monocytes to more than 500 per cu. mm. is frequently a non-specific sign of some occult disease and should lead to a thorough search for a cause. Before the antibiotic era, monocytosis usually meant tuberculosis, subacute bacterial endocarditis, or some other generalized infectious disease. Now, it more often is an early "preleukemic" manifestation of a hematologic malignancy. However, it may also herald a collagen disease or a cancer.

An increase in the number of tissue macrophages may reflect an appropriate response to foreign antigens, so-called "overwork hyperplasia." It can be seen under conditions of sustained, but low-grade invasion of microorganisms, such as in *Whipple's disease, kala azar, malaria* or

TABLE 22–18 CLASSIFICATION OF MONOCYTE-MACROPHAGE DISORDERS

Quantitative Abnormalities
Reactive monocytosis
Reactive mononuclear phagocytic response

Qualitative Abnormalities
Gaucher's disease
Niemann-Pick disease

Malignant Disorders
Monocytic leukemia
Histiocytic lymphoma
Letterer-Siwe disease
Histiocytic medullary reticulosis
Hand-Schüller-Christian disease
Eosinophilic granuloma

histoplasmosis. In these conditions, the macrophage proliferation causes splenomegaly and, to a lesser extent, lymphadenopathy. Cytopenias are frequently present, and it may be difficult to distinguish between increased blood cell destruction due to hypersplenism from decreased production due to encroachment by macrophages on available bone marrow space.

Qualitative Abnormalities

The lipid storage diseases include a number of rare autosomal recessive disorders, each characterized by a deficiency in one of the catabolic enzymes involved in the breakdown of the sphingolipids (Brady, 1972). The deficiency affects all tissues, but the macrophages, by virtue of their prominent role in the catabolism of the lipid-rich membrane, are particularly prone to accumulate undegraded lipid products. This leads to the production of lipid laden and probably "blocked" foamy macrophages, stimulation of further macrophage production and eventually to a tremendous expansion of the mononuclear phagocyte system.

In *Gaucher's disease,* there is a deficiency of β-glucosidase which normally splits glucose from its parent sphingolipids, globoside and ganglioside (Fig. 22–112). The accumulation of glycosphingolipids, derived chiefly from granulocytes, gives an onion skin appearance to the pale lipid laden macrophage cytoplasm. These cells, of course, also show a positive PAS stain for carbo-

SPHINGOLIPIDS

FATTY ACID – SPHINGOSIDE – SIDE CHAIN
[CERAMIDE   ]

GLOBOSIDE
CERAMIDE – GLUCOSE – GALACTOSE – GALACTOSE-N ACETYLGALACTOSAMINE
(1)   (3)

GANGLIOSIDE
CERAMIDE – GLUCOSE – GALACTOSE-N ACETYLGALACTOSAMINE – GALACTOSE
(1)   (4)   (5)

SPHINGOMYELIN
CERAMIDE – PHOSPHORYL CHOLINE
(2)

Figure 22–112 In the lysosomal degradation of glycolipid constituents of senescent cells, the carbohydrates or the phosphorylcholine constituents have to be removed sequentially before final hydrolysis of ceramide, the sphingosine-fatty acid complex. Absence of the following specific enzymes will lead to accumulation of their substrate in the macrophages.

1. β-Glucosidase deficiency: Gaucher's disease
2. Sphingomyelinase
   deficiency: Niemann-Pick
3. α-Galactosidase deficiency: Fabry's disease
4. Hexosaminidase deficiency: Tay-Sachs disease
5. β-Galactosidase deficiency: Gangliosidosis

hydrate. In its typical form, Gaucher's disease is a slowly progressive disease in which the accumulation of Gaucher's cells causes massive splenomegaly and hepatomegaly, bone marrow expansion, and pulmonary infiltration. In *Niemann-Pick disease,* the deficiency is in an enzyme that normally cleaves phosphoryl choline from its parent sphingolipid, sphingomyelin. The macrophages in this condition have the appearance of typical "foam cells" and do not stain with PAS. They cause a rapidly progressive hyperplasia of the mononuclear phagocyte system and the accumulation of undegraded sphingomyelin leads to neuronal degeneration and death within a few years of life.

Cells resembling Gaucher's cells and "foam cells" can also be seen in the marrow of patients with chronic granulocytic leukemia. Here the cause lies not in a deficiency of a catabolic enzyme, but, rather, in an increased lipid load from the sphingolipid-rich granulocyte membrane. "Foam cells" are also seen in the hyperlipidemias demonstrating that the plasma may be a source of lipid in the macrophage cytoplasm (Ferrans, et al., 1971).

Malignant Disorders

The acute monocytic or myelomonocytic leukemia is for diagnostic and therapeutic convenience treated as a myeloproliferative disorder closely related to acute myelogenous leukemia. *Chronic monocytic leukemia,* however, is logically a disorder of the monocyte-macrophage system. Chronic monocytic leukemia is a rare, often slowly progressive condition with minimal lymphadenopathy and moderate splenomegaly. The blood smear shows numerous promonocytes and mature monocytes, but the morphologic identification of the cells can be quite taxing.

A number of variations have been described under designations such as *histiocytic leukemia,* *leukemic reticuloendotheliosis, hairy cell leukemia,* or *reticulum cell leukemia.* These conditions have traditionally been assigned to the monocyte-macrophage system although basic phagocytic properties of the involved cells have not always been clearly demonstrated (Katayama and Finkel, 1974). Recent attempts to identify cellular surface markers have raised the possibility that some or all of the involved cells synthesize immunoglobulins and that these conditions actually belong to the lymphoproliferative system. Such taxonomic questions may appear clinically unimportant today. However, our progress in designing chemotherapeutic agents tailored to the metabolic functions of malignant cells is so rapid that we can anticipate to have future treatments for conditions belonging to the phagocytic system that are very different from treatments for conditions belonging to the immunocytic system.

Malignant proliferative disorders of the more differentiated macrophages may result in *histiocytic medullary reticulosis*. This is a rapidly progressive and fatal febrile disorder of adults with lymphadenopathy, hepatosplenomegaly, hemolytic anemia, thrombocytopenia and leukopenia. Its hallmark is erythrophagocytosis, and red cell laden macrophages are readily demonstrable in the pleomorphic cellular infiltrate. The childhood counterpart is termed *"Letterer-Siwe" disease,* but the phagocytic cells here are less erythrophagocytic and hemolytic anemia is not a prominent factor. Chronic unrestrained proliferation of completely differentiated macrophages are found locally as *eosinophilic granuloma* or more diffusely as *Hand-Schüller-Christian disease*. These diseases have been lumped together under the term *"histiocytosis X,"* but a thorough clinical and pathologic evaluation should provide a specific diagnosis and especially should separate these probably malignant disorders from benign reactive hyperplasia of the mononuclear phagocyte system.

IMMUNOCYTES

STRUCTURE

The immunocytes work together with the phagocytes to maintain the integrity of the whole organism against foreign invaders. With functional responsibilities in such close accord, it is natural that these two families of cells should share many common anatomic sites in the lymphoreticular system of the body. Lymphatic tissue is found throughout the body and, on cytogenetic grounds, is classified into primary and secondary types. Lymphocytes are first differentiated in the primary lymphatic tissue. They are then sent out to populate the secondary lymphatic tissue, where they function in specific immune responses. The primary lymphoid organs in mammals are the bone marrow and the thymus. The secondary lymphatic organs, consisting of the spleen and the lymph nodes along with subepithelial lymphoid tissue in the gastrointestinal tract, are characterized by a basic arrangement of lymphocytes into follicles with germinal centers. In the marrow the lymphocytes typically are scattered among the other cellular elements; germinal follicles are not seen in either thymus or marrow. A primary lymphoid organ equivalent to the "bursa of Fabricius" in the fowl has been postulated to exist in mammalian species, but whether such a "bursa

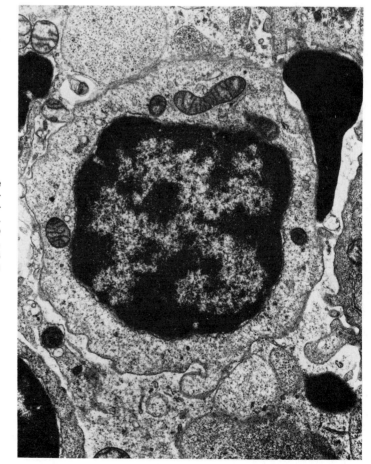

Figure 22–113 Electron microscope picture of a small mature human lymphocyte. Cytoplasm is scanty and contains mitochondria and ribosomes. Chromatin is densely packed into masses in a centrally placed nucleus. (Courtesy of Dr. A. Abraham, Divisions of Pathology and Research, Lankenau Hospital, Philadelphia, PA.)

equivalent" truly exists remains an open question. A circulating pool of lymphocytes is found in the blood, mixed with other cell types, as well as in lymph, which contains few cellular elements other than lymphocytes.

Immunocytes are subclassified morphologically as lymphocytes and plasma cells. The small lymphocyte, a nondividing cell (which therefore does not take up tritiated thymidine), is about 9 μ in diameter on fixed and stained peripheral blood films. It has a skimpy rim of pale blue homogeneous cytoplasm which may contain a few azurophilic granules. Its nucleus has a chromatin pattern tightly arranged in bluish-purple blocks, often with a small notch or indentation in the nuclear membrane (Fig. 22–113). The large lymphocyte has a more generous rim of cytoplasm which stains a deeper blue. Its nucleus is also larger, with nuclear chromatin blocks spaced somewhat further apart, giving the nucleus a more "loose"

appearance. Nucleoli may be seen. Large lymphocytes are proliferating and take up tritiated thymidine into their nuclei. The lymphoblast has a nuclear chromatin pattern which no longer exhibits a blocklike pattern but instead is finely divided, with a "grainy" texture in the midst of which one or two nucleoli are seen. Plasma cells (or "plasmacytes") are recognized in Wright-Giemsa stains by the eccentrically placed nucleus, with densely stained chromatin blocks close together, and a deep blue-green cytoplasm, with a clear zone containing the Golgi apparatus adjacent to one side of the nucleus (Fig. 22–114). The high level of secretory activity of plasma cells is reflected not only by the intense cytoplasmic basophilia but by the frequency of cytoplasmic inclusions (such as grapelike vacuoles or crystalloidal structures). "Proplasmacytes" and "plasmablasts" show increasing looseness of nuclear chromatin and prominence of nucleoli.

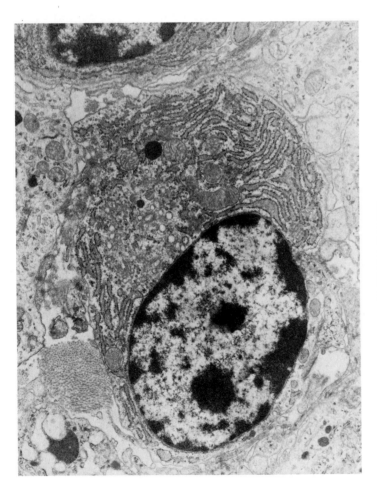

Figure 22–114 Electron microscope picture of a mature human plasma cell. Rough endoplasmic reticulum completely fills the cytoplasm of this immunoglobulin-secreting cell. The nucleus resembles that of the small lymphocyte but assumes an eccentric position. (Courtesy of Dr. A. Abraham, Divisions of Pathology and Research, Lankenau Hospital, Philadelphia, PA.)

FUNCTION

The immunocytes are an intelligence corps which gives *specificity* to the attack of the warrior phagocytes upon foreign antigenic foes. *Memory* of such specificity is another responsibility of the immunocytes, so that future defenses against a known antigenic opponent are more easily mustered. To a limited degree immunocytes may themselves participate directly in the attack.

Immune responses are of two types — one is cell-borne and mediated by "T" (for thymus-derived) lymphocytes, the other is humoral and mediated by "B" (for "bursa-equivalent" or "bone marrow"-derived) lymphocytes. This functional division of the immunocytes is paralleled by sepa-

rate developmental lines as well as by separate (although closely intermingled) anatomic sites of distribution.

As T and B lymphocytes follow their separate pathways of maturation and development, distinctive features appear on the cell surfaces which facilitate laboratory identification (Fig. 22–115).

T cells form "E rosettes" with normal sheep erythrocytes, develop specific surface antigens, and express on their surfaces genetically controlled factors that govern a variety of immune responses.

B cells synthesize intrinsic surface immunoglobulins and in addition they also develop surface receptors for the Fc region of immunoglobu-

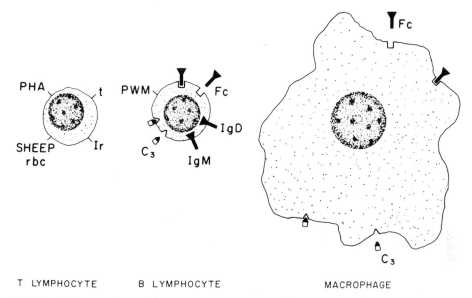

T LYMPHOCYTE   B LYMPHOCYTE   MACROPHAGE

Figure 22–115 Surface markers of lymphocytes and macrophages.

T lymphocytes are identified primarily by their tendency to form spontaneous sheep cell "E rosettes," presumably mediated by a surface receptor for sheep erythrocytes (sheep rbc). T lymphocyte specific surface antigens (t) can be identified by immunologic techniques. Indeed, antigenic differences in surface membrane may permit identification of T lymphocyte subpopulations (i.e., helper, suppressor, effector cells) in some species. Phytohemagglutinin (PHA) causes T lymphocytes to enter mitosis. Genetic factors, closely linked on the chromosome to the major histocompatibility complex, find expression on the T cell surface (Fudenberg, et al., 1978). One of these, the "immune response" (Ir) gene, controls cellular and humoral responses to many antigens. Another is responsible for cytotoxic and blastogenic reactions to lymphocytes of different histocompatibility type (graft versus host reaction, mixed lymphocyte culture).

B lymphocytes carry surface immunoglobulin IgM and IgD as intrinsic components of their membranes, identifiable by immunofluorescent methods. Other immunoglobulins present on the B cell surface may originate from the plasma through binding of their Fc regions to Fc receptor sites on the B cell membrane. (Intrinsic membrane immunoglobulin can be distinguished from bound immunoglobulin by in-vitro incubation techniques.) Attachment of aggregated IgG or of IgG coated erythrocytes or other immune complexes identify B lymphocytes via their Fc receptor sites. Complement coated erythrocytes attach at the complement (C_3) binding site to form "EAC rosettes." Pokeweed mitogen (PWM) induces blastogenesis of B lymphocytes. B lymphocytes also carry specific surface antigens.

Macrophages and monocytes have Fc and C_3 receptors and thus may be confused with B lymphocytes. However, they lack intrinsic surface immunoglobulin.

lins and for complement components (Fig. 22–116). B cells differ from T cells in their response to mitogens (Uhr, 1975).

The dividing line between T and B cells as identified by these surface markers is not as sharp as we would like. Complement and Fc receptors, for example, may be found on some subpopulations of T cells. Some T lymphocytes may carry a low-density coating of surface immunoglobulin. The fact that neutrophils and monocytes bear surface receptors for complement and the Fc fragment adds to the confusion of accurate identification. Changes in the specific antigenic composition of the surface membrane occur during normal immunocyte differentiation. Thus identification of differences in surface antigens among immunocytes by immunologic techniques may at times be more reflective of developmental stage than of any particular subpopulation. Finally, differences in surface appearance among lymphocytes have been shown by scanning electron microscopy, but the significance of this observation is still open to question (Fig. 22–117).

Cell-mediated immunity is responsible for delayed hypersensitivity, homograft rejection, graft-versus-host reaction, defense against viral, fungal, and certain bacterial infections, such as tuberculosis, and possibly even defense against the growth of neoplastic cells in the body. The T lymphocytes regulate humoral immunity but do not have the capacity to secrete circulating antibody. Their anatomic sites of distribution in the lymph nodes are in the deep cortical regions and in the periphery of the germinal follicles (Fig. 22–118). In the spleen they are found in the periarteriolar lymphatic tissue. They also constitute the majority of lymphocytes in the circulating pool of blood and lymph. The population of these specific anatomic sites with T lymphocytes is dependent upon the thymus gland, which in turn is dependent upon the marrow as the source of its stem cells. The thymus may directly "condition" a lymphocytic stem cell derived from the marrow or it may secrete a hormonal substance which conditions marrow lymphocytes at some distance from the thymus to function as T lymphocytes or both mechanisms may prevail.

The cell-mediated immune response differs from the humoral response in several important respects. After initial recognition and processing of specific antigen by phagocytes, T lymphocytes are programmed in a still unknown manner and become specifically "activated" (Fig. 22–119). This activation causes DNA synthesis, blast transformation, and subsequent cellular proliferation. It also causes the production of nonimmunoglobulin humoral factors called lymphokines which further amplify the immune response by recruiting other non-committed T lymphocytes to become specifically activated and to proliferate (David, 1973). Migration inhibition factor prevents macrophages from leaving the area, presumably

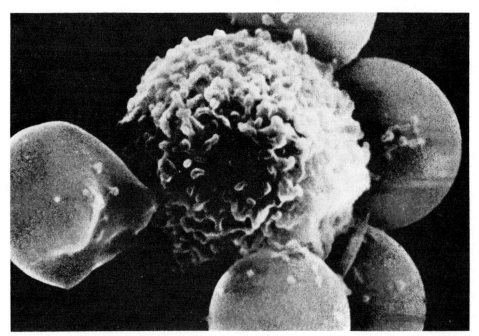

Figure 22–116 Complement coated erythrocytes adhere to a B lymphocyte to form an "EAC rosette." "E rosettes" have the same appearance but are formed by the adherence of normal uncoated sheep erythrocytes to T cells. (From Tsukada, M., et al.: Acta. Haematol. Jap., *39*, 43, 1976.)

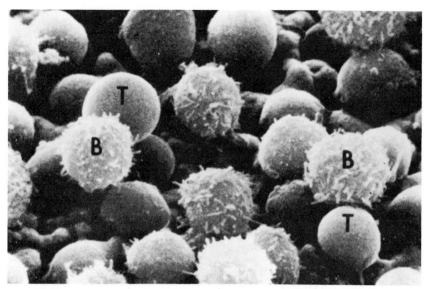

Figure 22–117 Scanning electron microscopic picture of lymphocytes, some showing roughened surfaces studded with microvilli (B) and others with smooth membrane surfaces (T). The significance of this difference in surface is uncertain, although it originally was thought to distinguish B from T lymphocytes. (From Polliack, A., et al.: J. Exp. Med., *138*:607, 1973.)

Figure 22–118 Diagram of lymph node. *TL* = T lymphocyte; *BL* = B lymphocyte; *M* = macrophage; *Ag* = antigen; *Ab* = antibody; *Af. D* = afferent lymphatic duct; *Ef. D* = efferent lymphatic duct; *PCV* = post-capillary venule. The crosshatched zones represent areas populated by B lymphocytes (superficial cortical zone, germinal centers, and medullary cords). Areas containing open circles represent T lymphocyte regions (deep cortical zone, follicle periphery). T lymphocytes circulate in close proximity to macrophages, allowing interaction between these cells and specific antigen. (From Craddock, C. G., et al.: N. Engl. J. Med., *285*:380, 1971. Reprinted by permission.)

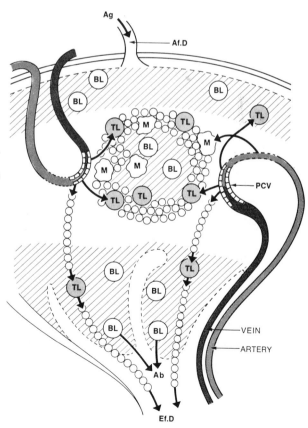

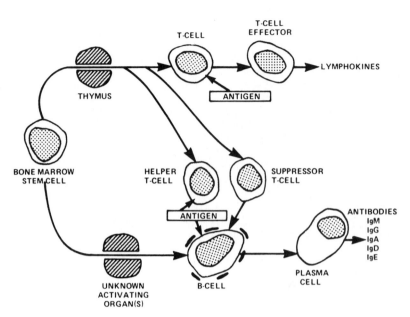

Figure 22–119   The cellular (T) and humoral (B) immune systems. The participation of macrophages is important both for antigen processing as well as for the afferent effector arm of the immune response. Lymphokines are non-immunoglobulin substances secreted by T lymphocytes. They include macrophage migration inhibition factor, transfer factor, and other active principles. (From Waldman, T. A.: Ann. Allergy, *39*:79, 1977, with permission.)

serving the cause of antigen localization and destruction. Most of the activated T lymphocytes serve as "effector" cells by exerting a cytotoxic effect, by complement activation, and by attracting macrophages. Some cytotoxic ("killer") lymphocytes directly attack cellular antigens. Others require antibody combined with antigen on the foreign cell surface in order to seek out the cell for destruction (Podleski, 1976). Some of the activated T cells produce a population of small nondividing lymphocytes which bear a "memory" of the event. These "memory cells" remain for very long periods of time, possibly even a lifetime, in a resting and nondividing state, ready to resume immediate proliferation upon re-exposure to the specific antigen. Subpopulations of T lymphocytes called helper and suppressor cells regulate the humoral immune response, as described below. Individuals may differ in their immune responsiveness to specific antigens because of inherited differences in the "immune response" gene, which is closely related on the chromosome to the major histocompatibility locus and plays an important role in regulating the T cell response (Paul and Benacerraf, 1977).

B immunocytes occupy the superficial cortical regions, the medullary cords, and the germinal centers of the follicles of the lymph nodes, spleen, gastrointestinal tract, and other tissues (Fig. 22–118). The B immunocytes form an immobile pool; the majority do not circulate. They are also derived from a bone marrow stem cell but their further development is not dependent upon the thymus. B lymphocytes must also be programmed with information about a specific antibody, and for many antigens they cooperate with T lymphocytes in this programming process (Fig. 22–119). Possibly the relatively immobile B lymphocytes require the cooperation of the freely circulating T cells to achieve rapid widespread activation throughout the body. Surface membrane immunoglobulins on B lymphocytes are exclusively of the IgM and IgD types and act as receptors for specific antigens. The formation of antigen-antibody complexes on the B lymphocytes causes them to proliferate and mature into antibody-secreting plasma cells. As B cells differentiate into plasma cells they lose their intrinsic membrane immunoglobulin. The plasma cell represents the most mature form of the activated B lymphocyte and no longer has the capacity to divide. The antibodies produced effect the immune response by virtue of their properties as agglutinins, lysins, and opsonins. Like T lymphocytes, some B lymphocytes have the capacity to develop into long-lived memory cells.

The secretion of antibodies of great diversity into plasma and extravascular fluids is the special prerogative enjoyed by the B cells. An understanding of the molecular structure of antibodies is necessary to appreciate how precise specificity yet wide diversity are combined in one family of closely related proteins. The immunoglobulins fall into five families of proteins. IgG immunoglobulins, of molecular weight 160,000 and sedimentation constant 7S, are normally present in serum at a concentration of about 1250 mg. per 100 ml., constituting by far the major type. Their relatively small molecular size permits transport across the placenta. IgA immunoglobulins (normal serum concentration 250 mg. per 100 ml.) are the major type found in body secretions (saliva, tears, colostrum, and gastrointestinal, respiratory, and urinary tract fluids). They form polymers of 9S, 11S, and 13S from the basic unit of 7S. IgM immunoglobulins (normal serum concentration 120 mg. per 100 ml.) are large 18S molecules, also an association of 7S units, especially well suited for agglutination and complement fixation. The IgM synthesized in the B cell membrane is monomeric, however. The other two families of immunoglobulins, IgD and IgE, are present in much lower concentrations, 3 mg. per 100 ml. and 0.03 mg. per 100 ml., respectively. IgD functions almost exclusively as a membrane-bound immunoglobulin; very little is secreted into the plasma. IgE exists primarily in complex formation with mast cells, where it awaits combination with antigen, triggering mast cell release of histamine and other active products. IgE is important in allergic reactions involving the skin, the lungs, and other tissues (Table 22–19).

All the immunoglobulin families have a basic structure in common (Fig. 22–120). This unit consists of two light (or "L") and two heavy (or "H") chains, so termed because of their difference in molecular weight (22,000 as opposed to 52,000). Disulfide bridges bind the H chains to each other and to the L chains. Hydrogen bonding also helps hold the molecular pieces together. The N-terminal ends of an L and H chain together form the antigen binding site. Since there are two such regions on the molecular surface, the immunoglobulin unit is divalent; i.e., it can combine with two antigen molecules. Univalent antibody can be artificially produced by cleavage of the molecule with papain. Such treatment produces one Fc fragment, which carries the C-terminal ends of

both H chains, and two Fab fragments, each of which carries the N terminal of one H and one L chain. The Fab fragments function as univalent antibodies. The Fc portion of the molecule is of particular importance in bringing about complex formation with phagocyte and lymphocyte Fc receptors. The molecule contains a variable amount of carbohydrate attached to the H chain.

The amino acid sequence of the H and L chains is governed by the same kinds of genetic controls that govern the structure of other body proteins. The H chains each contain about 450 amino acid residues, and the L chains about 214. About three fourths of the H chain and one half of the L chain are invariant in their amino acid structure. Specificity, however, lies in the remaining one fourth of the H chain and one half of the L chain where regions of the molecule show great variation in amino acid structure which determines their specificity for antigen. These two structural regions of H and L chains have been called "C" (for common) and "V" (for variant).

There are only two different types of L chains — κ and λ. Only one type is present in any given molecule, but both types are represented in all immunoglobulin families. Class specificity lies in the type of H chain.

There are four subclasses of IgG H chains (γ1, γ2, γ3, γ4). IgA has α heavy chains and is a polymer of two, three, or four 7S units plus a "secretory component" which facilitates transport into body secretions (Walker and Isselbacher, 1977). IgM, a pentamer of 7S units, has μ heavy chains (Fig. 22–121). Subclasses of α and μ heavy chains have also been described. IgA and IgM contain considerably more carbohydrate than IgG.

In basic respects the genetic control of immunoglobulin synthesis resembles that of hemoglobin. The major subunits of the molecule — L and H chains of immunoglobulin and α and β chains of hemoglobin — are under the control of gene regions which are separate and independent and

TABLE 22–19 COMPARISON OF IMMUNOGLOBULIN CLASSES

	IgG	IgA	IgM	IgD	IgE
Serum concentration (mg. per 100 ml.)	1250	250	120	3	0.03
Sedimentation constant S_{20}	6.6S	7S, 9S, 11S, 13S	18S	6.5S	7.9S
Carbohydrate (total %)	2.9	5–10	11.8	10–12	11
Heavy chains	γ	α	μ	σ	ϵ
Light-chain frequency kappa:lambda ratio	2:1	1:1	3:1	1:4	

IgD functions almost exclusively as a B lymphocyte surface immunoglobulin and IgG and IgA as plasma immunoglobulins. IgM serves both as a surface immunoglobulin and is secreted into the plasma in significant quantities. IgE is secreted by plasma cells but is mostly bound to mast cells, where it awaits complex formation with antigen.

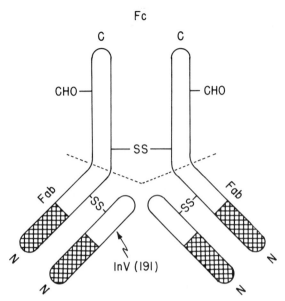

Figure 22–120   Diagram of the structure of the 7S immunoglobulin. C and N represent C-terminal and N-terminal amino acids, respectively. *CHO* = carbohydrate. Disulfide bonds connect the smaller L chains with the larger H chains, and the latter with each other. The interrupted line represents papain cleavage into Fc and Fab fragments. The Fc region may combine with Fc receptors on the surfaces of B lymphocytes and macrophages. The Fab fragments contain the antigen binding sites. The InV locus at the 191st amino acid residue of the L chain is shown. The crosshatched areas represent the variable regions, and the clear areas the common regions.

yet which must coordinate their efforts in order to produce balanced synthesis of the subunits, thus avoiding shortages or surpluses of unpaired polypeptide chains. The extraordinary molecular diversity of the immunoglobulins, however, is a major point at which genetic control of this system of body proteins differs from all others. The synthesis of specific immunoglobulin, including the common and variable region for each H and L chain, is under the control of one clone of B immunocytes. The body contains numerous such clones, leading to heterogeneous production of almost countless different immunoglobulin molecules. Both lymphocytes and plasma cells synthe-

size immunoglobulin, plasma cells producing about two thirds of the IgG. On the other hand, about 90 per cent of IgM is produced by lymphocytes. The gene regions controlling the common structural regions of L and H chains are inherited. Inherited amino acid substitutions may affect these common regions. Thus, INV-1 and INV-3 are genetic alleles affecting the κ chain at the 191st amino acid site, where either leucine or valine, respectively, is placed. Precisely how B immunocytes develop gene regions in different clones to control the variant regions of the L and H chains remains a mystery. A somatic theory postulates that the antigen, after being processed

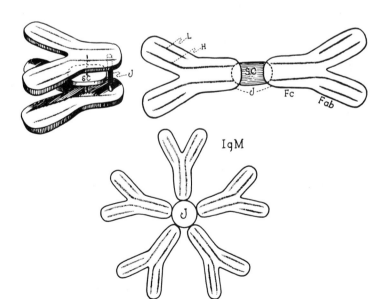

Figure 22–121   Assembly of 7S units in higher molecular weight immunoglobulins, IgA (*above*) and IgM, showing "secretory component" (*SC*) and "joining piece" (*J*). Joining piece is necessary to form polymers. Secretory component is produced by mucosal epithelial cells and is necessary for the transport of dimeric IgA into body secretions. It appears to protect IgA from the action of digestive enzymes. (Reprinted, by permission, from Tomasi, T. B.: The New England Journal of Medicine, *287*: 501, 1972.)

by a macrophage, somehow produces a "reverse flow" of information which thus establishes itself as a permanent record in the programmed genome of a given clone of B cells. The germ line theory postulates that all genetic information, common as well as variant, is obtained through inheritance.

KINETICS

The differentiation, proliferation, and fate of the body's lymphocytes contrast sharply with those of the other cellular elements of the blood. The maturation and proliferation processes which give rise to a specialized peripheral lymphatic tissue are not accompanied by significant morphologic changes other than that change which sets apart the large proliferating cells from the small non-proliferating cells. The marrow serves as the ultimate source of all lymphocytes and together with the thymus is considered a primary lymphatic structure concerned with the differentiation and proliferation of a peripheral population of mature, specialized lymphocytes in

the blood, lymphatics, lymphatic tissue, and spleen. The fully developed red cells, granulocytes, and platelets have a finite life span at the end of which the cell disintegrates. In the case of the peripheral lymphatic tissue, the cells retain the ability to undergo cell division once again by a process of "blastogenesis." The peripheral lymphatic system is also charged with the task of maintaining immunologic memory, which it does by means of a small population of exceedingly long-lived cells which may survive for many years and then once again re-enter cell division upon specific stimulation by antigen. Thus, the cell life span of lymphocytes varies tremendously.

The information which has been obtained about lymphocyte kinetics has relied heavily upon cytologic techniques of DNA labeling by tritiated thymidine. Lymphocytes identified by chromosomal markers have also been used.

The lymphocytes in the primary lymphatic tissue — the marrow and the thymus — undergo relatively rapid and continuous proliferation quite independently of specific antigenic stimulation (Fig. 22–122). For decades evidence has been

LYMPHOPOIESIS

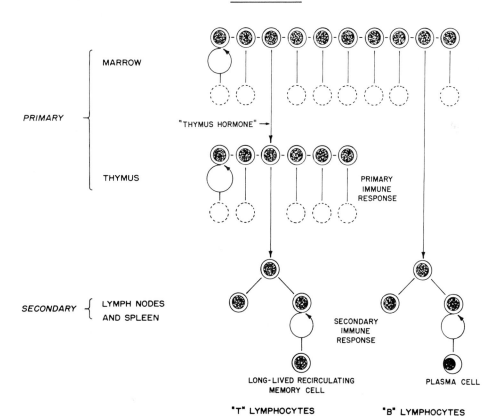

Figure 22–122 Diagram of lymphopoiesis. Interrupted circles represent effete cells in marrow and thymus which do not achieve perpetuity in the secondary lymphatic tissue. Proliferation takes place in both the primary and secondary tissues, in the latter as a result of specific immune response.

presented for and against the theory that the marrow lymphocytic stem cell is pluripotential and also gives rise to the diverse cells of the myeloid series. Indeed the recent observation that an acute lymphoblastic crisis may complicate the course of chronic myelogenous leukemia argues in favor of a common ancestral stem cell for the lymphoid and myeloid cell lines.

Marrow and thymic lymphopoiesis appears to be more active than a fully developed adult's peripheral lymphatic tissue would require for replenishment, and therefore it is reasonable to assume that the bulk of lymphopoiesis in these organs is wasteful, most of the proliferated cells undergoing destruction in order to prevent massive accumulation of unwanted numbers. Relatively few are directed to assume positions in peripheral secondary lymphatic tissue. Under normal conditions, the secondary lymphatic tissue is not actively proliferating, but upon exposure to antigen, specifically stimulated cells undergo rapid division, with germinal centers showing the greatest level of activity.

The bulk of the T lymphocytes of the peripheral lymphatic tissue recirculate. They follow a path from blood to lymph node and spleen through lymphatic channels back to blood. Egress from the blood into the lymphatic tissue occurs through the wall of the postcapillary venule, where the T cells percolate through the periphery of follicles and the deep cortical areas eventually to be collected into the efferent lymphatic (Fig. 22–118).

Approximately 10 hours are required for lymphocytes to leave the blood and appear in the thoracic duct. The T cells do not recirculate through the marrow or thymus to any significant degree. The T cell system can be lymphocyte-depleted by means of thoracic duct drainage or extracorporeal irradiation, leaving the T areas of the lymphatic tissue empty. The recirculating population consists of "short-lived" and "long-lived" cells. This conclusion is based on experiments in animals given continuous injections of tritiated thymidine over a period of many months. In rats, about 40 to 45 per cent of small lymphocytes take up label in 5 to 10 days. The labeling index continues to increase thereafter, but even after nine months, about 5 to 10 per cent of the small lymphocytes remain unlabeled. They are considered to be the long-lived memory cells. All large lymphocytes label within three days. The gradual slope of decline of the DNA labeled cells shows a slow replacement rate and a long survival time of most small lymphocytes.

The B cells are largely noncirculating. They maintain a fixed position in the germinal centers, medullary cords, and superficial cortical zones of the secondary lymphatic tissue. Apparently the majority of cells produced are short-lived. Mature plasma cells probably do not survive longer than two or three days. A small proportion of B cells

mature in the marrow because a few plasma cells are normally seen there.

PATHOPHYSIOLOGY

Classification and General Considerations

The system of fixed and circulating immunocytes which constitute the secondary lymphatic tissue provides a vital defensive function. Thus, the most common alterations occur in reactive response to the presence of foreign antigens, such as local or systemic infections. The reaction may consist of focal or generalized adenopathy, splenomegaly, the presence of large "young" lymphocytes or plasmacytoid cells in the circulation, or an elevation of the absolute lymphocyte count. Another common reactive change is a generalized increase in all immunoglobulin types.

Neoplastic alterations of the immunocytes represent inappropriate proliferative responses which produce an increase in the number of immunocytes and may be associated with either an increase or a decrease in the concentration of immunoglobulins. These conditions are often associated with functional impairment of cellular or humoral immune mechanisms which, in turn, leads to an abnormal susceptibility to a variety of infections which are often quite different from those commonly observed in patients with an intact immune system (Levine and associates, 1972). Autoimmune phenomena, such as hemolytic anemia or thrombocytopenia, are also observed in patients with lymphoproliferative disorders. In clinical practice the problem of distinguishing neoplastic from reactive conditions affecting the immune system may be difficult, and judgments must be made with great care because of the vast differences in prognosis and treatment between the two states.

An over-all classification of disorders of the immunocytes is summarized in Table 22–20.

Quantitative Disorders

Lymphocytopenia and Hypogammaglobulinemia. A reduction in the number of circulating lymphocytes below the normal level of 1000 to 1500 per cu. mm. comes about through either increased loss or decreased production. The alteration represents primarily a change in the T cells, which constitute the majority of circulating lymphocytes. Mechanical loss of lymphocytes can be produced by tapping the circulating stream at the thoracic duct and draining off the lymph. A similar mechanism may explain the lymphocytopenia of intestinal lymphangiectasia and other disorders associated with leakage of lymph into the gastrointestinal tract. Lymphocytes are extraordinarily radiosensitive and a fall in the lym-

TABLE 22–20   CLASSIFICATION OF
IMMUNOCYTE DISORDERS

I. *Quantitative Disorders*
    Lymphocytopenia and hypogammaglobulinemia
        Primary
            Congenital
            Acquired
        Secondary
    Lymphocytosis and hypergammaglobulinemia
        Reactive
        Immunoproliferative

II. *Qualitative Disorders*

III. *Immunoproliferative Disorders*
    Leukemia
        Chronic lymphatic
        Acute lymphatic
    Lymphoma
        Hodgkin's
        Non-Hodgkin's
    M-component disorders
        Plasma cell myeloma
        Macroglobulinemia
        Benign monoclonal gammopathy
    Other variants
        Leukemic reticuloendotheliosis
        Mycosis fungoides
        Sézary syndrome

phocyte count of the peripheral blood precedes the decrease in either granulocytes or platelets caused by radiation. Lymphocytopenia is often present in patients during acute stress or therapy with corticoids. The studies of Fauci and Dale have demonstrated that glucocorticoids produce lymphocytopenia by shifting the distribution of lymphocytes from the intravascular to the extravascular space. The effect is transitory. In patients with certain lymphoproliferative disorders, however, glucocorticoids may produce the opposite effect and temporarily raise the blood lymphocyte count by means of altering the body distribution from extra- to intravascular sites. Adrenal steroids also cause cell lysis and inhibit cell proliferation, but these actions are limited to certain sensitive lymphocyte subpopulations. Steroid sensitivity is highly species-dependent.

The secondary lymphatic tissue is the immediate source of the circulating lymphocytes. Ablation of this source by malignant replacement, as in the case of advanced Hodgkin's disease or widespread metastatic carcinoma, or its destruction by irradiation of the lymph node-bearing regions of the body, leads to an inability of these regions to return adequate numbers of lymphocytes into the blood through the lymphatics. Chemotherapeutic alkylating agents will also affect

lymphocyte replacement by interfering with the proliferating and the short-lived small lymphocyte pools.

Hypogammaglobulinemia occurs as an acquired or congenital syndrome, but it is not necessarily associated with lymphocytopenia, since the source of immunoglobulins is not T lymphocytes but rather the non-circulating B cells. In infants or children, hypogammaglobulinemia usually represents a congenital immune deficiency. In adults, the condition is acquired either by increased loss in the urine or the gastrointestinal tract as a complication of nephrotic syndromes or protein-losing enteropathy, or by decreased production, usually secondary to a lymphoproliferative disorder.

Primary acquired late onset hypogammaglobulinemia ("common variable") varies greatly in severity and in the pattern of immune deficiency (Geha and associates, 1974). Recurrent sinopulmonary infections and malabsorption are among the more common of the clinical complications. At least one variety is thought to be the result of increased activity of a subpopulation of suppressor T lymphocytes acting to inhibit the normal development of B cells into mature secretory plasma cells.

The *congenital immune deficiency syndromes* of childhood form an array of rare but intriguing conditions upon which much of our understanding of the normal immune mechanism is based. The *Bruton type of agammaglobulinemia* is a sex-linked developmental defect of the B system of lymphocytes and plasma cells. Those regions of the secondary lymphatic tissue populated by these cells are empty, whereas the thymic-dependent areas remain intact. Circulating lymphocytes are present in normal numbers, but the concentration of immunoglobulins in the plasma is very low. The numerous infections which occur, usually in the sinopulmonary tract, can be prevented by the therapeutic use of gamma globulin injections. The *DiGeorge syndrome* is a severe developmental defect of the third and fourth pharyngeal pouches with consequent thymic aplasia and a profound lack of the thymic-dependent system of T cells. The corresponding regions of the T system are depleted of lymphocytes, and this is associated with lymphocytopenia but normal plasma immunoglobulin concentrations. *Swiss type lymphocytopenic agammaglobulinemia* ("combined immunodeficiency") affects both systems of immunocytes and thus would appear to trace its origins back to the common stem cell of origin in the bone marrow. A number of cases of severe combined immunodeficiency have been associated with deficiency of the enzyme adenosine deaminase (Parkman and co-workers, 1975). The adenosine which accumulates is toxic to lymphoid cells. Combined immunodeficiency may be corrected by bone marrow transplantation, whereas thymic transplantation should suffice in the DiGeorge syndrome (Bortin and Rimm, 1977).

Other congenital immune deficiency syndromes have been described, some resembling the Swiss type, others of a more mixed nature, such as *Wiskott-Aldrich syndrome* and *hereditary ataxia telangiectasia*. The features of Wiskott-Aldrich syndrome include sex-linked inheritance, thrombocytopenia, eczema, and susceptibility to infection associated with impaired ability to form antibody in response to polysaccharide antigens. The level of IgM is low, but IgG is normal and concentrations of IgA are often very high. Death in childhood is the result, owing either to severe infection or to the development of malignant disease, often of a lymphoma-like character. Successful therapy with transfer factor has been reported. In ataxia telangiectasia, the immune deficiency affects IgA and IgE along with qualitative deficiency in cell-mediated response.

The physiologic hypogammaglobulinemia of infancy must be distinguished from the congenital immune deficiency syndromes. Following the gradual disappearance from the infant's circulation of maternal IgG, endogenous synthesis takes over, raising IgG and IgM levels to about three fourths the adult level by one year of age. IgA levels increase more slowly, reaching adult levels by about two years.

Lymphocytosis and Hypergammaglobulinemia. Lymphocytosis is defined as an increase in the absolute lymphocyte count above 4000 per cu. mm. in adults, above 7000 cu. mm. in young children, and above 9000 per cu. mm. in infants. In "relative" lymphocytosis, the proportion of lymphocytes in the peripheral blood is increased because of concomitant granulocytopenia, but the absolute number is not above the normal range.

The leukocyte response evoked by a particular infection varies with the particular organism and also with the stage of the infection. Some infections, mostly viral but including some bacterial, are noted for their ability to evoke a lymphocytic response. Pertussis and acute infectious lymphocytosis are two childhood illnesses with a particularly striking tendency to raise the blood lymphocyte count — predominantly small mature forms — to very high levels in the range of 15,000 to 50,000 per cu. mm., but occasionally to as high as 100,000 per cu. mm.

Infectious mononucleosis is associated with a more modest lymphocytosis, usually not in excess of 20,000 per cu. mm., but there is a greater proportion (usually about 20 per cent of the total) of young and "atypical" forms (Lai, 1977). These are as large as 15 to 25 μ in diameter, with a generous rim of cytoplasm, often deep blue, foamy, and containing vacuoles, with an irregular outline which tends to cling to adjacent red cells. The nucleus is also larger, its chromatin clumps are somewhat more widely spaced, and its outline is often indented, irregular, or lobulated into "monocytoid" forms. One or two nucleoli per nucleus are occasionally seen.

Infectious mononucleosis is caused by the Epstein-Barr virus (EBV). B lymphocytes become infected with EBV. T lymphocytes then undergo a reactive proliferative response, giving rise to the atypical lymphocytes in the peripheral blood. EBV antigen can be identified on B cell membranes but is absent from the T cells. The humoral response is also of use in establishing the diagnosis by means of a significantly positive heterophile antibody titer.

During this period of T cell response in infectious mononucleosis, as in other viral infections, there is a temporary period of anergy associated with loss of the delayed hypersensitivity response. The explanation for this transient decrease in immune reactivity is unknown.

The EBV also appears to be of importance in the causation of the African type of *Burkitt's lymphoma* and of nasopharyngeal carcinoma (Klein, 1975). It is constantly associated with both these neoplasias. Why certain individuals respond to EBV infection with a benign self-limited disorder and others are stricken with malignancy is a mystery. Presumably the immunologic T cell response differs in the two circumstances; its failure to contain the infection under certain circumstances leads to a neoplastic transformation. EBV is also associated with Hodgkin's disease, but its importance in the genesis of this neoplasia is questionable.

The heterophile antibody test is positive in the great majority of cases, distinguishing infectious mononucleosis from a large number of other infections which may give rise to a similar blood picture, although usually with fewer atypical lymphocytes. These infections include measles, mumps, adenovirus, viral hepatitis, cytomegalovirus, toxoplasmosis, brucellosis, typhoid fever, *Listeria monocytogenes,* and even tuberculosis. These infections sometimes cause only a relative lymphocytosis, the most prominent change being a reduction in circulating granulocytes. Relative lymphocytosis is also a feature of the very early (usually preclinical) stages of bacterial infection, as granulocytes begin to leave the circulation to go into the infected tissues, or the very late stages of severe and overwhelming bacterial infection after exhaustion of granulocyte reserves. In the latter circumstance, the relative lymphocytosis is an ominous prognostic indicator. As one would predict from the effect of adrenal steroids on lymphocytes, adrenal insufficiency may cause a rise in the blood lymphocytes.

An inappropriate increase in the absolute lymphocyte count, not explainable on the basis of either immunoreactive states or endocrine disease, is indicative of a lymphoproliferative disorder, usually lymphatic leukemia. Small mature lymphocytes predominate in chronic lymphatic leukemia. In the early stages of this disorder the elevation may be slight, but counts are usually in the range of 50,000 to 250,000 per cu. mm. when the diagnosis is first made. A rare patient may reach values as high as 1,000,000 per cu. mm. The leukocytosis of acute lymphatic leukemia is usually lesser in degree. Instead of the small mature lymphocyte, it features immature lymphoblasts.

One of the most important problems in clinical hematologic diagnosis is the distinction between leukemia and "leukemoid" reactions. The clinical course, whether benign and self-limited or persistent or progressive, is one obvious point of difference. The ability to distinguish the morphologic features of leukemic lymphoblasts from the young and atypical lymphocytes found in infectious states is another. The association of anemia, thrombocytopenia, and/or granulocytopenia suggests leukemia, but these findings singly or in combination are sometimes seen in infections. Perhaps the most salient pathophysiologic point of distinction lies in the fact that replacement of the primary lymphatic organ, the bone marrow, is a prominent feature of leukemia. Reactive states cause proliferation mostly in the secondary lymphatic tissue; the reactive young and "atypical" lymphocytes which characterize infectious

mononucleosis and other infections therefore do not replace the normal marrow cells to any significant degree. Lymphocytes and plasma cells may increase in the marrow as a reactive change, but they usually are in the range of 5 to 15 per cent of the total marrow cells, hardly ever above 30 per cent, and never replace the marrow tissue as leukemic proliferation usually does.

An increase in plasma immunoglobulin concentration above the normal range is a common response not only in many infectious diseases but also in other conditions, such as liver cirrhosis, carcinoma, sarcoidosis, and lupus erythematosus, to name a few. Such responses are polyclonal and affect a variety of immunoglobulins. This is reflected in the serum electrophoretic pattern by a diffuse increase, or "broad-band" hypergammaglobulinemia. Immunoelectrophoretic analysis shows increases in all immunoglobulin families, IgG, IgA, and IgM. In an acute immune response, the increase in IgM occurs first. The finding in a serum electrophoretic pattern of hypergammaglobulinemia due to a narrow dense band in the broad region where the gamma globulins are normally found has a different significance. It is the secretory product of a monoclonal line of B cells producing only one type of immunoglobulin. This narrow band is often referred to as a "spike," but the term "M-component," for monoclonal component, is more appropriate (Fig. 22–123). The pres-

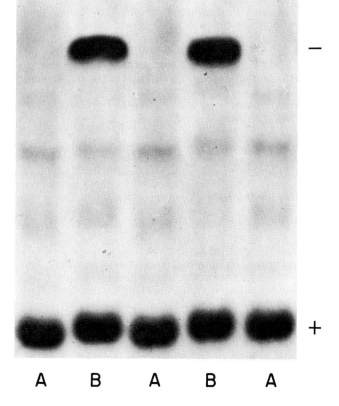

Figure 22–123 Electrophoretic separation of serum proteins on cellulose acetate. A is normal serum. B is abnormal serum containing an M-component located near the cathodal end of the strip in the gamma zone. (The cathodal end is at the top and the anodal at the bottom of the picture.)

A   B   A   B   A

ence of an M-component in the serum or urine requires investigation of the patient for a malignant proliferative disorder of the B cells, i.e., myeloma or primary macroglobulinemia. On the other hand, the mere presence of such a component does not by itself establish such a diagnosis.

Qualitative Disorders

There are several points in the immune response at which qualitative defects in lymphocyte function may be the primary factors responsible for a poor immune response. In contrast to the granulocytic series, however, it is difficult to separate functional defects of the lymphocyte from numerical deficiency, since the process of specific activation (with the assistance of modifying factors) sets off a series of cell proliferations of the specifically activated clone. Thus, a qualitative defect at the afferent level of the immune response will be reflected in deficient numbers at the efferent limb.

Malignant transformation of cells in the body is increasingly being viewed as a qualitative breakdown in the function of "surveillance" lymphocytes whose function it is to recognize specific "tumor" antigens on the surface of such cells and to bring about their destruction. The association of defective lymphocyte function with malignant transformation in the congenital immune deficiency states is indeed a striking example of a lack of surveillance. In a similar fashion, individuals who are under prolonged immunosuppressive therapy also show an increased tendency to develop malignant disease, often a lymphoma. Immune deficiency is a common feature of most of the lymphoproliferative disorders, but whether it precedes the development of the neoplasia or comes as a consequence of it — or both —remains a controversial subject.

Immunoproliferative Disorders

The neoplastic alterations of the lymphoid tissue produce an array of conditions quite distinct from but equally as rich in diversity as the myeloproliferative group of hematologic syndromes. The rapid expansion of basic knowledge about lymphocytes has produced a flurry of new concepts of lymphoproliferative disorders which rely on cell markers as well as traditional histopathology (Jaffe and co-workers, 1977). The rapidly emerging concepts are forcing reappraisal of old ideas.

The lymphatic leukemias primarily invade the bone marrow, with a prominent tendency to infiltrate the circulating bloodstream. The condition spreads to involve lymph nodes, spleen, and in-

deed many other tissues in the body. The lymphomas are a group of related conditions which affect the secondary lymphatic tissue first with tumor formation which subsequently spreads to the other tissues including the marrow, without much tendency in most cases to release significant numbers of malignant cells into the circulation. The third major group of immunoproliferative conditions, plasma cell myeloma and primary macroglobulinemia, cause extensive marrow replacement but show little tendency to infiltrate the blood. They do give rise to a high frequency of aberrations of immunoglobulin synthesis.

Lymphoproliferative disorders may be classified according to their origins from a T or B cell line and also with respect to the functional stage of cell differentiation from which the monoclonal neoplasia springs. The T cell neoplasias include acute lymphatic leukemia, lymphoblastic lymphoma, mycosis fungoides, and Sézary syndrome. The B cell disorders include the M-component disorders, chronic lymphatic leukemia, and most of the non-Hodgkin's lymphomas. Hodgkin's disease continues to elude a niche in this schema (Table 22–21).

Chronic Lymphatic Leukemia (CLL). This disease increases in frequency with advancing age, whereas acute lymphatic leukemia is mostly a disease of childhood. The terms "chronic" and "acute" were originally descriptive of the clinical courses, but therapeutic advances in the management of the acute variety have narrowed the gap in life expectancy between the two. As a result, the terms are now more indicative of the morphology of the leukemic cell than of the prognosis. The small mature lymphocyte is the hallmark of chronic lymphatic leukemia; the lymphoblast is the sign of the acute variety.

CLL is rare in childhood but not uncommon in mature and older adults; two thirds of patients are over the age of 60. There is a 2:1 sex predominance in favor of males. The diagnosis is usually easily made by the observation that large numbers of small mature lymphocytes have accumulated in the blood and bone marrow. In comparison with the normal these lymphocytes are often more friable, have deeper nuclear clefts, and sometimes have more cytoplasm. Immature lymphoid cells are less than 5 per cent of the total. The absolute lymphocyte count in the blood is usually elevated to 10,000 to 150,000 per cu. mm. or even higher at the time of initial diagnosis, although a "subleukemic" (or "aleukemic") variety may be seen in which the cellular infiltration is confined to the marrow. Generalized lymphadenopathy and splenomegaly are common. Lymphocytic infiltration of the liver and of other body tissues increases as the disease progresses. The median life expectancy is about five years, but the clinical course is variable. One fifth of the patients, often

TABLE 22–21 CLASSIFICATION OF IMMUNOPROLIFERATIVE DISORDERS
ACCORDING TO FUNCTIONAL STAGE OF DIFFERENTIATION
(EARLY, INTERMEDIATE, OR LATE)

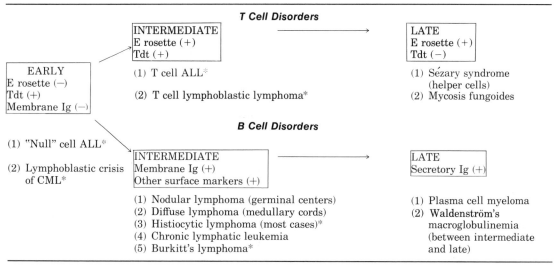

T Cell Disorders

INTERMEDIATE
E rosette (+)
Tdt (+)

(1) T cell ALL*

(2) T cell lymphoblastic lymphoma*

LATE
E rosette (+)
Tdt (−)

(1) Sézary syndrome
(helper cells)
(2) Mycosis fungoides

EARLY
E rosette (−)
Tdt (+)
Membrane Ig (−)

B Cell Disorders

(1) "Null" cell ALL*

(2) Lymphoblastic crisis
of CML*

INTERMEDIATE
Membrane Ig (+)
Other surface markers (+)

(1) Nodular lymphoma (germinal centers)
(2) Diffuse lymphoma (medullary cords)
(3) Histiocytic lymphoma (most cases)*
(4) Chronic lymphatic leukemia
(5) Burkitt's lymphoma*

LATE
Secretory Ig (+)

(1) Plasma cell myeloma
(2) Waldenström's
macroglobulinemia
(between intermediate
and late)

*Neoplastic cells predominantly transformed into large cells or "blasts."
Abbreviations: ALL = acute lymphatic leukemia   CML = chronic myelogenous leukemia
             Tdt = terminal deoxynucleotidyl transferase   Ig   = immunoglobulin
NOTE: "Null" cell ALL and lymphoblastic crisis of CML may originate from an undifferentiated marrow lym-
       phoid cell line or from early cell lines with incompletely developed T or B cell characteristics (Gralnick
       and associates, 1977). Hodgkin's disease is not included in this schema.

those in the somewhat younger age group, are resistant to therapy and die within a year. At the other extreme, one third of patients are still alive after 10 years.

From the pathophysiologic point of view this disorder is better described as an abnormality of cell accumulation rather than one of cell proliferation. The leukemic cell population is predominantly non-dividing and inert. Immunoglobulins of the IgM type and sometimes also of the IgD type are present on the lymphocyte membrane. They are monoclonal and indicate the origin of CLL from a single line of B lymphocytes. Etiology is obscure, but the rarity of CLL among individuals of Oriental extraction along with a significant occurrence of multiple cases within the families of affected patients suggests that genetic factors are important.

Although years may pass without the occurrence of significant symptoms, many patients have anorexia, fatigue, weight loss, and sweats. Growth of lymphatic tumors may cause mechanical symptoms. Anemia, thrombocytopenia, and granulocytopenia are unfavorable signs and usually indicate impending trouble in any one or a combination of the functions these respective cellular elements fulfill. The most important cause of this cytopenia is the crowding out from the marrow of the normal precursor cells by the closely packed lymphocytes. Massive splenic enlargement may add to the severity of the cytopen-

ia by trapping and sequestering or destroying any one or a combination of the blood cells. About 5 to 10 per cent of patients have an associated Coombs'-positive autoimmune hemolytic anemia, with spherocytosis, reticulocytosis, and erythroid hyperplasia in an otherwise lymphocytic marrow, along with the other usual signs of hemolysis. Death as a result of infectious complications runs high, since the disease fundamentally represents a breakdown in the normal defense mechanism. The susceptibility to infection may stem either from severe neutropenia or from the impediment to the production of circulating antibody. About half the cases show decreased serum immunoglobulin concentrations and about 5 per cent show an M-component in the serum electrophoretic pattern. The abnormal lymphocytes are poorly responsive to mitogenic stimulation with phytohemagglutinin, as would be expected of B lymphocytes.

The goal of therapy is to relieve symptoms and to improve anemia, thrombocytopenia, or granulocytopenia by reducing the size of the lymphocyte mass. Since cell proliferation is not a prominent feature, chemotherapeutic agents which depend on the DNA synthetic or mitotic phases of cycling cells are not useful. Chemotherapeutic destruction of the lymphocyte mass by alkylating agents (chlorambucil or cyclophosphamide) and adrenal glucocorticoids used singly or in combination are the mainstay of treatment.

Therapy has no doubt decreased morbidity and improved quality of life in CLL, but it seems likely that it has not dramatically increased life expectancy. Although peripheral blood counts improve, hypogammaglobulinemia is often not affected by treatment. The goal is to achieve "control" of the disease rather than "complete remission," as in the acute leukemias, since there is no evidence that added clinical benefit would accrue from the additional therapy that would be necessary. If properly managed, many patients may live out their normal life span with this disease. It rarely changes character, and the danger lies almost entirely in the immune deficiency and in bone marrow and organ impairment from lymphocyte encroachment.

Acute Lymphatic Leukemia (ALL). Primarily a disease of childhood with peak incidence at the age of four, ALL affects 20- to 30-year-old adults with a frequency about equal to that of acute granulocytic leukemia. Above that age, 90 per cent or more of the acute leukemias are granulocytic. The onset is relatively sudden, with symptoms of anemia, bleeding, or fever. Preleukemic manifestations are absent. Bone pain is not uncommon. The white blood cell count is usually increased, occasionally to values of 100,000 per cu. mm. or higher, with infiltration of the blood with lymphoblasts, but about one third of the cases present with a normal or low white cell count. Anemia and thrombocytopenia are the rule, but immunologic abnormalities are not observed, except inasmuch as they may come later as a result of the immunosuppressive effects of therapy. Intracranial hemorrhage is a life-threatening event, the likelihood of which is increased if severe thrombocytopenia occurs together with extreme elevations of the white cell count. Serum uric acid concentrations often are high, and precautions are necessary to avoid urate nephropathy. Neurologic manifestations due to infiltration of the central nervous system or of peripheral nerves are not uncommon. A slight to moderate degree of lymphadenopathy and hepatosplenomegaly are often present. Many other body tissues also become infiltrated with leukemic cells. Slow but unrestrained proliferation of the lymphoblasts crowds out normal blood precursor cells and produces death within a few months from hemorrhage or infection if the condition is not treated. Successful treatment eradicates all visible evidence of malignant tissue and allows the normal marrow cells to repopulate the marrow and to restore peripheral blood counts to normal, a state called "complete remission."

About a quarter of the cases of acute lymphatic leukemia (ALL) are positive for T cell membrane markers (Belpomme and associates, 1977). These tend to have a greater frequency of thymic and subcutaneous tumor formation, higher white cell count, greater likelihood of central nervous system involvement, and a generally less favorable outcome. Almost three quarters do not show any of the usual surface markers, and have therefore been called "null," or "non-T non-B" cell ALL. However, almost all ALL cells are positive for the marker enzyme "terminal transferase" (terminal deoxynucleotidyl transferase) (Greenwood and associates, 1977). This enzyme is highly characteristic of thymocytes and is also present in marrow, but it is absent from fully mature T cells. Its presence in almost all cases of ALL suggests that "null" cell ALL is in fact a neoplasia of an undifferentiated T cell line which has not yet developed the characteristic T cell surface markers. About one third of cases of acute blastic transformation of chronic myelogenous leukemia are also positive for terminal transferase. This finding indicates a lymphoblastic rather than a myeloblastic origin. Indeed, the morphologic appearance of these cells and their responsiveness to vincristine and prednisone treatment also support the concept of their lymphoid origin.

By means of experiments using tritiated thymidine, Mauer and his co-workers have found that the leukemic cells in patients with ALL do not proliferate in a uniform fashion. There appear to be two pools, one consisting of larger blasts which take up tritiated thymidine and are thus proliferating, while the other is made up of smaller blast cells which do not take up the DNA label and thus are not in a state of proliferation (Fig. 22–124). The cell cycle times of the proliferating leukemic cells generally vary in the range from three to ten days, although some apparently do not divide more often than once every 20 days. The large proliferating blasts predominate in the bone marrow; the small non-proliferating blasts are relatively more frequent in the circulating blood, where they have a relatively short life span with $T^{1/2}$ of about 25 hours. The importance of the non-proliferating pool of leukemic cells lies in its resistance to modalities of therapy which depend on cells being in a state of cycle, i.e., entering phases of DNA synthesis and/or mitosis. These non-dividing cells have the capacity to re-enter a proliferative phase after some period of dormancy, suggesting that they may be the bearers of the seeds of relapse, which is such a constant feature of the disease.

Chromosomal abnormalities, usually aneuploidy, are inconstantly present in ALL. They vary from case to case, but seem to remain constant in any given patient throughout the course of the disease. Their relationship to pathogenesis is unknown. Other aspects of cytogenetics and etiology of acute leukemia are discussed in the section on acute granulocytic leukemia.

The following concepts of chemotherapeutic strategy have been developed for the treatment of acute leukemia:

Induction — the initial stage of chemotherapy

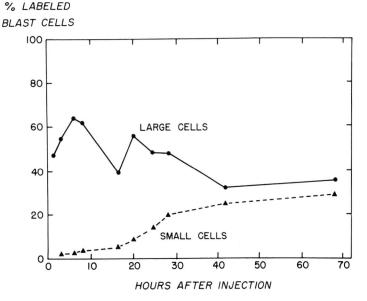

% LABELED
BLAST CELLS

Figure 22–124 The labeling of large and small blast cells in a patient with acute leukemia after an injection of tritiated thymidine. The large cells are proliferating and therefore immediately take up the label. Initially, small cells take up no label because they are not dividing. Large blasts, however, become small non-dividing blasts, causing a belated appearance of the label in these cells. (Redrawn from Mauer, A. M., et al.: Human Tumor Cell Kinetics. National Cancer Institute Monograph No. 30, p. 71.)

LARGE CELLS

SMALL CELLS

HOURS AFTER INJECTION

designed to bring about complete remission in leukemia, i.e., alleviation of the symptoms, restoration of normal blood counts, and a return to a normal bone marrow in which less than 5 per cent of the cells are blasts. In ALL, vincristine and prednisone given together produce complete remission in about 90 per cent of new cases. The two agents act on different phases of the cell cycle, vincristine on the M (mitotic) phase and prednisone chiefly on the G_1 (intermitotic) phase. This example illustrates an important principle which has proved itself in certain other oncologic circumstances, namely, that combinations of agents are more effective and have no more toxicity than when each of the agents is used singly. Meticulous supportive care during induction with such measures as platelet transfusion, protective isolation, and the judicious use of antibiotics is important to the attainment of a successful outcome, especially in acute granulocytic leukemia, in which remission is so much more difficult to achieve than in ALL.

Consolidation and Intensification—a relatively intensive phase of chemotherapy which may be administered for an arbitrary period of time after the induction of complete remission. The object is to further reduce the number of leukemic cells, already so few that they are clinically inapparent, and thus delay clinical relapse by increasing the number of cell doublings necessary to grow enough leukemic tissue to produce clinical signs and symptoms. During this phase the improved bone marrow function brought about by the remission induction markedly increases the patient's hematologic tolerance to the cytotoxic effects of the chemotherapy.

Maintenance — a prolonged therapeutic effort to maintain the patient in a continuous state of complete remission for as long a time as possible. Without such treatment the remission in ALL lasts only one to four months. Those patients who relapse sooner after unmaintained remission probably have a shorter leukemic cell cycle time than those who stay in remission longer. Single or multiple agents, given alone or together, continuously, sequentially, or in cycles, have been used. Methotrexate, 6-mercaptopurine, and cyclophosphamide have been particularly useful. Nonspecific immune stimulation with such agents as BCG vaccine also appears to be active in maintaining remission.

Reinforcement — the application during the period of maintenance therapy of treatments of the type with which remission was first induced. For example, in ALL, vincristine and prednisone given from time to time during maintenance therapy appear to lengthen remission duration significantly.

Total Therapy — the effort, in addition to all the above stratagems, to eradicate hidden nests of leukemic cells which otherwise escape the chemotherapeutic onslaught. The central nervous system is a favorite hideout for such nests, a fact amply documented by the 30 to 50 per cent incidence of meningeal leukemia in ALL, a complication which almost always arises when the patient is in bone marrow remission. Meningeal leukemia causes symptoms and signs of increased intracranial pressure — headache, nausea and vomiting, and papilledema. Leukemic cells are found in the cerebrospinal fluid along with an elevated pressure, a decreased glucose concentration, and often some elevation of the protein concentration. With the exception of prednisone and the nitrosourea derivatives, chemotherapeutic agents do not readily cross the blood-brain barrier. The response to intrathecal therapy with methotrexate or to irradiation of the craniospinal axis is prompt. Based on the frequency of this complication and on the efficacious nature of the therapy, the most recent addition to the therapeutic strategy in ALL is the prophylactic treatment of this body site, in the hope of eliminating secluded nests of leukemic cells, with either intrathecal chemotherapy or radiation therapy or both. Simone has recently summarized the experience with "total therapy" at St. Jude's Hospital in Memphis.

The development of therapeutic strategy over the years has been paralleled by a progressive increase in life expectancy in children with ALL (Fig. 22–125). Hope is turning to expectation that many children with ALL will be cured as a result of "total therapy." In adults with ALL, the results of treatment have not been as good, with the increase in life expectancy having been lengthened from a median of four to six months to about 18 months.

Malignant Lymphoma, Hodgkin's Type. Noted for its predilection for young adults, Hodgkin's lymphoma makes up about one third of all cases of lymphoma (Moran and Ultman, 1974). All age groups are affected, a low frequency in childhood rising to about 2.5 cases per 100,000 population in adolescents and young adults. After the age of 50, the frequency increases along with that of

other malignant disease. Males predominate 3:2, and females appear to have a better prognosis. In contrast to the other lymphomas, Hodgkin's is more likely to start in the low cervical or supraclavicular lymph nodes and to cause high fever and intense itching. A small percentage of cases arise outside of the lymphatic system. Sometimes it is the cause of fever of unknown origin, even in the absence of apparent external lymphadenopathy.

Often the peripheral blood is entirely normal, but a variety of different changes can be seen. Increases in the granulocyte and platelet counts are not uncommon. Monocytosis and eosinophilia are less frequent. Coombs'-positive acquired hemolytic anemia occurs in occasional patients, but anemia, when it is present, is usually the variety seen with chronic disease. Pancytopenia may be caused by any combination of the factors of bone marrow invasion, hypersplenism, and bone marrow suppression from treatment. Absolute lymphocytopenia is a sign of rather advanced involvement of the lymphatic system significantly associated with an impairment of delayed hypersensitivity and other cellular immune responses. T cell function is impaired while the ability to form specific antibody is usually preserved. The cellular immune defect leads to the occurrence of complicating infections which are often of an unusual nature, such as aspergillosis, moniliasis, and other fungal diseases; *Pneumocystis carinii* infection; and localized or generalized herpes zoster. Rare "epidemics" have suggested that it may be spread as an infectious disease with a low

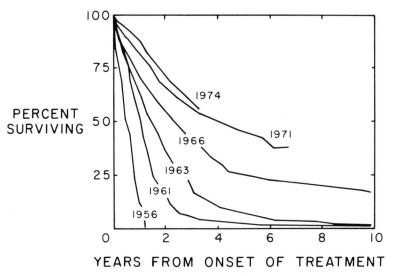

Figure 22–125 Improved survival in acute lymphatic leukemia between 1956 and 1977 in patients under age 20 at time of diagnosis. The years indicated are the start of treatment. A series of modifications in the treatment protocols over the years has been associated with progressive improvement in survival, with a significant proportion of long-term survivors off all treatment for several years. (Redrawn from data of Cancer and Leukemia Group B, by permission of Dr. James F. Holland)

order of contagion, but there is no proof that Hodgkin's disease is caused by an oncogenic infectious agent.

In contrast to the other lymphomas, Hodgkin's tends to begin in one site and to spread locally from one involved lymph node region to the next nearest group of lymph nodes, accounting for the high cure rate after local treatment and for the better results obtained by "extended field" as compared to "limited field" radiotherapy (Fig. 22–126). The other lymphomas are more likely to be "polycentric" rather than "unicentric" at the time of their origin. With the passage of time, however, the tendency is strong for relentless progression of lymphoma of any type, first within the lymphatic system, and then finally to extralymphatic structures such as liver, bone, lungs, and other organs. The course in any individual patient, however, is often unpredictable.

The Lukes-Butler system of classification for Hodgkin's disease has gained a large measure of acceptance, chiefly because it is clinically useful in terms of prognosis and management (Table 22–22). The presence of the Reed-Sternberg cell is a sine qua non for the diagnosis in any of the subgroups. Whether lymphocytes are preserved or depleted within the biopsied lymph node determines the favorable or unfavorable extremes of prognosis.

The evaluation of the extent of the disease by means of physical examination, radiographic procedures, and even exploratory laparotomy (or "staging") is essential in order to design a program of treatment properly. The stages into which Hodgkin's lymphoma is classified are shown in Figure 22–127. The presence of symptoms increases the probability that the disease is more disseminated. Splenic involvement increases the likelihood that the liver is also involved.

Extended field radiotherapy is the treatment of choice for patients with involvement confined to lymphatic tissue. When extralymphatic structures are involved, chemotherapy is preferred. Combined programs of radiotherapy plus chemotherapy are now under investigation. Although localized palliative radiotherapy occasionally is necessary, the major goal of radiotherapy is the cure of the patient. Chemotherapy has been traditionally considered to offer nothing more than temporary, although often very effective, palliation. Following in the footsteps of the experience gained with acute lymphatic leukemia, the chemotherapy of Hodgkin's disease has recently utilized combinations of agents, rather than single agents, given for a number of months to "induce" remission. The chemotherapeutic agents of greatest value are the alkylating agents (nitrogen mustard, cyclophosphamide, and chlorambucil); the vinca alkaloids (vincristine and vinblastine); the nitrosourea and anthracycline derivatives; procarbazine; bleomycin; and adrenal glucocorticoids. When these principles of chemotherapy are

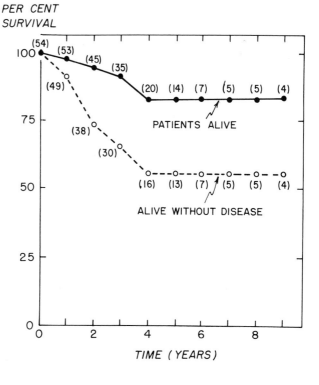

Figure 22–126 Survival in patients with localized Hodgkin's disease treated with radical radiation therapy. Most of the deaths and recurrences occurred within 3 years. A similar group of patients not treated radically had a 5-year survival of 35 per cent, but no survivor was free of disease. (Redrawn from Prosnitz, L. R., et al.: Amer. J. Roentgenol., *105*:618, 1969. Courtesy of Charles C Thomas, Publisher.)

TABLE 22–22   LUKES-BUTLER NOMENCLATURE: HODGKIN'S LYMPHOMA

Subgroup	Median Survival (Years)*	General Histologic Features
Lymphocyte predominant	9.2	Reed-Sternberg cells are seen in the midst of a sea of small mature lymphocytes arranged into a nodular or diffuse pattern.
Nodular sclerosis	4.2	A nodular pattern with the nodules separated by broad fibrous bands containing collagen bundles. The cellular pattern in the nodules may vary considerably, resembling that in any of the other three subgroups.
Mixed cellularity	2.5	A heterogeneous, usually diffuse cellular pattern containing lymphocytes, plasma cells, eosinophils, neutrophils, histiocytes, and fibroblasts, along with Reed-Sternberg cells, sometimes very numerous. Collagen bundles are absent.
Lymphocyte depletion	1.3	Undifferentiated histiocytes (or "reticulum cells") usually predominate in a diffuse pattern; at times Reed-Sternberg cells are very numerous. Fibrous obliteration of the entire lymph node is another variant of this subgroup.

*Lukes, R. J.: J.A.M.A., *222*:1294, 1972.

properly applied, as many as 40 per cent of patients with relatively advanced disease are alive and well for five years, a finding that encourages the hope that chemotherapeutic cure is being achieved in some cases.

Malignant Lymphoma Other Than Hodgkin's Type. Equally diverse in clinical manifestations and just as obscure etiologically, the non-Hodgkin's lymphomas are distinct from the Hodgkin's type and the principles of management and therapy differ (Patchevsky and associates, 1974). The most important difference is the greater tendency for the disease to be disseminated at the time of initial diagnosis by lymph node biopsy or histologic examination of an adequate piece of tissue from some extranodal site. Indeed, 90 per cent of patients with apparent Stage I or II disease show retroperitoneal node involvement by lymphography. This important point of difference no doubt explains why extended field radiotherapy does not clearly produce better results than more limited fields, as it does in patients with Stage I or II Hodgkin's disease. There is a slight male predominance. Most patients are older than 45 years of age. Systemic symptoms resemble those of Hodgkin's disease, but temperature elevations tend not to run as high. Their presence bears a similar poor prognostic significance.

A time-honored classification much used by cli-

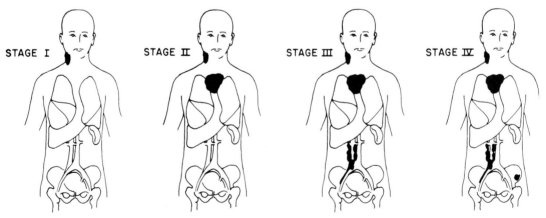

Figure 22–127   Stages of Hodgkin's disease. I to III represents progressively greater degrees of lymphatic involvement, while IV represents spread to extralymphatic structures.

nicians included three major categories: reticulum cell sarcoma, lymphosarcoma, and giant follicular lymphoma. This breakdown has been very useful from the clinical point of view because of the prognostic differences between these major groups. However, histologic classification has often proved difficult and even contradictory. This has been especially true for reticulum cell sarcoma because of the lack of uniform criteria and of a generally accepted nomenclature. The system of Rappaport has gained some measure of acceptance in recent years (Table 22–23). This system classifies the over-all node architecture as "diffuse" or "nodular" and the predominant cell type as a "well differentiated lymphocyte," a "poorly differentiated lymphocyte," or a "histiocyte." Controversy still surrounds the origin of the "histiocyte." Some consider it a close relative of the tissue macrophage and/or of cells capable of secreting reticulin fibers demonstrable by special silver stains. By the application of techniques for identifying surface markers, most "histiocytes" actually appear to be B lymphocytes, although many have no surface markers at all and a few are T cells. A nodular pattern and a well differentiated cell type are indicators of more favorable prognosis.

Traditional lymphoma histopathology has used the term "undifferentiated" to mean either a large transformed lymphoid blast cell, a lymphoid cell with an irregular or deeply cleaved nucleus, or both. The newer usage of the terms "undifferentiated" and "differentiated" refers to the level of functional development of the lymphoid cell, with allowance that a cell line derived from any level of functional development may enlarge and undergo transformation. Thus, for example, Burkitt's lymphoma arises from a B cell line that is moderately differentiated along functional lines, but the neoplastic cell population has transformed into blasts which traditional histopathology would consider morphologically "undifferentiated." Such differences of word usage are responsible for a certain amount of confusion in the current literature.

A life expectancy of eight to ten years is not an unreasonable hope for the majority of patients with nodular lymphoma. The course of this lymphoma may continue to follow a remarkably benign pattern even after the lymphatic system is rather generally involved. Lymph node enlargement may occur in very erratic fashion, first in one body region and then later in another near or distant region. The symptoms are often those of mechanical obstruction or of compression caused by the enlarged lymph nodes. After several years of disease the histologic pattern may change to a less differentiated cytologic type. Systemic symptoms intervene, relapses become more frequent, and resistance to treatment increases as the malignant cells spill beyond the confines of the lymphatic system. A fatal outcome is the ultimate rule, despite the initial symptom-free years.

The diffuse lymphocytic lymphomas are somewhat less benign, although individual cases may well follow a benign and protracted course (Pangalis and associates, 1977). About 50 per cent succumb within two years but 25 per cent are still alive after five years, and a significant number survive well beyond that. Focal or diffuse involvement of the marrow can be demonstrated in about one third of cases. When significant numbers of malignant cells infiltrate the circulating blood, the disorder is called lymphosarcoma cell leukemia, a condition which rather closely resembles chronic lymphatic leukemia. Lymphosarcoma cells have a more immature lacy nuclear chromatin pattern, a folded nucleus, and often irregular cytoplasmic outlines, but the distinction from chronic lymphatic leukemia may be difficult. A lymph node biopsy is not useful in the diagnosis of chronic lymphatic leukemia, but if one is obtained it will show a pattern indistinguishable from that of diffuse lymphocytic lymphoma.

Histiocytic lymphoma is the most malignant; 60 to 80 per cent of patients succumb within one year. However, even in this category individual patients not uncommonly defy over-all statistics and survive for five years or longer. Modern combination chemotherapy appears to have improved the over-all prognosis, and Fisher and co-workers report a five-year survival of 38 per cent of all patients treated. The tendency for the disease to first become apparent in extranodal sites — especially the gastrointestinal tract and bone — is most striking. Extensive involvement of the gastrointestinal tract or of the bone marrow predicts

TABLE 22–23 CLASSIFICATION OF NON-HODGKIN'S LYMPHOMA

Nodular Lymphoma (Follicular Lymphoma)
  Poorly differentiated lymphocytic
  Mixed histiocytic-lymphocytic
  Histiocytic

Diffuse Lymphoma
  Well differentiated lymphocytic (lymphosarcoma)
  Poorly differentiated lymphocytic (lymphosarcoma)
  Mixed histiocytic-lymphocytic
  Histiocytic (reticulum cell sarcoma)
  Lymphoblastic
  Undifferentiated
    Burkitt's
    non-Burkitt's

(Modified from Rappaport, with more traditional terms in parenthesis. (From Byrne, G. E., Jr.: Cancer Treat. Rep., *61*:935, 1977.)

a poorer outcome for the patient. Marked weight loss with little overt manifestation of tumor growth, occult hepatosplenomegaly, or an infiltrating tumor of the muscle, brain, or almost any tissue may be the presenting sign. A leukemic phase of the illness occurs much more rarely than in diffuse lymphocytic lymphoma.

For the most part pathogenetic mechanisms in non-Hodgkin's lymphomas resemble those in Hodgkin's. Although chronologic patterns of progression may be capricious, spread usually occurs from the lymphatic system to the liver, spleen, and other tissues. Death may be caused by the tumor itself or it may come as a result of infectious complications which follow in the footsteps of the damage done to the immunologic system. Autoimmune phenomena, such as hemolytic anemia or thrombocytopenia, occur in a minority of patients before, concomitant with, or following the first overt sign of lymphoma. About 5 per cent of sera from non-Hodgkin's lymphoma have an IgM or IgG M-component, a finding which is rare in Hodgkin's. Other abnormalities of immunoglobulin production, such as Bence Jones proteinuria or hypogammaglobulinemia, are observed in some patients with non-Hodgkin's lymphoma but not as a rule in Hodgkin's. The several principles of staging outlined in the management of Hodgkin's lymphoma appear also to represent sound approaches to the patient with non-Hodgkin's types.

Other non-Hodgkin's lymphomas with distinctive clinical and morphologic features include lymphoblastic T cell lymphoma and Burkitt's lymphoma. Lymphoblastic T cell ("convoluted cell") lymphoma is a close relative of T cell ALL. It affects younger adults with rapidly growing tumors, usually affecting the mediastinum, with early transition to a leukemic phase and central nervous system involvement. The neoplastic cells are positive for terminal transferase. Most are also positive for T cell surface markers. Some also have complement receptors. The term "convoluted cell" refers to the surface contour of the cell nuclei as seen in fixed preparations. This appearance however cannot be relied upon as a marker of T cell origin (Greenberg and co-workers, 1976). Burkitt's lymphoma also has a rapid rate of cell proliferation. It commonly forms jaw tumors in the endemic African variety, although in the U.S.A. intra-abdominal presentation is more the rule. Despite the blastic appearance of the neoplastic cells they are heavily coated with surface IgM, identifying this lymphoma as a B cell type (Mann and associates, 1976).

M-Component Disorder. An "M-component" is the secretory product of a single monoclonal line of immunoglobulin-producing immunocytes. The abnormal protein is recognized as a narrow homogeneous band or "spike" in the electrophoretic pattern of serum or concentrated urine. It is the product of a cellular clone which has undergone an unusual degree of proliferation, often of a neoplastic character. The absolute production rate of the M-component can be used as a measure of the mass of the abnormal cell line, assuming that each cell produces a fixed quantity of immunoglobulin per unit time. The production rate can be estimated from measurement of its concentration and a knowledge of its turnover rate. An imbalance in the production rates of the subunits which combine to make up the immunoglobulin molecule causes overproduction of one of the subunits, usually L chains, which spill out readily into the urine because of their low molecular weight. The L chains, called "Bence Jones protein" in the premolecular era, are either κ or λ in type, but not both, a further demonstration of the monoclonal character of the cell of origin. Excesses of H chains in the serum and urine are a much more seldom observed event.

The presence of these abnormal proteins is sometimes uncovered by sheer diligence on the part of physicians, but increasingly they are discovered accidentally because of the frequency with which serum electrophoresis is used as a routine test. The heat test for Bence Jones protein in the urine is unreliable and should be replaced by electrophoresis of sufficiently concentrated urine. Paper dip techniques in common use for the routine detection of albuminuria are not sensitive to the presence in the urine of other proteins, such as L chains. L chains may be detected in the serum, but since they are so rapidly excreted by the kidney, their concentration is very low unless there is renal insufficiency. The concentration of the serum M-component varies from the range of 1 gram per 100 ml. to more than 10 grams per 100 ml. The daily urinary excretion of L chains may vary from less than 1 gram per day to 15 to 20 grams per day. Immunoelectrophoretic techniques are now in common use to classify the M-components of the serum and urine. Quantitation of immunoglobulins show depressed serum concentrations of the uninvolved types. The ability to produce specific antibody is often impaired. Recurrent bacterial pneumonia and other infectious complications then appear.

M-components in the serum sometimes confer strange properties upon it which may be of pathophysiologic significance. Reversible precipitation or gelation in the cold (i.e., the M-component is a "cryoglobulin") may cause circulatory embarrassment in exposed body parts. Red cells readily aggregate into "rouleaux," and the erythrocyte sedimentation rate is often rapid, but significant hemolysis usually does not occur. Bleeding may stem from antagonistic effects on plasma coagulation factors, fibrin polymerization, and platelet function. The M-component, especially if it is an

IgM type, may increase plasma viscosity by eight- to tenfold. Block and Maki have reviewed the "hyperviscosity syndrome" that may develop, with visual disturbances, retinal venous congestion and a sausage-like periodicity of the vein walls ("boxcar effect"), mental confusion, stupor, and even coma. Since the patients are usually aged, prompt recognition is not always achieved. Symptoms are quickly ameliorated by plasmapheresis. The excretion in the urine of large amounts of L chains is significantly related to the development of renal insufficiency, presumably through tissue deposition of L chains as amyloid, or by a direct toxic effect of this small protein on the renal tubule epithelial cells (Stone and Frenkel, 1975). Hypercalcemia and hyperuricemia also contribute to the multifactorial renal disease which complicates plasma cell myeloma.

Plasma cell myeloma is a malignant proliferation of plasma cells, usually in the bone marrow, sometimes forming solitary or multiple tumors, but almost always going on to widespread dissemination as diffuse "myelomatosis." Destructive bone disease is the major pathologic consequence, possibly because of the secretion locally of an osteoclast-stimulating factor (Mundy and associates, 1974). Localized osteolytic punched-out lesions affecting the skull, ribs, pelvis, or proximal portions of the long bones, as well as diffuse osteoporosis of the whole skeletal system, are common. Extramedullary myelomas may rarely form almost anywhere. Lymphatic involvement is not a feature of the disease, and hepatosplenomegaly is generally not detected. Localized bone pain and pathologic fractures are the most fearsome consequences. Symptomatic hypercalcemia, apparently related to bone dissolution, is common and may require emergency treatment.

Amyloidosis associated with plasma cell myeloma usually assumes the clinical features of the primary rather than the secondary form. Fragments of the L chains are invariably found in the tissue deposits. Musculoskeletal involvement is impressive and causes symptoms of arthritis, carpal tunnel syndrome, myocardial weakness, and macroglossia.

A mild normocytic and normochromic anemia is common, and about one third of patients have pancytopenia related to replacement of the marrow by the neoplastic plasma cells. Morphologic confirmation of the diagnosis is always necessary, either by biopsy of a plasma cell tumor or by random aspiration of bone marrow. If sheets of immature plasma cells replace the normal marrow cellular elements, the morphologic picture is diagnostic, but if the plasma cells are fewer, great care must be exercised in morphologic interpretation. Reactive plasmacytosis may increase the marrow plasma cells to 25 to 30 per cent of the total, although usually a reactive plasmacytosis is not in excess of 10 to 15 per cent. *"Benign monoclonal gammopathy"* and *primary amyloidosis* must also be distinguished from plasma cell myeloma. Increasing degrees of plasma cell immaturity along with frequent polyploid forms favor the latter diagnosis.

Depressed concentrations of the normal serum immunoglobulins are a constant feature of plasma cell myeloma. For quite some time this has been explained mechanistically as a "crowding out" of normal plasma cells by the neoplastic clone. Modern immunology has offered more plausible theories. These include the possibility of deficiencies of B cell surface receptors for antigen; excessive negative feedback from the high level of monoclonal protein and/or plasma cell mass; and depression of humoral immunity by a population of suppressor cells (Broder and associates, 1975).

Three fourths of plasma cell myeloma patients have either an IgG or an IgA M-component in the serum, IgG occurring twice as commonly as IgA. Almost all the remaining one fourth who lack such a serum component will have an M-component in the urine, with decreased serum immunoglobulin concentrations. In all, about one half to two thirds have demonstrable L chains in the urine. Rare cases of IgD and IgE myeloma have been reported. A few plasma cells are commonly seen in the peripheral blood in myeloma, but overt plasma cell leukemia is a rare and rapidly fatal variant.

Primary macroglobulinemia of Waldenström typically affects older people in their eighth decade. The clinical picture overlaps that of chronic lymphatic leukemia and lymphocytic lymphoma, in which about 5 per cent of patients have an M-component, usually IgM. The typical presentation of primary macroglobulinemia is one of a dense infiltration of the bone marrow with small mature lymphoid cells, many of which have plasmacytoid features. A number of typical plasma cells may also be seen. There is no leukemic infiltration of the blood; generalized lymphadenopathy and splenomegaly are present but are not marked. The diagnosis is confirmed by demonstrating the presence in the serum of an IgM M-component in excess of 2 grams per 100 ml. L chains may be found in the urine. Anemia is common and may be severe. Pancytopenia is not uncommon. Osteolytic bone lesions are exceptionally rare.

Finding an M-component in the serum or urine alone cannot be considered diagnostic of either of the above immunoproliferative conditions without the assistance of supporting information. The term *"benign monoclonal gammopathy"* has been applied to those patients with an M-component in the serum, usually less than 2 grams per 100 ml., without decreases in the other serum immuno-globulins, significant abnormalities in blood counts, bone disease, or more than a minority of mostly mature plasma cells in the marrow as reviewed by Abramson and Shattil. In some instances the M-component spontaneously disappears, suggesting that it may have been evoked as a physiologic but monoclonal response to some undetermined but highly specific antigen. About 15 per cent of these patients are discovered to have an associated carcinoma. A low concentration of monoclonal IgM occurs with cold agglutinin hemolytic anemia. Amyloidosis is thought to bear some relationship to an underlying process of plasma cell proliferation either of a secondary reactive nature, as in chronic infections, Hodgkin's lymphoma, or rheumatoid arthritis, or of a primary nature (Glenner and associates, 1973). Indeed one school of thought contends that primary amyloidosis is an expression of plasma cell myeloma, even in the absence of osteolytic bone disease and other diagnostic criteria of myeloma. M-components and marrow plasmacytosis are common findings in primary amyloidosis, the diagnosis of which is most readily confirmed by biopsy of the gum or rectal mucosa. In the absence of these associated conditions, patients with "benign monoclonal gammopathy" commonly remain stable and asymptomatic for many years and require no treatment, but in some instances the condition exists as the asymptomatic preclinical stage of plasma cell myeloma.

Heavy chain diseases are rare, having been first described by Franklin, who observed γ type H chains in the serum and urine of a patient with a lymphoma-like illness. A peculiar variant of H chain disease is the α type, which presents as a lymphoma of the small intestine in association with the signs and symptoms of sprue (Seligmann, 1975). The relationship is particularly intriguing because of the known abundance of IgA-secreting plasma cells in the normal gastrointestinal tract.

Therapy of the symptomatic M-component disorders is often successful and may arrest progression of the disease for years (Alexanian and co-workers, 1975). The chemotherapeutic agents of greatest utility have been alkylating agents (melphalan and cyclophosphamide) and adrenal glucocorticoids. Palliative radiation therapy is helpful for local bone pain and for such dread complications as spinal cord compression, for which surgical decompression may also be necessary.

Other Variants. *"Leukemic reticuloendotheliosis"* is now often considered a variant of lymphocytic lymphoma or chronic lymphatic leukemia, although as the name implies the abnormal cell was originally perceived as a reticuloendothelial cell, or macrophage (Naeim and Smith, 1974).

Because of the characteristic fringed cytoplasm of the neoplastic lymphoid cell seen by conventional microscopy, the disorder has earned the nickname *"hairy cell leukemia."* The neoplastic lymphoid cells infiltrate the bone marrow, spleen, and peripheral blood, but lymph node enlargement is not prominent. Splenectomy may be helpful. Resistance to chemotherapy has been the rule.

Mycosis fungoides and *Sézary syndrome* are two cutaneous variants of T cell lymphoma, the former characterized by a distinctive histologic feature of the skin (the "Pautrier abscess") and the latter by the presence in the peripheral blood of somewhat atypical convoluted lymphocytes containing a rim of PAS positive vacuoles surrounding the nucleus (Long and Mihm, 1974). Broder and co-workers have found that the Sézary syndrome is a neoplasia of functionally differentiated helper T cells which, as expected, are no longer positive for terminal transferase but do retain the characteristic surface markers. The cutaneous predilection may be the result of a "homing" instinct of this T cell subpopulation for the skin. Therapeutic responses to topical applications of nitrogen mustard have been explained by the hypersensitivity reaction evoked in the skin.

Pseudolymphoma. Some patients present clinical syndromes that lie in a twilight zone between lymphoma and chronic inflammatory states. These may be of a chronic autoimmune nature with an occasional subsequent lymphomatous transformation (e.g., *Sjögren's syndrome*). Others are idiopathic or drug-induced hypersensitivity states. Both clinicians and pathologists are faced with confusion and consternation in trying to arrive at a definite decision that only time will resolve. The term *"pseudolymphoma"* conveys the uncertainty. Lukes and Tindall have described the syndrome of *"immunoblastic lymphadenopathy,"* with lymph node enlargement, fever, sweats, an increase in polyclonal immunoglobulin, and a characteristic histopathologic picture. They postulate that it is a hypersensitivity state but allow that neoplastic transformation occasionally takes place. Chronic pulmonary lymphocytic infiltrates also fall in this general category (*lymphomatoid granulomatosis, lymphoid interstitial pneumonitis*) (Israel and associates, 1977). Similarly, lymphocytic infiltrations in the stomach, parotid, thyroid, or orbit may occasionally cause confusion in correctly distinguishing between a chronic inflammatory state and a lymphocytic lymphoma. Immunofluorescent staining of tissue sections to determine whether the lymphocyte population bears monoclonal or polyclonal surface immunoglobulin may help in sifting out the neoplastic conditions (Warnke and Levy, 1978).

THROMBOCYTES

STRUCTURE

In 1906, Wright first proposed that the megakaryocyte, a well-known but mysterious bone marrow giant cell, produced blood platelets. Numerous subsequent morphologic and kinetic studies have supported this proposal and shown that this cell plays a key role in hemostasis. The average megakaryocyte measures about $5000\,\mu^3$ in volume (Fig. 22–11) but cells almost twice that size and with diameters of more than 100 μ are often seen. Like other differentiated precursor cells, the megakaryocyte descends from a committed stem cell (CFU-M) programmed to undergo blast transformation to a megakaryoblast. This blast cell is morphologically similar to other blast cells, but the nucleus is engaged in rapid DNA synthesis without cell cleavage, so-called endomitosis. Within a few days, the blast cell has grown considerably in size, and the single dense nucleus may contain 2, 4, 8 or even 16 times the normal diploid content of DNA. At that time, further DNA synthesis and nuclear endomitosis cease and cellular maturation commences. The nucleus becomes lobulated and the cytoplasm increases in volume, both processes occurring in rough proportionality to the ploidy of the cell. Specific cytoplasmic organelles appear and the cytoplasm takes on a pale blue granular appearance. At this stage the cytoplasm becomes burrowed out by invaginated surface membrane which transforms the cytoplasm into a honeycomb of granulated fragments. These are then peeled off in long ribbons into the bone marrow sinusoids where they finally break up into individual platelets. After the lobulated megakaryocytic nucleus has become depleted of cytoplasm it is rapidly disposed of by macrophages.

As is true for the red blood cells, the newly formed platelets are larger than more mature forms, and careful sizing of blood platelets on a peripheral blood smear may provide information about the rate of platelet production. The mature platelets are disk-shaped, measure about 2 to 3 μ in diameter and are pale blue with a granular core. On electron microscopy (Fig. 22–128), the core is found to consist of glycogen granules, mitochondria, vacuoles, and various dense particles. The glycogen and mitochondria provide energy essential for viability and function. The vacuoles appear to be part of a spongelike canalicular system covered by interiorized phospholipid-containing surface membrane. This system facilitates the absorption of and interaction with various coagulation factors and also serves as a conduit for substances released from cytoplasm. Some of the dense particles, are enzyme-containing lysosomes, whereas others contain ADP and serotonin, which are released during aggregation. The platelets also contain a network of microfilaments which are organized into microtubules under the platelet membrane. These structures contain contractile proteins and may be responsible for the conversion from discoid to spherical shape which takes place during aggregation and subsequent clot retraction.

FUNCTION

Platelets constitute our first and foremost line of defense against accidental blood loss. They accumulate almost instantaneously at the site of a vascular injury and attempt first to provide a temporary seal by plugging the vascular leak and second to promote the formation of a permanent seal by making available an essential coagulation factor. The aggregation of non-sticky, circulating platelets into a firm platelet plug is a remarkable feat which is triggered by contact of the platelets to exposed subendothelial tissue, resulting in turn in phospholipase activation, prostaglandin and thromboxane synthesis, and the release of ADP. Observations in vitro, summarized by Zucker and by Deykin, have shown that the addition of small amounts of ADP to platelet-rich suspensions causes a change in the suspension stability, with smooth disk-shaped granulated platelets being transformed reversibly into aggregates of spiny, sticky degranulated spheres (Fig. 22–129). Large amounts of ADP will result in an irreversible aggregation of platelets, whereas intermediate amounts cause a characteristic biphasic response with aggregation, disaggregation, and renewed aggregation (Fig. 22–130). The second wave of aggregation is believed to be induced by endogenous ADP released from storage granules in the platelet. The addition of collagen to a platelet-rich suspension causes degranulation but only one wave of aggregation corresponding in time to the second ADP wave and believed to be due in part to collagen-induced release of endogenous ADP from platelets.

Prostaglandins E_2 and $F_{2\alpha}$ are formed during platelet aggregation, and the addition of aspirin or indomethacin will impair both prostaglandin formation and platelet aggregation (Smith and Willis, 1971). This basic observation has led to extensive studies, reviewed by Smith and Silver, of the role of prostaglandins in platelet function. It has been found that platelet aggregation activates a phospholipase which makes free arachidonic acid available to a platelet cyclo-oxygenase, transforming it to the short-lived but potent aggregating cyclic endoperoxides PGG_2 and PGH_2 (Fig. 22–131). This enzymatic transformation is inhibited by aspirin or indomethacin. The cyclic endoperoxides are either transformed to very

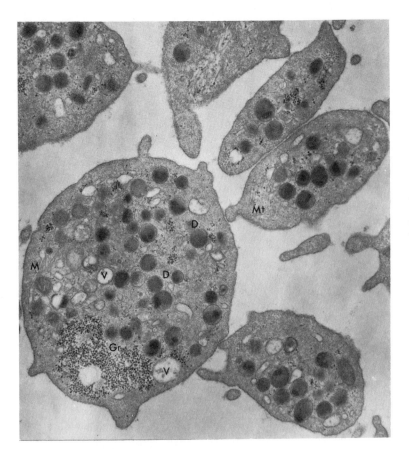

Figure 22–128 Electron microscopic picture of normal platelets showing dense particles (*D*), vacuoles (*V*), mitochondria (*M*), micro-tubules (*Mt*), and glycogen granules (*Gr*). (Courtesy of Dr. D. Zucker-Franklin.)

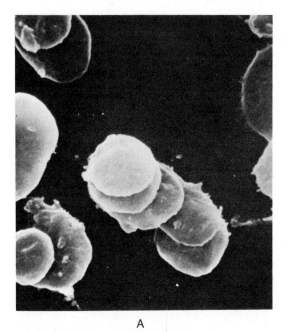

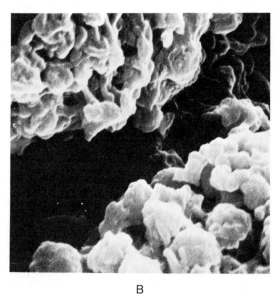

A   B

Figure 22–129 Pictures made by the scanning electron microscope of free disk-shaped platelets (*A*) and aggregates of spiny transformed platelets (*B*). (From Hovig, T.: Series Hematologica, *3*:47, 1970.)

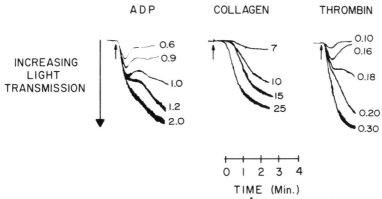

Figure 22–130 Aggregation of human platelets in citrated platelet-rich plasma at 37° C. ADP, collagen suspension, or thrombin was added (arrow) to give the fluid concentrations shown (μ moles/liter, μ liter/ml., or units/ml., respectively). Photometric recordings indicate the increase in light transmission as the platelets aggregate over a period of about 3 minutes. (Courtesy of Dr. D. C. B. Mills.)

small amounts of inactive prostaglandin PGE_2 or $PGF_{2\alpha}$ or by means of thromboxane synthetase to large amounts of another short-lived but potent aggregating agent, thromboxane TXA_2. These observations of in vitro activity provide the framework for our current concept of the mechanism responsible for the formation of a hemostatic platelet plug.

The initiating event in hemostasis is vascular injury with exposure of otherwise concealed collagen fibers to circulating blood (Fig. 22–132). Within a few seconds platelets passing by will adhere to the raw collagen fibers, become degranulated, and release ADP, prostaglandin intermediates, and serotonin, which in turn cause aggregation of new platelets, further ADP release, and further platelet aggregation. In this

fashion a chain reaction is established, with the formation of a firm platelet plug covering the vascular break. In addition, a phospholipoprotein, so-called platelet factor 3, is unmasked on the surface of the transformed platelets. This membrane-bound factor augments thrombin formation and results in the coating of the platelet plug with resilient fibrin and the formation of a white thrombus. Thrombin also causes platelet aggregation, prostaglandin synthesis, and ADP release and contributes to both the platelet and the fibrin phases in the formation of a hemostatic seal.

Recent studies by Moncada and co-workers have disclosed that normal vascular walls contain prostacyclin synthetase which transforms platelet endoperoxides into prostacyclin PGI_2 which actively inhibits platelet aggregation. The

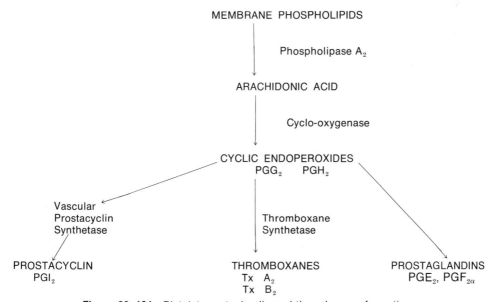

Figure 22–131 Platelet prostaglandin and thromboxane formation.

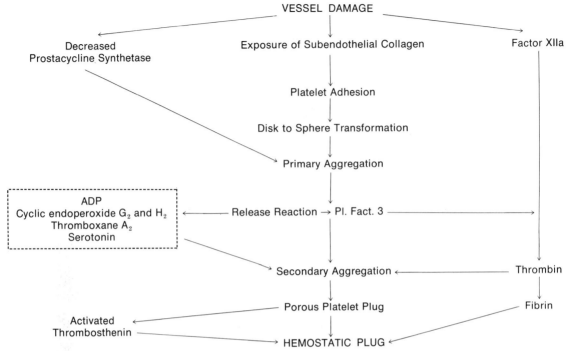

Figure 22–132 Formation of hemostatic platelet plug.

presence of this prostacyclin may provide a balance for the proaggregating endoperoxides and thromboxane A_2, and vessel injury could conceivably decrease the production of prostacyclin and thereby tilt the balance toward aggregation and clotting. A certain amount of intravascular coagulation and red thrombus formation takes place before the flow of blood has diluted and dissipated ADP, thrombin, and other procoagulants. Final clot retraction and consolidation are caused by thrombosthenin, a contractile platelet protein. Similar to other contractile proteins, it acts as an ATPase and requires ATP as an energy source. The release of prostaglandins, serotonin, and lysosomal enzymes during the early phase of platelet adhesion and aggregation is in part also responsible for the inflammatory reaction that may occur around a newly formed thrombus.

In addition to sealing vascular breaks, platelets appear to play an almost continuous role in maintaining normal vascular integrity. Patients with thrombocytopenia have a decreased capillary resistance, and petechiae appear following the slightest trauma or change in blood pressure. It seems probable that these petechiae are caused by superficial endothelial desquamations which under normal conditions are sealed immediately by platelets but in patients with thrombocytopenia remain open and permit the escape of a small amount of blood.

KINETICS

Until recently, kinetic studies of megakaryocytes and thrombocytes have appeared quite forbidding because of difficulties in quantitating the rate of production of platelets, the size of the circulating platelet mass, and the life span of individual platelets. However, careful planimetric measurements of megakaryocytes in bone marrow sections, the introduction of phase contrast microscopic measurements, automatic particle counting, and the use of random and cohort labeling with various isotopes have provided valuable and reproducible kinetic data. These data indicate that platelet production, like red cell production, is controlled by a feedback system which regulates the transformation of a committed but undifferentiated stem cell to a differentiated blast cell.

As previously emphasized, our current concept of the bone marrow stem cell pool is that it is made up of a multipotential compartment and several unipotential compartments, one of them committed to the megakaryocytic cell line (Fig. 22–7). The interrelationship between these compartments is not clear, but it appears that the multipotential stem cells are predominantly dormant (G_0) and are called into supportive action only if the committed stem cell compartments become depleted. Because increased erythropoiesis after blood loss or hemolysis is often associated with increased thrombopoiesis and under certain conditions with decreased granulocytopoiesis, questions have been raised, but not answered, about specific cooperation or competition among the committed stem cell compartments. In response to demands for platelets, the stem cells committed to megakaryocytes undergo blast transformation and differentiate to megakaryoblasts. During the next two to three days and before visible cytoplasmic maturation, the nucleus divides two to four times, resulting in the formation of a large blast cell. After the endomitotic division has ceased the nucleus becomes lobulated, the cytoplasm matures, granulated material segregates, and platelets are finally peeled off two to three days later. It has been estimated (Table 22–1) that the normal human bone marrow contains about 15×10^6 megakaryocytes per kg. body weight, with each megakaryocyte producing about 2000 to 7000 platelets. Since the average megakaryocytic volume is about 5000 μ^3, the total megakaryocytic mass is about $45 \times 10^9 \mu^3$ per kg. body weight, about one tenth the total mass of nucleated red cell precursors ($5 \times 10^9 \times 90\mu^3$). However, the daily production of platelets, about 2.5×10^9 per kg. body weight, is close to that of erythrocytes, about 3.1×10^9 per kg. body weight.

After the release from the bone marrow, the platelets will circulate for about eight to ten days before they are removed and destroyed by the macrophages, primarily in liver and spleen. During their circulating life span, the platelets are distributed between the spleen and the bloodstream. Aster has pointed out that, at any one time, about one third of the circulating platelets are present in the spleen, probably in a slow transit through the tortuous splenic cords rather than as trapped and starved cells. A transit time of merely 8 minutes would explain such a segregation of the total platelet mass between spleen and blood. It has been proposed that the youngest platelets are sequestered preferentially by the spleen but this may be due to a slower transit time of cells of larger size. Certainly, the sequestration of platelets in the spleen does not appear to last long enough to produce cellular injury, and splenic contraction induced by epinephrine will expel perfectly normal platelets into the circulation. The physiologic significance, if any, of the splenic pooling of platelets is not known, but its existence does explain that the platelet count almost invariably is higher in splenectomized than in normal individuals. In patients with splenomegaly, a significant proportion of the circulating platelets is slowly meandering through the large spleen, and although total platelet mass may be normal, the platelet count can be quite low. This splenomegalic thrombocytopenia is rarely as severe as thrombocytopenia caused by hypersplenic destruction of platelets. However, hemostasis depends on the number of circulating platelets, and if a large spleen cannot mobilize its content of platelets in time, the effect is the same as if the platelets had been permanently destroyed.

Since platelets are consumed during their function as hemostatic agents, it could have been anticipated that their destruction would be random rather than age-dependent. In other words, survival curves should be exponential rather than linear with time. Somewhat surprisingly, however, most studies of platelet life span utilizing random labels such as ^{51}chromium or cohort labels such as ^{32}phosphorus have indicated an age-dependent linear life span (Fig. 22–133). Furthermore, studies by Abrahamsen of individuals receiving anticoagulants have failed to show a change in the slope of the survival curve or a prolongation of the platelet life span. This would tend to rule out the existence of major continuous intravascular coagulation with random platelet utilization. However, the spread of the survival curve is wide enough to conceal the presence of some minor random utilization in addition to the major age-dependent destruction.

Under physiologic conditions, the platelet count and especially the platelet mass are kept constant, indicating the existence of a feedback system adjusting platelet production to platelet destruction. This feedback has a built-in delay that causes a considerable rebound thrombocytosis after induced thrombocytopenia and rebound thrombocytopenia after induced thrombocytosis (Fig. 22–134). The magnitude of this delay in humans can be estimated from careful measurements of the platelet count in patients who have undergone splenectomy. In such patients the platelet count tends to oscillate, with a period twice as long as the time it takes from the initiation of a signal for increased platelet production until the produced platelets have finished their life span. This oscillating pattern is occasionally very pronounced (Fig. 22–135), making it easy to discern a period which in most cases is quite uniform, about 28 days. Since the life span of platelets is about 10 days, the delay from the triggering effect of a stimulus until the platelet is released from the bone marrow must be around 4 days, which is about the time it takes for the megakaryoblast to mature into a megakaryocyte and release platelets. The stimulus could act either on the megakaryoblasts causing them to undergo additional endomitotic divisions, thereby increasing their volume, and producing more platelets, or it could act on committed stem cells causing the production of an increased number of megakaryoblasts. Since the megakaryocytes of patients with thrombocytopenia due to increased platelet destruction are both larger and more numerous than normal, Harker concluded that the

CIRCULATING PLATELET ^{51}Cr
(% of Maximum Value)

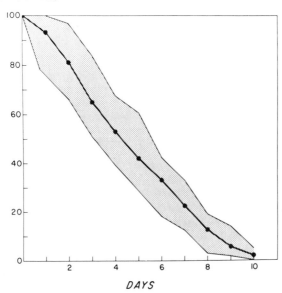

Figure 22–133   Survival of ^{51}Cr-labeled human platelets. Shaded area from 30 normal subjects. (From Aster, R. H.: J. Clin. Invest., 45:645, 1966.)

stimulus does both. It has also been suggested that the stimulus shortens maturation time, a suggestion more difficult to accept because the introduction of additional endomitotic divisions should lengthen the total maturation time, unless of course the generation time is cut way down.

Numerous investigators have suggested that the responsible stimulus is transmitted by a spe-cific humoral factor, a so-called thrombopoietin (Adams, et al., 1978). Evatt and Levin, followed by McDonald, were the first, however, to provide convincing experimental data in support of this suggestion. Utilizing ^{75}selenium methionine to label megakaryocytic cytoplasm, Levin and co-workers showed that injection into normal an-imals of serum from donors with thrombocyto-penia will cause a greater isotope incorporation

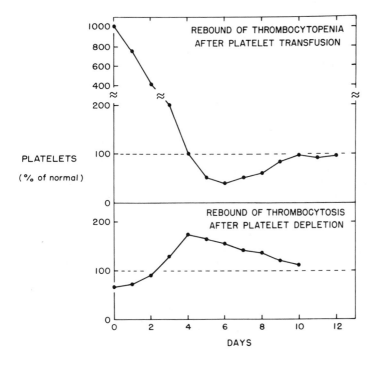

Figure 22–134   Rebound thrombo-cytopenia after platelet transfusion and rebound thrombocytosis after platelet depletion in normal rats. (Adapted from Odell, T. T., Jr., et al.: Acta Haematol., 38:34, 1967, and Odell, T. T., Jr., et al.: Acta Haematol., 27:171, 1962.)

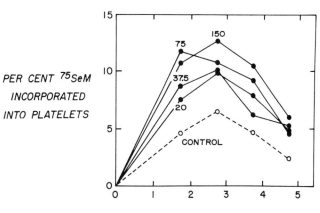

Figure 22-135 Effect of plasma from thrombocytopenic donor rabbits upon incorporation of selenomethionine-75 (^{75}SeM) into the platelets of rabbits previously transfused with platelet concentrates. The plasma, in volume from 20 ml. to 150 ml., was administered in three divided doses and ^{75}SeM was given 6 hours after the last infusion (solid lines). The broken line is the mean ^{75}SeM utilization in six platelet transfused control rabbits. (From Shreiner, D. P., and Levin, J.: J. Clin. Invest., *49*:1709, 1970.)

into new platelets than injections of serum from normal donors. The difference becomes more pronounced if endogenous thrombopoiesis of the recipient is suppressed by platelet transfusions (Fig. 22-135). Although the technique is similar to the technique which has been used successfully in the study of erythropoietin, the logistic problems of maintaining a preparatory thrombocytosis are so large that very little additional information about thrombopoietin has been obtained.

If a thrombopoietin controls the production of platelets, what controls the production of thrombopoietin? Obviously platelets are needed for the maintenance of vascular integrity and it would seem likely that impaired hemostasis causes the release of a thrombopoietin in the same way as impaired oxygenation of the kidney causes the release of erythropoietin. However, as shown by the age-dependent life span of platelets, most platelets do not get involved in hemostatic activities. Furthermore, hemostatic function remains normal until the platelet count is reduced far below the level at which a compensatory increase in platelet production is initiated. Finally, the patients with congestive splenomegaly in whom up to 80 per cent of the total platelet mass is in the spleen fail to show a compensatory increase in platelet production despite low circulating platelet count and impaired hemostatic function. These observations suggest that it is the platelet mass rather than the platelet count which triggers the release of thrombopoietin. On the other hand, it is very difficult to envision a sensor which can perceive the size of the platelet mass, distributed as it is between the spleen and the circulating blood. Furthermore, it seems possible that rather than being the number or mass, it is the surface area which is involved in sensing and adjusting the concentration of thrombopoietin. The platelet surface is well known to act as a sponge and absorb a variety of plasma factors. Actually, deGabriele and Penington have shown that thrombopoietic activity of plasma could be

removed by preincubation with normal platelets. Consequently, platelet function, mass, and surface have to be incorporated into the hypothetical model of the feedback circuit controlling platelet production and depicted in Figure 22-136.

PATHOPHYSIOLOGY

Classification and General Considerations

The thrombocytic disorders are usually classified according to number and function of platelets into "quantitative abnormalities" and "qualitative abnormalities" (Table 22-24).

In general, patients with platelets in inadequate numbers or with inadequate functional competence will have petechiae, hemorrhages, prolonged bleeding time, and impaired clot retraction. Since platelets are primarily responsible for hemostasis in small superficial vessels, petechiae are the hallmark of platelet deficiency disorders. Local pressure from tissue tension will tend to diminish blood loss from deep vessels, and the presence of many petechiae and hemorrhages on the skin or visible mucous membrane does not necessarily mean that similar bleedings are present throughout the body. Actually, deep bleedings into tissues or joint spaces are much more characteristic of a deficiency in coagulation proteins than of a deficiency in platelets. The minimal number of platelets needed for normal hemostasis is usually considered to be about 50,000 per cu. mm. However, spontaneous hemorrhages are rare until the platelet count is reduced to less than 20,000 per cu. mm. Observations by Karpatkin and others indicate that the hemostatic competence of young, large platelets is greater than that of old platelets, explaining that hemorrhagic problems tend to be less at a given platelet level for individuals with thrombocytopenia due to peripheral destruction than for those with thrombocytopenia due to decreased production.

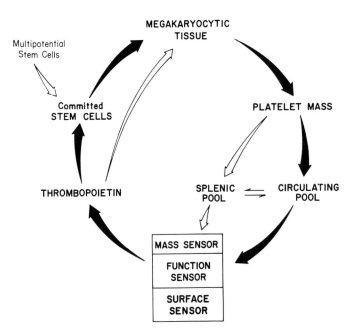

Multipotential
Stem Cells

Figure 22-136 Model of a feedback control system for platelets. (Adapted from Erslev, A. J.: Am. J. Pathol., 65:629, 1971.)

Elevated platelet counts are usually tolerated well but may cause either thrombosis or bleeding. The thrombotic tendency is probably related to an excessive hemostatic response to minor vascular injury, but the reason for the bleeding tendency in face of an increased number of functional platelets is still unknown.

Quantitative Abnormalities

Thrombocytopenia. *Decreased platelet production* occurs in a bewildering collection of congenital and acquired disorders. In some the pathogenesis has been unraveled but in most the

TABLE 22-24 CLASSIFICATION OF THROMBOCYTIC DISORDERS

I. *Quantitative Abnormalities*
    Thrombocytopenia
        Decreased production
            Congenital
            Acquired
                Megakaryocytic disorders
                Bone marrow replacement
        Increased destruction
            Immune
            Consumptive
        Uneven distribution
            Hypersplenism
    Thrombocytosis
        Reactive
        Myeloproliferative disorders
II. *Qualitative Abnormalities*
    Congenital
    Acquired

responsible dysfunction of the megakaryocytes awaits identification.

Of special interest among the many descriptions of individual cases is a report by Shulman and co-workers about a child with severe congenital thrombocytopenia who was found to respond to infusions of normal plasma with brief increases in platelet count and who for many years has been kept alive and functioning on regularly spaced plasma infusions. The responsible plasma factor was named thrombopoietin and was believed to cause maturation of existing megakaryocytes. Reevaluation of this case recently has suggested a link to thrombotic thrombocytopenic purpura and to the responsiveness of this disease to plasma.

Acquired abnormalities of megakaryocytes causing moderately severe thrombocytopenia are usually found in patients with megaloblastic anemia due to folic acid or B_{12} deficiency, and specific treatment causes a prompt return of platelet count to normal. Patients with chronic alcoholism also may have maturation problems of both nucleated red cells and megakaryocytes, but the cause is difficult to pinpoint, since such patients usually suffer from a multitude of nutritional deficiencies and hepatic abnormalities. Nevertheless, metabolic studies by Post and Des Forges have demonstrated that one cause may be alcohol itself, which apparently impairs megakaryocytic function directly. Although iron deficiency has been associated with thrombocytopenia, thrombocytosis is observed far more commonly. If decreased platelet production is found in iron-deficient patients, it is usually assumed that complicating deficiencies of folic acid or B_{12} are responsible.

Viral infections and exposures to certain drugs are often associated with megakaryocytic dysfunction and thrombocytopenia. During pregnancy, such infections and exposures may lead to neonatal thrombocytopenia, usually of short duration. However, if the bone marrow insult occurs during the first trimester, a specific syndrome characterized by *amegakaryocytic thrombocytopenia*, malfunction of the heart, and absence of the radius may occur. Since the megakaryocytes, heart, and radius all appear at about the sixth to eighth week of gestation, an infectious or toxic insult at that time may explain the development of this seemingly unrelated triad. In both children and adults, viral infections frequently cause thrombocytopenia. For example, inoculation with live measles vaccine will, as Oski and Naiman have shown, regularly cause a temporary decrease in platelet production. As a general principle, a self-limited viral infection should always be suspected as the etiology in every patient with unexplained thrombocytopenia. Despite this frequent association, drugs are actually the most common cause of defective platelet production. The many myelosuppressive agents used in the treatment of neoplastic and autoimmune disorders make up the majority of drugs causing thrombocytopenia. The anticipated response to such drugs is a general bone marrow suppression, but certain drugs such as cytosine arabinoside and busulfan have a reputation for causing particularly marked suppression of platelet production. More capricious and still unexplained is the mild megakaryocytic suppression which may follow the use of thiazide diuretics. It has recently been suggested that they may bring about a process of immunologic "rejection" of megakaryocytes akin to the "rejection" of nucleated red cells observed in patients with pure red cell aplasia. However, drug-induced immunologic injury of megakaryocytes is a far less common cause for thrombocytopenias than drug-induced, immunologic destruction of circulating platelets.

Among disorders of *increased destruction*, antibodies play a prominent role. Immunologic destruction of platelets can cause thrombocytopenia at any age. In the newborn the pathogenetic mechanism is similar to that causing erythroblastosis fetalis inasmuch as an antibody produced in the mother crosses the placenta and causes destruction of the infant's platelets. During pregnancy and at time of delivery, platelets from the fetus pass into the circulatory system of the mother, and if they contain antigens different from hers, they will evoke an antibody response. The subsequent transfer of the antibody across the placenta results in platelet destruction and thrombocytopenia. Such isoimmune thrombocytopenia does not depend on ABO or Rh incompatibility but on incompatibility in the platelet specific antigens (Pl^{A1}) or the more general HL-A tissue antigen system. Since tests for antigens and antibodies in this system are time-consuming and difficult, the diagnosis is usually made by exclusion. First, thrombocytopenia due to infections has to be ruled out immediately. Maternal viremia can cause changes in the fetal production and destruction of platelets, and bacteremia in the newborn may be associated with disseminated intravascular coagulation and thrombocytopenia. Other infectious etiologies to be excluded are congenital syphilis, toxoplasmosis, cytomegalic inclusion disease, and rubella. Second, the possibility that the mother has idiopathic thrombocytopenic purpura with an anti-platelet autoantibody crossing the placenta and non-specifically attacking the infant's platelets must be excluded by obtaining a thorough history and a platelet count on the mother. Finally, maternal drug ingestion must be looked into as a possible cause.

In children and adults, the cause for immunologic destruction of platelets is usually idiopathic, but the possibility that it is drug related should always be considered. Quinidine is the most widely recognized offender, and its mechanism of action is slowly being unraveled. When attached to a protein the drug acts as a hapten, causing the production of antibodies in sensitized individuals. It was first assumed that the hapten attached itself to a platelet protein and that this hapten-platelet complex elicited and responded to antibody. However, recent data suggest that the hapten is bound to a plasma protein carrier and that it is this complex which elicits and combines with antibody. The subsequent binding of the antigen-antibody complex to platelet membrane is due to a chance affinity between the immune complex and the membrane, and the platelet is actually an "innocent bystander" in the immunologic reaction (Fig. 22–137). Unfortunately for the platelets the coating with antigen-antibody complexes causes agglutination, complement-fixation, and destruction. A great number of drugs have been implicated in immunologic platelet destruction but only in a few instances have in-vivo and in-vitro testing convincingly shown a drug to be causative. (Miescher, 1973). In addition to quinidine, quinine, stibophen, digitoxin, methyldopa, sulfonamides, sedormid and gold have been so identified. The association of aspirin or birth control pills with thrombocytopenia has been of interest, but the possibility of a mere coincidence rather than a cause-effect relationship has not been ruled out. In order to establish a diagnosis of drug-induced thrombocytopenia several in-vitro tests have been developed. These are based on finding impaired platelet function after the addition of the drug to the patient's plasma. Inhibition of normal clot retraction is the easiest test (Fig. 22–138) but it is less sensitive than tests depending on agglutination,

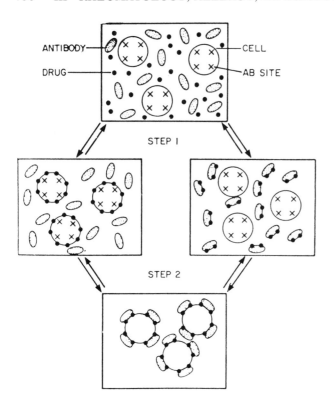

ANTIBODY

DRUG

CELL

AB SITE

STEP 1

STEP 2

Figure 22–137 Possible mechanism for drug-induced and other immunologic thrombocytopenias. *Left,* the platelets are directly involved by initially being coated by antigen. *Right,* the platelets act as "innocent bystanders." (From Shulman, N. R.: Ann. Intern. Med., *60:*506, 1964.)

lysis, complement fixation, or release of platelet factor 3.

Idiopathic thrombocytopenic purpura (ITP) is a disorder characterized by increased platelet destruction in an otherwise healthy individual. In childhood, ITP is usually acute and time-limited, and many studies have related it immunologically to a preceding viral infection. In adults, ITP is usually chronic and, although also believed to be immunologically determined, its etiology is still truly idiopathic.

Acute thrombocytopenia may follow well-established viral infections such as rubella, rubeola, or chicken pox, but in most cases the preceding illness consists merely of a mild respiratory or gastrointestinal upset, so frequently experienced in childhood that it is often overlooked. The thrombocytopenia is usually first noticed after the "viral symptoms" have subsided, suggesting that the platelet injury is caused by antibodies rather than by the virus itself. It has been proposed that platelet antibodies are elicited by platelet membranes antigenetically altered by the attachment of viral particles. However, similar to the mechanism believed to operate in drug-induced thrombocytopenia, the platelets may merely be "innocent bystanders" with a fatal affinity for viral antigen-antibody complexes. In either case, the antibody production and action would depend on the presence of a circulating viral antigen, and the disease would be of limited

duration. Complete recovery can be expected if the patient is carried through the dangerous thrombocytopenic period by the judicious use of careful observation, protection against trauma, platelet transfusions, and corticosteroids. Splenectomy, although undoubtedly effective, need rarely be contemplated in the acute time-limited ITP of childhood.

The chronic variety of ITP is a disease of adults, although children who fail to recover from acute ITP must be included. Like acute ITP, it is believed to be immunologically induced, but if a foreign antigen is involved, this antigen must be an almost permanent component of the body, since the disease despite remissions is rarely cured. The thrombocytopenia often found in association with disseminated lupus erythematosus is considered an ITP, since its pathogenesis is still clearly idiopathic.

The immunologic nature of this disorder was first suspected when Harrington and co-workers found that plasma or its gamma globulin fraction from patients with chronic ITP caused thrombocytopenia when infused into normal subjects. Supportive evidence for the existence of an autoimmune mechanism was provided by the fact that infants of mothers with chronic ITP often have transient thrombocytopenia at birth and that in-vitro immunologic tests indicate the presence of an antiplatelet antibody in plasma from a large number of patients with chronic ITP. So far the antibody has reacted with all platelets, regardless of antigenic composition, and it appears that it is directed against a common platelet component rather than a type-specific antigen. The agent responsible for the production of autoantibodies is unknown, but the life-long presence of certain viral antigens in tissue cells makes a viral etiology an attractive hypothesis.

The severity of chronic ITP and its response to splenectomy seems to be dependent on the amount of antibody coating the platelets. Heavy coating will cause agglutination with easy recognition, sequestration, and destruction by all macrophages, and splenectomy by removing merely a fraction of these will be of only moderate therapeutic benefit. Light coating, however, will not cause significant agglutination of circulating platelets, and only the spleen with its slow percolation of blood through vessels densely lined with macrophages will recognize, sequester and destroy coated platelets. In this condition, splenectomy will be of definite benefit, and the life span and function of lightly coated platelets will be almost normal after surgery. In a few cases the titer of antiplatelet antibodies has decreased

after splenectomy, suggesting that the spleen preferentially produces these antibodies and that splenectomy not only removes a filter but also eliminates a major site of antiplatelet antibody production (McMillan, et al., 1974).

One of the most controversial findings in chronic ITP has been the presence of megakaryocytes of unusual morphologic appearance. Not only are they increased in number, as would be expected as a compensation for increased destruction of mature platelets, but many are immature, devoid of intracytoplasmic demarcations, and show no evidence of active platelet production (Fig. 22–139). It has been suggested that the antibody to circulating platelets also reacts with megakaryocytes and prevents platelet formation. However, platelet turnover studies show an increased rate of platelet production, and it seems more likely that accelerated thrombopoietic activity causes an early release of platelets from still immature cells and a shift to the left in the megakaryocytic series. The presence of unusually large platelets in the blood of patients with chronic ITP also suggests a hurried production with the release of unfinished pieces of megakaryocytic cytoplasm.

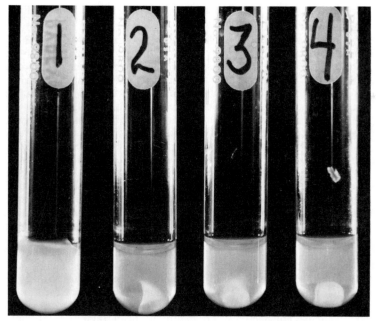

Figure 22–138 A positive clot retraction inhibition test in a patient with quinidine-induced purpura. The four test tubes were prepared as follows:

	Serum	Quinidine	Normal Platelet-Rich Plasma
(1)	Patient	+	+
(2)	Patient	−	+
(3)	Control	+	+
(4)	Control	−	+

After one hour of incubation, CaCl$_2$ was added, and the degree of clot retraction inhibition was observed one hour later. Inhibition of clot retraction is seen in tube 1.

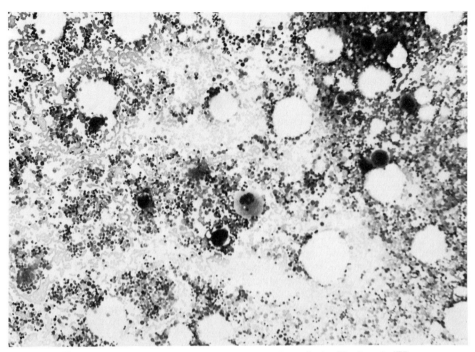

Figure 22–139 Megakaryocytic hyperplasia in patient with chronic ITP.

The clinical manifestations of chronic ITP are determined entirely by the number of available platelets, and the treatment is directed toward maintaining the number at an asymptomatic level. As expected, platelet transfusions are of very brief effect, since transfused platelets are destroyed as fast as endogenous platelets. Adrenocortical steroids are usually quite effective in increasing the platelet count in patients with chronic ITP. They may act by suppressing phagocytic activity, but the exact reason for their beneficial effect still has not been established (Claman, 1972). In patients who do not respond to steroids with an increase in platelet count, the bleeding manifestations are nevertheless reduced, as if the steroids in some way enhance capillary stability. In the treatment of chronic ITP, steroids usually are administered for a few months in the hope that the disease will remit spontaneously. If the thrombocytopenia recurs immediately after discontinuation of the drug or if the patient is only partly responsive, splenectomy is the treatment of choice. Splenectomy will result in a sustained improvement in 70 to 90 per cent of patients. In almost all, the operation will be followed by a brief thrombocytosis which reaches its peak at about the tenth day and then slowly decreases over the next few months (Fig. 22–140). This sequence corresponds well to the fact that in the absence of the spleen the platelets produced by the increased number of megakaryocytes live a normal 10-day life span, and it suggests that it must take some time to adjust the number of megakaryocytes in the bone marrow to the actual need for platelets in the circulation. Postsplenectomy thrombocytosis is of concern in patients in whom postoperative complications force them to rest immobile in bed, and in such patients the use of preventive anticoagulants or platelet antiaggregating agents may be indicated. It is assumed that platelets of patients who do not derive lasting benefit from splenectomy are so heavily coated with antibody that they are removed by the total mononuclear phagocyte system, not merely by the spleen. In such patients, immunosuppression has been attempted using drugs developed for the treatment of neoplastic disorders. In some patients gratifying remissions have been obtained especially after the use of vincristine, but the decision to use these potentially leukemogenic agents certainly has to be made with great reluctance and only if other methods of treatment fail.

Post-transfusion purpura is an unusual syndrome consisting of a temporary period of thrombocytopenia with onset about a week after blood transfusion. The disorder occurs only in individuals lacking the platelet-specific antigen (Pl^{A1}), a circumstance found in only 1 to 2 per cent of the population. The presence of this antigen in platelet material present in the transfused blood evokes the production of an antibody in the recipient. Immune complexes adhere to the patient's own platelets ("innocent bystanders") bringing

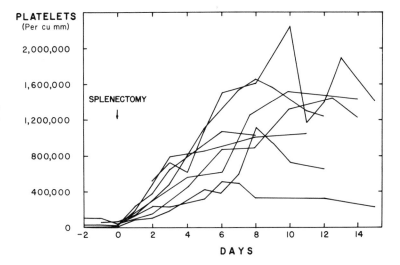

Figure 22–140 Thrombocytosis following splenectomy in patients with ITP.

about their destruction as in quinidine purpura. Spontaneous remission occurs when the immune complexes are cleared from the circulation.

Non-immunologic destruction of circulating platelets in bacterial or viral infections is often difficult to separate from immunologic destruction since these infections may be associated with both. However, non-immunologic destruction usually occurs at the height of the infectious illness and is accompanied by decreased levels of several coagulation proteins such as fibrinogen and Factors V and VIII. The pathogenesis is believed to be increased platelet consumption due to *disseminated intravascular coagulation* (DIC) (Deykin, 1970). Despite the presence of purpura and increased bleeding tendency, heparin may be the treatment of choice whenever laboratory studies indicate an increased rate of consumption of platelets and coagulation proteins. The thrombocytopenia characterizing *"thrombotic thrombocytopenic purpura"* or the *"hemolytic uremic syndrome"* is probably caused by excessive intravascular deposition of platelets in cerebral and renal vessels. However, there is little evidence of excessive consumption of coagulation proteins and it appears that these diseases are caused by a platelet or vascular wall dysfunction due to the absence of a plasma factor. The recent therapeutic use of exchange transfusions and of plasma infusions appears most promising in these otherwise highly fatal diseases (Byrnes and Khurana, 1977).

Thrombocytopenia is observed regularly in patients with splenomegaly, and in the past many explanations were given for the development of this *hypersplenic thrombocytopenia*. The most obvious explanation for the thrombocytopenia would appear to be increased platelet destruction by the large spleen, but this explanation was made untenable some years ago when Cohen,

Gardner, and Barnett found that the platelet life span in patients with hypersplenic thrombocytopenia was normal. The alternate explanation, that platelet production was decreased owing to the effect of megakaryocytic inhibitors released by the large spleen, was also found to be untenable because platelet turnover studies did not suggest a decreased rate of platelet production. Recent studies by Aster of platelet kinetics have provided a third and much more likely explanation.

As described earlier, the spleen, because of its tortuous vascular channels, always contains a considerable number of platelets in slow transit. In patients with splenomegaly, the transit time becomes longer, and instead of containing about 30 per cent of all circulating platelets, a large spleen may contain up to 80 per cent of the platelets. Since platelet production appears to be aimed at maintaining a constant total platelet mass, the uneven distribution of platelets between spleen and circulating blood is not being compensated for by an increased rate of platelet production, and the splenomegalic patient will stay thrombocytopenic. This explanation is supported by the observation that the infusion of platelets to patients with hypersplenic thrombocytopenia results in lower peripheral recovery than normal (Fig. 22–141) and that large numbers of viable platelets can be mobilized from an intact spleen by giving epinephrine and from an excised spleen by flushing its vascular system with saline. Supporting evidence is also provided by the fact that hypersplenic thrombocytopenia is not always proportional to the size of the spleen but is more closely related to its vascularity. For example, congestive splenomegaly secondary to liver cirrhosis is usually associated with lower platelet counts than "meaty" splenomegaly secondary to lymphomas or lipidosis. The potential availabili-

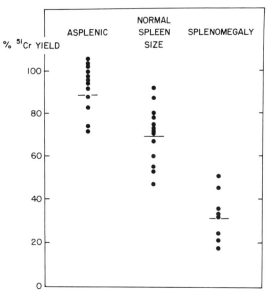

Figure 22–141   Recovery of transfused platelets in the circulating blood of asplenic patients, normal patients, and patients with congestive splenomegaly. (Gardner, F.: Clin. Haematol., *1*:307, 1972.)

ty of splenic platelets and the distributional limits to the number of platelets which can be present in the spleen make this thrombocytopenia rather mild and rarely in need of treatment per se.

Thrombocytosis. Thrombocytosis occurs as an obscure reactive response to a number of illnesses and as a manifestation of the myeloproliferative syndrome. A high platelet count is a useful diagnostic clue in patients with anemia, since iron deficiency regularly causes an increase in platelet production, and counts in excess of one million per cu. mm. may be found in children with nutritional iron deficiency anemia. Other conditions in which a high platelet count may be of diagnostic help are Hodgkin's disease, disseminated malignant diseases, and chronic inflammatory disorders (Schloesser, et al., 1965; Tranum and Haut, 1974; and Marchasin, et al., 1964). Pronounced thrombocytosis with levels of several millions per cu. mm. is usually seen only after splenectomy or in myeloproliferative disorders, such as polycythemia vera, myelofibrosis, chronic myelogenous leukemia, or essential thrombocytosis. The clinical manifestations of very high platelet counts consist of a capricious combination of thrombotic episodes and increased bleeding tendency. The thromboses are probably caused by aggregation and platelet factor 3 release by the expanded platelet mass, but the bleeding tendency is more difficult to explain. Cardamone and co-workers have found a platelet

dysfunction in some cases, but in most cases the only abnormality found has been an increase in the number of circulating platelets.

Qualitative Abnormalities

Qualitative abnormalities of platelet function have been found in a confusing collection of rare hereditary disorders and more commonly in uremia or after ingestion of certain drugs such as aspirin, antihistamines, and antiinflammatory agents. The inherited disorder most often found is *von Willebrand's disease* described in the next chapter. *Glanzmann's thrombasthenia* is seen more rarely and is characterized by a prolonged bleeding time, impaired clot retraction, and absent ADP-induced aggregation. The number and morphology of platelets and megakaryocytes are normal, but the patients suffer from a mild, lifelong increased bleeding tendency. Impaired platelet glycolysis with decreased ATP production and decreased reductive capacity has been found in some cases (Karpatkin and Weiss, 1972), whereas in others the adsorption of fibrinogen to platelets appears to be defective. *Storage pool disease* is a recently recognized congenital disorder of platelet formation (Holmsen and Weiss, 1972). The platelets respond to exogenous ADP with a normal first-phase aggregation, but fail to release endogenous ADP in response to collagen (second-phase aggregation). The number of ADP-containing dense particles is diminished, suggesting that the basic abnormality is a defect in the production, packaging, or storing of ADP. The clinical consequences are mild, and consist primarily of increased bruising and excessive bleeding after trauma or surgery. The so-called *thrombopathies* are congenital platelet disorders with even less of a common metabolic denominator than the thrombasthenias. The platelets may be larger than normal in size, so-called *Bernard-Soulier syndrome,* or they may be defective in platelet factor 3 activity, in ADP release, in adhesive capacity, and so on, but so far the cases are collectors' items and have failed to provide unifying clues.

Of the acquired disorders of platelet function, the clinically most important is the disorder found associated with chronic renal failure. Purpura and increased bleeding tendency are important manifestations of uremia and occur regularly despite normal platelet counts. Platelets from affected individuals have been found to be lacking in platelet factor 3 activation. However, of probably greater significance is the finding that these platelets fail to aggregate normally in response to ADP. Intensive dialysis rectifies this response and also normalizes the bleeding time, and it seems most likely that a retention product of small molecular size is responsible for the platelet defect. Horowitz has proposed that this chemical is guanidinosuccinic acid, a metabolite of urea, but definite proof is still lacking. The effect of aspirin on in-vitro platelet function is quite remarkable. The ingestion of only one to two aspirin tablets will cause a week-long impairment in the release of platelet ADP in response to collagen or other aggregating agents such as epinephrine. Studies by Roth and Majerus suggest that this impaired ADP release may be caused by irreversible aspirin-induced acetylation of platelet cyclo-oxygenase necessary for the transformation of arachidonic acid to prostaglandin endoperoxides. Although aspirin clinically has been associated with an increased bleeding tendency, it must be conceded that bleeding problems, despite the striking in-vitro changes, are rare among the millions who daily consume aspirin preparations.

PLASMA COAGULATION FACTORS

NORMAL STRUCTURE AND FUNCTION

WHITE AND RED THROMBI

The circulatory system is self sealing, thanks to the clotting ability of the blood and the contractility of the vascular wall. Leakages ranging from pinpoint hemorrhages to life-threatening exsanguination may occur when the coagulation mechanism breaks down. On the other hand, the pathologic formation of clots within the intact circulatory system is equally serious. The cause and nature of clot formation within the circulatory system vary with the site. The "white thrombus," consisting of platelets trapped in a fibrin meshwork, forms in rapid-flow arterial systems at points where the continuity of the endothelial lining is interrupted. The "red thrombus" has a white head with growth downstream of a red tail and is found in the venous system as a result of stasis of blood flow. Clots in large vessels are likely to undergo fibrous organization and recanalization, whereas those formed in the microvasculature are dissolved by virtue of the presence in the vascular wall of potent activators of the fibrinolytic system.

Although platelets are the "prime movers" in the formation of the white thrombus, the substance and strength of the clot, whether white or red, lie in the physical nature of the fibrin polymer which is formed as the end-product of a complex and controlled series of sequential reactions of the plasma coagulation factors. The nomenclature of the plasma coagulation factors has undergone revision over the years. Current and past usage is summarized in Table 22–25. Factors V and VII through XIII are in fact most commonly designated by their numbers today, while Factors I and II are generally called fibrinogen and prothrombin, respectively. There is no Factor VI. Factor III is tissue thromboplastin and should not be confused with platelet factor 3.

The cascade hypothesis has provided a conceptual framework that pictures the coagulation factors existing in an inactive (or procoagulant) and active state. The active form of one factor specifically activates the next one in line in a sequential series of controlled reactions, giving rise to a cascade, or "waterfall" effect. The process of activation is accomplished for most of the factors by the enzymatic splitting off of a small piece of the inactive procoagulant. There is progressive acceleration and amplification of the chain of reactions culminating in the formation of the fibrin clot. Most of the activated clotting factors (designated "a") are serine proteases, which are a family of protein-cleaving enzymes with serine at their active centers. Factors V, VIII, XIII, and fibrinogen are notable exceptions. Coagulation factor serine proteases have a high degree of substrate specificity. Plasmin is also a serine protease with the major function of cleaving fibrin and fibrinogen.

Fibrinogen

Fibrinogen, the raw material for the production of the clot, is a major constitutent of the plasma, with a normal concentration of 200 to 400 mg. per

TABLE 22–25 PLASMA COAGULATION FACTORS AND THEIR SYNONYMS

Factor I	Fibrinogen
Factor II	Prothrombin
Factor III	Tissue thromboplastin
Factor IV	Calcium
Factor V	Proaccelerin
Factor VII	Proconvertin; SPCA
Factor VIII	Antihemophilic Factor (AHF)
Factor IX	Plasma thromboplastin component (PTC), Christmas factor
Factor X	Stuart-Prower factor
Factor XI	Plasma thromboplastin antecedent (PTA)
Factor XII	Hageman factor
Factor XIII	Fibrin stabilizing factor

100 ml. The other plasma factors, present in much lower concentration, stand poised as the parts of a loaded gun with trigger cocked, aimed at fibrinogen. Most of the body pool of fibrinogen circulates in the plasma with a catabolic rate having a half-life of four days. The plasma concentration readily increases secondary to a large number of stimuli, including pregnancy, acute or chronic inflammatory states, and injury or surgical operation. The increase is entirely accounted for by increased synthesis, which takes place in the liver.

Fibrinogen spends an uneasy existence in the plasma, circulating between the forces of clot promotion, represented by thrombin, and those of clot dissolution, represented by plasmin. Its molecular weight of 340,000 is equally divided between two identical subunits centrally bound together to give the molecule a symmetrical mirror-image structure (Fig. 22–142). Each of the subunits consists of an Aα, a Bβ, and a γ polypeptide chain, the N-terminal ends of which are bound together into a "disulfide knot." Thrombin acts enzymatically on fibrinogen at arginyl-glycyl bonds by splitting off small pieces from the N-terminal ends of the Aα and Bβ chains amounting to about 3 per cent of the total molecular weight. The pieces split off are called fibrinopeptides A and B, respectively, with fibrinopeptide A released at a more rapid rate than B. Their cleavage from the parent molecule leaves behind "fibrin monomer," which then rapidly undergoes intermolecular association to form hydrogen-bonded polymers. The clot is finally strengthened by the action of Factor XIIIa. This causes strong linkage between adjacent fibrin strands through crosslinking peptide bonds which join γ and α chains in an intermolecular association. Such "stabilization" renders the clot insoluble in 5 M urea and rather more resistant to plasmin digestion.

Certain snake venoms resemble thrombin in their action on fibrinogen. Pit viper venom hydrolyzes only the Aα polypeptide chains, releasing fibrinopeptide A. The parent molecule, like fibrin monomer, polymerizes into a clot. However, the clot is weak and is readily dissolved through the action of plasmin.

In contrast to the limited fibrinogen degradation which sets off its polymerization into a firm clot, the degradative process of clot dissolution by plasmin involves a much more aggressive attack upon the molecule at multiple points in its structure. Plasmin (or "fibrinolysin") is an enzyme which resembles trypsin in its breadth of action as an endopeptidase which splits lysine and arginine bonds. Like trypsin, it attacks a variety of proteins, including plasma proteins. It is active at neutral pH; trypsin has a more alkaline pH optimum. The circulating plasma proteins are not physiologically exposed to its broadly destructive propensity, since it circulates as an inactive precursor, plasminogen, which is activated locally at the site of clot deposition. Plasmin attacks fibrinogen with the same fervor that characterizes its assault upon fibrin. The degradation products of the two cannot be distinguished and therefore are referred to as fibrinogen-fibrin degradation products, or "split products."

During the initial degradation of fibrinogen by plasmin, its molecular weight is reduced from 340,000 to 270,000 with the release of low molecular weight fragments from the carboxy-terminal ends of the Aα chains and the amino terminal ends of the Bβ chains (Fig. 22–143). The latter fragments contain the B fibrinopeptides. The macromolecular structure which remains, called fragment X, retains the property of engaging in clot formation after exposure to thrombin. However, in comparison to fibrin monomer, it clots slowly and its presence weakens the clot structure. Fragment X undergoes additional cleavage by

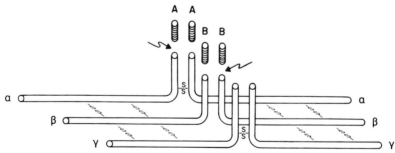

Figure 22–142 Schematic illustration of the molecular structure of fibrinogen. Three pairs of polypeptide chains (Aα, Bβ, and γ) are symmetrically arranged with their N-terminal regions joined in the "N-terminal disulfide knot." The C-terminal regions are represented here at opposite ends of the molecule, although they may actually be juxtaposed in the three dimensional orientation of the globular molecule. Thrombin cleavages release fibrinopeptides A and B, as shown by the arrows. Thus, the structure of fibrinogen is (AαBβγ)₂ and that of fibrin monomer is (αβγ)₂. Disulfide bonding is symbolically represented; the N-terminal disulfide knot alone has 12 bonds. (Adapted from Marder, V. J., and Budzynski, A. Z.: Schweiz. Med. Wochenschr. *104*:1338, 1974.)

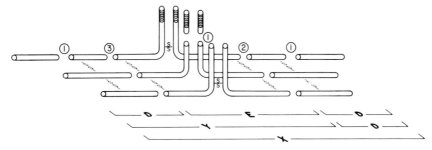

Figure 22–143 The degradation of fibrinogen by plasmin. The first stage (1) releases small fragments, including fibrinopeptide B, leaving behind fragment X. In the second stage (2) fragment X is asymmetrically reduced to fragments D and Y. The third stage (3) results in further breakdown of fragment Y to fragments D and E. The latter contains the N-terminal disulfide knot.

plasmin, with further reduction of molecular weight to derivatives designated fragment Y (MW 155,000) and fragment D (MW 90,000). Both of these fragments are nonclottable, but they interfere with fibrin strand formation and are potent anticoagulants. As degradation goes on to completion, fragment Y is further reduced to fragments D and E. The latter contains the N-terminal disulfide knot, has a MW of 55,000, and is relatively less active with regard to its anticoagulant effect.

Excessive action of plasmin in vivo is best detected by demonstrating elevated levels of fibrinogen-fibrin degradation products in serum from which all clottable material has been completely removed in the presence of a fibrinolytic inhibitor. Although excess plasmin activity most commonly occurs secondary to abnormal clotting, a high level of "split products" does not distinguish primary from secondary fibrinolysis. The presence of soluble complexes of fibrin monomer polymerized with fibrinogen-fibrin degradation products into higher molecular weight derivatives clearly signals that the increased plasmin activity was preceded by excessive action of thrombin on fibrinogen. These soluble complexes are demonstrated in plasma by tests for "paracoagulation." These include precipitation after addition of protamine sulfate, reversible insolubility in the cold (hence the term "cryofibrinogen"), and gelation after addition of ethanol. Nossel has proposed that excessive action of thrombin on fibrinogen in vivo might also be detected by an assay of the plasma for its content of fibrinopeptide A.

Plasminogen

Plasminogen is present in the plasma at a concentration of 10 to 20 mg. per 100 ml. Potent and specific plasminogen activators are present in many tissues and body fluids. As an example, the plasminogen activator of the urinary tract keeps this system free of clots and the potential disaster they could cause by obstructing the flow of urine. Especially large quantities of plasminogen activators are found in white cell lysosomes, from which they are released with difficulty, and also in the endothelial cells which line the vascular walls, from which release easily occurs. The development of a fibrin clot causes a rapid release of plasminogen activator into the clot, where it converts plasminogen to plasmin (Fig. 22–144). Plasmin thus appears mostly at the site of the clot, with relatively little spilling over into the general circulation. Plasmin is unstable and its activity soon disappears. Circulating plasmin inhibitors also contribute to the systemic protection of fibrinogen and other plasma proteins. Since the ratio of surface endothelium to cross-sectional area is greatest in the microcirculation, this is the site within the circulatory system with the greatest potential for plasminogen activation and complete clot dissolution.

A variety of influences other than fibrin deposition also bring about the release of plasminogen activators from the endothelium. These include exercise, acute stress of almost any kind, and pharmacologic and other kinds of vasoreactive stimuli. The increase in plasma fibrinolytic activity, however, is transient and mild, since the plasminogen activators are rapidly cleared from the plasma by the liver with a half-life of only 13 minutes. The impairment of this clearing mechanism will lead to somewhat less transient and less mild degrees of systemic fibrinolysis, a situation which arises in shock or in the presence of liver disease, as described by Hillenbrand and associates.

Surface Activation

Rupture of the endothelial lining of blood vessels exposes collagen and initiates thrombus formation. The fibrin clot is laid down as the end result of the recognition of the altered surface by Factor XII, which then becomes activated. Beyond its role in initiating clot formation, Fac-

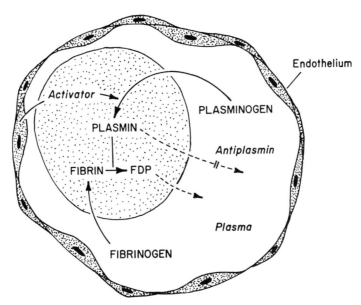

Figure 22–144 The local activation of plasminogen at the site of fibrin clot within a small blood vessel. (*FDP =* fibrin degradation products.)

tor XIIa also initiates reactions leading to the formation of vasoactive peptides (kinins) and plasmin and to the activation of the complement system. Despite the fact that Factor XII stands at the central point of this variety of events important to the defensive inflammatory response, inherited deficiency of this factor produces no clinical consequences, even though laboratory parameters such as the partial thromboplastin time are abnormal. A possible explanation may lie in the existence of "back-up" systems and "built-in safeguards," requirements of any skillfully engineered system which must be free from

failure. But the nature of these safeguards is still not understood.

Normal clotting in vitro is dependent on the kallikrein-kinin system, since deficiency of prekallikrein (Fletcher factor) or of high molecular weight kininogen (Fitzgerald factor) causes an abnormal prolongation of the partial thromboplastin time (Figure 22–145) (Donaldson and coworkers, 1976). Like Factor XII deficiency, lack of either of these factors causes no abnormal clinical effects, including bleeding. Although evidence indicates that kallikrein amplfies Factor XII activation in a feedback reaction, most of the details

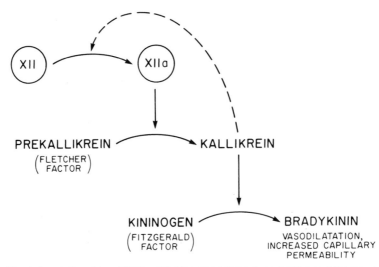

Figure 22–145 The interrelationship of Factor XII (Hageman factor), prekallikrein (Fletcher factor), and kininogen (Fitzgerald factor).

relating the kallikrein-kinin system to the initiation of the plasma coagulation factor cascade remain to be filled in.

Vitamin K Dependent Factors

The biologic activities of Factor II, VII, IX, and X depend upon an adequate supply of vitamin K, which comes mostly from the diet with a smaller proportion from bacterial synthesis in the gastrointestinal tract. These four factors share similar amino acids in certain areas of their structure and this homology has suggested a common genetic locus of origin early on in evolution, even though Factor IX is X-linked while the other three factors are autosomal. Vitamin K is not involved in the assembly of the amino acid backbones of these factors, but rather plays a key role in their post-synthetic transformation in the hepatocytes, as summarized by Davie and Fujikawa. This modification converts the factors from inert proteins to the biologically active forms present in normal plasma. Most of the investigations have dealt with prothrombin, but it is likely that the same mechanism applies to the others. Vitamin K mediates the carboxylation of ten glutamic acid residues clustered near the amino terminal end of the molecule. The carboxylation occurs at the γ position yielding γ-carboxyl glutamic acid derivatives. Calcium binding is dependent upon this cluster of carboxyl groups; without calcium binding the factor has no activity. In the vitamin K-depleted individual, prothrombin and presumably Factors VII, IX, and X in the plasma cannot be detected by their usual functional properties. However, they are present in adequate quantities if measured by their immunochemical properties.

Certain adsorbents, such as barium sulfate, selectively remove the vitamin K-dependent factors from plasma. This process, like calcium binding, is also dependent on carboxylation. Adsorption is useful in preparing test plasma deficient in the vitamin K-dependent factors for use in laboratory diagnosis. Elution from the adsorbent yields factor concentrates therapeutically useful in the management of patients with hemophilia B as well as in certain other hemorrhagic circumstances.

The coumarin anticoagulants compete with vitamin K in the body to bring on a deficiency of the vitamin K-dependent factors. They are of therapeutic value in the prevention of thrombosis. It takes about six hours before the effect is counteracted by the administration of vitamin K. Obviously, the coumarins are not active when added to plasma in vitro.

Factor VIII

The structure of Factor VIII has remained elusive for a long time, but recently the mystery has begun to unravel, giving rise to a picture of a most unorthodox molecule — or complex of molecules. It has a molecular weight of at least 1,200,000 and consists of identical subunits each with molecular weight of about 230,000 (Fig. 22–146). Three separate and distinct structural loci

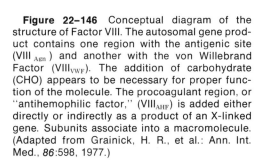

Figure 22–146 Conceptual diagram of the structure of Factor VIII. The autosomal gene product contains one region with the antigenic site (VIII $_{Agn}$) and another with the von Willebrand Factor (VIII$_{VWF}$). The addition of carbohydrate (CHO) appears to be necessary for proper function of the molecule. The procoagulant region, or "antihemophilic factor," (VIII$_{AHF}$) is added either directly or indirectly as a product of an X-linked gene. Subunits associate into a macromolecule. (Adapted from Grainick, H. R., et al.: Ann. Int. Med., 86:598, 1977.)

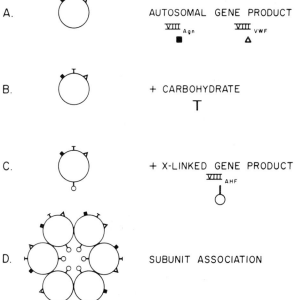

of the molecule have been identified: (1) a low molecular weight procoagulant piece (VIII_{AHF}) which contains the antihemophilic factor deficient in patients with hemophilia A; (2) a high molecular weight portion which contains the antigenic site (VIII_{Agn}) to which precipitating antibodies are formed; and (3) another locus on the high molecular weight piece with an activity necessary for normal platelet adhesion to vascular walls, designated VIII_{VWF}, or von Willebrand factor because it is deficient in patients with von Willebrand's disease. Quantitation of VIII_{AHF} is done biologically by specifically measuring its activity in VIII_{AHF} deficient plasma, and VIII_{Agn} is measured immunochemically by a precipitating antibody. A method has recently been described for measuring VIII_{VWF}, depending on the empiric observation that the antibiotic ristocetin causes aggregation of washed normal platelets in a reaction that depends on the plasma concentration of VIII_{VWF}. This reaction occurs with a specific VIII_{VWF} receptor present on the platelet membrane.

Whether these three Factor VIII principles should be considered as a complex molecule or as a multimolecular complex is still uncertain. Under certain in-vivo experimental conditions, to be discussed subsequently, they exhibit different metabolic behavior patterns, suggesting processes of association within the body. There is no doubt that Factor VIII is the product of at least two different genes, since VIII_{AHF} is an X-linked trait and VIII_{VWF} is autosomal.

Intrinsic and Extrinsic Clotting Systems

The terms "intrinsic" and "extrinsic" refer to clotting inside and outside the vascular system, respectively. The intrinsic system is relatively slow and the extrinsic somewhat faster, thanks to the action of tissue thromboplastin. In either case the final common pathway is the conversion of prothrombin to thrombin, the active enzyme which acts upon fibrinogen as its substrate.

The sequential reaction of clotting factors which brings about this conversion involves aspects of the cascade hypothesis as well as the concept of complex formation on phospholipid micelles (Fig. 22–147). The first phase of the intrinsic system is the surface activation of Factors XII and XI. Factor XIa then triggers coagulation by activating IX to IXa, a potent procoagulant. A complex is then formed of Factors IXa and VIII with platelet phospholipid. The formation of this "Factor VIII complex" is accelerated by the presence of small quantities of thrombin. This complex then converts Factor X to Xa, which by itself has "prothrombinase" activity. Its reaction rate with prothrombin, however, is markedly accelerated by the presence of Factor V and platelet phospholipid.

The extrinsic system short-circuits the first two phases of the intrinsic system by directly activating Factor X through the formation of a complex between Factor VII and tissue thromboplastin, which is composed of phospholipid and protein. Tissue thromboplastin is found in many tissues, but brain, lung, and placenta are particularly rich sources.

Calcium is required for most of the coagulation reactions, a point of considerable laboratory importance. Citrate, which complexes calcium, is the most commonly used anticoagulant for sample collection in coagulation testing. However, it is virtually impossible for hypocalcemia to be of sufficient magnitude in vivo to cause abnormal bleeding.

The thrombin formed as the end-product of this accelerating series of reactions not only causes formation of fibrin monomer and activates Factor XIII, but it also engages in positive feedback by promoting platelet aggregation and by increasing the activities of Factors V and VIII. It also increases its own rate of formation by activating prothrombin. The activated forms of the coagulation factors are cleared from the circulation rapidly, thereby keeping the process of clot formation under physiologic control.

Control of Coagulation Reactions: Heparin Cofactor

The key to keeping the forward forces of clot formation under control lies in prompt removal of the activated coagulation factors from the circulation. One important means of achieving this goal is the maintenance of rapid blood flow to wash away local concentrations from the site of thrombus formation. Given an adequate perfusion, the liver rapidly clears the activated factors with a half-life of only a few minutes. There they are rapidly degraded.

There are at least two plasma inhibitors of the activated factors. One is an α-2 macroglobulin. The other, of greater importance, is antithrombin III, identified by Rosenberg as the "heparin cofactor." Antithrombin III is an anti-serine protease (Fig. 22–148). The serine proteases seek out arginine residues where they cleave their protein substrates. In like fashion, the active serine site has an affinity for an arginine site on the antithrombin III molecule, but in this instance the product of the reaction is a stable complex rather than a cleavage. Originally antithrombin III was thought to inhibit only thrombin, but now it is known that it inhibits other serine proteases as well, including Factors XIIa, XIa, Xa, and plasmin.

The combination of heparin with antithrombin III enhances its affinity for serine proteases about 100 fold. The effect is immediate. In the absence of antithrombin III heparin has no effect on clot

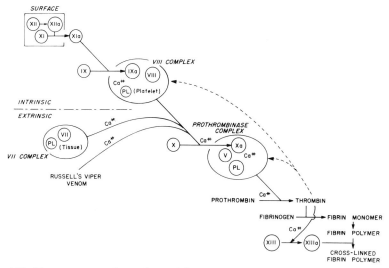

Figure 22–147 The sequence of reactions of the plasma coagulation factors. (PL = phospholipid)

formation, hence its identification as the "heparin cofactor." Heparin binds to a specific ε-amino lysyl group at a point on the molecule distant from the active arginine which forms the complex with serine proteases.

Heparin in plasma prolongs the prothrombin time by only a few seconds; its action on the activated partial thromboplastin time is much more pronounced. Its action is immediate and, in contrast to the coumarin anticoagulants, is present in vitro as well as in vivo. It is rapidly cleared from the circulation with a half-life of 90 minutes

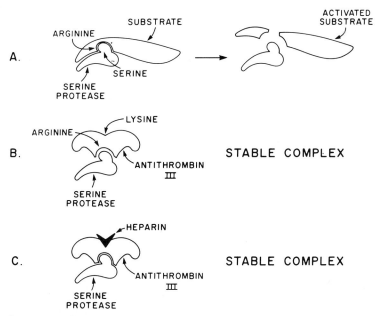

Figure 22–148 Conceptual diagram of the action of serine proteases and their inhibition by antithrombin III.
  A. Serine protease forms a complex with its specific substrate and cleaves it, producing activation (or degradation in the case of plasmin acting upon fibrin-fibrinogen).
  B. Serine protease forms a stable complex with antithrombin III.
  C. The binding of heparin with antithrombin III markedly enhances its affinity for serine protease, illustrated as a "better fit."

and its effect is dissipated within six hours. Although there is significant renal excretion, its metabolic fate is not thoroughly understood.

Synthesis and Turnover

Most of the coagulation factors are made in the liver, with the notable exception of Factor VIII. Jaffe has summarized evidence pointing to the endothelial cells as the source of Factors VIII_{Agn} and VIII_{VWF}, although not of VIII_{AHF}, the origin of which remains unknown. Fibrinogen and Factor VIII are "acute phase reactants," and their levels rise in response to inflammatory states, surgery, and pregnancy.

A significant proportion of the intravascular coagulation factor pool is associated with platelets, partly with the outer membrane and partly in the interior granules. The origin of the platelet coagulation factors is still open to question, but it has been suggested that the interior pool of Factor VIII_{Agn} and VIII_{VWF} is produced in megakaryocytes. If so, this would provide an intriguing functional link between the platelets and the vascular endothelium, which hitherto has often been looked upon as only an inert lining of the vasculature. An epinephrine response is rapidly followed by a transient rise in both the platelet count and the plasma Factor VIII level. The platelets are presumably released from the sequestered pool in the spleen. The mechanism of the Factor VIII increase is not clear.

The biologic half-lives of most of the clotting factors are relatively short (Table 22–26). Factor VII has the shortest and fibrinogen and Factor XIII have the longest. The disappearance of a plasma protein from the intravascular space is a complex function determined not only by its catabolism but also by its passage into extravascular spaces. Thus the meaning of "half-life" is open to considerable discussion. Nonetheless the value is useful in scheduling the frequency of replacement infusions in patients being treated for bleeding due to known factor deficiencies.

Coagulation Tests

Most of the tests of the clotting mechanism depend on the appearance of a fibrin clot in the test tube. The simplest of these is the whole blood clotting time, which is a crude measure of the intrinsic system. A much more convenient, accurate, and reproducible method of measuring the clotting time in the laboratory rather than at the bedside is to collect citrated plasma and subsequently measure the plasma clotting time in the laboratory by adding excess calcium. The normal "recalcification time" is about 100 to 240 seconds, compared to 5 to 15 minutes for the whole blood clotting time. The addition of various reagents to recalcified plasma gives considerable information

TABLE 22–26   BIOLOGIC HALF-LIVES OF PLASMA COAGULATION FACTORS

Factor VII	1.5 to 5 hours
Factor VIII	9 to 18 hours
Factor V	15 to 20 hours
Factor IX	20 to 24 hours
Factor X	1 to 2 days
Factor XI	1.7 to 3.5 days
Factor XII	2 days
Factor II	2.8 to 4.4 days
Factor I	3.2 to 4.5 days
Factor XIII	4.5 to 7 days

about the coagulation mechanism. The addition of a substitute for platelet phospholipid (a "partial thromboplastin") shortens the time to about 60 to 90 seconds; this is the "partial thromboplastin time," which reflects the status of the intrinsic system. The activation of Factors XII and XI by surface-active materials, such as kaolin, celite, or ellagic acid, shortens the time to about 25 to 40 seconds and gives a more reproducible test ("activated partial thromboplastin time"). If tissue (i.e., complete) thromboplastin is added, the plasma clotting time is about 13 seconds, and the corresponding test, somewhat erroneously called the "prothrombin time," is a measure of the extrinsic system. The addition of Russell's viper venom ("Stypven time") activates Factor X directly and thus eliminates Factor VII as a variable in the assessment of the extrinsic system. The addition of thrombin ("thrombin time") is a direct measure of the ability to form a fibrin clot in the test plasma and normally produces a clot so rapidly (about 6 seconds) that dilution of the thrombin is necessary in order to lengthen the time and thus to obtain more accurate and meaningful results. It is obvious that all tests which depend on the appearance of a fibrin clot require an adequate concentration of fibrinogen in the test plasma.

In summary, the initial evaluation of a hemostatic disorder requires an activated partial thromboplastin time (APTT) and a prothrombin time (PT) to evaluate the intrinsic and extrinsic systems. Deficiencies of Factors X, V, II, or fibrinogen, or the presence of heparin or "split products" prolong both the APTT and the PT. Factor VII lack prolongs the PT but not the APTT, while the reverse is true for deficiencies of Factors XII, XI, IX, or VIII. The thrombin time detects fibrinogen abnormalities, heparin, or "split products." Although the concentration of fibrinogen is readily measured, a rough index of fibrinogen level is easily obtained by inspecting the bulk of a retracted clot in a test tube. Rapid lysis of the incubated clot indicates pathologic fibrinolysis. The routine hemostasis evaluation is completed by a platelet count and sometimes by tests of platelet function, of which clot retraction and bleeding time are the most useful.

Tentative conclusions about the identity of a plasma factor deficiency are drawn from substitution tests in an "expanded" partial thromboplastin time. The reagents used for substitution are aged plasma (which lacks the labile Factors V and VIII), fresh adsorbed plasma (which lacks the vitamin K dependent Factors II, VII, IX, and X), and fresh serum (which lacks the consumable Factors II, V, VIII, and fibrinogen). For example, the prolonged APTT in a patient with VIII$_{AHF}$ deficiency (hemophilia A) is corrected by substitution of normal fresh adsorbed plasma, but not aged plasma or serum. In Factor IX deficiency (hemophilia B) the abnormality is corrected by normal serum or aged plasma, but not adsorbed plasma. Final confirmation and quantitation is accomplished by specific factor assays using a test plasma of known deficiency mixed with patient plasma.

ABNORMAL STRUCTURE AND FUNCTION

The hereditary abnormalities of the coagulation factors are readily classified because they are definable in terms of a single inherited abnormality in either the amount or the structure of a single protein. Acquired defects are more difficult to categorize in that they frequently affect many different aspects of the coagulation sequence as well as multiple coagulation factors (Table 22–27).

The general effects are those of bleeding and/or clotting. The clinical nature of the bleeding gives clues about its underlying cause. Intra-articular hemorrhage is highly characteristic of hemophilia and is only rarely seen in other disorders, while petechiae are strongly suggestive of thrombocytopenia. Ecchymoses and purpura are very nonspecific; deep hemorrhage into muscles or the retroperitoneum is more a feature of hemophilia or of adverse effects of anticoagulants. Intracranial hemorrhage, regardless of the underlying hemostatic defect, is the most dread complication. Bleeding from the umbilical stump or after circumcision may be the first sign of a hereditary disorder. Later in life, the onset of the menses, dental extraction, and surgical procedures are natural tests of hemostasis. Delayed hemorrhage several days after the completion of a procedure raises the index of suspicion that there is a disorder of plasma coagulation factors.

DISORDERS OF FIBRINOGEN AND RELATED FACTORS

A low level of circulating fibrinogen may be secondary to decreased production or more frequently to an increase in the rate of its degrada-

TABLE 22–27 CLASSIFICATION OF DISORDERS OF PLASMA COAGULATION AND VASCULAR FACTORS

I. *Disorders of Fibrinogen and Related Factors*
    Hereditary
        Afibrinogenemia
        Dysfibrinogenemia
        Factor XIII deficiency
    Acquired
        Disseminated intravascular coagulation
        Primary fibrinolysis
        Liver disease

II. *Disorders of the Intrinsic and Extrinsic Systems*
    Hereditary
        Hemophilia A
        Hemophilia B
        Deficiencies of surface active Factors XII or XI
        Other deficiencies: Factors VII, X, V, or II
        von Willebrand's disease
    Acquired
        Vitamin K deficiency
        Liver disease
        Hemorrhagic diseases of the newborn
        Exogenous anticoagulants
        Endogenous anticoagulants (antibodies to Factor VIII and other Factors)

III. *Vascular Disorders*
    Hereditary
        Hereditary hemorrhagic telangiectasia
        Ehlers-Danlos syndrome and other connective tissue disorders
    Acquired
        Superficial purpura
        Scurvy
        Cushing's syndrome
        Amyloidosis
        Allergic purpura

tion. The excess in fibrinogen consumption above its production rate is most often due to a process of intravascular coagulation. Rarely it is caused by the presence of a high level of circulating plasmin.

Several different terms have been used to describe the process of *extensive intravascular clotting,* none of them entirely satisfactory. "Consumption coagulopathy" emphasizes the depletion of the plasma coagulation factors, but not all the factors are consumed, and the "panel" of depressed factor levels is neither uniform nor predictable. "Disseminated intravascular coagulation" places major emphasis on the pathogenetic importance of the deposition of large quantities of fibrin throughout the microcirculation but does not fit those situations in which the fibrin deposition is extensive and yet mostly or entirely localized to the vascular beds of certain tissues.

If not fatal, the process may be acute and self-limited, subacute, or chronic, depending on the underlying cause as discussed by Colman and his associates. It may be set off by a pathologic activation of the extrinsic or the intrinsic clotting systems; in many circumstances the triggering mechanism is not known. The activation of the extrinsic system is caused by the entry into the circulation of large amounts of tissue thromboplastin. Examples are the hypofibrinogenemic states associated with pregnancy: abruptio placentae, amniotic fluid embolism, toxemia, and retained dead fetus. Since fibrinogen concentration normally increases in pregnancy, the finding of a plasma concentration within the normal range may be indicative of significant consumption if found late in pregnancy in association with one of the aforementioned complications. Widespread carcinoma may incite intravascular clotting, also presumably on account of the tumor content of tissue thromboplastin which finds its way into the circulation. The intrinsic system may be activated by bacterial septicemia and certain rickettsial and viral infections (Rocky Mountain spotted fever, epidemic hemorrhagic fever) which lay bare the vascular endothelium and expose collagen. Antigen-antibody complexes trigger intrinsic clotting by an unknown mechanism in massive transfusion reactions (although the thromboplastic properties of red cell membrane may play some role) and in anaphylactic reactions. It has been suggested that an immunologic mechanism underlies purpura fulminans, a serious and often fatal disorder primarily of children which characteristically follows shortly after recovery from a minor viral infection (Spicer and Rau, 1976). Properly timed injections of endotoxin given to animals have been experimentally used to produce the so-called generalized Shwartzman reaction, a disseminated intravascular coagulation syndrome, but in this model the precise initiating event also remains obscure. The classification of intravascular coagulation syndromes is given in Table 22–28.

Local factors may prepare the vascular bed of a certain organ or tissue for selective fibrin deposition. In pregnancy the kidney is particularly vulnerable, and the syndrome which may ensue is bilateral renal cortical necrosis with oliguric renal failure. In cavernous hemangiomas, a large vascular bed with a high ratio of endothelial surface area to vascular cross-sectional area accommodates a large volume of blood with static flow. This may be sufficient to set up a chronic process of extensive but localized fibrin deposition, the endothelium contributing high plasminogen activating activity and thus releasing fibrin degradation products into the circulation.

An adequate hepatic perfusion is necessary for rapidly clearing activated coagulation factors as well as fibrinogen-fibrin degradation products and their complexes from the circulation. Any impairment of this process will prolong and aggravate the severity of the coagulopathy. Clinical states of shock, whatever the underlying primary cause, lead to poor perfusion and may seriously

TABLE 22–28 CLASSIFICATION OF DISSEMINATED INTRAVASCULAR COAGULATION SYNDROMES

I. Pregnancy
  Abruptio placentae
  Amniotic fluid embolism
  Toxemia
  Retained dead fetus
  Saline abortion
  Septic abortion with septicemia
  Hydatidiform mole
II. Malignant Disease
  Metastatic carcinoma
  Acute leukemia (promyelocytic)
III. Infectious Disease
  Bacterial septicemia (meningococcal, other gram negative and gram positive)
  Rickettsial (Rocky Mountain spotted fever)
  Viral (epidemic hemorrhagic fever)
  Parasitic (malaria)
IV. Pediatric Syndromes
  Neonatal (respiratory distress syndrome, retained dead twin fetus, septicemia, rubella, abruptio placentae)
  Purpura fulminans
  Hemolytic uremic syndrome
V. Antigen-Antibody Complexes
  Anaphylactic reaction
  Massive transfusion reaction
VI. Miscellaneous
  Liver disease
  Aneurysm
  Vasculitis
  Postoperative (open heart and other thoracic surgery, prostatic surgery)
  Massive trauma (including burns)
  Heat stroke
  Drowning
  Snake bite
  Giant hemangioma

increase the magnitude of the syndrome. Macrophage blockade with substances such as Thorotrast contributes to the severity of intravascular coagulation syndromes experimentally in animals. A similar blockade may be of pathogenetic significance in septicemia or in massive hemolysis.

The ischemic consequences to local tissues of the blockage of the microcirculation are fortunately usually self-limited, owing to the local fibrinolytic efficiency, which rapidly removes the fibrin deposits. However, renal failure is one of the most dire of the ischemic effects. Cutaneous patches of gangrene and acrocyanosis are more externally visible effects seen in purpura fulminans and sometimes in septicemia. Erythrocyte fragmentation, occurring as red cells are forced through the obstructing fibrin meshwork, causes the morphologic appearance of microangiopathic hemolytic anemia on the peripheral blood film. The picture may be accompanied by clinical signs of hemolysis. Intravascular coagulation causing oliguric renal failure and erythrocyte fragmentation is therefore one of the "hemolytic uremic" syndromes.

Laboratory tests reflect the paradoxic circumstance that excessive intravascular clotting brings forth a hemorrhagic diathesis. The consumption of coagulation factors in vivo resembles the process of conversion of plasma to serum in vitro. The most consistent changes are decreases in the platelet count and in the levels of fibrinogen and Factors II, V, and VIII. Plasminogen activation releases fibrinogen-fibrin degradation products into the circulation. These form complexes with fibrin monomer and interfere with the normal polymerization of fibrin monomer during clot formation. The widespread derangements in the coagulation mechanism are reflected by abnormalities in all the routine laboratory tests. These include prolongation of the prothrombin time, the activated partial thromboplastin time, and the thrombin time. The concentration of "split products" in the serum is elevated, and tests of paracoagulation, as described earlier, may be positive. The test tube clot is small and easily broken up. Serial measurements of the routine coagulation tests, platelet count, fibrinogen concentration, and Factor VIII level may help to make the clinical decision about the presence of and the course of a suspected case of extensive intravascular clotting. Laboratory confirmation may be difficult in mild cases.

Treatment varies with the individual circumstances. In acute syndromes, the prompt and vigorous treatment of the primary underlying cause and the correction of shock are the most important measures. Heparin is sometimes used in order to arrest the deposition of fibrin, but not without fear of increasing the bleeding tendency. Repletion of coagulation factors and platelets may be indicated. Replacement therapy is best combined with heparin if the process has not been arrested and fibrin deposition is continuing. Inhibitors of fibrinolysis such as epsilon aminocaproic acid are contraindicated, since they will delay the physiologic resolution of the fibrin clots within the vasculature.

Primary fibrinolysis is an acute severe bleeding state which resembles intravascular clotting but must be distinguished from it because the treatments differ. The high levels of circulating plasmin which set up this state are sometimes secondary to metastatic carcinoma of the prostate, thoracic surgery, injury to the genitourinary tract with extravasation of urokinase-containing urine into tissues, or cirrhosis or shock with impaired ability to clear plasminogen activators from the circulation. Plasmin attacks circulating fibrinogen and causes a decrease in its concentration along with the appearance of fibrinogen degradation products in the circulation. These unfortunately cannot be distinguished from the fibrin degradation products of disseminated intravascular coagulation. Other coagulation factor levels may also be depressed. However, in contrast to intravascular coagulation syndromes, the test-tube clot which initially forms completely dissolves within one or two hours, the platelet count is normal, the red cell morphology does not show fragmentation, and the bleeding improves with the therapeutic use of fibrinolytic inhibitors. Since the syndrome is primarily associated with the action of plasmin rather than thrombin, tests of paracoagulation on the plasma are negative. Under certain circumstances, such as metastatic prostatic carcinoma, primary fibrinolysis occurs together with disseminated intravascular coagulation and laboratory distinction of the two states is not possible.

Inherited disorders of fibrinogen are rare. Afibrinogenemia is a quantitative deficiency secondary to a profound lack of synthesis, while dysfibrinogenemia refers to a variation in the structure of the molecule, as discussed by Ratnoff and Forman. Only trace quantities of fibrinogen are detectable in *hereditary afibrinogenemia,* an autosomal recessive condition which is of clinical significance only in the homozygous form. Whole blood or recalcified plasma clotting times are indefinitely long and are not corrected with the addition of thrombin. Successful arrest of hemorrhage is achieved by replacement therapy sufficient to raise the fibrinogen level above 60 mg. per 100 ml. *Hereditary dysfibrinogenemia* is a mild or even asymptomatic disorder. Several different types have been described, presumably differing in the specific amino acid substitution in the molecule. The detailed abnormalities involved and the molecular mechanisms with respect to the altered function of the molecule remain for the most part to be worked out. Plasma coagulation tests may be broadly deranged. Fibrinogen concentration measured by immunochemical or physical methods is normal, but methods which depend on "clottable fibrinogen" give low values. The condition is autosomal, and affected heterozygotes therefore have normal fibrinogen along with the variant molecule. *Acquired dysfibrinogenemia* occurs in patients with severe liver disease (Martinez, Palascak, and Kwasniak, 1978). It has also been found in association with hepatoma.

Hereditary deficiency of Factor XIII is properly included among disorders of fibrinogen, since Factor XIII also affects clot structure. Deficiency is detectable in the laboratory by virtue of the fibrin clot solubility in 5 M urea. The defect, also autosomal recessive, is clinically severe and, as in hereditary afibrinogenemia, may first come to attention because of bleeding at the site of the sloughed umbilical cord. Wound healing is impaired because fibroblastic organization of the clot is not normal. Affected homozygotes have less than 1 per cent of the normal concentration and respond particularly well to replacement therapy because Factor XIII has a relatively long half-life and only small quantities are required. Factor XIII is among the factors consumed in disseminated intravascular coagulation, another explanation for a lowered level. Consumption or decreased hepatic synthesis account for low levels in patients with liver disease.

INTRINSIC AND EXTRINSIC SYSTEM DISORDERS

Hemophilia A and *hemophilia B* are hereditary deficiencies of Factor VIII and Factor IX, respectively. The two disorders are clinically indistinguishable except by laboratory test. Both are sex-linked and thus transmitted by asymptomatic carrier females to half their sons. Female homozygotes, offspring of affected fathers and carrier mothers, are exceedingly rare. Hemophilia A occurs with a frequency of 1 per 10,000, 5 to 10 times the frequency of hemophilia B. Severe hemophilia is characterized by repeated hemarthroses and ultimately by chronic arthritis and joint destruction. Ankles, knees, and elbows are most susceptible. The normal ineffectiveness of the extrinsic clotting system in the articular structures may explain the particular susceptibility of this tissue to hemorrhage in the face of severe deficiencies of the intrinsic system. Patients with hemophilia of moderate severity may have only occasional joint hemorrhages, whereas mild cases usually have normal joints. Deep hematomas may dissect along fascial planes and cause nerve compression or compromise the vascular supply of an extremity. Even with intensive treatment the surgical risk is great, and intracranial hemorrhage, often provoked by minor head trauma, may be untreatable and have a fatal outcome.

In severe hemophilia A Factor VIII$_{AHF}$ is less than 1 per cent the normal level, in moderate cases 2 to 5 per cent, and in mild cases 6 to 30 per cent. The defect is limited to the procoagulant piece of Factor VIII molecule, VIII$_{AHF}$, which is either missing or is present but not functioning. Factors VIII$_{Agn}$ and VIII$_{VWF}$ are unaffected. It has been possible to classify patients with hemophilia A into two groups, based on reactions of their plasma with certain neutralizing antibodies to VIII$_{AHF}$. Plasma from about 10 per cent of patients with hemophilia A will neutralize these antibodies and is designated as cross-reacting material positive (CRM$^+$) or A$^+$. The remaining 90 per cent are CRM$^-$ or A$^-$. The pathogenetic significance of this observation and its possible relationship to genetic polymorphism are still not clear. Similar immunochemical approaches suggest that analogous pathogenetic mechanisms also apply to hemophilia B.

The accurate diagnosis and classification as to degree of severity of hemophilia A and B ultimately rest upon the direct measurement of the levels of Factor VIII and Factor IX activity. The treatment of major hemorrhagic episodes or the preparation of patients for surgery also requires the ability to measure the specific factor level to ensure that it remains in excess of 30 per cent at all times. The partial thromboplastin time is sensitive to levels below 20 per cent and thus is almost always prolonged in untreated patients of any degree of severity. The prothrombin time and the bleeding time are normal. Female carriers cannot be identified with certainty because their functional levels, 25 to 75 per cent for hemophilia A heterozygotes and 9 to 90 per cent for hemophilia B heterozygotes, overlap considerably with the range of normal, 50 to 150 per cent. Ratnoff and Jones report 94 per cent accuracy in identifying female carriers of hemophilia A with the use of newer methods which compare the ratios between the levels of procoagulant (VIII$_{AHF}$) and antigenic activity (VIII$_{Agn}$). In hemophilia A heterozygotes the ratio is about half the expected value in normals.

Replacement therapy with plasma or plasma derivatives is effective in both hemophilia A and hemophilia B (Fig. 22–149). Treatment must be specific, however, an axiom which has become of crucial importance since plasma fractionation procedures have come into common use. Cryoprecipitate and other Factor VIII-rich preparations lack Factor IX activity, whereas fractions containing Factor IX and the other vitamin K-dependent factors lack Factor VIII. Factor IX is relatively stable and is present in stored plasma which is a poor source of Factor VIII. The longer biologic half-life of Factor IX (about 24 hours as compared to 12 for Factor VIII) is also of importance in that less frequent infusions of Factor IX are required to maintain its functional activity at the desired level.

Von Willebrand's disease is also a hereditary disorder of Factor VIII but, in contrast to hemophilia A, it is inherited as an autosomal dominant and in addition has an associated defect of platelet adhesion to injured blood vessels, causing a prolonged bleeding time. Platelet adhesion to glass beads is also impaired, but other platelet functions, such as the usual aggregation reactions and ADP release, are typically normal. Epistaxis, menorrhagia, and gastrointestinal hemorrhage are common, but joint hemorrhage is rare. The Factor VIII$_{AHF}$ level is reduced below 50 per cent to as low as 1 to 5 per cent. The partial thromboplastin time is not adequate to detect those cases with less severely depressed levels. Factor VIII$_{AHF}$ levels fluctuate in individual cases,

FACTOR VIII LEVEL

(%)

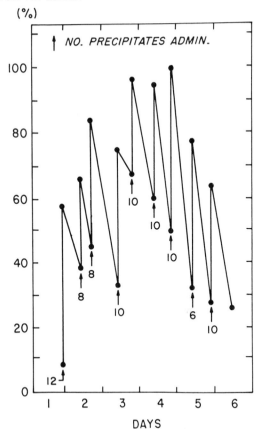

Figure 22–149 Plasma Factor VIII$_{AHF}$ levels measured during treatment of a patient with hemophilia A by repeated infusions of cryoprecipitate. (Redrawn from Pool, J. G., and Shannon, A. E.: N. Engl. J. Med., 273:1443, 1968. Reprinted by permission.)

in contrast to their constancy in hemophilia A. Pregnancy stimulates an increased Factor VIII$_{AHF}$ level, as in normal women, and thus may ameliorate hemorrhagic manifestations.

"Classic" von Willebrand's disease is associated with deficits in all three aspects of the Factor VIII molecule — procoagulant activity, antigenic level, and "ristocetin cofactor" concentration are reduced. However, Gralnick and his associates have summarized evidence that several variants can be characterized. The "classic" cases are considered to represent quantitative deficiency of the VIII$_{VWF}$ locus, which by the nature of the Factor VIII molecular structure described above requires an equal loss of VIII$_{Agn}$ and VIII$_{AHF}$. In one variant the levels of VIII$_{AHF}$ and VIII$_{Agn}$ are normal and only the bleeding time is long in association with a low level of "ristocetin cofactor." These cases are considered to represent a qualitative defect of the VIII$_{VWF}$ locus which is nonetheless structurally represented and thus unassociated with abnormalities of the other two aspects of the Factor VIII molecule. Another variant appears to be a combination of quantitative and qualitative defects in which the degree of reduction of VIII$_{Agn}$ and VIII$_{AHF}$ is not as profound as that of VIII$_{VWF}$.

One of the most intriguing differences between hemophilia A and von Willebrand's disease lies in their response to plasma infusions. The increase in VIII$_{AHF}$ level in hemophilia A is entirely accounted for by the amount of infused material; the maximum occurs immediately after infusion and the declining level thereafter follows the known biologic half-life of VIII$_{AHF}$, about 12 hours. Plasma infusions given to patients with von Willebrand's disease actually stimulate the production of VIII$_{AHF}$. Levels, reaching a peak at 4 to 24 hours, are higher than those which could be explained on the basis of the amount of infused material. The subsequent decline to original pretreatment levels occurs slowly over several days (Blatt and associates, 1976) (Fig. 22–150). Donor plasma taken from patients with hemophilia A indeed has more potent VIII$_{AHF}$ stimulating activity than normal plasma. The correction of the prolonged bleeding time, if it is corrected at all, is much more transient and may last only a few

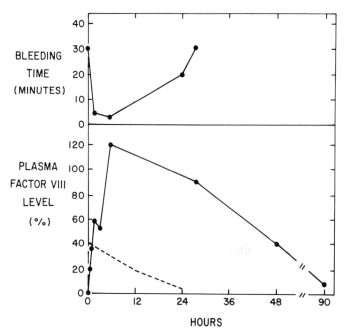

Figure 22–150 Response of Factor VIII$_{AHF}$ level and of bleeding time in a patient with von Willebrand's disease after, given at time zero, a single infusion of a fraction prepared from normal plasma. The interrupted line represents the response in Factor VIII$_{AHF}$ level to be expected in a patient with hemophilia A. (Modified from Williams, W. J.: *In* Williams et al. (Ed.): Hematology, McGraw-Hill Book Co., New York, 1972, p. 1340.)

hours. The persistence in the circulation of VIII$_{Agn}$ and "ristocetin cofactor" activity tends to be intermediate, less prolonged than the VIII$_{AHF}$ elevation but more prolonged than the period of bleeding time correction. The only sure conclusion that can be drawn from these observations is that the metabolic behavior of Factor VIII is complex. The explanation for the relative inefficacy of infusions in favorably influencing the bleeding time may point to the significance of intraplatelet and/or endothelial cell depots of VIII$_{VWF}$ which cannot be easily repleted by simple infusion of exogenous material. Platelet transfusion does not correct the bleeding time defect as it does in hereditary or acquired defects of platelet aggregation, further evidence that the poor platelet adherence in von Willebrand's disease is related to a plasma deficiency.

Ristocetin induced platelet aggregation is also deficient in the *Bernard-Soulier syndrome,* a hemorrhagic condition in which the intrinsically defective platelets are large, heavy, and decreased in number. In this disorder there is a deficiency in the platelet receptor for VII$_{VWF}$. There is no plasma deficiency of Factor VIII constituents.

Acquired defects in Factor VIII, other than those found in the intravascular coagulation syndromes, result from the pathologic production of autoantibodies directed against Factor VIII (Shapiro and Hultin). Somewhat paradoxically, about 5 to 20 per cent of patients with hemophilia A develop antibodies against Factor VIII after repeated replacement therapy. These greatly complicate successful therapy when they are present in high titer. Fortunately, the titer falls with time, and if the intervals between hemorrhagic episodes are sufficiently spaced, intensive replacement therapy may successfully arrest the bleeding before the anamnestic response to the infused Factor VIII raises the antibody titer to levels which would preclude successful treatment. Acquired antibodies to Factor VIII are also seen in association with such autoimmune disorders as lupus erythematosus, rheumatoid arthritis, ulcerative colitis, and regional enteritis. A third variant occurs days to weeks postpartum. A fourth type is found without obvious relationship to other coexisting factors, especially in older people. The antibody behaves as a natural circulating anticoagulant and its addition to normal plasma will delay its clotting time. Specific confirmation is made by measuring the neutralization of the Factor VIII activity of normal plasma by plasma containing the natural antibody. Therapy may be difficult if spontaneous disappearance does not alleviate the problem. Immunosuppressive therapy has been successfully used in a few instances. Concentrates of vitamin K dependent factors have been reported to be effective in the control of bleeding because of their content of Factor Xa, an artifact of the method of preparation, which bypasses Factor VIII. They are not without adverse effects, including thrombosis and hepatitis. Autoantibodies to other plasma coagulation factors have also been discovered, but the great majority have been directed against Factor VIII.

Hereditary deficiencies of the remaining plasma coagulation factors are uncommon. Of the surface-active factors, Factor XII deficiency is not associated with any bleeding abnormality, and the hemorrhagic diathesis of Factor XI deficiency is mild. Deficiency of Factor X, V, or II will prolong prothrombin and partial thromboplastin times. In Factor VII, only the prothrombin time is long. All are associated with mild to moderate bleeding manifestations.

Inadequate supplies of vitamin K cause depletion of the vitamin K-dependent factors: II, VII, IX, and X. Absorptive impairment secondary to gastrointestinal disease or to obstruction of the biliary tract causes clotting factor depletion which is correctable by parenterally administered vitamin K. The coumarin and indandione derivatives antagonize the hepatic synthesis of the vitamin K-dependent factors by competitive inhibition. A large number of medications interact with these anticoagulants by either increasing or decreasing their effects, as reviewed by Koch-Weser and Sellers. The Factor VII level is the first to fall because of its short biologic half-life. Factors II, IX, and X reach their nadir at about 5 to 10 days after anticoagulant therapy is begun. Vitamin K, occasionally required to arrest hemorrhage in patients treated with anticoagulant, will significantly increase the levels of the dependent factors within 6 hours. If more rapid correction is necessary, replacement therapy with plasma or with concentrates of the vitamin K-dependent factors can be given. Vitamin K therapy is ineffective if the low factor levels are the result of severe liver disease, which in addition to the vitamin K-dependent factors is associated with failure of synthesis of other factors, such as Factor V, fibrinogen, and Factor XIII along with a host of other defects (Walls and Losowsky, 1971).

The normal newborn infant has lower concentrations of the vitamin K-dependent factors than the adult, partially because of the immaturity of the fetal liver and partially because of low vitamin K stores. Prematurity exaggerates the phenomenon. Breast milk is a poor source of vitamin K, but cow's milk contains significant quantities. A hemorrhagic disease occurring two to three days after birth owing to low levels of the vitamin K-dependent factors has been associated with a sufficiently high mortality rate that prophylactic administration of a small quantity of vitamin K is considered warranted, even though only a partial correction of the coagulation abnormalities is achieved. The syndrome must be distinguished from other neonatal hemorrhagic syndromes, such as the thrombocytopenias, disseminated intravascular coagulation disorders, and hemophilia. The coumarin drugs cross the placental barrier and therefore are not given to pregnant women.

Hemorrhagic complications following heparin therapy are relatively infrequent, considering how extensively this drug is used. The duration of action of heparin is limited to 4 to 6 hours and thus the use of protamine, which neutralizes heparin, is rarely necessary in the management of hemorrhagic complications. Hemorrhagic complications may also occur following therapy with plasminogen activators, such as streptokinase or urokinase, but these agents are also rapidly removed if phagocytic clearing mechanisms are functioning normally.

Reviews on anticoagulant therapy have been written by Gurevich, by Rogers and Sherry, and by Wessler and Gitel. Bell has compared streptokinase and urokinase in a review of the status of fibrinolytic agents in therapy.

HYPERCOAGULABLE STATES

Pathologic thrombosis in the coronary or cerebral circulation, in the deep veins of the legs, in the heart interior, or in other vascular sites is among the most important of public health problems. Yet, with some exceptions to be discussed below, it has been impossible to predict which individuals will suffer this often devastating aberration of blood coagulation.

Table 22-29 lists a few selected conditions which are known to be associated with a thrombotic tendency, some to a striking degree. These are classified as diseases of the vascular integrity, of stasis of blood flow, cellular abnormalities of the blood, and plasma abnormalities, but overlap between categories frequently occurs. In several of these conditions the thrombotic tendency occurs concomitantly with a bleeding tendency.

Hereditary deficiency of antithrombin III is an autosomal dominant condition in which multiple members of affected families develop thrombotic tendencies in early or middle life. Since this is another one of the "consumable" plasma factors, low levels occur in disseminated intravascular coagulation. Antithrombin III lack is one of several possible explanations for heparin resistance.

HEMOSTASIS: VASCULAR FACTORS

The vascular wall stands closely juxtaposed to the normal process of hemostasis. Platelets adhere at cut surfaces and aggregate where collagen is bared. Serotonin is released by platelets, causing vasoconstriction which may assist the task of vessel plugging. Collagen also activates

TABLE 22-29 HYPERCOAGULABLE STATES

Altered Intravascular Surfaces
Atherosclerosis (and predisposing conditions such as
   diabetes mellitus, hypertension, the hyper-
   lipidemias, etc.)
Prosthetic heart valves
Vasculitis
*Thrombotic thrombocytopenic purpura
Homocystinuria
*Pseudoxanthoma elasticum

Stasis of Blood Flow
Deep venous thrombosis (and predisposing causes,
   such as immobilization, venous compression, valve
   incompetence, etc.)
Valvular heart disease
Congestive heart failure
Cardiac arrhythmia

Cellular Abnormalities of the Blood
*Polycythemia vera
*Thrombocythemia
Sickle cell disease
Paroxysmal nocturnal hemoglobinuria
*Leukemia

Plasma Abnormalities
*Disseminated intravascular coagulation
   (see Table 7–4)
Postoperative state
Pregnancy
Oral contraceptive use
Malignancy
Antithrombin III deficiency
*Dysfibrinogenemia
Plasminogen deficiency

---

*Also often associated with pathologic bleeding.

the intrinsic coagulation system. The vascular endothelium then finally initiates the process of clot lysis by releasing plasminogen activator. However, intrinsic defects of the vascular wall itself may be of pathogenetic importance in the etiology of hemorrhage. The supporting structures around the vessels may lose elasticity and turgor, an important factor in the *superficial purpura* commonly seen in the inelastic skin of normally aging individuals. This syndrome, somewhat injudiciously named "senile purpura," is clinically benign and is not associated with clinical bleeding, its most serious consequence being cosmetic. Hereditary disorders of connective tissues, such as *Ehlers-Danlos syndrome,* also decrease the compliance of perivascular tissues sufficiently to cause significant hemorrhage. *Scurvy,* usually seen in combination with alcoholic liver disease and other nutritional deficiencies, affects the integrity of connective tissue of the vascular wall. Perifollicular hemorrhages resembling pe-

techiae suggest vitamin C lack. Excessive amounts of adrenal glucocorticoids weaken the structure of the vascular wall. Purpura and ecchymoses of *Cushing's syndrome* are explained on this basis. Amyloid deposition within vascular walls is another example of an acquired intrinsic disorder of the vessel wall. The abnormality in *hereditary hemorrhagic telangiectasia,* an autosomal dominant condition, is still not understood in terms of primary etiology but leads to localized dilatations of small vessels which appear as tiny punctate vascular spots which blanch on pressure. These non-pulsatile spots are found commonly on the lips and mucous membranes of the mouth and nose as well as on the fingertips. However, internal involvement commonly occurs in the gastrointestinal tract as well as in other organs, including the lungs and the central nervous system. The telangiectasias usually do not develop until the fifth or sixth decade of life, when the weakened vascular wall finally becomes apparent. Epistaxis and gastrointestinal hemorrhage are the most common symptoms.

Damage to the vascular wall as a consequence of various infections has already been mentioned. Immunologic vascular damage leads to the syndrome of *allergic purpura,* which resembles thrombocytopenic purpura in the sense that a petechial eruption forms with predilection for the dependent portions of the body. The eruption appears more violaceous and more confluent than thrombocytopenic purpura, and also has a tendency to involve the buttocks and flexor surfaces of the legs. When the purpuric signs are combined in a triad together with gastrointestinal hemorrhage and arthritis, the term *"Henoch-Schönlein purpura"* is appropriate. The condition may affect the pediatric age group, in which a postinfectious cause appears to be most common, or adults, in which case drug reactions may be more likely trigger mechanisms (Cream, et al., 1970). In either group, nephritis is the most serious complication, as discussed by Meadow and associates.

The diagnosis of the primary vascular purpuric syndromes rests primarily on clinical recognition. Laboratory confirmation is at present unsatisfactory. The bleeding time and the tourniquet test (in which the appearance of petechiae is observed after inflation of a blood pressure cuff to the level sufficient to occlude venous return but not arterial filling) are primarily tests of adequacy of platelet numbers and function, and although abnormalities may be detected in the primary vascular disorders, the information is not of great assistance in establishing their presence. The fact that almost 10 per cent of normal people have a positive tourniquet test also diminishes the diagnostic value of this procedure.

IDENTITY OF BLOOD CELLS

One of the earliest and most fundamental events in the emergence of life must have been the packaging of complex molecules into cells separated from the environment by membranes. These membranes provided the cell with both physical protection and metabolic discrimination, and during the further evolutionary development, the cell membranes have become the biologic expression of cellular identity.

Cell membranes are, in general, made up of a 45 Å.-thick lipid bi-layer containing free-floating protein globules (Fig. 22–151). The lipid component consists primarily of tightly packed phospholipid molecules with their hydrophobic fatty acid tails intertwined in the center of the membrane and their hydrophilic phosphoglycerol heads providing the intrinsic and extrinsic boundaries (Danielli and Dawson, 1935). At body temperature, the lipid bi-layers exist in a semi-liquid form permitting considerable lateral movements within the membrane but owing to the layers of polar forces, little opportunity for movements across the membranes.

In nucleated cells, the lipid membrane can be renewed to compensate for loss from injury or from interiorization during processes of phagocytosis or pinocytosis (Fig. 22–102). In non-nucleated cells, such as in erythrocytes, considerable remodeling may take place through a dynamic exchange with extracellular neutral lipids, especially cholesterol. However, structural membrane lipids cannot be replaced and the senescence of the red cells is associated with or caused by a loss in surface area.

The physiologic role of the lipids in the transport of molecules across the membrane is not clear. The lipid bi-layer appears best suited to serve as an impenetrable insulator. Actually, the membranes with the least transport function, such as the myelin coating of the nerves, are the ones with the highest content of lipid, and the membranes with the most transport obligations, such as the mitochondrial membranes, contain very little lipid. Recent studies have suggested that most if not all membrane transport is mediated by protein globules floating like icebergs in the semi-fluid lipid matrix (Singer, 1974). These protein globules can be visualized directly by electron microscopy of freeze-cleaved red cell membranes (Fig. 22–152). It is assumed that these globules have a hydrophobic half deeply embedded in the hydrophobic lipid center and a hydrophilic half emerging from the surface. Some proteins may even be banded like woolly bears with their hydrophobic center band embedded in the hydrophobic lipid center and their hydrophilic ends emerging from both interior and exterior surfaces (Fig. 22–151). Such protein bridges would alone or in groups be well suited to mediate molecular transport across the membranes. In ma-

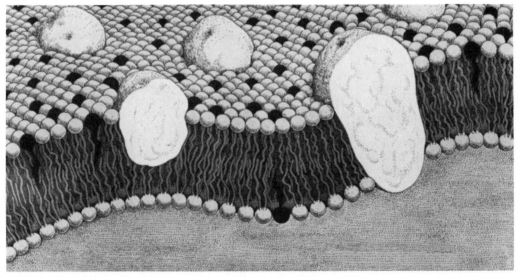

Figure 22–151 Floating iceberg model of cell membranes with globular proteins embedded in a bi-layer of lipids (grey) and cholesterol (black). The proteins make up the membrane's "active sites." Some pass entirely through and may contain transport pores. (From Singer, S. J.: Hosp. Practice, 81, May 1973.)

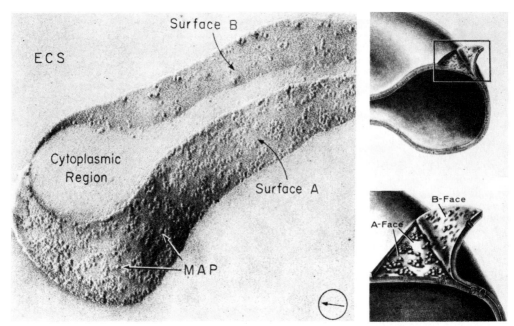

Figure 22–152 Artist's conception and actual electron microscopic view of a freeze-cleaved human red cell ghost membrane. Its A surface is oriented toward the extracellular space (ECS), and is partly covered with clusters of 100 Å membrane-associated particles (MAP). Surface B has fewer particles and faces the cell's interior. (From Weinstein, R. S., and McNutt, N. S.: Seminars Hematol., 7:259, 1970.)

ture red cells the transmembranous proteins are attached on the inner side of the membrane to rod-like proteins, spectrins (Fig. 22–153). These abundant proteins have so far not been identified with an enzymatic function and they may merely serve as a reinforcing scaffold for the lipid bi-layer. On the outer side of the membrane, the proteins serve as metabolic receptors and as anchors for sialic acid groups and for branching antigenic oligosaccharides.

The floating iceberg concept of membrane structure has been strongly supported by the observation that cross-linking antibodies to membranous proteins will move the proteins together into one spot, so-called capping. Because of the above-mentioned attachment of red cell transmembranous proteins to spectrin, this capping phenomenon is not observed in red cells (Singer 1974). In summary, it appears likely that all membranes consist of a lipid bi-layer that acts as a non-specific insulating component, and protein globules that act as receptors or transport enzymes, providing the cells with their functional identity.

In addition to functional identity, cells also have individual identity achieved by the presence and configuration of specific systems of sugar and protein molecules on the membranes. This fingerprint individuality of the membrane surface ap-

parently is needed for the phagocytes to distinguish between self and non-self and probably plays a major role in the recognition and destruction of altered or foreign cells. It is also of importance for blood transfusions and organ transplantations, and the unravelling of blood and tissue types has had both theoretic and practical rewards (Fudenberg and co-workers, 1978).

The ABO system was the first recognized system of specific, individual surface markers. This system is expressed on all cells in the body, but owing to its practical importance for blood transfusions, it has been identified with red blood cells (Marcus, 1969). The prime members of the system, the A, B, and H antigens, are branching carbohydrate chains that extend above the membrane and are attached to specific sphingolipid protein sites in the membrane. These sites begin to appear during the early maturation of nucleated red cells (Minio, et al., 1972) and, at the time of release from the bone marrow, each red cell has about 1 million ABH sites. The ABH antigens (Watkins, 1966) are derived from a common precursor substance consisting of a chain of four sugars terminating in a galactose (Fig. 22–154). A genetic locus with the allelic genes H and h determines the first step of differentiation (Fig. 22–155). The H gene codes for an enzyme that transfers fucose to the terminal galactose of the precursor substance producing the antigen H. Since this antigen is needed as substrate for the production of A and B antigens, individuals without the H gene, or in other words, homozygous for h, will not make any of the ABH antigens. People with this rare phenotype called "Bombay" will have all three isoantibodies, Anti A, Anti B, and Anti H, and the only compatible donors will be other individuals of the Bombay type.

After the production of H antigens, the final determination of the specific blood type is controlled by three allelic genes in the ABO chromosomal locus. The A gene codes for an enzyme that transfers acetylgalactosamine to the terminal galactose and changes the H antigen to an A antigen. The B gene codes for an enzyme that transfers galactose to the terminal galactose and changes the H antigen to a B antigen. The O gene does not code for any recognized transferase and the H antigen remains unchanged. (See reviews by Mollison and by Giblett.)

About 20 per cent of individuals with A antigens belong to the clinically important sub-group A_2 (Table 22–30). The difference between this antigen and the common A antigen, so-called A_1, is, in part, quantitative rather than qualitative. The transferase, coded by the A_1 gene, transforms almost all the H-substrate to A_1 antigen while the transferase coded by A_2 is less active and leaves considerable amounts of unchanged H on the surface. This explains why A_2 red cell agglutinates in vitro—both with Anti-A_1 and with Anti-H. The occasional but potentially dangerous presence of Anti-A_1 antibodies in the plasma of the A_2 individuals, however, cannot be explained merely by the low density of A_1 antigen on the cell surface; and it seems likely that there are additional subtle differences in transferases or substrates.

The same precursor substance attached to cell surfaces is also present in body fluids. In its soluble form, it is attached to a circulating lipo-

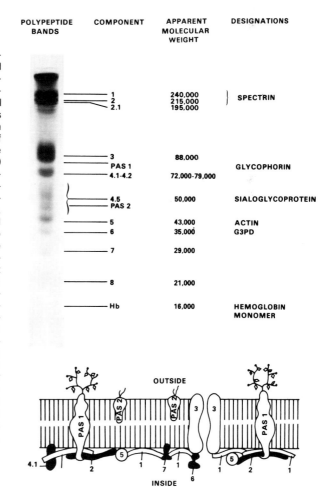

Figure 22–153 Characterization of the protein components of the red cell membrane and diagrammatic representation of its macromolecular architecture. Polyacrylamide gel electrophoresis after solubilization with sodium dodecyl sulfate shows a series of membrane components represented as numbers 1 to 8 with the addition of hemoglobin monomer at the lower portion of electrophoretic gel. Molecular weights of these components range from 240,000 down to 16,000 daltons. Several of the membrane protein components have been isolated and identified as indicated at right. Below is a diagram of a macromolecular model of the red cell membrane, showing the approximate locations of known red cell membrane protein components relative to the lipid bilayer. PAS-1, or glycophorin, is the transmembrane protein which bears the oligosaccharides and charged sialic acid groups at the external membrane surface. At the internal surface it presumably makes contact with spectrin components 1 and 2. These spectrin components form a continuous meshwork on the internal aspect of the membrane and interact with component 5, actin. Component 3 is a large-molecular-weight transmembrane protein which may contain a central aqueous core and serve in transmembrane transport of cations and other substances. Component 6 represents glyceraldehyde-3-phosphate dehydrogenase, an enzyme component localized to the internal membrane surface. (Courtesy of Lessin, L. S., and Bessis, M.: Hematology, 2nd Ed. McGraw-Hill, New York, 1977, p. 103.)

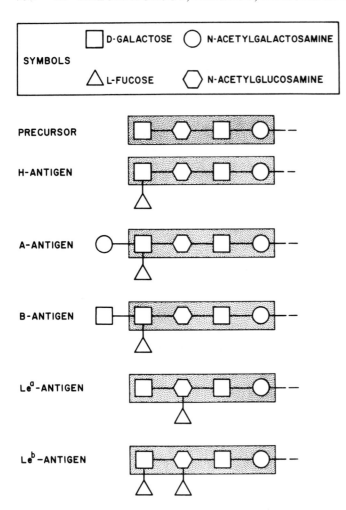

Figure 22–154   The biochemical configuration of the sugar chains in the closely linked group of ABH, Le^a, and Le^b antigens. They all have a common precursor skeleton and the addition of sugar is accomplished through the activity of genetically determined transfer enzymes. (Adapted from Watkins: Science, *162*:172, 1966.)

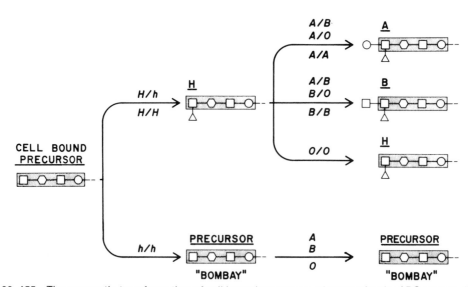

Figure 22–155   The enzymatic transformation of cell bound precursor substance for the ABO system. (See text.)

TABLE 22–30 ABO SYSTEM

Subgroups	Antigens	Antibodies
0	H	Anti A + Anti A₁ + Anti B
A₁	A₁	Anti B
A₂	A₁ + H	(Anti A₁ in 1% of subjects)
B	B	Anti A + Anti A₁
A₁B	A₁ + B	None
A₂B	A₁ + B	(Anti A₁ in 25% of subjects)

protein and serves as a substrate for the ABO determined transferases. The elaboration of soluble antigens, however, is more complex, since it involves the interaction of two closely related genetic loci—the "secretor" and the "Lewis" loci (Fig. 22–156).

About 20 per cent of all individuals lack the secretor gene (Se) and are homozygous se/se. In these individuals, the soluble precursor substance cannot be altered by the transferase produced by the H, A, and B genes. They are so-called non-secretors and have no ABH antigens

in their saliva, regardless of their capacity to produce ABH antigens on cell surfaces. If they are also Lewis negative (le/le), they do not secrete Lewis blood groups either. However, if they are Lewis positive (Le/le or Le/Le), as is 90 per cent of the population, the Lewis gene will code for a fucosyl transferase that transfers a fucose to the next to the last sugar molecule of the soluble precursor substance and changes it into a Lewis antigen — so-called Le^a substance. This substance in turn will be passively absorbed to the membrane of circulating red cells providing the cells with the phenotype $Le^{(a+b-)}$ (Table 22–31).

About 80 per cent of all individuals possess the secretor gene (Se/Se or Se/se), and in these individuals, the transferases coded by the H and the A and B genes can act on the soluble precursor substance and can make specific soluble antigens parallel to their action on the precursor substance on the red cells. Ten per cent of these individuals are Lewis negative, and no soluble Lewis substance will be produced or passed on to the red cells. In the 90 per cent who have the Lewis gene, however, the precursor substance will be exposed to two fucosyl transferases, one coded by the Lewis gene and capable of transferring a fucose to the next to the last sugar molecule, and the other coded by

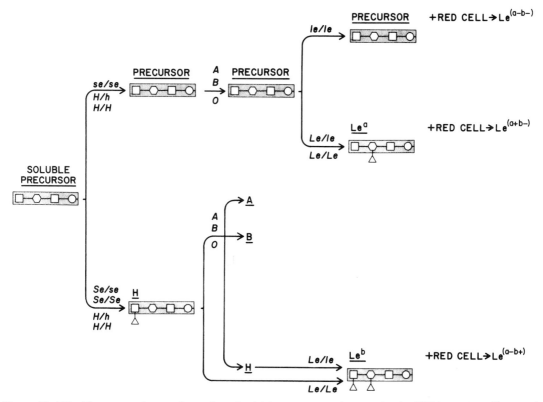

Figure 22–156 The enzymatic transformation of soluble precursor substance for the ABO Le system. (See text.)

TABLE 22–31 H-ABO-Se-Le SYSTEM

Genotype				Phenotype	
H (99.9%)*	ABO (100%)*	Se (80%)*	Le (90%)*	Soluble	Red Cells
+	+	−	−	−	ABO
					$Le^{(a-b-)}$
+	+	−	+	−	ABO
				Le^a	$Le^{(a+b-)}$
+	+	+	−	ABO	ABO
				−	$Le^{(a-b-)}$
+	+	+	+	ABO	ABO
				Le^b	$Le^{(a-b+)}$

*Incidence of genes in population.

the H gene and capable of transferring a fucose to the last sugar molecule. The result is the production of an Le^b substance that in turn will be absorbed to red cells, and render them $Le^{(a-b+)}$ (Table 22–31).

Of the other blood group systems, the Ii system is the most closely related to the ABO and Lewis systems. The antigens are carbohydrates; they are present in secretions as well as on cell membranes; they are present in close proximity to the ABH antigens on the red cell surface, and they are associated with naturally occurring isoantibodies. The phenotypic expression of the Ii system bears a remarkable resemblance to that of the fetal-adult hemoglobins. Antigen i is present during fetal development and is gradually replaced by antigen I at time of birth (Giblett and Crookston, 1964). In some individuals and in certain hematologic disorders, however, the antigen i reappears in a fashion analogous to that of fetal hemoglobin. Anti I is a cold reactive antibody present in small amounts in all adults and in large amounts in patients with atypical (mycoplasma) pneumonia, and in some patients with cold-reactive, acquired hemolytic anemia.

Naturally occurring isoantibodies may also be directed against antigens of the MN and P systems. The antigens in all systems with isoantibodies appear slowly during fetal maturation and are still not fully expressed at time of birth. The isoantibodies are usually not found until three to six months after birth, and if present earlier, are acquired passively from the mother. The isoantibodies of the ABO system are primarily of the complement-binding IgM type. Even isoantibodies of the IgG type, however, will bind complement and cause hemolysis, presumably due to the great density of the ABH sites on the red cell surface. Antibodies of the IgM type cause visible agglutination in vitro because their pentameric structure provides enough length to

bridge the gap between cells. The IgG antibodies, on the other hand, usually cannot do so unless the negative repelling charge of red cells is decreased by trypsin or papain treatment or by coating with albumin. Albumin may also cause clustering of antigenic sites, thereby facilitating IgG-induced agglutination of cells sparsely covered by antigens (Victoria, et al., 1975). The addition of antibodies against IgG molecules or complement (Coombs serum) leads to visible agglutination of IgG-coated red cells. The immunologic origin of the naturally occurring isoantibodies is still unknown. They may be genetically determined, but it seems more likely that they are acquired during early infancy in response to AB-like exogenous antigens absorbed through the immature gastrointestinal mucosa.

In a number of blood group systems, such as Rh, Kell, and Duffy, naturally occurring antibodies are absent, and sensitization occurs first after repeated parental exposures to their antigens. Of these systems, the Rh system is of most importance, since the strong antigenicity and early fetal emergence of the D antigen make it a frequent offender in transfusion reactions and in the development of erythroblastosis fetalis.

The Rh antigens are lipoproteins rather than glycolipoproteins, and they are present in a much smaller number on the red cell surface than the antigens of the ABO system. This low antigenic density, about 10–20,000 sites per cell, may explain the fact that IgG immune Rh antibodies rarely fix complement or cause intravascular hemolysis. The biochemical structure of the antigenic sites is poorly understood. They appear, however, to be integral parts of the lipid surface layer, rather than elevated above it as in the case of the branching polysaccharide chain of the ABH sites. This conclusion is supported by the fact that in the absence of all Rh sites, as found in the rare genetic condition, Rh null, the red cells

TABLE 22-32 NOMENCLATURE AND FREQUENCY OF Rh-Hr SYSTEM

Separate Gene Hypothesis (Fisher-Race) Gene and Agglutinogen	Single Gene Hypothesis (Wiener)		Frequency in Caucasians (Race and Sanger, 1962)
	Gene	Agglutinogen	
DCe	R'	Rh_1	41%
DcE	R^2	Rh_2	14%
Dce	R^o	Rh_o	3%
DCE	R^z	Rh_z	<1%
ce	r	rh	39%
Ce	r'	rh'	1%
cE	r''	rh''	1%
CE	r^y	rh_z	<1%

are defective and short-lived, while in the absence of all ABH sites, as found in the Bombay type, the red cell surface is presumably normal, since the red cells survive normally in the circulation (Levine, et al., 1973).

It has been proposed that the Rh sites in the surface layer of the membrane consist of three connected loci; the first containing either C (rh') or c (hr'), the second containing either E (rh") or e (hr"), and the third containing either D (Rh$_o$) or no known antigen. Only the D is a strong antigen and the antigenic behavior of the eight possible combinations (Table 22–32) is mostly determined by the presence or absence of D. Although the concept of three separate but connected loci (Fisher and Race) is attractive and easy to understand and remember, family studies indicate that each of the eight possible combinations behaves as the product of a single gene (Wiener), a finding justifying the use of the Rh-Hr terminology, at least by blood bankers. Since the blood type of each individual is determined by a pair of genes, 36 genotypes are possible resulting in the production of 18 different phenotypes. This multitude of types are of great importance for genetic mapping, but for transfusion reaction and erythro-

blastosis, the presence or absence of the D (Rh$_o$) antigen is still the prime concern.

Although the ABO and possibly also the Rh genes express themselves on all cell surfaces, the major antigens of the leukocytes and platelets do not belong to these systems. These antigens, also ubiquitous in distribution, are the histocompatibility antigens of the HL-A system (for Human Leukocyte Antigens) as well as a few antigens presumably specific for each cell type. During the last decade, histocompatibility antigens have become of prime importance for skin and organ transplantation and for platelet and leukocyte transfusions (reviewed by Bach and van Rood, 1976). They are glycoproteins and so numerous that about 1 per cent of all proteins found on the lymphocyte membrane are HL-A antigens. They undergo continuous production and turnover, and it seems likely that soluble HL-A antigens in tissue fluids originate from cell membranes. The genetic locus controlling the production of the HL-A antigens consists of a complex of subloci which in man are located in close proximity on chromosome No. 6 (Fig. 22–157).

The two major subloci HLA-A and HLA-B (new nomenclature) are serologically defined or, in

Figure 22–157 Chromosome #6 with the HLA D, B, C, and A regions and some established loci for other gene complexes (PGM-3 = Phosphoglucomutase-3, GLO = Glyoxylase, PG-5 = Urinary pepsinogen-5). Complement C2 is situated in a specific locus close to HLA-D while other complement loci are less defined although situated in the HLA region. (Adapted from McKusick, V. A. and Ruddle, F. H., 1977.)

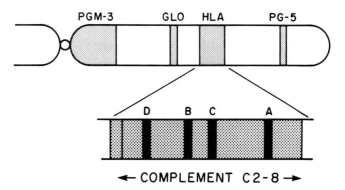

TABLE 22-33   THE HLA SYSTEM

Sublocus A	Sublocus B	Sublocus C	Sublocus D
Recognized Antigens, 1977			
HLA–A1	HLA–B5		
HLA–A2	HLA–B7		
HLA–A3	HLA–B8		
HLA–A9	HLA–B12		
HLA–A10	HLA–B13		
HLA–A11	HLA–B14		
HLA–A28	HLA–B18		
HLA–A29	HLA–B27		
Provisionally Identified Antigens, 1977			
HLA–Aw23	HLA–Bw15	HLA–Cw1	HLA–Dw1
↓	↓	↓	↓
HLA–Aw43	HLA–Bw42	HLA–Cw5	HLA–Dw6

other words, their numerous allelic antigens can be detected by specific antibodies. The antigens of sublocus HLA-C also produce circulating antibodies, but only a few alleles have been detected. The antigens of the important HLA-D locus are presently identified only by the mixed lymphocyte culture test (Table 22–33).

The serologic test, i.e., HLA microcytotoxicity test, depends on complement fixation to lymphocytes in the presence of a specific antibody. Complement fixation will damage the cell membrane and permit a dye to enter the cell or a ^{51}Cr-labeled cytoplasmic component to be released. Using a battery of antibodies obtained from multiparous women, patients with skin grafts or patients having received multiple transfusions of leukocytes, it has been possible to identify eight antigens determined by sublocus HLA-A and eight antigens by sublocus HLA-B (Table 22–33). A great number of additional antigens have been described and have received the designation w for workshop. In the inheritance of these HLA genes, the loci are so close together that there is rarely any crossover and the genes are passed on in fixed groups (Fig. 22–158).

The mixed lymphocyte culture or response test, so called MLC or MLR, is an in-vitro representa-tion of the in vivo lymphocyte response to foreign antigens. It consists of culturing lymphocyte suspensions from two individuals together for several days. The lymphocyte suspension from the unknown is "the responder," while the lymphocytes from an individual with a known HLA type serve as "the stimulator." The stimulating cells are prevented from responding by previous exposure to mitomycin C. The degree of DNA synthesis induced in the responding cells and measured by ^{3}H-thymidine incorporation is a measure of the genetic difference between individuals.

The antigens in the two serologically identifiable subloci of the HLA system underlie the matching grades in use for kidney transplantation (Table 22–34) and in case of cadaver transplant there is usually too little time for mixed lymphocyte culture matching. However, serologic matching alone is inadequate and immunosuppression is needed even for excellent A- and B-matches. In case of transplantation from live donors, more thorough tissue typing and cross-matching by means of a MLC test can be carried out. This is especially needed for bone marrow transplantation in which both host versus graft and graft versus host reactions play a role. Cross-matching or cross-culturing of lymphocytes from HLA-in-

INHERITANCE   OF   HISTOCOMPATIBILITY   ANTIGENS

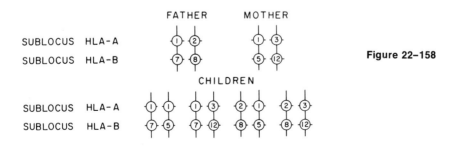

Figure 22–158

TABLE 22–34 MATCHING GRADES FOR HL-A SYSTEM

Grade

A	Identical siblings
B	Identical unrelated or no antigen in donor not present in recipient
C	1 Incompatibility
D	2 Incompatibilities
E	3 Incompatibilities
F	Positive crossmatch or ABO incompatibility

compatible individuals will, of course, result in DNA synthesis and blast transformation, but it may also be positive in perfectly matched individuals, suggesting the existence of additional genes not yet recognized by our serologic and MLC techniques for tissue typing. The enormous complexity of these systems has limited the therapeutic use of bone marrow transplantation and of platelet and leukocyte transfusions between unrelated individuals. Owing to the close genetic linkage of tissue types, however, such procedures carried out between matched siblings are often successful and, as summarized by Storb and co-workers, can provide dramatic therapeutic benefits.

REFERENCES

BONE MARROW

Baikie, A. G., Court Brown, W. M., Buckton, K. E., Harnden, D. G., Jacobs, P. A., and Tough, I. M.: A possible specific chromosome abnormality in human chronic myeloid leukaemia. Nature (London), *188*:1165, 1960.

Barr, R. D., and Whang-Peng, J.: Hemopoietic stem cells in human peripheral blood. Science, *190*:284, 1975.

Boggs, D. R., and Chervenick, P. A.: Hemopoietic stem cells. *In* Greenwalt, T. J., and Jamieson, G. A. (Eds.): Formation and Destruction of Blood Cells. J. B. Lippincott Co., Philadelphia, 1970, p. 240.

Clarke, B. J., and Houseman, D.: Characterization of an erythroid cell of high proliferative capacity in normal human peripheral blood. Proc. Nat. Acad. Sci. USA, *74*:1105, 1977.

Craddock, C. G., Longmire, R., and McMillan, R.: Lymphocytes and the immune response. N. Engl. J. Med., *285*:324, 1972.

Crosby, W. H.: Experience with Injured and Implanted Bone Marrow: Relation of Function to Structure. *In* Stohlman, F. Jr. (ed.): Hematopoietic Cellular Proliferation. Grune & Stratton, New York, 1970, p. 87.

Ebbe, S.: Thrombopoietin. Blood, *44*:605, 1974.

Erslev, A. J.: Feedback circuits in the control of stem cell differentiation. Am. J. Pathol., *65*:629, 1971.

Finch, C. A.: Pathophysiologic aspects of sickle cell anemia. Am. J. Med., *53*:1, 1972.

Finch, C. A., Harker, L. A., and Cook, J. D.: Kinetics of the formed elements of human blood. Blood, *50*:699, 1977.

Gregersen, M. I., and Rawson, R. A.: Blood volume. Physiol. Rev., *39*:307, 1959.

Gregory, C. J., and Eaves, A. C.: Human marrow cells capable of erythropoietic differentiation in vitro. Definition of three erythroid colony responses. Blood *49*:855, 1977.

Hudson, G.: Bone marrow volume in the human foetus and newborn. Br. J. Haematol., *11*:446, 1965.

Huggins, L., and Blockson, B. H.: Changes in outlying bone marrow accompanying a local increase of temperature within physiologic limits. J. Exp. Med., *64*:253, 1956.

Killmann, S. A., Cronkite, E. P., Fliedner, T. M., and Bond, V. P.: Mitotic indices of human bone marrow cells. III. Duration of some phases of erythrocyte and granulocytic proliferation computed from mitotic indices. Blood, *24*:267, 1964.

Kretchmar, A. L.: Erythropoietin: Hypothesis of action tested by analog computer. Science, *152*:367, 1966.

Nakeff, A., and Daniels-McQueen, S.: In vitro colony assay for a new class of megakaryocyte precursor: Colony-forming unit megakaryocyte (CFU-M). Proc. Soc. Exp. Biol. Med., *151*:587, 1976.

Ogawa, M., Grush, O. C., O'Dell, R. F., Hara, H., and MacEachern, M. D.: Circulating erythropoietic precursors assessed in culture: Characterization in normal men and patients with hemoglobinopathies. Blood, *50*:1081, 1977.

Reissmann, K. R., and Udupa, R. B.: Effect of erythropoietin on proliferation of erythropoietin-responsive cells. Cell Tissue Kinet., *5*:481, 1972.

Robinson, W. A., and Mangalik, A.: The kinetics and regulation of granulopoiesis. Seminars Hematol., *12*:7, 1975.

Till, J. E., and McCulloch, E. A.: A direct measurement of the radiation sensitivity of normal mouse bone marrow cells. Radiat. Res., *14*:213, 1961.

Trentin, J. J.: Determination of bone marrow stem cell differentiation by stromal hemopoietic inductive microenvironment (HIM). Am. J. Pathol., *65*:621, 1971.

Weiss, L.: The hemopoietic microenvironment of the bone marrow: An ultrastructural study of the stroma in rats. Anat. Rev., *186*:161, 1976.

Weiss, L.: The histology of the bone marrow. *In* Gordon, A. S. (Ed.): Regulation of Hematopoiesis. Appleton-Century-Crofts, New York, 1970, p. 79.

Weiss, L., and Chen, L. T.: The organization of hematopoietic cords and vascular sinuses in bone marrow. Blood Cells, *1*:617, 1975.

Wu, A. M., Till, J. E. Siminovitch, L., and McCulloch, E. A.: A cytological study of the capacity for differentiation of normal hemopóietic colony-forming cells. J. Cell. Physiol., *69*:177, 1967.

ERYTHROCYTES

Abramson, N., LoBuglio, A. F., Jandl, J. H., and Cotran, R. S.: The interaction between human monocytes and red cells. Binding characteristics. J. Exp. Med., *132*:1191, 1970.

Adamson, J. W., Fialkow, P. J., Murphy, S., Prechal, J. F., and Steinman, L.: Polycythemia vera: stem cell and probable clonal origin of the disease. N. Engl. J. Med., *295*:913, 1976.

Aisen, P., and Brown, E. B.: The iron binding function of transferrin in iron metabolism. Seminars Hematol. *14*, 31, 1977.

Alving, A. S., Johnson, C. F., Tarlov, A. R., Brewer, G. J., Kellermeyer, R. W., and Carson, P. E.: Mitigation of the haemolytic effect of primaquine and enhancement of its action against exoerythrocytic forms of the Chesson strain of plasmodium vivax by intermittent regimens of drug administration. Bull. WHO, *22*:621, 1960.

Arderman, S., Chanarin, I., and Doyle, J. C.: Studies on secretion of gastric intrinsic factor in man. Br. Med. J., *2*:600, 1964.

Bert, P.: La pression barométrique. Masson, Paris, 1878.

Bessis, M.: Life Cycle of the Erythrocyte. Sandoz Monographs, 1966.

Beutler, E., Yeh, M., and Fairbanks, V. F.: The normal human female as a mosaic of X-chromosome activity: Studies using the gene for G-6-PD deficiency as a marker. Proc. Nat. Acad. Sci., U.S.A., *48*:9, 1962.

Bookchin, R. M., and Nagel, R. L.: Interaction between hemoglobins: sickling and related phenomena. Seminars Hematol. *11*:577, 1974.

Bothwell, T. H., and Finch, C. A.: Iron Metabolism. Little, Brown & Co., Boston, 1962.

Brain, M. C.,: Microangiopathic hemolytic anemia. Ann. Rev. Med., *21*:133, 1970.

Brown, S. M., Gilbert, H. S., Krauss, S., and Wasserman, L. R.:

Relative polycythemia: a non-existant disease. Am. J. Med., 50:200, 1971.

Bull, B. S., and Kuhn, I. N.: The production of schistocytes by fibrin strands (a scanning electron microscopic study). Blood, 35:104, 1970.

Bunn, H. F., Forget, B. G., and Ranney, H. M.: Human Hemoglobins. W. B. Saunders Co., Philadelphia, 1977.

Bunn, H. F., and Jandl, J. H.: The renal handling of hemoglobin. II. Catabolism. J. Exp. Med., 129:925, 1969.

Castle, W. B.: Current concepts of pernicious anemia. Am. J. Med., 48:541, 1970.

Chanarin, I.: The Megaloblastic Anemias. F. A. Davis Co., Philadelphia, 1969.

Charache, S., Conley, C. L., Waugh, D. E., Ugoretz, R. J., and Spurrell, J. R.: Pathogenesis of hemolytic anemia in homozygous hemoglobin C disease. J. Clin. Invest., 46:1795, 1967.

Chisholm, J. J., Jr.: The continued hazard of lead poisoning. Hosp. Pract., 8:11, 127, 1973.

Chodos, R. B., Wells, R., Jr., and Chaffee, W. R.: A study of ferrokinetics and red cell survival in congestive heart failure. Am. J. Med., 36:553, 1964.

Condon, P. I., and Serjeant, G. R.: Ocular findings in homozygous sickle cell anemia in Jamaica. Am. J. Ophthalmol., 73:533, 1972.

Cooper, R. A.: Abnormalities of cell membrane fluidity in the pathogenesis of disease. N. Engl. J. Med., 297:371, 1977.

Cooper, R. A., and Jandl, J. H.: Bile salts and cholesterol in the pathogenesis of target cells in obstructive jaundice. J. Clin. Invest., 47:809, 1968.

Cooper, R. A., and Jandl, J. H.: The selective and conjoint loss of red cell lipids. J. Clin. Invest., 48:906, 1969.

Cronkite, E. P., and Bond, V. P.: Radiation Injury in Man. Charles C Thomas, Springfield, Illinois, 1960.

Davidson, R. J. L.: March or exertional hemoglobinuria. Seminars Hematol., 6:150, 1969.

deFuria, F. G., Miller, D. R., Cerami, A., et al.: The effects of cyanate in vitro on red blood cell metabolism and function in sickle cell anemia. J. Clin. Invest., 51:566, 1972.

Dhar, G. J., Bossenmaier, I., Petryka, Z. J., Cardinal, R., and Watson, C. J.: Effects of hemetin in hepatic porphyria. Further studies. Ann. Int. Med., 83:20, 1975.

Donohue, D. M., Reiff, R. H., Hanson, M. L., Betson, Y., and Finch, C. A.: Quantitative measurements of the erythrocytic and granulocytic cells of the marrow and blood. J. Clin. Invest., 37:1571, 1958.

Edwards, C. Q., Carroll, M., Bray, P., and Cartwright, G. R.: Hereditary hemochromatosis. Diagnosis in siblings and children. N. Engl. J. Med., 297, 7, 1977.

Erbe, R. W.: Inborn errors of folate metabolism. N. Engl. J. Med., 293, 753, 1975.

Erslev, A. J.: Humoral regulation of red cell production. Blood, 8:349, 1953.

Erslev, A. J.: The role of erythropoietin in the control of red cell production. Medicine, 43:661, 1964.

Erslev, A. J.: Anemia of chronic renal disease. Arch. Intern. Med., 126:774, 1970.

Erslev, A. J.: The renal biogenesis of erythropoietin. Am. J. Med., 58:25, 1975.

Filmanowicz, E., and Gurney, C. W.: Studies on erythropoiesis. XVI. Response to a single dose of erythropoietin in polycythemic mouse. J. Lab. Clin. Med., 57:65, 1961.

Finch, C. A.: Iron metabolism. Nutrition Today, Summer, 1969, p. 2.

Finch, C. A., Harker, L. A., and Cook, J. D.: Kinetics of the formed elements of human blood. Blood, 50:699, 1977.

Finch, C. A., and Lenfant, C.: Oxygen transport in man. N. Engl. J. Med., 286:407, 1972.

Finch, J. T., Perutz, M. F., Bertles, J. F., and Döbler, J.: Structure of sickled erythrocytes and of sickle cell hemoglobin fibers. Proc. Nat. Acad. Sci., U.S.A., 70, 718, 1973.

Freda, V. J., Gorman, J. G., Pollack, W., and Bowe, E.: Prevention of Rh hemolytic disease — 10 years' clinical experience with Rh immune globulin. N. Engl. J. Med., 292, 1014, 1975.

Gallo, R. C., Fraimow, W., Cathcart, R. T., and Erslev, A. J.:

Erythropoietic response in chronic pulmonary disease. Arch. Intern. Med., 113:559, 1964.

Gardner, F. H., Nathan, D. G., Piomelli, S., and Cummins, F. J.: The erythrocythaemic effects of androgen. Brit. J. Haematol., 14:611, 1968.

Gardner, F. H., and Pringle, J. C., Jr.: Androgens and erythropoiesis. II. Treatment of myeloid metaplasia. N. Engl. J. Med., 264:103, 1961.

Gemsa, D., Woo, C. H., Fudenberg, H. H., and Schmid, R.: Erythrocyte catabolism by macrophages in vitro. The effect of hydrocortisone on erythrophagocytosis and on the induction of heme oxygenase. J. Clin. Invest., 52, 812, 1973.

Giblett, E. R.: Genetic Markers in Human Blood. Oxford, Blackwell Scientific Publications Ltd., 1969, p. 349.

Gidari, A. S., and Levere, R. D.: Enzymatic formation and cellular regulation of heme synthesis. Seminars Hematol., 14, 145, 1977.

Gilette, P., Manning, J. M., and Cerami, A.: Increased survival of sickle cell erythrocytes after treatment in vitro with sodium cyanate. Proc. Nat. Acad. Sci., 68:2791, 1971.

Gordon, A. S., Cooper, G. W., and Zanjani, E. D.: The kidney and erythropoiesis. Seminars Hematol., 4:337, 1967.

Götze, O., and Müller-Eberhard, H. J.: Paroxysmal nocturnal hemoglobinuria. Hemolysis initiated by the C3 activator system. N. Engl. J. Med., 286:180, 1972.

Granick, S., and Levere, R.: Heme synthesis in erythroid cells. Progr. Hematol., 4:1, 1964.

Gräsbeck, R.: Intrinsic factor and the transcobalamins with reflections on the general function and evolution of soluble transport proteins. Scand. J. Clin. Lab. Invest., 19:(Suppl. 95), 1967.

Gräsbeck, R.: Intrinsic factor and other vitamin B_{12} transport proteins. Progr. Hematol., 6:233, 1969.

Hall, C. A.: Transcobalamins I and II as natural transport proteins of vitamin B_{12}. J. Clin. Invest., 56, 1125, 1975.

Harris, J. W.: Notes and comments on pyridoxine responsive anemia and the role of erythrocyte mitochondria in iron metabolism. Medicine, 43:803, 1964.

Harris, J. W., and Kellermeyer, R. W.: The Red Cell. Cambridge, Harvard University Press, 1970.

Haurani, F. I., Burke, W., and Martinez, E. J.: Defective reutilization of iron in the anemia of inflammation. J. Lab. Clin. Med., 65:560, 1965.

Herbert, V.: Experimental nutritional folate deficiency in man. Trans. Am. Assoc. Physicians, 75:307, 1962.

Hershko, C., Cook, J. D., and Finch, C. A.: Storage iron kinetics. II. The uptake of hemoglobin by hepatic parenchymal cells. J. Lab. Clin. Med., 80, 624, 1972.

Hillman, R. S., and Finch, C. A.: Erythropoiesis: normal and abnormal. Seminars Hematol., 4:327, 1967.

Hines, J. D., Hoffbrand, A. V., and Mollin, D. L.: The hematologic complications following partial gastrectomy. Am. J. Med., 43:555, 1967.

Hoffbrand, A. V.: Synthesis and breakdown of natural folates (folate polyglutamates). Progr. Hematol., 9, 85, 1975.

Horowitz, H. J., Stein, J. M., Cohen, B. D., and White, J. M.: Further studies on the platelet-inhibitory effect of guanidinosuccinic acid and its role in uremic bleeding. Am. J. Med., 49:336, 1970.

Hurtado, A.: Acclimatization to high altitudes. In Weihe, W. H. (Ed.): Physiological Effects of High Altitude. Pergamon Press, New York, 1964, p. 1.

Itano, H. A.: The human hemoglobins; their properties and genetic control. Adv. Protein Chem., 12:216, 1957.

Jacobs, A.: Iron balance and its disorders. Proc. Roy. Soc. Med., 63:1215, 1970.

Jacobs, A.: Iron overload — clinical and pathologic aspects. Seminars Hematol., 14, 89, 1977.

Jacobson, L. O., Goldwasser, E., Fried, W., and Plzak, L.: Role of the kidney in erythropoiesis. Nature (London), 179:633, 1957.

Jaffe, C. J., Atkinson, J. P., and Frank, M. M.: The role of complement in the clearance of cold agglutinin sensitized erythrocytes in man. J. Clin. Invest., 58, 942, 1976.

Jaffé, E. R., and Hsieh, H. S.: DPNH-dependent methemoglobin reductase deficiency and hereditary methemoglobinemia. Seminars Hematol., 8:417, 1971.

Jensen, W. N., and Lessin, L. S.: Membrane alterations associated with hemoglobinopathies. Seminars Hematol., 7:409, 1970.

Josephs, R., Jarosch, H. S., and Edelstein, S. J.: Polymorphism of sickle cell hemoglobin fibers. J. Mol. Biol., 102, 409, 1976.

Jourdanet, D.: De l'anémie des altitudes et de l'anémie en général dans ses rapports avec la pression de l'atmosphére. Braillere, Paris, 1863.

Kan, Y. W., Golbus, M. S., Trecartin, R. F., et al.: Prenatal diagnosis of β thalassemia and sickle cell anemia. Lancet, i:269, 1977.

Kansu, E., and Erslev, A. J.: Aplastic anemia with "hot pockets". Scand. J. Haematol., 17:326, 1976.

Kass, L. S.: Pernicious Anemia. W. B. Saunders Co., Philadelphia, 1976.

Kirschbaum, J. D., Matsno, T., Sato, K., Ishimarn, M., Tsucchmoto, T., and Ishimarn, T.: A study of aplastic anemia in an autopsy series with special reference to atomic bomb survivors in Hiroshima and Nagasaki. Blood, 38:17, 1971.

Knospe, W. H., Blom, J., and Crosby, W. H.: Regeneration of locally irradiated bone marrow. II. Induction of regeneration in permanently aplastic medullary cavities. Blood, 31:400, 1968.

Koenig, R. J., Peterson, C. M., Jones, R. L., et al.: Correlation of glucose regulation and hemoglobin A_{1c} in diabetes mellitus. N. Engl. J. Med., 295, 417, 1976.

Krantz, S. B., and Kuo, V.: Studies on red cell aplasia. II. Report of a second patient with an antibody to erythroblast nuclei and a remission after immunosuppressive therapy. Blood, 34:1, 1969.

Kushner, J. P., Barbuto, A. J., and Lee, G. R.: An inherited enzymatic defect in porphyria cutanea tarda. Decreased uroporphyrinogen decarboxylase activity. J. Clin. Invest., 58, 1089, 1976.

Kushner, J. P., Lee, G. R., Wintrobe, M. M., and Cartwright, G. E.: Idiopathic refractory sideroblastic anemia. Clinical and laboratory investigation of 17 patients and review of the literature. Medicine, 50:139, 1971.

Landaw, S. A., Callahan, E. W., Jr., and Schmid, R.: Catabolism of heme in vivo: comparison of the simultaneous production of bilirubin and carbon monoxide. J. Clin. Invest., 49:914, 1970.

Leblond, P. F., Chamberlain, J. K., and Weed, R. J.: Scanning electron microscopy of erythropoietin — stimulated bone marrow. Blood Cells, 1:639, 1975.

Lessin, L. S., and Bessis, M.: Morphology of the erythron. In Williams, W. J., et al. (Eds.): Hematology, 2nd Ed. McGraw-Hill Book Co., New York, 1977, p. 103.

Lessin, L. S., Jensen, W. N., and Klug, P.: Ultrastructure of the normal and hemoglobinopathic red blood cell membrane. Arch. Intern. Med., 129:306, 1972.

Lewis, S. M., and Dacie, J. V.: The aplastic anemia: Paroxysmal nocturnal hemoglobinuria syndrome. Br. J. Haematol., 13:236, 1967.

Lipschitz, D. A., Cook, J. D., and Finch, C. A.: A clinical evaluation of serum ferritin as an index of iron stores. N. Engl. J. Med., 290, 1213, 1974.

Logue, G., and Rosse, W.: Immunologic mechanisms in autoimmune hemolytic disease. Seminars Hematol., 13, 277, 1976.

Marks, P. A., and Rifkind, R. A.: Protein synthesis in erythropoiesis. Science, 175:955, 1972.

Marsh, G. W., and Lewis, S. M.: Cardiac hemolytic anemia. Seminars Hematol., 6:133, 1969.

Martland, H. S.: The occurrence of malignancy in radioactive persons. Am. J. Cancer, 15:2435, 1931.

Marver, H. S., and Schmid, R.: The Porphyrias. In Stanbury, J. B., Wyngaarden, J. B., and Frederickson, D. S. (eds.): The Metabolic Basis of Inherited Disease. McGraw-Hill, New York, 1972, p. 1087.

McIntyre, P.: Radioactive tracers in hematologic disease. Hosp. Pract., 7:3, 99, 1972.

Metcalfe, J., Dhindsa, D. S., Edwards, M. J., and Mordjinis, A.: Decreased oxygen affinity of blood for oxygen in patients with low-output heart failure. Circ. Res., 25:47, 1969.

Miller, M. E.: Thymic dysplasia ("Swiss agammaglobulinemia").

I. Graft vs. host reaction following bone marrow transfusion. J. Pediatr., 70:730, 1967.

Milner, P. F., Clegg, J. B., and Weatherall, D. J.: Hemoglobin H disease due to a unique hemoglobin variant with an elongated alpha-chain. Lancet, 1:729, 1971.

Modan, B., and Lilienfeld, A. M.: Polycythemia vera and leukemia — the role of radiation treatment. A study of 1,222 patients. Medicine, 44:305, 1965.

Mollin, D. L., Waters, A. H., and Harriss, E.: Clinical aspects of the metabolic inter-relationships between folic acid and vitamin B_{12}. Vitamin B_{12} and intrinsic factor, 2. In Heinrich, H. C. (Ed.): Europaisches Symposion, Hamburg. Stuttgart, Enke, 1961, p. 737.

Morley, A., and Stohlman, F., Jr.: Erythropoiesis in the dog: the periodic nature of the steady state. Science, 165:1025, 1969.

Motulsky, A. G.: Hemolysis in glucose-6-phosphate dehydrogenase deficiency. Fed. Proc., 31:1286, 1972.

Muirhead, H., Cox, J. M., Mazzarella, L., and Perutz, M. F.: Structure and function of haemoglobin III. A three-dimensional Fourier synthesis of human deoxyhaemoglobin at 5.5 A resolution. J. Mol. Biol., 13:646, 1965.

Muldowney, F. P., Crooks, J., and Wayne, E. F.: The total red cell mass in thyrotoxicosis and myxoedema. Clin. Sci., 16:309, 1957.

Müller-Eberhard, H. J.: Chemistry and Function of the complement system. Hosp. Pract., 12:8, 33, 1977.

Murayama, M.: Molecular mechanism of red cell "sickling." Science, 153:145, 1966.

Murray, J. F., Gold, P., and Johnson, B. L., Jr.: The circulatory effects of hematocrit variations in normovolemic and hypervolemic dogs. J. Clin. Invest., 42:1150, 1963.

Nienhuis, A. W., Barker, J. E., and Anderson, W. F.: Effect of erythropoietin on hemoglobin synthesis. In Fisher, J. (ed.): Kidney Hormones, Vol. 2. Academic Press, New York, in press.

Nienhuis, A. W., and Benz, E. J., Jr.: Regulation of hemoglobin synthesis during the development of the red cell. N. Engl. J. Med., 297, 1318, 1977.

Owren, P. A.: Congenital hemolytic jaundice: The pathogenesis of the "hemolytic crisis." Blood, 3:231, 1948.

Pape, L., Multani, J. S., Stitt, C., and Saltman, P.: In vitro reconstitution of ferritin. Biochemistry, 7:606, 1968.

Perutz, M. F.: Stero chemistry of cooperative effects in haemoglobin. Nature, 228:726, 1970.

Pillow, R. P., Epstein, R. B., Buckner, C. D., Giblett, E. R., and Thomas, E. D.: Treatment of bone marrow failure by isogeneic marrow infusion. N. Engl. J. Med., 275:94, 1966.

Piomelli, S., Lamola, A. A., Poh-Fitzpatrick, M. B., Seaman, C., and Harber, L. C.: Erythropoietic protoporphyria and lead intoxication: the molecular basis for difference in cutaneous photosensitivity. J. Clin. Invest., 56:1519, 1975.

Prchal, J. F., Adamson, J. W., Murphy, S., Steinman, L., and Fialkow, P. J.: Polycythemia vera: the in vitro response of normal and abnormal stem cell lines to erythropoietin. J. Clin. Invest., 1978 (in press).

Propper, R. D., Cooper, B., Rufo, R. R., Nienhuis, A. W., Anderson, W. F., Bunn, H. F., Rosenthal, A., and Nathan, D. G.: Continuous subcutaneous administration of deferoxamine in patients with iron overload. N. Engl. J. Med., 297, 418, 1977.

Pruzanski, W., and Shumak, K. H.: Biologic activity of cold-reacting auto-antibodies. N. Engl. J. Med., 297, 538, 1977.

Ratto, O., Brescoe, W. A., Morton, J. W., and Comroe, J. H., Jr.: Anoxemia secondary to polycythemia and polycythemia secondary to anoxemia. Am. J. Med., 19:958, 1955.

Reissmann, K. R.: Studies on the mechanism of erythropoietic stimulation in parabiotic rats during hypoxia. Blood, 5:372, 1950.

Ricketts, C., Jacobs, A., Cavill, I.: Ferrokinetics and erythropoiesis in man: The measurement of effective erythropoiesis, ineffective erythropoiesis and red cell life span using ^{59}Fe. Br. J. Haematol., 31, 65, 1975.

Rosenberg, L. E., Lilljeqvist, A-C., and Hsia, Y. E.: Methylmalonic aciduria: metabolic block localization and vitamin B_{12} dependency. Science, 162:805, 1968.

Rosse, W. F.: Quantitative immunology of immune hemolytic

anemia. II. The relationship of un-bound antibody to hemolysis and the effect of treatment. J. Clin. Invest., *50*:734, 1971.

Rosse, W. F., Dourmashkin, R., and Humphrey, J. H.: Immune lysis of normal and paroxysmal nocturnal hemoglobinuria (PNH) red blood cells. II. The membrane defects caused by complement lysis. J. Exp. Med., *123*:969, 1966.

Schmid, R.: Bilirubin metabolism in man. N. Engl. J. Med., *287*, 703, 1972.

Schroeder, W. A., Huisman, T. H. J., Shelton, R., Shelton, R. B., Kleihauer, E. F., Dozy, A. M., and Robberson, B.: Evidence for multiple structural genes for the γ chain of human fetal hemoglobin. Proc. Nat. Acad. Sci. U.S.A., *60*:537, 1968.

Shahidi, N. T., and Diamond, L. K.: Testosterone-induced remission in aplastic anemia of both acquired and congenital types. N. Engl. J. Med., *264*:953, 1961.

Shahidi, N. T.: Androgens and erythropoiesis. N. Engl. J. Med., *289*:72, 1971.

Skalak, R., and Brånemark, P. I.: Deformation of red blood cells in capillaries. Science, *164*:717, 1969.

Smith, J. R., and Landaw, S. A.: Smokers' polycythemia. N. Engl. J. Med., *298*:6, 1978.

Spaet, T. H., Bauer, S., and Melamed, S.: Hemorrhagic thrombocythemia. A blood coagulation disorder. Arch. Intern. Med., *98*:377, 1956.

Stamatoyannopoulos, G., Bellingham, A. J., Lenfant, C., and Finch, C. A.: Abnormal hemoglobins with high and low oxygen affinity. Ann. Rev. Med., *22*:221, 1971.

Stewart, W. B., Yuile, C. L., Claiborne, H. A., Snowman, R. T., and Whipple, G. H.: Radio iron absorption in anemic dogs. Fluctuations in the mucosal block and evidence for a gradient of absorption in the gastrointestinal tract. J. Exp. Med., *92*:375, 1950.

Storb, R., Prentice, R. L., and Thomas, E. D.: Treatment of aplastic anemia by marrow transfusion from HLA identified siblings. Prognostic factors associated with graft versus host disease and survival. J. Clin. Invest., *59*:625, 1977.

Streiff, R. R.: Folate deficiency and oral contraceptives. J.A.M.A., *214*:105, 1970.

Tabulation of reports compiled by the Panel on Hematology of the Registry on Adverse Reactions. Council on Drugs. American Medical Association, May, 1965, and June, 1967.

Thomas, E. D., et al.: Aplastic anemia treated by bone marrow transplantation. Lancet, *1*:284, 1972.

Thorling, E. B.: Paraneoplastic erythrocytosis and inappropriate erythropoietin production: A Review. Scand. J. Haematol., Suppl. 17, 1972.

Thorling, E. B., and Erslev, A. J.: The "tissue" tension of oxygen and its relation to hematocrit and erythropoietin. Blood, *32*:332, 1968.

Torrance, J., Jacobs, P., Restrepo, A., Eschbach, J., Lenfant, C., and Finch, C. A.: Intraerythrocytic adaptation to anemia. N. Engl. J. Med., *283*:165, 1970.

Valentine, W. N.: Hereditary hemolytic anemias associated with specific erythrocyte enzymopathies. Calif. Med., *108*:280, 1968.

Valentine, W. N., Paglia, D. E., Fink, K., and Madokoro, G.: Lead poisoning. Association with hemolytic anemia, basophilic stippling, erythrocyte pyrimidine-5'-nucleotidase deficiency, and intraerythrocytic accumulation of pyrimidines. J. Clin. Invest., *58*, 926, 1976.

Vincent, P. C., and de Gruchy, G. C.: Complications and treatment of acquired aplastic anemia. Br. J. Haematol., *13*:977, 1967.

Ward, H. P., Kurnick, J. E., and Pisarczyk, M. J.: Serum level of erythropoietin in anemias associated with chronic infection, malignancy and primary hematopoietic disease. J. Clin. Invest., *50*:332, 1971.

Waxman, S., Metz, J., and Herbert, V.: Defective DNA synthesis in human megaloblastic bone marrow: Effects of homocysteine and methionine. J. Clin. Invest., *48*:284, 1969.

Weatherall, D. J., and Clegg, J. B.: The Thalassemia Syndromes. Blackwell Scientific Publications Ltd., London, 1972.

Weed, R. I.: Hereditary spherocytosis. Arch. Int. Med., *135*, 1316, 1975.

Weed, R. I., LaCelle, P. L., and Merrill, E. W.: Metabolic dependence of red cell deformability. J. Clin. Invest., *48*:795, 1969.

Weed, R. I., and Reed, C. F.: Membrane alterations leading to red cell destruction. Am. J. Med., *41*:681, 1966.

Weintraub, L. R., Weinstein, M. B., Huser, H. J., and Rafal, S.: Absorption of hemoglobin iron: Role of heme-splitting substance in intestinal mucosa. J. Clin. Invest., *47*:531, 1968.

Wiley, J. S.: Red cell survival studies in hereditary spherocytosis. J. Clin. Invest., *49*:666, 1970.

Williams, D. M., Lynch, R. E., and Cartwright, G. E.: Drug-induced aplastic anemia. Seminars Hematol., *10*:195, 1973.

Wishner, B. C., Ward, K. B., Lattman, E. E., and Love, W. E.: Crystal structure of sickle cell deoxyhemoglobin at 5 Å resolution. J. Mol. Biol., *98*, 179, 1975.

Worwood, M.: The clinical biochemistry of iron. Seminars Hematol., *14, 3*, 1977.

Wood, W. G., Clegg, J. B., and Weatherall, D. J.: Developmental biology of human hemoglobins. Progr. Hematol., *10*, 43, 1977.

Yunis, A. A., Smith, U. S., and Restrepo, A.: Reversible bone marrow suppression from chloramphenicol. A consequence of mitochondrial injury. Arch. Intern. Med., *125*:272, 1970.

PHAGOCYTES

Baehner, R. L., and Nathan, D. G.: Quantitative nitroblue tetrazolium test in chronic granulomatous disease. N. Engl. J. Med., *278*:971, 1968.

Beeson, P. B., and Bass, D. A.: The Eosinophil. W. B. Saunders Co., Philadelphia, 1977.

Bizzozero, O. J., Johnson, K. G., and Ciocco, A.: Radiation-related leukemia in Hiroshima and Nagasaki, 1946–1964. N. Engl. J. Med., *274*:1095, 1966.

Blume, R. S., Bennett, J. M., Yankee, R. A., and Wolff, S. M.: Defective granulocyte regulation in the Chediak-Higashi syndrome. N. Engl. J. Med., *279*:1009, 1968.

Boggs, D. R.: The kinetics of neutrophilic leukocytes in health and disease. Seminars Hematol., *4*:359, 1967.

Brady, R. O.: Biochemical and metabolic basis of familial sphingolipidosis. Seminars Hematol., *9*:273, 1972.

Cline, M. J.: Biochemistry and function of monocytes and macrophages. *In* Williams, W. J., et al. (Eds.): Hematology, 2nd Ed. McGraw-Hill Book Co., New York, 1977, p. 861.

Cline, M. J., and Golde, D. W.: A review and reevaluation of histiocytic disorders. Am. J. Med., *55*:49, 1973.

Craddock, C. G., Perry, S., Lawrence, J. S., Buxbaum, L., and Pieper, G.: Production and distribution of granulocytes and the control of granulocyte release. *In* Wolstenholme, G. E. W., and O'Connor, M. (Eds.): Ciba Foundation Symposium on Haemopoiesis. Churchill, London, 1960, p. 237.

Dameshek, W.: Some speculations on the myeloproliferative syndromes. Blood, *6*:392, 1951.

Ferrans, V. J., Buja, M., Roberts, W. C., and Frederickson, D. S.: The spleen in Type I hyperlipoproteinemia. Am. J. Pathol., *64*:67, 1971.

Fialkow, P. J., Thomas, E. D., Bryant, J. J., and Neiman, P. E.: Leukaemic transformation of engrafted human marrow cells in vivo. Lancet, *1*:251, 1971.

Golde, D. W., and Cline, M. J.: Regulation of granulopoiesis. N. Engl. J. Med., *291*:1388, 1974.

Golde, D. W., Finley, T. N. and Cline, M. J.: The pulmonary macrophages in acute leukemia. N. Engl. J. Med., *290*:875, 1974.

Gralnick, H. R.: Classification of acute leukemia. Ann Int. Med., *87*:740, 1977.

Gross, L.: Viral etiology of leukemia and lymphomas. Blood, *25*:377, 1965.

Higby, D. J., and Henderson, E. S.: Granulocyte transfusion therapy. Ann. Rev. Med., *26*:289, 1975.

Hohn, D. C., and Lehrer, R. I.: NADPH oxidase deficiency in X-linked chronic granulomatous disease. J. Clin. Invest., *55*:707, 1975.

Holmes, B., Quie, P. G., Windhorst, D. B., and Good, R. A.: Fatal granulomatous disease of childhood: An inborn abnormality of phagocytic function. Lancet, *1*:1225, 1966.

Jarrett, W. F. H.: Viruses and leukemia. Br. J. Haematol., 25:287, 1973.

Karnofsky, M. L., Noseworthy, J., Simmons, S., and Glass, E. A.: Metabolic patterns that control the functions of leukocytes. In Greenwalt, T. J., and Jamieson, G. A. (Eds.): Formation and Destruction of Blood Cells. J. B. Lippincott Co., Philadelphia, 1970, p. 207.

Katayama, T., and Finkel, H. E.: Leukemic reticuloendotheliosis. A clinicopathologic study with review of the literature. Am. J. Med., 57:115, 1974.

Kennedy, B. J.: Cyclic leukocyte oscillations in chronic myelogenous leukemia during hydroxyurea therapy. Blood, 35:751, 1970.

Killmann, S. A.: Acute leukemia: the kinetics of leukemic blast cells in man. An analytical review. Series Haematol., 1(3):38, 1968.

Mahmoud, A. A. F., Stone, M. K., and Kellermeyer, R. W.: Eosinophilopoietin: a low molecular weight peptide stimulating eosinophil production in mice. Clin. Res., 25:519a, 1977.

March, H. C.: Leukemia in radiologists, ten years later. Am. J. Med. Sci., 242:137, 1961.

Metcalf, D., and Stanley, E. R.: Haematological effects in mice of partially purified colony stimulating factor (CSF) prepared from human urine. Br. J. Haematol., 21:481, 1971.

Meuret, G.: Disorders of the mononuclear phagocyte system. An analytical review. Blut, 34:317, 1977.

Miller, M. E., Oski, F. A., and Harris, M. B.: Lazy leucocyte syndrome. Lancet, 1:665, 1971.

Nowell, P. C., and Hungerford, D. A.: A minute chromosome in human chronic granulocytic leukemia. Science, 132:1497, 1960.

O'Riordan, M. L., Robinson, J. A., Buckton, K. E., and Evans, H. J.: Distinguishing between the chromosome involved in Down's syndrome (trisomy 21) and chronic myeloid leukemia (Ph^1) by fluorescence. Nature, 230:167, 1971.

Pederson, B.: The blast crisis of chronic myeloid leukemia. Acute transformation of a preleukemic condition? Br. J. Haematol., 25:141, 1973.

Pisciotta, A. V.: Studies on agranulocytosis X. A biochemical defect in chlorpromazine-sensitive marrow cells. J. Lab. Clin. Med., 78:435, 1971.

Pisciotta, A. V.: Immune and toxic mechanisms in drug-induced agranulocytosis. Seminars Hematol., 10:279, 1973.

Richard, K. A., Morley, A., Howard, D., and Stohlman, F., Jr.: The in vitro colony-forming cell and the response to neutropenia. Blood, 37:6, 1971.

Robinson, W. A., and Mangalik, A.: The kinetics and regulation of granulopoiesis. Seminars Hematol., 12:7, 1975.

Rosenthal, S., Canellos, G. P., DeVita, V., Jr., and Gralnick, H.R.: Characteristics of blast crisis in chronic granulocytic leukemia. Blood, 49:705, 1977.

Skipper, H. E.: Cellular kinetics associated with "curability" of experimental leukemia. In Dameshek, W., and Dutcher, R. M. (Eds.): Perspectives in Leukemia. Grune and Stratton, New York, 1968, p. 187.

Smalley, R. V., Vogel, J., Huguley, C. M., Jr., and Miller, D.: Chronic granulocytic leukemia: cytogenetic conversion of the bone marrow with cycle-specific chemotherapy. Blood, 50:107, 1977.

Spiers, A. S. D.: Chemotherapy of acute leukaemia. Clin. Haematol., 1:127, 1972.

Stohlman, F., Jr., and Quesenberry, P. J.: Colony-stimulating factor and myelopoiesis. Blood, 39:727, 1972.

Stossel, T. P.: Phagocytosis, N. Engl. J. Med., 290:717, 774, 833, 1974.

van Furth, R.: Origin and kinetics of monocytes and macrophages. Seminars Hematol., 7:125, 1970.

Wagner, H. N., Jr., and Iio, M.: Studies of the reticuloendothelial system (RES). III Blockade of the RES in man. J. Clin. Invest., 43:1525, 1964.

Ward, P. A.: Insubstantial leukotaxis. J. Lab. Clin. Med., 79:873, 1972.

Ward, P. A., Cochrane, C. G., and Müller-Eberhard, H. G.: Further studies of the chemotactic factor of complement and its formation in vivo. Immunology, 11:141, 1966.

Warner, H. R., and Athens, J. W.: An analysis of granulocyte kinetics in blood and bone marrow, in leukopoiesis in health and disease. Ann. N.Y. Acad. Sci., 113:523, 1964.

White, J. G.: The Chediak-Higashi syndrome: A possible lysosomal disease. Blood, 28:143, 1966.

Zucker-Franklin, D., Elsbach, P., and Simon, E. J.: The effect of the morphine analog levorphanol on phagocytosing leukocytes. Lab. Invest., 25:415, 1971.

Zuelzer, W. W., and Cox, D. E.: Genetic aspects of leukemia. Seminars Hematol., 6:228,1969.

IMMUNOCYTES

Abramson, N., and Shattil, J. J.: M-components. J.A.M.A., 223:156, 1973.

Alexanian, R., Balcerzak, S., Bonnet, J. D., Gehan, E. A., Haut, A., Hewlett, J. S., and Monto, R. W.: Prognostic factors in multiple myeloma. Cancer, 36:1192, 1975.

Belpomme, D., Mathé, G., and Davies, A. J. S.: Clinical significance and prognostic value of the T-B immunological classification of human primary acute lymphoid leukaemias. Lancet, i:555, 1977.

Block, K., and Maki, D.: Hyperviscosity syndromes associated with immunoglobulin abnormalities. Seminars Hematol., 10:113, 1973.

Bortin, M. M., and Rimm, A. A.: Severe combined immunodeficiency disease. Characterization of the disease and results of transplantation. J.A.M.A., 238:591, 1977.

Broder, S., Edelson, R. L., Lutzner, M. A., Nelson, D. L., MacDermott, R. P., Durm, M. E., Goldman, C. K., Meade, B. D., and Waldman, T. A.: The Sézary syndrome. A malignant proliferation of helper T cells. J. Clin. Invest., 58:1297, 1976.

Broder, S., Humphrey, R., Durm, M., Blackman, M., Meade, B., Goldman, C., Strober, W., and Waldman, T.: Impaired synthesis of polyclonal (non-paraprotein) immunoglobulins by circulating lymphocytes from patients with multiple myeloma. Role of suppressor cells. N. Engl. J. Med., 293:887, 1975.

Byrne, G. E., Jr.: Rappaport classification of non-Hodgkin's lymphoma. Histologic features and clinical significance. Cancer Treat. Rep., 61:935, 1977.

David, J. R.: Lymphocyte mediators and cellular hypersensitivity. N. Engl. J. Med., 288:143, 1973.

Fauci, A. S., and Dale, D. C.: The effect of hydrocortisone on the kinetics of normal human lymphocytes. Blood, 46:235, 1975.

Fisher, R. I., DaVita, V. T., Johnson, B. L., Simon, R., and Young, R. C.: Prognostic factors for advanced diffuse histiocytic lymphoma following treatment with combination chemotherapy. Am. J. Med., 63:177, 1977.

Franklin, E. C.: Some insights of clinical investigation on immunology. Surface IgD, IgE, and heavy-chain variants. N. Engl. J. Med., 294:531, 1976.

Fudenberg, H. H., Pink, J. R. L., Wang, A. C., and Douglas, S. D.: Basic Immunogenetics, 2nd ed. Oxford University Press, New York, 1978.

Geha, R. S., Schneeberger, E., Merler, E., and Rosen, F. S.: Heterogeneity of "acquired" or common variable agammaglobulinemia. N. Engl. J. Med., 291:1, 1974.

Glenner, G. G., Terry, W. D., and Isersky, C.: Amyloidosis: its nature and pathogenesis. Seminars Hematol., 10:65, 1973.

Gralnick, H. R., Galton, D. A. G., Catovsky, D., Sultan, C., and Bennett, J. M.: Classification of acute leukemia. Ann. Int. Med., 87:740, 1977.

Greenberg, B. R., Peter, C. R., Glassy, F., and MacKenzie, M. R.: A case of T-cell lymphoma with convoluted lymphocytes. Cancer, 38:1602, 1976.

Greenwood, M. F., Coleman, M. S., Hutton, J. J., Lampkin, B., Krill, C., Bollum, F. J., and Holland, P.: Terminal deoxynucleotidyl transferase activity in neoplastic and hematopoietic cells. J. Clin. Invest., 59:889, 1977.

Holland, J. F., and Glidewell, O.: Oncologists reply: survival expectancy in acute lymphocytic leukemia. N. Engl. J. Med., 287:769, 1972.

Israel, H. L., Patchevsky, A. S., and Saldana, M. J.: Wegener's granulomatosis, lymphomatoid granulomatosis, and benign lymphocytic angitis and granulomatosis of lung. Ann. Int. Med., 87:691, 1977.

Jaffe, E. S., Braylan, R. C., Nanba, K., Frank, M. M., and Berard, C. W.: Functional markers: a new perspective on malignant lymphoma. Cancer Treat. Rep., 61:953, 1977.

Klein, G.: The Epstein-Barr virus and neoplasia. N. Engl. J. Med., 293:1353, 1975.

Lai, P. K.: Infectious mononucleosis: recognition and management. Hosp. Pract., 12:8, 47, 1977.

Levine, A. S., Graw, R. G., Jr., and Young, R. C.: Management of infections in patients with leukemia and lymphoma. Current concepts and experimental approaches. Seminars Hematol., 9:141, 1972.

Long, J. C., and Mihm, M. C.: Mycosis fungoides with extracutaneous dissemination; a distinct entity. Cancer, 34:1745, 1974.

Lukes, R. J., and Tindle, B. H.: Immunoblastic lymphadenopathy. A hyperimmune entity resembling Hodgkin's disease. N. Engl. J. Med., 292:1, 1975.

Mann, R. B., Jaffe, E. S., Braylan, R. C., Nanba, K., Frank, M. M., Ziegler, J. L., and Berard, C. W.: Non-endemic Burkitt's lymphoma. A B-cell tumor related to germinal centers. N. Engl. J. Med., 295:685, 1976.

Mauer, A. M., Saunders, E. F., and Lampkin, B. C.: Possible significance of nonproliferating leukemic cells. In Perry, S. (ed.): Human tumor cell kinetics. Natl. Cancer Inst. Monogr. 30:63, 1969.

Moran, E. M., and Ultman, J. E.: Clinical features and course of Hodgkin's disease. Clin. in Haematol., 3:91, 1974.

Mundy, G. R., Raisz, L. G., Cooper, R. A., Schechter, G. P., and Salmon, S. E.: Evidence for the secretion of an osteoclast stimulating factor in myeloma. N. Engl. J. Med., 291:1041, 1974.

Mundy, G. R., Raisz, L. G., Shapiro, J. L., Bandelin, J. G., and Turcotte, R. J.: Big and little forms of osteoclast activating factor. J. Clin. Invest., 60:122, 1977.

Naeim, F. and Smith, G. S.: Leukemic reticuloendotheliosis. Cancer, 34:1813, 1974.

Pangalis, G. A., Nathwani, B. N., and Rappaport, H.: Malignant lymphoma, well differentiated lymphocytic. Its relationship with chronic lymphocytic leukemia and macroglobulinemia of Waldenström. Cancer, 39:999, 1977.

Parkman, R., Gelfand, E. W., Rosen, F. S., Sanderson, A., and Hirschhorn, R.: Severe combined immunodeficiency and adenosine deaminase deficiency. N. Engl. J. Med., 292:714, 1975.

Patchevsky, A. S., Brodovsky, H. S., Menduke, H., Southard, M., Brooks, J., Nicklas, D., and Hoch, W. S.: Non-Hodgkin's lymphoma: a clinico-pathologic study of 293 cases. Cancer, 34:1173, 1974.

Paul, W. E., and Benacerraf, B.: Functional specificity of thymus dependent lymphocytes. Science, 195:1293, 1977.

Podleski, W. K.: Cytodestructive mechanisms provoked by lymphocytes. Am. J. Med., 61:1, 1976.

Polliack, A., Lampen, N., Clarkson, B. D., and De Harven, E.: Identification of human B and T lymphocytes by scanning electron microscopy. J. Exp. Med., 138:607, 1973.

Prosnitz, L. R., Hellman, S., vonEssen, C. F., and Kligerman, M. M.: The clinical course of Hodgkin's disease and other malignant lymphomas treated with radical radiation therapy. Am. J. Roentgenol., 105:618, 1969.

Seligmann, M.: Immunochemical, clinical, and pathological features of α-chain disease. Arch. Int. Med., 135:78, 1975.

Simone, J. V.: Childhood leukemia: the changing prognosis. Hosp. Practice, 9:7, 59, 1974.

Stone, M. J., and Frenkel, E. P.: The clinical spectrum of light chain myeloma. A study of 35 patients with special reference to the occurrence of amyloidosis. Am. J. Med., 58:601, 1975.

Tomasi, T. B.: Secretory immunoglobulins. N. Engl. J. Med., 287:500, 1972.

Tsukada, M., Hanamura, K., Eguchi, M., Komiyama, A., and Akabane, T.: Scanning electron microscopic study of peripheral blood lymphocytes, thymic cells, and acute lymphoblastic leukemic cells in children. Acta Haematol. Jap., 39:43, 1976.

Uhr, J. W.: The membranes of lymphocytes. Hosp. Pract., 10:3, 113, 1975.

Waldman, T. A.: Disorders of suppressor cells in the pathogenesis of immunodeficiency, autoimmune and allergic diseases: human disease associated with disorders of an immunological breaking system. Ann. Allergy, 39, 79, 1977.

Walker, W. A., and Isselbacher, K. J.: Intestinal antibodies. N. Engl. J. Med., 297:767, 1977.

Warnke, R., and Levy, R. Immunopathology of follicular lymphomas. A model of B-lymphocyte homing. N. Engl. J. Med., 298:481, 1978.

THROMBOCYTES

Abrahamsen, A. F.: Platelet survival studies in man — with special reference to thrombosis and atherosclerosis. Scand. J. Haematol., Suppl. 3, 1968, p. 7.

Adams, W. H., Liu, Y. K., and Sullivan, L. W.: Humoral regulation of thrombopoiesis in man. J. Lab. Clin. Med., 91:141, 1978.

Aster, R. H.: Pooling of platelets in the spleen: Role in the pathogenesis of "hypersplenic" thrombocytopenia. J. Clin. Invest., 45:645, 1966.

Byrnes, J. J., and Khurana, M.: Treatment of thrombotic thrombocytic purpura with plasma. N. Engl. J. Med., 297:1386, 1977.

Cardamone, J. M., Edson, J. R., McArthur, J. R., and Jacob, H. S.: Abnormalities of platelet function in the myeloproliferative disorders. J.A.M.A., 221:270, 1972.

Claman, H. N.: Corticosteroids and lymphoid cells. N. Engl. J. Med., 287:388, 1972.

Cohen, P., Gardner, F. H., and Barnett, G. O.: Reclassification of the thrombocytopenias by the 51-Cr-labeling method for measuring platelet lifespan. N. Engl. J. Med., 264:1294, 1961.

deGabriele, G., and Penington, D. G.: Regulation of platelet production: "thrombopoietin." Br. J. Haematol., 13:210, 1967.

Deykin, D.: The clinical challenge of disseminated intravascular coagulation. N. Engl. J. Med., 283:636, 1970.

Deykin, D.: Emerging concepts of platelet function. N. Engl. J. Med., 290:144, 1974.

Erslev, A. J.: Feedback circuits in the control of stem cell differentiation. Am. J. Path., 65:629, 1971.

Evatt, B. L., and Levin, J.: Measurements of thrombopoiesis in rabbits using 75selenomethionine. J. Clin. Invest., 48:1615, 1969.

Gardner, F. H.: Platelet kinetics and lifespan. Clin. Haematol., 1:307, 1972.

Harker, L. A., and Finch, C. A.: Thrombokinetics in man. J. Clin. Invest., 48:963, 1969.

Harrington, W. J., Minnich, V., Hollingsworth, J. W., and Moore, C. V.: Demonstration of a thrombocytopenic factor in the blood of patients with thrombocytopenic purpura. J. Lab. Clin. Med., 38:1, 1951.

Holmsen, H., and Weiss, H. J.: Further evidence for a deficient storage pool of adenine nucleotides in platelets from some patients with thrombocytopathia — "storage pool disease." Blood, 39:197, 1972.

Horowitz, H. J.: Uremic toxins and platelet function. Arch. Intern. Med., 126:823, 1970.

Hovig, T.: Influence of various compounds on blood platelets and platelet aggregation. A scanning electron microscopic study. Series Haematol., 3:47, 1970.

Karpatkin, S.: Heterogeneity of human platelets. II. J. Clin. Invest., 48:1083, 1969.

Karpatkin, S., and Weiss, H. J.: Deficiency of glutathione peroxidase associated with high levels of reduced glutathione in Glanzmann's thrombasthenia. N. Engl. J. Med., 287:1062, 1972.

McMillan, R., Longmire, R. L., Yelenosky, R., Donnell, R. L., and Armstrong, S.: Quantitation of platelet-binding IgG produced in vitro by spleens from patients with idiopathic thrombocytopenic purpura. N. Engl. J. Med., *291*:812, 1974.

Marchasin, S., Wallerstein, R. D., and Aggeler, P. M.: Variation of the platelet count in disease. Calif. Med., *101*:95, 1964.

Miescher, P. A.: Drug-induced thrombocytopenia. Seminars Hematol., *10*:311, 1973.

Moncada, S., Gryglewski, S., Bunting, S., and Vane, J. R.: An enzyme isolated from arteries transforms prostaglandin endoperoxides to an unstable substance that inhibits platelet aggregation. Nature, *263*:663, 1976.

Odell, T. T., Jr., Jackson, C. W., and Reiter, R. S.: Depression of the megakaryocyte platelet system in rats by transfusion of platelets. Acta Haematol., *38*:34, 1967.

Odell, T. T., Jr., McDonald, T. P., and Asano, M.: Response of rat megakaryocytes to bleeding. Acta Haematol., *27*:171, 1962.

Oski, F. A., and Naiman, J. L.: Effect of live measles vaccine on the platelet count. N. Engl. J. Med., *275*:352, 1966.

Post, R. M., and Des Forges, J. F.: Thrombocytopenia and alcoholism. Ann. Intern. Med., *68*:1230, 1968.

Roth, G., and Majerus, P.: The mechanism of the effect of aspirin on human platelets. I. Acetylation of a particulate fraction protein. J. Clin. Invest., *56*:624, 1975.

Schloesser, L. L., Kipp, M. A., and Wenzel, F. J.: Thrombocytosis in iron-deficiency anemia. J. Lab. Clin. Med., *66*:107, 1965.

Shreiner, D. P., and Levin, J.: Detection of thrombopoietic activity in plasma by stimulation of suppressed thrombopoiesis. J. Clin. Invest., *49*:1709, 1970.

Shulman, I., Pierce, M., Lukens, A., and Currimbhoy, Z.: Studies on thrombopoiesis. I. A factor in normal human plasma required for platelet production; chronic thrombocytopenia due to its deficiency. Blood, *16*:943, 1960.

Shulman, N. R.: A mechanism of cell destruction in individuals sensitized to foreign antigens and its implications in autoimmunity. Ann. Intern. Med., *60*:506, 1964.

Smith, J. B., and Silver, M. J.: Prostaglandin synthesis by platelets and its biologic significance. *In* Gordon, J. L. (ed.): Platelets in Biology and Pathology. North Holland Pub. Co., Amsterdam, 1976, p. 331.

Smith, J. B., and Willis, A. L.: Aspirin selectivity inhibits prostaglandin production in human platelets. Nature, *231*:235, 1971.

Tranum, B. L., and Haut, A.: Thrombocytosis: Platelet kinetics in neoplasia. J. Lab. Clin. Med., *84*:615, 1974.

Wright, J. H.: The histogenesis of the blood platelets. J. Morphol., *21*:263, 1910.

Zucker, M. B.: Platelet function. *In* Williams, W. J., et al. (eds.): Hematology, 2nd ed. McGraw-Hill Book Co., New York, 1977, p.1200.

PLASMA COAGULATION FACTORS

Bell, W. R.: Thrombolytic therapy. A comparison between urokinase and streptokinase. Seminars in Thrombosis and Hemostasis, *2*:1, 1975.

Blatt, P. M., Brinkhous, K. M., Culp, H. R., Kraus, J. S., and Roberts, H. R.: Antihemophilic factor concentrate therapy in von Willebrand disease. J.A.M.A., *236*:2770, 1976.

Colman, R. W., Robboy, S. F., and Minna, J. D.: Disseminated intravascular coagulation (DIC): an approach. Am. J. Med., *52*:679, 1972.

Cream, J. J., Gumpel, J. M., and Peachey, R. D.: Schönlein-Henoch purpura in the adult. A study of 77 adults with anaphylactoid or Schönlein-Henoch purpura. Q. J. Med., *39*:461, 1970.

Davie, E. W. and Fujikawa, K.: Basic mechanisms in blood coagulation. Ann. Rev. Biochem., *44*:799, 1975.

Donaldson, V. H., Glueck, H. I., Miller, M. A., Movat, H. Z., and Habal, F.: Kininogen deficiency in Fitzgerald trait: Role of high molecular weight kininogen in clotting and fibrinolysis. J. Lab. Clin. Med., *87*:327, 1976.

Gralnick, H. R., Coller, B. S., Shulman, N. R., Andersen, J. C., and Hilgartner, M.: Factor VIII. Ann. Int. Med., *86*:598, 1977.

Gralnick, H. R., Sultan, Y., and Coller, B. S.: von Willebrand's disease. Combined qualitative and quantitative abnormalities. N. Engl. J. Med., *296*:1024, 1977.

Gurevich, V.: Guidelines for the management of anticoagulant therapy. Seminars in Thrombosis and Hemostasis, *2*:176, 1976.

Hillenbrand, P., Parbhoo, S. P., Jedrychowski, A., and Sherlock, S.: Significance of intravascular coagulation and fibrinolysis in acute hepatic failure. Gut, *15*:83, 1974.

Jaffe, E. A.: Endothelial cells and the biology of Factor VIII. N. Engl. J. Med., *296*:377, 1977.

Koch-Weser, J. and Sellers, E. M.: Drug interactions with coumarin anticoagulants. N. Engl. J. Med., *285*:487, 1971.

Marder, V. J., and Budzynski, A. Z.: Fibrinogen and its derivatives, hereditary and acquired abnormalities. Schweiz. Med. Wschr., *104*:1338, 1974.

Martinez, J., Palascak, J. E., and Kwasniak, D.: Abnormal sialic acid content of the dysfibrinogenemia associated with liver disease. J. Clin. Invest., *61*:535, 1978.

Meadow, S. R., Glasgow, E. F., White, R. H. R., Moncrieff, M. W., Cameron, J. S., and Ogg, C. S.: Schönlein-Henoch nephritis. Q. J. Med., *41*:241, 1972.

Nossell, H. L.: Radioimmunoassay of fibrinopeptides in relation to intravascular coagulation and thrombosis. N. Engl. J. Med., *295*:428, 1976.

Pool, J. G., and Shannon, A. E.: Production of high-potency concentrates of antihemophilic globulin in a closed bag system. N. Engl. J. Med., *273*:1443, 1965.

Ratnoff, O.D., and Forman, W. B.: Criteria for the differentiation of dysfibrinogenemic states. Seminars Hematol., *13*:141, 1976.

Ratnoff, O. D., and Jones, P. K.: The laboratory diagnosis of the carrier state for classic hemophilia. Ann. Int. Med., *86*:521, 1977.

Rogers, P. H., and Sherry, S.: Current status of antithrombotic therapy in cardiovascular disease. Progr. Cardiovasc. Dis., *19*:233, 1976.

Rosenberg, R. D.: Actions and interactions of antithrombin and heparin. N. Engl. J. Med., *292*:146, 1975.

Shapiro, S. S., and Hultin, M.: Acquired inhibitors to the blood coagulation factors. Seminars in Thrombosis and Hemostasis, *1*:336, 1975.

Spicer, T. E., and Rau, J. M.: Purpura fulminans. Am. J. Med., *61*:566, 1976.

Walls, W. D., and Losowsky, M. S.: The hemostatic defect of liver disease. Gastroenterology, *60*:108, 1971.

Wessler, S., and Gitel, S.: Control of heparin therapy. Progress in Thrombosis and Hemostasis, *3*, 311, 1976.

IDENTITY OF BLOOD CELLS

Bach, F. H., and van Rood, J. J.: The major histocompatibility complex — genetics and biology. N. Engl. J. Med., *295*:806, 872, 927, 1976.

Danielli, J. F., and Dawson, H.: A contribution to the theory of permeability of thin films. J. Cell. Comp. Physiol., *5*:495, 1935.

Fudenberg, H. H., Pink, J. R. L., Wang, A. C., and Douglas, S. D.: Basic immunogenetics, 2nd ed. Oxford University Press, New York, 1978.

Giblett, E. R.: Erythrocyte antigens and antibodies. *In* Williams, W. J., et al. (eds.): Hematology, 2nd ed. McGraw-Hill Book Co., New York, 1977, p. 1497.

Giblett, E. R., and Crookston, M. C.: Agglutinability of red cells by anti-i in patients with thalassemia major and other hematologic disorders. Nature, *201*:1138, 1964.

Lessin, L. S., and Bessis, M.: Morphology of the erythron. *In* Williams, W. J., et al. (eds.): Hematology, 2nd ed. McGraw-Hill Book Co., New York, 1977, p. 103.

Levine, P., Tripodi, D., Struck, J., Jr., Zmijewski, C. M., and Pollack, W.: Hemolytic anemia associated with Rh null but not with Bombay blood. Vox Sang., *24*:417–424, 1973.

McKusick, V. A., and Ruddle, F. H.: The status of the gene map of the human chromosomes. Science, *196*:390, 1977.

Marcus, D. M.: The ABO and Lewis blood-group system: immunochemistry, genetics and relation to human disease. N. Engl. J. Med., *280*:994, 1969.

Minio, F., Howe, C., Hsu, K. C., and Rifkind, R. A.: Antigen density on differentiating erythroid cells. Nature (New Biology), *237*:187, 1972.

Mollison, P. L.: Blood Transfusion in Clinical Medicine, 5th ed. Blackwell, Oxford, 1972.

Race, R. R., and Sanger, R.: Blood Groups in Man, 4th ed. Blackwell, Oxford, 1962.

Singer, S. J.: Architecture and topography of biologic membranes. Hosp. Pract., *8*:5, 81, 1973.

Singer, S. J.: Molecular biology of cellular membranes with applications to immunology. Adv. Immunol., *19*:1, 1974.

Storb, R., Prentice, R. L., and Thomas, E. D.: Treatment of aplastic anemia by marrow transplantation from HLA identical siblings. J. Clin. Invest., *59*:625, 1977.

Victoria, E. J., Muchmore, E. A., Sudora, E. J., and Masouredis, S. P.: The role of antigen mobility in anti-Rh_0(D)-induced agglutination. J. Clin. Invest., *56*:292, 1975.

Watkins, W. M.: Blood group substances. Science, *162*:172, 1966.

Weinstein, R. S., and McNutt, N. S.: Ultrastructure of red cell membranes. Seminars Hematol., *7*:259, 1970.

NORMAL ADULT LABORATORY VALUES*

		Old System	New System
Red cell count	Men:	4.6–6.0 (5.1) $\times 10^6$/mm.^{3}	$\times 10^{12}$/l.
	Women:	4.1–4.8 (4.5) $\times 10^6$/mm.^{3}	$\times 10^{12}$/l.
Hemoglobin	Men:	14.5–16.7 g./100 ml.	g./dl.
	Women:	12.2–15.0 g./100 ml.	g./dl.
Packed cell volume	Men:	42–49%	.42–.49 l./l.
	Women:	38–45%	.38–.45 l./l.
Erythrocyte indices:			
Mean corpuscular volume		82–92μ^3	fl.
Mean corpuscular hemoglobin		27–32$\mu\mu$g.	pg.
Mean corpuscular hemoglobin conc.		32–36 g./100 ml.	g./dl.
White cell count		5,000–10,000/mm.^{3}	5–10 $\times 10^9$/l.
Differential:			
Neutrophils (segs)		54–62%	%
Neutrophils (bands)		5–10%	%
Neutrophils (total)		3,000–7,000/mm^3	3–7 $\times 10^9$/l.
Eosinophils		0–3%	%
Basophils		0–1%	%
Lymphocytes		18–35%	%
Monocytes		3–7%	%
Platelet count	Men:	210,000–340,000/mm.^{3}	210–340 $\times 10^9$/l.
	Women:	208,000–380,000/mm.^{3}	208–380 $\times 10^9$/l.
Reticulocyte count		0.5–2.6%	%
Absolute reticulocyte count		25,000–125,000/mm.^{3}	25–125 $\times 10^9$/l.
†Prothrombin time		12–15 sec.	sec.
†Partial thromboplastin time		50–90 sec.	sec.
†Partial thromboplastin time, activated		25–46 sec.	sec.
†Thrombin time		20–26 sec.	sec.
Fibrinogen		198–434 mg./100 ml.	1.98–4.34 g./l.
Bleeding time (Ivy method)		2–7 min.	min.
Euglobulin lysis time		more than 2 hrs.	hrs.
Fibrin degradation products		0–4μg./ml.	mg./l.
Factor VIII and other coagulation Factors		50–150% of normal	0.5–1.5 U./ml.
†Serum iron		80–180μg./100 ml.	14–32μmol./l.
†Total iron binding capacity		250–425μg./100 ml.	45–76μmol./l.
% saturation		20–50 (35) %	%
†Serum ferritin	Men:	20–200 ng./ml.	μg./l.
	Women:	10–200 ng./ml.	μg./l.
†Serum B$_{12}$		200–1100 pg./ml.	ng./l.
†Serum folate		1.9–14 ng./ml.	μg./l.
†Schilling test	Stage I	10–40 (18)% of dose	%
	Stage II	10–42 (18)% of dose	%
Haptoglobin (hemoglobin binding capacity)		50–150 mg./100 ml.	.5–1.5 g./l.
Bilirubin (total)		0.1–1.2 mg./100 ml.	1–12 mg./l.
Bilirubin (direct)		0–0.3 mg./100 ml.	0–3 mg./l.
Serum lactic dehydrogenase		100–225 mU./ml.	0–90 I.U./l. 30° C.
Hemoglobin A$_2$		1.8–3.3%	%
Hemoglobin F		<2.0%	%
Erythropoietin (plasma)		3–20 mU./ml.	mU./ml.
Erythropoietin (urinary excretion)		2–5 U./24 hr.	U./24 hr.

*Ranges given in terms of ±2 standard deviations. Mean values in parentheses.
†Normal values vary with technique used.

23

The Spleen

Allan J. Erslev, and Thomas G. Gabuzda

STRUCTURE

The mature normal spleen — no longer involved in hematopoiesis — is the largest of the lymphoid organs. Yet it is also a unique filtration bed for the circulating blood well equipped with macrophages to remove undesired particles from the circulation. The parenchyma or "pulp" is partitioned by fibrous trabeculae, through which run the arteries, veins, and lymphatics. Arterioles run out from the trabeculae into the white pulp, branch at right angles into the marginal zone, and then terminate in the red pulp (Fig. 23–1). The venous drainage system originates in the sinus system of the red pulp. The blood then flows out through the trabecular veins and on into the portal system. The efferent lymphatic drainage runs into the thoracic duct.

In the white pulp, a sleeve of T lymphocytes — the "periarterial lymphatic sheath" — is wrapped around the central artery (Fig. 23–2). Nodular accumulations of lymphocytes, often at the sites of the right angled vascular branches, form follicles along the course of the central arteriole. These contain germinal centers rich in B lymphocytes surrounded by mantle zones of T lymphocytes and macrophages. The cellular structure is held together by a network of fibrillar reticular cells.

The marginal zone is an ill-defined boundary between the white and red pulp. Into its interstices, also held together by fibrillar reticular cells, empty many arteriolar branches filling the spongy network with blood cells. Under provocative stimuli, macrophages readily migrate into this area.

Blood from the marginal zone as well as from central arterial terminals drains into the red pulp, either directly into venous sinuses and on out through the efferent veins, or into the cords that lie between the sinuses (Fig. 23–3). The blood cells that enter the cords must pass through the fenestrated wall separating the cords from the sinuses before gaining access to the venous drainage system. They are thus delayed to varying degrees in their transit. The fenestrations in the wall separating the cords and sinuses are about 3 μ in diameter, so small that erythrocytes must be squeezed through with effort. They pass through because their pliability and deformability is normally very great (Fig. 23–4). The sinus side of the wall is lined by reticular endothelial cells lying upon the fenestrated basement membrane. The cordal side of the wall is made up of the adventitial network of reticular cells and macrophages surrounding and separating the sinuses.

Blood flow through the spleen, thus, is both fast and slow. Rapid transit is achieved by the fraction that bypasses the cords and enters directly into the sinuses. The slow transit fraction is temporarily detained in the cords. Normally, this detention is not very great; the time required for complete mixing of blood within the spleen as measured with tagged erythrocytes is only about 2 minutes. When the spleen enlarges, however, the detention time of the "slow flow" fraction may increase to as long as an hour, with potentially deleterious effects on the survival time of erythrocytes, particularly if they do not have their customary flexibility and become more easily entrapped in the splenic cords.

Plasma skimming is another important aspect of the splenic circulation. Laminar flow in the central arteries directs leukocyte-rich plasma into the perpendicular branches feeding the germinal follicles and the marginal zone. This leaves behind more viscous high hematocrit blood in the central artery to flow on into hemoconcentrated red pulp.

FUNCTION

The circulating blood passes through no more discriminating a filter than that of the spongy red pulp of the spleen. While the liver, by virtue of its larger blood flow, performs the lion's share of phagocytic clearance of unwanted particles from the circulation, the spleen is more discriminating

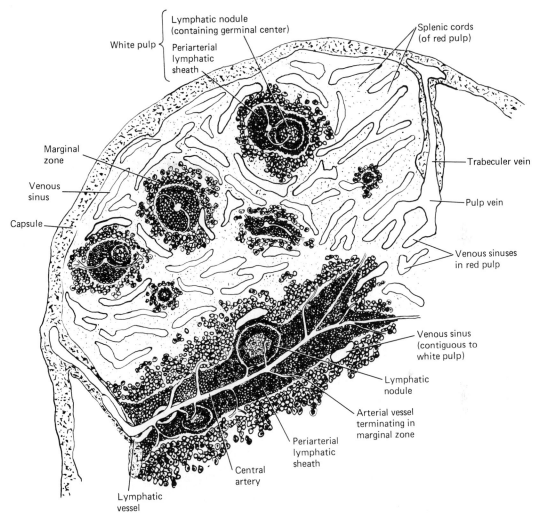

Figure 23-1 The structure of the spleen. The white pulp consists of the periarterial lymphatic sheath and lymphatic nodules with germinal centers. The red pulp contains the splenic cords and sinuses. The marginal zone is interposed between white and red pulp. The central artery sends branches out into the marginal zone and then terminates in the red pulp. Blood from the splenic cords passes through a fenestrated wall into the sinuses and is then collected into the splenic veins. (From Weiss, L., and Tavassoli, M.: Sem. in Hematol., 7, 372, 1970, Reprinted from Histology, by L. Weiss, and R. O. Greep, Copyright © 1977, McGraw-Hill Book Company.

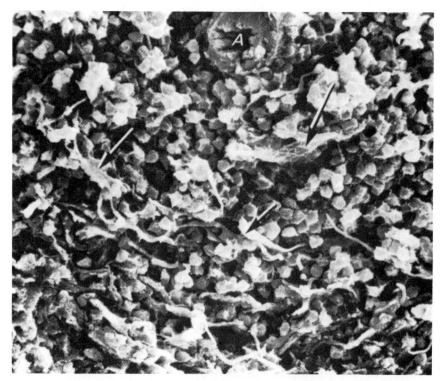

Figure 23–2 Scanning electron micrograph of the splenic white pulp in the region of the periarterial lymphatic sheath. A sea of lymphocytes is held together by reticular cells and their associated fibrils (shown by arrows). The central arteriole (A) is shown in cross section near the upper margin. (From Weiss, L. Blood *43*:665, 1974.)

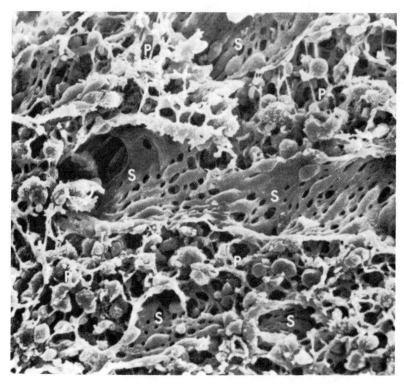

Figure 23–3 Scanning electron micrograph of the splenic red pulp, showing the fenestrated sinuses (S) and the spongy cords (P) that lie between the sinuses and consist of hematogenous cells enmeshed in an adventitial reticular network. (From Miyoshi, M., and Fujita, T. Arch. Histol. Japan *33*:225–246, 1971.)

776

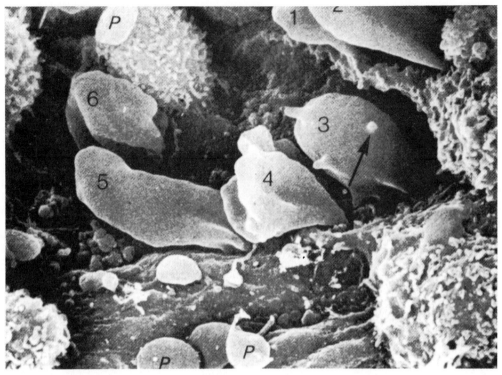

Figure 23-4 Scanning electron micrograph demonstrating erythrocytes (numbered 1 through 6) squeezing through the fenestrated wall in transit from the splenic cord to the sinus. The view shows the endothelial lining of the sinus wall, to which platelets (P) adhere, along with "hairy" white cells, probably macrophages. (From Weiss, L. Blood *43*:665, 1974.)

and is able to pick out for destruction more subtly altered cells. Warm antibody coated erythrocytes and the sensitized platelets of autoimmune thrombocytopenic purpura are examples of such altered cells usually missed by the hepatic macrophages past which they circulate too rapidly to be trapped, but selected for destruction in the spleen.

Erythrocytes undergo a certain degree of restructuring as they percolate through the splenic cords. Reticulocytes endure preferential splenic delay in transit, possibly because their transferrin coating makes them more "sticky" than mature erythrocytes. Intracytoplasmic inclusions left over after extrusion of the newly formed erythrocyte into the marrow sinusoid are plucked by splenic macrophages from the cell interior, usually without detriment to the integrity of the self sealing red cell membrane. These inclusions include iron granules, hemoglobin precipitates, fragments of DNA, or even the entire erythroid cell nucleus. They are not numerous unless bone marrow function is hyperactive or abnormal, such as in Cooley's anemia or sickle cell anemia. In these conditions, the asplenic state is characterized by large numbers of circulating normo-

blasts and inclusion-containing erythrocytes. Loss of membrane surface along with membrane cholesterol accompanies the cellular grooming during splenic transit.

In man, the spleen is an important reservoir of platelets, as reported by Aster. About 30 per cent of the body's platelets are sequestered there in slow transit and in dynamic equilibrium with the circulating pool. The splenic platelets are immediately moved into the circulation after stress or injection of epinephrine. The transitory platelet increase is accompanied by a parallel increase in Factor VIII level. Neither response is seen in the splenectomized individual. There is no significant storage pool of red or white cells in the human spleen, although in some animals, such as the dog, horse, or sheep, muscular contraction of the splenic capsule abruptly increases the peripheral hematocrit by means of "autotransfusion" of a reservoir of splenic blood.

The spleen is a dispensable organ in the adult, but young children may suffer sudden overwhelming infection in its absence, as reported by Erickson and co-workers in 1968. Children with Cooley's anemia or other severe systemic disorders are the most susceptible. There are even occasional reports of sudden fatal sepsis in splen-ectomized adults. The first immunologic response to antigen introduced directly into the circulation appears to take place in the spleen after phagocytosis by splenic macrophages. Possibly this function of the spleen is more vital in the early years of life. Likhite has reported that removal of the spleen is in fact followed by a significant drop in plasma concentration of IgM.

PATHOPHYSIOLOGY

ASPLENIA

The asplenic state is usually the result of surgical removal, performed either in the hematologically normal individual who has suffered traumatic rupture or for such hematologic indications as hereditary spherocytosis, idiopathic thrombocytopenic purpura, or staging operation for Hodgkin's disease. In sickle cell anemia repeated splenic infarctions lead to "autosplenectomy" during childhood. Atrophy of the spleen occurs in association with malabsorption syndromes (Wardrop and associates, 1975). Although true con-

genital asplenia is a rare condition, "functional asplenia" is found in normal neonates, especially the premature. Chronic hemolysis may also cause functional asplenia, presumably because erythrophagocytosis blocks the splenic macrophages.

The removal of the spleen is followed by a rise in platelet and granulocyte counts, often reaching peaks after about ten days of more than one million and 30,000 per mm³, respectively. The elevated counts gradually return to normal values in most cases. Late postsplenectomy effects include an absolute lymphocytosis, monocytosis, and the presence of occasional immature cells in the peripheral blood. Interaction between the spleen and bone marrow has been postulated to explain these changes, but experimental proof for this hypothesis has never come forth.

The asplenic state can usually be suspected by the presence of red cell inclusions, especially Howell–Jolly bodies, which otherwise are removed by the normal spleen (Fig. 23–5). In pathologic states these may be very numerous. Significant numbers of target cells and spiculated erythrocytes, or "burr" cells, are also present, along with a parallel increase in erythrocyte membrane surface, membrane cholesterol con-

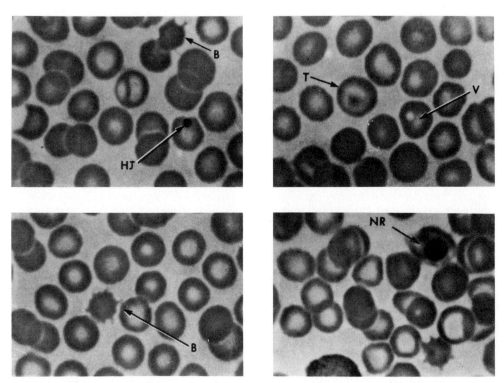

Figure 23–5 Morphologic signs in the peripheral blood of asplenia. HJ–Howell-Jolly body (fragment of DNA); T-target cell; V–vacuole; B–"burr" cell; NR–nucleated red cell. (From Holroyde, C. P. *In* Custer, R. P.: An Atlas of the Blood and Bone Marrow. Philadelphia, W. B. Saunders Co., 1974, p. 125.)

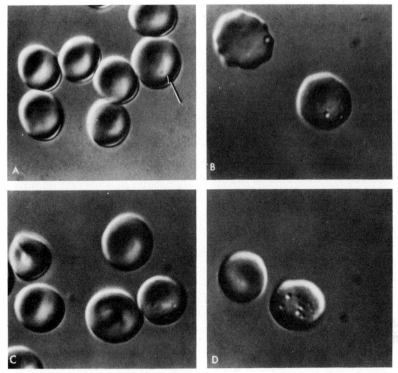

Figure 23-6 Interference contrast microscopy of erythrocytes. A. Normal adult with intact spleen. Only 1-2% of the cells have vacuoles; B. Normal adult after splenectomy performed because of ruptured spleen. About 50% of the cells contain vacuoles; C. Full term infant, and D. premature infant demonstrate an increased proportion of vacuole-containing cells, the latter to a more striking degree. (From Holroyde, C. P. *In* Custer, R. P.: An Atlas of the Blood and Bone Marrow. Philadelphia, W. B. Saunders Co., 1974, p. 134.)

tent, and osmotic resistance. Reticulocytes may be slightly increased and a few giant platelets are seen in the circulation. Special microscopic techniques demonstrate erythrocyte vacuoles which give the cell surface a pitted appearance (Fig. 23-6).

SPLENOMEGALY

Occasionally splenic enlargement is caused by a disorder intrinsic to the spleen, such as a cyst, but more often it occurs as a feature of a systemic disease process (Table 23-1). A reactive response of the lymphoid white pulp is seen in infections, especially viral, while neoplastic proliferation is responsible for the splenomegaly of the lymphoproliferative disorders. The splenic pool of macrophages hypertrophies when subjected to a chronic work load. This may be caused by bacterial infections, such as subacute bacterial endocarditis or miliary tuberculosis, or from the state of chronic hemolysis itself. Hypertrophy of the

splenic pool of lipid-laden macrophages is responsible for the splenomegaly of the lipidoses.

The spleen may return to shades of its past developmental history and become swollen with hematopoietic myeloid tissue. Severe chronic hemolytic anemia is one stimulus for extramedullary hematopoiesis, especially in Cooley's anemia. Splenic infiltration with hematogenous elements also occurs as a common feature of the myeloproliferative syndromes. In temperate zones, some of the largest spleens occur in patients with myelofibrosis and myeloid metaplasia.

Vascular congestion — "congestive splenomegaly" — is seen most often as a consequence of portal hypertension secondary to hepatic cirrhosis, but obstructions of the portal or splenic vein are other etiologic considerations. Marked splenomegaly in patients living in tropical regions — "tropical splenomegaly" — apparently is caused by chronic malarial infestation or other infections endemic to the region. "Non-tropical idio-

TABLE 23–1   CLASSIFICATION OF SPLENOMEGALY

Lymphatic Disorders
 Reactions to infections, especially viral (e.g., infectious mononucleosis)
 Reactions to connective tissue disorders (e.g., disseminated lupus erythematosus)
 Lymphoproliferative disorders (e.g., lymphatic leukemia, lymphoma)

Macrophage Disorders
 Reactions to infections (e.g., subacute bacterial endocarditis, miliary tuberculosis, tropical splenomegaly)
 "Work hypertrophy" secondary to chronic hemolytic anemia
 Lipidoses (e.g., Gaucher's disease)
 Proliferative disorders (e.g., histiocytic medullary reticulosis, Letterer-Siwe disease)

Infiltrative Disorders
 Myeloproliferative disorders
 Extramedullary hematopoiesis secondary to chronic hemolytic anemia (e.g., Cooley's anemia)
 Amyloidosis

Increased Splenic Vein Pressure (Congestive Splenomegaly)
 Splenic or portal vein thrombosis
 Liver cirrhosis

Miscellaneous
 Sarcoidosis
 Congenital cyst ("true", epithelial lined, "primary")
 Post traumatic cyst (not lined, "secondary")
 Rare tumors, primary and metastatic
 Non-tropical idiopathic splenomegaly

pathic splenomegaly" was so designated by Dacie and associates because of the non-diagnostic histology of the spleen after its removal in patients without evidence of other coexisting disease. A significant proportion of such patients subsequently develop lymphoma.

ACCESSORY SPLEENS

Small accessory spleens are found in the splenic hilum, the mesentery, the region of the tail of the pancreas or elsewhere in about 10 per cent of normal individuals. They may enlarge after splenectomy and cause relapse of the hematologic condition for which the operation was originally done. This is, however, an unusual occurrence. "Splenosis" follows the seeding of multiple small implants of spleen tissue in the peritoneal cavity as a result of rupture of the splenic capsule. The spleen cells colonize and develop into nodules of spleen tissue studded on serosal surfaces.

THE SPLEEN AS A TRAP

"Hypersplenism" is a term honored by both time and usage, but in the light of present concepts of the interactions of the hematogenous cells with the spleen, it lacks pathophysiologic precision. It is characterized by (1) reduction in erythrocytes, platelets, granulocytes, or any combination of these cellular elements of the peripheral blood; (2) splenomegaly; (3) a cellular marrow implying adequate marrow compensation in response to the cytopenia; and (4) correction of the cytopenia by splenectomy. Strictly speaking the term should thus not be used until successful response to splenectomy has been documented.

The splenic blood volume, normally about 50 ml., may increase to such a degree in splenomegalic states that it contains as much as 25 per cent of the total blood volume, and up to 90 per cent or more of the total pool of platelets. However, the platelets, if otherwise untainted, withstand this altered distribution quite nicely. They easily escape from the splenic cords into the sinuses, where they are found temporarily adhering to the vascular wall, happily bathed by flowing blood with excellent preservation of their viability. Granulocytes, if otherwise normal, also seem to endure sequestration in the enlarged spleen without suffering undue damage. Red cells, dependent upon glycolysis for energy, are susceptible to deterioration during repeated passages through the splenic cords. The depressed glucose concentration in the splenic red pulp, as low as a third the level in the blood, and the inhibitory action of the low pH, the result of lactic acid accumulation, severely limit glycolysis. Hemoconcentration and low Po_2 add insult to injury — especially in sickle cell disorders. The larger the spleen the greater the likelihood of clinically significant sequestration phenomena, but precise correlation with the degree of splenomegaly is not always possible. Differences in the extent of cell entrapment in the splenic cords among patients with comparable degrees of splenomegaly may be explained by differences in the partition of splenic blood flow into rapid and slow transit streams.

The rigid inelastic cells of sickle hemoglobinopathy, homozygous Hemoglobin C disease, or the Heinz body hemolytic anemias are more easily trapped and damaged in the spleen than normal erythrocytes. The erythrocyte in hereditary spherocytosis, by virtue of its high glycolytic requirement, is exquisitely sensitive to erythrostasis, and the stress of repeated passages through the splenic environment produces fragmentation at the membrane surface with sphering and ultimately entrapment and lysis. The state of chronic hemolysis provokes work hypertrophy of the spleen which in turn may adversely reciprocate and worsen the hemolysis. In Cooley's anemia, the spleen may enlarge so massively that transfused erythrocytes do not survive sufficiently long to enable the patient to maintain adequate hemoglobin levels. Splenectomy then becomes mandatory. If the massive splenomegaly in the patient with myelofibrosis and myeloid metaplasia is responsible for intolerable transfusion requirements or for bleeding due to severe thrombocytopenia, splenectomy may be beneficial even in the face of marrow failure.

THE SPLEEN AND AUTOANTIBODIES

Erythrocytes or platelets coated with 7S antibody are selectively taken up and destroyed in the spleen. In autoimmune hemolytic anemia and thrombocytopenic purpura, the antibody is of endogenous origin. During splenic transit the antibodies on the cell surfaces cause adhesion to macrophages, the instruments of cell damage and destruction. The notion that an autoantibody is responsible for granulocyte destruction in the spleen in patients with splenic neutropenia or Felty's syndrome is still inferential. When cells are more grossly affected with autoantibody and such phenomena as agglutination or complement mediated membrane damage occur in the circulation, cell destruction in extrasplenic sites predominates.

The observation that some patients achieve permanent remission after splenectomy with eventual disappearance of the autoantibody has led to the hypothesis that in these instances the spleen is the major or even the sole site of its synthesis. If this is true, the concentration of the autoantibody would be much higher in the splenic plasma, possibly leading to instantaneous cell destruction, with little or no evidence of the presence of antibody coated cells in the circulation. Indeed, the concentration of antibody in the plasma may be so much less in the general circulation than in the spleen that its detection would be difficult. Such phenomena would explain instances in which laboratory detection of such autoimmune states has been elusive. The recent experiments of Karpatkin and associates, corroborated by those of McMillan and coworkers, have provided direct evidence that spleen cells prepared from the excised spleens of patients with autoimmune idiopathic thrombocytopenic purpura do indeed synthesize an anti-platelet antibody, leading to platelet destruction by the splenic macrophages.

THE SPLEEN, INTRAVASCULAR VOLUME, AND PORTAL HYPERTENSION

In patients with massive splenomegaly (Table 23–2), the blood flow through the organ increases from its normal value of 5 per cent to as much as 50 per cent of the cardiac output. The large volume of blood draining out through the splenic vein distends the portal vascular tree with two important consequences, "dilutional" anemia and portal hypertension.

Although anemia in the presence of massive splenomegaly may be primarily related to pooling of a quarter or more of the red cell mass along with varying degrees of hemolysis, measurement of the total red cell mass may reveal that it is actually normal or even increased with an even greater expansion of total plasma volume and blood volume, i.e., there is a dilutional anemia. The mechanism of these changes in intravascular volume has been described by Hess and coworkers. The portal vascular bed is expanded at the expense of the remainder of the intravascular space, including the renal circulation. Stimulation of the renin-angiotensin-aldosterone system retains salt and water. Reduced colloid osmotic pressure then stimulates albumin synthesis. Normal albumin concentrations are restored and the total albumin pool is expanded.

Massive splenomegaly is also associated with high cardiac output, hypermetabolism, and a wide pulse pressure. Decreased peripheral vascular resistance, necessary to meet the needs of heat dispersion, also compromises the renal circulation and stimulates renin secretion to expand intravascular volume.

If the spleen is surgically removed, the expanded blood volume only gradually returns to normal

---

TABLE 23–2 SOME CAUSES OF CHRONIC MASSIVE SPLENOMEGALY

Myelofibrosis with myeloid metaplasia
Chronic granulocytic leukemia
"Hairy cell" leukemia
Chronic lymphocytic leukemia
Lymphosarcoma
Cooley's anemia
Gaucher's disease
Kala-azar
Malaria

over a matter of several months. The reason for this slow reversal probably is the long time necessary for normal catabolic processes to dispose of the excess in the total body albumin pool.

Portal hypertension secondary to massive splenomegaly may be complicated by esophageal and gastric varices and risks of upper gastrointestinal hemorrhage. Varices may also form secondary to splenic vein thrombosis because of the increased blood flow from splenic accessory veins into the venous system of the greater curvature of the stomach and lower esophagus. When the spleen is the cause of serious portal hypertension, its removal may be the cure. However, outflow obstruction due to hepatic cirrhosis is by far the commonest cause of portal hypertension, for which splenectomy is almost never helpful except perhaps when bleeding occurs in association with unusually severe thrombocytopenia.

REFERENCES

Aster, R. H.: Pooling of platelets in the spleen. Role in the pathogenesis of "hypersplenic" thrombocytopenia. J. Clin. Invest. 45:645, 1966.

Dacie, J. V., Brain, M. C., Harrison, C. V., Lewis, S. M., and Worlledge, S. M.: Non-tropical idiopathic splenomegaly ("primary hypersplenism"); a review of ten cases and their relationship to malignant lymphomas. Br. J. Haematol. 17:317, 1969.

Erickson, W. D., Burgert, E. O., Sr., and Lynn, H. B.: The hazard of infection following splenectomy in children. Am. J. Dis. Child. 116:1, 1968.

Fujita, T. Application of scanning electron microscopy to hematological studies. Acta Haematol. Jap. 35:453, Aug. 1972.

Hess, C. E., Ayers, C. R., Sandusky, W. R., Carpenter, M. A., Wetzel, R. A., and Mohler, D. N. Mechanism of dilutional anemia in massive splenomegaly. Blood, 47, 629, 1976.

Holroyde, C. P. Asplenia. In Custer, R. P.: An Atlas of the Blood and Bone Marrow. Philadelphia, London, Toronto, W. B. Saunders Co., 1974, p. 123.

Karpatkin, S., Strick, N., and Siskin, G. W.: Detection of splenic antiplatelet antibody synthesis in idiopathic autoimmune thrombocytopenic purpura (ATP). Br. J. Haematol. 23:167, 1972.

Kevy, S. V., Tefft, M., Vawter, G. F., and Rosen, F. S.: Hereditary splenic hypoplasia. Pediatrics 42:752, 1968.

Likhite, V. V. Immunologic impairment and susceptibility to infection after splenectomy. J.A.M.A., 236, 1376, 1976.

McMillan, R., Longmire, R. L., Tavassoli, M., Armstrong, S., and Yelenosky, R.: In vitro platelet phagocytosis by splenic leukocytes in idiopathic thrombocytopenic purpura. N. Engl. J. Med. 290:249, 1974.

Wardrop, C. A. J., Lee, F. D., Dyet, J. F., Dagg, J. H., Singh, H., and Moffat, A.: Immunological abnormalities in splenic atrophy. Lancet, 2, 4, 1975.

Weed, R. I., and Weiss, L.: The relationship of red cell fragmentation occurring within cell to cell destruction. Trans. Assoc. Am. Physicians, 79:426, 1966.

Weiss, L.: A scanning electron microscopic study of the spleen. Blood. 43:665, 1974.

Weiss, L., and Tavassoli, M.: Anatomical hazards to the passage of erythrocytes through the spleen. Seminars Hematol. 7:372, 1970.

GASTROENTEROLOGY, ENDOCRINOLOGY, AND METABOLISM

24

The Esophagus

DAVID B. SKINNER

INTRODUCTION

The primary function of the esophagus is the transportation of ingested material from the pharynx to the stomach. A second function is the prevention of involuntary regurgitation of stomach contents. Abnormalities of the esophagus can be considered in relation to the four major components contributing to normal esophageal function. These components are the cricopharyngeal sphincter at the upper end, the muscular layers of the esophagus, the mucosal lining of the esophagus, and the sphincter mechanism at the cardia. The esophagus plays no important role in the digestion or absorption of food, although the initial breakdown of starches by salivary gland secretions may occur during the transportation of food through the length of the esophagus.

STRUCTURE

The cricopharyngeal sphincter consists of skeletal muscle fibers, which are arranged obliquely in its upper portion and blend into those of the inferior pharyngeal constrictor muscle. In the lower portion of the sphincter the fibers are arranged transversely and are continuous with the muscle layers of the esophagus. The muscle bundles composing the sphincter arise from the back and sides of the cricoid cartilage anteriorly and insert into a fibrous raphe in the posterior midline. In the resting state the sphincter is contracted, maintaining a mean pressure of approximately 30 mm. Hg. During swallowing, relaxation occurs. When studied by intraluminal pressure recordings, the sphincter ranges from 3 to 5 cm.

in length, but appears somewhat shorter in radiographic examinations. It is located at the level of the sixth cervical vertebra.

Esophageal muscle fibers are of the striated or skeletal type in the upper one third of the esophagus and are of smooth muscle in the lower esophagus. The transition between skeletal and smooth muscle is indistinct and somewhat variable in location. Esophageal muscle is arranged in two layers, the outer layer running longitudinally, and the inner layer positioned transversely or obliquely around the lumen. There is no true serosal layer on the surface of the esophagus, but the outer longitudinal muscle fibers blend into the overlying fibrous tissue of the pleura and pericardium and the fibrofatty tissue of the mediastinum.

The mucosa of the esophagus is squamous epithelium continuous with that of the pharynx at the upper end. At the distal esophagus there is a sharp transition to simple columnar epithelium which may be visible during esophagoscopy as the ora serrata or "Z" line. Scattered unevenly throughout the esophageal submucosa are intrinsic glands. These produce mucus which reaches the lumen through small excretory ducts and provides lubrication for the passage of ingested material. Simple tubular glands similar to those at the cardia of the stomach may be located at the upper and lower ends of the esophagus and are confined to the lamina propria mucosae. In some individuals there may be islands of gastric columnar epithelium replacing squamous epithelium. These are more commonly encountered in the distal esophagus. Occasionally, acid-secreting or oxyntic cells are encountered in these patches of columnar epithelium. The esophageal mucosa is separated from the muscle layers by a submucosal layer which permits considerable movement of the mucosa in relation to the muscle.

In man, a lower esophageal sphincter cannot be identified by anatomic dissection. However, functionally, the distal esophagus behaves as a sphincter, in that the resting luminal pressure at the gastroesophageal junction is greater than in the esophagus above or the stomach below. This contracted segment relaxes in response to a swallow. The characteristics of this sphincter are described by manometric studies. Normally the sphincter straddles the gastroesophageal mucosal junction and ranges in length from 2 to 4 cm. Resting pressure is generally 8 or more mm. Hg greater than gastric pressure. The reversal of pressure deflections caused by respiration occurs in the cephalad portion of this high pressure zone. Below the pressure reversal point, inspiration causes an increase in pressure similar to that in the abdomen, whereas proximal to this level inspiration causes a decrease in pressure similar to the intrathoracic pattern. When manometric studies and cineradiography are performed simultaneously, the lower portion of the distal esophageal sphincter corresponds to the submerged or closed segment within the diaphragmatic hiatus and upper abdomen while the upper portion of the sphincter zone corresponds to the distal half of the phrenic ampulla radiographically.

The junction of the esophageal and gastric mucosa is located at the level of the tenth thoracic vertebra within the esophageal hiatus of the diaphragm. The hiatus is a muscular tunnel, 2 to 3 cm. long, through which pass the esophagus, vagus nerves, and extensions of endo-abdominal fascia. The endo-abdominal fascia and endothoracic fascia join together to form the phreno-esophageal membrane. This sheet of fibrous and elastic tissue extends from the muscular margins of the hiatus to the esophagus circumferentially and inserts into the esophageal submucosa slightly above the upper margins of the hiatus and above the mucosal junction.

Disease of the esophagus may be classified and understood by considering its effect upon the two primary functions of the esophagus — transportation of ingested material and the prevention of reflux — and the four above-mentioned major components which contribute to normal function: the cricopharyngeal sphincter, the muscle layers, the mucosal lining, and the lower esophageal sphincter. Since dysphagia or difficulty in swallowing is almost a universal complaint in patients with any disease interfering with esophageal function, this symptom must be regarded as non-specific. However, dysphagia must be regarded as a strong indication for complete diagnostic evaluation of esophageal structure and function.

Only in this way will a precise diagnosis of the individual pathologic condition be made at a time when therapy can be instituted to restore esophageal function to normal.

TRANSPORTATION OF INGESTED MATERIAL

Normal Swallowing

When food or liquid is swallowed, the bolus is transmitted from the pharynx to the stomach by the coordinated action of all four esophageal components. Instantaneously, with the onset of swallowing, the cricopharyngeal sphincter relaxes and luminal pressure level falls to that in the body of the esophagus. This sphincter relaxation lasts for a short time, often one second or less, and is followed by a contraction of the sphincter which may produce a luminal pressure of up to 80 mm. Hg.

The arrangement of circular and longitudinal esophageal muscle fibers allows both constriction of the lumen and shortening of the esophagus which are essential for effective peristalsis. A primary peristaltic wave triggered by a swallow is characterized by a progressive contraction which moves down the body of the esophagus at the rate of 2 to 4 cm. per second and generates intraluminal pressures which generally range between 30 and 60 mm. Hg above resting pressure. Preceding the peristaltic contraction, relaxation occurs. The arrangement of mucosal folds, their loose adherence to the muscle, and the marked ability of the relaxed muscle to stretch permit distention of the esophagus to several centimeters without disruption. A single swallow generates a peristaltic contraction which progresses completely down the full length of the esophagus. However, if a second swallow is performed immediately, the initial peristaltic wave is interrupted and a second wave begins in the upper esophagus and progresses downward. In older persons the proportion of swallows followed by a primary progressive peristaltic contraction is diminished when compared to that of younger individuals.

Other types of esophageal contractions are observed. Secondary peristalsis is a progressive peristaltic wave that occurs without initiation by a swallow. These may be triggered by a bolus in the esophagus or may occur spontaneously. Tertiary or segmental contractions are non-peristaltic and may follow a swallow in an older patient with disordered esophageal function, may result from stimulation by an oversized bolus, or may be initiated by irritants such as regurgitated acid in the lumen. High-amplitude tertiary contractions are considered spastic and may persist for prolonged periods.

In response to a swallow, the lower esophageal sphincter segment relaxes promptly, permitting intraluminal pressure to drop to gastric level. This relaxation lasts until the peristaltic wave reaches the lower esophagus. As the peristaltic wave reaches the upper portion of the sphincter, it participates in the contraction with a marked increase in pressure, whereas the lower portion of the sphincter simply regains its resting tone of approximately 8 mm. Hg above intragastric pressure. The concentric contraction of the distal esophagus is useful in differentiating between esophagus and stomach radiographically, since the latter does not contract in coordination with esophageal peristalsis. The termination of the peristaltic contraction can be employed to locate the muscular junction between esophagus and stomach.

The entire action of the esophagus in response to a swallow is coordinated by vagal or parasympathetic nerve fibers which provide the major innervation of the esophagus. Both central and local neural pathways appear to be involved in the peristaltic contraction. Anticholinergic drugs or vagotomy causes a decrease in the strength of the peristaltic contraction and diminishes the resting pressure in the lower esophageal sphincter. Sympathetic innervation has been demonstrated anatomically, but the function of these nerve fibers is not completely understood.

Disorders of the Cricopharyngeal Sphincter

Failure to Relax. Precise neuromuscular coordination of swallowing is most critical at the level of the cricopharyngeal sphincter. Since this sphincter normally remains in the tonic or contracted state, it must relax to permit a swallowed bolus to enter the esophagus. As previously noted, the time of relaxation is short and must precede and overlap the time of pharyngeal contraction. Relaxation is controlled by branches from the vagus nerves. A number of neurologic disorders may interfere with this coordinated function and cause faulty timing or failure of sphincter relaxation, which in turn prevents passage of the bolus into the esophagus and favors the likelihood of aspiration of swallowed material through the larynx into the tracheobronchial tree. Failure of the sphincter to open may cause symptoms of obstruction in the throat, with periodic choking or frequent cough accompanying swallowing. In some patients the symptoms are not very dramatic and the disorder may lead to chronic pulmonary damage from aspiration of small quantities without the patient being aware of difficulty in swallowing. Underlying diseases which may interfere with neuromuscular coordination include minor or major vascular occlusions in the brain stem, myasthenia gravis, amyotrophic lateral sclerosis, peripheral neuropathies involving the vagus nerve, and skeletal abnormalities such as cervical osteoarthritis.

Spasm. A second source of failure of the cricopharyngeal sphincter to relax is spasm of this muscle. Radiographic studies have demonstrated that patients with disorders lower in the esophagus such as severe gastroesophageal reflux may have regurgitation or retention of material in the upper esophagus. This in turn irritates the sphincter and causes spasm. In addition to aspiration during swallowing, such patients may be aware of a chronic irritation in the throat and may develop a fear of swallowing which has been previously categorized as "globus hystericus." Some patients with neurologic or muscular dysfunction of the cricopharyngeal sphincter will develop secondary laryngeal changes, causing symptoms of hoarseness and chronic pharyngitis. Inflammatory polyps of the vocal cords and trachea may be found.

Cricopharyngeal(Zenker's)Diverticulum. Zenker's diverticulum is the most common type encountered in the esophagus. It is a false or acquired diverticulum characterized by pouching of the mucosal or submucosal layers through a defect in the muscular wall. The defect is located just proximal to the cricopharyngeal sphincter in the posterior wall of the inferior pharynx. Recent studies suggest that the pouch is secondary to dysfunction of the cricopharyngeal sphincter. When a bolus is forced into the lower pharynx against a closed sphincter, high pressures build up just above the sphincter. There is a weak place posteriorly in the musculature of the inferior pharynx where the oblique muscle fibers of the inferior constrictor blend into the transverse fibers of the sphincter. At this point a blowout of mucosa or diverticulum may develop.

In patients with a fully developed cricopharyngeal diverticulum it is common to elicit a history of swallowing difficulty dating back several years prior to awareness of the pouch. Initially the symptoms are cervical dysphagia and occasional bouts of aspiration or choking. As the pouch enlarges, solid particles and fluid become trapped and later regurgitate into the pharynx. When the patient lies down or stoops forward he may notice undigested food eaten hours earlier now regurgitating back into the mouth. The swallowing of large solid particles such as pills, capsules, or pieces of meat may be particularly difficult, as these routinely lodge in the pouch. A patient with a fully developed pouch finds that he must eat slowly and carefully to avoid aspiration. Friends and family frequently notice gurgling noises when the patient eats or swallows.

Complications of this disorder include chronic or acute aspiration, the risk of a large solid bolus lodging in the larynx that may cause asphyxiation, an increased risk of perforation from foreign bodies, and the development of ulcerations in the pouch from retained irritating particles. Carcinomas have developed within such pouches. There is a particular risk of perforation during endoscopic or intubation procedures for patients with this disorder.

Disorders of Esophageal Muscle

Esophageal muscular disorders may interfere with transmission of a swallowed bolus in several ways.

Other Esophageal Diverticula. Pulsion diverticula may occur at levels in the esophagus other than the cricopharyngeal region. The next most common site is the lower esophagus. These epiphrenic diverticula also consist of mucosal protrusions through the muscular layer that develop just proximal to the lower esophageal sphincter or just proximal to a segment of spastic esophageal muscle. The mechanism for development of such a diverticulum appears similar to that for the cricopharyngeal diverticulum. Although aspiration and laryngeal irritation do not occur, other symptoms from retention of swallowed material are similar.

When studied manometrically, the esophagus distal to the pulsion diverticulum characteristically demonstrates spastic or tertiary contractions, or failure to relax as the peristaltic wave progresses down the esophagus. When viewed radiographically, the usual finding is a segment of tonic or contracted muscle just beyond the opening of the pouch. Dysphagia frequently accompanies pulsion diverticulum. This has been attributed to the large size of the pouch hanging in a dependent position and compressing the adjacent lower esophagus. However, dysphagia may accompany a small diverticulum, in which case such a mechanical explanation cannot be invoked. It is now thought that the dysphagia represents a primary disorder in the esophageal muscle rather than a secondary effect of the diverticulum.

More rare are true diverticula which may occur at any level and in which the body of the esophagus appears to be normal above and below the opening of the pouch. The wall of the true diverticulum consists of both mucosal and muscular layers. Distinction is sometimes made between those diverticula which appear rounded and have a narrow orifice similar to that of pulsion diverticula and are considered of congenital origin, and those with broad openings, generally in the midesophagus, which are commonly called traction diverticula. This latter term derives from the theory that the esophagus is pulled out of its normal course by contractions of adhesions to adjacent inflammatory lymph nodes or chronic mediastinal infection; however, clear evidence of this is frequently not demonstrable. These diverticula cause no or few symptoms unless they reach a large size.

Systemic Sclerosis. Systemic sclerosis or scleroderma is a generalized disease involving smooth muscle and connective tissues throughout the body. Esophageal involvement is the most common alimentary tract manifestation and may precede other clinical evidence of the disease. The esophageal changes consist of atrophy of the smooth muscle in the lower two thirds of the organ distal to the segment of skeletal muscle. The smooth muscle is gradually replaced by fibrosis. The muscle atrophy causes a failure of the peristaltic wave to progress into the lower esophagus and causes weakness or obliteration of the lower esophageal sphincter mechanism. This in turn permits increased gastroesophageal reflux which may lead to secondary esophagitis. The fibrosis of the muscle may lead to a stricture of the distal esophagus, or stricture may develop owing to the severity of the esophagitis accompanying gastroesophageal reflux. The effects of reflux in such patients may be particularly severe because of the inability of the esophagus to respond by secondary peristalsis and empty itself of regurgitated gastric contents. Either aperistalsis or stricture may cause the symptom of dysphagia.

The absence of peristalsis when observed manometrically or by radiographic techniques and systemic manifestations of the disease differentiate this disorder from abnormal gastroesophageal reflux due to an incompetent lower esophageal sphincter in an otherwise healthy patient. The common radiographic finding is failure of ingested barium to pass the level of the carina when the patient is in a supine position. When the patient sits upright, the barium falls under the influence of gravity. When a stricture develops in such patients the esophageal disease may become the most prominent feature of systemic sclerosis and lead to progressive weight loss and starvation. Because of the atrophic esophageal wall and frequent secondary esophagitis, attempts to treat this disorder by dilatation may be difficult and the risks of esophageal perforation are high.

Esophageal Spasm. When esophageal spasm is encountered, it is generally secondary to another esophageal disorder. The majority of patients who demonstrate spasm will be found to have either abnormal gastroesophageal reflux which appears to trigger spasm, particularly in the lower esophagus, or a partial obstruction such as a ring, web, hypertensive lower esophageal sphincter, or tumor. Occasionally, patients are encountered in whom none of these disorders can be identified, and spasm on a primary neurogenic or functional basis must be diagnosed. Whenever this diagnosis is made, careful search for an underlying cause should be undertaken.

Characteristically, spasm is localized or segmental in distribution, with the most prominent spastic contractions occurring repeatedly at the same level. Complete or partial obstruction to the passage of ingested food may result from spasm. A prominent feature of this disorder is severe substernal pain which may be suggestive of the symptoms accompanying ischemic heart disease. Since the spasm may be reduced by the use of nitrites, response to nitroglycerin is not a useful way to differentiate between this disease and coronary heart disease. The diagnosis of esophageal spasm is made by the characteristic radiographic appearance of a corkscrew esophagus or multiple constrictive rings which do not dilate during fluoroscopic observation. Another useful diagnostic technique is manometry, which shows high-pressure contractions occurring spontaneously or in response to a swallow and located at the same level in the esophagus on repeated studies.

Leiomyoma. Benign tumors of smooth muscle in the esophagus are occasionally encountered. Normally, these are incidental findings in the course of barium swallow radiography, but occasionally these tumors may reach sufficient size to interfere with the passage of ingested food and cause dysphagia. They are not normally fixed to the esophageal mucosa and cannot be diagnosed endoscopically. When a leiomyoma is suspected from radiographic findings, a biopsy should not be attempted through the esophagoscope because of the dangers of introducing infection and causing inflammatory adhesion of the tumor to the mucosa, which interferes with later surgical removal.

Disorders of Mucosa

Neoplasm. Benign neoplasms of the esophageal mucosa are infrequent and generally of little clinical importance. Occasionally, squamous polyps or papillomas may be encountered. Adenomas arising in the esophageal glands are rare. The most common esophageal neoplasm is carcinoma. This most frequently causes the symptom of dysphagia and occurs with sufficient frequency that any patient complaining of persistent dysphagia should be thoroughly investigated for the possibility of this disease.

Carcinoma of the esophagus is a virulent neoplasm causing approximately five deaths per hundred thousand population in the United States each year. The disease is more frequent in males than in females, and in non-white than in white Americans. It occurs more commonly in the sixth, seventh, and eighth decades of life. Carcinoma may develop in association with conditions contributing to esophageal retention or irritation such as excessive use of alcohol or tobacco, and among patients having achalasia or lye strictures. Patients with the Plummer-Vinson syndrome (see below) are susceptible to squamous cell carcinoma of the cervical esophagus and hypopharynx.

Carcinoma may present a variety of appearances, including ulceration, fungating tumor, or diffuse scirrhous strictures. The most common site of origin appears to be in the middle third of the esophagus. Microscopically, squamous cell carcinoma is by far the most common type. Adenocarcinoma truly arising in the esophagus separated from the stomach is rare. Adenocarcinoma at the cardia is more common and probably arises from gastric mucosa. Carcinomatous change in esophageal mucosa may be multifocal. The disease spreads by direct extension, lymphatic invasion, and blood-borne metastases. The rich lymphatic network of the esophageal submucosa permits early and extensive spread of the tumor up and down the length of the esophagus. It is not uncommon to encounter malignant cells 5 cm. or more from the visible margins of a tumor. Direct invasion of adjacent structures such as the trachea or aorta is common and a frequent cause of life-threatening complications. One reason for the poor prognosis of these tumors is the advanced state which they reach before causing symptoms. Because of the ability of smooth muscle to stretch, involvement of the esophageal lumen must be nearly circumferential before dysphagia and obstruction develop.

Although the patient may recall a sensation of substernal fullness or poorly localized chest pain, the usual presenting complaint is dysphagia or difficulty in swallowing. The level of the obstruction may be quite accurately localized by the patient's symptoms. Rapid weight loss and emaciation accompany the dysphagia. As the obstruction becomes more complete, regurgitation of swallowed food, vomiting, or choking and aspiration are noted. Hoarseness may develop from recurrent nerve involvement by the primary tumor or lymph node metastases. Horner's syndrome, hematemesis, or melena may occur. When the tumor invades the trachea or bronchus, cough, hemoptysis, or dyspnea results. Complications of the tumor may be heralded by the presence of lymph nodes in the neck, bone pain from metastases, hemorrhage from invasion of mediastinal vessels, fever from perforation or abscess, and severe cough from tracheobronchial involvement. Tracheo-esophageal fistula may develop in advanced cases and be the terminal event.

Because the obvious symptoms from carcinoma of the esophagus represent complications of the disease at an advanced stage, it is especially important that the diagnosis be made whenever possible at any earlier stage, when treatment is more favorable and symptoms are less apparent. Any patient complaining of symptoms which might arise from the esophagus should undergo radiographic examination and have specimens of esophageal washings submitted for cytologic examination. In addition to the standard barium swallow observed fluoroscopically and recorded on permanent x-ray films, it is often helpful to examine the esophagus by cineradiographic techniques, so that the course of the barium may be examined repeatedly if questionable regions in the esophagus are observed. Just as the pathologic presentation of esophageal carcinoma is variable, the radiographic manifestations may take many forms such as a fungating mass, ulcerations, stricture, or polypoid tumor. In some patients the radiographic appearances may be more suggestive of benign disease.

Cytologic examination of cells obtained from esophageal washings offers a high diagnostic yield in patients with this disease. In addition to the patients whose symptoms or x-ray findings suggest a possible neoplasm, those who may have a high risk of the disease such as individuals with longstanding lye stricture, achalasia, or the Plummer-Vinson syndrome are good candidates for repeated cytologic examinations at six-month or yearly intervals.

To confirm or establish the diagnosis of carcinoma in patients whose symptoms or x-ray findings are suggestive, esophagoscopy is an essential diagnostic procedure. A biopsy will provide confirmatory evidence of the diagnosis and indicate the cell type. Because of the tendency for esophageal neoplasms to spread up and down the mucosa, biopsies are generally taken above the level of the tumor to ascertain whether submucosal spread has occurred. This has great importance in planning treatment for the disease. In patients whose neoplasm is located in the middle third of the esophagus, bronchoscopy should also be performed to detect evidence of tracheal or left main bronchial invasion or vocal cord paralysis.

Web or Ring. Benign rings or webs of the esophageal mucosa may cause symptoms by obstructing the passage of solid food through the lumen. Although these mucosal constrictions may occur at any level in the esophagus, there are two specific clinical forms in which this lesion is more frequently encountered.

The Plummer-Vinson syndrome, when fully developed, includes a hypochromic microcytic anemia, spoon-shaped fingernails, atrophy of the tongue and of the pharyngeal and esophageal mucosa, fissures at the corners of the mouth, and dysphagia. This syndrome occurs more frequently in fair-complexioned females of Northern European descent. The dysphagia may result from a hypopharyngeal or upper esophageal mucosal web. These patients have a higher than normal incidence of carcinoma of the upper esophagus and must be carefully observed for a change in symptoms suggesting the development of a neoplasm. Such patients are candidates for periodic cytologic examination of esophageal washings.

Schatzki and Gary (1953) and Ingelfinger and Kramer (1953) independently described the condition of lower esophageal ring causing dysphagia. This clinical syndrome often occurs in older male patients and is manifested by sudden severe dysphagia after ingestion of a large bolus of solid food. The sensation of food sticking under the lower sternum and severe pain are prominent symptoms. As the food digests or is gradually propelled through the narrow segment, the symptoms subside and may not recur for prolonged periods until a large bolus is once again ingested. The symptoms of severe pain which may accompany this disorder are due to spasm of the esophageal muscle above the ring as the esophagus contracts upon the impacted bolus. In this regard the symptoms of pain come from a mechanism similar to that which causes pain lower in the intestinal tract, namely, vigorous contraction of gut muscle above an obstructing point.

Pathologically, the "Schatzki" ring is found to have esophageal squamous mucosa on the superior surface and columnar mucosa on the inferior surface. A thin layer of fibrous tissue may be seen in the submucosa between the two layers of mucosa. Deeper layers of the esophagus are normal. Occasional cases are described in which the ring is located completely within the zone of esophageal squamous epithelium.

The effect of the ring is to limit esophageal distention. Thus, when the esophagus is empty, no ring is visible. It is only when the lumen of the esophagus is distended beyond the diameter of the ring that it becomes noticeable. For this reason the ring may be missed in radiographic examinations unless the lower esophagus is studied in the dilated condition. The diameter of the ring has a strong correlation with the presence of symptoms. Patients whose rings measure less than 13 mm. in diameter almost always have symptoms of dysphagia, whereas those whose rings are larger than 13 mm. may be asymptomatic. Rings of large diameter are frequent findings in routine barium swallow examinations but those which progress to a narrow aperture and cause symptoms are uncommon. Because the ring represents a zone of restricted distensibility rather than a constant weblike defect in the esophagus, it may be easily missed by esophagoscopy. The diagnosis is generally made only on radiographic study.

Stricture. Stricture or abnormal narrowing with contraction of the esophagus may occur from a variety of causes. Malignant neoplasms may present as a stricture. The ingestion of corrosive substances such as lye may cause destruction of the esophageal wall, with stricture formation. The most common type of benign esophageal stricture is caused by reflux esophagitis. The diagnosis of a stricture is made by x-ray examination demonstrating a persistent narrowing or contraction of the esophagus. However, the specific type of stricture generally cannot be diagnosed solely by x-ray but is determined by the clinical history and esophagoscopic findings.

Strictures secondary to gastroesophageal reflux are thought to occur through the following mechanisms: An incompetent lower esophageal sphincter permits free reflux of upper gastrointestinal secretions, including acid, pepsin, bile, and pancreatic secretions, into the lower esophagus. Prolonged contact of these substances with the esophageal mucosa causes penetration and breakdown of the mucosa, superficial ulceration, submucosal inflammation, edema and muscle spasm. The damage is repaired by deposition of inflammatory tissue followed by collagen deposition and fibrosis, just as injured tissue heals elsewhere in the body. If the reflux decreases, the mucosa may be restored by migration and regeneration of columnar epithelial cells rather than the squamous epithelium which normally lines the lower esophagus. Continuous or repeated insults to the mucosa lead to increasing amounts of tissue destruction and fibrosis. Initially this occurs in the superficial layers, but as the condition becomes more severe the muscle fibers are damaged and replaced by fibrous tissue as well. As the collagen matures, it contracts, causing rigidity, narrowing, and shortening of the esophageal wall until a tight stricture develops. As the lumen is gradually occluded by the contracting fibrous tissue, the amount of reflux diminishes, and the mucosa and esophagus above the level of the stricture are spared from further insult and appear normal. The development of a stricture through these steps has been documented sequentially in individual patients and has been seen in various stages in numerous patients, providing evidence for this theory of stricture development.

At the time when a stricture is apparent radiographically, the fibrosis may still be limited to the submucosal layers, with edema and spasm causing much of the narrowing, or the x-ray finding of a stricture may represent far advanced disease, with total breakdown and replacement of the esophageal wall by fibrosis and granulation tissue. Thus, the clinical and radiographic diagnosis of esophageal stricture may represent pathologic conditions of varying degrees of severity. This must be taken into account when therapy is planned and the results of treatment are assessed.

The physiologic effects of reflux esophagitis and stricture are initially those of disordered peristalsis. Partial esophageal narrowing as well as esophageal reflux can disrupt or alter progression of the peristaltic wave and cause synchronous or tertiary contractions. Inability of the esophagus to empty permits prolonged contact of refluxed material with the mucosa and aggravates the esophagitis. It is only when the stricture becomes far advanced that the bolus of food is mechanically obstructed by the narrowing. By this time, the patient's intake of solid food is markedly restricted. As the stricture tightens, the reflux may be less, so that the symptoms of heartburn and regurgitation are diminished. Dysphagia may be the only complaint. This leads to a paradox in which the most severe stages of esophagitis may be associated with few symptoms of reflux, although this is thought to be the underlying cause of the inflammation and stricture. In patients whose esophagus is relatively insensitive to reflux or in whom reflux occurs mainly while supine and asleep, dysphagia may be the earliest complaint leading the patient to the physician.

In addition to symptoms of reflux, dysphagia, and inanition, the patient with a stricture is likely to have pulmonary complaints of nocturnal cough, or choking or coughing when eating, and may develop pulmonary infection secondary to aspiration. Other complications of a stricture include hemorrhage, usually from ulceration in areas of ectopic columnar mucosa, or perforation of the esophagus, again usually due to ulceration in areas of ectopic gastric epithelium.

Between the two common types of benign esophageal strictures — those due to reflux esophagitis and those secondary to ingestion of caustic materials — important differences exist. The stricture secondary to reflux is almost always rather short and localized to the region just above columnar epithelium, whether this be at the gastroesophageal junction or high in the esophagus in patients whose esophagus is lined with columnar or gastric epithelium. Thus, the patient with a short stricture in the midesophagus caused by reflux will have columnar epithelium below the stricture. On the other hand, a patient whose stricture is due to ingestion of lye or other corrosives will often have long segments of esophagus damaged by the chemicals and replaced with fibrous tissue. Damage may be particularly severe at the levels of the esophagus where there is a shelf or transient holdup of the bolus, such as the cricopharyngeal region, the level of the aortic arch, and just above the diaphragm.

A second distinction between the reflux and corrosive strictures is that the cause of the reflux stricture persists, so that the condition continues to worsen rather than improve with time. Methods of therapy which do not prevent the underlying reflux may fail to provide relief from further stricture development. On the other hand, the stricture secondary to ingestion of corrosives is caused by a single injury. Taking this into account, one may employ methods of therapy which differ from those used in treatment of a reflux stricture.

Malignant strictures of the esophagus are considered in a preceding section and will not be discussed further here. The secondary effects and complications of the malignant stricture may be similar to those of the benign stricture.

Disorders at the Cardia Interfering with Transportation of Ingested Material

Achalasia. Achalasia is an uncommon disease of unknown etiology in which the lower esophageal sphincter fails to relax in response to a swallow, and there is an absence of peristalsis in the body of the esophagus. Findings on visual or radiographic examination include a normally contracted distal esophageal segment of approximately 2 to 4 cm. in length composed of normal muscle. The body of the esophagus is generally dilated and may distend to a very large size sufficient to contain several quarts of fluid. Generally, the muscle of the esophageal wall in its midportion is thickened, but in far advanced cases it may become atrophic and fibrotic. Microscopically, the distinctive feature of achalasia is the absence or decrease in number of the ganglion cells in Auerbach's plexus. Fibrosis of the plexus may be noted. These changes are found throughout the esophagus but are more conspicuous in the lower portion. The inner circular muscle layer may be hypertrophied or sclerotic, and scarring of the muscle cells may be noticed microscopically. Although several reports have suggested that there may be abnormalities of the vagus nerves or the central nervous system in patients with achalasia, these findings have not been thoroughly substantiated or generally accepted.

While the etiology of achalasia is unknown, a similar type of mega-esophagus with similar pathologic changes in the muscle and Auerbach's plexus may be seen in Chagas' disease. This disease occurs in South America and is caused by *Trypanosoma cruzi*. Evidence suggests that the organism secretes a neurotoxin which affects the ganglion cells. Although this disease is clinically similar to achalasia, the organism has not been found in the vast majority of patients suffering from typical achalasia in North America or Europe.

The physiologic disorder of achalasia may best be studied by esophageal manometry. The characteristics of the lower esophageal sphincter segment in the resting state are the same as in normal individuals. However, in the body of the esophagus the resting intraluminal pressures are generally high and may exceed the pressures of the gastric fundus. The manometric abnormalities of achalasia are most striking when the response to a swallow is studied. The lower esophageal sphincter fails to relax following a swallow, and contraction may occur prematurely in the upper portion of the sphincter, so that the sphincter is effectively closed when the peristaltic wave would normally reach the lower esophagus. In addition to the failure of the sphincter to relax, passage of the bolus is further impeded by the absence of peristalsis in the body of the esophagus. Following the swallow, a simultaneous contraction generally occurs throughout the length of the esophagus with no progression of the pressure waves. In far advanced cases in which the muscle has become sclerotic, atrophic, and fibrotic, no contraction at all may be observed.

A further physiologic abnormality in the patient with achalasia is the response to methacholine. In the normal subject, injection of this drug generally causes no change in pressure in the body of the esophagus. In a patient with achalasia, subcutaneous injection of 5 to 10 mg. of methacholine chloride may cause an increase in resting esophageal pressure of 20 cm. of water or more. This may be associated with severe substernal pain, similar to that in patients with esophageal spasm. The methacholine response may be abolished by administration of atropine sulfate.

The symptoms caused by these specific pathologic and physiologic changes are sufficiently distinctive to separate this disease from other esophageal disorders. Initially, the patient will notice intermittent obstruction to swallowing localized to the lower substernal region. The obstruction is generally less when a meal is taken slowly and the food is warm. The obstruction may be intermittent and may be more severe when the patient is tense or nervous. As the symptoms become more pronounced, the patient becomes aware of regurgitation whenever he stoops forward. Unlike gastroesophageal reflux, the regurgitated material is not acid or sour, and undigested food can often be identified. Pain is generally not associated with the regurgitation. The pain which occurs with achalasia, if any, is usually of the spastic type, rather than heartburn. It may be quite severe, is located substernally, and persists for a long time.

When esophageal retention becomes marked, pulmonary symptoms secondary to aspiration become prominent. The patient may awaken to find ingested food material regurgitated onto the pillow. Secondary pulmonary complications including lung abscess may occur. Nutrition may be impaired and the patient suffers weight loss and vitamin deficiency. Although bleeding is quite uncommon in these cases, a retention esophagitis may develop and cause chronic anemia from blood loss. In addition to these complications from obstructed swallowing, patients with achalasia are thought to have a higher than normal incidence of squamous cell carcinoma in the mid-portion of the esophagus.

Hypertensive Lower Esophageal Sphincter. A rare variation of the spastic esophageal motor disorders may be increased tone in the lower esophageal sphincter, causing dysphagia and severe pain. Generally, retention of ingested food in the esophagus is not prominent in these patients. This finding differentiates it from achalasia, as does the finding of increased sphincter pressure during manometric studies. In other respects, this syndrome is similar to that of esophageal spasm described above. Whether the hypertensive sphincter syndrome occurs as secondary manifestation of a gastroesophageal reflux remains uncertain.

Other Diseases Affecting Transportation of Ingested Material

A variety of diseases which involve the esophagus may have a secondary effect of blocking transportation of ingested material. Extrinsic conditions such as neoplasm metastatic to the mediastinum or esophageal wall may interfere with swallowing in a manner similar to that of primary carcinoma of the esophagus. An enlarging thoracic aortic aneurysm may compress the esophagus and cause secondary dysphagia. Primary bronchogenic carcinoma adjacent to the esophagus may involve the esophageal wall and block ingestion of food. A foreign body lodged in the esophagus generally interrupts swallowing, owing to both its physical presence and the edema and inflammation it causes in the wall of the esophagus.

Esophageal atresia with tracheo-esophageal fistula is a fairly common abnormality of the newborn which obviously interferes with transportation of ingested food. Following surgical correction of the atresia and fistula, function of the esophagus will generally return to normal unless a stricture develops at the anastomosis. Acquired tracheo-esophageal fistulas may occur from malignant disease in the mediastinum or rarely from inflammatory diseases such as tuberculosis or histoplasmosis. Such fistulas permit transportation of food material from the esophagus directly into the lungs, with resulting severe cough and pulmonary infection.

Rupture of the esophagus may occur spontaneously, from penetrating wounds or external trauma, from foreign bodies, or during the course of esophageal intubation. This catastrophic event occurs most commonly during esophagoscopy or gastroscopy. When perforation accompanies endoscopy, the common sites are just distal to the cricopharyngeal sphincter and in the lower esophagus. Spontaneous rupture of the esophagus is almost always caused by vomiting and occurs most frequently along the left lateral aspect of the lower esophagus. During vomiting, the antrum of the stomach contracts and the upper stomach and esophagus relax, permitting increased intra-abdominal pressure to force the gastric contents cephalad. The distal esophagus may increase dramatically in diameter fivefold or more. The left lower esophageal wall is the weakest point of the organ and can be ruptured by pressures of 5 lbs. per square inch or less, providing the setting for spontaneous rupture during vomiting.

Following esophageal rupture, the patient experiences a sudden severe substernal or epigastric pain. If the rupture occurs when the patient is anesthetized or sedated for endoscopy, this initial symptom may be absent. Following rupture, mediastinal dissection of air or pneumothorax develops. This is manifested by crepitus felt in the neck or a mediastinal crunching sound heard on auscultation over the back. If the rupture does not penetrate the pleura, an effusion secondary to the mediastinitis develops in the pleura within the course of several hours. Free perforation into the pleura causes a hydropneumothorax and empyema. A tension pneumothorax may occur. The patient rapidly becomes gravely ill, with signs of shock. This illness may be mistaken for perforated duodenal or gastric ulcer, acute pancreatitis, acute myocardial infarction, or dissecting aortic aneurysm. The diagnosis can be resolved by abdominal and thoracic roentgenograms, serum amylase levels, electrocardiogram, and x-ray visualization of the esophagus by a swallow of radiopaque water-soluble substance.

PREVENTION OF GASTROESOPHAGEAL REFLUX

The second major function of the esophagus is the prevention of involuntary regurgitation of stomach contents. The responsibility for this function is vested in the esophagogastric junction or cardia.

Mechanisms for Competency of the Cardia

In normal individuals the mechanism which permits unimpeded passage of swallowed material into the stomach while preventing regurgitation of gastric contents back through the esophageal orifice is remarkably effective. Withdrawal of a pH electrode across the cardia often reveals a 5 unit change in pH over a distance of approximately 0.5 cm. This represents a 100,000-fold difference in hydrogen ion concentration across this short distance. In spite of a great deal of investigation as to the structure and function of the esophagogastric junction, precise understanding of the mechanism which prevents reflux remains incomplete.

A variety of factors have been suggested as contributing to competency of the cardia. The strength or resting pressure of the lower esophageal sphincter has a statistical correlation with the control of reflux. Yet, in individual patients a high pressure in the sphincter may be present, and free reflux occurs. Conversely, a low sphincter pressure may be found in a patient without reflux. Since no anatomic sphincter can be demonstrated in humans, the source of the pressures recorded in the distal esophagus remains uncertain. The high-pressure zone probably represents a summation of intrinsic pressure generated from the lower esophageal muscle, extrinsic pressure resulting from the diaphragmatic hiatus, and positive abdominal pressure exerted against the endo-abdominal fascia, which inserts at or above the level of the sphincter. An active role of the distal esophageal muscle in generating the measured sphincter pressure and in the prevention of reflux is suggested by the observation that pressures in the lower esophageal sphincter rise markedly when the hormone gastrin is administered. The ability of the sphincter to adapt its tension to changes in abdominal pressure further suggests an intrinsic role of the lower esophageal muscle in preventing reflux. Most investigators now accept the lower esophageal muscle as being at least partially responsible for competency of the cardia.

The esophageal hiatus of the diaphragm may play a role in the normal control of reflux, but it is not essential. Some patients with a hiatal hernia have a competent cardia, whereas others in whom a hiatal hernia cannot be demonstrated may have an incompetent cardia.

The location of a portion of the lower esophageal sphincter within the positive pressure abdominal environment appears to be important in the prevention of reflux. The pressure gradient across the diaphragm is usually 10 mm. Hg or more and increases during inspiration. The compressing effect of abdominal pressure during all phases of respiration supplements the intrinsic pressure generated by the lower esophageal muscle segment. Intra-abdominal pressure may remain effective even in patients with hiatal hernia if the extension of endo-abdominal fascia through the hiatus inserts into the esophagus above the sphincter. Thus, compression by the right crus of the diaphragm or muscular contraction of the diaphragm does not appear important, but an intra-abdominal location of the distal esophageal segment probably does contribute to competency of the cardia.

Other suggested factors for which there is less evidence of effectiveness include an acute esophagogastric angle of entry and the plugging of the esophageal orifice by redundant gastric folds. Further investigations are necessary to determine precisely how competency of the cardia is achieved in the normal human being.

Hiatal Hernia.   Hiatal hernia is one of the most common disorders of the alimentary tract. Its significance varies greatly, depending upon type, size, and associated complications. It is essential to understand that gastroesophageal reflux and hiatal hernia, which often appear together, are separate entities, each of which may occur without the other. For this reason, it is important to differentiate the symptoms, diagnosis, and complications for each of the two conditions.

Hiatal hernia is defined as stomach passing into the thorax through the esophageal hiatus of the diaphragm. There are two basic types of hiatal hernia which can be differentiated by the anatomic and physiologic abnormalities of each. Combinations of the two types constitute a third group of hiatal hernias, and the presence of other organs in addition to the stomach passing through the esophageal hiatus makes up a fourth category of hiatal hernia.

In Type I, the axial or sliding hiatal hernia, the esophagogastric junction is displaced through the diaphragm as the leading point of the hernia. In Type II, the paraesophageal or rolling hernia, the esophagogastric junction remains fixed at the level of the hiatus, but a portion of the gastric fundus advances above the cardia into a hernia sac. It is the Type I hiatal hernia which may be accompanied by gastroesophageal reflux and its distinctive symptoms and complications. Type II hiatal hernia is rarely associated with abnormal reflux. The combined Type III hiatal hernia, in which the esophagogastric junction is herniated through the diaphragm but a portion of the gastric fundus is more cephalad than the cardia, may be associated with the symptoms and complications of both Type I and II hernias.

The diagnosis of a hiatal hernia is established primarily by radiographic study and is confirmed by surgical dissection. Diagnostic methods such as manometry, mucosal potential difference measurements, and pH recordings are more useful in diagnosing gastroesophageal reflux and its complications than in establishing the presence of a hiatal hernia.

Generally, the common small Type I hiatal hernia is asymptomatic and causes no complications unless abnormal gastroesophageal reflux is present. The symptoms and complications often attributed to this hernia are really those of reflux and will be described in the next section.

The Type II hiatal hernia may be asymptomatic, even though quite large, or may cause symptoms related to the abnormal position of the stomach in the hernia sac. These symptoms are most commonly mild discomfort or fullness in the epigastrium or chest after eating. This may be relieved by belching or vomiting. Dysphagia may occur because of extrinsic compression of the esophagus by the adjacent large hernia pouch. This type of hernia is associated with a substantial incidence of serious mechanical complications involving the gastric pouch. Complications include hemorrhage from ulcers or gastritis in the supradiaphragmatic stomach, gastric obstruction, or volvulus, which may lead to strangulation and gastric infarction. Very large Type II hernias are commonly combined with displacement of the cardia proximally and may be associated with reflux and its complications. Large hernias introduce a risk of intrathoracic gastric dilatation with respiratory embarrassment. When the sac is sizable, other organs such as colon, small intestine, or spleen may herniate and provide a further source of complications.

Gastroesophageal Reflux. Regurgitation of gastric contents through the esophagogastric junction probably occurs at times in everyone. Manometric study has shown that newborn infants lack a lower esophageal high pressure zone, and they frequently regurgitate. During the first year of life, competency of the cardia is acquired and regurgitation ceases. Although occasional reflux may occur as a normal event in older patients, frequent reflux into an esophagus sensitive to the irritating gastrointestinal secretions may cause symptoms and complications. When this occurs, the clinical condition of abnormal gastroesophageal reflux results. This rarely develops in the interval between infancy and late teen age. Thereafter the incidence of abnormal reflux rises, and the problem is most common in patients over 40 years of age. There seems to be an increased tendency for reflux to occur in obese individuals.

Although abnormal reflux commonly is associated with Type I or sliding hiatal hernia, a causal relationship between these two conditions is not established. Individuals without a hiatal hernia demonstrated radiographically or at surgery may experience reflux through an incompetent cardia, and, as mentioned in the preceding section, patients having a hiatal hernia do not necessarily experience abnormal reflux.

In the typical patient with gastroesophageal reflux, manometric studies often demonstrate a decreased resting pressure in the lower esophageal sphincter. Generally, the sphincter segment will be of normal length unless a large hiatal hernia is present which distorts the pressure recordings. Relaxation to swallowing is normal. As described above, however, there is not a precise one-to-one relationship between sphincter pressure and competency of the cardia, so that man-

ometric studies alone are not acceptable as diagnostic evidence of abnormal reflux.

Radiography is the most useful technique for detecting a hiatal hernia, but it is less successful in demonstrating reflux. The diagnosis of abnormal reflux can be made by the radiologist, if he sees reflux at a time other than when the patient swallows. If reflux is suspected as the cause of the patient's complaint but cannot be demonstrated radiographically, the use of pH recordings is a more sensitive and reliable method for making the diagnosis. In patients with severe reflux there may be a disorder of esophageal motor function manifested by an increased proportion of simultaneous contractions rather than progressive peristalsis. A bolus of acid placed in the esophagus in such subjects may not be cleared normally.

The typical symptoms caused by gastroesophageal reflux are pain and regurgitation aggravated by postural positions such as stooping or lying down. Discomfort is usually felt beneath the sternum and in the subxiphoid region, with occasional radiation to one side. The pain may radiate to the shoulders, neck, arms, ears, or between the scapulae, but it nearly always includes the substernal region. The nature of the pain is a burning sensation and is frequently called "heartburn" by the patient. Regurgitation may be noted as a sour or bilious taste in the mouth or as the "repeating" of food. Effortless vomiting after meals may occur in severe cases. Aggravation of the symptoms by bending over or lying flat permits the diagnosis of reflux clinically. If the patient's complaints are not related to posture, heartburn or regurgitation may be the result of other causes and cannot be attributed to abnormal reflux on the basis of symptoms alone.

Other symptoms which may be caused by reflux include vague epigastric or substernal discomfort, a foreign sensation, fullness or tightness in the neck, hoarseness, change in voice, chronic pharyngitis from reflux through the cricopharyngeal sphincter, or symptoms which mimic those of angina pectoris. When atypical symptoms are noted, the diagnosis cannot be made on clinical grounds and must depend on objective evidence of reflux and exclusion of other causes. Recordings of pH in the esophagus to document reflux may be especially helpful. In patients with atypical symptoms, the perfusion of acid and saline alternately into the esophagus may be useful in determining whether the symptoms are of esophageal origin. Reproduction of the patient's spontaneous symptoms by infusion of acid and not with saline represents a positive acid perfusion test.

The complications of gastroesophageal reflux include esophagitis, stricture, bleeding, ulceration, spasm, and aspiration of regurgitated material into the lungs. Esophagitis is the most common complication of reflux. Since the severity of the patient's symptoms correlate poorly with esophagitis, this diagnosis can be made with certainty only by esophagoscopy. Patients who present with advanced esophagitis and stricture may have minimal or no symptoms of reflux prior to the onset of obstruction, whereas some who complain most bitterly of heartburn and regurgitation are found on esophagoscopy and biopsy to have no or minimal esophagitis. The reason for such variability in sensitivity of the esophagus to reflux is not completely understood. One symptom which does suggest the presence of esophagitis and mediastinal inflammation is soreness between the scapulae following ingestion of hot or alcoholic liquids. When dysphagia develops, esophagitis is more likely to be present. However, reflux alone may trigger esophageal muscle spasm, causing dysphagia in the absence of esophagitis, and therefore this symptom is not diagnostic.

Because of the lack of specific symptoms for reflux esophagitis, esophagoscopy is essential in diagnosing this condition. The esophagoscopic findings may be categorized based upon severity. These include no visible esophagitis and Grade I esophagitis, when the mucosa is reddened but not ulcerated. In such cases, biopsy may show only thinning of the mucosa and perhaps dilatation of epithelial vessels without other change. Grade 2 esophagitis is recorded when superficial erosions and ulcerations are noted. When the wall of the esophagus becomes somewhat stiffened and fibrotic in addition to being ulcerated, Grade 3 esophagitis is present. When the fibrosis and contraction has caused a stricture, Grade 4 esophagitis is observed. Stricture is discussed in detail in a preceding section. Ulceration of the esophageal mucosa commonly takes the form of circumferential destruction of the squamous epithelium just above the columnar epithelial border. Localized penetrating ulcers into the wall of the esophagus, particularly in islands of ectopic gastric mucosa, may occur and cause rapid hemorrhage. Bleeding may also be severe in milder forms of esophagitis when diffuse oozing of blood from the mucosal surface is encountered.

Another common complication of an incompetent cardia is aspiration. Mild degrees manifested by nocturnal cough and occasional hoarseness are frequently noted in the histories of patients who prove to have reflux. When aspiration becomes more severe, pulmonary complications such as recurring pneumonitis or lung abscess may occur.

REFERENCES

Allen, T.H., and Clagett, O.T.: Changing concepts in the surgical treatment of pulsion diverticula of the lower esophagus. J. Thorac. Cardiovasc. Surg., 50:455, 1962.

Belsey, R.: The pulmonary complications of oesophageal disease. Br. J. Dis. Chest, 54:342, 1960.

Belsey, R.: Functional disease of the esophagus. J. Thorac. Cardiovasc. Surg., 52:164, 1966.

Bennett, J.R., and Hendrix, T.R.: Diffuse esophageal spasm: A disorder with more than one cause. Gastroenterology, 59:273, 1970.

Bernstein, L.M., Fruin, R.C., and Pacini, R.: Differentiation of esophageal pain from angina pectoris: Role of the esophageal acid perfusion test. Medicine (Balt), 41:143, 1962.

Bombeck, C.T., Dillard, D.H., and Nyhus, L.M.: Muscular anatomy of the gastroesophageal junction and role of phrenoesophageal ligament. Autopsy study of sphincter mechanism. Ann. Surg., 164:643, 1966.

Botha, G.S.M.: The Gastro-oesophageal Junction. Little, Brown and Co., Boston, 1962.

Castell, D.O., and Harris, L.D.: Hormonal control of gastroesophageal sphincter strength. N. Engl. J. Med., 282:866, 1970.

Cauthorne, R.T., VanHoutte, J.J., Donner, M.W., and Hendrix, T.R.: Study of patients with lower esophageal ring by simultaneous cineradiography and manometry. Gastroenterology, 49:632, 1965.

Cohen, B.R., and Wolfe, B.S.: Roentgen localization of the physiologically determined esophageal hiatus. Gastroenterology, 43:43, 1962.

Cohen, S., and Harris, L.D.: The adaptive response of the lower esophageal sphincter. Clin. Res., 17:300, 1969.

Cohen, S., and Harris, L.D.: Does hiatus hernia affect competence of the gastroesophageal sphincter? N. Engl. J. Med., 282:866, 1970.

Delahunty, J.E., Alonso, W.A., Margulies, S.I., and Knudson, D.H.: Relationship of reflux esophagitis to pharyngeal pouch (Zenker's diverticulum) formation. Laryngoscope, 81:570, 1971.

Ellis, F.H., Jr., and Olsen, A.M.: Achalasia of the Esophagus. W.B. Saunders Co., Philadelphia., 1969.

Foster, J.H., Jolly, P.C., Sawyers, J.D., and Daniel, R.A.: Esophageal perforation: Diagnosis and treatment. Ann. surg., 161:701, 1965.

Fyke, F.E., Jr., Code, C.F., and Schlegel, J.G.: The gastroesophageal sphincter in healthy human beings. Gastroenterologia (Basel), 86:135, 1956.

Gephart, T., and Graham, R: The cellular detection of carcinoma of the esophagus. Surg. Gynecol. Obstet., 108:75, 1959.

Gryboski, J.D., Thayer, W.R., Jr., and Spiro, H.M.: Esophageal motility in infants and children. Pediatrics, 31:382, 1963.

Harris, L.D., and Pope, C.E., II: "Squeeze" vs. resistance: An evaluation of the mechanism of sphincter competence. J. Clin. Invest., 43:2272, 1964.

Hayward, J.: The lower end of the oesophagus. Thorax, 16:36, 1961.

Hiebert, C.A., and Belsey, R.: Incompetency of the gastric cardia without radiologic evidence of hiatal hernia. J. Thorac. Cardiovasc. Surg., 42:352, 1961.

Holder, T.M., and Ashcraft, D.W.: Esophageal atresia and tracheoesophageal fistula. Curr. Probl. Surg., August, 1966.

Hunt, P.S., Connell, A.M., and Smiley, T.B.: The cricopharyngeal sphincter in gastric reflux. Gut, 11:308, 1970.

Ingelfinger, F.J.: Esophageal motility. Physiol. Rev., 38:533, 1958.

Ingelfinger, F.J., and Kramer, P.: Dysphagia produced by contractile ring in lower esophagus. Gastroenterology, 23:419, 1953.

Ismail-Beigi, F., Horton, P.F., and Pope, C.E., II: Histological consequences of gastroesophageal reflux in man. Gastroenterology, 58:163, 1970.

Just-Viera, J.O., Morris, J.D., and Haight, C.: Achalasia and esophageal carcinoma. Ann. Thorac. Surg., *3*:526, 1967.

Katz, D., and Hoffman, F. (Eds.): The Esophagogastric Junction. Excerpta Medica, Amsterdam, 1971.

Mackler, S.A.: Spontaneous rupture of the esophagus, an experimental and clinical study. Surg. Gynecol. Obstet., *95*:345, 1952.

Mossberg, S.M.: The columnar lined esophagus (Barrett syndrome): An acquired condition? Gastroenterology, *50*:671, 1966.

Olsen, A.M., and Schlegel, J.F.: Motility disturbances caused by esophagitis. J. Thorac. Cardiovasc. Surg., *50*:607, 1965.

Schatzki, R.: The lower esophageal ring: Long-term followup of symptomatic and asymptomatic rings. Am. J. Roentgenol., *90*:805, 1963.

Schatzki, R., and Gary, J.E.: Dysphagia due to diaphragm-like localized narrowing in lower esophagus ("lower esophageal ring"). Am. J. Roentgenol., *70*:911, 1953.

Skinner, D.B., and Booth, D.J.: Assessment of distal esophageal function in patients with hiatal hernia and/or gastroesophageal reflux. Ann. Surg., *172*:627, 1970.

Skinner, D.B., and DeMeester, T.R.: Gastroesophageal reflux. Current Problems in Surgery, Vol. 13, 1976.

Skinner, D.B., Belsey, R.H.R., Hendrix, T.R., and Zuidema, G.D. (Eds.): Gastroesophageal Reflux and Hiatal Hernia. Little, Brown and Co. Boston, 1972.

Sutherland, H.E.: Cricopharyngeal achalasia. J. Thorac. Cardiovasc. Surg., *43*:114, 1962.

Terracol, J., and Sweet, R.H.: Diseases of the Esophagus. W.B. Saunders Co., Philadelphia, 1958, p. 247.

Wilkins, E.W., Jr., and Skinner, D.B.; recent progress in surgery of the esophagus: I. Pathophysiology and gastroesophageal reflux. II. Clinical entities. J. Surg. Res., *8*:41, 90; 1968.

Wynder, E.L., and Fryer, J.H.: Etiologic considerations of Plummer-Vinson (Paterson-Kelly) syndrome. Ann. Intern. Med., *49*:1106, November, 1958.

25

The Stomach

JOSEPH B. KIRSNER AND CHARLES S. WINANS

ANATOMIC VARIATIONS

The form and position of the stomach vary in different persons and in the same person at various times, depending on the degree of filling, the size and position of the adjacent organs, the condition of the anterior abdominal musculature, and the physical habitus. In the relatively short, obese person with a tense abdominal wall, the stomach often lies high in the left upper abdomen and is steer-horn in shape; whereas in the tall, thin person the greater curvature may extend to the brim of the true pelvis and the stomach is in the shape of the letter J. Such variations in the position of the stomach are of no clinical significance; they do not produce symptoms. The important consideration is not the location, but rather the structure and the physiologic activity of the stomach.

CONGENITAL ANOMALIES

Congenital absence of the stomach has been reported but is extremely rare.

Hypertrophic Stenosis of the Pylorus

Obstructive narrowing of the pylorus by hypertrophy of the pyloric muscle is most common in infants two or three weeks old, although it may be observed at any time between the ages of ten days and three or four months. Males are involved four times more often than females, and the condition affects first-born children more commonly. A genetic predisposition is suggested by the fact that more than one family member occasionally is affected. Indeed, hypertrophic pyloric stenosis is ten times more common among first-degree relatives of male index cases and 25 times more common among first-degree relatives of female index cases than in the general population. The condition generally is attributed to congenital hypertrophy, with or without spasm. The stenotic pylorus is represented by an oval tumor of muscular tissue approximately 3 cm. long and 1.5 cm. in diameter, with hypertrophy, especially of the circular layer of the muscularis propria, and fibrotic thickening of the submucosa. Microscopically, the hypertrophic muscular layer may be edematous and infiltrated with leukocytes. Decreased numbers of myenteric plexus ganglion cells, sometimes having an immature or degenerated appearance, have been described, suggesting that the primary defect is in the innervation of the muscle. Symptoms usually begin during the second to fourth weeks after birth, and consist of non-bilious projectile vomiting after feeding, constipation or obstipation, and rapid loss of weight. The nutritional depletion may be pronounced. Dehydration and alkalosis develop as a consequence of the loss of fluid and electrolytes in the gastric content.

Rarely, apparently primary hypertrophic pyloric stenosis becomes symptomatic only in adulthood. The congenital origin of such cases is less certain, although similar histologic patterns and the mixture of both infantile and adult-onset cases in some families support this possibility. More commonly, however, pyloric stenosis in adults is acquired in association with peptic ulcer disease of duodenum or pyloric channel, extrinsic adhesions, or infiltrative neoplasms and inflammatory disorders. In such instances there is little

798

or no true circular muscle hypertrophy and the increase in pyloric mass is due to fibrosis, inflammation, or tumor.

Diverticula

Diverticula of the stomach are infrequent, being seen once in about 2000 radiologic examinations of the upper digestive tract. Seventy-five per cent of gastric diverticula are located near the cardia, high on the posterior wall of the stomach. Such diverticula classically have been considered congenital in origin and to be "true" diverticula, possessing all coats of the stomach wall. Many, however, in reality have little or no muscular coat, suggesting the possibility that they are of the acquired, "pulsion" type. The characteristic juxtacardiac location in a weakened area where the longitudinal muscle fibers are divided and the muscular wall is formed mainly of circular and oblique fibers is consistent with this possibility. The next most common location for gastric diverticula is the prepyloric area, where about 15 per cent are found. Most of these probably are acquired as a result of gastric or extragastric disease. Some antral diverticula, especially the "partial" or intramural diverticula, are associated with ectopic pancreatic tissue, implying a congenital origin. Gastric diverticula are not more common in individuals with diverticula of other portions of the digestive tract. They do not often cause symptoms except, unusually, in the presence of inflammation or ulceration, or unless they are huge and so situated as to fill readily with food and secretions. Endoscopic examination will differentiate gastric diverticula from ulcerations or excavated tumors in those instances where radiographic studies are unclear.

Gastric Torsion and Volvulus

The stomach may rotate about its long axis so that the greater curvature turns upward or at 90° to this axis, when the pylorus turns forward to the left and cardia passes backwards. Torsion is present when the degree of rotation is less than 180° and obstruction is not complete. Some degree of rotation of the stomach is a common radiologic finding and probably of little clinical significance. Volvulus is an extension of torsion in which the degree of rotation is more than 180°, so that obstruction occurs at each end of the twisted segment. Volvulus may develop as an exacerbation of torsion or it may occur in a previously normally situated stomach. Diaphragmatic anomalies, including large paraesophageal hernias, contribute to the development of volvulus. The onset of gastric volvulus is sudden and acutely painful. The exciting cause may be a large meal, a minor injury, or a sudden movement. Pain is severe and continuous and is experienced chiefly in the epigastric and left subcostal regions. It then may radiate through to the back or remain retrosternal in site. There may be repeated attempts at vomiting but only with the emission of small amounts of mucoid material. These symptoms are accompanied by the rapid development of very severe epigastric distention. Perhaps the most important clinical observation is inability to pass a nasogastric tube to relieve the gastric distention. The triad of acute distention, frequent futile retching, and inability to pass a tube is pathognomonic of gastric volvulus.

SENSORY DISTURBANCES

Appetite and Hunger

The sensations of appetite and hunger are closely related. Appetite is a pleasant sensation, conditioned by previous agreeable experiences with the smell, taste, and appearance of food. Hunger is an unpleasant sensation of abdominal emptiness, epigastric discomfort, or pangs of dull pain produced by the intermittent contractions of the empty stomach and/or intestine and arising from the physiologic need for food. The distinction between hunger and appetite is not always sharp, and accentuation of the appetite often is interpreted as a part of the total complex of hunger. The following sensory components may be enumerated:

1. Pleasant olfactory and gustatory sensations with their associated pleasant memories of the taste and smell of food are the classic features of appetite.

2. Painful hunger pangs result from contractions of the empty stomach and intestines.

3. An indefinite, unpleasant, generalized, steady and continuous sensation is interpreted as hunger and is vaguely referred to the abdomen.

4. Accessory phenomena such as lassitude, weakness, drowsiness, faintness, irritability, restlessness, and headache may occur concomitantly.

As summarized by Janowitz:

At the physiologic level of regulation of intake, deficits of the body's stores of calorically significant nutrients activate feeding reflexes which are facilitated by areas in the lateral hypothalamus and are inhibited by the ventromedial hypothalamus. These deficits concomitantly give rise to hunger sensations which may be cues for food intake. These hypothalamic centers are sensitive to local temperature and appear to be influenced by body stores of water. Day-to-day regulation of the amount of food consumed is regulated in part by oropharyngeal receptors; and the size of an individual meal is controlled by gastric and upper intestinal receptors responding to distention, probably mediated by the vagus nerve. The hypothalamic areas also are believed to be influenced by the metabolic consequences of food absorbed and assimilated. The specific dynamic action of food, the utilizable blood glucose, the concentration of other metabolites in the blood, the level of protein in the diet and depot fat, all have been proposed as cues to the central nervous system, but none has been firmly established as governing short or long-term control.

Excessive appetite and hunger occur in various conditions, as in convalescence from an acute infectious disease, but the mechanism is unexplained. A similar situation obtains in thyrotoxicosis, in which the requirement of food is maintained at a high level because of the excessive metabolism. In diabetes mellitus the glucose in the blood is not available to the tissues; hunger and polyphagia result. Excessive appetite also may be a feature of the emotionally disturbed individual. In peptic ulcer the distress may be interpreted as hunger, because the patient fails to differentiate it from a hunger pang or because it occurs when the stomach is thought to be empty and is relieved by eating.

Anorexia is a loss of appetite or lack of desire for food. Loss of appetite is a variable but common symptom in various diseases. It is an early and prominent feature of hepatitis and of gastric or pancreatic neoplasm. Anorexia also accompanies advanced renal disease, congestive heart failure, alcoholism, thiamine deficiency and endocrine disorders such as Addison's disease and panhypopituitarism. Loss of appetite may also be a manifestation of an emotional disturbance, usually depression. As such it is the outstanding symptom of *anorexia nervosa*, a psychoneurotic state observed chiefly in adolescent girls but infrequently in males. The age of onset usually is within a year or two of the advent of puberty, but it occurs during the "teens" and occasionally in early adult life. The problem is regarded as a "self-inflicted" starvation disorder, pivoting around the maturational changes of puberty and their psychosocial implications for the patient. The clinical features include cachexia, amenorrhea, constipation, and hypothermia. Laboratory findings include hypoproteinemia, anemia, and various manifestations of abnormal endocrine function. The mortality rate is considerable, ranging from 5 to 15 per cent. The diagnosis is established principally in terms of differentiation from panhypopituitarism. Death occurs from inanition or suicide, especially when the disorder is of 10 years' duration or longer. According to H. Bruch, primary anorexia nervosa is characterized by "body-image disturbances of delusional proportion; with a distortion in the accuracy of perception or recognition of bodily states, regression of ego, and a pervading sense of ineffectiveness, conceived as the outcome of a transactional pattern between mother and child which is deficient in confirmation of child-initiated behavior." Anorexia nervosa patients have an overwhelming feeling of help-lessness and ineffectiveness in planning their lives and managing their feelings.

Vomiting

Vomiting is defined as the forceful expulsion of gastric and intestinal contents through the mouth. Immediately preceding vomiting are tachypnea, copious salivation, dilatation of the pupils, sweating, pallor, and rapid heartbeat — all signs of widespread autonomic stimulation. Vomiting begins with deep inspiration. The glottis is closed and the nasopharynx is shut off partly or completely. Inspiration is converted to an expiratory effort, with simultaneous contraction of the abdominal muscles. Because the glottis is closed, the increase in intrathoracic and intra-abdominal pressure is transmitted to the stomach and esophagus. The body of the stomach and the muscle of the esophagus relax. At the same time a strong annular contraction at approximately the angulus of the stomach nearly divides the body from the antrum. While the body of the stomach remains flaccid, peristaltic waves sweep aborally over the antrum. The positive intrathoracic and intra-abdominal pressures force expulsion of the gastric contents through the mouth. Finally the voluntary muscles relax and respiration resumes.

The vomiting center is located in the dorsolateral border of the lateral reticular formation, immediately ventral to the tractus solitarius and its nucleus, near the sensory nucleus of the vagus. It may be excited directly by mechanical stimuli, such as increased intracranial pressure; by impulses mediated by the chemoreceptor trigger zone (lying superficially in the floor of the fourth ventricle) as in emesis from motion sickness, irradiation or such emetic drugs as apomorphine, morphine and digitalis; by afferent impulses produced by distention of the stomach and duodenum; or by impulses from any region of the body. The diversity of the causes of vomiting is reflected in its association with such metabolic problems as renal failure, hyperparathyroidism, and alkalosis and in situations such as migraine and labyrinthine disorders. Vomiting may be produced in susceptible persons by impulses from the higher cerebral centers, as when unpleasant subjects are discussed or when offensive odors are encountered. The afferent impulses reach the center along many routes, the chief ones being the vagal and sympathetic nerves from the stomach and other abdominal viscera. The efferent fibers are contained chiefly in the phrenic, vagus, and sympathetic nerves.

Nausea

Nausea denotes an unpleasant sensation, ordinarily referred to the back of the throat, the epigastrium, or both, and often culminates in vomiting. It may be accompanied by vasomotor manifestations of autonomic stimulation, such as salivation, sweating, faintness, vertigo, and tachycardia. The clinical significance of nausea is identified with that of vomiting. It may be produced by gastric or pancreatic disease, by pyloric or intestinal obstruction, by emotional disturbances, unpleasant visual, olfactory or gustatory stimuli, by various biochemical abnormalities associated with metabolic disorders, or by intense pain from any source. Nausea (and anorexia) often are associated with gastric hypofunction: hypotonicity, hypoperistalsis, and hyposecretion.

Belching

Belching is the eructation of swallowed air. Normally a small amount of air is swallowed in the process of eating, with the rapid swallowing of food, the chewing of gum, or excessive smoking. Most of the swallowed air does not reach the stomach, but is regurgitated immediately from the lower esophagus as a part of the act of belching. Some of the gas passes into the stomach and accumulates in the gastric air bubble until it is eliminated in a more or less spontaneous belch. The chronic belcher then renews the cycle of swallowing more air, most of which he regurgitates with each belch, but some of which passes on into the stomach, until once more a spontaneous belch occurs. In time, the act becomes almost involuntary. Belching is not related specifically to disease of the gallbladder, stomach, or any other organ. It is primarily a functional event often induced by a sensation of abdominal fullness or discomfort, which the patient attempts to relieve by the gastroesophageal expulsion of air.

MOTOR DISTURBANCES

Physiologic Considerations

Although structurally a single organ, functionally the stomach must be viewed as having two distinct portions. Proximally, the fundus and body of the stomach serve primarily as a reservoir, increasing in volume as it fills with food and secretions in a fashion so as to maintain intragastric pressure unchanged. This process has been termed *receptive relaxation*. Distally, the antrum of the stomach subserves the process of mixing, trituration, and emptying. Contraction waves originating in the midportion of the stomach proceed peristaltically toward the pylorus, creating an "antral pump" mechanism, the efficiency of which in emptying the stomach presumably is determined not only by the frequency and strength of peristaltic contractions, but also by the dimensions of the antrum.

Electromyography of gastric muscle recently has allowed the beginning of an understanding of antral motor activity. Arising from a pacemaker high on the greater curvature, electrical *slow waves* are propagated through the longitudinal muscle layer toward the pylorus. The electrical slow wave (also termed gastric pacesetter potential) is a cyclical wave of partial depolarization and repolarization of the muscle membrane which, in humans, occurs at a frequency of three per minute. Under physiologic circumstances this frequency is extremely constant and the slow waves are generated continuously regardless of the presence or absence of muscular contractions. At times, presumably under appropriate conditions of stimulation, bursts of *fast wave* depolarizations are superimposed upon the nadir of slow wave depolarization. These depolarization spikes initiate muscular contractions which, being phase-linked to the moving slow waves, move peristaltically through the antrum.

The precise mechanisms for the control of fast wave activity, and thereby gastric peristalsis, are not known. The stomach may be viewed, however, as a pump which is constantly under varying degrees of restraint. Indeed, with the exception of gastric distention which speeds emptying, all other influences on gastric motor activity are inhibitory. Receptors within the duodenal mucosa sensitive to osmolarity, acidity, and fat content of the duodenal content initiate enterogastric nerve reflexes which inhibit gastric emptying. Additionally, secretin, cholecystokinin, enterogastrone, and perhaps other hormones liberated from the duodenum and gastrin, released from the antral mucosa, result in delay in gastric emptying. Thus, in a complex fashion gastric motor activity and emptying are the integrated result of central nerve impulses, local and central nerve reflexes, and hormonal influences acting upon the intrinsic gastric neuromuscular apparatus.

Although the muscular thickening that characterizes the pylorus strongly suggests a sphincteric function which might influence the rate of gastric emptying, such a function for the pylorus has been difficult to establish. Indeed, recent evidence suggests that the pyloric sphincter, like most other gastrointestinal tract sphincters, functions mainly to prevent retrograde flow of intestinal content. Thus, in health, the pyloric high pressure zone, as determined by intraluminal manometry, is increased by the presence of acid or fat within the duodenum, presumably by the action of endogenously released secretin and cholecystokinin. If marker substances such as phenol red are infused into the duodenum together with acid, a markedly reduced recovery of the marker from the stomach accompanies the increased pyloric sphincter pressure, suggesting that pyloric contraction indeed abolishes duodenogastric reflux. Gastrin antagonizes the effect of the duodenal hormones on the pyloric sphincter. Failure of secretin and cholecystokinin to augment pyloric sphincter pressure in gastric ulcer patients has been suggested as an important pathophysiologic defect in that disorder.

Pathophysiologic States

When vagotomy is performed therapeutically to reduce gastric acid secretion, gastric tonus also is reduced, the peristaltic waves are shallower, and gastric emptying is delayed. With the passage of time, there is more or less recovery, attributable perhaps to control regained by the intrinsic gastric neurogenic mechanism. Gastric peristalsis also may be decreased in patients with diabetes mellitus, presumably due to autonomic neuropathy, as well as in progressive systemic sclerosis where the gastric musculature is atrophic. Studies indicate that the rate of gastric emptying is increased in patients with uncomplicated duodenal ulcer and is reduced in those individuals with gastric ulcer, functional changes which may be important in the pathophysiology of peptic ulcer disease.

Spasm of the entire stomach or of a portion of the stomach has been described in lesions of the central nervous system and also in the presence of cholelithiasis or pancreatic disease. The relationship of such spasm to abdominal pain is questionable. Painful gastric spasms are noted occasionally in the apparently normal stomach. Localized muscular spasm occurs not infrequently with gastric lesions, as in hourglass contracture with a benign ulcer, the contracture disappearing when the ulcer heals. Contraction of the stomach along the greater curvature also has been observed in emotionally disturbed patients who ruminate. The incisura-type indentation is presumably spastic in nature but it is not accompanied by pain. Painless spasm of the pylorus, as evidenced by rather persistent closure, occurs with intrapyloric peptic ulcer, with gastric and duodenal lesions adjacent to the pylorus, and occasionally with gastric ulcers located proximal to the pylorus on the lesser curvature.

GASTRIC SECRETION

PHYSIOLOGIC CONSIDERATIONS

The secretion of hydrochloric acid physiologically is a composite of three interrelated phases: neurogenic (vagal), gastric (gastrin), and, to an extent less well understood, intestinal. The neurogenic phase is initiated by stimuli such as the sight, smell, or taste of food acting upon receptors in the cerebral cortex and the subsequent stimulation of the vagal nucleus. The process presumably is mediated chemically by acetylcholine

from postganglionic parasympathetic nerve endings acting upon gastric parietal cells. Vagal excitation also releases gastrin from the antrum and sensitizes the parietal cells to stimulation by gastrin. Chief cell secretion is also augmented by vagus nerve stimulation, which elicits a copious secretion of gastric juice rich in acid and pepsin. Truncal division of the vagi is followed by a pronounced reduction in the volume and acidity of the gastric secretion in all patients but which is quantitatively most impressive in hypersecreting duodenal ulcer patients. The production of hydrochloric acid, however, is not eliminated completely by vagotomy and remains demonstrable with sufficient stimulation of the secretory mechanism. Stimulation of the splanchnic nerves evokes an alkaline secretion, chiefly from the pyloric glands, rich in mucus and poor in peptic activity. Emotional disturbances exert an important influence upon the secretory and motor functions of the stomach. Prolonged anxiety, hostility, and resentment can cause engorgement of the gastric mucosa and increased secretion, whereas depression and fear induce pallor of the mucosa and a reduction in acid output. These changes are related, respectively, to increased and decreased rates of blood flow through the gastric vasculature.

The gastric phase of secretion is mediated by the hormone gastrin, released from the antrum in response to distention by food and fluid, by vagal stimulation, and by exposure of the mucosa of the antrum to the products of protein digestion. Release of gastrin by these stimuli is reduced or eliminated when the antral mucosa is exposed to a low pH. Multiple molecular species of gastrin now have been identified (Fig. 25-1). First to be described was the heptadecapeptide (G-17), which exists in two forms (I and II) depending on the absence or presence of an esterified SO_3H attached to the tyrosine in position 12. Both terminals are blocked, the N-terminal with pyroglutamyl and the C-terminal with an amide. The C-terminal four amino acids of the gastrin molecule (TRY-MET-ASP-PHE-NH$_2$) possess the full physiologic range of actions of the parent molecule. This material, with 4-butyloxycarbonyl-beta-alanine attached to the N-terminus, now is available commercially as the gastrin-like pentapeptide, pentagastrin. It is noteworthy that cholecystokinin, which shares many physiologic actions with gastrin, possesses five C-terminal amino acids in common with gastrin.

The other major circulating form of gastrin is "big gastrin" or G-34. Amino acid sequencing indicates it to have 34 amino acids, the C-terminal heptadecapeptide sequence of which is identical with that of G-17. Like G-17, G-34 exists in sulfated and non-sulfated forms. An even larger gastrin molecule ("big-big gastrin"), the amino acid sequence of which has not yet been identified, and

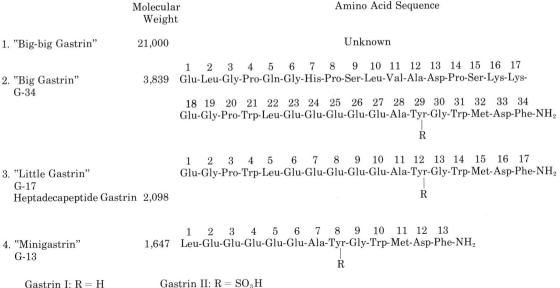

	Molecular Weight	Amino Acid Sequence

1. "Big-big Gastrin"   21,000   Unknown

2. "Big Gastrin"   3,839
   G-34

```
  1   2   3   4   5   6   7   8   9  10  11  12  13  14  15  16  17
Glu-Leu-Gly-Pro-Gln-Gly-His-Pro-Ser-Leu-Val-Ala-Asp-Pro-Ser-Lys-Lys-

 18  19  20  21  22  23  24  25  26  27  28  29  30  31  32  33  34
Glu-Gly-Pro-Trp-Leu-Glu-Glu-Glu-Glu-Glu-Ala-Tyr-Gly-Trp-Met-Asp-Phe-NH₂
                                            |
                                            R
```

3. "Little Gastrin"
   G-17
   Heptadecapeptide Gastrin 2,098

```
  1   2   3   4   5   6   7   8   9  10  11  12  13  14  15  16  17
Glu-Gly-Pro-Trp-Leu-Glu-Glu-Glu-Glu-Glu-Ala-Tyr-Gly-Trp-Met-Asp-Phe-NH₂
                                            |
                                            R
```

4. "Minigastrin"   1,647
   G-13

```
  1   2   3   4   5   6   7   8   9  10  11  12  13
Leu-Glu-Glu-Glu-Glu-Glu-Ala-Tyr-Gly-Trp-Met-Asp-Phe-NH₂
                          |
                          R
```

Gastrin I: R = H   Gastrin II: R = SO₃H

Figure 25–1   The molecular species of gastrin.

a smaller tridecapeptide gastrin ("minigastrin," G-13) have been isolated by chromatographic techniques. G-17 has a greater molar potency for acid secretion, but a shorter half-life in serum than G-34. As the immunologic methods commonly employed for the quantitation of gastrin in serum specimens do not distinguish between these two major molecular forms, little information is yet available concerning potentially important differences between the relative proportions of serum G-17 and G-34 in health and disease.

Gastrin exerts a wide spectrum of motor and secretory actions involving multiple target organs. These include strong stimulation of acid gastric secretion from parietal cells, weak to moderate stimulation of pepsin secretion, increased gastric intrinsic factor secretion, increased blood flow in the stomach, stimulation of gastric motor activity, and a trophic action upon the gastric fundal mucosa. Gastrin also has important extragastric actions. Thus, it stimulates water and electrolyte secretion by the pancreas, liver, and small intestine and enzyme secretion by the pancreas. Gastrin stimulates release of insulin and calcitonin, and stimulates smooth muscle contraction in the lower esophageal sphincter, small intestine, colon, and gallbladder. Absorption of glucose, electrolytes, and water by the small intestine is inhibited by gastrin, as is contraction of smooth muscle of the pyloric sphincter, ileocecal sphincter, and the sphincter of Oddi.

By use of fluoresceinated antibodies to human gastrin I, gastrin has been localized in greatest concentration within special mucosal cells in the gastric antrum. These cells, termed "G-cells," are most abundant in the midportion of the pyloric glands. They have a flasklike shape with a broad base and narrow apex which extends to the mucosal surface. Electron microscopy reveals characteristic secretory granules 150 to 250 nm. in diameter within the G-cells as well as microvilli at the mucosal surface that may contain receptors for inhibition and stimulation of the G-cells by stomach contents. Gastrin also can be extracted from the mucosa of the proximal duodenum. Indeed, although its concentration here is much less than that in the antrum, because of the larger mass of duodenal mucosa, the duodenum contains nearly as much gastrin as the antrum. Tiny amounts of gastrin also have been found by some investigators in the delta cells of the pancreas. The identity of the G cells, the factors which control their proliferation, and their possible relationship to the pancreatic delta cells remain to be determined.

Radioimmunoassay techniques for the measurement of serum gastrin content indicate normal fasting levels to be from 20 to 200 pg. per ml. It must be recognized, however, that the gastrin antibodies used in this measurement detect not only G-17 but also other of the various molecular subtypes of gastrin, in some cases with varying affinities. It is possible, therefore, that specimens containing the same measured level of "gastrin" may differ markedly in gastrin sub-type composition. Although potentially important, the actual significance of such gastrin heterogeneity is uncertain. The fasting serum gastrin concentration of duodenal ulcer patients in the majority of studies has not differed significantly from that of normal controls, whereas the fasting serum gastrin of gastric ulcer patients usually is moderately elevated. In general, there has been recognized an inverse relationship between gastric acid outputs and serum gastrin, although this relationship appears to pertain only to subjects with relatively low levels of maximal gastric acid output below 10 mEq. per hour. The higher serum gastrin levels in patients with low levels of acid secretion presumably reflect the absence of inhibition of antral gastrin release by acid antral content in the hyposecretors. Elevation of serum gastrin, often to levels in excess of 1000 pg. per ml., is seen in certain clinical situations. The hypergastrinemia of the Zollinger-Ellison syndrome arises not from the antral G cells but from the hyperfunctioning, gastrin-secreting pancreatic tumor cells. In contrast, in the other diseases where hypergastrinemia is associated with acid hypersecretion the gastrin arises from the antrum itself. For example, in a few duodenal ulcer patients, study of antral mucosal biopsy tissue with fluoresceinated antibody to gastrin has revealed a marked increase in the number of antral G cells, a condition termed antral G-cell hyperplasia. The cause of this hyperplasia remains obscure, but marked elevation of serum gastrin is seen following a protein meal. Rarely, surgical error will leave a portion of the antrum attached to the afferent duodenal loop when partial gastrectomy with Billroth II gastroenterostomy is performed. Distention of the retained antrum with highly alkaline biliary and pancreatic secretions will lead to hypergastrinemia. These latter two conditions can be distinguished from the Zollinger-Ellison syndrome by the fact that antral gastrin release is inhibited following the intravenous injection of secretin, resulting in a fall in serum gastrin, whereas gastrin release from gastrin-secreting pancreatic tumors is augmented by secretin. Hypergastrinemia without acid hypersecretion is seen in pernicious anemia and atrophic gastritis. About one third of pernicious anemia patients develop hypergastrinemia in the range characteristic of the Zollinger-Ellison syndrome, apparently because chronic achlorhydria leads to hyperplasia of the antral G cells. Increased serum gastrin levels also are demonstrable in atrophic gastritis associated with antibodies to parietal cells but with adequate absorption of vitamin B_{12}, but not in simple atrophic gastritis without parietal cell antibodies. Hypergastrinemia thus may be characteristic only of gastritis associated with autoimmune reactions to gastric antigens. Simple atrophic gastritis appears to be a different disease and the non-elevated serum gastrin levels may reflect disease of the antral mucosa with loss of G-cells, whereas "autoimmune gastritis" selectively affects the parietal cell bearing mucosa, and the antral mucosa is spared. Anephric patients, those with advanced renal failure, and patients with extensive resection of small intestine may demonstrate gastric hypersecretion or hypergastrinemia or both. As the kidneys and small intestine are both active sites of gastrin removal, the hypergastrinemia in these conditions results from delay in gastrin metabolism. Hypergastrinemia is sometimes seen in hyperparathyroidism, particularly when a gastrinoma is present, as in the multiple endocrine adenoma, type I, syndrome. In this instance, the elevated level of serum calcium appears to stimulate gastrin release. Epinephrine-induced gastrin release presumably is the mechanism for the hypergastrinemia observed with pheochromocytoma.

In addition to acetylcholine and gastrin, it has been known for more than 50 years that histamine elicits from parietal cells a large amount of hydrochloric acid secretion. Paradoxically, the conventional antihistamine drugs (now termed H_1-receptor antagonists), although capable of blocking many of the actions of histamine on smooth muscle and vascular permeability, are ineffective in reducing gastric acid secretion. Recently, however, it has been determined that the parietal cell possesses a special H_2-receptor and that blocking this receptor with a specific antagonist markedly reduces parietal cell acid secretion as stimulated by all known stimulants of human gastric acid secretion. It is not yet certain whether histamine is the final common mediator of acid secretion elicited by other stimulants such as gastrin and acetylcholine or if the parietal cell possesses receptors for multiple agonists. It is currently believed most likely, however, that receptors for gastrin and acetylcholine as well as histamine exist, but that blocking one receptor type modifies the interaction between the other receptors and their agonists in a way which makes the parietal cell less responsive to all stimulants. Various congeners of histamine show preferential stimulation of the H_1 or H_2 type of receptor. Thus betazole, an isomer of histamine, has preferential effects on gastric secretion and has been used clinically as a stimulant of gastric acid secretion when it is desired to test the maximal acid secreting capacity of a patient's stomach. Most recently, however, pentagastrin has become the stimulant of choice for use in gastric analysis. The gastric acid hypersecretion sometimes seen in patients with systemic mast cell disease is associated with hyperhistaminemia. Similarly, the gastric hypersecretion seen following portacaval anastomosis involves the effect of a secretory stimulant, produced in the alimentary canal and not inactivated within the liver as a consequence of the shunt. High levels of blood histamine, in fact, have been reported in one such patient with intractable peptic ulcer disease.

The physiologic activity of the gastric chief and parietal cells appears to depend also upon adequate circulating quantities of pituitary, adrenal, thyroid and parathyroid hormones. In their insufficiency or absence, gastric secretory activity is greatly diminished. The growth of the gastric mucosa probably depends upon growth hormone from the pituitary gland and a normal pituitary gland is essential to the structural integrity of the gastric mucosa and to the normal secretory function.

The third or intestinal phase of gastric secretion begins with the entrance of partly acidified or neutralized food into the small intestine, initiating a humoral mechanism, with the release of gastrin and other hormones. The resting serum gastrin concentration of partial gastrectomy patients with Billroth I gastroduodenostomies is about half that of unoperated duodenal ulcer patients, presumably owing to the loss of antral gastrin. Following an oral homogenized beef meal, a slow rise in serum gastrin occurs in Billroth I patients, with peak values at about two hours — strikingly later than the peak serum gastrin in normal subjects, which is seen between 30 and 45 minutes after the meal — suggesting that the rise in serum gastrin in the former group is of small intestinal origin. If the beef meal is instilled directly into the duodenum, the rise in serum gastrin is identical in magnitude and duration in both Billroth I and normal subjects. When serum gastrin and gastric acid secretion are measured simultaneously following intraduodenal administration of the test meal to duodenal ulcer patients, a significant rise in acid output with peak secretion coinciding with peak gastrin level occurs, suggesting that intestinal gastrin release may be of physiologic significance. In addition to gastrin, there may be other intestinal mechanisms for stimulation of gastric acid secretion and there are also a number of hormonal and neural intestinal mechanisms for the inhibition of acid secretion, making the intestinal phase of gastric secretion quite complex.

Gastric secretion may be inhibited under various circumstances, such as emotional disturbances, presumably via inhibitory fibers in the vagus and splanchnic nerves. Gastric secretion also is influenced by at least two major autoregulatory mechanisms. All stimulants for gastrin release are inhibited by acid in contact with the antral mucosa, presumably by a direct effect on the G cell. A pH of about 1.0 produces maximal suppression, with lesser degrees of inhibition resulting from the presence of less acid gastric content. Additionally, the presence of acid or fat in the upper small intestine releases inhibitory hormones, termed enterogastrones, which inhibit both the release of gastrin from the G cells and the action of gastrin upon the acid-secreting parietal cells. Two hormones best known to be liberated under these circumstances are secretin and cholecystokinin, both of which are capable of inhibiting gastrin-stimulated acid secretion. Other peptide hormones, including glucagon, vasoactive intestinal peptide, gastric inhibitory peptide, and calcitonin, similarly inhibit the action of gastrin, although their possible physiologic significance in the inhibition of acid secretion has not been determined. A depressant of gastric secretion, gastrone, has been identified in the mucous secretion of the stomach, particularly in patients with achlorhydria. Its physiologic role, if any, is undetermined.

The volume of gastric juice secreted under fasting conditions in the average normal adult ranges from 1000 to 1500 ml. per day. The principal components of this gastric secretion are hydrochloric acid; various mucosubstances (acid amino polysaccharides, fucomucins, sialomucins); proteolytic enzymes, including at least seven pepsins; rennin, cathepsins, gastric intrinsic factor, water-soluble blood group substances and other biologically active materials; nonproteolytic enzymes; the anions chloride, phosphate, and sulfate; and the cations sodium, potassium, calcium, and magnesium. The alkaline component of gastric secretion is a mixture of various constituents, including mucus from the surface mucous cells, cytoplasm of desquamated cells, and a transudate of interstitial fluid. The known sources of various gastric secretory products are listed in Figure 25-2.

Pepsin is the major proteolytic enzyme found in human gastric juice. It is synthesized and stored within the chief cells of the oxyntic gland area in an inactive form, pepsinogen. Following secretion into the gastric lumen it is converted autocatalytically in the presence of acid to pepsin by the

Cells	Products
Fundic gland area:	
Parietal	acid, intrinsic factor
Chief	Group I and II pepsinogens
Mucous	Group I and II pepsinogens, mucus
Argentaffin	Serotonin, histamine
Antral gland area:	
Mucous	Mucus
Gastrin (G)	Gastrin
Pyloric gland mucous	Group II pepsinogens, mucus

Figure 25-2 Gastric cells and their secretory products (after Isenberg, 1975).

cleavage of several small basic peptides. In general, pepsinogen secretion is stimulated by the same factors that augment gastric acid secretion, with the exception that secretin, which inhibits acid secretion, is a strong stimulant of pepsinogen. Immunochemical studies of pepsinogen have revealed that there are, in fact, at least seven electrophoretically distinct pepsinogens which can be divided immunologically into two unrelated groups. Group I includes pepsinogens 1-5, which are limited to the oxyntic gland mucosa where they are identified by immunofluorescent studies within the chief and mucous neck cells. Group II pepsinogens 6 and 7 are found in the fundal (oxyntic), pyloric, and duodenal mucosa. Whether quantitative or qualitative differences in pepsinogen secretion are seen in disease states remains to be determined, although the relative proportions of the different pepsinogens in human gastric mucosa apparently vary from person to person.

Hydrochloric acid is secreted by the parietal cell, found in the oxyntic gland mucosa just below the mucous neck area. Parietal cells are pyramidal in shape, with the apex extending toward the lumen of the gland and the broader base placed against the basement membrane of the glands. Electron microscopy demonstrates numerous intracellular mitochondria, an extensive secretory canalicular system lined with microvilli, and numerous tubulovesicular structures. With secretory stimulation, the tubulovesicles are transformed into a microvillus membrane, resulting in a marked increase in the area of the parietal cell's secretory surface. The peak acid output following maximal acid stimulation is directly related to the total number of parietal cells which, in adult human males, averages about one billion cells. The parietal cell mass in duodenal ulcer patients is 1.5 to 2 times greater. Whereas the trophic effect of chronic hypergastrinemia may explain the parietal cell hyperplasia in the Zollinger-Ellison syndrome, the cause of the increased parietal cell mass in duodenal ulcer patients is not known.

The biochemical events leading to acid secretion are not fully understood. There is some evidence, however, to suggest that acetylcholine, histamine, or gastrin acts upon cell membrane receptors to stimulate guanylate cyclase, resulting in the production of cyclic GMP which, in turn, stimulates intracellular activity. The hydrogen ion presumably results from the hydrolysis of water in the presence of carbonic anhydrase. The hydroxyl reacts with carbon dioxide, producing bicarbonate which leaves the basal portion of the cell. The resulting increase in venous pH has been termed the "alkaline tide." The hydrogen ions are secreted into the secretory canaliculi in a process involving at least two types of ATPases. The secretion of the parietal cell contains hydrochloric acid in an initial acid concentration of 160 to 170 mEq. per liter, has a pH of slightly less than 1.0, and is isosmotic or slightly hyperosmotic in relation to the blood. Because gastric juice is a mixture of both parietal and non-parietal secretions, the actual hydrogen ion concentration of gastric juice is much lower, averaging about 40 mEq. per liter in fasting normal humans. Variations in the acid concentration of gastric juice presumably are due to changes in the ratio of the acid and non-acid components (Hollander's 2-component hypothesis).

DISTURBANCES IN GASTRIC SECRETION

Pathologic alterations in gastric secretion involve changes in total volume, acid concentration, or both. Consequently gastric acid secretion is most commonly expressed as acid output (mEq. per unit time), the product of volume and concentration (see Table 25-1). Variations in acid output do not correspond exactly with anatomic changes in the mucosa, although true anacidity occurs most frequently in association with atrophy of the stomach. Normal persons with apparently normal mucosa exhibit a wide variety of secretory responses, ranging from achlorhydria with a pH of approximately 8.0 to a highly acid juice with a pH of 1.0. These differing secretory rates are not correlated with specific symptoms or dis-

TABLE 25–1 REPRESENTATIVE OUTPUTS OF HYDROCHLORIC ACID IN DIFFERENT CLINICAL STATES

	Basal (mEq./hr.)	Maximal after Histamine or Pentagastrin Stimulation (mEq./hr.)	Nocturnal (mEq./12 hrs.)
Normal	2–3	16–20	18
Gastric Ulcer	2–4	16–20	8
Duodenal Ulcer	4–10	25–40	60
Zollinger-Ellison Syndrome	30	45	120

ease, except that chronic peptic ulcer does not occur in the continued absence of acid gastric juice. The complete absence of all gastric juice (achylia gastrica) is rare, for some secretion containing enzymes in small amounts is almost always present. The terms "achlorhydria" and "anacidity" therefore may be preferable. Anacidity may be defined as a decrease in pH of gastric content of less than one unit or a pH above 6.0 following maximal stimulation of the gastric secretory mechanism with histamine, betazole, or pentagastrin. The pH of the gastric secretion in pernicious anemia usually ranges between 7.0 and 8.0; the pH in atrophy of the gastric mucosa unaccompanied by other disease is similar, although more variable; values between 3.5 and 7.0 may be observed in gastric carcinoma. Anacidity is not a normal variant, since it is associated with an almost total loss of functioning parietal cells, as in severe gastric atrophy. The gastric content in "true" gastric atrophy is characterized by progressive secretory failure involving initially hydrochloric acid, then pepsin, and, finally, intrinsic factor. Maximal stimulation tests indicate that anacidity occurs in no more than 20 per cent of patients with gastric carcinoma and with gastric polyps. Patients with true anacidity who do not have pernicious anemia require careful observation for the later development of pernicious anemia or gastric carcinoma. In gastric carcinoma the stomach content is characterized by reduced acid secretion and by elevation of certain enzyme constituents, including beta glucuronidase, lactic dehydrogenase, glutamic oxaloacetic transaminase, and phosphohexose isomerase. Whether these alterations precede as a reflection of a vulnerable mucosa or accompany the neoplasm remains unclear. Histologic studies indicate that the number of parietal cells in the fundus of the stomach is relatively high in patients with duodenal ulcer and decreases progressively in benign gastric ulcer and in gastric cancer, especially in patients without acid; parietal cells are virtually absent in pernicious anemia.

The clinical conditions associated with gastric hypersecretion are duodenal ulcer, stomal ulceration after partial gastrectomy, the Zollinger-Ellison syndrome, antral G-cell hyperplasia and the retained-excluded antrum after gastric surgery. An excessive output of hydrochloric acid is observed in approximately 50 per cent of patients with duodenal ulcer. In such instances the basal acid output as well as the acid output after maximum stimulation is elevated, although the ratio of basal to maximal acid output is less than 0.4. In contrast, the Zollinger-Ellison syndrome is characterized by extremely high basal outputs of hydrochloric acid in response to continuous stimulation by hypergastrinemia. The rise in acid output following administration of exogenous stimulants, therefore, is relatively small, and the ratio of basal to maximal acid output usually exceeds 0.6. The mechanism for the gastric hypersecretion which characterizes patients with duodenal ulcer has been the subject of intense scientific investigation during the past decade.

MECHANISM OF PAIN

The normal gastric mucosa is insensitive to touch, cutting, pinching, tearing, and exposure to solutions of varying hydrogen ion concentration. Heat and cold are experienced as such. Vigorous pressure on the gastric wall elicits a steady, dull, gnawing pain, experienced approximately in the region of the stimulus. This pain, like that produced by distention or by powerful contractions, arises from stretching of the muscular and peritoneal layers of the stomach. Its mechanism involves a local rise in smooth muscle tension produced by spasm, obstruction or rapid distention, and subsequent contraction or stretching of the nerve terminals lying between the circular muscle fibers. The intensity of the distress is proportional to the state of contraction of the stomach at the time and to the rapidity of the stimulus. The entire reflex involved in the transmission of such impulses may be via the afferent visceral fibers accompanying the sympathetic pathways; the cerebrospinal nerves need not participate. The threshold for pain in the stomach and, therefore, for the development of symptoms is influenced by the condition of the gastric mucosa at the time. Vascular engorgement and acute inflammation diminish the threshold for pain, and in their presence stimuli such as hydrochloric acid or gastric contractions not causing discomfort when the mucosa is normal elicit painful sensations. Vascular ischemia causes pain presumably by altering the motor activity of the stomach. The stomach is in proximity to numerous other organs with differing nerve supplies; their involvement contributes additional components to the symptomatology of gastric disease.

The pain of peptic ulcer is caused primarily by the hydrochloric acid in the gastric content. The acid evokes a chemical inflammation and thereby lowers the pain threshold of the nerve endings present in the base and in the edges of the ulcer. The pain is a true visceral sensation, arising directly at the site of the lesion. It is not dependent on hyperperistalsis, gross spasm of the musculature, pylorospasm, or distention of the antrum. However, the acid may activate not only the pain mechanism but also gastric motor activity; under these circumstances, ulcer pain originating in a sensitive ulcer may be increased by motility or muscle spasm. The importance of acid in the development of ulcer pain is further indicated by the occurrence of the distress only when the gastric content is acid. The concentration of hydrochloric acid at the time of distress is not necessarily excessive, nor does it exceed that present in the same stomach without pain when the ulcer is healed or in the healing phase. The threshold of acidity necessary to evoke pain varies from one patient to another and in the same patient from time to time. The presence of pain is dependent, therefore, on the presence of both an inflamed lesion lowering the pain threshold and an adequate stimulus, acid gastric juice. The pain is relieved by emesis or aspiration of the stomach, which removes the acid, or by the ingestion of food or alkali, which neutralizes hydrochloric acid. When the pain mechanism is sensitive, pain may be induced by the introduction of hydrochloric acid in physiologic concentrations (0.1N.) or by acid gastric juice; it is alleviated by withdrawal or neutralization of the acid. The pain induced by the hydrochloric acid is not prevented by prior parenteral or oral administration of anticholinergic compounds. Pain sensitivity disappears quickly with treatment, presumably as the acute inflammatory process in the ulcer subsides and long before appreciable healing of the ulcer could occur. Furthermore, gastroscopic studies demonstrate that many peptic ulcers occur in the absence of symptoms. In at least a quarter of patients whose ulcers are complicated by hemorrhage or perforation, no history of antecedent ulcer pain can be elicited. The absence of pain in these instances is difficult to explain, except on the vague basis of an individually high pain threshold, protection of the ulcer crater from the hydrochloric acid by blood during the course of hemorrhage, and the very rapid formation of an acute perforating ulcer encompassing development and penetration into a blood vessel within hours.

Location of Pain

The pain of peptic ulcer is almost always located in the epigastrium and usually is limited to an area several centimeters in diameter. With gastric ulcer, pain is most likely to be experienced in the midline high in the epigastrium below the xiphoid process, or sometimes to the left of the midline. When the ulcer is in the upper portion of the stomach, pain occasionally will be perceived in the anterior or left lateral portion of the chest. Such shifts of pain usually occur with progressive deepening of the ulcer. So long as gastric ulcers remain shallow and do not actively penetrate or perforate, the distress usually is indistinguishable from that of duodenal ulcer. In duodenal ulcer, the pain ordinarily is located in the midepigastrium or slightly to the right of the midline. In jejunal ulcer, it is located in a periumbilical loca-

tion, but may be in the left midabdomen and also in the left lower abdominal quadrant. The pain may be referred laterally to the left chest in the area supplied by the sixth and seventh thoracic nerves or may extend through to the back at the level of the eighth to tenth dorsal vertebrae. This latter radiation is more common in duodenal ulcer located on the posterior wall of the duodenum. Sudden, severe abdominal pain frequently indicates an acute perforation. Perforation of an ulcer on the posterior wall of the duodenum causes pain in the location characteristic of pancreatic pain, i.e., in the region between the twelfth thoracic and second lumbar vertebrae. The pain is characteristic in its occurrence at night, aggravation by the supine position, partial relief by sitting or by lying with the trunk flexed, or by pressure over the midabdomen while the patient leans forward over folded arms or a pillow. Perforation of an ulcer on the anterior wall of the duodenum may cause pain in the right lower abdominal quadrant, where the lesion may be confused with acute appendicitis, or it may produce pain in the right groin or testis, simulating right ureteral pain. Its distribution also depends partly on the course taken by the escaping gastric contents. Gravitation of the contents to the right paracolic gutter produces pain in the right lower abdominal quadrant. Pain in front, behind, or on top of the shoulder and at the base of the neck denotes involvement of the diaphragm and irritation of the phrenic innervation. When an ulcer on the lesser curvature of the stomach perforates into the lesser omental tissues, lesser omental sac, undersurface of the liver, anterior aspect of the pancreas, or the diaphragmatic crura, there may develop an upward and left shift of pain into the anterior part of the thorax and left hypochondrium, and a referred or somatic pain often is present in the interscapular region, usually at about the level of the sixth thoracic vertebra. If pain is transmitted to the left shoulder cap, the lesion usually is located high in the stomach. If perforation occurs into the peritoneal aspect of the pancreas and into the anterior surface of the pancreas, the pain usually is at the umbilical level anteriorly and at the level of the twelfth thoracic vertebra to the second lumbar vertebra posteriorly.

Pain in Gastric Carcinoma

The pain originating from gastric carcinoma may be of several types. In the presence of hydrochloric acid, the pain often is undistinguishable from that produced by benign peptic ulcer, because the mechanism is the same: acid irritation. An ulcerating carcinoma perforating the greater curvature may simulate a benign ulcer and also may cause pain in the left shoulder cap, pancreatic pain, and pain in the left lower abdominal quadrant, secondary to involvement of the left transverse mesocolon, perisplenitis, and parietal involvement of peritoneum in the eleventh or twelfth thoracic segment. In the absence of acid and peptic activity, gastric cancer is painless until the tumor progresses beyond the confines of the stomach and involves somatic tissue. The pain then becomes constant, is unrelated to the nature of the gastric content, and is relieved only by opiates. This pain is attributable to malignant infiltration of both the somatic and splanchnic nerves. Benign gastric tumors, e.g., polyps and leiomyomas, do not produce pain unless they obstruct the pylorus or the cardioesophageal orifice.

Transmission of Pain

At least three distinct mechanisms may be involved in pain originating within the abdomen: true visceral pain with impulses transmitted over afferent visceral fibers accompanying the sympathetic trunks; referred pain, with impulses carried over both afferent visceral and cerebrospinal nerve fibers; and the peritoneocutaneous reflex of Morley, with impulses transmitted only via cerebrospinal nerves. True visceral pain alone may be present, or all three mechanisms may participate, as in the perforation of peptic ulcer with peritonitis.

Pain impulses arising in the stomach and duodenum are conducted along sensory fibers in the splanchnic branches of the sympathetic nerves. The splanchnic nerves enter first the celiac ganglion, travel via the greater splanchnic nerves to the spinal cord, probably to the corresponding posterior roots of the eighth through thirteenth thoracic spinal nerves, and thence to the higher centers by way of the spinal thalamic tract. The parasympathetic supply of the stomach and duodenum arises in the dorsal vagal nucleus in the floor of the fourth ventricle, and the afferent fibers end in the same nucleus, which is a mixture of visceral efferent and afferent cells. The fibers are conveyed to and from the abdomen through the vagus nerves, esophageal plexus, and vagal trunks. The reproduction of ulcer pain after complete section of the vagi by introducing hydrochloric acid into the stomach of a patient with a sensitive ulcer demonstrates that pain impulses travel via the splanchnics. The skin area to which visceral pain is referred is determined by the segment of the cord receiving the visceral afferent (sympathetic) fibers. Ulcer distress arising from lesions not penetrating to the serosa has a cutaneous reference, indicating that visceral nerves are capable of mediating pain referred to somatic segments.

GASTRITIS

In health, the mucosa of the gastric fundus and body consists of the gastric pits or foveolae, comprising the superficial 25 per cent of mucosal thickness, and the deeper, glandular portion forming the remaining 75 per cent. The surface and pits are lined by columnar mucus-producing cells which originate at the base of the pits and eventually are extruded into the gastric lumen after migrating upward along the epithelial basement membrane. These surface mucous cells have a relatively rapid turnover time of about four to six days. Into each pit enter three to seven gastric glands, which are more or less straight tubular structures extending downward to the muscularis mucosa. In the superficial portions of the glands are found the parietal cells, while the chief cells are located predominantly in the deeper portions of the glands. A lamina propria extends throughout the mucosa and contains capillaries, collagenous fibers, and cellular elements, predominantly mononuclear cells. An absolutely normal mucosa is found only during infancy or in the first decade of life. Subsequently, there is a progressive interstitial infiltration with lymphocytes, plasma cells, and eosinophils sometimes accompanied by metaplasia of the glandular epithelium in virtually every adult stomach. These changes, which probably reflect local inflammatory and possibly immunologic influences, are descriptively termed "gastritis."

The diagnosis of gastritis is based most satisfactorily on the objective histologic criteria outlined below. Indeed, much confusion has arisen in the medical literature about the diagnosis and classification of gastritis based on gross endoscopic appearance. Even worse, the term "gastritis" also has been used loosely to describe vague dyspeptic symptoms of uncertain cause with the implication that these symptoms are attributable to gastric mucosal inflammation. Such an implication often is without foundation and many times cannot be verified objectively in patients with such non-specific complaints. Indeed, the majority of patients whose gastric mucosal biopsies evidence objective changes of gastritis are asymptomatic or suffer from gastrointestinal hemorrhage.

Acute gastritis is said to be present when histologic examination of the gastric mucosa reveals a patchy, superficial, local cell necrosis, often with small areas of cellular exfoliation. Associated features include vascular congestion, sometimes with extravasation of blood into the lamina propria, acute inflammatory cell infiltration, and edema. The changes are generally superficial and the deeper layers of the mucosa are not involved. Although the mucosal appearance may be normal endoscopically, frequently the endoscopist notes erythema, petechial or confluent intramucosal hemorrhage, multiple small erosions or acute ulcerations, and increased amounts of surface mucus. Some special terms, for instance acute hemorrhagic gastritis and acute erosive gastritis, are occasionally used when one or another of the above pathologic features is especially prominent. All of the changes, however, presumably represent the acute mucosal reaction to a wide variety of endogenous or exogenous injurious factors. Examples of such agents include alcohol, salicylates and a variety of other medications, bile acids, bacterial and fungal infections, and metabolic states such as uremia. Again, descriptive terms such as "acute alcoholic gastritis," "caustic gastritis," and "phlegmonous gastritis" are sometimes used to emphasize a presumed etiology.

Current concepts suggest that most causes of acute gastritis have in common the breakdown of the gastric mucosal barrier. In health, gastric acid secreted into the lumen of the stomach stays there, and very little diffuses back through the mucosal surface cells, which are protected by their lipid-protein surface membrane and tight intercellular junctions, and, perhaps, by the thin surface layer of gastric mucin. According to Davenport, hydrogen ion diffuses rapidly back into the mucosa when this barrier is broken. There it releases histamine from mast cells, which stimulates additional acid secretion and causes dilatation of mucosal capillaries with an increase in their permeability. There ensues transudation of plasma and red cells into the interstitial spaces, producing edema and increased interstitial pressure. The interstitial fluid containing electrolytes, proteins, and glucose is filtered across the mucosal surface and, as modified by the filtration process, enters the gastric lumen. The back-diffusion of hydrogen ions may also cause rapid release of vasoactive substances, including, in addition to histamine, serotonin, kinins, and other products of cellular injury.

Among agents which may potentially injure the mucosal barrier, aspirin has been studied in greatest detail. At a pH of 2, aspirin is more than 95 per cent in the non-ionized, fat-soluble form which can diffuse readily across the lipid mucosal membrane. In this circumstance, it breaks the tight junctions between cells, leading to their exfoliation and enhancing the back-diffusion of hydrogen ions. In addition to salicylates, other potentially injurious substances include alcohol, bile salts, steroids, indomethacin, antibiotics, digitalis preparations, xanthine derivatives, potassium chloride, and thiazides. The breakdown of the normal gastric mucosal barrier also has been demonstrated in critically ill human patients and in dogs subjected to experimental hemorrhagic shock. An alteration in gastric mucosal

blood flow may be of importance in these situations.

Acute gastritis often develops suddenly in a previously healthy gastric mucosa and is capable of healing completely within the short period of a few days. Clinically, acute gastritis is of greatest importance when the mucosal injury includes extensive erosions and is complicated by severe hemorrhage. Indeed, 25 to 30 per cent of patients with severe hemorrhage from the upper gastrointestinal tract are found to be bleeding from acute hemorrhagic gastritis. Treatment includes the restoration of blood volume, removal of noxious agents such as aspirin and low temperature gastric lavage. Uncontrolled bleeding requires surgical intervention — often near-total gastrectomy if the hemorrhagic process is an extensive one. In view of the presumed importance of continued gastric acid secretion and its back-diffusion to perpetuate mucosal injury, it is possible that the new H_2-receptor antagonist drugs, which can virtually abolish gastric acid secretion, will be of great use clinically to interrupt this vicious circle of acid-induced mucosal injury.

Chronic gastritis is also best defined and classified on the basis of mucosal histology. Although the literature again is confused by classifications of chronic gastritis based on gastroscopic and/or clinical features, Morson recognizes three basic histologic patterns: chronic superficial gastritis, atrophic gastritis, and gastric atrophy.

The major features of *chronic superficial gastritis* include a mucosa of normal thickness with abnormalities of the mucus-producing cells lining the surface and pits with preservation of the deeper tubular structures without loss of glandular elements. The surface cells may be decreased in number and may assume a cuboidal rather than a columnar appearance. Their mucin content is decreased and their nuclei hyperchromatic. The lamina propria is infiltrated by increased numbers of lymphocytes and plasma cells. There is variable edema and vascular congestion. The clinical significance of chronic superficial gastritis is uncertain, although it is sometimes seen in association with peptic ulcer and gastric carcinoma. The relationship, if any, to acute gastritis also is unclear. Although chronic superficial gastritis may regress, long term follow-up of such patients indicates that the majority progress to the stage of *atrophic gastritis*. In this condition the over-all mucosal thickness may or may not be decreased, but in addition to changes in the superficial epithelial cells, there is damage to the gastric glands, with loss of greater or lesser numbers of chief and parietal cells which are replaced by mucus-secreting cells. In the superficial mucosa, and sometimes also in the deeper zones, a metaplastic change toward an intestinal type of epithelium is seen. This includes the appearance of mucus-containing goblet cells, not normally found in the stomach. In addition, the columnar cells of the metaplastic epithelium may have a prominent brush border and Paneth cells may be found in large numbers. Mitotic activity is increased. Histochemically, alkaline phosphatase and aminopeptidase are found in the superficial columnar cells, together with a marked increase in thiamine pyrophosphatase and beta-glucuronidase. Finally, in atrophic gastritis an infiltrate of lymphocytes and plasma cells, often marked, is found within the lamina propria. *Gastric atrophy* may be the end-result of chronic gastritis and usually involves extensive areas of the gastric mucosal surface. The mucosal thickness is greatly decreased, and the chief and parietal cells are virtually absent from the mucosa of the body and fundus; in the antrum only a few pyloric gland elements may remain. The changes of intestinal metaplasia are extensive. The inflammatory cell infiltrate in the lamina propria usually is minimal.

The cause of chronic gastritis and of gastric atrophy is not well understood, although these conditions are more common with increasing age. In one study chronic atrophic gastritis appeared to be associated with blue eyes, low socioeconomic class, cigarette smoking, heavy consumption of alcohol, and the drinking of hot tea. In general, however, there is little evidence that the exogenous agents associated with acute gastritis are responsible for the chronic disorders. All types of chronic gastritis are observed in association with gastric ulcer, while atrophy of the gastric mucosa is invariably present in pernicious anemia and gastric polyposis and not infrequently in patients with sprue, pellagra, and iron-deficiency anemia.

There is growing evidence that in many instances chronic atrophic gastritis may be the consequence of chronic mucosal injury by bile salts and other components of intestinal juice regurgitated through the pylorus, perhaps by disruption of the gastric mucosal barrier as outlined above. Extensive chronic gastritis is seen in the distal stomach of patients with gastric ulcers, a group where duodenogastric bile reflux is known to be unusually frequent and severe. Following partial gastrectomy with Billroth II gastrojejunostomy, there ensues both extensive bile reflux into the gastric remnant and a severe and progressive chronic gastritis extending proximally from the stoma, where it is most severe. Experimentally, atrophic gastritis develops in tubes of canine gastric mucosa exposed to constant bile flow. Although these facts suggest a relationship between bile reflux and chronic gastritis, the hypothesis that this relationship is a causal one clinically remains to be proved.

A possible immune mechanism in the development of gastric atrophy has been suggested on the basis of a series of interesting observations in patients with pernicious anemia: resemblance of the gastric mucosal lesion in pernicious anemia to that of the thyroid in autoimmune thyroiditis; the frequent clinical interrelations of pernicious anemia with autoimmune disease of the thyroid (thyroiditis, myxedema, Hashimoto's disease), the high incidence of circulating thyroid antibodies in patients with pernicious anemia, and, conversely, the high incidence of gastric antibodies in serum from patients with these thyroid diseases; the infiltration of the atrophic mucosa by lymphocytes and plasma cells which contain immunoglobulins reactive with gastric antigens; the frequent presence of circulating antibodies reacting specifically with parietal cell cytoplasmic antigen and/or gastric intrinsic factor in patients with pernicious anemia; and the presence of the same parietal cell antibody in serum from patients with atrophic gastritis without pernicious anemia who are presumably candidates for the later development of that disease. Treatment with corticosteroids may permit regeneration of gastric mucosal glands, with recovery of acid and intrinsic factor secretion and normal absorption of Vitamin B_{12}. Those who respond tend to have the highest titers of circulating parietal cell antibodies. There is no correlation in this regard with the presence of antibodies to intrinsic factor. Patients with extensive intestinal metaplasia of the gastric mucosa are least likely to benefit from steroid therapy.

Parietal cell antibodies are circulating antibodies of the IgG variety with an affinity for the cytoplasm of parietal cells. They are demonstrable in 80 to 90 per cent of patients with pernicious anemia and in 60 per cent of patients with other forms of gastritis without hematologic abnormality. Parietal cell antibodies also are more common in older patients. However, their presence is not necessarily correlated with the severity of the gastritis. The presence of parietal cell antibodies suggests that such patients have a genetically determined ability to form antibodies, but there is no evidence in such patients that the gastritis is the result of these antibodies or that antibodies predispose to the severity and the chronicity of the gastritis. Interestingly, gastric antibodies are not found in patients with postgastrectomy gastritis, and damage to the gastric mucosa by chemical or physical agents does not stimulate the appearance of these immunologic phenomena. Although these facts are all consistent with the hypothesis that in at least some patients immunologic mechanisms are of etiologic importance in atrophic gastritis, this possibility remains unproved and must be confirmed by additional evidence.

The evaluation of symptoms in patients with

chronic gastritis is difficult. Experimentally, acute inflammation and sustained hyperemia of the gastric mucosa lower the threshold for pain. Chronic inflammation, therefore, may be expected to facilitate the occurrence of gastric symptoms. Clinically, however, chronic gastritis is noted gastroscopically quite often in the absence of abdominal distress. In other patients with chronic gastritis, the symptoms are varied and vague; their incidence, type, or severity cannot be correlated with the character or degree of gastritis. The most frequent complaints of such patients are loss of appetite, fullness, belching, vague epigastric pain, nausea, and vomiting. These are also the symptoms of functional gastrointestinal distress.

The consequences of chronic gastritis are not completely known. Although minor surface alterations, such as erosions and hemorrhages, usually heal completely, severe and complete atrophy of the stomach generally tends to persist unchanged. The association of chronic atrophic gastritis and gastric ulcer, and the fact that the gastritis persists even after the ulcer heals, suggest that the gastritic mucosa is more vulnerable to chronic peptic ulceration. Benign gastric polyps of a regenerative or adenomatous nature may occur in patients with atrophic gastritis, and the risk of development of gastric cancer appears to be considerably increased in patients with chronic gastritis, particularly in the group with gastric atrophy and pernicious anemia. Other than surveillance of the patient for the development of these complications, no treatment is at present available for chronic gastritis.

Finally, a number of gastritis syndromes not included in the preceding classification have been described. *Giant hypertrophic gastritis* (Ménétrier's disease) is a disorder of unknown cause, characterized by conspicuous increases in the height and thickness of the gastric folds, especially along the greater curvature of the body of the stomach. The hypertrophy is limited to the mucosa, the submucosa and the muscle layers of the stomach remaining normal. The disorder is restricted to the body and fundus of the stomach and usually stops abruptly at the margin of the antrum. Microscopically, there is a marked hyperplasia of the surface epithelial cells which line elongated, tortuous, and cystic gastric pits that may extend to or even through the muscularis mucosae. An intense inflammatory cell infiltrate may be present in the lamina propria. The gastric mucosa is abnormally permeable, and the pronounced exudation of serum proteins into the gastric content and their subsequent digestion may lead to hypoproteinemia. The clinical manifestations in addition to the edema associated with the protein loss include vague, non-specific gastrointestinal complaints. Gastric bleeding

may be the sole manifestation. While gastric secretion may be normal, low, or even increased, many patients have achlorhydria. The gross appearance of the mucosa in *hypertrophic glandular gastritis* (hypertrophic hypersecretory gastritis) is somewhat similar. The mucosa in this condition is greatly thickened because of the glandular hyperplasia with great increases in the numbers of parietal and chief cells. Inflammatory changes may be present, together with cysts and collections of lymphocytes. Both types of hypertrophic gastritis must be differentiated from the mucosal hypertrophy of the Zollinger-Ellison syndrome and from infiltrating adenocarcinoma or lymphoma. *Eosinophilic gastroenteritis* is a disorder of the intestinal tract characterized by infiltration of one or more layers of the gut wall by large numbers of eosinophilic leukocytes accompanied by a striking increase in the number of eosinophils in the peripheral blood. Most commonly the gastric antrum is involved. Symptoms are non-specific and include intermittent nausea, vomiting, and abdominal pain. Although the pathogenesis of eosinophilic gastroenteritis is not clearly understood, its frequent occurrence in patients with a history of asthma, allergic rhinitis, and atopic eczema, and its dramatic relief by corticosteroid therapy suggest an allergic or immunologic etiology. *Granulomatous gastritis* may occur as a manifestation of Crohn's disease, tuberculosis, syphilis, or sarcoidosis.

PEPTIC ULCER

Pathogenesis

A peptic ulcer develops as a result of a localized area of necrosis and digestion of the lining of the digestive tract. The process is a penetrating one, beginning in the mucosa and gradually extending through the muscularis mucosa into or through the muscularis propria. In some cases the ulcer penetrates into blood vessels, resulting in hemorrhage or completely through the gut wall into adjacent organs or as a free perforation into the peritoneal cavity. Regenerative activity is almost always present and at any time may lead to the healing of the ulcer, especially if it is protected from gastric juice. Healing occurs from below upward with the growth of granulation tissue and fibroblasts. In small superficial lesions, healing is complete. In large, chronic ulcers, healing is slower; new glands are not formed, and tissue is replaced by fibrous and elastic tissue.

Clinically, chronic peptic ulcer occurs only in those portions of the digestive tract exposed to the action of acid juice: the lower portion of the esophagus, the stomach, the upper portion of the small intestine, or the small bowel adjacent to a patent gastroenterostomy or a Meckel's diverticulum containing ectopic gastric glands. The majority of peptic ulcers, however, occur along the lesser curvature of the stomach and in the first three or four centimeters of the duodenum, the "duodenal bulb."

Although a common disorder, the exact incidence of peptic ulcer has been difficult to establish because of inaccuracies in diagnosis and the failure to distinguish between gastric and duodenal ulcer in many reports. It has been generally believed, however, that one out of every ten American males will suffer from duodenal ulcer during his lifetime, whereas the peak prevalence of duodenal ulcer in females is about 40 per cent that of males. The frequency of gastric ulcer is only about 25 per cent that of duodenal ulcer, and again males predominate over females with a ratio of about three to one. Interestingly, over the past several decades there has been a substantial decrease in the frequency with which duodenal ulcer is diagnosed, with a decline in incidence of 40 to 50 per cent, particularly among the younger members of the population. The cause of this important change is unknown, although it has been suggested that the data are consistent with the effect of an environmental factor, maximal around the turn of the century and now disappearing. Peptic ulcer disease is more common in patients with rheumatoid arthritis, chronic obstructive lung disease, and patients with hepatic cirrhosis who have been treated by portacaval shunt. Both gastric and duodenal ulcer are significantly more common in cigarette smokers than in non-smokers, and gastric ulcer appears to be more prevalent among habitual users of aspirin. Although it is commonly believed that corticosteroids, alcohol, coffee, indomethacin, phenylbutazone, and reserpine predispose to peptic ulceration by virtue of their ability to alter the characteristics of gastric mucus, interfere with epithelial cell replication, or increase gastric acid secretion, critical evaluation of available data has failed to substantiate this belief. A significant relationship is present between blood group status and peptic ulcer. Duodenal ulcer appears to be 35 per cent more common in individuals of blood group O than among individuals of groups A, B, and AB. Patients who fail to secrete blood group substances into their gastric juice are 50 per cent more liable to duodenal ulceration, while those of blood group O who are also non-secretors are most susceptible, with a liability about 2.5 times that of secretors of groups A and B. Gastric ulcers, on the other hand, are significantly more common in individuals of blood group A. Contrary to popular opinion, studies have failed to demonstrate that any particular personality type is common to ulcer patients. A number of psycho-

analytic studies, however, have concluded that a basic abnormality of the peptic ulcer patient is a marked dependency need, often in conflict with an adult aspiration for independence and achievement. The psychosomatic theory of peptic ulcer proposes that such long-standing psychic conflict or anxiety predisposes to peptic ulceration by increasing gastric secretion or damaging mechanisms of mucosal homeostasis. Presumably, these effects are mediated via the vagus nerve and render the individual vulnerable to acute ulceration shortly after some stressful emotional event. Although gastric secretory studies as well as direct observation of the gastric mucosa in patients with gastrostomies have confirmed the assumption that emotional events can alter mucosal function, studies designed to test the assumptions of the psychosomatic theory have in general been poorly controlled and, therefore, inconclusive.

The term "peptic ulcer" carries the implication that the lesion is the result of the action of the acid peptic juice. Pure gastric secretion is capable of destroying and digesting all living tissues, including the stomach. Current concepts emphasize the importance of the destructive effect of the peptic juice in the development of peptic ulcers, particularly in the many duodenal ulcer patients who are acid-hypersecretors. Indeed, peptic ulcer does not occur in patients whose gastric glands are incapable of secreting acid. Conversely, especially severe peptic ulcer disease is frequently seen in patients with extreme hypersecretion, such as those with the Zollinger-Ellison syndrome. Experimentally, peptic ulcer may be produced by various operations that interfere with the neutralization of acid by the intestinal content, by the administration of acid, or by the continuous stimulation of highly acid gastric secretion.

Also of presumably great importance in the development of peptic ulcer is the vulnerability of the mucosa to digestion by the acid-peptic juice. Tissue resistance depends on multiple factors, including the integrity of the gastric and duodenal mucosal cells, the rapid and continuous regeneration of epithelial cells to replace those lost by exfoliation, the quality of the mucus layer overlying the epithelial cells, the tight junctions linking each cell to its neighbor, and the mucosal vascular supply. Failure of one or more of these aspects of mucosal resistance may explain the development of gastric ulcers, which characteristically occur in patients with normal or reduced acid secretory capacity, and may be of importance in the development of duodenal ulcer in patients who do not possess gastric acid hypersecretion. Because little can be done to bolster weakened mucosal defenses beyond the removal of harmful exogenous substances such as aspirin, most current medical and surgical therapies for peptic ulcer are directed toward preventing the secretion of gastric acid or removing it by intraluminal neutralization after it has been secreted.

During the past decade detailed investigations have led to a better understanding of physiologic abnormalities found in ulcer patients which might be of importance in the development of their lesions. For *duodenal ulcer* the outstanding characteristic is the increase in parietal cell mass accompanied by augmented secretory capacity. Although the cause of this hyperplasia of the acid-secreting mucosa is really unknown, it often has been assumed that increased stimulation by the vagus nerve mechanism is responsible. Because "vagal tone" is impossible to measure, this concept is difficult to substantiate. Furthermore, because the reduction in acid secretion percentage-wise following vagotomy is no greater in duodenal ulcer patients than in normosecretors, some other as yet undiscovered mechanism may be important. The parietal cell in duodenal ulcer patients also seems to be abnormally sensitive to stimulation by gastrin. Thus, the dose of pentagastrin required to produce one half maximal secretion in such patients is only about one third that needed in patients without duodenal ulcer. Although the fasting serum gastrin level in duodenal ulcer is, if anything, slightly lower than normal, following a meal an abnormally large rise in serum gastrin ("integrated gastrin response") characterizes the duodenal ulcer patient. A possible explanation for this is the failure of normal mechanisms to inhibit release of gastrin from the antrum of patients with duodenal ulcer. For example, similar degrees of antral acidification inhibit gastrin release much less in duodenal ulcer patients than in normal subjects. The most important buffer in food is found in its protein content. The rate of gastric emptying is increased in duodenal ulcer patients and this leads to an increased duodenal acid load, particularly during the second half-hour after the meal when much of the protein buffer has been consumed or emptied from the stomach. It often has been postulated that duodenal ulcer subjects have a defect in secretin release from the duodenal mucosa or diminished pancreatic bicarbonate output following entry of acid into the duodenum. However, recent studies have failed to substantiate these hypotheses. Although the abnormalities of gastroduodenal function catalogued above are interesting, it has not been possible to combine them into a logical pathophysiologic sequence for the development of duodenal ulcer disease.

Patients with *gastric ulcer* are perhaps best characterized by their lack of gastric acid hypersecretion and by the almost universal presence of chronic superficial or atrophic gastritis around and distal to the location of the ulcer in the stomach. Indeed, a gastric ulcer most often occurs in the gastritic mucosa adjacent to the more normal parietal cell-bearing, acid-secreting mucosa. The presence of excessive duodenogastric reflux and an increased bile acid concentration within the gastric content are also typical of gastric ulcer. These latter abnormalities are possibly explained by malfunction of the pyloric sphincter which fails to tighten in a normal fashion following entry of acid, protein, or fat into the duodenum. Because all these abnormalities persist after healing of the gastric ulcer, it is unlikely that they are merely secondary phenomena. These observations can be interpreted to suggest that the pyloric sphincter abnormality is a major factor in the pathogenesis of gastric ulcer in that it permits harmful duodenogastric bile reflux. This may result in damage to the gastric mucosa, rendering it more susceptible to ulceration by even reduced amounts of gastric acid secretion. The strength of this argument is somewhat weakened by the fact that the addition of acid to the stomach is reported to restore pyloric sphincter function in gastric ulcer patients to normal. Thus, hyposecretion may somehow be responsible for the pyloric malfunction. Clarification of these relationships and their importance, if any, in the pathogenesis of gastric ulcer awaits further study.

Although ulcerative lesions of the gastrointestinal tract in regions exposed to acid are grouped together under the term peptic ulcer, it is quite probable that all ulcers, even those in a similar location, may not be of a single etiology. For example, there is considerable evidence that, although a hereditary predisposition exists for both, gastric and duodenal ulcers represent separate diseases. Relatives of gastric ulcer patients have a threefold increased prevalence of gastric ulcer as compared to the population at large, but a normal prevalence of duodenal ulcer. Similarly, relatives of duodenal ulcer patients experience a threefold increase in risk for development of duodenal ulcer, but no increased risk of gastric ulcer. Differences in blood group distribution mentioned above between the two types of ulcer patients also suggest that they are separate disorders with a hereditary predisposition. It is also likely that duodenal ulcer is merely the common clinical result of a variety of separate diseases of different etiologies, both genetic and non-genetic. For example, duodenal ulcer associated with the multiple endocrine adenoma syndrome, Type I (Wermer syndrome), appears to be inherited as a distinct autosomal dominant disorder, whereas such simple Mendelian inheritance patterns cannot explain the familial aggregation in ordinary duodenal ulcer disease. Clinically, duodenal ulcer patients can be separated into at least two groups based upon the degree of acid secretion and upon certain clinical characteristics. A bimodal distribution of serum pepsinogen concentrations among duodenal ulcer patients also suggests the presence of at least two distinct disorders. These observations are consistent with the hypothesis that peptic ulcer disease in fact represents a heterogeneous group of diseases which result from a variety of genetic and/or environmental causes. The failure to recognize such heterogeneity may explain the failure of investigations to identify a likely cause for "peptic ulcer." Future studies of clinically and biochemically well defined homogeneous groups of ulcer subjects may be more fruitful.

Endocrine Relationships

There is no known etiologic relationship between the ordinary peptic ulcer and primary endocrine disorders. However, certain endocrine (humoral) abnormalities may be associated with refractory peptic ulcer and gastric hypersecretion. The *Zollinger-Ellison (Z-E) syndrome* is characterized by single or multiple non-beta islet cell adenomas of the pancreas; enormous outputs of hydrochloric acid and pepsin; single or multiple ulcers in the esophagus, second, third, and fourth portions of the duodenum, and in the jejunum, in addition to the stomach and duodenal bulb; and refractoriness to medical or to surgical treatment short of total gastric resection. The parietal cell mass is sixfold greater than normal and threefold larger than in patients with the usual duodenal ulcer. Gastric rugae and the mucosal folds in the small intestine often are enlarged. The Z-E syndrome is relatively uncommon but not rare. The disorder is more common in men, the ratio being six males to four females. It occurs in all age groups, but especially during the third to fifth decades.

Ulcer pain is present in approximately 95 per cent of patients. Symptoms exceed one year in duration in more than 80 per cent, and range from five to ten years in duration in 30 per cent. Atypically located and multiple peptic ulcers strongly suggest the disorder. However, three fourths of the ulcers in the Z-E syndrome are not located atypically and they are not multiple, at least as determined by conventional barium x-ray examination. While case reports often describe the severe, occasionally dramatic complications of atypically located peptic ulceration, the symptoms often are indistinguishable from those of ordinary peptic ulcer until operation removes the anatomic integrity of the stomach and duodenum and disrupts normal homeostatic mechanisms controlling acid gastric secretion. The course then usually, although not invariably, is more complicated, with severe recurrent ulcer pain, bleeding, and perforation, the entire sequence occasionally developing very rapidly after ulcer surgery.

Diarrhea occurs in approximately one third of patients with the Z-E syndrome and can be regarded as the consequence of gastric acid hypersecretion and the presence of large amounts of acid within the upper small intestine, for removal of gastric acid by nasogastric suction markedly alleviates or eliminates the diarrhea. Steatorrhea is not uncommon and is attributable to multiple factors: acid inactivation of pancreatic lipase, precipitation of bile salts leading to defective micelle formation, direct injury to the intestinal mucosa by the excessive hydrochloric acid, and acid injury to the vitamin B_{12}-intrinsic factor complex.

Aside from the damage to the gastrointestinal tract, the most striking anatomic finding in the Z-E syndrome is the presence of the adenomas within the pancreas. They may occur anywhere within the pancreas but especially in the body and tail. Aberrant adenomas may be found in the hilus of the spleen, in the gastric wall, and along the curvature of the second portion of the duodenum. In about 10 per cent of patients no distinct adenoma is discovered, but rather an increased number of pancreatic islets containing a higher than usual proportion of non-beta cells is found. Despite the frequently benign histologic characteristics of the adenoma cells, approximately 60 per cent are malignant, as evidenced by the presence of metastases. Extracts of pancreatic adenoma in the Z-E syndrome contain large quantities of gastrin, and ultrastructural studies indicate that the secretory granules within the adenoma cells generally resemble those of the G-cells of the gastric antrum. Because the delta cells of normal pancreatic islets have been shown to contain gastrin by immunofluorescence studies, it is believed that the pancreatic "gastrinomas" of the Z-E syndrome originate from the delta cells.

The fasting serum from the majority of patients with the Z-E syndrome contains gastrin levels in excess of 300 pg. per ml. and usually tenfold or higher than the normal mean serum gastrin of 100 pg. per ml. In contrast, the fasting serum gastrin of patients with ordinary duodenal ulcer disease averages less than 100 pg. per ml. Thus, measurement of serum gastrin provides a useful technique for the detection of the Z-E syndrome when it is suspected. As physicians have become more alert to the recognition of patients with the Z-E syndrome, it has become apparent that some patients have fasting serum gastrin levels within the normal range. Measurement of serum gastrin following stimulation of gastrin release from the pancreatic tumor by calcium infusion or intravenous secretin injection, described above, will allow diagnosis of these cases as well.

The other characteristic laboratory finding in the Z-E syndrome is the enormous "basal" secretion of hydrochloric acid by the fasting stomach. Volumes in excess of 200 ml. per hour are common; one half of patients have a basal acid output of more than 15 mEq. per hour and two thirds have a basal acid output of greater than 10 mEq. per hour. This basal hypersecretion results from the constant near-maximal stimulation of the parietal cells by the elevated levels of circulating serum gastrin. In fact, additional stimulation of the parietal cells by exogenous histamine, betazole, or pentagastrin produces relatively little augmentation of gastric acid secretion, so that the ratio of basal to maximal (post-stimulation) acid output is usually 0.6 or greater.

Although frequently metastatic, the pancreatic tumors of the Z-E syndrome, like many carcinoid tumors, are quite indolent and progress very slowly. Death seldom results from the neoplasm itself, but rather from complications of the severe peptic ulcer disease it produces. Thus, treatment is directed toward the peptic ulcer disease rather than directly toward the tumor. Unfortunately, the severe ulcer diathesis is not controlled by the usual antacid and anticholinergic therapy; by gastric irradiation; or by conventional peptic ulcer surgery, including vagotomy with pyloroplasty, gastroenterostomy, or resection of the antrum. Only total gastrectomy with ablation of the parietal cell mass has been shown to be successful in controlling peptic ulcer diseases associated with the Z-E syndrome, and this is currently the treatment of choice. In some instances H_2-receptor antagonist drugs have been used with great success, at least short term, as a nonsurgical treatment for the Z-E syndrome. The long term efficacy of such treatment remains to be established.

Multiple endocrine adenomatosis, Type I, (Wermer's syndrome) is a familial disorder characterized by the concomitant presence of multiple tumors or hyperplasia of several endocrine glands. The parathyroid glands are most frequently involved, followed by the pancreatic islets, pituitary, adrenals, and thyroid glands. Bronchial and intestinal carcinoid tumors, pheochromocytomas and lipomas are included in the syndrome. The adenomas may or may not be hormonally active in one or more glands and in any combination. Peptic ulcer is present in more than 50 per cent of cases; the sexes are affected equally; and the disease has been described in all age groups after the first decade, with the peak occurrence in the third and fourth decades. Multiple endocrine adenomatosis appears to have a genetic basis attributable to the action of an autosomal dominant gene of high penetrance. Approximately one half of the ulcers are multiple and in atypical locations. The most common presenting feature of the syndrome is peptic ulcer

and its complications. Symptoms of hypoglycemia are next in frequency. Acromegaly, pituitary dwarfism, hypogonadism, Cushing's syndrome, hyperaldosteronism, and hyperthyroidism may occur alone and in any combination. Complications of perforation, obstruction, and hemorrhage are common. Diarrhea and steatorrhea occur in 10 per cent of patients in association with ulcer. Although gastrin has been extracted from the pancreatic adenomas, all attempts to isolate gastrin or a gastric secretagogue from adenomas of other endocrine glands have failed. The peptic ulcer associated with multiple endocrine adenomatosis seems identical in all respects to that of the Zollinger-Ellison syndrome. On the basis of present information, therefore, it perhaps is justifiable to regard the Z-E syndrome as the "gastrin-secreting, pancreatic islet-cell tumor component" of multiple endocrine adenomatosis. Treatment of each endocrine abnormality follows the usual measures; management of the ulcer in multiple endocrine adenomatosis is the same as for the Z-E syndrome.

Peptic ulcers are not more frequent in patients with adrenocortical hyperfunction. However, an association between duodenal ulcer and hyperparathyroidism, especially among men, has been frequently suspected. This suspicion is based on the fact that in one series of 300 duodenal ulcer patients, hyperparathyroidism was simultaneously present in four (1.3 per cent), a prevalence somewhat higher than one would expect from chance alone. Similarly, in some reported series as many as 30 per cent of patients with hyperparathyroidism have been noted to suffer from peptic ulcer disease. In other reports, however, the prevalence of peptic ulcer disease has not been increased among patients with hyperparathyroidism, and the matter must still be regarded as uncertain and controversial. If such a relationship exists, however, the mechanism is unclear, as, despite the fact that gastric hypersecretion has been noted to fall to normal following removal of parathyroid tumors in a few patients, the majority of patients with hyperparathyroidism possess normal rates of both basal and maximal acid secretion.

There are, however, a number of observations which might lead one to suspect an association between hyperparathyroidism and hypercalcemia and peptic ulcer disease. Calcium has an important influence on gastric acid secretion. In hypoparathyroid patients with serum calciums under 7.0 mg./dl., the stomach is usually achlorhydric. Conversely, as little as 2 gm. of oral calcium carbonate or an intravenous infusion of calcium will increase the rate of gastric acid secretion temporarily. Indeed, the calcium-containing antacids, although potent neutralizers of acid, enjoy little current use clinically because of the "rebound" gastric hypersecretion which follows their use. The mechanism of this calcium associated hypersecretion appears to be the release of gastrin by calcium. The situations cited, however, are acute ones; with chronic hypercalcemia, gastric acid secretion usually appears to adapt to normal levels.

One special relationship between hyperparathyroidism and peptic ulcer disease has been well documented. Patients whose hyperparathyroidism is part of the multiple endocrine adenomatosis, type I, syndrome who also have pancreatic gastrinomas have a particularly severe ulcer diathesis. In such patients the hypercalcemia stimulates marked release of gastrin from the pancreatic tumor and extreme hypersecretion of acid by the stomach, in contrast to normal subjects or ordinary duodenal ulcer patients in whom calcium infusions result in relatively modest rises in serum gastrin and gastric acid secretion.

Symptoms

The outstanding symptom of peptic ulcer is pain, characterized by its chronicity, periodicity, and relation to the ingestion of food. The average duration at the time the patient is first seen by the physician is six or seven years; in occasional cases the symptoms have been present for 40 or 50 years. The periodicity of the distress is striking, the symptoms lasting from a few days to a few months, followed by periods of remission of similar duration. The explanation for this intermittent pattern remains unknown, but presumably it is the symptomatic reflection of spontaneous cycles of ulceration and healing. Exacerbations of peptic ulcer occur at all times of the year, but in some patients they may be confined to the spring and fall seasons. In some patients the tendency is for the periods of distress to become more frequent and of longer duration, whereas the remissions are less frequent and shorter. On the other hand, progression is not inevitable; in many individuals recurrences become less frequent and eventually the ulcer may heal completely.

The pain is usually a gnawing or aching sensation, sometimes described as burning, boring, "heartburn," or pressure in the upper abdomen, cramplike, or, indeed, as hunger. It differs from the intermittent pangs of true hunger in that ulcer distress is almost always steady and continuous for 15 minutes to an hour or more unless relieved, whereas the hunger pang lasts for only a minute or so. The rhythm of pain in peptic ulcer is related to the digestive cycle; it is the same for both gastric and duodenal ulcer. Pain attributable to peptic ulcer usually is absent before breakfast, appears one to four hours after breakfast, and lasts 30 minutes or more, perhaps until relief

is obtained at the noon meal. The distress recurs one to four hours later and usually is more severe than in the forenoon. The afternoon pain likewise may disappear spontaneously, but more often food or alkali is required to obtain relief. In the evening, the pain may recur one to four hours after eating; it may be less severe than in the afternoon. The patient may be awakened with pain, usually between midnight and 3:00 in the morning. Rarely does nocturnal pain appear unless pain has been present in the evening, and rarely indeed does pain attributable to ulcer develop later in the night, unless it has been present earlier. The presence of nocturnal pain often is interpreted as evidence of pyloric obstruction or high-grade stenosis, but occurs also in non-obstructive, acutely inflamed, or penetrating lesions. In young children with peptic ulcer the distress may lack the usual rhythmicity and periodicity, the pain is vague, and vomiting is common. In older children, the symptoms resemble those of adults. Nausea, vomiting, anorexia, and weight loss in older patients with gastric ulcer initially may suggest the presence of malignancy.

Nausea is not a common symptom. Vomiting may result from severe pain, but usually indicates pyloric obstruction. Painless vomiting may occur with non-obstructive ulcer, and is more common with gastric than with duodenal ulcer. The appetite and weight usually are well preserved, but severe loss of weight may result from continued vomiting or the patient's fear of eating. The frequent ingestion of food to relieve pain, on the other hand, more often produces a gain of weight. Constipation and flatulence reflect an associated irritable colon. Diarrhea may result from various causes: the excessive use of laxative antacids; gastric hypersecretion, the acid inactivating intestinal and pancreatic enzymes and thus interfering with normal digestive processes; and a gastrojejunocolic fistula, short-circuiting the gastrointestinal content.

Complications

Bleeding occurs in the life history of at least 25 per cent of patients with peptic ulcer; the ulcers associated with bleeding vary in size and duration, with all gradations from superficial erosions to huge penetrating lesions. They may be located in the esophagus, stomach, duodenum, or in the jejunal stoma after a gastroenterostomy. The ulcers usually are on the posterior wall. The anterior surfaces of the stomach and duodenum do not contain major vessels, and the vascular channels are smaller than on the posterior wall. The associated symptoms are determined by the rapidity and severity of the blood loss. The manifestations of severe hemorrhage include sudden weakness, faintness, perspiration, dizziness, headache, palpitation, chilliness, abdominal cramps, thirst, dyspnea, syncope, and collapse as a consequence of the pronounced decrease in blood volume and diminished cardiac output. These symptoms respond promptly to the transfusion of whole blood and other supportive measures. Ulcer pain may be absent or infrequent.

In the absence of a definite diagnosis of peptic ulcer, upper gastrointestinal bleeding requires differentiation from a variety of other conditions associated with bleeding. These include erosive gastritis, esophageal varices, carcinoma of the stomach, vascular abnormalities, and the Mallory-Weiss syndrome. The latter condition is characterized by longitudinal lacerations in the cardioesophageal region varying from 3 to 20 mm. in length and from 2 to 3 mm. in width. They occur during the retching and straining associated with intense vomiting. The mucosal tears are attributed to unequal distensibility of the mucosa and musculature and severe pressure in the cardioesophageal area.

Pyloric or duodenal obstruction results from spasm, edema, and inflammation in an active pyloric or duodenal ulcer, from cicatricial stenosis, or from a combination of these changes. The obstruction in the majority of patients is temporary and disappears during medical treatment as the inflammation and edema subside. Permanent narrowing may result from frequent recurrences of ulcer. Each episode results in the proliferation of connective tissue, followed eventually by cicatricial contraction. The end-result is a firmly contracted scar narrowing the lumen. Obstruction in gastric ulcer may result from inflammation and narrowing of the gastric antrum, and from shortening of the lesser curvature of the stomach, with upward retraction of the antrum and distortion of the pylorus. The most significant symptoms of obstruction are the vomiting of retained food and gastric content, loss of weight, and weakness. In addition, the pain may become continuous rather than periodic, and the usual pain relief from food and alkali may be absent.

The loss of large quantities of chloride ion and a smaller but significant amount of sodium, as well as of potassium and fluid, in the vomitus produces an alkalosis characterized by an increase in the carbon dioxide content and pH and a decrease in the concentration of chloride, potassium and sodium ions in the plasma. The consequent diminution in blood volume, reduction in the flow of blood through the kidneys, and tissue dehydration lead to a temporary impairment of renal function. The symptoms of the electrolyte imbalance (alkalosis) include loss of appetite, distaste for food, increased nausea, weakness, lassitude, headache, nervous irritability, and occasionally coma. Tetany is rare, since the carbon

dioxide tension of the blood usually is maintained above the critical level, but muscular twitchings and hyperirritability of the reflexes may be present. These manifestations disappear rapidly with correction of the biochemical disturbance by the intravenous administration of appropriate amounts of chloride, sodium, potassium, and water.

Perforation complicates 1 to 2 per cent of all ulcers, and perforations recur in 1 to 2 per cent of these cases. Pyloroduodenal perforations exceed gastric perforations in a proportion of 20:1 for men and 5:1 for women. Perforations in males exceed those in females by a ratio of 50:1. The ulcers usually are on the anterior wall of the stomach or duodenum, unsupported by contiguous structures. Ulcers on the posterior wall tend to penetrate rather than perforate, and their further extension is limited to adjacent solid organs. Perforations occur more often after eating and during the latter part of the afternoon or evening. Ulcers perforate at all times of the year, but probably less often during the summer and more frequently during the winter. The symptoms begin with sudden, extremely severe pain in the upper abdomen, extending rapidly throughout the abdomen as a consequence of the escape of the irritating gastric and intestinal contents and the development of a chemical peritonitis. The pain may be referred to one or both shoulders because of irritation of the diaphragm, which is innervated by the phrenic nerves. The sudden severe pain is replaced within six to 12 hours by a dull discomfort, and may disappear within 24 hours. The subsequent development of a bacterial peritonitis produces fever, tachycardia, increasing abdominal distention, and toxemia. Death occurs within five to seven days if surgical and medical management prove inadequate.

Jejunal ulcer is a complication of the surgical treatment of peptic ulcer developing under circumstances of ineffective control of gastric secretion and exposure of the vulnerable jejunal mucosa to the acid-pepsin gastric content. Jejunal ulcers are most frequent in the efferent loop, approximately 1 cm. beyond the anastomosis. Jejunal ulcer also may develop in the absence of surgery in patients with the Zollinger-Ellison syndrome. Males predominate 10:1. The pain of jejunal ulcer may be in the left lower quadrant or in the lower abdomen. It often is more severe than previously and less responsive to treatment. The characteristic relationship to the intake of food may disappear and nocturnal distress is frequent. Nausea and vomiting may signify an associated malfunction or obstruction of the stoma. Loss of weight is common but is not pronounced unless a jejunocolic fistula develops.

A gastrojejunocolic fistula may develop from penetration of an ulcer at the anastomosis between the stomach and jejunum into the adjacent transverse colon, or a gastrocolic fistula may complicate a penetrating gastric ulcer. The principal symptoms are the pain of peptic ulceration and diarrhea of varying intensity. The diarrhea and the bypass of small intestine result in rapid and severe loss of weight, electrolytes, and water. Regurgitation of colonic contents into the stomach produces fecal vomiting. The associated malnutrition often is pronounced. Rarely, duodenal ulcer may cause an obstructive jaundice as a consequence of ulceration into the common bile duct; inflammatory obstruction of the duct; penetration into the head of the pancreas, causing pancreatitis; or penetration into the gastrohepatic ligament, obstructing the common bile duct proximally.

Various surgical procedures are available for the management of peptic ulcer. These are designed to limit the acid-secreting capacity of the stomach by severing its vagal connections with the central nervous system and limiting antral gastrin release by antral resection or drainage. They include partial gastric resection; truncal or "selective" vagotomy combined with pyloroplasty, antral resection or gastrojejunostomy; and the so-called "super selective" vagotomy wherein only the vagal innervation of the acid-secreting mucosa is severed. Important post-surgical problems, both gastrointestinal and metabolic, follow gastric resection. These include the mechanical difficulties of reduced gastric capacity, stomal dysfunction, jejunogastric intussusception, diarrhea, uncovering of a latent malabsorption (gluten-sensitive enteropathy), chronic obstruction of the afferent loop, recurrent ulcer formation, and the dumping syndrome. The nutritional and metabolic problems after gastric secretion occur later, sometimes many years later, as in the disordered calcium metabolism with demineralization of bone, associated with deficiency of vitamin D, resulting from the combination of diminished oral intake and impaired absorption. The late difficulties also include deficiencies of vitamin B_{12} and folic acid, decreased absorption of iron, intestinal leakage of albumin, increased susceptibility to infections including pulmonary tuberculosis, and, in emotionally vulnerable patients, addiction to alcohol or drugs or psychotic episodes. Late gastrointestinal problems may include the development of gastric carcinoma involving the gastric stump, bezoar formation and milk intolerance. The evidence for an increased incidence of cholelithiasis after gastric resection or vagotomy is inconclusive.

The dumping syndrome is caused by accelerated gastric emptying following gastric surgery, especially partial gastric resection but also after gastroenterostomy, pyloroplasty, and vagotomy, with the rapid entrance of large amounts of gastric content into the proximal jejunum. The hyperosmolar intestinal content initiates the movement of extracellular fluid from the plasma to the bowel lumen to achieve isotonicity, decreasing the circulating blood volume and inducing compensatory vasoconstriction. The distention of the jejunum and the presence of a hypertonic solution also activate a humoral mechanism that stimulates the production and release of serotonin from the argentaffin cell mass in the proximal jejunum. The serotonin presumably acts upon target organs, including the circulatory system. Bradykinin has been implicated in the early vasomotor symptoms and serotonin in the delayed response. The early manifestations, within five to 30 minutes after eating, include such vasomotor phenomena as a sense of warmth, sweating, weakness, palpitation, vertigo, desire to lie down; and such digestive complaints as abdominal discomfort, nausea, and explosive diarrhea. The late manifestations relate to the rapid entrance of glucose into the blood, producing hyperglycemia before sufficient insulin has been mobilized to facilitate its metabolism. The hyperglycemia elicits an overproduction of insulin, causing hypoglycemia two to three hours after a meal. Recent studies suggest that postgastrectomy hypoglycemia is caused by an inducible gastrointestinal insulin-secretory factor, possibly related to glucagon, potentiating glucose-mediated insulin release. Dumping may be precipitated by any food but especially by those rich in glucose and disaccharides when fluids are taken simultaneously, and by nervous tension. Dumping is more frequent after surgery for duodenal ulcer in women and among emotionally labile patients.

BENIGN GASTRIC TUMORS

Gastric neoplasms may be classified pathologically as of epithelial, mesenchymal, or endothelial origin. Their clinical differentiation, however, is difficult. The benign epithelial tumors include tubular adenomas and villous adenomas, which appear grossly as sessile or pedunculated mucosal polyps. The mesenchymal tumors include leiomyoma, leiomyoblastoma, lipoma, osteoma, and osteochondroma. Endothelial tumors include hemangioma, lymphadenoma, and endothelioma. Gastric teratomas arise from the visceral wall, the embryonic splanchnopleure, and are composed of tissues representing all three embryonic germ layers. They apparently occur exclusively among males. Tumors originating in the neural tissue, such as neurofibroma, neuroepithelioma, and neurilemoma, also may occur. The pathogenesis of most benign gastric tumors is as obscure as that of carcinoma of the stomach.

Tubular adenomas are most commonly associated with chronic atrophic gastritis or gastric mucosal atrophy. They may be single or multiple; they vary in size from a few millimeters to 7 cm. in diameter. Their surface is smooth and lobulated, or the epithelium may be thrown into frondlike processes if the lesion is a villous adenoma. Histologically,. the proliferating epithelial tubulae are packed closely together, and there may be crowding of the nuclei with variable degrees of hyperchromatism and increased numbers of mitotic figures — all features of a neoplastic process. There is some liability to malignant change, which is uncommon in growths less than 1.5 cm in diameter and becomes increasingly frequent with polypoid lesions of larger size.

Leiomyomas are the most frequently seen tumors of mesenchymal origin, constituting about 2 per cent of all gastric tumors. They originate from the smooth muscle of the gastric wall and may remain for some time as an intramural structure. As the tumor enlarges, it may grow either into the gastric mucosa toward the lumen, or outward toward the serosa; sometimes taking both directions to assume an hourglass appearance. About one third present as an ulcerated intragastric polypoid tumor and one fourth as a polypoid lesion covered by intact mucosa. The risk of evolution to leiomyosarcoma is small. Because of their tendency to remain silent, leiomyomas may grow to a very large size. They may outgrow their blood supply, leading to central necrosis and large cavities in the tumor connected by fistulous tracts to the gastric lumen. The most common symptom is hemorrhage, either acute or chronic. Abdominal discomfort, partially suggestive of peptic ulcer, may be present. Leiomyomas situated close to the pylorus induce symptoms of obstruction.

A variety of non-neoplastic disorders may simulate benign or malignant neoplasms of the stomach. Heterotopias, most frequently consisting of aberrant pancreatic tissue, are not uncommon in the distal antrum and pyloric canal. Rarely polypoid hamartomas including the genetically transmitted polyps of the Peutz-Jeghers syndrome and "juvenile" polyps are seen in the stomach, although such hamartomas are more frequently present in the small intestine and colon. Occasionally, inflammatory pseudotumors consisting of collections of lymphocytes, lymphoblasts, histiocytes, or plasma cells together with a mixed inflammatory infiltrate and reactive changes are found within the gastric mucosa. In the past these have sometimes been erroneously diagnosed as malignant lymphoma and so are commonly termed "pseudolymphomas." The most important feature distinguishing pseudolymphomas from true malignant lymphomas is the presence of follicle formation with true germinal centers. Pseudolymphomas are commonly associated with chronic

gastritis and with peptic ulcer. Also arising in stomachs involved with chronic atrophic gastritis are "regenerative" or "hyperplastic" polyps. Microscopically, there is overgrowth of the tubules of the superficial epithelium, sometimes with a degree of cystic change. The lamina propria is edematous and infiltrated with inflammatory cells.

CARCINOMA OF THE STOMACH

Malignant neoplasms of the stomach may be squamous cell carcinomas, carcinoid tumors, lymphomas, leiomyosarcomas or other sarcomas, but approximately 95 per cent are adenocarcinomas. Gastric cancer is the fifth most common cause of cancer death in the United States and afflicts primarily the older segment of the population, with the average patient being in his mid-50s at the time of diagnosis. Males develop gastric cancer slightly more frequently than females and there is an inverse relationship between cancer risk and socioeconomic status. Between 1930 and 1967, the age-adjusted mortality rate from gastric cancer in the United States decreased from 29 to 10 per 100,000 in men and from 22 to 5 per 100,000 in women. This appears to be a true decrease in incidence as, despite the increasing application of surgical treatment, the over-all five-year survival rate for patients with gastric cancer remains stable at about 13 per cent. No reasonable explanation for this fortunate trend in gastric cancer mortality is apparent. Similar trends have been noted in Canada and Australia, but not in other major countries. For example, in Japan, Finland, and Chile, gastric carcinoma has been and remains the most common gastrointestinal carcinoma and one of the major causes of death.

The cause of adenocarcinoma of the stomach is unknown. It is certainly not directly inherited, although a hereditary predisposition to its development is suggested by a clear familial aggregation of gastric cancer cases demonstrated in many studies and by the fact that individuals of blood group A appear to be slightly, but significantly, at greater risk. Furthermore, there seems to be some ethnic relationship in that the incidence of gastric cancer is unusually high in Japan, Chile, Finland, and Iceland. In Sumatra, the incidence is high among the Chinese population, but rare among the Javanese; in Israel, gastric carcinoma appears to be more common among Jews of Northern European ancestry than among Jews of Mediterranean or Asian origin.

These ethnic and geographic differences in gastric cancer incidence also suggest the possibility of an environmental influence. Indeed, the death rate from gastric carcinoma among Japanese-born migrants to the United States is lower than that in Japan, while among Japanese born in the United

States the risk of gastric cancer is essentially the same as that of other native-born Americans. Although one study suggests a relationship between gastric cancer and air pollution, in that gastric cancer rates correlated well with levels of suspended particulate matter in the air, the search for carcinogenic environmental factors has centered primarily around dietary factors and other ingested substances. The use of alcohol, tobacco, coffee, and condiments apparently is of no etiologic significance. In Japan smoked meats, sake, and rice treated with talc contaminated with asbestos have been suggested as possible carcinogenic influences. In other geographic areas, fish, cabbage, potatoes, superheated fats, soybean products, and rye bread have been suggested. Most recently the ingestion of nitrites and nitrates as water contaminants or food additives has been investigated as a possible carcinogenic factor as these substances are easily converted to nitrosamines which are potent carcinogens. In Colombia, a positive correlation has been found between the risk of gastric cancer and the nitrate concentration of well water. Nitrates and nitrites also are used as preservatives in bacon, cured meats, and in fish preparations. They may react with amines to produce nitrosamine in the process of cooking. There is an inverse relationship between the hydrogen ion concentration of the gastric content and its nitrite content, and achlorhydric gastric juice contains metabolically active bacteria capable of generating nitrites from nitrate and of nitrosating amines. Thus, the characteristic hypochlorhydric or achlorhydric intragastric environment of the gastric cancer patient is most suitable for the formation of carcinogenic nitrosamines. Despite this intriguing circumstantial evidence, however, it must be stressed that no single substance has yet been identified with certainty as an important gastric carcinogen.

The relationship of atrophic gastritis to carcinoma is obscure. Some degree of atrophy is observed in almost all cancer-bearing stomachs. Extensive atrophy of the gastric mucosa is invariably present in pernicious anemia and gastric polyposis, diseases in which the incidence of gastric carcinoma is distinctly higher than among similar age groups of the general population. In pernicious anemia the severe gastric atrophy affects the mucosa of the body of the stomach. Yet where cancer develops it may be in either the body or the antrum, suggesting that some factor other than the gastritis may be responsible for predisposing to the development of the tumor. The transitional changes from atrophic gastritis with small areas of hyperplasia to papilloma and to carcinoma have been demonstrated. On the other hand, atrophic gastritis occurs in association with gastric disease other than carcinoma and in the absence of any other apparent disorder. Perhaps the associated intestinal metaplasia of the gastric epithelium is more significant than the atrophy as a vulnerable substrate for gastric neoplasia. Possibly the gastritis is associated with a high cell turnover, creating an unstable cellular situation and increasing the vulnerability to neoplasia.

The possible role of achlorhydria in the development of gastric carcinoma is closely related to that of atrophic gastritis. Complete anacidity is present in only a very small proportion of patients with carcinoma; in many, the output of hydrochloric acid is reduced; but in some instances the acidity is high. Neither the atrophy nor the anacidity appears to be of direct etiologic significance; rather, they represent detectable abnormalities produced by some as yet undefined defect in the cells of the gastric mucosa. The apparently increased incidence of gastric carcinoma in the residual stomach after operations (especially gastrojejunostomy) for peptic ulcer, especially among males with blood group A, represents still another clinical situation reflecting an increased tissue vulnerability to neoplasia. Gastric carcinoma thus may be regarded as an acquired disease, developing in an abnormal gastric mucosa and probably arising on the basis of cellular reaction to continued injury, presumably from unknown chemical carcinogens.

Carcinoma may involve any part of the stomach but develops most frequently from the mucus-secreting cells of the antrum and pylorus, especially along the lesser curvature, an area probably more exposed to carcinogenic influences. As noted, the majority of gastric cancers are adenocarcinomas, and these originate in the mucus-secreting cells of the mucosa. The tumor does not necessarily begin with a single cell, but many cells throughout an area of variable size may undergo neoplasia, as in multiple polyposis and frank multicentric carcinoma. Gastric carcinoma, like other neoplasms, varies enormously in its rate of growth, from the "acute" rapidly metastasizing tumors to "subacute" and "chronic" neoplasms. Nothing is known of the factors accelerating its progress in some instances and retarding it in others, nor of the conditions inhibiting growth in some directions and favoring it in others. Some cancers project into the lumen with little penetration into the wall, others extend directly through the gastric wall, and still others spread chiefly along the wall, primarily along the mucosa, the so-called "superficial spreading carcinoma." This latter neoplasm extends no deeper than the muscularis mucosae,. and surgical removal offers an excellent prognosis for long-term survival. Acid gastric juice can digest neoplastic as well as non-neoplastic mucosa, submucosa, and muscularis, producing a lesion closely resembling a benign ulcer. Metastatic spread occurs by direct extension through the stomach to involve adjacent organs. Lymphatic spread involves the regional nodes along the lesser curvature, in the greater omentum, the hilum of the spleen, and in the subpyloric and suprapancreatic nodes.

The resistance of the body to cancer is not well understood, but it exists, as indicated in part by the sharp circumscription of some tumors, with atrophy and pyknosis of cancer cells at the margins of the lesion and the proliferation of fibrous tissues. Other histologic features associated with a favorable prognosis include the presence of an inflammatory reaction around the tumor, good cellular differentiation and, of course, the absence of lymph node metastases. Some lesions are associated with early ulceration; in others it is a late manifestation, and in some ulceration never occurs. The immunologic aspects of gastric (and other) carcinoma only now are attracting attention.

Symptoms

There are no symptoms pathognomonic of early gastric carcinoma. The onset of the disease usually is so insidious and its course so latent that it is seldom suspected by the patient or the physician until it is advanced. An interval of six to 12 months usually elapses between the initial manifestations and establishment of the diagnosis. The development and nature of the symptoms depend chiefly on the location of the growth, the presence of hydrochloric acid, the size and extent of the carcinoma, and its tendency to ulcerate, bleed, or metastasize. A tumor at the cardiac end of the stomach, sufficiently large to narrow the lumen of the esophagus, causes the progressive difficulty in swallowing characteristic of an esophageal neoplasm. Severe vomiting often is the first indication of neoplasm obstructing the pylorus. On the other hand, a carcinoma on the lesser or greater curvature of the stomach, or the body, may not cause symptoms until ulceration, bleeding, secondary infection, or metastases develop.

Symptoms include some type of indigestion, such as vague upper abdominal discomfort, a sense of fullness, ulcer-like distress but without the usual relief after the taking of food or antacid, or continuous epigastric pain. Anorexia is common, although in many instances the appetite initially may be unimparied. The patient experiences a sense of fullness after eating less than the customary amount of food. The cause of the anorexia is not known. Loss of appetite in later stages is attributed generally to a diminution of gastric tone and peristalsis secondary to neoplastic infiltration, but this explanation is not entirely satisfactory. The decreased desire for food reduces the total caloric intake and results in progressive loss of weight. The inadequate diet and the loss of nutrient substances by vomiting or diarrhea may lead to protein and vitamin deficiencies; in patients with pyloric obstruction, the malnutrition may become extreme.

Pain may occur early or late in the disease, or occasionally not at all. It seldom is severe until the carcinoma has ulcerated or invaded the wall of the stomach. The distress may be only a vague sensation of fullness or burning in the epigastrium. When hydrochloric acid is present, the pain often is indistinguishable from that of benign peptic ulcer. In general the pain tends to appear earlier and to be more severe in patients with acid gastric secretion than in those with anacidity, presumably because of peptic ulceration. In many cases, however, the distress of carcinoma differs from that of peptic ulcer in that it is aggravated by the ingestion of food and relieved partially or not at all by alkali or emesis. With progression and extension of the carcinoma to involve the celiac plexus and the spinal nerves, the pain may become severe, constant, and relieved only by opiates.

Nausea and vomiting may occur relatively early in the disease, regardless of the location of the lesion, but are much more frequent when the tumor obstructs the pylorus. The vomitus may or may not contain food, bile, or blood, but the so-called "coffee-ground emesis" is common. Dysphagia and substernal distress are characteristic of a tumor involving the cardiac orifice of the stomach and the lower end of the esophagus. Ulceration of a comparatively small tumor located in a "silent" area, with penetration into the wall of a blood vessel, may cause hematemesis or melena before other symptoms appear. Anemia is frequent, usually hypochromic and microcytic in type, and is caused by the occult loss of blood. However, the hematologic picture may be that of a true pernicious anemia, owing probably to coexistence of the two diseases. The anemia very occasionally results from carcinomatous infiltration of the bone marrow and displacement of the hematopoietic cells. Weakness, increasing fatigue, and lack of energy are related usually to the loss of weight and anemia, but they may precede these latter manifestations. Diarrhea is not uncommon, and in patients with diffusely infiltrating linitis plastica of the stomach may be ascribed to rapid gastric emptying, in addition to increased bacterial invasion of the upper gastrointestinal tract as a consequence of the diminished acid secretion. Infrequently, the "initial" manifestations are those of metastatic lesions such as carcinomatosis of the peritoneum, massive enlargement of the liver, or severe backache caused by extension of the neoplasm into the celiac plexus or the spine. Severe progressive dyspnea results from diffuse pulmonary lymphatic spread of gastric carcinoma.

REFERENCES

Anton, A. H., and Woodward, E. R.: High levels of blood histamine and peptic ulcer in a patient with portacaval shunt. Arch. Surg., *92*: 96-97, 1966.

Ballard, H. S., Frame, B., and Hartsock, R. J.: Familial multiple endocrine adenoma-peptic ulcer complex. Medicine, *43*: 481-516, 1964.

Beaven, M. A.: Histamine. N. Engl. J. Med.,*294*: 30-36, 320-325, 1976.

Berenson, M. M., Sannella, J., and Freston, J. W.: Menetrier's Disease. Serial morphological, secretory, and serological observations. Gastroenterology, *70*: 257-263, 1976.

Bruch, H.: Eating Disorders: Obesity, Anorexia Nervosa and the Person Within. Basic Books Inc., New York, 1973.

Code, C. F.: Reflections on histamine, gastric secretion and the H_2-receptor. N. Engl. J. Med., *296*: 1459-1462, 1977.

Davenport, H.: The digestive tract, 3rd ed. Yearbook Publishers Inc., Chicago, 1971.

Davenport, H. W.: Salicylate damage to the gastric mucosal barrier. N. Engl. J. Med., *276*: 1307-1312, 1967.

Davenport, H. W.: Back diffusion of acid through the gastric mucosa and its physiological consequences. In Progress in Gastroenterology, Jerzy-Glass, G. (ed.) Vol. II. Grune & Stratton, New York, 1970.

Deering, T. B., and Malagelada, J. R.: Comparison of an H_2-receptor antagonist and a neutralizing antacid on postprandial acid delivery into the duodenum in patients with duodenal ulcer. Gastroenterology, *73*: 11-14, 1977.

Dragstedt, L. R., Woodward, E. R., Seito, T., Isaza, J., Rodriguez, J. R., and Samijan, R.: The question of bile regurgitation as a cause of gastric ulcer. Ann. Surg., *174*: 548-559, 1971.

Edward, F. C., and Coghill, N. F.: Aetiological factors in chronic atrophic gastritis. Br. Med. J., *2*: 1409-1415, 1966.

Ellison, E. H., and Wilson, S. D.: The Zollinger-Ellison syndrome: reappraisal and evaluation of 260 registered cases. Ann. Surg., *160*: 512-530, 1964.

Fritsch, W. P., Hausamen, T. U., and Rick, W.: Gastric and extragastric gastrin release in normal subjects in duodenal ulcer patients and in patients with partial gastrectomy (Billroth I). Gastroenterology, *71*: 552-557, 1976.

Grossman, M. I., Guth, P. H., Isenberg, J. I., Passaro, E. P., Roth, B. E., Sturdevant, R. A. L., and Walsh, J. H.: A new look at peptic ulcer. Ann. Int. Med., *84*: 57-67, 1976.

Grossman, M. I., Kirsner, J. B., Gillespie, I. E., and Ford, H.: Basal and histalog-stimulated gastric secretion in control subjects and in patients with peptic ulcer or gastric cancer. Gastroenterology, *45*:14-26, 1963.

Holmes, K. D.: Mallory-Weiss syndrome. Review of 20 cases and literature review.: Ann. Surg., *164*: 810-820, 1966.

Isenberg, J. I.: The parietal cell. Viewpoints on Digestive Diseases 7: No. 2, 1975.

Ivey, K. J.: Gastric mucosal barrier. Gastroenterology, *61*: 247-257, 1971.

Janowitz, H. D.: Hunger and appetite — physiologic regulation of food intake. Am. J. Med., *25*: 327-332, 1958.

Keller, R. T., and Roth, H. P.: Hyperchlorhydria and hyperhistaminemia in a patient with systemic mastocytosis. N. Engl. J. Med., *283*: 1449-1450, 1970.

Kirsner, J. B.: Peptic ulcer. In Beeson, P. B., and McDermott, W. (eds.): Cecil-Loeb Textbook of Medicine, 13th ed. W. B. Saunders Co., Philadelphia, 1971, p. 1259.

Kirsner, J. B., Levin, E., and Palmer, W. L.: Observations on the excessive nocturnal gastric secretion in patients with duodenal ulcer. Gastroenterology, *11*: 598-617, 1948.

Lipkin, M.: The development of gastrointestinal cancer. Viewpoints on Digestive Diseases, *4*: No. 4, 1972.

Longstreth, G. F., Go, V. L. W., and Malagelada, J. R.: Cimetidine supression of nocturnal gastric secretion in active duodenal ulcer. N. Engl. J. Med., *294*: 801-804, 1976.

Mendeloff, A. I.: What has been happening to duodenal ulcer?. Gastroenterology, *67*: 1020-1022, 1974.

Morson, B. C., and Dawson, I. M. P.: Gastrointestinal Pathology. Blackwell Scientific Publications, London, 1972.

Overholt, B. F., and Jeffries, G. H.: Hypertrophic, hypersecretory protein losing gastropathy. Gastroenterology, *58*: 80-87, 1970.

Palmer, W. L.: The mechanism of pain in gastric and duodenal ulcers. II. The production of pain by means of chemical irritants. Arch Int Med. *38*: 694-000, 1926.

Paulino, F., and Roselli, A.: Carcinoma of the stomach; with special reference to total gastrectomy. Curr. Probl. Surg., 1973, pp. 1-72.

Pearse, A. G. E., and Bussolati, G.: Immunofluorescence studies of the distribution of gastrin cells in different clinical states. Gut, *11*: 646-648, 1970.

Prolla, J. C., Kobayashi, S., and Kirsner, J. B.: Gastric cancer. Arch. Int. Med., *124*: 238-246, 1969.

Rotter, J. I., and Rimoin, D. L.: Peptic ulcer disease — a heterogeneous group of disorders? Gastroenterology, *73*: 604–607, 1977.

Rovelstad, R.: The incompetent pyloric sphincter bile and mucosal ulceration. Am. J. Dig. Dis., *21*: 165-173, 1976.

Smith, B. M., Skillman, J. J., Edwards, B. G., and Silen, W.: Permeability of the human gastric mucosa. N. Engl. J. Med., *285*: 716-721, 1971.

Snyder, N., III., Scurry, M. T., and Deiss, W. P., Jr.: Five families with multiple endocrine adenomatosis. Ann. Int. Med., *76*: 53-58, 1972.

Strickland, R. G., and MacKay, I. R.: A reappraisal of the nature and significance of chronic atrophic gastritis. Dig. Dis., *18*: 426-440, 1973.

Tatsuta, M., and Okuda, S.: Location, healing and recurrence of gastric ulcers in relation to fundal gastritis. Gastroenterology, *69*: 897-902, 1975.

Taylor, K. B.: Gastritis. N. Engl. J. Med., *280*: 818-820, 1970.

Twomey, J. J., Jordan, P. H., Jr., Laughter, A. H., Mauwissen, H. J., and Good, R. A.: The gastric disorder in immunoglobulin-deficient patients. Ann. Int. Med., *72*: 499-504, 1970.

Te Velde, K., Hoedemaekerm, P. J., Anders, G. J. P. A., Arends, A., and Nieweg, H. O.: A comparative morphological and functional study of gastritis with and without autoantibodies. Gastroenterology, *51*: 138-148, 1966.

Van Wayjen, R. G. A., and Linschoten, H.: Distribution of ABO and Rhesus blood groups in patients with gastric carcinoma, with reference to its site of origin. Gastroenterology, *65*: 877-883, 1973.

Walker, I. R., Strickland, R. G., Ungar, B., and MacKay, I. R.: Simple atrophic gastritis and gastric carcinoma. Gut., *12*: 906-911, 1971.

Walsh, J. H., and Grossman, M. I.: Gastrin. N. Engl. J. Med.,*292*: 1324-1377, 1975.

Walsh, J. H., Trout, H. H. III, Debas, H. T. and Grossman, M. I.: Immunochemical and biological properties of gastrins obtained from different species and of different molecular species of gastrins. In Chey, W. Y., and Brooks, F. P. (eds): Endocrinology of the Gut. Charles B. Slack, Inc., Thorofare, N. J., 1974, pp. 277-289.

Weiner, H.,: Duodenal Ulcer, Vol. 6 (ed.). Advances in Psychosomatic Medicine, S. Karger, Basel, London, New York, 1971.

Wellmann, K. F., Kagan, A., and Fang, H.: Hypertrophic pyloric stenosis in adults. Gastroenterology, *46*: 601-608, 1964.

Wermer, P.: Endocrine adenomatosis and peptic ulcer in a large kindred. Am. J. Med., *35*: 205-212, 1963.

Wright, L. F., and Hirschowitz, B. I.: Gastric acid secretion. Am. J. Dig. Dis., *21*: 409-418. 1976.

Yalow, R. S.: Gastrins: Small, big, and big-big. In Chey, W. Y., and Brooks, F. P. (eds)./ Endocrinology of the Gut. Charles B. Slack, Inc., Thorofare, N. J., 1974, pp. 261-276.

Zollinger, R. M., and Ellison, E. H.: Primary peptic ulceration of the jejunum associated with islet cell tumors of the pancreas. Ann. Surg., *142*: 709-728, 1955.

26

The Small Intestine

DAVID W. WATSON, AND WILLIAM A. SODEMAN, JR.

The small intestine is a complex tube whose structure is well designed to subserve such seemingly diverse but related functions as the aboral transport of luminal contents, the secretion of enzymes and hormones, the digestion and absorption of ingested materials, and the mounting of an immune response. These functions are modified by neurohumoral influences and are materially aided by contributions from the pancreas and hepatobiliary system. The primary function of the small bowel, however, is digestion and absorption. All other activities either regulate or facilitate this process.

The pathophysiologist seeks to explain the signs or symptoms of intestinal disease in terms of an alteration in this structure and these functions. Implicit in such an undertaking is an understanding of normal structure and function and the manner in which they are modified by those processes which we call disease. In the small intestine, as elsewhere, structure and function are intimately though not always obviously related, and the greater our knowledge of how this relationship operates to ensure the gut's contribution to health the easier it will be to predict the consequences of changes induced by disease.

Although our understanding of small intestinal pathophysiology has increased, many unanswered questions remain. This discussion is based upon information that is firmly established for the human small intestine and does not present concepts based solely upon presumably parallel animal models, however applicable they may appear. Sufficient species differences in small bowel structure and function exist so as to make such carte blanche applications hazardous.

We will present an outline of normal structure from the gross to the electron microscopic level and discuss normal function and abnormal structure-function relationships as they apply to motor function, digestion and absorption, secretion, and immune responses. Circulatory disturbances have wide-ranging effects involving several of the aforementioned functions and will be discussed separately.

NORMAL STRUCTURE

By means of postmortem measurements the length of the small intestine has been estimated to be 6.5 to 7.0 meters. In life, however, tubes 3 meters long may pass into the cecum. Its caliber diminishes slightly from duodenum to terminal ileum, in part accounting for the fact that foreign bodies such as gallstones more frequently obstruct the lower ileum. The division of the small bowel into duodenum (20 to 30 cm.), jejunum (2.5 meters) and ileum (3.5 meters) is imprecise and based upon rather slight modifications of structure and relatively more important differences in function. Certain of the latter, such as the absorption of monosaccharides, amino acids, and β-monoglycerides, occur mainly in the jejunum. Other portions of the small intestine, however, can to a large extent compensate for loss of this segment. On the other hand, the physiologic absorption of vitamin B_{12} and the active transport of bile salts are exclusive functions of the terminal ileum.

The wall of the small bowel is composed of four basic layers: the mucosa, submucosa, muscularis externa, and serosa. The mucosa is composed of an epithelial cell layer with its filamentous basement membrane, a lamina propria containing blood vessels, lymphatics, smooth muscle cells, nerve fibers, plasma cells, lymphocytes, fibroblasts, eosinophils, macrophages, reticular cells, mast cells, collagen, and reticular fibrils and is separated from the submucosa by the muscularis mucosa. The submucosa contains larger blood vessels, lymphatics, more connective tissue, nerves and ganglia, and more lymphoid elements. The muscularis externa is divided into an inner circular layer and an outer longitudinal layer of smooth muscle, with the myenteric plexus interspersed between the two. In the past the longitudinal muscle has been described as a long, drawn-out spiral and the circular layer as a tight spiral. More recent studies indicate that fibers in both layers deviate from a strictly longitudinal or circular orientation at random, both right and left, so that the net direction in the two layers is axial and circumferential.

The small intestine is distinguished by four structural features which together enormously increase its luminal surface area. The valvulae conniventes are circumferential folds of mucosa and submucosa absent from the duodenal bulb but prominent in the duodenum and jejunum, and disappearing in the mid-ileum. They are responsible for the feathery appearance of the small bowel on barium studies and constitute the transverse folds seen in plain x-rays of air-filled intestine. The villi are projections of mucosa, readily discernible with a hand lens, which are usually finger-like or leaflike but under some conditions

appear as ridges or convolutions. Figure 26–1 is an illustration of villi as viewed with the scanning electron microscope. The individual cells of the villi and to a lesser extent the crypts possess filamentous microvilli, which in turn are coated with a finely filamentous material or "fuzz." The surface area of the adult small intestine has been estimated at from 5100 to 5900 square centimeters.

The mucosal crypts lie between the villi and extend basally to the muscularis mucosa. This relationship is depicted in Figure 26–2. In normal Americans and Europeans the villi constitute two thirds to three fifths of the mucosal thickness and the crypts two fifths to one third. As many as 20 crypts surround each villus but a functional ratio of 3:1 seems likely. Recently it also has been appreciated that the intestine is coated with a relatively thick layer of water molecules through which other molecules move by diffusion. This is a stagnant layer wherein bulk mixing caused by intestinal motility is unimportant. This "unstirred layer" constitutes an important determinant of the kinetics of absorption.

The surfaces of the villi and the linings of the crypts are covered by a continuous single layer of five different types of columnar cells: goblet cells, Paneth cells, enterochromaffin cells, undifferentiated crypt cells, and the differentiated villous epithelial cells (enterocytes or absorptive cells).

The majority of cells in the crypts are undif-

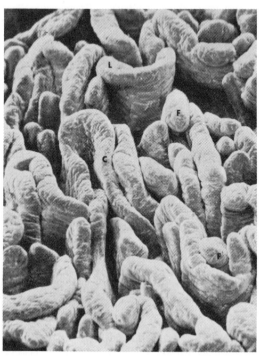

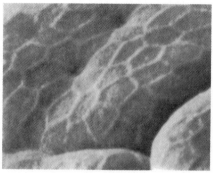

Figure 26–1 *A,* Human jejunal biopsy. Scanning electron micrograph (SEM) showing a leaf-shaped villus, *L;* finger-shaped villi, *F;* and a convolution, *C.* Surface creases can be distinguished (× 110). *B,* Human jejunal biopsy. SEM of part of the surface of a single villus. The mouths of two goblet cells are prominent and the hexagonal cell outlines are clearly seen (× 2300). (Toner, P. G., and Carr, K. E.: J. Pathol., *97*:611, 1969.)

A

B

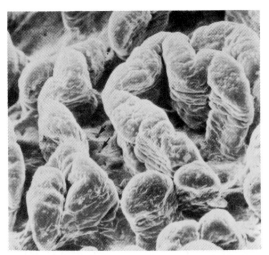

Figure 26–2 Human duodenal biopsy. SEM showing various shapes of villi. The mouths of intestinal crypts opening into the circumvillar basin are arrowed (× 210). (Toner, P. G., and Carr, K. E.: J. Pathol., 97:611, 1969.)

ferentiated cells which have a high mitotic index. They have numerous ribosomes and polysomes but little endoplasmic reticulum, scant microvilli, and undeveloped terminal webs. Although they contain what appear to be secretory granules no secretory function has been established and their main purpose is to serve as a source of the differentiated epithelial cell types. Newly formed cells migrate up the crypts and as they reach the junction of the crypt and villus they undergo morphologic, biochemical, and functional maturation to become villous absorptive cells, goblet cells, or Paneth cells. The origin of the enterochromaffin cells is less certain. During this migration-maturation process the differentiating cells develop larger and more numerous microvilli, a well-demarcated terminal web, more numerous mitochondria and rough endoplasmic reticulum, a decrease in free ribosomes and polysomes, loss of secretory granules, and the formation of large apical dense bodies which represent lysosomal derivatives. As these cells differentiate into villous absorptive cells they acquire enzymes, receptors, and carriers essential for the final phases of digestion and the processes of absorption. Cells migrating up the villus continually push the older, more differentiated cells toward the villous tip, from which they are eventually extruded into the lumen. This renewal process is accomplished in a period of three to seven days.

The absorptive cells are the most numerous and functionally most important cells on the villous surface. They are simple columnar cells in which the luminal surface is specialized to form a striated or brush border. This brush border is composed of microvilli ranging in length from 0.75 to 1.5 μ and in width from 0.10 to 0.20 μ. They number 3000 to 6500 per cell and are closely and regularly spaced with an intervillous distance of 0.01 to 0.05 μ. They are enclosed by an extension of the same trilaminar-appearing plasma membrane that surrounds the remainder of the cell. The microvillous core contains a central zone of 10 to 50 closely packed parallel filaments or tubules extending from the microvillous tip to the terminal web, which is the area just basal to the microvilli. It contains no organelles but only nonparallel tubular filaments similar to those in the microvilli and a few structures termed apical vesicles, thought to represent lysosomes. These tubular filaments are smaller and quite distinct from the cytoplasmic microtubules which lie roughly parallel to the long axis of the absorptive cell in the supranuclear cytoplasm. The microvillous plasma membrane is coated with a strongly adherent, filamentous "fuzz" termed the glycocalyx. It is composed of a sulfated, weakly acidic mucopolysaccharide which appears to be continuously synthesized by the Golgi apparatus of the epithelial cell, transported to the microvillous surface, and eventually shed into the lumen. The glycocalyx is most prominent on the absorptive cells, especially at the villous tips. Figure 26–3 illustrates the fine structural relationships of these cells.

The microvillous plasma membrane and its glycocalyx constitute a digestive-absorptive unit. Several enzymes have been localized to this structure, including alkaline phosphatase, the disaccharidases, aminopeptidases, dipeptidases, adenosine triphosphatase, thiamine triphosphatase, and folic acid conjugase. The active transport of glucose, galactose, and amino acids as well as the uptake of the vitamin B_{12}-intrinsic factor complex is mediated by receptors and carriers localized to this region.

The epithelial cells covering the villi and lining the crypts are joined at their lateral margins by a junctional complex composed of three parts. Just basal to the origin of the microvilli the outer leaflets of the lateral plasma membranes fuse to form the tight junction (zonula occludens). Just basal to this lies the intermediate junction (zonula adherens) and beneath it the desmosome (macula adherens), so named because the cytoplasm underlying the plasma membrane at this point is condensed. These latter two structures represent only close approximations of the plasma membranes, not fusion. The epithelial cells with their junctional complexes form a tight unbroken membrane lining the luminal surface of the small intestine.

This epithelial membrane is a complex dynamic "organ" regulating the flux of materials be-

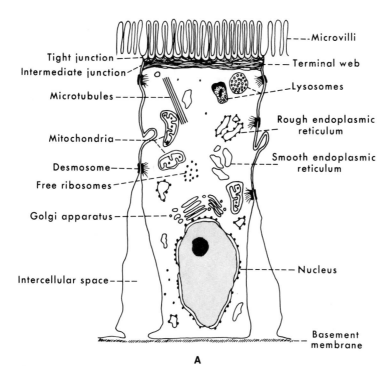

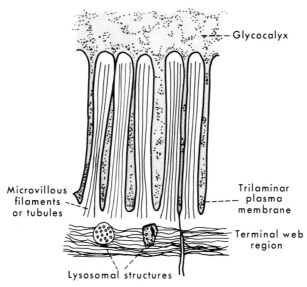

Figure 26–3 Schematic representation of *A*, differentiated villous absorptive cell, and *B*, the glycocalyx-microvillus structure.

tween the lumen and the lamina propria. Its integrity depends upon the continual replication, maturation, and metabolism of its cells. Interruption of any of these vital processes will lead to a failure of this organ, which will usually be expressed as a malabsorption syndrome.

MOTOR FUNCTION

Normal Motor Function

The over-all concept of small intestinal motor activity becomes more meaningful when it is not viewed as the primary function of the small bowel but rather as complementary to the organ's major activity. To facilitate the digestive-absorptive process, small intestinal movements must do two things: mix ingested materials with pancreatic and hepatobiliary secretions and propel luminal contents from one end to the other at a rate suitable for both optimal absorption and the continuing entry of gastric contents. Normally this rate is approximately 1 cm. per minute, and as a result the residue from the previous meal leaves the ileum at about the same time the next meal enters the stomach. An understanding of how these two activities are accomplished requires a consideration of the electrical and contractile events taking place in the small intestine.

Intestinal smooth muscle exhibits spontaneous contractions, can be stimulated by stretch, and will conduct impulses independently of nerves. Its resting membrane potential is unstable and varies irregularly with basal tension and the general level of contractile activity, but it also fluctuates in two consistent patterns. The first is a rhythmically occurring, omnipresent fluctuation arising in the longitudinal muscle and identified as either the slow wave, the basic electrical rhythm (BER), or the pacesetter potential. As visualized by Code, et al., if at any one instant the electrical activity of the small bowel could be stopped or frozen in place, each slow wave or pacesetter potential would be fixed in the wall

and would extend over a distance which may be termed its cycle length or wavelength for that particular segment. The bowel beneath each cycle would then represent a physiologic motor unit, with the slow wave prescribing its dimensions and controlling the nature of motor activity occurring within it at any one instant. These pacesetter potentials evoke no muscular contractions themselves but instead govern the rate at which the second type of electrical activity may take place. These are termed spike potentials and are responsible for the contractions of the circular muscle. Spike potentials can occur only during the periods of maximal depolarization of the pacesetter potentials. This relationship between pacesetter potentials, spike potentials, and circular muscle contraction is presented in Figure 26–4.

The pacesetter potential passes caudally as a sheath or ring whose front constitutes a rapid depolarization reaching all circumferential points simultaneously. An intact intrinsic nerve plexus is required for this to occur. Its frequency is rather constant with time but displays a declining gradient over the small bowel from 11.8 cycles per minute in the duodenum and first 10 cm. of the jejunum to 9.0 cycles per minute in the ileum. This decline may be stepwise through a sequence of frequency plateaus, each representing the distance traversed by the pacesetter potentials originating in that segment, but there is no agreement on this point. Since pacesetter potentials of a given frequency pass over relatively long segments and exhibit this declining frequency, they serve to integrate the activity of the whole organ.

The conduction of either pacesetter or spike potentials is made possible by tight side-to-side or end-to-end junctions between the individual muscle cells. These nexuses represent a partial fusion of the outer leaflets of the trilaminar plasma membranes and provide low resistance electrical shunts between cells.

The pacesetter potential therefore sets the frequency but not the magnitude of circular muscle contraction. An alteration in frequency of the pace-

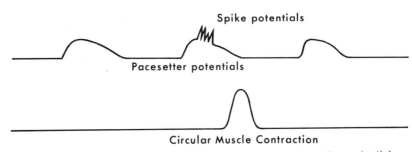

Figure 26–4 Digrammatic presentation of the relationship between pacesetter potentials, spike potentials, and circular muscle contraction.

setter potential may be brought about in several ways. Duodenal compression or transection causes a decrease in frequency distal to the injury. A decrease in frequency is also seen with hypothermia, hypothyroidism, hypoglycemia, malabsorption syndromes, substances interfering with active membrane transport, and damage to the intrinsic nerve plexuses. Serotonin, Pituitrin, and Pitressin also cause a decrease in frequency, the latter two by reducing blood supply to the longitudinal muscle. An increase in frequency occurs with pyrexia, hyperthyroidism, adrenergic stimulation, and morphine administration. Pacesetter potentials are relatively insensitive to cholinergics, anticholinergics and topical anesthetics. Extrinsic nerve stimulation, the ingestion of food, and changes in electrolyte concentrations also have little or no effect on the frequency of pacesetter potentials.

Spike potentials are the electrical counterparts of circular muscle contraction and therefore are associated with luminal pressure changes. They are not propagated and their sequential occurrence in successive segments (peristalsis?) is due rather to propagation of the pacesetter potentials to which they are coupled. Not every pacesetter potential need evoke a spike potential but the frequency of spike potentials can never exceed the frequency of pacesetter potentials. The latter are conducted from their origin in the longitudinal muscle to the circular muscle probably via the nexuses.

The electrical response, if any, of the circular muscle to a given pacesetter potential is governed by an interplay of influences provided by the activity of the intrinsic nerve plexuses acting as part of local or central reflexes and various circulating or locally produced hormones. The amplitude of circular muscle contraction is proportional to the number, duration, and amplitude of the spike potentials. The factors which influence the generation of spike potentials are somewhat different from those that alter the frequency of pacesetter potentials. Spike potentials are initiated by rapid radial stretch or distention of the bowel wall, vagal stimulation, and ingestion of food. In contrast to pacesetter potentials, spike potentials are relatively sensitive to the effects of drugs, hormones, and other pharmacologically active substances. They are initiated by cholinergic drugs, hydrochloric acid, serotonin, and morphine and are eliminated by anticholinergics, ganglionic blocking agents, barbiturates, and sympathomimetics. Mechanical obstruction at first results in an increase in spike potentials proximal to the obstruction and a decrease distally. Anoxia causes an initial stimulation but eventually results in their disappearance.

Although coordinated intestinal motor activity may occur in the absence of extrinsic autonomic innervation this system is important in modify-ing motor activity in relationship to other physiologic responses within the body. Unfortunately, its structure and function are still not well understood. The vagi contain motor preganglionic parasympathetic fibers making synaptic connections with secondary parasympathetic motor neurons in the subserosal, myenteric, and submucosal plexuses. Postganglionic sympathetics also traverse the vagi but their termination is unclear. Motor fibers in the splanchnic nerves are preganglionic sympathetic fibers terminating in the abdominal sympathetic ganglia and postganglionic sympathetic fibers arising in the paravertebral ganglia. Postganglionic sympathetic fibers are then distributed to the gut with branches of the associated arteries. Their sites of termination are not known, although some catecholamine-containing fibers form meshes around cholinergic ganglion cells and others enter the muscle layers. Sensory nerves travel in both systems, with vagal fibers originating in the unipolar cells of the nodose ganglion. The nerve cells lying within the gut are postganglionic parasympathetic or internuncial neurons and perhaps cells with sensory function, although no specialized neural structures have been identified as sensory. The enteric plexuses appear to be interconnected but the anatomic relationship between fibers originating in them and secretory and smooth muscle cells is unknown.

The influence of extrinsic nerve stimulation on spike potentials is imperfectly understood, and for the present only the following generalization can be made. In the absence of significant small intestinal activity both parasympathetic and sympathetic stimulation initiate spike potentials, whereas an actively contracting bowel tends to be inhibited. The small intestine contains both alpha- and beta-adrenergic receptors. Alpha receptors have an affinity for epinephrine and act to eliminate spike potentials. Beta receptors bind isoproterenol and, in the duodenum at least, their stimulation tends to elicit spike potentials, but the remainder of the intact human small intestine has not been adequately studied. Alpha receptors predominate in the small bowel, and the net effect of either alpha or beta stimulation is an inhibition of small intestinal smooth muscle activity. How this is mediated in the case of beta receptors is not clear.

Apart from serving as a source of pacesetter potentials, the contribution of the longitudinal muscle layer to small intestinal motor function is not well understood. No electrical events corresponding to its contraction have been recorded. Current views suggest that is serves largely to regulate the overall "tone" of the bowel wall and the caliber of its lumen. Its contraction produces a net increase in luminal diameter and thereby a decrease in pressure.

Little is known about the electrochemical

events involved in the contractile process. It appears that the release of calcium ions from a site of storage triggers contraction. The term "smooth" is not strictly apt, however, since faint striations are in fact present as uniform small filaments of actin. Myosin has also been identified in "smooth" muscle but its location is unknown.

The interaction of these electrical and contractile events under the direction of various local and systemic neurohumoral influences results in intestinal *motility*. This is an ambiguous term at best, however, and may refer to movements of the bowel wall, smooth muscle contraction, luminal pressure changes, or propulsion of luminal contents. Since circular muscle contraction and the rate of flow of luminal contents may have an inverse relationship, the term becomes self-contradictory. The ambiguity is further compounded by adding the prefixes hyper and hypo. From the standpoint of small intestinal function, only two types of motor activity are important — mixing and propulsion, which correspond grossly to Type I and Type III waves, as seen in motility records.

Mixing is accomplished predominantly by Type I waves occuring either as isolated stationary "standing ring" contractions of circular muscle involving a 1 to 2 cm. segment of bowel or as a series of such contractions, referred to as rhythmic segmentation. This latter type of motor pattern is represented diagrammatically in Figure 26–5. Segmenting activity decreases in frequency from the duodenum to the ileum, and although it is the predominant type of activity recordable, it is present only 2 per cent of the time in the resting small intestine. Segmenting contractions are more frequent after a meal or following morphine administration and have the effect of slowing transit. In patients with rapid transit, segmenting activity is decreased.

Flow through the alimentary canal can be thought of as analogous to flow through the vascular system, albeit more complex and less well understood. Both systems possess pacemakers, pressure receptors, and osmoreceptors, and flow is enhanced as viscosity decreases. The rate at which intestinal contents move through the small intestine is dependent upon a pressure gradient generated by the bowel wall and the peripheral resistance of the gut. The resistance varies with the diameter of the lumen and the contractility or tone of the intestinal wall. The prime regulator of transit, however, is peripheral resistance. Precisely how this resistance is varied and in what manner contractile activity is ordered to bring about the required pressure differential for transit to occur is still largely undefined. Peristalsis, a moving ring contraction, is controversial. It must occur infrequently and over short distances, if at all, since normally it takes several hours for contents to traverse the small bowel. There is no quantitative information about the frequency, velocity, or range of movement of peristalsis in the human small intestine. The so-called "peristaltic rush" connotes a vigorous ring contraction progressing rapidly from the duodenum to the ileum. Its existence is debated and if it does occur it is probably always pathologic. Some aboral movement of contents will occur with isolated or rhythmic segmenting contractions. As Texter has pointed out, the aboral transport of luminal contents is more closely related to the pressure gradient between proximal and distal segments than to the activity of any single type of contraction. With the probable exception of waves that progress over a considerable distance (peristalsis) and of rhythmic sequences, pressure

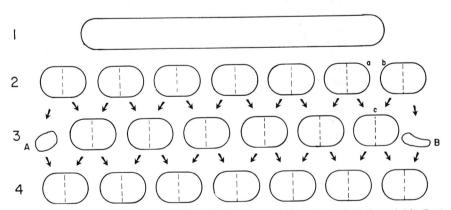

Figure 26–5 Diagram representing process of rhythmic segmentation. Rows 1, 2, 3, and 4 indicate sequence of appearances in loop. Dotted lines mark regions of division. Arrows show relation of particles to segments they subsequently form. (Hightower, N. C., Jr.: *In* Code, C. F. (ed.): Handbook of Physiology. Vol. IV. American Physiological Society, Washington, D.C., 1968.)

waves contribute more to the increase of peripheral resistance than to the promotion of propulsion. Since there is a progressive decrease in the level of activity in sequentially more distal segments of the small intestine, the resulting gradient probably constitutes the most important mechanism for transit. It is therefore the total motor pattern of the entire small bowel that underlies transit rather than any one or another specific kind of contractile activity. A generalized increase in activity will just as effectively retard transit as complete atony, since in neither case will a pressure gradient be produced.

Abnormal Motor Function

Without a satisfactory knowledge of normal motor function an understanding of pathologic processes must also be incomplete. Furthermore, the definition of abnormal motor function depends upon one's point of view. To the physiologist it is an alteration of smooth muscle contractility; the radiologist finds it reflected in some abnormality of the distribution and movement of barium; those interested in "motility" patterns will be impressed by unusual fluctuations in intraluminal pressures, while the physician at the bedside wonders about the origin of abdominal pain, constipation, and diarrhea. Unfortunately it is not possible to describe any consistent or reproducible relationship between these different kinds of measurements, and in many instances signs and symptoms of altered function remain largely unexplained.

On the clinical level, disturbed motor function will be manifest primarily as abdominal pain or some alteration in transit perceived as constipation or diarrhea. The only known stimulus for pain production in the small bowel is an increase in intramural tension. Distention therefore will produce pain only when accompanied by significant tone in the intestinal wall or a strong contraction involving a relatively broad segment. The intensity of pain is proportional to the rapidity with which the tension develops and its magnitude. Any stimulus capable of eliciting such increases in tension may produce pain. Most commonly they arise as a result of luminal obstruction, vascular insufficiency, ulceration, increased levels of certain pharmacologically active substances or the administration of drugs such as parasympathomimetics or codeine. Whether ulceration and ischemia produce pain by causing secondary intramural tension changes or by some other mechanism is not clear. Like other visceral forms of pain, that arising in the small intestine is not sharply localized. The sensory innervation of the small intestine derives largely from the tenth thoracic spinal segment, and small bowel pain is perceived in the corresponding somatic dermatome. Since pain originating in midline-derived structures tends to be referred to the midline, small bowel pain is characteristically periumbilical, with some spillover into the adjacent supra- and infra-umbilical areas. The increased intramural tension, regardless of cause, tends to wax and wane episodically and therefore the pain is usually described as cramping or colicky. In the presence of a pain-causing lesion, the superimposition of factors contributing to increased motor activity will lead to intensification; for example, the pain of intestinal obstruction or mesenteric vascular insufficiency is more prominent after eating. This classic description is often modified, however, by individual variations in pain threshold, prior abdominal surgical procedures, and the presence of concurrent disease. Although bilateral vagotomy has no effect on pain perception, it appears that bilateral abdominal sympathectomy, like midthoracic cord lesions, may reduce or abolish it.

Diarrhea and constipation as expressions of altered motor function cannot be as readily interpreted in terms of small intestinal disease or transit times. They are described by events occurring or not occurring at the anal opening, and interposed between this point of awareness and the small bowel are the colon and rectum. Transit times through the small bowel vary within a wide range under presumably normal conditions and only extremes will be manifest as an alteration in bowel habit. Complete obstruction of the small bowel eventually will lead to constipation. Partial obstruction may do so as well, but not infrequently the process causing the partial obstruction leads to more rapid emptying of the small bowel and colon distal to the obstruction, causing diarrhea.

The small intestine may initiate diarrhea in two ways: by exposing the colon to intestinal contents at a rate-volume relationship which exceeds its absorptive capacity or by allowing the entry into the colon of substances stimulating rapid emptying as may occur in the malabsorption syndromes. Small intestinal causes of diarrhea which are the result of abnormalities involving secretion (for example, cholera) or malabsorption (for example, nontropical sprue) will be discussed in relationship to the pathophysiology of those disorders.

Lesions which do reflect primarily, although not exclusively, abnormal motor function include obstruction, ileus, and humoral influences provided by the products of certain tumors and endocrine disorders.

Obstruction and Ileus. The term obstruction should be reserved for partial or complete occlusion of the intestinal lumen, regardless of cause. Simple obstruction implies luminal occlusion only, whereas a strangulating obstruction involves both luminal occlusion and interference with blood supply. Closed loop obstruction implies a segment of intestine with its lumen occluded at both ends. Ileus, on the other hand, refers to an adynamic state of the intestine occurring either segmentally or throughout its entire length.

Small intestinal obstruction may follow external compression from tumors or abscesses, torsion or volvulus usually in relationship to a fibrous adhesion, herniation, intussusception, intramural fibrosis as in Crohn's disease, intramural hemorrhage or edema, and intraluminal tumors, or foreign bodies such as gallstones. The manifestations of an obstruction depend upon its site, degree, duration, rapidity of development, and whether or not it is a simple, closed loop or strangulating obstruction.

When the obstruction is in the duodenum or proximal jejunum, distention is slight and there is early vomiting of large amounts of bile-stained fluid. With lesions of the lower jejunum and ileum, distention is often marked by the time vomiting of fecal-appearing material occurs. Periumbilical, cramping pain is the most prominent symptom. With complete obstruction, constipation is usual, but with partial obstruction, diarrhea or constipation may be present. Bowel sounds are more frequent and often of higher pitch in partial obstructions and early in complete obstruction, with increases in intensity often coinciding with crescendos of pain. Abdominal examination in the patient with early simple obstruction usually discloses only distention, occasional visible contractile activity, and the auscultatory findings mentioned. Percussion may reveal increased resonance but this will depend on the relative amounts of fluid and gas within the bowel lumen. Signs of peritonitis appear rapidly with strangulating obstructions, somewhat later in untreated closed loop obstructions, and relatively late in untreated simple obstructions. Although rigidity of the abdominal wall signifies peritonitis, rebound tenderness may be elicited with a distended, inflamed bowel in the absence of actual peritoneal inflammation.

Acute obstructions are usually the result of torsion or volvulus, intussusception, or herniation. Chronic obstructions are more often due to inflammatory strictures or tumors. The more slowly the obstruction develops, the more indolent and less pronounced the symptoms will be. In acute, high-grade obstruction as distention progresses, even in a localized segment, the initial intestinal hyperactivity is replaced by generalized ileus. This is due to the activation of alpha- and beta-adrenergic receptors by a sympathoadrenal discharge, with inhibition of contractile activity.

Chronic partial obstruction leads to generalized protein-calorie malnutrition, but acute obstruction causes marked abnormalities of fluid and electrolyte balance.

In contrast to obstruction, ileus represents inadequate or absent propulsive motor activity. It occurs with such regularity following abdominal operations that postoperative ileus has been referred to as physiologic ileus, even though at times it may represent a mortal complication. More severe and protracted ileus results from bacterial and chemical peritonitis or sudden and usually painful distention of other hollow structures such as the bile ducts, ureters, and urinary bladder. It may also be a sequel to complete or near complete luminal occlusion, intestinal ischemia, or hypokalemia. Ileus under these circumstances has been termed paralytic as opposed to physiologic but the difference is in degree rather than kind. All true ileus can properly be described as adynamic. Reference has occasionally been made to something called "dynamic ileus," supposedly representing functional obstruction due to intestinal spasm. This is a contradiction in terms and it is doubtful that such a condition exists, at least within the small intestine.

In the case of postoperative ileus the stomach may remain atonic for several days but the small intestine usually exhibits activity within a few hours. If the ileus persists, the bowel becomes progressively distended with gas and fluid. The gas is largely swallowed air but colonic bacteria may contribute significant amounts, especially if the small bowel has become colonized.

The most prominent findings in the patient with ileus are those related to the postoperative abdomen or the underlying disease process, usually peritonitis. There is abdominal distention, and bowel sounds are minimal or absent. Signs of dehydration and evidence of ineffective circulating plasma volume may also be present.

It has been known for some time that the gut is not intrinsically paralyzed but is capable of contraction when properly stimulated. Neely and Catchpole have redrawn attention to this fact and have proposed that ileus is due to inhibition of contractile activity by sympathetic overactivity brought about by increased levels of circulating adrenal catecholamines and/or sympathetic nerve stimulation. As previously pointed out, this reaction is mediated by adrenergic stimulation. The experimental observation that postoperative or paralytic ileus can be prevented by abdominal sympathectomy or splanchnic anesthesia has strengthened this view.

Such a mechanism readily suggests a rational approach to management, first utilizing drugs to block the sympathetic overactivity, followed by parasympathetic stimulation of the "liberated" intestine. Guanethidine and bethanechol, guanethidine and prostigmine, or phentolamine and prostigmine have been utilized with good results. Since guanethidine blocks the release of norepinephrine rather than causing alpha blockade, phentolamine, an alpha blocker, may be required if there are already increased circulating levels of epinephrine and norepinephrine. Since alpha receptors predominate in the small intestine, beta blockers appear not to be required. Patients selected for this therapy must fulfill certain criteria. Hypovolemia must be corrected first to prevent hypotension from sympathetic blockade; electrolyte balance, especially hypokalemia, must be managed and intestinal obstruction carefully excluded. Nasogastric suction also remains a useful adjunct to minimize distention. Long tubes of the Miller-Abbott type have been employed but it is often difficult to obtain passage through an adynamic gut.

Radiologic examinations utilizing plain films of the abdomen may be of help in substantiating the presence of obstruction or ileus and occasionally in differentiating the two. Dilated air-filled loops of bowel with air-fluid levels are characteristic of both. In ileus the air-filled bowel may not be as dilated as in obstruction but many exceptions will be found. Perhaps most helpful is the distribution pattern of intestinal gas. With ileus, gas is characteristically found throughout the small and large bowel, although not necessarily in a continuous column, whereas in obstruction, gas may not be present distal to the occlusion. A localized ileus may mimic obstruction, however, and it must be remembered that as the fluid-gas ratio increases, little of note may be seen radiologically.

The consequences of acute obstruction or ileus are reflected in marked alterations of fluid and electrolyte distribution. The severity of fluid loss and the extent of acid-base derangement depend not only on the anatomic portion and extent of bowel involved but also on the duration of the process. In proximal obstruction there is external loss through vomiting of large amounts of gastric, pancreatic, biliary, and duodenal secretions, with a lesser amount remaining sequestered within the gastrointestinal lumen. As much as 5 liters may be lost within a 24-hour period. Most commonly a metabolic acidosis develops, since the amount of bicarbonate lost usually exceeds the loss of hydrogen ion. With lower obstructions or generalized ileus, as much as 40 per cent of the circulating blood volume may accumulate within the gut without evidence of external fluid loss. As the bowel distends, there is increasing fluid and electrolyte accumulation within its lumen, representing a shift from the extracellular compartment. This loss is nearly isosmotic with plasma with regard to the concentrations of major ions. It represents both a decrease in insorption and an increase in exsorption. Elevations of intraluminal pressure up to 20 cm. of water increase insorption, but above this level insorption falls off while exsorption continues to increase. The mechanism underlying this effect is unknown. Initially, the serum sodium concentration remains relatively normal but gradually hyponatremia develops as sodium loss exceeds that of water. The reason for this also is not clear. Both clinical and experimental observations indicate that hypotonic dehydration leads to more profound circulatory abnormalities than does isotonic dehydration. The resulting decrease in plasma volume is at first compensated for by generalized vasoconstriction, so that blood pressure and pulse rate remain normal for a time. When these homeostatic mechanisms are interfered with by generalized anesthesia, precipitous drops in blood pressure may occur, underscoring the need for preoperative fluid replacement in all patients. Depending on the stage of the process and the rapidity of its development, various degrees of dehydration and circulatory collapse will be observed. Because of starvation, dehydration, ketosis, loss of alkaline secretions, and declining renal function, a metabolic acidosis develops. If ischemia is present, as in a strangulating obstruction, a profound and often fatal lactic acidosis may occur. Losses of potassium are high and the resulting hypokalemia may contribute to atonicity and distention. The fully developed clinical picture is one of an acutely ill patient exhibiting signs of dehydration, abdominal distention, tachycardia, hypotension, diaphoresis, hemoconcentration, normal or low serum concentrations of sodium and potassium, normal or elevated BUN and serum creatinine, and metabolic acidosis.

Strangulating obstructions develop the same pattern of fluid and electrolyte abnormalities but because of the associated intestinal ischemia also exhibit signs of tissue necrosis. Closed loop obstructions also commonly result in ischemia of the bowel wall, as do simple obstructions if they remain untreated for a sufficient length of time. As pointed out by Bynum and Jacobson, however, it is doubtful that increased intraluminal pressure per se can cause ischemic necrosis of the intestine. Decreased blood flow, mainly involving the mucosa, occurs at pressures above 30 mm. Hg but marked anoxia is prevented by the phenomena of autoregulation and autoregulatory escape (see section on mesenteric vascular disease). Additional factors such as decreases in plasma volume and reflex vasoconstriction probably are of material importance in the production of ischemia in untreated simple obstruction. In simple and closed loop obstructions, venous outflow is usually impeded first, whereas in strangulating obstructions, both arterial and venous occlusion occur early. The result is tissue anoxia, increased capillary permeability, and intramural and mucosal hemorrhage. Intramural edema and marked losses of protein develop and the integrity of the epithelial membrane is disrupted, resulting in bacterial invasion with peritonitis and bacteremia. Progressive ischemia, gangrene, and peritonitis rapidly ensue. This stage is accompanied by fever and leukocytosis in addition to the previously discussed fluid and electrolyte disturbances. With tissue necrosis and compromised renal function, hypokalemia may be replaced by hyperkalemia. Materials produced by tissue necrosis, hemorrhage, and infection accumulate in the peritoneal cavity and their absorption is a major factor in the profound cardiovascular collapse which too often characterizes the terminal phase of this condition.

Management of patients with intestinal obstruction or ileus requires early recognition of the problem, prompt differentiation of various forms of obstruction and ileus, replacement of fluid and electrolyte losses, correction of acidosis, nasogastric suction to minimize distention, and prompt surgical correction in the case of obstruction. Therapy with adrenergic blocking agents and parasympathomimetics may prove to be helpful adjuncts to the successful management of the patient with simple ileus.

Motor Dysfunction Due to Humoral Mechanisms. The electrical and contractile processes which underlie normal intestinal motor function are integrated and modified by various humoral substances, the concentrations of which under certain circumstances may be markedly altered. Hyperthyroidism, hypoparathyroidism, adrenal insufficiency, carcinoid tumors, medullary carcinomas of the thyroid, gastrin-producing tumors of the pancreas (Zollinger-Ellison syndrome), certain nongastrin-producing pancreatic tumors (Verner-Morrison syndrome), and neural crest tumors may be associated with crampy abdominal discomfort and diarrhea, while hypothyroidism and hyperparathyroidism are often characterized by constipation. Carcinoid tumors and medullary carcinomas of the thyroid may be taken as examples of this type of abnormality. It is to be emphasized, however, that most of the above conditions affect small bowel secretion as well as motor activity, so that the clinical expression observed is a net effect of the two processes.

Carcinoids may appear in any entodermally derived tissue or teratomas. In the small intestine they arise from enterochromaffin cells (Kulchitsky cells or argentaffin cells). The appendix is the most frequent site of origin (53 per cent), but carcinoids are the most common neoplasm of the small intestine, most arising in the ileum. They also may develop in other portions of the gastrointestinal tract, biliary tree, pancreas, ovary, and bronchi. They are generally small, 95 per cent being less than 2 cm. in diameter. Most appear cytologically benign, and the only reliable criteria of malignancy are invasion and metastasis. The majority are asymptomatic, being discovered in the course of investigating and treating other conditions such as appendicitis.

Clinical manifestations may be due to ulceration or obstruction or to the carcinoid syndrome.

This syndrome occurs most commonly with tumors of the jejunum or ileum which have metastasized to the liver. The pharmacologically active principles of these tumors are inactivated by hepatic enzyme systems, and therefore no systemic symptoms will be produced unless they are released into the systemic circulation. Systemic manifestations include characteristic attacks of flushing involving the head, neck, and upper trunk, at times precipitated by eating, alcohol, emotion, or pressure on the tumor; abdominal cramping pain and diarrhea; bronchoconstriction; and right-sided heart failure, pellagra-like skin lesions and ascites. Usually only a few of these features are present intermittently in any one patient.

The tumors are known to contain serotonin, 5-hydroxytryptophan, kallikreins, histamine, and ACTH. Increased serotonin levels probably are responsible for the increased intestinal motor activity and diarrhea as well as the endocardial fibrosis leading to pulmonary and tricuspid valve deformity. The metabolic pathway of serotonin is presented in Figure 26–6. Serotonin lowers the excitation threshold of intestinal smooth muscle, resulting in increased responsiveness to otherwise inadequate stimuli. In keeping with this mechanism is the sometimes beneficial effect of serotonin antagonists such as methysergide or cyproheptadine and the deleterious response to monoamine oxidase inhibitors. Improvement may also occur with p-chlorophenylalanine, which inhibits the hydroxylation of tryptophan, the rate-limiting step in serotonin synthesis, or, with methyldopa, a decarboxylase inhibitor. Serotonin is known to produce fibroblastic proliferation and its administration to experimental animals has resulted in endocardial lesions simi-

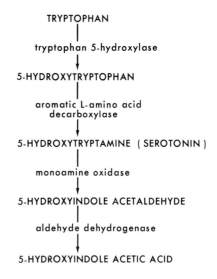

TRYPTOPHAN

tryptophan 5-hydroxylase

5-HYDROXYTRYPTOPHAN

aromatic L-amino acid decarboxylase

5-HYDROXYTRYPTAMINE (SEROTONIN)

monoamine oxidase

5-HYDROXYINDOLE ACETALDEHYDE

aldehyde dehydrogenase

5-HYDROXYINDOLE ACETIC ACID

Figure 26–6 Outline of tryptophan metabolism.

lar to those encountered in patients. Serotonin is metabolized primarily in the liver and lungs to 5-hydroxyindoleacetic acid, and increased urinary excretion of the latter is presumptive evidence for the presence of a functioning carcinoid. Slight increases in urinary 5-hydroxyindoleacetic acid, however, may be found after the ingestion of foods high in serotonin such as bananas, tomatoes, avocados, red plums, walnuts, and eggplant. Cough syrups containing glyceryl guaiacolate may cause false positive reactions for 5-hydroxyindoleacetic acid, and patients with nontropical sprue may exhibit slight elevations. The pellagra-like syndrome seen in some patients results from the diversion of large amounts of tryptophan to serotonin synthesis.

The substances responsible for the attacks of flushing and bronchoconstriction are less certain. Serotonin appears to be a less likely cause than histamine or bradykinin. Since epinephrine may provoke flushing as well as release kallikreins from tumor tissue, alpha-adrenergic blocking agents may ameliorate flushing by blocking their release.

Efforts to treat the various components of the syndrome are worthwhile even if only partially successful, since the average duration of life from the onset of symptoms to death is 8 years, with a 21 per cent 5-year survival for patients with liver metastases.

The most recent substances to be incriminated in disturbances of intestinal motor activity are the prostaglandins. They are derivatives of prostanoic acid and occur in four forms, designated E, F, A, and B, which differ in the structure of the attached 5-membered carbon ring. Although no clear role for prostaglandins in normal gut motor physiology has been demonstrated, types E and F do affect intestinal smooth muscle function. Prostaglandins $F_{1\alpha}$ and $F_{2\alpha}$ generally cause contraction of both longitudinal and circular muscle, and prostaglandins E_1 and E_2 produce contraction of longitudinal muscle and inhibition of circular muscle. The intravenous infusion of E_1 in man causes abdominal cramps and $F_{2\alpha}$ results in diarrhea. The F series act via a direct effect on circular muscle, while the E compounds affect longitudinal muscle directly as well as stimulate cholinergic nerve fibers within the small intestine. The resulting net effect is smooth muscle contraction. Some medullary carcinomas of the thyroid and neural crest tumors contain large amounts of prostaglandins E_1 and $F_{2\alpha}$ and patients often exhibit increased blood levels of these substances and have diarrhea. Since the prostaglandins probably also augment intestinal secretion via cyclic AMP, this may further contribute to the diarrhea in such patients.

Some conditions, such as scleroderma, appear to interfere with normal intestinal motor responses by structurally altering smooth muscle. Others, like diabetes mellitus, may affect function by way of lesions involving the autonomic nerve supply.

DIGESTIVE-ABSORPTIVE FUNCTION

Advances in our knowledge of normal digestive and absorptive mechanisms have enabled the physician to understand better the pathophysiology of the different malabsorption syndromes. The terms "digestion" and "absorption" merely emphasize different phases of a single continuing process initiated by events taking place within the small intestinal lumen and completed by the specialized functions of the villous absorptive cell. Its plasma membrane maintains differences in composition and electrical charge between the luminal and intracellular environment by influencing the rates at which molecules enter the cell. The differences between the function of this membrane at the cell's apical and basal surfaces result in a net movement of molecules through the cell which we call absorption.

Substances traverse this membrane by processes having different kinetics and energy requirements. These transport mechanisms include passive diffusion, nonionic diffusion, carrier-mediated transport, facilitated transport, and exchange diffusion. The term active or "uphill" transport is best used in a general sense to refer to a process requiring energy and coupled directly to cellular metabolism. Net movement is usually but not invariably against a concentration gradient and electrochemical potential difference. In this sense, only carrier-mediated processes constitute true active transport. Carrier-mediated transport is coupled to cell metabolism and exhibits substrate specificity, saturation kinetics, competitive inhibition, and counter transport. The transported substance binds reversibly to a carrier on one side of the membrane and is released on the opposite side. Solutes such as hexoses, amino acids, and pyrimidines are absorbed by this mechanism. Passive diffusion is movement due solely to the kinetic energy and electrical charge of molecules and the electrical field in which they exist. Free fatty acids and beta-monoglycerides are examples of substances absorbed by this mechanism. Nonionic diffusion involves the association between an anion and cation on one side of a membrane with the complex then crossing the membrane and dissociating on the side opposite to the original anion and cation. The net effect is the transfer of ionized compounds. In contrast to passive diffusion, nonionic diffusion accounts for the movement of a charged species independent of the electrical potential difference. Such processes are, however, highly dependent on the H^+ concentration. This type of transport characterizes the absorption of unconjugated bile salts and many drugs. Facilitated transport refers to a process that also exhibits substrate specificity, saturation kinetics, competitive inhibition, and counter transport and results in net movement of substrate but is not directly coupled to cell metabolism and cannot produce net transport against an electrochemical potential difference. Fructose absorption is in part accomplished in this way. Exchange diffusion implies the obligatory exchange of a molecule on one side of a membrane for a molecule of the same species on the opposite side. It is not directly coupled to cell metabolism and cannot produce net transport but may result in substantial fluxes across membranes. Sodium transport under certain conditions may constitute an example of exchange diffusion.

Normal Digestion and Absorption

The digestion of dietary lipids, carbohydrates, and proteins is initiated in the lumen of the duodenum and proximal jejunum and completed at the glycocalyx and microvillous plasma membrane of the jejunal absorptive cells. Normally, the resulting fatty acids, beta-monoglycerides, monosaccharides, and amino acids as well as water- and fat-soluble vitamins (with the exception of vitamin B_{12} are absorbed predominantly in the jejunum. The ileum is capable of transporting these substances but absorption is usually complete before this portion of the intestine is reached. Ileal absorption may become quantitatively important when the jejunum is abnormal

or no longer present. Figure 26–7 outlines the basic steps involved in the digestion and absorption of fat, carbohydrates, and protein.

Fat Absorption. The average American and Northern European diet contains 60 to 100 grams of fat, the majority of which is in the form of neutral fat or triglyceride. Most is hydrolyzed in the proximal small intestine by pancreatic lipase, which preferentially splits the ester bonds in the α and α' positions, forming free long-chain fatty acids and beta-monoglycerides. Pancreatic juice also contains a protein, termed colipase, which helps the lipase adhere to the lipid droplets. Pancreatic lipase has a pH optimum between 6 and 7 and is inactivated by higher H^+ concentrations. Cephalic stimulation via the vagus causes the release of cholecystokinin-pancreozymin from the duodenal and jejunal mucosa which in turn increases the secretion of lipase and other enzymes from the pancreas. Fatty acids and especially essential amino acids further augment this hormonal response, which also causes contraction of the gallbladder, increasing the delivery of bile salts and other biliary constituents to the intestinal lumen. Lipolysis does not directly alter dietary lipid solubility but the resulting fatty acids and beta-monoglycerides differ from triglycerides in being amphipaths. The bile salts are detergent-like molecules which when present in a concentration greater than 1 to 2 millimoles per liter (the critical micellar concentration) aggregate into macromolecular complexes known as micelles. The fatty acids and beta-monoglycerides, being amphipaths, will dissolve into the micelle structure of the bile salts to form mixed micelles

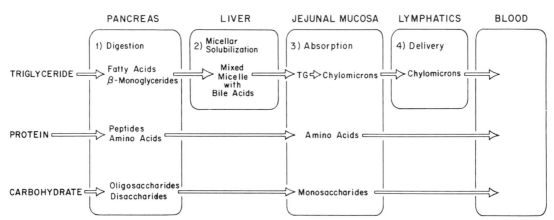

Figure 26–7 A comparison between the four major steps of fat digestion and absorption and the corresponding processes involved in the assimilation of protein and carbohydrates. This diagram emphasizes that the processes of micellar solubilization and delivery of chylomicrons through the intestinal lymphatics are not involved in the absorption of these latter two nutrients. Thus, diseases that cause dysfunction at level of step 2 or 4 result in the malabsorption only of fat, i.e., isolated steatorrhea, whereas diseases that exert their effect at the level of step 1 or 3 may produce significant malabsorption of fat, protein, and carbohydrate. (Wilson, F. A., and Dietschy, J. M.: Gastroenterology, *61*:911, 1971.)

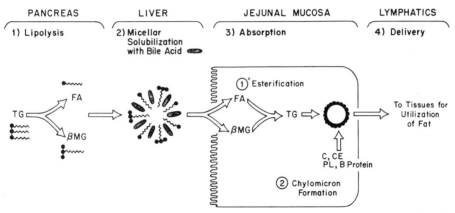

Figure 26–8 Diagrammatic representation of the major steps in the digestion and absorption of dietary fat. These include (1) the lipolysis of dietary triglyceride (TG) by pancreatic enzymes; (2) micellar solubilization of the resulting long-chain fatty acids (FA) and beta-monoglycerides (βMG) by bile acids secreted into the intestinal lumen by the liver; (3) absorption of the fatty acids and beta-monoglyceride into the mucosal cell, with subsequent re-esterification and formation of chylomicrons; and finally (4) movement of the chylomicrons from the mucosal cell into the intestinal lymphatic system. During the process of chylomicron formation small amounts of cholesterol (C), cholesterol ester (CE), and phospholipid (PL) as well as triglyceride are incorporated into this specific lipoprotein class. (Wilson, F. A., and Dietschy, J. M.: Gastroenterology, 61:911, 1971.)

and so achieve aqueous solubilization. Micelle formation accelerates the diffusion of lipolytic products through the unstirred layer to the absorptive cells. It also indirectly increases the rate of lipid hydrolysis by removing the end products of the reaction. An important characteristic of the bile salts participating in this process is their conjugation with either taurine or glycine. Normally there are no unconjugated bile salts in bile. Unconjugated bile salts are weaker detergents and less efficient contributors to micellar solubilization.

When the mixed micelle reaches the epithelial cell membrane the fatty acids and betamonoglycerides enter the cell by passive diffusion. There is then rapid re-esterification to triglyceride, which becomes associated with protein, cholesterol, cholesterol esters, and phospholipid to form a specific class of lipoproteins called chylomicrons. The chylomicrons are then released from the basal portion of the epithelial cell, cross the interstitial space and enter the lacteal. The chylomicrons are coated with apoproteins which potentiate the action of lipoprotein lipase in the systemic circulation. The chylomicrons enter the systemic circulation via the thoracic duct and are hydrolyzed as they pass through capillaries by lipoprotein lipase coating the capillary surface. The resulting fatty acids are then solubilized by being bound to albumin and transported to sites of uptake. The important steps involved in the digestion and absorption of fat are oulined in Figure 26–8.

The lacteal has a blind distal end at the villous tip and proximally anastomoses with the submucosal lymphatics. The manner in which chylomicrons gain entry into the lacteal is still debated. Electron microscopy has demonstrated no pores in the lacteal wall, but pinocytotic vesicles appear to occupy approximately 15 per cent of the endothelial cell cytoplasm, suggesting to some that this is a major pathway of chylomicron uptake. Others, however, maintain that these macromolecular aggregates enter the lacteal through gaps at the endothelial cell junctions.

The flow of lymph through the lacteal appears to be dependent on the "pumping" action of the villus, which occurs independently of intestinal motor activity. The smooth muscle fibers of the villus are responsible for this movement and may be under the control of a hormone, villikinin, found only in small intestinal mucosa and released in response to mechanical and chemical stimuli.

Some deconjugation of bile salt molecules occurs normally in the intestinal lumen and the unconjugated bile salts are absorbed largely by non-ionic diffusion throughout the small bowel. Conjugated bile salts are taken up by an active transport mechanism in the terminal ileum. Approximately 96 per cent of the bile salt pool is reabsorbed during each cycle of the enterohepatic circulation, and each day the pool is cycled 6 to 10 times. This results in a normal daily loss of only 500 mg. of bile salts in the feces. This loss is exactly compensated for by hepatic synthesis and to an extent increased losses can be balanced by increased production. Active ileal absorption is crucial, however, to maintaining the integrity of the total bile salt pool and normal micellar solubilization.

In contrast to dietary fat, the medium-chain triglycerides now widely used as dietary supplements in certain gastrointestinal disorders are composed of fatty acids of 6 to 12 carbon atoms and are handled by the gut in a somewhat different manner. They are hydrolyzed largely by pancreatic lipase, which is more active against triglycerides composed of short-chain fatty acids. Effective hydrolysis appears to occur in the presence or absence of bile salts and the hydrolytic products are mainly free fatty acids with little monoglyceride. They are not incorporated into chylomicrons but are transported by the portal venous system. Micelle formation is probably not obligatory for their effective absorption, since bile diversion has little effect on their uptake by the epithelial cells. Furthermore, a small but significant amount of medium-chain triglycerides is absorbed intact. In some patients with defective lipolysis and/or fat absorption they may constitute important forms of diet therapy because they are more efficiently handled by the gut.

Carbohydrate Absorption. Western diets contain approximately 350 grams of carbohydrate, with an average composition of 60 per cent starch, 30 per cent sucrose, and 10 per cent lactose. The conversion of these substances to monosaccharides is a necessary process for normal absorption. Salivary and to a greater extent pancreatic α-amylase attack the interior 1,4 α-linkage of amylase (starch), producing maltose and maltotriose. Amylopectin, a branched-chain carbohydrate having similar 1,4 α-linkages but in addition 1,6 α-linkages at the branching points, yields maltose, maltotriose, and branched saccharides called α-dextrins containing an average of eight glucose molecules. Isomaltose, the disaccharide with 1,6 α-linkages, is not a physiologic substrate in the small intestine. Since amylase has little or no activity for the outer 1,4 α-linkages in these molecules, no glucose is formed in the intestinal lumen under physiologic conditions. Although the intestinal mucosa is the site of some intrinsic and adsorbed amylase activity, most hydrolysis takes place within the lumen. The resulting maltose, maltotriose, and α-dextrins as well as ingested lactose and sucrose are then presented to the brush border, where they are converted to their component monosaccharides by enzymes (maltase, sucrase, lactase, and α-dextrinase) located in the glycocalyx-plasma membrane structure. From a pathophysiologic point of view, lactase is the most important of these enzymes. Lactase activity has been demonstrated to reside in three different beta galactosidases: enzyme I, a neutral lactase with a pH optimum of 5.5 to 6.0, located in the brush border

and active against lactose and synthetic beta galactosides; enzyme II, an acid beta galactosidase with a pH optimum of 4.5, located in the cellular lysosomal fraction and active against lactose and synthetic beta galactosides; and enzyme III, a cytoplasmic neutral hetero beta galactosidase, having a pH optimum of 5.5 to 6.0 and hydrolyzing only synthetic beta galactosides. Enzyme I is responsible for most normal intestinal lactase activity.

Some monosaccharides diffuse back into the lumen, but most of the glucose, galactose, and fructose is absorbed. Existing data are compatible with the hypothesis that glucose and galactose are transported from the intestinal lumen across the brush border into the epithelial cell by a shared carrier-mediated process and that the rate and direction of movement depend on the distribution ratio of Na^+ and possibly K^+ across this membrane. Sodium is therefore required for absorption and this asymmetrical distribution of cations depends directly on energy production. Fructose, however, appears to be absorbed to a large extent by facilitated transport, since it does not accumulate against its own concentration gradient, but the mechanism is saturable and its absorption is more rapid than pentoses but slower than that of glucose or galactose. The events involved in the digestion and absorption of carbohydrates are schematically summarized in Figure 26–9.

An important concept, not yet fully developed, involves the dietary regulation of small intestinal enzyme activity. Rosensweig has studied the adaptive responses of disaccharidase and glycolytic enzymes (common to all cells) in man following dietary manipulation. Sucrose or fructose feeding increases the activities of sucrase and maltase but not lactase, whereas glucose and galactose also enhance glycolytic enzyme activity, but the increase is less than that observed after feeding isocaloric amounts of noncarbohydrate calories. In the case of disaccharidases, the adaptive response occurs within a 2- to 5-day period (the time required for intestinal cell renewal), suggesting an action on the undifferentiated crypt cells. In the experimental animal, lactase activity adapts in a period of 8 to 10 weeks, but short-term experiments in man have failed to show lactase adaptation.

The full implication of this phenomenon is not yet apparent, but it is obvious that dietary habits must be taken into consideration when abnormalities of epithelial enzyme activity are present.

Protein Absorption. The usual dietary intake of 70 to 90 grams of protein presents the digestive-absorptive mechanism with a more complex task than that presented by fat or carbohydrate. A much larger group of enzymes is required to re-

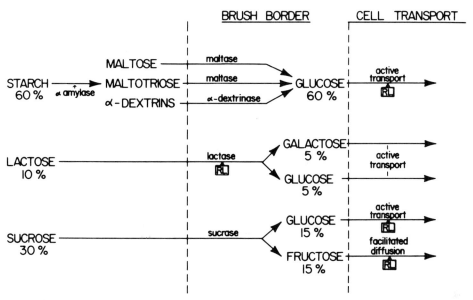

INTRALUMINAL

INTESTINAL

Figure 26–9 Schematic representation of the events involved in the digestion and absorption of carbohydrates. RL is the rate-limiting step in the particular reaction. (Gray, G. M.: Gastroenterology, *58*:96, 1970.)

duce native proteins to their amino acid components. This process is initiated in the gastrointestinal lumen by pepsin, which is dispensable for adequate protein assimilation, and the numerous pancreatic proteases including trypsinogen, chymotrypsinogen, procarboxypeptidase A, procarboxypeptidase B, leucine aminopeptidase, proelastase, and nucleases. They are released largely in response to vagal influences and the action of cholecystokinin-pancreozymin. These mechanisms are described more fully in the chapter dealing with the pancreas and in the portion of this section discussing the endocrine function of the small intestine. The inactive trypsinogen is converted to active trypsin by enterokinase, and the trypsin then acts to complete the conversion of the other proenzymes to their active forms. Trypsin and chymotrypsin are endopeptidases which split the peptide bonds within the protein molecule, while the carboxypeptidases are exopeptidases acting only on the terminal peptide bonds. These various enzymes differ in both topographical activity and amino acid specificity, and because of their restricted sites of action, protein digestion occurs only by virtue of their sequential activity.

A large proportion of the pancreatic proteases are adsorbed onto the epithelial cell surface, and whether their activity is exerted mainly within the lumen or in the region of the microvilli is

uncertain. In either case, peptides that are 3 to 6 amino acid residues long are released and presented to the brush border and intracellular enzyme systems, where three groups of peptidases complete the process of amino acid liberation. The amino-oligopeptidases have been partially localized to the brush border and hydrolyze the longer peptides probably to amino acids, dipeptides, and tripeptides. The amino-tripeptidases, also partially localized to the brush border, split the N-terminal residues from tripeptides. Lastly, there are several dipeptidases including glycylglycine peptidase, leucyl-glycine peptidase, glycylleucine peptidase and imino and imido peptidases hydrolyzing proline-containing peptides. Their location is not known.

From studies comparing normal and cystinuric patients it is clear that both free amino acids and dipeptides can enter the epithelial cell and significant dipeptidase activity probably takes place within the cytoplasm. Only certain amino acids are in fact readily released within the lumen in free form. Appreciable amounts of the basic amino acids (arginine and lysine) and neutral amino acids (valine, phenylalanine, tyrosine, methionine, and leucine) are released and transported by the epithelial cell membrane. In contrast, glycine, the imino acids (proline and hydroxyproline), the hydroxyl-substituted amino acids (serine and threonine), and the dicarboxylic amino acids (aspartic and glutamic) remain about 90 per cent peptide-linked until their disappearance from the lumen, and they presumably enter the cell as constituents of small peptides. It is clear that glycine is more rapidly and efficiently absorbed as the di- and tripeptide than as the free amino acid. The physiologic importance of oligopeptide absorption, however, remains unclear. Most peptides are hydrolyzed by several electrophoretically distinct enzymes and, conversely, each enzyme hydrolyzes several different peptides. The specificity and localization of the many intestinal peptidases are still uncertain and their role in protein digestion is obviously more complex than the brush border disaccharidase system.

The manner in which peptides cross the plasma membrane is unknown. It has been proposed that amino acids are transported via a carrier-mediated process that, like hexose absorption, is stimulated by Na^+. Amino acid influx is not tightly coupled to Na^+ influx, however, and in the absence of Na^+ amino acid transport still exhibits saturation kinetics and competitive inhibition. Sodium does not affect the maximum velocity of amino acid influx but does increase the apparent affinity of the carrier system. Hereditary defects of amino acid transport have provided evidence for several different transport systems, each having different affinities for different groups of amino acids. These are presented in Table 26–1.

Somewhat analogous to carbohydrate digestion, it is apparent that the absorption rates of essential amino acids at least can be influenced by dietary, caloric, or protein deprivation in man. Adibi and Allen subjected patients to a 14-day period of either protein or protein-calorie deprivation and found a decreased rate of jejunal amino acid transport with a corresponding increase in fecal nitrogen, which could not be correlated with any light or electron microscopic changes. This sort of observation again emphasizes the potential modifications in intestinal absorptive function that may follow dietary manipulation.

Folic Acid and Vitamin B$_{12}$ Absorption. Folic acid is 2-amino,4-hydroxypteridine joined to a p-aminobenzoic acid residue and linked to one molecule of L-glutamic acid. Naturally occurring folates contain additional L-glutamic acid molecules linked by the unusual γ-peptide bond, with pteroylheptaglutamic acid being the principal species in most plant and animal tissues. This conjugated form is converted in the small intestine to the free monoglutamate by γ-glutamyl carboxypeptidase ("conjugase"), an enzyme associated with the mucosal cell but of which the precise site of action is unknown. Absorption of pteroylmonoglutamic acid occurs largely in the proximal small intestine but its transport mechanism has not been defined. Within the intestinal cell the monoglutamate is converted by dihydrofolate reductase and a methylating mechanism to reduced methyl folate (largely 5-methyltetrahydrofolate) prior to entry into the portal circulation. Tetrahydrofolic acid functions as a cofactor in various important enzyme systems.

Vitamin B$_{12}$ in food is bound to protein by peptide bonds which are hydrolyzed by cooking, acidification, and proteolytic enzymes. In the presence of the free vitamin, intrinsic factor produced by the gastric parietal cells dimerizes and one

TABLE 26–1   INTESTINAL AMINO ACID TRANSPORT MECHANISMS

Type	Amino Acids Transported	Type of Transport	Rate
Neutral (monoamino-monocarboxylic)	Aromatic (tyrosine, tryptophan, phenylalanine) Aliphatic (glycine,* alanine, serine, threonine, valine, leucine, isoleucine) Methionine, histidine, glutamine, asparagine, cysteine	Active, Na^+-dependent	Very rapid
Dibasic (diamino)	Lysine, arginine, ornithine, cystine	Active, partially Na^+-dependent	Rapid (10% of neutral)
Dicarboxylic (acidic)	Glutamic acid, aspartic acid	Carrier-mediated, ?active, partially Na^+-dependent	Rapid
Imino acids and glycine	Proline, hydroxyproline, glycine*	Active, ?Na^+-dependent	Slow

*Shares both the neutral and imino mechanism with low affinity for the neutral.
From Gray, G. M., and Cooper, H. L.: Gastroenterology, *61*:535, 1971.

mole of the dimer binds two moles of the vitamin. In addition to being essential for its active ileal absorption, intrinsic factor probably serves to protect vitamin B_{12} from digestion and to a limited extent from bacterial utilization. The free vitamin can be absorbed by passive diffusion throughout the small intestine but only 1 per cent is handled in this way. The absorption of physiologic amounts (> 2 mg.) is intrinsic factor-mediated and takes place only in the terminal ileum where 60 to 80 per cent is absorbed. The B_{12}-intrinsic factor complex attaches to receptors located in the glycocalyx-plasma membrane complex of the terminal ileal absorptive cells. This attachment requires the presence of Ca^{++} and/or Mg^{++} and a pH above 5.6. The vitamin B_{12} is released from intrinsic factor in or on the ileal absorptive cell and is transported to the portal blood bound to a carrier, transcobalamin. Vitamin B_{12} has an enterohepatic circulation with two thirds to three fourths of biliary B_{12} reabsorbed in the ileum, provided that intrinsic factor is adequate. The fate of intrinsic factor is not clear but it does not appear to be absorbed (see Chapter 27).

The absorption of other water-soluble vitamins has been little studied and the manner in which ascorbic acid, riboflavin, and other members of the B group are handled by the small intestine is largely unknown. Absorption of the fat-soluble vitamins A, D, E, and K in general parallels that of lipid absorption. Vitamin A deserves special comment here, since its absorption has been utilized as a form of lipid tolerance test. It is ingested largely in an esterified form which requires hydrolysis by pancreatic and brush border enzymes prior to micellar solubilization. After entering the epithelial cell it is re-esterified with long-chain fatty acids and transported via the lymph in association with the chylomicrons. It has recently been appreciated, however, that significant absorption occurs by way of the portal vein. Consequently, vitamin A transport is a more general index of absorption and is not strictly equatable with lipid tolerance. The absorption of the other fat-soluble vitamins as well as iron and calcium is discussed in those sections dealing with their overall metabolism and pathophysiology.

The digestive-absorptive process therefore involves not only the handling of a wide range of ingested materials but numerous enzymes and hormones, each requiring its own optimal environment, as well as highly specialized cellular structure-function relationships. Although such physiologic complexity quite naturally predisposes to pathophysiologic diversity, it is in most instances possible to understand the different malabsorption syndromes in terms of one or more alterations in this overall process.

Abnormalities of Digestion and Absorption

Many disease processes directly or indirectly alter gastrointestinal physiology in such a manner that normal absorptive mechanisms are compromised and maldigestion or malabsorption of one or more dietary constituents occurs. There may be malabsorption of fat alone or of protein and carbohydrate as well. A defect may be so severe and widespread that it precludes the normal absorption of any ingested nutrient, or so circumscribed that only single substances are affected. Furthermore, some disorders cause malabsorption by more than one pathophysiologic mechanism.

A large number of tests have been utilized in the differential diagnosis of malabsorption syndromes. However, many are of little value despite their continued use. The physician who has a sound understanding of the normal mechanisms of digestion and absorption as well as the tests useful in their investigation will be able to arrive at a correct diagnosis in the vast majority of cases by correlating clinical information with the following diagnostic procedures: the quantitative determination of stool fat, the quantitative determination of stool nitrogen, the xylose absorption test, the lactose tolerance test, the vitamin B_{12} absorption test, and peroral intestinal biopsy. Hemoglobin concentrations and red cell morphology as well as serum levels of albumin, cholesterol, carotene, prothrombin activity, iron, calcium, phosphorus, and alkaline phosphatase are *nutritional indices* and not tests of absorption. Abnormalities may reflect not only malabsorption but inadequate intake and increased utilization or loss by other routes.

The quantitative chemical determination of fecal fat is the most reliable measure of steatorrhea. The amount of fat appearing in the stool of normal individuals is usually less than 7 per cent of the dietary intake. With the usual intake of 60 to 100 grams, this will result in the excretion of less than 6 grams per 24 hours. Even with intakes as high as 200 grams, only 8.7 plus or minus 0.7 grams will appear in the stool. With zero fat intake, approximately 3 grams will still be present, presumably from sloughed epithelial cells and bacterial lipids. In the patient with compromised digestive or absorptive capacity the amount of fat excreted in the stool is more directly related to the amount ingested. The van de Kamer method is most commonly employed for quantitating fecal fat, but this procedure must be modified for the patient receiving medium-chain triglycerides, since medium-chain fatty acids will otherwise be underestimated.

The normal fecal nitrogen excretion is in the range of 2.0 and 2.5 grams in persons with intakes between 80 and 100 grams. Desquamation of epithelial cells, secretory proteins, and leakage of plasma proteins contribute to the intraluminal nitrogen pool and, provided that significant protein-losing enteropathy is not present, fecal nitrogen determinations are a useful measure of protein malabsorption.

Xylose, a 5-carbon monosaccharide, is absorbed primarily by passive means in the proximal small intestine. The amount excreted in the urine during the first five hours following an oral dose of 25 grams should be greater than 4.5 grams. Artifactually low values may be due to vomiting, delayed gastric emptying, dehydration, impaired renal function, or the presence of massive ascites. The mean normal excretory rate also decreases with advancing age and probably is reflective of declining renal function. Values less than 2.5 to 3.0 grams are encountered in disease states in which there is significant loss of the functional integrity of the jejunum or massive bacterial overgrowth in the proximal small intestine, resulting in bacterial utilization. The administra-

tion of antibiotics may correct abnormal values due to the latter condition.

Vitamin B_{12} absorption usually is assessed by some variation of the standard Schilling test. Excretion of greater than 5 to 8 per cent in 24 hours of the orally administered radiolabeled B_{12} is generally regarded as normal. Provided that the patient has or has been given adequate amounts of intrinsic factor, excretory rates below 1 to 3 per cent per 24 hours are found in two situations: (1) in the presence of massive bacterial overgrowth or infestation with certain tapeworms involving the proximal small intestine, in which there is binding of both free B_{12} and the B_{12}-intrinsic factor complex by the microorganisms; and (2) disease states or surgical procedures that lead to significant loss of the functional integrity of the terminal ileum. The administration of appropriate antibiotics will often correct the Schilling test in the former but not the latter situation.

Peroral intestinal biopsy has considerably facilitated the diagnosis of certain malabsorption syndromes. Knowledge of normal histology at var-

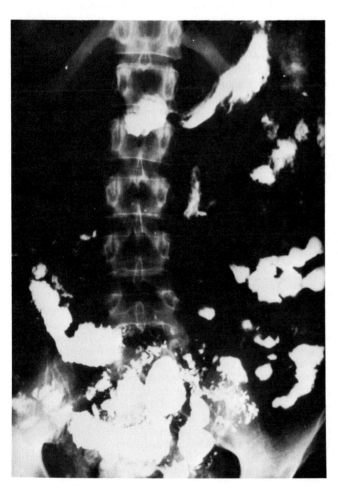

Figure 26–10 Barium meal demonstrating a typical malabsorption pattern, consisting of segmentation, localized dilatation, and moulage formation.

ious levels of the intestine as well as variations encountered in different populations is a definite requisite for making comparisons with diseased tissues. In at least five specific disorders the histologic findings are sufficiently unique to be diagnostic: nontropical sprue, Whipple's disease, a-beta-lipoproteinemia, amyloidosis, and mastocytosis. In radiation enteritis, lymphangiectasia, tropical sprue, nongranulomatous ulcerative jejunitis, scleroderma, eosinophilic gastroenteritis, dermatitis herpetiformis, hypogammaglobulinemia, and some parasitic infestations the changes are usually compatible with but not diagnostic of the particular disorder. In most other conditions leading to maldigestion and malabsorption small intestinal histology is normal, at least to light microscopy.

The signs and symptoms exhibited by the patient with a malabsorption syndrome quite naturally will vary with the disease responsible. The manifestations of the malabsorption itself will depend on the nature and amount of the substances involved and the duration of the process. Weight loss, muscle wasting, anemia, tetany, edema, bleeding tendencies, osteomalacia, osteoporosis, fatigue, abdominal distention, multiple vitamin deficiencies, steatorrhea, and diarrhea are commonly observed in various combinations. Classically, with steatorrhea the stools are described as voluminous or bulky, foul smelling, greasy, frothy, pale yellow, and floating. Unfortunately, not all such descriptions by the patient will be associated with an increase in fecal fat, and significant steatorrhea may exist in the absence of any of these characteristics. True diarrhea may be produced by disorders causing a decrease in transit time, the malabsorption of water and electrolytes, the malabsorption of bile salts, or the cathartic action of hydroxylated fatty acids. Hypocalcemia and hypophosphatemia result from the formation of insoluble calcium soaps with unabsorbed fatty acids, vitamin D deficiency, and loss of calcium-binding protein normally located in the glycocalyx.

Radiologic examination of the small intestine with a barium meal may be helpful in disclosing a "malabsorption pattern" but is rarely capable of providing an etiologic diagnosis. The characteristic features are illustrated in Figure 26–10 and include localized dilatations, segmentation of the barium column, loss of mucosal detail (moulage), flocculation of the barium due to the presence of increased amounts of water and mucus in the intestinal lumen, and thickening of the valvulae conniventes.

The presence of a malabsorption syndrome therefore must be suspected under a variety of clinical circumstances. An understanding of the pathophysiologic mechanisms that may be responsible is essential to the proper interpretation

of clinical signs and symptoms as well as abnormalities reported by the clinical laboratory. A classification of malabsorption syndromes based upon the type of defect responsible is presented in Table 26–2. The normal digestive-absorptive process may be disrupted by abnormalities occur-

TABLE 26–2 A PATHOPHYSIOLOGIC CLASSIFICATION OF DISORDERS ASSOCIATED WITH MALABSORPTION

Abnormalities of intraluminal events
  Inadequate digestion
    Pancreatic insufficiency
    Acid hypersecretion
    Gastric resection
  Altered bile salt metabolism
    Intraluminal binding of bile salts
    Hepatobiliary disease
    Ileal resection or disease
    Bacterial overgrowth
Abnormalities of mucosal transport
  Generalized defects
    Nontropical sprue (celiac disease, gluten enteropathy)
    Tropical sprue
    Crohn's disease
    Intestinal resection or bypass
    Nongranulomatous ulcerative jejunitis
    Radiation enteritis
    Whipple's disease
    Drug-induced malabsorption
    Hypothyroidism
    Addison's disease
    Hyperthyroidism
    Hypoparathyroidism
    Parasitic disease
    Mast cell disease
    Dermatitis herpetiformis
    Intestinal ischemia
    Intestinal lymphoma
    Protein malnutrition
    Amyloidosis
  Selective defects
    A-β-lipoproteinemia
    Disaccharidase deficiency
    Monosaccharide malabsorption
    Amino acid malabsorption
    Vitamin B_{12} malabsorption
Abnormalities of lymphatic transport
    Primary intestinal lymphangiectasia
    Whipple's disease
    Crohn's disease
    Radiation enteritis
    Intestinal lymphoma
    Constrictive pericarditis
    Congestive heart failure
Unclassified abnormalities
    Carcinoid syndrome
    Dysgammaglobulinemias
    Diabetic gastroenteropathy
    Scleroderma

ring within the intestinal lumen, at the level of the mucosa (involving the absorptive cells or the lamina propria) or the intestinal lymphatics.

Intraluminal Abnormalities. The intraluminal phase of the digestive-absorptive process is concerned with the digestion of fats, carbohydrates, and proteins, and the micellar solubilization of free fatty acids and beta-monoglycerides. Maldigestion will result from any disorder interfering with *effective* pancreatic enzyme activity. This may be due to abnormalities of pancreatic exocrine function secondary to chronic pancreatitis, carcinoma of the pancreas, mucoviscidosis, or pancreatic resection, which reduce the absolute amount of enzyme available, or to acid hypersecretion and gastric resection, which result in ineffective activity of otherwise adequate amounts of enzyme.

Several factors appear to play a role in the malabsorption associated with the acid hypersecretion of the Zollinger-Ellison syndrome. The low intraluminal pH denatures or inactivates pancreatic enzymes, especially lipase, and conjugated bile salts may be precipitated from solution. It is also possible that the absorptive capacity of the mucosal cells may be impaired by acid injury. Pancreatic exocrine insufficiency results in severe steatorrhea and nitrogen loss, but xylose absorption, and jejunal histology are normal. Mild, variable decreases in vitamin B_{12} absorption may occur. The cause is unknown. Since micelles are present in most instances the absorption of fat-soluble vitamins is less affected. Patients with the Zollinger-Ellison syndrome exhibit moderate increases in fecal fat and slight impairment of xylose absorption. B_{12} absorption and jejunal histologic findings are normal. No values for fecal nitrogen have been reported.

Following gastric resection particularly with a Billroth II-type anastomosis, malabsorption may involve interference with absorptive processes at several steps. Duodenal bypass leads to a poor secretory response of the pancreas and inadequate mixing of food with bile salts and pancreatic enzymes. Rapid intestinal transit also may occur, with a reduction of contact time between the intestinal contents and the mucosal absorptive cells. The reasons for the abnormal transit time are essentially unknown. An additional factor in certain patients is massive bacterial overgrowth in the afferent loop, giving rise to an intestinal stasis syndrome (see below). Steatorrhea is generally mild, and nitrogen excretion and xylose absorption are usually normal, although the latter may be reduced in the presence of a stasis syndrome. Jejunal biopsy usually is normal but occasionally reveals mild villous atrophy of doubtful functional significance. Vitamin B_{12} absorption may be reduced for three possible reasons: (1) inadequate intrinsic factor secretion

by the gastric remnant; (2) rapid passage of B_{12} through the gastric remnant, preventing the formation of the B_{12}-intrinsic factor complex; or (3) the presence of an afferent loop stasis syndrome. Correction of an abnormal Schilling test with exogenous intrinsic factor or antibiotics will help in determining the precise cause. Although many inconsistencies are encountered, malabsorption tends to occur with a decreasing order of severity subsequent to the following surgical procedures: total gastrectomy with esophagojejunostomy, subtotal gastrectomy with gastrojejunostomy, subtotal gastrectomy with gastroduodenostomy, and vagotomy and pyloroplasty.

Altered bile salt metabolism with failure to achieve adequate micellar solubilization may result from one or more different mechanisms. Intraluminal binding of bile salts occurs with the administration of cholestyramine, a nonabsorbable anion exchange resin used in the management of intractable pruritus due to increased tissue levels of bile salts. In general, steatorrhea is present only in patients receiving in excess of 12 grams per day and fecal fat losses are relatively mild. Portal-systemic shunts that lower the extraction of bile salts from portal venous blood, hepatocellular disease that reduces bile acid synthesis, and intra- or extrahepatic cholestasis with or without jaundice which limits biliary excretion all may contribute to a micellar defect. The result is an isolated, mild steatorrhea. The reason why the steatorrhea is not more severe is that the two most important steps in fat absorption remain intact: lipolysis and epithelial cell uptake. Furthermore, the ileum, which does not normally participate significantly in fat absorption, in part compensates for decreased jejunal uptake. In patients with an external biliary fistula, for example, fat absorption is little impaired on a low fat intake and as much as 75 per cent of an intake of 120 grams may be absorbed. With increasing intake, however, there is increasing steatorrhea. More severe disturbances in the absorption of the fat-soluble vitamins occur since they are not detectably absorbed in the absence of micelles.

Blind loop or intestinal stasis syndromes may be due to a variety of anatomic or motor disturbances of the intestine including afferent loops following gastric resection, enteroenterostomy or internal fistulas with bypass of a segment of small bowel, multiple strictures, jejunal diverticulosis, scleroderma, diabetic enteropathy, and gastrocolic fistula. The common denominator is stasis and bacterial colonization of the small intestine with a more fecal type of flora. Bacterial counts in luminal fluid from the duodenum, jejunum, and proximal ileum normally are low, in the range of less than 10^4 per ml., and consist primarily of streptococci, aerobic lactobacilli, and diphtheroids as well as fungi. The distal ileum represents a transitional zone, with bacterial counts between 10^5 and 10^8 per ml. In two thirds of cases there are appreciable numbers of gram-negative organisms, largely aerobic coliforms with very few anerobic bacteria such as bacteroides. The two most important factors controlling the "relative sterility" of the proximal small intestine are gastric acid secretion and the cleansing action of propulsive motor activity. It is also probably important that bacterial generation times are much longer in the intestinal lumen than under in-vitro conditions. An alteration in these protective mechanisms may permit the establishment of a colonic type of flora containing large numbers of bacteroides, coliforms, and clostridia. This bacterial overgrowth has several important metabolic effects. First, and most important, there is deconjugation and dehydroxylation of bile salts resulting in decreased micelle formation. Second, the bacteria are capable of binding the B_{12}-intrinsic factor complex, preventing its absorption, and of metabolizing xylose. The characteristic findings in patients with an intestinal stasis syndrome therefore include mild steatorrhea and abnormal B_{12} absorption. Fecal nitrogen values and jejunal histologic findings usually are normal, while xylose absorption may be normal or decreased. The abnormal values for fecal fat and the diminished B_{12} and xylose absorption most often return to normal after several days of antibiotic therapy, especially with lincomycin.

Bacterial stasis syndromes may result in some additional effects unrelated to malabsorption: (1) increased serum folate levels due to bacterial synthesis and release of folic acid; (2) increased urinary indican excretion from the conversion of tryptophan to indole which is hydroxylated and sulfated in the liver to indoxysulfate or indican; and (3) increased ammonia production by the deamination of dietary protein to form urea, with subsequent conversion to ammonia by intestinal ureases.

Abnormalities of Mucosal Transport. Most disorders affecting the small intestinal mucosa result in widespread defects characterized by malabsorption of most normally transported materials. Any process causing structural or functional abnormalities of the glycocalyx-plasma membrane digestive-absorptive unit, the remainder of the epithelial cell proper, or the surrounding lamina propria may produce a generalized malabsorption syndrome. Most, if not all, tests of absorption will be abnormal and the fecal losses of fat and nitrogen are often severe. On the other hand, highly specific defects may occur with only single substances exhibiting abnormal transport.

Nontropical sprue (celiac disease, gluten-sensitive enteropathy) provides a good example of generalized primary intestinal malabsorption. Jejunal biopsies of patients with untreated celiac

disease almost always show total or near total villous atrophy. In order for this to be apparent it is important that the sections be properly oriented so that they are cut perpendicular to the luminal surface. The total mucosal thickness is relatively normal and as a result the crypts appear elongated. The surface epithelial cells exhibit several abnormalities: (1) their vertical height is decreased and they assume a more cuboidal shape; (2) the simple columnar orientation is replaced by a stratified configuration; (3) cytoplasmic degenerative changes are apparent; (4) the brush border structure is attenuated or even inapparent; (5) there is a relative decrease in goblet cells; and (6) there is infiltration of the epithelial cell layer by lymphocytes. The crypt cells generally appear normal by both light and electron microscopy but there is a relative increase in the number of Paneth and enterochromaffin cells, and the undifferentiated cells at the bases of the crypts exhibit increased mitoses. In fact, Trier and Browning, using tissue cultures of intestinal epithelium from untreated patients, found an increased proliferation and migration of crypt cells similar to the recovery phase of sublethal ionizing radiation. The cells also reverted to a more normal appearance after only 24 hours in a gluten-free medium. The lamina propria contains increased numbers of plasma cells and eosinophils and the interstitial spaces appear to be filled with a lightly staining amorphous material. Morphologic changes are most marked in the duodenum and jejunum and tend to be less prominent in the ileum.

Although the cereal protein gluten (wheat, rye, barley, and oats) is firmly established as the offending agent, the mechanism of its noxious effect remains unknown. Gluten is the starch-free portion of the cereal grain, and the toxic factor is contained in its 70 per cent alcohol-soluble fraction (gliadin). This consists of a complex mixture of several electrophoretically and chromatographically separable proteins of varying molecular weight. Clinical challenge with peptic-tryptic digests suggests that the toxic factor is a polypeptide of molecular weight less than 1000. Efforts to demonstrate abnormal peptidase activity in treated patients, however, have failed. Antibodies to gluten fractions are present in the serum and intestinal secretions of untreated and to a lesser extent of treated patients, but their significance is debated. No antibodies in the diseased tissue itself react with gluten fractions and no complement-fixing immune complexes have been demonstrated. Interestingly enough, however, the celiac jejunal epithelial cells uniquely bind gluten fractions in vitro. Whatever the reason, the basic problem appears to be an inadequately compensated, shortened life span of the villous absorptive cells.

The net result is a decrease in intestinal surface area, a loss of enzymes and carriers, and compromised absorptive cell function. The main physiologic defect is a failure of transport by the epithelial cell. The result is malabsorption of most dietary constituents, including fat, carbohydrate, protein, vitamins, iron, and calcium. The fecal losses of fat and nitrogen tend to be relatively severe and the absorption of xylose is markedly impaired. Jejunal histology in the untreated case is essentially diagnostic. Vitamin B_{12} absorption may be normal or low, depending upon the severity of the ileal abnormality. The anemia which develops is most commonly due to iron deficiency, but macrocytic anemias due to folic acid and less often to B_{12} deficiency are also frequent. With the loss of brush border enzymes, disaccharidase deficiencies occur, of which lactose intolerance is clinically the most prominent. Water and electrolyte transport also are affected, and perfusion of the jejunum with isotonic electrolyte solutions results in a net secretion of water, sodium, and potassium instead of absorption.

Improvement of absorption coincides with the removal of gluten-containing cereals and cereal products from the diet. Cytologic abnormalities begin to disappear within a matter of days, whereas villous architecture reverts toward normal over a period of weeks and months. It is doubtful, however, whether villi ever achieve a totally normal appearance.

Other clinical entities which are characterized by abnormal villous architecture and distorted morphology of intestinal absorptive cells include tropical sprue, dermatitis herpetiformis, and nongranulomatous ulcerative jejunitis. The absorptive defect therefore is qualitatively similar to that of celiac disease.

In contrast, the morphologic changes in Whipple's disease are most striking in the lamina propria, where the normal cellular elements are replaced by macrophages containing periodic acid-Schiff positive glycoprotein within their cytoplasm. In addition, rod-shaped structures can be seen in the lamina propria that under the electron microscope have the features of bacteria. The villous absorptive cells and mucosal surface area, however, are relatively well preserved. Nonetheless, in-vitro studies of tissue biopsy specimens have demonstrated impaired amino acid transport and fatty acid esterification. There is also morphologic evidence suggesting an impaired delivery of triglyceride to the lymphatics. Precisely how the observed structural abnormalities are translated into functional defects is not clear. Characteristically, patients with Whipple's disease exhibit severe malabsorption of fat and protein but very little alteration of xylose or B_{12} absorption.

The malabsorption associated with intestinal resection can be divided into three essentially distinct syndromes: massive resection or bypass; removal of the jejunum; and ileectomy. It is patently obvious why the first of these results in severe malabsorption of fat and protein as well as of xylose and vitamin B_{12}. On the other hand, removal of the jejunum causes only a mild defect in fat absorption, presumably because the ileum can almost totally compensate for its loss. This may simply represent the expression of functions not normally called upon in the presence of an intact jejunum. The jejunum, however, is selectively important for the absorption of iron, calcium, and folic acid, and extensive jejunal resection commonly results in severe deficiencies of these nutrients. Conversely, loss of the ileum leads to a more severe malabsorption of fat and B_{12}. This is because disruption of the enterohepatic circulation of bile salts results in ineffective micellar solubilization. Ordinarily this would produce only a modest steatorrhea, because the ileum would partially compensate for the resulting reduced jejunal absorption. When the ileum is missing or diseased, however, this cannot occur. Furthermore, the coexisting B_{12} deficiency itself appears to affect the maturation of villous absorptive cells, thereby contributing to the absorptive defect. Loss of the ileum is also frequently associated with watery diarrhea which is due to the cathartic action of the large amount of unabsorbed bile salts entering the colon.

Adaptive changes in the remaining intestine leading to increased absorption are well documented in experimental animals but have been little studied in man. It has been shown in man that a gradual improvement in fat, carbohydrate, and nitrogen absorption occurs after extensive small bowel resection, and intestinal biopsies have revealed an increase in the number of epithelial cells per unit length of the villus, suggesting mucosal cell hyperplasia.

A number of drugs have been implicated in the production of mucosal transport defects primarily involving fat. Cholestyramine has been discussed in relation to its effect on micelle formation. Colchicine produces a diffuse alteration of absorptive function manifested by slightly increased fecal losses of fat and nitrogen and decreased xylose absorption. It probably exerts this effect by disturbing epithelial cell function and inhibiting cell renewal. A variety of cathartic agents may also cause slight steatorrhea, hypokalemia, and protein-losing enteropathy, but no satisfactory explanation of their effect has been put forward. Neomycin, the most widely studied of the drugs producing malabsorption, has been shown to produce morphologic changes in intestinal villi, to inhibit the intraluminal hydrolysis of triglycerides, and to precipitate bile salts. Neomycin is a polybasic aminoglucoside, and it has been suggested that an interaction between its cationic amino groups and the anionic fatty acids and bile acids leads to precipitation of the whole micellar complex. Triparanol produces an intestinal lesion indistinguishable from celiac disease and results in mild fat and nitrogen losses. High doses of para-aminosalicylic acid also have induced a reversible defect in fat and xylose absorption.

The remainder of the mucosal transport defects listed in Table 26–2 lead to malabsorption by even less well understood mechanisms. Some disorders such as amyloidosis, radiation enteritis, parasitic infection, and mast cell disease are associated with morphologic abnormalities, whereas the various endocrinopathies appear to represent mucosal cell dysfunction induced by metabolic influences.

In contrast to these generalized absorptive defects, a few conditions represent defective transport of a single substance. Except for a-beta-lipoproteinemia they are not characterized by any morphologic abnormalities, and only lactase deficiency and pernicious anemia occur with any frequency.

A-beta-lipoproteinemia is a rare disorder involving a partial or total absence of plasma beta-lipoprotein. It is probably inherited as an autosomal recessive, and total deficiency is associated with lipid malabsorption, acanthocytosis, peripheral neuropathy, and retinal lesions. The defect in lipid absorption and the absence of beta-lipoproteins appear to be due to an inability of the epithelial cell to synthesize the protein moiety of chylomicrons. Jejunal biopsies reveal a normal villous architecture, but in the fasting state numerous cytoplasmic fat droplets are found in the absorptive cells. Mild steatorrhea is the only absorptive abnormality observed.

Isolated vitamin B_{12} deficiency is most commonly due to inadequate intrinsic factor activity in association with pernicious anemia, chronic atrophic gastritis, and subtotal or total gastrectomy. As discussed previously, gastrectomy may or may not be associated with the malabsorption of other substances. Resection or disease of the ileum is seldom if ever characterized by defective B_{12} transport alone. A condition referred to as selective B_{12} malabsorption (Imerslund's syndrome) has been described, however, which may represent absence of ileal B_{12}-intrinsic factor receptors. Those affected are most often children of North African non-Ashkenazic origin who have renal abnormalities with proteinuria, normal intrinsic factor activity, and no intrinsic factor antibodies.

Abnormalities of hexose transport may also involve a single substance. Congenital glucose-galactose malabsorption presents in infancy as intractable diarrhea until these monosaccharides or their disaccharide precursors are excluded from the diet. In some, there is an associated glycosuria, suggesting a coexisting renal tubule transport defect. It seems likely that the specific carrier involved in glucose-galactose transport is lacking or defective, since sodium flux and other sodium-dependent processes such as amino acid absorption are normal.

Spontaneously occurring defects of amino acid transport have contributed important information to our understanding of the different types of carrier systems involved in normal amino acid transport. They have also emphasized the great similarity between intestinal and renal tubule transport systems. Cystinuria, an inherited disorder of basic amino acid transport, is perhaps the best studied of such defects. These patients have defective renal and intestinal transport systems for cystine, arginine, ornithine, and lysine. Three forms have been described, depending on the type of intestinal transport defect: Type I, in which there is absent intestinal transport of both cystine and the dibasic amino acids; Type II, in which there is absent intestinal transport of both cystine and the dibasic amino acids; Type II, in which only dibasic amino acids are improperly absorbed; and Type III, in which there is abnormal transport only by the renal tubule. Patients with Hartnup's disease have defective renal tubule transport systems for neutral amino acids but only tryptophan malabsorption has thus far been demonstrated in the small intestine. This accounts for the increased urine indican characteristic of such patients. Joseph's syndrome (prolinuria, iminoglycinuria) involves the urinary loss of proline and glycine with a variable defect present in the intestine; some individuals demonstrate transport defects for both amino acids, some for proline alone, and others have no intestinal transport defect. Patients with Lowe's syndrome (oculocerebrorenal syndrome) have a renal tubule defect involving neutral and dibasic amino acids but apparently only dibasic amino acids are handled abnormally by the intestine.

Isolated deficiencies of the various disaccharidases have also been described, lactase deficiency being the most frequent and best understood. Its prevalence remains disputed, but it may appear as a congenital or presumably acquired abnormality affecting Negroes, Orientals, and Cypriot Greeks somewhat more frequently than Caucasians. Its more frequent occurrence in patients with ulcerative colitis, Crohn's disease (uninvolved intestine), and even viral hepatitis has been alleged by some and denied by others. A previously asymptomatic lactase deficiency may become manifest when combined with other gastrointestinal disease, however, because of (1) an increased lactose load contained in an ulcer diet, (2) an increased rate of gastric emptying following gastric resection, or (3) the concurrent development of intestinal disease. Several criteria have been proposed for diagnosis of lactase deficiency: (1) diarrhea, cramping abdominal pain, and flatulence upon ingesting lactose; (2) absent or diminished lactase activity in mucosal biopsy specimens; (3) a flat lactose tolerance curve after the oral administration of 50 grams of lactose, with normal tolerance curves for glucose and galactose; (4) a fall in the stool pH after ingestion of lactose due to the conversion of the unabsorbed lactose to lactic acid by the colonic bacteria; and (5) disappearance of symptoms upon the removal of lactose from the diet. The severity of the defect varies widely, and since there is a gradient of lactase activity in the small bowel with peak levels in the jejunum and proximal ileum, it is not possible to measure total intestinal lactase activity using biopsy specimens and this information therefore may be misleading. Spuriously flat lactose tolerance curves may occur in the presence of delayed gastric emptying or a rapid rise and fall of the blood glucose during the first 30 minutes of the test. Direct instillation of lactose into the duodenum will resolve the first problem and the measurement of capillary rather than venous blood glucose will obviate the latter.

Abnormalities of Lymphatic Transport. Any condition interfering with the normal flow of lymph from the lacteal through the abdominal lymphatic systems to the thoracic duct and thence to the general circulation may result in increased losses of lymph constituents, namely, plasma proteins, chylomicron fat, and small lymphocytes. From a pathophysiologic point of view, such conditions are not, strictly speaking, absorptive defects as much as they are disorders of lymph flow. However, fat does tend to accumulate in the villous absorptive cells, in the intercellular spaces between absorptive cells, in the extracellular space of the lamina propria, and in the endothelial cells of the lacteals; from the standpoint of lipid absorption, these conditions can be considered as exit blocks.

Disorders of lymphatic transport may be congenital, as in the case of primary intestinal lymphangiectasia, or acquired secondary to structural abnormalities occurring as part of other primary intestinal disease or to an increase in lymphatic pressure due to increases in central venous pressure. Because of the associated loss of plasma proteins, lymphatic abnormalities also represent one type of protein-losing gastroenteropathy. Pure lymphatic abnormalities result in mild steatorrhea, modest elevations of fecal nitrogen, hypoalbuminemia, hypogammaglobulinemia and, not infrequently, lymphocytopenia. Circulating immunoglobulins may therefore be low and cellular immune responses impaired. Clinical manifestations related to the lymphatic abnormality may include diarrhea, edema, and sometimes repeated infections and cutaneous anergy, including the ability to accept homografts. The edema in patients with primary intestinal lymphangiectasia may be asymmetrical since there is often an asymmetrical hypoplasia of peripheral lymphatics as well. Small intestinal x-ray examination shows thickening of the mucosal folds and sometimes suggestive features of a mild malabsorption pattern. Lymphangiography will demonstrate the structural lymphatic defect and occasionally puddling of the dye in the intestinal lumen. Mucosal biopsy reveals the dilated mucosal lymphatics but cannot provide an etiologic diagnosis. Ideally, therapy should be directed toward relief of the responsible lymphatic obstruction; however, this may be possible in only a few situations, such as constrictive pericarditis or congestive heart failure. In the other conditions, especially primary intestinal lymphangiectasia, a reduction in lymph flow and pressure can be achieved by reducing the dietary intake of long-chain triglycerides and replacing them with medium-chain triglycerides which are absorbed by the portal vein.

It is evident that management of a patient with a malabsorption syndrome must proceed from a definition of the mechanism(s) involved whenever possible. In many instances treatment of the responsible disease process, such as nontropical sprue or Whipple's disease, will restore adequate absorption. When specific therapy is not possible, alternative measures must be employed. In some cases simply increasing the intake of nutrients may suffice, unless increasing diarrhea from increased steatorrhea becomes a problem. Simple bile acid deficiency probably is best treated by a low-fat diet for this reason. Bile acid replacement is not practical; the amount required (4 to 8 gm. per meal) leads to diarrhea, since dihydroxy bile acids are potent cathartics. When indicated, pancreatic enzyme replacement is helpful but inefficient owing to inactivation by gastric acid. In both situations medium-chain triglycerides may be useful. They are more rapidly and efficiently hydrolyzed by lipase, and the principal resulting fatty acid, octanoic acid, is fully water soluble. It is absorbed via the portal circulation and does not form chylomicrons. When bacterial overgrowth is present, long-term continuous or intermittent therapy with antibiotics may be beneficial. Total parenteral nutrition is also an important adjunct in many patients, providing nutritional support while more definitive and lasting treatment is being developed. Finally, some patients, especially those with extensive intestinal resection, may require permanent home parenteral nutrition.

Protein-Losing   Gastroenteropathies. Although not strictly disorders of absorption it is convenient to discuss other aspects of the protein-losing gastroenteropathies at this point, since they do represent states of increased intestinal nitrogen loss. A classification of the major protein-losing states is presented in Table 26–3. Over 40 disorders have been associated with abnormal protein loss, many representing only single case reports, and the reader is referred to the review by Waldmann for a more complete listing of these conditions. Generally, protein-losing states fall into one of the following categories: (1) benign or malignant tumors largely of the stomach or colon; (2) any condition associated with gastrointestinal inflammation with loss of epithelial cell integrity; (3) primary or secondary structural abnormalities of lymphatic channels from the lacteal to the termination of the thoracic duct; and (4) a sustained and significant increase in central venous pressure, which is then transmitted to the thoracic duct. Fecal nitrogen is often mildly elevated but is not diagnostically helpful because of the digestion and absorption of variable amounts of the protein lost and the inability to distinguish between increased loss and malabsorption. Therefore, techniques using radiolabeled macromolecules are utilized in an attempt to document and quantitate gastrointestinal protein loss.

An ideal substance should fulfill the following requirements: (1) the labeled substance should have a normal metabolic behavior; (2) there should be no excretion of the label into the gastrointestinal tract unless it is bound to protein; and (3) there should be no absorption of the label from the gastrointestinal tract after its catabolism. None of the readily available substances completely fulfills these requirements.

Using intravenously administered ^{131}I-labeled albumin, one may determine the plasma volume, the total albumin pool, the rate of albumin degradation, and, in the steady state, the rate of albumin synthesis. Patients with protein loss, regardless of the mechanism involved, have reduced circulating and total body pools of albumin, a normal or slightly increased rate of albumin synthesis, and a markedly shortened albumin survival. Data obtained from serum and urinary radioactivity curves, however, indicate only that hypercatabolism or increased loss is the cause of the hypoproteinemia but do not necessarily implicate the gastrointestinal tract. The fecal output of ^{131}I cannot be used as an estimate of protein loss, since most of the label entering the intestinal tract is removed, reabsorbed, and excreted in the urine. Also there is active secretion of ^{131}I into the gastrointestinal tract regardless of where in the body it is removed. Amberlite IRA-400, an ion exchange resin, has been utilized in an effort to trap the ^{131}I in the lumen but with only partial success. The half-life of ^{131}I-albumin is 14 to 22 days.

[131]I-labeled polyvinylpyrrolidone is a synthetic polymer with an average molecular weight of 40,000 that is unaffected by digestive enzymes and is poorly absorbed. Normal subjects excrete 0 to 1.5 per cent of an intravenous dose, while patients with protein loss excrete 2.9 to 32.5 per cent. Variable but significant amounts of the label are removed and absorbed; nevertheless, it can be of great value as a screening test.

[51]Cr-labeled albumin is perhaps the most useful of the readily available substances, since the label is neither significantly absorbed from nor secreted into the gastrointestinal tract. Normals excrete 0.1 to 0.7 per cent of an intravenous dose, while patients with protein loss excrete 2 to 40 per cent of the radioactive substance. A disadvantage is its short apparent half-life of three to 10 days owing to the elution of the label from the protein. For this reason, ^{51}Cr-albumin cannot be used to determine pool sizes or rates of protein synthesis and catabolism.

A more complete analysis of protein metabolism can be achieved by the simultaneous use of ^{51}Cr-albumin and ^{125}I-albumin. The size of the albumin pool and rates of albumin catabolism and synthesis can be determined from the ^{125}I data and the magnitude of gastrointestinal protein loss estimated by ^{51}Cr-albumin.

WATER AND SOLUTE TRANSPORT

The usual concentrations of electrolytes in small intestinal fluid vary somewhat between the jejunum and the ileum. Sodium and potassium concentrations are similar in the two areas, the former being approximately 140 mEq. per liter

TABLE 26–3 CLASSIFICATION OF PROTEIN-LOSING GASTROENTEROPATHIES

Loss of epithelial integrity
    Menetrier's giant hypertrophic gastritis
    Gastric carcinoma
    Carcinoma of the colon
    Nontropical sprue
    Crohn's disease
    Gastrointestinal lymphoma
    Acute gastroenteritis
    Ulcerative colitis
    Gastrointestinal polyposis syndromes
Lymphatic hypertension
    Primary intestinal lymphangiectasia
    Retroperitoneal tumors
    Retroperitoneal fibrosis
    Constrictive pericarditis
    Congestive heart failure
    Whipple's disease
    Crohn's disease
    Gastrointestinal lymphomas

and the latter 7 mEq. per liter. Jejunal chloride concentrations, however, are higher than in the ileum (129 mEq. per liter as compared to 81 mEq. per liter), while the reverse is true for bicarbonate (17 mEq. per liter versus 63 mEq. per liter). The manner in which water and ion fluxes are regulated to maintain these differences as well as to accomplish the efficient absorption of large volumes of fluid and electrolytes is imperfectly understood. The following general prnciples, although lacking incontrovertible experimental support, are consistent with present information. For a more detailed discussion and reference to the literature the reader is referred to the excellent discussion by Krejs and Fordtran.

It is generally accepted that crypt cells secrete and villous cells absorb, but it must be appreciated that what is measured in most instances is net transport, not unidirectional fluxes. Since cell membranes are lipoidal structures, solutes such as glucose and electrolytes must pass the epithelial layer either via pores or some carrier-mediated mechanism. Pores appear to exist at the tight junctions and are larger in the jejunum than in the ileum. They are more permeable for cations than anions, and approximately 80 per cent of sodium, potassium, and chloride is transported by this route in the jejunum and ileum. The brush border contains a mobile carrier binding both sodium and glucose, and each increases the affinity of the carrier for the other. Thus, in the presence of intraluminal glucose, sodium is actively absorbed. Amino acids have a similar but weaker effect mediated by a different carrier. The most important specialized activity of the brush border membrane, however, is the neutral sodium chloride entry mechanism. This double ion exchange mechanism allows sodium to be absorbed in exchange for hydrogen and chloride in exchange for bicarbonate.

In both the jejunum and ileum the basolateral membrane of the absorptive cells contains a sodium pump which actively secretes sodium into the intercellular space. In the jejunum, bicarbonate exits with sodium; in the ileum, chloride accompanies the sodium ions. This sodium pumping generates a potential difference (PD), especially in the jejunum, so that the intercellular and subserosal spaces are positive compared to the luminal surface and intracellular compartment. This PD causes intercellular sodium to diffuse to some extent back into the lumen, thus resulting in a final PD near zero. A portion of this intercellular sodium also enters the plasma accompanied by an anion.

In the jejunum, active sodium transport is achieved by both the glucose-sodium carrier mechanism and sodium-hydrogen exchange. No chloride-bicarbonate exchange mechanism appears to operate here, and chloride absorption is passive, being absorbed with sodium via pores.

In the ileum the same mechanisms are operative plus the chloride-bicarbonate exchange mechanism. The secreted hydrogen and bicarbonate form CO_2 and water in the lumen and are absorbed. In the ileum the luminal contents equilibrate at about pH 7.8. Often there is net bicarbonate secretion due to more rapid anion than cation exchange.

All water transport is passive secondary to osmotic or hydrostatic forces. The active ion transport mechanisms discussed increase the concentration of solute in the intercellular space, and as a result water moves across the basolateral membrane and through the tight junctions. The hydrostatic pressure in this space increases, forcing fluid into the capillaries. The fluid finally absorbed is isotonic, but the combined activities of the ion transport and hydrostatic mechanisms make possible the absorption of water against a concentration gradient (lumen to plasma).

An important observation is that increases in hydrostatic pressure at the mucosal surface have relatively little effect on water and solute transport. At the serosal surface, however, such increases may result in increased secretion and decreased absorption. This effect becomes significant at venous pressures more than 15 cm. of water above normal.

Water absorption in turn has an effect on solute transport termed "solvent drag." Small solutes may be caught in the moving stream of water and absorbed, especially in the jejunum with its larger pore size. Movement of water out of one compartment also may increase the concentration of some solutes and, therefore, their electrochemical potential.

Present evidence indicates that potassium movement in the small intestine is passive and dependent on concentration and electrochemical differences generated by the mechanisms already discussed.

The fasting intestine contains little fluid. After a meal between 2 and 3 liters of exogenous and endogenous fluid are presented to it, with the daily load amounting to about 8.5 liters. It is truly remarkable that man can ingest a diet which varies markedly in its water and solute content without causing osmotic disequilibrium. This is prevented largely because: (1) the gastric mucosa is relatively impermeable to bulk water flow; (2) gastric emptying is controlled by osmoreceptors; (3) nutrients in the small bowel lumen are largely macromolecules with relatively lower osmotic activity; (4) these nutrients are rapidly broken down and absorbed; and (5) ingested fat, a significant component of most diets, is not osmotically active.

The diarrhea of cholera, almost entirely of small bowel origin, offers an impressive demonstration of abnormal fluid and electrolyte fluxes in this organ. In the adult with acute cholera the secretory capacity amounts to 1 to 2 liters per hour. The fluid is approximately isosmotic with plasma and is nearly protein-free. The predominant cation is sodium and the predominant anions are chloride and bicarbonate, the latter two exhibiting the same relationships in the jejunum and ileum as under normal circumstances. The *Vibrio cholerae* does not invade the intestinal wall, and as a result there is no disruption of the epithelium or significant inflammation. Consistent with the absence of epithelial cell damage is the fact that glucose absorption and glucose-coupled sodium transport remain normal. Once this was realized, the oral administration of glucose to stimulate fluid absorption became an important adjunct to therapy. The epithelium of the small intestine can be triggered to secrete chloride actively by both cholera exotoxin and cyclic AMP. Furthermore, the exotoxin results in an increase in the cyclic AMP concentration in the intestinal mucosa. Despite its gradual development, secretion is difficult to reverse once the toxin has come into contact with the epithelium. There are two possible driving forces for the massive intestinal secretion encountered in cholera: active transport by the epithelium and a hydrostatic pressure difference from the interstitial tissue to the lumen. On the basis of present evidence it is highly probable that the fluid loss results from an active secretory process. The massive diarrhea characteristic of acute cholera ensues because the absorptive capacity of the colon is readily overwhelmed by the large quantity of water and electrolytes presented to it.

The products of several other bacteria also elicit small intestinal fluid secretion, including *E. coli*, Shigella, and *Clostridium perfringens*. The massive diarrhea occasionally occurring in association with several hormone-secreting tumors such as malignant carcinoids, medullary carcinomas of the thyroid, and some nonbeta cell tumors of the pancreatic islets may also in part be due to an enhancement of cyclic AMP activity. This possibility rests upon the concept of a two-messenger system of hormone action. The first messenger is a hormone stimulating adenylate cyclase activity within the target cell. This results in the formation of increased amounts of cyclic AMP (the second messenger) from ATP. In view of the large number of agents that increase cyclic AMP concentrations in this way, it is likely that this secretory mechanism plays an important part not only in cholera but in other disorders associated with diarrhea.

THE SECRETION OF HORMONES AND ENZYMES

The gut has been known for some time to contain a large number of endocrine cells. Immunocytochemical and ultrastructural techniques have

permitted the localization of several peptide hormones to these cells. Table 26–4 lists the cell types as presently designated, their location, and the hormones they contain. Physiologic roles have so far been demonstrated only for gastrin, cholecystokinin-pancreozymin, and secretin. Several of the remainder are of sufficient interest, however, to warrant some discussion.

Although most small bowel enzymes are fixed in that they function at sites in the glycocalyx-plasma membrane structure or epithelial cell cytoplasm, one enzyme is released into the lumen in physiologic concentrations (enterokinase).

Secretin and Cholecystokinin-Pancreozymin

Secretin is released from the duodenum and probably the proximal jejunum in response to H^+, the magnitude of response being proportional to the amount rather than to the concentration of the H^+. It shares a 14 amino acid sequence with glucagon, but no fragment with superior biological activity has been identified. Cholecystokinin-pancreozymin is secreted from the duodenum and jejunum following vagal stimulation, but especially in response to free fatty acids and essential amino acids in the intestinal lumen. It contains the same C-terminal pentapeptide as gastrin but most of its activity is contained in the C-terminal heptapeptide. The activities of these two hormones are summarized in Table 26–5. Their func-

TABLE 26–4 ANATOMIC AND CELLULAR LOCALIZATION OF SMALL INTESTINAL HORMONES

Hormone	Cell	Distribution
Gastrin	G	Upper duodenum
	G1	Duodenum and jejunum
GIP	K	Duodenum and jejunum
Motilin	EC2	Duodenum and jejunum
Somatostatin	D	Duodenum and jejunum
Enteroglucagon	L	Duodenum and jejunum Ileum and colon
Secretin	S	Duodenum
CCK-PZ	I	Duodenum and jejunum
VIP	D1(H)	Duodenum and jejunum Ileum and colon

Modified from the Revised Wiesbaden Classification of Human Endocrine Cells. Solcia, E., Pearse, A. G. E., Grube, D., et al.: Revised Wiesbaden classification of gut endocrine cells. Rendic. Gastroenterol., 5:13–16, 1973.

TABLE 26-5 PHYSIOLOGIC EFFECTS OF SECRETIN AND CHOLECYSTOKININ-PANCREOZYMIN

	Cholecystokinin-Pancreozymin (CCK–PZ)	Secretin
Gallbladder contraction	S	0
Stomach		
H+	Sw	I
Pepsin	Sw	S
Motility	S	I
Exocrine pancreas		
HCO_3^-	Sw	S
Enzymes	S	Sw
Endocrine pancreas		
Insulin	S	S
Glucagon	S	0
Intestine		
Brunner's glands	S	S
Motility	S	I
Hepatic bile		
HCO_3^-	Sw	Sw

S — Stimulates
Sw — Stimulates weakly
I — Inhibits
Iw — Inhibits weakly
0 — No effect

Modified from Go, V.L.W., and Summerskill, W.H.J.: Am. J. Clin. Nutr., 24:160, 1971.

tion in coordinating the various phases of the digestive-absorptive process is related to their effects on gastric emptying, gastroduodenal motor responses, and the secretion of acid, bile, and pancreatic juice.

No primary disorders of their secretion have been reported. In diffuse mucosal lesions of the small intestine such as nontropical sprue, however, their activities may be reduced. These patients often exhibit delayed emptying of the gallbladder; decreased luminal concentrations of pancreatic lipase, bile acids, and micellar lipid; and decreased intestinal motor activity. Furthermore, the secretion of bicarbonate by the pancreas is impaired following duodenal acidification.

The physiology and pathophysiology of gastrin are discussed elsewhere. As yet no physiologic role for duodenal gastrin has been determined.

Gastric Inhibitory Peptide (GIP)

GIP shares structural similarities with secretin and glucagon, and the highest concentrations are found in the jejunum, with significant amounts in the duodenum and upper ileum. It inhibits gastric acid secretion, pepsin secretion, and antral and fundic motility and stimulates small intestinal secretion. Plasma concentrations rise rapidly after a meal, and fat, glucose, and amino acids appear to be effective stimuli for its release. It is of interest that acidification of the duodenum has no effect on GIP release, thus eliminating it from a negative feedback role. The most significant physiologic action of GIP, however, probably is the postprandial enhancement of insulin release. This most likely accounts for the greater insulin release following oral as compared to intravenous glucose. Its most potent insulin-releasing action is seen in conditions of hyperglycemia. A role for GIP in reactive hypoglycemia at present remains undefined.

Motilin

Motilin is confined to a distinct population of enterochromaffin cells of the duodenum and upper jejunum. Levels rise after acidification of the duodenum and after fat ingestion. It causes marked contractions in isolated gastric and upper small intestinal tissue, an increase in lower esophageal sphincter pressure, and delayed gastric emptying. No physiologic role has been established.

Enteroglucagon (EG)

Enteroglucagon appears to be chemically and biologically different from pancreatic glucagon but shares immunoreactivity. It is found in highest concentrations in the lower ileum and colon. Plasma EG rises after a meal, and its release is stimulated primarily by carbohydrate and long-chain triglycerides. Owing to its distal localization its release is enhanced by rapid transit, and it is greatly increased in the dumping syndrome. Little is known of its physiology but one patient with an EG-producing tumor exhibited intestinal stasis and increased mucosal growth.

Vasoactive Intestinal Peptide (VIP)

VIP is structurally related to secretin, glucagon, and GIP. It is not only produced by an endocrine cell in the gut, but also is found in fine nerve fibers in the lamina propria and in the cell bodies of the myenteric plexus. VIP inhibits gastric acid production, stimulates insulin release, has a glucagon-like action, and stimulates both pancreatic and small intestinal secretion. It is not significantly released after a meal and probably functions as a local hormone. Its production by pancreatic islet cell tumors and ganglioneuromas has implicated it in the clinical expression of the Verner-Morrison or watery diarrhea syndrome.

Somatostatin

Most somatostatin-containing cells are located in the gastric antrum, with fewer cells in the duodenum and jejunum. It exhibits a wide range of inhibitory activities including growth hormone and TSH release, insulin and glucagon release, gastrin release, gastric acid production, gallbladder contraction, and pancreatic enzyme production. It also suppresses motilin and VIP production. For this reason it has been suggested that it functions as a local rather than a circulating hormone.

Several other poorly characterized peptides have been collectively referred to as "candidate hormones." These include such designated substances as urogastrone, gastrone, bulbogastrone, and substance P. Little or nothing is known of their precise localization or biologic activity.

Enterokinase

As previously discussed, enterokinase is concerned with the conversion of pancreatic proenzymes to their active forms. The enzyme is located in the proximal duodenum in relationship to the microvilli, but its mechanism of release into the duodenal lumen has not been established. Bile salts appear to constitute one effective stimulus, and in their presence enterokinase activity is increased. Recently, several cases of enterokinase deficiency have been recognized in infants presenting with diarrhea from birth, showing failure to thrive, and exhibiting a good clinical response to pancreatic extracts.

IMMUNOLOGIC FUNCTION

Normal Structure and Function

Unlike most other organs such as the heart or kidney, the gastrointestinal tract is replete with immunologically competent tissue. It is capable not only of experiencing but also of mounting an immune response. In this respect it maintains functional identity with other peripheral lymphoid tissues such as the lymph nodes and spleen. Little is known, however, regarding either the qualitative or quantitative contributions of the gut to the body's immune responses. Of further importance is the realization that all the currently recognized, so-called central lymphoid tissues such as the thymus and avian bursa of Fabricius, which determine the immunological capabilities of the whole organism are lymphoepithelial derivatives of the gut. The small intestine, therefore, assumes a position of considerable importance to the immunologist as well as to those who seek an understanding of its more classic functions. Any attempt to relate abnormalities of the small bowel to concurrently observed immunologic changes must proceed from an awareness of the potential of the small intestine as both a central and peripheral lymphoid organ as well as an immunologic target.

The lymphoid elements of the small bowel are arranged in different ways, but the functional implications of these structural variations are unknown. The Peyer's patches lie in the lamina propria and submucsoa and consist of lymphoid follicles containing germinal centers. The lymphocytes in the follicular cortex appear to represent a separate population when compared to similar areas of spleen and lymph nodes. Small lymphocytes from thoracic duct lymph preferentially "home" to the Peyer's patches as well as lymph nodes and spleen. These structures are well developed by the fifth month of fetal life, increase in size and number until the age of 10 or 12, and gradually atrophy thereafter. Although Peyer's patch cells are capable of antibody synthesis and probably of both primary and secondary immune responses, the importance of this function in relation to their location is unclear. The means of antigen uptake by the small intestine is unknown. The epithelium over the dome area of Peyer's patches differs in being cuboidal. This specialized epithelial cell has been termed an M-cell and may play a role in antigen transport. The lamina propria also contains a second population of lymphoid cells differing in certain respects from the Peyer's patches. Its lymphocytes and plasma cells also contain various immunoglobulins but they are not arranged in any structured fashion. Large lymphocytes from the thoracic duct lymph preferentially seed the lamina propria as do lymphoblasts formed in lymph nodes following antigenic stimulation. It is not known, however, whether primary or secondary immune responses occur in situ within this nonaggregated lymphoid tissue of the lamina propria. Peyer's patches and the lamina propria both contain T and B lymphocytes. B lymphocytes are responsible for local antibody production, but the role of T cells in this location is not firmly established. Some probably are helper T cells, modulating B cell function, and others are engaged in cell-mediated immune reactions. The presence of F_c-receptor cells and C'-receptor lymphocytes in the normal small intestine remains controversial. The third type of lymphoid elements found in the small intestine are the theliolymphocytes. They lie within and between the mucosal epithelial cells and have been identified as activated T cells. Their source, function, and fate, however, are unknown.

The lymphoid tissues of the Peyer's patches and lamina propria are sparse and appear undeveloped prior to birth and in the germ-free state. With the development of an intestinal flora, lymphocytes and plasma cells become more numerous and germinal centers develop.

It is apparent that all three of these lymphoid "structures" maintain a lymphoepithelial relationship which is similar to that of the thymus and the avian bursa of Fabricius. The former is responsible for the development of the cellular immune system and the latter, in avian species at least, regulates the development of the humoral immune system. This has led to considerable speculation concerning which, if any, of the small intestinal lymphoid elements constitute a human bursal equivalent.

The gut-associated lymphoid tissue like the spleen and lymph nodes is on the route of recirculating lymphocytes. Present evidence suggests that only activated T and B cells (immunoblasts) gain access to this compartment. While these cells may originate in any of the organized peripheral lymphoid tissues, it seems clear that a significant proportion arise within the aggregated lymphoid tissue of the gut as a result of the interaction of lymphocytes with intraluminal antigen. This accounts for most of the immunoblasts in thoracic duct lymph, and a high proportion of these migrate back to the large and small intestine. Indeed thoracic duct lymphocytes activated by histocompatability antigens migrate preferentially to the gut and have been traced to Peyer's patches, the lamina propria, and intraepithelial sites. It has been postulated that immunoblasts cross the capillaries in the intestinal mucosa in a random fashion, and, under the influence of intraluminal antigen, appropriately primed effector cells are inhibited from returning to the general circulation as a consequence of antigen-driven stimulation to final differentiation or multiplication. An important consequence of this recirculating and homing mechanism is the propagation throughout the gut and the dissemination throughout the body of a local immune response by means of mobile effector cells.

Most immunoglobulin-containing cells in the small intestine are mature plasma cells, although some immunoglobulins are found within immature plasma cells and lymphocytes. It is well established that IgA is the predominant immunoglobulin in the lymphoid cells and secretions of the small intestine. IgM, IgG, and IgD are also present in that order. Recently, IgE has been identified in the small intestine but its relative amount has yet to be established. The IgA found in the small intestine and its secretions differs from 7S serum IgA in that it is an 11S globulin with a molecular weight of 390,000. This secretory IgA appears to represent a dimer of the 7S serum IgA coupled to a nonimmunoglobulin glycoprotein, referred to as secretory piece or T (transport) component. This secretory component has been identified as a product of the epithelial cells and is associated with the mucus-containing area of intestinal goblet cells. Its precise function is not known, although it no doubt confers some biological advantage on IgA in the external secretions. There are two subclasses of IgA—IgA$_1$ and IgA$_2$. IgA$_2$ appears to predominate in the intestinal secretions and differs from IgA$_1$ in that it contains no disulfide bonds linking the light and heavy chains, and contains a genetic marker, Am$_2$, within its heavy chain structure.

The human infant is born totally lacking IgA in serum and external secretions, and secretory IgA appears sooner and reaches adult levels more quickly than serum IgA. The small intestine therefore has been regarded as a potentially important source not only of secretory but also of serum IgA. Secretory IgA has been demonstrated to possess antiviral and antibacterial activity as well as the properties of isohemagglutinins. Although the precise role played by secretory IgA in the external secretions remains unsettled, it probably constitutes an important defense against certain microorganisms and perhaps other potentially harmful substances.

Abnormal Structure and Function

Gastrointestinal symptoms consisting usually of diarrhea, malabsorption, and malnutrition are found in patients with primary immunodeficiency syndromes, occurring in 20 to 50 per cent of those with adult onset but rarely in the congenital disorders. Table 26–6 presents a classification of these syndromes developed by a group of the World Health Organization. They are more fully discussed in Chapter 3, and our attention here is focused on their impact on the small intestine. Although the syndromes are not discussed in the following chapter, the colon and rectum also participate in many of the histologic and functional alterations described here.

Two distinctive histologic patterns have been described in the small intestine of patients with immunodeficiency syndromes and gastrointestinal symptoms: The first, nodular lymphoid hyperplasia of the small intestine, has been so named because of the multiple small lymphoid nodules present within the mucosa. These nodules contain hyperplastic germinal centers but plasma cells are sparse throughout the intestine and the epithelial and villous architecture usually remain well preserved. The second pattern has been referred to as hypogammaglobulinemic "sprue" because there is villus atrophy and the mucosa often presents a flat appearance. These patients differ, however, from those with gluten-sensitive enteropathy not only in the presence of the immunodeficiency but also in failing to respond in many instances to a gluten-free diet. Plasma cells are also nearly completely absent in the small intestine of patients with this type of pattern.

In their initial report, Hermans and his associates described five characteristic features of patients with nodular lymphoid hyperplasia: (1) dysgammaglobulinemia, consisting of the virtual absence of IgA and IgM, with a moderate reduction in IgG; (2) susceptibility to sinopulmonary infections; (3) diarrhea; (4) *Giardia lamblia* in the

TABLE 26-6 CLASSIFICATION OF PRIMARY IMMUNODEFICIENCY SYNDROMES AND INCIDENCE OF GASTROINTESTINAL (GI) DISEASE

Type of Immunodeficiency	Incidence of GI Disease	Characteristic GI Symptoms, Findings, and Morphologic Abnormalities
1. B-cell defects:		
infantile X-linked agammaglobulinemia	(+)	*Giardia lamblia* (rare), absence of plasma cells in mucosa, early crypt abscesses
X-linked immunodeficiency with hyper-IgM	−	−
selective IgA deficiency	++	celiac sprue, nodular lymphoid hyperplasia, *Giardia lamblia,* malignancy
transient hypogammaglobulinemia of infancy	−	−
immunodeficiency syndrome with normal serum immunoglobulin levels	(+)	diarrhea, malabsorption
variable immunodeficiency (acquired hypogammaglobulinemia)	+++	nodular lymphoid hyperplasia, celiac sprue, severe B_{12} malabsorption, *Giardia lamblia,* colitis, malignancy
2. T-cell defect		
DiGeorge syndrome (thymic hypoplasia)	(+)	recurrent diarrhea, failure to thrive
3 B- and T-cell defects		
immunodeficiency with ataxia-telangiectasia	(+)	vitamin B_{12} malabsorption, carcinoma of stomach
immunodeficiency with thrombocytopenia and eczema (Wiskott-Aldrich syndrome)	+++	severe recurrent bloody diarrhea, malabsorption
immunodeficiency with short-limbed dwarfism	+	diarrhea, crypt abscesses
cartilage-hair hypoplasia	+	recurrent diarrhea, failure to thrive, steatorrhea, vacuolated, lipid laden macrophages
immunodeficiency with thymoma	(+)	frequently diarrhea
severe combined immunodeficiency (a) autosomal recessive (with or without red blood cell adenosine deaminase deficiency; with reticuloendotheliosis) (b) X-linked (c) sporadic	+++	severe diarrhea, malabsorption, absence of plasma cells, vacuolated and lipid-containing macrophages

Reproduced from: Gastrointestinal Tract and Immunodeficiency. Ochs, H. D., and Ament, M. E. *In* Immunological Aspects of the Liver and GI Tract. A. Ferguson and R. N. M. MacSween, Eds., MTP Press, Ltd., Lancaster, 1976, p. 85.

stools; and (5) nodular lymphoid hyperplasia of the small intestine. Additional cases have been described with idiopathic acquired hypogammaglobulinemia, and two subjects have been reported with a selective absence of IgA. In those patients studied, cellular immune mechanisms appear to be intact. Mild steatorrhea is often present and in many instances both the diarrhea and steatorrhea respond favorably to treatment of the Giardia infection. The radiographic findings in nodular

lymphoid hyperplasia are characteristic, demonstrating innumerable small filling defects measuring only a few millimeters in diameter which are uniform in size and smooth in contour. Segmental involvement of the small intestine and colon may be present or the entire small bowel may be involved, and a mild malabsorption pattern is at times superimposed.

In so-called hypogammaglobulinemic sprue, steatorrhea is often more marked. These patients also frequently harbor *Giardia lamblia* in the small intestinal secretions, and in many instances the associated diarrhea and steatorrhea are improved after treatment of the giardiasis. These patients generally exhibit an acquired type of hypogammaglobulinemia, although again selective IgA deficiency has been encountered.

The relationship between the immunodeficiency and the structural and functional abnormalities present in the small intestine is unknown. It should be noted that selective IgA deficiency is not uncommon in the general population, occurring in approximately one of every 700 individuals. Many of these patients are without any intestinal symptoms and many patients with acquired hypogammaglobulinemia fail to demonstrate structural abnormalities or symptoms related to the small intestine. At the present time, therefore, these various structural and functional changes cannot be understood in pathophysiologic terms.

VASCULAR DISORDERS OF THE SMALL INTESTINE

Normal Physiology

The splanchnic circulation receives 28 per cent of the cardiac output and contains 20 per cent of the total blood volume, with 65 per cent distributed to the mucosa. After eating, there is a 30 per cent increase in splanchnic flow which correlates with the processes of secretion and absorption. This effect is probably in part mediated by the release of gastrin, secretin, and cholecystokinin-pancreozymin, all of which act to increase superior mesenteric artery flow.

Intestinal blood flow is regulated primarily by the sympathetic nervous system via alpha receptor activity. Stimulation can virtually interrupt flow, especially to the mucosa, while the elimination of normal constrictor activity results in a 20 to 40 per cent increase. When all factors capable of augmenting blood flow are operative, the maximal possible increase is in the range of 500 per cent. A decrease in splanchnic flow may result from a number of influences, including exercise, standing, intraluminal pressures above 30 mm. Hg, and increased sympathetic neurohumoral activity. Although muscle contraction leads to a decrease in flow, the net effect of intestinal motor activity is to increase flow probably as a result of increased cholinergic activity and the release of various metabolites.

Intestinal blood flow also exhibits autoregulation and autoregulatory escape. Autoregulation involves the coordination of physiologic mechanisms to maintain blood flow in the face of a decrease in arterial pressure, while autoregulatory escape is the intrinsic ability of the intestinal vasculature to "escape" from persistent vasoconstrictor activity imposed by alpha-adrenergic stimulation. It therefore represents a protective mechanism within the intestinal circulation to counter ischemia during prolonged sympathetic activity.

An additional concept important to an understanding of intestinal ischemia is that of countercurrent exchange (Fig. 26–11). The effect of such an arrangement is that arterial substances (for example, oxygen) entering at the base of the villus will progressively decrease in concentration toward the villous tip, whereas absorbed materials entering at the villous tip will leave the villus more slowly. Countercurrent exchange operates

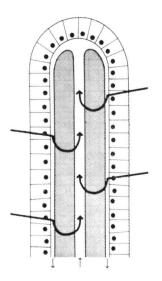 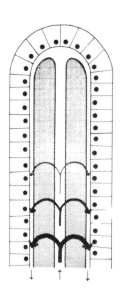

Figure 26–11 The functional implications of the mucosal countercurrent exchanger schematically illustrated. *A*, Absorbed materials are delayed in their egress from the villus, and *B*, arterial O_2 achieves a progressively lower concentration at the villous tip.

at low perfusion rates and aggravates mucosal ischemia.

Intestinal Ischemia and Infarction

A compromise in the arterial supply of the small intestine may result in either chronic intestinal ischemia or infarction. Approximately 60 per cent of infarctions result from nonocclusive disease, while 30 per cent are due to either thrombosis or embolism, the former probably being more frequent. The remaining 10 per cent follow venous occlusion.

Chronic intestinal ischemia is best understood as a series of recurring attacks of acute ischemia which do not result in infarction. Although any disease process which results in a decrease in arterial flow may be responsible, the vast majority of cases are a result of atherosclerotic narrowing of the celiac axis and superior or inferior mesenteric arteries. The constriction is asymmetrical and most evident in the first centimeter of the involved vessel. The most prominent manifestation is cramping, periumbilical pain (intestinal angina) which characteristically occurs 10 to 15 minutes after eating and lasts two to three hours. Larger meals produce more pain and there is a tendency for it to become worse with the passage of time. As noted previously, ischemia causes increased contractility of smooth muscle and the mechanism responsible for pain production is probably smooth muscle spasm. Patients tend to restrict their food intake in an effort to avoid these episodes of pain, and as a result weight loss may be marked. Not uncommonly, mild diarrhea with or without a slight increase in stool fat and nitrogen occurs, probably as a result of impaired epithelial cell function and an increase in propulsive motor activity.

It must be recognized, however, that symptom production cannot always be correlated with anatomic abnormalities demonstrated by arteriography. Even occlusion of all three major arterial branches of the abdominal aorta has been encountered in the absence of apparent symptoms. Granting such inconsistencies, the general view is that a patient with characteristic abdominal pain and weight loss not explained by a primary disorder of the gut, pancreas, or hepatobiliary system and who has significant (> 50 per cent of the lumen) narrowing in two of the three mesenteric arteries should be regarded as having a clinical disturbance of the mesenteric arterial circulation. If a gradient of >35 mm. Hg is present at the time of operation, this assumption is strengthened. Surgical correction will result in relief of pain in 90 per cent of such patients and reversal of the malabsorption in 75 per cent. Protection from future fatal infarction, however, is less well established.

Main stem occlusion of the superior mesenteric artery is characterized by two phases: initially there is mucosal ischemia, necrosis, and hemorrhage, with associated intestinal muscle spasm; this is followed by paralysis of smooth muscle, intestinal dilatation, and necrosis of the entire bowel wall, with peritonitis and major fluid and blood loss into the gut. Significant inflammatory changes are characteristically absent, with hemorrhage and edema being the predominant features. Patients at first complain of colicky periumbilical pain which gradually becomes continuous, severe, and poorly localized. Initially there is a disproportionate lack of physical findings followed by signs of sympathetic overactivity, peritonitis, and cardiovascular collapse. Occlusion by an embolus may occur at different levels. In the presence of significant atheromatous disease, the main stem of the superior mesenteric artery may be involved (18 per cent) but 55 per cent of emboli lodge at the origin of the middle colic artery.

Nonocclusive infarction results from an interplay of several factors. The common denominator is a decrease in splanchnic flow resulting in a reduced perfusion pressure. This may be due to a reduced cardiac output or a decrease in the fraction entering the mesenteric circulation. A further decrease in flow, especially to the mucosa, is brought about by the activation of alpha-adrenergic receptors and the renin-angiotensin mechanism. The gut is therefore placed in an impossible situation. Autoregulatory escape will not maintain flow, and continued sympathetic activity reduces flow especially to the mucosa. An increase in blood viscosity and the collapse of small vessels at low perfusion pressure no doubt provide aggravating factors. Furthermore, many patients are taking digitalis, which has a mesenteric constrictor effect, and this may be a contributing influence. The result is mucosal necrosis and hemorrhage and, if the process is severe enough, transmural infarction.

In patients suspected of having acute intestinal ischemia the role of early arteriography is controversial. Its proponents point out that it offers the only means of establishing the presence of arterial embolization or thrombosis — conditions often amenable to prompt surgical correction. Also, although of unproven benefit, the intra-arterial administration of vasodilators has some theoretical basis. The prognosis of nonocclusive acute intestinal ischemia is poor, the mortality approaching 100 per cent. This is true because extensive amounts of bowel are usually involved, the patients are poor surgical risks, and no correctable lesion is present.

Venous occlusion affects the superior mesenteric vein 20 times more frequently than it affects the inferior mesenteric vein, but it is doubtful that occlusion of the latter leads to symptoms. Venous occlusion is associated with the gradual onset of vague abdominal discomfort, anorexia, and a change in bowel habits associated with slight abdominal tenderness and diminished bowel sounds. Intramural edema is marked and the sequence of events described previously takes place, albeit more slowly. Most often it represents a complication of hypercoagulable states, polycythemia, carcinomas, portal hypertension, sepsis, or surgical injury.

REFERENCES

Adibi, S. A., and Allen, E. R.: Impaired jejunal absorption rates of essential amino acids induced by either dietary caloric or protein deprivation in man. Gastroenterology, 59:404, 1970.

Asp, N. G., and Dahlqvist, A.: Multiplicity of intestinal beta-galactosidases. Contribution of each enzyme to the total lactase activity in normal and lactose intolerant patients. Acta Paediat. Scand., 60:364, 1971.

Asp, N. G., Dahlqvist, A., and Koldovsky, O.: Small intestinal beta-galactosidase activity. Gastroenterology, 58:591, 1970.

Balcerzak, S. P., Lane, W. C., and Bullard, J. W.: Surface structure of intestinal epithelium. Gastroenterology, 58:49, 1970.

Bass, P.: In vivo electrical activity of the small bowel. In Code, C. F. (Ed.): Handbook of Physiology. Vol. IV. American Physiological Society, Washington, 1968, p. 2051.

Bayless, T. M., Swanson, V. L., and Wheby, M. S.: Jejunal histology and clinical status in tropical sprue and other chronic diarrheal disorders. Am. J. Clin. Nutr., 24:112, 1971.

Bennett, A., and Fleshler, B.: Prostaglandins and the gastrointestinal tract. Gastroenterology, 59:790, 1970.

Bentley, D. W., Nichols, R. L., Condon, R. E., et al.: The microflora of the human ileum and intra-abdominal colon: Results of direct needle aspiration at surgery and evaluation of the technique. J. Lab. Clin. Med., 79:421, 1972.

Binder, H. J.: A comparison of intestinal and renal transport systems. Am. J. Clin. Nutr., 23:330, 1970.

Bloom, Stephen R., and Polak, Julia M.: The new peptide hormones of the gut. In Glass, G. B. (ed.): Progress in Gastroenterology, Vol. III. Grune and Stratton, New York, 1977, p. 109.

Braddock, L. E., Fleisher, D. R., and Barbero, G. J.: A physical chemical study of the van de Kamer method for fecal fat analysis. Gastroenterology, 55:165, 1968.

Brandborg, L. L.: Structure and function of the small intestine in some parasite diseases. Am. J. Clin. Nutr., 24:124, 1971.

Brooks, F. P.: Absorption. In Control of Gastrointestinal Function. The Macmillan Co., London, 1970.

Bynum, T. E., and Jacobson, E. D.: Blood flow and gastrointestinal disease. Digestion, 4:109, 1971.

Bynum, T. E., and Jacobson, E. D.: Blood flow and gastrointestinal function. Gastroenterology, 60:325, 1971.

Christensen, J.: The control of gastrointestinal movements: some old and new views. N. Engl. J. Med., 285:85, 1971.

Code, C. F., Szurszewski, J. H., and Kelly, K. A.: A concept of motor control by the pacesetter potential in the stomach and small bowel. Am. J. Dig. Dis., 16:601, 1971.

Corcino, J. J., Waxman, S., and Herbert, V.: Absorption and malabsorption of vitamin B₁₂. Am. J. Med., 48:562, 1970.

Cornes, J. S.: Number, size and distribution of Peyer's patches in the human small intestine. I. The development of Peyer's patches. Gut, 6:225, 1965.

Daniel, E. E., Robinson, K., Duchon, G., et al.: The possible role of close contacts (nexuses) in the propagation of control electrical activity in the stomach and small intestine. Am. J. Dig. Dis., 16:611, 1971.

Demling, L.: The motility of the gastrointestinal tract. Digestion, 2:362, 1969.

Dixon, J. A., Harman, C. G., Nichols, R. L., et al.: Intestinal motility following luminal and vascular occlusion of the small intestine. Gastroenterology, 58:673, 1970.

Dobbins, W. O., III: Morphologic and functional correlates of intestinal brush borders. Am. J. Med. Sci., 258:150, 1969.

Dobbins, W. O., III: Intestinal mucosal lacteal in transport of macromolecules and chylomicrons. Am. J. Clin. Nutr., 24:77, 1971.

Donaldson, R. M., Jr.: Small bowel bacterial overgrowth. Adv. Intern. Med., 16:191, 1970.

Dowling, R. H.: The enterohepatic circulation. Gastroenterology, 62:122, 1972.

Editorial: Ileus: Paralytic or sympathetic? Lancet, 1:329, 1971.

Editorial: "Enterogastrone(s)." Lancet, 1:1224, 1971.

Eggermont, E., Molla, A. M., Rutgeerts, L., et al.: The source of human enterokinase. Lancet, 2:369, 1971.

Elsas, L. J., Hillman, R. E., Patterson, J. H., et al.: Renal and intestinal hexose transport in familial glucose-galactose malabsorption. J. Clin. Invest., 49:576, 1970.

Farrar, J. T., and Zfass, A. M.: Small intestinal motility. Gastroenterology, 52:1019, 1967.

Fasel, J., Hadjikhani, H., and Felber, J. P.: The insulin secretory effect of the human duodenal mucosa. Gastroenterology, 59:109, 1970.

Fichtelius, K. E.: The gut epithelium — a first level lymphoid organ? Exp. Cell Res., 49:87, 1968.

Field, M.: Intestinal secretion: Effect of cyclic AMP and its role in cholera. N. Engl. J. Med., 284:1137, 1971.

French, A. B.: Protein-losing gastroenteropathies. Am. J. Dig. Dis., 16:661, 1971.

Freter, R.: Locally produced and serum derived antibodies in "local immunity." N. Engl. J. Med., 285:1375, 1971.

Go, V. L. W., and Summerskill, W. H. J.: Digestion, maldigestion, and the gastrointestinal hormones. Am. J. Clin. Nutr., 24:160, 1971.

Gorbach, S. L.: Intestinal microflora. Gastroenterology, 60:1110, 1971.

Gray, G. M.: Carbohydrate digestion and absorption. Gastroenterology, 58:96, 1970.

Gray, G. M., and Cooper, H. L.: Protein digestion and absorption. Gastroenterology, 61:535, 1971.

Greenberger, N. J.: The intestinal brush border as a digestive and absorptive surface. Am. J. Med. Sci., 258:144, 1969.

Hall, J. G., and Smith, M. E.: Homing of lymph-borne immunoblasts to the gut. Nature, 226:262, 1970.

Harrison, L. A., and Jacobson, E. D.: Gastrointestinal hormones. J. Okla. Med. Assoc., 63:157, 1970.

Hellier, M. D., Perrett, D., and Holdsworth, C. D.: Dipeptide absorption in cystinuria. Br. Med. J., 4:782, 1970.

Hellier, M. D., Perrett, D., Holdsworth, C. D., et al.: Absorption of dipeptides in normal and cystinuric subjects. Gut, 12:496, 1971.

Hendrix, R. T., and Bayless, T. M.: Digestion: Intestinal secretion. Ann. Rev. Physiol., 32:139, 1970.

Henry, C., Faulk, W. P., Kuhn, L., et al.: Peyer's patches: Immunologic studies. J. Exp. Med., 131:1200, 1970.

Hermans, P. E., Huizenga, K. A., Hoffman, H. N., et al.: Dysgammaglobulinemia associated with nodular lymphoid hyperplasia of the small intestine. Am. J. Med., 40:78, 1966.

Hightower, N. C., Jr.: Motor action of the small bowel. In Code, C. F. (Ed.): Handbook of Physiology. Vol. IV. American Physiological Society, Washington, 1968, p. 2001.

Hofmann, A. F.: Fat absorption and malabsorption: physiology, diagnosis and treatment. In Isenberg, J. I. (ed.): Viewpoints on Digestive Diseases, Vol. 9, Number 4, 1977.

Holt, P. R.: Medium chain triglycerides: Their absorption, metabolism and clinical applications. In Glass, G. B. J. (ed.): Progress in Gastroenterology. Grune and Stratton, New York, 1968, p. 277.

Hughes, W. S., Cerda, J. J., Holtzapple, P., et al.: Primary hypogammaglobulinemia and malabsorption. Ann. Intern. Med., 74:903, 1971.

Jacobson, E. D., Brobmann, G. F., and Brecher, G. A.: Intestinal motor activity and blood flow. Gastroenterology, 58:575, 1970.

Jeffries, G. Y. H., Weser, E., and Sleisenger, M. H.: Malabsorption. Gastroenterology, 56:777, 1969.

Jordan, P. H., Jr., Boulafendis, D., and Guinn, G. A.: Factors other than major vascular occlusion that contribute to intestinal infarction. Ann. Surg., 171:189, 1970.

Kraft, S. C., and Kirsner, J. B.: Immunological apparatus of the gut and inflammatory bowel disease. Gastroenterology, 60:922, 1971.

Krejs, G. T., and Fordtran, J. S.: Physiology and pathophysiology of ion and water movement in the human intestine. In Sleisenger, M. H., and Fordtran, J. S. (eds.): Gastrointestinal Disease. W. B. Saunders Co., Philadelphia, 1978, p. 297.

Kriebel, G. W., Jr., Kraft, S. C., and Rothberg, R. M.: Locally produced antibody in human gastrointestinal secretions. J. Immunol., 103:1268, 1969.

Lenz, H., Blomer, A., and Dux, A.: Analysis of the propulsive movements of the small intestine. Cineradiographic and experimental studies. Am. J. Dig. Dis., 16:1107, 1971.

Lundgren, O.: Countercurrent exchange in the small intestine. Am. Heart. J., 79:285, 1970.

Marsh, M. N., and Swift, J. A.: A study of the small intestinal mucosa using the scanning electron microscope. Gut, 10:940, 1969.

Neely, J., and Catchpole, B.: Ileus: The restoration of alimentary tract motility by pharmacologic means. Br. J. Surg., 58:21, 1971.

Nordstrom, C., and Dahlqvist, A.: Intestinal enterokinase. Lancet, 1:1185, 1971.

Ochs, H. D., and Ament, M. E.: Gastrointestinal tract and immunodeficiency. In Ferguson, A., and MacSween, R. N. M. (eds.): Immunological Aspects of the Liver and Gastrointestinal Tract. MTP Press Ltd., Lancaster, England, 1976, p. 83.

Parrott, D. M. V.: The gut associated lymphoid tissues and gastrointestinal immunity. In Ferguson, A., and MacSween, R. N. M. (eds.): Immunological Aspects of the Liver and Gastrointestinal Tract. MTP Press Ltd., Lancaster, England, 1976, p. 1.

Pearse, A. G. E., Coulling, I., Weavers, B., et al.: The endocrine polypeptide cells of the human stomach, duodenum, and jejunum. Gut, 11:649, 1970.

Peters, T. J.: Intestinal peptidases. Gut, 11:720, 1970.

Pettersson, T., and Wegelius, O.: Biopsy diagnosis of amyloidosis in rheumatoid arthritis. Malabsorption caused by intestinal amyloid deposits. Gastroenterology, 62:22, 1972.

Phillips, S. F., and Gaginella, T. S.: Intestinal secretion as a mechanism in diarrheal disease. In Glass, G. B. J. (ed.): Progress in Gastroenterology. Vol. III. Grune and Stratton, New York, 1977, p. 481.

Porter, H. P., Saunders, D. R., Tytgat, G., et al.: Fat absorption in bile fistula in man. A morphological and biochemical study. Gastroenterology, 60:1008, 1971.

Rosenberg, I. H., and Godwin, H. A.: The digestion and absorption of dietary folate. Gastroenterology, 60:445, 1971.

Rosenweig, N. S., Herman, R. H., and Stifel, F. B.: Dietary regulation of small intestinal enzyme activity in man. Am. J. Clin. Nutr., 24:65, 1971.

Rubin, W.: Celiac disease. Am. J. Clin. Nutr., 24:91, 1971.

Rubin, W.: The epithelial "membrane" of the small intestine. Am. J. Clin. Nutr., 24:45, 1971.

Sadikali, F.: Dipeptidase deficiency and malabsorption of glycylglycine in disease states. Gut, 12:276, 1971.

Savilahti, E., Visakorpi, J. K., and Pelkonen, P.: Morphological and immunohistochemical findings in small intestinal biopsy in children with IgA deficiency. Acta Paediat. Scand., 60:363, 1971.

Schiff, E. R., and Dietschy, J. M.: Steatorrhea associated with disordered bile acid metabolism. Am. J. Dig. Dis., 14:432, 1969.

Scratcherd, T., and Case, R. M.: The role of cyclic adenosine-3',5'-monophosphate (AMP) in gastrointestinal secretion. Gut, 10:957, 1969.

Sessions, J. T., Jr., de Andrade, S. R. V., and Kokas, E.: Intestinal villi: Form and motility in relation to function. In Glass, G. B. J. (ed.): Progress in Gastroenterology. Grune and Stratton, New York, 1968, p. 248.

Shanbour, L. L., and Jacobson, E. D.: Autoregulatory escape in the gut. Gastroenterology, 60:145, 1971.

Shih, V. E., Bixby, E. M., Alpers, C. S., et al.: Studies of intestinal transport defect in Hartnup disease. Gastroenterology, 61:445, 1971.

Storer, E. H.: The pharmacologic and biochemical nature of carcinoid tumors. Curr. Probl. Surg., November, 1970, p. 41.

Tarlow, M. J., Hadorn, B., Arthurton, M. W., et al.: Intestinal enterokinase deficiency. A newly recognized disorder of protein digestion. Arch. Dis. Child., 45:651, 1970.

Texter, E. C., Jr.: Pressure and transit in the small intestine. The concept of propulsion and peripheral resistance in the alimentary canal. Am. J. Dig. Dis., 13:443, 1968.

Thompson, G. R., Barrowman, J., Guterrez, L., et al.: Action of neomycin on the intraluminal phase of lipid absorption. J. Clin. Invest., 50:319, 1971.

Tidball, C. S.: The nature of the intestinal epithelial barrier. Am. J. Dig. Dis., 16:745, 1971.

Tomasi, T. B., Jr., Tan, E. M., Solomon, A., et al.: Characteristics of an immune system common to certain external secretions. J. Exp. Med., 121:101, 1965.

Toner, P. G., and Carr, K. E.: The use of scanning electron microscopy in the study of the intestinal villi. J. Pathol., 97:611, 1969.

Toner, P. G., Carr, K. E., Ferguson, A., et al.: Scanning and transmission electron microscopic studies of human intestinal mucosa. Gut, 11:471, 1970.

Toner, P. G., and Ferguson, A.: Intraepithelial cells in the human intestinal mucosa. J. Ultrastruct. Res., 34:329, 1971.

Trier, J. S., and Browning, T. H.: Epithelial-cell renewal in cultured duodenal biopsies in celiac sprue. N. Engl. J. Med., 283:1245, 1970.

Trier, J. S., Phelps, P. C., Eidelman, S., et al.: Whipple's disease: Light and electron microscope correlation of jejunal mucosal histology with antibiotic treatment and clinical status. Gastroenterology, 48:684, 1965.

van de Kamer, J. H., ten Bokkel, H., and Weyers, H. A.: Rapid method for determination of fat in feces. J. Biol. Chem., 177:347, 1949.

Waldmann, T. A.: Protein-losing enteropathy. Gastroenterology, 50:422, 1966.

Watson, D. W.: Immune responses and the gut. Gastroenterology, 56:944, 1969.

Weser, E.: Intestinal adaptation to small bowel resection. Am. J. Clin. Nutr., 24:133, 1971.

Weser, E.: Intestinal adaptation after small bowel resection. In Isenberg, J. I. (ed.): Viewpoints on Digestive Diseases. Vol. 10, Number 2. American Gastroenterological Association, Thorofare, New Jersey, 1978.

Weser, E., and Sleisenger, M. H.: Pathophysiology of sprue syndromes. Adv. Intern. Med., 15:253, 1969.

Williams, L. F., Jr.: Vascular insufficiency of the bowels. D. M., August, 1970.

Williams, L. F., Jr.: Vascular insufficiency of the intestines. Gastroenterology, 61:757, 1971.

Williams, L. F., Jr., and Wittenberg, J.: Vascular insufficiency of the intestine. In Isenberg, J. I. (ed.): Viewpoints on Digestive Diseases. Vol. 5, Number 2, 1973.

Wilson, F. A., and Dietschy, J. M.: Differential diagnostic approach to clinical problems of malabsorption. Gastroenterology, 61:911, 1971.

Wilson, H.: Carcinoid syndrome. Curr. Probl. Surg., November, 1970, p. 36.

Wilson, H., Cheek, R. C., Sherman, R. T., et al.: Carcinoid tumors. Curr. Probl. Surg., November, 1970, p. 4.

27

The Large Intestine

WILLIAM A. SODEMAN, JR.
AND DAVID W. WATSON

INTRODUCTION

The colon, including the rectum, forms the multifunctional termination of the gastrointestinal tract. Its anatomy is substantially differentiated from the relatively simple muscular tube of the small intestine. The colon is approximately 150 cm. long. It is highly variable in diameter, though as a general rule the cecum is the widest part and the angulation at the rectosigmoid juncture forms its narrowest constriction. The cecum, ascending colon, and proximal one half of the transverse colon are derived from the midgut and share innervation and vascular supply with the small intestine. The distal colon is a hindgut derivative and utilizes the inferior mesenteric artery and sacral parasympathetic innervation. There is substantial anastomosis between the two vascular beds and considerable overlap of innervation, so that these embryonic divisions are indistinct. In adult life, the left and right colon perform distinctly different tasks, though there is no evidence that this is a reflection of embryonic origin.

The wall of the colon has the same four layers as the small intestine: mucosa, submucosa, muscularis externa, and serosa. The mucous membrane is not thrown into villous extensions. Scanning electron microscopy (Fig. 27–1) shows a flat epithelial surface broken into polygonal units by a cleft. Openings of the numerous goblet cells are apparent, and the center of each polygonal unit is perforated by a crypt of Lieberkühn that is lined with goblet cells and penetrates down to the muscularis mucosa. Cells lining the crypt have been observed to be oriented in spiraling lines. A second unit consisting of 20 to 100 crypts has been observed by the scanning electron microscope and suggested by cell turnover studies. Both the small and the large units seem to be defined by mucosal vascular patterns. On conventional microscopic examination the surface epithelial cells that are presumably engaged in absorption present a striated border similar to that of small intestinal cells. Under the electron microscope the striated border resolves into microvilli complete with a fuzzy coat. There are scattered argentaffin cells. Cell renewal is initiated in the crypts, and cells migrate upward to the surface where they are extruded at the midpoint between crypts. The cell renewal time, based on cultured biopsy specimens of the rectum, averages 90 hours. Crypts disappear in the anal canal and the mucosa is replaced by stratified squamous cell epithelium. The lamina propria is represented by a thin layer of connective tissue that extends between the crypts. The submucosa resembles that of the small intestine and it contains nerves, plexuses, larger blood vessels, and scattered lymphoid follicles.

The muscular wall of the colon consists of two layers: an inner circular and outer longitudinal layer. Muscle fibers of the inner circular layer deviate from a strict circular orientation; however, because of close attachment to the taeniae it has, thus far, been impossible to identify a helical orientation. The longitudinal layer is gathered into three strips or bundles, the taeniae coli. The taeniae are spaced approximately equally around the circumference of the bowel. One taenia follows the mesenteric attachment. A thin layer of longitudinal muscle bridges the gap between the taeniae. The colon wall presents the appearance of being drawn into multiple loose sacculations,

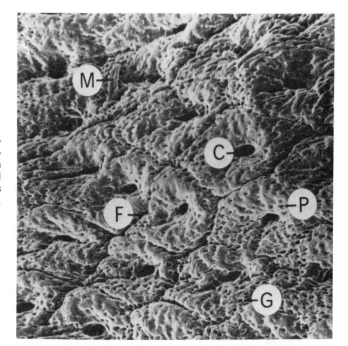

Figure 27–1 Scanning electron micrography of normal rectal mucosa. Each polygonal unit is surrounded by a furrow *(F)* with the crypt lumen *(C)* opening centrally. Filled *(P)* and empty *(G)* goblet cells and a mucus thread *(M)* can be identified (× 240). (Kavin, H., et al. Gastroenterology, 59:426, 1970.)

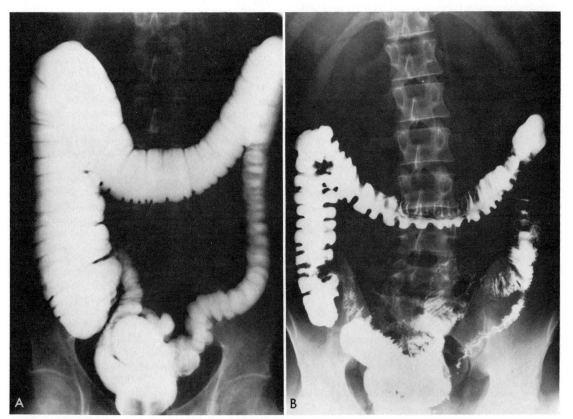

Figure 27–2 *A,* Normal barium enema examination showing both inter- and intrahaustral folds. *B,* Postevacuation film of the same patient showing the position of interhaustral folds.

the haustra. Haustrations are most apparent in the transverse colon and may be absent from the descending colon and sigmoid. The haustral folding is a dynamic process that is a result of circular muscle contraction, not puckering by taenial shortening. Each individual apparently has some points of regular haustral folding that are marked histologically by a concentration of muscular tissue and bridging by the serosa; however, intrahaustral folding can occur, so that the x-ray appearance of haustration may seem to vary from time to time (Fig. 27–2).

The mesenteric attachments permit substantial mobility of the colon. Only the descending colon and rectum are relatively fixed structures. The colon is supplied with external sympathetic and parasympathetic innervation and an extensive ganglionic plexus that permits intrinsic reflex innervation. Classic teaching holds that sympathetic innervation is inhibitory and parasympathetic innervation is stimulatory toward colonic musculature. Although there is extensive support from animal experimentation, it is difficult to apply to man. Neurogenic tumors that secrete epinephrine have been noted to result in intractable diarrhea in children. Truncal vagotomy may result in diarrhea. While it is reasonable to accept the concept of parasympathetic stimulation and sympathetic inhibition, it must be remembered that the final expression of any sort of stimulation in terms of motility will depend upon the state of the intrinsic innervation and that paradoxic responses may occur. From the anatomic standpoint, parasympathetic fibers to the right colon are carried in the vagus and those that arrive at the left colon come from the second through fourth sacral segments by way of the pelvic nerves. Sympathetic innervation is derived from cord segments thoracic 11 through lumbar 2 and arrives from the mesenteric ganglia in mesenteric and hypogastric nerves.

Integration of motility is the responsibility of the myenteric and submucosal plexuses. When they are absent, as in megacolon, contractions may continue in the aganglionic segment, but integrated motility is absent. As in the small intestine, the colon contains α and β receptors, with β receptors predominating; however, their function remains poorly elucidated. Central innervation may modify the ganglia activity but it cannot substitute for it. There also is substantial evidence for some degree of humoral control of intestinal activity. Although this is poorly understood at the present time, it clearly implies further difficulty in assigning roles to the various components of intestinal innervation.

The normal function of the colon encompasses controlled transit, absorption, and, to a limited degree, secretion. These culminate in defecation, a mechanism for elimination of metabolic wastes

and dietary residue. It is customary to speak in relatively laudatory terms of the colon's ability to desiccate and evacuate fecal contents, but it seems to us that the task, relative to the magnitude of small intestinal function, is unimpressive. The degree of mixing of intestinal content in the colon makes transit time only a relative approximation. Material ingested as a bolus will become dispersed over a substantial length of bowel and aliquots may appear over several days. When glass beads are ingested, a different color at each of the three meals, their appearance in the stool, including their distribution in the fecal pellet, is completely mixed and it is impossible to tell which color was ingested first. The colonic lumen may contain, alone or in a mixture, material behaving as a solid, liquid, or gas. Transit times do vary with the differing phases. Intestinal gas may transit, mouth to anus, in one to two hours, with liquids and solids lagging hours to days behind. Actual transit intervals in individuals are affected by a variety of factors, with the quantity of nonabsorbable residue in intestinal contents as the primary factor.

NORMAL MOTOR FUNCTION

Electrical Activity

All evidence suggests that the membrane electrical properties of colonic smooth muscle, including the rectum and anal sphincter, resemble those of the remainder of the gastrointestinal tract. Innervation, both extrinsic and intrinsic, plus circulating humoral substances must combine to provide integrated function in the colon. The pacesetter potential or basic electric rhythm (BER) in the small intestine seemingly acts as a governor initiating and integrating its function. The decreasing aboral gradient of the rhythm of slow wave deplorization integrates the pattern of flow of small intestinal content, resulting in transit down the intestine. Net flow down the colon is slower than in the small intestine and is modified by a degree of voluntary control. A simple gradient of BER has not been established in the colon; rather, there is the suggestion that the colon may be divided into several functionally distinct segments. There have been few studies in man, largely because of technical difficulties. Slow waves have been recorded throughout the colon, in the rectum and anal sphincter in man. No BER has been identified in the ascending colon. The slow waves are irregular in occurrence. A BER of 9 to 16 cycles per minute has been identified in the transverse and descending colon. No gradient has been identified. Results in the sigmoid have been variable. A rhythm ranging from 8.4 to 10.6 cycles per minute has been recorded; however, such rhythmic activity has been present for only brief intervals in one study, averaging 5 per cent of the total observation time. BER in the rectum has been recorded with a major component of 6 cycles per minute and a minor component of 3 cycles per minute. Spike waves have also been recorded, frequently appearing in bursts. In the small intestine, spikes appear related to circular muscle contraction and can result in intraluminal pressure changes. No such relationship has been identified in the colon. The internal anal sphincter claims a BER with the highest frequency thus far identified in the intestinal tract, averaging 17 cycles per minute. This has been correlated with high resting tone suggesting active closure of the sphincter. Sphincter relaxation correlates with inhibition of the BER. Curiously, the internal anal sphincter represents the only identification of BER in circular muscle thus far. Our sketchy knowlege of BER in the colon provides us little insight concerning integration of colonic motor activity.

Motility Mechanisms

Bayless and Starling initiated manometric studies of colonic motility in 1899. Cannon performed contrast studies of the colon in cats in 1902. Holzknecht described mass movement in man in 1909. To the present, no completely satisfactory description of motility mechanisms in the colon has been forthcoming. A number of technical problems remain. Access to proximal colon has been difficult and the lumen size plus the character of its contents make motility recording either by a balloon or by open-tip manometry difficult. Radiologic study utilizing contrast material has been hampered by the over-all slowness of colonic mechanisms. Transit is regularly measured in days, yet motility events may be of short duration, with long quiet intervals. It is difficult to identify a decisive moment. The definitive combined radiologic and manometric studies have been burdened with both sets of technical difficulties and too few such studies have been performed.

It is important for the interpretation of available information concerning colonic motility to identify the strengths and weaknesses of the methods utilized in its study. The classic approach to motility study utilized liquid-filled open-tipped tubes or liquid-filled balloon-tipped tubes which are connected to strain gauge manometers. Balloon-tipped tubes not only introduce the artifactual stimulus of the balloon itself, but they seem to vary in their response, depending on the proximity of the balloon to the wall of the colon. Open-tipped tubes, even if perfused, face artifactual hazards from the semisolid colonic contents. Finally, in the saccular colon it is clear

that pressure changes do not always reflect contraction of muscle immediately adjacent to the sensor tip. A capsule containing a miniature radiomanometer has been devised but its localization has been difficult. A series of wave patterns of the classic types I, II, III, and IV have been described but they have been difficult to translate into motility events. From the standpoint of manometry, colonic activity is best separated into segmentation or kneading by alternate formation and relaxation of haustral-like folds, and transportation, which implies peristaltic-like movement over longer segments of bowel. From the clinical standpoint, manometry's most significant contribution has been the identification of the negative relationship between colonic activity and motility. Segmenting activity produces in the colon a state of high resistance to flow. Normal, that is, slow or controlled, transit is associated with a substantial degree of manometric activity, much of which is segmenting. Peristalsis and mass transit, which can sweep colonic contents over distances of 10 to 100 cm., are found only in the absence of segmenting activity. Colons are manometrically quiet except presumably at the instant when the wave of mass movement passes down the bowel. For this reason drugs, particularly anticholinergics that quiet the bowel and reduce segmenting activity, are likely to worsen simple diarrhea. Drugs that increase tone and thus trigger spike activity will retard transit, reducing stool frequency in simple diarrhea.

Radiologic assessment of motility likewise has its strengths and weaknesses. Roentgenograms of hollow viscera all produce negative shadows that depend upon the use of contrast material. Both the physical and chemical qualities of the contrast can modify motility. Most contrast media will form a diffuse nonparticulate shadow and one must be satisfied with several assumptions to interpret changes in size, shape, and density of the opacified masses in terms of motility. Changes in density may as easily be the result of dilution by non-opacified material as of the loss of material by transit. Finally, colonic movements are slow and ill-suited to cine recording. The static films are poor records of dynamic events. Recently, several groups of investigators, most notably Ritchie and co-workers, have utilized time-lapse roentgenography to identify motility mechanisms. They administered a suspension of barium orally and on the following day performed a time-lapse x-ray study, taking films at intervals of one a minute for a period of 1 to 3 hours. Both control observations and a variety of stimuli have been utilized.

Ritchie's analysis has demonstrated two separate classes of activity (Table 27-1). The first is produced by haustral systole. It may involve one or several haustra. It may or may not result in

TABLE 27–1   COLONIC MOTILITY, TYPES OF CONTRACTIONS

Type of Movement	Frequency of Occurrence		Distance Traveled	Rate
	At Rest (%)	Postprandial (%)		
Haustral shuttling	38	13	0	0
Haustral propulsion	36	57	5 to 10 cm.	2.5 cm./min.
Haustral retropulsion	30	52	5 to 20 cm.	2.5 cm./min.
Multihaustral propulsion				
Systolic ⎫	9	17	Variable	5 cm./min.
Serial ⎬				2.5 cm./min.
Peristaltic ripples	Not Reported	Not Reported	5 to 10 cm.	0.1 to 2.0 cm./min.
Peristalsis	6	8	18 to 20 cm.	1 to 2 cm./min.
Mass propulsion	Rare	12	30 cm.+	5 to 35 cm./min.

(Data taken from Ritchie, J. A.: Gut, *9*:442, 1968.)

transit and transit may be in either direction. The second is progressive contraction of the bowel, a ringlike wave of activity that is propulsive and may go in either direction. These are not the exact equivalents of manometric segmentation and transit. These two broad classes of activity have been further subdivided on the basis of their apparent mechanical effect. The simplest activity is haustral shuttling. This consists of successive formation of a constriction at the midpoint of the haustra, with relaxation of the immediately preceding and following folds. Colonic content in effect shuttles back and forth from haustra to haustra, with mixing but without a net aboral or adoral transit. Ritchie's observations were based on studies of 190 individuals. This sort of activity was observed in 38 per cent of individuals at rest but in only 13 per cent after a meal. As an extension of this simple activity there is haustral propulsion and retropulsion. This is simple, successive, sequential contraction of single haustra that does result in movement in one or the other direction. This occurred in 36 per cent of the individuals as aboral movement and in 30 per cent as adoral movement at rest. After a meal, aboral movement occcurred in 57 per cent of individuals and adoral movement in 52 per cent. Some individuals experienced movement in both directions during the period of observation. The distances covered ranged from 5 to 20 cm. at a rate of 2 to 2.5 cm. per minute. A more complex variety of movement was termed multihaustral propulsion. This could be systolic or serial. Systolic movement occurred when three or more haustra merged. Transit occurred by the addition of single haustra to the head of the mass, with formation of empty haustra at the tail. Multihaustral propulsion was termed serial when three haustra would join. The contents merged and then subsequently one empty haustra re-

formed, with the net transfer of its contents to the remaining two.

Activity involving either of these mechanisms was observed in 9 per cent of these individuals at rest and 17 per cent postprandially. Transit could be in either direction and at rates up to 5 cm. per minute. Systolic activity appeared best suited to moving fluid contents either alone or around more solid contents without displacement of the solid stool.

Progressive contractions appeared to occur with several degrees of magnitude. Peristaltic ripples are ring contractions that are progressive and that do move contents over 5 to 10 cm. lengths. They move at a rate that is usually less than 1 cm. a minute. At their maximum they merge with peristalsis proper, which is a propagated ring contraction carried over a distance of 18 to 20 cm. It is preceded by relaxation and often followed by tonic contraction of the bowel. Some sort of peristalsis was noted to occur in 6 per cent of colons at rest and 8 per cent postprandially. Contractions of this sort have been noted to move both aborally and adorally. Finally, there is mass propulsion, which is thought to be peristaltic movement of the colon contents of a magnitude that may empty up to one half the length of the large bowel. This sort of activity was observed in only a few of the nearly 190 individuals studied. Mass propulsion seemed rare in the resting state and in most cases was observed postprandially. Mass propulsion has been noted to move aborally only and at a rate of progression which is rapid, in the range of 5 to 35 cm. per minute. Progressive waves depend on relaxation of interhaustral folds. If the relaxation fails, progressive waves are aborted. Progressive waves move the entire intestinal content, solid or liquid.

There are two other components in motility, the significance of which is not clearly defined.

The first is colonic shortening by taenial contraction. This does occur in combination with many of the activities mentioned above, but its role in transit is not clear. Secondly, there are the postural or gravity effects. In an organ in which the lumen is partially open, such as the colon, and which is filled with gaseous, fluid, and semisolid contents, gravity and postural changes have observable effects, but these have been difficult to define and their significance remains unclear. They are important, however, in pathologic states. Those individuals suffering from diarrhea may achieve some control over their bowel action by simple bed rest. The constipation which plagues many patients upon admission to the hospital with enforced bed rest probably has its origin in the same mechanism.

Transit

Contractile mechanisms not only are complex but also have segmental or regional expression. It is rare to observe a completely inactive colon. It is similarly rare to observe a normal colon that is active throughout its entire length. There are nearly always inactive portions. In general, the right colon is responsible for the largest absorption of water and solute. Haustral shuttling and systolic propulsion yield the maximum mucosal contact necessary to make this process efficient.

The left colon is faced with semisolid colonic contents, which it stores and evacuates. This is carried out most economically in terms of effort by serial propulsion and peristalsis. While this is generally true if viewed as a net response, all varieties of activity have been observed throughout the colon. Again the clearest documentation of the spectrum of segmental activity has come from the work of Ritchie (Table 27–2). He noted marked changes in activity postprandially, with haustral activity most notable in the right colon. Other investigators have suggested that the activity of the distal colon, as measured by the motility index, is enhanced by eating. Stimula-

tion of motor activity in the human sigmoid colon by exogenous cholecystokinin and inhibition of activity by exogenous secretin has been reported. A similar effect has been observed with endogenous release of cholecystokinin. This would support the suggestion that at least some of the integration of colonic activity may rest upon hormonal basis though the hormone responsible remains unclear.

In Western man with normal bowel habits, colonic activity is punctuated three times a day by a change in activity that follows eating. Activity as a general rule is enhanced in the postprandial state but transit down the colon as a whole remains unchanged. Retropulsion apparently balances increased propulsion. Following the ingestion of a meal there is an increase in ileal activity, with resultant slow filling of the cecum and ascending colon. The ileal influx is shuttled and propelled by systolic haustral contractions. Fluid contents may flow around masses of solid material, which accounts for mixing and the apparent length of transit time. Peristaltic movements may occur. Gradually, as the prandial stimulus subsides, areas of inactive bowel reemerge. Retropulsive movements occur in the right colon under the stimulus of a meal but are uncommon at rest. In this fashion the fluid contents of the right colon are rocked back and forth over the absorptive epithelium with each fresh surge of ileal influx. At rest the net propulsion amounts to about 1 cm. per hour. The contents are desiccated and as the left colon is approached the character of the colonic activity changes. At 18 to 24 hours, some portion of the ileal influx will have entered the rectum, but because of mixing, the colon clearance times for the entire bolus will be much longer. Retropulsion increases as the sigmoid region is approached. Gradually the sigmoid fills and periodically material passes on into the rectum. This distention initiates a defecatory urge. Response to this is governed, as will be discussed, by a number of physiologic and environmental variables. Defecation may result in

TABLE 27–2 COLONIC MOTILITY, DISTRIBUTION OF ACTIVITY

	Proportion of Section Remaining Inactive		Proportion of Colon Showing (Nonpropulsive Segmentation)	
	At Rest (%)	Postprandial (%)	At Rest (%)	Postprandial (%)
Cecum and ascending colon	42	16	38	45
Transverse colon	8	5	44	20
Descending colon	25	19	31	18
Pelvic colon	34	26	22	28
Rectum	60	59	20	22
Whole colon (mean)	32	21	35	25

(Data taken from Ritchie, J. A.: Gut, 9:502, 1968.)

simply local rectal emptying or it may lead to mass propulsion emptying the entire distal colon.

Variations of this normal sequence result not only from changes in the stimulus in the muscle, as by inflammation or distention, but also from changes in the character of the colonic content. This explains why a response to a barium enema bears so little relationship to normal function. The propulsion of gas through the colon and its passage reflect its relatively unaltered state during its passage down the large intestine.

Defecation

The rectum constitutes the distal 15 cm. of the large intestine. The rectosigmoid junction is indistinct, but the caudal level is well marked by the junction of mucous membrane with the anal canal's transitional epithelium. The rectum below its junction with the sigmoid enlarges to form the rectal ampulla. Above the peritoneal reflection, the rectum is bound to the pelvis by a fibrous sheath and below the support is provided by the muscles of the pelvic diaphragm. The musculature of the rectum is formed by a continuation of the colonic muscular coats. The outer longitudinal layer spreads from the taeniae of the sigmoid to form a continuous even coat. The superficial fibers insert into the perineal body and merge with the levator. The deep fibers insert into the perianal skin. The circular muscle differentiates into the internal sphincter surrounding the anal canal. The anus forms the terminal 2 to 4 cm. of the intestinal tract. The pectinate line marks the boundary between the anal canal and the rectum. The anus is lined with stratified squamous epithelium.

The external sphincter is made up of striated muscle which lies outside the internal sphincter and extends down below it to encircle the terminal portion of the anal canal. This muscle arises in the central perineum and inserts into the coccyx. The integrated function of the colon, rectum, and sphincters depends upon both sensory and motor innervation. Sensory endings are provided with both somatic and autonomic pathways. Sensory pathways for the anal canal and the perianal skin ascend through the somatic nerves to segments S2, S3, and S4. Proprioceptive spindles are present in the striated muscles of the external sphincter. Autonomic sensory innervation for the rectum passes to the same segments, though along parasympathetic pathways. A wide variety of sensory endings are present in both the rectum and anal canal. Motor fibers to the striated external sphincter arrive through the pudendal nerve and the coccygeal plexus, and originate in segments S2 to S5. Parasympathetic motor nerves to the internal sphincter descend from L5 and S1 to S3 through the pelvic nerves. These stimuli are inhibitory. Sympathetic fibers arrive via the hypogastric nerve and are excitatory motor stimuli. Sympathetic innervation of the rectum is drawn from L2 to L4 and parasympathetic fibers arrive from S2 to S4.

A variety of mechanisms combine to maintain fecal continence. These include a variety of mechanical factors resulting from rectosigmoid angulations and the valves of Houston and reflex sphincter responses. None is as important as the variety of reflex responses that are capable of operating without central control. A degree of basal tone is the feature of both rectum and sphincter. Flow of feces into the rectum gives rise to immediate increase in pressure, which at a critical volume stimulates rectal contraction and produces an urge to defecate. If this is denied, the rectum will relax and accommodate the feces, as evidenced by a fall in pressure. When defecation is denied, some feces may be returned to the sigmoid or higher. Both sphincters are in a continuous state of contraction. BER identified in the internal sphincter is inhibited by sphincter relaxation. Of the two, the internal sphincter seems to contribute the largest share of the squeeze closing the anal canal. The external sphincter is variably contracted with posture and other activities which stress continence. Distention of the rectum results in relaxation of the internal sphincter. This relaxation is short-lived, but it will allow rectal contents to descend into the anal canal far enough to permit their identification by sensory receptors. Voluntary contraction of the external sphincter can maintain continence during the short interval of internal sphincter relaxation. There is a prompt (but poorly understood) increase in external sphincter squeeze which defends continence against increases in intraabdominal pressure from straining and other activity. Micturition results in reflex relaxation of the external sphincter.

With such a wide variety of reflex controls, anorectal function is susceptible to many sorts of neurologic lesions. These may be grouped into three broad categories: (1) Loss of central innervation with intact sensation. This results in defecatory urge, which, while it cannot be denied, does remain under some local voluntary control. (2) Loss of both sensory and motor control above the sacral outflow results in a reflex colon. (3) Loss of the sacral cord or peripheral nerves results in an absence of reflex control.

Defecation is initiated in a continent man when the central nervous system accepts the information that the left colon and rectum are primed for defecation and when the environment is deemed acceptable for this activity. Intraabdominal pressure increases, the sphincters relax, the pelvic floor tenses, and the colon contracts. Evacuation of the distal rectum may be coupled with mass peristalsis which can empty the colon as high as the splenic flexure, but as often as not it seems to be related to multihaustral movement that empties only the distal end of the colon. Edwards and Beck obtained pre- and postdefecation films of individuals with radiopacified feces. They noted that small quantities of feces moved in and out of the rectum regularly and that a "call to stool" is initiated only when a critical volume to which the individual person is habituated is reached. This differs from the established teaching that the rectum remains empty until immediately prior to defecation but it confirms the regular clinical observation of feces palpable at the rectal examination. Some individuals empty the rectum only partially but others empty it completely. A number of factors remain to be defined to understand completely the controls of normal defecation.

NORMAL ABSORPTION AND SECRETION

In addition to transportation and elimination of dietary and metabolic waste, the colon is charged with the task of defending fluid and electrolyte homeostasis in the gastrointestinal tract. Fine regulation of electrolyte and fluid balance belongs to the renal and respiratory systems, yet the flux of liquid and electrolytes across the gastrointestinal mucosa is of such a magnitude that highly developed gastrointestinal regulation is essential.

Water and Electrolytes

Under ordinary circumstances the gastrointestinal tract is presented with a volume of 8 to 9 liters of combined secretion and ingested fluid daily. Absorption by the small intestine will reduce this to a volume of 500 to 600 ml. This daily volume will pass the ileocecal valve carrying an electrolyte load of 40 to 70 mEq. of sodium, 3 to 6 mEq. of potassium, 20 to 40 mEq. of chloride, and 30 to 35 mEq. of bicarbonate. Passage through the colon will reduce the volume to 100 ml.

Electrolyte concentrations, based on fecal dialysis studies by Wrong and colleagues, will average sodium 30 mEq. per liter, potassium 75 mEq. per liter, chloride 15 mEq. per liter, and bicarbonate 30 mEq. per liter. Approximately 50 per cent of the anion in fecal water will be made up of organic anion which results from bacterial action on carbohydrates. The resultant stool will be hyperosmolar (376 mOsm.).

The absorptive work is not uniformly distributed down the colon and there is evidence of regional specialization. The largest fluid volume and electrolyte absorption occurs in the right colon. The rectum is apparently impermeable to electrolytes and water. These values for absorption and secretion represent the net result and underlying this net result there may be a substantial effort in terms of flux of electrolytes in both directions across the mucosa (Table 27–3).

In terms of mechanisms, the absorption of water seems to be passive following the osmotic gradient produced by the absorption of sodium. The absorption of sodium is an active process. Absorption may be accomplished against a significant concentration gradient. Absorption has been noted from colonic luminal concentrations as low as 25 mM. sodium. Sodium is absorbed along an electrical gradient of 30 to 40 mv., mucosa negative.

Potassium can be secreted into the colon. Several mechanisms may be involved in the entry of potassium into the lumen. Mucus secreted by goblet cells in the colon may contain extraordinary quantities of potassium. Concentrations of up to 140 mEq. per liter have been noted. The potassium is not bound and may be reabsorbed, so that the contribution of mucus to potassium secretion will vary with the rapidity of transit and the total quantity of mucus secreted. The majority of potassium passing into the colon does go passively down an electronegative gradient. When luminal potassium concentrations rise above 15 mEq. per liter, the flux of potassium changes to absorption rather than excretion. There is no apparent interaction between the transfer of sodium and potassium.

TABLE 27–3 COLONIC ABSORPTION AND SECRETION FROM THE COLON

| | | Maximum Capacity/24 Hours | | |
| | | Flux | | |
	Average/24 Hours	Absorbed	Secreted	Net
Water	400 ml.	10,800 ml.	7800 ml.	3000 ml.+
Na+	66 mEq.+	878	418	460+
K+	3 mEq.−	26	58	32−

(Data taken from Shields, R., and Miles, J. B.: Postgrad. Med. J., 41:435, 1965.)

The colon is sensitive to aldosterone and other mineralocorticoids. The effect, increased sodium absorption and potassium secretion, resembles the steroid action on the kidney. A cyclic AMP-dependent mechanism for Na secretion similar to small intestinal response has been suggested.

Chloride has a net absorption which exceeds that of sodium. Chloride transport itself is not active and it seems to be absorbed as a paired ion with sodium. The absorption of chloride and the secretion of bicarbonate are coupled. In the absence of chloride, bicarbonate will be absorbed as a paired ion with sodium. When chloride is present, bicarbonate will be secreted apparently in exchange for chloride. Some secreted bicarbonate will combine with organic acids produced by bacteria in the feces. The absorptive capacity of the colon is limited. Calculations based on extrapolations of perfusion results are indicated in Table 27–3, along with the magnitude of the flux and the usual daily load.

Nutrients and Metabolic Products

The large intestine also has a meager digestive and synthetic role which only rarely may achieve clinical significance but should be remembered. Ordinarily, ingested cellulose passes through the intestinal tract largely unaltered. Bacterial digestion does break down some but this contribution is minimal. In constipated individuals with markedly prolonged transit times, colonic digestion of cellulose and absorption can become a significant factor in the diet. This circumstance is one that Davenport terms the "greedy colon." In addition to cellulose digestion, colonic bacteria can synthesize a number of vitamins, most notably folic acid but including riboflavin, biotin, vitamin K and nicotinic acid. Failure to produce these compounds can occasionally result in a clinical deficiency. An enterohepatic circulation involving the colon has been identified for several compounds. A urea-ammonia cycle is apparently limited to the colon. The colon also participates, though to a much more limited degree, in the enterohepatic circulation of bile acids. Urea is synthesized by the liver and enters the systemic circulation. The small intestinal mucosa is permeable to urea which may diffuse into the lumen, but quantitatively the amount involved is small, less than 500 mg. of the 7 grams normally degraded by the gut daily. The colonic mucosa is relatively impermeable to the diffusion of urea in either direction. Circulating blood urea is hydrolyzed in the colonic epithelial wall by bacterial ureases that either penetrate or are closely applied to the mucosa. Most of the ammonia that is produced is absorbed by the circulation. The alkaline pH in the lumen favors the dissociation of any ammonium that may diffuse into it. Free ammonia readily penetrates the mucosa and the nitrogen is returned to the liver for resynthesis of urea or use in protein synthesis. This colonic conservation of nitrogen may achieve clinical importance in the face of protein malnutrition. The apparent involvement of blood urea rather than luminal urea helps to explain the success of systemic urease inhibitors such as acetohydroxamic acid in treatment of hepatic encephalopathy.

Synthesis of bile acids by the liver is limited. The bile acid pool which varies from 1.2 to 6.0 grams is conserved by cycling through the enterohepatic circulation. In the course of 6 to 10 cycles a day, a small amount escapes the small intestinal absorption mechanism. The daily fecal excretion amounts to an average of 500 mg. of bile acid. Chenodeoxycholic acid escaping into the colon is dehydroxylated by bacteria to form lithocholic acid, which is nonabsorbable and is excreted. It accounts for 300 mg. of the 500 mg. of bile acid lost daily. Cholic acid is dehydroxylated to desoxycholic acid and about half of this will be reabsorbed by the colon. Since 200 mg. is lost in the feces, there must be addition to the bile acid pool of approximately 200 mg. of this secondary bile acid daily from the colon.

Drugs

A wide variety of drugs are regularly administered by enema or suppositories. Salicylates, sedatives, antiemetics, opiates, bronchodilators, tranquilizers, and selected antibiotics all have significant absorption and systemic effect. A number of agents administered for local action, such as corticosteroids, may have significant systemic absorption which will limit their use. Neomycin is also in this category.

A seemingly endless number of drugs have been administered rectally without success. Chloramphenicol, tetracycline, and sulfonamides are erratically absorbed by the rectal mucosa, though they may be well absorbed by the oral route. There are no identified carrier mechanisms in the colonic mucosa. Absorption depends on several factors. Small molecules may diffuse through the pores in the colonic epithelium. They could be carried in by water during its passive absorption. Rectal absorption of water and electrolytes is markedly restricted if it occurs at all, and hence the absorption of a drug by diffusion will depend on the level to which the preparation is carried in the colon. Its retention time will also be a critical factor that determines absorption. This may well account for the erratic absorption of many of the antibiotic compounds. As a general rule, compounds which remain in a lipid-soluble state at colonic pH are better absorbed. They presumably dissolve through the lipid-containing cell membrane. Some drugs such as neomycin are as well absorbed rectally as they are orally and the absorption appears completely unaffected by retention time or other identifiable factors. The mechanism of their absorption remains to be defined. An additional avenue for absorption may be available for those agents which are used topically in the treatment of inflammatory bowel disease. The ulcer bed and denuded mucosa expose deeper, perhaps barrier-free areas which may permit absorption.

Gas

The gastrointestinal tract contains an average of 100 ml. of gas. This may be subject to wide variation with changes in diet. While gas may be distributed down the entire length of the intestinal tract, a substantial percentage of it accumulates in the colon. Gas passed by rectum is made up of swallowed air, gas diffusing across the mucosa from the circulation, and gas produced by bacteria in the small intestine and colon. Its final composition will obviously reflect the activity of these various sources. In addition to oxygen, nitrogen, and carbon dioxide, methane and hydrogen may be major components of flatus. A number of gaseous components are present in trace amounts. Swallowed air contains small quantities of the rare gases and a number of volatile metabolic products may be present. These can include ammonia, hydrogen sulfide, skatole, indole, and fatty acids. Ordinarily, these represent less than 1 per cent of flatus.

Hydrogen is produced by bacteria, and in the absence of bacterial overgrowth of the small intestine it is derived primarily from the colon. There is no other source for production of gaseous hydrogen in the human body. Methane is similarly produced by bacterial fermentation in the intestine. Bacteria utilize only substrate found within the lumen, and production of gas is related to the numbers of gas-forming bacilli and the dietary availability of suitable substrate. Carbon dioxide may be swallowed but more significant amounts are produced in the intestinal tract as a consequence of neutralization of acid by bicarbonate. Free carbon dioxide is in equilibrium with bicarbonate and with circulating carbon dioxide. It can diffuse across the mucosa. A similar equilibrium exists for nitrogen and oxygen. In the colon, bacterial utilization of oxygen may result in extremely low or negligible concentrations of oxygen. In this fashion, an anaerobic environment may be maintained within the colon.

Passage of gas through the colon may be far more rapid than liquid or semisolid feces. Resistance to flow by haustration is substantially less effective for gases than it is for liquids. Also, colonic activity is usually sufficient to prevent layering of fluid and solid fecal contents into separate phases but it is insufficient to prevent the separation of a gaseous phase. This makes possible the differential motility of gas in the colon.

DISORDERS OF MOTOR AND ABSORPTIVE FUNCTIONS

DIARRHEA WITH NORMAL-APPEARING COLON

Diarrhea may be a result of a wide variety of stimuli. The final common path resulting in frequent stools lies with an increase in the volume load, a decrease in the absorptive capacity, or in rapid transit. On occasion, stimulation of colonic secretion may be a factor. The number of pathophysiologic mechanisms that may lead through one or several of these pathways is huge and a comprehensive discussion is beyond the limits of this chapter. In this and subsequent sections, examples utilizing each of the pathways will be presented and it should be remembered that these are illustrative and not a complete portrayal. It is rare to find only a single mechanism operative, and even in an apparently pure disorder, there may be secondary involvements of several mechanisms ultimately producing the diarrhea. This feature has important therapeutic implications. Without this concept clearly in mind, the use of some agents in the treatment of diarrhea (and their success) may seem paradoxic. This is particularly true with regard to the use of hydroscopic, bulk-producing materials in the treatment of diverticulosis and irritable bowel syndrome.

The primary causes of most diarrheal disease without structural abnormality remain either hidden, i.e., idiopathic, or beyond any reasonable hope of control, i.e., viral gastroenteritis, and one relies on a number of nonspecific agents to obtain symptomatic relief. There are a few circumstances in which the primary pathologic condition is identifiable and susceptible to modification. Diarrhea associated with hyperthyroidism presumably represents an extension of the general hypermetabolic state. Control of excess circulating thyroid hormone, medically or surgically, offers primary control of diarrhea. Similarly, epinephrine-producing neurogenic tumors offer an identifiable mechanism. In addition, the case for an excitatory role for sympathetic innervation is strengthened by the clinical observation of the result of these tumors. Although resection of the tumor may not always be feasible, the use of epinephrine-blocking agents offers a therapeutic avenue. Diarrhea may be associated with certain medullary tumors of the thyroid. This is thought to be related to release of a prostaglandin. The identity of the diarrheogenic hormone found in some nonbeta islet cell tumors of the pancreas is not clear. It may well be a secretory agent similar to the prostaglandin released by medullary tumors of the thyroid. The syndrome of watery diarrhea and hypokalemia has occurred in individuals with the Zollinger-Ellison syndrome, but it does also appear in a pure form unrelated to gastric hypersecretion. Primary mechanisms of this sort deserve specific therapy. However, in absolute numbers they form a relatively insignificant proportion of the diarrheal diseases. One identifiable primary mechanism that does seem to form a significant portion of diarrheal diseases is related to lactose malabsorption. Many individuals on a constitutional or acquired basis will have a decline in lactase activity in the small intestine following weaning. The final level of lactase activity seems to vary from individual to individual. When the small intestinal mucosa is stressed with a lactose load beyond its metabolic capacity, the unsplit dissaccharide will be carried down the small intestine and discharged into the colon. In the colon, lactose can serve as a substrate and it will be fermented by a variety of bacteria. The fermentation process produces lactic acid and gas. The combination of volume and the acid stimulus produces intestinal hyperactivity that may be manifested by audible intestinal sounds, cramping abdominal pain, and occasionally diarrhea. Small intestinal lactase does appear to be an inducible enzyme in some animals. However, it remains to be demonstrated that the enzyme level is inducible in man. The only effective therapy at this time is the elimination of lactose from the diet to produce a reduction to levels that an individual may tolerate.

Simple Diarrhea

Volume overload of the colon resulting in frequent stools probably represents the commonest of gastrointestinal afflictions. The colonic overload in simple diarrhea is a product of disturbed small intestinal function. Cholera is a classic example. Exposure of small intestinal mucosa to cholera toxin results in activation of the adenylate cyclase system regulating sodium secretion. Massive flux of sodium and fluid into the bowel lumen is the result. This secretion exceeds the reabsorptive capacity of the small intestine and the colon. The colon simply fills to capacity and watery diarrhea ensues. The radiologists can ordinarily fill a colon at the time of barium enema with 1500 ml. of barium suspension. Patients with full-blown cholera ordinarily produce watery stools at the rate of 500 ml. per hour. Cholera as a clinical entity is exotic. The diarrhea of travelers, enteropathogenic *E. coli* infection, viral gastroenteritis, Clostridium and staphylococcal enterotoxin-containing food, and the use of saline cathartics represent more practical clinical ex-

tensions of the concept of simple volume overload of the colon. Although the colon is capable of absorbing up to 3000 ml. of fluid daily (Table 27–3), this represents a relatively meager absorption capacity of 125 ml. per hour or slightly more than 2 ml. a minute. It is not difficult for a volume load to exceed these limits in a short period of time. One effect of the volume load is a change in the composition of the stool. As the volume increases so does the sodium concentration and the potassium content of the stool decreases. Gradually, at a volume of approximately 3000 ml. of stool a day, the composition approaches that of normal plasma. Clearly, there must also be some alteration in intestinal motility; however, this is less impressive in simple diarrhea than in the irritable colon syndrome and inflammatory bowel disease. Perhaps the absence of the motility components is more apparent than real, since, as will be discussed, the motility alterations associated with diarrhea produce a quiet colon.

Irritable Colon Syndrome

A great deal of human emotion is expressed by conscious voluntary activity such as a smile, clearing of the throat, or a nod of the head. Often, the translation of the emotional content into activity, such as applause, will vary from culture to culture. There is a similar body of reflex emotional expression, such as blushing or weeping, over which voluntary control has never been remarkably effective. Some reflex emotional responses cross the rather indistinct boundary that separate physiologic from pathologic response. It is not uncommon to identify individuals who respond to stress with urticaria, asthma, or emesis. When the emotional expression alters intestinal motility and absorption, producing pain and/or diarrhea, often alternating with constipation, the condition is described as the irritable colon syndrome.

The stringent limits that we as individuals set to identify as our normal bowel habits are more often culturally than physiologically inspired. Much, but not all, of what is diagnosed as irritable bowel syndrome is hardly disease. If public defecation at the roadside were considered a poetic expression rather than vulgar display, individuals with an irritable bowel would be the laureates of the land.

Three other factors seem to have a strong impact on the expression of irritable colon. One is an ill-understood constitutional or familial factor, about which little more can be said than that it exists. Second, the observation has been made that individuals with irritable bowel syndrome have a preponderance of a fast BER (3 cycles per minute) in the distal colon when contrasted with normal individuals. Hormonal stimuli such as

CCK produce a contractile response that matches the 3 cycles per minute BER. The last is related to irritants. These may be infections, respiratory as well as gastrointestinal, or, more commonly, food irritants. Food as an irritant seems as often as not to represent an idiosyncratic response of an individual rather than the expression of a toxic food. The kind of food which precipitates symptoms varies widely from individual to individual. This brings the full circle back to emotional factors.

There is, to be sure, an element of emotional overlay that will accompany any of the colonic afflictions discussed in this chapter. Also, there is great individual variation in terms of colonic response to emotional stress. The various appellations applied to the irritable colon syndrome, i.e., spastic gut, psychophysiologic gastrointestinal reaction, functional bowel syndrome, and mucous colitis, indicate that in many people it represents an emotional disturbance alone. When irritable colon syndrome is seemingly not an extension of organic disease, that is, when it is truly idiopathic, it poses a challenge to physicians to continue symptomatic control. It is true that irritable colon syndrome must once have included those individuals with lactose intolerance, amebiasis, and a wide variety of other identifiable colonic diseases and there probably remain some primary mechanisms yet to be identified and extracted. However, this does not make it a wastebasket diagnosis. Clearly, an exaggerated response to stress can, alone and unaided, be responsible for both the spastic and diarrheal varieties of irritable colon syndrome.

From the standpoint of pathologic physiology, irritable colon syndrome may be separated into two varieties — spastic and diarrheal. The spastic variety presents clinically with an alteration in bowel habits and abdominal pain. Diarrhea may alternate with constipation. The cramping abdominal pain seems to be the key clinical feature in determining the pathophysiology. These individuals experience a stimulation of haustral contractions. Vigorous segmental contractions produce closed chambers containing trapped fluid and gas. Further contractions result in increased tension in the colonic wall and cramping abdominal pain. Increased segmentation yields a high resistance state within the colon and there will be little effective transit. As the increased segmentation subsides, haustral transit may occur and peristaltic activity may be stimulated; thus, the cramping abdominal pain may terminate in a diarrheal rush. The diarrheal variety is relatively more simple in clinical appearance. Patients do not have cramping abdominal discomfort, though there may be ample audible intestinal activity. The call to stool may be precipitated and result in passage of a liquid stool. A sequence of response with a number of watery stools in progressively smaller volume, beginning in the morning and terminating in the forenoon, with the patient remaining relatively symptom-free for the remainder of the day, is not uncommon.

With this variety the mechanism seems to be related to a quiet colon. Manometrically, there is an absence of the phasic contractions that are usually identified with segmentation. In this case, small changes in pressure may result in substantial flow down the lower resistance colon. Absence of haustral activity sets the stage for peristalsis and mass movement. The response by the sigmoid colon to the ingestion of food may be a normal increase in phasic contraction, but this quickly fades at the termination of the meal and the colon returns to its basic hypotonic state.

Either variety of irritable colon syndrome may be associated with increased mucus secretion. Occasionally, this may present as spectacular ropy strands of mucus passed in the stool without apparent associated feces. More often, small amounts of mucus will collect in the rectum, just above the sphincter. The quantity will be too small to act as a stimulus, but the patient quickly learns that the passage of flatus may prove embarrassing. This additional anxiety and the necessity to retreat to the toilet to pass flatus further compound the irritable colon syndrome.

Each mechanism implies specific therapy. In the spastic variety, anticholinergics, which have been noted manometrically to inhibit phasic activity, may give a measure of control over the cramping abdominal pain. To do this the dose must be carried to a critical level. The inhibition of phasic activity carried to completion may exacerbate the diarrheal component as the colon is reduced to a low resistance state. It takes great patience to direct anticholinergic therapy in this situation. Irritable bowel of the diarrheal variety obviously responds poorly to anticholinergics alone. The addition of opiates, which enhance tone and may stimulate phasic activity, and the use of hydroscopic bulk agents, which act to increase resistance to fluid flow, constitute a better and more effective regimen. In either case, the thoughtful selection of sedatives and tranquilizers may support the regimen.

Bile Acid Diarrhea

Bile acid diarrhea illustrates a third general response to the development of diarrhea in a normal-appearing colon. Suitable concentrations of conjugated and unconjugated dihydroxy bile acids in the colon stimulate secretion of sodium and water. This produces diarrhea by a volume overload that has its primary genesis within the colon itself.

Disorders of the enterohepatic circulation of bile acids may lead to diarrhea by a number of mechanisms. When the bile acid circulation is broken and the pool size falls, the concentration of bile entering the duodenum may be insufficient to permit complete fat absorption. Steatorrhea, often with diarrhea, may result. In small intestinal stasis syndrome, bacterial deconjugation of bile acids may lead to similarly insufficient levels of bile acid for the formation of micelles and fat absorption. The diarrhea under these circumstances is a result of hepatic and small intestinal failure. When the enterohepatic circulation is broken because of ileal dysfunction and failure of active ileal absorption of bile acids, larger than normal quantities of bile acids may pass into the colon. Experimentally, perfusion of the human colon with deconjugated dihydroxy bile acids in a concentration of 3 to 5 mM. produces a marked secretion of sodium and water. A cyclic AMP-dependent Na secretory mechanism has been suggested. Equimolar mixtures of conjugated bile acids cause similar secretion of sodium and water plus additional secretion of potassium and bicarbonate. The magnitude of secretion is sufficient to explain diarrhea associated with an enterohepatic circulation broken at the ileal level. Inhibition of absorption of water and electrolyte by bile acid has also been observed. Successful therapy of bile acid diarrhea has been described using cholestyramine, a resin which binds bile acid. Successful application of cholestyramine requires a careful selection, for though its reduces bile acid effects, it increases steatorrhea. There is a relatively limited zone in which the net result is an effective reduction of diarrhea.

DIARRHEA WITH STRUCTURAL CHANGES IN THE COLON – INFLAMMATORY BOWEL DISEASE

Specific Inflammatory Disease

Inflammatory disease of the wall of the colon results in diarrhea by one or a combination of several mechanisms. Mucosal erosion and ulceration destroy the epithelial barrier and leave a raw exuding surface. When the stool content is primarily exudate, blood, and necrotic epithelium, the clinical diagnosis of dysentery is appropriate, and widespread colonic disease may be suspected. Shigella, amebae, and Staphylococcus that produce pseudomembranous enterocolitis are perhaps the commonest specific agents producing dysenteric symptoms. Pathologic changes are not limited to the mucosal inflammation. Inflammatory cell infiltration and ulceration may extend into the submucosa and the muscularis. Rarely, septic perforation will occur. The extension of inflammatory disease to deeper levels, with resultant infiltration and edema, changes

the physical characteristics of the wall, particularly the stiffness, and, because of irritation of nerve plexuses, may alter motility mechanisms. In the presence of active inflammation it is common to see absence of haustration, with resultant low resistance to flow down the colonic lumen. As inflammation subsides and healing occurs, several varieties of derangement are possible, depending on the pattern of fibrosis that evolves. If the fibrotic reaction is diffuse, the pattern of absent haustration may solidify. This is best exemplified in the hosepipe appearance of the colon in burnt-out chronic ulcerative colitis and is a less frequent but not unheard of sequela of specific infectious colitis. Changes of this sort require rather massive involvement of the colon or prolonged repetitive bouts of inflammation. When fibrosis is localized, a partial or complete stricture may result. Complete obstruction in the large intestine, whether by stricture or volvulus or whatever mechanism, results in changes similar to those described in the small intestine. In individuals with a competent ileocecal valve, the added complication of closed loop obstruction with toxic dilatation can occur. When stricture produces only partial obstruction, the distention may result in an irritable focus with a distal increase in transit, producing diarrhea.

Several agents which produce inflammatory bowel changes do not ordinarily present with widespread colonic disease. Amebic, tuberculous, and fungal infections typically present with a regional involvement. The usual involvement is cecal and is thought to be related to stasis in the cecal segment. For most organisms this location represents the first point of slowing of the intestinal stream, affording an opportunity for prolonged contact by multiple organisms that is necessary for penetration of the epithelial barrier. It is also possible that the relative fluidity and concentration of nutrients plus the favorable redox potential in the cecum play an important role in the establishment of infection in this area. Regional infection is also common in the rectosigmoid, the other point of relative stasis of the fecal stream. In addition to an ulcerative inflammatory response, a proliferative granulomatous response to most of these agents may occur. These infectious pseudotumors can disorder motility and result in diarrhea. Several of the parasites, particularly schistosomes, produce colonic lesions by embolization or deposition of ova in the intestinal wall. With the development of delayed immune sensitivity, a granulomatous reaction surrounds these lesions, which may ulcerate through the mucosa or may produce proliferative granulomatous polyps. In all these cases, specific and effective chemotherapy can halt progression of these lesions. However, their resolution may lead to significant structural changes and to the production of additional symptoms.

Diverticular Disease of the Colon

Diverticula in the colon represent outpouchings or herniations of mucosa and submucosa between fasciculi of the circular muscle of the colonic wall. True diverticula contain all coats of the colon wall, similar to Meckel's diverticula in the small intestine. These do occur, but they are exceedingly rare. The usual diverticula form in response to two sets of circumstances. In the colon there are, in effect, two kinds of diverticular disease. These two varieties are simple diverticulosis and spastic diverticulosis. Both may eventuate in inflammatory bowel disease; however, in both the inflammation is a late phenomenon complicating the end stage of the disease. In the absence of inflammation, simple diverticula are silent and usually unassociated with any symptoms. Some workers have felt that they are the sequelae of the diarrheal variety of irritable bowel syndrome. The diverticula of spastic diverticulosis are not asymptomatic. Here the disease is felt to be an extension of the spastic variety of irritable bowel syndrome. Thus, pain and alteration of bowel habits will precede the development of diverticula. Simple diverticula are outpouchings through weakened portions of an otherwise normal circular muscle. They increase in frequency with age and after age 40, 5 per cent or more of the population of the United States will have demonstrable diverticula. Constitutional and environmental factors are thought to be major factors in their occurrence. Diverticula are rare among African and Asian populations. Simple diverticula represent herniations at points of anatomic weakness, often at points of penetration of the musculature by arteries. While single scattered diverticula are common, occasional individuals may present with massed simple diverticula. With massed diverticula, each herniation is thought to be the result of increased pressure pushing the mucosa through the muscular defect. The result is an apparent shortening of the colon, because the total area of the mucosa remaining to line the lumen is inadequate. This apparent shortening is unassociated with inflammation and is a simple mechanical phenomenon. Simple diverticula may become inflamed, just as any outpouching of the gut may in a fashion similar to the appendix develop intraluminal inflammation. This sort of inflammation seems to be a rare occurrence. However, rupture of inflamed simple diverticula with peritonitis, abscess, and fistula have been reported. Inspissated contents may produce ulceration of the diverticulum neck. Because of the close association of many simple diverticula with small arteries, the ulceration can lead to spectacular lower gastrointestinal bleeding. Right-sided diverticula may bleed for this reason as readily as those on the left. Selective angiography is apparently the most reliable method of identifying the bleeding diverticula. Bleeding diverticula are notoriously inapparent at surgery and may require multiple colostomies for their identification. Selective infusion of epinephrine or vasopressin through arterial catheters offers some hope for medical therapy of massive bleeding from this source. It certainly represents a step up over blind resection of portions of the colon in the therapeutic armamentarium for bleeding diverticula. Evidence has begun to accumulate that would suggest that many colonic bleeds in elderly patients are secondary to the development of submucosal vascular ectasias. These apparently are degenerative lesions which increase in frequency with aging. Commonly they are multiple.

Spastic diverticulosis, which is limited in distribution to the sigmoid and distal descending colon, is an entirely different entity in terms of its pathologic physiology. The circular muscle in the distal colon is organized into fasciculi or rings. There are fibers that bridge from one ring to another ring, but the general structural orientation remains and is visible in a longitudinal cross section of the bowel. In certain individuals with a spastic variety of irritable colon syndrome, these rings of sigmoid musculature begin to undergo remarkable muscular hypertrophy with a crowding together of the muscle fibers. This hypertrophy may be eccentric and usually will involve only a portion of the circumference of the ring. The portion of the colonic wall running between the mesenteric taenia and the two antimesenteric taeniae is involved. The remaining one third of the circumference of the wall lying between the two antimesenteric taeniae is relatively spared. The muscular hypertrophy permits the formation of multiple closed chambers from the lumen of the sigmoid, and within these chambers there may be significant increase in intraluminal pressure as a result of contraction of the hypertrophied circular muscle (Fig. 27–3). This increase in tension results in cramping abdominal pain. The muscular thickening and crowding of the circular muscle yields a characteristic pattern on radiographic examination, often termed a sawtooth deformity (Fig. 27–4). The wall thickening may also present as a palpable mass. All these features — the pain, the mass, and the radiologic abnormality — may present in the absence of inflammation and have been reported in the absence of diverticula. Diverticula form in a fashion similar to simple diverticula as herniations of mucosa blown out through weakened areas between the hypertrophied fasciculi of the circular muscle. On occasion the increased pressure generated in the closed chamber will cause a perforation of the tip of the diverticulum. This can give rise to the formation of pericolitis, abscess, peritonitis, and fistula formation. This then represents true diverticulitis and will also give rise to

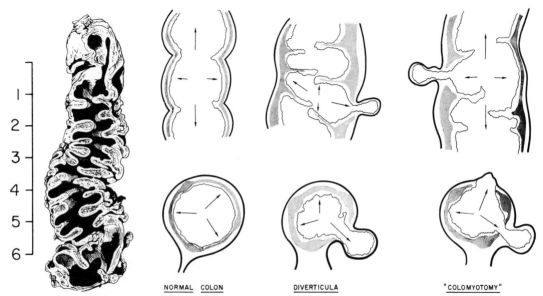

NORMAL COLON   DIVERTICULA   "COLOMYOTOMY"

Figure 27–3   Figure on left is a drawing of a gross specimen of sigmoid colon which is involved in sigmoid diverticulitis. The hypertrophied rings of circular muscle which give rise to the saw-tooth deformity on x-ray are clearly apparent. The remainder of the illustration indicates the mechanism of formation of diverticula and their relief by colomyotomy. (See also Figure 27–4.) (Ranson, J. H. C., et al.: Am. J. Surg., *123*:185, 1972.)

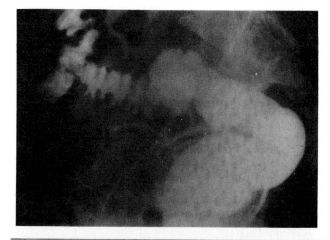

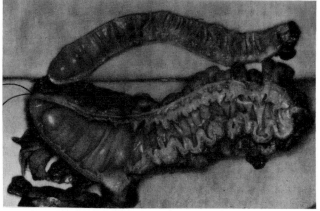

Figure 27–4 Photograph of a gross specimen of sigmoid colon *(bottom)* and a preoperative barium enema of this colon *(top)* showing the abrupt change from normal sigmoid to that involved with hypertrophy of the circular muscle. The saw-tooth or serrated deformity is easily visible on x-ray. (Arfwidsson, S.: Acta Chir. Scand., Supplement *342*:40, 1964.)

TABLE 27–4 PATHOLOGIC FEATURES OF CROHN'S DISEASE AND ULCERATIVE COLITIS

	Crohn's Disease	*Ulcerative Colitis*
Gross Features		
Anal and perianal lesions	Major and common	Minor and uncommon
Bowel wall	Thickened	Normal to slight increase
Strictures	Common	Uncommon
Fistulas	Common	Rare
Pseudopolyps	Rare	Common
Ulcers	"Fissure"	Punctate to troughlike
Distribution	More proximal	More distal
Continuity	Often "skip" areas	Always contiguous
Toxic megacolon	Uncommon	More common
Carcinoma	Rare	Increased
Microscopic Features		
Primary impact	Submucosa	Mucosa
Type of reaction	Productive	Exudative
Lymphoreticular hyperplasia	Marked and transmural	Minimal and superficial
Granulomas	40 to 80%	Ocassionally
Crypt abscesses	Occasionally	Usual
Vascular ectasia and edema	Marked	Related to acute inflammation
Epithelial regeneration	Rare	Common

(Watson, D. W.: Calif. Med., *117*:25, 1972.)

a palpable mass and pain. It may be distinguished from the noninflammatory "diverticulitis" by the presence of fever, leukocytosis, and the finding of extravasated barium at the time of enema. Treatment will vary with the stage of the disease. When perforation and pericolitis occur, the patient must be treated as any perforated viscus is treated. Recurrent diverticulitis may be a management problem. Connell treats recurrent pericolitis with intermittent courses of nonabsorbable sulfa for periods of four to five days each month. In the absence of inflammation, two courses are currently open. Long sigmoid myotomy dividing the hypertrophied rings of muscle but without penetrating the mucosa has been reported to give symptomatic relief (Fig. 27–3). Recently, the use of high-residue diets based largely on bran content has been reported to yield relief of symptoms that is maintained indefinitely. Critical evaluation and controlled trials of bran have not been performed. If the relationship between spastic irritable bowel and spastic diverticulitis is verified, earlier and more aggressive therapy of the former may be preventative.

Idiopathic Chronic Inflammatory Bowel Disease

On the basis of certain clinical and histopathologic features, two distinct forms of chronic inflammatory bowel disease are currently recognized. The utility of this separation derives from differences in histologic appearances and clinical events which reflect different patterns of morbidity and mortality. The terms ulcerative colitis and

Crohn's disease have been most frequently applied to these disorders, but in the colon the latter has also been frequently referred to as granulomatous colitis, transmural colitis, or ileocolitis when disease is present in both small and large bowel. The differential features of the two conditions are summarized in Table 27–4. This separation into two seemingly distinct conditions, however, should not obscure their obvious interrelationship, which is expressed most fully in the colon, in which the distinction between ulcerative and granulomatous colitis at times may not be possible. If the morbid anatomy characteristic of each form is kept in mind, the clinical differences between the two are more readily appreciated. In classic Crohn's disease the submucosal edema and fibrosis and the deep fissure ulcers often lead to partial intestinal obstruction and fistulae, whereas the mucosal ulceration characteristic of ulcerative colitis more commonly results in hemorrhage and perforation. In the colon, however, chronic inflammatory bowel disease often presents a mixed histologic appearance, with a corresponding overlapping of clinical manifestations.

Ulcerative Colitis

Although occurring most frequently in Great Britain, North America, New Zealand, and Australia, ulcerative colitis has a worldwide distribution, as evidenced by reports from Costa Rica, Africa, and India. The peak incidence occurs in the second and third decades with a smaller peak after age 60. A genetic predisposition appears likely for the following reasons: (1) the higher incidence in Jews and the less common occurrence among blacks; (2) a familial occurrence ranging between 5 and 12 per cent which is interdependent with Crohn's disease; (3) an association with ankylosing spondylitis, which itself has genetic determinants; and (4) the presence of anticolon antibodies in healthy relatives. With respect to ankylosing spondylitis it should be noted that the prevalence of the histocompatability antigen, HLA-B27, found in that disorder, does not occur in ulcerative colitis except in association with spondylitis.

Efforts to determine cause have emphasized infectious, psychogenic, and immunologic factors. An infectious origin appears highly unlikely and the potential influence of psychogenic factors probably has been overemphasized. It has been widely held that patients with ulcerative colitis exhibit a characteristic personality type, but the few controlled studies available fail to demonstrate a relationship between ulcerative colitis and various psychologic parameters. Some type of immune reaction involving small lymphocytes and bacterial or colonic antigens appears most likely, but present evidence is inconclusive. Circulating lymphocytes have been demonstrated to be cytotoxic for colon epithelial cells and this effect can be modified by bacterial extracts. Recent evidence suggests these may be Fc-receptor cells "armed" by antigen-antibody complexes containing colonic or bacterial antigens.

Although primarily a disorder of the colon, it is clear that ulcerative colitis is often a systemic disease exhibiting a wide range of extracolonic manifestations. These are listed in Table 27-5.

The colon's contribution to the clinical picture is in the form of some combination of diarrhea, hematochezia, and cramping lower abdominal pain. The intensity of these symptoms varies widely between patients and from time to time in the same patient. Onset may be gradual or fulminant and the course chronic and continuous or remittent and relapsing. Asymptomatic intervals vary from a few weeks to many years, but eventual relapse is the rule, the rate varying between 27 and 50 per cent per year. Fever and leukocytosis may occur with acute attacks and hypoalbuminemia and anemia is common. The latter is most often due to blood loss but other causes include malabsorption of iron, autoimmune hemolytic anemia, microangiopathic hemolytic anemia, G-6-PD deficiency, and Heinz body anemia related to Azulfidine therapy.

Diagnosis depends upon observing characteristic features of the disease by proctosigmoidoscopy or barium enema. Since both gross and microscopic features are non-specific, it is also important to exclude bacterial and parasitic infections, especially in patients with acute disease of recent onset. Classically the muscosa appears hypere-

mic, edematous, granular, and friable, often with fine ulcerations and active bleeding. Involvement is always continuous over the length involved. Rectal biopsy may reveal characteristic but non-specific changes and will always be abnormal in the presence of active disease or demonstrable disease elsewhere in the colon. A histologically normal rectum in the presence of more proximal disease is highly unlikely in ulcerative colitis and favors a diagnosis of Crohn's disease. The radiologic appearance of ulcerative colitis is well known and only a few comments are appropriate here. In more acute phases there will be rather broad-based mucosal ulcerations, edema of the mucosa, and often loss of haustrations. More chronic involvement is manifested by loss of mucosal detail, loss of haustrations, shortening of the colon, widening of the retrorectal space, pseudopolyps, and occasionally rectovaginal or rectovesical fistulae. The terminal ileum may be involved with a superficial "backwash" ileitis in about 10 per cent of cases. Involvement begins distally and proceeds proximally always in a continuous fashion without skip areas. There is little or no fibrosis even with long-standing disease, and the majority of radiologic findings, including shortening and loss of haustrations, are potentially reversible.

TABLE 27-5 EXTRACOLONIC MANIFESTATIONS OF ULCERATIVE COLITIS

Skin lesions
  Erythema nodosum
  Erythema multiforme
  Pyoderma gangrenosum
  Nonspecific pustular dermatosis
Mucous membrane lesions
  Aphthous stomatitis
  Ulcerative esophagitis
Eye lesions
  Episcleritis
  Uveitis
  Iritis
  Conjunctivitis
  Marginal corneal ulceration
Bone and joint lesions
  Arthralgias
  Sacroiliitis
  Arthritis of ulcerative colitis
  Ankylosing spondylitis
  Rheumatoid arthritis
Hepatobiliary lesions
  Active chronic hepatitis
  Pericholangitis
  Unclassified inflammatory changes
  Cirrhosis (postnecrotic and biliary)
  Carcinoma of extrahepatic bile ducts
  Primary sclerosing cholangitis
Pericarditis
Renal calculi

Complications include severe hemorrhage, perforation, toxic megacolon, malnutrition, carcinoma of the colon, and, in children, failure of sexual development and growth retardation. Three high-risk factors have been identified with respect to the development of carcinoma of the colon: (1) onset in childhood, (2) total or near total colonic involvement, and (3) duration of disease longer than 10 years. Obstruction and fistulization are seldom encountered in patients with ulcerative colitis.

All non-surgical treatment is empirical and symptomatic. Emphasis has been placed upon the administration of Azulfidine (salicylazosulfapyridine), measures to control diarrhea, and the use of systemic or topical steroids. Both Azulfidine and corticosteroids may suppress active disease, but only the former has demonstrated prophylactic value in continuing remissions. The aforementioned complications are frequent indications for colectomy, but the most frequent reason for surgical intervention in patients with ulcerative colitis continues to be intractability and failure of medical management. Although some continue to employ subtotal colectomy, there is a growing emphasis upon one-stage total proctocolectomy and permanent ileostomy.

The outcome of the disease is most dependent on the age of the patient, the extent of the involvement, and the severity of the current attack. Mortality is highest in those above the age of 60, those with total involvement and the severest attacks. The single most important factor governing prognosis is the severity of a given attack. The reported mortality for severe attacks varies between 11 and 26 per cent and that for mild or moderate attacks is less than 1 per cent. The late outcome or long-term mortality remains inadequately defined, since most studies are based upon projected values involving relatively small numbers of patients.

Crohn's Disease

Crohn's disease most frequently is confined to the small intestine with 90 per cent of cases involving the terminal ileum. It may occur however in a segmental distribution anywhere in the small bowel and has even been described in the esophagus and stomach. The colon may be the only site of involvement in some 10 to 17 per cent of patients or may be involved as part of an enterocolitis in 17 to 40 per cent. It has an ethnic and age distribution similar to ulcerative colitis except for the lack of a secondary peak in the older age group. Reliable data concerning its incidence and prevalence in the general population and its geographic distribution are not available, however, owing to the uncertain frequency of granulomatous colitis, since a firm diagnosis of the latter often requires surgical material. Again

a genetic predisposition seems probable, but hypotheses concerning etiology are even less well formulated than in the case of ulcerative colitis. Similar to the latter, these patients frequently possess anticolon antibodies and circulating lymphocytes which are cytotoxic for allogenic colon epithelial cells. The presence of anergy in a significant proportion of patients has been found by some but not by others and this question remains unsettled.

The proclivity to transmural involvement with edema and fibrosis often results in chronic partial intestinal obstruction. The mucosa may become secondarily involved to a lesser extent, so that hemorrhagic ulceration is not as frequently encountered as in patients with ulcerative colitis. Similarly, the thickened bowel wall rarely is the site of a free perforation. Instead, the deep cleft-like fissure ulcers, characteristic of this disease, lead to fistulization and abscess formation. The relative sparing of the muscosal layer probably also accounts for the less frequent development of carcinoma in these patients compared to those with ulcerative colitis.

Sigmoidoscopic examination presents a variable appearance. Fully one half of patients with large bowel involvement and all the patients with disease limited to the small bowel will have a normal rectum, both grossly and histologically. In the known presence of more proximal inflammatory disease this in itself strongly favors a diagnosis of Crohn's disease as compared to ulcerative colitis. A small proportion of patients have rectal involvement that will be grossly or microscopically distinguishable from ulcerative colitis as assessed by rectal biopsy. The remainder exhibit features suggesting the presence of Crohn's disease. These include skip areas, large ulcerations and various anal and perianal lesions. The latter may present as indolent, undetermined anal fissures, sometimes extending to involve the perineum and even to the inguinal regions; enterocutaneous fistulae; solitary ulcers; and edematous anal tags. These anal lesions at times are the initial manifestation of disease, and biopsy of an ulcer, fissure, or fistulous tract may demonstrate granulomas and greatly assist in diagnosis. The point of demarcation between normal and abnormal bowel is relatively sharp in contrast to ulcerative colitis. Opinions differ regarding the usefulness of rectal biopsy in establishing a diagnosis, since the major thrust of the disease is in the submucosa and therefore a biopsy, to be helpful, must be deep enough to include a substantial portion of this area. This is often safe only on the rectal valves or the margin of an ulcer, and if characteristic changes are observed, including marked submucosal fibrosis and in inflammation with granulomas, a diagnosis of Crohn's disease may be possible.

Radiologically, the presence of certain features

strongly suggests a diagnosis of Crohn's disease as opposed to ulcerative colitis. These include strictures, asymmetrical involvement of the bowel wall, fissure ulcers, enteric or enterocutaneous fistulae, disease limited to the more proximal portions of the colon, skip areas, and the presence of similar abnormalities within the small intestine. Many cases, however, will be indistinguishable from ulcerative colitis on radiologic grounds and many of these will exhibit overlapping histologic features. The spectrum of extraintestinal manifestations seen in patients with ulcerative colitis is also encountered in patients with Crohn's disease, although they are seen somewhat less frequently. Nonsurgical therapy in Crohn's disease follows the same general pattern of that utilized in patients with ulcerative colitis except that both Azulfidine and corticosteroids have a much less profound effect on patients with Crohn's disease, and the evidence presented by Cooke and Fielding suggests that mortality and complications are actually increased in patients with Crohn's disease receiving long-term steroid therapy. The surgical management of Crohn's disease is less satisfactory than in the case of ulcerative colitis. This is due to the frequent necessity for resection of physiologically important amounts or areas of bowel and the relatively high recurrence rate. Recurrence rates vary from 30 to 65 per cent, depending upon the distribution of disease at the time of surgery. Recurrence is least frequent with disease limited to small bowel, especially terminal ileum, is somewhat more frequent with colon involvement, and is most likely in the presence of ileocolitis. Some 30 per cent of patients will require more than one operation, with the risk of recurrence rising somewhat with each successive procedure. Resection is preferable to bypass procedures, the latter being carried out only when resection is technically unfeasable.

The prognosis of Crohn's disease has been difficult to define, since it often depends on confirmation of the diagnosis by surgical means and the length of observation. It has generally been considered to be a chronic disease of high morbidity and low mortality, with physicians often trying to recall when they had last witnessed an autopsy on a patient with the disorder. Chronic and recurrent intestinal obstruction and malnutrition dominate the clinical picture. Malnutrition may be due to inadequate intake or malabsorption. The latter may result from loss of absorptive surface due to disease or resection (short bowel syndrome), loss of bile salts with defective micellar solubilization, bacterial overgrowth, or stasis secondary to blind loops or strictures. The underlying mechanisms are discussed in Chapter 31. Total parenteral nutrition is often required to correct nutritional defects prior to surgical thera-

py, and in patients in whom surgery is not possible long-term management may include home hyperalimentation. The over-all mortality is probably in the range of 15 per cent. In a study by Prior et al. of 295 patients followed for 1 to 38 years there were 53 deaths, more than twice the number expected for either sex. There was also a tendency for mortality to be higher in those with onset before age 40 and when corticosteroids had been employed.

It is obvious from the foregoing discussion that in many, probably most, instances ulcerative colitis and Crohn's disease appear to be distinct and separable entities, clinically, radiologically, and histopathologically. It is also true that they share many familial, ethnic, and immunologic similarities and as many as 20 per cent of cases of large bowel disease cannot be fitted into one of the two available types. Whether we are dealing with distinct entities having overlapping manifestations or a spectrum of a single disease remains unclear. In either case, differences exist which have prognostic and therapeutic relevance. Although the clinical course and complications encountered in the classic forms of the two extremes of chronic inflammatory bowel disease are readily understood in terms of histopathologic events characteristic of each, the latter cannot at present be understood in etiologic or pathogenetic terms.

CONSTIPATION

There is remarkably wide variation in human bowel habits. Diarrhea is present when stool frequency increases to the point at which formed stools are no longer produced. The end-point for constipation is less easy to define. Davenport reports human tolerance for fecaliths of up to 100 lbs. and intervals between defecation as long as one year. Under normal circumstances failure to defecate regularly at intervals of at least seven days probably requires prompt investigation. Many individuals may be appropriately diagnosed as constipated with smaller changes in bowel habit. Except for the emotional turmoil, the only pathologic changes that may regularly be associated with constipation are the development of hemorrhoids, anal fissure, and the consequences of straining at stool.

Constipation may occur by several mechanisms. Congenital failure of the formation of intramural ganglia will result in a constricted colonic segment. Failure of integrated contraction causes a functional obstruction, with the back-up of feces and the presentation of megacolon. Excision of the offending segment results in return of transit and a resumption of bowel function. The pathophysiology of simple constipation is substantially less clear. Two varieties are recognized. In spastic or colic constipation, individuals demonstrate a motility abnormality of the sigmoid and descending colon. In the resting state there is a substantial increase in segmentation and non-propulsive activity and there is delay of transfer of feces into the rectum. Rectal examination reveals a relatively empty rectum containing at best a few small lumps of hard feces. The underlying cause of the motility abnormality remains unclear. There has been a demonstration of the failure of normal physiologic mechanisms such as the effect of eating to stimulate a change of activity in the sigmoid colon. Stool softeners and a thoughtful use of contact laxatives orally or in suppository form and the use of bulk agents may effect a return to normal bowel habits.

Sensory constipation is an extension of the normal social inhibition of bowel action necessary to control defecation. When the rectum is distended to a critical volume, the urge to defecate is initiated. If it is denied, the rectum will relax and distend to accommodate the feces. The addition of larger quantities of feces will be required to reactivate the reflex. When voluntary denial is frequent, the rectum may become desensitized and a failure of call to stool by rectal distention results. On examination, these individuals will be found to have a rectum full of soft feces. This resembles the circumstances that result from cord transection with sensory failure. Therapy is more difficult with sensory constipation and requires re-education of the patient to achieve normal bowel habits.

Local pain and fear of its recurrence can inhibit defecation. Careful evaluation for rectal inflammatory lesions is an essential part of the therapy of constipation.

DISORDERS OF SECRETORY FUNCTION

Normal function of the colon includes net absorption of sodium and chloride and absorption of water. Potassium and bicarbonate may be absorbed or secreted. Because there is a substantial flux of sodium and potassium into and out of the lumen, it often is difficult to identify a disorder that is the result of enhanced secretion. The net secretion of sodium and water when the colon is exposed to conjugated bile acids may as well be the result of decreased active sodium absorption as an increase in secretion. There are two disorders in which abnormal electrolyte secretion seems to be a primary defect — chloridorrhea and the hypokalemia associated with villous adenoma of the rectum. In addition, the colon shares with the small intestine a role in the immune system. The colon may mount its own immune response, secreting coproantibodies into the lumen.

Chloridorrhea

Chloridorrhea occurs in both a congenital and an acquired form. Normal handling of chloride in the colon results in passive absorption as paired ion with sodium. In the absence of chloride in the lumen, bicarbonate is absorbed. When chloride is present in the lumen, the chloride absorption seems to be coupled with an exchange for bicarbonate. The acquired form of chloridorrhea occurs in individuals who suffer from both diarrhea, due to some primary colonic disease, and severe hypokalemia. It is thought that the potassium deficiency affects the permeability of the mucosa, and the chloride-bicarbonate exchange is interrupted. Increased delivery of chloride into the gut is postulated. While the chloride secretion may be reabsorbed in individuals with normal colons, in individuals with some primary colonic disease absorptive failure due to mucosal abnormality or increased transit results in chloridorrhea. In congenital chloridorrhea, a similar mechanism exists. The primary colonic lesion is the congenital inability to absorb chloride adequately through the colonic mucosa. The excess fecal chloride acts as an osmotic cathartic. With development of hypokalemia, additional chloride loss by secretion results. Fecal chloride concentrations regularly exceed the sum of fecal sodium and potassium concentrations. Correction of potassium defect by supplementation and by limiting dietary chloride results in a significant improvement in diarrhea and electrolyte balance. Similar therapy should prove effective in acquired chloridorrhea.

Villous Adenoma

Villous adenomas are benign tumors of the colon. They may occur throughout the colon, though they are most common in the rectosigmoid. Their gross and microscopic appearance is that of multiple frondlike extensions. The folds are lined with numerous goblet cells and may produce truly astounding quantities of mucus secretion. Villous adenomas are distinguished clinically by a well-established potential for malignant transformation and for the production of mucus diarrhea which may on occasion lead to severe hypokalemia. Although the frequency of carcinomatous change has been reported to be as high as 50 per cent, the biologic activity of this tumor is low and successful secondary resections are reported. Mucus secretion is a result of the large number of goblet cells contained in the tumor. The occasional villous adenoma that is found in the colon higher than the rectosigmoid does not result in diarrhea, since reabsorption of electrolytes secreted in the mucus may occur. As was indicated earlier, there is little or no reabsorption from the rectum and therefore tumors in the rectal segment are the prime offenders. Colonic mucus generally contains concentrations of sodium which are isotonic with plasma, 140 mEq. per liter. Concentrations of potassium are very much higher than serum concentrations. Concentrations as high as 140 mEq. per liter have been reported. However, the potassium concentration in mucous diarrhea usually remains only 3 to 10 times the serum level. The resultant loss of potassium will involve not only electrolyte changes but can precipitate kaliopenic nephropathy, digitalis toxicity, muscle weakness, and fatigue. Losses of a magnitude sufficient to cause death have been reported. The proper treatment is surgical removal of the tumor.

TUMORS OF THE COLON

The colon may play host to a full range of neoplasms, both benign and malignant. By far the most common benign tumor is the adenomatous polyp and the most common malignant tumor is adenocarcinoma. Villous adenomas have been presented under disorders of secretion. The benign adenoma, whether sessile or pedunculated, rarely produces significant symptoms. Occasionally, a benign tumor will bleed significantly or a low-lying polypoid adenoma will cause enough rectal irritation to produce diarrhea, but for the most part they are silent lesions. Extensive discussion of polyps would be unrewarding were it not for the controversy over whether benign adenomatous polyps are inclined to develop into adenocarcinoma. Hyperplastic polyps frequently occur in the colon. The simple adenomatous polyp is a neoplasm. Studies by Lane and coworkers of small polyps reveal distinct changes in glands with absence of papillary infolding and increase in cellularity. Mitotic figures may be found well above their normal zone of occurrence in the crypts and there are distinct changes in nuclei and distribution of cell types. In addition there are changes in the pattern of secretion and the basement membrane. Studies suggest that hyperplastic polyps are a result of hypermaturation of an area of colonic epithelium. Cell turnover and invagination are delayed but the above features serve to distinguish adenomatous polyps from them. The question of whether they are prone to undergo malignant transformation is controversial. There are two views: One suggests that adenomatous polyps have no greater potential for becoming carcinomatous than any of the remaining colonic epithelium. The latter do admit that the cytologic appearance of cellular atypia may develop in polyps but state that regardless of cytologic appearance their biological behavior remains that of a benign tumor. They further admit the presence of polypoid carcinomas. These are felt to represent cancers from the time of their origin and not malignant degeneration in a polyp. Generally, all cancers are felt to be larger than 1.5 cm. in diameter. Thus risk of operation has been felt to be greater than the risk that a polypoid lesion less than 1.5 cm. in diameter is a carcinoma. Long pedicles tend to favor slow-growing tumors of longer duration (Fig. 27–5). Both groups agree that villous adenomas can undergo malignant degeneration. The other group, believing in malignant potential of an adenomatous polyp, has yet to demonstrate unequivocally that a metastasizing carcinoma has developed from a benign adenomatous polyp in any individual. The group favoring no malignant potential appears to have the balance in their favor; however, a barium enema never permits one to make a cytologic differentiation between villous adenoma, polypoid carcinoma, and adenomatous polyp. The resolution of the problem at this time lies with the endoscopist. Flexible fiberoptic colonoscopes are available in lengths suitable to permit examination of the entire colon from the cecum to the anus. As experience broadens, it appears technically feasible to reach the cecum in 75 to 85 per cent of cases. Snares with electrocoagulation and forceps are available to permit biopsy at any level. The safety of the procedure contrasts favorably with the alternative direct surgical approach. Overholt has collected figures for 3793 polypectomies. Perforations occurred in 0.23 per cent of patients, bleeding in 0.9 per cent, and death in less than 0.03 per cent. The estimated economic savings of colonoscopic polypectomy over surgery are significant. At the present time colonoscopy represents the most reasonable approach to the diagnosis and therapy of small polypoid lesions. If one accepts the suggestion that adenomatous polyps remain benign, even fragmentary biopsy will provide the necessary differentiation of the polypoid lesions. There will of course always be individuals for whom colonoscopy, for medical, technical, or emotional reasons, cannot be performed. A like group for similar reasons will not be operable. With regard to carcinoma proper, several additional points bearing on the pathologic physiology of their presentation should be mentioned. Carcinomatous lesions remain silent until they encroach on the lumen, bleed, or present with metastasis. The fluid contents in the right colon make obstruction a late occurrence. Right-sided lesions characteristically come to attention because of blood loss from the ulcerated and friable tumor surface or because of distant metastasis. The semisolid contents of the left colon, particularly the rectum and sigmoid, permit obstruction with smaller, earlier tumors. The critical feature of the colonic cancer and practically any cancer is not its size or location as much as its biological activity. Cancers of low biologic activity may remain resectable after long intervals and after reaching large size. Tumors of high biologic activ-

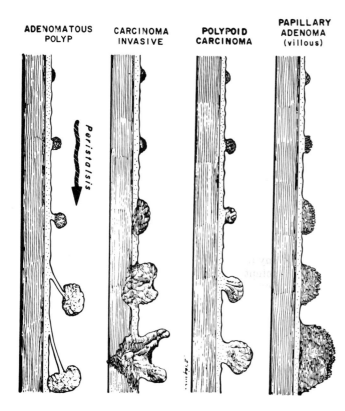

ADENOMATOUS POLYP **CARCINOMA INVASIVE** **POLYPOID CARCINOMA** **PAPILLARY ADENOMA (villous)**

Peristalsis

Figure 27–5 Castleman's conception of pedicle formation. With papillary adenomas, the broad base prevents prolapse, so that pedicles are rare. Polypoid cancer may develop with a short pedicle. Invasive cancer rapidly fixes mucosa to muscularis, so that pedicle formation becomes impossible. Simple adenomas, by proliferation at the tip, develop large heads, so that the underlying mucosa is soon pulled into a pedicle by peristalsis. (From Welch, C. E.: Polypoid Lesions of the Gastrointestinal Tract. Philadelphia, W. B. Saunders Co., 1964.)

ity will metastasize before any hope of identification is present. There is no practical measure of biologic activity that may be used clinically at this time. Some hope exists for the use of quantitative determination of fetal intestinal tract proteins and other endogenous substances produced by cancer. Apparently gastrointestinal tumors, particularly colonic cancer plus a number of nongastrointestinal tumors, undergo regression to an embryonic cellular activity at the time of malignant transformation. Gold and co-workers have described a radioimmunoassay for carcinoembryonic antigen (CEA), one of these fetal intestinal tract proteins. The full range of the specificity and sensitivity of testing for this protein is yet to be identified. LoGerfo and co-workers have utilized a similar assay for a tumor associated antigen (TAA) which may be different from CEA. It is similarly incompletely evaluated. CEA and TAA testing remain the current hope for any increase in sensitivity for the diagnosis and management of colon carcinoma.

COLONIC MICROFLORA

The colon is best known for the lush growth of bacteria that inhabits the lumen. The difference in numbers of microorganisms in samples aspirated from the distal ileum in the cecum may be in the order of 4 to 6 $\log_{10}$. The bacterial flora of

the large intestine does not represent an uncontrolled growth of a mass of organisms, for there appear to be a variety of mechanisms for qualitative and quantitative control of the flora. Normal flora performs several "functions." The digestion of cellulose and the production of a variety of vitamins have been discussed. Balanced normal flora may inhibit the overgrowth of pathogenic organisms, particularly staphylococci. The risk of staphylococcal overgrowth with enterocolitis is always present when normal flora is rendered unstable by antibiotic therapy. There also is an apparent necessity for specific bacterial flora to be present for full clinical expression of ameba infection. Normal flora may contribute to local and systemic pathologic changes in a number of other ways. Fermentation of lactose produces symptoms in lactase deficiency, and bacterial metabolism of bile acids may alter the enterohepatic circulation. The urea-ammonia cycle is also dependent upon bacterial action and may achieve significance in protein malnutrition and hepatic encephalopathy. Specific infections such as Shigella have been discussed. The colon may also harbor a range of other pathogenic organisms, particularly *Vibrio cholerae* and Salmonella, contributing to the carrier state. The full significance in terms of the pathologic physiology of colonic disease of alterations of controls over bacterial flora remains to be identified.

REFERENCES

Allen, F. D.: Essentials of Human Embryology. 2nd ed. New York, Oxford University Press, 1969.

Ammon, A. V., and Phillips, S. F.: Inhibition of colonic water and electrolyte absorption by fatty acids in man. Gastroenterology, 65:744–749, 1973.

Bentley, D. W., Nicols, R. L., Condon, R. E., and Gorbach, S. L.: The microflora of the human ileum and intraabdominal colon: Results of direct needle aspiration at surgery and evaluation of the technique. J. Lab. Clin. Med., 79:421, 1972.

Bleiberg, H., Mainguet, P., Galand, P., Chretien, J., and Dupont-Mairesse, N.: Cell Renewal in the Human Rectum. In vitro autoradiographic study on active ulcerative colitis. Gastroenterology, 58:851, 1970.

Bloom, A. A., LoPresti, P., and Farrar, J. T.: Motility of the intact human colon. Gastroenterology, 54:232, 1968.

Boley, S. J., Sammartano, R., Adams, A., DiBiose, A., Kleinhaus, S., and Sprayregen, S.: On the nature and etiology of vascular ectasias of the colon. Degenerative lesions of aging. Gastroenterology, 72:650, 1977.

Breen, K. J., Bryant, R. C., Levinson, J. D., and Schenker, S.: Neomycin absorption in man. Studies of oral and enema administration and effect of intestinal ulceration. Ann. Intern. Med., 76:211, 1972.

Casarella, W. J., Kanter, I. E., and Seaman, W. B.: Right-sided colonic diverticula as a cause of acute rectal hemorrhage. New Eng. J. Med., 286:450, 1972.

Castleman, B., and Krickstein, H. I.: Do adenomatous polyps of the colon become malignant? New Eng. J. Med., 267:469, 1962.

Castleman, B., and Krickstein, H. I.: Current approach to the polyp-cancer controversy. Gastroenterology, 51:108, 1966.

Chaudhary, N. A., and Truelove, S. C.: The irritable colon syndrome. A study of the clinical features, predisposing causes, and prognosis in 130 cases. Quart. J. Med., 31:307, 1962.

Christensen, J.: The controls of gastrointestinal movements: Some old and new views. New Eng. J. Med., 285:85, 1971.

Christensen, J.: Myoelectric control of the colon. Gastroenterology, 68:601, 1975.

Connell, A. M.: The motility of the pelvic colon. Part II. Paradoxical motility in diarrhoea and constipation. Gut, 3:342, 1962.

Connell, A. M.: Motor action of the large bowel. In Code, C. F. (Ed.): Handbook of Physiology. Vol. IV. Washington, D.C., American Physiological Society, 1968.

Cooke, W. T., and Fielding, J. F.: Corticosteroids or corticotrophin therapy in Crohn's disease (regional enteritis). Gut, 11:921, 1970.

Couturier, D., Roze, C., Couturier-Turpin, M. H., and Debray, C.: Electromyography of the colon in situ. An experimental study in man and in the rabbit. Gastroenterology, 56:317, 1969.

Crane, C. W.: Observations on the sodium and potassium content of mucus from the large intestine. Gut, 6:439, 1965.

Davenport, H. W.: Physiology of the Digestive Tract. 3rd ed. Chicago, Year Book Medical Publishers, Inc., 1971.

deDombal, F. T.: Ulcerative colitis. Epidemiology and aetiology, course and prognosis. Brit. Med. J., 1:649, 1971.

Derjanecz, J. J., and Clarke, C. W.: Papillary adenomas of the colon and rectum: Clinical and pathological behavior. A plea for more conservative treatment. Canad. J. Surg., 7:389, 1964.

Devroede, G. J., and Phillips, S. F.: Conservation of sodium, chloride and water by the human colon. Gastroenterology, 56:101, 1969.

Devroede, G. J., and Phillips, S. F.: Failure of the human rectum to absorb electrolytes and water. Gut, 11:438, 1970.

Dinoso, V. P., Jr., Meskinpour, H., Lorbin, S. H., Gubierry, J. G., and Clay, W. Y.: Motor responses of the sigmoid colon and rectum to exogenous cholecystokinin and secretin. Gastroenterology, 65:438–444, 1973.

Dowling, R. H.: The enterohepatic circulation. Gastroenterology, 62:122, 1972.

Edwards, D. A. W., and Beck, E. R.: Fecal flow, mixing and consistency. Amer. J. Dig. Dis., 16:706, 1971.

Edwards, D. A. W., and Beck, E. R.: Movement of radiopacified feces during defecation. Amer. J. Dig. Dis., 16:709, 1971.

Elsen, J., and Arey, L. B.: On spirality in the intestinal wall. Amer. J. Anat., 118:11, 1966.

Evanson, J. M., and Stanbury, S. W.: Congenital chloridorrhoea or so-called congenital alkalosis with diarrhoea. Gut, 6:29, 1965.

Feldman, F., Cantor, D., Soll, S., and Bachrach, W.: Psychiatric study of a consecutive series of 34 patients with ulcerative colitis. Brit. Med. J., 3:14, 1967.

Fenoglio, C. M., Richart, R. M., and Kaye, G. I.: Comparative electron-microscopic features of normal, hyperplastic and adenomatous human colonic epithelium II. Gastroenterology, 69:100, 1975.

Field, M.: Intestinal secretion: Effect of cyclic AMP and its role in cholera. New Eng. J. Med., 284:1137, 1971.

Field, M.: Intestinal secretion. Gastroenterology, 66:1063, 1976.

Fleischner, F. G.: Diverticular disease of the colon; new observations and revised concepts. Gastroenterology, 60:316, 1971.

Fordtran, J. S., and Ingelfinger, F. J.: Absorption of water, electrolytes and sugars from the human gut. In Code, C. F. (Ed.): Handbook of Physiology. Vol. III. Washington, D.C., American Physiological Society, 1968.

Goligher, J. C., deDombal, F. T., Watts, J. M., and Watkinson, G.: Ulcerative Colitis. Baltimore, Williams and Wilkins Co., 1968.

Gorbach, S. L.: Intestinal microflora. Gastroenterology, 60:1110, 1971.

Hayashi, T., Yatami, R., Apostol, J., and Stemmermann, G. N.: Pathogenesis of hyperplastic polyps of the colon: a hypothesis based on ultrastructure and in vitro cell kinetics. Gastroenterology, 66:347–356, 1974.

Hellmans, J., Vantrappen, G., Valembois, P., Janssens, J., and Vandenbroucke, J.: Electrical activity of striated and smooth muscle of the esophagus. Amer. J. Dig. Dis., 13:320, 1968.

Hofmann, A. F.: The syndrome of ileal disease and the broken enterohepatic circulation: Cholerheic enteropathy. Gastroenterology, 52:752, 1967.

Hofmann, A. F., and Poley, J. R.: Cholestyramine treatment of diarrhea associated with ileal resection. New Eng. J. Med., 281:397, 1969.

Holzknecht, G.: Die normale Peristaltick der Kolon. Muench Med. Wschr., 56:2401, 1909.

Ivey, K. J.: Are anticholinergics of use in the irritable colon syndrome? Gastroenterology, 68:1300, 1975.

Lane, N., Kaplan, H., and Pascal, R. R.: Minute adenomatous and hyperplastic polyps of the colon: Divergent patterns of epithelial growth with specific associated mesenchymal changes. Contrasting roles in the pathogenesis of carcinoma. Gastroenterology, 60:537, 1971.

Levitan, R., and Ingelfinger, F. J.: Effect of d-aldosterone on salt and water absorption from the intact human colon. J. Clin. Invest., 44:801, 1965.

Levitt, M. D., and Bond, J. H., Jr.: Volume, composition, and source of intestinal gas. Gastroenterology, 59:921, 1970.

LoGerfo, P., Herter, F., and Hansen, H. J.: Tumor associated antigen in patients with carcinoma of the colon. Amer. J. Surg., 123:127, 1972.

Matsumoto, K. K., Peter, J. B., Schultze, R. G., Hakim, A. A., and Franck, P. T.: Watery diarrhea and hypokalemia associated with pancreatic islet cell adenoma. Gastroenterology, 50:231, 1966.

Mekhjian, H. S., Phillips, S. F., and Hofmann, A. F.: Colonic secretion of water and electrolytes induced by bile acids: Perfusion studies in man. J. Clin. Invest., 50:1569, 1971.

Mendeloff, A. I., Monk, M., Siegel, C. I., and Lilienfeld, A.: Illness experience and life stresses in patients with irritable colon and with ulcerative colitis. New Eng. J. Med., 282:14, 1970.

Meshkinpour, H., Dinoso, V. P., and Lorber, S. H.: Effect of intraduodenal administration of essential amino acids and sodium oleate on motor activity of the sigmoid colon. Gastroenterology, 66:373, 1974.

Morson, B. C.: The muscle abnormality in diverticular disease of the sigmoid colon. Brit. J. Radiol., 36:385, 1963.

Morson, B. C.: Current concepts of colitis. Trans. Med. Soc. London, 86:159, 1970.

Overholt, B. F.: Colonoscopy. Gastroenterology, 68:1308, 1975.

Painter, N. S., Almeida, A. Z., and Colebourne, K. W.: Unprocessed bran in treatment of diverticular disease of the colon. Brit. Med. J., 2:137, 1972.

Phillips, R. A.: Cholera in the perspective of 1966. Ann. Intern. Med., 65:922, 1966.

Phillips, S. F.: Absorption and secretion by the colon. Gastroenterology, 56:966, 1969.

Phillips, S. F., and Edwards, D. A. W.: Some aspects of anal continence and defecation. Gut, 6:396, 1965.

Prior, P., Waterhouse, J. A., Fielding, J. F., and Cooke, W. T.: Mortality in Crohn's disease. Lancet, 1(3):1135, 1970.

Provenzale, L., and Pisano, M.: Methods for recording electrical activity of the human colon in vivo. Amer. J. Dig. Dis., 16:712, 1971.

Reilly, M.: Sigmoid myotomy — interim report. Proc. Roy. Soc. Med., 62:715, 1969.

Ritchie, J. A.: Colonic motor activity and bowel function. Part I. Normal movement of contents. Gut, 9:442, 1968.

Ritchie, J. A.: Colonic motor activity and bowel function. Part II. Distribution and incidence of motor activity at rest and after food and carbachol. Gut, 9:502, 1968.

Ritchie, J. A.: Movement of segmental constrictions in the human colon. Gut, 12:350, 1971.

Ritchie, J. A., Truelove, S. C., Ardran, G. M., and Tuckey, M. S.: Propulsion and retropulsion of normal colonic contents. Amer. J. Dig. Dis., 16:697, 1971.

Rosch, J., Gray, R. K., Grollman, J. H., Jr., Ross, G., Sterkel, R. J., and Weiner, M.: Selective arterial drug infusions in the treatment of acute gastrointestinal bleeding. A preliminary report. Gastroenterology, 59:341, 1970.

Samuel, P., Saypol, G. M., Meilman, E., Mosbach, E. H., and Chafizadeh, M.: Absorption of bile acids from the large bowel in man. J. Clin. Invest., 47:2070, 1968.

Schanker, L. S.: Absorption of drugs from the rat colon. J. Pharmacol. Exp. Ther., 126:283, 1959.

Schultz, S. G., and Curran, P. F.: Intestinal absorption of sodium chloride and water. In Code, C. F. (Ed.): Handbook of Physiology. Vol. IV. Washington, D.C., American Physiological Society, 1968.

Schuster, M. M.: The riddle of the sphincters. Gastroenterology, 69:249, 1975.

Shields, R., and Miles, J. B.: Absorption and secretion in the large intestine. Postgrad. Med., 41:435, 1965.

Shorter, R. G., Huizenga, K. A., Spencer, R. J., Aas, J., and Guy, S. K.: Cytophilic antibody and the cytotoxicity of lymphocytes for colonic cells in vitro. Amer. J. Dig. Dis., 16:673, 1971.

Snape, W. J., Jr., Carlson, G. M., and Cohen, S.: Colonic myoelectric activity in the irritable bowel syndrome. Gastrenterology, 70:326, 1976.

Snape, W. J., Jr., Carlson, G. M., Matuango, S. A., and Cohen, S.: Evidence that abnormal myoelectrical activity produces colonic motor dysfunction in the irritable bowel syndrome. Gastroenterology, 72:383, 1967.

Solomon, S. S., Moran, J. M., and Nabseth, D. C.: Villous adenoma of rectosigmoid accompanied by electrolyte depletion. J.A.M.A., 194:5, 1965.

Stobo, J. D., Tomasi, T. B., Huizenga, K. A., and Shorter, R. G.: In vitro studies of inflammatory bowel disease: surface receptors of the mononuclear cell required to lyse allogeneic colonic epithelial cells. Gastroenterology, 70:171, 1976.

Thompson, D. M. P., Murphy, J., Freedman, S. O., and Gold, P.: The radioimmunoassay of circulating carcinoembryonic antigen of the human digestive system. Proc. Nat. Acad. Sci., 64:161, 1969.

Torsoli, A., Ramorino, M. L., and Crucioli, V.: The relationships between anatomy and motor activity of the colon. Amer. J. Dig. Dis., 13:462, 1968.

Ustach, T. J., Tobon, F., Hambrecht, T., Bass, D. D., and Schuster, M. M.: Electrophysiological aspects of human sphincter function. J. Clin. Invest., 49:41, 1970.

Waller, S. L., and Misiewica, J. J.: Colonic motility in constipation or diarrhoea. Scand. J. Gastroent., 7:93, 1972.

Watson, D. W.: The problem of chronic inflammatory bowel disease. Calif. Med., 117:25, 1972.

Williams, I.: Changing emphasis in diverticular disease of the colon. Brit. J. Radiol., 36:393, 1963.

Wolpert, E., Phillips, S. F., and Summerskill, W. H. J.: Transport of urea and ammonia production in the human colon. Lancet, 4:1387, 1971.

Wrong, O., Metcalfe-Gibson, A., Morrison, R. B. I., Ng, S. T., and Howard, A. V.: In vivo dialysis of faeces as a method of stool analysis. I. Technique and results in normal subjects. Clin. Sci., 28:357, 1965.

Zamcheck, N., Moore, T. L., Dhar, P., and Kupchik, H.: Immunologic diagnosis and prognosis of human digestive-tract cancer: Carcinoembryonic antigens. New Eng. J. Med., 286:83, 1972.

Zetzel, L.: Granulomatous (ileo) colitis. New Eng. J. Med., 288:600, 1970.

28

Normal and Pathologic Physiology of the Liver *

F. L. Iber

Direct physical examination of the whole liver is impossible because it is well protected by the ribs. Secretion is difficult to sample; therefore, examination of the stool, urine, and changes in the blood must be relied upon for information about the liver. Liver biopsy reveals infiltrations and cell changes; scintiscans reveal over-all shape; and visualization of the blood vessels and bile ducts within the liver is possible by radiologic and sonographic techniques.

ANATOMIC CONSIDERATIONS AND TECHNIQUES FOR GAINING INFORMATION (TABLE 28–1)

Liver Size and Shape

There is marked variation in liver shape but very little variation in liver weight (2 per cent of body). Palpation primarily provides information about the inferior descent of the anterior edge of the liver; it is not surprising that the location of the palpable edge correlates poorly with liver mass. Percussion reveals the span and the anterior projection of the liver. Scintiscanning, or isotope imagery, is the best technique to outline the liver in two or more dimensions; it not only accurately estimates liver mass, but reveals large collections of a non-liver mass (such as cancer) within the liver substance.

---

*Recognition is given to Mr. Barry O'Neil for the artwork done in preparation of this chapter.

Scans

Rose bengal, an anionic dye, can be readily labeled with radioiodine. This dye, when administered intravenously, is taken up by the liver cells, as is bilirubin, and is actively excreted into the biliary passages. Ten to 45 minutes after intravenous administration, the dye is uniformly distributed throughout the hepatic parenchymal cells. A scintillation camera will show a homogeneous distribution of radioactivity. Thirty to 90 minutes after administration, dye is in the biliary passages and in the intestinal tract. Approximately two hours after administration no radioactivity remains in the liver. Radioactive rose

TABLE 28–1 APPRAISAL OF LIVER STATUS

Gross Anatomic Measurements
1. Scans
a. Liver cell uptake
b. Serial uptake, biliary passage filling, and excretion ^{131}I-Rose bengal, ^{93}Tc-cationic dyes, Gallium citrate
c. Reticuloendothial uptake, ^{93}Tc-sulfur colloid
2. Ultrasound (also CAT scans)
a. Gallbladder
b. Enlarged bile ducts
3. Arteriography
a. Hepatic and splenic arteries
b. Portal vein and branches
4. Cholangiography
a. Oral and intravenous radiopaque dyes
b. Percutaneous transhepatic
c. Via endoscope in retrograde fashion

TABLE 28–2 USES OF SCANS*

1. Size, shape, and volume of liver.
2. Presence of non-liver nodules within image.
3. Identification of chest or abdominal mass as liver.
4. Showing impaired or irregular vascularity of liver.
5. Patency of common bile duct — serial rose bengal.
6. Enlargement of hilar bile ducts — rose bengal and colloid.
7. Size, shape, and volume of spleen.
8. Abscess or cancer — gallium

*Colloid, unless specified.

bengal is now utilized to show patency of the biliary passages by serial scanning but is not used for liver scanning because anionic dye uptake is impaired in liver disease and the scans are poor. Cationic substances are also excreted by the liver and are not impaired by the presence of elevated levels of bilirubin or bile salts. A derivative of xylocaine, hydroxyindole diacetic acid can be readily chelated with ^{93}technetium and provides a very useful scanning agent for use in subjects with jaundice. Its uptake by the liver and passage into the biliary tree and subsequently into the intestinal tract can be followed with serial scans.

Most forms of liver disease injure liver cells and stimulate the reticuloendothelial system of the liver. This feature may be utilized to provide clearer images in the presence of liver damage. Colloidal substances (technetium or iodine on either sulfur colloid or denatured albumin) of the correct molecular size or range are preferentially taken up by the reticuloendothelial cells of the liver and spleen. These cells remain active in the presence of major hepatic cellular disease, and therefore the scans are adequate. These scanning agents are widely utilized for determining the size, shape, and homogeneity of the liver. Table 28–2 indicates the utilization of scanning. Scanning materials specific to certain types of tissue now are increasingly utilized. Thus, gallium citrate accumulates in leukocytes (i.e., an abscess) or tumors, whereas iodinated albumin remains in the vascular space, indicating blood-filled masses.

Ultrasound

Bursts of sound of specific wavelength may be released into the abdomen through sensitive transducers and the reflected echo recorded to provide information about the sound transmission properties of the underlying structures. Fluid-filled spaces such as the gallbladder and biliary passages, the portal vein, and, occasionally, abnormal masses are clearly delineated.

Aberrant and abnormal collections within the liver such as abscesses or cancer are also recognized.

Arteriograms

The splenic or hepatic artery may be directly cannulated by percutaneous introduction of catheters. In the early phase, arteriograms will outline the arterial vessels of the liver or spleen and, in the late phase, the portal or hepatic veins. By employing this technique, the patency and anatomic course of all groups of blood vessels may be determined. Nodularity, erosion, new blood vessel formation, tumor blush, and collateral circulation may also be indicated. Portovenograms are made either by injecting radiopaque dye into the spleen (the dye is subsequently picked up and returned via the splenic and portal veins) or by cannulating the vestigial umbilical vein or a branch of the mesenteric vein.

Cholangiography

Three methods exist to fill the bile ducts and gallbladder with radiopaque dyes in order to permit x-ray examination to detail the ducts and their branches. Oral cholecystography usually demonstrates the gallbladder. When ingested orally, several iodinated anionic dyes are absorbed, excreted by the liver and concentrated by the gallbladder sufficiently to permit the gallbladder to be seen radiographically. In about 25 percent of normal persons even the larger biliary passages will show. Intravenous dyes of similar properties but not undergoing absorption are given to provide even more opacification of the ducts, and usually the ducts and gallbladder may be visualized. Neither process is adequate in the patient with disease of either the liver or major biliary passages.

Transhepatic cholangiography is useful when the ducts are blocked and dilated following continued secretion by the liver. A long, very thin needle is inserted blindly into the liver and a duct entered by chance. Radiopaque dye is injected under fluoroscopic control until sufficient dye is present to demonstrate the blocked portion. A highly trained operator can cannulate the ampulla of Vater directly and in retrograde fashion fill the biliary passages via a flexible endoscope inserted into the duodenum. This process is called endoscopic retrograde cholangiography.

Peritoneoscopy

The peritoneal cavity is distended with air, and a lighted telescope is inserted to inspect the surfaces of the anterior organs. The liver, a portion of the gallbladder, some of the mesenteric circulation, and portions of the intestine are nearly always seen. A great expanse of peritoneal surface may also be observed. Nodular lesions of the liver are usually seen and biopsy specimens may be taken if indicated.

Histology

Approximately two thirds of the liver consists of hepatocytes arranged in highly ordered plates. Each 8- to 12-surfaced cell has surface contact with blood vessels called sinusoids, but one or two surfaces remain in close contact with an adjacent cell and contain a minute bile duct or bile canaliculus (Fig. 28–1). The sinusoids are lined with endothelial cells and large reticuloendothelial cells called Kupffer cells. Proper polygonal cell function is highly dependent upon a rich intimate blood supply and adequate bile capillary drainage. The wall of the sinusoid is probably the most permeable capillary in the body, as indicated by the crossing of large proteins synthesized by the liver. The reticuloendothelial system of the liver, one of the most active in the body, offers optimal opportunity for phagocytosis, owing to the slow flow of blood through the sinusoids.

Pathologic processes may directly affect the liver polygonal cells or the Kupffer cells. They may alter the blood supply or the biliary drainage. The invasion of inflammatory cells may produce major pathologic changes. The liver is normally undergoing constant repair, and it is estimated that liver cell renewal occurs each 50 to 75 days. A newly formed liver cell is less enzymatically mature than an older one and cannot perform efficiently many liver functions.

Regeneration

The mammalian liver possesses a remarkable capacity both to regenerate its polygonal cells when portions are damaged and to cease regeneration when the proper mass is present. (Regeneration occurs in areas receiving portal blood.) Any form of dietary deficiency, particularly folic acid B_{12} and protein, will restrict regeneration, but no known material will stimulate it. Animal perfusion studies clearly indicate that a humoral factor stimulates hepatic mitosis — perhaps arginine, pituitary hormones, insulin, or glucagon may be such a substance. Regeneration is much more striking in the young than in the old. There is no evidence that regeneration is impaired in liver disease, and most data support an increased destructive activity.

In all forms of hepatic damage, the bile ducts and large blood vessels seem to emerge more intact than the other hepatic elements. Mesenchymal elements (connective tissue) grow predominantly following certain types of liver damage (alcoholic, as an example). New blood vessel formation is far more prominent in tumor nodules than in regenerative liver nodules.

CLINICALLY IMPORTANT BIOCHEMISTRY OF THE LIVER

If one looks at the emergence of the liver by means of comparative physiology, it is apparent that processing of food, conversion of food from one form to another, food storage, and formation of an important digestive fluid are activities com-

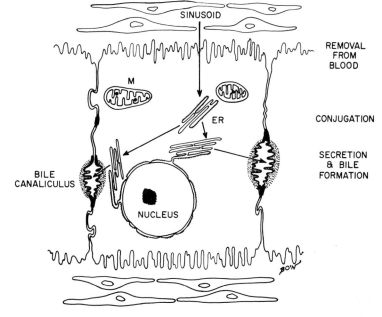

Figure 28–1 Schematic model of liver cell, indicating the smooth and rough endoplasmic reticulum (*ER*), the mitochondria (*M*), and other structures.

mon to nearly all species. Removal of noxious substances, both those in the environment and those produced metabolically, is another major function. Finally, most species use the liver to make substances used elsewhere in the body.

The Great Toxin Remover — Heme, Ammonia and Purine Metabolism

Three substances are produced in quantity each day in the human body, and all seem to be toxic, since they are excreted. These are ammonia, porphyrins, and purines. The body has developed complex mechanisms that involve the liver and the kidney working in conjunction to remove these substances, without producing harm and with a great deal of energy expenditure. Thus, ammonia is converted to urea, porphyrins are converted to bilirubin, and purines are converted to uric acid. The liver has a major role in the removal of all these substances from the body. Many other molecules are modified and removed by the liver. Ammonia and purine metabolism will be briefly considered in this section.

Ammonia arises metabolically from the breakdown of amino acids when they are used for energy production and as a by-product of renal production of ammonia to conserve base. Additional ammonia arises from the intestinal tract. The intestinal production is usually the most important. Intestinal ammonia is predominantly the result of action of intestinal bacteria on dietary nitrogen-containing food and of metabolically produced urea. The portal blood contains from 4 to 50 times the ammonia content of other blood of the body, yet the liver so successfully removes it that hepatic venous blood is the lowest in content of any in the body. The liver contains the enzyme machinery that condenses ammonia with bicarbonate in the presence of carbamyl phosphate synthetase as the first step in the formation of urea. Despite the predominant role of the liver in urea formation, impairment of ammonia uptake is more prominent in liver disease than is over-all urea synthesis, although urea formation is significantly impaired in cirrhosis of the liver. Increased peripheral blood ammonia is frequently found in liver disease. It arises most notably from the shunting of portal blood directly to the systemic circulation. Increased production of ammonia is also due to the increased small intestinal flora in liver disease and to the diminished uptake of ammonia by damaged liver cells.

Purines are progressively oxidized to uric acid in primates and the final enzyme in this oxidation, xanthine oxidase, is contained solely in the liver. As far as can be determined, there seem to be no clinical consequences of mild impairment of this system in liver cell disease.

Bilirubin Metabolism (Fig. 28–1)

The liver plays a varied and intimate role in bilirubin metabolism. The prominent and unique yellow color of the patient with liver disease (jaundice) invites attention to those factors basic to an understanding of liver physiology.

All bilirubin in the body results from the breakdown of cyclic tetrapyrroles, functioning as electron transport pigments. Hemoglobin is the most significant of these pigments in the production of bilirubin, but myoglobin, P-450, and various cytochromes all contribute cyclic tetrapyrroles which are catabolized and eliminated via the bilirubin pathway.

The liver plays no apparent role in the destruction of erythrocytes, and although its reticuloendothelial cells will occasionally ingest a damaged erythrocyte, there is evidence that the red cell is not broken down. On the other hand, lysed red cells and hemoglobin bound or not bound to haptoglobin are taken up by specialized Kupffer cells and converted successively to biliverdin and free bilirubin. For each molecule of cyclic tetrapyrrole converted to bilirubin, a molecule of CO is released and eventually eliminated through the lungs. A precise measure of the rate of formation of CO is an exact measure of bilirubin formation.

The majority of free bilirubin is formed in the reticuloendothelial system of the body outside the liver. The iron and globin are stripped from the hemoglobin before the ring is opened. Free bilirubin is formed and is released into the bloodstream. Free bilirubin, although containing several polar groups, is highly insoluble in water or body fluids owing to a tight intramolecular arrangement that renders the active groups unavailable. Free bilirubin is tightly bound to serum albumin to be soluble in blood; the binding constant is about the same as that between albumin and free fatty acids. Because of this nearly total association with albumin, the volume of distribution is identical to that of albumin. Free bilirubin is lipid soluble and over several days is extracted into body fat. This extraction and subsequent tissue staining is responsible for jaundice; bilirubin confined to the blood is not apparent to an external observer regardless of the level.

Functions of the Liver. Three separate functions of the liver are commonly distinguished: (a) uptake of albumin-bound free bilirubin by the liver cell, (b) combination of free bilirubin with glucuronide into conjugated bilirubin, and (c) active secretion of conjugated bilirubin into the bile. Each of these operations illustrates important liver physiologic characteristics, and abnormalities of each occur that result in a disease (Fig. 28–1).

UPTAKE.   The liver contains a protein of about

30,000 m.w. that binds bilirubin in the liver cell and seems responsible for the transfer of albumin-bound bilirubin into the liver cell. This process occurs at the cell surface, the albumin does not enter the liver cell, and no energy is required in this transfer. It seems to maintain an equilibrium in which bilirubin moves from tightly bound to albumin to slightly tighter binding on this intrahepatic transport and storage protein, called Y protein or ligandin; movement continues from blood to liver because the Y protein in the liver cell is constantly being freed of its bilirubin load.

Normal albumin is saturated with 2 moles of free bilirubin per mole of albumin; thus, each gram of albumin can convey about 8 mg. of free bilirubin, a state seldom reached in disease. Many molecules share the same binding sites on albumin as bilirubin and if present in sufficient concentration may lessen bilirubin binding. Synthetic vitamin K and certain salicylates are examples. The rate of transfer of free bilirubin into the liver cell is dependent upon (a) the concentration of bilirubin in the blood, (b) the concentration of albumin in the blood, (c) the blood flow to the liver, (d) the concentration of Y protein in the liver cell, and (e) the concentration of bilirubin on the Y protein in the liver cell. Two- or threefold increases in this transport may be achieved over a period of time, probably by increasing (e) and (d), but abrupt lesser increases or chronic increases exceeding this range can be accomplished only by increasing the level of bilirubin in the blood. At levels of bilirubin of 6 or 7 mg. per 100 ml. any achievable amount of free bilirubin may be transported. If serum free bilirubin level is above this, the transport machinery is defective.

The Y protein has a short half-life, and its rate of restoration is impaired by protein starvation. Thus, any form of free hyperbilirubinemia is exaggerated by a 24-hour fast or in chronically starved patients in whom this form of jaundice may be apparent. The same transport system is utilized by a number of albumin-bound organic acids. Sulfobromophthalein, bile salts, fatty acids, and many acidic drugs removed by the liver initially enter the liver cell bound to Y protein.

CONJUGATION. Conjugation occurs inside the liver cell. This process combines two proprionic acid side chains on the bilirubin molecule with glucuronide molecules. In this fashion the tight intramolecular arrangement of bilirubin is destroyed and a water soluble molecule called conjugated bilirubin is produced. Conjugation occurs on the smooth endoplasmic reticulum (ER) and requires activated glucuronic acid to combine with bilirubin through the intervention of an enzyme called glucuronyl transferase. There is evidence that portions of the ER adjacent to the bile canaliculus are principally responsible for this enzyme activity.

Conjugation enzymes mature late in the development of the fetus and are not fully developed until the tenth month after conception. Thus, premature infants have impaired conjugation, and varying degrees of impairment may be commonly found in underweight newborns. This is emphasized by the abrupt destruction of erythrocytes that occurs at the time of birth (hemoglobin decreases from about 19 to 14 gm. per 100 ml.) and its concomitant pigment load. Under this circumstance, free bilirubin accumulates in the blood in large amounts. When the level exceeds 20 mg. per 100 ml., the possibility of entry into central nervous tissues and subsequent brain damage is quite high. Birth brain anoxia due to birth injury makes this possibility a likelihood. Such brain damage resulting from free bilirubin is called kernicterus after the yellow staining of basal ganglia of the brain. The abnormal hemolysis produced by maternal anti-Rh positive serum reaching the Rh-positive fetus most often produces such damage. If the hazard arises *after* birth, the level of bilirubin may be monitored; if above 20 mg. per 100 ml., it may be lowered by removing about one fifth of the patient's blood and replacing it with normal blood. This exchange transfusion is highly effective in lowering the circulating free bilirubin. A series of circumstances combine to make bilirubin brain damage feasible in childhood but nearly impossible later in life. These are ERYTHROBLASTOSIS FOETALIS

(a) Physiologic or abnormal breakdown of red cells in large amounts.

(b) Conjugation impairment due to prematurity.

(c) Failure of immature blood-brain barrier to exclude bilirubin.

(d) Anoxic birth injury.

Conjugation of bilirubin is impaired by several experimental drugs, by a steroid occasionally occurring in maternal milk, and by certain plant toxins. Two inborn errors of metabolism are associated with impairment of bilirubin conjugation. The first of these, Crigler-Najjar syndrome, is present at birth, is associated with a high degree of brain damage (two thirds of cases), and is unresponsive to any known treatment. The second, the Arias type of Crigler-Najjar, appears shortly after birth, does not result in brain damage, and is apparently controlled by inducing microsomal enzymes with phenobarbital, lowering the bilirubin to normal. The diagnostic features of both forms are very high free bilirubin (more than 10 mg. per 100 ml.), presence early in and throughout life, and absence of any apparent bilirubin conjugation in liver biopsy specimens. In acquired disease, conjugated impairment almost never accounts for jaundice.

SECRETION.   Conjugated bilirubin is produced in proximity to the bile canaliculus and is rapidly secreted into the bile. Under normal conditions it does not escape from the hepatic cell. However, if there is necrosis of liver cells, conjugated bilirubin in the bile ducts may reach the space of Disse. Accumulation of conjugated bilirubin in the liver cells for any reason may also lead to conjugated bilirubin in the blood and in the urine. Conjugated bilirubin passes freely into all the fluids of the body; it is partially bound to albumin, so that its distribution is influenced by the protein content. Conjugated bilirubin stains most protein-containing subcutaneous fluids and is readily observed in the sclerae of the eye and in the loose connective tissue beneath the tongue. It enters urine, spinal fluid, ascites, and most edema fluid. The most clinically useful difference between free and conjugated bilirubin is the regular appearance of conjugated bilirubin in the urine, whereas free bilirubin cannot reach the urine. If no bilirubin is excreted at all, the daily production rate (250 mg. per day) will raise the serum bilirubin 4 to 6 mg. per 100 ml. per day. Conjugated bilirubin is the only form in the bile.

Urobilinogen. Intestinal bacteria reduce conjugated bilirubin progressively to compounds called stercobilin or urobilinogen. These products, which number approximately 20 different substances, account for the color of stool. If intestinal bacterial reduction occurs normally, no bilirubin is found in the stool. Several of these products undergo extensive enterohepatic circulation. The sum of all known tetrapyrrole products does not equal the amount of bilirubin excreted; other small metabolic products occur. The determination of urobilinogen in the urine and the stool is a useful assessment of over-all pigment metabolism.

Normally the stool contains 125 to 200 mg. urobilinogen and the urine 0.5 to 4 mg. in 24 hrs.; about 70 mg. of urobilinogen is absorbed via the portal vein and excreted almost entirely via the liver. Less than 5 per cent of this absorbed urobilinogen reaches the urine. Urobilinogen is a weak acid and as such is more concentrated in alkaline urine than an acid one. Normally, fresh urine with a pH of 5.5 or more contains urobilinogen, reflecting that conjugated bilirubin is reaching the gut and normal bacterial reduction and intestinal absorption of the urobilinogen are occurring. The total absence of urobilinogen in fresh urine of pH 5.5 or higher indicates that this cycle is broken. Most commonly, total obstruction of the biliary passages is present; less commonly, bacterial reduction (such as after extensive antibiotic use) is interrupted. Marked increase in urine urobilinogen suggests an increased production of urobilinogen, inefficient hepatic cell removal (such as in liver cell disease), or abnormal vascular communications between the portal and systemic circulation, bypassing the liver.

Tests of Bilirubin Metabolism.   *Total bilirubin* in blood and urine may be accurately measured. However, partition into free and conjugated may be only crudely approximated by the "direct reacting" and "indirect reacting" bilirubin. Pure free bilirubin will almost always be less than 20 per cent direct reacting. Conjugated bilirubin, on the other hand, may be as much as 50 per cent indirect reacting. In clinical situations, if less than 25 per cent of the bilirubin is direct reacting, it may be presumed that *all* the bilirubin is free. If 50 per cent or more of the bilirubin is direct reacting, it should be assumed that all is conjugated. Determination of bilirubin in a fresh urine sample is the most precise method of determining whether bilirubin is entirely in the free form or not; in such cases the Ictotest or Harrison spot test will show it to be absent from the urine.

Aside from the serum and urine bilirubin, assessment of bilirubin metabolism either is available in only a limited number of highly specialized laboratories or is indirect. Table 28–3 indicates the problems and the direct and indirect tests commonly used in diagnosis. These tests and their utility in certain clinical examples are discussed below.

SULFOBROMOPHTHALEIN (BSP) AND INDOCYANINE GREEN (ICG) TESTS.   These materials behave similarly in assessing liver metabolism. Both are intravenously administered anionic dyes. Both travel tightly adherent to albumin, both are taken up by the Y protein of the liver (in direct competition with bilirubin), and BSP but not ICG is conjugated by an enzyme on the endoplasmic reticulum with glutathione. Conjugated BSP and ICG are then secreted by the anion pump into the bile. In clinical use, a fixed dose of the dye is administered intravenously (5 mg. per kg. BSP– 0.5 mg. per kg. ICG) and a blood sample is taken 45 minutes later for BSP (20 minutes for ICG) to determine how much dye has persisted in the blood. If more than 6 per cent is found, liver cell uptake is considered defective. Any form of jaundice competes with the removal of both dyes, but in the nonjaundiced patient the removal from blood is mainly a measurement of the uptake and storage of the liver cell. On a research basis, both tests may be modified to measure maximal storage and maximal transport by the anion pump. Less damage is required to produce BSP or ICG retention than bilirubin retention.

URINE UROBILINOGEN.   A fresh urine sample should be used and the pH determined; only if the pH is 5.5 or higher should urobilinogen be measured. The serial dilution which contains detectable material should be ascertained. The important questions are (a) is there some urobilinogen

TABLE 28–3 TESTS OF BILIRUBIN METABOLISM

I. Increased Production
   A. Direct and specific
      1. CO production   1 mol. CO for each mol. bilirubin, any source
      2. Fecal urobilinogen   Only about 2/3 total measured
      3. ^{51}Cr RBC survival   Adult RBC only
   B. Indirect but useful
      1. Serum haptoglobin   Only detects hemoglobin release
      2. Reticulocyte levels   Marrow reaction
   C. Indirect and rarely helpful
      1. Coombs' test   ⎫ Only 1 or 2 specific diseases detected
      2. Osmotic fragility   ⎬ with these
      3. Hemoglobin electrophoresis   ⎭
II. Impaired Conjugation
   A. Assay of glucuronyl transferase activity in liver biopsy   ⎫
   B. Comparison of glucuronide excretion of other agents   ⎬ Require special laboratory procedures
III. Impaired Excretion of Conjugated Bilirubin Associated
   with Extensive Malfunction of Liver Cells
   A. BSP maximal excretory rate   ⎫
   B. I.V. cholangiography   ⎬ Useful if bilirubin less than 3
   C. Serial rose bengal scans
   D. Urobilinogen in the urine
   E. Tests of protein, or injury of cells   See Table 28–6
IV. Impaired Excretion of Conjugated Bilirubin with
   Preservation of Other Liver Cell Function (Cholestasis)
   A. Tests of anion pump (also abnormal if severe and
      prolonged impaired biliary flow)
      1. Appearance of conjugated BSP in venous blood
         after 90 minutes
      2. BSP maximal excretory rate
      3. Accumulation of bile salts in serum
      4. Lipoprotein of cholestasis
   B. Intermediate bile ductule disease
      1. Antimitochondria antibody
      2. Liver biopsy
   C. Patent large biliary passages
      1. I.V. cholangiography
      2. Transhepatic cholangiography
      3. Operative cholangiography
      4. Rose bengal scans, serial
      5. Sonography

present and (b) is it present in a dilution of 1 to 50 or greater? Absence of urobilinogen indicates either (a) absence of conjugated bilirubin reaching the intestine or (b) absent bacterial conversion to urobilinogen usually due to antibiotics but occasionally due to colectomy or rapid diarrhea preventing sufficient numbers of the correct bacteria. An excess of urobilinogen indicates one of the following: increased production of bilirubin, an impaired removal of urobilinogen from portal blood due to damaged liver cells, or increased shunting of portal blood into the systemic circulation.

Classification of Jaundice. The problems of jaundice in the first year of life and much later are sufficiently different that the approach is usually kept separate. Table 28–4 indicates the major classification and cause of jaundice in the first year of life.

TABLE 28–4 CLASSIFICATION OF JAUNDICE IN FIRST YEAR OF LIFE

I. Predominantly Indirect Reacting
   A. Increased breakdown of red cells
      1. Physiologic
      2. Hemolysis, Rh and other
   B. Conjugation defects
      1. Prematurity
      2. Lack of glucuronyl transferase, permanent Crigler-Najjar
      3. Lack of glucuronyl transferase, inducible, Arias type
      4. Inactivation of glucuronyl transferase, abnormal breast milk steroid
II. Predominantly Direct Reacting
   A. Hepatic cell defect
      1. Giant cell hepatitis
   B. Cholestasis
      1. Giant cell hepatitis
      2. Biliary atresia

Some jaundice in the first days of life is normal as a function of transfer from the anoxic intra-uterine existence to the open world. About one third of the hemoglobin is destroyed, and this sudden pigment load is sufficient to produce jaundice. If the child weighs under 3000 grams (an index of fetal maturity), bilirubin conjugation is probably impaired and will enhance greatly the level of indirect reacting bilirubin. Several acquired blockages of normal glucuronyl transferase have been reported; one of the most interesting is due to an abnormal steroid in mothers' milk absorbed by nursing babies. An occasional congenital defect is failure of bile ducts to develop. This may be a defect in just small segments in the large bile ducts, which is amenable to surgical repair, or total absence of intralobular ducts.

Jaundice in the older child and adult may be approached in a similar way. It is useful to divide the problems into those which have predominantly unconjugated or free bilirubin in the serum in contrast to those which have predominantly direct reacting pigment. Table 28–5 indicates a useful classification along these lines. Two predominant forms of unconjugated hyperbilirubinemia occur — those due to increased production and those due to inborn errors of metabolism. Unless some of the specialized tests indicated in Table 28–3 are applied, it may prove very diffi-cult to specifically assign a case to one or the other.

Patients with predominantly direct reacting pigment are most conveniently divided into those with multifunctional liver cell impairment and those with cholestasis, which is predominantly failure of excretion of bilirubin and bile salts. This distinction, although it includes some overlapping diseases, is the way in which one must approach clinical problems.

Protein Synthesis — A Function of the Rough Endoplasmic Reticulum

Granular or rough endoplasmic reticulum receives RNA from the nucleus and is the site at which the extensive protein synthesis of the hepatocyte occurs. Table 28–6 indicates the wide variety of proteins that are made almost exclusively by the liver and many are subsequently released into the blood. To support this extensive synthetic factory there is a rich array of systems in the liver cell which store amino acids, convert an amino acid present in excess to one present to a lesser degree, and are sources of energy. Because of these many complex interrelated functions, protein synthesis will be completely normal only when there are adequate numbers of completely normal liver cells, few or no inhibitors of protein synthesis affecting this complex function, and an adequate supply of dietary protein to assure availability to those amino acids that cannot be adequately synthesized within the body.

The blood level of a given protein is a function of both its rate of synthesis and its rate of removal. Some proteins persist a very short time in the blood after release. Factors operative in disease may hasten the removal of the protein from blood (such as loss of albumin into the intestinal tract

TABLE 28–5 CLASSIFICATION OF JAUNDICE IN OLDER CHILDREN AND ADULTS

I. Predominantly Indirect Reacting Bilirubin
  A. Increased production of bilirubin
    1. Chronic — Hemoglobin or red cell membrane abnormality
    2. Acute — Red cell damage, drug, thermal, or immunologic
  B. Impaired transfer albumin to Y-protein
    1. Familial unconjugated hyperbilirubinemia — Gilbert's
    2. Nonfamilial cases
    3. Acquired cases
  C. Conjugation defects (rare)
    1. Toxins
    2. Crigler-Najjar
    3. Arias type
II. Predominantly Direct Reacting Bilirubin
  A. Associated with multifunctional impairment of the liver
    1. All forms of hepatitis
    2. Infiltrative liver disease
      a. Tumor
      b. Amyloid, lipid
  B. Cholestasis
    1. Anion pump injury — hepatitis
    2. Bile capillary injury — drugs
    3. Obstruction to large hepatic and common bile ducts

TABLE 28–6 PROTEINS MADE PREDOMINANTLY BY THE LIVER

1. Albumin
2. Coagulation Proteins
  a. Fibrinogen (Factor I)
  b. Prothrombin (Factor II)
  c. Factors III, V, VIII, IX, X, and XI
3. Transport Proteins
  a. Haptoglobin
  b. Transferrin
  c. Ceruloplasmin
  d. Hormone transport proteins
  e. Y protein
  f. Alpha-lipoprotein
  g. Beta-lipoprotein
4. Reaction to Injury
  a. Alpha-globulin
  b. Beta-globulin

or the urine, or depletion of serum fibrinogen due to accelerated coagulation).

Under normal circumstances, serum proteins synthesized in the liver vary widely in removal rates. Thus, albumin persists in the serum with a half-time of approximately 30 days; fibrinogen with a half-time of approximately 4 days, and prothrombin with a half-time of approximately 12 hours. This means that total cessation of hepatic manufacture and release would result in a fall of prothrombin to 5 per cent, of fibrinogen to 60 per cent, and of albumin to 92 per cent of initial level in two days. The small change in albumin might well be overlooked. Use of the persistence time of these several proteins is helpful in dating the onset of severe liver cell failure.

The wide variety of proteins made by the liver and present in the serum is of less use in diagnosing than in comprehending the many changes present in long-standing liver cell disease.

Albumin. A lowering of the serum albumin level (often to less than one half normal) is common in cirrhosis and is clinically apparent in fluid retention of edema and ascites. Many physiologic substances and drugs are tightly bound to albumin and are altered in their effective blood levels and in their hepatic and renal transport by this lowering.

Coagulation Abnormalities. These are common in acute and long-standing liver disease. The four liver-made proteins requiring vitamin K as a cofactor for synthesis (II, VII, IX, X) and measured as the one-stage prothrombin time are the most frequently abnormal. Substantial hemorrhage may be a complication of liver disease. Absorptive defects of vitamin K, increased activation of intravascular clotting with subsequent consumption of coagulation factors, and platelet defects due to persistence of products of fibrinolysis are additional commonplace problems of coagulation that require detailed evaluation.

The most frequent coagulation abnormality in liver disease comes about because of inadequate absorption of vitamin K, a fat soluble vitamin. Any form of cholestasis (with or without jaundice) interferes with the efficient absorption of all fat soluble vitamins. This problem is best detected by measurement of the one-stage prothrombin time; if this is abnormal by more than 2 seconds, the test should be repeated 12 or more hours after the parenteral injection of 1 to 5 mg. of vitamin K. A return of the prothrombin time to normal indicates impaired absorption.

The second most frequent coagulation abnormality in liver disease is an inability to manufacture coagulation proteins. Both the one-stage prothrombin time and the partial thromboplastin times are prolonged and respond little or not at all to parenteral vitamin K replacement.

An infrequent but treatable coagulation abnor-

mality is excessive activation of the coagulation cascade, with consumption of the platelets and coagulation proteins. This is best detected by a low platelet count (under 50,000), a reduced level of total fibrinogen, and often is associated with prolonged prothrombin time and partial thromboplastin time. Split products of fibrinogen breakdown are detectable if methods are available to you. Treatment consists of use of heparin.

The many transport protein abnormalities in liver disease suggest the wide groups of functions that may be abnormal in liver disease. Thus, iron transport is often abnormal in hepatic disease; haptoglobin (used to assess the amount of free hemoglobin being formed to diagnose hemolysis) may be misleading. Lipoproteins and lipid transport may be quite abnormal. The liver produces specific binding proteins for most non-peptide hormones and in liver disease the level produced may be less than normal. Many tissue effects of hormones depend upon the amount of free or non-protein-bound hormone, therefore there is an alteration of the hormone status. Disorders of menstruation and fertility are quite common with liver disease.

Alcohol, many antibiotics, a few cancer chemotherapy drugs, and some toxins impair protein synthesis as their means of action. Nearly all affect lipoprotein synthesis by hepatic cells and result in an accumulation of fat within the liver cell.

Function of the Smooth Endoplasmic Reticulum

Large numbers of enzymes are bound to the smooth endoplasmic reticulum. Figure 28–2 illustrates a widely utilized electron transport scheme used in the metabolism of many drugs. Each enzyme used is bound to the membranes of the endoplasmic reticulum so that an insoluble molecule can be sequentially acted upon by enzymes attached adjacent to one another. The substrates are usually of limited solubility and are often combined by these enzymes with highly polar molecules (such as sulfate, glucuronide, glutathione, glycine, acetate) to permit subsequent excretion by liver or renal tubular cells.

A few normal substances are metabolized using these membrane-bound enzymes. Most steroid hormones are made inactive by this system. Fatty acids are oxidized by this system. The system is also important for many trace materials and particularly important in drug metabolism. Many drugs are fairly insoluble in water and resist excretion. The liver is a major organ responsible for biotransformation — the chemical modification of a drug that usually alters its biologic activity and renders it more susceptible to

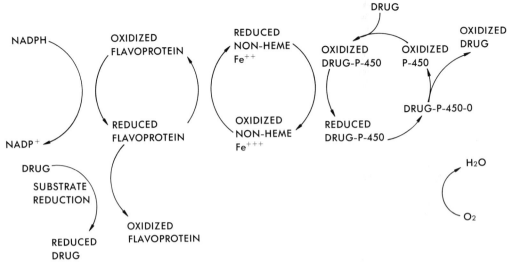

Figure 28–2 Endoplasmic reticulum electron transport used for drug oxidation and reduction.

excretion by both the kidney and the liver. Oxidation reactions such as N- and O-dealkylization, aromatic ring and side chain hydroxylation, N-oxidation, N-hydroxylation, and deamination of primary and secondary amines are common. Reduction of nitro groups, reductive cleavage of azo groups, and reduction of ring double bonds may occur. Conjugation of phenols, alcohols, carboxylic acids, and amines with glucuronides, sulfates, acetates, or glycine is a common mode of rendering molecules more polar for excretion. Specific enzymes for each reaction are usually necessary to activate the drug or to carry out portions of the chemistry. However, certain of the enzymes in the endoplasmic reticulum are used in common by many systems. NADPH and cytochrome P-450 are common requirements for most of these. Figure 28–2 indicates a common relationship between these.

Lipid solubility seems an important determinant of which drugs utilize the endoplasmic reticulum enzymes. The rates of reaction vary markedly and, similarly, the effect of liver disease on these drug removal reactions varies. Steroid inactivation is usually slow in almost any form of liver cell disease, and sex hormone, adrenal cortical hormone, and aldosterone may persist in liver cell disease. Bilirubin conjugation is usually not altered in liver cell disease, bile salt conjugation is often impaired, and the normal threefold increase of glycine conjugations over taurine is reduced.

Antibiotics, hypnotics, and hypoglycemic agents all show unusual persistence in the presence of liver disease. One can best generalize by stating that any drug using the hepatic endoplas-

mic reticulum should be used with caution and its blood level or biologic effects observed in the presence of liver disease.

An important and unique aspect of the endoplasmic reticulum is its near total hypertrophy (with all the contained enzymes) after treatment with certain agents that saturate one or more of its enzymes. Most substances (nearly all common drugs and many environmental trace elements) are Type I inducers of endoplasmic reticulum and cause an increased activity of nearly all drug and steroid metabolizing enzymes. A less frequent type of inducer (Type II), exemplified by many carcinogenic molecules (such as methylcholanthrene) leads to hypertrophy of only the enzymes for Type II molecules. There is some evidence that activation of the Type II system renders a person more prone to carcinoma. Type I inducers (example, phenobarbital) are best known and most widespread. Drug removal rates are accelerated for nearly all agents using enzyme on the ER. For this reason, many patients with hepatic disease may have increased rather than impaired endoplasmic reticulum enzymes. This may be from drugs they have received in the course of treatment or it may be from alcoholism.

Carbohydrate Metabolism

The liver has an active role in glucose and carbohydrate metabolism. The liver stores glucose as glycogen in the absorptive period, preventing the blood glucose from reaching a diabetic level. Even in a well-nourished person the glycogen supply is adequate to maintain the blood glucose for only a few hours. The liver constantly converts lactic acid and amino acids into glucose to maintain adequate glucose in the blood; this process is called gluconeogenesis. Gluconeogenesis is stimulated by glucagon and epinephrine, both of which act by stimulating formation of cyclic-AMP within the liver cell.

Disorders in the enzymes rapidly converting glycogen to glucose are known and produce glycogen storage disease, usually limited to children.

Acute damage to large numbers of liver cells may result in substantial amounts of lactic, pyruvic, citric, and alphaketoglutaric acids in the serum; these may replace other anions and result in both acidosis and a 10 to 30 mEq. per liter increase in the undetermined anion (the numerical difference between the sum of the sodium and potassium and the sum of the bicarbonate and chloride).

Injury to liver cells usually results in elevated levels of circulating amino acids. All except valine and leucine are highly stimulatory to the release of glucagon which in turn promotes gluconeogenesis. Both insulin and glucagon are released into the portal vein flow and therefore reach the liver in much higher concentrations than in the peripheral blood — both have different sensitivities on liver cells than on peripheral tissues. When portal hypertension develops and there is collateral flow, the peripheral levels of these hormones may be elevated and the liver levels diminished, resulting in hyperglycemia or hypoglycemia depending upon which hormone predominates. In very severe liver cell injury, symptomatic hypoglycemia may result. This is found most often in heart failure with circulatory congestion of the liver or in alcoholics — particularly after a prolonged fast.

Lipid Metabolism

The liver cell actively takes up free fatty acids from albumin binding in the plasma into the cell — associated with the y and z protein (also called ligandin) or to the mitochondrial membranes. Mitochondrial oxidation is readily possible, resulting in acetyl-CoA which enters the tricarboxylic acid cycle or may be converted to ketone bodies. The cytosol of the liver can readily synthesize fatty acids. Esterification of free fatty acids is almost uniquely a liver function. Triglycerides are packaged with protein and carbohydrate portions made by the rough endoplasmic reticulum into very low density lipoproteins (VLDL) which are extruded via the Golgi apparatus into the space of Disse.

Cholesterol is synthesized by the liver (as well as the intestine, adrenal cortex, and arterial wall) from acetyl-CoA using endoplasmic reticulum bound enzymes. The rate-limiting step in this synthesis is in the formation of the intermediate mevalonic acid. Cholesterol is utilized by the liver for the synthesis of bile acids and other products and is excreted into the bile. Cholesterol is the principal component of radiolucent gallstones.

BILE FORMATION, BILE FLOW, AND CHOLESTASIS

Bile contains water and electrolytes in amounts approximately the same as those in plasma, but in addition contains four major organic components (bile salts, lecithin, cholesterol, bilirubin) and many others. Bile is formed initially in the bile canaliculus at the juncture of two hepatocytes as a result of active secretion of anions by the liver cell. Water diffuses passively to maintain isotonicity. The thick epithelium of intermediate-sized bile ducts may add or remove water and/or electrolytes, about two thirds of the initially formed bile is reabsorbed in the small bile ducts. The gallbladder markedly concentrates hepatic bile by the removal of water and electrolytes. Remarkably, the contents of the biliary tree remain nearly isotonic throughout all these alterations, largely owing to the propensity of the organic molecules to form loose molecular complexes (called micelles). These micelles serve principally to keep the more insoluble components (cholesterol) in solution. Many substances are secreted by the liver into bile for excretion; almost any organic acid may be so excreted. The normal composition of the major components of bile are indicated in Table 28–7.

Mechanism of Bile Formation

The wall of the bile canaliculus, with the likely participation of adjacent endoplasmic reticulum and possibly components of the Golgi apparatus, is capable of actively secreting a variety of materials into the lumen. The most active transport system excretes a number of organic anions; bile salts are by far the most important single material secreted by this system. This is commonly called the anion pump. Table 28–8 indicates the variety of substances actively transported into bile, at the level of the liver cell. The wall of the bile canaliculus seems freely permeable to water and uncharged molecules up to a molecular weight of about 900, but charged molecules seem retarded in their passage. As a result of the active secretion of bile salt and other molecules, water moves to preserve isotonicity and bile flow begins. Bile volume is highly dependent upon total bile salt secretion; normal flow is 450 to 700

TABLE 28–7 COMPOSITION OF HUMAN HEPATIC BILE

Component	mg. per 100 ml.	% Total Solids	mEq./L.
Bile salts	140–2230	8–53	3–45*
Lecithin	140–810	9–21	2–8*
Cholesterol	97–320	3–11	2–6*
Bilirubin	12–70	0.4–2.0	less than 1
Urobilinogen	5–45	0.2–1.5	less than 1
Sodium			146–165
Potassium			2.7–4.9
Chloride			88–115
Bicarbonate			27–55

*Variability due to micelle formation.
(After Thureborn, E.: Acta Chir. Scand. (Suppl.) *303*:1, 1962.)

ml. per 24 hr. The epithelium of intermediate bile ducts is capable of both absorbing and secreting into bile; water, electrolytes, and possibly glucose seem to be the principal substances transported. Similar to the pancreas, these epithelial cells are responsive to the hormone secretin; a voluminous secretion elevated in bicarbonate results.

Enterohepatic Circulation

Many of the organic molecules contained in the bile are reabsorbed by the intestine into the portal venous blood and are transported to the liver, where they are re-excreted. Intestinal reabsorption may be highly efficient (95 per cent for bile salts), of intermediate efficiency (30 to 50 per cent for urobilinogen), or very slight (bilirubin). The process of liver bile excretion, gut absorption, and liver re-excretion is called enterohepatic circulation. The hepatic extraction of the reabsorbed material may be so efficient that little reaches the peripheral venous blood. This recycling of substances through the biliary tree is employed to treat biliary tract infections. An antibiotic which is recycled through the biliary tract many times is chosen. Enterohepatic circulation assumes substantial importance when interrupted. In intestinal disease, bile salt conservation is impossible and depletion occurs. When inefficient liver cell extraction occurs, products normally removed by the liver appear in the urine, as, for example, urobilinogen. If portal blood is shunted to the periphery, higher peripheral blood levels may occur. Cholestyramine, an insoluble resin taken orally, binds certain materials undergoing enterohepatic circulation (bile salts, digitalis glycosides, cholesterol) in the intestine and thus depletes the body of them.

TABLE 28–8 REPRESENTATIVE COMPOUNDS ACTIVELY EXCRETED BY HEPATIC CELLS

Organic Acids
  Naturally occurring: Used Diagnostically:
    bile salts*   sulfobromophthalein**
    bilirubin   indocyanine green
    urobilinogen*   iopanoic acid**
    lecithin**   iodipamide
  Therapeutic agents:
    sulfonamides**
    penicillin**
    ampicillin*
    chlorthiazide**
    streptomycin*
    tetracycline*
Bases
  procaine amide ethobromide
  xylocaine
Neutral
  adrenal and sex sterols
  cholesterol*
  digitalis glycosides**

*Highly active enterohepatic circulation.
**Mildly active enterohepatic circulation.

Bile Salts and Bile Salt Metabolism

Bile salts are synthesized exclusively by the liver from cholesterol. Cholic acid and chenodeoxycholic acid are the two bile salts made by the liver of man. Adult man forms about 200 to 300 mg. of cholic acid per day and a similar amount of chenodeoxycholic. Under stimulation cholic acid synthesis can increase seven-to tenfold and chenodeoxycholic acid synthesis two- or threefold. Bile salts are conjugated in the acid group with either glycine or taurine, with two to three times as much in the glycine form.

Conjugation of bile salts is important for both hepatic excretion and distal ileal reabsorption. If intestinal bacteria deconjugate large quantities of bile salts in the intestine, they are lost via the stool, because reabsorption becomes inefficient.

The human adult body contains 3 to 4 gm. of

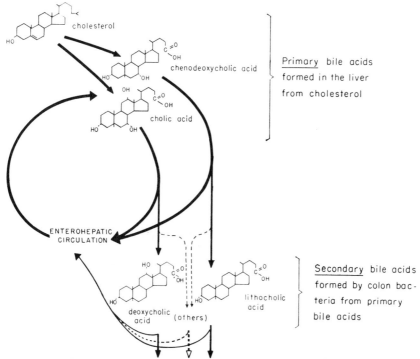

Figure 28-3 Formation of primary and secondary bile acids from cholesterol. (Reproduced from Carey, J.: *In* Schiff, L. (ed.): Diseases of the Liver, 3rd ed., J. B. Lippincott Co., Philadelphia, 1969.)

bile salts, and these are completely excreted into the intestine and reabsorbed six to ten times each day. This excretion and reabsorption is so remarkably complete that only about 0.1 gm. of bile salt or less is lost from the body during each "enterohepatic circulation." Disorders of liver cell function retard the rate at which the bile salts can be returned to the intestine, but disorders of terminal ileal function or disorders of bacterial overgrowth which cause deconjugation increase the amounts lost from the body. About 0.5 gm. of bile salt is normally lost from the body each day. The liver synthesizes and replaces this amount. Intestinal bacteria reduce bile acids (see Fig. 28-3) to new ones called "secondary bile acids." The product of cholic acid reduction, deoxycholic acid, acts as a normal bile salt and undergoes enterohepatic circulation. The product of chenodeoxycholic acid reduction, lithocholic acid, is reabsorbed once, but is then sulfated by the liver and can no longer be reabsorbed.

Bile salts are the principal component of bile, making up 90 per cent of the non-electrolyte solutes. Bile is formed by the active transport of bile salts from the liver, with water following passively. Bile salts have two, three, or four polar groups all on one surface; the remainder of the molecule is water insoluble, lipid soluble. This amphoteric property provides a major function in forming micelles which keep insoluble materials in contact with a water surface in the biliary passages and in the intestine. In the former, bile salts facilitate the excretion of cholesterol; in the latter, they facilitate the absorption of long chain triglyceride and other lipid soluble materials.

Alteration of Bile Salts in Disease. Too little bile salt reaching the intestine results in malabsorption of fat and fat soluble materials. This arises most frequently from interference with either the patency of biliary passages or with the efficient reabsorption of bile salts from the gut. This can be caused by disease, loss of the terminal ileum, or bacterial overgrowth resulting in the deconjugation of the bile salts. Accumulation of bile salts in the blood stream produces pruritus. Liver cell diseases result in both elevated bile salt levels in the serum due to inefficient hepatic removal and maldigestion of fatty meals due to failure to rapidly recycle the available bile salt to the intestine.

The formation of cholesterol gallstones is the result of an imbalance between the amount of cholesterol in the bile and the amount of bile salt, producing a bile supersaturated with cholesterol. This condition over many years may produce gallstone formation. Treatment with one bile salt, chenodeoxycholic acid, seems to correct the balance by altering hepatic synthesis and excretion so that less cholesterol comes into the bile and more bile salt is there, causing the stones to dissolve slowly.

Since the liver manufactures bile acids and salts, abnormalities due to liver cell disease might be anticipated. The most prominent abnormality seems to be a decrease in cholic acid and a relative increase in deoxycholic acid and chenodeoxycholic acid. The reasons for this shift are obscure, but it has been observed in a wide variety of different forms of hepatocellular disease.

Although conjugation of bile acids is mildly impaired in disease, it seems less important than the increased production of dihydroxy acids.

Cholestasis

Clinically, bilirubin and bile salts are the two most prominent components of bile. Whenever

there is evidence that adequate amounts of *both* of these substances have failed to reach the intestinal tract and have accumulated in the blood, the condition is designated cholestasis. This concept is useful, since there are marked similarities in patients with jaundice from the extremes of disease of the liver cell to mechanical obstruction at the level of the ampulla of Vater (Fig. 28–4).

Cholestasis is ordinarily diagnosed with evidence from three different sources (Table 28–9). Lack of bilirubin and bile salts in the stool produces steatorrhea, vitamin K deficiency and its prolongation of the prothrombin time, light stools, and lack of urobilinogen in the urine. Accumulation of bilirubin and bile salts in the blood produces pruritus and jaundice. If the cholestasis is severe and prolonged for months, the blood cholesterol and phospholipid levels will rise markedly. The cholesterol may deposit in the skin as xanthomas. The high cholesterol is caused by increased rate of hepatic and intestinal manufacture. Bile salts reaching the gut normally repress hepatic and intestinal synthesis of cholesterol. Finally, in cholestasis some evidence of stimulation or injury to the hepatic and biliary epithelial cells is present. This is demonstrated most prominently by marked elevation of the enzyme, alkaline phosphatase, due to induction of hepatic production. The result of bile salt injury of liver cell membranes is a modest elevation of serum transaminase. Injury and mild inflammation are also apparent on liver biopsy. This takes the form of distorted bile canaliculi, bile lakes (lysed cells due to bile accumulation), and occasional inflammatory cells.

In practice, cholestasis is diagnosed when there

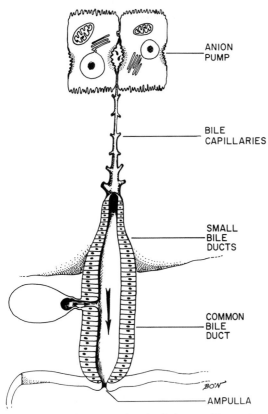

Figure 28–4 Various levels of abnormality producing cholestasis. Changes within the liver cells and the smallest bile capillaries produce similar clinical presentations. Bile ducts 1 mm. in diameter and larger are capable of secretion and absorption, and dilate markedly with distal obstruction. Blockage of the drainage at any level produces cholestasis.

TABLE 28–9   FINDINGS SOMETIMES PRESENT IN CHOLESTASIS

Clinical	Laboratory
Due to Accumulation in Blood	
Jaundice	Elevated bilirubin
Itching	Elevated bile salts
Due to Lack in Intestine	
Bulky, loose stools	Increased stool fat and weight
Ecchymoses	Prolonged prothrombin time
White or light stools	No bile pigment, no urobilinogen
	Decreased urine urobilinogen
Xanthoma	Elevated serum cholesterol (after prolonged cholestasis)
Injurious Effects on Liver	
Mild hepatomegaly	Elevated serum alkaline phosphatase
	Elevated SGOT, SGPT
	Liver biopsy changes

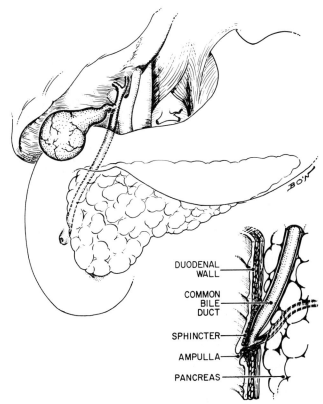

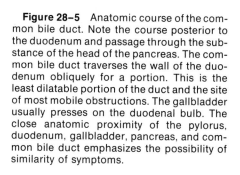

Figure 28–5 Anatomic course of the common bile duct. Note the course posterior to the duodenum and passage through the substance of the head of the pancreas. The common bile duct traverses the wall of the duodenum obliquely for a portion. This is the least dilatable portion of the duct and the site of most mobile obstructions. The gallbladder usually presses on the duodenal bulb. The close anatomic proximity of the pylorus, duodenum, gallbladder, pancreas, and common bile duct emphasizes the possibility of similarity of symptoms.

DUODENAL WALL

COMMON BILE DUCT

SPHINCTER

AMPULLA

PANCREAS

is jaundice, elevation of the serum alkaline phosphatase, and little or no evidence of major hepatocellular damage. If the stools are light (owing to both increased fat content and reduced pigment) and there is no urine urobilinogen, the syndrome is even more firmly established.

The practical problem of cholestasis is to determine at what level from the liver cell to the ampulla the block has occurred (Fig. 28–4). Studies of bile salt and bilirubin metabolism are usually not helpful in this determination. From the level of the bifurcation of the hepatic ducts distally, surgical removal or bypass of the lesion producing cholestasis is indicated; at higher levels, surgical intervention is not practical and often exaggerates the underlying condition.

Two little-known factors about the common causes of cholestasis often permit one to suspect correctly the proper cause: (1) bile ducts larger than 1 mm. in diameter are capable of tremendous dilatation with the secretory pressure of the liver and (2) cholestasis at the level of the anion pump or the bile capillaries rarely is complete for more than a few days. Each factor is useful in several ways. If cholestasis is caused by a surgical lesion, dilatation of the many ducts and moderate to marked enlargement of the liver must be present. If a patient with cholestasis has a normal-sized liver, a surgical lesion is very unlikely. The most common cause of surgical cholestasis is a gallstone impacted in the common bile duct. This most often lodges in the narrowest and least distensible portion of the common bile duct, which is the portion of the duct traversing the wall of the duodenum (Fig. 28–5). Dilatation proximal to such an obstruction will usually produce a 2- to 4-cm. turgid tube passing beneath the duodenal bulb (Fig. 28–6). A standard barium meal will usually reveal this garden-hose-like mass, producing a silhouette as it passes posteriorly. Such a mass clearly indicates a distended common bile duct. Occasionally the ducts in the hilum are sufficiently enlarged to produce a defect on colloid scan of the liver. Sometimes the turgid distended gallbladder is clearly and diagnostically palpable, indicating this problem. Visualization of the ducts by direct or radiologic means (direct laparotomy or peritoneoscopy, transhepatic or direct cholangiography) should indicate substantial dilatation beyond the normal 8 to 10 mm. in diameter. Ultrasound or sonography has become sufficiently precise to detect the fluid-filled and enlarged bile ducts within the hepatic parenchyma and to provide an excellent measure of the size of the gallbladder. This technique, of no harm to the patient, has enhanced the ability to detect a dilated gallbladder and the

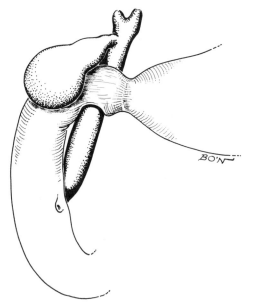

Figure 28-6   Detail of a common duct obstructed in the wall of the duodenum in the area of the ampulla. Note the marked dilatation of the common duct compared to Figure 28–5 and the filling defect produced in the duodenal area by the turgid dilated duct.

bile ducts markedly. Computer assisted tomography of the liver area (CAT scan) provides information of a similar nature.

The lack of complete obstruction in medical cholestasis is best appreciated by serial observations over several days. If small amounts of pigment appear in the stools or urobilinogen in the urine, incomplete obstruction is present. Newer radiopharmaceuticals excreted by the liver into the bile may be used both for scans and for demonstrating the patency of the common bile duct. A trace of these given intravenously is completely taken up by the normal liver in 30 to 60 minutes and completely excreted into the bile within two hours. In cholestasis, the uptake by the liver is normal but the subsequent excretion is retarded. However, in surgical cholestasis the obstruction is usually complete, so that scans done 1 hour and 24 hours after a single dose of radioactive rose bengal are essentially identical; in contrast, in the less complete intrahepatic cholestasis the scan at 24 hours is decreased in intensity usually by 50 per cent or more and often all the dye has passed into the gut. Newer radioactive molecules make this differentiation even more precise. If the cause of the jaundice is not clear by this time, some procedure to demonstrate either the detailed anatomy of the biliary passages by x-ray examination or histologic studies of the liver is necessary. Radiocontrast dye can be introduced into the normal biliary passages by the retrograde cannulation of the ducts via a duodenoscope; or it can be injected into the dilated ducts by blindly puncturing the liver with a very fine needle and injecting under fluoroscopic control. A liver biopsy can be taken for histologic examination. Sometimes the likelihood of a surgically relievable cause is so high that an exploratory operation is undertaken.

HEPATIC BLOOD FLOW AND PORTAL HYPERTENSION

Blood Flow Through the Liver

All portal venous blood and all hepatic arterial blood combine into a single capillary bed that drains from the liver via the hepatic veins. The total blood flow in the liver is the same as the hepatic venous blood flow or the sum of the hepatic arterial and portal venous flow. About 20 per cent (or 1 to 2 liters per min.) of the resting cardiac output reaches the liver, one third via the hepatic artery and two thirds via the portal vein. The portal venous flow varies markedly during the day because the arterial flow to the stomach and intestines varies. Stimulation of gastric or pancreatic secretion enhances both arterial flow and venous drainage. Similarly, food in the intestine stimulates motility and blood flow. Inflammation of these organs or of the spleen also increases blood flow.

The hepatic artery seems more responsive to the needs of the liver. Hepatic anoxia lowers intrahepatic resistance and increases arterial flow. Hepatic inflammation also increases hepatic arterial flow. The hepatic, splenic, and superior mesenteric arteries are similarly responsive to many regulatory agents. Bradykinin, low doses of epinephrine and some prostaglandins are arterial vasodilators, whereas serotonin, pitressin, high doses of epinephrine, norepinephrine, and other prostaglandins diminish arterial flow.

Both the portal and hepatic arterial supply come together in the sinusoids. These are highly permeable capillaries which surround three to six surfaces of each liver cell. The blood comes into sufficient contact with the reticuloendothelial cells (Kupffer cells) and liver cells to assure that more than 99 per cent of substances taken up by either cell will be removed in a single passage through the liver. In the resting state, blood actively flows in only about one fifth of the sinusoids. The remaining four fifths are temporarily static but the actual flow into the sinusoids can change from moment to moment. A higher proportion of the total number of sinusoids is conducting blood when the total liver blood flow increases. The liver resistance changes with flow, so that a doubling of portal venous flow is associated with only a slight rise of pressure in the portal vein.

TABLE 28-10 METHODS TO MEASURE PORTAL PRESSURE AND LIVER BLOOD FLOW AND TO ASSESS LIVER COLLATERAL FLOW

---

1. Liver Blood Flow
   a. Sulfobromophthalein or indocyanine green constant infusion with samples from hepatic venous catheter.*
   b. Radioactive colloid injection intravenously and determine the rate of removal from peripheral blood.
   c. Infuse substance into hepatic artery and sample at hepatic vein. Calculate dilution.*
2. Portal Pressure Measurement
   a. Catheterize the occluded umbilical vein.*
   b. Splenic pulp manometry.*
   c. Wedged hepatic venous pressure.*
3. Collateral Veins
   a. All methods in part 2.
   b. Venography phase of splenic and superior mesenteric artery injection.*
   c. Esophageal varices:
      (1) Esophagoscopy
      (2) Barium swallow

---

*Skilled operator required.

Liver blood flow may be measured in man by three methods (Table 28–10). The dyes sulfobromophthalein (BSP) and indocyanine green (ICG) are almost entirely removed by the liver. If either is infused at a constant rate for 30 to 45 minutes, the blood level rises and increases until the liver removal rate can keep up with the rate of infusion. At this time, simultaneous samples of mixed hepatic venous blood and peripheral arterial blood are obtained by appropriately placed catheters. The arterial level of dye represents that entering both the hepatic artery and the portal vein, and the hepatic venous level represents the concentration after some dye removal from the liver. The difference represents the amount of dye removed from each ml. of blood perfusing the liver. Since the rate of infusion and the rate of hepatic removal are the same, the infusion rate for the dye may be utilized to determine the liver blood flow.

The reticuloendothelial system of the liver specifically removes particles within a narrow range of size; the RE system of other organs will not remove such particles. If a trace dose of such particles is injected intravenously, the removal rate is a function of how much of the cardiac output is actually reaching the liver. Isotopic techniques have been so defined that an estimate of liver flow may be made from external counting.

A precise third method of determining liver flow, particularly applicable when shunts are present and liver cell function is diminished, is available by constant infusion of labeled albumin into the hepatic artery and constant sampling via the hepatic vein through appropriately positioned catheters. The dilution of the infused albumin reveals the total hepatic blood flow.

In practice, liver blood flow is of limited value in diagnosis. All forms of stable chronic liver disease seem to alter blood flow when need for oxygen is present. Any form of splenic disease and most forms of pancreatic, small intestinal, gastric, and colonic inflammatory disease are associated with enhanced portal blood flow. Inflammatory liver diseases increase liver flow but diseases associated with loss of total numbers of available liver cells are associated with diminished flow.

Portal Pressure

The pressure measured in the portal vein, or its feeding veins, fluctuates not only with each respiration but also with intra-abdominal pressure and modestly increases following each meal. Knowledge of the pressure at only one point in time may be misleading or unrepresentative; one desires to know whether the pressure is persistently above normal levels.

The pressure may be persistently elevated because of an obstruction in the portal vein or at any point retarding flow of blood from the portal vein to the heart. In the presence of a totally normal liver increased liver blood flow usually will not result in an elevated pressure. Minor abnormalities of the liver, however, along with an increased portal blood flow, may be responsible for some forms of portal hypertension.

Measurement of portal pressure is complex and requires a highly skilled physician and complex apparatus (Table 28–10). One accurate procedure is to dissect out the occluded umbilical vein in the umbilicus under local anesthetic and pass a catheter into the portal vein for direct measurement. Less directly, a needle may be passed into the pulp of the spleen and the pressure in the splenic sinusoids will indicate a close approximation of the portal pressure. Still more indirect is the pressure recorded when a straight catheter is passed retrograde into a hepatic vein until it occludes the lumen. The pressure in the occluded vein will rise until blood is forced through available collateral channels proximal to this blockage; these are at the level of hepatic sinusoids. If such a recorded pressure is normal, this indicates that the resistance to flow from sinusoids is normal. In some diseases the pressure recorded in this manner is much elevated, indicating an increased resistance to the escape of blood from the sinusoids. This pressure, called the wedged hepatic venous pressure, is a measurement of postsinusoid resistance.

The detailed evaluation of portal pressure requires the measurement of pressure in the portal

TABLE 28–11   CAUSES OF PORTAL PRESSURE ELEVATION AND ANATOMIC LOCATION

Disease	Frequency	Anatomic Level of Block	Comment
Extrahepatic portal vein occlusion	Infrequent	Portal vein	
Schistosomiasis	Common	Tiny portal veins	Endemic areas
Cancer nodules			
Extramedullary hematopoiesis			
Fat, lipid, amyloid accumulation	Common	Sinusoids	
Hypertrophy of endoplasmic reticulum			
As above plus increased portal blood flow due to splenomegaly or inflammation	Rare	Sinusoids	
Cirrhosis	Common	Postsinusoid	
Budd-Chiari syndrome	Rare	Hepatic veins	
Veno-occlusive disease	Rare	Hepatic veins	Endemic areas
Inferior vena cava	Rare		
Constrictive pericarditis	Rare		
Heart failure	Common	Right auricle	

vein or one of its branches. If it is elevated, the site of increased resistance must be determined. Wedged hepatic venous pressure may be measured to determine whether the elevation arises between that point and the heart or on the portal vein side of the sinusoid. Peripheral venous pressure may sometimes indicate a cardiac or periph-eral localization of the resistance producing portal hypertension. Table 28–11 indicates some forms of portal pressure elevation and the anatomic localization of the increased resistance. Figure 28–7 emphasizes these anatomic locations.

Consequences of Portal Hypertension.   There are many abnormalities that result from portal hyper-

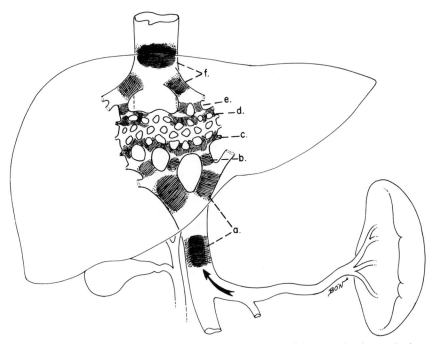

Figure 28–7   Schematic representation of the levels of obstruction of the portal vein producing portal hypertension. (*a*) Blockage of the extrahepatic or large intrahepatic branches of the portal vein. (*b*) Blockage of the tiny portal veins, such as is found in noncirrhotic portal hypertension of India. (*c*) Blockage immediately presinusoidal, as produced by embolism and granuloma with schistosomiasis. (*d*) Postsinusoidal block common in alcoholic cirrhosis. (*e*) Block as in veno-occlusive disease. (*f*) Hepatic vein, subhepatic vein, and inferior vena cava blockage.

TABLE 28–12 SEQUELAE OF PORTAL
HYPERTENSION

1. Splanchnic Sequestration
   a. Increases portal pressure after meal.
   b. Diminishes nonsplanchnic blood volume.
   c. Enhances renal retention of sodium.
   d. Increases over-all plasma volume.
   e. Impairs vascular homeostasis in bleeding.
2. High Portal Pressure
   a. Promotes development of collaterals — esophageal
      varices common.
   b. Promotes hemorrhage from varices.
   c. Promotes flow of blood through collaterals —
      shunting of portal blood promotes liver coma.
3. Congestion of Viscera
   a. Splenomegaly — hypersplenism.
   b. Impaired intestinal and stomach function.
   c. Thrombosis of spleen and mesenteric veins.
   d. Enhanced liver and mesenteric lymph formation
      — ascites.

tension regardless of the basic cause. The severity
and duration of portal hypertension seem more
important determinants than the exact level of
obstruction. The level of obstruction is of greatest
importance in the mode of treatment and prognosis. The sequelae of portal hypertension are conveniently divided into three groups — splanchnic
sequestration of blood, high pressure and development of collaterals, and congestion (Table 28–
12).

It is apparent that the portal pressure rises in
order to permit blood to leave the splanchnic bed
(all blood vessels which normally drain into the
portal system). If for any reason there is an increased entry of blood into the portal system (such
as following a meal or any temporary boost in the
cardiac output), this blood cannot promptly return
to the heart. It must pool in the splanchnic bed to
raise the pressure slightly and then the return
flow to the heart will increase. This increase in
portal volume and pressure occurs concomitantly
with a diminution in the blood volume available to
the remainder of the body. As a result, the renal
mechanisms to increase blood volume become operative and a portion of the sodium retention is a
direct result of this maldistribution of the blood
volume. Because of this, every patient with portal
hypertension develops an increased blood volume
compared to normal. The increase is entirely sequestered behind the obstructed portal circulation. No matter how large the volume, each time
more blood enters the splanchnic circulation there
is a temporary maladjustment. Should hemorrhage occur, this portion of the blood volume is
only slowly available to the heart because of the
high resistance before entering the systemic circulation.

The elevated pressure, over weeks or months,
promotes formation of collaterals to permit blood
to return to the heart through other channels.
Rarely, if ever, do these collateral channels restore the pressure to normal. Collaterals prevent
pressure from reaching levels that would rupture
vessels but are constantly associated with marked
elevation as compared to normal. Wherever the
inferior vena cava and portal vessels have a common distribution, significant anastomoses may
occur. The more important clinical areas are (a)
directly from the portal vein along the stomach, up
the esophagus, and anastomosing with the intercostal veins; (b) the area of the spleen between the
diaphragm and the posterior abdominal wall; (c)
along the umbilical vein or the mesentery through
adhesions with the anterior abdominal wall; (d)
posterior from branches in the area of the pancreas to the lumbar veins; and (e) around the rectum
in the area of the hemorrhoidal vessels. These
various collateral channels may be seen by various techniques. Sometimes they are visually
prominent (abdominal, periumbilical, hemorrhoidal areas) or loud bruits (over the umbilicus) are
detectable. They often produce large protrusions
into the esophagus (opacified by a barium sulfate
swallow) or similarly into the stomach. They are
sometimes seen in the esophagus (esophagoscopy)
or in the peritoneum (peritoneoscopy) and may
also be demonstrated radiographically by the injection of a radiocontrast medium into the portal
vein or its branches. The same techniques may be
used to measure portal pressure directly, or large
quantities of radiopaque media may be injected
into the splanchnic arteries and thus opacify the
portal veins and its branches (see Table 28–10).

Finally, the presence of collateral channels may
sometimes be suspected when divergence of large
amounts of materials normally limited to the portal circulation appear in the systemic circulation.
Extremely high levels of glucose (postprandially),
high levels of ammonia and amino acids, and
extremely high levels of urinary urobilinogen
may be produced by large quantities of portal
blood bypassing the liver and directly reaching
the systemic circulation. The role of ammonia in
liver coma is discussed in a later section.

Enlarged submucosal veins of the esophagus,
known as esophageal varices, serve as collateral
vessels between the portal venous system and the
inferior and superior venae cavae. These vessels
are tortuous and distended up to 8 mm. in diameter. The submucosa of the esophagus has little or
no supportive-connective tissue. Esophageal
varices are produced when portal pressure of more
than 20 mm. Hg above right heart pressure persists for months. At pressures above 35 mm., they
tend to rupture and bleed profusely. Bleeding almost always occurs in the vicinity of the transition
from intra-abdominal pressure to intrathoracic
and is mainly caused by a temporary elevation in

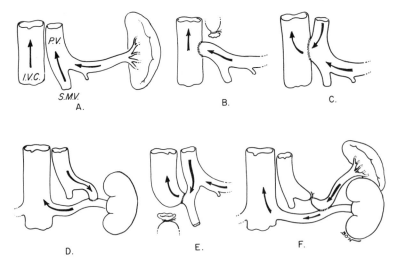

Figure 28-8 Types of portal systemic shunts constructed surgically. *A*, Normal. *I.V.C.*, inferior vena cava; *P.V.*, portal vein; *S.M.V.*, superior mesenteric vein.

B, End-to-side portacaval shunt—the portal vein is transected and the intestinal side anastomosed to I.V.C.

C, Side-to-side portacaval shunt.

D, Splenorenal shunt—usually the spleen is resected.

E, Mesocaval shunt. The I.V.C. is transected and the proximal portion anastomosed to the S.M.V. A prosthesis is often used and called an H graft.

F, Reverse splenorenal shunt, used to preserve S.M.V. blood flow to liver but decompress varices by permitting splenic venous flow and the variceal collaterals to drain through the renal circulation.

portal pressure. Surface irritation in the esophagus occasionally plays a role. Once bleeding begins, it is kept active by the sustained pressure, and the consequences of such hemorrhage are serious in that at least one sixth of such episodes produce death. Significant bleeding from other collateral beds in portal hypertension is infrequent. The surgical construction of a large low-resistance communication between the portal bed and the vena cava (portacaval shunt) will eliminate portal hypertension. Shunting, if adequate, is effective in removing the hazard of variceal bleeding and may facilitate disappearance of varices (Fig. 28–8).

Techniques for demonstrating collateral vessels and particularly esophageal varices are indicated in Table 28–10. Congestion of viscera is prominent in portal hypertension and occurs more frequently when the inflow to the splanchnic bed increases. In a few months' time this leads to prominent splenomegaly. Over many months, it is rare for a patient with portal hypertension not to have an enlarged spleen, usually apparent on palpation but invariably demonstrated by scanning. Infarction, a common occurrence in portal hypertension, may develop owing to an enlarged, congested spleen and the slow turnover of blood. The congested sinusoids of the spleen and the prolonged contact of the active RE cells of the spleen with the formed elements of the blood (platelets, erythrocytes, leukocytes) may injure and destroy some or all three of these. The loss of any of these formed elements due to enlarged spleen is sometimes called hypersplenism. This is most apparent in the lowering of the peripheral counts. Platelets are often lowered from a normal of 250,000 to half that level or less; leukocytes are lowered to less than

4000, mostly owing to loss of polymorphonuclear leukocytes. Lowering of the red blood cells is less frequent. Despite the frequent occurrence of these lowered levels, this is rarely of clinical consequence in producing bleeding (due to platelet lack), increased infection (due to leukocyte lack), or symptoms of anemia. The lowering is reversed both by splenectomy and a portacaval shunt to correct the congestion and stasis.

Congestion of the mesenteric vessels may lead to mesenteric infarction. Small thromboses of the mesenteric veins seem frequent in portal hypertension. They produce altered motility of the small intestine and occasionally damage the wall, producing peritonitis and septicemia, but they are difficult to recognize unless they are major. Whenever there are abrupt changes in congestion, intestinal function and motility may be temporarily impaired and edema of the gut and impaired absorption may result. This congestion is one of the factors contributing to ascites, which is discussed in a later section.

Lymph Flow.   The hepatic sinusoid is possibly the most permeable capillary in the body; it is estimated that normally 0.3 per cent of the blood flow through the liver passes through the walls of the sinusoid and appears as liver lymph (compared to approximately 0.01 per cent for muscle). This lymph mainly follows the bile channels in lymphatic vessels, exits from the liver in the porta hepatis, and joins the cisterna chyli along with the mesenteric and large leg lymphatics. Any process which increases sinusoidal pressure (such as cirrhosis) may markedly increase liver lymph formation. In patients with cirrhosis this increased lymph may exude from the surface of the liver and flow into the peritoneal cavity as ascites. This happens only when the rate of production exceeds the ability of the lymphatics to convey it back into the circulation. Protein elevation in lymph content reflects protein production by the liver (above 3.0 mg. per 100 ml.). Any interruption of hepatic lymphatics, such as may occur in biliary tract surgery or during surgery on the portal veins, may lead to large lymph fistulas into the peritoneal cavity.

In a similar fashion, any form of portal hypertension will increase the forces forming intestinal lymph in all parts of the bowel. If the increase is only slight, the lymphatics can convey it at about the same rate that it is formed. If the formation is acute or extremely rapid, it will produce edema of the cells of the bowel and may cross into the peritoneum and appear as ascites. Intestinal lymph is lower in protein content but may contain large amounts of lipid (chyle), particularly after fatty meals. Chylous ascites may result in patients with portal hypertension, though it is more frequent in patients with blockage of the lymphatics from obstruction. It has been observed that in all forms of portal hypertension the flow of lymph in the thoracic duct is markedly increased from 3 to 60 times the normal level.

Portacaval Shunts. A surgical collateral between the portal vein and the inferior vena cava may be constructed to lower portal pressure. Figure 28–8 indicates the forms that are frequently used. If properly constructed, all the pressure, congestion, and adverse effects disappear (Table 28–12), except the amount of portal blood shunted to the systemic circulation, which increases markedly. Shunts are most widely used to prevent subsequent hemorrhage from esophageal varices in patients in whom this has occurred at least once. Shunts produce some additional morbidity largely from the increased shunting of blood to the systemic circulation (liver encephalopathy), and this has led to a modification of procedures (see *F* in Fig. 28–8). These modified procedures have the advantage of preventing bleeding without producing such a total shunt of intestinal blood.

LIVER FUNCTION TESTS

A wide variety of tests assess aspects of the liver. Those tests listed in Tables 28–1, 28–3, 28–6, and 28–10 are liver function tests. Usually one restricts the term "liver function test" to those blood and urine tests indicated in Table 28–13. The meaning and method of performance of each of these will now be discussed. Of the several thousand known biochemical functions of the liver only a few are abnormal during the early stages of liver disease. Some tests have been abandoned because they are abnormal too frequently, others because the patient must be close to death before an abnormality appears.

TABLE 28–13 TESTS OF LIVER CELL DAMAGE

A. Cell Necrosis
  1. SGOT
  2. SGPT
  3. Cephalin cholesterol flocculation
  4. Bilirubinuria
  5. Biopsy*
  6. Serum Fe
  7. Serum B_{12}
B. Too Few Functioning Liver Cells
  1. Bilirubin
  2. Sulfobromophthalein, indocyanine green
  3. Albumin
  4. Prothrombin
  5. Fibrinogen
  6. Urine urobilinogen
  7. Amino acidemia and aciduria
  8. Increased undetermined anion
C. Inflammation
  1. α, γ immunoglobulin, IGM, IGG
D. Specific Etiology
  1. Hepatitis A, B antigen and antibody
  2. Antimitochondrial antibody
  3. Amebae, hydatid complement fixation
  4. Eaton-Barr agent antibody
E. Intrahepatic or Extrahepatic Shunts
  1. Ammonia

*Increased risk.

Liver Biopsy

A special needle is inserted into the liver and a core of tissue 1 to 2 mm. in diameter is removed for histologic or other examination. Continued hemorrhage accounts for some mortality (1 per 10,000) during this procedure. The cellular injury and nature of inflammatory response are revealed in all diffuse processes. If there is diffuse cancer, metabolic storage disease, or infection, it will be seen. Focal conditions such as tumor metastases or diseases affecting only some of the hepatic lobules (such as congenital fibrosis or biliary cirrhosis) are often missed completely. A biopsy examination is the most definite of the commonly employed procedures and is used in almost every patient with liver disease in whom the diagnosis is unknown or the prognosis uncertain. Even in liver clinics 10 to 20 per cent of biopsies performed reveal a major unsuspected diagnosis. Table 28–14 lists the utility of liver biopsy in making clinical decisions.

Tests of Cellular Necrosis

Intact hepatocytes contain a number of substances in the cystosol in concentrations much higher than in the circulating blood. These substances may be released into the serum following damage to the cell wall. Persistence of each abnor-

TABLE 28–14   CLINICAL DECISIONS
FOLLOWING LIVER BIOPSY

	False-Positive (%)	False-Negative (%)
Is there cancer in liver?	0	30
Hepatitis decision		
Is disease hepatitis?	0	2
Is it active?	0	5
Will cirrhosis or		
CAH follow?	2	1
Drug or virus	20	20
Cirrhosis		
Is there cirrhosis?	5	5
Active?	0	0
Etiology?		
Alcohol	5	5
Virus, Iron	15	15
Inherited	5	5
Cholestasis		
Is it extrahepatic?	5	10
What is the nature of		
the liver disease?	0	15

mal substance is determined by a balance between its rate of release and its duration of survival in the bloodstream. Serum glutamic pyruvic transaminase is the most specific and widely used measure of hepatocellular necrosis. In a person in good nutritional state, with good stores of intracellular enzyme, damage to as little as 1 per cent of the liver cells will raise the serum level. Serum glutamic oxaloacetic transaminase acts similarly but is less specific, for all forms of striate muscle contain this material. Serum iron and vitamin B_{12} behave similarly but remain elevated longer than the transaminase.

In severe necrosis, amino acids are released from the liver cells and appear in high concentration in the blood; the more insoluble ones (tyrosine and cysteine) appear in the urine as crystals.

The cephalin-cholesterol flocculation test, now rapidly disappearing because of the delay of 48 hours for its final reading, is a sensitive test for liver necrosis. Suspensions of cephalin and cholesterol are stabilized by normal serum but sera containing minute quantities of protein released from necrotic liver cells will produce flocculation. A positive test indicates acute liver necrosis. High gammaglobulin levels also produce flocculation. Thymol turbidity, Takata-Ara flocculation, colloidal gold flocculation, and Weltmann tests are all similar to the cephalin-cholesterol flocculation test.

The liver biopsy may reveal damaged cells with pyknotic nuclei or feathery degeneration, but more commonly it reveals inflammatory cells surrounding the place where the cell was or distorted liver cords due to loss of many cells or rapid regeneration, indicating their replacement. Very active necrosis may leave cellular debris in the form of eosinophilic or hyaline bodies (Mallory body, Councilman body).

Tests of Insufficient Functioning Liver Cell Mass

It is apparent from partial hepatic ablation studies in animals and in man needing major liver surgery that most of these liver tests are normal until about half the liver is gone. At this level the BSP test (sulfobromophthalein test) or the indocyanine green test becomes abnormal. Alterations of liver blood flow alter this transport only if the normal flow is reduced by more than 50 per cent.

When 60 per cent or more of the liver cells are not functioning, jaundice occurs. If the pigment load is enhanced for any reason (hemolysis or transfusion), lesser amounts of liver damage are needed. The principal cause of jaundice is impairment at the level of the anion pump. Conjugation is usually adequate.

The liver makes many proteins that are released into the bloodstream and can serve as liver function tests; albumin and prothrombin are the most useful. If the liver ceased to function totally, the albumin level on the third day would be reduced only about 10 per cent, but the prothrombin level would be about 5 per cent of normal. Prothrombin (half-time 12 hours) and fibrinogen (half-time 4 days) reflect acute liver damage more readily than does albumin, with its 30-day half-life. Prothrombin requires adequate amounts of vitamin K as a cofactor in its hepatic synthesis; vitamin K malabsorption is common in cholestasis. Any patient with a prolonged prothrombin time should have the level checked again 12 hours after administration of 5 mg. of parenteral vitamin K. A marked change in the circulating level is seen if the cause is malabsorption. The liver regulates the plasma amino acid level by taking up elevated levels and converting one amino acid into another. If these functions are lost, elevated amino acid levels result, particularly levels of alanine and the aromatic amino acids, and deficiencies of some of the branched-chain ones follow. Similarly, removal of lactate, alphaketoglutaric and citric acid levels are liver functions that become impaired. This is manifested by a rise in the undetermined anion analogous to that found in lactic acidosis.

Tests of Inflammation

The globulin level is the most widely used test of inflammatory response and antibody formation.

This is prominently elevated in any form of liver disease infiltrated with round cells. This is usually gamma globulin on electrophoresis.

Tests of Specific Etiology

Hepatitis-B Antigen. A portion of the long-incubation hepatitis virus may be detected with sensitive antisera. This is called the hepatitis-B antigen, sometimes called Australia antigen, and seems diagnostically specific. It appears in the serum of 90 per cent or more of all patients weeks or months before the onset of active disease. At the time of hepatocellular manifestations it is present in about 60 per cent of such patients and persists for about 15 additional days and then disappears. It persists in the serum of about 20 per cent of the patients with chronic hepatitis. Because all transfused blood is tested for Hepatitis B, when an infection occurs it is usually not B. Antibody to hepatitis B indicates previous infection and is less clearly associated with existing disease; an antibody to hepatitis A now exists.

Antimitochondrial Antibody. Antibody to mitochondria of a variety of species (rat or guinea pig liver mitochondria are commonly used) seems a feature of primary biliary cirrhosis. This test is of great value if the techniques are sensitive and the limit of normal is set sufficiently high to exclude many common inflammatory diseases. There is no clear understanding of its meaning.

Fetoglobulin, Placental Alkaline Phosphatase, and Carcinoembryonic Antigen. These three substances, produced by carcinoma in the adult, seem a part of the development of embryonic cells but are lost by normal adult tissues. Fetoglobulin found in an adult nearly always indicates liver carcinoma; placental alkaline phosphatase in a person without a placenta indicates a carcinoma of entodermal origin; colon and pancreatic carcinomas seem responsible for production of the carcinoembryonic antigen. Sensitive serologic tests for etiologic agents are useful in detecting amebiasis, hydatid disease, and certain fungus disorders.

APPROACH TO THE PROBLEM OF CLINICAL LIVER DISEASE

Liver disease may start predominantly as a focal process; such processes use the rich blood supply of the liver but interfere little with the hepatocyte function. In contrast, liver disease may indicate diffuse involvement of the hepatocytes. These two types of initial disease are quite distinct in typical cases but may completely overlap as they advance. There is some value in having a clear understanding of each.

Focal Liver Disease and Its Typical Syndromes

Two prototypes of focal liver disease must be considered. One is a single abscess or metastasis within the liver that progressively grows but, even when massive, interferes but slightly with overall liver function. The other consists of myriad small foci (such as miliary tuberculosis or extramedullary hematopoiesis) which similarly may grow without affecting liver function.

Systemic symptoms are a function of the basic pathologic condition invading the liver but are important to keep in mind. Abscesses, specific infectious agents (amebae, hydatid, tuberculosis), and cancer with necrosis may produce impressive systemic signs of fever and weight loss; however, these signs may not reveal themselves in the history, physical examination, or laboratory screening to indicate that the liver is the host to the problem. This is particularly true in the diseases mentioned and in some cases of lymphoma.

Modest hepatomegaly is most readily detected by scanning. Uniform distribution of an increased mass of 20 per cent throughout the liver would result in an average increase in each dimension of 1 cm. and this amount cannot be detected upon ordinary physical examination. If the increase is not uniformly distributed or produces symptoms (fullness in the abdomen, pulling on the side), hepatomegaly might well be found. Tight clothing in women often brings about the finding of abdominal masses, and hepatomegaly is also found in this way. If the enlargement is rapid or if the underlying process is one that may hemorrhage into itself, pain may result.

Painful sensations in the liver seem to arise from receptors lying in the liver capsule and along the fibrous tissue following the portal veins and its branches. These sensations pass from the liver via the sympathetic nerves, through the celiac plexus, and on to the seventh through twelfth paravertebral ganglia. These nerve endings seem particularly sensitive to distention but are not affected by penetration, heat, or cold. Acute distention of the capsule, as produced by vascular or bile congestion or rapid infiltration of inflammation, produces exquisite pain and tenderness. Pain and tenderness will disappear after a few days of steady distention. Other innervated portions include the hepatic veins and bile ducts, which produce the sensation of pain when they are acutely distended or in spasm. The parietal peritoneum overlies much of the liver capsule and is particularly sensitive after inflammation or occurrence of fibrin deposits. Thus, focal processes may alter the capsule, vessels, or overlying peritoneum and produce pain and tenderness.

Slow-growing, usually benign tumors or infiltrations of the liver may remain indefinitely silent. Moderate infiltrations of fat, amyloid, Gaucher's lipid, or hamartomas may remain silent during life. Sonograms, CAT scans (computer assisted tomography), and radioisotope scans with specific substances (gallium localizing in abscesses or tumors) often specifically assist in identifying focal liver disease.

Generalized Liver Disease and Its Typical Syndromes (Table 28–15)

Jaundice. In liver cell disease, jaundice is due to either damage to the anion pump or cholestasis. Both produce jaundice in which the serum bilirubin is more than half direct-reacting. If there is no increased production of bile pigments, the degree of jaundice is a general reflection of the severity of the disease, and the level of jaundice may increase as its course progresses. Stable jaundice of liver cell origin is usually an indication of increased destruction of liver cells exceeding their replacement rate. If there is no evidence of liver cell destruction, cholestasis is usually prominent, owing to the huge regenerative capacity of the liver.

Acute Liver Cell Failure. Destruction of about 90 per cent or more of liver cells within a few weeks or less results in a rapid, devastating, often fatal syndrome in which jaundice and confusion are nearly always present but often mild, and in which metabolic changes, hemorrhage, and cardiovascular collapse may be so prominent as to produce death. Many of the common manifestations of liver disease, such as jaundice, require time to occur while material accumulates in the blood; and the course, until death due to liver failure, may be so rapid that these manifestations do not occur prominently.

The totally failing liver is unable to clear amino acids or the citric acid cycle intermediates from the blood (lactate, pyruvate, alphaketoglutarate), and these materials are acidic. Prominent acidosis and a marked increase in the undetermined anion may be observed. The undetermined anion is the numerical difference between the sum of the sodium and potassium minus the sum of the chloride and bicarbonate. It is usually less than

TABLE 28–15 SYNDROMES OF GENERALIZED LIVER DISEASE

1. Jaundice, including cholestasis
2. Acute liver failure
3. Fluid retention
4. Portal hypertension
5. Confusion, including hepatic encephalopathy and hypoglycemia
6. Systemic wasting

16 mEq. per L. but may be as high as 60 mEq. per L. in acute liver failure.

The liver manufactures nearly all coagulation proteins and many of these are diminished in any form of liver disease. The one-stage prothrombin time measures a complex relationship of Factors I (fibrinogen), II (prothrombin), V, VII, and X, all of which are manufactured by the liver. Activated coagulation with further removal of clotting factors by consumption may occur in acute inflammatory liver disease, and this may result in prominent oozing into all tissues.

In animals it has been noted that when liver tissue is removed and permitted to autolyze under sterile conditions and is then reinjected, peripheral vasodilatation and increased cardiac output result. It is likely that the sudden release of destroyed liver tissue is responsible for some cardiovascular changes. In addition, acute liver failure may have manifestations in all the other areas.

Fluid Retention. Any form of liver cell disease is associated with prominent fluid retention mediated via sodium retention by the kidney. Any experimental design leading to congestion within the liver results in profound sodium retention. It is possible that a portion of this is due to sequestration of an important proportion of the plasma volume behind the liver, but other factors may also be important. Sodium retention is mediated by the renin-angiotensin-aldosterone mechanisms, but after a few days a fundamental alteration in blood distribution occurs within the kidney and is probably hormonally mediated (third factor). The common pathway of sodium retention by the kidney is clearly understood. Most patients with liver cell failure have 6 to 30 lb. of increased extracellular fluid and will secrete increasing amounts of sodium and water as the liver disease improves.

This increased extracellular fluid will distribute itself in a variety of places. It will be manifest as edema or ascites, dependent upon local factors. If there is mostly erect posture or venous stasis of the legs, the fluid will be most visible in the legs. If there is portal hypertension, the venous pressure in either the hepatic or mesenteric bed must exceed that in the legs, and ascites results. Fluid retention usually corrects itself when the disease improves. If this is unlikely or complications are feared, it is appropriate to stimulate sodium excretion by the kidney.

The important relationship between plasma volume and portal pressure was discussed earlier. An ambulatory patient with fluid is often put to bed, the result being redistribution of leg fluid, increased portal pressure, and finally hemorrhage. Patients exhibiting increased fluid stores should be gently controlled before bed rest is enforced.

Portal hypertension has been discussed in an earlier section, including its major complications — hypersplenism and esophageal varices with hemorrhage — and its indirect complications — ascites and increased collateral circulation.

Confusion, Including Hepatic Encephalopathy and Hypoglycemia. Hypoglycemia occurs so frequently that it should be the first problem suspected when a patient with liver disease becomes confused. Hypoglycemia usually arises from impaired gluconeogenesis in (a) severe liver cell damage; (b) congestive heart failure; and (c) alcoholics, particularly after a prolonged fast.

Liver encephalopathy is an altered metabolic state of the central nervous system. It is brought about by the direct shunting of some material from the intestinal tract bypassing the liver to the brain. This material seems to be present in proteins in the intestinal tract and may be ammonia. Once encephalopathy is present, a variety of noxious materials seem to affect the central nervous system adversely in a similar manner. The signs and symptoms of liver encephalopathy are aggravated by ammonia, hypokalemia, anoxia, sedative drugs, and central nervous system depressants (such as morphine).

The shunting of intestinal blood through or around the liver cells seems more important in the production of liver coma than does the presence of damaged liver cells. This syndrome is known to occur in the presence of a normal liver cell mass.

In its mildest form there is a slight disturbance of thought processes and a disturbance of the diurnal sleep rhythm, so that the patient is awake at night and dozes all day. At the next stage there is mental-motor dissociation, which shows far more impairment than is revealed by any routine neurologic testing. Thus, if the patient is asked to copy a simple line drawing or to write his name, it cannot be done, even though the patient tries. Still later, the "flapping tremor" or asterixis becomes apparent. This tremor is elicited by asking the patient to hold the arms and hands extended maximally against gravity and encouraging him to hold them perfectly still. Periodically, the sustained stimulus to hold them against gravity will be relaxed owing to a temporary block in the signal, and despite the will of the patient the hand will drop; the patient, in trying to comply, will quickly jerk the limb back into position, and a flapping effect is produced. Subsequently, stages are progressive loss of memory and then unconsciousness. Finally, deep coma may intervene and death occurs. The level of consciousness has been raised by treatments aimed at interrupting the supply of ammonia reaching the brain. This is achieved by discontinuing oral intake of all protein- and nitrogen-containing materials. The G.I. tract is purged to remove blood and other foodstuffs and to lessen the stasis that promotes accumulation of ammonia-forming bacteria. Nonab-

sorbed antibiotics, particularly neomycin, are highly effective in inhibiting the function of intestinal flora. Lactulose, a disaccharide that cannot be absorbed, therefore produces lactate from bacterial action and osmotic diarrhea, interferes with ammonia absorption, and is useful in treating liver encephalopathy.

An alternative hypothesis on the cause of liver coma (and also the hepatorenal syndrome) is the false transmitter hypothesis. Biological amines, related structurally to norepinephrine, may accumulate in liver disease and make the usual neurotransmitter substance norepinephrine less effective owing to the accumulation of these false transmitters at the synapse. Such a problem could be overcome by providing the nerve cells with more precursor for norepinephrine synthesis such as dopa or dopamine. Animal and human data consistent with this hypothesis exist, but there is not yet sufficient proof to warrant widespread application in treatment.

REPRESENTATIVE HEPATIC DISEASES

Vascular Impairment

An example of vascular impairment is congestive heart failure due to myocardial disease. The liver has two vascular supplies and either is sufficient to maintain a fully functioning liver. However, when the venous drainage is blocked from the liver owing to either intrahepatic or extrahepatic disorders, it produces a profound derangement of liver function which is largely due to damage from anoxia. Initially, there is vascular stasis throughout the liver without death of liver cells, but all metabolic function of the liver is inefficient. The liver becomes enlarged owing to vascular congestion and may become very tender. Fluid retention, a result of sodium retention, usually is present. After several weeks, liver cells die with prominent transaminase elevation. Lack of liver cells is apparent from marked BSP retention, jaundice, hypoalbuminemia, and low prothrombin time. In order for blood to continue to flow through the liver, portal hypertension, splenomegaly, and in extreme cases even portal collateral circulation must develop. Healing following correction of the circulatory problem is rapid and dramatic.

Hepatitis

Viral hepatitis, alcoholic hepatitis, and allergic or idiosyncratic hepatitis (from drugs or other environmental agents) are the principal forms of hepatitis. Coincidental with the injury to liver cells are systemic symptoms such as fever, nausea and vomiting, and malaise. The exact cause of these symptoms is unclear. The liver soon becomes enlarged from edema of injury which is caused by the infiltration of inflammatory and regenerative cells (they are larger than the destroyed cells). Tenderness may be prominent at this stage. Jaundice, a cumulative phenomenon, becomes most marked usually after healing has started. Transaminase elevation is most prominent during the maximal injury phase.

Self-limited hepatitis from the preceding causes is usually not associated with either hyperglobulinemia or hypoalbuminemia. The majority of all forms of hepatitis completely heal and at a subsequent time the liver is completely normal. In cases of viral hepatitis among previously healthy young people, 85 per cent recover completely within 3 months and in total 95 per cent recover completely. In cases of alcoholic hepatitis, about 50 per cent later develop cirrhosis; in cases of viral hepatitis, about 3 per cent have cirrhosis and about 2 per cent have a chronically active (destructive) form of the disease that may persist for years or until death.

There are hepatotoxic substances in nature and medicine but the latter have usually been eliminated with the advent of safer agents. A hepatotoxic substance is an agent that, if given in a sufficient amount, will cause liver damage; the toxic pattern is readily reproduced in animals but not in all species. Idiosyncratic or allergic hepatitis is the most common and troublesome form of liver disease. It develops only in a small number of people, is not dose related, and cannot be predicted from animal testing. Nearly every drug and many environmental chemicals have produced this form of hepatitis. Some drugs, such as phenothiazine tranquilizers, isonicotinic acid hydrazide, and halothane, are very frequent causes.

Cirrhosis

The term cirrhosis as used in medicine has two definitions; occasionally they are synonymous, but very often they are quite different. The most precise description is a pathologic entity which has three features: (1) Present or deduced major hepatic necrosis sufficient to destroy total lobules in at least two thirds of the liver. This may occur in a single wave or many small waves of necrosis. (2) Major scarring as a result of this necrosis which becomes a permanent type of connective tissue. (3) Formation of new liver through the process of regeneration. As a result, the architecture of the liver is completely destroyed and is largely formed of scars and regenerative nodules. To the clinician the term cirrhosis refers to any form of long-standing liver disease in which the features of portal hypertension are prominent. Although these conditions are usually presumed to be synonymous, only with some element of proof is this actually the case.

The cirrhotic liver (in pathologically confirmed cases) is strikingly different from the normal or precirrhotic liver in the following ways:
— The necrosis usually continues and may be the most prominent feature.
— The new liver cells have a very inefficient relationship to the blood supply. They are usually very deficient and much less subject to increase with need. There is little to no portal blood supply, and if the perfusion pressure is not maintained high, the blood supply, already marginal, will drop precipitously and may produce additional ischemic damage. A regenerative nodule grows concentrically like a berry, and the blood supply and drainage come in from the outside like fingers surrounding a ball. The growth of a nodule is dependent upon its success in developing a blood supply. Soon competition develops for space, and the growing nodule presses against the contracting scars. This pressure is detrimental to the veins. The nodule, if successful, becomes totally arterially dependent. Because the venous drainage is under high pressure, there is increased lymph flow from the sinusoids. This interferes with efficient cellular exchange and thus causes postsinusoidal resistance or outflow obstruction which is found in cirrhosis.
— Regeneration is rarely complete — there is always liver cell deficiency.
— Major shunts of portal blood exist in vascularized scars, portal collaterals, and plexuses surrounding bile ducts.
— Sequestration of additional portions of the plasma volume behind the liver due to portal hypertension impairs vascular homeostasis.

Despite the fact that on the average there is 20 per cent increase in total blood volume, the blood volume available to perfuse the kidneys, heart, and brain is less than normal. These features explain many of the problems that patients with cirrhosis have in common, but in varying degrees. These features are (a) Liver destruction (activity) and liver cell insufficiency. (b) Usually inefficient metabolism of food — mild malabsorption (reflecting bile salt insufficiency), frequent glycosuria, and weight loss despite adequate calorie intake. (c) Portal hypertension, esophageal varices, and enlarged spleen with hypersplenism are frequently present. The collateral circulation is responsible for elevated urinary urobilinogen, extremely high postprandial blood sugar, and often hyperammonemia. (d) Poor tolerance of hemorrhage or electrolyte depletion resulting from impaired vascular homeostasis. The frequent postural hypotension and impaired renal function may be features of this problem. (e) Prominent ascites.

Patients with cirrhosis show a propensity for the complications of gastrointestinal hemorrhage (usually from esophageal varices), liver encephalopathy, liver cell failure, and renal insufficiency. It is likely that the poor vascular homeostasis and possibly a small hemorrhage are the principal precipitants of the additional liver cell failure and renal insufficiency.

In the cirrhotic liver there is an increased tendency for a primary tumor called a hepatoma to form. This tumor often produces a primitive protein made in the fetus (fetoglobulin), which enters into the blood. This is found in about 50 per cent of the patients with hepatoma and seems to occur in no other tumor.

Cirrhosis may result from many different causes of liver damage. Viral hepatitis, alcoholic liver damage, biliary cirrhosis, and hemochromatosis are the principal forms. In approximately one third of all cases a cause cannot be assigned. Prognosis is far more dependent upon continuation of destructive activity and upon the maximal functioning liver cell mass that can be attained from the specific complication. Except for hepatoma and renal insufficiency, highly effective treatments exist for the other complications, including portal hypertension, hypersplenism, bleeding esophageal varices, liver coma, and ascites.

EFFECT OF LIVER DISEASE ON OTHER ORGANS

Cardiovascular Effects

Acute hepatic necrosis may release vasodilating substances into the blood. Wide pulse pressure, warm palms, and high cardiac output may be manifestations of this. An inflamed liver may have such a high blood flow that it creates cardiac overload by acting as an arterial venous shunt. Most forms of active liver disease cause a 20 to 50 per cent increase in cardiac output.

Plasma volume is usually increased by one third in chronic liver disease; this increased volume is entirely sequestered in the obstructed splanchnic circulation. It has no influence on cardiovascular function except that the return of blood to the systemic circulation is retarded and occasionally leads to hypovolemia and postural hypertension. Regulation of plasma volume following hemorrhage is limited.

Lowered arterial Po_2 commonly accompanies liver disease, particularly when associated with ascites. Many patients regain normal Po_2 by breathing high concentrations of oxygen. This suggests ventilatory perfusion abnormalities brought about by the large liver or the prominent ascites. Rarely, an unresponsive lowering of the Po_2 after oxygen inhalation is found and is caused by anatomic shunts within the substance of the lung. This is most prone to occur after 3 to 7 years

of cirrhosis, and clubbing of the fingers is often seen at this stage.

Many hepatic alterations of pH are possible. Liver disease is often associated with nausea, vomiting, or diarrhea, and large depletions of potassium may occur. Depletion may be accompanied by an intracellular acidosis and an extracellular alkalosis. Severe impairment of renal acidification is often present in chronic hepatic disease and further accentuates potassium depletion. In any form of hepatocellular damage, acidic products of metabolism, amino acids, and carbohydrate intermediates may be released into the blood and produce acidosis. This is most commonly seen as a persistent lowering of the serum bicarbonate.

In liver encephalopathy, hyperventilation due to an altered central threshold is common and alkalosis results.

Renal Changes

Renal blood flow and glomerular filtration are well preserved in most cases of mild and moderately severe liver disease. Chronic sodium retention by the kidney in association with liver disease initially involves the aldosterone mechanism, but when severe or prolonged it involves a different system. A far higher proportion of the glomerular filtrate is reabsorbed by the proximal loop of Henle (as high as 99.6 per cent), thus limiting the amount of sodium that reaches the distal convoluted tubule. A hormone called "third factor" is postulated to be the cause. Severe limitation of sodium on the distal convoluted tubule impairs excretion of free water and impairs responsiveness to diuretics acting on the distal convoluted tubule (spironolactones, thiazides).

In cirrhosis, a higher than normal portion of renal blood flow goes to the medulla. This high flow cleanses the high concentration of medullary solutes, so that in the water-deprived person with cirrhosis there is only about a twofold increase in medullary osmolality compared to the three- or fourfold increase in the normal subject. This makes urine concentration more difficult for the patient with cirrhosis.

It may be concluded that the person with chronic hepatic disease excretes sodium poorly and is unable either to excrete large volumes of free water or to concentrate the urine as markedly as the normal person in order to conserve water.

Renal tubule acidosis is commonly observed in the presence of liver disease. This condition is simply an expression of the kidney's production of an inappropriately alkaline urine, even in the presence of a large acid load and systemic acidosis. This reflects the limited ability of the cirrhotic kidney to make and excrete hydrogen ion. To compensate for this defect, there are increased losses of potassium into the urine and increased formation of ammonia. Thus, if hydrogen ions cannot be excreted, an acid load is excreted which is largely neutralized with sodium, potassium, or ammonium. Since sodium cannot be easily secreted, potassium is the predominant ion and losses of 150 mEq. per day have been observed. Ammonia for the urine is manufactured in the renal tubular cells from glutamate. Increased ammonia due to an acid pH and rapid flow is diffused into both urine and blood. In these patients approximately twice as much ammonia is delivered into the renal venous blood as into the urine, further increasing the load to be removed by the liver.

The hepatorenal syndrome is progressive oliguria and azotemia occurring without apparent cause in patients with liver disease. There is an abrupt increase in glomerular filtration resistance, with the maintenance of normal renal histology and over-all blood flow. There is shunting of blood from the glomeruli, the cause of which is unknown but is probably a hormone.

Studies of arteriography and of the washout curves of radioactive krypton indicate that glomerular flow to such kidneys is markedly reduced but that tubular and medullary flow is preserved. If the urine is carefully examined, its sediment is normal but the urine sodium content is extremely low (less than 5 mEq. per L.). If the kidney from such a patient who has died is transplanted into a normal recipient, it functions normally, indicating that it was the original environment that caused the malfunction.

Since there are oliguria and azotemia, the principal differential diagnosis is shock kidney or necrosis of the tubule epithelium. In the hepatorenal syndrome the amount of urinary sodium is less than 5 mEq. per L. and the ratio of urine to blood creatinine or urea is greater than 1:3 and usually greater than 1:15. In contrast, in the disease with renal tubular damage the urinary sodium is rarely less than 30 mEq. per L. and the ratio of urine to plasma creatinine or urea is 1:3 or less, indicating that there is little tubular function.

Endocrine Changes

The liver is not considered an endocrine organ, yet it plays a significant role in hormone metabolism, because most nonpeptides are biotransformed by the liver into an inactive form. Most non-peptide hormones are bound to a carrier protein in the plasma that limits the level of free hormone; the liver usually manufactures these carriers. These two functions may lead to increases in the circulating level of the free hormone which may persist longer than normal. If the production of the hormone is under careful feedback regulation (that is, the rate of release of hormone is also controlled by the tissue level of the hormone), this will have no effect. However, if this regulatory mechanism is insensitive, the hormone levels may be altered in liver disease.

Peptide hormones may be inactivated by the liver. Careful study of blood hormone levels in patients with liver cell disease often reveals many abnormalities.

Coagulation Difficulties

The release of coagulation protein was discussed earlier. The liver seems to be the principal organ responsible for the removal of activated coagulation factors from the plasma and for the removal of fibrinogen degradation released by the action of fibrinolysin or fibrin. The persistence of activated coagulation factors in the blood may account for consumptive coagulopathy. All aspects of coagulation may be affected; even platelet levels may be reduced owing to hypersplenism or consumptive coagulation. Additionally, platelets may be less active in contraction, owing to release of serotonin. Although the final pattern of abnormality in liver disease is not settled, it is apparent that many possible coagulation difficulties exist in the presence of liver disease.

REFERENCES

GENERAL

Popper, H., and Schaffner, F. (eds.): Progress in Liver Diseases, Vol. 1. Grune & Stratton, New York, 1961; Vol. 2, 1965; Vol. 3, 1970; Vol. 4, 1973; Vol. 5, 1976. In-depth monographs on a single topic.

Schiff, L. (Ed.): Diseases of the Liver, 4th ed. J. B. Lippincott Co., Philadelphia, 1975. A multiauthored, extremely accurate collection of monographs for details on all areas of liver disease.

Sherlock, S.: Diseases of the Liver and Biliary System, 5th ed. Blackwell Scientific Publications, Oxford, 1975. A text that makes clinical problems clear and accurate. Clear pictures and concise prose often make it the best source for further reading.

ANATOMY AND TESTING

Baum, S.: Hepatic Angiography. In Popper, H., and Schaffner, F. (Eds.): Progress in Liver Diseases, Vol. 3. Grune & Stratton, New York, 1970, p. 444.

Castell, D. O., O'Brien, K. D., Muench, H., and Chalmers, T. C.: Estimation of liver size by percussion in normal individuals. Ann. Intern. Med., 70:1183, 1969.

Eyler, W. R., Schuman, B. M., Du Sault, L. A., and Hinson, R. A.: Rose Bengal I[131] liver scan. J.A.M.A., 194 (No. 9):990, 1965.

McAfee, J. G., Ause, R. G., and Wager, H. N.: Diagnostic value of scintillation scanning of the liver. Arch. Intern. Med., 116:25, 1965.

Wagner, H. N., Jr., McAfee, J. G., and Mozley, J. M.: Diagnosis of liver disease by radioisotope scanning. Arch. Intern. Med., *107*:324, 1961.

BIOCHEMISTRY

Arias, I. M., Gartner, L. M., Cohen, M., Ben-Ezzer, J., and Levi, A. J.: Chronic nonhemolytic unconjugated hyperbilirubinemia with glycuronyl transferase deficiency. Evidence for genetic heterogeneity. Trans. Assoc. Am. Physicians, *81*:66, 1968.

Arias, I. M., and London, I. M.: Bilirubin glucuronide formation in vitro. Demonstration of a defect in Gilbert's disease. Science, *126*:563, 1957.

Bloomer, J. R., Berk, P. D., Howe, R B., and Berlin, N. I.: Interpretation of plasma bilirubin levels based on studies with radioactive bilirubin. J.A.M.A., *218*:216, 1971.

Bourke, E., Milne, M. D., and Stokes, G. S.: Mechanism of renal excretion of urobilinogen. Br. Med. J., *2*:1510, 1965.

Collins, J. R., and Crofford, O. B.: Glucose intolerance and insulin resistance in patients with liver disease. Arch. Intern. Med., *124*:142, 1969.

Combes, B., and Schenker, S.: Laboratory tests. *In* Schiff, L. (Ed.): Diseases of the Liver. 4th ed. J. B. Lippincott Co., Philadelphia, 1975, p. 204.

Fingl, E., and Woodbury, D. M.: *In* Goodman, L. S., and Gilman, A. (Eds.): The Pharmacological Basis of Therapeutics. The Macmillan Co., New York, 1970.

Grace, N. D., and Powell, L. W.: Iron storage disease and the liver. Gastroenterology, *67*:1257, 1974.

Gray, C. H., and Nicholson, D. C.: Recent developments in our knowledge of the urobilins. Medicine, *46*:83, 1967.

Hecker, R., and Sherlock, S.: Electrolyte and circulatory changes in terminal liver failure. Lancet, *2*:1121, 1956.

Levi, A. J., Gatmaitan, Z., and Arias, I. M.: Deficiency of hepatic organic anion binding protein as a possible cause of nonhemologic unconjugated hyperbilirubinemia in the newborn. Lancet, *2*:139, 1969.

Levi, A. J., Gatmaitan, Z., and Arias, I. M.: Two hepatic cytoplasmic protein fractions Y and Z and their possible role in hepatic uptake of bilirubin, sulphobromophthalein and other anions. J. Clin. Invest., *48*:2156, 1969.

McFadzean, A. J., and Yeung, R. T. T.: Further observations on hypoglycemia in hepatocellular carcinoma. Am. J. Med., *47*:220, 1969.

Odell, G. B., Ryan, W. B., and Richmond, M. D.: Exchange transfusion. Pediat. Clin. North Am., *9*:605, 1962.

Powell, L. W., Hemingway, E., Billing, B. H., and Sherlock, S.: Idiopathic unconjugated hyperbilirubinemia (Gilbert's syndrome). N. Engl. J. Med., *277*:1108, 1967.

Remmer, H.: Detoxification of drugs in the liver. *In* Popper, H., and Schaffner, F. (eds.): Progress in Liver Diseases, Vol. 2. Grune & Stratton, New York, 1965, p. 116.

Schoenfield, L. J.: Sulfobromophthalein transport and metabolism. Gastroenterology, *48*:530, 1965.

Summerskill, W. H. J.: Ammonia metabolism in the gastrointestinal tract. *In* Glass, B. J. (Ed.). Progress in Gastroenterology, Vol. 2. Grune & Stratton, New York, 1970.

BILE FORMATION, BILE FLOW, AND CHOLESTASIS

Carey, J. B., Jr.: Bile salts and hepatobiliary disease. *In* Schiff, L. (Ed.): Diseases of the Liver, 3rd ed. J. B. Lippincott Co., Philadelphia, 1969.

Coyne, M. J., and Schoenfield, L. J.: Gallstone Formation and Dissolution. *In* Popper, H., and Schaffner, F. (ed.): Progress in Liver Diseases, Vol. V. Grune & Stratton, 1976, New York, p. 622.

Danzinger, R. G., Hofmann, A. F., Schoenfield, L. J., and Thistle, J. L.: Dissolution of cholesterol gallstones by chenodesoxycholic acid. N. Engl. J. Med., *286*:1, 1972.

Gorbach, S. L.: Intestinal microflora. Gastroenterology, *60*:1110, 1971.

Hanson, R. F., and Pries, J. M.: Synthesis and enterohepatic circulation of bile salts. Gastroenterology, *73*:611, 1977.

Havel, R. J.: The abnormal lipoprotein of cholestasis. N. Engl. J. Med., *285*:578, 1971.

Javitt, N. B.: Symposium on bile salt. Am. J. Med., *51*:565, 1971.

Javitt, N. B.: Bile Acids and Hepatobiliary Disease. *In* Schiff, L. (ed.): Diseases of the Liver, 4th ed. J. B. Lippincott Co., Philadelphia, 1975, p. 111.

Kaplan, M. M., and Righalli, A.: Induction of rat liver alkaline phosphatase. Mechanism of serum elevation in duct obstruction. J. Clin. Invest., *49*:508, 1970.

Mistilis, S. P., and Lam, K. C.: Extrahepatic Biliary Obstruction. *In* Schiff, L. (ed.): Diseases of the Liver, 4th ed., J. B. Lippincott Co., Philadelphia, 1975, p. 1388.

Seidel, D.: The abnormal lipoprotein of cholestasis. N. Engl. J. Med., *285*:1538, 1971.

Small, D. M.: The Formation and Treatment of Gallstones. *In* Schiff, L. (ed.): Diseases of the Liver, 4th ed. J. B. Lippincott Co., Philadelphia, 1975, p. 146.

Strack, P. R., Newman, H. K., Lerner, A. G., Green, S. H., Meng, C., Del Guercio, L. R. M., and State, D.: Integrated procedure for rapid diagnosis of hepatobiliary disorders. N. Engl. J. Med., *285*:1225, 1971.

Thureborn, E.: Human hepatic bile. Composition changes due to altered enterohepatic circulation. Acta Chir. Scand. (Suppl.) *303*:1, 1962.

Wheeler, H. O.: Secretion of Bile. *In* Schiff, L. (ed.): Diseases of the Liver, 4th ed. J. B. Lippincott and Co., Philadelphia, 1975, p. 87.

HEPATIC BLOOD FLOW, PORTAL HYPERTENSION

Chiandussi, L.: Umbilical-portal catheterization in diagnosis of liver disease. *In* Popper, H., and Schaffner, F. (eds.): Progress in Liver Diseases, Vol. 3. Grune & Stratton, New York, 1970, p. 466.

Dumont, A. E., and Mulholland, J. H.: Hepatic lymph in cirrhosis. *In* Popper, H., and Schaffner, F. (eds.): Progress in Liver Diseases, Vol. 2. Grune & Stratton, New York, 1965, p. 427.

Kimber, C., Deller, D. J., Ibbotson, R. N., and Lander, H.: The mechanism of anemia in chronic liver disease. Q. J. Med. (new series), *34*:33, 1965.

Liebowitz, H. R.: Pathogenesis of ascites in cirrhosis of the liver. N. Y. State J. Med., I. *69*:1895; II. *69*:2012; July, 1969.

Reynolds, T. B.: Portal hypertension. *In* Schiff, L. (ed.): Diseases of the Liver. 4th ed. J. B. Lippincott Co., Philadelphia, 1975, p. 333.

Reynolds, T. B., and Redeker, A. G.: Hepatic hemodynamic and portal hypertension. *In* Popper, H., and Schaffner, F. (eds.): Progress in Liver Diseases, Vol. 2. Grune & Stratton, New York, 1965, p. 457.

LIVER FUNCTION TESTS

Discombe, G.: Flocculation tests. Lancet, *1*:1005, 1959.

Edmonson, H. A. and Schiff L.: Needle Biopsy of the Liver. *In* Schiff, L. (ed.): Diseases of the Liver, 4th ed. J. B. Lippincott Co., Philadelphia, 1975, p. 247.

Feizi, T.: Immunoglobulins in chronic liver disease. Gut, *9*:193, 1968.

Moore, T. L., Kupchik, H. Z., Marcon, N., and Zamchek, N.: Carcino-embryonic antigen assay in cancer of the colon and pancreas and other digestive tract disorders. Am. J. Dig. Dis., *16*:1, 1971.

Paronetto, F.: Immunologic aspects of liver diseases. *In* Popper, H., and Schaffner, F. (eds.): Progress in Liver Diseases, Vol. 3. Grune & Stratton, New York, 1970, p. 299.

Rachmilewitz, N., Stein, Y., Aronovitch, J., and Grossowicz, N.: The clinical significance of serum cyanocobalamine in liver disease. Arch. Intern. Med., *102*:1118, 1958.

Ratnoff, O. D.: Disordered hemostasis in hepatic disease. *In* Schiff, L. (Ed.): Diseases of the Liver, 3rd ed. J. B. Lippincott Co., Philadelphia, 1969, p. 147.

Smith, J. B., and O'Neill, R. T.: Alphafetoprotein occurrence in germinal cell and liver malignancies. Am. J. Med., *41*:767, 1971.

Stolbach, L., Krant, M. J., and Fishman, W.: Ectopic production of an alkaline phosphatase isoenzyme in patients with cancer. N. Engl. J. Med., *281*:757, October, 1969.

Wright, R., McCollum, R. W., and Klatskin, G.: Australia antigen in acute and chronic liver disease. Lancet, *2*:117, 1969.

Zieve, L., Hill, E., Hanson, M., Falcone, A. B., and Watson, C. J.: Normal and abnormal variations and clinical significance of the one minute and total serum bilirubin determinations J. Lab. Clin. Med., *38*:446, 1951.

CLINICAL LIVER DISEASE

Davidson, C. S., and Gabuzda, G. J.: Hepatic coma. *In* Schiff, L. (Ed.): Diseases of the Liver. 4th ed. Philadelphia, J. B. Lippincott Co., 1975, p. 466.

Leevy, C., et al.: Liver Disease of the Alcoholic: Role of Immunologic Abnormality in Pathogenesis, Recognition, and Treatment. *In* Popper, H., and Schaffner, F. (eds.): Progress in Liver Diseases, Vol. V. Grune & Stratton, New York, 1976, p. 516.

Losowsky, M. D., Jones, D. P., Lieber, C. S., and Davidson, C. S.: Local factors in ascites formation during sodium retention in cirrhosis. N. Engl. J. Med., *268*:651, 1963.

Mistilis, S. P.: Chronic Active Hepatitis. *In* Schiff, L. (ed.): Diseases of the Liver, 4th ed., J. B. Lippincott Co., Philadelphia, 1975, p. 787.

Rake, M. O., Panneli, G., Flute, P. T., and Williams, R.: Intravascular coagulation in acute hepatic necrosis. Lancet, *1*:533, 1970.

Shear, L., Cheng, S., and Gabuzda, G. J.: Compartmentalization of ascites and edema in patients with hepatic cirrhosis. N. Engl. J. Med., *282*:1391, 1970.

Zuckerman, A.: Hepatitis B: Nature of the Virus and Prospects for Vaccine Development. *In* Popper, H., and Schaffner, F. (eds.): Progress in Liver Disease, Vol. V. Grune & Stratton, New York, 1976, p. 326.

EFFECT OF LIVER DISEASE ON OTHER ORGANS

Abelmann, W. H., Kramer, G. E., Verstraete, J. M., Gravallese, M. A., Jr., and McNeely, W. F.: Cirrhosis of the liver and decreased arterial oxygen saturation. Arch. Intern. Med., *108*:34, 1961.

Baldus, W. P., and Summerskill, W. H. J.: Liver-Kidney Interrelationships. *In* Schiff, L. (ed.): Diseases of the Liver, 4th ed. J. B. Lippincott Co., Philadelphia, 1975, p. 445.

Baldus, W. P., Summerskill, W. H. J., Hunt, J. C., and Maher, F. T.: Renal circulation in cirrhosis. Observations based on catheterization of the renal vein. J. Clin. Invest., *43*:1090, 1964.

Fischer, J. E., and Baldessarini, R. J.: Pathogenesis and Therapy of Hepatic Coma. *In* Popper, H., and Schaffner, F. (eds.): Progress in Liver Diseases, Vol. V. Grune & Stratton, New York, 1976, p. 363.

Maddrey, W. C., Sen Gupta, K. P., Basu Mallick, K. C., Iber, F. L., and Basu, A. K.: Extrahepatic obstruction of the portal venous system. Surg. Gynecol. Obstet., *127*:989, 1968.

Murray, J. F., Dawson, A. M., and Sherlock, S.: Circulatory changes in chronic liver disease. Am. J. Med., *24*:358, 1958.

Ratnoff, O. D.: Disordered Hemostasis in Hepatic Disease. *In* Schiff, L. (ed.): Diseases of the Liver, 4th ed. J. B. Lippincott Co., Philadelphia, 1975, p. 184.

Schenker, S., Breen, K. J., and Hoyumpa, A. M.: Hepatic encephalopathy: current status. Gastroenterology, *66*:121, 1974.

Shear, L., Bonkowsky, H. L., and Gabuzda, G. J.: Renal tubular acidosis in cirrhosis. A determinant of susceptibility to recurrent hepatic precoma. N. Engl. J. Med., *280*:1, 1969.

Shorr, E.: *In* Liver Injury. Transactions of the Sixth Conference. Edited by F. W. H. Offbauer. Sponsored by Josiah Macy, Jr., Foundation, 1947, p. 33.

Summerskill, W. H. J.: Hepatic failure and the kidney. Gastroenterology, *51*:94, 1966.

Summerskill, W. H. J., and Baldus, W. P.: Ascites. *In* Schiff, L. (ed.): Diseases of the Liver, 4th ed. J. B. Lippincott Co., Philadelphia, 1975, p. 424.

Walls, W. D., and Losowsky, M. S.: The hemostatic effort of liver disease. Gastroenterology, *60*:108, 1971.

29

Pathophysiology of Gallbladder Disease

ROBERT J. BOLT, M.D.

NORMAL STRUCTURE

The gallbladder is a pear-shaped distensible organ with an average length of 10 cm. and a width of 3 to 5 cm. It is attached to the inferior surface of the liver, occupying a position between the right and quadrate lobes. It is joined to the rest of the biliary tree by the cystic duct at the point where the common hepatic duct becomes the common bile duct. The common bile duct enters the second portion of the duodenum. In this region there is a neuromuscular sphincter, the sphincter of Oddi. The body of the gallbladder is normally in contact with both the duodenum and colon. Its impression on the duodenum often can be seen by the radiologist during barium contrast examinations. Its position is variable and the tip may be below the level of the iliac crest, especially when the patient is erect. An inflamed gallbladder can thus be mistaken for an inflamed appendix. The mucosa of the gallbladder consists of an epithelial layer of tall columnar cells overlying a lamina propria. It is thrown into multiple irregular folds that increase its absorptive area. A fibromuscular layer lies deep to the mucosa and is surrounded by a subserous adventitia and a serosa continuous with the serosa of the liver.

The cystic artery arises from the right hepatic artery and passes posterior to the common bile duct before dividing into superior and inferior branches which supply the gallbladder and cystic duct. The venous drainage begins in capillary plexuses which drain into superficial veins on the surface of the liver and then directly into the liver.

The gallbladder has an extensive lymphatic network which communicates with lymphatic channels draining the adjacent liver. These join the lymphatics of the cystic duct and the proximal portions of the extrahepatic duct system and drain into the nodes at the porta hepatis.

The biliary tree is innervated by both the sympathetic and parasympathetic systems. Preganglionic sympathetic fibers are derived from the seventh to the tenth thoracic segments and postganglionic fibers chiefly from the celiac ganglia. The hepatic division of the anterior vagal trunk supplies parasympathetic preganglionic fibers which synapse with postganglionic fibers in the gallbladder wall. Afferent fibers course with the splanchnic nerve as the right phrenic nerve; the latter relationship explains the occurrence of right shoulder pain in some patients with gallbladder disease. Parasympathetic stimulation causes gallbladder contraction.

NORMAL FUNCTION

Although the gallbladder concentrates and stores bile, the physiologic importance of this function is unknown. Hepatic bile (prior to entry into the gallbladder) has a specific gravity of 1.008 and a pH of 5.9 to 8.6 (usually 8 to 8.6). It is an isosmotic solution containing approximately 97 per cent water. Its solids consist largely of cholesterol, bile salts, phospholipids (especially lecithin), mucin, conjugated bilirubin, and electrolytes. The major electrolytes are sodium, potassium, chloride, and bicarbonate. Bile also contains significant amounts of calcium as well as many enzymes and drug metabolites (Table 29–1).

TABLE 29-1

Composition of Normal Hepatic Bile

pH	5.7–8.6
Bile salts	30–50 mM.
Phospholipids	10–15 mM.
Cholesterol	2–4 mM.
Bilirubin	0.25–1.25 mM.
Electrolytes	Na^+, K^+, Ca^{++}, Mg^{++}, Fe^{++}, Cl^-, HCO_3^-, PO_4^-, $SO_4^=$

Organic anions, drugs, hormones, etc.
H_2O–97%

Concentration of Major Electrolytes

	mEq/L.
Sodium	145–165
Potassium	2.7–4.9
Calcium	2.5–4.8
Magnesium	1.4–3.0
Chloride	88–115
Bicarbonate	27–55

In adults, the liver secretes 250 to 1500 ml. (average 700 ml.) of bile per day. Bile is secreted continuously, but its flow (choleresis) is augmented after meals. The volume of bile secreted is determined largely by the amount of bile salts synthesized within the liver. This in turn depends on the integrity of their enterohepatic circulation. Conjugated bile salts are secreted by the hepatocytes, providing an osmotic driving force for the movement of water into bile. As bile flows through the biliary tree its volume increases because of the act of secretion by the biliary epithelium of an electrolyte solution rich in bicarbonate.

Choleresis is under the control of neural and humoral mechanisms. It is increased by vagal stimulation and the action of secretin, cholecystokinin-pancreozymin (CCK-PZ), gastrin, and glucagon. Other choleretic agents include exogenously administered bile salts, acetylsalicylic acid, cincophen, pilocarpine, acetylcholine, choline, insulin, and histamine. Most of these agents cause an increase in hepatic bile output and contraction of the gallbladder. Vagal stimulation and CCK-PZ also cause relaxation of the sphincter of Oddi.

The gallbladder is a reservoir and concentrates hepatic bile four- to tenfold by absorbing electrolytes and water. This concentrating mechanism proceeds rapidly and helps to prevent large increases of pressure within the system. The bile salts, bile pigments, lecithin, and cholesterol, to which the gallbladder wall is essentially impermeable, become highly concentrated. Under fasting conditions, the gallbladder is relaxed and may contain 50 to 60 ml. of bile. During this time the sphincter of Oddi is closed.

A knowledge of bile salt metabolism is important for two reasons. Bile salts are necessary for micellar solubilization in the absorption of dietary lipids and also to maintain biliary cholesterol in solution. The latter function is important to an understanding of cholesterol gallstone formation.

In man, two "primary" bile acids, cholic (trihydroxy) and chenodeoxycholic (dihydroxy), are synthesized in the liver from cholesterol and conjugated with glycine and, to a lesser extent, with taurine. They then form salts with sodium and potassium. Most of the primary bile salts reaching the gut are absorbed; a relatively small amount throughout the small intestine by nonionic diffusion, but most importantly by an active transport process in the terminal ileum. Bile salts not absorbed enter the colon, where bacterial enzymes deconjugate and dehydroxylate them to form the "secondary" bile acids. Thus, deoxycholic (dihydroxy) is derived from cholic acid and lithocholic (monohydroxy) from chenodeoxycholic acid. Deoxycholic acid is absorbed, reconjugated in the liver, and secreted into bile. Lithocholic acid is poorly absorbed and only minute quantities normally appear in bile.

Bile therefore contains sodium or potassium salts of six different conjugated bile acids. Cholic and chenodeoxycholic acids account for 80 per cent of the total bile salt pool, with deoxycholic making up most of the remaining 20 per cent. This pool contains approximately 4 to 5 gm. of bile salts and has a half-life of three to five days. It is recirculated six to ten times each day, and the daily hepatic synthesis of new bile acids accounts for about 10 per cent of the total pool. This is roughly equivalent to the amount lost in the feces (200 to 500 mg. daily).

DISEASES

CHOLELITHIASIS/CHOLECYSTITIS

Prevalence

In 1959, Wilbur and Bolt presented figures indicating that 14.6 per cent of "normal Caucasian men" with an average age of 46.8 years had evidence of gallbladder abnormalities, past or present. Previous reports based on autopsy evidence had placed the incidence in this age group at somewhat lower figures. However, it is now generally accepted that approximately 10 to 15 per cent of adults residing in the United States do indeed have cholelithiasis. If one were to accept previous studies that indicated that at least 50 per cent of patients harboring gallstones are asymptomatic, then the true prevalence could be estimated on the basis of the clinical prevalence as reported in the Framingham study. Thus, there must be approximately 20 million or more individuals carrying gallstones in the United States. Approximately 800,000 new cases develop each year, and half of these ultimately will have surgery. Small states that gallstone disease accounts for 5000 to 8000 deaths per year and that the total cost of morbidity from this disease approaches one billion dollars.

Recent studies of population surveys reveal interesting trends and patterns of gallstone disease prevalence with geographic locations and race. Sampliner's startling epidemiologic survey of Pima Indians showed that 70 per cent of females over the age of 30 and males over 55 harbored gallstones. Subsequent surveys have shown that native American Indians of other tribes have a similarly high prevalence of gallstones. Inhabitants of Sweden approach these astounding figures, with 57 per cent incidence in females and 32 per cent incidence in males over the age of 20. This compares with an incidence of under 5 per cent in Japan. The incidence in England and Wales is only slightly lower than that quoted for the United States: 6.2 per cent in males and 12.1 per cent in females aged 45 to 69. These figures are based on routine cholecystograms obtained on 1442 inhabitants. It is obvious that gallstones assume importance both medically and financially throughout the world and reach epidemic proportions in certain populations.

PATHOPHYSIOLOGY

Types of Stones

In discussing gallstones, one should clearly differentiate the bilirubin line from the cholesterol line. Not only is the basic pathophysiology different in these two groups, but clinical manifestations, including prognosis and management, are different. This statement should be modified by the clause that bilirubinate stones on the one hand, and cholesterol stones on the other, are rarely, if ever, pure pigment or pure cholesterol. There are multiple variations in percentage composition embracing the entire spectrum from almost pure pigment to almost pure cholesterol. In the United States, approximately three fourths of patients with gallstones will prove to have cholesterol as the primary component and approximately one fourth have been shown to be of the pigment type. Table 29–2 demonstrates the primary points of difference between the bilirubin line and the cholesterol line of stones.

Calcium bilirubinate stones are a dark reddish-brown, are fragile, and their surface areas are quite irregular. The cut surface is amorphous, and stones are frequently formed within the biliary tree as well as within the gallbladder. As a result, residual stones as well as recurrent stone formation is more common with the bilirubinate line than with the cholesterol line of gallstones. It has become increasingly important to differentiate these two types in view of newer methods for medical dissolution of the cholesterol line. It has been suggested that this differentiation can be made on the basis of radiolucency or radiopacity of the stone on plain films of the abdomen. Unfortunately this differentiation is far from precise, and Trotman has demonstrated that although 86 per cent of radiolucent stones were found to be of the cholesterol line, 14 per cent were of the pigment line. On the contrary, 67 per cent of radiopaque stones were found to be primarily of the pigment line and 33 per cent of the cholesterol. Radiopacity is related to calcium content, and bilirubinate stones generally contain more calcium than do cholesterol stones. Bilirubinate stones are found more commonly in Asian countries than in the United States or in European countries. In addition, they are associated with specific diseases — particularly hemolytic anemias (sickle cell, thalassemia major, congenital spherocytosis) and are seen in infants with severe erythroblastosis fetalis. Of interest is the report of an apparent increase in pigment stones following insertion of prosthetic mitral valves. Gallbladders containing stones removed from patients with alcoholic cirrhosis have been reported to be primarily of the bilirubin line. Sex and age differences are also noted in that the average age for clinical presentation of pigmentary stones is in the 50s and the average age for cholesterol stones is in the 40s. Males are as commonly af-

TABLE 29–2 TYPES OF GALLSTONES

	Pigment Line	Cholesterol Line
Distribution	Asia	Europe, United States
Appearance	Jagged edge	Smooth surface
Color	Dark reddish-brown	Light
Formation	Intraductal	Intragallbladder
Post cholecystectomy	May recur	Seldom recur
Associated disease	Hemolytic states	See text
	Cirrhosis	
	Parasitic infestation	

flicted with pigment stones as females, in contrast to cholesterol stones in which there is a predominance of females.

Pigment Stones. Maki undoubtedly has been the most authoritative investigator into the pathogenesis of calcium bilirubinate stones. Table 29–3 summarizes the factors involved in bilirubin precipitation in bile.

In stone formation of either type, the initial step is precipitation of a substance that is normally soluble in bile. Maki has postulated that β-glucuronidase, perhaps of bacterial origin, hydrolyzes bilirubin glucuronide to free bilirubin and glucuronic acid. Calcium, a normal constituent of bile, combines with the carboxyl radical of liberated bilirubin to form calcium bilirubinate. The excess unconjugated bilirubin forms column-like complexes which precipitate to form calculi that are opaque radiographically. This postulate is supported by studies which show that bile infected with *E. coli* do indeed exhibit intense β-glucuronidase activity in vitro and the addition of commercially prepared β-glucuronidase to normal bile results in precipitates similar to those of infected bile. Maki further postulates that the cause of cholangiohepatitis in southeast Asia is not *E. coli* reaching the liver by the portal vein but an "ascending infection" possibly with duodenitis. Hypo- or achlorhydria "common in Japan" may facilitate bacterial growth in the duodenum and result in ascending infection of the biliary system, thus accounting for the high incidence of both pigmentary stones and cholangiohepatitis in these population groups.

Maki's proposals have received further support as the result of studies by Boonyapisit and others at the University of Pennsylvania. Their data revealed that normal human gallbladder bile does indeed contain low concentrations of unconjugated bilirubin and no evidence of detectable hydrolysis of conjugated bilirubin. Further, they demonstrated that an abnormally increased concentration of unconjugated bilirubin in gallbladder bile is associated with formation of pigment calculi. Moreover, lithogenic biles with elevated concentrations of unconjugated bilirubin also exhibited abnormal hydrolysis of conjugated bilirubin. However, hydrolysis was unrelated to the presence of bacteria. This would support previous studies indicating that the gallbladder bile surrounding pigment gallstones is usually sterile. They suggest that β-glucuronidases produced by the gallbladder epithelium or secreted into bile by the liver may be the basic cause. An alternative explanation is that the inhibitor glucaro-1-4-lactone, normally present in bile, may be decreased, allowing the small amount of β-glucuronidase present to act. It has been shown that oral administration of glucaric acid inhibits β-glucuronidase activity. Once calcium bilirubin is precipitated in the form of bilirubin crystals, further aggregation, concretion, etc. occur, resulting in the formation of stones. Although this stage is poorly understood, work by Sutor suggests that inhibitors of crystal growth play a role in radiopaque stone aggregation and stone formation.

Cholesterol Line. Cholesterol is normally maintained in clear solution by a remarkably precise control of the relative proportions of bile acids – phospholipids (lecithin) – cholesterol. Cholesterol is relatively insoluble in a solution of bile salts alone, but its solubility is greatly increased in the presence of appropriate concentrations of both bile acid and lecithin, at which point micelle formation occurs. The development of "critical micelle concentration" was elegantly summarized by Hofmann and Small in 1967. Subsequently, the method for presenting the three major components of bile on triangular coordinates has been widely accepted (Figure 29–1).

When the percent molar concentrations are determined in vitro and when counter ion concentrations, pH, temperature, biliary solid content, etc., are maintained under standard conditions,

TABLE 29–3   BILIRUBIN STONE FORMATION

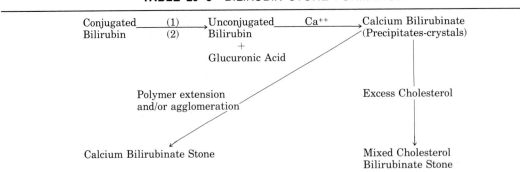

(1). β-Glucuronidase
(2). Glucaro-1,4-lactone

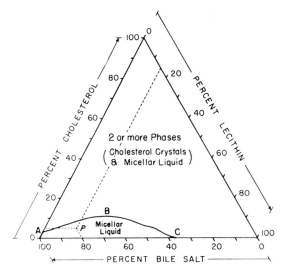

Figure 29–1 Method for presenting the three major components of bile (bile salts, lecithin, and cholesterol) on triangular coordinates. Each component expressed as percentage mole of total bile salt, lecithin, and cholesterol. Line ABC represents the maximum solubility of cholesterol and varying mixtures of bile salt and lecithin. Point represents bile composition containing 5% cholesterol, 15% lecithin, and 80% bile salt and falls within the zone of the single phase of micellar lipid. Expressed in other terms, the line ABC represents the metastable limit for cholesterol. (From Redinger, R. N. and Small, D. M., Arch. Int. Med. *130*:618, 1972. Reprinted by permission.)

TABLE 29–4 BILE ACID SYNTHESIS AND METABOLISM

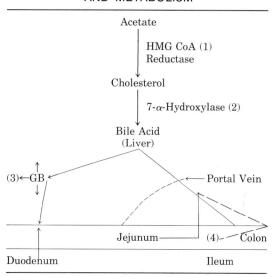

(1) Hydroxymethylglutaryl CoA reductase – rate limiting enzyme in cholesterol synthesis. Increase = lithogenicity.

(2) Rate limiting enzyme in conversion of cholesterol to bile acid. Decrease = lithogenicity.

(3) Gallbladder mucosa inflammation = increased bile acid absorption = lithogenicity.

(4) Malabsorption = bile acid loss = lithogenicity.

plotting the determinations in the triangle by lines parallel to sides of the triangle will differentiate bile that is supersaturated from bile in which cholesterol is fully solubilized. Supersaturated or lithogenic bile would be represented by all intercepts outside the ABC line. Metzger and co-workers have proposed the use of a simple calculation, expressed as the lithogenic index, to denote the degree of saturation. Regardless of the manner of expression, the first step in cholesterol stone formation involves a change in bile acid/lecithin/cholesterol ratios sufficient to exceed the capability of bile to solubilize cholesterol. Thus, factors causing a decrease in total bile acid (quantitative or qualitative), a decrease in phospholipid concentration, or an increase in relative concentration of cholesterol will favor stone formation. Similarly, factors tending to increase the total pool of bile acids and phospholipids or tending to decrease the cholesterol in bile will favor dissolution of stones.

Bile Acids. Alteration of bile acid metabolism at any one of several points as indicated in the numbers on Table 29–4 could result in formation of lithogenic bile. Factors enhancing HMG CoA reductase activity or depressing 7-α-hydroxylase

activity would favor supersaturation of bile with cholesterol (lithogenic bile). Depression of 7-α-hydroxylase activity or enhancement of HMG CoA reductase has been reported in patients with cholesterol stones. Enterohepatic cycling of bile acid has been described earlier in this chapter. The following situations interfering with this cycle might be expected to reduce the effective total bile acid pool and thus lead to lithogenicity.

1. Impaired intestinal absorption from any cause.
2. Administration of bile acid-binding drugs such as cholestyramine.
3. Ileal inflammation or bypass surgery (since the majority of bile acids are actively absorbed in the terminal ileum).
4. Bacterial overgrowth in the proximal small bowel resulting in qualitative ineffectiveness.
5. Marked reduction of enterohepatic cycling, as in fasting.

During fasting the impaired enterohepatic cycling may itself result in greater inhibition of bile acid synthesis relative to cholesterol. Thus, Redinger and co-workers have suggested that, for several weeks following surgery, bile acid synthesis is decreased leading to supersaturation with cholesterol. Finally it should be remembered that gallbladder mucosa is virtually impermeable to conjugated bile acids, bilirubin, cholesterol, and cholecystographic contrast media. However, any interference with the integrity of the gallbladder mucosa could result in absorption of bile acids in amounts inappropriate to cholesterol, leading to supersaturation.

Cholesterol.   Cholesterol synthesis and metabolism is depicted in Table 29–5.

The rate limiting enzyme is, as previously stated, β-hydroxy- β-methyl, glutaryl CoA reductase (HMG CoA reductase). Factors stimulating HMG CoA reductase activity increase endogenous cholesterol synthesis. This endogenous cholesterol is believed to be the primary source for both cholic and chenodeoxycholic acid formation. To what degree endogenous (synthesized) and exogenous (dietary) cholesterol is compartmentalized (i.e., contributes primarily to bile acid formation) is excreted unchanged in bile or is transported in plasma to peripheral tissues deserves further investigation.

Phospholipids.   The precise role of phospholipid metabolism in the alteration of non-lithogenic to lithogenic bile is unclear. The relative proportions of lecithin in bile of patients with cholesterol stones has been reported as normal. Moreover, direct measurements of phospholipid secretion in patients with cholesterol stones have failed to detect significant abnormalities. Thus, the role of altered phospholipid metabolism in production of bile lithogenicity appears to be, at best, minimal.

Gallbladder.   Elsewhere in this chapter, it is pointed out that cholesterol stones, in contrast to bilirubin (pigment) stones, form almost exclu-

sively within the gallbladder. Moreover, recurrent cholesterol stones following cholecystectomy are the exception rather than the rule. On this basis, it would seem logical to conclude that gallbladder function or dysfunction might play a major role in promoting lithogenicity by one or more methods:

1. Inappropriate absorption of bile acids as compared to cholesterol. This alternative may be operative in an uncommon situation such as vascular insufficiency of the gallbladder associated with periarteritis nodosa or other instances of non-calculous cholecystitis. Certainly this factor does not appear to play a role in most situations.

2. Support of nucleation and growth as a result of stagnation.

3. Secretion of a substance inducing the liver to increase its synthesis of cholesterol and/or decrease synthesis of bile acid.

Several investigators have confirmed the finding that bile secreted by the liver in patients with gallstones is already supersaturated with cholesterol. Whether cholecystectomy corrects this, as claimed by Shaffer and co-workers, or whether hepatic secretion of a supersaturated bile continues as suggested by McDougall's and Kimball's groups, remains controversial. Perhaps more than one factor is involved. That is, secretion of supersaturated bile by the liver aided by stagnation in the gallbladder whereby crystallization and growth of gallstones would more readily occur.

There are certain clinical situations favoring lithogenicity. Both depression of bile acid synthesis and/or increased secretion of cholesterol in

TABLE 29–5   CHOLESTEROL METABOLISM

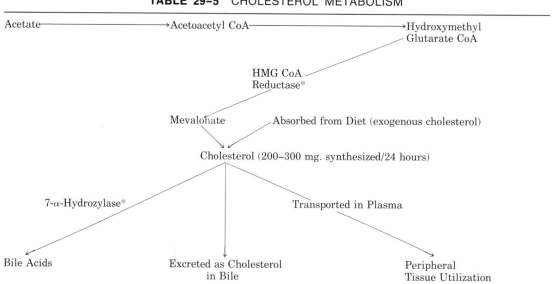

*Rate limiting enzymes

bile appear to play a role in the following situations:

1. Heredity (70 per cent lithogenic bile in Pima Indians, 0 per cent lithogenic bile in Masai).
2. Increasing age.
3. Obesity. It should be noted that during fasting the bile tends to become more lithogenic. However, after weight reduction, the bile has been demonstrated to again become non-lithogenic.
4. Increased cholesterol intake in the diet.
5. Pregnancy, oral contraceptives, and postmenopausal estrogen therapy.
6. Clofibrate therapy.

Literature concerning the effect of a polyunsaturated fat diet is confusing. In at least one retrospective study, the suggestion is made that there is an increased prevalence of stones in men on long-term polyunsaturated fat diets. This finding is not, as yet, confirmed by other studies. Finally, the increased prevalence of stones in patients with cirrhosis is apparently due to an increase in the number of pigment stones and is not related to cholesterol metabolism.

Dissolution

Much of the knowledge regarding stone formation has resulted from the discovery that administration of chenodeoxycholic acid will dissolve cholesterol stones. The concept of dissolving stones by medical means has been entertained ever since 1896, when Naunyn first demonstrated that gallstones dissolved when placed in dog bile. Substances used in attempts to dissolve gallstones include lecithin plant sterols, medium chain glycerides, phenobarbital, Zanchol, Bilron, wheat bran, and chenodeoxycholic acid. Of these substances, chenodeoxycholic acid has been the most promising. Table 29–6 summarizes these results. It should be emphasized that use of this bile acid poses potential problems:

1. Although it has been demonstrated to alter bile constituents so that super saturated is converted to unsaturated bile (lithogenic to non-lithogenic), this acid does not correct the basic defect underlying formation of supersaturated bile by the liver. Hence, it must be continued, in all probability, for the lifetime of the patient.
2. Its breakdown to lithocholic acid may cause liver damage. Indeed this has been reported to occur in baboons.
3. Its use during pregnancy (when bile tends to become supersaturated) may be dangerous to the fetus since it has been shown that chenodeoxycholic acid can cross the placental barrier.

Because studies in experimental animals suggested hepatotoxicity, clinical trials have been discontinued in Britain.

NEOPLASMS

Tumors of the gallbladder are rare. Most adenocarcinomas that do appear are solitary, hard, fibrous masses in the wall of the gallbladder.

TABLE 29–6

Investigator	Number of Patients	Agent and Dose (daily)	Length of Study (mos.)	Number with Stones Unchanged	Number (%) Reduced	Number (%) Dissolved
Danzinger	7	CDCA* 0.75–4.5 gm.	6–22	3(43)	3(43)	1(14)
Bell	12	CDCA 0.75–1.5 gm.	6	6(50)	3(25)	3(25)
Thistle	18	CDCA 18 mg./kg.	6	7(39)	11(61)	0
	17	Cholic 18 mg./kg.	6	17(100)	—	—
	18	Placebo	6	18(100)	—	—
Dowling	26	CDCA 0.75–1.0 gm.	6	11(42)	4(15)	11(42)
Coyne	10	CDCA 9 mg./kg.	12	6(60)	4(40)	—
	8	Phenobarb 1.5 mg./kg.	12	8(100)	—	—
	8	Placebo	12	8(100)	—	—
Iser	25	CDCA 0.25–12.5 gm.	6–42	9(36)	6(24)	10(40)
Tompkins	7	Commercial Soy Bean Lecithin 48 gm./daily	24	7(100)	—	—

*Chenodeoxycholic acid.

They spread by direct extension to the liver and by the lymphatics to cystic and periportal lymph nodes. They practically always develop in a gallbladder which contains stones. Their incidence is so low that this possibility is not an indication for prophylactic cholecystectomy in a patient with otherwise asymptomatic stones. The prognosis is poor (in large part because of late diagnosis), and survival is rare despite any form of therapy. Cholesterolosis and adenomyomatosis may be confused with benign or malignant polypoid lesions of the gallbladder. Most patients with either cholesterolosis or adenomyomatosis are asymptomatic. However, in the presence of symptoms compatible with biliary colic, surgical intervention is indicated in selected instances.

SCLEROSING CHOLANGITIS

Primary sclerosing cholangitis is a rare disease of unknown cause. It is frequently associated with ulcerative colitis or other chronic inflammatory bowel disease. It may simulate a very slowly growing bile duct carcinoma and is difficult to distinguish from other extrahepatic causes of biliary obstruction. Only the chronicity of the process militates against a diagnosis of neoplasm. Clinically, it manifests itself as a progressively obstructive jaundice, and the usual differential diagnostic procedures are necessary. If a localized sclerosis is found, resection and/or bypass procedures may be possible. Some have recommended the use of corticosteroids and broad-spectrum antimicrobial agents, but results have been unpredictable. As with carcinoma of the biliary tree, the prognosis is poor, and death generally occurs within a few years after the appearance of symptoms.

CONGENITAL LESIONS

Congenital lesions of the gallbladder involving variations in size, shape, and location are of little or no clinical significance. The only clinically significant congenital lesions are those which involve the bile ducts themselves, including partial absence or atresia of one or both of the hepatic ducts or common bile ducts. Depending on the degree of absence or atresia, jaundice usually is noted after the first week of life and is progressive. Surgical exploration and correction must be carried out relatively early, but the condition is amenable to relief in only about 15 per cent of patients.

CLINICAL EVALUATION

The gallbladder is studied primarily by the use of radiopaque substances given orally, intravenously or, in selected patients, by percutaneous transhepatic injection of the bile ducts or retrograde cannulation of the common bile duct under endoscopic control. The latter two techniques are used when there is need to visualize the biliary duct system in the presence of jaundice.

The drugs presently used are all substituted triiodobenzoic acid compounds. Those excreted by the liver and used to evaluate the gallbladder are of high molecular weight and have at least one side chain at the five position of the benzene ring. They are moderately lipid-soluble and, when absorbed from the duodenum or administered intravenously, become tightly bound to plasma albumin and are transported to the liver. Within the liver, they are conjugated with glucuronic acid, rendering them water soluble, and then excreted into the biliary tree. When given orally, they are administered 12 hours before the radiographs are taken and fatty foods are prohibited to prevent emptying of the gallbladder. The gallbladder mucosa is normally impermeable to the drug, absorption does not occur, and thus visualization of the gallbladder is made possible.

There are four reasons for nonvisualization of the gallbladder by oral cystography:

1. The patient did not take the tablets; the tablets were vomited; or the drug was not absorbed.
2. The material was absorbed but could not be excreted owing to liver disease or obstruction of the biliary tree.
3. The drug was absorbed and excreted but the gallbladder was inflamed and absorption through the gallbladder wall occurred.
4. The cystic duct was blocked and the drug could not enter the gallbladder.

It must be emphasized that if, for any reason, the liver is unable to excrete bilirubin it also will be unable to excrete contrast material. Thus, it is seldom worth attempting an oral examination when the serum bilirubin is above 2 mg. per 100 ml. Complications of oral cholecystography include bowel irritation and, rarely, reaction to the drug itself.

Intravenous cholangiography presents the liver with a large amount of drug in a shorter period of time. It is rapidly excreted by the liver, filling the gallbladder and biliary ducts; therefore the entire extrahepatic biliary tree can be visualized, especially when tomography is utilized. Since the gallbladder need not concentrate the drug, it will visualize even when its wall is damaged by inflammation. Cholangiography carries some risk; hepatic damage and acute renal failure due to tubular necrosis have been reported. Less serious reactions consist of nausea, vomiting, and a fall in blood pressure. Slow injection reduces the chances of such complications.

The failure of either oral or intravenous cholangiography to visualize the gallbladder in the preence of jaundice, occasionally poor intestinal absorption of oral contrast agents, and occasional reactions to intravenous injection have stimulated a search for alternative methods for visualizing the gallbladder and biliary duct system. Recently the use of technetium-99m pyridoxylidene glutamate (99m-Tc-PG) has been advocated. This is a new radiopharmaceutical that is taken up by hepatocytes and rapidly excreted into the bile canaliculi entering the gallbladder through the cystic duct. The concentration of 99m-Tc-PG in the bile is sufficient to allow satisfactory imaging of the biliary tree and gallbladder. Satisfactory images of the biliary tract can be obtained using small doses (2 to 5 m Ci). Under normal conditions this radioactive drug reaches the liver in approximately five minutes and the gallbladder in 10 to 20 minutes. Confirmed nonvisualization by any of the preceding means, in the presence of symptoms suggestive of gallbladder disease indicates abnormality in over 90 per cent of patients. No figures are available as to the incidence of gallbladder disease in asymptomatic persons with nonvisualization.

In the presence of jaundice, percutaneous transhepatic or retrograde cholangiography must be carried out. Evaluation can be further refined by performing duodenal drainage or ultrasound study or both. Duodenal contents are aspirated with or without stimulation of gallbladder contraction by CCK-PZ and examined for cholesterol crystals and/or calcium bilirubinate granules. The gallbladder and gallstone can be accurately demonstrated by ultrasound. No preparation is needed except for a fat-free diet for some hours (an empty gallbladder cannot be located). Stones of any size can be demonstrated with about the same accuracy as by radiography, and the greatest value of the technique therefore is in the jaundiced patient in whom nonvisualization would be expected by oral or intravenous cholecystography.

MANAGEMENT

It must be remembered that for every patient presenting with an acute episode of cholecystitis/cholelithiasis there are one and possibly two patients whose gallbladders contain stones but who have no symptoms whatever. Thus, the average practitioner is dealing only with the "tip of the iceberg" when he is faced with the management of an individual patient suffering an acute episode of gallbladder disease. Moreover, this group of patients may present symptoms at any point on a severity spectrum — from very mild, right upper quadrant distress without fever and with minimal tenderness, to severe, excruciating right upper quadrant pain accompa-

nied by diaphoresis and shock. Chills, rigor, and fever frequently accompany this latter syndrome. Therefore, treatment must be individualized. Management of patients presenting with an acute episode is surgical, but controversy exists whether operative treatment should be immediate or delayed. The great frequency of remission with conservative treatment suggests that surgery can be delayed until the patient is in the best possible state of health. Exceptions to this rule are made when the patient presents with a complication such as bile peritonitis or ascending cholangitis with septicemia. Routine medical management of an acute episode consists of the following:

1. Use of analgesics for relief of pain.
2. Attempts to decrease the rate of enterohepatic cycling by removing gallbladder and pancreatic stimuli. This involves intermittent suction and nothing by mouth.
3. Careful intravenous rehydration and electrolyte repletion.

Early relief of pain is desirable, and parenteral morphine sulfate (15 mg.) continues to be an effective drug. Some have recommended the use of sublingual glyceryl trinitrate (0.5 mg.) to reduce the spasmogenic effect of morphine. Other synthetic drugs such as meperidine (50 mg.), believed by many to have less spasmogenic effects, may be substituted for morphine. The use of local heat to the abdomen in addition to the above measures, often is helpful.

Patients in the early state have variable degrees of inflammatory change in the gallbladder. The importance of bacterial rather than chemical inflammatory change in the gallbladder wall is impossible for the clinician to measure. Fever and leukocytosis are, at best, crude indices of bacterial inflammation and may be quite misleading, particularly in the aged. In view of this, antibiotic coverage should not be routine, but should be individualized.

Fluid replacement during the period of nasogastric suction is essential. In most situations alkalosis is relatively mild, and acidifying agents are rarely necessary. Sufficient fluid must be given to rehydrate the patient and keep up with both urinary and insensible water loss. Discretion must be used in fluid replacement particularly in older individuals. Certainly a hypertonic glucose solution and physiologic saline will form the basis for replacement therapy. Calcium, sodium, potassium, and other electrolytes should be replaced as indicated by serum electrolyte values. The vast majority of patients will demonstrate gradual improvement under the above regimen permitting the removal of the nasogastric tube after approximately 48 hours and initiation of feeding by mouth. Repeated use of morphine sulfate and/or sublingual glyceryl trinitrate should be unnecessary.

As soon as removal of the nasogastric tube is indicated the patient may be started on clear liquids for the first few meals. Following this, progression to a low fat diet, containing no more than 20 gm. of fat, relatively high carbohydrate levels, and of average protein content may be instituted. If the diagnosis of cholelithiasis and/or cholecystitis is firm, cholecystectomy should be advised. Certainly if rapid and complete recovery has occurred, and the patient is in acceptable condition, cholecystectomy may be carried out any time during the two weeks following the initial attack. If, however, the patient is markedly overweight or other surgical contraindications exist, the patient should be discharged and continued on a low-fat, low-cholesterol diet, with cholecystectomy planned at the time optimal conditions exist.

Continued treatment is required for those patients in whom symptoms persist or progress after 48 hours of therapy. Nasogastric suction and intravenous fluid should be continued. If progression is marked by onset of fever or leukocytosis, or both, antibiotic therapy should be started. Multiple choices exist, but one should choose a drug not only effective against a wide spectrum of bacteria, but specifically effective against coliform organisms. Ampicillin (1 gm.) intravenously every six hours, or tetracycline (250 mg.) intravenously every six hours, may be used. Some have recommended doxycycline; others have preferred to use a combination of penicillin and gentamicin. If progression is marked by increasing episodes of biliary colic, chills, and fever, emergency cholecystectomy may be necessary between 48 and 72 hours. A small percentage of patients under treatment may progress and/or may develop a complication. Complications include the following:

1. Pancreatitis.
2. Empyema.
3. Emphysematous cholecystitis.
4. Fistula Formation (gallbladder-bowel).
5. Ascending cholangitis.
6. Perforation, abscess, peritonitis.
7. Common duct obstruction.

Pancreatitis rarely has its onset while treatment is being carried out. However, this possibility should be entertained whenever a patient develops increasing abdominal pain despite treatment. It becomes more obvious if the location of the pain changes from the right upper quadrant or epigastric region to the back. Serum amylase and lipase determinations should be obtained in these patients to verify the diagnosis. The use of morphine sulfate can cause elevation of these enzymes and may be misleading. Failure

to respond to the above outlined treatment may require emergency exploration.

Empyema of the gallbladder most often occurs in the older age group. Symptoms in this group may be inconspicuous and the diagnosis difficult. If the development of empyema is recognized, institution of intravenous penicillin G (20 million units daily) as well as gentamicin is indicated. Emergency cholecystectomy is indicated.

A rare patient will manifest continued symptoms, and plain films of the abdomen may reveal collections of gas, either in the wall or within the gallbladder itself. With the patient in the erect position, a fluid level may be seen in the gallbladder. This is diagnostic of acute gaseous (emphysematous) cholecystitis. Colon bacilli, some forms of streptococci, and clostridia are the chief bacterial infections producing sufficient gas to be seen on x-ray examination. Again, emergency cholecystectomy is indicated.

An equally serious circumstance occurs when a patient suddenly develops spiking fever, chills, and rigor. This is usually associated with increasing jaundice, elevation of alkaline phosphatase, and leukocytosis. This triad of leukocytosis, increasing jaundice, and chills is strongly suggestive of ascending cholangitis. A shocklike state may ensue. Blood cultures must be obtained since antibiotic therapy should be instituted and may be modified, depending on results of the blood cultures. Shock accompanying ascending cholangitis is distressing. When this occurs steroids should be instituted in high doses. Dexamethasone-21-phosphate in doses of 20 to 40 mg. intravenously and 4 to 20 mg. every four to six hours are recommended. The mortality rate is excessively high. Metaraminol or levarterenol bitartrate may be necessary to maintain blood pressure.

Rupture or perforation of the gallbladder is extremely rare when the patient is under treatment for an acute episode of cholecystitis. However, when it does occur, bile salts released in the abdominal cavity irritate the peritoneum. The result is an outpouring of fluid and in some instances hypovolemic shock. Bile is a good culture medium, gram-negative and clostridia organisms are commonly found. The patient must be prepared for immediate surgery, and fluid loss into the peritoneal cavity may require replacement of as much as 2 to 8 L. within a brief period. Electrolyte loss is usually uniform, so an imbalance is unusual. It is recommended that plasma and whole blood, as well as intravenous saline and glucose be used. Antibiotics, nasogastric suction, narcotics, vasopressors, and steroids must be used as indicated. The prognosis is worse in those patients over 50 years of age, but the mortality rate is significant at any age.

Common duct obstruction can occur initially or

any time during the course of an attack of cholecystitis. Its occurrence is a straightforward indication for surgical intervention.

Discussion thus far has concerned treatment of acute cholecystitis or acute episodes of chronic cholecystitis/cholelithiasis. When the diagnosis of chronic cholecystitis is unequivocal the treatment of choice remains surgical. Conservative treatment is reserved for the debilitated and aged or for patients with associated conditions definitely contraindicating operation. Moreover, a few patients refusing surgery will require long term treatment. In this group of patients one of the stone dissolving substances previously discussed can be tried. It should be reemphasized that medical dissolution should be attempted only in those patients with cholesterol stones and is ineffective for pigment or bilirubin stones. Concomitant measures have been recommended regardless of the type of stones present. The degree of efficacy of these concomitant measures remains unproved. However, it seems reasonable that the diet should be low in fat with protein and carbohydrate dependent on the caloric requirements of the individual. Reduction diets are frequently necessary. Overeating at any one meal should be avoided. Protein supplements in the form of skim milk powder, 120 gm. in 1,000 ml. of skim milk taken in amounts of 120 to 240 ml. with and between meals is often a helpful supplement in the older age patient. Hydrocholeretic drugs such as Zanchol have been recommended.

As previously noted, this has been shown to have an effect on altering bile composition toward the non-lithogenic side. Evaluation of the effectiveness of drugs of this type on symptoms is difficult owing to the unpredictability of the disease process. Zanchol (Florantyrone) is a gamma-oxy-gamma-(8-fluoranthene) butyric acid. It is supplied in tablets of 250 mg. and can be given before each meal. Unfortunately side-effects of this drug include the very symptoms for which the drug is being used: that is, nausea, vomiting, and diarrhea. Moreover, changes in liver profile have been reported. Taking these factors into consideration, the use of hydrocholeretic drugs of this type cannot be strongly recommended. Finally, an anticholinergic sedative combination such as Donnatol or Butibel may be prescribed before each meal. On occasion pharmacologic side-effects such as sleepiness, tiredness, blurring of vision, or difficulty on urination may occur. Used in the usual dosage of one tablet before each meal, these side-effects are mild. An occasional hypersensitivity reaction may be seen. This is manifested primarily as a mild dermatitis medicamentosa.

To summarize, the treatment of proved acute or chronic cholecystitis continues to be surgical. Medical attempts at control of symptoms and/or dissolution of cholesterol gallstones, if present, should be reserved for those patients in whom surgery is strongly contraindicated or refused by the patient.

REFERENCES

Bainton, B., Davies, G. T., Evans, K. T., and Gravelle, I. H.: Gallbladder disease: prevalence in a South Wales industrial town. N. Engl. J. Med., 294:1147–1149, 1976.

Balint, J. A., Beeler, D. A., Kyriakides, E. C., and Treble, D. H.: The effect of bile salts upon lecithin synthesis. J. Lab. Clin. Med., 77:122–133, 1971.

Bell, C. C., Vlahcevic, Z. R., and Swell, L.: Alterations in the lipids of human hepatic bile after the oral administration of bile salts. Surg. Gynecol. Obstet., 132:36–42, 1971.

Bell, G. D., Whitney, B., and Dowling, R. H.: Gallstone dissolution in man using chenodeoxycholic acid. Lancet, 2:1213–1219, 1972.

Bennion, L. J., and Grundy, S. M.: Effects of obesity and caloric intake on biliary lipid metabolism in man. J. Clin. Invest. 56:996–1011, 1975.

Biss, K., Ho, K. J., Mikkelson, B., Lewis, L., and Taylor, C. B.: Some unique biologic characteristics of the Masai of East Africa. N. Engl. J. Med., 284:694–700, 1971.

Boonyapisit, S. T., Trotman, B. W., and Ostrow, J. D.: Unconjugated bilirubin and the hydrolysis of conjugated bilirubin in gallbladder bile of patients with cholelithiasis. Gastroenterology, 74(1):70–74, 1978.

Boston Collaborative Drug Surveillance Program: Oral contraceptives and venous thromboembolic disease, surgically confirmed gallbladder disease and breast tumors. Lancet, 1:1399–1404, 1973.

Boston Collaborative Drug Surveillance Program: Surgically confirmed gallbladder disease, venous thromboembolisms, and breast tumors in relation to postmenopausal estrogen therapy. N. Engl. J. Med., 290:15–19, 1974.

Comfort, M. W., Gray, H. K., and Wilson, J. M.: The silent gallstone: ten to twenty year followup study of 112 cases. Ann. Surg., 128:931–937, 1948.

Cooper, J., Geizerova, H., and Oliver, M. F.: Clofibrate and gallstones. Lancet, 1:1083, 1975.

Coyne, M. J., Bonorris, G. G., Chung, A., Goldstein, L. I., Lahana, D., and Schoenfield, L. J.: Treatment of gallstones with chenodeoxycholic acid and phenobarbital. N. Engl. J. Med., 292:604–607, 1975.

Coyne, M. J., Bonorris, G. G., Goldstein, L. I., and Schoenfield, L. J.: Effect of chenodeoxycholic acid and phenobarbital on the rate-limiting enzymes of hepatic cholesterol and bile acid synthesis in patients with gallstones. J. Lab. Clin. Med., 87:281–291, 1976.

Danzinger, R. G., Hofmann, A. F., Schoenfield, L. J., and Thistle, J. L.: Dissolution of cholesterol gallstones by chenodeoxycholic acid. N. Engl. J. Med., 286:1–8, 1972.

Danzinger, R. G., Hofmann, A. F., Thistle, J. L., and Schoenfield, L. J.: Effect of oral chenodeoxycholic acid on bile acid kinetics and biliary lipid composition in women with cholelithiasis. J. Clin. Invest., 52:2809–2821, 1973.

DenBesten, L., Conner, W. E., and Bell, S.: The effect of dietary cholesterol on the composition of human bile. Surgery, 73:266–273, 1973.

Dowling, R. H.: Chenodeoxycholic acid. The British experience. Hosp. Prac., 9(12):85–93, 1974.

Friedman, K. K., Kannel, W. B., and Dawler, T. R.: Epidemiology of gallbladder disease: observations in the Framingham study. J. Chron. Dis., 19:273–292, 1966.

Gerdes, M. M., and Boyden, E. A.: The rate of emptying of the human gallbladder in pregnancy. Surg. Gynecol. Obstet., 66:145–156, 1938.

Goswitz, J. T.: Bacteria and biliary tract disease. Am. J. Surg., 128:644–646, 1974.

Grundy, S. M., Duane, W. C., Adler, R. D., Aron, J. M., and Metzger, A. L.: Biliary lipid outputs in young women with cholesterol gallstones. Metabolism, 23:67–74, 1974.

Grundy, S. M., Metzger, A. L., and Adler, R. D.: Mechanisms of lithogenic bile formation in American Indian women with cholesterol gallstones. J. Clin. Invest., 51:3026–3043, 1972.

Herman, A. H., Redinger, R. N., and Small, D. M.: The effects of surgery on bile secretion and composition. Surg. Forum, 22:378–380, 1971.

Heywood, R., Palmer, A. K., Foll, C. V., and Lee, M. R.: Pathological changes in fetal Rhesus monkey induced by oral chenodeoxycholic acid. Lancet, 2:1021, 1973.

Hofmann, A., and Small, D. M.: Detergent properties of bile salts. Correlation with physiological function. Ann. Rev. Med., 18:333–376, 1967.

Iser, J. H., Dowling, R. H., Mok, H. Y. I., and Bell, G. D.: Chenodeoxycholic acid treatment of gallstones. A follow-up report and analysis of factors influencing response to therapy. N. Engl. J. Med., 293:378–383, 1975.

Kerner, M., Raicht, R. F., Mosbach, E. H., and Zimmon, D. S.: Zanchol, a potential litholytic agent in man. Gastroenterology, 69:836, 1975.

Kimball, A., Pertsemlidis, D., and Panveliwalla, D.: Composition of biliary lipids and kinetics of bile acids after cholecystectomy in man. Am. J. Dig. Dis., 21:776–781, 1976.

Lewis, R., and Gorbach, S.: Modification of bile acids by intestinal bacteria. Arch. Int. Med., 130:545–549, 1972.

Lieber, M. M.: Incidence of gallstones and their correlation with other diseases. Ann. Surg., 135:394, 1952.

Ludlow, A. I.: Autopsy incidence of cholelithiasis based on records of Institute of Pathology, Western Reserve University and University Hospital. Am. J. Med. Sci., 193:481, 1937.

Mabee, T. M., Meyer, P., DenBesten, L., and Mason, E. E.: The mechanism of increased gallstone formation in obese human subjects. Surgery, 79:460–468, 1976.

Maki, T.: Pathogenesis of calcium bilirubinate gallstones: Role of E. coli, β-glucuronidase and coagulation by inorganic ions, polyelectrolytes and agitation. Ann. Surg., 164:90, 1966.

Matolo, N.: Gallbladder and biliary tract scanning with ^{99m}Tc–PG. West. J. Med., 126:386–387, 1977.

McDougall, R. M., Walker, K., and Thurston, O. G.: Prolonged secretion of lithogenic bile after cholecystectomy. Ann. Surg., 182:150–153, 1975.

McSherry, C. K., Morrissey, K. P., Swarm, R. L., May, P. S., Niemann, W. H., and Glenn, F.: Chenodeoxycholic acid induced liver injury in pregnant and neonatal baboons. Ann. Surg., 184:490–499, 1976.

Merendino, K. A. and Manhas, D. R.: Man-made gallstones: a new entity following cardiac valve replacement. Ann. Surg., 177:694–704, 1973.

Metzger, A. L., Heymsfield, S., and Grundy, S. M.: The lithogenic index — a numerical expression for the relative lithogenicity of bile. Gastroenterology, 62:499–500, 1972.

Miettinen, T. A.: Cholesterol production in obesity. Circulation, 44:842–850, 1971.

Nakayama, F., and van der Linden, W.: Bile composition. Sweden versus Japan. Its possible significance in the difference in gallstone incidence. Am. J. Surg., 122:8–12, 1971.

Naunyn, B.: A Treatise on Cholelithiasis. (Translated by A. E. Garrod.) The New Syndenham Society, London, 1896, p. 22.

Nicholas, P., Rinaudo, P. A., and Conn, H. O.: Increased incidence of cholelithiasis in Laennec's cirrhosis. Gastroenterology, 63:112–121, 1972.

Nicolau, G., Shefer, S., Calen, G., and Mosbach, E. H.: Determination of hepatic cholesterol 7α-hydroxylase activity in man. J. Lipid Res., 15:146–151, 1974.

Nicolau, G., Shefer, S., Galen, G., and Mosbach, E. H.: Determination of 3-hydroxy-3-methylglutaryl CoA reductase. J. Lipid Res., 15:94–98, 1974.

Nicolau, G., Shefer, S., Galen, G., and Mosbach, E. H.: Hepatic

3-hydroxy-3-methylglutaryl CoA (HMG CoA) reductase and cholesterol 7α-hydroxylase in man. Gastroenterology, 64:887, 1973 (Abstract).

Northfield, T. C., and Hofmann, A. F.: Biliary lipid output during three meals and an overnight fast. I. Relationship to bile acid pool size and cholesterol saturation of bile in gallstone and control subjects. Gut, 16:1–17, 1975.

Pertsemlidis, D., Panveliwalla, A., and Ahrens, E. H.: Effects of clofibrate and of an estrogen-progestin combination on fasting biliary lipids and cholic acid kinetics in man. Gastroenterology, 66:565–573, 1974.

Pomare, E. W., Low-Beer, T. S., and Heaton, K. W.: The Effect of Wheat-Bran on Bile Salt Metabolism and Bile Composition. In: Advances in Bile Acid Research. F. K. Schattauer Verlag, Stuttgart, New York, 1974, pp. 355–360.

Redinger, R. N., Herman, A. R., and Small, D. M.: The effects of surgery on hepatic physiology in the primate. Gastroenterology, 60:795, 1971 (Abstract).

Rosenak, B. D., and Kohlstaedt, K. S.: Bile salt therapy in liver and gallbladder disease. Am. J. Dig. Dis. & Nutrition, 3:577–580, 1936.

Sampliner, R. E., Bennett, P. H., Comess, L. J., Rose, F. A., and Burch, T. A.: Gallbladder disease in Pima Indians. N. Engl. J. Med., 283:1358–1364, 1970.

Schreibman, P. H., Pertsemlidis, D., Liu, G. C. K., and Ahrens, E. H.: Lithogenic bile, a consequence of weight reduction. J. Clin. Invest., 53:72a, 1974 (Abstract).

Schwartz, C. C., Vlahcevic, Z. R., Halloran, L. G., Gregory, D. H., Meek, J. B., and Swell, L.: Evidence for the existence of definitive hepatic cholesterol precursor compartments for bile acids and biliary cholesterol in man. Gastroenterology 69:1379–1382, 1975.

Scott, G. W., Smallwood, R. E., and Rowlands, S.: Flow through the bile duct after cholecystectomy. Surg. Gynecol. Obstet., 140(1):912–918, 1975.

Shaffer, E. A., Braasch, J. W., and Small, D. M.: The influence of cholecystectomy and obesity on biliary lipid secretion in cholesterol gallstone disease. Gastroenterology, 70:A–78/936, 1976.

Small, D. M.: Gallstones 1971. Viewpoints on Dig. Dis., 3:3, 1971.

Sturdevant, R. A. L., Pearce, M. L., and Dayton, S.: Increased prevalence of cholelithiasis in man ingesting a serum-cholesterol-lowering diet. N. Engl. J. Med., 288:24–27, 1973.

Sutor, D. J., and Percival, J. M.: Presence or absence of inhibitors of crystal growth in bile. I. Effect of bile on the formation of calcium phosphate, a constituent of gallstones. Gut, 17:506–510, 1976.

Sutor, D. J., and Wooley, S. E.: The nature and incidence of gallstones containing calcium. Gut, 14:215–220, 1973.

Swell, L., Bell, C. C., and Vlahcevic, Z. R.: Relationship of bile acid pool size to biliary lipid excretion and the formation of lithogenic bile in man. Gastroenterology, 61:716–722, 1971.

Tangedahl, T. N., Matseshi, J. W., Thistle, J. L., and Hofmann, A. F.: Plant sterols increase effectiveness of chenodeoxycholic acid therapy in lowering cholesterol saturation of fasting state bile in patients with radiolucent gallstones. Gastroenterology, 72:2, 1977 (Abstract).

The Coronary Drug Project: Clofibrate and niacin in coronary heart disease. J.A.M.A., 231:360–381, 1975.

Thistle, J. L., Carlson, G. L., Hofmann, A. F., and Babayan, V. K.: Medium chain glycerides rapidly dissolve cholesterol gallstones in vitro. Gastroenterology, 72:2, 1977 (Abstract).

Thistle, J. L., Eckhart, K. L., Nensel, R. E., Nobrega, F. T., Poehling, G. G., Reimer, M., and Schoenfield, L. J.: Prevalence of gallbladder disease among Chippewa Indians. Mayo Clinic Proc., 46:603–608, 1971.

Thistle, J. L., and Hofmann, A. F.: Efficacy and specificity of chenodeoxycholic acid therapy for dissolving gallstones. N. Engl. J. Med., 289:655–659, 1973.

Tompkins, R. K.: The systemic treatment of gallstones. Adv. Surg., 10:87–98, 1976.

Trotman, B. W., and Soloway, R. D.: Pigment vs. cholesterol

cholelithiasis: clinical and epidemiological aspects. Am. J. Dig. Dis., *20*:735–740, 1975.

Trotman, B. W., Soloway, R. D., Sanchez, H. M., Morris, T. A., and Miller W. T.: Evaluation of radiographic lucency or opaqueness of gallstones as a means of identifying cholesterol or pigment stones. Gastroenterology, *68*:1563–1566, 1975.

Wenckert, A., and Robertson, B.: The natural course of gall-stone disease. Eleven-year review of 781 nonoperated cases. Gastroenterology, *50*(3):376–381, 1966.

Wilbur, R. S., and Bolt, R. J.: Incidence of gallbladder disease in "normal" men. Gastroenterology, *36*:251–255, 1959.

Winch, J., Burnett, W., Banks, M., and Cranvitch, B.: Factors concerned in the pathogenesis of gallstones. Gut, *10*:954–955, 1969 (Abstract).

Yamaguchi, I., Sato, T., Sato, H., and Matsushiro, T.: Quantitative determination of D-glucaric acid in bile in relation to the inhibitory effect upon bacterial B glucuronidase. Tokyo J. Exp. Med., *87*:123–132, 1965.

30

Pathophysiology of the Pancreas

P. J. SNODGRASS, M.D.

INTRODUCTION

The key to understanding the pathophysiology of diseases of the human pancreas is a knowledge of its biochemistry and physiology. The mechanism of injury in acute pancreatitis is generally agreed to be *autodigestion* which depends on factors that activate or inhibit within the gland the enzymes normally secreted into pancreatic juice. Diagnosis of diseases like acute pancreatitis, chronic pancreatitis, and cancer of the pancreas depends on study of these enzyme activities in serum, urine, or pancreatic juice and their responses to physiologic stimulants. Treatment of pancreatic disease also depends on knowledge of how enzymes can damage tissue and of the results of enzyme deficiency in the gut. More than in almost any other organ, diseases of the pancreas are manifestations of disordered physiology and biochemistry.

ENZYMES OF THE HUMAN PANCREAS

Electrophoretic studies on human pancreatic juice indicate that at least 18 different proteins can be detected. Table 30–1 reviews the composition of human pancreatic juice. The key to the activation of the pancreatic zymogens is *enterokinase,* a proteolytic enzyme found in the mucosa of the duodenum, both bound to the brush border and also present in the soluble fraction of the duodenal mucosa cells. The enzyme is released into the lumen of the duodenum by a number of stimuli, such as the polypeptide hor-

mones cholecystokinin, secretin, gastin, and glucagon, and by bile salts as well. As shown in Table 30–1, enterokinase converts both trypsinogens of human pancreatic juice to *trypsins 1 and 2.* Enterokinase cleaves the lysine-isoleucine bond of residues 6 and 7 of bovine trypsinogen, splitting off the N-terminal activation peptide and allowing the generation of active trypsin. Enterokinase does this much better than trypsin can autocatalytically generate itself because it binds trypsinogen six times stronger and produces trypsin 2000 times faster than trypsin acts on trypsinogen. Enterokinase recognizes the N-terminal sequence of trypsinogen and is tailored to act specifically on trypsinogen. However, it cannot activate chymotrypsinogen or other zymogens. Calcium stabilizes the trypsin molecule at alkaline pH and retards its autodigestion by trypsin and other proteases. Another reason for the effectiveness of enterokinase in the activation process is that it is not inhibited by the trypsin inhibitor of human pancreatic juice. Enterokinase synthesis may be induced by feeding trypsinogen to a mutant mouse (CBA/Jepi) which lacks pancreatic acinar cells. The essential nature of enterokinase is best demonstrated by congenital enterokinase deficiency, in which children afflicted with this disease develop severe protein maldigestion because they are not able to activate zymogens and thus digest proteins

Trypsin rapidly activates chymotrypsinogen to *chymotrypsins,* proelastases to *elastases,* procarboxypeptidase to *carboxypeptidases,* and prophospholipase A to *phospholipase A.* In human pancreatic juice, two separate trypsinogens have been identified, and each gives rise to a separate

928

TABLE 30–1 ENZYMES IN HUMAN PANCREATIC JUICE

Zymogen	Enzyme*	Activator	Co-Factors, Stabilizers	Substrates, Products, Bonds Cleaved
	(PROTEOLYTIC)			
Trypsinogen-1	Trypsin-1 (cationic)	Enterokinase Trypsin	Ca^{++}	Internal peptide bonds of protein whose carbonyl group is contributed by arg or lys
Trypsinogen-2	Trypsin-2 (anionic)	Enterokinase	Ca^{++}	Same as Trypsin-1
Chymotrypsinogen	Chymotrypsin-1 Chymotrypsin-2	Trypsin	Ca^{++}	Internal peptide bonds of proteins whose carbonyl group is from try, phe, tyr, leu, met
Proelastase-1	Elastase-1 (cationic)	Trypsin		Internal bonds of elastin or other proteins formed from neutral amino acids, esp. ala
Proelastase-2	Elastase-2 (anionic)	Trypsin		Same as Elastase-1 but digests proteins better than elastin
Procarboxypeptidase A	Carboxypeptidase A	Trypsin	Zn	All C-terminal amino acids except arg and lys or penultimate pro
Procarboxypeptidase B	Carboxypeptidase B	Trypsin	Zn	C-terminal arg, lys
	(LIPOLYTIC)			
	Lipase (Glycerol ester hydrolase;) (Bile salt-inhibited lipase)		Co-lipase Ca^{++} Emulsifying agents, any interface	Primary ester bonds of water-insoluble, aggregated carboxylic esters (triglyceride → fatty acids + 2-monoglyceride)
	⌈ Non-specific lipase ⌉ ⌊ Bile salt-dependent lipase ⌋		Bile salts	Water-insoluble carboxyl esters of primary and secondary alcohols in micellar solution (Vitamin A palmitate → Vit A alcohol + palmitic acid)
	Cholesterol esterase (Sterol ester hydrolase)		Trihydroxy-bile salts	Esters of sterol ring with β-OH on 3 position, in micellar solution
Prophospholipase A_2	Phospholipase A_2	Trypsin	Bile salts Ca^{++}	Fatty acid ester bond at 2-position of 1,2 diacylphosphoglyceride (lecithin → fatty acid + 1-lysolecithin)
	(OTHER)			
	α-Amylase (α-1,4 glucan-4-glucanohydrolase)		Cl^- Ca^{++}	Endoamylase, cleaves α-1,4 bonds of polyglucosides (starch) to maltose, maltotriose and limit dextrins; exists at 6 isoenzymes
	Ribonuclease		Phosphate Citrate	Endonuclease, cleaves ribonucleic acid adjacent to cytidine nucleotide phosphodiester bonds to produce oligonucleotides
	Deoxyribonuclease I		Mg^{++} plus Ca^{++} or Mn^{++}	Endonuclease, splits between purine and phosphate of pyrimidine nucleotide; specificity controlled by divalent cations. Products are oligonucleotides
	(INHIBITORS) Pancreatic secretory trypsin inhibitor			Inhibits trypsin incompletely and reversibly as 1:1 complex (Kazal-type)

*The enzymes in brackets [ ] have not been identified or characterized in human pancreatic juice, only in the juice of the cow or pig.

trypsin: one which is cationic in its electrophoretic migration and one which is anionic. The anionic protein is much less stable than the cationic, even in the presence of calcium. Chymotrypsinogen is usually seen as one band, giving rise to two chymotrypsins. Elastolytic activity resides in two different proteins in human pancreatic juice. The first one, proelastase 1, is classic elastase, which works primarily on the internal bonds of elastin and of other proteins. Another enzyme, called proelastase II or protease E, splits elastin poorly and digests protein well. The two carboxypeptidases which act upon different C-terminal amino acids are both zinc metalloenzymes and contain one mole of firmly-bound zinc per mole of enzyme; the zinc is essential for catalytic activity. There is no good evidence for a true collagenase in human pancreatic juice.

From the point of view of digestion of calorically important foods, the key lipolytic enzyme is *lipase,* also called glycerol ester hydrolase. This enzyme acts by splitting the primary (alpha) ester bonds of water-insoluble, emulsified carboxylic esters, particularly esters of glycerol. Thus, triglyceride is cleaved to yield fatty acids from the two alpha positions, leaving the 2-(beta) monoglyceride. Lipase functions by binding the hydrophobic side of the molecule to particles of triglyceride, which are water-insoluble. The activity is a direct function of the particle size: the more interface available for the enzyme to bind, the faster the activity. Emulsifying agents for water-insoluble substrates are therefore essential for this enzyme activity. These emulsifying agents exist in the duodenum but their exact nature has not been defined. Bile salts are often said to be the duodenal emulsifying agents, but bile salts, rather than being activators of lipase at the critical micellar concentration found in the duodenum, are actually inhibitors. Bile salts shift the pH optimum of lipase from 8–9 to 6–7, the pH found in the duodenum. Evolution has resulted in the development of a small molecular weight protein of about 10,000 molecular weight called *co-lipase,* which is secreted in pancreatic juice, forms a 1:1 complex with lipase, protects it against inhibition by bile salts, and also protects lipase against denaturation when it is spread out on an interfacial surface. Calcium ions are also essential for lipase activity in the presence of bile salts and allow the enzyme to bind to water-insoluble substrates.

Another lipase exists in mammalian pancreatic juice, but it has not been purified or carefully studied in man. It requires bile salts for activity, and acts upon water-insoluble carboxylesters of primary and secondary alcohols in micellar solution. An example of the enzyme activity of this *non-specific lipase-esterase* is the splitting of vitamin A esters to vitamin A alcohol and fatty acids. The third important lipolytic enzyme in

human pancreatic juice is *cholesterol esterase* or *sterol ester hydrolase.* This enzyme requires as a cofactor trihydroxy-bile salts such as taurocholic acid. Although it can split other esters, it is the only one of the lipolytic enzymes which can cleave esters of cholesterol. This enzyme is crucial in cholesterol absorption because ingested cholesterol is in the form of cholesterol esters which cannnot be absorbed by man unless they are first cleaved to free cholesterol and then taken up out of micellar solution.

The next lipolytic enzyme is the only one known to exist as a proenzyme — *phospholipase A_2*. It cleaves fatty acids from the 2 position of a phospholipid such as lecithin, giving rise to a fatty acid and lysolecithin. Its zymogen is activated by trypsin, which cleaves off an N-terminal activation peptide to yield the active enzyme, which is activated by bile salts and stablized by calcium.

The only enzyme in human pancreatic juice able to digest polysaccharides is *amylase*, which cleaves the α-1,4 bonds of polymers of glucose, such as starch. It is activated by chloride ions and contains one firmly bound mole of calcium per mole of enzyme, which is essential for activity. It produces the disaccharide, maltose, a trisaccharide, maltotriose, and a core of starch resistant to amylase, called a limit dextrin. Pancreatic amylase is the product of a gene located on human chromosome 1 and is closely linked to a locus on the same chromosome which produces the amylase found in salivary glands and many other human tissues. The most purified form of human pancreatic amylase had six bands on electrophoresis. These result from two families of amylases, with or without glycosyl groups. The families are further modified by loss of amide groups. Salivary amylase also exists as 6 to 8 isoenzymes, but the pancreatic and salivary isoenzyme families can be distinguished by electrophoresis or electrofocusing techniques.

Ribonuclease requires phosphate or citrate for activation and cleaves internal bonds of a ribonucleic acid molecule adjacent to cytidine to produce oligonucleotides. *Deoxyribonuclease I* is also an endonuclease and it splits the phosphate diester bond joining the purine and pyrimidine nucleotide. The exact bonds on double-stranded or single-stranded DNA which it cleaves are controlled to a great extent by the binding of divalent cations. Thus, its activity differs whether magnesium or manganese is bound, and its activity is markedly increased when calcium is bound along with magnesium.

Lastly, a significant part of the protein content of human pancreatic juice is a low molecular weight pancreatic secretory trypsin inhibitor. This small molecule binds strongly to both cationic and anionic human trypsins and inhibits their activity. However, it does not completely inhibit trypsin, even when present in excess, and the inhibition is reversible, owing to digestion of the inhibitor by bound trypsin plus calcium ions. It does not inhibit enterokinase and cannot prevent the rapid release of excess trypsin, which reverses any inhibition in the intestinal lumen. Within the pancreatic cells and ducts, however, it acts as a major protective mechanism against inappropriate activation of trypsinogen molecules. There are actually 2–4 variants of this inhibitor in human juice.

The pancreatic proteolytic enzymes represent a great danger to the organism should they be activated within the substance of the pancreas. Evidence accumulated over many years indicates that acute pancreatitis results from activation of these zymogens within the pancreas and that the disease is due to autodigestion. Different protective mechanisms have evolved to prevent such a catastrophe. The first is that the proteolytic enzymes are synthesized as zymogens and require activation before they can carry out their functions. Although all but one of the lipolytic enzymes are made as active enzymes, not zymogens, they cannot act upon the lipid membranes of the pancreatic cell unless bile salts are present or unless the lipids are presented to them in an emulsified or micellar form.

Another protective mechanism is that these enzymes are not freely dispersed within the cell cytoplasm but are always contained within lipoprotein membranes. Attached to the N-terminus of each enzyme is a hydrophobic signal peptide which somehow attaches the nascent protein and ribosome to the membrane of the endoplasmic reticulum. The proteins are secreted into the lumen where these signal peptides are removed and the proenzymes assume their tertiary structures. They migrate to the Golgi region of the cell, where they are invested in a membrane, glycosidic groups added to some, and condense as zymogen granules, which accumulate at the apex of the cell. Upon proper stimulation, the membrane of the zymogen granule fuses with the apical cell membrane of the acinar cell of the pancreas, and the enzymes are secreted into the lumen.

In addition to the secretory trypsin inhibitor in pancreatic juice, there are proteolytic enzyme inhibitors in many body fluids and tissues which probably play a role in protecting against the uncontrolled activity of these pancreatic enzymes within the gland or when the enzymes gain access to the blood stream and lymphatics (Table 30–2). In species other than primates, such as the cow, there is present in the acinar cell (but not in the juice) a trypsin inhibitor (Kunitz type) which is a very potent inhibitor of trypsin, chymotrypsin, kallikrein, plasmin, and thrombin. The human pancreas does not have this trypsin inhibitor. In the cow this trypsin inhibitor has been found in salivary gland, lung, and liver. If man is found not to have this protein in his tissues, he lacks an important safety factor which protects against protease injury.

Circulating in the plasma of man are a number of protease inhibitors which are effective in inhibiting the activity of any pancreatic protease which might inadvertently gain entrance to the plasma or extracellular fluids. Alpha-1-antitrypsin is a glycoprotein molecule of 120,000 molecular weight which very potently inhibits both cationic and anionic trypsin, chymotrypsin, and elastase as well as plasmin and thrombin.

TABLE 30–2   PROTEASE INHIBITORS IN MAN#

Human Proteases	Plasma Inhibitors*			Tissue Inhibitors*	
	$\alpha_1 AT$	$\alpha_2 MG$	C-1 INH	PSTI	Bovine Basic TI (Aprotinin)
Trypsin 1	+++	+++	+++	++	+++
Trypsin 2	+++	+++	+++	++	+++
Chymotrypsin	+++	+++	+	0	+
Elastase	+++	+++	?	0	+
Carboxypeptidase A	0	0	?	?	?
Carboxypeptidase B	0	0	?	?	?
Kallikreins	0	++	+++	0	+++
Plasmin	++	+++	+	0	+++
Thrombin	+++	++	0	+++	++
C-1 esterase	?	?	+++	?	?
Factor XIIa	0	0	+++	?	?
Factor XIa	0	0	+++	?	?
Enterokinase				0	0

#Inhibition is defined as ability to prevent activity vs. usual protein substrates. May not prevent cleavage of synthetic ester or peptide substrates. Relative inhibitory potency is given as a qualitative scale: 0 = none, + = slight, ++ = moderate, +++ = strong.

*$\alpha_1 AT = \alpha_1$-antitrypsin; $\alpha_2 MG = \alpha_2$-macroglobulin; C-1 INH = C-1 esterase inhibitor; PSTI = pancreatic secretory trypsin inhibitor.

Alpha-2-macroglobulin, an 800,000 molecular weight glycoprotein, binds both forms of trypsin and prevents it from digesting proteins. When this inhibitor is bound to the trypsin molecule, trypsin can still split small, synthetic peptide or ester substrates. Thus, a benzoyl arginine esterase activity is found in plasma even when added trypsin is bound to α_2-macroglobulin.

Finally, there is an inhibitor to the complement protein, C-1 esterase, in plasma and it also has the ability to inhibit chymotrypsin, kallikrein and plasmin (Table 30–2). Other proteolytic inhibitors have been described but not well characterized in human plasma. The physiologic role of these plasma protease inhibitors is thought to be control of enzymatic processes like clotting, fibrinolysis, and kinin production. They may play a secondary protective role when enzymes from the pancreas enter the extracellular fluids.

An important biochemical and clinical phenomenon having to do with the pancreatic enzymes is the exocrine-endocrine partition. This term is used to describe the fact that although 99.9 per cent of the enzymes secreted by the acinar cells of the pancreas enter the ducts and pass down into the duodenum, a small fraction diffuses back into the extracellular fluid and then into the plasma. It has been known for many years that there is amylase activity in normal human plasma which is derived from the pancreatic form of amylase. There is also a normal or basal lipase, phospholipase, ribonuclease, and deoxyribonuclease activity in human plasma. Proteolytic enzymes are difficult to identify in plasma because they are bound to inhibitors. There is little evidence to suggest that in the physiologic state the proteases bound to alpha-1-antitrypsin or alpha-2-macroglobulin are in fact trypsin, chymotrypsin or elastase. In acute pancreatitis, however, there is evidence that these enzymes are bound to these inhibitors. One point that may be of importance clinically is that no protease inhibitors for carboxypeptidases A or B have been detected, and it is possible that in pathologic states these enzymes might be able to act uncontrolled by peptidase inhibitors.

Feedback Inhibition of Pancreatic Secretion

Considerable evidence is available that if pancreatic enzymes, particularly trypsin and chymotrypsin, are not present in the intestinal lumen in their active form there is some form of feedback stimulation of pancreatic acinar cell function. In rats fed soybean trypsin inhibitor, which inactivates pancreatic trypsin, the animals develop marked hyperplasia and hypertrophy of the pancreas as well as excessive pancreatic secretion. In humans, rats, and pigs, if pancreatic secretion is removed from the intestine, an immediate increase in secretion rate occurs. Replacement of bile into the intestine reduces this hypersecretion. It appears that bile prevents rapid degradation of trypsin and chymotrypsin in the lumen of the bowel and that any situation in which the concentration of active enzyme is maintained sustains the feedback. It is known that bile stabilizes human trypsin in vitro. The clinical significance of these findings, if they can be extended to man, is that diseases in which there are decreased bile salts in the intestine may be associated with decreased pancreatic enzyme function and a hypersecretion of the pancreas.

STIMULUS-SECRETION COUPLING IN THE PANCREAS

As a result of studies on various pancreatic model systems, including isolated acinar cells, pancreatic lobules, pancreatic slices and intact animals, we can summarize the relative roles of various stimuli and of intracellular mechanisms for enzyme secretion as follows:

When a secretagogue like CCK binds to the plasma membrane on the acinar cell, there is a sudden influx of sodium into the cell and a decrease in the transmembrane potential, which normally is positive on the outside and negative internally. Shortly thereafter there is a release of membrane-bound calcium into the cytoplasm of the cell. In a manner not understood, this increased cytoplasmic calcium leads to fusion of the membranes of the zymogen granules with the apical cell membrane and, by a process of exocytosis, enzyme secretion results. At the same time that calcium is released, the intracellular level of cyclic GMP rises rapidly, but there is little evidence that the cyclic GMP plays a role in enzyme secretion, because a number of conditions have been described where cyclic GMP increased and secretion did not occur, or vice versa. It was surprising to find that rat acinar cells also have receptor sites for secretin and for vasoactive intestinal peptide (VIP). When secretin binds to the cell membrane, it results in an increase in intracellular cyclic AMP (cAMP) which causes both secretion of bicarbonate into the ductal lumen and a potentiation of enzyme secretion in man. We do not know in man whether secretin binds to acinar cells; it has been assumed that the centroacinar and ductal cells were the main source of bicarbonate in man and the major target of secretin binding. In summary, the second messenger of CCK and of acetylcholine in acinar cells is calcium, and the second messenger of secretin and of VIP is cAMP. The microtubules and microfilaments at the apical end of the cell also may play a role in secretion, because injuring the microtubules with colchicine or vinblastine or the microfilaments with cytochalasin B inhibits secretion of amylase stimulated by carbachol, an acetylcholine analogue, CCK, secretin, or VIP. Thus, the microtubules and microfilaments probably play a role beyond the point where calcium or cAMP stimulates the discharge of secretory granules.

HORMONAL CONTROL OF PANCREATIC SECRETION

In Table 30–3 are summarized the hormones which are known to play a role in stimulating human exocrine pancreatic secretion and those hormones which are postulated to play such a role. The first hormone ever described, *secretin,* is secreted by cells found in the duodenal mucosa, called S cells. Since the advent of reliable radioimmunoassays for secretin, it has been possible to prove what releases secretin into the plasma of man. Hydrochloric acid and bile in the duodenum does this; amino acids, fatty acids, and hypertonic solutions do not. Studies in animals and man indicate that the release of secretin is a function of the surface area of the duodenum which is titrated below a pH of 4.5. After a mixed meal, the pH of gastric contents is initially above 4.5 and the plasma secretin level rises little, yet secretion of pancreatic water and bicarbonate is brisk. This finding has raised doubts about the physiologic role of secretin. The current explanation is that a low basal level of plasma secretin is adequate because it is strongly potentiated by CCK to produce the water and bicarbonate secretion seen after a meal.

Another mechanism of secretin release is that by ethanol: two ounces of 86-proof vodka will release secretin into the plasma of man, presumably by its stimulation of gastric acid secretion. Secretin has a half-life in the plasma of man of three to four minutes. It is not removed significantly by the liver, but the kidneys remove both secretin and CCK.

When secretin stimulates the pancreas there is an increased output of cAMP in pancreatic juice which correlates well with evidence in isolated pancreas fragments that secretin results in an increased cAMP level in pancreatic cells. Previously secretin was thought to stimulate only centroacinar and ductal cells to secrete bicarbonate, and the protein that poured out during early secretin stimulation was considered a "wash-out" phenomenon, a flushing out of proteins that had accumulated in the duct system. However, dose response curves in man show a linear increase of output as a function of the log dose of secretin for volume, bicarbonate, *and* for protein. Trypsin output also increases in a linear fashion as the secretin dose is increased logarithmically. The main evidence that bicarbonate comes from ductal cells is that carbonic anhydrase is present only in ductal cells, not acinar cells. This enzyme is thought to play a role in bicarbonate secretion by forming bicarbonate from plasma CO_2 which diffuses into the cell and combines with OH^- groups. Diamox, a carbonic anhydrase inhibitor, decreases volume and bicarbonate output by 50 per cent in man. Micropuncture studies have not been done in man, but the results of those done in animals vary with the species. In the rabbit, the findings suggest that the small duct cells secrete bicarbonate while in the cat the acinar cells may also secrete bicarbonate.

Sodium is transported into the lumen after secretin stimulation in vitro. The unanswered question is whether sodium transport in the pancreas is active or whether it follows active bicarbonate transport. The potential difference between the plasma or extracellular fluid and the lumen of the pancreatic ducts of animals is negative, with the plasma positive and the ductal lumen negative. During secretin stimulation the net potential difference becomes even more negative. These results are most consistent with active bicarbonate secretion. The human mechanism again is not known.

Antidiuretic hormone in large doses can reduce the volume and bicarbonate concentration of secretin-stimulated juice; thus, the permeability to water is increased in pancreatic ductal cells as it is in renal collecting duct cells. Dibutyryl-cAMP or theophylline increases protein and amylase secretion from pancreas slices 30 to 50 per cent in species like the rabbit and mouse. In all species, secretin stimulation increases cAMP output into pancreatic juice. CCK increases cAMP transiently. Secretin also binds to adipose tissue, increases adipose tissue cAMP, and stimulates lipolysis.

VIP is in parentheses in Table 30–3 because at the present time there is little evidence that it plays a physiologic role in human pancreatic secretion. The hormone is present throughout the intestine, is found in D-1 cells of the pancreas, in the central nervous system, and in peripheral nerves. There are receptor sites on acinar cells of the rat pancreas for VIP which are different from those for secretin. Because the amino acid sequence of VIP is very similar to that of secretin, it binds weakly to secretin receptors and does produce water and bicarbonate secretion. However, VIP blood levels are very low, and it is not known what the normal stimuli for its release might be.

Glucagon, which also resembles structurally both secretin and VIP, does not stimulate exocrine pancreatic secretion, but inhibits enzyme

TABLE 30–3   HORMONAL CONTROL OF PANCREATIC SECRETION

Hormone #	Origin*	Stimuli for Release	Pancreas Target Cells	Second Messenger	Effects on Exocrine Pancreas
Secretin	Duodenum, S cells	Duodenal pH <4.5 and length of gut acidified; bile in the duodenum	Acinar, centro-acinar cells pancreas; ductal cells pancreas, and bile ducts	cAMP	Bicarbonate and water secretion (+++); potentiates CCK
[VIP]	Intestine; ?H cells; pancreas D_1 cells	Physiologic release mechanisms unknown; possible local tissue hormone	Ductal cells, acinar cells	cAMP	Bicarbonate and water secretion (+); in large doses, vasodilation, smooth muscle relaxation; augments CCK effect
Glucagon	A cells, pancreas islets	Hypoglycemia; secretin, CCK, GIP	Ductal cells acinar cells	cAMP	Inhibits enzyme secretion and volume output
CCK	Duodenum, jejunum, I cells	Essential amino acids, esp. phe, met, val; HCl to duodenal pH <3; fatty acids, soaps; Ca^{++}, K^+, Mg^{++}. Bile salts inhibit release	Acinar cells	Ca^{++}	Increases enzyme secretion (+++) and synthesis; potentiates secretin; stimulates acinar hyperplasia
Gastrin	Stomach antrum, duodenum, G cells	Antrum or duodenum >pH3; postganglionic vagal stimulation	Acinar cells	Ca^{++}	Increases enzyme secretion (+); potentiates secretin
Acetylcholine	Postganglionic cholinergic fibers	CNS stimulation to vagal nucleus, smell, taste, hypoglycemia; local reflexes like gastric distention	Acinar cells	Ca^{++}	Increases enzyme secretion (+++) and synthesis
[Somatostatin]	Pancreas islets, stomach antrum, upper intestine, D cells	Probable local tissue hormone; release factors unknown	?	?	Inhibits secretin and CCK release and volume response to secretin
[Pancreatic polypeptide]	Nonislet D_2 cells, acinar and ductal cells	Mixed gastric meal and duodenal HCl; probably CCK, secretin; insulin hypoglycemia	Acinar cells	?	Suppresses enzyme secretion; low doses augment and high doses inhibit secretin responses
[Chymodenin]	?	Unknown	Acinar cells	?	Specific stimulation of chymotrypsinogen secretion

*Revised Wiesbaden classification for endocrine cell types.
#VIP = vasoactive intestinal peptide, CCK = cholecystokinin-pancreozymin. Hormones in brackets [ ] have not been proved to have a physiologic role in pancreatic secretion.

secretion and volume output in the presence of secretin. Studies in man indicated that an infusion rate of glucagon of 40 μg./kg./hr. decreased volume and enzyme output by 90 per cent. A later study in man showed that with a basal stimulation with secretin and CCK, an IV bolus of glucagon, 5 μg./kg., would decrease volume and protein by 90 per cent.

In the isolated dog pancreas, glucagon given against a background of secretin stimulation did not change volume or enzyme output, nor did it change the output of enzymes or volume on a background of secretin and CCK. Glucagon does not decrease amylase output from pancreas cells in-vitro. However, there are interactions between secretin and glucagon because when glucagon release is stimulated by intravenous alanine infusions, intravenous secretin will decrease portal vein glucagon levels. Morever, CCK is known to release glucagon from the alpha cells and secretin cannot suppress this.

Cholecystokinin, which has the same C-terminal pentapeptide sequence as gastrin (Table 30–4), is the most potent stimulus of pancreatic enzyme secretion, and on prolonged stimulation also increases pancreatic enzyme synthesis. It strongly potentiates secretin action, and secretin weakly potentiates enzyme secretion by CCK. There is also evidence that, on prolonged stimulation, CCK promotes DNA synthesis and acinar cell hyperplasia.

Immunofluorescent studies with an antibody to CCK in man indicate that the hormone is found in cells scattered throughout the duodenum and jejunum in the crypts and occasionally in the villi. The cells are not found in the ileum, pancreas, stomach, or colon. The release of CCK from these cells occurs with exposure to essential amino acids, fatty acids, or HCl below pH 3. Bile does not appear to stimulate, but probably inhibits CCK release. Radioimmunoassays of CCK combined with chromatography show that intestinal CCK exists in multiple molecular forms, 60 per cent reacting like the C-terminal octapeptide and 18 per cent reacting like CCK $_{33}$, CCK $_{39}$ or larger. By one plasma radioimmunoassay, the normal level is 60 $\pm$ 17 pg./ml., but after meals there is a tremendous increase to nanogram levels. In chronic pancreatitis with exocrine insufficiency, there is a persistent fasting hypersecretion to levels as high as 8000 pg./ml. This finding suggests that CCK release is inhibited by some feedback mechanism which has not been defined.

The amino acids which are most potent in releasing CCK in man are L-phenylalanine, tyrosine, valine and tryptophan. Nonessential amino acids do not release CCK. Raising the serum calcium by calcium infusions increases fasting trypsin output in man and increases the response to a low dose of CCK. CCK isolated from pork duodenum has an activity of 3000 Ivy dog units per mg. in the purest preparation thus far available. On a molar basis, the C-terminal octapeptide of CCK has a threefold greater activity on the pancreas than does the whole molecule, and caerulein, which is a decapeptide, has 1.4 times the activity on a molar basis (Table 30–4). Gastrin-I is 1/34 as potent as CCK in stimulating pancreatic secretion, and Gastrin II, which lacks the sulfate group on the tyrosine sulfate, is only 1/1000 as strong as CCK. The C-terminal pentapeptide of gastrin, which lacks a tyrosine sulfate, has only 1/3400 of CCK activity. Studies of a series of CCK fragments showed that the shortest one with CCK activity on the gallbladder and pancreas is the heptapeptide which has the sulfated tyrosine as its N-terminus. Maximal activity is achieved with the decapeptide, and activity falls off thereafter with the entire CCK sequence. The active site as far as gallbladder contraction and pancreatic secretion are concerned must be the c-

TABLE 30–4 THE STRUCTURAL BASIS FOR THE SIMILAR EFFECTS ON THE PANCREAS OF CHOLECYSTOKININ, GASTRIN II AND CAERULEIN

PORCINE CHOLECYSTOKININ

$$\begin{array}{cccccccccc} & 24 & 25 & 26 & 27 & 28 & 29 & 30 & 31 & 32 & 33 \\ \text{NH}_2\text{-Lys-(22 residues)-Glu-} & \text{Glu-} & \text{Asp-} & \text{Tyr-} & \text{Met-} & \text{Gly-} & \text{Try-} & \text{Met-} & \text{Asp-} & \text{Phe-NH}_2 \\ & & & \underset{\text{SO}_3}{} & & & & & & \end{array}$$

NH$_2$-Lys-(22 residues)-Glu-Glu-Asp-Tyr(SO$_3$)-Met-Gly-Try-Met-Asp-Phe-NH$_2$ (residues 24–33)

LITTLE HUMAN GASTRIN I

pyroGlu-Gly-Pro-Try-Leu-(Glu)$_4$-Glu-Ala-Tyr(SO$_3$)-Gly-Try-Met-Asp-Phe-NH$_2$ (residues 1 2 3 4 5 … 10 11 12 13 14 15 16 17)

CAERULEIN, from skin of Australian hylid frog, Hyla caerulae

pyroGlu-Glu-Asp-Tyr(SO$_3$)-Thr-Gly-Try-Met-Asp-Phe-NH$_2$ (residues 1 2 3 4 5 6 7 8 9 10)

terminal end of the molecule, and the N-terminal residues therefore must lend specificity to the CCK action. CCK also has effects on the endocrine pancreas: it releases insulin from isolated rat islet cells even without glucose in the medium. CCK release from the duodenum is prevented by atropine, suggesting that there is an intramucosal reflex susceptible to muscarinic receptor blockade. Essential amino acids and glyceryloleate, a product of triglyceride digestion, increase enzyme secretion and contract the gallbladder. Adding various bile salts to either acids or glyceryloleate decreases this CCK effect.

During the purification of CCK from porcine duodenal extracts, Jorpes and Mutt found that the activities on the gallbladder and on the pancreas increased in constant proportion and proved once and for all that cholecystokinin and pancreozymin are one hormone. All surface anesthetics such as cocaine or procaine will prevent release of secretin, CCK or gastrin when stimulators of the mucosal lumen are used, suggesting that there is some kind of receptor site on the plasma membrane which must be triggered in order to release these hormones from their secretory granules.

Jorpes developed a hypothesis for the release of secretin and cholecystokinin based on their structure and charge. At physiologic pH, the net charge of the 27 amino acids of secretin is + 4, i.e., it is a very basic amino acid. Jorpes suggested that when hydrochloric acid enters the duodenum it titrates the ionized carboxyl groups of proteins that bind secretin by ionic bonds to the basic groups on the peptide. CCK is also a basic protein, having a net charge of +2, so its release by a pH <3 in the duodenum could be by the same mechanism. Gastrin, on the other hand, is a very acidic molecule and is released by titrating the contents of the stomach to a pH of 5.5 to 6.5, suggesting that basic groups on proteins bind the gastrin via the carboxyls of its aspartate groups. When these are neutralized and the carboxyl groups on the proteins are ionized, gastrin is released. The general theory has never been tested in an in-vitro system.

Inactivation of CCK or gastrin is minimal on transit through the liver, and only 25 per cent of secretin is inactivated. The short half-lives of these hormones in plasma may result from deamidation of the C-terminal phenylalanine amide of CCK and gastrin and of the valine amide of secretin, since the amide groups are essential for activity. As the dose of CCK is increased logarithmically, secretion of protein in man increases in a sigmoid curve to a maximum. Although alkaline phosphatase activity increases in the juice after CCK or secretin stimulation, this may be a wash-out phenomenon from the duct cells, which are known to contain alkaline phosphatase in their luminal membranes. Secretin and vagal stimulation together increase the volume response synergistically. Similarly, CCK increases secretin bicarbonate output more than the sum of the two separate responses. The output of the enzymes with CCK and secretin was only additive. All investigators find that secretin and CCK together give a greater volume and bicarbonate response than do secretin and CCK separately. Secretin and gastrin given simultaneously show only an additive effect.

Gastrin, given in pharmacologic doses, can produce enzyme secretion much as CCK does, but there is controversy whether after normal meals serum gastrin rises high enough in man to stimulate the pancreatic acinar cells. The weight of the evidence at present is that it does so, and gastrin should be considered a normal stimulant of pancreatic enzyme secretion. The C-terminal pentapeptide of gastrin (Pentavlon) also stimulates volume and bicarbonate and enzyme output when there is a secretin background infusion. The standard subcutaneous dose of pentagastrin, 6 μg./kg., which gives a maximum acid output, increases the volume and bicarbonate and lipase output of the pancreas as well. A linear log dose-response of protein, volume, and bicarbonate output occurs in the dog on stimulation with gastrin, caerulein, or CCK. The relative molar potencies as far as enzyme output is concerned are 1.0 for CCK, 2.8 for caerulein, and 0.25 for gastrin.

Pure gastrin II (17 amino acids) in man gives a maximal trypsin output and empties the gallbladder at a dose of 60 picomoles/kg./hr., whereas it takes 540 picomoles/kg./hr. to get a maximal acid output. Gastrin levels found after a meal are those which give a 50 per cent maximal acid response. All of this strongly supports the physiologic effect of gastrin on the human pancreas.

Acetylcholine released from the postganglionic cholinergic fibers plays a major role in pancreatic secretion via the pathways of the vagus nerve.

Somatostatin, a hormone widely dispersed in the central nervous system and intestinal tract, has been found to be an inhibitor of the release of many hormones including growth hormone, insulin, glucagon, secretin, CCK, and pancreatic polypeptide. When CCK is given intravenously, somatostatin in relatively large doses can block the effect of CCK on enzyme secretion. Its physiologic role in the function of the pancreas is still not defined, so it is shown in parentheses in Table 30–3.

Pancreatic polypeptide has been isolated and its amino acid sequence determined. It does not resemble any of the above hormones, and its role in mammalian physiology is not yet known. Its plasma level increases after a mixed meal, on adding HCl to the duodenum or on stimulating the vagus nerve. Relatively large doses suppress enzyme secretion of the pancreas, while low doses augment and high doses inhibit secretin responses. Lastly, a hormone called *chymodenin* has been isolated and its amino acid sequence determined. It is alleged to show a specific stimulation of chymotrypsinogen secretion by the pancreas of the rabbit in comparison to other hormones. These findings have not been confirmed, and its physiologic role is still questionable.

Calcium plays a crucial role as a second messenger of CCK, gastrin, and acetylcholine as well as stabilizing or activating certain of the pancreatic proteases and lipases. About 20 per cent of the calcium in pancreatic juice is bound to some of the enzymes, as discussed previously. The rest of the calcium is ionized, is thought to enter the pancreatic juice via the tight junctions between cells, and does not travel through the cytoplasm of the cell.

The mechanism by which sodium is secreted into the pancreatic juice may involve a sodium-potassium ATPase, because addition of ouabain or ethacrynic acid to the extracellular fluid surrounding pancreatic cells inhibits sodium output into the juice. Micropuncture studies in the cat indicate that the acinar cells secrete a chloride concentration of approximately 47 mEq./L., which is very similar to the concentration of chloride found within the cells. As the pancreatic juice moves down the ductal system, the sodium bicarbonate concentration reaches 100 to 140 mEq./L. owing to ductal cell bicarbonate secretion. In the larger ducts chloride-bicarbonate exchange results in a decreasing bicarbonate. The situation is different in other species, however, and it is not known at the present time which mechanism pertains in man, i.e., whether the acinar secretion is high in bicarbonate or whether the bicarbonate is predominately secreted by the ductal cells.

NEUROSTIMULATION

In man there is good evidence for a *cephalic phase* of pancreatic secretion mediated by the vagus nerve and triggered by the sight, smell, taste, and chewing of food. The main result is to increase enzyme output, and this may be achieved by both acetylcholine and vagally-released gastrin acting on acinar cells. Surprisingly, volume and bicarbonate secretion also increase even when acid is excluded from the duodenum, suggesting that a low level of secretin release is present and is potentiated by acetylcholine and gastrin. Fasting duodenal bicarbonate concentrations are equal to those in plasma, while enzyme output is one tenth of the peak cephalic response, suggesting that resting vagal tone or hormone release is very low in fasting

man, accounting for the basal volume of 2 to 10 ml. per hour. There is also a *gastric phase* which is twofold in origin. Secretion is stimulated by distention of the antrum of the stomach, which releases gastrin, and by distention of the fundus, which stimulates by a vago-vagal reflex. This response is blocked by atropine or vagotomy. The character of the pancreatic juice from vagal or gastrin stimulation is one high in enzymes and low in volume and bicarbonate. When the HCl enters the duodenum, the release of secretin can be blocked by atropine, whereas atropine has no effect on the intravenous secretin response. Atropine does partially block the effect of exogenous CCK.

An important clinical question is whether operations for peptic ulcer disease involving a truncal vagotomy and drainage procedures influence pancreatic secretion. Vagotomy with a pyloroplasty or a gastroduodenostomy decreases basal enzyme output and also decreases the release of secretin by HCl or the release of CCK by amino and fatty acids. High-dose exogenous CCK or secretin give a normal response, however. The output of enzymes after a test meal is decreased in vagotomized man. In spite of these findings, there is little clinical evidence that truncal vagotomy causes a clinically significant impairment of digestion. However, when vagotomy is combined with a gastrojejunostomy a mild degree of fat malabsorption occurs similar to that which occurs in a subtotal gastrectomy and gastrojejunostomy.

The vagus nerve has an influence on pancreatic acinar mass. Stimulation over a period of days by the cholinergic agent bethanechol causes hypertrophy of the pancreas. In contrast, prolonged stimulation with CCK also causes hypertrophy and in addition increases DNA synthesis, i.e., causes hyperplasia.

DIAGNOSTIC TESTS IN PANCREATIC DISEASE

The exocrine-endocrine partition of pancreatic enzyme activity serves as the most important basis of diagnosis of pancreatic disease. Because the normal activities of amylase and of lipase were detected in human serum many years ago, these have become by tradition the mainstays of diagnosis of pancreatic inflammation or neoplasia. There is no intrinsic reason why these particular enzymes should have been selected, since plasma activity of phospholipase A, ribonuclease, and deoxyribonuclease also have been detected and found to be useful. The proteolytic enzymes cannot be assayed by enzymatic means in plasma with reliability because they are bound to the plasma protease inhibitors. Although the bound trypsin, chymotrypsin, or elastase may cleave small molecular weight synthetic substrates while bound to α_2-macroglobulin, for example, the enzyme bound to α_1 antitrypsin is not active. Moreover, much of the cleavage of synthetic trypsin substrates in human serum is due to thrombin and plasmin bound to α_2-macroglobulin during the process of blood clotting. Therefore, arginine amidase activity does not represent serum trypsin activity, and during acute pancreatitis, the increase in arginine amidase activity is not a measure of pancreatic trypsin release into plasma.

Serum amylase activity remains the most widely used diagnostic serum pancreatic enzyme assay, in spite of the fact that amylase is also found in the salivary glands and many other tissues and that there are many isoenzymes of amylase. Many methods are used to assay serum amylase. Each one must have its normal values defined and must be tested to make certain that it can accurately measure amylase activity in urine and in other body fluids where inhibitors may be present. The classic amyloclastic method involves the cleavage of starch, which causes fading of the blue color of starch stained with iodine. The saccharogenic method involves the measurement of the reducing substance, maltose, which is produced when amylase cleaves starch. Another method uses a dye which is bound to the starch molecule and released during amylase digestion. Lastly, there are coupled enzyme reactions in which the maltose released is split to glucose by added maltase, and the glucose is converted by hexokinase to glucose-6-phosphate, which is used to reduce NAD to NADH by glucose-6-phosphate dehydrogenase. The differing normal ranges resulting from these different methods are confusing to the clinician.

The isoenzymes of amylase have also been separated by different methods including polyacrylamide gel, agarose gel, cellulose acetate electrophoresis, DEAE-Sephadex column separation, and recently by isoelectric focusing. The problem with these methods is that none of them distinguishes all the salivary from the pancreatic isoenzymes, and none is simple and rapid enough to use in a clinical chemistry laboratory. A promising method uses an inhibitor protein from wheat which inhibits the human salivary isozyme 100 times more potently than the pancreatic isozyme. Out of a total amylase activity in males of 132 ± 50 I.U./L., pancreatic isozyme equals 82 ± 30 and salivary 50 ± 30, using the Phadebas blue starch method and the inhibitor.

One of the best methods available for simultaneous resolution of the various bands in body fluids is polyacrylamide gel slab electrophoresis. After the enzymes have been separated they are incubated with a starch solution and the color developed with iodine. This method of separation allows the two main bands of salivary amylase (2 and 4) and of pancreatic amylase (2 and 4) to be seen in normal serum and urine. Salivary isozyme band 2 overlaps pancreatic band 4, salivary band 4 overlaps pancreatic band 6, and genetic variants occur where a slowly moving salivary amylase overlaps pancreatic band 2, so complete separation of the total salivary from total pancreatic amylase activity is difficult. During disease states, where either the pancreatic or the salivary isoenzymes are increased in amount, more of the bands become visible in serum or urine so that qualitative judgment as to which type of amylase is increased becomes easier. The electrofocusing methods also resolve a number of these isoenzymes, but there is overlap between pancreatic and salivary bands.

The advantage derived from separating the isoenzymes is that one can tell whether changes in total serum amylase activity are due to the pancreas or to the salivary glands and other tissues which contain the salivary isoenzymes. Patients with mumps, carcinoma of the ovary or lung, or acute salpingitis have been found to have an increased salivary amylase activity. Patients with severe pancreatic exocrine insufficiency due to chronic pancreatitis or cystic fibrosis have a decreased pancreatic isoamylase activity, whereas the total activity remains normal because the salivary isoenzymes are increased.

All methods for measuring amylase in serum are interfered with when there is a lipemic serum due to a high concentration of chylomicrons or very low density lipoproteins, such as occurs in some patients with acute pancreatitis. The true activity is revealed by dilution of the serum. The serum inhibitor, which is not the triglyceride molecules themselves, also appears in urine.

A controversy existed as to whether there is a true α-amylase in liver and whether any of the serum amylase is from liver. An α-amylase has been clearly demonstrated in isolated rat liver cells and it is released by perfused rat liver. The enzyme isolated from rat liver has been found to differ greatly from pancreatic and salivary amylase in its structure, however. There is still no proof that an α-amylase exists in human liver or that a liver isozyme can be found in serum or urine.

Evocative Serum Enzyme Tests

When the serum enzymes are not elevated by a disease process at the time the patient is being studied, pancreatic disease may be revealed by stimulating the pancreas with CCK and secretin to cause maximal secretion. If areas of ductal obstruction exist, increased regurgitation of amylase or other enzymes into the plasma may occur, i.e., the endocrine-exocrine partition ratio will be increased. Normal individuals given CCK plus secretin show no changes in serum amylase or lipase activities over a period of four to six hours, whereas patients who have functioning but obstructed pancreatic acinar tissue usually show a change in either the serum amylase or lipase from normal to abnormal levels and usually a rise twofold or more above the basal activity. This so-called "evocative test" has been useful in patients who have early pancreatic disease with an obstructive component as in chronic pancreatitis and cancer.

When a patient has exocrine insufficiency, proved by an output of less than 10 per cent of normal lipase or bicarbonate into the duodenum on CCK-secretin stimulation, he rarely responds with any increase in serum enzyme activities because the acinar tissue is mostly destroyed. A similar negative response can be expected in a patient whose disease has led to islet damage and diabetes. In patients with functioning tissue and chronic pancreatitis, the test is positive about 75 per cent of the time. The test has been criticized because patients who have biliary tract disease and no known pancreatic disease occasionally have had positive tests, but this may be due to obstruction at the sphincter of Oddi by fibrosis. One of the most valuable corroborative findings is to reproduce the patient's pain syndrome at the time that the pancreas is stimulated and to correlate that with an increase in enzyme activities.

Another kind of evocative serum enzyme test involves stimulation of the pancreas with a parasympathomimetic agent, such as Prostigmin, while giving an agent which obstructs flow of pancreatic juice by causing spasm of the sphincter of Oddi, such as morphine. In this test, normal individuals show an increased serum amylase or lipase activity, whereas the test does not elevate the activity in patients who have no duct obstruction and advanced acinar destruction. The highest serum enzyme activities occur in normal subjects and in patients with moderate acute pancreatitis. This reflects competent secretory function in the presence of high grade obstruction, but is not of great differential diagnostic value. Surprisingly none of these evocative tests has been reported to cause attacks of acute pancreatitis.

Urinary Amylase Secretion

The molecular weight of amylase is 55,000. Proteins of this size are cleared by the glomerulus at a slow rate, and some of the proteins are reabsorbed by the renal tubules, resulting in an overall amylase renal clearance of 1 to 3 ml. per minute. Some years ago it was found that urinary amylase excretion in acute pancreatitis increased as expected when the serum amylase rose, but, when the serum amylase returned to normal, urinary amylase excretion remained elevated for some days. Urinary amylase excretion proved to be a more sensitive index of pancreatitis than did the serum amylase test. When this was investigated by calculating urinary amylase clearance over a two-hour period and comparing it with creatinine clearance, it was found that in acute pancreatitis the clearance of amylase rose on the average 3.8-fold, the clearance of creatinine 1.9-fold, and the amylase:creatinine clearance ratio rose 1.9-fold. Subsequent research has established the mechanism for this increased urinary amylase:creatinine clearance ratio. There is no increase in glomerular permeability nor in a serum isoenzyme which is more easily cleared during acute pancreatitis. The clearance ratio of pancreatic amylases is 3 per cent normally, and that of salivary amylases is 0.5 per cent. During acute pancreatitis, the clearance of pancreatic amylases goes to 7.3 per cent and that of salivary amylases to 4.6 per cent. When B_2-microglobulin, a small molecular weight protein, is infused, the clearance of this protein increases 80-fold in acute pancreatitis. This finding suggests that it is the reabsorption by the renal tubule cells of small molecular weight proteins which is impaired in acute pancreatitis. In other situtations such as massive burns, diabetic ketoacidosis, or following open-heart surgery with bypass, the clearance of amylase also is increased, yet no pancreatitis is apparent. An increased amylase:creatinine clearance ratio can be produced in animals by poisoning the renal tubule cells with maleate. Thus the phenomenon can occur with various forms of renal tubule cell injury.

Although the mechanism of this increased clearance is reasonably well established, the clinical usefulness is still a matter of argument. Most investigators find that the clearance ratio is increased above the upper limits of normal in acute pancreatitis, but many find that it is not sufficiently increased in chronic pancreatitis or in carcinoma of the pancreas to be of diagnostic help. During evocative tests with CCK and secretin, amylase excretion into the urine and the amylase:creatinine clearance ratio are increased more than the serum activity. In acute and chronic renal failure, the clearance ratio should remain normal if the loss of renal function affects amylase proportionately to creatinine. The data are conflicting on this point, some giving normal and some elevated clearance ratios. In general, a serum amylase above 300 Somogyi units/dl. is more consistent with acute pancreatitis than with renal failure. Another problem results from the fact that the amylase:creatinine clearance ratio varies with the method used to assay the amylase. Using an iodometric method, the normal mean ratio is 1.5 per cent, using a saccharogenic method it is 2.2 per cent, and using a dyed-starch method it is 0.8 per cent. Therefore, every laboratory has to establish its own normal clearance ratios, using the method of the laboratory. When separate amylase and creatinine clearances are analyzed before the ratio is calculated, it is clear that the amylase clearance gives the same information as the ratio. The only reason that the ratio has become so popular is that it can be done on a random voided urine specimen and a simultaneous serum value. A timed urinary collection is not necessary. Since convenience reigns in clinical medicine, the clearance ratio seems to be with us.

Assay of serum lipase eliminates many of the problems which occur with the serum amylase. First, serum lipase activity is elevated in pancreatitis as often as is the serum amylase. Second, lipase activity is elevated in chronic renal failure only when the BUN is above 250 mg./dl. Third, the serum lipase is not elevated in burns or diabetic ketoacidosis. Previous methods were slow, but rapid methods have been developed using stabilized triglyceride emulsions at alkaline pH and titrating the mEq. of hydrogen ion produced as the fatty acids are released. These tests can be performed as rapidly as the serum amylase assays. Urinary lipase measurements have been done only rarely, and little is known about their usefulness.

Macroamylases

Patients have been found with elevated serum amylase activities, but normal-to-low activities in the urine. The clearance ratios calculated in these patients are low. When the amylase was studied by methods which allow measurements of molecular weight, it was found that instead of the amylase migrating as a protein with a molecular weight of 55,000, it was now migrating with proteins of molecular weights 200,000 to a million. These large molecular weight amylases are bound to immunoglobulins (IgG or IgA), or in some cases they are polymers of amylase. Because they cannot be filtered by the glomerulus, their renal clearance is decreased and they persist in plasma. The best way to detect macroamylases is to filter the serum over Sephadex to get approximate molecular weights. The polymers of amylase can be depolymerized under certain conditions by treating with guanidine hydrochloride or by incubating the material with starch, suggesting that the binding of the amylase to other proteins is via the polysaccharides of a glycoprotein. Patients with macroamylasemia rarely have any significant diseases. It is a harmless curiosity unless the patient is erroneously treated for pancreatitis.

DIGESTION-ABSORPTION TESTS OF PANCREATIC FUNCTION

One of the standard approaches toward estimating pancreatic function is to administer orally to a patient a material which requires pancreatic enzymatic activity to make the products absorbable by the intestine. The appearance of the digested product is measured either in the plasma or the urine, and the undigested substrate can be measured in the stool. The most common manifestation of exocrine pancreatic insufficiency is steatorrhea, so the commonly used tests are those involving lipids. The secondary motive for these tests is to avoid if possible the unpleasant handling and analysis of fecal samples. Man has such a great excess of lipase in pancreatic juice that when triglyceride is substituted for carbohydrate there is no increase in fecal fat excretion over an intake range of 90 to 170 grams per day. Lipid excretion is 2 grams per day on a lipid-free diet; this lipid probably is bacterial in origin. In an animal after total pancreatectomy, 60 per cent of fecal fat is absorbed without pancreatic enzymes. In patients with severe pancreatic insufficiency, aspiration of ileal contents revealed that 75 per cent of the lipid was in the form of neutral fat and 25 per cent was fatty acids. Analysis of their stool fat indicated that 30 per cent of the fat was in the form of triglycerides and 70 per cent was split fat. The partial digestion of triglyceride in the colon was due to bacterial and fungal lipases.

The standard method for analyzing fecal fat involves saponification of the neutral fat to fatty acids, followed by titration of the fatty acids. The results are given as total fatty acids and not as neutral vs. split fat, so the degree of digestion of the fat is not assessed quantitatively. Qualitative methods, to be described later, are necessary to estimate relative amounts of triglyceride and fatty acids. The total excretion of fat still remains the baseline against which all other fat tolerance or excretion tests are measured. In normal man on a diet of approximately 100 grams of fat per day, the fat excretion should not exceed 5 to 7 grams. As a general rule, stool fat should not exceed 7 per cent of intake.

One of the lipid absorption tests which has received the most evaluation is the comparison of absorption of a tracer dose of ^{131}I-labeled triolein vs. that with labeled oleic acid. Blood samples are taken hourly for eight hours and the radioactivity of plasma determined. The stools are also collected for 72 hours until only trace levels of radioactivity are present, and the percentage of the dose administered found in the stool is measured rather than doing a fat analysis. The total radioactivity in stool should be less than 5 per cent in 72 hours and the peak blood radioactivity greater than 10 per cent of the dose. The fate of absorbed long-chain fatty acids is complex. They are re-esterified in the intestinal mucosal cell; the triglycerides are incorporated into chylomicrons, which are secreted into lymph; and the chylomicron triglycerides are removed by liver and peripheral tissues by lipoprotein lipase. The level of labeled triglyceride at any time is not only a function of absorption but may be high or low because of abnormalities at any later step in metabolism.

In patients with severe exocrine pancreatic insufficiency, abnormal stool and blood levels are usually obtained but the correlation between the chemical and radioactive fecal fat excretion is not close. When mild to severe cases of steatorrhea are evaluated, the incidence of false-positives plus false-negatives is about 25 per cent for both the blood and fecal measurements. The errors occur in the patients who have borderline pancreatic insufficiency. The oleic acid absorption in patients with pancreatic insufficiency is often abnormal and has been improved by pancreatic extracts, a finding which questions whether the difference between the absorption of triolein vs. oleic acid is an adequate test for defects in digestion. Perhaps the 2-monoglycerides are required to form mixed micelles from which fatty acids are absorbed.

A recent extension of this approach is the administration of ^{14}C-labeled palmitic acid or glycerol tripalmitate. The excretion of ^{14}C-CO_2 in the breath is measured for two-minute periods hourly for eight hours. Palmitic acid is oxidized to CO_2 in mitochondria of tissues which take up triglyceride, but the rates vary with other substrate availability. The results of such tests indicate that normal individuals reach a specific radioactivity in their breath CO_2 at least 60 per cent of the activity of the label given. In a mucosal disease such as celiac disease, both palmitic acid and glyceryl tripalmitate give low results but the ^{14}C-CO_2 levels in the breath after ingestion of ^{14}C-tripalmitate or palmitic acid are equally depressed and the ratio remains normal. In severe pancreatic insufficiency the ^{14}C-CO_2 excretion is low after tripalmitate and near normal with palmitic acid, so the ratio of the neutral fat over the split fat excretion is low. When correlations between chemical fecal fat excretion and the breath test with tripalmitate have been performed, it turns out that there is a good correlation in the normal range or above 20 grams per day, but between 7 and 20 grams per day there is a 20 per cent incidence of false-positives and false-negatives.

The same approach can be used without radioactive material by administering vitamin A acetate or vitamin A alcohol orally and comparing the blood levels of vitamin A over the ensuing six hours. Vitamin A esters cannot be absorbed until a pancreatic esterase releases the vitamin A al-

cohol. In pancreatic insufficiency the peak increment above the fasting level after the vitamin A alcohol is normal, whereas that after the acetate is low. In celiac disease both give low results. The correlation between fecal fat excretion and depression in vitamin A acetate absorption indicates that false-positives and false-negatives total about 25 per cent. The main conclusion from fat tolerance tests is that they lack the sensitivity to detect early pancreatic damage, because more than 90 per cent of the lipase output of the pancreas must be absent before the tests become abnormal. They are accurate in gross steatorrhea and avoid the unpleasant chemical analysis of stools for fat, but they sacrifice accuracy for convenience. The major defect is their inability to tell reliably whether the steatorrhea is due to maldigestion or malabsorption.

Similar tests have been done to test protein digestion. The physiology which underlies these tests will be reviewed briefly. Digestion of bovine serum albumin when mixed with a normal mixed meal is much slower than previously thought, so that at four hours protein still remains undigested in the ileum, and amino acids, di- and tri-peptides are still found throughout the jejunum and ileum. The peptides are more rapidly absorbed than the free amino acids, and are split in the mucosal or liver cells to amino acids. Stool nitrogen content, which should not exceed 2 grams per day, does not become abnormal until more than 90 per cent of pancreatic protease secretion is lost. Thus, one approach has been to measure the enzyme activity in the stool assuming that it bears a constant relation to the duodenal protease secretion. The results are confused by the presence of bacterial proteases which have activities that mimic those of chymotrypsin for example.

A protein tolerance test used in past years involved the administration of gelatin which, when digested, is absorbed to a great extent as peptides containing hydroxyproline which are excreted and measured in the urine. After 28 grams of gelatin, the increment in urinary hydroxyproline excretion in 24 hours is below control levels in advanced but not in mild pancreatic insufficiency. If the gelatin is fed along with 25 grams of D-xylose, a defect in mucosal absorption can be detected as well. A normal D-xylose excretion in the urine, which is usual in chronic pancreatitis, and a low hydroxyproline excretion after gelatin would indicate a defect in protein digestion.

The best indirect approach to assessing pancreatic proteolytic activity has been the administration in the test meal of a synthetic substrate for chymotrypsin. Benzoyl-tyrosine-para-amino-benzoic acid (Bz-Tyr-PABA) is cleaved by chymotrypsin, releasing the PABA, which is absorbed through the intestinal mucosa and excreted in the urine. After administration of 1 gram of the compound, at least 50 per cent should be excreted in the urine in six hours. In advanced chronic pancreatitis, the excretion usually is low, and the percentage excreted correlates well with the degree of abnormality of the Lundh test. However, since this test requires not only digestion but absorption, severe mucosal disease may give abnormal values. PABA must be excreted in the urine; therefore, severe renal disease invalidates the test. Patients with a serum creatinine above 2 mg./dl. are usually excluded. It still is not known how much pancreatic damage must occur for this test to become abnormal; i.e., its sensitivity is undefined.

There have also been attempts to evaluate starch digestion by tolerance tests. Patients with severe pancreatic insufficiency excreting 12 to 50 grams per day of fat in their stools have a 90 per cent reduction in the rate of starch hydrolysis in the jejunal lumen. In spite of this, their total ability to utilize the starch they have been fed is still adequate. This is not due to salivary amylase, of which very little can be detected in the duodenal lumen, but apparently is due to the large excess activity of pancreatic amylase in the juice which allows 10 per cent to digest the amount of starch available. This finding suggests that starch is an excellent caloric source for a patient with pancreatic insufficiency.

Starch tolerance tests usually are performed by the administration of 100 grams of starch orally, with measurement of blood sugars over a period of three hours. The peak blood sugar is compared with that after a dose of 100 grams of glucose given the next day. Surprisingly, the peak blood glucose usually is somewhat higher after starch than after glucose. The increment after glucose administration, minus the increment after starch divided by the increment after starch multiplied by 100, normally is less than 70 per cent. Higher values occur when starch is maldigested. There are a large number of false-negative results in patients with proved pancreatic disease owing to the tremendous reserve capacity of amylase. For this reason, this test is rarely used.

The future role of digestion and absorption tests in the evaluation of patients with possible pancreatic insufficiency will be as simple screening procedures. If such tests prove to have less than 10 per cent false-negatives, they will lead to the more specific and complicated tests such as duodenal intubation and measurement of pancreatic enzymes.

Figure 30–1 shows a simplified algorithm for the evaluation of patients with possible steatorrhea. The intent is to confirm steatorrhea if present and to differentiate that due to pancreatic insufficiency from other forms. If a patient's history, his physical examination, or the gross appearance of his stools suggest he may have steatorrhea

and this history indicates an adequate fat intake, the simplest and most directive test that can be done is to stain a fresh stool sample obtained at rectal examination with a saturated solution of Sudan 3 dye in methanol, homogenized with the stool in water or saline. This should detect neutral fats (triglycerides). Emulsifying another fragment of stool with 33 per cent acetic acid and Sudan stain, covering the emulsion with a cover slip, and warming to the point where bubbles appear (about 80° C.) will change fatty acid soaps into undissociated fatty acids and melt them so that they can take up Sudan stain. As the slide cools, fatty acids will crystallize out in long colorless, needle-like sheaves. A qualitative Sudan stain is positive when more than 10 globules 20 μ or more in diameter are seen per high power field. A test showing 0-trace neutral or split fat contains less than 7 gm./day; one showing 4+ split fat or neutral fat usually contains more than 20 gm./day by analysis. A 1+ to 3+ grade may contain normal to elevated values. Thus, only the qualitative extremes are reliable guides to amounts of fat in the stool.

Both slides can be used to look for partially digested meat fibers which still contain cross striations and sharp edges. If neutral fat is present and partially digested meat fibers are apparent, it is very probable that a defect in digestion is present. Neutral fat is present in normal stool only as a few 5 to 10 μ particles. Undigested meat fibers are not seen in other situations unless the patient has very rapid peristalsis. Split fat, of course, is seen whenever neutral fat is present because of bacterial lipases in the colon. Such a patient has presumed pancreatic insufficiency and should be placed on 100 grams of fat a day for three days to assess the quantitative severity of the steatorrhea. A D-xylose test and a small bowel barium study, looking for a malabsorption pattern, are screening tests which, when negative, point toward a diagnosis of pancreatic disease. If they are normal, there is unlikely to be a mucosal lesion and a secretin or Lundh test is worth doing. If available, either a ^{14}C-glycerol palmitate breath test or a Bz-tyrosine-PABA urine test would be a good screening test, justifying a duodenal intubation test if found abnormal. If the screening test is normal, it does not rule out pancreatic disease.

An abnormal secretin or Lundh test justifies a therapeutic trial of a potent pancreatic extract, such as Ilozyme, along with an agent which prevents gastric acid and pepsin inactivation of the enzymes, such as cimetidine. If the patient has pancreatic insufficiency as the only cause of steatorrhea, he should cease to have diarrhea and should gain weight, and his stool should show no significant fat on Sudan stain. If no significant fat is seen on the initial examination, the patient should be placed on 100 grams of fat per day for

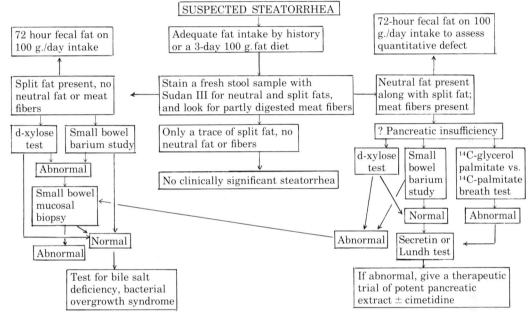

Figure 30–1 A simplified algorithm for evaluation of patients with pancreatogenous vs. other forms of steatorrhea.

three days and then return for another microscopic examination. A negative examination rules out clinically significant steatorrhea as a cause of diarrhea or weight loss.

The usefulness of the 72-hour fecal fat determination is to decide whether the fat losses can account for weight loss. They rarely do so if they are below 20 grams per day, but 7 to 20 grams of fat per day may contribute to diarrhea via the effect of fatty acids on colonic absorption of sodium and chloride. If the stool contains split fat in large amounts and no neutral fat or meat fibers, the patient's steatorrhea has either a mucosal or luminal cause. Here the D-xylose test and small bowel barium study should be abnormal, leading to small bowel biopsy. The biopsy may show evidence of villous atrophy, as seen in gluten enteropathy, or it may lead to a diagnosis of Whipple's disease and other rare diseases. If the pancreatic studies and small bowel biopsy are both normal, the patient probably has a bile salt deficiency due to liver disease, ileal disease or bacterial overgrowth. Every physician should obtain experience with the Sudan examination of stool. It takes only five minutes and leads to an efficient evaluation of steatorrhea if present.

RADIOLOGIC AND NUCLEAR METHODS OF DIAGNOSIS

The major methods for diagnosis of diseases of the pancreas requiring the help of radiologists and nuclear medicine specialists are barium meals, seleno-methionine scanning of the pancreas, ultrasound, angiography, endoscopic retrograde cholangiopancreatography, and transhepatic cholangiography. Few prospective comparisons of these methods are available. One by Eaton in 1968 compared four of them in the same group of patients. The traditional barium contrast studies were found to have a low true positive ratio or sensitivity for pancreatic lesions. Considering all pancreatic diseases, a barium examination of the stomach and duodenum gave a sensitivity of 52 per cent and an overall diagnostic accuracy of 57 per cent because the stomach and duodenum are affected only secondarily by a mass effect or mucosal edema. The sensitivity of duodenal barium contrast studies is increased by giving an anticholinergic agent, which allows detailed mucosal studies undisturbed by peristalsis. This procedure is called a hypotonic duodenogram. It can be done by placing a tube in the duodenum, or, without a tube, by using effervescent tablets to give the air contrast part of the study. Eaton's study of hypotonic duodenography in diseases of the pancreas gave a sensitivity of 55 per cent and an accuracy of 56 per cent. The test obviously is most useful in diseases of the head of the pancreas; it cannot detect cancer in the body or tail. The problem is in telling whether mucosal swelling or compression along the pancreatic border of the duodenum is due to invasion by carcinoma or to inflammation from pancreatitis. These procedures are, however, inexpensive and non-invasive and should serve as early screening procedures in suspected disease of the pancreaticoduodenal area.

Because the pancreas avidly takes up amino acids and synthesizes them into pancreatic enzymes, attempts have been made to label the pancreas with radioactive amino acids, the most successful of which has been substituting ^{75}Se, a gamma-emitting isotope, for the sulfur of methionine. When this is administered intravenously, after a meal, there is immediate uptake of the isotope into the pancreas, incorporation of the amino acid into pancreatic proteins, and eventually discharge of the radioisotope into the duodenum. Over a period of approximately one hour, repeated gamma camera scans usually allow a visualization of the normal pancreas, although it is often difficult to separate it from the overlying liver, which also takes up seleno-methionine. The signal-to-noise ratio for a seleno-methionine scan of the pancreas is poor because of uptake of the amino acid in the blood stream and in other tissues, and the pancreatic image is less well defined than hepatic scans.

Eaton found the scan in various pancreatic diseases had a sensitivity of 86 per cent and an accuracy of 72 per cent. It was most useful when it was normal. A prospective comparison of diagnostic tests in cancer of the pancreas from Mayo Clinic showed that the scan had a sensitivity of 90 per cent but its specificity, the per cent having negative results when the disease was absent, was only 33 per cent. Some reports have been more enthusiastic about the scan and have found a good correlation between a normal scan and a normal Lundh test, or a good correlation when the pancreas was not visualized due to cancer of the head of the pancreas or diffuse chronic pancreatitis and a low trypsin output on the Lundh test. Others who have compared the seleno-methionine scan with the CCK-secretin test find that in in chronic pancretitis the scan is abnormal 95 per cent of the time, whereas the bicarbonate output, the most reliable part of the function test, was abnormal 89 per cent of the time. In cancer of the pancreas, the scan was abnormal in 79 per cent and the function test abnormal in 85 per cent of patients. Unfortunately, the detection of a tumor mass on a scan has had no effect on the resectability rate, which remains very low in cancer of the pancreas.

Angiography of the pancreas is technically difficult because the splenic, gastroduodenal, and superior mesenteric arteries must be cannulated in order to visualize all the blood vessels. Subselective cannulation of either of the pancreaticoduodenal vessels or the dorsal pancreatic is sometimes necessary, and this is even more difficult to do. Vessels of the pancreas are not arranged in a constant order, and it is difficult to tell whether they have been displaced by a mass. Furthermore, cancer of the pancreas infiltrates tissue and does not push vessels aside. It is a hypovascular tumor and does not cause a tumor stain. Its major angiographic characteristics are encasement of an artery by a process of fibrosis or edema and occlusion of large veins, such as the splenic or superior mesenteric. There is a 25 per cent incidence of false-positives for cancer due to atherosclerosis or chronic pancreatitis and a 25 per cent false-negative rate because small lesions cannot be seen. In Eaton's study the sensitivity for various pancreatic diseases was 55 per cent, the specificity 60 per cent and overall accuracy 56 per cent. Once disease had been detected by other means, the Mayo Clinic study showed that the sensitivity for the diagnosis of pancreatic cancer was 70 per cent but the specificity was 95 per cent. There is no evidence that angiographically detectable tumors are resectable more often than those detected by other means. The usefulness of the angiogram is in confirming the diagnosis of cancer of the pancreas or of a pseudocyst.

Ultrasound is a non-invasive and relatively inexpensive technique. Using the B-mode scan and the gray scale display method, lesions as small as 2 cm. can be detected as long as their density is different from that of the pancreas. The thickness of the normal pancreas has now been well defined by ultrasound, and 82 per cent of the time the gland can be visualized. Cysts are clearly identified, and a swollen edematous gland also can be seen. Sixty per cent of the time ultrasound findings modified the management of patients, whereas endoscopic retrograde pancreatography was correct and helpful 86 per cent of the time and computerized tomography 74 per cent of the time. The Mayo Clinic study referred to previously showed that, as a screening test for detection of pancreatic disease, the ultrasound had a sensitivity of 75 per cent, and a specificity of 82 per cent. With the instruments available at present, an enlarged edematous gland in acute pancreatitis can be seen in 83 to 90 per cent of cases, and a pseudocyst larger than 2 cm. can be seen 90 per cent of the time. In 50 per cent of the cases of acute pancreatitis followed serially, a cystic lesion is identified, but 20 to 40 per cent of the time these resolve spontaneously. There is a considerable disagreement about whether chronic pancreatitis can be identified by ultrasound. A cystadenoma is seen as a quite characteristic, multiloculated cystic tumor. Lesions as small as 2 cm. have been detected, but the major problem is that a tumor looks very much like localized chronic pancreatitis. Compared to computerized tomography, which fails to see the pan-

creas only 7 per cent of the time, ultrasound fails to visualize it 10 to 20 per cent of the time because of overlying gas or technical considerations. However, ultrasound is better able to distinguish the differences in density between a normal pancreas, an edematous pancreas, and cancer than is computerized tomography.

Endoscopic retrograde pancreatography (ERP) is a demanding procedure requiring an expert endoscopist, a radiologist, a radiologic suite, and technical help. It requires from 15 to 60 minutes, is very expensive, and gives the patient a moderate radiation exposure. In spite of these problems, in centers where this special expertise is available it has turned out to be one of the most reliable means of confirming pancreatic disease. The success rate, for example, in the hands of experts is around 92 per cent for pancreatography and 87 per cent for cholangiography. The complication rate is 2 to 3 per cent and the mortality 0.1 to 0.2 per cent. Because of overdistention of the ductal system, acute pancreatitis has been reported in about 1 per cent of total studies, although death rarely results. Sepsis occurring behind an obstructed ductal system is the most lethal complication. It is seen in 0.7 per cent of patients and has caused death in 0.1 per cent. Filling of a pseudocyst by ERP is a serious error because it almost always results in infection and requires immediate drainage. Ultrasound should always be done before ERP to avoid this complication. Some investigators give antibiotics in the contrast medium and intravenously when they feel that a risk may be present. The amount of filling of the pancreatic ductal system usually is monitored by fluoroscopy, but some investigators have used manometry and find that the main and second order ducts are visualized by 3 to 5 ml. injected at a pressure of 110 mm. Hg.

One of the most disturbing facts about the procedure is that it is not only difficult to do but difficult to interpret. Observer variation is between 5 and 55 per cent. One reason is that many anomalies of the ductal system mimic disease. Carcinoma of the pancreas is rarely detected early, and a normal exam is seen in 2 to 12 per cent of cases of advanced cancer because the lesion does not affect the ductal system. Chronic pancreatitis causes dilatation of the ducts, variability in their caliber, and filling defects in 50 per cent of cases where there have been two or more attacks. Early cases of chronic pancreatitis usually show normal ducts or minor variations in the caliber of the secondary branches. The changes in the ducts in chronic pancreatitis do not correlate well with changes in parenchymal function. The experts agree that it is difficult to tell cancer of the pancreas from chronic pancreatitis by radiographs alone, but, using available clinical data and ancillary tests, the interpretation becomes much more accurate. Cytologic tests of the endoscopically-obtained juice have been disappointingly poor in the yield—less than 50 per cent sensitive—and rarely are critical in making the diagnosis.

Many investigators feel that pancreatic drainage surgery or resection should be based on ERP. In postoperative follow-up, there may not be a correlation between the patency of the duct-to-gut drainage procedure and the patient's symptomatic relief. The ERP has been useful in diagnosing the site of a leak of pancreatic ascites, allowing the surgeon to direct his attention to that area. In chronic relapsing pancreatitis, 50 per cent of the examinations have indicated what is called a "surgical lesion" — that is, a stricture, a compressive obstruction, a mass, a cyst, or a stone. CCK and secretin tests were performed in 10 cases where the ducts were normal; the bicarbonate and enzyme output was normal in four, borderline in one, and abnormal in five. The Mayo group concluded that ERP in cancer detection gives a sensitivity of 95 per cent, and a specificity of 90 per cent. Therefore, after ultrasound or pancreatic function testing suggests that something is wrong with the pancreas, ERP is the best way to confirm it. The differentiation between cancer and chronic pancreatitis remains difficult and requires other means of support. There is no question but that surgery on the pancreas of a patient with chronic pancreatitis should be guided by preoperative ERP.

Computerized tomography is the most recent and least studied of these diagnostic procedures. Improvement in instrumentation has now reached the point where scans can be done in two minutes or less, reducing the amount of artifact due to peristalsis, gas, and movement of the patient. Good figures cannot be given from a prospective study for the sensitivity, specificity, or predictability of this procedure in diseases of the pancreas. The pattern in chronic pancreatitis is that of a patchy, heterogenous absorption of the x-ray beams, often with calculi. In cancer of the pancreas there is also evidence of a heterogenous mass which sometimes distorts adjacent structures. With the early and less precise scanners, only 64 per cent of proved cancers of the pancreas demonstrated a mass and the tumor had to be greater than 10 cm. in diameter. Recently, only 7 per cent of a large series of examinations were technically unsatisfactory, and the sensitivity for cancer detection is being reported in the 75–88 per cent range. One difficulty is that when an abnormality is found it may not be a part of or within the pancreas. One of the most effective of the new instruments gave false-positive rates of one of 12 normals, four of 32 cancers, and six of 19 cases of chronic pancreatitis—the problem again being that inflammation cannot be differentiated from cancer.

Although transhepatic cholangiography is technically not a study of the pancreas, it is often used to confirm or deny the presence of a tumor or stone obstructing the distal common duct. Its success rate and its complication rate are approximately equal to those of ERP, although it is easier to perform than ERP when using the Chiba or skinny needle.

To summarize the best application of these radiologic and nuclear medicine methods in detecting pancreatic disease, ultrasonography should be done first, with or without support from a pancreatic function test. If disease is thought to be present and cancer is possible, then retrograde pancreatography is the procedure of choice, adding cytology with its yield. If ERP is technically unsuccessful or not available, angiography is the next step. An obstructing lesion of the common duct can be evaluated successfully by transhepatic cholangiography as well as by ERP. The sensitivity and specificity of computerized tomography may turn out to be such that it will replace ultrasound as a scanning procedure, but it is unlikely to substitute for other tests as a means of confirming the diagnosis of cancer versus chronic pancreatitis.

DUODENAL DRAINAGE TESTS OF PANCREATIC FUNCTION

The most reliable method of determining the functional capacity of the exocrine pancreas is to measure its ability to secrete water, bicarbonate, or enzymes into the duodenal lumen after an appropriate stimulus. Over the last 40 years, repeated attempts have been made to develop the perfect or "best" duodenal drainage test, i.e., the most sensitive and specific test of exocrine pancreatic secretion. This should be applicable on a routine clinical level and should show a high level of predictability in the diagnosis of exocrine insufficiency, chronic pancreatitis, or cancer of the pancreas. To the present time, this goal has not been achieved. The reason seems to be that the goal was not realistic. The reserve capacity of the exocrine pancreas is so great that early alcoholic pancreatitis may still give enzyme or bicarbonate outputs within the wide normal range. On the other hand, if only patients with advanced pancreatic insufficiency are studied, any test of secretion will give abnormal values in all such cases. Secretory tests for cancer of the pancreas cannot be expected to be abnormal unless the main duct is blocked in the head or body of the gland, causing a measurable reduction in secretory mass. The pancreas may not function normally because it has lost secretory tissue or because it is not being stimulated normally by the gut hormones. In the latter case, a test meal that requires release of gastrin, CCK, and secretin, as well as vagal stimulation, provides a better approach than exogenous CCK + secretin. The "best test" may differ with the question being asked. If the question is whether a reduction in pancreatic acinar or ductal secretory mass has occurred, as in chronic pancreatitis, we can design an ideal test to answer this question, but it may not be applicable in every physician's hands.

First of all, a tube must be positioned in the duodenum to collect pancreatic juice and a separate tube or another lumen of the same tube must be positioned in the stomach to remove gastric acid, which might destroy bicarbonate in the duodenum. Because no duodenal tube gives 100 per cent recovery of duodenal fluid, the duodenum must be perfused with physiologic saline containing a nonabsorbable marker, such as polyethylene glycol, that will allow correction for volume losses.

The next decision is what physiologic stimulus should be used and in what manner it should be delivered. The best stimulation would be one that gave an evaluation of the functioning secretory mass of the pancreas. Reasoning from studies done to measure parietal cell mass in the stomach with histamine or gastrin, we should develop dose-response curves in normal males and females of varying ages. If a maximal response occurs, we will assume that it is proportional to the functioning mass of certain secretory cells, since we cannot count them or weigh the gland in normal humans. In the pancreas, the acinar cell secretion of enzymes could be assessed by a maximal stimulation by CCK or by a cholinergic stimulus, whereas the centroacinar and ductal cells of the pancreas could be maximally stimulated to produce bicarbonate by secretin. A measurement of maximum response is most easily accomplished if the stimulus is applied by a constant intravenous infusion, so that the output of the pancreas rises to a plateau response and remains there over a period of time. The best bicarbonate stimulus has been found to be an infusion of pure secretin at a dose of 4 to 6 clinical units/kg./hr. intravenously. The maximal enzyme response is obtained by a constant infusion of pure CCK at a rate of 4 to 8 Ivy dog units/kr./hr., or, alternatively, the synthetic C-terminal octapeptide of CCK (Syncalide), which gives a maximal response at a dose of 20 ng./kg./hr. Caerulein, a decapeptide which has almost the same structure as the 10 C-terminal amino acids of CCK, stimulates enzyme secretion maximally at a dose of 75 ng./kg./hr. Using polyethylene glycol as a marker of water flux, it is apparent that some duodenal fluid is lost beyond the tube and that there is some reabsorption of water and bicarbonate in the duodenum, so that over-all recovery by a duodenal tube is about 80 per cent. Maximal stimulation of both the acinar and ductal tissues would mean that volume output, maximal bicarbonate concentration, or hourly bicarbonate output could be measured as well as the concentration or output of any of the pancreatic enzymes.

The enzymes that are most accurately measured are trypsin and chymotrypsin. Lipase and amylase require careful control of assay conditions, and activities may not be linear on dilution. There is evidence that in the normal human the outputs of each of these enzymes are parallel, but in pancreatic disease the outputs of trypsin or chymotrypsin are reduced more than that of amylase. The output of lipase correlates most closely with the degree of steatorrhea. When less than 10 per cent of the normal lipase output is obtained, steatorrhea is always present. One of the problems in measuring proteolytic enzymes is that the activation of trypsinogen to trypsin relies upon endogenous enterokinase, and this should be circumvented by addition of purified enterokinase to the collected juice. The assay of chymotrypsin is best accomplished by addition of bovine trypsin to insure complete activation. Duodenal contents contain bile, which tends to inhibit lipase, so the assay should be carried out immediately in the presence of an optimal calcium concentration and after addition of a well-emulsified substrate, preferably triolein. The lipase activity will be a function not only of the amount of lipase, but also of the amount of colipase present. This molecule reverses the inhibition by bile acids and stabilizes the lipase molecule. The assay should properly be called a lipase-colipase activity. Measurements of amylase activity are accurate only if salivary amylase is excluded from the duodenum during the study.

It should now be apparent that the measurement of pancreatic secretory mass requires at least two hours, meticulous care in doing the test, and accurate enzyme assays. Each laboratory must perform its standard pancreatic function test on a series of normal individuals in order to establish normal ranges. Maximal pancreatic responses to these stimuli apparently do not decrease with age.

Different methods of collection will give different outputs and concentrations of bicarbonate and enzymes. If CCK and secretin are used, the sphincter of Oddi will remain open and bile will constantly dilute the pancreatic juice. Bile contains bicarbonate produced from biliary duct epithelium by the secretin stimulus. Brunner's gland secretion is said to be stimulated by secretin. Thus, the duodenal tube collects a mixture of at least three secretions, in which only the enzyme outputs are reliable markers of pancreatic function. This problem can be avoided by the more invasive and difficult procedure of cannulating the pancreatic duct through an endoscope. Secretin given alone leaves the sphincter of the bile duct closed and bile goes into the gallbladder unless it is nonfunctional. Duodenal bile is minimal, so bicarbonate output more certainly reflects pancreatic function. Thus, normal values for a secretin test in individuals who have been cholecystectomized would have to be determined separately.

The endoscopic method has given us our first reliable data on pure pancreatic juice secretion in normal humans. Secretin infusions produce a maximal rate of secretion at a dose of 0.5 clinical units per kg./hr. The maximal bicarbonate concentration of this juice is 135 ± 9 mEq./L. and the bicarbonate output reaches a maximum of approximately 0.37 mEq./hr./kg. body weight. Secretin leads to a constant protein output in pure pancreatic juice resulting from the rise in volume and a matched decrease in protein concentration, suggesting that secretin in man does release enzyme. Cyclic AMP output also correlates closely with bicarbonate concentration, supporting the studies which show that secretin stimulates via cAMP. The technical problems involved with cannulating the pancreatic duct, however, make it unlikely that this will ever become a routine method of assessing human pancreatic function.

A major problem for all who wish to measure pancreatic exocrine function is the plethora of different units employed for standardizing the hormones. The purest preparation of secretin available is that from the GIH Laboratory of the Karolinska Institute in Sweden. This is calibrated in clinical units, one of which is equal to four Crick-Harper-Raper units, which is the way Boots Pure Drug Company in England assays its secretin. Over the years, as the manufacturers have changed their methods, their standards, and their assays, the relative potencies of clinical to C-H-R units also have changed. One clinical unit also equals, at the present time, 20 Hammersten cat units, an older method of expressing secretin potency. Synthetic secretin is now available; its potency has been compared to that of the GIH secretin. One μg. of synthetic secretin is equivalent to about four clinical units; the vial of GIH secretin containing 75 clinical units contains 19 μg. of secretin (four clinical units/μg.). In duodenal juice, the maximal bicarbonate secretory rate is achieved at a dose of four to six clinical units/kg./hr., whereas the maximal concentration of bicarbonate is achieved at a lower dose, one clinical unit/kg./hr. Secretin has been given for years as a single bolus intravenously, which results in a rise and fall in rate of flow over a 60- to 80-minute period. This method of testing measures the total amount of bicarbonate put out in 60 or 80 minutes and, by short intervals by collection, looks for the maximal bicarbonate concentration. One of the best of such studies used a dose of GIH secretin of 2 units/kg. body weight, which gave a volume greater than 1.8 ml./kg./hr., a maximal

bicarbonate concentration of 100 ± 10 (lower limit of normal, 82) mEq./ L., and a bicarbonate output of 15 ± 7 (lower limit, 6.2) mEq./ hr. For reasons given previously, these results do not apply to patients without a gallbladder.

There is evidence in animals for dietary adaptation of the enzymes in pancreatic juice. Thus, rats fed a high-carbohydrate, low-protein diet have an increase in amylase and a decrease in protease outputs. The reverse is true on a high-protein, low-carbohydrate diet. However, no adaptation occurs in man for amylase, lipase, trypsin, chymotrypsin, or ribonuclease on isocaloric diets varying from one to 350 gm. of protein per day over a period of two weeks.

For a routine test of pancreatic secretory mass, the simplest method is to do a secretin test, using a constant infusion of four clinical units/kg. secretin over a period of an hour, collecting the juice in 10-minute periods, ignoring the losses, and measuring the maximal bicarbonate concentration and the output for 60 minutes. Since enzyme output is weakly stimulated by secretin and enzyme activities are difficult to quantitate, bicarbonate should be the mainstay. Any hospital laboratory can accurately measure bicarbonate concentrations.

In cirrhosis of the liver, the volume output usually is increased on a secretin test, and the bicarbonate concentrations are therefore low, partly because of a great increase in volume output from the pancreas and from the biliary tree. Bicarbonate outputs are low when both the pancreas and the liver are diseased, but are normal when only the liver is diseased. The information derived from measuring volume, bicarbonate concentration, and output after secretin gives as much useful clinical information in the diagnosis of chronic pancreatitis and carcinoma of the pancreas as do added measurements of enzyme activities or outputs.

In 1962, Lundh suggested another test of pancreatic secretion which evaluates the entire sequence of events that follows ingestion of a meal. A single-lumen tube is passed into the duodenum, and no attempt is made to remove gastric juice. The patient drinks a mixed liquid meal containing carbohydrate, protein, and fat. As the meal empties into the duodenum, endogenous CCK, secretin, gastrin, and other GI hormones are released and act upon the exocrine pancreas. The variables which influence this test are: (1) the rate of emptying of the test meal from the stomach; (2) the gastric acid output, which acidifies the meal and releases secretin; (3) the release of hormones from duodenal and jejunal mucosa; (4) the response of the acinar cells and ductal cells to gut hormones. Lundh chose to measure peak enzyme activity in the duodenal secretion over a period of two hours by collecting at 10-minute intervals in the first hour and at 20-minute intervals in the second hour. The enzyme outputs show a rise, a fall, and a second rise over the two-hour period. Most investigators collect the entire two-hour period and measure average trypsin, amylase, or lipase activity. Although bicarbonate and volume are not measured, secretin plays a role by diluting the enzymes and reducing enzyme concentration. This tube only leads to collections of 20 to 50 per cent of the total duodenal secretion, so outputs of enzymes cannot be measured. The maximal enzyme activities are close to those obtained with maximal CCK stimulation.

The Lundh test has been compared with secretin and CCK function tests in a small number of patients. There are no significant differences in diagnostic sensitivity or specificity, except that abnormal results occur in the Lundh test when disease is present in small bowel mucosa, the liver, or the biliary tree — not just in the pancreas. In patients who have a gastrojejunostomy, there is good correlation in the Lundh test between the lipase activity in the efferent loop and the degree of fat malabsorption. In enterogenous malabsorption due to gluten enteropathy and other small bowel diseases, the Lundh test shows decreased concentrations of enzymes in about one third of patients. This is due to dilution with excessive fluid in the duodenum, to decreased CCK release, and to decreased acinar cell function. In a CCK test, protein malnutrition also interferes, as it does in the test meal. Thus, in patients with protein malnutrition the amylase output correlates very well with serum albumin, which is a good marker for protein malnutrition. In patients with gastrojejunostomies, it is difficult to study pancreatic secretion because the water and bicarbonate are reabsorbed as they travel down the duodenum and jejunum and falsely low values are obtained. Studies comparing output at the papilla of Vater with that at the efferent loop from the stomach indicate there is a loss of 65 per cent of volume, 70 per cent of the bicarbonate, and 50 per cent of the enzymes.

The sensitivity of the CCK-secretin test was evaluated by Sarles in 1963 in a small group of patients who underwent multiple biopsies of the pancreas at the time of surgery for chronic pancreatitis. In these patients, studied with a combination of secretin and CCK, the average maximal bicarbonate concentration in patients with minor damage on biopsy was 79 mEq./L. Those with diffuse and moderate damage had a mean value of 41 mEq./L., and those with diffuse major damage 23 mEq./L. The average normal bicarbonate was 100, with a lower limit of normal of 75 mEq./L. Maximum fasting lipase activity also declined from 29 to 8.7 to 8.1 units/min./L. as the degree of damage increased. This is the only study in the literature in which there is a correlation of func-

tion by duodenal intubation with structural damage. We interpret these results as meaning that in chronic pancreatitis there is an impairment in the function of the cells that produce water and bicarbonate as well as that of the cells that produce enzymes.

In summary, then, an ideal exocrine pancreatic function test is difficult to carry out and probably never will be widely applied clinically. The two most reasonable compromises that have evolved are: (1) the secretin test with measurement of bicarbonate and volume after constant infusion of maximal secretin; (2) a test meal with measurement of trypsin activity over a two-hour period.

ACUTE PANCREATITIS

Pathogenesis and Etiology

The major clinical setting in which human acute pancreatitis occurs is that of stones in the gallbladder, usually with passage of stones through the common duct into the duodenum. Attempts to explain this association have led to an extensive literature testing the hypothesis that a common channel between the common bile duct and pancreatic duct of Wirsüng, combined with obstruction of the papilla of Vater by a stone, leads to reflux of bile into the pancreatic ducts. The mixture of bile and pancreatic juice is postulated as causing acute pancreatitis by initiating autodigestion. The observation that triggered this theory was that of Eugene Opie, a pathologist at Johns Hopkins Hospital, who in 1901 performed an autopsy on a patient who had died with acute pancreatitis and found a gallstone impacted in the ampulla of Vater. Opie postulated that a common channel allowed bile to reflux into the pancreatic duct and set off pancreatitis. He aspirated gallbladder bile and injected it under high pressure into the pancreatic duct of seven dogs and produced an acute hemorrhagic pancreatitis in all seven animals.

Over the years investigators have tried to create various animal models to assess the role of bile reflux in human pancreatitis. We will summarize the important findings and indicate whether or not any animal model has reproduced a form of acute pancreatitis which closely resembles that seen spontaneously in man. One model in the dog allowed bile from the common duct to reflux into the pancreas by connecting the main pancreatic duct end-to-side to the common duct. Such animals tended spontaneously to have attacks of acute pancreatitis, but they were also triggered by treating with morphine, which causes spasm of the sphincter of Oddi. In the Opie model, which involves a high pressure injection of bile (above 40 to 50 cm. of water), an immediate acute hemorrhagic pancreatitis resulted, but histologically it consisted primarily of a bile necrosis unlike that seen in human pancreatitis. If, on the other hand, purified pancreatic enzymes are injected into the pancreatic duct under low pressures (less than 40 cm. of water), different histologic patterns occur. When trypsin is injected, a pancreatic edema with occasional areas of necrosis occurs that resembles human edematous pancreatitis. When elastase is injected, an acute hemorrhagic pancreatitis occurs in which the major damage involves blood vessel walls. Such hyaline necrosis of vessels is seen in human pancreatitis. If enterokinase is injected, acute pancreatitis can be produced, but again it is not severe and looks like that obtained with trypsin. A widely used dog model incubates sterile gallbladder bile and pancreatic juice together at room temperature for 24 hours; this mixture is then infused into the pancreatic duct under low pressure. Almost uniformly, a severe hemorrhagic pancreatitis occurs.

The two elements in bile which are critical for this incubation to be effective are bile salts and lecithin. The element in pancreatic juice that seems to be most crucial is phospholipase A. Activated by bile salts, phospholipase A cleaves a fatty acid from lecithin to produce *lysolecithin*. When lysolecithin itself is injected into the pancreatic duct, a necrotizing pancreatitis occurs that resembles the human lesion. The cell membranes of the pancreas, of course, contain lecithin and are an adequate substrate without the addition of lecithin from bile. Thus, the simplest model that closely mimics human pancreatitis is the infusion of trypsin and a single bile salt into the pancreatic duct at physiologic concentrations and at pressures below 40 cm. of water for 30 minutes. Trypsin produces the phospholipase A, which is activated by the bile salt, and cell membrane lecithin serves as the substrate.

In confirmation of these experimental studies it has been found that a normal human pancreas at autopsy contains only a trace of lysolecithin, whereas in a patient with acute pancreatitis there is a high concentration of free lysolecithin. In addition, in the normal postmortem human pancreas there is usually found to be no free elastase activity, but there is some free chymotryptic and trypsin activity. In acute pancreatitis, all of the elastase is free and the chymotrypsin and the trypsin activities are increased. These findings support the hypothesis that acute pancreatitis in man is associated with activation of trypsin, which activates the other zymogens, most importantly prophospholipase A to phospholipase A. This enzyme produces lysolecithin, which then lyses cell membranes, releasing more zymogens to be activated. A positive feedback process occurs that perpetuates the pancreatitis.

Another form of experimental pancreatitis also bears on the human situation. If the duodenum of a dog is ligated proximally and distally to the papilla of Vater and the lesser papilla of Santorini, stimulation of pancreatic secretion by feeding these animals results in severe hemorrhagic pancreatitis, the so-called "closed-loop" pancreatitis. There is good evidence that this is due to reflux of duodenal contents into the pancreatic duct. This process of duodenal reflux has been postulated as occurring after the passage of a gallstone through the sphincter of Oddi, when there is temporary damage to the smooth muscle fibers.

One simple but effective approach toward understanding the pathogenesis of gallstone pancreatitis has been to filter the feces for eight days after an attack of pain which was consistent with pancreatitis. In two series, 84 per cent of patients found to have acute pancreatitis and gallstones had gallstones recovered from their stools, whereas only 11 per cent of patients with gallstones and no evidence of pancreatitis had stones recovered. Operative cholangiograms showed reflux into the pancreatic duct in 67 per cent of those who had gallstone pancreatitis, whereas among the controls only 18 per cent refluxed. At surgery, gallstones in those with pancreatitis were found in the gallbladder, occasionally in the common duct, and rarely impacted in the ampulla. Patients who had gallstones without pancreatitis had few common duct stones. Therefore, gallstones and pancreatitis seem to be associated with the passage of stones through the cystic duct into the common duct and through the sphincter of Oddi. This finding strengthens the theory of those who postulate that acute pancreatitis is due to reflux into the pancreas, and it makes reflux of duodenal contents through a damaged sphincter a much more likely theory than simple reflux of bile. When enterokinase mixes with pancreatic juice, it is thought to lead to activation of trypsin from trypsinogen in amounts which overwhelm the available pancreatic secretory trypsin inhibitor, thus setting off acute pancreatitis. Moreover, enterokinase is not inhibited by the trypsin inhibitor in pancreatic juice.

When cholangiograms are carried out at the time of gallbladder surgery, contrast medium injected into the common bile duct refluxes into the pancreatic duct 60 to 80 per cent of the time. In autopsy specimens in humans, 80 to 90 per cent of specimens show a common channel of 5 mm. or less in length which allows reflux into the pancreas if the papilla is obstructed. Reflux from the common duct into the pancreatic duct is rarely seen during ambulatory intravenous cholangiograms, suggesting that anesthesia creates an abnormal relationship between the two ductal pressures.

The pressure in the duct of Wirsung has rarely been measured in normal humans. In one of the few studies, basal pressures in the pancreatic duct were found to be 7 to 12 cm. of water; pressures rose as high as 30 cm. of water for 20 minutes after secretin and as high as 30 cm. for one hour after a meal. Pressures in the human common duct rarely exceed 30 cm. except at the peak of gallbladder contraction.

Because the secretory pressure in the pancreatic duct is higher in the resting and secretory states than it is in the comon duct, reflux does not occur in vivo unless a decreased resistance to pancreatic ductal filling occurs. Preincubation of pancreatic juice and bile in the gallbladder of dogs creates a condition where the pancreas takes up bile at a normal bile duct pressure. Pancreatic enzyme activity is detectable in 10 per cent of elective cholecystectomies, so many patients have the anatomic and biochemical setting for reflux of activated bile to occur. When the entire pancreatic reflux literature is considered with a jaundiced eye, we must admit that it remains a plausible but unproved theory to account for acute pancreatitis.

The other factor important in experimental pancreatitis in animals is *obstruction* of the ductal system. Intense stimulation of the pancreas produces no lesions, but in the presence of ductal obstruction pancreatic edema can be produced in most species. Obstruction of the ductal system combined with feeding of mice results in the appearance of zymogen granules in the extracellular fluid and lymphatics at the basal portion of the cells and the appearance of the enzymes in plasma. Whether the granules pass through the basement membranes or through tight junctions from acinar lumina is not known. Occasionally some fat necrosis is seen, but hemorrhagic pancreatitis is rare in uncomplicated ductal obstruction in animals. The lesion can be changed from edema to necrosis by decreasing blood flow to the pancreas via 15 minutes of occlusion of the pancreaticoduodenal artery or by venous occlusion. How does impaired blood flow convert edema to necrosis? The lesion is not simply ischemic necrosis but also autodigestion, so it may be that the plasma protease inhibitors are the critical missing items. When the pancreatic alpha-1-antitrypsin and alpha-2-macroglobulin in pancreatic exudate and in ascitic fluid of a dog with experimental pancreatitis become saturated with proteolytic enzymes there is a sudden worsening of the animal's condition and it dies rapidly. In human pancreatitis, pancreatic edema often leads to severe plasma loss, hypotension, and impaired pancreatic perfusion, which may help transform edematous into necrotic pancreatitis as in the animal model.

When the large or small pancreatic ducts are obstructed, enzymes reach the blood stream by absorption into the lymphatics. These channels also carry enzymes throughout the retroperitoneum, through the posterior parietal peritoneum into the ascitic fluid, and across the diaphragm into the pleural spaces. In dogs there are connections of the lymphatics between the gallbladder, cystic duct, common duct, lymph nodes of the duodenum, and the pancreatic lymphatic system. Thus, India ink injected into the lymphatics of the gallbladder can be found in the interstitium of the pancreas, particularly if there is any obstruction to main lymph flow via the thoracic duct. Acute cholecystitis produced in a dog can result in associated local areas of acute pancreatitis, and injection of lipase into the obstructed pancreatic duct has resulted in acute cholecystitis. These lymphatic connections are postulated as being another mechanism for the occurrence of acute pancreatitis in patients with a single large gallstone which does not enter the common duct. In addition, acute cholecystitis has been seen as a complication of acute pancreatitis in man.

Evidence for the appearance of pancreatic proteases in blood is now available with the advent of radioimmunoassays for trypsin, chymotrypsin, and elastase. In pancreatitis these are present, bound primarily to alpha-1-antitrypsin and alpha-2-macroglobulin. When alpha-2-macroglobulin binds to these enzymes, small synthetic peptide or ester substrates can still reach the active site of trypsin, chymotrypsin, or elastase, which can hydrolyze such synthetic substrates at a rate close to that seen in the free state. Moreover, trypsin bound to alpha-2-macroglobulin is still able slowly to digest intact or denatured proteins, and, in particular, it is able to activate trypsinogen or chymotrypsinogen quite rapidly. It also can act on fibrinogen to lead to clot formation and eventual lysis by digestion of the fibrin clot. Alpha-1-antitrypsin is a more important inhibitor in plasma because it binds strongly and irreversibly to the active site of these three proteases. During acute pancreatitis in man, free trypsin, chymotrypsin, and elastase have been measured in the juice. After recovery only the zymogens are present, raising the possibility that acute pancreatitis is associated with a relative decrease in the synthesis or release of the secretory trypsin inhibitor.

The conclusion from studies of animal models for acute pancreatitis is that the critical factor seems to be activation of trypsinogen to trypsin, which leads to subsequent activation of prophospholipase A and the other zymogens. Bile salts are necessary for phospholipase activity. Trypsin and bile salts alone are enough to initiate intraductal pancreatic digestion, but the process is circumscribed unless there is impaired blood flow to the pancreas or impaired delivery of the plasma protease inhibitors, particularly alpha-1-antitrypsin. Ductal obstruction resulting from edema may intensify the process, as can venous thrombosis in and about the pancreas. The key factor still remains activation of trypsinogen to trypsin.

For some reason the idea has been accepted that hypercalcemia itself is able to activate trypsinogen to trypsin. This theory is used to explain why patients with hyperparathyroidism have a marked increase in the incidence of acute and chronic pancreatitis. In hospital controls, about 0.3 per cent of patients have had acute or chronic pancreatitis, whereas 6 per cent of patients with hyperparathyroidism have had pancreatitis. Acute pancreatitis is also seen in other diseases in which hypercalcemia occurs, such as multiple myeloma or sarcoidosis. It is true that calcium is necessary to stabilize trypsin and prevent autodigestion of the enzyme, but calcium itself is not able to activate trypsinogen to trypsin. Thus, the reason why pancreatitis is more frequent in hypercalcemic states is still unknown. There is no question that the concentration of ionized calcium in pancreatic juice increases in proportion to the increase in ionized calcium in the plasma, and pancreatic secretion is stimulated by hypercalcemia both directly and indirectly by the release of gastrin. Yet there is no reason why stimulation of secretion in a normal gland should lead to pancreatitis. Another theory states that the high ionized calcium concentration in the pancreatic juice leads to precipitation of proteins in the ducts, leading to obstruction. How obstruction leads to activation of trypsin or to more than pancreatic edema is not explained.

Another hypothesis which has been proposed to explain the formation of trypsin within the gland is the autoactivation of trypsinogen by trypsinogen. This hypothesis is based on the fact that highly concentrated solutions of trypsinogen, completely free of trypsin, incubated over a period of time, result in a slow generation of trypsin molecules. It is known that the active center of trypsin is present in an incomplete state in the trypsinogen molecule, requiring a folding process that brings a serine and histidine into apposition to create the active site. When the concentration of trypsinogen is high enough, as exists in the zymogen granules or in the small pancreatic ducts, this theory predicts that two molecules of trypsinogen become apposed to one another and that the serine of one and the histidine of the other complete an active site of trypsin, which will split the activation peptide off the N-terminus of trypsinogen. This is only speculation at present, but at least it is based on experimental fact and implies that within the pancreas a constant, slow rate of activation of trypsinogen to trypsin goes on and that the secretory trypsin inhibitor is the key to protecting against the accumulation of free trypsin. A transient impairment in synthesis or secretion of the inhibitor, or digestion of the inhibitor such as occurs in the presence of calcium ions, could set the stage for autodigestion.

There are four key facts which have been es-

tablished over the years from experiments in animals. First, bile alone does not cause pancreatitis unless it is injected into the pancreatic duct at a pressure well above the physiologic range. Second, pancreatic pressure normally exceeds biliary pressure. Third, the presence of active trypsin alone in the pancreatic duct does not cause pancreatitis. Fourth, active trypsin alters the properties of gallbladder bile so that, when they are incubated together, the pancreas more readily accepts the mixture and pancreatitis is more likely to occur. The best explanation for this is the effect of the lysolecithin produced by bile salts and phospholipase A.

In addition, certain facts have been established in man. First, an anatomic common channel exists in over 80 per cent of individuals, thus allowing for potential reflux in both directions. Second, reflux of pancreatic juice into the biliary tree does occur. Third, the evidence for biliary reflux into the pancreatic duct in an intact pancreatobiliary tree is circumstantial and rests on the occasional finding of bile in the pancreatic duct postmortem.

Specific Causes of Acute Pancreatitis

Listed in approximate order of frequency in Table 30–5 are the generally accepted causes of acute pancreatitis. In most of these, the mechanisms for the pancreatitis are not understood. The controversies about the mechanism for *gallstone pancreatitis* do not diminish its paramount importance in the etiology of the disease. *Trauma* due to blunt or penetrating injuries appears to be a sim-

TABLE 30–5 CAUSES OF ACUTE PANCREATITIS

Gallstone disease, with or without common duct stones
Trauma, blunt or penetrating
Postoperative
Peptic ulcer, penetrating into the pancreas
Hyperlipemia, types 1 or 5
Hypercalcemia, esp. hyperparathyroidism
Hereditary, with or without aminoaciduria
Drugs (see Table 30–6)
Mumps
Infectious hepatitis
Coxsackie B virus
Mycoplasma pneumoniae
Atheromatous embolism
Vasculitis (systemic lupus, periarteritis nodosa)
Thrombotic thrombocytopenic purpura
Behçet's disease
Primary tumors
Metastatic tumors
Ascariasis of the biliary tree
Scorpion bite
Hypothermia
Idiopathic

ple mechanism, but *how* trauma activates the zymogens is unexplained. One hypothesis incriminates release of lysosomal proteases. Often the pancreatitis is minimal and the patient ends with a pancreatic fistula which drains externally or into a gut lumen.

Pancreatitis after *surgery* usually follows procedures in the region of the gland such as a gastrectomy, but it may occur without obvious trauma to the pancreas or interference with its blood supply. It is a particularly lethal form of pancreatitis. A *peptic ulcer* which penetrates into the pancreas usually causes no more than a localized pancreatitis in the region of the ulcer bed.

Hyperlipoproteinemias of types I and V are associated with acute attacks of pancreatitis. Both are associated with grossly elevated levels of chylomicrons and very low density lipoproteins. The current hypothesis states that the chylomicrons lodge in the capillaries of the pancreas, where they are digested by pancreatic lipase or by endothelial lipoprotein lipase, releasing fatty acids at such a rapid rate that they exceed the capacity of circulating serum albumin to bind them. Unbound fatty acids somehow damage cell membranes and release enzymes. This theory needs better experimental verification, but it is empirically true that reducing the chylomicron level with a low-fat diet in type I or with insulin in a diabetic with type V hyperlipemia prevents attacks of pancreatitis.

Hyperchylomicronemia may play a role in the pathogenesis of other patients with pancreatitis. As many as 40 per cent of patients with acute pancreatitis have elevated triglyceride levels, and 10 to 20 per cent have grossly milky serum. No relationships with postheparin lipolytic activity (lipoprotein lipase activity) or a circulating inhibitor of liproprotein lipase have been found with the triglyceride levels. All hyperlipemic patients during the acute disease have been found to have lipoprotein electrophoretic patterns that resemble type I or V.

After these patients have recovered and are asymptomatic, they have been studied again, and at this time their fasting triglyceride patterns show types IV or V, occasionally normal patterns, and, rarely, type I or III. Their postheparin lipolytic activities are the same as controls. A single load of ethanol or carbohydrate does not increase their serum lipids, but feeding of a meal containing 250 gm. of corn oil along with a small amount of carbohydrate and protein shows in almost all these patients a marked increase in plasma triglycerides, and the free fatty acid levels are much higher than normal between six and ten hours after the meal. In two such patients, ingesting the high lipid meal precipitated another attack of pancreatic pain — one in an alcoholic patient, the other in a patient with type V hyperlipemia.

Three criteria must be fulfilled in order to label an individual as having *hereditary pancreatitis:* (1) at least three members of his family must have the disease; (2) painful attacks must be traceable back to childhood; (3) there should be no other definable etiologic factors. It is usual to separate out of this classification types I and V hyperlipemia. The renal tubule abnormality that has been associated with a minority of cases of hereditary pancreatitis results in the loss of lysine, cystine, ornithine, and arginine in the urine. The renal tubule absorption of lysine is normally about 99 per cent, but falls to 90 per cent in patients with this syndrome. There is no evidence in these patients of a basic amino acid absorption defect in the gut as there is in genetic cystinuria. It is postulated that the basic defect in hereditary pancreatitis is some anatomic defect in the ductal system of the pancreas or in the sphincter of Oddi. The occurrence of the aminoaciduria in a few of these patients is not thought to have an etiologic role in the pancreatitis, but simply to be a linked genetic defect to whatever the defect is which results in the pancreatitis.

Many *drugs* (Table 30–6) have been reported as causing acute pancreatitis, but often they have been implicated on the basis of case reports confused by the presence of other drugs. When the case reports are multiple, involve only one drug, and when drug challenges were positive, we grade the level of confidence as 3+. When there are more than one or two case reports of reasonable quality, the grade is 2+, and when there are only isolated case reports, the grade is only 1+.

Certain specific *infections* can involve the pancreas and cause an inflammatory process, such as mumps, infectious hepatitis, Coxsackie B viruses, and mycoplasma. *Atheromatous emboli* from the aorta go to the pancreas with a frequency secondary only to the kidney. When they lodge in small pancreatic vessels they may elicit localized areas of pancreatitis about them, but rarely cause diffuse pancreatitis. The end-result is usually pancreatic atrophy and fibrosis. In a similar way, localized pancreatitis can occur with any form of *vasculitis* which obstructs blood flow, such as periarteritis nodosa, systemic lupus erythematosus, Behčet's disease, and thrombotic thrombocytopenic purpura. *Primary tumors*, such as adenocarcinoma of the pancreas, or metastatic tumors such as oat cell carcinoma of the lung can obstruct pancreatic ducts and lead to localized pancreatitis behind the obstruction. *Ascaris lumbricoides*, the roundworm, may migrate up into the biliary radicals from the duodenum and has been associated with acute pancreatitis in adults and children. *Scorpion bite* is a fairly common cause of pancreatitis in Jamaica. The toxin of this arachnid produces an increased pancreatic volume and enzyme secretion, while at the same time causing spasm of the sphincter of Oddi. It might be

TABLE 30–6 DRUGS IMPLICATED IN THE ETIOLOGY OF ACUTE PANCREATITIS

Drug	Level of Confidence	Presumed Mechanism
Corticosteroids, ACTH	+++	? ductular obstruction by secretions
Synthetic or natural estrogens	+++	Hypertryglyceridemia in type I or V hyperlipemics
Azathioprine	+++	?
Thiazide diuretics	++	Toxic to mouse acini
Furosemide	++	Pancreatic hypersecretion
Ethacrynic acid	+	?
Tetracycline	.++	Toxic to rat acini
Rifampin	++	?
Phenformin	++	Only with lactic acidosis
Propoxyphene	+	?
Clonidine	+	?
Asparaginase	+	?
Salicylate	+	?
Indomethacin	+	?
Warfarin	+	?
Salicylazosulfapyridine	+	?

+++ many good case reports ± animal models
++   some fair case reports
+   one or two case reports

the form of pancreatitis which best supports the obstruction and secretion theory. Lastly, patients have been reported to develop pancreatitis after accidental *hypothermia*. After all possible causes have been considered, 10 to 20 per cent of patients in every series must be called *idiopathic* at our present state of knowledge. There is still room for astute bedside observation to help uncover the causes of these cases.

Conspicuously absent from Table 30–5 is *alcoholism* as a cause of acute pancreatitis. As we will discuss in greater detail in the section on chronic pancreatitis, alcohol seems to play its role by creating a chronic obstructive disease of the pancreas which eventually results in acute symptoms. The first attack should not be called acute pancreatitis, but should be called the first symptomatic episode of chronic pancreatitis. There is little clinical evidence that a human with a normal pancreas who indulges in an alcoholic debauch can suffer acute pancreatitis. The effect of acute alcohol ingestion on normal man is to produce transient increases in volume, bicarbonate, and enzyme secretion and then to inhibit pancreatic secretion as the blood alcohol level rises above 100 to 150 mg./dl. There is no evidence that alcohol produces spasm of the sphincter of Oddi.

The Pathogenesis of Clinical Findings in Acute Pancreatitis

The natural history of acute pancreatitis varies with its etiology. Patients who have a chronic alcoholic pancreatitis tend to have severe first episodes and less severe episodes thereafter. The mortality rate from alcoholic pancreatitis in most countries is less than it is from gallstone pancreatitis.

Since typical acute pancreatitis is that associated with gallstones, we will use this as the model for the natural history of acute pancreatitis. As a general rule, the pathologic changes in the pancreas are a function of the duration of the acute pancreatitis. For example, patients who die within the first week usually show pancreatic edema and some fat necrosis. During the second week, the gland shows an increase in the amount of hemorrhage. Severe necrosis and autodigestion of the gland and its surrounding tissues usually are not seen until the third week, and by then (or later) abscess formation is common. All of this is consistent with an ongoing autodigestive process that progresses until finally a complication results that kills the patients. Those who die within the first 14 days of the disease (75 per cent) usually die with irreversible shock, yet the changes in the gland may be quite minimal, showing only pancreatic edema. This suggests that even though fluid replacement is adequate, shock persists, causing many observers to believe that some hypotensive factors are produced in acute pancreatitis. The late deaths (25 per cent) occur because of complications of the pancreatitis and deterioration of the patient's nutrition.

The risk factors that make pancreatitis more lethal are older age (over 60 years), coincident cardiovascular disease, or pre-existing diabetes mellitus. The physical findings with the worst prognostic import are persisting lack of peristalsis (ileus), the appearance of a mass, or Grey Turner's sign. The latter is the appearance of bluish-brown discoloration in the flanks due to retroperitoneal hemorrhage dissecting out subcutaneously between the muscle layers.

The complications of this disease that lead to late death are pseudocyst formation, abscess formation, duodenal obstruction due to ileus, gastroduodenal ulcerations, and pulmonary failure.

Evidence that persisting autodigestion leads to the late complications and mortality in this disease has come from autopsy findings in patients in the fourth to 14th week after onset of illness in which areas of relatively normal pancreas have been found in a sea of necrotic material, the normal tissue being connected with large areas of autodigestion retroperitoneally. This suggests that the remaining functioning pancreas is now a source of great danger to the patient, since it has been disconnected from its ductal system by necrosis of other areas of the gland. The patient theoretically would be better off if all functioning and necrotic pancreas could be removed at the time the collections of debris are drained. Studies are underway to evaluate this surgical approach. Generally speaking, surgery is avoided in acute pancreatitis unless the diagnosis is in doubt. If the patient has an acute abdominal syndrome with an elevated amylase, it may be due to acute cholecystitis, a perforated ulcer of the anterior duodenal wall, or intestinal obstruction with strangulation, all of which can lead to increased serum amylase activities. To allow a patient to go untreated surgically with a perforated or ischemic gut may be fatal. Therefore, any patient in whom the diagnosis of acute pancreatitis is not secure should undergo a diagnostic laparotomy to settle the diagnosis and to repair other lesions. The mortality in a simple exploration of a patient was not greater than that of no laparotomy in some rather poorly controlled studies.

It should also be remembered that in acute pancreatitis about 25 per cent of the patients develop *jaundice*, but only 10 per cent have their jaundice on the basis of obstruction of the common duct. Only 2 to 3 per cent have obstruction due to stones. The rest are obstructed by swelling of the head of the pancreas, compressing the common duct. The 15 per cent who have non-obstructive jaundice have some cholestatic form of liver disease, usually alcoholic. In these latter two situations surgical drainage would not be helpful. Abscesses which arise within or outside the pancreas are usually infected by bowel organisms, commonly *E. coli*, other gram-negative organisms, sometimes anaerobic bacteria, and occasionally *Staphylococcus aureus*. There is no evidence from controlled studies that treatment with antibiotics from the beginning improves survival or reduces morbidity, but once infection is established aggressive treatment with antibiotics is important. Unfortunately, proof of secondary infection often requires positive blood cultures or x-ray signs showing evidence of gas formation in the retroperitoneal area by gas-forming organisms. The only effective treatment for an abscess is surgical drainage.

Follow-up studies in patients with acute pancreatitis due to gallstone disease indicate that if they do not have the gallstones removed they are likely to have recurrences of acute pancreatitis. Those whose gallstones are removed, leaving none behind in the common duct, are cured of recurrent attacks of pancreatitis in 95 per cent of cases. Recurrences of pancreatitis after gallstone surgery is a good indication that stones have been left behind in the common duct. There is very little evidence in follow-up studies that patients with acute gallstone pancreatitis, even after a number of attacks, develop chronic pancreatitis. The pancreas, though severely damaged by an attack of acute pancreatitis, has the ability to regenerate by hypertrophy and hyperplasia. Many patients with abnormal pancreatic function in the post-acute stage have returned to normal function after one to three months. It is therefore exceedingly important that any patient with acute pancreatitis have gallstone disease ruled in or out and treated definitively. It is a medical tragedy to suffer recurrent and possibly lethal pancreatitis because of neglect to remove gallstones.

The mechanism of *disseminated fat necrosis* has never been defined. The usual hypothesis states that lipase or phospholipase is released into the blood stream and travels to the peripheral tissues, where it digests triglycerides and phospholipids. However, the bile salts necessary to activate phospholipase A or the emulsifying agents necessary to break up triglycerides into tiny droplets so that lipase can act are not present in the periphery. One possible mechanism by which the enzymes reach the periphery is that they may be carried by white cells inside their granules, the enzymes having been taken up into granules by endocytosis. Another hypothesis suggests that the lipase of the adipose tissue is being activated by something released during acute pancreatitis, since glucose plus insulin will prevent disseminated fat necrosis in the epididymal fat pad of a rat with acute pancreatitis.

Another complication of acute pancreatitis is *pancreatic ascites*. This occurs in both acute and chronic pancreatitis and is almost always due to a rupture in the substance of the pancreas so that pancreatic secretions escape into the peritoneal cavity. This results in 85 per cent of cases from leakage from a pancreatic pseudocyst which still connects to the ductal system. Most of the patients in whom this has been described have had chronic pancreatitis due to alcoholism. Pancreatic ascites can occur after an attack of pancreatitis or as a presenting symptom, coming on insidiously. The patient is plagued with increasing abdominal girth, weight loss, and varying amounts of abdominal pain. The ascites usually is massive. Such patients often have erythema nodosa or other signs of subcutaneous fat necrosis. The ascitic fluid contains very high levels of amylase and lipase, averaging 20,000 Somogyi units/dl. of amylase. The protein content is usually greater than 3 gm./100 dl. The clinical picture is such that many patients are thought to have cirrhosis of the liver with ascites. At laparotomy, fat necrosis is infrequent; in most cases only chronic inflammation is found in the peritoneum. The fluid usually is serous or serosanguinous, occasionally turbid, and rarely chylous. Other causes of ascites must be excluded, including cancer, cirrhosis, and tuberculous peritonitis. In none of these is the amylase or lipase activity as high as in pancreatic ascites. One way of determining preoperatively the source of the leak is to perform endoscopic retrograde pancreatography (ERP), which often demonstrates the area of the leak and allows the surgeon to plan his procedure. Since ERP may cause sepsis when an obstructed pancreatic ductal system or pseudocyst is entered, the surgeon should be ready to perform immediate surgery when ERP is done in a patient with pancreatic ascites. The cause of the fluid accumulation is not understood. The fluid is not all pancreatic exocrine secretion; it is partly an exudate due to the action of the pancreatic enzymes on the peritoneal surface. Sometimes with parenteral hyperalimentation, resting of the pancreas, and removal of the ascitic fluid the problem will resolve on its own. When this does not occur, surgical correction of the problem is necessary. The ascitic fluid contains no bilirubin unless jaundice occurs and shows no bacteria on Gram stain. The differential points between this fluid and that in a perforated ulcer, mesenteric vascular obstruction, or strangulation-obstruction is that in these cases bacteria can often be seen on Gram stain, and in a perforated ulcer bilirubin appears in the fluid. The amylase activity of ascites can be elevated in infarcted or perforated bowel, so this is not a diagnostic differential point. Flecks of digested fat sometimes can be seen in the ascites of acute pancreatitis. The finding of an elevated amylase activity in pleural fluid is, however, much more specific for acute pancreatitis. It apparently reaches the pleural cavity via lymphatic connections.

The possibility that vasoactive peptides are being released into the peritoneal cavity in acute pancreatitis has lead to therapy by peritoneal dialysis. Partly controlled studies indicate that the blood pressure returned to normal and the non-cardiac pulmonary edema and renal failure improved. Bovine glandular trypsin-kallikrein inhibitor (Aprotinin, Trasylol) has been given intravenously to treat severe cases of pancreatitis, but without consistent effects on survival rates or other signs of improvement. This small peptide is excreted very rapidly by the kidneys, and high plasma levels are difficult to achieve. Glucagon, which suppresses pancreatic function, has failed to help in controlled trials. Although autodigestion seems to be critical in the pathogenesis of pancreatitis, at the present time we have no therapy capable of blocking either the proteases or the lipases once they become active within the pancreas and surrounding tissues. In the best positive Aprotinin study, 7.5 per cent of those given the trypsin inhibitor died and 25 per cent died with the placebo (P <0.05). It appeared that the older patients were protected in the inhibitor group.

In an American series of pancreatitis, primarily alcoholic, 60 per cent developed respiratory problems, with 20 per cent of these being acute respiratory failure; 20 per cent developed renal failure; and 20 per cent developed other complications. Studies of patients with shock and acute pancreatitis indicate that it is primarily due to a critical reduction in plasma volume. Large volumes of colloid and crystalloid restored hemodynamic findings to normal in most patients. It is in those who are resistant to volume that bradykinin or other hypotensive peptides may be playing a role. The volume needs may be as great as 6 liters in the first 24 hours.

Another problem rarely encountered in acute pancreatitis is that of excessive *bleeding* and *clotting*. During the acute attack it is not unusual for thrombosis to occur in the large veins about the pancreas, such as in the splenic vein. Occasionally, diffuse clotting occurs, and in a rare number of patients disseminated intravascular coagulation (DIC) results in diffuse bleeding. When patients have been followed serially with a number of clotting parameters during acute pancreatitis, DIC is actually rare. Some patients show an increase in fibrin split products or show a positive ethanol gel test for fibrinolysis, but rarely does fullblown DIC occur with decreased platelet counts, decreased fibrinogen levels, and prolonged prothrombin or thrombin times. In spite of the fact that trypsin can activate factors 2 and 11 and can digest fibrinogen and fibrin, thereby precipitating clotting or bleeding, the problem of DIC is surprisingly low clinically. As a model of blood clotting problems in pancreatitis, low concentrations of trypsin given intravenously to animals led to clotting, and high concentrations led to uncoagulable blood. Thrombin is formed at low doses of trypsin and fibrinogen is degraded at high doses. The prothrombin activation cannot be blocked by the plasma trypsin inhibitors. Trypsin can activate factor 11 (PTA) directly without the mediation of factor 12.

The adult *respiratory distress syndrome*, also called noncardiac pulmonary edema, is one of the most serious complications of acute pancreatitis. It is associated with a decreased compliance and a decreasing arterial pO_2. It is due to accumulation of interstitial edema fluid, which eventually breaks out into the alveoli. The factors in acute pancreatitis that cause increased permeability of the pulmonary capillaries are not known. The usual speculation is that pancreatic lipases and proteases enter the blood and digest the membranes of the pulmonary capillaries, but there is no proof for these theories. The end-result is a severe pulmonary edema, which results in decreased gas exchange, shunting of blood to unventilated segments, and a decreased pO_2 with a normal pCO_2. In addition, there is almost always atelectasis, which is postulated as being due to decreased surfactant in the alveoli. The surfactant, a phospholipid, is thought to be destroyed by phospholipase A. Finally, pleural effusions occur on both sides as a result of the subdiaphragmatic inflammatory process.

Another major complication of acute pancreatitis is *pseudocysts*. A pseudocyst is defined as a collection of fluid and necrotic debris surrounded or walled-off by peritoneal membranes or by a fibrous pseudocapsule. It results from active enzymes escaping into surrounding tissues, usually through breaks in the capsule of the pancreas. These can occur in the lesser sac, anywhere in the retroperitoneum, or between the leaves of the mesentery. When the ductal system dilates within the substance of the pancreas, it is a true or retention cyst. When these retention cysts or pseudocysts become infected, they then are described as abscesses. Since the advent of ultrasound it is apparent that many patients with acute pancreatitis develop pseudocysts. Eighty per cent of these cystic collections resolve in two weeks according to ultrasound. Those that do not resolve may cause complications. As they expand they press upon adjacent tissues, resulting in pain, compression of the common bile duct and jaundice, thrombosis of the portal or splenic vein, or even gastric outlet obstruction. If a pseudocyst ruptures suddenly into the peritoneal cavity, it results in a shocklike state and a death rate of 14 per cent in one series. Chronic leakage usually results in pancreatic ascites. Cysts may erode through the diaphragm and rupture into the thorax, leading to pleural effusion, chylothorax, or a pleural abscess. One of the most severe complications is hemorrhage into the cyst due to erosion of an arterial vessel in the wall. Management of hemorrhage is most difficult. Some have been controlled by using vasopressin infusions into the surrounding vessels or controlled hypotension. Surgical drainage is often unsuccessful in the acute stage when the wall is friable. After six weeks, pseudocysts develop a thick fibrous capsule which allows an anastomosis with the intestinal tract for internal drainage. If they are drained after six weeks when a good capsule is formed, the mortality is 9 per

cent. If attempts are made to drain them in the acute stage, the mortality is quite high — as much as 60 per cent. According to controlled studies, there is no evidence that prophylactic antibiotics prevent infection of necrotic collections, nor do they prevent the infection of pseudocysts. Once infection does occur, early drainage of the infected cyst or abscess is critical to the patient's survival.

The pancreas often is injured during upper abdominal trauma, such as penetrating wounds due to a knife, a bullet or shotgun pellets, or blunt trauma due to a steering wheel injury. The pancreas is especially susceptible to crushing injury against the unyielding vertebral bodies. The mortality rate with trauma to the upper abdomen varies with the mode of injury. In one series, stab wounds had a mortality rate of 8 per cent, gunshot wounds 25 per cent, shotgun injuries 60 per cent, and steering wheel injuries 50 per cent. Injuries involving the head of the pancreas are more severe than in the body or tail, i.e., 28 per cent versus 16 per cent mortality, respectively, because injuries to the head often involve the liver, duodenum, bile duct, major vessels, and colon. Penetrating trauma usually damages other organs, whereas in blunt trauma one third of cases involve isolated damage to the pancreas. Injury to the pancreas alone rarely kills, but it often results in complications and morbidity. For example, in blunt injury to the pancreas, pseudocysts appear in 33 per cent of cases. When this occurs, the mortality is 20 per cent and the complication rate is 37 per cent. The major complications are a fistula, which results from the opening up of the ductal system, and abscess formation, which occurs later. After blunt injury, there may be a delay in development of symptoms of hours to days. One way of detecting damage early is peritoneal lavage and assay of pancreatic enzymes. A decision not to explore such patients surgically requires a radiologic study with swallowed contrast material (Gastrografin) to prove that there has not been a breach in the integrity of the intestinal lumen. The optimal management at the present time seems to be immediate surgery and removal, not drainage, of the damaged pancreas and anastomosis of the remaining functioning pancreas to a small bowel loop. This allows the pancreatic juice to drain into the intestine, where it belongs, and removes the contused, damaged gland, which often is the site of pancreatitis and fistula or cyst formation. When first operating after blunt trauma, the surgeon sees an edematous pancreas with patchy hemorrhage. It is a difficult decision whether to resect injured areas. Postoperatively, 30 per cent of these patients will develop a fistula, acute pancreatitis, or a pseudocyst. It is interesting that, in spite of a severe crushing injury to the pancreas, diffuse acute pancreatitis is relatively uncommon, testifying to the effective protective mechanisms against autodigestion in a normal gland.

Pathogenesis of Laboratory Findings in Pancreatitis

The laboratory findings are characteristic in most surviving patients, and not finding the usual pattern may have serious prognostic implications. For example, the serum amylase, which is elevated at the onset, falls rapidly within the first few days, regardless of whether the disease process is mild or severe. The serum or urinary amylase tests are useful as diagnostic tools, but have no relation to prognosis unless a late rise or a persistent elevation of the amylase occurs, suggesting pseudocyst formation.

The hematocrit is usually elevated on admission because of loss of plasma from the intravascular space. When the plasma volume is repleted and the hematocrit falls below normal, it means that bleeding has occurred within or around the pancreas or into the gastrointestinal tract from erosions. The white count is usually elevated between 10,000 and 20,000 on admission and falls slowly as the patient improves. A white count that remains elevated or rises again is evidence that severe pancreatitis or a septic complication has occurred.

The appearance in serum of methemalbumin has been proposed as a test for digestion of blood and therefore a clue to the transition from edematous to hemorrhagic pancreatitis. When hemorrhage occurs in or around the pancreas, blood is digested, ferroheme is split from the globin by pancreatic enzymes, and the heme is oxidized to ferriheme or metheme. Metheme binds both to albumin to form methemalbumin and to a protein called hemopexin. Methemalbumin can be measured in serum by a number of methods and its presence is always abnormal. It is not specific for pancreatitis, however, being seen in other situations where blood is being digested by enzymes of white cells or macrophages, as in a large hematoma, or where blood is being digested in the wall of the bowel, as in strangulation-obstruction, or where hemoglobin is being released in large amounts by hemolysis. The differentiation between hemolysis and pancreatitis as a source of methemalbumin can be made because in hemolysis the hemoglobin released binds to the serum protein, haptoglobin, and the complex is removed, leading to a low serum haptoglobin level. In acute pancreatitis the haptoglobin usually is elevated as an acute phase reactant. Experience with this test over a period of years has indicated that it is not reliable for hemorrhagic pancreatitis, being falsely negative in proved cases. The most important false-positive situation is in gut necrosis, where

the finding of methemalbumin may mislead the physician away from exploratory surgery.

Hyperglycemia is observed commonly in patients undergoing their first attack of pancreatitis, and they may develop or present with diabetic ketoacidosis. The serum insulin levels are inappropriately low for the level of blood sugar. Plasma glucagon levels are markedly elevated compared to patients undergoing stress for other reasons. This low insulin:glucagon ratio, plus elevated blood catecholamine and cortisol levels, appears to account for the hyperglycemia. Almost always the diabetes of acute pancreatitis is transient, unless chronic alcoholic pancreatitis has permanently damaged the islets.

Among patients with severe acute pancreatitis, up to 30 per cent have a serum calcium that falls below 8.5 mg./dl., the lower limits of normal. The calcium begins to fall within a day or two of onset, reaches its nadir at about five to seven days, and then usually returns to normal. A number of studies have indicated that a low total calcium is a bad prognostic sign associated with high mortality. One of the problems in the interpretation of the low serum calcium is that approximately 50 per cent of calcium is protein bound in the plasma and there is frequently a decrease in serum albumin during the course of acute pancreatitis. In addition, many of these patients never show signs of tetany or of a decreased *ionized* calcium. Therefore, the crucial question has been whether there is a decrease in serum ionized calcium and, if so, what the mechanism for this might be. When the pancreatic and peripancreatic tissues were analyzed in patients dying of acute pancreatitis, a considerable amount of calcium was present as calcium soaps in the areas of fat necrosis. The total calcium in fat was 1 to 2 grams and was considered to be the explanation for the early fall in serum calcium. However, other states associated with a falling ionized calcium set off parathyroid hormone secretion and mobilization of calcium from bone. Why does this not happen in acute pancreatitis and why does a prolonged period of low ionized calcium occur in some patients?

Glucagon levels are increased in severe acute pancreatitis, and glucagon can increase serum urinary calcium excretion and decrease serum calcium in animals to a small extent after large doses. Glucagon might be releasing calcitonin, although calcitonin's role in reducing serum calcium in man is not clear. Glucagon in large doses decreased the serum calcium in dogs only about 0.4 mg./dl. Parathyroid extract increased both the serum calcium and magnesium in man or dogs with acute pancreatitis. Understanding of the problem had to await the development of radioimmunoassays for many of these hormones. In 1976 Robertson at the Medical College of Virginia studied patients with severe relapses of chronic alcoholic pancreatitis. In these patients, the serum glucose, radioimmunogastrin, serum magnesium, and tubular reabsorption of phosphate all were normal. The albumin concentration fell from a normal average of 4.5 to 3.6 gm./dl. per cent, and the serum phosphate fell from a normal of 3.6 to 2.4 mg./dl. The ionized calcium measured with an ion electrode fell from a normal range of 1.10 to 1.22 mM. to 0.9 to 1.05 mM. in all the patients, even though the total serum calcium was still normal in two of these patients. In many of these patients the glucagon and calcitonin levels were increased, but there was no correlation between the ionized calcium and the calcitonin levels. Glucagon given in a large dose of 1 mg. parenterally to these patients caused no change in the serum calcium. Parathyroid hormone levels were measured with a radioimmunoassay sensitive to the carboxyl-terminal end of the peptide, and might have reacted with biologically inactive fragments. All but one of the patients had low parathormone levels, whereas in a group of patients with chronic hypocalcemia due to other conditions, most had an elevated parathormone level. The administration of a large dose of parathormone increased the serum calcium in these patients and increased urinary cAMP secretion; moreover, basal cAMP activity was higher than normal. This study shows that there was an inappropriately low parathyroid hormone response for the reduction in serum ionized calcium, that there was no evidence of failure of the kidney to respond to PTH, and there was no evidence that bone was responding to the PTH available. Other studies have shown that the parathormone level by a different assay was elevated in six of 11 patients; calcitonin was low in seven of 11; ionized calcium was low to low-normal; the total calcium, magnesium, and phosphorus were low to low-normal; gastrin levels were normal; and glucagon levels usually were increased two- to four-fold.

Studies from England with another parathormone assay in a large number of patients showed that some with severe pancreatitis have a markedly elevated parathormone level, which falls to the normal range in four or five days, whereas another group of severe cases showed a low PTH level throughout. The tubular reabsorption of phosphate and the serum phosphate were low, suggesting renal responsiveness to parathormone. The albumin usually was low, but the ionized calcium in this series was rarely decreased. The best conclusion from these conflicting studies seems to be that parathormone secretion in some patients with acute pancreatitis is inappropriately low considering the decrease in serum ionized calcium. The initial decrease in serum calcium probably does relate to sequestration of calcium as soaps in and about the pancreas, but thereafter the persistent hypocalcemia in some patients is not ex-

plained. Probably the problem has been overemphasized since ionized calcium is rarely measured and total calcium depends greatly on the albumin concentration. Lack of bone response to parathormone could be due to resistance to parathormone due to magnesium deficiency or vitamin D deficiency, but there is little evidence for either. One source of confusion is that different antisera to parathormone measure different parts of the molecule and do not necessarily correlate with biologic activity. From a clinical point of view, the important fact is that patients who develop a low serum ionized calcium have a poor prognosis, but there is no evidence that treating the calcium, which is relatively easy to do, is going to restore these patients to a good prognosis. It is mostly an index of severity of the disease process.

CHRONIC PANCREATITIS

The different clinical types of pancreatic inflammatory disease were delimited as follows by a panel of experts in Marseilles, France in 1962: (1) acute pancreatitis; (2) recurrent acute pancreatitis; (3) chronic relapsing pancreatitis; and (4) chronic (persistent) pancreatitis. The clinical differentiation between acute and chronic disease was based on the presence of continuing pancreatic dysfunction after the acute attack was over. After recovery, pancreatic function tests in patients with acute or recurrent acute pancreatitis return to normal, whereas patients who have chronic pancreatitis have persisting abnormalities of function. Chronic relapsing pancreatitis is the familiar syndrome where recurrent attacks of pain are experienced at weekly to monthly intervals. "Chronic pancreatitis" is used to define patients with daily episodes or constant pain and to describe a small group, 10 per cent of the total, in whom pain is absent but who show progressive loss of function, eventually resulting in exocrine pancreatic insufficiency. This latter type is more precisely called "chronic persistent pancreatitis" to contrast with the relapsing form.

Pathology of Chronic Pancreatitis

Classification of pancreatitis can also be done on the basis of gross and microscopic pathology. The commonest type of chronic pancreatitis is calcifying pancreatitis, which is quite distinct from the pancreatitis that occurs secondary to obstruction of the main pancreatic duct by a slowly growing cancer. The first characteristic of calcific pancreatitis is patchy lobular distribution of lesions. An affected lobule can be surrounded by normal ones, and even at advanced stages of the disease some more or less intact lobules persist. Within the affected lobule the following features are seen: (1) dilatation of the acini, leading to the formation of rounded cavities surrounded by atrophic cuboidal epithelium; (2) atrophy of the ductal epithelium; (3) eosinophilic protein plugs within the ductal lumina which subsequently calcify; these plugs consist of precipitated pancreatic zymogens and enzymes, often with calcium coprecipitated; (4) perilobular and intralobular fibrosis; and (5) perineural inflammation and fibrosis. In the beginning, the main pancreatic duct of Wirsung is normal, but later it may become dilated if calculi accumulate in the head of the gland or stenosis occurs near the ampulla of Vater, leading to the generalized ductal dilatation. Part of the dilatation also may result from loss of surrounding parenchymal tissue and fibrotic retraction. The protein plugs or stones which occur in the small ducts precede the large ductal calculi. This pathology of calcifying pancreatitis is found associated with certain conditions: (1) chronic alcoholic pancreatitis; (2) idiopathic chronic pancreatitis; (3) familial pancreatitis; (4) chronic pancreatitis in regions where protein-calorie malnutrition is prevalent; (5) chronic pancreatitis in cases of hyperparathyroidism. On a cellular basis, in early calcifying pancreatitis there is an increase in the number of prozymogen granules and a decrease in the number of mature zymogen granules. The rough endoplasmic reticulum and Golgi apparatus are dilated. These findings are consistent with hyperfunction of the acinar cells.

During an acute attack of relapsing pancreatitis, the gross findings at surgery are pancreatic and peripancreatic edema, variable amounts of fat necrosis, and, rarely, some hemorrhage and necrosis. The lesion usually is patchy at the beginning. As the disease progresses, the normal elasticity of the gland is lost and it becomes hard, even woody, to palpation. The lobular architecture is lost in affected areas. On section the tissue is firm and pale and does not bleed much, reflecting the increased fibrosis. Healthy areas of parenchyma can be seen surrounded by fibrosis. The surface is marked by the presence of sacculations, which are dilated ducts. The disease can be quite severe and yet show little effect on the main ductal system. Large ductal cysts may develop which contain proteinaceous or calcified precipitates identical to those seen in the small ducts. The calculi consist primarily of protein and calcium carbonate and may grow to be as large as 200 grams. Retention cysts are ductal sacs containing cloudy or bloody fluid. They communicate with the ductal system and usually are found in the head or neck of the pancreas where they may obstruct the main duct. Rarely these become infected.

The pathology of chronic pancreatitis involves the common bile duct secondarily and leads to stenosis of the intrapancreatic course of the bile duct. Other pathologic consequences are compression and sometimes thrombosis of the splenic vein with splenic enlargement. Rarely migratory thrombophlebitis in peripheral veins is present in chronic pancreatitis. Pleural effusions and ascites are also rare complications. The ascites may be chylous owing to obstruction of lymphatics in the retroperitoneum. Disseminated fat necrosis is a rare but puzzling complication of chronic pancreatitis. Subcutaneous fat necrosis resembles erythema nodosa or Weber-Christian disease. The joints may be involved by a periarticular inflammation, mimicking gout or rheumatoid arthritis. Punched-out areas of bone loss or linear calcifications in the medullary cavities of the long bones may be seen. The frequency of cancer of the pancreas is increased in chronic pancreatitis; in some series, as high an incidence as 2 per cent has been recorded, whereas the overall incidence in white males is 0.01 per cent.

In areas involved with acute exacerbations, edema, necrosis, hemorrhage, and fat necrosis can be seen microscopically. Polymorphonuclear leukocytes and plasma cells are uncommon inflammatory cells; lymphocytes and fibroblasts predominate. The nerves become involved in this chronic inflammatory, sclerosing process, and this may account for the severe pain. The islets of Langerhans tend to be spared, appearing as islands in a sea of fibrosis without any exocrine cells remaining.

There are two patterns of calculus deposits in the pancreas. One is associated with heavy alcohol ingestion, and the calculi are small, diffuse, and spread throughout the gland, with some larger calculi in the ductal systems. Another group of patients who do not have alcohol as an etiologic factor have large calculi which usually are found in the head and body of the gland. These larger calculi are frequent in females, sometimes with a familial incidence. They may be related in some cases to malnutrition or primary hyperparathyroidism. Therefore, chronic calcifying pancreatitis is not always a sign of alcoholism.

Non-specific ductular ectasia is seen in a number of chronic wasting diseases, such as uremia, and is not a specific lesion for the pancreas. The initial change is proliferation or hyperplasia of centroacinar and intercalated ductal cells. Later, there is swelling of these hyperplastic cells, some necrosis, and atrophy leading to ductular dilatation. It is a common, non-specific lesion possibly due to inspissation of secretory protein.

Another form of chronic pancreatic degeneration not related to alcoholism is that due to atheromatous embolization. The pancreas is often involved by emboli of cholesterol and lipid material from an atheromatous aorta or other large vessels, third only in frequency to involvement of the kidney and spleen. It is characterized by cholesterol clefts in the thrombosed vessels. As a result, focal atrophy and fibrosis can result in the areas of ischemia. Rarely an inflammatory process of pancreatitis may be generated. Some individuals have been found to have enough destruction of the pancreas to result in pancreatic exocrine insufficiency. Hemochromatosis also leads to fibrosis and atrophy of the exocrine pancreas as well as the islets of Langerhans.

Effects of Ethanol on Pancreatic Secretion of Normal Man and of Patients with Chronic Pancreatitis

Because the commonest etiology of chronic pancreatitis world-wide is alcohol abuse, the effects of alcohol on the pancreas of man and animals deserve review. The major contributor to these studies is Henri Sarles and his group from Marseilles, France. The general conclusions which have emerged from these studies are as follows:

(1) Intravenous ethanol sufficient to elevate the blood alcohol level to 100 mg./dl. or above causes a decrease in the *outputs* of bicarbonate, enzymes, and bile salts into the duodenum. This inhibition occurs in normal controls and in patients with chronic alcoholic pancreatitis. Since volume of juice is not reduced much, the concentrations of solutes are also decreased, enzymes more than bicarbonate. A jejunal infusion which raises the blood alcohol to this level accomplishes the same effect. Inhibition by intravenous alcohol can be blocked by atropine, suggesting that it is mediated by the vagus.

(2) An intragastric ethanol meal stimulates secretion of gastric acid by a cholinergic mechanism and by release of gastrin. Radioimmunoassays of secretin confirm the rise after *oral* ethanol, but there is no secretin release when the ethanol is placed in the duodenum, confirming that it is the HCl which releases the secretin. Oral ethanol also increases plasma radioimmunogastrin levels by a small amount, but duodenal alcohol does not increase gastrin release.

The Pathogenesis of Alcoholic Pancreatitis

The clinical history underlying chronic alcoholic pancreatitis in man is similar to the conditions required to produce lesions in the animal models. First of all, the intake of alcohol must be at a moderate level for a long period of time. The diagnosis of chronic pancreatitis occurs at an average age of 38 years in subjects with an average daily consumption of 200 ml./day, which equals a pint of 80 proof liquor, two liters of wine, or 4 quarts of beer. In Marseilles, surveys of chronic pancreatitis patients showed that prior to onset of pain they ingested an average of 180 gm. of alcohol per day compared to controls without the disease who drank an average of 70 gm./day. There are strong differences in individual susceptibility, however. Some develop the disease on 50 gm./day and some escape it on 300 gm./day. Duration of ingestion is an important variable: it takes eight to 15 years to develop full-blown pathologic lesions. Thus, heavy social drinkers who do not meet current definitions of alcohol addiction can develop chronic pancreatitis. Only 7 per cent had a painless course. The first attack was similar to acute pancreatitis, although autopsy studies in patients who died showed established lesions of chronic pancreatitis as well as acute autodigestion. The average age of onset of acute pancreatitis due to gallstones and other causes was 51 years, which is evidence against recurrent acute attacks causing chronic pancreatitis.

Protein plugs similar to those seen in animals appear in the pancreatic juice of the patients with chronic alcoholic pancreatitis when at surgery a polyvinyl drainage tube is left in the main pancreatic duct. These plugs in man are also made up of precipitated pancreatic enzymes. The hypothesis has therefore been proposed by Sarles that chronic alcohol ingestion superimposed on a diet rich in proteins and lipids results in secretion of a pancreatic juice high in protein and that the enzymes tend to precipitate out in the ductal system.

Lactoferrin is an iron-containing protein present in human milk and in a wide variety of exocrine secretions. It resembles transferrin and binds two atoms of iron per molecule. Its physiologic role is not known. Lactoferrin has been identified in a very low concentration in normal human pancreatic juice by radioimmunoassay, but its concentration is much higher in patients with chronic pancreatitis. The lactoferrin in pancreatic juice probably is not derived from the plasma, where it is also found, but seems to be secreted by acinar cells of the pancreas. The concentration in the juice rises after injection of cholecystokinin. Lactoferrin's postulated role in chronic pancreatitis derives from the fact that it can bind to acidic proteins, forming precipitates which could block the pancreatic ducts.

About 10 per cent of patients with relapses of alcoholic pancreatitis are found to have lactescent serum, i.e., with triglyceride concentrations above 300 to 400 mg./dl. Feeding these patients a high-fat meal elevated their serum triglycerides above 500 mg./dl. and occasionally precipitated an attack of pain. Cameron postulates that certain alcoholics have an underlying hyperlipemic trait and that a fatty meal or alcohol can acutely increase the triglyceride level. Infusing an isolated dog pancreas with triglyceride caused it to swell and release enzymes into the blood. The pancreas of an alcoholic already has many areas of ductal obstruction and regurgitates lipase during fat ingestion or alcohol ingestion. He is therefore more likely to release free fatty acids at a lower triglyceride level than is a patient with no obstructive process. The ensuing activation of trypsinogen is unexplained by this theory.

Other Causes of Chronic Pancreatitis

Hypercalcemia, as occurs in hyperparathyroidism, vitamin D intoxication, multiple myeloma, sarcoidosis, and milk-alkali syndrome, has been associated with calcifying chronic pancreatitis. The concentration of free, non-protein bound calcium in the juice is controlled by the ionized calcium level in the plasma. In patients with chronic alcoholic pancreatitis the basal concentration of calcium in the juice is higher than normal, and after secretin stimulation the concentration increases even further. Without in vitro experimental support, the theory has been proposed that the excess free calcium precipitates the proteins in the ducts.

Hereditary pancreatitis can present over an age range of 11 months to 61 years. The average age of onset is 11 years, and the average age at the time of diagnosis is 31 years. Most patients have an Anglo-Saxon background, but some cases have been reported from Japan. The mode of inheritance is autosomal dominant with incomplete penetrance. An increased incidence of pancreatic calcification and pancreatic carcinoma among affected individuals has been reported. The incidence of carcinoma is one series was 21 per cent within these kindred. Some hereditary pancreatitis is associated with hypertrophy of the sphincter of Oddi and with marked dilatation of the pancreatic duct. The genetic abnormality in this sub-group may encompass a wide variety of structural defects in the sphincter or duct system.

Malnutrition also can result in a form of pancreatic exocrine failure, but not a true inflammatory lesion. Studies on the pathology of kwashiorkor indicate that patients who die with the disease show atrophy of the acinar cells, dilatation of the ducts, fine bands of fibrosis, little inflammation, and, rarely, loss of islets. This seems to be primarily an atrophic lesion due to protein malnutrition. Early in the course of the disease, these patients can be treated with a normal protein diet, and the lesion is reversible and secretory protein output returns to normal. In the acute stage, when essential amino acids are absent, protein output in the juice is decreased and the pancreas contains few zymogen granules. Volume and bicarbonate output are normal.

Thus, kwashiorkor is not a cause of chronic pancreatitis as much as a cause of chronic pancreatic atrophy.

There is also a syndrome in countries where kwashiorkor exists wherein patients have calcifying pancreatitis with inflammation resembling that seen with alcoholism. Some of these patients have alcoholism and malnutrition, but some do not drink alcohol. For example, in Indonesia, a chronic pancreatitis is seen which is associated with calcification of the gland, usually with diabetes, but is not associated with ethanol ingestion. The patients often have a painless course. The only etiologic factor recognized is chronic poor nutrition; yet protein deficiency alone does not cause this lesion. Which macronutrients or micronutrients are important in the development of this disease is unknown.

Many surgeons believe that *obstruction of the sphincter of Oddi* by chronic inflammation can cause chronic pancreatitis. But is there such an entity as "Odditis"? Histology of biopsies of the papilla of Vater and the sphincter of Oddi does show mucosal proliferation, chronic inflammation and submucosal fibrosis in a few patients with pancreatitis. Usually this is seen in patients who have passed common duct stones, not in chronic alcoholic pancreatitis. The same histology also can be seen in patients with no pancreatic or biliary disease. Studies of the sphincter's resistance to passage of probes or of infused saline are suspect because they are done under anesthesia. Often a tight sphincter relaxes with a physiologic stimulus such as CCK. The conclusion drawn from reviewing a large and poorly controlled series of reports in the literature is that obstructive lesions of the sphincter of Oddi are rare as a primary lesion. The evidence that chronic Odditis or sphincter fibrosis causes chronic pancreatitis is unconvincing. Physiologic perfusion studies of sphincter function during endoscopic cannulation of the ducts may finally give us reliable evidence for unyielding obstruction or for spasm in patients with postcholecystectomy syndromes or acute pancreatitis without biliary tract stones.

Clinical Associations of Chronic Pancreatitis

Chronic pancreatitis is not associated with severe calcium malabsorption or osteomalacia as it is in diseases in which the intestinal mucosa is diseased (celiac sprue) or where the small bowel is resected. The nutritional defect of pancreatic insufficiency rarely results in a hemoglobin below 10 gm. The albumin is reduced in only 16 per cent of cases, the serum calcium in 9 per cent, and the prothrombin time in 34 per cent, whereas low values for these are seen in 60 to 89 per cent of patients with sprue. The key to the mild nutritional deficiency in patients with chronic pancreatitis is the fact that (1) they have a normal small bowel mucosa and can absorb many nutrients in spite of poor digestion; (2) they have an increased food intake compared to patients with malabsorption; (3) they have less accumulation of fatty acids in their small intestine which tend to bind calcium and magnesium and lead to losses in the stool. *Iron absorption* was originally thought to be increased in certain patients with chronic pancreatitis, but studies with radioactive isotopes of iron indicate that there is no correlation between iron absorption or storage pools and the degree of pancreatic insufficiency.

Vitamin B malabsorption occurs in a minority of patients with pancreatic insufficiency. This can be improved by feeding pancreatic extract, the active principle of which is trypsin and the other proteases. Vitamin B_{12} is bound in the stomach to salivary proteins, so-called "R-proteins," which prevent intrinsic factor from competing for B_{12} in the acid pH of the stomach. It is not until these R-proteins are digested in the small bowel lumen by pancreatic proteases that the B_{12} is released and intrinsic factor can bind it, therefore allowing it to be absorbed in the ileum.

Patients with acute gallstone pancreatitis or first attacks of alcoholic pancreatitis have an increased plasma glucagon, averaging ninefold above control patients, but at the same time only a twofold increase in insulin. This is a diabetogenic ratio of glucagon to insulin and helps explain their transient diabetes. In patients with chronic pancreatitis, however, the glucagon level is not elevated during relapses. Patients with pancreatic insufficiency show no glucagon response to alanine, whereas the genetic diabetic shows a brisk response to alanine infusion. The clinical significance of this is that the brittleness of diabetes in chronic pancreatitis may be due to an inability to secrete glucagon under stress and thus to increase gluconeogenesis. Chronic pancreatitis patients show an increased blood glucose during intravenous glucose testing, combined with a delayed and poor insulin output. Their diabetes is therefore due to impaired insulin secretion and requires insulin administration.

Pancreatic ascites is almost inevitably due to a leak from a pancreatic duct. If this occurs in the anterior wall of the pancreas, it drains into the peritoneal cavity via the lesser sac or greater peritoneal surface. If this leak is walled off, a pseudocyst is formed. If the leak occurs posteriorly from the pancreas and enters the retroperitoneum, juice moves by least resistance into the mediastinum and sometimes breaks through into the pleura. The fluid contains very high amylase activity and a high albumin concentration owing to a low grade enzymatic inflammation of the peritoneal membranes.

Only about one half of the patients in series of pancreatic ascites have acute pancreatitis. The other half have chronic pancreatitis, where pain is not frequently a part of the syndrome. Massive distention is the main complaint. Occasionally, subcutaneous fat necrosis occurs. The fluid is clear, yellow, occasionally chylous, and rarely bloody. The localization of the leak can be found by endoscopic retrograde pancreatography, and, once the site is apparent, it is possible to close it surgically when conservative drainage of the ascitic fluid or effusions has not been successful in allowing the leak to close spontaneously.

In some patients with chronic pancreatitis, *stenosis of the distal common duct* occurs. During relapses, these patients are prone to become jaundiced, and infection of the partially obstructed common duct can occur with ascending cholangitis.

Gastric emptying is much faster in patients with pancreatic insufficiency, and it returns toward normal when pancreatic extracts are fed. The reason for this is unknown. Patients in whom the CCK-secretin evocative serum enzyme test is positive usually are found at surgery to have obstruction at the level of the sphincter or the main pancreatic duct.

Exocrine function has been studied repeatedly in patients with diabetes, and the consensus is that some patients who have no evidence of exocrine insufficiency may show impaired responses to secretin or cholecystokinin. It is juvenile-onset diabetics who have impaired pancreatic function, not adult-onset diabetics. Age-matched controls were compared with juvenile-onset diabetics who had had the disease from one to ten years. There was a decrease in bicarbonate output after cholecystokinin and secretin proportional to the duration of diabetes and to the insulin dosage.

Patients with chronic pancreatitis and diabetes had the expected low bicarbonate values, whereas those with adult-onset diabetes had normal values. This suggests that the viral or autoimmune injury currently thought to be the etiology of juvenile-onset diabetes also damages the acini and ductal cells and that this is progressive with time. None of the patients showed a reduction in secretion greater than 90 per cent, so they did not exceed the exocrine reserve of the pancreas and did not show pancreatic insufficiency.

The Natural History of Alcoholic Pancreatitis

A series of 113 patients were followed for four years or more after the onset of their first symptoms of chronic alcoholic pancreatitis. The clinical course showed improvement in 42 per cent, remained stable in 32 per cent, and showed worsening of signs and symptoms in 26 per cent. The onset of diabetes and steatorrhea usually began nine years after the onset of pain. Only two of these 113 patients died of their disease during the follow-up period. Four of every five continued to work. These results indicate that chronic pancreatitis is a painful but not life-threatening disease.

Figure 30–2 shows the sequence of events in a typical patient with chronic alcoholic pancreatitis. The graph includes a period of 15 years of drinking at a level of 150 to 180 gm./day. In those patients who are destined to develop the disease, the average time of onset of various symptoms is shown.

For eight years after the onset of heavy drinking, pancreatic damage is asymptomatic and subclinical, but during that time functioning acinar and ductal mass is being destroyed by the process described previously. At the same time, the output of enzymes and bicarbonate after stimulation with CCK or secretin is also slowly declining, although there are few data on patients in this asymptomatic stage. At an average of eight years, the patients begin to have acute painful episodes, the first being the most severe. It often results in transient diabetes. Thereafter, the episodes are less severe, resembling pancreatic edema, and usually follow resumption of alcohol intake. Somewhere in the middle of the course of the disease stimulation of the patient with CCK and secretin in 50 to 80 per cent of patients will elicit an elevation in the serum amylase or lipase. It is not until functioning pancreatic mass is reduced to about 10 per cent and the enzyme and bicarbonate output to about 10 per cent that symptoms and signs of exocrine insufficiency develop. The onset of diarrhea is due to steatorrhea; then, shortly thereafter or at the same time, clinical diabetes becomes permanent. Tolerance tests begin to become abnormal once less than 10 per cent of functioning mass is left, and steatorrhea and creatorrhea make their appearance.

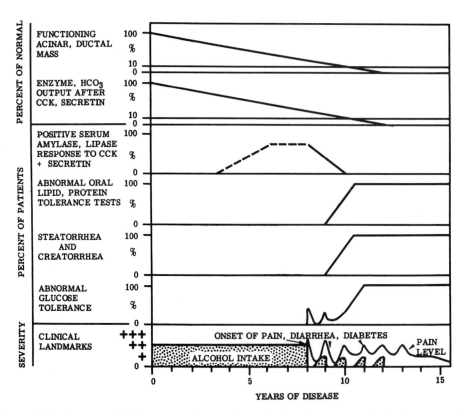

Figure 30–2 The natural history of a typical patient with chronic relapsing alcoholic pancreatitis.

CYSTS OF THE PANCREAS

Two types of cysts are associated with pancreatic disease. The first is the true *retention cyst* of the pancreas, which is lined with an epithelial layer derived from the pancreas and presumably is a result of the dilatation of the ductal system. These retention cysts usually are in the head of the gland, communicate with the ductal system and usually are small and therefore cannot be palpated externally or cannot be detected by barium contrast studies of the duodenum or by angiography. They are best detected by endoscopic retrograde pancreatography. Occasionally these true retention cysts can be massive and may develop as a congenital abnormality. On the other hand, the so-called *pseudocyst* is lined with a fibrous capsule or with the peritoneal membranes of adjacent peripancreatic structures.

The pseudocyst may or may not communicate with the ductal system. These cysts usually are large and therefore can be detected either by palpation externally or by barium contrast studies or angiography. They can occur anywhere in the gland. The best screening test for a pseudocyst is ultrasonography. The pseudocysts enlarge and spread into almost any area surrounding the pancreas. By far the most common site is the lesser sac. If they perforate posteriorly, they enter the retroperitoneum and can go up into the mediastinum or can dissect down over the kidneys all the way to the groin. Occasionally, they have dissected up the mediastinum as far as the neck. They have been known to rupture into the pericardium or into the pleural cavity. Some pseudocysts dissect between the leaves of the mesentery of the small bowel or the mesocolon. Occasionally, pseudocysts become secondarily infected with bacterial organisms, and this results in a sudden rise in temperature and white count, tenderness, and signs of sepsis. The bacteria found in infected pseudocysts are single organisms in about one half of the patients, and multiple organisms are found in the other half. The commonest organisms are staphylococcal species, *E. coli*, streptococcal species, and Proteus species. The presence of gas within a cystic cavity on plain film of the abdomen is diagnostic of an infected pseudocyst. If the pseudocyst ruptures into the peritoneal cavity, mortality is high. If it merely leaks into the peritoneal cavity, massive pancreatic ascites usually is the sequela. Rarely these pseudocysts have ruptured into vessels such as the portal vein, leading to generalized fat necrosis of the skin, bone marrow and tissues throughout the body.

The serum amylase tends to be elevated in about 50 per cent of patients with a pseudocyst. Since many of them do not contain significant amounts of pancreatic enzymes, the elevation is thought to result from compression of the adjacent pancreas. Rarely, the course of pseudocysts is a wasting, downhill course. Spontaneous remission, sepsis, bleeding, and obstructive jaundice may all occur. Rarely, hematobilia may result from bleeding from a pancreatic pseudocyst into the pancreatic ductal system.

Chronic pancreatic ascites is usually associated with a pseudocyst. The protein varies between 2.2 to 2.6 gm./dl., and the ascites fluid almost always has a higher amylase activity than the serum. In 65 per cent of patients, the serum amylase was greater than 200 Somogyi units/dl., and the ascites amylase was greater than 1500 in 13 per cent.

The causes of a pseudocyst vary from acute pancreatitis due to biliary disease to trauma to chronic pancreatitis. About 10 to 20 per cent of patients with alcoholic chronic pancreatitis will develop a pseudocyst; therefore, repeated ultrasound studies at the time of acute attacks pay dividends.

THE PATHOPHYSIOLOGY OF CARCINOMA OF THE PANCREAS

Carcinoma of the pancreas has become an increasingly serious problem in oncology. The age-adjusted death rate in males is approximately nine per 100,000 and for females six per 100,000, ranking this disease as number 4 and number 6 respectively among cancer causes of death. An estimated 20,000 deaths from cancer of the pancreas occurred in the United States in 1978. Between 1920 and 1965 the incidence increased from 2.9 to 8.2 per 100,000, a change not due to improved reporting of the disease. The incidence is rising at a rate of 15 per cent per every 10-year period. The average age of patients with cancer of the pancreas is approximately 64 years, but it can occur in people as young as 30, the rate increasing progressively with increasing age.

The etiologic factors for cancer of the pancreas are mostly unknown, and the candidate causes are poorly documented. For example, there is a 2.5-fold higher incidence of cancer of the pancreas in heavy smokers, and the onset is 10 years earlier on the average than in non-smokers. However, there is some confusing evidence that heavy smoking actually results in a lower incidence, possibly because these patients die of cancer of the lung before they can die of cancer of the pancreas. The presumed mechanism by which smoking causes cancer of the pancreas is thought to be the absorption of carcinogens which are taken up by the pancreas. There is an increased incidence of cancer of the pancreas and of lymphoma among chemists in the United States, and this fact has been interpreted to mean that industrial carcinogens may play a role in the disease. There is no question that tumors of the pancreas can be induced by feeding or injecting rats with benzanthracene or methylcholanthrene analogs and, in particular, various forms of nitrosamines. The pancreas is only one of many organs in which these agents will cause an adenocarcinoma.

There appears to be an increased incidence of cancer of the pancreas in patients with diabetes mellitus, particularly in patients who have had diabetes for some years. The Joslin Clinic reported an incidence of 256 cases of cancer of the pancreas in 10,000 diabetic patients, an exceedingly high incidence compared to the normal population, which is approximately 1 per 10,000. Chronic pancreatitis is alleged to have a relationship to cancer of the pancreas, particularly if there are calcifications in the pancreas. One review of the literature suggests that 3.6 per cent of patients with calcified chronic pancreatitis developed cancer of the pancreas, but adequate controls are lacking. Patients with hereditary pancreatitis of the mendelian-dominant form which results in calcification of the pancreas appear to have an increased incidence of carcinoma of the pancreas. One third of the disease-related deaths in patients with hereditary pancreatitis are due to cancer of the pancreas.

A study carried out with age-matched controls indicated that a high intake of alcohol was related to an increased incidence of cancer of the pancreas. Sixty-five per cent of patients with cancer of the pancreas at a VA Hospital had a moderate to heavy ethanol intake for an average of 15 years, whereas only 14 per cent of the age-, sex-, and race-matched controls were moderate to heavy alcoholics, and these had been drinking an average of 10 years. Unfortunately the incidence of chronic pancreatitis in these heavy drinkers was not established.

The clinical features of cancer of the pancreas are well described in textbooks, and will not be reviewed here. One of the most discouraging aspects of cancer of the pancreas is its almost total resistance to therapy. Over the period 1960 to 1970, there was no increase in one-year survival, which is only 14 per cent. There is no evidence that radical surgery, chemotherapy, radiation therapy, or any other form of therapy can cure or prolong life to a greater extent than palliative procedures. One of the reasons for this terrible mortality rate is the tendency of the tumor to spread before it becomes locally symptomatic. By the time of surgery, 90 per cent of patients show spread to regional lymph nodes and to the liver. There is a hypothesis that if we could detect the tumor when it is smaller it might be possible to increase the cure rate, but this has not been proved. The five year survival, adjusted for normal life expectancy, remains at 1 per cent for males and 2 per cent for females.

The combination of ultrasound as the initial screening test, a CCK pancreatic function test as the second screen, and ERCP as the confirming test will detect 90 per cent of patients with pancreatic disease and 80 per cent of those with cancer of the pancreas. Patients without pancreatic disease will be reliably shown not to have it. The usual secretin pancreatic function test cannot be considered to give similar results until this is demonstrated by a prospective study. The accuracy of cytologic examination of duodenal fluid has been investigated repeatedly in patients with pancreatic-biliary-duodenal cancers. Three large series which we have analyzed gave a positive predictive capacity of 90 per cent, a negative predictive capacity of 93 per cent, a sensitivity of 60 per cent, and a specificity of 99 per cent. Such success rates require expert cytologists.

Another approach to diagnosis is to test for circulating tumor antigens, such as carcinoembryonic antigen (CEA), alpha-fetoprotein, and pancreatic oncofetal antigen in patients with cancer of the pancreas. The pancreatic oncofetal antigen is a crude fraction of fetal pancreas which produces antibodies that cross-react with serum antigens in patients with many tumors. It is elevated occasionally in acute pancreatitis, in other carcinomas invading the pancreas, and in stones impacted in the common duct. The CEA level is elevated in many carcinomas, as well as in alcoholic hepatitis and heavy smokers. One investigation of pancreatic cancer showed that CEA was a positive predictor in 48 per cent and a negative predictor in 75 per cent of cases; alpha-fetoprotein gave values of 33 per cent and 71 per cent; pancreatic oncofetal antigen gave 60 per cent and 94 per cent predictabilities. When CEA and pancreatic fetal antigen were combined, the positive predictive capacity rose to 73 per cent. This would mean that a negative pancreatic fetal antigen test reliably rules out cancer of the pancreas, whereas positive CEA and pancreatic fetal antigen tests are good predictors that a patient has carcinoma, possibly of the pancreas. The unfortunate part of this study was that all the patients who had positive results had large tumors, with or without liver metastases. Studies using CEA indicate that, by the time the CEA is elevated, the tumor is large, outside the pancreas, and therefore inoperable.

Measurements of serum amylase, serum lipase, or urinary amylase excretion are not helpful in the diagnosis of cancer of the pancreas. Only 13 per cent of the serum amylases, 11 per cent of lipases, and 27 per cent of the hourly urinary amylase excretions were elevated in a large series from the Mayo Clinic. There is no evidence that the amylase:creatinine clearance ratio improves these statistics. The results of duodenal intubation and secretin tests by many investigators have indicated that the usual finding in cancer of the head of the pancreas is a decreased volume of pancreatic juice which contains a normal concentration of bicarbonate and enzymes. This results from a block of the duct of Wirsung in the head of the gland. Enzyme output was decreased in 90 per cent of patients with cancer of the head of the pancreas and proportionately less as the tumor blocked the duct in the body and in the tail of the gland. The most discriminating test was the output of trypsin or lipase after CCK infusion.

A more direct diagnostic procedure is percutaneous aspiration biopsy of the pancreas, using a long 23-gauge needle and aspirating with saline vigorously to obtain cells, which are then examined cytologically. The guiding of the needle into a mass in the pancreas is done by ultrasound.

Angiography has other advantages. It allows one to predict the size of the tumor, often allows one to predict whether it is resectable, and it can help distinguish whether a positive ERCP is due to cancer or chronic pancreatitis. Combining ERCP with cytology has improved diagnostic yields. In one series, ERCP detected 65 per cent of the cases, and cytology taken at ERCP detected 54 per cent. When both were combined, the detection rate over-all was 92 per cent. Dreiling has performed over 5000 pancreatic function tests, using a bolus of secretin alone and measuring volume, bicarbonate, and amylase. For the ability to detect abnormalities of the pancreas by this test, he reports a positive predictive value of 93 per cent and a negative predictability of 95 per cent. In a series of 400 patients with cancer of the pancreas, he was able to detect a quantitative defect, i.e., decreased volume and outputs but normal concentrations of bicarbonate and enzymes, in 95 per cent of patients with carcinoma of the head of the pancreas. The yield was only 17 per cent in cancer of the body and 19 per cent in cancer of the tail. His cytology examinations gave a sensitivity of 83 per cent. By Dreiling's data, the secretin test could be substituted for the CCK-secretin test.

The diagnostic accuracy of computerized tomography is in the process of being evaluated. At the present time it shows remarkable ability to visualize pancreatic masses and to tell whether or not they are within the gland or have invaded surrounding structures. The lower limit of detection is around 2 cm., which would be an early carcinoma of the pancreas and possibly lead to better survival rates. The false-positive problem in computerized tomography of the abdomen has not yet been well evaluated. If ultrasound and computerized tomography turn out to be sensitive enough, then patients with minimal complaints could be screened reliably for cancer of the pancreas before undergoing invasive and specific diagnostic studies such as ERCP, angiography, and surgery. If this approach gives a high level of accuracy, then a prospective study of the radical surgery of small lesions of the pancreas would be possible.

The natural history of the disease involves intraductal spread of the tumor, multifocal occurrence of the malignancy, and a tendency for lymph node spread over a wide area. Total pancreaticoduodenectomy with splenectomy overcomes some of these problems and permits wider lymphatic resection. It also avoids the need for pancreaticojejunal anastomosis, which is a source of much of the postoperative morbidity in a partial pancreatectomy, the Whipple operation. Patients who have undergone a total pancreatectomy can live in good health if their tumor does not recur. Their digestion is well managed by potent pancreatic extracts combined with cimetidine to prevent inactivation of the oral pancreatic enzymes. Diabetes is managed with 30 to 40 units of lente insulin per day, but the diabetes is somewhat brittle.

CYSTIC FIBROSIS

This is the commonest lethal *genetic* disease of white populations, occurring in one in 2000 live births of populations of Caucasian descent. Cystic fibrosis is inherited as an autosomal recessive trait, which means that about 5 per cent of the population are carriers. It is characterized clinically by chronic pulmonary disease, pancreatic achylia, and abnormally high sweat electrolytes. Other symptoms that can complicate the picture are meconium ileus, hepatic cirrhosis, and rectal prolapse. Cystic fibrosis is a generalized disorder that involves the pancreas seriously in 80 to 90 per cent of patients.

Two main defects lead to the pathologic damage. The first is an abnormality in the glycoprotein-rich secretions of most exocrine glands which leads to precipitation of secretions in the ductal system of these glands. The cause of the precipitation has never been explained. As a result, the pancreas, the lungs, the biliary tree, and the crypts of the gastrointestinal tract suffer primarily from this abnormality. The second major abnormality is an electrolyte defect of the eccrine sweat glands that results in high sodium and chloride concentrations in the sweat. Its clinical significance is that salt depletion may occur in hot weather. The diagnosis rests on the demonstration of an elevated sweat chloride concentration in a patient who has either a history of cystic fibrosis in the family or has chronic pulmonary disease, malabsorption, or failure to grow. The standard method of measuring sweat sodium and chloride is now pilocarpine iontophoresis with collection of the sweat in a cellulose sponge. Values of sweat chloride above 70 mEq./L. are diagnostic, and values between 50 to

60 mEq./L. are suggestive of cystic fibrosis. The upper normal value for sweat sodium is 70 mEq./L.

After the age of 20, sweat sodium and chloride values are not much different than in the younger age group. The upper limits of normal, i.e., two standard deviations above the mean, are 52 mEq./L. for chloride and 70 mEq./L. for sodium. Potassium concentrations are also slightly elevated in cystic fibrosis. An abnormal sweat test alone is not sufficient for a diagnosis of cystic fibrosis because there are other conditions in pediatrics in which these sweat electrolytes may be elevated. In these cases, duodenal drainage to assess pancreatic function is useful.

At the present time, there is no method by which heterozygotes can be identified by any chemical tests, including sweat electrolytes. Adult patients with chronic obstructive pulmonary disease have been repeatedly studied to see if some of them represent subclinical or primarily pulmonary forms of cystic fibrosis. The evidence at the present time is that this is a rare occurrence and that most patients with chronic obstructive pulmonary disease have normal sweat electrolytes. Those who have slight elevations return promptly to normal with the stimulus of salt restriction in the diet or a salt-retaining hormone. Patients with cystic fibrosis are not able to reduce their sweat electrolytes by either form of stress.

Pancreatic insufficiency is not the major clinical problem in cystic fibrosis because it can be treated adequately. Progressive lung disease determines the fate of the patient. At the present time, about 50 per cent of patients live to their 10th birthday, 30 per cent to their 20th birthday, and few beyond the age of 30. An increasing number of patients are coming into adult medicine and require the treatment of internists.

Pancreatic achylia is present in 80 to 90 per cent of patients. The pancreatic ducts are obstructed by inspissated pancreatic secretions, leading to distention and dilatation of the ducts, atrophy and degeneration of the acini, and severe fibrosis which eventually results in almost total destruction of acinar tissue, fatty replacement of pancreatic parenchyma, and persistence of the islets of Langerhans surrounded by fibrous tissue. Meconium ileus is due to the accumulation of thick, sticky material in the lumen of the bowel. This material is predominately sloughed mucosa and precipitated protein. Previously this was thought to accumulate because of lack of pancreatic enzyme digestion, but pathologic studies indicate that meconium ileus can occur in the newborn when the pancreas is still normal or mildly affected, whereas the crypts of Lieberkühn are always severely affected in the intestinal mucosa of patients with meconium ileus.

The pancreatic secretory abnormality has been studied with CCK-secretin tests in children with early pancreatic insufficiency. These children produce a small volume of juice containing high enzyme concentrations but a low bicarbonate content, suggesting that the initial damage is much more severe to the ductal cells than to the acinar cells. Eventually, acinar function is lost as well.

Pancreatic achylia produces the expected syndrome of maldigestion, but there is some evidence of malabsorption as well. Although the D-xylose test is normal and peroral biopsies of the small intestine have shown normal histologic patterns in the majority of cases, disaccharidase activities are sometimes decreased, usually lactase. Moreover, a fascinating abnormality in bile acid metabolism has been reported in which patients with cystic fibrosis and pancreatic insufficiency are found to excrete excessive amounts of bile acids into the stool, with losses as large as those seen in patients with ileal resection. Patients without steatorrhea do not excrete excessive bile acids. Although fat loss is improved by adding sodium bicarbonate to the pancreatic enzymes, it does not change the excessive bile acid loss. Administration of pancreatic enzymes in large amounts eventually will correct both the bile acid loss and the fat loss. This puzzling situation has been further investigated in cystic fibrosis patients who have normal intestinal function, biopsies, disaccharidase levels, and functioning gallbladders. It was found that such patients have a low bile acid pool, which doubles on administration of pancreatic enzymes. The secondary bile acids are reduced somewhat by treatment, from 57 per cent of the total to 40 per cent. Surprisingly, total bile acid synthesis remains the same before and after treatment. The fractional turnover rate of the untreated patients is very high, 0.6 or 0.7 per day for cholic and chenodeoxycholic acid; this turnover is reduced by treatment with pancreatic enzymes to 0.2 or 0.4 per day. One hypothesis that has been advanced to explain this is that the bile acids are bound to undigested protein or carbohydrate, leading to increased stool losses. The data are consistent with rapid cycling of the bile acid pool through the intestine, as is seen in patients who have a non-functioning gallbladder or who have had their gallbladder removed. There is no correlation between fat loss and bile acid loss in these patients. Bile acid concentrations in the duodenum, either fasting or after stimulation of gallbladder contraction, are normal both before and after pancreatic enzyme treatment.

One possible explanation for the increased cycling and functional cholecystectomy in such patients might be the constant and excessive secretion of large amounts of cholecystokinin, which is known to be secreted in chronic pancreatitis due to some unexplained lack of feedback signal to the cells which secrete CCK due to lack of pancreatic enzymes in the gut. Improvement in the bile salt metabolic picture with pancreatic enzymes may simply represent decreased CCK release. Confirmation of this speculation will require the development of a reliable plasma radioimmunoassay for CCK. Adults who have pancreatic insufficiency or patients with cystic fibrosis who survive to adulthood have steatorrhea but do not show these huge bile acid losses.

The gallbladder also can be involved in cystic fibrosis, leading to atrophy and obstruction in up to 25 per cent of patients. This would lead to increased cycling of bile salts but would not explain the loss in the stool.

Oral glucose tolerance tests in patients with cystic fibrosis show abnormal findings in 40 per cent of patients. As the glucose intolerance becomes more severe, the release of insulin into the peripheral plasma is more delayed and blunted. A small number of these patients eventually end with true diabetes. The striking fact is that when these patients are stimulated with glucagon or tolbutamide they show a sudden increase in release of insulin, suggesting that there is not a deficiency in number of beta cells or in stored insulin but an abnormality in stimulation or release by the normal stimulus, elevated blood glucose. Further studies have indicated that both insulin and glucagon release are impaired after a standard stimulation, such as intravenous arginine infusion. As long as the patients maintain a normal glucagon/insulin ratio they do not show much glucose intolerance. In addition, cystic fibrosis patients are not insulin-resistant as are adult-onset obese diabetics. Therefore, the conclusion has been that the islet cells encased in their fibrotic pancreas may not receive stimuli such as glucose normally or that the release of glucagon or insulin may be impaired because of the anatomic situation. Fortunately, clinical diabetes is an unusual complication in this disease.

The pathogenesis of cystic fibrosis has not been explained — either the precipitation of exocrine secretions or the impairment in sodium and chloride loss from eccrine glands. At present, it is important to differentiate a few rare disease entities from cystic fibrosis in children. There is a condition called aplasia of the exocrine pancreas in which there is complete replacement of the exocrine parenchyma by fat, normal islets of Langerhans, and no fibrosis or dilatation of the ducts. There is also a syndrome of pancreatic deficiency and bone marrow dysfunction in which the patients have pancreatic achylia, shortness of stature, a normal sweat test, no pulmonary involvement, and a variety of hematologic abnormalities including thrombocytopenia, neutropenia, and anemia. Fecal fat is only slightly increased, and malabsorption not marked.

REFERENCES

GENERAL REVIEWS

Delmont, J. (Ed.): The Sphincter of Oddi. Karger, Basel, 1977.

Howat, H. T. (Ed.): Clinics in Gastroenterology, Vol. 1. W. B. Saunders, Philadelphia, 1972.

BIOCHEMISTRY, PHYSIOLOGY

Boden, G., Wilson, R. M., Essa-Koumar, N., and Owen, O. E.: Effects of a protein meal, intraduodenal HCl, and oleic acid on portal and peripheral venous secretin and on pancreatic bicarbonate secretion. Gut, 19:277, 1978.

Borgstrom, B., and Erlanson, C.: Pancreatic juice co-lipase: physiological importance. Biochim. Biophys. Acta, 242:509, 1971.

Elmslie, R., White, T. T., and Magee, D. F.: The significance of reflux of trypsin and bile in the pathogenesis of human pancreatitis. Brit. J. Surg., 53:809, 1966.

Feinstein, G., Hofstein, R., Koifmann, J., and Sokolovsky, M.: Human pancreatic proteolytic enzymes and protein inhibitors. Eur. J. Biochem., 43:569, 1974.

Guy, O., Lombardo, D., Bartelt, D. C., et al.: Two human trypsinogens. Purification, molecular properties, and N-terminal sequences. Biochemistry, 17:1669, 1978.

Harper, A. A.: The control of pancreatic secretion. Gut, 13:308, 1972.

Kassell, B., and Kay, J.: Zymogens of proteolytic enzymes. Science, 180:1022, 1973.

Keller, P. J., and Allan, B. J.: The protein composition of human pancreatic juice. J. Biol. Chem., 242:281, 1967.

Lightwood, R., and Reber, H. A.: Micropuncture study of pancreatic secretion in the cat. Gastroenterology, 72:61, 1977.

Maroux, S., Baratti, J., and Desnuelle, P.: Purification and specificity of porcine enterokinase. J. Biol. Chem., 246:5031, 1971.

Merritt, A. D., and Karn, R. C.: The human α-amylases. Adv. Hum. Genet., 8:135, 1977.

Pearse, A. G. F., Polak, J. M., and Bloom, S. R.: The newer gut hormones. Cellular sources, physiology, pathology, and clinical aspects. Gastroenterology, 72:746, 1977.

Pubols, M. H., Bartelt, D. C., and Greene, L. J.: Trypsin inhibitor from human pancreas and pancreatic juice. J. Biol. Chem., 249:2235, 1974.

Rehfeld, J. F.: Immunochemical studies on cholecystokinin. II. Distribution and molecular heterogeneity in the central nervous system and small intestine of man and hog. J. Biol. Chem., 253:4022, 1978.

Schmitz, J., Preiser, H., Maestracci, D., et al.: Subcellular localization of enterokinase in human small intestine. Biochim. Biophys. Acta, 343:435, 1974.

Singh, M., and Webster, P. D. III.: Neurohumoral control of pancreatic secretion. Gastroenterology, 74:294, 1978.

Stiefel, D. J., and Keller, P. J.: Preparation and some properties of human pancreatic amylase, including a comparison with human parotid amylase. Biochim. Biophys. Acta, 302:345, 1973.

DIAGNOSTIC TESTS

Arvanitakis, C., and Cooke, A. R.: Diagnostic tests of exocrine pancreatic function and disease. Gastroenterology, 74:932, 1978.

Burrows, P. J., Fleming, J. S., Garnett, E. S., et al.: Clinical evaluation of the ^{14}C-fat absorption test. Gut, 15:147, 1974.

Burton, P., Hammond, E. M., Harper, A. A., et al.: Serum amylase and serum lipase levels in man after administration of secretin and pancreozymin. Gut, *1*:125, 1960.

Cotton, P. B.: Progress report. ERCP. Gut, *18*:316, 1977.

Eaton, S. B., Fleischli, D. J., Pollard, J. J., et al.: Comparison of current radiologic approaches to the diagnosis of pancreatic disease. N. Engl. J. Med., *279*:389, 1968.

Gyr, K., Stalder, G. A., Schiffmann, I., et al.: Oral administration of a chymotrypsin-labile peptide — a new test of exocrine pancreatic function in man (PFT). Gut, *17*:27, 1976.

Levitt, M. D., Ellis, C., and Engel, R. R.: Isoelectric focusing studies of human serum and tissue isoamylases. J. Lab. Clin. Med., *90*:141, 1977.

O'Donnell, M. D., FitzGerald, O., and McGeeney, K. F.: Differential serum amylase determination by use of an inhibitor, and design of a routine procedure. Clin. Chem., *23*:560, 1977.

ACUTE PANCREATITIS

Acosta, J. M., and Ledesma, C. L.: Gallstone migration as a cause of acute pancreatitis. N. Engl. J. Med., *290*:484, 1974.

Creutzfeldt, W., and Schmidt, H.: Aetiology and pathogenesis of pancreatitis (current concepts). Scand. J. Gastroenterol. (Suppl.), *6*:47, 1970.

Drew, S. I., Joffe, B., Vinik, A., et al.: The first 24 hours of acute pancreatitis. Changes in biochemical and endocrine homeostasis in patients with pancreatitis compared to those in control subjects undergoing stress for reasons other than pancreatitis. Am. J. Med., *64*:795, 1978.

Elliott, D. W.: Appraisal of the usefulness of various experimental models for the study of acute pancreatitis. *In* Beck, I. T., and Sinclair, D. B. (Eds.): The Exocrine Pancreas. Williams & Wilkins, Baltimore, 1971, p. 86.

Geokas, M. C., Rinderknecht, H., Swanson, V., and Haverback, B. J.: The role of elastase in acute hemorrhagic pancreatitis in man. Lab. Invest., *19*:235, 1968.

Popper, H. L., Necheles, H., and Russell, K. C.: Transition of pancreatic edema into pancreatic necrosis. Surg. Gynecol. Obstet., *87*:79, 1948.

Robertson, G. M., Moore, E. W., Switz, D. M., et al.: Inadequate parathyroid response in acute pancreatitis. N. Engl. J. Med., *294*:512, 1976.

Weir, G. C., Lesser, P. B., Drop, L. J., et al.: The hypocalcemia of acute pancreatitis. Ann. Int. Med., *83*:185, 1975.

CHRONIC PANCREATITIS

Allen, R. H., Seetharam, B., Podell, E., and Alpers, D. H.: Effect of proteolytic enzymes on the binding of cobalamin to R protein and intrinsic factor. J. Clin. Invest., *61*:47, 1978.

Cameron, J. L., Capuzzi, D. M., Zuidema, G. D., and Margolis, S.: Acute pancreatitis with hyperlipemia. Evidence for a persistent defect in lipid metabolism. Am. J. Med., *56*:482, 1974.

Cameron, J. L., Zuidema, G. D., and Margolis, S.: A pathogenesis for alcoholic pancreatitis. Surgery, *77*:754, 1975.

Cameron, J. L.: Chronic pancreatic ascites and pancreatic pleural effusions. Gastroenterology, *74*:134, 1978.

DiMagno, E. P., Go, V. L. W., and Summerskill, W. H. J.: Relations between pancreatic enzyme outputs and malabsorption in severe pancreatic insufficiency. N. Engl. J. Med., *288*:813, 1973.

Donowitz, M., Hendler, R., Spiro, H. M., Binder, H. J., and Felig, P.: Glucagon secretion in acute and chronic pancreatitis. Ann. Int. Med., *83*:778, 1975.

Frier, B. M., Saunders, J. H. B., Wormsley, K. G., and Bouchier, I. A. D.: Exocrine pancreatic function in juvenile-onset diabetes mellitus. Gut, *17*:685, 1976.

Gross, J. B., and Jones, J. D.: Hereditary pancreatitis: analysis of experience to May 1969. *In* Beck, I. T. and Sinclair, D. G. (Eds.): The Exocrine Pancreas. Williams & Wilkins, Baltimore, 1971, p. 247.

Levrat, M., Descos, L., Moulinier, B., and Pasquier, J.: Evolution au long cours des pancréatites chroniques. Arch. Franc. des Malad. de l'Appareil Digest., *59*:5, 1970.

Llanos, O. L., Swierczek, J. S., Teichmann, R. K., et al.: Effect of alcohol on the release of secretin and pancreatic secretion. Surgery, *81*:661, 1977.

Marin, G. A., Ward, N. L., and Fischer, R.: Effect of ethanol on pancreatic and biliary secretions in humans. Am. J. Digest. Dis., *18*:825, 1973.

Sarles, H., Sarles, J-C., Camatte, R., et al.: Observations on 205 confirmed cases of acute pancreatitis, recurring pancreatitis, and chronic pancreatitis. Gut, *6*:545, 1965.

Sarles, H.: Chronic calcifying pancreatitis — chronic alcoholic pancreatitis. Gastroenterology, *66*:604, 1974.

Strum, W. B., and Spiro, H. M.: Chronic pancreatitis. Ann. Int. Med., *74*:264, 1971.

CANCER OF THE PANCREAS

DiMagno, E. P., Malagelada, J-R., Taylor, W. F., and Go, V. L. W.: A prospective comparison of current diagnostic tests for pancreatic cancer. N. Engl. J. Med., *297*:737, 1977.

Mainz, D., and Webster, P. D. III.: Pancreatic carcinoma. A review of etiologic considerations. Am. J. Digest. Dis., *19*:459, 1974.

Morgan, R. G. H., and Wormsley, K. G.: Progress report. Cancer of the pancreas. Gut, *18*:580, 1977.

Wood, R. A. B., and Moossa, A. R.: The prospective evaluation of tumour-associated antigens for the early diagnosis of pancreatic cancer. Br. J. Surg., *64*:718, 1977.

CYSTIC FIBROSIS.

di Sant'Agnese, P. A.: Cystic fibrosis and other genetic pancreatic diseases in childhood. *In* Beck, I. T. and Sinclair, D. G. (Eds.): The Exocrine Pancreas. Williams & Wilkins, Baltimore, 1971, p. 227.

Handwerger, S., Roth, J., Gorden, P., et al.: Glucose intolerance in cystic fibrosis. N. Engl. J. Med., *281*:451, 1969.

Weber, A. M., Roy, C. C., Chartrand, L., et al.: Relationship between bile acid malabsorption and pancreatic insufficiency in cystic fibrosis. Gut, *17*:295, 1976.

31

Nutritional Factors in Disease

George A. Bray

The nutritional factors in human physiology include all the necessary as well as all the usable environmental elements taken in through the mouth. Carbohydrates, proteins, and lipids are the dietary elements ingested in large quantity, but the vitamins and minerals, although small in quantity, are of equal importance in maintenance of normal health. Nutrition deals with the composition and utilization of dietary components. The nutritional disorders which result from the interaction of diet and the human body are the subject of this chapter. Certain aspects of biochemistry and physiology will be reviewed as they relate to the mechanisms by which deviations from normal nutrition produce their pathologic consequences.

An over-all view of the interaction of nutrition and metabolism is presented in Figure 31-1. In this figure, the dietary or storage forms of triglycerides, polysaccharides, and proteins are shown at the top, their circulating forms in the middle, and the final common pathway for metabolism at the bottom. Dietary intake of macro- and micronutrients varies considerably between individuals in a given population. They also change from day to day in the same individual and even more strikingly between cultural or population groups. In spite of this, the requirements for operation of the "human machine" are essentially the same. The body is thus confronted with a series of metabolic problems: (1) Ingestion and digestion of diverse nutrients. (2) Absorption of the simple products for storage. (3) Utilization of nutrients for body needs. (4) Disposal or storage of excesses. (5) Attempts to remedy deficiencies by interconversion of nutrients.

The essential nature of vitamins and minerals has been clearly established and these will be discussed in detail below. There is no clearly es-tablished requirement for carbohydrates since in their absence, glucose can be obtained from amino acids, provided that sufficient quantities of protein are available. However, most diets provide a mixture of polysaccharides and simple carbohydrates which are usually a major dietary source of calories. The polyunsaturated fatty acids (i.e., linoleic or linolenic acids) cannot be synthesized in the body. A requirement of approximately 1 to 3 per cent of total caloric intake as essential fatty acids is necessary for maintenance of health. When essential fatty acids are

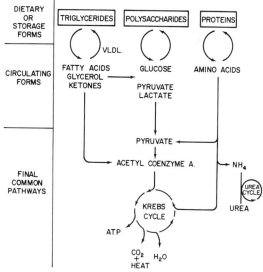

Figure 31–1 An overview of metabolism. This figure provides a view of the flow of nutrients from their dietary sources and their stored forms into the final common pathway of acetyl-CoA formation and metabolism through the tricarboxylic acid cycle.

Chemical Structure: CH_3—$(CH_2)_{14}$—$COOH + 23\ O_2 \rightarrow 16\ CO_2 + 16\ H_2O$

(palmitic acid)

Molecular Weights: 256   736   704   288

Figure 31–2 Oxidation or complete combustion of palmitic acid to CO_2 and water. During this oxidation, a compound weighing 256 g./mole is burned. Since the CO_2 and O_2 will equilibrate with the environment, 288 g. of water remain after the combustion of only 256 g. of fatty acid. This explains how the oxidation of fat can lead to the temporary accumulation of weight in individual patients.

absent, changes in the skin are seen clinically. Deficiencies in essential fatty acids are most easily demonstrated in growing children but can also be manifested in adults if they are fed a diet deficient in these acids for several weeks. A number of amino acids are also required in the diet since they cannot be synthesized in the body. These nine essential amino acids include lysine, methionine, valine, leucine, isoleucine, tryptophan, phenylalanine, threonine, and histidine. Deficiency of essential amino acids impairs protein synthesis. There is great variability in the amino acid composition of dietary proteins. Vegetable proteins, for example, tend to be relatively deficient in one or another amino acid compared to amino acid composition of human proteins. Thus, wheat is deficient in lysine, whereas corn is deficient in tryptophan. Of the vegetable proteins, soy beans and other beans provide the highest quantities of essential amino acids.

OBESITY

Obesity is appropriately defined in terms of body fatness. In its extreme forms, obesity can be recognized at a glance. The round-jowled, puffing, often red-faced individual weighing in excess of 300 pounds is a familiar sight. However, quantitative assessment of the degree of obesity in these individuals and in lesser degrees of obesity is difficult for the physician. Neither the usual recording of body weight nor the criteria based upon weight in relation to height are sufficiently accurate in many instances. For example, above average muscle development of an unusually large skeleton could be mistaken for obesity. It is fair to say, however, that when weight exceeds the norm by more than 30 per cent in any but the most athletic male, there is almost certainly obesity, i.e., an above-normal percentage of fat.

Measurement of body weight on a scale does not distinguish between mass occurring as excess fat, as bone, as muscle, or as water, and this lack of distinction can have significant clinical implications. Obese patients often fail to lose weight and may even gain weight when put on a diet. This is usually attributed to "cheating" by the patient when it may, in fact, be the result of the wrong measurement. This can happen even when caloric intake is severely restricted, and careful measurements shown that food intake is less than that required to maintain weight. This paradox is explained in terms of the oxidation of fatty acids (Fig. 31-2). This equation shows that when 256 grams of palmitic acid are completely oxidized, 288 grams of water are produced. When gaseous exchange of O_2 and CO_2 is completed, the body is left with a net gain in weight of 32 grams of water for every mole of palmitic acid which is oxidized. Until this excess water is excreted, a patient may gain weight when fatty acids are the principal metabolic fuel. Such a phenomenon has been observed frequently and has been known to persist for more than 30 days, even when patients have been hospitalized under strictly controlled conditions. Measuring body weight on a scale would be misleading under these circumstances, since the scale could not assess changes in the various components of the body weight. For this reason, more sophisticated techniques are necessary to understand the nature of the weight in obesity and its relation to the normal composition of the human body.

Analysis of Human Body Components

Several techniques have been used to assess the components of the human body (Table 31-1). The most direct method is analysis of individual cadavers for lipid, water, protein, and ash components. Technical difficulty in such analyses and the rarity of opportunities to obtain cadavers for

TABLE 31–1 TECHNIQUES FOR MEASURING "FATNESS"

A. Direct carcass analysis
B. Indirect methods
  1. Densitometric
  2. Dilutional
    a. Radioactive (^3H_2O, ^{40}K)
    b. Chemical (cyclopropane)
  3. Anthropometric
    a. Height and weight
    b. Skin folds
    c. Ultrasound
    d. Soft-tissue x-rays

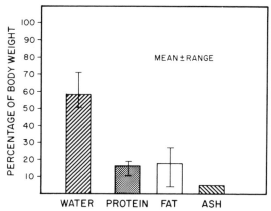

Figure 31-3 Analysis of body composition in five cadavers. The heights of individual bars are the mean for five patients, and the vertical lines represent the range. Body components are plotted as per cent of total body weight. (Adapted from Widdowson, E. M.: *In* Brozek, J. (ed.): Human Body Composition: Approaches and Application. Pergamon Press, New York, 1965.)

this purpose have led to publication of only seven complete studies. The data from five of these analyses of total body composition are shown in Figure 31-3. Water represented just under two thirds of the total body weight. Fat and protein were at least 15 per cent of body weight. Since direct analyses cannot be performed on the living subject, three alternative methods have been used. Measurement of density of the human being is the first of these. This can be accomplished by weighing the subject in and out of water, a principle that Archimedes discovered centuries ago. It allows an assessment of the fraction of body weight which is fat and that which is nonfat. Measurement of body density has been widely applied, since it is simple and highly accurate.

The second approach to measurement of body composition in vivo is the use of isotope dilution. When a known quantity of isotope is injected into the bloodstream and its concentration is measured after allowing for equilibration with the body stores of that compound, the ratio of radioactivity in plasma to the quantity injected will give a measure of the apparent volume of distribution for the substance. Radioactively labeled water (^3H_2O), potassium (^{42}K or ^{40}K), and sodium (^{22}Na or ^{24}Na) have been among the most widely used substances for obtaining measurements of body composition by this technique. The data from the measurements obtained by isotopic dilution are similar to those obtained using body density and direct carcass analysis. However, measurements by isotopic dilution provide additional information, since they allow for an estimate of intra- and extracellular fluid compartments.

Studies on humans during gain and loss of weight have provided important insights into the nature of the components which are accumulated or lost. In normal volunteers gaining 10 to 20 kg. over a period of six months, nearly two thirds of the increase in weight is fat; the remainder is extracellular fluid and cellular components. Direct measurements of the size of fat cells from such individuals have shown that the size of the fat cells has increased with weight gain. Conversely, when obese patients lose weight in a hospital, the initial weight loss is predominantly water and protein, but with prolonged caloric restriction the largest fraction of the loss is fat. These data therefore illustrate the complexity of body composition and the difficulties in assigning a diagnosis of obesity based on body weight alone.

Measuring the thickness of skin folds is another approach to assessing the amount of body fat. Criteria have been developed for assessing fatness by measuring the triceps skinfold, the combined triceps and subscapular skinfold, or a group of skinfolds in four regions including biceps, triceps, subscapular, and suprailiac. A mid-triceps skinfold greater than 25 mm. in females and 18 mm. in males is defined in some studies as obesity, and a combined triceps plus subscapular of 37 mm. as obesity in other studies. Criteria for other skinfolds and their relationships to body fat can be obtained by consulting the monograph by Bray (1976).

Despite all its limitations, the scale is still the best tool available for patients and most physicians to use in determining the degree of excess weight. When this overweight is sufficiently great, i.e., 30 per cent or more above values in standard tables for height and weight (Table 31-2), one can assume that the patient is obese.

An even more adequate way to relate height and weight for assessing the magnitude of overweight is with the body mass index. This index also is defined as the ratio of the body weight in kilograms divided by the height in meters squared (Wt/[Ht]²). When the body mass index (BMI) is 27, this is usually defined as overweight, and when the body mass index is 30 or more, it is in a range associated with excess risk of disease. A table for obtaining body mass index from measurements of height and weight can be obtained in the reference by Bray, Jordan, and Sims (1976).

Imbalance Between Caloric Intake and Expenditure

There is little argument at present that obesity results from an excess intake of food in relation to body needs. The basis for this proposition resides in the work published in 1783 by Lavoisier and Laplace using the guinea pig. The "law of the conservation of energy" gave this early work a

TABLE 31–2 DESIRABLE WEIGHT IN RELATION TO HEIGHT*

Height	Men		Women	
	Average	Range	Average	Range
4 10″			102	92–119
4′ 11″			104	94–122
5′ 0″			107	96–125
5′ 1″			110	99–128
5′ 2″	123	112–141	113	102–131
5′ 3″	127	115–144	116	105–134
5′ 4″	130	118–148	120	108–138
5′ 5″	133	121–152	123	111–142
5′ 6″	136	124–156	128	114–146
5′ 7″	140	128–161	132	118–150
5′ 8″	145	132–166	136	122–154
5′ 9″	149	136–170	140	126–158
5′ 10″	153	140–174	144	130–163
5′ 11″	158	144–179	148	134–168
6′ 0″	162	148–184	152	138–173
6′ 1″	166	152–189		
6′ 2″	171	156–194		
6′ 3″	176	160–199		
6′ 4″	181	164–204		

*Adapted from data courtesy of the Metropolitan Life Insurance Company.

theoretical basis. That this law applies to species other than the guinea pig was readily shown. In classic experiments, Rubner found that the amount of heat produced by a dog in the absence of food equals the heat from combustion of the fat and protein which were burned during starvation minus the heat of combustion in the urine. Atwater and Benedict made similar observations in man and concluded that "for practical purposes we are, therefore, warranted in assuming that the law of conservation of energy obtains in general in the living organism as indeed there is every a priori reason to believe that it must." A demonstration that this law applied to the obese subject was delayed until the 20th century. It has been amply demonstrated that obese subjects, like their lean counterparts and all other known living systems, obey the law of conservation of energy.

Measurements of the energy contained in food are expressed in calories or joules (joule=4.18 kcal.). A calorie measures the quantity of heat required to raise the temperature of 1 gram of water from 15° to 16° C. As noted above, the quantity of heat obtained by the combustion of a foodstuff outside the body is equal to the quantity of heat obtained by combustion of the same foodstuff to the same end products. In the case of carbohydrate and lipid, the end products are carbon dioxide and water and the heat produced

during their combustion in vitro is directly related to the heat produced in vivo. Since protein is incompletely oxidized in the living organism, a correction is required. The end products of protein catabolism are carbon dioxide, water, and urea. The urea excreted in the urine represents a significant number of calories. Thus, to obtain an accurate assessment of total caloric utilization, the quantity of urea must be known.

Measurement of O_2 consumption and CO_2 production with a correction for urinary nitrogen allows an indirect quantitation of energy expenditure. This technique of indirect calorimetry (measurement of oxygen consumption and carbon dioxide production) has been widely used in assessing the caloric needs of the human organism. Figure 31-4 is a presentation of the energy expenditure for a reference man and a reference woman as estimated by the National Research Council in 1974. The male, aged 22 and weighing 70 kilos, required 2800 calories; the female, aged 22 and weighing

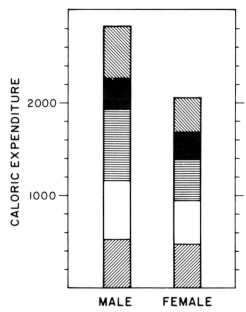

Figure 31–4 Estimated average energy expenditure of men and women. The lower hatched bars represent the energy expended during sleeping and reclining (1.0 to 1.1 kcal./min.). The unshaded open portion represents the average energy expended during sitting (1.1 to 1.5 kcal./min.). The horizontally shaded section represents the energy expenditure during standing (1.5 to 2.5 kcal./min.). The solid segment represents the energy expended during walking (2.5 to 3 kcal./min.). The top portion of each bar represents other activities (3 to 4.5 kcal./min.). The lower value within each preceding set of parentheses represents the average value for females and the upper value the average for males. (Adapted from Recommended Dietary Allowances.)

58 kilos, required 2000 calories. The total requirements for the reference subjects in 1974 are about 10 per cent lower than a decade earlier. Yet, even these current estimates are probably too high. The increased use of the automobile and decreased amount of physical activity have accounted for a steady reduction in total caloric requirements of men and women. Since these are "reference" figures, they must be modified before being applied to a given individual. Factors such as age, the degree of activity, pregnancy, and the presence of certain diseases all serve to modify energy requirements. There are convincing data that the caloric needs decline with age at approximately 5 per cent per decade. Since activity also declines, the actual caloric need declines even more rapidly. Pregnancy, as well as several hormones, can increase the body's oxygen consumption. Thyroid hormone was the first hormone shown to have a calorigenic action. In conditions of thyroid hormone excess, total energy requirements are increased, and in the absence of this hormone, total caloric requirements drop sharply. Other hormones which have a calorigenic action include the catecholamines (epinephrine and norepinephrine), human growth hormone, and the androgenic steroids.

Regulation of Energy Balance

As noted earlier, obesity represents an imbalance between caloric intake and caloric expenditure. It now appears that the regulation of food intake, as well as the utilization of calories, is defective in the obese individual. This net effect appears as an increase in the efficiency for food utilization. Efficiency may be defined in a number of ways. We will consider efficiency from the point of view of food storage. The more weight gained for a given food intake, the greater the efficiency. Thus, a more efficient animal or human being will store a greater fraction of total calories ingested. For every 1000 calories ingested, the efficient animal might store 20 per cent, while the inefficient animal would store only 10 per cent. This means that for the same caloric intake, it is possible for one animal to become considerably heavier and more obese than another. Such considerations have obvious commercial significance and it has been observed that animals bred for obesity will store a larger fraction of their calories in their carcass than will lean animals. Differences in efficiency have also been noted in laboratory animals in which obesity is inherited as a recessive trait. In these obese animals, more fat will accumulate per gram of food ingested than in lean littermates. Although few measurements are available, the current data would suggest that this form of efficiency results from inactivity of the fat animal. Thus, for any given food intake, fewer calories are used for activity than in the lean animal. We must conclude that the efficiency of the fat animal may be substantially greater than for lean animals.

Regulation of Food Intake

Control of food intake involves several factors. These include components of the central nervous system, metabolic factors, and the external environment.

Central Nervous System. The classic experiment of Hetherington and Ranson demonstrated that injury to a portion of the hypothalamus near the midline in the so-called "ventromedial nucleus" would consistently induce increased food intake and obesity in laboratory animals. This syndrome in experimental animals is analogous to the development of obesity noted by Fröhlich in his classic case report in 1903. Hypothalamic obesity resulting from injury to the ventromedial nucleus is accompanied by a number of alterations. The animals are consistently and uniformly hyperphagic and prefer a diet with a high fat content rather than a high carbohydrate or a high protein diet. They will avoid eating food which tastes bad or which has an unpalatable consistency. They show increased levels of insulin and enlargement of the pancreatic islets of Langerhans. Finally, these animals, though initially hyperactive following introduction of these lesions, become hypoactive, although they can easily be aroused to rage. Injury to this region of the brain is followed by a period of rapid weight gain (dynamic phase) and then by a plateau weight (static phase), at which they will again regulate their food intake and body weight.

Lateral to this ventromedial nucleus is a second hypothalamic area, destruction of which leads to total, but temporary, aphagia. If animals are tube-fed following this initial injury, eventually they will begin eating again but will maintain weight at a level lower than normal. Animals with this lateral hypothalamic lesion will no longer eat in response to insulin-induced hypoglycemia but will eat in response to cold or to other metabolic stimuli. Thus, there appear to be two hypothalamic centers involved in the regulation of food intake: a ventromedial system, which is involved in controlling signals for satiety, and a lateral system, which is involved in regulating the drive for food intake.

Studies on the distribution of adrenergic fibers in the brain stem have added significantly to our understanding of the relationship between the ventromedial and lateral regions of the hypothalamus. The ventromedial region of the hypothalamus is rich in dopaminergic fibers and also contains significant fibers from the ventral noradrenergic bundle. Destruction of the ventral noradrenergic bundle can reproduce many of the symptoms of the syndrome of hypothalamic obesity, suggesting that the noradrenergic fibers may mediate many of the phenomena associated with the ventromedial hypothalamus. The lateral hypothalamic area is traversed by the dopaminergic fibers which pass through this region from the brain stem. An injury to the lateral hypothalamus that causes a substantial reduction in dopamine will produce total aphagia (cessation of eating). Smaller reductions will produce graded decreases in food intake and loss of weight. It thus appears that the ventromedial and lateral hypothalamic regions are associated with bundles of adrenergic nerve fibers which have a predominantly anterior, posterior, or rostral caudal orientation, with little or no direct medial-lateral connection. Further evidence for the importance of adrenergic control of the hypothalamic centers in feeding has been provided by the injection of small quantities of norepinephrine into these regions. Norepinephrine will elicit feeding behavior in satiated animals, whereas the injection of isoproterenol into the hypothalamus will lead to inhibition of food intake. In current terminology, the regulation of food intake may be described as an "alpha-adrenergic" feeding center and "beta-adrenergic" satiety center.

There is now substantial evidence in studies of human fat that incorporation of radioactivity into long chain fatty acids can occur in this tissue and that the rate of this process is dependent upon the nutritional state of the individual from whom the fat is obtained. Comparison of adipose tissue and liver as sites of fatty acid synthesis had indicated that in human beings the liver is the principal site of fatty acid synthesis. The fatty acids formed in the liver are incorporated into triglycerides and thence into lipoproteins which are secreted into the circulation as very low-density lipoprotein (VLDL) particles. The fatty acids in these lipoproteins are cleaved from the triglyceride in peripheral tissue by the action of lipoprotein lipase. The process of lipogenesis in liver as in peripheral adipose tissue is modulated by the nutritional state, by the concentration of insulin, and by the fraction of dietary calories which are provided as carbohydrate.

Metabolic Factors. Metabolic factors are a second group of regulatory mechanisms for food intake. In most animals, body fat is a fairly constant fraction of total body weight. Although there is a tendency for the human being to gain weight with increasing age, the number of calories stored in fat in relation to the total calories eaten is very small. This is illustrated in Figure 31-5. No more than 0.34 per cent of calories need be stored to gain 1 pound per year. The nature of the mechanism involved in providing information about the quantity of metabolic energy is unknown. Several theories have been put forward, but they are as yet too limited to provide a sufficient explanation. That the body does regulate its food intake based on metabolic stores is, however, clearly shown by two kinds of experiments. In the first, the available food is diluted with various indigestible substances such as cellulose. In normal animals, the total amount of nutritional value is maintained constant, although the quantities of diluted food that are ingested varies. A similar result has been obtained by giving part of the food by stomach tube. As the quantity of food provided through a tube is increased, the amount ingested orally is decreased. Thus, there are mechanisms by which the feeding centers discern the metabolic needs of the organism and respond by food-seeking behavior.

The External Environment. The external environment provides a third category of factors which regulate food intake. As noted above, animals with injury to the hypothalamus become finicky in what they will eat. A similar observation has been made in obese human subjects. When exposed to ice cream adulterated with small amounts of quinine, the obese will eat less than the lean, though they eat much more normal ice cream. Similarly, other factors in the external environment also influence food intake. The experiments of Shachter and his colleagues have shown that the obese individual eats more when food is readily available. It appears from these and other experiments that the obese subject is more responsive to external cues than he is to metabolic cues. In contrast, the lean subject eats largely in response to metabolic needs, with

$$2800 \text{ cal/d} \times 365 \text{ days/year} \times 20 \text{ yrs.} = 20.5 \times 10^6 \text{ cal}$$

$$\text{Gained 20 lbs.} \times 3500 \text{ cal/lb.} = 70 \times 10^3 \text{ cal}$$

$$\text{or } 0.3\% \text{ of ingested calories stored}$$

Figure 31-5 Caloric intake and expenditure to accumulate 20 pounds. This figure assumes the average caloric intake of the standard male to be 2800 kcal./day and calculates the total number of calories expended during a period of 20 years. If 20 pounds are gained and if each pound is assumed to have 3500 calories, only 70,000 calories, or less than 0.34 per cent of the total calories, are stored. This shows the high efficiency of the human body in regulating energy intake and expenditure over prolonged periods of time.

external cues from taste, smell, and sight playing a much smaller role.

Caloric Storage and Utilization

Triglycerides represent the primary form of energy storage in most mammalian species (Table 31-3). Whether the excess caloric intake occurs as protein, fat, or carbohydrate seems to be of little importance. The storage form is primarily triglyceride. This has obvious advantages. A gram of triglyceride contains 9 calories. The adipocyte has about 7 to 7.5 calories per gram, with the aqueous components making up the difference. The caloric value of a gram of lean body mass, in contrast, is in the range of 1.5 calories, since approximately two thirds of this weight is fluid. Storage of carbohydrate as glycogen, though of importance as an immediate source of glucose, has the disadvantage of requiring a substantial addition of water and therefore a substantial addition of total weight relative to caloric storage. The rapid storage and subsequent utilization of large stores of triglyceride are of prime importance in two situations — the migratory bird and the hibernating mammal. Prior to the flight across the Gulf of Mexico, birds will eat enormous quantities of food and store it as fat which can be released and burned during long-distance flight. A similar mechanism is involved in energy storage for the hibernating animal.

Three mechanisms are available for the storage of excess calories as triglycerides. The triglyceride can be stored by an increase in the size of the existing fat cells. It is also possible for the number of fat cells to increase, with little or no change in the size of individual cells. Finally, it is possible for both the size and number of adipocytes to increase. The adipocyte is a highly differentiated cell which arises from a mesenchymal precursor. During the process of growth and development, a number of these precursor cells differentiate into fat cells. The mature fat cell does not divide and does not dedifferentiate into fat-free cells. Thus, once developed, the fat cell appears to remain throughout the life of the organism. Almost all forms of obesity are accompanied by an increased size of fat cells. This form of adaptation to glyceride storage is probably the principal mechanism when obesity develops in adult life (Fig. 31-6, top panel). In the forms of obesity which develop in early years of life, however, an increase in the total number of fat cells appears to be a major mechanism for adapting to the increased demands for triglyceride storage. Thus, individuals with gross obesity which begins in the early years of life show an increased mass of fat cells which do not subsequently dedifferentiate, although significant amounts of weight may disappear (Fig. 31-6, lower panel).

A series of biochemical reactions are involved in the formation of fatty acids and their conjugation with α-glycerophosphate (sn-glycerol-3-phosphate) to form triglycerides. Lipogenesis, i.e., the formation of fatty acids, appears to be controlled by nutritional state, by the presence of hormones, and by the size of the adipocyte. There is now substantial evidence in studies of human fat that incorporation of radioactivity into long-chain fatty acids can occur and that this process is dependent upon the nutritional state of the individual from whom the fat is obtained. Rapid formation of fatty acids is observed in adipose tissue taken from overfed patients. With caloric restriction, the rate of lipogenesis is severely depressed. Of the hormonal factors, insulin is of primary importance in controlling the rate of lipogenesis both in vivo and in vitro. The size of the adipose cell is also a determining factor in the rate of lipogenesis. With large fat cells, the rate of fatty acid synthesis is reduced. However, overfeeding for a short period of time will increase lipogenesis in large fat cells to a striking degree. The frequency with which food is ingested is a final factor which seems to be of importance in controlling lipogenesis. In experimental animals and in man, the ingestion of food in one or two large meals produces significant changes in the metabolic and biochemical function. When an individual eats a few large meals, he tends to have an impaired ability to metabolize glucose, to have a higher level of plasma cholesterol, to be more obese, and to show a greater rate of fatty acid formation in adipose tissue than is observed in individuals eating more frequent meals, but of smaller size.

The triglyceride stores in adipose tissue generally serve the body's needs during the intermeal periods. Thus, storage of carbohydrate as fatty acids in adipose tissue represents a storage form for fatty acids which are produced following food ingestion. Following food ingestion, there is an increase in the output of insulin which is stimu-

TABLE 31-3 METABOLIC FUELS IN MAN*

Fuel Supply	Normal Man (70 kg.)		Obese Man (140 kg.)	
Fat	15.00 kg.	141,000 kcal.	80.000 kg.	752,000 kcal.
Protein	6.00 kg.	24,000	8.000 kg.	32,000
Glycogen				
Muscle	0.12 kg.	480	0.160 kg.	640
Liver	0.07 kg.	280	0.700 kg.	280
Glucose	0.02 kg.	80	0.025 kg.	100
		165,840 kcal.		785,020 kcal.

*Adapted from Cahill, G. F., and Owen, O. E.: *In* Rowland, C. V., Jr.: Anorexia and Obesity. Little, Brown & Co., Boston, 1970.

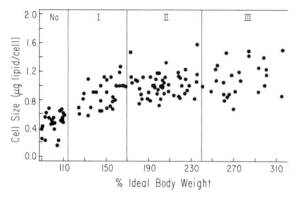

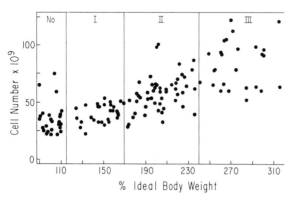

Figure 31–6 Body weight and fat cell size and number. The top panel displays data obtained by Dr. Hirsch on the relation of fat cell size to body weight. Essentially all overweight individuals showed an increase in the size of fat cells. The lower panel shows the relation of fat cell number to body weight. An increase in number of fat cells was more common among the more obese individuals. However, there were some with childhood onset obesity who had a normal number of fat cells and others with adult onset obesity who had an increased number of fat cells. (From Hirsch, J., and Batchelor, B.: Clin. Endocrinol. Metab., 5:No. 2, 1976. Reproduced by permission of the author and publisher.)

lated both by ingestion of glucose and by the presence of amino acids and, in turn, there is stimulation by gastrointestinal factors which facilitate the release of insulin. As the nutrients absorbed from the gastrointestinal tract enter the blood, the concentration of insulin is rising and this augments the storage of glucose in the liver as glycogen and of fatty acids and glucose in adipose tissue as triglycerides. As the concentration of glucose returns toward normal, there is a concomitant decline in the concentration of insulin and a return of the concentration of fatty acids toward their initial levels. This transition from the fed to the fasting state is facilitated by a reduction in insulin and may also be facilitated by the rise in growth hormone which is frequently observed four to five hours after ingesting a meal. The release of fatty acids from adipose tissue is essential to provide for the metabolic needs of peripheral tissues during the intermeal period. Studies from several laboratories originally suggested that obese patients had an impaired ability to release and utilize fatty acids. The evidence supporting this hypothesis came from two observations. First, it was observed that with fasting there was a very small rise in the concentration of free fatty acids. Second, it was observed that the injection of hormones which tend to increase

free fatty acids and to enhance lipolysis in adipose tissue had less effect in obese patients than in normal subjects. This conclusion has not been supported by testing with more sophisticated techniques. Measurement of the turnover and metabolism of fatty acids has shown that obese patients release and metabolize fatty acids more rapidly than lean subjects. Supporting evidence has also come from studies of adipose tissue in vitro which have shown that the breakdown of triglycerides with the formation of free fatty acids and glycerol in vitro occurs at a higher rate with large adipose cells of the kind obtained from obese subjects, as compared with adipocytes from normal-weight subjects. Present evidence would thus suggest that the utilization of adipocyte triglycerides is normal or supernormal in obese individuals.

Endocrine Consequences of Obesity

The consequences of obesity can be divided into several groups, but we will consider only those of hormonal or metabolic origin. The most frequent endocrine change is hyperinsulinemia. Figure 31-7 shows that the level of insulin in the fasting state has a highly significant, positive correlation with the degree of obesity. The more obese an

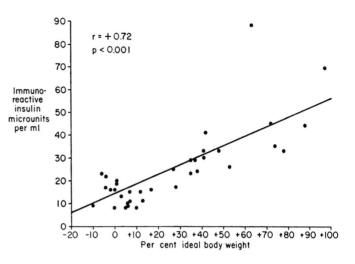

Figure 31–7 Relation of immunoreactive insulin to body weight. Fasting levels of immunoreactive insulin have been plotted against the percentage of ideal body weight. Thus, body weight is a primary factor in determining the fasting serum insulin. (Reproduced with permission from Bagdade, J. D., et al.: J. Clin. Invest., *46*:1549, 1967.)

individual, the higher his fasting insulin. Similarly, the release of insulin in response to such stimuli as glucose, leucine, and tolbutamide is greater in obese individuals than in lean subjects. Thus, not only are their basal levels of insulin elevated, but output of insulin in response to several stimuli is increased. Moreover, when glucose utilization and insulin are related, the obese individual requires more insulin to stimulate the utilization of glucose than normal. This implies that obese people are resistant to insulin. Studies by Salans and his collaborators have suggested that the adipocyte may be one site for this resistance. Other studies have shown, however, that muscle membrane is also resistant to insulin. With a technique for perfusing the human forearm, it is possible to examine the response of muscle and adipose tissue simultaneously. The muscle of the obese individual behaves as does the muscle of a normal individual after exposure to high concentrations of insulin. Thus, the obese individual has an induced resistance to insulin in muscle and adipose tissue and probably liver.

The initial step in the response of tissues to insulin is the interaction of circulating insulin with receptors for insulin located on the cell surface. Measurement of the binding of insulin to insulin receptors has now been examined in adipose tissue and liver membrane from obese and normal humans and experimental animals. The numbers of insulin-binding receptors on the plasma membranes of adipocytes from obese humans are significantly reduced when compared with fat cells from normal weight subjects. Evidence from tissue culture studies suggest that the number of receptors which bind insulin on a cell surface can be reduced by incubating the tissue in a high concentration of insulin. This type of feedback reduction in the number of receptors in the pres-

ence of high concentrations of insulin has important value in preventing excessive response to insulin in peripheral tissues. Current concepts about the mechanism of insulin resistance thus favor the theory that insulin resistance results from decreased numbers of receptors on peripheral tissues resulting from exposure of these tissues to high concentrations of insulin.

A second consistent alteration in obesity is an impaired output of growth hormone. Basal concentrations of growth hormone are normal or slightly reduced. Most striking is the impaired response to stimuli which usually increase growth hormone. The concentration of this hormone can usually be increased four to five hours after the administration of glucose orally by the induction of hypoglycemia with insulin and by the administration of arginine by the intravenous route. In the obese individual, the output of growth hormone is impaired to all these stimuli.

The third consistent alteration in endocrine function of obese subjects is the increased production rate of adrenocortical steroids. Although the concentrations of plasma cortisol remain normal, the production rate of cortisol by the adrenal gland and the excretion of its metabolites in the urine are increased in obesity.

These three endocrine adaptations are ones that would be expected from an internal milieu which favored the synthesis of fatty acid and deposition of triglycerides. It might be supposed that these endocrine alterations were causally related to obesity. However, it is possible that they are the consequence of overeating rather than a cause of corpulence. To gain insight into this question, Sims and his collaborators induced a weight gain of 30 to 40 pounds in a group of normal volunteers and studied their endocrine

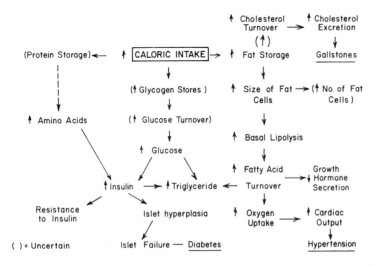

Figure 31–8 Consequences of ingesting an excess number of calories. An increased intake of calories will increase the size of the storage forms of protein, glycogen, and fat. However, since triglyceride can expand far more than the others, it is the principal storage site for extra calories. The ingestion of a surfeit of calories is associated with a number of metabolic changes, increasing lipolysis and reesterification, increased insulin secretion, and increased concentration of five amino acids.

and metabolic responses. In all cases, the pattern of endocrine adaptation was similar to that observed in the patients with spontaneous obesity. That is, normal volunteers who gained weight by overeating demonstrated hyperinsulinemia, a reduced output of growth hormone in response to arginine, and increased production of cortisol by the adrenal gland. They also demonstrated insulin resistance of the muscle in the forearm similar to that observed in patients with spontaneous obesity. It would thus seem that the endocrine alterations in obesity are probably a consequence rather than a cause of the disease.

Figure 31-8 presents a diagram of the metabolic consequences of ingesting excess calories. This diagram shows on the right side the effects on fat tissue; in the middle, the effects on carbohydrate; and on the left, the effect on protein metabolism. Increased caloric ingestion from whatever cause leads to increased storage of fat, enlarged fat cells, increased basal lipolysis, and increased turnover of free fatty acids. This sequence of events may be responsible for the increased secretion of cholesterol which occurs in obesity and thus in turn makes obese patients more susceptible to the development of gallstones. The increased turnover of glucose and secretion of insulin may be related to the tendency of obesity to be the precipitating factor for diabetes mellitus. The increased circulating concentrations of the branch chain amino acids may be one in stimulating insulin secretion.

PROTEIN AND/OR CALORIE DEFICIENCY

Several clinical syndromes result from the deficiency of proteins and/or calories. These condi-

tions can occur when there is an insufficient supply of food, as in times of war or famine, or when the quality of the available food is inadequate for human needs. The presence of severe disease of the gastrointestinal tract may also impair absorption of nutrients. Finally, voluntary reduction in or abstinence from food has been used as a treatment of obesity. Our knowledge of the consequences of starvation increased rapidly during the first and second World Wars and more recently with the introduction of fasting as a treatment for obesity. Several clinical and pathologic features of the syndromes with caloric or protein deprivation are presented in Table 31-4. Three of these — starvation, anorexia nervosa, and marasmus in children — represent deficiencies of both protein and calories and may more appropriately be named protein-calorie malnutrition, although there are some features unique to each. Kwashiorkor develops when protein is the element which is deficient in the diet.

Starvation

Death is the ultimate consequence of total starvation and is frequently observed during periods of acute famine or in concentration camps during international conflagrations. The duration of survival following restriction of intake depends upon the severity of the deprivation, upon the quantity of reserve energy (i.e., fat), and upon the adaptive mechanisms of the body. The presence of concurrent diseases accelerates deterioration. In classic studies on animals, Howe showed that dogs could be trained to starve. After 45 days during an early fast, his champion dog was near death. After a period of recovery with refeeding, the same animal was able to "learn" to starve for more than 117 consecutive days. In each case the

TABLE 31-4 A COMPARISON OF SOME FORMS OF MALNUTRITION

	Starvation	Anorexia Nervosa	Kwashiorkor	Marasmus
Primary deficiency	Calories	Calories	Protein	Calories
Age	Any age	10 to 30	At weaning	Children
Sex	Either	90% Female	Both	Both
Growth retardation	–	–	Slight	Significant
Body water	Decreased	Decreased	Increased	Decreased
Subcutaneous fat	Decreased	Decreased	May be normal	Decreased
Skin and hair lesions	–	–	Increased	Absent
Edema	Late	Late	Present	None
Diarrhea	Late	None	Present	Marked
Weight loss	Marked	Marked	Mild or absent	Marked
Serum albumin	Normal	Normal	Decreased	Normal
Hemoglobin	Normal	Normal	Decreased	Normal
Mg	Decreased	Decreased		Decreased
Liver	Normal	Normal	Enlarged and fatty	Normal
Pancreatic enzyme	–	–	Decreased	Normal

nutritional needs during this period were supplied by the stores in the body. The distribution of calories in fat, protein, and carbohydrate in a normal and an obese individual is shown in Table 31-3. Carbohydrates stored in the form of glycogen in liver and muscle, or as circulating glucose, represent only a small fraction of total body calories. The mechanisms by which the body adapts to the deficiency of carbohydrate intake are examined in detail below. Although the maintenance of blood glucose is essential for survival, it is clear that the triglycerides in adipose tissue are the principal source of calories. These represent nearly 80 per cent of the total caloric stores of the normal individual and well over 95 per cent in an obese subject. With a caloric requirement of 2000 calories daily, a normal man would be expected to survive between 30 and 60 days of starvation. In contrast, the obese subject exemplified in Table 31-3 could survive for nearly a year. Indeed, obese individuals have been starved for therapeutic purposes in excess of 250 days without apparent ill effects.

The supply of glucose is clearly limited, yet it is an obligatory substrate for the brain under normal circumstances and is the primary fuel used by red cells, leukocytes, the renal medulla, and peripheral nerves. If glycogen were supplying total caloric needs, the available supply would provide the body for only 10 hours. In the absence of carbohydrate intake, therefore, protein or fat must provide for most of the caloric needs. In addition, glucose must be formed from one of these substances. There is no net conversion of fatty acids or acetate to carbohydrate and, therefore, essentially all the new glucose formed during starvation comes from alanine, lactate, or pyruvate. This process of gluconeogenesis occurs primarily in the liver, with the kidney participat-

ing to a small extent. The oxidation of fatty acids activates the conversion of amino acids to glucose. In the short-term fast, lasting several hours to 2 to 3 days, the needs of the body for glucose are supplied from protein and Cori cycle intermediates (lactate) and are stimulated by the release of free fatty acids from the adipose tissue. Evidence from studies of Cahill and his collaborators suggest that insulin is the principal hormone concerned with regulating the initial process of adaptation to fasting. This is most clearly seen by comparing the period of food ingestion with the intermeal period. Following the ingestion of food, insulin is released from the pancreas and serves to increase the uptake of glucose into muscle and adipose tissue and to enhance the conversion of glucose to glycogen in the liver. Insulin similarly diminishes the release of free fatty acids from adipose tissue by inhibiting lipolysis and simultaneously accelerating the conversion of glucose into long-chain fatty acids within the adipocytes. Thus, the outpouring of insulin following the ingestion of foods containing carbohydrate or amino acids accelerates the storage of fuels for the coming period without food. With fasting, the concentration of insulin declines and the entry of glucose into tissues falls. Triglycerides are hydrolyzed and the fatty acids are released into the circulation to be metabolized in liver and peripheral tissues. The low levels of insulin similarly reduce the conversion of carbohydrate to glycogen in muscle. Thus, in a short-term fast, reduction in the concentration of insulin increases the release of free fatty acids from adipose tissue and of amino acids from muscle. In this way the substrates for gluconeogenesis and energy metabolism in peripheral tissues are supplied. This is shown schematically in Figure 31-7.

As fasting is continued, the excretion of nitrogen falls, indicating that mobilization of amino acids has diminished. In time, the supply of carbon precursors for the formation of glucose from amino acids falls below the metabolic requirements of the brain, red cells, and renal medulla. Two possibilities exist to permit survival. One is that the glucose-requiring tissue can adapt to utilize other substrates; the other is that glucose could be formed from long-chain fatty acids. There is, at present, no evidence for the latter possibility. There is, however, evidence to indicate that with prolonged fasting the brain can adapt to utilize ketone bodies to provide a significant fraction of the total caloric needs. Thus, after a prolonged period of fasting (i.e, five to six weeks), a number of adaptations have occurred in fuel consumption by the organism. The brain which was previously consuming 140 grams of glucose has decreased its consumption to 80 grams, the remainder being derived by oxidation of ketone bodies. Release of ketogenic amino acids is significantly reduced. With prolonged fasting, gluconeogenesis from the liver is decreased and the kidney becomes a more significant source of new glucose (Fig. 31-9). Indeed, during prolonged fasting the kidney provides as much or more glucose than the liver primarily because of the renal ammonia production. With fasting there is also a reduction in total caloric requirements by 15 to 20 per cent.

One mechanism for the decreased metabolism in starvation may be the reduced concentration of triiodothyronine. Approximately 75 per cent of the circulating triiodothyronine is formed from thyroxine in peripheral tissues. In starvation, the production of triiodothyronine falls significantly. Reverse (i.e., 3,3′,5′-triiodothyronine) is increased in reciprocal fashion to the reduction in triiodothyronine. Since triiodothyronine is the most potent calorigenic hormone, reduction in the concentration of this hormone during starvation might account for the lower consumption of oxygen. Other hormonal changes also occur.

The decreased concentration of insulin appears to provide the principal signal for the early responses to fasting. Insulin, however, remains low during prolonged fasting and does not seem to be a signal for the adaptive processes observed primarily in the brain and liver. Human growth hormone, glucocorticoids, and glucagon have also been explored as possible agents in the adaptation of fasting but do not appear to provide the needed hormonal signal. The major differences between the fed state and short- or long-term fasts is shown in Figure 31-9.

In addition to the endocrine and metabolic changes already described, fasting produces a number of other alterations that warrant brief comment. A thorough discussion of this subject, however, is beyond the purpose of this chapter.

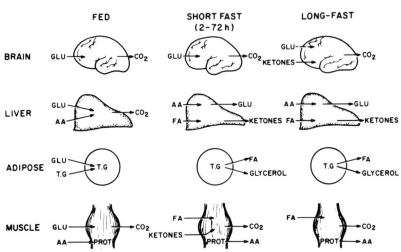

Figure 31–9 Effect of fasting on substrate utilization. Effects of substrate utilization by brain, liver, adipose tissue, and muscle in the fed state after short fast of 2 to 72 hours and following a prolonged fast. In the fed state and during a short fast, glucose is the principal substrate for the brain. With prolonged fasting, however, the brain adapts to the use of ketones for a significant fraction of its total energy requirements. With fasting, the liver adapts from burning glucose and amino acids to converting amino acids to glucose and converting free fatty acids to ketones, which are then used in the peripheral tissues. In the fed state, adipose tissue stores fatty acids as triglyceride, and in the short- and long-term fast it releases these triglycerides as their fatty acid and glycerol moieties. Muscle during the fed state utilizes glucose and amino acids, but with fasting uses free fatty acids or ketones. (Adapted from Cahill, G. F., Jr., and Owen, O. E.: In Rowland, C. V., Jr. (ed.): Anorexia and Obesity. Little, Brown and Co., Boston, 1970.)

The decrease in circulating levels of insulin and glucose already has been noted. Changes in the concentration of growth hormone are variable, but it is frequently increased. The excretion of 17-hydroxycorticosteroids and 17-ketosteroids is decreased. Concentrations of gonadotropins and testosterone show no change with fasting. Plasma levels of amino acids undergo a variety of changes. Alanine, which is an important precursor for gluconeogenesis, falls to one third of its normal level. Valine, leucine, and isoleucine initially increase in concentration but subsequently decline. Glycine, on the other hand, rises significantly with continued fasting. In addition to these changes in amino acids, there are significant losses of sodium, potassium, and magnesium from the body. The changes in magnesium are particularly interesting, since plasma magnesium remains normal, yet magnesium depletion can amount to 20 per cent. A mild ketoacidosis is uniformly found along with hyperuricemia. The increased concentrations of uric acid probably result from an increase in concentrations of keto acids, primarily β-hydroxybutyrate. This has been supported by the fact that the excretion of uric acid is reduced by the infusion of lactate or β-hydroxybutyrate. Riboflavin is decreased most rapidly but there is also a delayed fall in pantothenic acid, pyridoxine, and thiamine.

Some of the consequences of starvation are diagrammed in Figure 31-10. It shows the decreased fat content, decreased fat cell size, and increased fatty acid and ketone production which results from the mobilization of triglycerides in adipose tissue depots. The changes in metabolism of glucose and insulin, whose concentrations decline, and of glucagon, whose concentration goes up, are also depicted. The hyperuricemia observed during starvation can be largely accounted for by the increased concentration of beta-hydroxybutyrate, which competes with the renal tubule for secretion of uric acid. One hypothesis for the increased sodium excretion is that increased concentrations of glucagon stimulate sodium loss during fasting. The alterations in protein and amino acid metabolism have been described earlier.

Several significant consequences can occur during fasting. Postural hypotension and collapse have been observed. Gouty arthritis and precipitation of uric acid stones have been reported and can be prevented by treatment with the appropriate drugs. The most serious consequence, however, is death. It has been reported in several patients undergoing therapeutic starvation and indicates that such treatment should only be undertaken with careful medical supervision.

Anorexia Nervosa

Anorexia nervosa represents a second form of protein-calorie deficiency with loss of tissue. Although this is a clinically defined entity, it represents a physiologic pattern of change similar to that observed with caloric restriction or total starvation. This disease affects primarily females in the age range of 10 to 30 years. Not infrequently, these individuals have been modestly overweight and suddenly go into a catabolic phase. Patients with anorexia nervosa show little concern about their relatively cachectic state. Weight loss is marked and subcutaneous fat is often nearly absent. Adipocytes can be expected to be very small indeed. Breast development remains little changed and there is no loss of axillary or pubic hair and no development of skin lesions. The concentration of adrenocortical hormones in the plasma remains normal, but it is reduced in the urine. Menstrual cycles are absent in these individuals. Plasma growth hormone is elevated.

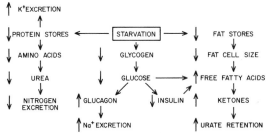

Figure 31–10 Effects of starvation on body function. This diagram shows the effects of starvation on body stores of fat, carbohydrate, and protein. There is a reduction in fat stores and fat cell size, and an increase in free fatty acids as the primary energy source. This increased ketone concentration impairs uric acid excretion by the kidney, with urate retention in the blood and the occasional precipitation of gouty arthritis. Starvation also depletes glycogen and glucose and, through the increase in glucagon, may lead to a rise in sodium excretion. Protein stores that initially are mobilized to provide glucose are conserved as the body adapts to using more fatty acids and to conserving protein stores.

Marasmus and Kwashiorkor

The findings in the various forms of starvation are to be contrasted with those observed when protein deficiency is the principal defect. This illness, known as kwashiorkor, is seen in its relatively pure form occasionally but is more frequently observed with various degrees of simultaneous caloric deficiency. In its relatively pure form, kwashiorkor begins at the time of weaning when the infant is deprived of protein intake but supplied with an adequate number of calories. Growth retardation is slight in comparison with the significant growth retardation observed with caloric restriction. Subcutaneous fat may be normal in the individual with kwashiorkor but is uniformly reduced in patients with marasmus or caloric deficiency. This is readily explained in terms of the alterations in the ingested fuel mixture. When protein is deficient but calories are adequate, these calories must be either carbohydrate or fat. The ingestion of carbohydrate as noted above stimulates the release of insulin and serves as a stimulus for the production and storage of triglyceride and glycogen. It is thus not surprising that body fat stores are relatively well preserved in kwashiorkor.

A second consequence is that body weight loss is mild or absent in contrast to starvation, in which marked weight loss occurs. Edema, however, is a common feature in kwashiorkor and can be attributed largely to the striking reduction in serum albumin. Since the intake of protein is reduced, the supply of amino acids to the liver from the gastrointestinal tract is inadequate. In the presence of normal carbohydrate intake, the release of amino acids from muscle sources is reduced, and consequently the supply from this source is also lower than normal. Thus, protein supplies to the liver are insufficient for the synthesis of normal amounts of serum albumin. With the reduction in serum albumin to levels of 1 to 2 grams per 100 ml. blood (20 to 30 per cent of normal), the oncotic pressure in plasma is reduced. Plasma osmotic pressure becomes insufficient to counterbalance the hydrostatic and osmotic forces in the extracellular fluid, and there is a tendency for fluid to accumulate in the extravascular compartment. This has been confirmed by the measurements of increased quantities of total body water and of extracellular fluid in patients with kwashiorkor. The deficiency in protein is also accompanied by an enlarged, fatty liver which is usually not seen when both calories and protein are deficient. The appearance of skin and hair lesions in kwashiorkor may be a reflection of vitamin deficiencies which are often observed when protein is deficient. Diarrhea, a late event in starvation, is less common in the patients with kwashiorkor. It is thus possible to distinguish between the various forms of protein-calorie malnutrition on clinical grounds and using laboratory measurements. Particularly prominent in the patient with protein depletion but adequate caloric intake are the marked reduction in albumin, the enlarged fatty liver, and nearly normal amounts of subcutaneous fat. With starvation, however, adipose stores are mobilized to provide energy for body stores and to spare protein and carbohydrate.

Accelerated Starvation

There are important differences between the physiologic adaptation to starvation alone and the sequence of food deprivation when it is associated with trauma, injury, or infection. First, stressful situations associated with injury, burns, or infection activate the autonomic nervous system. Many of the differences between starvation and injury can be attributed to enhanced activity of the sympathetic nervous system. Among these are enhanced glucagon secretion, impaired insulin secretion, and increased epinephrine release. This sequence of events leads to a relative decline in insulin and a rise in glucose resulting from enhanced glycogen mobilization and accelerated gluconeogenesis. The inhibition of insulin secretion and increased concentrations of catecholamines from sympathetic discharge would also be associated with increased release of free fatty acids. In addition to the marked hyperglycemia, there is an increase in vasopressin and corticosteroid secretion which are responsible for decreased water excretion by the kidneys and increased sodium reabsorption by the renal tubule. In addition, elevated levels of corticosteroids may be responsible for the accelerated rates of protein breakdown which have been observed in stress. These metabolic differences resulting from neural and endocrine disturbances associated with stress are important when considering the use of nutrient replacement during stress and starvation. This field of parenteral nutrition is of growing importance as the availability of amino acid and lipid containing solutions becomes widespread. For more detailed discussions of the intricacies of parenteral nutrition, the reader is referred elsewhere.

LIPIDS

Interest in the role of lipids in human disease has been continually reinforced by the observations that cardiovascular disease, particularly acute myocardial infarctions, occurs with significantly higher frequency in individuals with high serum cholesterol. The major lipid components of blood are listed in Table 31-5. Cholesterol is a 25-carbon molecule with four rings and is a normal constituent of animal and plant fats. Triglyc-

TABLE 31–5   LIPID COMPONENTS OF BLOOD

Serum Lipids	Concentration
Total cholesterol mg./100 ml.	230 ± 35*
Phospholipids mg./100 ml.	220 ± 30
Triglycerides mg./100 ml.	105 ± 25
Free fatty acids μEq./L.	400 to 800

*Mean ± S.D.

erides are esters of fatty acids and glycerol. Phospholipids are a class of diglycerides with a phosphate ester on the third hydroxyl of glycerol. Fats or lipids account for approximately 40 per cent of the calories available for consumption in the retail market of the United States. Over the past 20 years there has been a gradual decrease in the sources of animal fat from 75 to 66 per cent, while the fraction of fats available from vegetable sources has increased from 25 to 34 per cent. This transition has been accelerated by observations that the quality of fats in the diet, as well as their total quantity, may play a role in the development of human cardiovascular disease. A relationship between changes in serum cholesterol and the intake of fats and cholesterol has been derived by Keys from the data of many investigators (see formula below). From this formula it can be seen that a reduction in saturated fats in the diet would have a more significant effect on serum cholesterol than increasing unsaturated fats. The effect of dietary cholesterol is small, since it appears as the square root of its concentration.

Fat Ingestion and Metabolism

The ingestion of fats is followed by their cleavage into smaller moieties prior to absorption. Considerable interest has been focused on the mechanism for hydrolysis, absorption, and transport of dietary lipids. Triglycerides are cleaved by a pancreatic lipase into monoglycerides or glycerol and fatty acids. In the presence of bile acids and phospholipids, water/soluble micelles composed of fatty acids and monoglycerides are formed. These micellar aggregates are then absorbed into the mucosal cells of the ileum. The bile acids are recycled into the portal circulation, taken up by the liver, and secreted into the bile again. The fate of the fatty acids depends upon their chain length. For fatty acids with less than 12 carbon atoms, the triglycerides formed in the intestinal epithelium are released into the portal circulation and transported directly to the liver. With the long-chain fatty acids of more than 12 carbon atoms, however, transport is more complex. These fatty acids, after conversion to triglycerides, are surrounded by a protein coat to form chylomicrons. Although chylomicrons consist predominantly of triglycerides, they also contain small amounts of cholesterol and phospholipid. These aggregates are secreted into the lacteals of the intestinal villi and enter the general circulation through the thoracic duct. In high concentration they give the serum a creamy appearance. Chylomicrons are removed from the circulation after hydrolysis of the triglyceride by lipoprotein lipase, which is present in many tissues. This enzyme is increased by insulin and

glucose and is activated by heparin. The fatty acids and glycerol thus formed enter adipose or muscle cells for metabolism or storage.

In addition to the chylomicrons formed in the gastrointestinal tract, pre-beta-lipoproteins can also be assembled in the liver and secreted into the circulation. The fatty acids in these lipoproteins can be synthesized from glucose in the liver or from fatty acids taken up from the blood. The fate of the lipoproteins is similar to that of the chylomicrons, i.e., the triglycerides are hydrolyzed by lipoprotein lipase. The cholesterol and phospholipid remaining after cleavage of the triglycerides are partly transferred to higher density lipoproteins, with the remainder becoming β-lipoproteins. There are thus two sources of the large triglyceride-rich lipoproteins: (1) chylomicrons formed from dietary lipid and (2 hepatic lipoproteins formed from fatty acids synthesized in the liver or taken up from the circulation.

Our understanding of lipid metabolism was greatly expanded by the introduction of techniques for separating the various serum lipoproteins by electrophoresis. By using this technique along with measurements of triglyceride and cholesterol, and in some instances using flotation methods in the ultracentrifuge, it is possible to distinguish chylomicrons from alpha-, beta-, and pre-beta-lipoproteins. A typical electrophoretic pattern of normal serum is shown in Figure 31–11. When analyzed quantitatively, the compo-

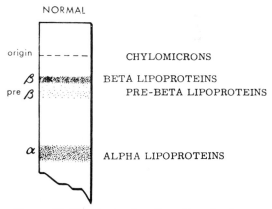

Figure 31–11 Electrophoretic pattern for lipoproteins. This schematic diagram shows the pattern obtained during electrophoresis of normal serum. The sample applied at the origin undergoes electrophoresis in an albumin buffer. Chylomicrons, if present, remain at the origin. The first band contains β-lipoproteins and the faint band running just in front of the β-lipoproteins contains the pre-β-lipoproteins. The high density α-lipoproteins migrate farthest on paper electrophoresis.

$$\Delta \text{ Cholesterol} = 1.2[2(\Delta S) - \Delta U] + 1.5\Delta \left(\sqrt{\text{Chol } \frac{\text{mg.}}{1000 \text{ cal.}}} \right)$$

ΔS = Glycerides of saturated fatty acids (C_{12} to C_{16}) as a percentage of total calories.

ΔU = Glycerides of polyunsaturated fatty acids in the diet as a percentage of total calories.

---

nents of these various lipoproteins differ. The cholesterol content is highest in the alpha-lipoprotein and lowest in chylomicrons and pre-beta-lipoproteins, with the beta-lipoprotein being intermediate. In contrast, the triglyceride concentration is highest in chylomicrons and lowest in the alpha-lipoproteins.

Defects in Fat Metabolism and Their Determination by Electrophoretic Techniques

At least two proteins make up the envelope for the circulating lipoproteins. These are an A protein associated in highest concentration with the alpha-lipoproteins and a B protein associated in highest concentration with the beta-lipoproteins. Deficiency of the B protein has been described in more than 30 individuals and presents a characteristic clinical picture. As might be expected, the concentrations of chylomicrons and beta-lipoproteins are very low, since the protein which provides the principal coating is absent. Indeed, some patients have no detectable beta-lipo-proteins. Serum cholesterol is also strikingly reduced. These patients also demonstrate neurologic abnormalities and an irregularity of the red blood cells called acanthocytosis. Persons lacking the B protein manifest their disease in infancy as a failure to grow and the appearance of fat in the stools. The basic pathophysiology is failure to form the protein coat by which triglycerides of long-chain fatty acids can be transported. Since triglycerides formed from short- and medium-chain fatty acids do not require a protein coat for transport, they have proved useful in treating patients with a beta-lipoproteinemia.

A second defect in transport of lipoproteins is observed with absence of the A protein. This disease was orginally found on Tangier Island in Chesapeake Bay and has since been called Tangier disease. The defect is an absence of A protein associated with a reduction in the concentration of cholesterol and phospholipid in the plasma, but triglyceride shows only mild changes. The most striking abnormality in individuals with this disease is the large orange-colored tonsils which result from the deposition of cholesterol esters in this tissue. Similar esters are also deposited in the reticuloendothelial cells of liver and spleen. In the absence of alpha-lipoprotein, lipid is carried primarily by the beta-lipoproteins which appear to be normal by immunoelectrophoresis.

Absence of lipoprotein lipase from peripheral tissues produces a third defect in lipid metabolism and is inherited as an autosomal recessive trait. This enzyme is essential for the hydrolysis of triglycerides carried on chylomicrons and pre-beta-lipoproteins prior to their entry and storage in adipose cells and other peripheral tissues. Absence of this enzyme would lead to an accumulation of these lipoproteins in the serum. On visual examination the serum from such patients is creamy. The marked elevation in serum triglycerides and chylomicrons results from the dietary intake of triglyceride. If fat is excluded from the diet, the chylomicrons disappear and lipid levels return almost to normal. Thus, exclusion of fat from the diet represents the principal mode of treatment for individuals with this disease. The symptom complex observed is also susceptible to treatment by dietary restriction of fat and therefore probably results from the high levels of chylomicrons. These symptoms include abdominal pain, a creamy color to the retinal vessels, and the appearance of reddish-yellow lipid-containing plaques in the skin.

By using the technique illustrated in Figure 31-11 along with measurement of cholesterol and triglyceride, the lipoprotein patterns can be segregated into six groups, as illustrated in Table 31-6, which is adapted from the currently recommended international classification.

Type I results from deficiency of lipoprotein lipase and was described above. As would be expected with a deficiency of this enzyme, the pattern on electrophoresis shows a marked increase in concentration of chylomicrons.

The second type of pattern observed with this technique is a marked increase in the beta-lipoprotein fraction without elevation of triglycerides (IIa) or when this moiety is also elevated (IIb). This protein carries a significant fraction of the total cholesterol and is accompanied by significant elevations in concentration of plasma cholesterol. The familial form is inherited as an autosomal dominant and Types IIa and IIb appear in the same families. The defect in removal of low-density lipoproteins which characterize this disease was described earlier. This disease is often associated with accumulations of lipid (xanthomas) in tendons. Early cardiovascular

TABLE 31–6 CLASSIFICATION OF HYPERLIPOPROTEINEMIA BASED ON LIPOPROTEIN PATTERN

	Lipoprotein					Lipids		
Type	Chylo-microns	LDL β	VLDL pre-β	Floating β	Appearance of Standing Plasma	Cholesterol	Tri-glyceride	Chol./TG
I	+				Creamy	↑	↑ ↑	<0.2
IIa		+			Clear	↑ ↑	N	>15.0
IIb		+	+		Clear or faintly turbid	↑	↑	Variable
III				+	Turbid	↑	↑	Frequently >1.0
IV			+		Clear or turbid	N or ↑	↑	Variable
V			+		Creamy	↑	↑ ↑	>0.15; <0.06

Key:

+ = Present
↑ = Increased
↑ ↑ = Greatly Increased
N = Normal

death has often been associated with this syndrome. Recent evidence indicates that high levels of cholesterol can be detected in up to 0.5 per cent of newborns, making it an easily detectable and optimistically treatable affliction.

The third abnormality in the electrophoretic pattern (Type III) is known by its description as broad beta disease. This is observed when the beta band is increased in width and streaks over into the pre-beta region but without a separate band. This a rare disease and must be distinguished from IIb by showing that the lipoprotein floats at a density of 1.006. The familial form of this disease is inherited as an autosomal recessive and is manifested mainly in adult life. The increased amounts of triglyceride and cholesterol often result in lipid deposition in the skin. Such individuals are also plagued by coronary artery disease at an early age. Glucose metabolism is often abnormal in patients with this disease.

The fourth type of electrophoretic abnormality (Type IV) shows a striking increase in the concentration of pre-beta-lipoproteins and is among the two most common types. This disease is inducible by a high-carbohydrate diet and is often termed endogenous or "carbohydrate-inducible" hyperlipoproteinemia. This abnormality and that of Type II are frequently seen as complications of other diseases including diabetes, hypothyroidism, and the nephrotic syndrome. The serum from patients is usually cloudy. Glucose tolerance is often abnormal and these patients are frequently obese.

The final syndrome (Type V) is manifested by an elevation in both chylomicrons and pre-beta-lipoproteins. The activity of lipoprotein lipase is frequently low in patients with Type V disease and may account for their increased level of chylomicrons. As with Type I, patients suffering from Type V abnormalities frequently have abdominal pain and usually show abnormal metabolism of glucose. Progestational and anabolic steroids have been found to enhance the activity of lipoprotein lipase and to lower levels of triglyceride.

With the technique of lipoprotein electrophoresis and measurements of cholesterol and triglyceride, sophisticated genetic studies have been performed on the prevalence of lipoprotein types in the population, and a new classification based on this information has been introduced (Table 31-7). This classification is based on a study of 157 survivors of myocardial infarction and their relatives. The monogenic hyperlipidemia which is transmitted as an autosomal dominant trait could be subdivided into three genetic groups. Familial hypercholesterolemia, familial hypertriglyceridemia, and a combined hyperlipidemia. In addition to these monogenic types, there was a

TABLE 31–7 GENETIC CLASSIFICATION OF HYPERLIPIDEMIA°

	Prevalence in Population
Monogenic Hyperlipidemia*	
Familial hypercholesterolemia	~0.1–0.2%
Familial hypertriglyceridemia	~0.2–0.3%
Combined hyperlipidemia	~0.3–0.5%
Polygenic Hypercholesterolemia	
Sporadic Hypertriglyceridemia	

°Adapted from Goldstein, et al., 1973.
*Inherited as an autosomal dominant.

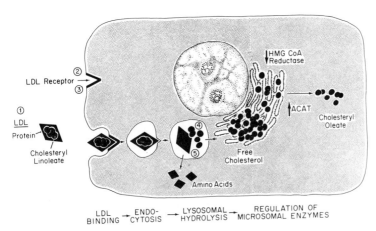

Figure 31–12 A diagram of the metabolism of cholesterol. This figure illustrates the entry of low density lipoproteins into the cell after interaction with cell receptors. The cholesterol esters are then broken down, and the cholesterol that is released inhibits the synthesis of new cholesterol and increases the rate of esterification of cholesterol. States of hypercholesterolemia can occur when the receptors for lipoproteins are reduced. (From Brown, M. S., and Goldstein, J. L.: N. Engl. J. Med., 294:1387.)

polygenic inheritance of hypercholesterolemia and the sporadic appearance of hypertriglyceridemia.

Recent studies by Brown and Goldstein (1976) have provided new insight into the pathogenetic sequence involved in the manifestation of hypercholesterolemia. This is shown in Figure 31-12. Using tissue cultures of fibroblast from normal and hypercholesterolemic individuals, they found that cells from heterozygotes had a reduction and cells from homozygotes had a nearly complete absence of receptors which bind low density lipoprotein. The mechanism for increased hypercholesterolemia could thus be explained by the loss of inhibition of cholesterol synthesis because the circulating cholesterol was unable to enter the cell and inhibit the key regulatory HMG CoA-reductase. In the normal individual, the low density of lipoprotein binds to a receptor on the cell surface and the receptor and LDL are incorporated into the cell. The cholesterol is then released and serves to inhibit further cholesterol synthesis within that cell. When these low-density lipoprotein receptors are reduced or absent, the quantity of LDL entering the cell is reduced and intracellular cholesterol synthesis is enhanced. The sites of abnormalities in this scheme for production of cholesterol are shown in Figure 31-12.

To summarize, the absorption, digestion, transport, and storage of the lipid components of the diet represent a complex and well-integrated system. Lipoproteins represent the principal form for transporting lipids in plasma. The introduction of electrophoretic techniques for separating the lipoproteins in plasma has provided significant new insights into the pathogenesis of a number of disease states. The two principal lipoproteins, alpha- and beta-lipoproteins, are associated primarily with A and B proteins in their coats. Disease syndromes have been described which result from the deficiency of one or the other of these proteins. Elevated chylomicrons

result from a deficiency of lipoprotein lipase, the enzyme which hydrolyzes circulating triglycerides, so that they can be absorbed and stored in adipose tissue. Four other types of abnormality in lipoprotein patterns have also been described which can occur as genetically transmitted forms or in association with other diseases.

VITAMINS

Vitamins may be defined as small chemical molecules which are essential for maintenance of normal metabolic processes but which cannot be synthesized within the body. These substances must therefore be provided in adequate amounts from dietary sources. Over the past 70 years, a number of vitamins have been elucidated and their clinical correlates put into focus. A listing of

TABLE 31–8 RECOMMENDED DAILY ALLOWANCES FOR VITAMINS

Vitamins	Recommended Daily Allowances
Water-Soluble Vitamins	
Thiamine (B_1)	0.2 to 1.5 mg.
Riboflavin (B_2)	0.4 to 1.7 mg.
Pyridoxine (B_6)	0.2 to 2.0 mg.
Niacin	5.0 to 20.0 mg.
Pantothenic acid	—
Folacin (folic acid)	0.05 to 0.4 mg.
Cyanocobalamin (B_{12})	1.0 to 5.0 μg.
Biotin	—
Ascorbic acid (C)	35 to 55 mg.
Fat-Soluble Vitamins	
Vitamin A	5000 I.U.
Vitamin D	400 I.U.
Vitamin E	5 to 25
Vitamin K	—

these vitamins is presented in Table 31-8. They can be divided into two groups: the water-soluble vitamins, comprising the B-complex vitamins and vitamin C, and the fat-soluble vitamins, A, D, E, and K. The precise metabolic role of some vitamins has been clearly described, but the role of others is less well understood. The B-complex vitamins as a group are involved in the metabolism of carbohydrate as cofactors either for the transfer of hydrogen or for decarboxylation or transamination. Pyridoxine is involved in transfer of amino groups and biotin in the fixation of CO_2 during fatty acid synthesis and gluconeogenesis. Folic acid and vitamin B_{12} are involved in nucleic acid synthesis. The precise role for vitamin C is unclear. Vitamin A has several functions but its role in the visual cycle has been most clearly defined. Vitamin D has an essential role in bone metabolism. Vitamin K will be dealt with in more detail in the chapter on hematology.

Defining the requirements for these nutritional factors has occupied considerable research effort. Since most of them are intimately involved in intermediary metabolism, their requirements in general vary with the overall rate of metabolism. It would thus be expected that diseases which altered metabolism would alter the rates at which the vitamins are metabolized and thus increase or decrease their requirements. Hyperthyroidism, which increases oxygen consumption, enhances the need for thiamine and riboflavin. When thyroid function is decreased, the requirements for these vitamins fall. The definition of requirements for many vitamins must, therefore, be stated in terms of total caloric requirement. In general, however, the minimum daily requirements are high enough to allow a reasonable margin of safety for individual variation.

Water-Soluble Vitamins

Thiamine (Vitamin B₁). Thiamine was among the first of the B-complex vitamins to be chemically identified and serves as an important cofactor in the decarboxylation of pyruvic and α-ketoglutaric acids. Deficiency of this vitamin is manifested by defective metabolism of carbohydrates. One of the cardinal biochemical alterations accompanying the clinical states of thiamine deficiency is an increase in circulating levels of pyruvic acid. The inability to utilize pyruvate in thiamine deficiency is accompanied by the development of two clinical syndromes, one involving the peripheral nervous system and the other the cardiovascular system. Peripheral involvement of the nervous system, known as peripheral neuritis, is manifested as increased pain, a loss of sensation, or an aching or burning sensation. Significant alterations in the central

nervous system also occur and are most commonly observed in patients ingesting large quantities of alcohol. The cardiovascular manifestations are primarily those of inadequate energy supply to the myocardium and the periphery with an increase in cardiac output. Arterioles are dilated, leading to an increased flow of blood between the arterial and venous circulation. As a result of the high cardiac output and defective carbohydrate metabolism, heart failure occurs associated with shortness of breath, increased heart rate, subjective feelings of palpitation, and objective findings of irregular rhythms. The heart is usually enlarged and, as might be expected in a heart which is unable to pump blood at a sufficient rate, there is an increase in venous pressure. These neurologic and cardiovascular symptoms are most prominent in severe deficiencies, but careful studies of hospitalized patients have revealed significantly reduced levels of thiamine in approximately one third of such patients. Since the requirements for thiamine are related to the metabolic rate, both deficient food intake and hypermetabolism can produce symptoms of disease. Patients with prolonged alcoholic intake or people eating hypocaloric diets can suffer from mild symptoms of thiamine deficiency, while individuals with hypermetabolism (usually hyperthyroidism) will suffer from similar symptoms even though thiamine intake may be adequate normally.

Riboflavin (Vitamin B₂). Although riboflavin was chemically identified for the first time in 1879, its role in the production of disease was not appreciated for some years thereafter. Normal subjects on a riboflavin-deficient diet developed characteristic lesions within three months. Among the pathologic changes were vascularization of the cornea and cheilosis. Riboflavin and its two active nucleotides, flavin mononucleotide (FMN) and flavinadeninedinucleotide (FAD), are the hydrogen-accepting cofactors for several enzymes including xanthine oxidase, succinate dehydrogenase, triphosphopyridine nucleotide, and mitochondrial glycerophosphate oxidase. Like thiamine, the requirements for riboflavin depend on over-all metabolic activity and have been defined as 0.25 to 0.30 mg. per 1000 kcal. of food oxidized. Thyroid hormones play a major role in the control of flavoprotein metabolism. Hyperthyroidism clearly produces an increased metabolic rate and enhances the metabolism of riboflavin. This latter effect is manifested as an increase in the enzymes which convert riboflavin to its active form, flavin mononucleotide. Hypothyroidism, on the other hand, produces a decrease in hepatic flavin-containing enzymes which are similar to those produced by riboflavin deficiency. The metabolic rate is reduced in riboflavin-deficient animals as it is in hypothyroidism. Similarly, α-glycerophosphate dehydrogenase, a mitochondrial enzyme, is decreased in hypothyroidism and in riboflavin deficiency. These observations suggest that certain clinical features of hypothyroidism may be attributable to the inability to metabolize riboflavin in a normal manner.

Niacin (Nicotinamide). Deficiency of niacin produces pellagra, or black tongue. This illness is characterized by symptoms referable to the skin, gastrointestinal tract, and central nervous system. In experimentally induced deficiency in man, the earliest manifestations are a red eruption on the skin resembling sunburn which first appears on the back of the hand. Other areas which are exposed to light are subsequently involved. The lesions, which are symmetrical, may darken, shed skin, and eventually scar. Sores on the mucocutaneous membranes, a swelling of the tongue, nausea, and vomiting are present in a significant number of individuals. Symptoms referable to the central nervous system include headache, insomnia, depression, dizziness, and difficulty with memory. The presence of a nutritional factor which could cure these symptoms was demonstrated in the classic work of Goldberger and his colleagues, and this substance was subsequently found to be nicotinamide or niacin. This vitamin is a critical part of two cofactors, NAD and NADP, which are involved in the transfer of hydrogen in most biological oxidations. Although the role of NAD and NADP in biological oxidations and biochemical synthesis are well known, the mechanism by which the symptoms observed with deficiency of niacin relate to the levels of these cofactors remains unclear. One thing is known, however — the administration of nicotinic acid to patients suffering from pellagra produces dramatic alterations within 24 hours.

Pyridoxine (Vitamin B_6). After the identification of thiamine, riboflavin, and niacin, it became clear that other water-soluble nutritional factors were also necessary for normal metabolic function. In the period between 1930 and 1935 several groups of workers described an additional factor, vitamin B_6, subsequently called pyridoxine. This compound is activated by conversion to pyridoxal phosphate and is involved in a number of metabolic reactions with amino acids, including decarboxylation and transamination. Pyridoxine deprivation can produce symptoms in man and other species. These include changes in the skin, central nervous system, and production of red blood cells. In man, the skin lesions consist of seborrheic changes around the eyes, nose, and mouth and of swelling and redness of the tongue. With prolonged deficiency, convulsive activity in the central nervous system has been demonstrated. The anemia which accompanies pyridoxine deficiency is microcytic and hypochromic in type. All these symptoms can be promptly relieved by the administration of small doses of pyridoxine. The recommended dose of pyridoxine is related to protein intake, since its principal role is in the metabolism of amino acids. The range is between 1.25 and 2.00 mg. with protein intakes of 100 grams or less. With high protein intake, more pyridoxine may be needed.

In addition to the symptoms of deficiency which are cured by low doses of pyridoxine, there are a group of clinical states in which symptoms can be cured by much higher doses of this vitamin. These include some forms of convulsions, particularly in children; vitamin B_6-dependent anemia; xanthinuric aciduria; cystathionuria; and homocystinuria. The doses of vitamin B_6 required for control or amelioration of these conditions are in the range of 200 to 600 mg. daily as compared to a range of 1.5 to 2.0 mg. per day for normal maintenance. The convulsive activity in the brain would appear to be related to altered levels of gamma-amino butyric acid (GABA). This amino acid is produced by decarboxylation of glutamate, a process involving transamination and requiring pyridoxal phosphate. A reduction in the level of GABA increases the tendency for convulsive activity and probably accounts for the convulsions observed in such patients. The physiologic basis for the effect of pyridoxine in the other conditions is unknown at present.

Pantothenic Acid and Biotin. These two water-soluble agents are important cofactors in the metabolism of fats. Pantothenic acid was first identified in 1933 and was clearly associated with a nutritional deficiency disease in fowl by Wooley and his collaborators in 1939. Pantothenic acid is an essential component of coenzyme A, which is of prime importance in both synthesis and degradation of fatty acids. The presence of biotin was demonstrated from studies showing the production of a disease by feeding egg white. It is now known that raw egg white contains avidin, a glycoprotein of high molecular weight which irreversibly binds biotin. The structure of biotin was established in 1942. It is an important enzyme in the fixation of CO_2 during synthesis of fatty acids and during gluconeogenesis. Although specific syndromes can be produced in man by feeding synthetic diets deficient in pantothenic acid or biotin, these are almost unknown under natural conditions because of the wide availability of these two substances in foods.

Folic Acid and Vitamin B_{12} (Cobamide). These two vitamins are essential for the maintenance of normal hematopoiesis. Because of their integral relationship with the blood, discussion of vitamin B_{12} and folic acid is included in Chapter 22.

Vitamin C. Vitamin C or ascorbic acid, the last water-soluble vitamin, is essential for the prevention of scurvy. The existence of a nutritional factor which would prevent scurvy was recognized in 1753 by Lind, who demonstrated that oranges, lemons, and limes could prevent and cure scurvy among sailors, hence the nickname "limey" for British sailors. The chemical identification of this antiscurvy or antiscorbutic factor was not made for nearly 200 years. Progress was greatly aided by the demonstration that guinea pigs could be made scorbutic, i.e., develop scurvy. With this bioassay, several groups of workers demonstrated the essential nature of ascorbic acid. It was a hexuronic acid present in high concentrations in the adrenal gland, as well as in citrus fruits and cabbages.

The physiologic and biologic functions for ascorbic acid are far less clearly defined than for the other water-soluble vitamins. Most of the other vitamins function as cofactors for a specific enzymatic step in a chain of biochemical reactions. No such enzymatic step has been defined which requires ascorbic acid as a cofactor. The vitamin rather appears to function in its reduced form, dehydroascorbic acid, in oxidation-reduction reactions. Its role in the metabolism of tyrosine has been studied in some detail. The first step in metabolism is the transamination of tyrosine to p-hydroxyphenylpyruvic acid. The next step is conversion to homogentisic acid by parahydroxyphenylpyruvic acid oxidase, an enzyme which is inhibited by its substrate unless ascorbic acid is present. This effect occurs when the quantities of tyrosine are large. The functional role of the high concentrations of ascorbic acid found in the adrenal gland and in the ovary are unclear at present.

When vitamin C deficiency is produced, two groups of symptoms occur: those involving growth of bones and those involving blood vessels. During periods of rapid growth, a separation of the periosteum from the cortex occurs and subperiosteal hemorrhages may result. When growth is less rapid, the lesions in the epiphyseal-diaphyseal junction may lead to disunion and/or fragmentation. Changes in the capillary walls are also prominent, and hemorrhages into the space around hair follicles are common. All these symptoms are rapidly reversed by the administration of ascorbic acid, which is required in the range of 50 to 75 mg. per day. It is of interest that only man, certain primates, and the guinea pig have a requirement for vitamin C; other mammals are able to synthesize the vitamin by a series of reactions involving the glucuronic acid pathway. The correlation between the clinical symptoms and the biochemical reactions is unclear. Definition of this area again awaits further understanding of the biochemical mechanisms by which ascorbic acid acts at the cellular level.

Fat-Soluble Vitamins

The vitamins A, D, E, and K differ from the group discussed previously because they are soluble in fat. Toxicity from overdosage has been reported for vitamins A and D because body fat serves as a storage depot. Toxicity is not observed with the water-soluble vitamins because any excess is excreted in the urine.

Vitamin A. The discovery of vitamin A stemmed from studies on the skin lesions and xerophthalmia in rats fed artificial diets containing lard. The chemical factor which prevented this deficiency was identified in 1929 as beta-carotene and its structure was proved in 1931. Subsequent work on the physiologic role of beta-carotene and other carotenoid pigments has taken two lines: (1) studies on its effect on vision and (2) studies on growth and development. The actions in the visual cycle have been clearly elucidated by work from several laboratories. Deficiency of vitamin A impairs adaptation of the retina to the dark. It also impedes growth. The mechanism for the stimulation of growth by vitamin A has not yet been clearly established. Retinoic acid, an oxidation product of retinal, is a potent promoter of growth in the vitamin A-deficient animal, yet it is ineffective in restoring visual function. It may thus be that the components of vitamin A which are essential for growth may not be those which are involved in maintenance of the visual response to dark. The nature of this growth-promoting component of vitamin A awaits further investigation.

Induction of vitamin A deficiency requires prolonged periods of a deficient intake due to the fat solubility of this vitamin. The clinical symptoms which eventually appear involve desiccation and ulceration of the cornea and conjunctiva in the eye, increased frequency of respiratory infection, and keratinization and drying of the skin, with an occasional papular eruption. Kidney stones and alterations in the pancreatic ducts are frequently found. These symptoms of vitamin A deficiency are most commonly seen in patients suffering from impaired intestinal fat absorption. Thus, pancreatic disease, disease of the biliary tract, sprue, and ulcerative colitis are the primary causes of vitamin A deficiency; only rarely does dietary deficiency alone produce symptoms.

Overzealous treatment with preparations containing vitamin A can, however, induce symptoms of toxicity. These symptoms, which usually take six months or more to develop, require doses in excess of 50,000 units of vitamin A per day and consist of irritability, loss of appetite, and itching of the skin. Fatigue, myalgia, changes in body hair, and enlargement of the liver and spleen have also been observed. Withdrawal of the vitamin leads to rapid regression of most of the symptoms. The one exception is the bony hyperostoses which develop in the extremities and in the occipital region of the skull.

Vitamin D, Calcium, Magnesium, and Their Control. *Vitamin D* is a fat-soluble sterol which can prevent rickets. Much of the early work on this disease was prompted by the significant numbers of afflicted children in urban areas of the temperate zones. By 1920 it had been established that the disease was the result of a dietary deficiency and lack of sunlight. Irradiation of dietary rations and the skin were effective in preventing the disease. Demonstration of an antirachetic factor in various fish oils was followed by intensive chemical studies leading to the identification and elucidation of the structure of vitamin D_2 by 1937. The next major advance in the physiology of vitamin D was the synthesis of radioactively labeled vitamin D_2 of high specific activity. With radioactive vitamin D_2, it was shown that orally administered vitamin D_2 is converted to an active metabolite now known to be 25-hydroxycholecalciferol. This metabolite is active in vitro, whereas the native vitamins D_2 and D_3 require conversion. In the presence of parathyroid hormone renal tissue converts 25-hydroxylcholecalciferol to 1,25-dihydroxycholecalciferol, which acts even more rapidly than its precursor. The dihydroxy derivative may thus be the "active" form of vitamin D.

Figure 31–13 shows a diagram of the pathways involving metabolism of vitamin D. Absorption of this hormone from the gut is followed by transport to the liver and hydroxylation at the 25 position (middle, Fig. 31–13). This hydroxylation can be modified by drugs that influence the microsomal drug metabolizing enzyme system in liver, such as diphenyhydantoin. Such an effect is probably the basis for the development of osteomalacia (i.e., reduced calcification of bone matrix) in some individuals treated with this drug. The 25-hydroxylated vitamin D is then transported from the liver to the kidney where further hydroxyla-

tion occurs, producing an active 1,25-dihydroxyvitamin D_3 or an inactive 24,25-dihydroxyvitamin D_3. These processes are influenced by the concentration of parathyroid hormone, serum phosphorus, and calcium, as indicated in the accompanying figure.

Vitamin D has two principal actions. The first is to increase the absorption of calcium from the intestine and the second is to facilitate the reabsorption of calcium from bone in the presence of parathyroid hormone. The effects of vitamin D on the absorption of calcium from the gastrointestinal tract are dependent upon the formation of a transport protein in the gastrointestinal mucosa. When isolated intestine is perfused with solutions of vitamin D, it takes four hours or more to increase calcium absorption. The active metabolite 1,25-dihydroxycholecalciferol produces an increase in calcium transport in less than one and one-half hours. This effect is blocked by actinomycin D, an inhibitor of nucleic acid synthesis, suggesting that the synthesis of new protein is involved. Parathyroid hormone also plays a role in calcium absorption from the gut. In the hypoparathyroid animal, normal intake of vitamin D does not produce a normal rate of calcium absorption, although increased intake of vitamin C can restore calcium absorption to normal. Injections of parathyroid hormone lead to normal calcium absorption in the presence of normal intake of vitamin D. Similarly, in vitamin D-deficient animals, absorption of calcium is deficient, although there is excess secretion of parathyroid hormone. In the mechanisms of calcium absorption from the gut, vitamin D would appear to have the primary role, with parathyroid hormones making a secondary or minor contribution.

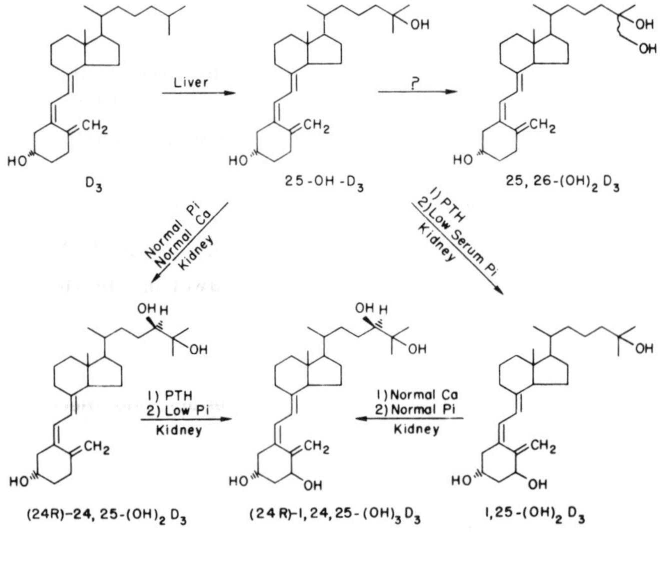

Figure 31–13 Metabolism of vitamin D. The initial hydroxylation of vitamin D occurs in the liver. Subsequent metabolism in the kidney is modulated by the levels of serum phosphorus and calcium and the concentrations of parathyroid hormone (PTH). The active metabolite is primarily the 25-$(OH)_2$-vitamin D_3. (Reproduced from DeLuca, H. F.: Ann. Int. Med., *88*:369, 1976, with permission of the author and publisher.)

The actions of vitamin D on bone have been less extensively studied, but an essential interaction with parathyroid hormone is again evident. In tissue cultures of bone, the addition of 25-hydroxycholecalciferol will stimulate bone reabsorption in a manner similar to that observed with parathyroid hormone. Moreover, this metabolite of vitamin D acts synergistically with parathyroid hormone. Although recent evidence suggests that parathyroid hormone acts on the kidney and bone to increase the production of cyclic-AMP, vitamin D does not influence this system. Thus, the synergism of parathyroid hormone and vitamin D on the reabsorption of bone appears to occur at different sites. Raisz has suggested that "the synergism could be explained if parathyroid hormone controlled entry of calcium into the nucleus and thus controlled the nuclear events of transcription and cellular transformation."

The maintenance of normal levels of circulating *calcium* is of prime importance for neuromuscular transmission and for cellular transport. The control mechanisms involved in maintaining the normal levels of serum calcium are determined not only by vitamin D but by parathyroid hormone, phosphorus, magnesium, and calcitonin. It is beyond the scope of this chapter to review these interactions in detail, but certain effects of pathologic derangements are worthy of note. Osteomalacia and rickets are the consequences of vitamin D deficiency which result from lack of sunlight, from deficiency of this vitamin in the diet, from resistance at the cellular level, or from malabsorption in the gastrointestinal tract. Pathologic consequences also occur with increased amounts of vitamin D. When parathyroid hormone is present, the ingestion of markedly increased amounts of vitamin D can induce a pathologic state similar to that observed with an excess excretion of parathyroid hormone. The state of vitamin D intoxication increases the concentrations of serum calcium and reduces the level of circulating phosphate. Calcium absorption from the gastrointestinal tract is increased, and bony abnormalities can be induced by increased absorption of calcium from bones. The consequences of hypercalcemia on the electrocardiogram and on neuromuscular conduction can be observed. Finally, persistent hypercalcemia can produce renal failure by damaging the kidney.

In the metabolism of *magnesium,* increased concentrations of parathyroid hormone can increase magnesium excretion and induce a state of magnesium deficiency. Such a change would tend to reduce the effects of parathyroid hormone. Magnesium deficiency can also be induced by dietary means and by alcoholism, and such a state is usually associated with hypocalcemia. The pathologic mechanism by which magnesium deficiency leads to hypocalcemia is unclear, although it has been attributed to resistance of the skeleton to the action of parathyroid hormone. One would expect that with hypomagnesemia the output of parathyroid hormone would be increased, as observed under in vitro and in vivo conditions, yet serum calcium is usually below normal. Support for diminished effectiveness of parathyroid hormone with magnesium depletion has been shown in studies with bone cultures and in measurements of cyclic-AMP excretion in the urine. By use of the technique of bone culture, it was shown that the effect of parathyroid hormone on calcium mobilization was reduced when the concentration of magnesium was low. Similarly, magnesium-deficient patients failed to excrete normal amounts of cyclic-AMP after the administration of parathyroid hormone. Since the action of parathyroid hormone on bone and kidney appears to involve cyclic-AMP, this may be the essential biochemical defect in this interaction. It is known from other studies on this membrane-bound enzyme complex that magnesium is essential for the conversion of ATP to $3',5'$-AMP (cyclic-AMP). Thus, in magnesium deficiency the impaired response of parathyroid hormone might be due to the slowed rate of conversion of ATP to cyclic-AMP in the absence of this divalent cation.

Vitamin E. The place of vitamin E, or alphatocopherol, in human nutrition is still unsettled. It was originally discovered as an essential factor for the maintenance of pregnancy in rats. Because this is a fat-soluble vitamin, depletion of the body stores occurs very slowly. Prolonged feeding of diets deficient in vitamin E to adults failed to produce clear-cut evidence of a deficiency state. However, in infants with protein-calorie malnutrition, vitamin E could reverse the hemolytic anemia which was often present. A similar hemolytic anemia occurs in monkeys fed a diet free of alpha-tocopherol, suggesting that this vitamin may play a role in hematopoiesis.

Vitamin K. Vitamin K is a fat-soluble vitamin essential for hepatic synthesis of clotting factors II, VII, IX, and X (see Chapter 22). Because it is a fat-soluble quinone, it is often deficient in states of malabsorption. Indeed, this is one of the observations which led to its discovery. Although the quinone structure was rapidly elucidated, it is still not known how the vitamin acts to enhance the synthesis of clotting factors. Of pathophysiologic importance is that this vitamin is competitively antagonized by such drugs as aspirin. Thus, bleeding disorders from deficiency of vitamin K can occur with hepatic disease or malabsorption or by use of drugs which are competitive antagonists.

Pathophysiologic Mechanisms of Disease States Resulting from Vitamin Deficiencies

Several pathogenetic mechanisms can lead to deficiencies of one vitamin or another and thus to the production of clinical or subclinical syndromes.

Deficient dietary intake is the first such mechanism. This can result from selective absence of one or more vitamins or its precursor in the diet, or to a generalized deficiency of all vitamins as observed in malnutrition or during total starvation. In other diseases such as alcoholism, dietary intake is frequently reduced but loss of vitamins is also accelerated. Absence of vitamin D in the diet or inadequate exposure to sunlight is associated with rickets. The failure to calcify bony matrix which characterizes this disease is now rare in this country because vitamin D is added to most milk supplies and because most infants receive supplements of vitamins. However, rickets is still seen occasionally when vitamin D is insufficient or when the response is impaired by genetic defects. Although relatively rare, it must be pointed out that cases of rickets due to vitamin deficiency are still seen even in the major metropolitan centers of the United States.

Generalized malnutrition and *therapeutic starvation* are also mechanisms for producing vitamin deficiency. Over the past decade, the use of starvation as therapy for human obesity has become widespread. During starvation there is a marked reduction in the circulating concentration of many vitamins. Thiamine, niacin, biotin, pantothenic acid, folate, riboflavin, and pyridoxine are among the vitamins which are lost. The decline in pyridoxine is progressive with the duration of starvation and reaches very low levels by 5 to 6 months. With starvation, riboflavin also drops progressively but rises promptly when food is returned to the diet. Thiamine is also reduced. In one particular patient with hypotension, vomiting, and weakness occurring after three weeks of fasting, the symptoms disappeared following the intravenous administration of thiamine. Other vitamin supplements had no effect.

Total absence of food, however, is not the only mechanism for nutritional reduction in vitamin levels. Surveys of hospitalized patients, particularly children, have shown that up to 45 per cent had lowered serum concentrations of one or more vitamins. This reduction varied with the ethnic origin of the patients. For example, Puerto Rican children showed lower circulating levels of thiamine, niacin, vitamin B_{12}, and folate than children from other ethnic groups in New York City. In contrast, Chinese children showed many instances of higher levels than other groups. Protein intake was of primary importance in determining the levels of many vitamins. When less than 38 grams of protein was ingested daily, there were marked reductions in the levels of biotin, thiamine, and ascorbic acid. Supplements with oral vitamins did not raise the serum levels to normal until protein intake was increased. Thus, protein deficiency per se influences the circulating levels of vitamins in a manner which is as yet poorly understood.

Alcoholism is a third pathologic state associated with reduced serum levels of some vitamins. These individuals frequently have a deficiency of folic acid and they are often deficient in thiamine. The deficiency in folic acid probably accounts for the frequent association of hematologic abnormalities and megaloblastic anemia. However, folic acid deficiency may also impair the ability of the liver to regenerate, since it is necessary for synthesis of DNA and for cell replication. The deficiency of thiamine in alcoholics is associated with a characteristic group of symptoms which include a wobbling gait, inability to move the eye muscles appropriately, and confusion. This symptom complex can be rapidly reversed by the intravenous administration of thiamine.

Malabsorption is another pathologic mechanism that induces vitamin deficiency. A number of disease states are associated with ineffective absorption of one or more vitamins and/or minerals from the gastrointestinal tract. Thus, food intake may be normal, but body supplies of essential elements may be deficient. This is more often seen when the pathologic alteration leads to increased loss of fat in the stools. As might be expected with increased fat excretion, the amount of fat-soluble vitamins A, D, and K is most frequently affected.

Similarly, calcium, which complexes with fatty acids formed during hydrolysis of triglyceride, is also lost with fatty acids. Thus, deficiencies of vitamin D and calcium lead to impaired formation of bone, with decreased circulating levels of calcium. This complex of symptoms in adults is known clinically as osteomalacia and is analogous to rickets in children. It is characterized by a loss of mineral from the skeleton with ensuing deformities of the weight-bearing bones. Pseudo-fractures may be detected on x-ray films as symmetrical lines at bony areas of reabsorption where nutrient arteries penetrate the bone. There is relative impairment of normal bone reabsorption and histologically defective mineralization of the newly formed bony matrix. The hypocalcemia which is usually present is relatively unresponsive to the injection of parathyroid hormone. Urinary excretion of calcium and increased secretion of phosphate from the kidney are observed. As a result of the lowered levels of circulating calcium, parathyroid hormone is secreted from the parathyroid gland in increased amounts but appears to be relatively less active than normal in improving calcium reabsorption from bone.

In addition to osteomalacia which results from loss of vitamin D and calcium, malabsorption also produces a loss of vitamin A. As noted earlier, vitamin A affects visual function and growth.

Impaired adaptation of the retina to the dark is the principal effect of vitamin A deficiency. The chemical process of dark adaptation requires the synthesis of rhodopsin, a combination of a protein opsin and a prosthetic group, 11-cis-retinal, which is derived from vitamin A. After exposure to light, this pigment undergoes a number of changes which lead to initiation of the nerve impulse. When vitamin A is deficient, the essential prosthetic group 11-cis-retinal is reduced and the production of rhodopsin, the photosensitive pigment, is impaired. Thus, malabsorption of fat can impair both bone formation and visual adaptation to darkness.

The third effect of malabsorption is the loss of vitamin K. This is an essential vitamin for the synthesis of prothrombin. In its absence, prothrombin levels are reduced and coagulation of blood is impaired, with a tendency to hemorrhage. In contrast to the other two fat-soluble vitamins, water-soluble forms of vitamin K can be administered and overcome this defect in formation of prothrombin.

Specific forms of malabsorption can also influence vitamin absorption. Pernicious anemia is a case in point in which vitamin B_{12} is not absorbed because intrinsic factor is lacking from the gastrointestinal mucosa. Injections of vitamin B_{12} will bypass this abnormality.

Although vitamin ingestion and absorption are normal, the *administration of antimetabolites or drugs* which compete directly or indirectly with vitamins for their active sites on enzymes may lead to symptoms of vitamin deficiency. Antimetabolites of folic acid are among the best known examples of this type of induced vitamin deficiency. Megaloblastic anemia responsive to folate therapy can be produced by two classes of drugs. The first class includes the anticonvulsants such as phenytoin (Dilantin) or phenobarbital. Both these drugs induce folate deficiency presumably by interfering with its reduction to dihydrofolic acid or by interfering with its role in the formation of DNA. A second group of antifolic acid metabolites includes those used in the treatment of certain cancers. These drugs interfere directly with folic acid metabolism. Aspirin is an example of the second group of drugs which will inhibit the effects of a vitamin. Salicylates compete with vitamin K and thus lower the production of prothrombin. Hypoprothrombinemia is frequently observed in patients treated with high doses of aspirin, and this effect can be overcome by administering supplements of vitamin K. Isoniazid (INH) is the final example of a drug which inhibits vitamin metabolism. This drug is widely used for the treatment of tuberculosis and has been observed to increase the excretion of pyridoxine (vitamin B_6). With high doses of isoniazid, a peripheral neuropathy, convulsions, and anemia have been observed. All three of these untoward effects resulting from the administration of isoniazid can be prevented or treated by supplements of pyridoxine.

Increased vitamin utilization in the presence of a normal dietary intake is another mechanism by which the effects of vitamin deficiency can be produced. This can occur in hypermetabolic states, such as those due to prolonged fever or other causes. There are three such common clinical states. The first is increased levels of thyroid hormone (hyperthyroidism or administration of exogenous thyroid hormone), the second is pregnancy, and the third is childhood. In hyperthyroidism, the metabolic rate is significantly increased. As noted earlier, the requirement for thiamine, riboflavin, niacin, and possibly the other water-soluble B-complex vitamins is a function of the total caloric expenditure. As caloric expenditure rises in hyperthyroidism, the daily requirements for each of these vitamins increases. To avoid induction of nutritional deficiency, it is often wise to treat patients with hyperthyroidism with supplements of B vitamins during the period of time when their disease is being controlled. A second physiologic state of hypermetabolism is observed during pregnancy and a third in the growing child. Caloric requirements per kilogram body weight are increased in children, and vitamin requirements for this age group are similarly higher than for adults. Many illnesses in children are accompanied by vitamin deficiencies as shown by low circulating levels of vitamins. Vitamin requirements are also increased in pregnancy. During gestation, a second body is formed and the increased metabolism required by this procedure demands more vitamins. It is customary to give vitamin supplements during this period to prevent depletion of maternal supplies, with potential pathologic consequences for the developing infant.

TRACE ELEMENTS

Improvements in analytical methods within the past decade have expanded our understanding of the role of trace elements in human nutrition and disease. In this section some of these elements and their role in the production of disease will be examined. The ability to induce pathologic changes by selective removal of one element from the diet provides one of the best examples of the correlation between pathologic and physiologic alterations. We will illustrate, when possible, the biochemical basis of these changes. In many instances, however, such a fundamental understanding is not yet possible because our knowledge of the role of these trace elements is as yet incomplete. A summary of the data concerning

TABLE 31-9 TRACE ELEMENTS

		Concentration			
Element	Body Content	Whole Blood	Plasma or Serum	Average Intake	Absorption
Calcium	1000 g.	9–10.5 mg./100 ml.	9–10.5 mg./100 ml.	0.2–1.5 g./d.	0.1–0.5 g.
Magnesium	25 g.	3.0 mEq./liter	1.8–2.5 mEq./liter	400 mg./d.	100 mg.
Iron	5 g.	43 mg./100 ml.*	70–180 μg./100 ml.	12–15 mg./d.	0.6–1.5 mg.
Zinc	2	800 μg./100 ml.	120 μg./100 ml.†	10–15 mg./d.	1 mg.
Copper	100–150 mg.	98 μg./100 ml.	109 μg./100 ml.	2.5–5 mg./d.	0.6–1.6 mg.
Iodine	10–20 mg.	–	4–8 μg./100 ml.	50–1000 μg./d.	50–1000 μg.
Manganese	12–20 mg.	9.8 μg./100 ml.	1.4 μg./100 ml.	2–8 mg./d.	
Molybdenum	10–20 mg.	1.4 μg./100 ml.	1.4 μg./100 ml.	100 μg./d.	90 μg.
Chromium	6 mg.	15 μg./100 ml.	1–6 μg./100 ml.	50 μg./d.	0.5 μg.
Cobalt	1 mg.	53	4.3 μg./100 ml.	300 μg./d.	30–60 μg./d.

*As iron in hemoglobin (0.34% $\times$ 12.7 g./100 ml.).

†Serum 16% higher than plasma (lysis of platelets releases zinc).

body content, plasma concentration, functional role, and deficiency appears in Table 31–9. Calcium, magnesium, iron, and zinc are quantitatively the largest, present in gram quantities. Copper, chromium, manganese, iodine, and fluoride, on the other hand, are found in only milligram quantities.

Zinc

The content of zinc is approximately 1.4 to 2.3 grams in a 70-kg. man, with 20 per cent of this amount in the skin. Circulating concentrations can be readily measured and average 121 μg. per 100 ml. in serum and somewhat more than ten times this concentration in red blood cells. Although intake is between 10 and 15 mg. per day, absorption is usually low, representing less than 10 per cent, and is decreased by certain binding agents, particularly phytates, which are present in various cereals. Zinc is a factor in a number of enzymes including alkaline phosphatase, found in liver and bone; carbonic anhydrase; carboxypeptidase from the pancreas; as well as lactate, malate, and alcoholic dehydrogenase. Zinc is also of importance in the beta cells of the pancreas and may be involved in the crystallization of insulin in the granules within these cells. This element also has an important role in the synthesis of DNA and protein, as shown by the reduced incorporation of radioactivity from thymidine into nuclear DNA in zinc deficiency. This impairment can be overcome by injecting zinc a short time before giving thymidine. The effects of zinc on the activity of ribonuclease offer one explanation for these effects on nucleic acid synthesis. Zinc is an inhibitor of this enzyme and in the deficient state the activity of ribonuclease might be enhanced.

Experimental zinc deficiency has been produced in several experimental animals and has been documented with reasonable certainty in human beings. Zinc deficiency in man is characterized by dwarfism and hypogonadism. Most cases have come from villages in Egypt and Iran where the ingestion of clay and diets high in cereal might impair the absorption of zinc. The subjects in question are usually males and show a marked delay in onset of sexual development. Pubic hairs are sparse or absent, and the testes are small. Facial hair is sparse and hepatosplenomegaly is frequent. Administration of zinc accelerated growth of these boys and led to an enhanced rate of sexual development. On this basis, it appears that zinc might be a causative factor of human disease.

The mechanism by which zinc impairs growth is unclear. It is known to be an essential part of the enzyme alkaline phosphatase, which is found in bone but its role in bone growth and development is still unsettled. Zinc deficiency is also accompanied by slow rates of growth in experimental animals, an effect which is independent of growth hormone. Although reproductive function is impaired in zinc-deficient dwarfs, the mechanism has not been established. Pituitary function, as indicated by thyroid status, is normal, and adrenal function is only slightly impaired. From the failure to develop sexually, one presumes that the output of gonadotropins is deficient.

Zinc deficiency also impairs the healing of wounds. Over 20 per cent of the total zinc stores are located in skin. Zinc supplements were shown to acclerate the rate of wound healing in groups of apparently normal men. Detailed studies of this phenomenon, however, showed that the effects of zinc were only detectable in those individuals with mild degrees of zinc deficiency. Little or no effect was present in individuals with normal levels of this element. A mild zinc deficiency thus occurs in a significant number of people. Among the groups in which the levels of zinc are reduced are cirrhotics, who show enhanced urinary zinc levels, and patients with the nephrotic syndrome.

Copper

Although copper has been known for centuries, its importance in nutrition has only been appreciated since 1930. At that time, an anemia in rats due to copper deficiency was clearly demonstrated. Since that time, it has been possible to show that patients with protein-calorie malnutrition have copper deficiency. The body stores approximately 80 mg. of copper. The largest fraction of this is in the liver and significant abnormalities in liver and brain occur in Wilson's disease, in which the transport protein for copper is markedly reduced. In this disease, the copper content of the liver and of brain is increased, with the development of neurologic symptoms and hepatic failure. Copper is part of several enzymes including cytochrome oxidase, tyrosinase, and uricase. Deficiency of copper produces three changes. The first is a hypochromic, microcytic anemia. Although copper is not known to be an important element in the production of the enzymes involved in hemoglobin synthesis, it appears to play a critical role in the overall process for utilization of iron. Copper-deficient infants recovering from protein-calorie malnutrition develop an anemia which is cured by administration of copper. These infants also have brittle bones. Leukopenia is the second principal manifestation of copper deficiency. Induction of this state in adults is difficult because of the ubiquity of copper. However, in severe malnutrition in which initial replacement is with milk for sustained periods, a deficiency in copper can be observed.

Chromium

Interest in the element chromium has been stimulated by the work of Mertz and his collaborators, who demonstrated that chromium deficiency in experimental animals was accompanied by abnormalities in the metabolism of glucose. This diabetes-like syndrome could be reversed by the administration of chromium. The body only contains 6 mg. of chromium. It is transported in blood by a specific protein known as siderophilin. Most, if not all, chromium is present with a valence of +3. This element appears to be an integral part of membranes and is contained in the enzyme phosphoglucomutase. The induction of experimental chromium deficiency impairs glucose tolerance in rats, in addition to lowering the sensitivity to the effects of insulin in vitro. The suggestion that chromium acts at the cell membrane is supported by the observation that the addition of certain chromium-containing compounds restores the response to insulin in vitro. These observations in experimental animals may be relevant to diabetes in man. It has been established that the concentration of chromium declines with age, paralleling reduced metabolism of glucose. There is suggestive evidence that in some individuals with impaired glucose tolerance, supplements of chromium can restore their metabolism of glucose toward normal. The possibility thus exists, and presents a fascinating challenge to medical science, that chromium deficiency may play a significant role in certain types of human diabetes.

Fluoride Metabolism

Fluoride is widely distributed in nature and is present in small concentrations in most supplies of soil and water. Whether this element is essential for nutrition, however, has not yet been established. Animals fed diets with very low levels of fluoride show little difference in growth rate and metabolic characteristics from animals fed diets supplemented with this element. The principal interest in fluoride has come from its inhibition of dental decay and the toxic state of fluorosis, i.e., the disease of excess fluoride intake. The initial studies demonstrating that fluoride had an effect on dental caries were conducted in the 1930s. The results of one such experiment are shown in Table 31–10. It is clear from this table that in a five year period there was a significant reduction in the number of carious teeth in children receiving fluoride supplements but no significant change in the control groups. This effect of fluoride was most striking in younger children and decreased with age. These data and many other controlled experiments clearly demonstrate that fluoride sup-

TABLE 31–10 EFFECT OF FLUORIDE ON DENTAL CARIES IN CHILDREN*

Age in Years	Control Areas		Areas with Fluoride Added in 1956		Per cent Reduction with Fluoride
	1956	1961	1956	1961	
3	3.53	3.32	3.80	1.29	66
4	5.18	4.83	5.39	2.31	57
5	5.66	5.39	5.81	2.91	50
6	6.32	6.22	6.49	4.81	26
7	7.08	6.89	7.06	6.05	14

*Fluoride added to drinking water of one area in 1956 at 1 part per million. Adapted from British Ministry of Health: Roy. Soc. Health J., 82:173, 1962.

plements at a level of 1 part per million (ppm.) in drinking water are capable of reducing dental caries. The mechanism by which this occurs, however, is unclear. Fluoride is found in its highest concentrations in bone and teeth and appears to be involved in the formation of bone matrix. An intake of water of 1 to 2 liters per day with a fluoride concentration of 1 ppm. will provide an intake of 1 to 2 mg. of fluoride. This appears to be optimal for reducing dental caries. At higher levels, fluoride poisoning or fluorosis occurs. This is primarily observed in animals but can be seen in man following industrial accidents. The symptoms develop after the compensatory mechanisms for disposition of fluoride have been exhausted. When the intake of fluoride increases sharply, the urinary excretion also rises until the maximum is achieved. Bone uptake also increases but has a finite capacity. When the capacities of the kidney and bone have been saturated, the extra fluoride is stored in tissue and induces the symptoms of fluorosis, which consist of a loss of appetite and a loss of body weight. Symptoms referable to the gastrointestinal and neuromuscular systems also occur, as do pulmonary congestion and respiratory and cardiac failure. It must be noted, however, that such levels of fluoride are hardly ever reached in man.

One of the principal sources of fluoride in the human diet is tea. This plant absorbs large quantities of fluoride from the soil and is in this sense unique. For most other foods, concentrations of 1 to 2 ppm. of fluoride are maximal. Fluoride concentrations in tea, however, can be up to 100 ppm. or 100 times that usually seen in almost all other sources of food.

Iodine

The importance of iodine in human metabolism has been known for over 50 years. This element which was discovered in the early part of the 19th century was studied extensively by Chatin, who correlated the prevalence of goiter with availability of iodine supplies in the soil, food, and water. His work in the middle of the 19th century strongly suggested that the regions with a high incidence of thyroid enlargement (goiter) were those regions with low iodine in food and water. His analytical methods were relatively crude by present standards and his work went largely unnoticed. Revival of interest in iodine came from the observations by Baumann that the thyroid gland contained iodine. Within a short time, the presence of thyroxine was demonstrated by Kendall, and in 1927 the structure and synthesis of this hormone were reported by Harrington. At the same time, studies by Marine and his collaborators demonstrated the efficacy of iodine supplements as a treatment for thyroid enlargement. In

a series of studies carried out in the school system of Akron, Ohio, in 1916 to 1920, these investigators showed that supplements of iodine significantly reduced the incidence of goiter among school children. From their work and the observations of many since that time, the essential nature of iodine intake for prevention of goiter and the need to supplement iodine intake in regions with low iodine content in the food and water has become clear. The principal supplementary sources of iodine in diet have come by the addition of iodide to salt in the form of iodized salt and more recently by the use of iodates in bread.

The iodide ingested in the diet is absorbed and circulates at a concentration of 0.06 to 0.80 μg. per ml. of serum. This iodide has two principal exit routes from the serum: (1) into the thyroid gland and (2) into the urine by filtration at the glomerulus. The fraction of iodide concentrated by the thyroid gland and converted to hormone is related to the total quantity of iodine already present in the thyroid. In areas of iodine deficiency, i.e., when intake is less than 75 μg. per day on the average, the iodine stores in the thyroid become deficient, since the daily requirements for hormone synthesis are approximately 80 μg. Thus, as deficiency develops, compensatory mechanisms increase the fraction of circulating iodine which is trapped by the thyroid gland and decrease the fraction which is excreted in the urine. Conversely, when iodine intake is high, the thyroid stores become saturated and further uptake of iodine is inhibited, and the relative fraction concentrated by the gland falls as the fraction appearing in the urine increases. This reciprocal relationship between uptake of iodine by the thyroid gland and its excretion in the urine has been used by Oddie, Fisher, and their collaborators to evaluate levels of iodine intake in various parts of the United States. Regional differences in dietary intake are clearly apparent (Fig. 31–14). It is the regions with low iodine intake where the incidence of endemic goiter is highest.

Severe iodine deficiency occurs in several regions of the world. One of the earliest studies of the pathophysiologic consequences of iodine deficiency was carried out by Stanbury and his collaborators in the Mendoza region of Argentina. More recent studies have been conducted in the Congo, in New Guinea, and in portions of South America and the Middle East. The more severe the lack of iodine, the greater the frequency of enlarged thyroid glands. However, even in the most severely deficient areas, enlargement of the thyroid gland does not occur in all persons. This observation suggests significant variability between individuals in their ability to compensate for severe iodine deficiency. Several mechanisms are involved in this compensation. The first of these is an increase in the fraction of ingested iodine which is trapped

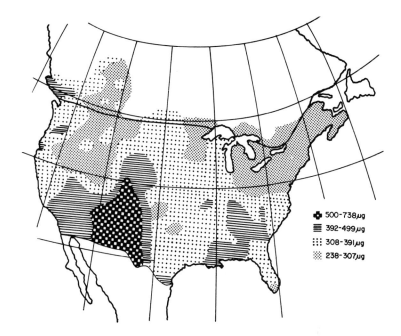

Figure 31–14 Iodine intake in the United States. These data on iodine intake in the United States were calculated from data on the regional uptake of radioactive iodine. The areas of highest iodine intake are in the southwest United States and the lowest regions are in the midwest, along the east coast and in some sections of the upper Rocky Mountains. (Reproduced with permission from Oddie, T. H., et al.: J. Clin. Endocrinol., 30:659, 1970.)

500-738µg
392-499µg
308-391µg
238-307µg

by the thyroid gland. In many areas, iodine uptake is frequently above 70 per cent and may reach 100 per cent of an administered dose. The iodide which is trapped by the thyroid is attached to tyrosine to form mono- and diiodotyrosine, which are in turn coupled to form thyroxine and triiodothyronine. As iodine becomes scarce, the percentage of monoiodotyrosine is increased in the thyroid gland relative to diiodotyrosine. Similarly, the proportion of 3,5,3'-triiodothyronine increases relative to thyroxine. Thus, the quantities of monoiodotyrosine and triiodothyronine are increased and the concentrations of diiodotyrosine and thyroxine are reduced in areas of iodine deficiency. Because the iodine stores are low, the turnover rate of thyroid iodine increases. Thus, triiodothyronine becomes a larger fraction of the circulating thyroactive hormone in iodine deficiency than when iodine stores are adequate. Finally, the thyroid gland itself enlarges in an attempt to compensate for the low iodine intake. Two underlying mechanisms are thus involved in the adaptation to iodine deficiency. The first are the intrathyroidal mechanisms of autoregulation. By this term one means that the responsiveness of the thyroid to the thyroid-stimulating hormone from the pituitary gland is increased in iodine deficiency. Thus, the uptake of iodide, the conversion to hormone, the release of hormone, and enlargement of the thyroid gland are all increased in an iodine-deficient thyroid. The second mechanism for regulating thyroidal iodine stores is the increase in the concentrations of thyroid-stimulating hormone (TSH). This mechanism presumably is activated

by a reduction in the concentration of circulating thyroxine and triiodothyronine detected by the hypothalamic receptors which control the output of thyrotropin-releasing hormone from the pituitary.

The enlarged thyroid which occurs in iodine-deficient areas can be reduced in size in many individuals given iodine supplementation. This has been shown repeatedly by giving iodine supplements to deficient groups. Thus, iodine is an essential element for human nutrition and in its absence compensatory processes occur which lead to thyroid enlargement. Failure of the compensatory mechanism to provide a reasonable circulating level of thyroid hormone is accompanied by hypothyroidism and failure to grow normally. Areas of severe iodine deficiency show an increase in the number of such goiterous cretins suffering from deficiency of thyroid hormones.

In some regions of the world, iodine supplies occur in excess. In these regions, thyroid glands tend to be smaller than normal, but in some individuals, thyroid enlargement occurs. This consequence of high intake of iodine has been termed iodide myxedema. The mechanism for this effect appears to be suppression of thyroid function by high iodide intake resulting in a drop in circulating thyroid hormone and compensatory increase in the output of thyrotropin by the pituitary. This, in turn, stimulates the thyroid gland to enlarge. A comparable effect of high iodide intake was observed in animals by Wolff and Chaikoff, and the mechanism of this effect is currently under intensive investigation.

REFERENCES

OBESITY

Albrink, M. J. (ed.): Clinics in Endocrinology and Metabolism, Vol. 5, No. 2. W. B. Saunders Co., Philadelphia, 1976.

Bagdade, J. D., Bierman, E. L., and Porte, D., Jr.: The significance of basal insulin levels in the evaluation of the insulin response to glucose in diabetic and nondiabetic subjects. J. Clin. Invest., 46:1549, 1967.

Bray, G. A.: The Obese Patient. (Vol. IX in the series: Major Problems in Internal Medicine.) W. B. Saunders Co., Philadelphia, 1976a.

Bray, G. A.: The Overweight Patient. Adv. Intern. Med., 21:267, 1976b.

Bray, G. A. (Chairman), Cahill, G., Jordan, H., Horton, E. S., Salans, L. B., and Sims, E. A. H. (Editorial Board): Obesity in Perspective. Fogarty Int. Ctr. Series on Preventive Med., Vol. 2, Part 1 and Part 2 (Bray, G. A., ed.). U.S. Government Printing Office, Washington, D.C., 1976.

Bray, G. A., Jordan, H. A., and Sims, E. A. H.: Evaluation of the obese patient. 1. An algorithm. J.A.M.A., 235:2008, 1976.

Bruch, H.: The Frohlich syndrome. Am. J. Dis. Child., 58:1282, 1939.

Garrow, J. S.: Energy Balance and Obesity in Man. American Elsevier Publishing Company, Inc., New York, 1974.

Goldman, R. F., Haisman, M. F., Bynum, G., Horton, E. S., and Sims, E. A. H.: Experimental obesity in man. Metabolic rate in relation to dietary intake. In Obesity in Perspective. Fogarty Int. Ctr. Series on Preventive Med., Vol. 2, Part 2. (Bray, G. A., ed.), U.S. Government Printing Office, Washington, D.C., 1976, p. 165.

Gordon, E. A.: Metabolic Aspects of Obesity. In Levine, R., and Luft, R., (eds.): Advances in Metabolic Disorders, Vol. 4. Academic Press, New York, 1970, p. 229.

Hetherington, A. W., and Ranson, S. W.: Hypothalamic lesions and adiposity in the rat. Anat. Rec., 78:149, 1940.

Hirsch, J., and Batchelor, B.: Adipose tissue cellularity in human obesity. Clin. Endocrinol. Metab., 5:299, 1976.

Hollenberg, C. H., Vost, A., and Patten, R. L.: Regulation of adipose mass: control of fat cell development and lipid content. Recent Progr. Horm. Res., 26:463, 1970.

Horton, E. S., Danforth, E., Jr., Sims, E. A. H., and Salans, L. B.: Endocrine and metabolic alterations in spontaneous and experimental obesity. In Bray, G. A. (ed.): Obesity in Perspective. Fogarty Int. Ctr. Series on Preventive Med., Vol. 2, Part 2. U.S. Government Printing Office, Washington, D.C., 1976, p. 323.

Lusk, G.: The Elements of the Science of Nutrition. W. B. Saunders Co., Philadelphia, 1928.

Moore, F. D., Olesen, K. H., McMurrey, J. D., Parker, H. V., Ball, M. B., and Boyden, C. M.: The Body Cell Mass and Its Supporting Environment. W. B. Saunders Co., Philadelphia, 1963.

Powley, T. L.: The ventromedial hypothalamic syndrome, satiety, and a cephalic phase hypothesis. Psychol. Rev., 84:89, 1977.

Recommended Dietary Allowances, 8th Ed. National Academy of Sciences, Washington, D.C., 1974.

Salans, L. B., Horton, E. S., and Sims, E. A. H.: Experimental obesity in man: cellular character of the adipose tissue. J. Clin. Invest., 50:1005, 1971.

Schachter, S., and Rodin, J.: In Festinger, L., and Schachter, S. (eds.): Obese Humans and Rats, Lawrence Erlbaum Associates, Washington, D.C., 1974.

Sims, E. A. H., Danforth, E., Jr., Horton, E. S., Bray, G. A., Glennon, J. A., and Salans, L. B.: Endocrine and metabolic factors of experimental obesity in man. Recent Progr. Horm. Res., 29:457, 1973.

Widdowson, E. M.: Chemical analysis of the body. In Brozek, J. (Ed.): Human Body Composition: Approaches and Applications. New York, Pergamon Press, 1965, pp. 31–55.

PROTEIN AND/OR CALORIE DEFICIENCY

Cahill, G. F., Jr., Herrera, M. G., Morgan, A. P., Soeldner, J. S., Steinke, J., Levy, P. L., Reichard, G. A., Jr., and Kipnis, D. M.: Hormone-fuel interrelationships during fasting. J. Clin. Invest., 45:1751, 1966.

Cahill, G. F., Jr., and Owen, O. E.: Body fuels and starvation. In Rowland, C. V., Jr. (ed.): Anorexia and Obesity. Little, Brown & Co., Boston, 1970, pp. 25–36.

Crisp, A. H.: Anorexia nervosa—"feeding disorder," "nervous malnutrition," or "weight phobia"? World Rev. Nutr. Diet., 12:452, 1970.

Latham, M. C.: Protein-calorie malnutrition in children and its relation to psychological development and behavior. Physiol. Rev., 54:541, 1974.

McCance, R. A., and Widdowson, E. M.: Calorie deficiencies and protein deficiencies. Little, Brown & Co., Boston, 1968.

Owen, O. E., Morgan, A. P., Kemp, H. G., Sullivan, J. M., Herrera, M. G., and Cahill, G. F., Jr.: Brain metabolism during fasting. J. Clin. Invest., 46:1589, 1967.

Vigersky, R. A., Loriaux, D. L., Andersen, A. E., and Lipsett, M. B.: Anorexia nervosa: Behavioral and hypothalamic aspects. Clin. Endocrinol. Metab., 5:517, 1976.

Young, V. R., and Scrimshaw, N. S.: The physiology of starvation. Sci. Am., 225:14, 1971.

LIPIDS

Brown, M. S., and Goldstein, J. L.: Receptor-mediated control of cholesterol metabolism. Science, 191:150, 1976.

Cuthbertson, W. F. J.: Essential fatty acid requirements in infancy. Am. J. Clin. Nutr., 29:559, 1976.

Fredrickson, D. S., Levy, R. I., and Lees, R. S.: Fat transport in lipoproteins. An integrated approach to mechanisms and disorders. N. Engl. J. Med., 276:32, 94, 148, 215, 273, 1967.

Goldstein, J. L., Schrott, H. G., Hazzard, W. R., Bierman, E. L., and Motulsky, A. G.: Hyperlipidemia in coronary heart disease. II. Genetic analysis of lipid levels in 176 families and delineation of a new inherited disorder, combined hyperlipidemia. J. Clin. Invest., 52:1544, 1973.

Glueck, C. J., Heckman, F., Schoenfeld, M., Steiner, P., and Pearce, W.: Neonatal familial type II hyperlipoproteinemia: Cord blood cholesterol in 1800 births. Metabolism, 20:597, 1971.

Levy, R. I., Fredrickson, D. S., Shulman, R., Bilheimer, D. W., Breslow, J. L., Stones, N. J., Lux, S. E., Sloan, H. R., Krauss, R. M., and Herbert, P. N.: Dietary and drug treatment of primary hyperlipoproteinemia. Ann. Intern. Med., 77:267, 1972.

Meng, H. C.: Fat Emulsions in Parenteral Nutrition. In Fischer, J. E. (ed.), Total Parenteral Nutrition. Little, Brown & Company, Boston, 1976, pp. 305–334.

VITAMINS

Baker, H., and Frank, O.: Vitamin status in metabolic upsets. World Rev. Nutr. Diet., 9:124, 1968.

Darby, W. J., McNutt, K. W., and Todhunter, E. N.: Niacin. Nutr. Rev., 33:289, 1975.

DeLuca, H. F.: Vitamin D endocrinology. Ann. Intern. Med., 85:367, 1976.

Frimpter, G. W., Andelman, R. J., and George, W. F.: Vitamin B_6-dependency syndromes. Am. J. Clin. Nutr., 22:794, 1969.

Gubler, C. J.: Thiamine. Wiley Press, New York, 1976.

Horwitt, M. K.: Vitamin E: a reexamination. Am. J. Clin. Nutr., 29:569, 1976.

Irwin, M. I.: A conspectus of research on vitamin C requirements in man. J. Nutr., 106:821, 1976.

Kleeman, C. R., Massry, S. G., and Coburn, J. W.: The clinical physiology of calcium homeostasis, parathyroid hormone, and calcitonin. Calif. Med., 114:16, 1971.

Lutwak, L., Singer, F. R., and Urist, M. R.: Current concepts of bone metabolism. Ann. Intern. Med., 80:630, 1974.

Stewart, C. P., and Guthrie, D.: Lind's Treatise on Scurvy. The Edinburgh University Press, Edinburgh, 1953.

Terris, M.: Goldberger on Pellagra. Louisiana State University Press, Baton Rouge, 1964.

TRACE ELEMENTS

British Ministry of Health: Report on the five year fluoridation studies in the United Kingdom, July 3, 1962. Roy. Soc. Health J., 82:173, 1962.

Mertz, W., Toepfer, E. W., Roginski, E. R., and Polansky, M. M.: Present knowledge of the role of chromium. Fed. Proc., 33:2275, 1974.

Oddie, T. H., Fisher, D. A., McConahey, W. M., and Thompson, C. S.: Iodine intake in the United States: a reassessment. J. Clin. Endocrinol., 30:659, 1970.

Sandstead, H. H.: Zinc nutrition in the United States. Am. J. Clin. Nutr., 26:1251, 1973.

Underwood, E. J.: Trace Elements in Human and Animal Nutrition. Academic Press, New York, 1977.

32

Endocrinology

Thomas W. Burns

INTRODUCTION

The endocrine system is composed of glands which secrete one or more hormones directly into the bloodstream. The ductless glands of the endocrine system are in contrast to the exocrine glands, the secretions of which pass into the lumen of the gastrointestinal tract or onto the skin. Over 100 years ago Claude Bernard introduced a fundamental concept of biology — homeostasis of the internal milieu. Survival of mammalian species has required mechanisms to maintain the constancy of the internal environment despite wide fluctuations in the physical environment and in the availability of essential nutrients. The endocrine system provides many of these mechanisms.

If a principal function of the endocrine system is the preservation of homeostasis, its method of accomplishing this is communication. Increasingly it appears that the nervous system and the endocrine system form a complementary "wire" and "wireless" communications network regulating a broad array of metabolic processes. Neural transmitters from higher centers impinge on the hypothalamus, thereby modulating the synthesis and secretion of neurohumoral substances which either regulate the release of anterior pituitary hormones or pass directly to the posterior pituitary. Once these hormones are released into the circulation, they in turn stimulate the secretion of hormones by specific target glands or act directly on other tissues of the body. At the distal end of the communications circuit, these hormones powerfully affect intracellular events. At the proximal end, many of these hormones, including those secreted by the thyroid, gonads, parathyroids, and pancreas, are essential for the

proper development and function of the central nervous system. While in no instance has the precise mechanism of action of the hormone on a tissue been elucidated, recent work suggests that hormone action commences with the interaction of the hormone with a specific receptor protein in either the cell membrane or cytosol. The hormone-receptor protein complex then activates the first of a series of enzymatic steps leading to the overt expression of the hormone's biologic activity. Thus, the central nervous system, the endocrine system, and the intracellular enzymatic systems form an interlocking triad of regulation, each element capable of directing and responding to appropriate signals which allow the transfer of information from the integrated center of the organism to its smallest operating unit.

BASIC PHYSIOLOGIC CONCEPTS

ELEMENTS OF THE ENDOCRINE SYSTEM

The principal components of the endocrine system are the hypothalamus, the anterior and posterior pituitary, the thyroid, the parathyroids, the pancreas, the adrenal cortex, the adrenal medulla, and the gonads (ovaries and testes). The endocrine function of the human pineal gland has not been established and will not be considered. The placenta elaborates several hormones, but there are few data implicating the endocrine placenta in human disease and it will not be commented upon further. Another endocrine "organ" that will not be discussed is the gastrointestinal tract. The so-called "gut hormones" are of both historical interest (see below) and the subject of

1002

intensive current investigation; however, the physiologic role of these substances has yet to be determined.

The secretory activity of the adrenal cortex, the thyroid, and the gonads is subservient to the tropic hormones of the anterior pituitary. The secretion of parathyroid hormone is regulated by the level of plasma ionized calcium, and that of insulin principally by the serum glucose concentration. The secretion of epinephrine by the adrenal medulla is controlled by the sympathetic nervous system.

HORMONES: DEFINITION AND BASIC CHARACTERIZATION

The term "hormone" was first used by Starling and Bayliss in 1906 to describe secretin and gastrin. They defined hormones as chemical substances released into the circulation by one group of cells and affecting one or more different groups of cells. A more useful definition, proposed by Huxley in 1935, emphasizes the biologic function of hormones rather than their means of transport. According to Huxley, hormones are molecules whose essential purpose is the transfer of information from one set of cells to another to meet the needs of the total organism.

At the present time it is possible to distinguish at least two groups of hormones. Those in the first group clearly subserve the transfer of information role of Huxley's definition. Examples include epinephrine, parathyroid hormone, insulin, and most of the hormones of the anterior pituitary. In general, the response of the body to these hormones is rapid and proportionate to the quantity of hormone present. The response promptly ceases when the concentration of hormone falls below a critical level. These hormones appear to act through the adenylate cyclase-cyclic AMP system to be described later. The second group of hormones is exemplified by the steroids, thyroxine, and growth hormone. The response of cells to these hormones is slow and may persist after the plasma concentration of the hormone has fallen below a physiologically effective level. Their primary function appears to be growth and maintenance. Since, in their absence, cells may not be able to respond to the first group of hormones, hormones of the second group have been termed permissive. Their mechanism of action appears to involve modification of protein synthesis. Thus far, there has been no demonstration that they activate the cyclic AMP system. The terms "neurocrine" and "paracrine" are being used to indicate cells that release a humoral substance capable of modifying the function of adjacent cells. Neurocrine cells release neurotransmitters. Examples of paracrine cells are the alpha cells of the pancreatic islets of Langerhans. These cells

release glucagon which, besides its systemic effects, may act locally to influence the secretion of insulin and somatostatin by beta and delta cells, respectively.

FEEDBACK CONTROL IN THE REGULATION OF HORMONE SECRETORY ACTIVITY

The concept of negative and positive feedback control is basic to a clear understanding of the normal and pathologic physiology of the endocrine system. The interrelations between the anterior pituitary and the thyroid, spelled out in more detail below, exemplify the principles involved. The secretory rate of thyroid hormone is increased by plasma thyroid-stimulating hormone (TSH) which is secreted by the anterior pituitary. [*Note:* Throughout this chapter, the term "thyroid hormone" is intended to include thyroxine (T_4) and triiodothyronine (T_3)]. As the level of thyroid hormone in the plasma increases, it reaches a concentration called the "set point," which causes the cessation of TSH secretion and hence of the secretion of thyroid hormone itself. The plasma concentration of thyroid hormone then falls, and when it declines below the set point, TSH secretion resumes. An analogy may be drawn between this process and the control of room temperature by the interaction of a thermostat and a furnace. The thermostat setting, for example 70°, is similar to the set point. Heat from the furnace will be delivered until the room temperature exceeds 70°. At that point, the thermostat signals the furnace to shut off and delivery of heat ceases. When the temperature falls below the set point, the thermostat is activated and signals the furnace to turn on. In this analogy, the furnace represents the thyroid gland, heat represents plasma thyroid hormone, the thermostat represents the anterior pituitary, and the electrical signal between the thermostat and the furnace is analogous to TSH. As will be seen subsequently, the regulation of thyroid hormone secretion is more complicated than this analogy suggests; it involves a third hormone, thyrotropin-releasing hormone (TRH), secreted by the hypothalamus.

The control of parathyroid hormone secretion is based on a simpler negative feedback. The principal stimulus to its secretion is a fall in plasma calcium concentration below a set point of approximately 10 mg. per dl. The increase in plasma parathyroid hormone, by its action on kidney and bone, increases serum calcium until the set point is reached. The relationship between insulin secretion by the pancreas and the plasma concentration of glucose exemplifies a positive feedback system. When glucose concentration exceeds a level of about 120 mg. per dl, insulin secretion increases and diverts glucose into the liver and peripheral tissues, thus reducing the blood glucose. The advantages of these feedback systems, which have many counterparts in the servomechanisms in industry, are obvious. They permit maintenance of closely controlled concentrations of hormones, metabolites, and nutrients in the plasma, and thus preserve the homeostasis of the internal milieu. As will be repeatedly emphasized, the diagnosis of an endocrine disease frequently is based on the interpretation of laboratory data in light of the feedback concept.

CHEMICAL NATURE, ELABORATION, SECRETION, AND TRANSPORT OF HORMONES

If hormones are classified on the basis of chemical structure, four broad categories emerge:
1. Small peptides.
2. Large polypeptides.
3. Steroids.
4. Derivatives of amino acids.

The structures of some neurohumoral substances elaborated by the hypothalamus are only now being elucidated. They appear to be small peptides with only a few amino acid residues. Vasopressin, also formed in hypothalamic nuclei, has 8 amino acids. The hormones of the anterior pituitary are large polypeptides, as are insulin, glucagon, and parathyroid hormone. The steroid hormones include secretions of the adrenal cortex, the ovaries, and the testes. Both thyroxine and epinephrine are amino acid derivatives.

Much information is accruing regarding the molecular events involved in the biosynthesis, storage, and release of hormones, especially thyroid hormone, insulin, and the steroid hormones. The fabrication of a hormone requires a number of enzymatic steps, and many diseases are now recognized which are due to a deficiency of a biosynthetic enzyme. This leads either to the absence of hormone production by the involved gland or to the synthesis of a defective hormone. It should be recalled that many hormones have the secondary function of interacting with either the hypothalamus or the pituitary to assist in the regulation of their own secretion. The structural requirements for both of these functions of a hormone are thought to be the same. The consequences of a target endocrine gland secreting a biologically inactive hormone are predictable from the negative feedback concept. An affected individual will display not only the effects of hormonal deficiency but also enlargement of the affected gland, because of an increase in the specific circulating tropic hormone. Examples of this phenomenon involving deficiencies in the biosynthesis of thyroid hormone will be discussed later.

After their release into the circulation, many hormones quickly combine with a carrier protein.

In general, the structure of the carrier protein is highly specific for its client hormone. Since only the free hormone is metabolically active, the binding of hormone to a specific protein provides another means of regulating its activity. The concentrations of carrier proteins are influenced by various factors including sex hormones, drugs, and certain diseases. Instances of both genetically induced deficiency and excess of the thyroid-binding protein (thyroid-binding globulin or TBG) have been observed. As discussed below, carrier proteins are being used as reagents in the laboratory for the measurement of the specific hormones they bind.

MECHANISM OF ACTION OF HORMONES

It is gratifying to students of biology when a unifying concept becomes established as fact. Such was the case when the nucleotide adenosine-triphosphate (ATP) was identified as the final donor of energy in almost all biologic reactions. A similar event has occurred concerning the mechanism of hormone action, since most, if not all, appear to act through one of two pathways.

Adenylate Cyclase – Cyclic AMP System

Largely through the patient and creative investigations of Sutherland and coworkers 15 years ago, the nucleotide cyclic AMP was recognized as a key mediator of the action of epinephrine on liver glycogen. Since then, research on the role of cyclic AMP has proliferated at a fantastic rate. Some of the hormone-tissue interactions in which cyclic AMP has been implicated are summarized in Table 32–1. Not only has cyclic AMP been found in cells of all animal species studied, but Pastan demonstrated its necessity for the induction of certain enzymes in the bacterium *E. coli*. Cyclic AMP has also been identified as the attractant substance that signals individual cells of the social ameba, the slime mold, to aggregate. Thus, the significance of cyclic AMP in biology rivals that of ATP.

The manner in which cyclic AMP mediates hormonal action appears constant for all hormones and animal species thus far studied. It is depicted schematically in Figure 32–1. The hormone circulating in plasma interacts with a receptor in the plasma membrane of the cell. The receptor may be an integral part of the enzyme adenylate cyclase or may merely be linked to it. In any event, the hormone-receptor interaction leads to activation of adenylate cyclase. This enzyme catalyzes the formation of cyclic AMP from ATP. Cyclic AMP then triggers the response that is recognized as the hormone's biologic action. In this scheme, the hormone is frequently designated as the "first messenger" and cyclic AMP as the "second messenger." The intracellular level of cy-

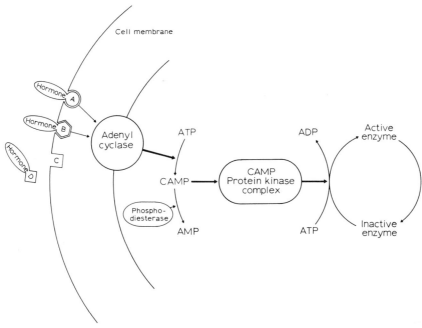

Figure 32–1 Cyclic AMP-mediated hormone action. Circulating hormones ("first messengers") interact with specific receptor sites on the plasma membrane of responsive cells, causing stimulation of adenylate cyclase. Adenylate cyclase catalyzes the conversion of ATP to cyclic AMP (CAMP). The nucleotide activates a protein kinase which, in turn, causes the activation of the enzyme(s) responsible for the expression of the hormone. Free cyclic AMP is quickly destroyed by a specific phosphodiesterase (see text).

clic AMP is decreased by the activity of a potent, specific esterase, phosphodiesterase. This enzyme is inhibited by xanthine derivatives such as theophylline and caffeine. These agents cause an increase in cyclic AMP and tend to mimic hormone action in in-vitro systems. Additional details are now known regarding the mechanism by which cyclic AMP initiates the cellular response to a hormone. The nucleotide interacts with protein kinase. This enzyme has two components: a receptor and a catalytic unit. In its unstimulated state, the receptor component prevents action by the catalytic unit. Interaction of the receptor with cyclic AMP removes the former, allowing the catalytic unit to act. This active form of protein kinase stimulates another enzyme or enzymes, presumably by phosphorylation, and this secondary enzyme (or enzymes) catalyzes the final step leading to the hormone's action and is thought to be inactivated by a phosphatase.

Sutherland and his co-workers have suggested four criteria which ideally should be met if cyclic AMP is to be considered the "second messenger" for a given hormone. These are (1) The hormone should be capable of stimulating adenylate cyclase in broken cell preparations from appropriate tissue. (2) A physiologic concentration of hormone should be able to increase the cyclic

AMP concentration of intact cells, and this increase in cyclic AMP should precede the physiologic response. (3) Phosphodiesterase inhibitors such as theophylline should potentiate the response to the hormone. (4) The activity of the hormone should be mimicked by cyclic AMP or its more soluble dibutyryl derivative.

A question that naturally arises when one views Table 32–1 is how can the same compound, cyclic AMP, mediate the highly specific responses of such a diverse array of hormones? There are at least two sites at which specificity could be endowed. Presumably all cells of the body (exclusive of those in the central nervous system) are equally exposed to a hormone circulating in the plasma. However, only the cells of responsive tissue have receptor sites that "recognize" the hormone. The receptor site has a conformational structure complementary to that of the hormone, permitting the latter to bind to the former with high affinity. Additional specificity is imparted by the nature of the substance(s) available to serve as substrates for the cyclic AMP protein kinase catalytic unit. In adipose tissue, the substance is a lipase; in liver, it is a phosphorylase. Specificity could also result if cyclic AMP were compartmentalized within the cell, but this has not been demonstrated thus far.

TABLE 32–1   HORMONES WHICH
UTILIZE CYCLIC AMP AS A SECOND
MESSENGER

Hormone	Tissue
Catecholamines	Various tissues
Glucagon	Liver, pancreatic islets, adipose tissue
ACTH	Adrenal cortex and adipose tissue
LH or ICSH	Ovarian and testicular tissue
Vasopressin	Various epithelial tissues
Parathyroid hormone	Kidney and bone, gut
TRH	Anterior pituitary
TSH	Thyroid tissue
MSH	Frog skin
Prostaglandins	Various tissues
Histamine	Brain
Serotonin	Fasciola hepatica

(From Robison, G. A., Butcher, R. W., and Sutherland, E. W.: Cyclic AMP. Academic Press, New York,
1971.)

Interaction of Hormones with Cytoplasmic Receptor Protein and Nuclear Acceptors

At present it appears that the steroid hormones
(testosterone, estradiol, progesterone, aldosterone, and cortisol) all exert their metabolic effects in a similar fashion (Fig. 32–2). Each appears to combine with a specific receptor protein
located in the cytoplasm; the steroid-receptor
complex is translocated to the nucleus, where it
combines with specific acceptors located on chromatin. The steroid-receptor-acceptor complex
causes the nuclear genetic material to produce
messenger RNA, which in turn signals the fabrication of the enzyme which is more directly responsible for the biologic expression of the hormone's activity. Specificity results from the
conformational structure of the receptor protein
and the nuclear acceptor sites.

The Role of Receptor Abnormalities in the Pathophysiology of Endocrine Disease

Many years ago one of the great pioneers in
endocrinology, Fuller Albright, predicted the existence of endocrinopathies in which the relevant
endocrine gland and its secretion are normal but
the tissues normally responsive to the hormone
are, in fact, resistant to it. Albright cited the
Seabright bantam as an animal model of his hypothesis. The Seabright rooster demonstrates
normal androgen effects in every respect except
for an underdeveloped comb. The comb tissue in
this species is insensitive to androgen. The first
clinical example of end organ resistance, pseudohypoparathyroidism, was described by Albright
and his colleagues in 1942.

Mechanisms underlying the resistant state are
beginning to be clarified in some of these dis-

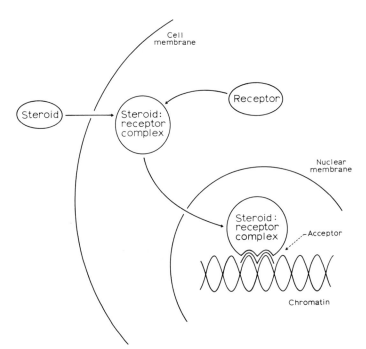

Figure 32–2   Mechanism of action of
steroid hormones. Steroid hormones
penetrate the cell membrane and combine with highly specific receptor molecules in the cytosol. The steroid-
receptor complex then enters the nucleus and binds to an acceptor. The
aggregate stimulates the production of
messenger RNA which stimulates the
synthesis of the protein substances that
are responsible for the hormone's action
(see text).

orders. From the work of Roth and his colleagues and a number of other workers, it appears that both the number of receptors and their affinity for hormone may be altered in disease. In the case of insulin, both in-vivo and in-vitro studies suggest that a major determinant of the number of receptors on insulin-sensitive cells is the ambient concentration of insulin itself. Thus, in maturity onset diabetes, one may find the combination of obesity, hyperglycemia, increased levels of circulating insulin and a *decrease* in insulin receptors on the cells of peripheral tissues. Very rarely, autoantibodies to insulin receptors may develop, producing a profound state of insulin resistance. This is seen in the disease acanthosis nigricans. Some of the receptor abnormalities in disease are discussed by Kahn and co-workers.

MANIFESTATIONS OF ENDOCRINE DISORDERS

The majority of endocrine diseases are secondary to either an excess or a deficiency of one or more hormones. Commonly, the clinical description of an endocrine disorder has antedated by many years an appreciation of the gland and hormone involved. Progress in relating clinical syndromes to deficient or excessive hormone was relatively slow until techniques became available for the measurement of hormones and their metabolites in blood and urine. The protean modes of presentation of endocrine disease are best appreciated by considering the specific examples in the following sections. However, it is important to appreciate the close symbiosis that exists between bedside medicine and laboratory physiology in the field of endocrinology. Perhaps in no other field of medicine has clinical observation been more important in shaping the direction of physiologic experimentation, and similarly there is no area in which the physician is more dependent on an understanding of physiologic principles in diagnosing and treating his patient.

Generally, the clinical manifestations of hormone excess and deficiency are extremely slow in evolving. With few exceptions, even the abrupt loss of a given hormone causes no immediate distress. Thus, when one recognizes clear-cut evidence of excessive or deficient endocrine function, one can usually conclude that the patient's condition began many months or even years earlier. Before he becomes critically ill, the patient passes through a prolonged period of increasing disability. Unfortunately, the early symptoms of the underlying disease are often vague and not very convincing to either patient or physician. Early diagnosis is further handicapped by the not

infrequent occurrence of predominantly psychiatric symptoms, which distract the physician from a realization of the organic basis of the patient's illness.

LABORATORY PROCEDURES

Although the presence of an endocrine problem is frequently suggested by symptoms, signs, or an abnormal finding among screening laboratory procedures, establishing the diagnosis usually requires one or more relatively sophisticated laboratory procedures. Increasingly, the latter include direct measurement of the hormone under suspicion.

Capability in this area has been greatly enhanced by the development of radiobinding assay methods. These methods have in common the use of a binding reagent (i.e., antibody, binding protein, or cellular receptor) that is highly specific for the substance to be measured. In the radioimmunoassay, the reagent is an antibody generated by a laboratory animal in response to injections of the foreign, human hormone to be measured. In the competitive protein-binding procedure, the binding reagent is a protein which in most cases is the protein that normally transports in plasma the hormone to be measured. Similarly, the binding reagent can be membrane or cytosol receptor material as in the radio-receptor assay.

Radioimmunoassay was first applied to the measurement of insulin in human serum by Berson and Yalow. At the present time, satisfactory procedures for most of the polypeptide hormones and many of the steroid hormones have been developed. The technique requires not only a specific antiserum of high affinity, but also a small supply of pure hormone to serve as a standard. In addition, a small quantity of pure hormone is labelled with a radioactive tracer. To perform an assay, a fixed titer of antiserum and fixed amount of tracer are added to a series of tubes. The amount of tracer is selected to provide a statistically significant number of counts; a titer of antiserum is chosen that will bind 30 to 60 per cent of the total radioactivity. For the definition of a dose-response relationship or standard curve, known quantities of highly purified, *non-labeled* hormone are added to a portion of the tubes (Equation 1 below). Aliquots of unknown serum are added to the remaining tubes (Equation 2). All tubes are incubated, during which time there is a partitioning of tracer between the bound (i.e., attached to antibody) and free state. The quantitative aspects of this partitioning are determined by the amount of unlabeled hormone (either standard or that contained in the unknown specimen) present in the tube. The kinetics are illustrated in the following equations:

Free (F)   *Bound (B)*

H_S + H^* + Ab $\rightleftharpoons$ H^*Ab + H_SAb (Equation 1)

H_u + H^* + Ab $\rightleftharpoons$ H^*Ab + H_SAb (Equation 2)

H^* = Radioactive labeled hormone
H_S = Pure hormone standard
H_u = Hormone in unknown
Ab = Antibody

Since both unlabeled and labeled hormones compete for a fixed number of antibody binding sites, an increase in the amount of unlabeled hormone results in fewer sites available to bind the tracer, and consequently more tracer remains unbound or free. For quantitation, it is necessary to separate bound hormone from free. A number of satisfactory methods (physical, chemical, and immunologic) have been developed. Following the separation, the radioactivity of either (or both) fraction(s) of each tube is counted. The relationship of response versus dose for the standards is plotted, often as B/F versus log dose, and the response of the unknown specimens is calculated from this standard curve. The procedure outlined for radioimmunoassay is also applicable for competitive protein-binding (CPB) and radioreceptor techniques.

Radioreceptor techniques to measure the serum concentration of hormones such as insulin and growth hormone are currently being performed in select research laboratories; others are in the developmental stages. These assays utilize the hormone receptors found either on cell membranes or in the cytosol and consequently are potentially more representative of biologic activity than are radioimmunoassay procedures. However, these assays are demanding in regard to both material preparation and technologic skill.

In summary, the advantages of radioimmunoassay and competitive protein-binding assays are these:

1. *Sensitivity.* The ability to measure the microgram, nanogram, and even picogram quantities of hormone that normally are present in the plasma.

2. *Simplicity.* Once the assay has been established, hundreds of samples per week can be processed.

3. *Specificity.* Because of the high binding affinity the reagent, (be it antibody or transport protein) great specificity is inherent in these methods.

One potential disadvantage of these assays is that they measure the immunologically active portion of the hormone rather than the biologically active portion. Some peptide hormones undergo fragmentation after they are secreted into the circulation. Since these fragments may have different rates of disposal, it is theoretically possible to have a high level of a fragment measurable by radioimmunoassay concomitantly with a normal concentration of fragments with biologic activity. Radioreceptor assays may ultimately prove more desirable due to their capability in identifying biologically active hormone.

HYPOTHALAMUS

One of the most exciting advances in endocrinology in recent years has been the discovery that the secretory activity of the anterior pituitary, long viewed as the "master gland" of the endocrine system, is subservient to humoral substances elaborated by the hypothalamus. The concept that neurosecretory cells could function both as neurons and hormone-secreting cells was not new. For some time it had been appreciated that the hypothalamic superoptic and paraventricular neurons elaborated vasopressin and oxytocin, which are transmitted down the axons of the cells to the posterior pituitary. Comparable neural connections between the hypothalamus and the anterior pituitary were searched for but not found. However, it is now established that there are vascular connections between the hypothalamus and the anterior pituitary. The median eminence of the hypothalamus contains a capillary network that drains into the hypophyseal portal veins. The latter enter the anterior pituitary and subdivide into a second capillary network. Thus, substances produced by neurosecretory cells of the median eminence and adjacent areas have ready access to the cells of the anterior pituitary via the hypophyseal portal system.

In 1969, two groups working independently established the identity of the first hypothalamic factor, thyrotropin releasing hormone (TRH). The leaders of these two groups, Dr. Roger Guilleman and Dr. Andrew Schally, were the recipients of the 1977 Nobel Prize in physiology and medicine. TRH is a tripeptide, pyroglutamyl histidylproline amide, which has been synthesized and is now being applied in the diagnosis of thyroid disease in man (see below). It is generally accepted that the secretion of each of the anterior pituitary hormones is controlled by a specific hypothalamic releasing hormone or an inhibiting factor or both. A 10-amino acid peptide (LHRH) that prompts release of LH has been identified and is available on a limited basis for clinical use. This substance stimulates the release of FSH as well as LH and hence is often referred to as gonadotropin releasing hormone (GNRH). An inhibitory substance appears to be involved in the control of MSH, prolactin, and growth hormone secretion. A 14-

amino acid peptide that suppresses the release of growth hormone has been isolated and identified by Guilleman. This substance, termed somatostatin, not only effects growth hormone secretion, but also when injected intravenously into normal man drastically curtails the secretion of insulin and glucagon.

If one assumes that anterior pituitary secretion is regulated by humoral substances from the hypothalamus, the question arises as to what, in turn, regulates the release of the latter? It has long been known that the hypothalamus is a major relay station within the central nervous system. Presumably, neural signals from many parts of the brain could activate the neurosecretory cells of the hypothalamus. Using neuropharmacologic agents known either to stimulate or block specific neurotransmitters, it has been shown that the monoamines norepinephrine, dopamine, serotonin, acetylcholine, and histamine have important influences on the secretion of the hypothalamic releasing and inhibiting factors. Obviously, much remains to be learned concerning the interactions among the higher centers of the brain, the hypothalamus and the pituitary.

Another question that arises is how the hypothalamic factors interact with the target gland hormones which have been known, or thought, to inhibit anterior pituitary secretion in a negative feedback fashion. The mode of interaction may be unique for each pituitary hormone. For example, thyroid hormone appears to oppose TRH at the level of the TSH-producing cells of the anterior pituitary. Cortisol, on the other hand, may act by inhibiting the production and/or release of corticotropin-releasing factor (CRF) at the level of the median eminence.

From the foregoing, it is clear that the central nervous system has a profound influence on the endocrine glands, the interface being the hypothalamus. Although less well documented, the converse may also be true, that is, the endocrine system may have profound influences on the central nervous system. For example, it has been shown that if newborn male rats are castrated and male hormone withheld for only four or five days, they will subsequently fail to exhibit normal male mating behavior as adult animals even though they are given androgen replacement therapy. This observation suggests an intriguing, though unproved, explanation for some instances of human homosexual activity. Impaired testicular function during a critical perinatal period conceivably could prevent the induction of the normal male behavior pattern in the central nervous system. Consistent with such a hypothesis is the fact that the testes of the newborn male are normally adult-like histologically; later in infancy, the testes regress to the prepubertal pattern and remain so until adolescence. Perhaps in

man, as in the rat, male hormone is required in the neonatal period to induce modification in the central nervous system necessary for the development of male behavior in later life. It has long been held that testicular function in adult homosexuals is normal. However, recent studies of large numbers of males with varying degrees of homosexuality revealed an inverse relationship between serum testosterone concentration and homosexual behavior. Subjects who were overtly homosexual had distinctly lower testosterone values.

NEUROENDOCRINE DISORDERS

In light of the new knowledge regarding the dominant role of the hypothalamus in regulating pituitary function, it seems likely that some diseases previously attributed to malfunction of the pituitary may actually be due to disordered function of the hypothalamus. For example, Cushing's syndrome results from prolonged excessive secretion of cortisol by the adrenal cortex. In a large number of cases, the abnormal secretion of cortisol is associated with adrenal hyperplasia secondary to abnormal, excessive secretion of ACTH. It may well be that the latter is also a secondary phenomenon, i.e., that the anterior pituitary is being subjected to an excessive stimulation by CRF. With this possibility in mind, one might consider adrenal hyperplasia a disease of the hypothalamus or of even higher loci in the central nervous system. This reasoning will remain speculative until the cause of the excessive secretion of ACTH is elucidated.

However, in some states of hormonal deficiency, the problem clearly resides at the level of the hypothalamus rather than at the target gland or the pituitary. Kallman's syndrome is a form of hypogonadism without evidence of other endocrine problems that illustrates the phenomenon of hypothalamic deficiency. In this disorder, young males fail to undergo puberty. They enter adulthood with a eunuchoid habitus and other evidences of androgen lack, such as immature genitalia, absence of facial hair, feminine body contour, female escutcheon, and the absence of libido and potentia. As expected, the plasma level of testosterone is very low; however, the gonadotropins are also very low in these patients, and the administration of LHRH results in increases in both LH and FSH, indicating that the pituitary is intact. Treatment of these individuals with LH in the form of human chorionic gonadotropin (HCG) and FSH (human menopausal gonadotropin, HMG) stimulates both Leydig cell function (as reflected by a dramatic increase in plasma testosterone) and the germinal epithelium of the testes (as indicated by the appearance of spermatozoa in the seminal fluid). Thus, therapy can result in normal sexual function including the ability to conceive. Interestingly, in the classic form of the syndrome, the patient has an impaired sense of smell, either hyposmia or anosmia. Less commonly, these patients may have other congenital anomalies such as cleft lip or palate and deafness.

ANTERIOR PITUITARY

PHYSIOLOGY

The pituitary is a small gland, weighing approximately 0.6 grams and measuring about 1 cm. in diameter. The anterior lobe, derived from endodermal tissue embryologically, makes up about 75 per cent of the gland by weight. It is contained in a bony socket, the sella turcica ("Turkish saddle"), situated at the base of the brain above the sphenoid sinus.

The anterior pituitary elaborates a number of peptide hormones, of which six have clearly defined functions in man. Adrenocorticotropic hormone (ACTH, corticotropin) stimulates the biosynthesis and release of cortisol by the adrenal cortex. Thyroid-stimulating hormone (thyrotropin, TSH) stimulates the uptake of iodide and the release of thyroid hormone by the thyroid. Follicle-stimulating hormone (FSH) stimulates the development of the graafian follicle and secretion of estrogen in the ovary and spermatogenesis in the testes. Luteinizing hormone (LH) prompts ovulation and the luteinization of the mature follicle in the ovary. In the male, this hormone, formerly called the interstitial cell-stimulating hormone (ICSH), stimulates the production and release of testosterone by the Leydig cells of the testes. Prolactin (lactogenic hormone, LTH) stimulates the secretion of milk by the breast of the postpartum female. Growth hormone (GH, somatotropin) promotes growth of all tissues in the immature subject. Its physiologic function in the adult, if any, is not clear. Melanocyte-stimulating hormone (MSH) promotes pigmentation in many species but its role in human physiology has not been definitely established.

In addition to these six hormones with defined functions, there are others whose role is less clear-cut. One of these is beta lipotropic hormone (β-LPH). This substance, which has been isolated and purified, stimulates lipolysis in rats but not in man. There is speculation that β-LPH undergoes cleavage to yield peptides such as MSH and the endorphins. The latter peptides, derived from the carboxyl portion of the parent molecule, have potent morphine-like properties that have recently excited great interest.

On the basis of their staining characteristics, the cells of the anterior pituitary have classically been characterized as chromophobic (without granules), eosinophilic, and basophilic. With more sophisticated techniques, cells previously believed to be chromophobes have been found to contain small basophilic or eosinophilic granules; these cells have been labeled amphophils. In the traditional view, chromophobe cells were believed to be either precursor or supportive cells without secretory activity; eosinophilic cells were considered responsible for the secretion of growth hormone and prolactin; and basophilic cells for the secretion of ACTH, TSH, and MSH. Such a schema is undoubtedly greatly oversimplified. For example, some pituitary tumors producing excessive quantities of ACTH, growth hormone, or prolactin have consisted of chromophobe cells. It should be remembered, however, that stained granules represent stored hormone. Conceivably, tumor cells could release hormone as rapidly as it is formed and thus be agranular when stained. Using the electron microscope, attempts have been made to relate the hormone secreted to granule size. Basophilic cells with granules of about 50 mμ in size are thought to elaborate TSH, while those with larger granules (200 mμ or more) are believed to produce gonadotropins. Much work remains to be done in this area before hormone-cell type relationships of the anterior pituitary are clearly established.

Control of Anterior Pituitary Secretion

The fact that anterior pituitary hormone secretion is under dual control has already been stated. These control mechanisms are (1) negative feedback, in which the target gland hormone, acting at the level of the pituitary or hypothalamus, inhibits secretion of its tropic hormone; and (2) control by hypothalamic hormones arising from neuronal cells in or near the median eminence and secreted into the hypophyseal portal circulation.

These mechanisms are so important from both conceptual and pragmatic points of view that their repeated emphasis is warranted. The interaction among the three hormonal elements controlling thyroid hormone secretion is the most firmly established and can serve to illustrate the principles involved.

The evidence suggests that the normal pituitary can secrete TSH at a low level *independent* of influences from high centers. Presumably, TRH tonically maintains the secretory rate of TSH at a basal level that constitutes the set point. The rate of TRH release is thought to be determined by neural signals, but the source of such signals and their relationship to physio-

Figure 32–3 Pathways of iodine metabolism and the relationships among the hypothalamus, pituitary, and thyroid. Ingested iodine is assimilated as iodide ion which is selectively taken up or "trapped" by the thyroid. Normally, the gradient between intrathyroidal and plasma iodide is about 25 to 1. Once in the thyroid, iodide is rapidly oxidized and combined with tyrosyl residues in a series of steps, collectively termed "organification," which take place in thyroglobulin molecules. Thyroglobulin is stored as colloid in the lumina of follicles. Iodine from the thyroid hormone precursors (diiodotyrosine [DIT] and monoiodotyrosine [MIT]) is recycled. Thyroid hormone (T_4 and T_3) is released from thyroglobulins by enzymatic cleavage. Both thyroid hormone release (X_1) and iodide "trapping" (X_2) are TSH dependent. Nearly all circulating T_4 and most T_3 is bound to proteins such as thyroid-binding globulin (TBG). Thyroid hormone interferes with the action of TRH on the TSH-synthesizing cells of the anterior pituitary. Whether thyroid hormone has a direct action on the hypothalamus is not known (see text).

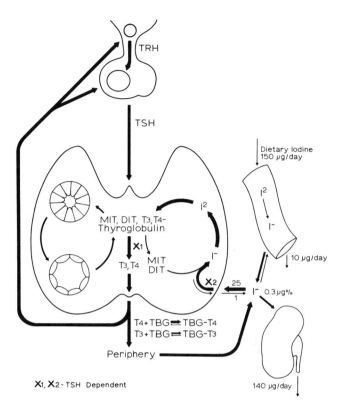

X_1, X_2 - TSH Dependent

logic phenomena such as temperature regulation is poorly understood. The evidence for a diurnal variation in circulating TSH is conflicting; if such a variation occurs, it is small in magnitude.

TRH stimulates both the synthesis and the release of TSH; these two actions can be dissociated. The latter is very prompt; in man, an increase in plasma TSH is detectable within minutes of an intravenous infusion of TRH. This release process appears to be mediated by the adenylate cyclase-cyclic AMP system. Thyroid hormone blocks the releasing action of TRH on the pituitary *if* the thyroid hormone is

administered some time before TRH is given. If the two hormones are administered simultaneously, or thyroid hormone just a few minutes before TRH, no block occurs. There is evidence that thyroid hormone stimulates the synthesis of a protein within the pituitary that inhibits TRH action. Whether thyroid hormone also acts on the hypothalamus or higher in the central nervous system to inhibit the formation or secretion of TRH is not known. These interrelations are illustrated in Figure 32–3.

The very marked biologic activity of TRH illustrates the phenomenon of amplification, in which a relatively minute amount of hormone

TABLE 32–2 SIZE, PITUITARY CONTENT, SECRETORY RATE, PLASMA LEVEL, CLEARANCE RATE, AND ESTIMATED ACTIVITY OF THE ANTERIOR PITUITARY HORMONES

Hormone	Molecular Weight	Pituitary Content (μg.)	Secretory Rate (μg./day)	Plasma Level (ng./ml.)	Clearance Rate (L./day)	Estimated Specific Activity of Pure Hormone (units/mg.)
ACTH	4,500	300	10	0.03	300	200
HGH	21,500	8,500	500	1.0–5.0	280	2
TSH	26,000	300	110	1.0–2.0	61	30
LH	30,000	80	30	0.5–1.5	36	14,000
FSH	41,000	35	15	0.5–1.0	19	14,000

(From Catt, K. J.: Lancet, *1*:830, 1970.)

acting as a primary signal stimulates the secretion of a much larger amount of a second hormone. It has been estimated that this amplification factor is about 100,000 in the case of the TRH-TSH interaction, i.e., 10 ng. of TRH will cause the secretion of 1 mg. of its tropic hormone.

Data tabulated by Catt which depict pituitary hormone size, storage, secretion rate, and other parameters are contained in Table 32–2.

CLINICAL ENTITIES

Pituitary Tumors

The pathophysiology of pituitary tumors involves two basic considerations: (1) the effects of a space-occupying mass in the strategic area above and lateral to the sella turcica and (2) the effects of excess or deficiency of one or more pituitary hormones.

From the standpoint of the first consideration, all pituitary tumors are similar in that presenting symptoms may be headache and visual impairment. The latter manifestation usually results from pressure of the tumor on the decussating fibers of the optic chiasma. Characteristically, the first pattern of visual field loss is the upper outer quadrant followed by the lower outer quadrant. The resulting defect, bitemporal hemianopsia may be apparent when the visual fields are assessed by gross confrontation at the bedside.

From the standpoint of the second consideration, pituitary tumors may be divided into four groups: (1) craniopharyngiomas; (2) chromophobe adenomas; (3) eosinophilic tumors; (4) the tumors of Nelson's syndrome. Hormonal deficiencies may arise in any of these four groups because of (a) the pressure of the tumor on normal cells; (b) the consequence of treatment; or, rarely, from (c) apoplexy or hemorrhage into the tumor. When hypopituitarism does occur, typically, growth hormone is the first hormone affected, followed, in sequence, by deficiency of gonadotropins, TSH, and ACTH. Thus, declining sexual function is an early clinical clue suggesting the presence of a pituitary tumor. Of the four groups, only craniopharyngiomas never elaborate hormones. Chromophobe adenomas were, until recently, believed to be nonsecretory. It is now known that as many as 25 per cent of chromophobes secrete excessive amounts of prolactin. A serum level of 200 ng./dl or greater is highly suggestive of the presence of a pituitary tumor. Serum prolactin not only serves as a marker in the diagnosis of pituitary tumor, but it is also a useful guide in assessing the effectiveness of treatment. The consequences of deficiencies of anterior pituitary hormones are discussed below, as are the consequences of excessive growth hormone produced by an eosinophilic tumor.

Nelson's Syndrome. Because of the underlying mechanisms it illustrates, the fourth group of tumors deserves additional comment. In 1960 Nelson and co-workers reported the occurrence of intense pigmentation in patients who were previously subjected to bilateral adrenalectomy for Cushing's disease. Each patient was found to have a chromophobe adenoma of the pituitary and a very high level of plasma ACTH. Clinical experience since Nelson's original report indicates that as many as 20 per cent of all patients undergoing adrenalectomy for adrenal hyperplasia due to Cushing's disease will develop this complication. The chromophobe tumor in these patients is more aggressive than the usual variety. Complications due to pressure on the surrounding structures are frequent, as is pituitary apoplexy. According to one hypothesis, the syndrome is best explained by assuming that the initial pathologic event is excessive secretion of CRF that is inadequately suppressed by the resultant abnormally high levels of plasma cortisol. Over a period of many months, the latter leads to Cushing's disease, which can be treated by removal of the hyperplastic adrenal glands and replacing their secretions with an exogenous glucocorticoid in physiologic amounts. The manifestations of Cushing's disease regress over a period of time. Unfortunately, the diminished, now normal levels of plasma cortisol permit a further increase in CRF secretion. The long-term excessive stimulation of the ACTH-producing cells of the anterior pituitary by CRF leads to tumor formation and to extremely high levels of plasma ACTH. It is the latter event that leads to pigmentation which may be so intense that a Caucasian may be mistaken for a black. It has been established that ACTH has pigmenting capability, which is very likely a result of the similarity of its N-terminal amino acid sequence to that of melanocyte-stimulating hormone. Thus, despite receiving appropriate therapy for Cushing's disease, these unfortunate patients may trade the severe disabilities of Cushing's disease for those of a pervasive pituitary tumor.

Multiple Endocrine Adenomata (MEA I; Wermer's Syndrome). In a small number of patients with pituitary tumors there is also a tumor or hyperplasia of the parathyroids and/or an islet cell adenoma of the pancreas or both. In 1954, Wermer described such tumors in four siblings and a parent; a number of similar reports have followed and there is generally agreement that neoplasia arising out of two or more endocrine glands represents a distinct entity. While isolated cases have been reported, more often, when appropriate studies are carried out, it is found to be familial with an autosomal dominant mode of inheritance. The combination of pituitary, parathyroid, and pancreatic neoplasia has been labelled MEA, Type I, to distinguish it from a second condition, MEA, Type II or Sipple's syndrome, in which medullary carcinoma of the thyroid is found in association with pheochromocytoma and hyperplasia or adenoma of the parathyroids. Needless to say, the dramatic presentation of three endocrine tumors occurring in the same individual, has invited much speculation as to the pathogenesis of the syndrome. Practically speaking, a patient who has any one of the three tumors should be assessed for the other two, and his close relatives should be screened. Since the second or third tumor can emerge years after the first, appropriate screening tests should be done periodically.

The Empty Sella Syndrome. The empty sella syndrome is an interesting condition in which there is partial loss of the glandular substance of the pituitary, permitting entry of air into the sella during pneumoencephalography. In life, the diagnosis can only be made with certainty with this procedure. The sella is often enlarged, suggesting the presence of a pituitary tumor and leading to the performance of the pneumoencephalogram. While a number of exceptions have been noted, in general, these patients do not have deficiencies of pituitary hormones. The question that immediately comes to mind is, if the sella is empty, why doesn't the patient manifest hypopituitarism? The answer is that the sella is not completely empty; a shell-like remnant of tissue, sufficient to permit normal secretory activity, remains. In fact, Ganglual and co-workers have reported a patient with Cushing's disease secondary to a microadenoma of the pituitary associated with an "empty" sella. The pathophysiologic basis for the development of the empty sella syndrome is not clear. One plausible hypothesis is that cerebral spinal fluid pressure is transmitted into the sella through a defect in the diaphragma sella. Probably only in a small percentage of affected individuals is the condition recognized. In one postmortem study, 40 cases were found in 788 consecutive autopsies. The clinical and radiographic features of a large number of patients with the disorder were reviewed by Neelon and co-workers in 1975. The possibility that the empty sella syndrome might be present should be kept in mind during the evaluation of a patient suspected of having a pituitary tumor. Unfortunately, empty sellas have been discovered in patients undergoing surgery directed at a misdiagnosed pituitary tumor. Preoperative pneumoencephalograms should obviate these tragic errors.

Acromegaly and Gigantism

Acromegaly (excessive size of the distal parts of the body) results from sustained, excessive secretion of growth hormone in the adult. The source of the growth hormone is an eosinophilic, or less often a chromophobic, tumor of the anterior pituitary. When such a tumor develops in childhood or adolescence before closure of the epiphyses, growth in height is greatly accelerated with resulting gigantism. In this circumstance, the disease process usually continues into adult life, so that the typical patient with gigantism also has the striking features of acromegaly. Massive enlargement of the hands, feet, and skull, particularly the mandible, occurs. The broadened nose together with the large head has suggested the term "leonine facies" to describe some acromegalic patients. Acromegaly is an outstanding example of an endocrine disorder that recognized decades before the hormone involved was discovered. The classic features of acromegaly were first described in 1886 by Pierre Marie. The metabolic effects of long-standing growth hormone excess are often surprisingly mild. Impairment of glucose tolerance is commonly seen, and frank diabetes mellitus occurs in perhaps 15 per cent of cases.

The normal hypothalamic-pituitary-target tissue interrelations of human growth hormone (HGH) are poorly understood. It is known that there is a hypothalamic HGH-releasing factor that stimulates the growth hormone-producing cells of the anterior pituitary. Perhaps some of the tumors in acromegalics arise from chronic overstimulation of the pituitary by this HGH-releasing factor — a mechanism comparable to that postulated for the ACTH-secreting tumor of Nelson's syndrome. The occurrence in some acromegalic individuals of tumors which are chromophobic or of mixed histology suggests an unusually low storage and rapid discharge of growth hormone. As discussed below, a number of stimuli capable of increasing plasma growth hormone have been identified, but relatively few inhibitors are known. One of these, hyperglycemia, is of practical value in the diagnosis of acromegaly. When a glucose load is administered to normal subjects, the ensuing hyperglycemia is associated with a decline in HGH to normal or undetectable levels. The basal HGH level of the acromegalic individual not only is typically elevated but can not be suppressed to within normal limits by hyperglycemia.

Pituitary Infantilism

The outstanding manifestation of pituitary deficiency which develops prior to puberty is failure to grow. This is true whether the deficiency is restricted to HGH alone or includes deficiencies of other tropic hormones. The term pituitary infantilism implies dwarfism and immaturity of the secondary sexual characteristics. The latter finding, of course, can only be appreciated clinically in the post-adolescent patient. The most common cause of pituitary infantilism is the craniopharyngioma; frequently, however, no organic lesion can be demonstrated. In pituitary infantilism, impaired secretion of tropic hormones other than HGH can almost always be demonstrated. There are uncommon forms of pituitary dwarfism studied extensively by McKusick and Merimee and collaborators in which only HGH secretion or peripheral responsiveness to HGH is deficient (see Table 32–3).

Before discussing these, we should consider briefly what is known about the mechanism of action of growth hormone. In terms of promoting growth, the hormone acts in the intact, immature animal to stimulate cartilage formation. One can study this process in vitro by incubating cartilage from immature rats with isotopically-labeled sulfate and measuring the incorporation of the label, as chondroitin sulfate, into cartilage. When one adds growth hormone itself to such a system, no increase in sulfate incorporation occurs. Similarly, serum from an animal that has undergone hypophysectomy has little activity. However, serum from such an animal *treated with growth hormone* is very active.

These findings led Daughaday to speculate that growth hormone does not affect growth directly; rather, it interacts with receptors that in turn generate a "sulfation factor" (now called somatomedin) which actually stimulates cartilaginous growth. More recently, such receptors have been found in the liver. Relevant to this hypothesis are findings from patients with a rare form of dwarfism first described in oriental Jews in Israel by Laron. These individuals resemble pituitary dwarfs in their physical characteristics. However, there are abundant levels of growth hormone in their sera as determined by radioimmunoassay. Like true pituitary dwarfs they have very low levels of sulfation factor in the sera. Unlike pituitary dwarfs, however, the administration of therapeutic amounts of growth hormone fails to induce an increase in somatomedin and promotes relatively little increase in stature. One explanation for these findings is that these patients have a defect in the proposed somatomedin generation system that cannot be overcome by the administration

of even large amounts of growth hormone. Alternatively, their pituitary glands could be elaborating an abnormal growth hormone which lacks biologic activity but is antigenically normal and thus measurable by radioimmunoassay. It is conceivable that such a molecule could interfere with exogenous growth hormone by competitive inhibition.

There is now evidence that both phenomena occur. Dwarfism related to the release of biologically inactive HGH is termed Loran dwarfism, Type I; when the defect is in the production of somatomedin (HGH being normal), the term Loran dwarfism, Type II is used. In attempting to explain the possible value of the somatomedin mechanism, Daughaday has pointed out that growth hormone is secreted in bursts throughout the day in response to a host of metabolic and neurogenic stimuli. This irregular and intermittent pattern of secretion would seem inappropriate for the gradual progressive processes involved in orderly cell growth. The interaction of growth hormone with a system generating the actual growth substance, e.g., somatomedin, would provide an attractive mechanism to explain the normal regulation of skeletal growth.

Recently, it has been found that the structure of somatomedin is very similar to that of another protein with biologically active, nonsuppressible insulin-like activity (NSILA). Whether or not NSILA is, in fact, somatomedin, is an intriguing question.

Sexual Ateliotic Dwarfism

As mentioned, Merimee and co-workers have described a variety of familial dwarfism due to a selective inability of the pituitary to secrete growth hormone; in these patients, all other anterior pituitary hormones are secreted normally. These authors applied the term sexual ateliotic (*ateliosis* = imperfect development) dwarfism to this disorder to denote normal sexual development in an individual with short stature. Theoretically, many mechanisms involving growth hormone synthesis, secretion, and tissue interaction might occur which would interfere with normal growth. Some of these are as follows:

— An absence or reduction in the hypothalamic growth hormone-releasing factor.
— An absence or abnormality of the growth hormone-producing cells of the anterior pituitary.
— Deficiency of the enzyme(s) required for the release of stored growth hormone.
— Production of a biologically abnormal growth hormone molecule, that is, one without metabolic activity but antigenical-

ly intact and thus measurable by immunoassay.
— Production of an abnormal growth hormone molecule with partial biologic activity which may or may not be measurable by immunoassay.
— A circulating antagonist(s) to growth hormone in the bloodstream.
— Increased destruction of normally secreted growth hormone.
— A defect in the somatomedin generation system.
— End-organ resistance to growth hormone or the growth principle (somatomedin).

Obviously a number of these proposed mechanisms could overlap, and most, it should be emphasized, are hypothetical. Similarly, the classification proposed by Merimee and coworkers in 1969 and contained in Table 32–3 should be regarded as tentative. Patients with Types I and II dwarfism have undetectable levels of plasma growth hormone which remain low during hypoglycemia or arginine infusion. They differ, however, in their mode of inheritance and in their responsiveness to insulin. Type I dwarfism is inherited as an autosomal recessive, while Type II is transmitted as an autosomal dominant trait. Patients with Type I dwarfism are highly sensitive to administered insulin, while those with Type II are resistant to it. Type III dwarfism is characterized by a high plasma level of HGH, as determined by radioimmunoassay, which may or may not be suppressed by hyperglycemia. In Type IV dwarfism, exemplified by the Pygmies of central Africa, growth hormone appears to be secreted normally. The administration of HGH, however, fails to elicit the expected changes in plasma free fatty acids and blood urea nitrogen. This could be due either to peripheral tissue unresponsiveness to normal growth hormone or to the secretion of a biologically defective but antigenically intact growth hormone molecule which saturates peripheral receptors. Current evidence supports the former explanation, i.e., peripheral tissue resistance.

To evaluate the ability of the anterior pituitary to secrete growth hormone three stimuli are commonly used. The first is hypoglycemia induced by the intravenous administration of 0.1 to 0.2 units of regular insulin per kg. of body weight to a fasting patient. The second is the infusion of 30 grams of the amino acid arginine monohydrochloride. In these tests, blood samples are obtained every 15 to 30 minutes over a one to two hour period for growth hormone and blood sugar determinations. Most normal individuals respond to these stimuli with a maximum plasma HGH of 20 ng per ml. or more. The third stimulating agent used is L-dopa which has the advantage that it can be used orally.

It should be emphasized that most of the current information concerning growth hormone was obtained in the last ten years following the development of a highly sensitive radioimmunoassay and the availability of purified growth hormone suitable for administration to man. Unfortunately, growth hormone is highly species specific. Preparations from domestic animals do not elicit metabolic effects in man. Since human growth hormone is necessarily prepared from pituitary glands obtained at autopsy, the supply available is obviously limited. Perhaps a metabolically active preparation can be synthesized after the precise identification of the amino acid sequence(s) which governs the hormone's biologic expression.

TABLE 32–3 SOME FEATURES OF SEXUAL ATELIOTIC DWARFISM

Type	Basal HGH	GH Response to I.V. INS/ARG	Response to HGH	Response to Insulin	Insulin Response to I.V. GLU/ARG	Mode of Inheritance	Nature of Defect
I	0	0	+	Sensitive	Decrease	Autosomal Recessive	Inability to produce HGH
II	0	0	+	Normal	Increase	Autosomal Dominant	Inability to produce HGH
III	High (Non-suppressible)	0 or +	0	Sensitive	Decrease	?(Yemenite Jews)	"Warped HGH" plus end-organ resistance
IV	Normal	Normal	0	Sensitive	Decrease	Pygmy	End-organ resistance

HGH = Human growth hormone
INS = Insulin
ARG = Arginine
GLU = Glucose
(Modified from Merimee, T. J., et al.: Lancet, *1*:963, 1969.)

Panhypopituitarism (Postpubertal)

The term panhypopituitarism signifies a deficiency of all anterior pituitary hormones. The most common cause in the adult is an expanding, chromophobe adenoma. In females, it may also occur as a sequela of hemorrhagic shock at the time of delivery. For reasons which are not entirely clear, the pituitary of the pregnant female at term is highly vulnerable to hypotension. When excessive blood loss occurs during delivery, a definite risk of pituitary necrosis is present. The resulting panhypopituitarism bears the eponym Sheehan's syndrome. Less common causes of adult hypopituitarism include craniopharyngioma and long-standing pituitary tumors associated with acromegaly.

The peripheral manifestations of panhypopituitarism in the adult are largely the consequence of deficiencies of four hormones: the gonadotropins (LH and FSH), ACTH, and TSH. Characteristically, evidence of target gland deficits appear in that order, i.e., gonadal, adrenal cortical, and thyroidal. Thus, loss of libido in the male and amenorrhea in the female are early symptoms. Loss of thyroid function causes dry skin, cold intolerance, somnolence, bradycardia, and constipation. Decrease in adrenal cortical function causes symptoms of hypovolemia and hypoglycemia and, in the female, loss of axillary and pubic hair. Typically, the patient with panhypopituitarism has pale skin and premature, fine wrinkles about the eyes and mouth. The loss of pigment has been attributed to ACTH deficiency.

As is so often the case in endocrinology, the definitive diagnosis of panhypopituitarism requires the judicious selection of certain laboratory procedures. The traditional approach has been the demonstration of hypofunction of the adrenal cortex and thyroid, which is reversed by the administration of ACTH and TSH, respectively. The advent of radioimmunoassays for several anterior pituitary hormones has permitted a more direct approach to the diagnosis. The use of arginine infusion, induced hypoglycemia or L-dopa to provoke growth hormone secretion has already been mentioned, as has the use of TRH to stimulate TSH release. In panhypopituitarism, the responses of HGH and TSH to these stimuli would be severely impaired or absent.

Much less common than panhypopituitarism are instances of isolated deficiency of a single pituitary hormone, so-called monotropic hypopituitarism. Monotropic growth hormone deficiencies (sexual ateliotic dwarfism) have already been described as has familial hypogonadotropic hypogonadism (Kallman's Syndrome), a deficiency of both pituitary gonadotropins. It is a relatively common cause of hypogonadism in the male and may also afflict females. Selective deficiencies of LH, TSH, ACTH, and prolactin have also been well documented.

POSTERIOR PITUITARY

PHYSIOLOGY

Vasopressin (antidiuretic hormone, ADH), the octapeptide which is the principal secretion of the posterior pituitary, has a major physiologic role in regulating water metabolism. Unlike anterior pituitary hormones, this hormone is actually produced in the hypothalamus by the supraoptic and paraventricular nuclei. It is transported down the axons of the hypothalamic-hypophyseal tracts to the posterior pituitary, where it is stored until secreted. It has been established, however, that the storage of ADH in the posterior pituitary is not essential for normal function. Normal water metabolism can persist after complete destruction of the posterior pituitary *if* the hypothalamus and proximal pituitary stalk are not damaged.

The usual stimulus to ADH secretion is an increase in plasma osmolality. Normally, the latter is closely maintained at 280 mOsm. per liter. When extracellular water is lost, plasma osmolality increases, causing the activation of osmoreceptors which signal the release of ADH. The precise location of the osmoreceptors and the manner in which they stimulate the release of ADH are not known. Increased plasma osmolality also stimulates the thirst center, which is anatomically adjacent to, or connected with, the supraoptic nuclei.

The action of ADH to conserve water is exerted primarily on the cells of renal collecting ducts. At this site, ADH exerts its unique ability of changing permeability of the epithelial cell membranes to enhance the egress of water from the tubules to the hypertonic fluid of the peritubular or interstitial space. This action of ADH is mediated by the adenylate cyclase-cyclic AMP system. The consequent shift of water reduces urine volume and increases its concentration. Thus, an increased serum osmolality tends to correct itself by reducing water loss and increasing water intake as depicted in Figure 32–4.

The integrated activity of ADH and thirst is highly effective in maintaining the osmolality of the body fluids within very narrow limits. These interrelations provide an ideal example of the precision with which the endocrine system normally functions to maintain the constancy of the internal milieu. Although plasma osmolality is the most important regulator of ADH secretion, other factors also influence it. For example, an abrupt decrease in plasma volume due to acute

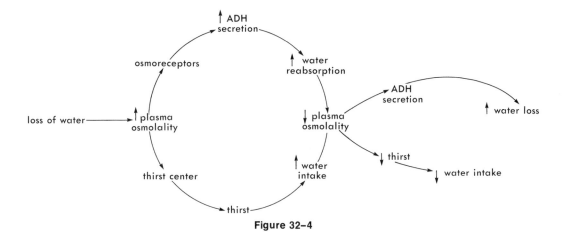

Figure 32-4

blood loss stimulates ADH secretion. Neural signals triggered by painful stimuli may also prompt ADH release, as do certain drugs such as nicotine. The posterior pituitary also secretes oxytocin. Although large doses of this substance will induce contractions of the gravid uterus, its physiologic importance in man has not yet been established.

CLINICAL ENTITIES

Diabetes Insipidus

Diabetes insipidus is the clinical condition that results from an impaired or absent capacity to secrete ADH. The term diabetes (from the Greek word meaning "siphon") signifies copious amounts of urine. The causes of diabetes insipidus are numerous. In one large series, one third of the cases were due to tumor, one third were of unknown cause, and one third were of a variety of causes including trauma, inflammation, and granuloma (Thomas). The principal manifestation of diabetes insipidus is the excretion of large volumes of urine — 5 to 15 liters or more daily — of low spe-

cific gravity (1.007 or less). To compensate for this prodigious water loss, the patient must drink large volumes of fluid. These two symptoms are particularly troublesome during the sleeping hours. Frequent urination and the need to satisfy thirst substantially encroach on the patient's rest, and loss of sleep is frequently his presenting complaint. For reasons that are not clear, the onset of symptoms is typically dramatically abrupt. The patient often recalls the precise day or hour when polyuria and thirst began. Another peculiar feature of the disease is the patient's marked preference for chilled fluids. He will go to considerable trouble to relieve his thirst with ice water.

A number of other disorders associated with the passage of large volumes of urine may simulate diabetes insipidus. An abbreviated differential diagnosis of polyuria is summarized in Table 32–4.

The presence of diabetes mellitus, chronic renal failure, or disturbances in calcium and potassium metabolism is easily established. Patients with psychogenic thirst should theoretically respond to water deprivation in a normal manner, that is, by decreasing urine volume and increasing urine concentration. Thus, after water is withheld from the patient who is an obsessive water drinker, the specific gravity of his urine should rise above 1.012 within a few hours and reach 1.020 or more after 12 hours. Unfortunately, the results of this procedure may be obscured by the patient's ability to obtain water surreptitiously and, conversely, by the ability of some patients with *partial* diabetes insipidus to concentrate urine to a specific gravity of 1.012 or 1.014. Lastly, water deprivation in a patient with unequivocal, total diabetes insipidus is potentially dangerous.

A second method of diagnosing diabetes insipidus involves the use of hypertonic saline and vasopressin. After the patient is well hydrated, with a urine flow rate of at least 5 ml. per min., a 3 per cent sodium chloride solution is infused for 45

TABLE 32-4   DIFFERENTIAL DIAGNOSIS OF POLYURIA

Cause	Mechanism
1. Diabetes insipidus	Decreased ADH secretion
2. Diabetes mellitus	Osmotic diuresis
3. Nephrogenic diabetes insipidus	End-organ resistance to ADH
4. Hypercalcemia	Impaired concentrating ability
5. Hypokalemia	Impaired concentrating ability
6. Psychogenic thirst	Obsessive water drinking

minutes. If no antidiuresis occurs within the next 30 minutes, aqueous vasopressin (ADH) is given, and urine collection is continued for another 30 minutes. If both kidney function and neurohypophyseal function are normal, the hypertonic saline infusion should cause a prompt fall in urinary flow and an increase in urinary specific gravity and osmolality. If ADH secretion is impaired, the saline infusion will be ineffective, but there will be a prompt decline in urine volume in response to vasopressin. If the defect is caused by an inability of the renal tubules to respond to ADH (i.e., nephrogenic diabetes insipidus), neither hypertonic saline nor vasopressin infusion will influence the rate of urine flow.

The Syndrome of Inappropriate Antidiuretic Hormone Secretion (SIADH)

This syndrome was first described by Schwartz in 1957 in patients with cancer of the lung. It has subsequently been noted as a complication of various underlying conditions, including head trauma, myxedema, tuberculosis, and meningitis, to name a few. A number of drugs have also been found to cause SIADH. In all instances, the manifestations are those which would be expected from the inappropriate release of ADH into the circulation. (In some instances, e.g., cancer of the lung, presumably the tumor does indeed elaborate and release autonomously an ADH-like peptide. In contrast to the anterior pituitary, no example of a hormone-producing tumor of the posterior pituitary or hypothalamus has been described.) There is retention of water and consequently dilution of body fluids. The increase in plasma volume leads to an increase in glomerular filtration and a decrease in aldosterone secretion, both factors that increase loss of sodium into the urine. Thus, the concentration of serum sodium is decreased by at least two mechanisms: (1) dilution by inappropriate water retention and (2) failure to reduce urinary sodium excretion.

When evaluating a patient for this syndrome, one should carefully rule out conditions that would *appropriately* lead to an increase in ADH secretion or to sodium wasting such as absolute or relative intravascular volume depletion (e.g., congestive heart failure) and adrenal cortical insufficiency. The symptoms of SIADH, essentially those of water retention proceeding to water intoxication, vary depending how low the serum sodium is and how fast it has fallen. As sodium falls below 120 mEq./L., there is the insidious appearance of headache, apathy, somnolence, and muscle weakness. With a rapid fall in sodium, nausea and vomiting may be the first symptoms. When the sodium concentration falls below 110, marked changes in the patient's sensorium occur. With further reduction, delirium, convulsions and coma

may occur. Besides removing the underlying cause, therapy consists of reducing the intake of free water.

THYROID

PHYSIOLOGY

Essential to understanding thyroid disorders is an appreciation of normal iodine metabolism and the normal interrelations between the thyroid and the pituitary-hypothalamic unit (see Figure 32–3). The latter has been discussed (see above).

Iodine Metabolism

A daily absorption of approximately 100 to 200 μg. of dietary iodine is required to ensure adequate thyroid hormone synthesis. Because of the use of iodine compounds in the production of flour in some parts of the United States, the daily ingestion of iodine may be 500 to 600 μg. With the exception of that contained in organic compounds, ingested iodine is reduced to ionic iodide (I⁻) before being assimilated into the bloodstream. During the first hour after absorption, iodide is distributed in a space representing approximately 35 per cent of body weight, or about 25 liters in a 70 kg. man. The concentration of circulating iodide has been estimated at less than 0.1 μg. per 100 ml. of plasma.

Uptake (Trapping). Normally, the thyroid has an iodide clearance rate between 10 and 35 ml. of plasma per minute. This uptake by the thyroid is an active, energy-requiring process, sometimes referred to as the "iodide pump." It is stimulated by TSH and is blocked by a number of anions such as thiocyanate and perchlorate. Normally, a concentration gradient of 1 to 25 exists between plasma and thyroidal I⁻. This gradient may be increased 10-fold or more in toxic goiter. Iodide ion constitutes approximately 10 per cent of the total intrathyroidal iodine which normally amounts to 5000 to 7000 μg. The iodide pool may be increased when organification is impaired by drug action, inflammation, or genetically determined enzyme defects. Careful studies have revealed that there are in fact two independent iodide pools within the thyroid gland. The first, normally about 10 μg., is composed by newly trapped iodide. Its uptake can be blocked by perchlorate or thiocyanate. The second pool, estimated at about 490 μg., consists of iodide released by enzymatic dehalogenation of monoiodotyrosine (MIT) and diiodotyrosine (DIT). This pool, apparently part of an internal recycling process which conserves iodide, is not directly affected by agents that block trapping. One can view the action of perchlorate or thiocyanate in "discharging" iodide as one of inhibition of inward transport of iodide while outward diffusion is unaffected.

Oxidation and Organification. After being trapped, iodide ions are rapidly transported into the luminal space of follicles and are either incorporated into an organic molecule or diffuse out of the follicles unchanged. Oxidation of iodide to molecular iodine (I_2) occurs prior to its displacement of hydrogen at the C_3 position of tyrosine. These reactions which lead to the formation of MIT and DIT occur rapidly, and their exact sequence has not been established. The oxidation step is probably catalyzed by a perioxidase. MIT is then iodinated at the C_5 position to form DIT. Probably the tyrosyl residues are attached to thyroglobulin or to other iodoproteins during these reactions. The oxidation-organification steps can be blocked by thiourea drugs such as propylthiouracil and are stimulated by TSH. The formation of the iodothyronines, thyroxine (T_4), and triiodothyronine (T_3), probably results from the condensation of iodotyrosines, either two DIT molecules or one DIT and one MIT molecule, with the extrusion of one side chain. DIT and MIT molecules that are not utilized in the formation of T_4 and T_3 undergo catalytic deiodination by a dehalogenase. The regenerated iodide (the second iodide pool) is subsequently reutilized in hormone synthesis in the thyroid (see earlier discussion). T_4 and T_3 are not susceptible to deiodination in the thyroid.

Storage and Release. Most of the iodinated compounds of the thyroid are in combination with thyroglobulin, a 650,000 M.W. protein, which is the principal iodoprotein in thyroidal colloid. Analysis of the globulin-bound iodinated compounds reveals the following relative amounts: MIT, 17 to 28 per cent; DIT, 25 to 42 per cent; T_3, 5 to 8 per cent; and T_4, 35 per cent. The quantity of these stored compounds is sufficient to maintain normal metabolism in an adult for several months. The large size of thyroglobulin precludes its escape from the intraluminal colloid under normal circumstances. The secretion of the thyroid hormone (T_3 and T_4) requires that it first be cleaved from thyroglobulin by proteolytic enzymes. T_3 and T_4, being freely diffusible, then readily enter the circulation. This process is stimulated by TSH and may be inhibited by large amounts of iodine. While the principal secretion of the thyroid is thyroxine (90 per cent or more), there is a small amount of T_3 in the venous effluent of the thyroid. It is estimated that approximately 80 to 90 μg. of thyroxine is secreted per day.

Transport of Thyroid Hormones. Once released, free thyroxine and triiodothyronine quickly bind with one of several carrier proteins. The protein with the strongest affinity for T_4 and T_3 is thyroxine-binding globulin (TBG), an interalpha (α_1-α_2) glycoprotein. The normal concentration of

TBG is about 1 mg. per 100 ml. of serum, a quantity sufficient to bind 10 to 26 μg. of T_4. A second protein, thyroxine-binding prealbumin (TBPA), also effectively binds thyroxine. Lastly, serum albumin binds T_4 but with less affinity than either TBG or TBPA. The equilibrium between TBG and bound and free T_4 is reversible, as illustrated by the equation

$$TBG \cdot T_4 \rightleftharpoons TBG + T_4$$

The concentration of free T_4 is normally about 1.0 to 2.0 ng. per 100 ml. (less than 1.0×10^{-10} Molar), representing about 0.05 per cent of total T_4. The binding affinity of T_3 for the protein carriers is substantially less than that of T_4. However, since it is the free hormone that penetrates cells to regulate metabolism, the metabolic contribution of T_3 is in fact important. Despite an absolute concentration, which is small compared to that of total T_4, the amount of free T_3 approaches that of free T_4 because of the weaker affinity of T_3 for its carrier proteins. Moreover, recent evidence indicates that T_4 can be converted to T_3 in peripheral tissues. In fact, 80 to 90 per cent of circulating T_3 is derived from the peripheral deiodonation of T_4. Monodeiodonation of T_4 leads to biologically active T_3 (3,5,3'-triiodothyronine) *and* to the biologically inactive compound, reverse T_3 (3,3',5'-triiodothyronine, rT_3). Normally, approximately equal quantities of T_3 and reverse T_3 are produced. However, the rT_3 pathway is favored in certain circumstances, such as during starvation and in the presence of chronic disease, whereas the T_3 pathway is favored in others: for example, in the presence of a high carbohydrate diet. From the work of Chopra (1976) and others, the details of the peripheral deiodonation of T_4 are emerging; it appears to be an important regulatory process in over-all metabolism. Recognition that a large proportion of secreted thyroxine is converted to T_3 peripherally has furthered speculation that T_4 is a prohormone.

There are numerous drugs that affect either the binding capacity or the amount of circulating thyroid-binding proteins. For example, diphenylhydantoin competes with T_4 for TBG binding sites, and salicylates displace T_4 from TBPA. Estrogenic compounds increase the amount of carrier protein. Familial deficiencies and excesses of TBG have been well documented. However, the concentration of *free* thyroxine is normal in these patients, hence, they are euthyroid.

It is estimated that the total extrathyroidal content of thyroxine-iodine in the normal adult is about 500 μg. Assuming a normal plasma volume and a T_4 concentration of 5 μg. per 100 ml. of plasma, only 150 μg. can be accounted for in the bloodstream. The large amount of remaining thyroxine-iodine is presumed to be bound to tissue protein. According to recent studies the liver is the major storage organ, containing up to 30 per cent of total body thyroxine-iodine. Normally the fractional turnover of thyroxine-iodine is about 10 per cent per day, reflecting a biologic half-life of 6.7 days. The fractional turnover rate is increased in hyperthyroidism and decreased in hypothyroidism. These findings are consistent with the observation that the fractional turnover rate may be regulated by the plasma concentration of *free* thyroxine. An alternate hypothesis proposes that the content of exchangeable cellular T_4 is the factor which determines turnover rate.

Cell Entry, Intracellular Metabolism, and Fate of Thyroxine. *Free* thyroxine and triiodothyronine appear to cross most cellular membranes; however, thyroxine is not present in cerebral spinal fluid and it crosses the human placenta slowly and in small amounts. Factors which control the entry of thyroxine into cells are poorly understood. The presence within the cell membrane of one or more proteins with a high binding affinity for T_4 is one possibility. Once in the cell, the manner in which thyroxine or an active derivative acts to increase cellular metabolism is yet another enigma. A once widely held hypothesis implicates the stimulation of uncoupling of oxidative phosphorylation. In contradiction to this possibility is the failure of other uncoupling agents such as 2,4-dinitrophenol to mimic the full spectrum of physiologic actions of T_4. Currently, studies are being conducted to test the hypothesis that changes in mitochondrial membrane function and alterations in nuclear RNA, RNA polymerase, and protein synthesis represent the initial manifestations of T_4 action within the cell. Three principal pathways for disposal of T_4 have been described: (1) conjugation of the phenolic portion of the molecule with formation of the glucuronide or sulfate; (2) degradation of the alanine side chain, and (3) deiodination.

Excretion of Iodide. Nearly all the iodide circulating through the kidneys is filtered by the glomeruli. However, much of the filtered iodide is reabsorbed, so that the renal iodide clearance rate is about 40 ml. per minute. In man, iodide reabsorption appears to be a passive, unregulated process. As indicated in Figure 32–3, urinary loss of iodine normally nearly balances iodine ingestion, with only small quantities of iodine being excreted in the feces.

TESTS OF THYROID FUNCTION

In recent years, radioimmunoassays for serum TSH and T_3 as well as for T_4 have become available. The first biochemical marker of a failing thyroid is elevation of the serum TSH. The serum T_4 may be maintained in the normal range (and the patient eumetabolic) because of an increase in TSH. The determination of TSH is valuable in assessing the significance of a borderline T_4 determination and to rule out pituitary deficiency when the T_4 is definitely low. Infrequently, serum T_3 elevation precedes an increase in T_4 in hyperthyroidism. Measurement of T_3 (RIA) confirms the diagnosis in such cases. The resin T_3 uptake (RT_3U) reflects the level of circulating thyroid binding globulin (TBG). When TBG is elevated, as in pregnancy, the patient usually has a high level of T_4 but is not hyperthyroid since *free* T_4 is not elevated. Determination of the RT_3U will demonstrate an increase in TBG and allow for the correction of the T_4 value.

To discuss the pathophysiology of thyroid disease in a meaningful fashion, it is useful to refer to other tests that are used in assessing thyroid function. In general, these fit into one of two categories: (1) those that depend on thyroidal iodine kinetics; and (2) those that reflect the impact of thyroid hormone on body metabolism.

The first group of tests is illustrated by the 24-hour uptake of radioactive iodine by the thyroid gland. In this procedure, a small (approximately 10 microcuries) amount of radioactive iodine (^{131}RAI) is administered orally and radioactivity over the thyroid gland is determined 24 hours later. As already mentioned, both the normal uptake of iodine and the discharge of thyroid hormone require TSH and a functioning thyroid gland. The second category is exemplified by the basal metabolic rate (BMR). In this procedure, the patient's rate of oxygen consumption is measured and compared to normal values based on the patient's age, size, and sex. Although the BMR is not in use now, it is conceptually useful since it reflects the over-all metabolic status of the patient.

The value of these procedures in defining the pathophysiology of thyroid disease is best conveyed by citing examples of their application:

Example	Serum T_4 (RIA)	RAI	BMR
1. Hyperthyroidism	Increased	Increased	Increased
2. Primary Hypothyroidism	Decreased	Decreased	Decreased
3. Goitrous cretinism	Decreased	Increased	Decreased
4. Normal subject on 0.15 mg. thyroxine	Normal	Decreased	Normal

The results in examples 1 and 2 are straightforward and require no comment. In the third example, goitrous cretinism due to either a severe dietary deficiency of iodine or an abnormality in the biosynthesis of thyroid hormone, the patient is unable to secrete an adequate amount of thyroid hormone. As a result, the level of circulating hormone is low and the patient is hypothyroid. The low concentration of hormone stimulates an increase in TSH release from the pituitary which, in turn, causes an increase in iodine uptake and, over a period of time, thyroid enlargement or goiter. In the fourth example, a patient with normal thyroid function has been placed on a therapeutic dose of thyroxine. Because of the negative feedback relation between the thyroid and anterior pituitary, this exogenous thyroid is not additive; rather it suppresses TSH release as reflected by a low to absent uptake of radioactive iodine, and endogenous thyroid hormone secretion virtually ceases. The normal metabolic rate (BMR) and T_4(RIA) reflect the euthyroid condition associated with the ingestion of physiologic quantities of thyroxine.

CLINICAL ENTITIES

Primary Adult Hypothyroidism (Myxedema)

The cause of adult hypothyroidism is usually unknown. The pathologic findings are quite nonspecific, the thyroid being atrophic and largely replaced by fibrous tissue. In some cases, the presence of high titers of serum antithyroglobulin antibodies suggests that at least in these instances the disease resulted from autoimmune thyroiditis. Not infrequently, hypothyroidism follows the treatment of Graves' disease with either radioactive iodine or surgery. The onset of the clinical disease in the idiopathic variety is extremely gradual. Thus, one can be reasonably confident that the manifestation of florid myxedema is the result of a condition that has been slowly developing for many years. Since all cells of the body are affected by the deficiency of thyroid hormone, the physician may encounter manifestations of the disease which arise from any major organ or system. As one might expect, these manifestations are often the opposite of those seen in hyperthyroidism (Table 32–5). The term "myxedema" refers to the infiltration of the dermis by a mucinous substance containing a mucopolysaccharide. The hypothyroid patient may be hypothermic, and his skin is usually dry and cold. He is comfortable during the hot days of summer and distressed by cool weather. His slow mentation and poor memory are often erroneously attributed to aging. The generalized decline in metabolic activity is reflected in the cardiovascular system by bradycardia and in the gastrointestinal tract by constipation.

The biochemical consequences of myxedema are formidable. Although cholesterol synthesis is decreased, its disposal rate is slowed to an even greater extent, resulting in a high level of cholesterol in the plasma. It is likely that chronic hypercholesterolemia is responsible at least in part for the increase in coronary artery disease encoun-

TABLE 32–5 CONTRASTING FEATURES OF HYPERTHYROIDISM AND HYPOTHYROIDISM

	Hyperthyroidism	Hypothyroidism
Appetite	Increased	Decreased or no change
Weight	Decreased	No change
Cold tolerance	Increased	Decreased
Perspiration	Excessive	Absent
Menses	Amenorrhea	Menorrhagia
Skin	Satin smooth	Coarse, dry
Pulse	Rapid	Slow
Mentation	Rapid	Sluggish
Reflexes	Brisk	Slow

tered in patients with hypothyroidism. These patients are also extremely sensitive to most drugs and anesthetic agents, presumably because of marked slowing of the metabolic pathways involved in drug disposal.

Cretinism and Juvenile Hypothyroidism

Since both the skeletal and nervous systems are profoundly dependent on thyroid hormone for normal development, it is predictable that the consequences of thyroid hormone deficiency in childhood are more severe with early onset. Hypothyroidism in the infant may result from congenital absence of the thyroid (athyreotic cretinism) or from abnormal biosynthesis of thyroid hormone. In the latter circumstance, there is compensatory goiter formation. Occasionally, thyroid function is normal during infancy, but then fails for unknown reasons during childhood or adolescence. As with the infant, a marked retardation in skeletal and mental development is observed. The importance of making an *early* diagnosis of hypothyroidism at any age cannot be overly stressed. An intriguing exception to the over-all impairment in growth and development in juvenile hypothyroidism was described by Vanwyke and Grumbach in 1960. This is the occurrence of sexual precocity, manifested by menstruation and breast development in the female and penile and testicular enlargement in the male. A popular hypothesis invoked to explain this manifestation is that normally in children there is an "overlap" in the suppressive effect of thyroid hormone on the anterior pituitary and hypothalamus, i.e., thyroid hormone suppresses not only TSH but also pituitary gonadotropin release. Thus, when there is a deficiency of circulating thyroid hormone, not only TSH but also the gonadotropins are secreted in increased quantities, the latter leading to the premature development of secondary sexual characteristics.

Toxic Diffuse Goiter (Graves' Disease)

The most common cause of thyrotoxicosis or hyperthyroidism (the terms are used interchangeably) is Graves' disease, a syndrome in which there is diffuse enlargement of the thyroid gland associated with autonomous excessive secretion of thyroid hormone. Exophthalmos is a common but not invariable feature of the syndrome. However, the eye signs may appear before thyrotoxicosis is evident, or not until after the thyrotoxicosis has been treated and the patient is euthyroid. The degree of enlargement of the gland is highly variable. It may be so slight that no goiter is evident. Thus, the three major components of the syndrome — diffuse thyroid enlargement, thyrotoxicosis, and exophthalmos — need not be present concurrently.

Although its cause is unknown, Graves' disease is characterized by certain features which may be clues to the underlying cause. It is a common disease, second only to nontoxic sporadic goiter as the most frequent disorder of the thyroid gland. As in most thyroid diseases, women are afflicted much more commonly than men; among patients with Graves' disease, the ratio of women to men is approximately 9:1. A family history of thyroid disease is often present; close relatives have a high incidence of nontoxic goiter, thyroiditis, or Graves' disease itself. It is a common clinical observation that symptoms of the disease often begin shortly after a major psychologic or physical stress. Until recently, it was believed that the diffuse enlargement and increased function of the thyroid might be due to an excessive secretion by the pituitary of TSH. If this were so, Graves' disease would be analogous to Cushing's disease, in which an excessive secretion of ACTH leads to adrenal hyperplasia and elevation in plasma cortisol. With the availability of a highly sensitive radioimmunoassay for TSH, it is now clear that the serum concentrations of TSH in patients with Graves' disease are decreased or undetectable; thus, the anterior pituitary and hypothalamus are eliminated as the primary pathogenic sites.

The diffuse hyperplasia of the gland in Graves' disease does suggest that it is being stimulated by some extrathyroidal substance. Some years ago, Adams and Purves reported that sera from patients with Graves' disease contained a factor with TSH-like activity. This substance was capable of discharging thyroid hormone from the glands of experimental animals. Unlike the response to TSH which was evident within one hour, the serum factor did not cause detectable changes until four to six hours after administration. Because of this characteristic it was labeled "long-acting thyroid stimulator," or LATS. Subsequent investigations have disclosed that LATS is a 7S gamma globulin antibody which is capable of interacting with thyroid cells. It has the capability to stimulate protein synthesis and glucose metabolism of thyroid tissue and to effect the release of thyroid hormone. Although LATS cannot be detected in the sera of many patients with Graves' disease, it is now felt that the sera of all patients with this disease contain an abnormal IgG of one kind or another. These IgG moieties are collectively termed Human Thyroid Stimulators (HTS). These immunoglobulins are antibodies directed against the TSH receptors of thyroid follicular cells. Binding of the antibody to the receptor stimulates the cell leading to hypertrophy of the gland and increase in hormone production. In-vitro studies indicate that both TSH and HTS act via adenylate cyclase and cyclic AMP. The autoimmune hypothesis of the pathogenesis of Graves' disease just described leaves unexplained the cause of the abnormal autoantibody production.

Other common causes of hyperthyroidism include multinodular toxic goiter and toxic adenoma. In these disorders, autonomously functioning thyroid tissue secretes excessive amounts of thyroid hormone. If one administers radioactive iodine to a patient with toxic adenoma and then scans over the neck, radioactivity is found only over the adenoma. This occurs because the excessive thyroid hormone secreted by the adenoma has suppressed TSH secretion and hence iodine trapping by the normal tissue surrounding the adenoma (Fig. 32–5).

Since all cells of the body are influenced by thyroid hormone, it is not surprising that, as in hypothyroidism, manifestations of thyroid hormone excess may involve all systems of the body. The clinical picture of florid thyrotoxicosis is distinctive. Typically, the patient is thin, hyperkinetic, and impatient with the relatively slow pace of those around him. Palpitation, increased cold tolerance, and diarrhea are common symptoms. On physical examination, characteristic eye signs and goiter are usually present. The skin is satiny smooth and warm; the pulse rate is elevated and the pulse pressure widened. The latter results

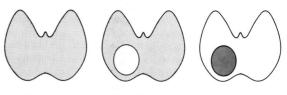

Normal   "Cold" nodule   Toxic adenoma

Figure 32–5 Thyroid scans. The *normal thyroid gland* picks up radioactive iodine (RAI) uniformly, resulting in a homogeneous distribution of radioactivity as shown. *"Cold" nodule:* Lesions such as cysts or tumors that occupy space but lack normal biologic activity appear as deficits on scan. *Toxic adenomas ("hot" nodule):* Occasionally adenomas develop which produce thyroid hormone autonomously; when the production of thyroid hormone from this source exceeds physiologic quantities, the patient becomes mildly toxic, TSH production is curtailed, and uptake of iodide by the surrounding normal thyroid virtually ceases.

from mild systolic hypertension and a decrease in diastolic pressure due in part to dilatation of peripheral vessels. There is often evidence of muscle wasting, particularly of the temporalis, shoulder girdle, and quadriceps. The deep tendon reflexes are very brisk. Infrequently, the manifestations of hyperthyroidism are markedly exaggerated. In this condition, termed "thyroid storm," the patient becomes agitated, delirious, and febrile and has a sustained tachycardia. Such an occurrence is a true medical emergency which often terminates fatally despite prompt and appropriate therapy.

The description of thyrotoxicosis as presented in the foregoing paragraphs is applicable to patients of middle age or younger. When patients over 60 develop the disease, the clinical picture is often not so clear-cut. Frequently a second disease such as congestive heart failure obscures the underlying thyrotoxicosis. The older person may not respond to excessive thyroid with the marked increase in energy and physical activity that is characteristic of the younger patient. The terms "masked hyperthyroidism" and "apathetic hyperthyroidism" are thus frequently appropriate for the disease as it presents in the older patient.

Usually, the determination of serum T_4(RIA) confirms the presence of hyperthyroidism suspected on clinical grounds. There are circumstances in which additional laboratory data are helpful in establishing the diagnosis. Two such situations will be described because they illustrate facets of the pathophysiology underlying thyrotoxicosis.

The first circumstance is exemplified by a young woman with weight loss, nervousness, palpitations, and a small goiter. Laboratory examinations reveal a T_4(RIA) of 11μg. per dl (normal, 5.0 to 11.6) and a radioactive iodine uptake of 20 per cent in 24 hours (normal, 8 to 15). The question then is whether the patient's thyroid function is within the normal range, albeit near the upper limit, or if it is definitely but minimally elevated. To answer this question, the physician can make use of the thyroid suppression test in which the radioactive iodine uptake is repeated after administering physiologic amounts of thyroid hormone for 10 days, e.g., 75μg. of triiodothyronine daily. If the patient is normal, the second radioactive iodine uptake should be significantly reduced compared to the first; if the patient has early hyperthyroidism, the RAI uptake will be virtually unchanged, since the gland is no longer being normally regulated by TSH. The availability of TRH has provided an alternate approach to this problem. In thyrotoxicosis, the level of serum TSH is not only suppressed, but it also fails to rise in response to intravenously administered TRH.

The second circumstance concerns the finding of a normal T_4(RIA) in a patient who by clinical appearance is clearly thyrotoxic and in whom the radioactive iodine uptake is abnormally high.

When the sera of such patients have been analyzed for triiodothyronine as well as thyroxine, abnormally high concentrations of the former thyroid hormone have been found coexistent with normal levels of thyroxine. In hyperthyroidism usually both triiodothyronine and thyroxine are increased. In this variant, which has been termed "T_3 toxicosis," only triiodothyronine is elevated. If left untreated, the patient with "T_3 toxicosis" will eventually manifest an increase in T_4(RIA).

Thyroid Carcinoma

While a detailed discussion of thyroid cancer is beyond the scope of this chapter, the pathophysiologic aspects of two varieties of malignancy are of sufficient interest and importance to warrant brief comment.

Post-Irradiation Thyroid Carcinoma. For a number of years it was common medical practice to use irradiation to treat a number of benign conditions in infants and young children. Thus, until approximately 20 years ago, x-ray therapy was applied to children with breathing difficulties, enlarged lymphoid tissue in the nasopharynx (adenoids) and other conditions. Recently, it has been discovered that a number of such patients have developed carcinoma of the thyroid. It is now appreciated the low levels of ionizing irradiation applied in the area of the head, neck, and shoulders, particularly to the very young, is carcinogenic to the thyroid. Individuals with a history of such irradiation should be carefully evaluated for the presence of thyroid tumor. The use of radioiodine imaging may disclose "cold nodules" that are not evident on physical examination (see Figure 32–5).

Medullary Carcinoma of the Thyroid. This malignancy arises from the parafollicular or C cells of the thyroid. These cells are responsible for the elaboration of the calcium lowering hormone, calcitonin, and individuals with medullary carcinoma characteristically have high serum levels of calcitonin. Medullary carcinoma tends to be familial and it may be associated with neoplasia of the adrenal medulla (pheochromocytoma) and parathyroid hyperplasia or adenoma.

ADRENAL CORTEX

PHYSIOLOGY

The classic description by Addison in 1849 of the disease caused by the destruction of the adrenal cortex first attracted attention to the critical importance of this gland in the maintenance of life. Many years later, cortisol and aldosterone, the principal secretions of the adrenal cortex, were identified as steroid molecules of basically similar structure. It is of interest that the other endocrine glands of mesodermal origin, the testis and ovaries, also elaborate steroidal hormones which have structures and modes of action similar to those of the adrenal cortex.

Regulation of Cortisol Secretion (Fig. 32–6)

The negative feedback control of cortisol secretion has already been alluded to (see earlier discussion). Normally, a rising level of plasma free cortisol inhibits the release of CRF from hypothalamic sites into the hypophyseal portal circulation, thereby causing a decrease in ACTH release by the anterior pituitary. This fall in plasma ACTH leads to a decline in cortisol secretion by the adrenal glands and, hence, a corresponding reduction in its plasma concentration; thus, the negative feedback loop is completed. This mechanism is modulated by several additional factors.

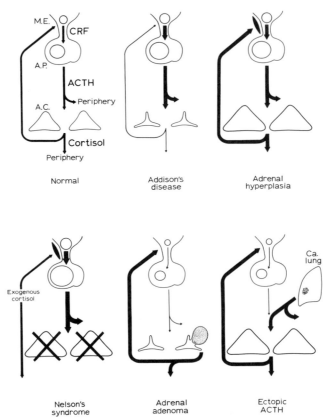

Figure 32–6 Hypothalamic, pituitary, and adrenal cortical relationships.

Normal: CRF elaborated by the median eminence *(M.E.)* stimulates the secretion of ACTH by the anterior pituitary *(A. P.)*. ACTH triggers the synthesis and release of cortisol, the principal glucocorticoid of the adrenal cortex *(A.C.)*; a rising level of cortisol inhibits CRF release, completing the negative feedback loop.

Addison's disease: In primary disease of the adrenal cortex, the level of plasma cortisol falls drastically and CRF release proceeds without inhibition, causing a marked increase in secretion of ACTH. High levels of the latter hormone promote the pigmentary changes characteristic of Addison's disease.

Adrenal hyperplasia: The primary lesion is probably at the level of the hypothalamus or higher. Production of CRF is excessive, leading to increased ACTH and cortisol secretion. The latter causes the peripheral manifestations of the disorder (Cushing's disease). Cells of the M.E. are resistant to the high levels of circulating cortisol.

Nelson's syndrome: When Cushing's disease is treated by bilateral adrenalectomy, the physiologic quantity of cortisol used to treat the patient is a relatively weak brake on CRF production. The latter increases substantially, causing intense stimulation of the ACTH-producing cells of the A.P., eventually leading to tumor formation and extreme pigmentation, which are characteristic features of the syndrome.

Adrenal adenoma: An adenoma or carcinoma of the adrenal may produce cortisol autonomously. When the rate of production exceeds physiologic quantities, Cushing's syndrome results; CRF release is inhibited by the high level of circulating cortisol, with resultant diminished ACTH secretion and atrophy of the normal adrenal tissue.

Ectopic ACTH: In this syndrome, an ACTH-like peptide is elaborated by a tumor such as carcinoma of the lung. The adrenals are stimulated; circulating cortisol increases inhibiting CRF production.

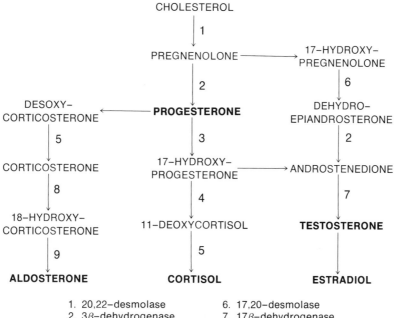

CHOLESTEROL

1

PREGNENOLONE ——————————→ 17–HYDROXY–
                                                            PREGNENOLONE

2   6

DESOXY–   ←———— **PROGESTERONE**   DEHYDRO–
CORTICOSTERONE   EPIANDROSTERONE

5   3   2

CORTICOSTERONE   17–HYDROXY– ——————→ ANDROSTENEDIONE
                     PROGESTERONE

8   4   7

18–HYDROXY–   11–DEOXYCORTISOL   **TESTOSTERONE**
CORTICOSTERONE

9   5   5

ALDOSTERONE   **CORTISOL**   **ESTRADIOL**

1. 20,22–desmolase   6. 17,20–desmolase
2. 3β–dehydrogenase   7. 17β–dehydrogenase
3. 17α–hydroxylase   8. 18–hydroxylase
4. 21–hydroxylase   9. 18–dehydrogenase
5. 11β–hydroxylase

Figure 32–7

There is evidence that elevations of ACTH in the plasma perfusing the median eminence of the hypothalamus suppress CRF release, creating a "short loop" negative feedback control. Since the plasma concentration of cortisol required to inhibit CRF release (the so-called "set point") varies diurnally, presumably on the basis of neural signals reaching the CRF-synthesizing neurons, ACTH and, in turn, cortisol are secreted in a cyclic fashion. Thus, the peak level of cortisol in the plasma normally occurs between 6 and 8 A.M. By 5 P.M. the concentration has decreased by about 50 per cent, and the fall continues until the nadir is reached around midnight, following which plasma cortisol increases. This normal circadian rhythm is lost in Cushing's syndrome. Other neural signals such as those triggered by various forms of "stress" can also override the normal feedback control and transiently increase cortisol secretion. CRF, which can cause ACTH release within minutes, is thought to be a small peptide similar to TRH, but its structure has not been positively established. ACTH is a 39-amino acid peptide with all biologic activity, including MSH-like activity, residing in the first 24 amino acids. This sequence has been synthesized and is available commercially. The amino acids from 25 to 39 vary from one species to another and account for the molecule's immunologic specificity.

ACTH is thought to exert its action through the adenylate cyclase-cyclic AMP system. The interaction of ACTH with receptors linked to the adenylate cyclase of adrenal cortical cell membranes leads to an increase in intracellular cyclic AMP which then promotes the synthesis of a protein capable of catalyzing the conversion of cholesterol to 20-α-hydroxycholesterol. The latter compound in turn is converted to pregnenolone, the precursor of all steroidal hormones of the adrenal cortex. A simplified schema for the biosynthesis of cortisol, aldosterone, testosterone, and estradiol from cholesterol is contained in Figure 32–7.

Regulation of Aldosterone Secretion (Fig. 32–8)

The principal regulator of aldosterone secretion is the renin-angiotensin system. Renin, a proteolytic enzyme of approximately 40,000 M.W., is produced in the kidney by specialized cells of the juxtaglomerular apparatus. Although the complete details regarding its synthesis and release are not yet clear, it is known that a decrease in plasma volume causes an increase in renin release and, conversely, an increase in plasma volume inhibits its release. Apparently, the juxtaglo-

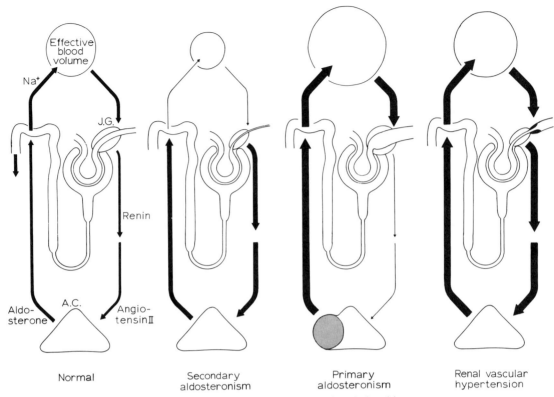

Figure 32–8 Normal and deranged aldosterone-renin-angiotensin relationships.

Normal: An increase in blood volume suppresses renin release by the juxtaglomerular apparatus (JGA) of the kidney whereas a decrease in volume stimulates its release. In the plasma, renin reacts with renin substrate to form angiotensin I; the latter is converted to angiotensin II in the lung. Angiotensin II stimulates aldosterone release from the adrenal cortex (AC) and (not shown in the diagram) causes vasoconstriction by direct action on the arterial bed. Changes in angiotensin II and aldosterone reflect those of plasma renin activity (PRA). Alterations in plasma aldosterone cause changes in sodium reabsorption and, in turn, in blood volume, completing the feedback loop. See text for details.

Secondary aldosteronism caused by restriction of dietary sodium: In the face of chronic inadequate dietary sodium, hypovolemia gradually ensues, leading to increased blood levels of PRA, angiotensin II, and aldosterone. Because of sodium deficiency, the increased aldosterone is ineffective in restoring plasma volume. Congestive heart failure is another cause of secondary aldosteronism on a different basis. Because of a decrease in cardiac output, there is a relative decrease in effective blood volume that is refractory to reexpansion by increased sodium reabsorption.

Primary aldosteronism: Here the initial pathologic event is the excessive, unregulated secretion of aldosterone from an adenoma or from hyperplastic adrenal glands. The high level of aldosterone causes hypervolemia and suppressed PRA.

Renal vascular hypertension: Significant narrowing of the renal arteries from any cause results in activation of the juxtaglomerular baroreceptors and an increase in PRA, angiotensin and aldosterone. The hypertension in these disorders is due not only to an increase in sodium reabsorption, but also to the direct vasopressor effect of angiotensin.

merular apparatus contain special cells capable of reacting to changes in renal perfusion pressure.

Once in the plasma, renin interacts with a substrate produced in the liver, angiotensinogen, to form angiotensin I, a decapeptide. In the lung, angiotensin I is converted to angiotensin II, which stimulates aldosterone secretion. Aldosterone, by promoting sodium retention, causes plasma vol-

ume expansion which then shuts off renin release, and the feedback loop is completed.

Aldosterone release is also influenced by potassium. An increase in plasma potassium promptly increases aldosterone secretion. Conversely, depletion of body potassium inhibits aldosterone release. ACTH administration also increases aldosterone secretion but this effect is transient;

aldosterone production declines to normal within 48 hours despite continued ACTH administration.

Biologic Actions

In man, cortisol and aldosterone are the principal representatives of gluococorticoids and mineralocorticoids, the two main classes of adrenal cortical steroids. The biologic activities of these steroids can be inferred from the descriptions of the classic clinical entities in which they are either deficient or in excess. An important action of cortisol is to promote the conversion of protein into glucose by induction of the enzymes of gluconeogenesis. In its role in regulating glucose homeostasis, cortisol frequently acts in opposition to insulin. The primary functions of aldosterone are interlinked: regulation of extracellular fluid volume and potassium metabolism. Unlike cortisol, which affects all cells of the body, the action of aldosterone appears limited to the kidney and the sweat and salivary glands. In the kidney, aldosterone acts on the distal tubule to promote the absorption of sodium ions in exchange for potassium and hydrogen ions. In excess, aldosterone initially stimulates sodium reabsorption by the proximal renal tubules, but after a short time "escape" from this effect occurs. Escape from the action of aldosterone on the distal tubule does not occur. Thus, in chronic aldosterone excess (primary aldosteronism) there is expansion of the extracellular fluid volume and profound potassium depletion, but no edema. In the female the androgenic steroids constitute a third functional group of steroids elaborated by the adrenal cortex. The androgenic steroids have anabolic effects and are thought to be required for the development of libido and the capacity to achieve orgasm. At least part of their effect on female sexuality depends on their tropic action on the clitoris. The mechanism of action of all steroid hormones probably involves interaction with specific protein receptors in the cytosol and nucleus, leading to modification of a portion of the genome, transcription of messenger RNA, and protein synthesis.

Biosynthesis, Transport, and Metabolism of the Adrenal Steroids (Fig. 32–6)

Cholesterol is the basic precursor of steroid biosynthesis. It is initially converted to its 20-α hydroxyl derivative in a reaction stimulated by ACTH via the adenylate cyclase-cyclic AMP system. There is then cleavage of the terminal, 6-carbon side chain of cholesterol, resulting in pregnenolone. Pregnenolone is transformed to progesterone by the action of a 3-β-hydroxysteroid dehydrogenase and an isomerase. Thereafter, a series of hydroxylations occur, each catalyzed by a specific hydroxylase and requiring NADH to form successively compounds with a hydroxyl group at C_{17}, C_{21}, and finally C_{11}, the last being cortisol. As discussed below, inborn errors of metabolism exist in which these enzymes are deficient.

In the mineralocorticoid pathway, progesterone is hydroxylated at the C_{21} position to form 11-desoxycorticosterone. There is then hydroxylation at the 11 position to form corticosterone, followed by hydroxylation at the 18 position to form 18-hydroxycorticosterone. Oxidation of this C_{18} hydroxyl group yields the final product, aldosterone. Another principal pathway involves the formation of dehydroepiandrosterone, a major metabolite of the adrenal cortex. This compound is formed by dehydroxylation of pregnenolone and cleavage of the C_{20}, C_{21} side chain to form the C_{19} steroid. Dehydroepiandrosterone is converted to androstenedione by a 3-β-hydroxysteroid-dehydrogenase and an isomerase. The latter steroid is the immediate precursor of testosterone. In females, testosterone is derived from the peripheral conversion of circulating androstenedione rather then from secretion by the adrenal gland.

Following its secretion, cortisol is transported and bound to an alpha-2-globulin called transcortin or cortisol-binding globulin (CBG). It is estimated that approximately 45 per cent of circulating cortisol is thus bound and only 5 per cent is in the biologically active, free form; the remainder conjugated with glucuronide is not included in the usual procedures used to measure plasma cortisol. Aldosterone circulates loosely

TABLE 32–6 SECRETORY RATES AND CONCENTRATIONS IN BODY FLUIDS OF THE ADRENAL CORTICAL HORMONES

	Plasma Level ($\mu g/dl$)		Secretion Rate (mg./day)	Urinary Metabolites (mg./day)
	Total	Free		
Cortisol	15	1	15–30	4–8
Aldosterone	0.003–0.015	0.003	0.050–0.250	0.025–0.035
Dehydroepiandrosterone	65	65	15–30	4–8

(Modified from Catt, K. J.: Lancet, *1*:1279, 1970.)

bound to albumin. Both hormones are metabolized in the liver by the reduction of ring A to tetrahydro derivatives which are conjugated with glucuronide. These water-soluble biologically inactive derivatives are excreted by the kidneys. The biologic half-life of cortisol, normally about two hours, is prolonged in liver disease and decreased in thyrotoxicosis; the half-life of aldosterone is 30 minutes. Adrenal steroid secretory rates and concentrations in body fluids are listed in Table 32–6.

CLINICAL ENTITIES

Addison's Disease

As mentioned above, the clinical features of chronic adrenal insufficiency were first described by Addison over a hundred years ago. The underlying pathologic process may be tuberculosis or other granulomatous disease such as histoplasmosis, metastatic carcinoma, or, most commonly, simple atrophy. Although the cause of the latter is unknown, there is reason to believe that it may be the consequence of an autoimmune reaction. Typically, the clinical manifestations of primary adrenal insufficiency are extremely insidious; rare exceptions are the acute adrenal insufficiency of meningococcemia (the Waterhouse-Friderichsen syndrome) and that due to adrenal hemorrhage secondary to anticoagulation therapy.

The manifestations of chronic adrenal insufficiency, regardless of cause, are attributable to deficiencies of cortisol and aldosterone and, in the female, androgenic steroids. Cortisol deficiency results in loss of appetite, weight loss, severe weakness, gastrointestinal disturbances, and emotional lability. Because of impaired gluconeogenesis, patients may become hypoglycemic after an overnight fast. The persistently low or absent plasma concentrations of cortisol lead to hypersecretion of ACTH and MSH, resulting in a characteristic increased pigmentation of the skin and mucous membranes. Aldosterone deficiency results in unregulated loss of body sodium and retention of potassium, with consequent reduction in plasma volume and hyperkalemia. The hypovolemia leads to prerenal azotemia, orthostatic hypotension, and ultimately shock. Because of its deleterious effect on cardiac rhythm, hyperkalemia is potentially a lethal complication of Addison's disease. Although the course of Addison's disease is typically prolonged, it may abruptly worsen if the patient is stressed by trauma or infection. Under these conditions, acute adrenal crisis may develop, manifested by vomiting, shock, high fever, and coma.

The laboratory findings in Addison's disease include a reduction in serum sodium, elevation in serum potassium, a reduced fasting blood glucose, and mild azotemia. These findings are of course not diagnostic of Addison's disease. To establish the diagnosis, it is necessary to demonstrate the inability of the adrenal glands to respond normally to ACTH stimulation. This may be done by analyzing the response of 17-hydroxycorticoids in 24-hour urine samples to the administration of ACTH over a three- to five-day period. In Addison's disease the control excretion of 17-hydroxycorticoids is typically less than 2 mg. per day and does not increase by more than 2 to 3 mg. during ACTH administration. In contrast, when adrenal insufficiency is secondary to hypopituitarism, the control values of urinary 17-hydroxycorticoids may be very low but will progressively increase with each day of stimulation to values which equal or exceed 8 to 10 mg. per day.

One particularly common form of secondary adrenal insufficiency deserves special comment. Large doses of cortisone and related glucocorticoids are often used in the chronic treatment of a variety of diseases such as asthma and rheumatoid arthritis. When such treatment is extended beyond four or five weeks, prolonged suppression of CRF and ACTH secretion ensues. If the steroid is then abruptly discontinued, the hypothalamic-pituitary axis is unable to respond normally to the reduction in circulating cortisol. The result is a mild degree of hypoadrenocorticism, which can become particularly significant if the patient is subjected to stress. This potential problem is minimized by using alternate day therapy whenever possible.

Cushing's Syndrome

Cushing's syndrome is the clinical condition that results from chronic exposure to excessive circulating levels of glucocorticoids. Four etiologic subsets of the disorder have been identified. First, the primary lesion may be either an adenoma or a carcinoma within the adrenal cortex which elaborates cortisol autonomously. Alternatively, the disease may be due to disordered hypothalamic-pituitary function, with a persistent overproduction of CRF and in turn ACTH, resulting in hyperplasia and hyperfunction of both adrenal glands. Characteristic of this disorder is a loss of the diurnal or circadian rhythm of ACTH secretion and a relative inability of cortisol to suppress ACTH secretion. The pituitary itself may be normal morphologically, or it may contain small basophilic tumors, as did the pituitary glands of the patients originally described by Cushing. This variety of Cushing's syndrome is often called "Cushing's disease." Thirdly, the adrenal cortex may be stimulated excessively by ACTH or an ACTH-like peptide elaborated by a nonpituitary tumor. This variety of Cushing's syndrome has been called the "ectopic ACTH syndrome." Carcinoma of the lung is perhaps the most frequent

TABLE 32–7 TYPICAL LABORATORY FINDINGS IN CUSHING'S SYNDROME DUE TO HYPERPLASIA, ADENOMA, CARCINOMA, AND ECTOPIC ACTH PRODUCTION

	Normal	*Adrenal Pathologic Condition*			
		Hyperplasia	*Adenoma*	*Carcinoma*	*Ectopic ACTH*
Plasma:					
Cortisol (μg./100 ml., A.M./P.M.)	17/8	30/25	35/35	50/50	35/35
ACTH (pg./ml.)	< 150	50 to 500	< 50	< 10	500 to 1000
Urine: 17 OHC (mg./24 hr.)					
Basal	2 to 10	15	30	50	30
After ACTH stimulation	2 to 5× ↑	3 to 5× ↑	↑/↔	↔	2× ↔
Dexamethasone suppression (2 mg./day)	< 3	> 4	30	50	30
Dexamethasone suppression (8 mg./day)	< 3	< 3	30	50	30

↑ = increase
↔ = no change
(Modified from Williams, G. H., and Lauler, D. P.: Laboratory evaluation of adrenocortical function. *In* Harvey, J. C. (Ed.): Practice of Medicine. Vol. II. W. F. Prior Co., Hagerstown, Maryland, 1966.)

neoplasm responsible. Fourthly, the most common form of Cushing's syndrome is that resulting from long-term therapy with pharmacologic doses of glucocorticoids for an illness such as rheumatoid arthritis, asthma, or ulcerative colitis.

The clinical manifestations of Cushing's syndrome are explicable on the basis of known effects of cortisol. Principal actions of cortisol include the promotion of protein catabolism and the diversion of amino acids into gluconeogenesis. When these physiologic processes are exaggerated by chronic cortisol excess, marked loss of protein occurs. The clinical consequences are muscle wasting, thinning of the skin, easy bruisability, abdominal striae, and osteoporosis. Cortisol, in addition to promoting glucose formation in the liver, also antagonizes the action of insulin in transporting glucose into cells. Predictably, diabetes mellitus is a common complication of Cushing's syndrome. In a number of ways, cortisol alters the normal response to infection and injury. Antibody formation is suppressed, and the accumulation and migration of polymorphonuclear cells at inflammatory sites are inhibited. Some manifestations of the disease are much less well understood: for example, the characteristic redistribution of adipose tissue causing moon facies, buffalo hump, supraclavicular fat pads, and truncal obesity. Also obscure is the basis of the mental aberrations commonly seen in Cushing's syndrome.

Because cortisol has some mineralocorticoid activity, a few patients with Cushing's syndrome have elevations in blood pressure and hypokalemia, findings typical of primary aldosteronism.

Although clinical findings may strongly suggest the diagnosis of Cushing's syndrome, laboratory confirmation is essential. One such approach entails the estimation of the 17-OHC content of 24-hour urine samples collected in the basal state

and then during the sequential administration of intravenous ACTH and oral dexamethasone, 2 mg. daily for three days, followed by 8 mg. per day for three days. The results of these procedures should establish the presence of Cushing's syndrome and, moreover, provide information regarding its cause. Illustrative data are summarized in Table 32–7 and shown graphically in Figure 32–6. It should be noted that the basal urinary excretion of 17-OHC in Cushing's syndrome due to hyperplasia may be normal (15 per cent of cases) or only slightly elevated. The hyperplastic glands ordinarily respond very briskly to ACTH stimulation.

Congenital Adrenal Hyperplasia (CAH)

The term CAH embraces a fascinating spectrum of disorders, each of which results from an inherited deficiency of a specific enzyme involved in the biosynthesis of adrenal steroids (see Fig. 32–7). In considering the pathophysiology of CAH, two basic facts need to be kept in mind: (1) of the various steroids elaborated by the adrenal cortex, cortisol, and only cortisol, suppresses ACTH secretion; (2) the rate-limiting step in cortisol biosynthesis is the ACTH-dependent conversion of cholesterol to pregnenolone. If a block exists between cholesterol and cortisol, excess pregnenolone will be produced because of increased plasma ACTH and the large amount of available cholesterol. Pregnenolone then flows down the pathway(s) available to it. Thus, we can anticipate the possibility of overproduction of some intermediaries (with or without biologic activity). Excess of one hormone may be coupled with deficiency of cortisol and possibly other hormones. In general, the clinical presentation is predictable if the site of the block is known; conversely, the clinical picture provides reliable clues as to the locus of the enzymatic defect.

C$_{21}$ Hydroxylase Deficiency.   Deficiency of C$_{21}$ hydroxylase is by far the most common cause of CAH. The deficiency of this enzyme results in impaired cortisol production and an increase in 17-OH progesterone, androstendione and testosterone. When the enzymatic deficiency is partial, as it is in about 70 per cent of cases, impaired cortisol production is corrected to a normal or near-normal rate by a compensatory increase in pituitary secretion of ACTH prompted by the initially low level of plasma cortisol. This increase in stimulation of the adrenals leads to hyperplasia and an increase in production of androgens. When the defect is more severe, this compensatory mechanism is inadequate and adrenal insufficiency ensues. Marked salt wasting is the hallmark of such patients. Besides cortisol deficiency, these individuals also produce inadequate amounts of aldosterone.

C$_{21}$ hydroxylase deficiency is perhaps the commonest cause of female pseudohermaphroditism (a term denoting the presence of male or ambiguous external genitalia in an individual with female karyotype and gonads). All newborn infants with ambiguous genitalia should be suspected of having CAH, and karyotypes should be done to determine genetic sex. The sex chromatin pattern, using buccal mucosal scrapings, is unreliable in early infancy. The presence of a phallus-like clitoris and a partially fused labia folds in a genetic female strongly suggests a C$_{21}$ defect. Urinary 17-ketosteroids and pregnanetriol (the principal metabolite of 17-OH progesterone) are both elevated in C$_{21}$ hydroxylase deficiency; however, urinary collections are difficult in the newborn. It is now possible to determine plasma 17-OH progesterone, and a marked elevation in this intermediary provides biochemical confirmation of the diagnosis. The diagnosis may be missed in infancy. The youngster with unrecognized CAH due to C$_{21}$ hydroxylase deficiency has an accelerated growth rate and an advanced bone age. Young girls with this deficiency will fail to menstruate or to develop feminine secondary sexual characteristics. Very mild degrees of deficiency probably account for the development of hirsutism in some adult females.

In a minority of newborn patients the defect is severe. Virilization, present in females, is overshadowed by life-threatening salt wasting. Such patients have reduced plasma sodium concentrations and elevated levels of plasma potassium; blood volume is reduced and blood pressure is difficult to maintain.

C$_{21}$ hydroxylase deficiency appears to be inherited as an autosomal recessive trait with variable penetrance. Parents of affected patients are presumably heterozygous for the trait. In one study,

when individuals were infused with ACTH, and 17-OH progesterone measured at frequent intervals thereafter, the rise noted in heterozygotes was substantially greater than that seen in control subjects, suggesting some limitation of the C$_{21}$ hydroxylation step in the former.

Once the diagnosis is established, the management of CAH is both straightforward and gratifying. A glucocorticoid such as cortisone acetate is given orally in physiologic doses. This exogenous replacement supplies the need of the peripheral tissues for cortisol. At the same time, ACTH secretion is suppressed, adrenal hyperplasia regresses, and the excessive production of androgens ceases. If salt-wasting is present, an aldosterone-like mineralocorticoid such as fluorohydrocortisone must be included in the therapeutic regimen.

Other Defects in Adrenal Steroidogenesis.   In addition to 21-hydroxylase deficiency, CAH may arise from lack of 11-β-hydroxylase, 17-hydroxylase, 3-β-hydroxysteroid dehydrogenase or cholesterol desmolase. The latter two conditions are extremely rare. Deficiency of 11-hydroxylase constitutes about 10 per cent of the cases of CAH. In this form of the disease, hypertension is a prominent clinical feature. Impairment of hydroxylation of C$_{11}$ leads to the accumulation of both 11-desoxycortisol and, by loss of the C$_{17}$ hydroxyl group, desoxycorticosterone. Whereas 11-desoxycortisol is biologically inactive, excessive serum levels of desoxycorticosterone cause hypertension by a mechanism which has not been fully elucidated. Confirmation of a clinical diagnosis of 11-hydroxylase deficiency requires the demonstration of excessive quantities of tetrahydrodesoxycortisol (the excretory product of 11-desoxycortisol) in the urine or of increased serum levels of 11-desoxycortisol. It is of interest that the pharmacologic agent, metyrapone, used to test for pituitary ACTH reserve, acts by inhibiting 11-hydroxylase, thus transiently simulating the inborn error of metabolism under discussion. CAH due to 11-β-hydroxylase deficiency also responds to physiologic doses of glucocorticoid.

Primary Aldosteronism (Conn's Syndrome)

Primary aldosteronism is the clinical condition caused by excessive, unregulated secretion by the adrenal cortex of the potent, salt-retaining steroid, aldosterone. The underlying pathologic lesion is usually a small adenoma. The history of both the clinical entity and the hormone is brief but instructive. By 1950 the research of many investigators had indicated that certain known actions of the adrenal cortex could not be attributed to cortisol alone. Greep and Deane were among those who postulated that there was an unidentified substance responsible for the powerful effect exerted by the adrenal cortex on mineral metabolism. In search of this missing "mineralocorticoid," Tait and co-workers isolated a factor they termed "electrocortin." This substance was soon characterized chemically and named aldosterone because of the aldehyde group on C_{18}. In 1955 the first case of primary aldosteronism was reported by Conn, who stated: "When in April, 1954, I was confronted with a patient who exhibited a most fascinating disturbance in electrolyte metabolism similar to a few cases which had been reported as potassium-losing nephritis, it could not have been presented to anyone more conscious of the possibility of aldosteronism in man than I was at that moment." Dr. Conn modestly goes on to say, "It actually required little imagination."

Chronic excessive secretion of aldosterone leads to hypertension and hypokalemia, the two characteristic findings in primary aldosteronism. Although the hypertension is usually mild or moderate in severity, it may result in manifestations of sustained hypertension such as left ventricular hypertrophy and narrowing of the retinal arterioles. The hypokalemia causes muscle weakness that may be so severe that an ascending neuritis such as that found in the Guillain-Barré syndrome is suggested. The electrolyte disturbance also leads to other symptoms such as polyuria, muscle cramps, intestinal atony, and paresthesias. On laboratory examination, the serum potassium is typically below 3.6 mEq. per L., serum sodium is normal or slightly elevated, bicarbonate is increased, and choloride is decreased (hypokalemic, hypochloremic alkalosis). There are inappropriately large amounts of potassium in the urine. The electrocardiogram reflects alterations in serum potassium.

Although the occurrence of hypokalemia in a hypertensive patient should suggest the diagnosis, confirmation requires the demonstration of both increased aldosterone secretion and low plasma renin activity. Urinary aldosterone should exceed 20 μg. per day in a patient with primary aldosteronism who is receiving ample dietary sodium, e.g., greater than 120 mEq. per day. In addition, the plasma renin activity should be low and remain suppressed despite a low sodium diet and several hours of ambulation. Patients with malignant hypertension, or hypertension due to chronic renal disease or renal artery stenosis, will also excrete large amounts of aldosterone, but in contrast the plasma renin activity will be elevated. The most common form of hypertension is termed "essential," since no specific etiologic factor can currently be identified. Although these patients have normal urinary aldosterone levels, approximately one third will display suppressed plasma renin values for reasons

which are not yet clear. A scheme recommended by Conn and coworkers for the evaluation of primary aldosteronism is given below:

Procedures
1. Two weeks: Unrestricted diet, no diuretics
2. Day 1: 120 mEq. Na diet.
   Day 2: 120 mEq. Na diet.
   Day 3: 120 mEq. Na diet; collect 24-hour urine for aldosterone; take fasting blood for plasma renin activity (PRA) after 2-hour ambulation.
3. Day 4: 10 mEq. Na diet.
   Day 5: 10 mEq. Na diet.
   Day 6: 10 mEq. Na diet; collect 24-hour urine for aldosterone; take fasting blood for plasma renin activity (PRA) after 2-hour ambulation.

Results
Aldosterone Excretion (μg./24 hr.)

	(120 mEq. Na diet)	(10 mEq. Na diet)
Normals	10.7 ± .6	39.5 ± 3.9
Patients (n = 13)	21 to 72	16 to 75

Plasma Renin Activity (ng./100 ml.)

	(120 mEq. Na diet)	(10 mEq. Na diet)
Normals	370 ± 36	1181 ± 117
Patients (n = 13)	0 to 372	0 to 446

The treatment of primary aldosteronism consists of surgical extirpation of the adenoma. Preoperative localization of the tumor may be made by the use of isotopically labeled cholesterol which concentrates in the involved adrenal or by arteriography. The prognosis is variable; if the process has been going on for many years, the cardiovascular complications of long-standing hypertension are usually irreversible and the hypertension itself tends to be fixed.

PARATHYROIDS

PHYSIOLOGY

Parathyroid Hormone, Vitamin D, and Calcitonin

The parathyroid glands are minute, with a total mass of only 200 mg.; they are of endodermal origin, being derived from the pharyngeal pouches. In the adult, they are usually located either in close proximity to or within the thyroid gland. They secrete parathyroid hormone, a polypeptide with a molecular weight of approximately 8500, which has the principal function of maintaining calcium homeostasis. The narrow range within which the serum calcium concentration is normally maintained attests to the importance of calcium homeostasis in higher life forms. Calcium plays an important role in such vital processes as neuromuscular excitability, muscular contraction, membrane permeability, and coagulation of blood. Furthermore, it is required for the activation of many critical enzymes and provides the major structural support for the organism. In the plasma, calcium circulates in three forms: bound to protein; complexed with anions, such as citrate; and ionized. Only the latter, normally about 4 mg. per dl, is metabolically active. In skeleton and in the plasma, calcium is chemically linked to phosphate. Like calcium, phosphate has great importance outside the skeleton. Phosphorylated compounds (e.g., ATP) are the currency of energy in cellular metabolism. Although parathyroid hormone is important in the regulation of plasma phosphate, there is no evidence that plasma phosphate has any direct effect on parathyroid hormone secretion. Apparently the release of parathyroid hormone in man is determined by one factor only — the level of ionized calcium perfusing parathyroid tissue.

A second substance, vitamin D, has a major role in the maintenance of calcium homeostasis. A naturally occurring vitamin D is produced by the conversion of 7-dehydrocholesterol to cholecalciferol (CC, vitamin D_3). This reaction takes place in the skin and requires ultraviolet light. A second form of the vitamin, D_2, is produced commercially by the irradiation of the plant sterol, ergosterol. It now appears clear the neither vitamin D_3 nor D_2 is itself metabolically active. Through the patient efforts of a number of workers, particularly DeLuca and his colleagues, the fascinating and complex metabolism of vitamin D has been greatly illuminated. The first step takes place in the liver; it is the hydroxylation of vitamin D_3 to 25-hydroxycholecalciferol (25 HCC). The latter metabolite is transported to the kidney bound to a specific carrier protein. In the kidney, 25 HCC is hydroxylated to 24,25 dehydroxycholecalciferol (DHCC) and 1,25 DHCC. It is 1,25 DHCC that is now believed to be the active metabolite. It also requires a specific carrier protein for transportation to its target tissues, bone and gut, where it stimulates calcium mobilization and absorption, respectively. The synthesis of 1,25 DHCC in the kidney appears to be a closely regulated process, the details of which are beginning to emerge. Both low calcium and low phosphate stimulate the synthesis while elevated calcium and high phosphate depress it. Interestingly, PTH enhances the production of 1,25 DHCC. Whether this is a direct effect or an indirect one involving, for example, phosphate, remains to be seen.

On the basis of these recent developments it might be appropriate to consider 1,25 DHCC a hormone rather than a vitamin. A vitamin is traditionally defined as a substance that is required in trace amounts for one or more vital metabolic processes. Except for those deprived of sunshine, 1,25 DHCC fails to fit this definition. On the other hand, it does have attributes of a hormone. Its synthesis is tightly controlled to prevent overproduction and its sites of action are remote from its site of production.

Besides PTH and Vitamin D, a third hormone, calcitonin, has been implicated in maintaining calcium homeostasis. Calcitonin, first described by Copp in 1962, is elaborated by the parafollicular or C cells of the thyroid. Calcitonin lowers plasma calcium by inhibiting calcium mobilization from bone. While calcitonin may be critical in lower life forms, its importance in human physiology is doubtful. The fact that patients who have undergone total thyroidectomy (and are thus without a source of calcitonin) have normal plasma calcium concentrations argues against a significant role for calcitonin in man.

Gastrointesinal Tract

The gastrointestinal tract is a critical site in the regulation of calcium metabolism. Intestinal absorption of calcium occurs either from the duodenum by active transport or at any point along the entire small bowel by simple diffusion. The latter movement of calcium across the intestinal mucosa is bidirectional; hence, fecal calcium consists of calcium excreted into the gut, as well as nonabsorbed dietary calcium. Although vitamin D has effects on other tissues, its primary action is to promote calcium absorption from the gastrointestinal tract by stimulation of its active transport. The absorption of intestinal phosphate is probably linked to that of calcium. The optimum ratio of intestinal calcium to phosphate for calcium absorption is 2 to 1. Absorption of calcium is impaired by diseases of the small bowel such as sprue and celiac disease and by hepatic disease such as biliary cirrhosis. It is also influenced by the acidity of the intestinal content and by dietary factors such as acetic acid, phytic acid, and oxalates.

Calcium absorbed from the gastrointestinal tract enters the extracellular pool of calcium, estimated at about 950 mg. in the adult. Extracellular calcium is in dynamic equilibrium with calcium in the intracellular component of soft tissue (about 11,000 mg), and with the so-called exchangeable calcium pool of the skeleton. The latter pool is estimated to turn over 40 to 50 times each day. The precise quantity and even the location of this exchangeable pool of bone calcium are not known. Some believe that it is contained within partially calcified bone, and others contend that it is calcium released from bone undergoing active resorption.

TABLE 32–8 SITES OF ACTION OF PARATHYROID HORMONE AND RELATIVE IMPORTANCE OF EACH ACTION IN MAINTAINING CALCIUM HOMEOSTASIS

	Action	Degree of Influence
Renal tubule	PO_4 Excretion	++++
	Ca^{++} Reabsorption	+
Bone	Bone Resorption	++++
Gut	Ca^{++} Absorption	±

Bone

In the adult in calcium balance, approximately 300 mg. of calcium per day is resorbed from bone and the same amount deposited each day. This turnover largely reflects the continuous process of bone remodeling. While a number of factors influence bone remodeling, such as age, bone disease and deficiency of calcium or phosphate, the principal controlling factors are (1) parathyroid hormone and vitamin D and (2) the effects of mechanical stress on the skeleton. The actions of parathyroid hormone and vitamin D on bone resorption subserve calcium homeostasis. Thus, when a conflict arises between maintenance of a normal serum calcium and skeletal integrity, bone is sacrificed to provide the needed calcium. Mechanical stress, the second factor, causes a remodeling of bone to meet changing requirements for structural strength. Within physiologic limits, it appears that parathyroid hormone is the prinicpal determinant of the magnitude of remodeling, while mechanical stresses are the principal determinants of the location where remodeling occurs.

The mechanism of action of parathyroid hormone on bone at the cellular level has not been determined. One line of evidence suggests that parathyroid hormone stimulates both the osteolytic activity of osteocytes, causing an early rise in plasma calcium, and also the differentiation of mesenchymal cells into osteoclasts, the cells responsible for bone resorption.

The Kidneys

The normal kidney is extraordinarily efficient in its conservation of calcium. Despite filtration by the glomeruli of an estimated 10,000 mg. of calcium daily, no more than 300 mg. of this is normally excreted in the urine. Calcium virtually disappears from the urine when plasma calcium falls below 7 mg. per dl. Tubular reabsorption of calcium is enhanced by parathyroid hormone, but this effect is small compared to hypercalcemia caused by the action of parathyroid hormone on bone. Vitamin D has a weak calciuric effect. The

kidney's efficiency in conserving calcium is not matched by an equal ability to excrete it when the need arises. Even with continued severe hypercalcemia, the 24-hour urinary excretion of calcium will rarely exceed 500 mg. This limitation is detrimental if calcium is being absorbed from the gut or mobilized from bone in an excessive and unregulated fashion as occurs, for example, in vitamin D intoxication or metastatic bone disease. A major renal action of parathyroid hormone is to inhibit the reabsorption of phosphate by the tubule. In the absence of parathyroid hormone, about 90 per cent or more of filtered phosphate is reabsorbed, whereas in hyperparathyroidism this value usually is less than 70 per cent. Parathyroid hormone may also stimulate the secretion of phosphate by the tubules as well as decrease its reabsorption. The major actions of parathyroid hormone are summarized in Table 32–8. The mechanism of action of parathyroid hormone on the renal tubules involves the adenylate cyclase-cyclic AMP system. Following the injection of parathyroid hormone, the urinary excretion of cyclic AMP is markedly increased.

CLINICAL ENTITIES

Hypoparathyroidism

By far the leading cause of parathyroid hormone deficiency is inadvertent removal or damage to the parathyroids during thyroid surgery. Permanent hypoparathyroidism is a serious complication of thyroidectomy, occurring with a frequency of about 1 per cent. Idiopathic hypoparathyroidism, a rare disorder, is noteworthy in several respects. It may be familial and be associated with generalized moniliasis and deficiencies of other endocrine glands. The sera of some patients with idiopathic hypoparathyroidism have high titers of antibody to human parathyroid tissue, suggesting an autoimmune cause.

The manifestations of hypoparathyroidism are directly attributable to impaired calcium homeostasis due to parathyroid hormone deficiency. Both total and ionized serum calcium are low, and serum phosphate is high. Hypocalcemia causes an increase in neuromuscular irritability. When the total serum calcium falls below 7 to 8 mg. per dl., the patient develops symptoms such as numbness, tingling, formication, and muscle cramping. With a further depression in serum calcium, the physical manifestations of hypocalcemia termed tetany, ensue. These include carpopedal spasm, laryngeal spasm and stridor, muscle twitching, and generalized convulsions. The latter occasionally lead to the erroneous diagnosis of epilepsy. This tragic mistake can be avoided by routinely determining the serum calcium in all patients undergoing their initial evaluation for a seizure disorder. The altered myocardial contractility due to hypocalcemia is reflected in the electrocardiogram by prolongation of the Q-T interval. Such a finding on a routine electrocardiogram should always arouse suspicion of occult hypocalcemia. Factors that alter the protein binding of calcium in the serum can either enhance or diminish the symptoms of hypocalcemia. For example, alkalosis will increase the quantity of calcium bound to protein with a corresponding reduction in ionized calcium; thus, hyperventilation can cause mild symptoms in the presence of a normal total serum calcium. Conversely, acidemia increases the dissociation of bound calcium, and thus may prevent tetany even when the total calcium is 5 or 6 mg. per dl.

Chronic hypocalcemia results in cataract formation and calcification within the central nervous system. The basal ganglia and cerebellum appear to be especially vulnerable. It has been thought that such calcification is the result of supersaturation of body fluids with calcium phosphate. Although the calcium × phosphate product may indeed be elevated in hypoparathyroidism, this fails to explain the peculiar distribution of calcification in hypoparathyroidism, which differs strikingly from that found in other diseases with a high calcium × phosphate product.

Pseudohypoparathyroidism

In 1942, Albright and his colleagues introduced the term pseudohypoparathyroidism to describe a 28-year-old female with a seizure disorder, short stature, and the serum calcium and phosphate findings of hypoparathyroidism. Large quantities of parathyroid hormone administered to this patient failed to correct the serum chemical abnormalities and did not cause an increase in phosphate excretion. These findings suggested that the basic problem was an inability to respond to parathyroid hormone rather than a deficiency of the hormone. Subsequently, similar patients have been reported and have manifested, in addition to hypocalcemia and an elevated serum phosphate, short stature and a short neck, a rounded fact, short metacarpal and metatarsal bones, extraosseous calcification, and mental retardation. The syndrome appears to be inherited as an X-linked dominant trait with partial penetrance. Patients with the characteristic physiognomy but without serum chemistry abnormalities have been identified and labeled with the rather awkward term "pseudopseudohypoparathyroidism." Since pseudopseudohypoparathyroidism and pseudohypoparathyroidism have occurred in the same

kindred and also in the same patient at different times, the former condition is regarded as a less severe genetic expression (or "forme fruste") of the latter.

Considerable evidence now supports Albright's thesis that pseudohypoparathyroidism is a disorder involving end-organ unresponsiveness to parathyroid hormone rather than a deficiency of the hormone. Hyperplastic parathyroid glands have been demonstrated in these patients at surgery, and their sera have been shown to contain abnormally high levels of immunoassayable parathyroid hormone. As mentioned above, the action of parathyroid hormone on the renal tubular cells is mediated by the adenylate cyclase-cyclic AMP system. When parathyroid hormone is administered to normal subjects or patients with hypoparathyroidism or pseudopseudohypoparathyroidism, the urinary content of cyclic AMP is greatly increased; contrariwise, no increase in cyclic AMP occurs in patients with pseudohypoparathyroidism. Thus, unresponsiveness of the renal tubule cells to parathyroid hormone is clearly implicated in the pathogenesis of the hypocalcemia and hyperphosphatemia of pseudohypoparathyroidism. This observation also tends to localize the biochemical defect in the kidneys to either the interaction of parathyroid hormone with adenylate cyclase or of adenylate cyclase with cyclic AMP. An additional question of importance in pseudohypoparathyroidism concerns the responsiveness of the other parathyroid hormone-sensitive tissues, especially bone. Since occasional patients with pseudohypoparathyroidism have developed osteitis fibrosa cystica, it would appear that bone is at least partially responsive to parathyroid hormone in some patients with this disorder. As is so often true in endocrinology, studies undertaken to clarify the nature of a relatively obscure disorder, pseudohypoparathyroidism, have yielded information of basic importance to an understanding of hormone action.

Primary Hyperparathyroidism

Primary hyperparathyroidism refers to the disorder in which parathyroid hormone is secreted autonomously and excessively by one or more of the parathyroid glands. It is to be distinguished from secondary hyperparathyroidism which occurs in response to chronic renal disease, malabsorption, and other disorders characterized by long-standing hypocalcemia. The underlying pathologic disorder in primary hyperparathyroidism is either one or more adenomas (about 90 per cent of cases), hyperplasia of all four glands (about 10 per cent), or carcinoma (less than 1 per cent). Infrequently, when hyperparathyroidism is familial, there is a high incidence of neoplasms involving other endocrine glands, especially the pituitary and the pancreas, or the thyroid and adrenal medulla. These pluriglandular syndromes are termed multiple endocrine adenomatosis (MEA). Certain neoplasms arising in other organs, especially the lung, liver, and genitourinary tract, occasionally elaborate a peptide with parathyroid hormone activity. The resulting biochemical disturbance which may closely mimic primary hyperparathyroidism is often referred to as the ectopic PTH syndrome.

The major manifestations of primary hyperparathyroidism are due to (1) the physiologic effects of hypercalcemia, (2) the effects of chronic hypercalcemia on the kidney, and (3) the effects of chronic excessive parathyroid hormone on bone. Hypercalcemia per se impairs the concentrating ability of the kidney and polyuria is an early symptom of hyperparathyroidism. Precipitation of fine crystals of calcium salts in the renal tubules (nephrocalcinosis) impairs both glomerular and tubular function. Renal stone formation occurs commonly in patients with hyperparathyroidism. A vicious cycle may ensue in which renal calculi predispose to infection, and alkalinization of the urine by infecting organisms in turn leads to further stone formation. If uninterrupted, this sequence of events may progress to uremia and death. Clearly, any patient who has or has had a renal stone should be investigated for hyperparathyroidism.

For reasons that are not yet clear, bone involvement in hyperparathyroidism sufficient to cause symptoms or to be detected by x-ray is becoming increasingly rare. An unproved hypothesis attempting to explain this trend has implicated the protective effect provided by the high calcium content of the typical American diet.

The high incidence of peptic ulcer disease which has been observed in patients with primary hyperparathyroidism may be a consequence of hypercalcemia. It has been shown experimentally that increasing the level of serum calcium stimulates an increase in circulating gastrin and an increased rate of secretion of hydrochloric acid by the stomach. Hypertension is also a frequent finding in hyperparathyroidism; although it is usually a reversible complication which disappears after correction of the primary disorder, it often persists following surgery in those patients with nephrocalcinosis.

Metabolic Bone Disease

The concept of metabolic bone disease was introduced over 30 years ago by Albright. The term applies to those disorders of bone in which — at the molecular level — all parts of the skeleton are involved. The qualification "at the molecular level" is important, since clinically, radiographically, and even histologically the disease may appear to be limited to only one or several sites. As might be predicted from its generalized nature, the identified causes of metabolic bone disease are usually hormonal or nutritional. Features of the three "classic" examples of metabolic bone disease — osteitis fibrosa cystica, osteoporosis, and osteomalacia—are given in Table 32–9. Other forms of bone disease may

TABLE 32–9 COMPARISON OF THE MAJOR METABOLIC BONE DISEASES

	Osteitis Fibrosa Cystica	Osteoporosis	Osteomalacia
Etiology	Excessive PTH	Varied but usually unknown	Vitamin D deficiency; malabsorption; etc.
Serum			
Calcium	Increased	Normal	Decreased or normal
Phosphate	Normal or decreased	Normal	Decreased
Alkaline phosphatase	Normal or increased	Normal	Increased
Pathophysiology	Increased bone resorption	Decreased bone mass (resorp. > accret.)	Decreased mineralization
Histopathology	Cysts; fibrosis; "Brown" tumor	Normal histology	Increased osteoid tissue
Radiology	Subperiosteal resorption; cysts	Rarefaction of axial skeleton; "codfish" vertebrae compression fractures	Rarefaction of appendicular skeleton; pseudofractures (Looser's zones)

be widely disseminated, as for example in metastatic cancer, but between metastatic sites the bone will be normal, and thus the process is not considered under the above classification.

Renal Osteodystrophy. Although it has long been appreciated that chronic hypocalcemia can lead to hyperplasia of the parathyroids, the full implications of this phenomenon as it applies to chronic renal disease are just beginning to emerge. The term "renal osteodystrophy" embraces a syndrome in uremic patients that includes profound disturbances in divalent ion metabolism, metabolic bone disease including osteomalacia, osteitis fibrosa cystica, and osteosclerosis, hyperplasia of the parathyroids and soft tissue calcification. In the past, the brief life span of a patient with severe renal failure precluded the development of advanced metabolic bone disease. With the advent of chronic dialysis and renal transplantation, the patient with uremia may survive for extended periods, providing the time required to develop severe renal osteodystrophy. It is estimated that 25 per cent of uremic patients treated with conventional therapy and 80 per cent of those in chronic dialysis programs have this bone disease.

The pathophysiology of renal osteodystrophy is complex; at least three independent factors are involved. These are: (1) phosphate retention; (2) a decrease in responsiveness of bone to the calcium mobilizing action of PTH and; (3) an acquired defect in vitamin D metabolism wherein formation of the active metabolite, 1,25 DHCC, is diminished. These factors have in common the propensity to reduce plasma calcium and cause parathyroid hyperplasia. Probably the earliest event in the pathogenic sequence leading to renal osteodystrophy is phosphate retention, commencing when the creatinine clearance falls to approximately 75 ml. per minute. The inverse relationship between the concentrations of calcium and phosphate in the plasma, emphasized many years ago by Fuller Albright, appears valid today. Thus, an elevation in phosphate causes a decrease in calcium so that the product of the two remains unchanged. The slight decline in calcium, however, causes an increase in PTH secretion; the latter prompts an increase in urinary phosphate excretion and a return of phosphate and calcium to normal. Thus, normal plasma levels of calcium and phosphate are achieved at the expense of an increase in PTH secretion. With advancing renal failure, plasma PTH continues to rise (as calcium and phosphate remain normal). However, when the creatinine clearance falls below 20 ml. per minute, few nephrons remain to respond to PTH; phosphate excretion decreases, plasma phosphate rises and calcium falls. At this point, hypocalcemia may be worsened by the relative resistance of the skeleton to PTH and diminished intestinal absorption of calcium secondary to impaired synthesis of 1,25 DHCC. The latter events lead to a diminished miscible pool of calcium and reduced calcification of osteoid tissue (osteomalacia). The chronic state of hypocalcemia prompts an extraordinary degree of parathyroid hyperplasia and extremely high levels of plasma PTH. The combined weight of glands may be several grams and the PTH concentrations are considerably higher than those seen in primary hyperparathyroidism. Whether or not hyperparathyroidism can become truly autonomous in renal failure (so-called "tertiary hyperparathyroidism") is controversial. There have been reports of hypercalcemia persisting after renal failure has been corrected by successful renal transplant. In any event, levels of plasma PTH sufficient to overcome resistance to its calcemic action on bone are reached. The bone pathology that results from prolonged exposure to very high levels of PTH is osteitis fibrosa cystica. Typically, bone pain occurs in renal failure in patients whose lives have been prolonged by repeated dialysis. In fact, it may be the patient's major complaint, other manifestations of uremia being controlled by dialysis. Not surprisingly, the skeleton of these patients, weakened by the overlapping processes of osteomalacia and osteitis fibrosis cystica, is subject to fracture with little or no trauma. Calcium mobilized from the bone in late renal failure tends to normalize the plasma calcium; however, the high levels of phosphate remain unchanged. As a result the product of the two rises, increasing the likelihood of deposition of calcium precipitates in non-osseous tissues. Soft tissue calcification is often widespread involving the subcutaneous tissue of the skin, the conjunctivae, joints, and blood vessels. Treatment of renal osteodystrophy is directed at reducing the amount of phosphate available for absorption by the gut and at increasing intestinal absorption of calcium. To meet the first objective, dietary phosphate is reduced and non-absorbable phosphate binding agents such as aluminum hydroxide are prescribed. Calcium as gluconate or carbonate is given to supplement dietary calcium. The highly potent vitamin D metabolite 1,25 DHCC is being used successfully in patients with severe bone disease and hypocalcemia. The principal difficulty encountered with this agent has been hypercalcemia which, fortunately, has persisted for only a few days after therapy has been discontinued. Lastly, total parathyroidectomy has been done in patients with hypercalcemia unassociated with prior vitamin D therapy. It is particularly important to correct hypercalcemia before implanting a new kidney.

To simplify postparathyroidectomy management, all four glands have been removed from the neck and the substance of one of the four cut into small fragments. These are implanted beneath the skin of the forearm where they are readily accessible if hypercalcemia develops in the future.

Osteoporosis. Osteoporosis is by far the most frequently encountered form of metabolic bone disease. It occurs most commonly in postmenopausal Caucasian females and in males over 60 years of age. The Negro race is infrequently affected. The basic abnormality is loss of bone substance which is seen radiographically as demineralization. The principal symptom is low back pain. Serum calcium, phosphate, and alkaline phosphatase are normal, as is the histologic and biochemical examination of biopsy samples of the bone itself.

The cause of primary or idiopathic osteoporosis is not known. As discussed earlier, maintenance of normal skeletal integrity requires a balance between bone formation and bone resorption. In osteoporosis, the latter exceeds the former. Whether resorption is pathologically increased or formation abnormally decreased, or both, is not clear. In recent years sophisticated methodology has been applied to the problem. Calcium kinetics, using ^{45}Ca, have been determined in patients with osteoporosis; in addition, their bones have been analyzed by microradiography and morphometric techniques using tetracycline labeling. Unfortunately, these different approaches have not yielded consistent results, and the cause (or causes) of primary osteoporosis remains unknown. Deficiency in dietary calcium may cause osteoporosis experimentally but its role in the development of the disease in man is uncertain. Deficiencies of estrogenic and androgenic hormones have long been considered to play important roles in the development of this disease. This view is supported by the high incidence of osteoporosis in postmenopausal women, young women with ovarian agenesis, and older men. However, long-term treatment with estrogens has not caused a detectable increase in bone mass in women with postmenopausal osteoporosis. At the present time, it appears likely that primary osteoporosis may be the result of several coexistent factors.

A number of specific conditions are recognized that lead to osteoporosis. These include Cushing's syndrome, prolonged treatment with glucocorticoids, immobilization, thyrotoxicosis, and pregnancy. In hyperparathyroidism, there may be osteoporosis coexistent with the more specific lesions of subperiosteal bone resorption and cyst formation.

Low back pain is the most frequent symptom of osteoporosis. Typically, it is insidious in onset. Occasionally the onset is acute or there is an acute exacerbation of pain superimposed on the chronic discomfort. These latter events are associated with compression fracture of a vertebral body. Not infrequently, advanced osteoporosis is discovered in x-rays taken for an unrelated condition in a patient who is free of back pain. Progressive shortening of stature due to collapsed vertebrae may occur with little or no pain.

The diagnosis depends on finding characteristic changes in the x-ray films of the skeleton, particularly the spine. The end plates of the vertebrae are less rarefied than the bodies, causing an increased contrast between the two. The end plates may be depressed centrally, leading to the so-called "codfish" appearance of the spine. With further advance in the disease, the nucleus pulposus herniates through the end plate, producing an irregular area of increased density in the central portion of the vertebral body, a finding known as the "Schmorl node." When compression fracture occurs, typically the anterior portion of the body gives way, producing a "wedgelike" deformity of the vertebral body. Cortical bone is less affected than cancellous bone in osteoporosis. One can grossly assess the long bones by comparing the combined thickness of the bone's cortices with its total thickness. Normally, the former accounts for approximately 45 per cent of the latter.

ADRENAL MEDULLA

PHYSIOLOGY

The primary function of the adrenal medulla is to secrete catecholamines. These are substances with diverse effects on intermediary metabolism, contractility of cardiac and smooth muscle, and neurotransmission. To accomplish these effects, the catecholamines reach target cells by two different routes: (a) epinephrine is secreted by the adrenal medulla into the circulation to perfuse peripheral tissues and (b) norepinephrine is released by nerve endings of the sympathetic nervous system to act on neighboring cells. Strictly speaking, only case (a) fulfills the criteria for a hormone; however, from an operational point of view, it is helpful to discuss metabolic responses to catecholamines regardless of their origin. The following discussion will consider the biosynthesis, metabolic actions, and degradation of the catecholamines.

Biosynthesis

The primary precursor in the biosynthesis of the catecholamines is phenylalanine. Successive hydroxylations, decarboxylation, and methylation yield norepinephrine and epinephrine as follows:

phenylalanine → tyrosine → dihydroxyphenylalanine (Dopa) → dopamine → norepinephrine → epinephrine

Epinephrine is the principal circulating catecholamine elaborated by the adrenal medullary cells, but they also secrete small quantities of norepinephrine. Norepinephrine is the principal neurotransmitter of the sympathetic nervous system and one of the principal ones of the central nervous system as well.

Mechanism of Action

The concept of alpha- and beta-adrenergic receptors is basic to an understanding of the mechanism of action of epinephrine and norepinephrine. As mentioned in the introduction to this chapter, the response to a hormone begins when it combines with a specific receptor in either the cell membrane or the cytosol. No example of this phenomenon has been studied more thoroughly than the interaction of catecholamines with their receptor sites.

The characterization of adrenergic receptors as alpha and beta originated with pharmacologic studies designed to measure the relative potencies of epinephrine, norepinephrine, and synthetic catecholamines such as isoproterenol on selected responses, including myocardial and smooth muscle contractility. Isoproterenol possessed the greatest potential for stimulating the myocardium, and norepinephrine the least; contrariwise, norepinephrine was the most effective vasoconstrictor, and isoproterenol the least effective. It was postulated that the stimulatory effect of these agents on myocardial contractility was mediated by alpha sites. The significance of this hypothesis was strengthened following the discovery of phentolamine, an agent that blocks alpha-site activity, and propranolol, a beta-site blocker. Extensive studies with these and similar drugs demonstrated that epinephrine and norepinephrine are agonists for both alpha and beta sites, while isoproterenol is essentially a beta agonist. The effect of epinephrine on adipose tissue and pancreatic islet cells, two tissues of fundamental metabolic importance, will illustrate the concept of adrenergic receptor sites.

Epinephrine has long been known to stimulate lipolysis via the adenylate cyclase-cyclic AMP system. Recent studies with isolated human fat cells which were incubated with epinephrine alone, or epinephrine with phentolamine or propranolol, indicate that both alpha- and beta-adrenergic sites are present on the adipocyte and that they mediate divergent effects on lipolysis. Epinephrine alone stimulates lipolysis and causes an increase in cyclic AMP,

effects that are greatly enhanced if phentolamine is also present. Contrariwise, the addition of propranolol to epinephrine causes a sharp fall in both intracellular cyclic AMP and lipolysis. Thus, stimulation of beta sites increases the lipolytic response, while the activation of alpha sites has the opposite effect. The beta effect predominates, since epinephrine alone causes an increase in lipolysis.

Similar in-vitro studies have been performed with isolated pancreatic islets of the rat. Epinephrine alone sharply decreases insulin release by the islets, and a further reduction occurs when the cells are exposed to both epinephrine and propranolol. Conversely, the addition of phentolamine to epinephrine causes a marked increase in insulin release. Thus, islet cells appear to have both alpha and beta sites which mediate divergent effects on insulin release. In contrast to adipose tissue, the alpha effect predominates, since epinephrine alone decreases insulin release.

The major actions of the catecholamines include:

— Inotropic and chronotropic action on the myocardium
— Blood vessel constriction and dilatation
— Bronchodilatation and constriction
— Contraction and relaxation of smooth muscle of gut and uterus
— Neurotransmission in the central nervous system
— Metabolic effects including those on lipolysis, insulin secretion, and hepatic glycogenolysis

The major metabolic effects of epinephrine result from its action on four major tissues: adipose tissue, pancreas, liver, and muscle. Catecholamine interactions with the first two have already been mentioned. In the liver, epinephrine stimulates adenylate cyclase, and the resultant increase in cyclic AMP promotes glycogenolysis and an increase in gluconeogenesis. It has not been firmly established that adrenergic receptor sites are involved in the initiation of these effects. In muscle, epinephrine stimulates glycogenolysis by beta-site activation. Unlike liver, muscle does not have a phosphatase capable of dephosphorylating glucose-6-phosphate. Hence, the products of glycogenolysis are either CO_2 and water or, in the presence of hypoxemia, lactate.

The principal metabolic effects of epinephrine in the intact organism are hyperglycemia and an increase in plasma free fatty acids. Hyperglycemia results from the release of glucose by the liver, the suppression of insulin release, and the stimulation of muscle glycogenolysis resulting in a release of lactic acid into the circulation. The latter serves as substrate for gluconeogenesis by the liver. Lipolysis is increased by direct stimulation of adipose tissue by epinephrine and also by the decline in plasma insulin. Thus, the responses of these four tissues to epinephrine are complementary in that each promotes an increase in the available supply of circulating free fatty acids and glucose. The increased levels of these two metabolic fuels ensure that the nervous system and muscle will have ample substrate during physiologic stress. The catecholamines have thus been characterized as the hormones of "flight or fight," since they are discharged most conspicuously at times of great threat to the animal's survival. Similarly, the cardiovascular and smooth muscle responses to catecholamines assist the organism in meeting such an emergency successfully. It is likely that the changes that occur during stress are but exaggerations of responses that take place continuously as the sympathetic nervous system and adrenal medulla act to modulate the flow of nutrients to and from the liver, adipose tissue, and muscle.

Degradation of the Catecholamines

The two principal pathways for the biochemical disposal of epinephrine and norepinephrine involve methylation and oxidation:

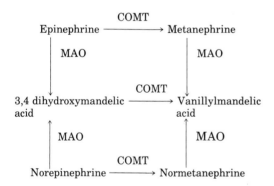

COMT (catechol-O-methyltransferase) is widely distributed throughout the body and acts rapidly to inactivate circulating catecholamines. MAO (monoamine oxidase) catalyzes the oxidative deamination of the catecholamines; it is located within nerve endings and acts to prevent excessive storage of norepinephrine.

CLINICAL ENTITIES

Loss of adrenal medullary function appears to cause little or no disability. Thus, patients who have undergone bilateral adrenalectomy respond satisfactorily to treatment with only adrenal cortical hormones. Such a procedure, of course, leaves the sympathetic nervous system

intact. However, the function of the latter has been reduced both surgically and pharmacologically in the treatment of hypertension. Although patients who undergo such treatment are subject to orthostatic hypotension, impaired metabolism among such patients has not been reported.

Pheochromocytoma

Pheochromocytomas (from the Greek, meaning "darkly staining cells") are tumors arising from chromaffin cells that secrete excessive amounts of epinephrine or both epinephrine and norepinephrine. Although usually located in the adrenal medulla, they may develop anywhere in the body where rests of chromaffin cells are found. The pre-eminent manifestation of pheochromocytoma is hypertension. In a series of 507 cases reviewed by Hermann and Mornex, 26 per cent of patients had paroxysmal hypertension, 61 per cent showed sustained hypertension, and 4 per cent were found to be hypertensive during pregnancy. In 9 per cent of cases, hypertension was not present. Among all patients with hypertension, however, pheochromocytoma is exceedingly rare, probably less than 0.1 per cent. Nevertheless, in most cases pheochromocytomas are benign and accessible to the surgeon and are an important cause of curable hypertension.

Most of the manifestations of pheochromocytoma can be anticipated from the known actions of epinephrine and norepinephrine. Often, they occur in paroxysmal fashion, as in the patient who has had normal or moderately elevated blood pressure but who suddenly becomes severely hypertensive, blanches, and complains of headache, chest pain, and palpitation. The metabolic effects of excessive circulating catecholamines, hyperglycemia and an increase in free fatty acids, can usually be demonstrated. In most patients, however, the presentation of pheochromocytoma is less dramatic, consisting of sustained hypertension and nonspecific symptoms such as weakness, tremor, palpitation, and anxiety. In either event, a firm diagnosis can be established only by appropriate laboratory testing.

In the past, reliance was placed on pharmacologic tests. For example, the prompt attenuation of severe hypertension by the administration of the alpha blocker phentolamine was highly suggestive of pheochromocytoma. The usefulness of phentolamine has now shifted from the sphere of diagnosis to that of therapy. Diagnosis is currently dependent on the demonstration of abnormally high concentrations of epinephrine, norepinephrine, or their metabolites in the urine. The upper limits of normal for the daily excretion of these substances in the adult are as follows:

epinephrine, 20 μg.

norepinephrine, 80 μg.

metanephrines, 1.3 mg.

vanillylmandelic acid (VMA), 6.5 mg.

However, to be meaningful, these tests must be performed by a competent laboratory on specimens which are free of interfering drugs or dietary constituents. If the patient has paroxysmal hypertension, urine must be collected during such an episode and the amount of catecholamine present expressed per gram of urinary creatinine.

PANCREAS

PHYSIOLOGY

The principal function of the endocrine pancreas is the secretion of insulin, a hormone necessary for the orderly intracellular storage and retrieval of dietary nutrients such as glucose, amino acids, and triglyceride. It is not difficult to perceive the survival value of insulin. With food supply erratic, the animal capable of storing nutrient fuel during times of plenty had a great advantage over the species that could not. Furthermore, since muscle and adipose tissue require insulin for glucose transport while nervous tissue does not, the insulin regulatory mechanism provides for the adequate development and function of the central nervous system, which is dependent on glucose for its metabolism. Without insulin, glucose would flow into muscle and adipose tissue cells in an unregulated fashion resulting in recurrent hypoglycemia.

Biosynthesis and Release of Insulin

Insulin is elaborated by the beta cells of the islets of Langerhans. These cells of endodermal origin occur in clusters throughout the pancreas. It has been estimated that the human pancreas contains about 1.5 million islets with a total weight of about 1 gram. Approximately 75 per cent of the cells of human islets are beta cells. The remainder are either alpha cells, which elaborate glucagon, or delta cells, which secrete gastrin. The average adult pancreas contains approximately 200 units of insulin (equivalent to 8 mg.); the average daily secretion of insulin is estimated at between 35 and 50 units. Insulin has a molecular weight of 6000 and is composed of two chains; the A chain has 21 amino acids, the B chain has 30. Steiner and co-workers demonstrated that insulin is derived from a larger molecule, termed proinsulin. Proinsulin contains a connecting peptide, the C chain, composed of 33 amino acids which join the N terminus of chain A to the carboxyl terminus of the B chain. Proinsulin is not biologically active and normally little of it is secreted; the C peptide is cleaved off by trypsin-like enzymes as part of the biosynthetic process. C peptide and insulin enter the circulation in equimolar quantities. The rate of disposal of C peptide is slower than insulin, however, so that its plasma concentration tends to be greater than that of insulin. Diabetic patients receiving insulin therapeutically develop antibodies that interfere with the measurement of plasma insulin by RIA. There is now available, however, a radioimmunoassay for the C peptide that is not interfered with by insulin antibodies. Newly discovered insulin-dependent diabetics have demonstrable levels of C peptide in their serum, indicating the presence of residual islet cell function. In most diabetics, the level of C peptide eventually declines over a period of several years.

Although numerous physiologic events may alter insulin secretion, the most important regulatory factor is the concentration of glucose in the plasma perfusing the pancreas. When blood glucose levels exceed approximately 100 mg. per 100 ml., insulin release is stimulated; as glucose falls, so does the rate of insulin secretion. However, even during prolonged fasting when the plasma level of glucose remains low, a continuing basal secretion of insulin can be demonstrated. Certain amino acids such as leucine and arginine can also stimulate insulin release, as can the intestinal hormones gastrin, secretin, pancreozymin, and glucagon-like peptide. Release of these intestinal hormones during digestion appears to intensify the pancreatic insulin response to glucose and amino acids. Insulin secretion is also influenced by catecholamines interacting with islet cell adrenergic receptor sites as described earlier. Depending on the method of analysis, the fasting level of insulin ranges from 10 to 20 μU. per ml. and increases 50 to 150 μU. per ml. following a meal or a glucose load. Its biologic half-life is less than 10 minutes, being rapidly cleared from the circulation by the liver and kidneys. The peak effect of intravenously administered insulin occurs between 30 and 60 minutes after infusion.

In addition to insulin, two other hormones are elaborated in the islets of Langerhans: glucagon in the alpha cells and somatostatin in the delta cells. Glucagon is also produced by cells in the gastrointestinal tract; the possible role of glucagon in the pathogenesis of diabetes is commented on below. Somatostatin, a tetradecapeptide, first identified in hypothalamic tissue, has a wide range of biologic effects in addition to suppression of growth hormone release, the first action attributed to it. The infusion of somatostatin suppresses both glucagon and insulin secretion. The significance of the close proximity of the cells producing these three hormones is not yet clear. Unger has suggested that the three hormones act to control the flow into and out of the circulation of nutrients such as glucose and amino acids by affecting their absorption and peripheral disposal. As part of this process, somatostatin and glucagon appear to influence the secretion of one another and of insulin.

Action of Insulin

The primary mechanism(s) by which insulin exerts its metabolic effects is not known despite intense efforts aimed at answering this question. A great deal is known about *what* insulin does, but relatively little is known regarding *how* it does it.

The action of insulin on three metabolically important tissues — adipose tissue, muscle, and liver — is summarized below. These actions are illustrated more graphically in subsequent paragraphs in which the consequences of insulin deficiency are discussed.

Adipose Tissue. Insulin stimulates the transport of glucose into the fat cell or adipocyte and probably the initial phosphorylation of glucose to glucose-6-phosphate. The ensuing metabolism of glucose-6-phosphate to acetyl-CoA affects fat metabolism in several ways:

1. Metabolism of glucose via the hexose monophosphate shunt generates NADH, the coenzyme required for fatty acid synthesis.

2. Metabolism of glucose via the Embden-Meyerhof pathway generates α-glycerol phosphate which is necessary for the esterification of fatty acids to form triglyceride. Unphosphorylated glycerol is not reactive. Since adipose tissue does not contain a glycerol kinase, glycerol derived from hydrolysis of triglyceride cannot be used in re-esterification.

3. The metabolism of glucose provides two carbon fragments for fatty acid synthesis.

Unrelated to its effect on glucose metabolism, insulin has two additional effects on fat metabolism:

1. Regulation of triglyceride in the peripheral tissues.

2. Regulation of lipolysis.

Circulating triglyceride does not enter the fat cell as such; it is hydrolyzed by a lipoprotein lipase present between the basement membrane of the capillary and the plasma membrane of the adipocyte. This enzyme, necessary for the clearing of exogenous and endogenous triglyceride particles from the plasma, is insulin-dependent. The regulation of fat mobilization or lipolysis is incompletely understood. Lipolysis is stimulated by norepinephrine released by sympathetic nerve endings, which acts via the adenylate cyclase-cyclic AMP system to activate the hormone-sensitive lipase which hydrolyzes triglyceride. Lipolysis is also stimulated by a fall in plasma insulin concentration and is inhibited by an increased concentration of insulin. The mechanism of action of insulin in altering lipolysis is not clear. It is tempting to speculate that it acts by inhibiting adenylate cyclase, but this has not been established.

In summary, insulin affects adipose tissue metabolism by promoting transport of glucose into the cell, stimulating fatty acid synthesis, inhibiting lipolysis, and inducing the enzyme necessary for the disposal of plasma triglyceride.

Muscle. Insulin is necessary for the transport of glucose into muscle cells in the resting state. Once in the cell, glucose is oxidized either completely to CO_2 or, if oxygen is limited, to lactic acid. Lactic acid then diffuses into the circulation, from which it is extracted by the liver and used as a substrate for glucose formation. The movement of carbon from the liver to muscle in the form of glucose and its return as lactic acid is known as the Cori cycle. It should be emphasized that muscle metabolizes ketones and fatty acids in preference to glucose, and that fatty acids are the principal fuel of muscle. In the process, both fatty acids and ketones are oxidized to CO_2 and water.

Muscle serves as the major reservoir of amino acids for the body. Insulin stimulates the transport of amino acids into muscle cells and their conversion into protein. Cortisol opposes this action. During fasting, the cortisol influence predominates, and alanine and glutamine are released from muscle and circulate to the liver, where they serve as a substrate for gluconeogenesis.

Liver. Insulin is not necessary for the transport of glucose into the liver, since hepatic cells are freely permeable to it. However, insulin powerfully influences glucose metabolism within the cell. Insulin promotes the formation of glycogen and stimulates the disposal of glucose via glycolytic pathways. It suppresses those enzymes necessary for gluconeogenesis and glycogenolysis. Thus, insulin antagonizes the hepatic effects of cortisol, epinephrine, and glucagon. The overall effect of insulin is to increase glucose utilization by the liver. During fasting, plasma insulin concentration falls, the influence of the gluconeogenic hormone cortisol predominates, and the liver releases the glucose required for the metabolism of the central nervous system.

During fasting and in insulinopenic diabetes mellitus, the release of fatty acids from adipose tissue is greatly increased. Fatty acids reaching the liver are metabolized via one of two major pathways. Some are converted to triglycerides, phospholipids, and cholesterol in the cytosol of the hepatocyte. Others are transported into mitochondria by carnitine acyl transferase and then oxidized to acetyl-CoA. The latter intermediary undergoes oxidation to CO_2 in the Krebs cycle or is converted to acetoacetate via the HMG-CoA cycle. Acetoacetate, the primary ketone body, is converted to beta hydroxybutyrate and acetone (the other ketone bodies) by reduction and decarboxylation, respectively. In diabetic ketoacidosis, the "metabolic set" of the liver favors the latter pathway and huge quantities of ketones are formed. Some investigators believe that the change in "set" in ketoacidosis favoring the shunting of fatty acids into the mitochondria is caused by an elevation in glucagon. If this premise is borne out, it would be consistent with the thesis that diabetes mellitus is a bihormonal disease characterized not only by a deficiency of insulin but by an excess of glucagon.

Two important differences between the liver, on one hand, and muscle and adipose tissue, on the other, deserve emphasis. Insulin is not required for glucose transport into the liver, and hepatic cells have a phosphatase capable of cleaving glucose-6-phosphate to produce free glucose, which readily diffuses into the plasma.

CLINICAL ENTITIES

Diabetes Mellitus

A relative or absolute deficiency of insulin results in the disease, diabetes mellitus. (The term *diabetes,* from the Greek, meaning "a siphon," denotes excessive urine formation; *mellitus* is derived from the Greek word mel, meaning honey). Diabetes mellitus is by far the most important disorder of the endocrine system, afflicting several million people in the United States alone. The term covers a wide spectrum of disability from the elderly asymptomatic individual with mild glucose intolerance to the youthful patient dependent on exogenous insulin. The pathophysiology of the disease is more clearly illustrated by the insulin-dependent diabetic and, unless otherwise specified, it is this variety of the illness that will be referred to in the following discussion. The manifestations of diabetes mellitus are divisible into two groups: (1) the acute diabetic syndrome characterized by hyperglycemia, ketoacidosis, and, if untreated, death; and (2) the chronic diabetic syndrome characterized by diffuse microangiopathy involving vital tissues and organs such as the kidney, retina, and nervous system and premature atherosclerosis of the large vessels.

At the present time, controversy exists as to whether insulin lack causes these vascular changes or whether they occur independently. One school of thought, for example, contends that thickening of the capillary basement mem-

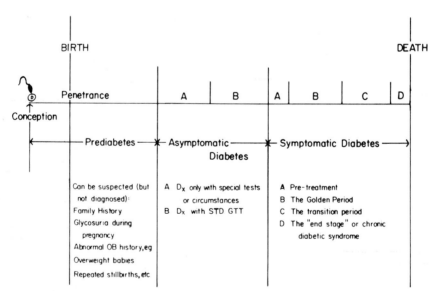

Figure 32–9 Natural history and sequelae of diabetes mellitus. Progression from one stage of the disease to another is unpredictable. Many individuals remain at the "prediabetic" or asymptomatic stage throughout life. The course of patients with symptomatic diabetes is also variable; with proper management they may remain free of significant complications throughout life. Whether or not attempts at very rigid control of the blood glucose level improves prognosis remains a controversial question (see text).

brane is responsible for both the acute manifestations and the chronic complications of diabetes mellitus. It is generally agreed that diabetes mellitus is an inheritable disease. If this is so, one can formulate the conflicting views regarding the pathogenesis of the vascular complications as follows:

(A) Genetic defect → Insulin deficiency and hyperglycemia → Acute diabetic syndrome, Basement membrane thickening → Chronic diabetic syndrome

(B) Genetic defect → Basement membrane thickening → Hyperglycemia → Acute diabetic syndrome, Chronic diabetic syndrome

The question is of more than academic interest, because if hypothesis A is correct, intensive effort to minimize hyperglycemia would be justified to prevent late vascular complications, whereas if B is correct, the argument for rigid control of the blood glucose concentration would be considerably weakened.

If indeed diabetes mellitus arises from one or more genetically determined defects, one can consider that the disease begins at conception. From that point on, one can divide its natural history as illustrated in Figure 32–9.

The manifestations of diabetes mellitus are predictable from the known actions of insulin discussed earlier. Insulin deficiency results in hyperglycemia, the central biochemical feature of the disease. It is due to impaired transport of glucose into muscle and adipose tissue and to the release of glucose by the liver. Above a blood level of about 160 mg. per 100 ml., the renal tubules are unable to absorb all the glucose filtered by the glomeruli. The renal excretion of glucose requires concomitant excretion of water and thus produces an osmotic diuresis.

Loss of water causes an increase in the serum osmolality, which stimulates the thirst center in the hypothalamus. The three "polys" of diabetes mellitus (polyuria, polydipsia, and polyphagia) are thus explicable by the body's loss of large quantities of glucose and water with a compensatory increase in hunger and thirst.

Ketoacidosis. As a more severe insulin deficiency ensues, hyperglycemia and glycosuria intensify, and ketonemia develops. The possible role of glucagon in the pathogenesis of ketoacidosis was mentioned above. Both acetoacetic acid and beta-hydroxybutyric acid dissociate to yield hydrogen ions, depressing the plasma pH. At a pH level of 7.2, the respiratory center is stimulated and the patient's breathing becomes deep and rapid (Kussmaul respirations). This hyperventilation is a defensive effort to prevent a further decline in plasma pH. It will be recalled from the Henderson-Hasselbalch equation that pH is determined by the ratio of plasma bicarbonate to carbonic acid $\frac{HCO_3^-}{H_2CO_3}$, which normally is about 20 to 1. With loss of bicarbonate (utilized to buffer hydrogen ions derived from ketone bodies), this ratio decreases, as does the pH. The increased loss of CO_2 from the lungs reduces plasma carbonic acid and tends to restore the ratio to normal. A further decline in the pH is associated with increasing depression of cerebral function, eventually culminating in coma and death. The major components in the pathogenesis of ketoacidosis are depicted schematically in Figure 32–10. At several points the consequences of ketonemia and hyperglycemia act synergistically with one another to accelerate the course of events. For example, the cations sodium and potassium are lost into the urine secondary to the osmotic diuresis and in association with the acidic ions acetoacetate and beta-hydroxybutyrate. Hyperosmolality, de-

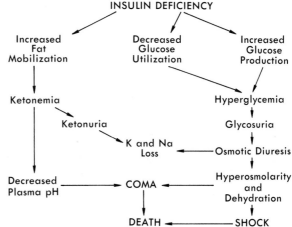

Figure 32–10 The pathogenesis of diabetic ketoacidosis (see text).

hydration, hypotension, and acidosis abet one another in causing deterioration of cerebral function.

Insulin deficiency prompts protein catabolism which results in the release of nitrogen and potassium into the circulation. Late in the course of ketoacidosis, when dehydration and hypovolemia have occurred, renal perfusion falters. Urinary water loss exceeds that of electrolytes so that plasma sodium and potassium concentrations may be increased in spite of the total body deficiency of these ions. It is not uncommon to see hyperkalemia, followed by hypokalemia during the initial hours of therapy of diabetic ketoacidosis. With the administration of insulin, potassium re-enters cells along with glucose. Fluid therapy causes expansion of plasma volume and a return of normal renal function. In the past, patients often did well initially only to develop profound muscle weakness and cardiac dysfunction without apparent cause. With the advent of frequent monitoring of plasma electrolytes, hypokalemia was soon identified as the cause of these complications. They are now readily prevented by the judicious administration of potassium.

Although initially ketonemia is the only cause of acidosis, the subsequent occurrence of hypotension and tissue hypoxia leads to lactate accumulation and a further lowering of the plasma pH. Lactate accumulation sufficient to produce acidosis can also occur in non-diabetic patients severely ill from a variety of causes in which tissue hypoxia is found.

Hyperosmolar Nonketotic Coma. In recent years a variant of hyperglycemic diabetic coma has been recognized. In this syndrome, descriptively named hyperosmolar nonketotic coma, hyperglycemia is usually extreme, between 900 mg. and 3000 mg. per 100 ml., while ketonemia is mild or undetectable, and acidosis is absent. It usually affects patients with mild diabetes not requiring insulin. Characteristically, the diabetic state worsens insidiously, often associated with the stress of unrelated illness or trauma. Initially the increasing fluid loss due to glycosuria can be balanced by an increase in the patient's fluid intake. Ultimately, however, this intake becomes insufficient, and progressive dehydration develops. The large loss of water in the urine continues but is no longer matched by a commensurate oral intake of water. Because the loss of water exceeds that of glucose, the serum rapidly becomes hyperosmolar. Associated with this rise in serum osmolality, and probably because of it, the patient becomes increasingly obtunded and unable to respond to his thirst. Thus, a vicious cycle ensues which rapidly leads to coma and, if not treated, to death.

TABLE 32–10 HORMONAL AND METABOLIC DIFFERENCES BETWEEN DIABETIC KETOACIDOSIS AND HYPEROSMOLAR NONKETOTIC COMA

	Hyperosmolar Nonketotic Coma (9 Patients)	Diabetic Ketoacidosis (6 Patients)
Blood Sugar (mg./100 ml.)	1058	798
CO_2 (mEq./L.)	22	9.6
Osmolarity (mOsm./L.)	368	327
Free Fatty Acids (mEq./L.)	880	2053
Immunoreactive Insulin (μU./ml.)	0 to 15	0 to 15
Growth Hormone (ng./ml.)	2	12
Cortisol (μg./100 ml.)	21	40

(Data adapted from Gerich, J. E., Martin, M. M., and Recant, L.: Diabetes, 19:354, 1970.)

The puzzling feature of the syndrome is that the affected diabetic patients are severely hyperglycemic but not acidotic. This apparent paradox may be due to the relatively greater potency of insulin in inhibiting fat mobilization as compared to its effect on glucose transport. Thus, patients with hyperosmolar nonketotic coma seem to have sufficient circulating insulin to retard the massive release of fatty acids that occurs in ketoacidosis but not enough insulin to stimulate the entry of glucose into peripheral tissues. This view is supported by data such as those reported by Gerich et al. and summarized in Table 32–10.

Hyperlipidemia. Although ketoacidosis and hyperosmolar nonketotic coma are the most dramatic life-threatening manifestations of acute insulin deficiency, others deserve mention. Infrequently, the uncontrolled diabetic will present with evidence of hyperlipidemia as the major manifestation of his disease. On physical examination there may be a widespread skin eruption of recent origin. These lesions, which are yellow-orange in color, papular, and about 2 to 4 mm. in diameter, are eruptive xanthomas. On funduscopic examination, the color of the venules is startling; instead of being deep red, they are white, gray, or light pink. This finding, lipemia retinalis, is directly related to the character of the patient's blood, which is pink or rose when aspirated by venipuncture. After clotting, the appearance of the supernatant serum obtained from the fasting patient is indistinguishable from cream. Chemical analysis reveals a marked increase in triglycerides to several thousand mg. per 100 ml. Analysis by ultracentrifugation reveals that the increased triglyceride consists mostly of dietary chylomicrons, although endogenous triglycerides are usually present as well. This impaired disposal of triglyceride results from relative inactivity of the insulin-dependent lipoprotein lipase, described earlier. Treatment with insulin promptly increases the activity of this enzyme; the plasma triglyceride level falls to normal in a short time, and the skin and retinal changes disappear. It is curious that hyperlipidemia does not occur more often in untreated diabetics. Other factors, in addition to insulin, must be important in influencing the activity of the lipoprotein lipase of peripheral tissues.

Hypoglycemia

Although a wide array of human ills are presently being attributed to hypoglycemia, well-documented, significant hypoglycemia is not very common. Principal causes of hypoglycemia are listed in Table 32–11. The time of day at which hypoglycemia occurs provides a clue to the underlying cause. Since hepatic production of glucose sustains the blood level during periods of fast, impaired glycogen storage and gluconeogenesis will lead to fasting hypoglycemia, which typically occurs in the early morning after eight or nine hours of fasting. This pattern also is seen with hypoglycemia due to insulin-secreting islet cell adenomas; hypoglycemia, controlled during the waking hours by constant eating, becomes apparent during the hours of sleep. The diagnosis of an insulinoma is strongly suggested by Whipple's triad: symptoms of hypoglycemia promptly relieved by intravenous glucose and associated with a blood sugar of less than 40 mg. per dl. A further finding, a level of serum insulin inappropriate for the blood glucose concentration, gives additional weight to the diagnosis.

In contrast to these "fasting" hypoglycemias are those that are reactive, that is, triggered by the assimilation of glucose following a meal. Normally, the secretion of insulin is approximately commensurate with the degree of hyperglycemia. However, following gastrectomy and, occasionally in the absence of surgery, glucose is very rapidly assimilated into the circulation. The resulting excessive hyperglycemia stimulated a brisk release of insulin which causes hypoglycemia as assimilation from the gastrointestinal tract wanes. The situation in the prediabetic is somewhat different. In this case, glucose is assimilated at a normal rate, but the insulin secretory response is delayed, as if the sensing mechanism or "glucostat" were not functioning properly; when the response does occur, it is excessive, causing hypoglycemia three to five hours after a meal.

The most frequent cause of clinically significant hypoglycemia is insulin self-administration by the diabetic patient. This may be the result of an improper insulin regimen or, as very often happens, dietary omission or excessive physical activity. Overnight hypoglycemia secondary to insulin overdose is frequently not recognized because the patient is asleep and therefore unaware of the early subjective symptoms of mild hypoglycemia. Furthermore, hypoglycemia occurring at 2 A.M., for example, stimulates increases in the hormones that counter hypoglycemia — epinephrine, cortisol, and possibly growth hormone. These hormones cause the blood glucose to rise at an accelerated rate when the level of plasma insulin falls, and consequently the patient finds glucose in his urine prior to breakfast. This overshoot or rebound in glucose concentration that follows hypoglycemia, first emphasized by Somogyi, has great clinical significance; it is often misinterpreted as evidence of insufficient insulin rather than too much insulin. Thus, the dosage of insulin is increased, the overnight hypoglycemia is more marked, and the rebound in blood glucose greater. The latter finding, of course, tends to perpetuate the mistake.

Regardless of its underlying cause, the manifestations of hypoglycemia tend to evolve in a characteristic pattern. With mild hypoglycemia, the patient experiences hunger, tremor, perspiration, weakness, blurred vision, and impaired mentation. Mental confusion is often followed by bizarre behavior. The patient may become bellicose and resistant to help. Neuromuscular function be-

TABLE 32–11 PRINCIPAL CAUSES OF HYPOGLYCEMIA

Underlying Condition	Mechanism
I. FASTING	
A. Addison's disease, panhypopituitarism	Impaired gluconeogenesis
B. Liver disease	Impaired gluconeogenesis, glycogen storage
C. Fasting + Alcohol	Impaired gluconeogenesis, depleted glycogen
D. Mesothelial tumors	Unknown
E. Insulin-dependent diabetes	Excessive insulin, iatrogenic
F. Islet cell adenoma	Excessive, unregulated insulin release
II. FED (Reactive)	
G. Postgastrectomy	Tachyalimentation of glucose
H. Functional	Tachyalimentation of glucose
I. Early ("chemical") diabetes	Abnormal "glucostat" ($\uparrow$ insulin secretion)

TABLE 32–12 DIFFERENTIAL DIAGNOSIS OF COMA DUE TO DIABETIC KETOACIDOSIS AND HYPOGLYCEMIA

	Acidosis	*Hypoglycemia*
Onset	Hour to days	Minutes
Background events	Intercurrent disease, omission of insulin	Exercise, omission of meal
Symptoms	Thirst, polyuria, headaches, nausea, vomiting, abdominal pain	Hunger, headache, perspiration, *confusion*, stupor
Physical findings	Kussmaul respirations, dehydration, flushed face, fast pulse: *appears ill*	Normal pulse, respirations: appears well
Typical laboratory findings		
Urine		
Glucose	5%	0 to 5%
Ketones	Strongly positive	0 to positive
Serum		
Glucose	400 mg./100 ml. or more	Less than 40 mg./100 ml.
Ketones	Positive, 1:8	Negative
HCO_3	Less than 10 mEq./L.	26 mEq./L.
Response to 50% glucose, I.V.	None	Dramatic

comes impaired. Staggering gait and irrational hostile behavior are frequently misinterpreted as drunkenness. Finally, the patient becomes comatose. If the hypoglycemia is profound, seizures may occur; if severe hypoglycemia remains untreated, permanent brain damage or death results. The sequence of events just described is typical, but the exact pattern varies among patients and even in the same patient from one episode to another. For example, on one occasion the patient may wander about in a confused state for two to three hours at approximately the same level of function; another time, he might pass from an alert and rational state to coma in a half hour or less.

The correct diagnosis of coma in the diabetic patient is critical, since the two commonest causes — too much or too little insulin — require diametrically opposite therapy. The major features that distinguished the two disorders, listed in Table 32–12, are explicable in terms of the pathophysiologic consequences of insulin deficiency and excess described previously.

TESTES

PHYSIOLOGY

The dual role of the testes in procreation and maintenance of male attributes has been appre-

ciated from antiquity. Throughout history, castration has been practiced in many societies, usually with the goal of rendering the victim devoid of both the desire and capability of sexual activity. Thus, in contrast to pituitary, thyroid, or adrenal deficiencies which occurred as the result of various diseases, one form of male gonadal deficiency, eunuchism, was deliberately induced. If the history of the involvement of the testes in reproduction is an old one, it is far from complete. In the following paragraphs, the current status of our knowledge of testicular physiology will be briefly reviewed.

In 1949, Barr and Bertram described a darkly staining chromatin material located at or very near the inner side of the nuclear membrane of neural tissue from female cats. This clump was conspicuously absent in tissue from males. In the ensuing years, comparable findings were obtained with human tissues. Properly stained material obtained from the buccal mucosa of the female was found to contain nuclear sex chromatin in 50 to 60 per cent of cells examined. Cells derived from males contained nuclear sex chromatin, presumably artefactual, in 1 to 2 per cent of cells counted. Davidson and Smith (1954), studying smears of human blood cells, found several clumps of chromatin lying beyond the main mass of nuclear material of the polymorphonuclear leukocytes of females but not of males. The ovoid clump was attached to the nucleus by a fine strand, producing a characteristic "drumstick" form. It is now generally accepted that the female nuclear sex chromatin of buccal mucosal cells (the "Barr" body) and the "drumstick" of the polymorphonuclear leukocyte represent the same phenomenon, presumably an inactivated X sex chromosome. The Lyon hypothesis, which attempts to explain the presence of female chromatin material, is discussed in Chapter 3.

Normal Human Sex Determination

Gametogenesis. Using the technique of tissue culture coupled with mitotic arrest, Tjio and Levan in 1956 were able to correct a long-standing misconception about the actual number of human chromosomes in somatic cells. Their work, which was soon amply confirmed, indicated that each somatic cell (i.e., all cells other than germ cells) normally contains 46 chromosomes, 22 pairs of autosomes and two sex chromosomes. This number is double (or diploid) the basic complement (termed the haploid number) contained in mature germ cells. In the normal female, the sex chromosomes are both X; in the normal male, there is one X and one Y chromosome. When the cell divides in the process of mitosis, these 23 pairs are replicated, producing two sets of 23 pairs. The germ cell or gamete, however, must contain the basic complement or haploid number of chromosomes to match an equal haploid number of the gamete of the opposite sex at time of fertilization (see Chapter 3). This reduction in the number of chromosomes occurs during the first maturation division. In the testes, the primary spermatocyte with 44 autosomes, plux X and Y sex chromosomes, divides to form two secondary spermatocytes, each containing 22 autosomes and either a Y or an X chromosome. This process of reduction division is termed meiosis. The comparable reduction division in the ovary occurs when a primary oocyte divides to produce a daughter cell, the secondary oocyte, containing 22 autosomes plus one X sex chromosome and a functionless polar body. In meiosis, homologous chromosomes line up in pairs. Before the cell actually divides, members of each pair separate and each complement moves away, one from the other, migrating toward the new central locus of the cell to be. This separation and migration of equal complements of chromosomes is termed disjunction. Disjunction thus is the basic process responsible for the haploid number of chromosomes of the mature gamete, be it spermatozoon or ovum. The ovum contains 22 autosomes plus one X chromosome; the spermatozoon contains 22 autosomes and either an X or a Y chromosome. At the time of conception, the union of ovum with spermatozoon produces a fertilized ovum with the diploid number of chromosomes, i.e., 44 autosomes (22 pairs) with either

two X chromosomes or one X and one Y chromosome. A male develops in the latter instance (44 + XY), and a female in the former (44 + XX). Thus, the sex of the fetus is determined by the chromosomal constitution of the spermatozoon; if it carries an X sex chromosome, a female results (44 + XX); if it contains a Y chromosome, the issue is male (44 + XY). The role of the female at this point is notably passive.

Fetal Development of the Gonads, Genital Ducts, and External Genitalia

Until about the seventh week of fetal life, the primitive gonads have no histologic features that would permit them to be identified as male or female. If the genotype of the fetus is XY, a testes-determining gene is present, causing the gonad to transform into a testis; if the genotype is XX, the gonad continues to grow but remains undifferentiated until about the 10th or 11th week, when primordial germ cells become transformed into oogonia. By the 8th week, the fetal testis contains functioning Leydig cells that secrete testosterone. The presence of the latter hormone stimulates the development of the genital ducts, precursors of the epididymis, vas deferens, and seminal vesicles. Somewhat later, about the 11th week, the primordial structures of the external genitalia (the genital tubercle, urethral folds, labial swellings, and urogenital sinus) commence maturation. Current evidence suggests that these latter structures are relatively insensitive to testosterone per se but are responsive to dihydrotestosterone (DHT). These target tissues contain a 5-α reductase that converts testosterone to DHT. Normal sexual development in the fetal male requires not only maturation of the male genital ducts and external genitalia, but also regression of the female or mullerian ducts (precursors of the fallopian tubes, uterus and upper vagina). This process commences about the eighth week and appears to be prompted by a non-steroidal, high molecular substance, mullerian duct regression factor, elaborated by the Sertoli cells of the testes.

Apparently, ovarian function plays little or no role in the fetal sexual development of the female. In the absence of testicular influences, the fetal internal and external genitalia mature into female structures. Patients with Turner's syndrome, in which the karyotype is XO and gonads primitive clusters of cells, invariably have a female phenotype.

The presence of testosterone in the fetal life is not only required for normal male sexual development; it also has an important influence on the developing central nervous system. Animal studies have shown that testicular deficiency at a critical time in the fetal life results in impaired male sexual behavior in adult life.

Postnatal Testicular Function

The secretory activity of the testes in utero is probably stimulated by the high levels of placental chorionic gonadotropin. Not surprisingly, the fetal testis resembles the adult gonad histologically.

Following delivery, the testes become quiescent but probably not completely inactive. Recent careful studies indicate that there are measurable levels of both gonadotropins and androgens beginning in early childhood. The mechanisms that initiate pubescence are poorly understood. Presumably, the primary signal arises from the hypothalamus or higher sites in the central nervous system. In any event, at an average age of 11 to 12 years LH plasma levels increase (FSH increases occur at an earlier age) and the testes enlarge, mainly owing to an increase in the volume of the seminiferous tubules. Leydig cell function is stimulated by LH, resulting in a marked increase in plasma testosterone. The latter is responsible for the development of male secondary sexual characteristics, including changes in external genitalia, body hair, voice, musculature, libido, and potentia. Eventually, this surge of androgens causes closure of the epiphyses of the long bones and growth ceases, but only after a pubescent growth spurt of 6 or more inches. If the sex steroid is deficient, epiphyseal closure is delayed and growth of the long bones continues. The result is the eunuchoid habitus characteristic of hypogonadism. In normal adults, span is approximately equal to height, and the lower segment of the body (measured from the top of the symphysis to the floor) equals the upper segment. In the eunuchoid subject, span and the lower segment exceed height and the upper segment, respectively.

The Adult Testis; Biosynthesis, Transport, and Action of Testosterone

The adult testis is approximately 4.5 cm. by 2.5 cm. and weighs between 15 and 20 grams. It comprises two major elements: (a) Leydig or interstitial cells, which make up approximately 10 per cent of testicular volume, and (b) the seminiferous tubules, lined with the spermatogonia and Sertoli cells, composing about 75 per cent of the volume of the testes. Each day the Leydig cells elaborate approximately 7 mg. of testosterone and 2 mg. of its immediate precursor, androstenedione, and the seminiferous tubules release about 150,000,000 spermatozoa.

The biosynthesis of testosterone follows the same basic pathway as that of the adrenal cortical steroids (see Figure 32–6). Either acetate or cholesterol can serve as the basic precursor; pregnenolone and 17-alpha-hydroxyprogesterone are important intermediaries. Once secreted, 95 per cent

of testosterone circulates in the plasma bound to a specific beta globulin. The normal range of testosterone in young adults is 440 to 1000 ng. per 100 ml. of plasma. There is a progressive decline in plasma testosterone after middle age. In females, the normal range is from 34 to 100 ng. per 100 ml. In the peripheral tissues, testosterone is converted to dihydrotestosterone. The relative roles of these two androgens in the development and maintenance of the sexual characteristics of the male has been clarified by studies on patients with familial incomplete male pseudohermaphroditism Type II described below. The proposed mechanism of action of the sex steroids including testosterone has already been alluded to.

Regulation of Testicular Function
(Fig. 32–11)

The evidence for a negative feedback relationship between the Leydig cells and the hypothalamic-pituitary axis is quite convincing. In 1968, Masao et al. reported on the effects of partially purified FSH-releasing factor prepared from beef hypothalami. Kastin et al. have now identified the hypothalamic substance capable of initiating LH release from the anterior pituitary; this factor has been termed the LH-releasing hormone (LHRH). LH acts on the testes to increase the conversion rate of cholesterol to pregnenolone, the rate-limited step in the formation of testosterone. Cyclic AMP appears to function as an intermediary or second messenger in this reaction. Above a critical concentration (the set point), plasma testosterone interferes with the release of LH. It is not clear whether this is accomplished by inhibition of LHRH secretion or by a direct inhibitory effect of testosterone on the anterior pituitary. In either event, the decline in plasma LH results in a decrease in testosterone secretion, completing the negative feedback loop.

The relationship between the anterior pituitary and the seminiferous tubules is not clear-cut. It appears certain that FSH is required for spermatogenesis. In the absence of FSH, the germinal epithelium desquamates and the seminiferous tubules become fibrotic or remain infantile. Contrariwise, in those circumstances in which there is primary injury to the germinal epithelium, there is an increase in FSH secretion. This occurs even when Leydig cell function (and hence testosterone production) remains normal, as, for example, in primary seminiferous tubule failure. Such observations suggest that a substance capable of retarding FSH secretion is elaborated by the germinal epithelium. Indeed, a number of investigators have labeled this hypothetical material "inhibin." Unfortunately, attempts to prepare an extract from testicular tissue capable of suppressing FSH release have been unsuccessful.

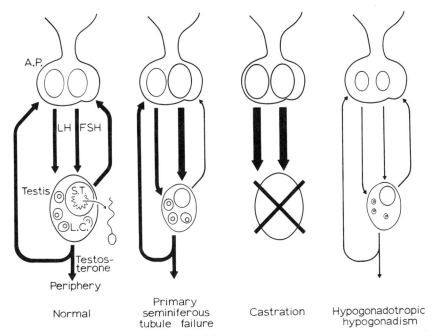

Figure 32–11 Anterior pituitary-testicular relationships.
Normal: The anterior pituitary *(A.P.)* secretes LH, which stimulates the Leydig cells *(L.C.)* to secrete testosterone. Rising levels of testosterone inhibit further LH secretion, completing the negative feedback loop. The anterior pituitary also secretes FSH, which stimulates the seminiferous tubules *(S.T.)* and spermatogenesis. The release of a humoral substance by cells of the seminiferous tubules (right hand arrow) is suspected but not established.
Primary seminiferous tubule failure: For unknown causes the seminiferous tubules undergo atrophy, and spermatogenesis ceases; urinary excretion of FSH is high. Leydig cell function remains intact.
Castration: When both Leydig cell and seminiferous tubular elements of the testes are lost, gonadotropin secretion is markedly increased.
Hypogonadotropic hypogonadism: Isolated loss of gonadotropin secretin by the pituitary in the pubescent male results in both sterility and underdeveloped male secondary sexual characteristics.

CLINICAL ENTITIES

Klinefelter's Syndrome (Seminiferous Tubule Dysgenesis)

Klinefelter's syndrome is among the most common causes of male infertility and hypogonadism. Although reports of this entity had been published earlier, Klinefelter, Reifenstein, and Albright in 1942 emphasized the features of the syndrome in a paper significantly entitled "A Syndrome Characterized by Gynecomastia, Aspermatogenesis without A-Leydigism and Increased Excretion of Follicle-Stimulating Hormone." This report described nine patients with small testes, gynecomastia, and increased FSH titers. The stature of the patients varied from normal to slightly eunuchoid, but all had good muscular development and masculine secondary sexual characteristics. The histologic alterations in the testes consisted of hyalinization of the seminiferous tubules with loss of Sertoli cells and spermatogonia elements, while interstitial cells appeared normal. Subsequent experience with large numbers of patients has revealed that impaired Leydig cell function, reflected by subnormal levels of circulating testosterone, and eunuchoid habitus underdeveloped secondary sexual characteristics, is a common feature of the syndrome.

The realization of the etiologic role of chromosomal abnormalities in the manifestations of Klinefelter's syndrome represents one of the most exciting events in the history of endocrinology. Plunkett and Barr reported chromatin-positive cells in patients with Klinefelter's syndrome. The disparity between the chromatin sex pattern ("female") and the physiognomy of the patients (male) was clarified when the chromosomal constitution of patients with classic Klinefelter's syndrome was identified as 44 + XXY. Thus, it now appears certain that the pathogenesis of Klinefelter's syndrome begins with an abnormal meiotic phase in one of the parents. The most common abnormality consists of failure of the sex chromosomes of the dividing cell to move away from one another and is termed nondisjunction. In the male parent, the

		Father	Mother	Offspring, genotype	Offspring, phenotype
I. Nondisjunction in the father:	(a)	22 + O	22 + X	44 + XO	Turner's
	(b)	22 + XY	22 + X	44 + XXY	Klinefelter's
II. Nondisjunction in the mother:	(c)	22 + X	22 + XX	44 + XXX	"super female"
	(d)	22 + X	22 + O	44 + XO	Turner's
	(e)	22 + Y	22 + XX	44 + XXY	Klinefelter's
	(f)	22 + Y	22 + O	44 + YO	—

gamete that results from nondisjunction has a chromosomal constitution of either 22 + XY or 22 + O; in the female, it is 22 + XX or 22 + O. The possible chromosomal constitutions of fertilized ova resulting from union of an abnormal with a normal gamete are summarized above.

Thus, Klinefelter's syndrome can arise from abnormal meiosis either in the father, as in (b) above, or in the mother, as in (e) above.

Although classic Klinefelter's syndrome is usually associated with a karyotype of 44 + XXY, a number of variants of the syndrome have been reported. For example, if there is mosaicism (or more than one stem line) of the sex chromosomes (e.g., XXY/XY), there may be few clinical abnormalities. On the other hand, when there is more than one abnormality of chromosomal division, as rarely occurs, there may be more than one supernumerary X chromosome, such as 44 + XXXY and 44 + XXXXY. In general, these patients have more profound disturbances of gonadal function. The spectrum of Klinefelter's syndrome from both the clinical and chromosomal standpoints was reviewed by Paulsen et al. in 1958.

The "Fertile Eunuch" Syndrome

Patients have been reported with eunuchoid habitus and decreased libido but with normal fertility and normal or near normal height. Histologic examination of testicular biopsy specimens has revealed normal seminiferous tubules but greatly reduced numbers of Leydig cells. The presumed pathogenesis of this uncommon condition — an isolated deficiency of pituitary LH, with normal FSH secretion — has recently been confirmed by radioimmunoassay determinations of plasma gonadotropins.

Hypogonadotropic Hypogonadism

When the gonadotropins, FSH and LH required to maintain normal testicular function in the male, are deficient or absent, as frequently occurs in patients with pituitary tumors, both the germinal and Leydig cell elements of the testes become atrophic. Spermatogenesis ceases, and the level of circulating testosterone falls dramatically. The consequences of the latter event emerge slowly; the patient's libido falters, and there is loss of muscle mass and eventually loss of facial and body hair. For a time, the testicular changes are reversible, as demonstrated by their response to the administration of replacement therapy such as human chorionic gonadotropin (HCG). However, after a period estimated at one to five years, the testes become unresponsive to hormonal stimulation.

If the gonadotropins are deficient at the time of pubescence, the changes characteristic of that period do not take place. The external genitalia remain infantile; body form, hair distribution, and voice remain feminine; and the epiphyses of the long bones remain open, permitting an increase in eventual height.

An interesting familial variety of prepubertal hypogonadotropin deficiency in which the affected patients have a greatly impaired or absent sense of smell (hyposmia or anosmia) was described earlier in this chapter.

Hereditary Male Pseudohermaphroditism (MPH)

The term male pseudohermaphroditism refers to individuals who have male karyotypes and gonadal tissue but ambiguous or femine external genitalia. Such patients are rather uncommon, but the elucidation of the mechanisms underlying their problem has done much to clarify the normal sexual differentiation and the mode of action of testosterone. From the known sequence of events in normal male sex development in the fetus, one can predict loci of defects that could lead to male pseudohermaphroditism. Firstly, failure of elaboration of mullerian duct regression factor by the Sertoli cells could result in the development of female internal genitalia. Uteri and fallopian tubes have been unexpectedly found in male patients undergoing surgery for cryptorchidism or inguinal hernia. Since the external genitalia of these patients are essentially normal male, they are not strictly speaking examples of male pseudohermaphroditism. Second, there could be failure of androgen-mediated virilization of the wolffian ducts and/or the external genitalia analagen. Abnormalities in this sequence can be divided into two categories: (1) defects in testosterone biosynthesis; (2) target tissue resistance to testosterone. In the first category, five distinct enzymatic deficiencies have been described. These are: cholesterol desmolase, 3-β-OH dehydrogenase, 17 hydroxylase, 17,20 lyase, and 17-β-OH reductase. The reactions catalyzed by these enzymes are shown in Figure 32–6.

In the second category, four entities have been delineated. These are: (1) the Syndrome of Complete Testicular Feminization; (2) the Syndrome of Incomplete Testicular Feminization; (3) Familial Incomplete Hereditary Male Pseudohermaphroditism Type I (Reifenstein's Syndrome); (4) Familial Incomplete Male Pseudohermaphroditism Type II (pseudovaginal perineoscrotal hypospadias). In all four of these conditions, plasma testosterone levels are increased. The pathophysiologies of entities 1 and 4 are reasonably well established and are of sufficient interest to warrant a brief description.

Syndrome of Complete Feminine Testicular Feminization. In this rare disorder, the external genitalia and physiognomy are completely feminised, in fact, floridly so. The testes, located either intraabdominally or in the inguinal canals, are normal histologically. The absence of female internal genitalia (fallopian tubes, uterus, and upper vagina) indicate that the fetal testes produced the mullerian duct regression factor normally. Thanks in large measure to the careful studies of Wilson and his colleagues, it appears quite certain that the basic defect in some patients with the syndrome is the absence of the receptor protein required to bind dihydrotestosterone (DHT) in the cytosol. Park and co-workers have found normal cytosol binding of DHT. They feel that the defect in these patients is deficiency in the nuclear acceptor protein that interacts with the DHT-receptor moiety. In either case, circulating testosterone is completely devoid of androgenic effect and fails to suppress LHRH, causing an increase in LH and, in turn, further increase in testosterone. A portion of the testosterone is converted to estradiol; it is elevated plasma estradiol that accounts for the hyperfeminization of the syndrome. Tissue from patients with the syndrome of incomplete testicular feminization and Reifenstein's syndrome (entities 2 and 3 above) also have deficient or defective DHT binding protein. Precisely how such abnormalities relate to the highly variable phenotype included in these two diagnostic categories remains to be elucidated. Patients with the first syndrome are basically female in appearance but have clitoral enlargement and labial scrotal fusion; at puberty, breast development occurs but virilism may also emerge. The clinical expression of Reifenstein's syndrome varies from a patient who has only gynecomastia and sterility to the more typical phenotype of the gynecomastia, sterility, and perineoscrotal hypospadias.

Familial Incomplete Male Pseudohermaphroditism Type II. The pathophysiology of this syndrome has been established by the elegant studies of

Peterson and co-workers. These workers have studied the clinical presentation and biochemical abnormalities in 38 patients with this disorder. In affected male children, the abnormality is limited to the external genitalia. There is a diminutive clitoral-like phallus, a bifid scrotum, and a urogenital sinus containing urethral and vaginal orifices. The vagina ends in a blind pouch. Internally, the wolffian structures are normally differentiated, and no mullerian structures are present. At puberty, virilization occurs with deepening of the voice, increase in muscle mass and growth in the external genitalia. The phallus grows to 4 to 6 cm, the bifid scrotum enlarges, and the testes enlarge and descend into the scrotum. Erection and ejaculation occur but because of the location of the urethra, insemination cannot take place. Postpubertal males have little or no beard, no temporal hair line recession, no acne, and greater muscle mass than do their unaffected counterparts. Thus far, no prostatic enlargement has been seen in the older affected males. The plasma testosterone of affected subjects is greater and DHT lower than the values found in control subjects; plasma LH and FSH are higher than in normal subjects. Peterson and co-workers feel that all these findings can be explained on a deficiency of 5, α reductase, the enzyme required for the conversion of testosterone to DHT. Apparently, the latter hormone is required for complete development of the fetal external genitalia. After birth, sensitivity of the external genitalia to testosterone develops, accounting for the virilization at puberty. The findings suggest that certain male attributes (baldness, acne, and prostatic enlargement) are dependent on dihydrotestosterone rather than testosterone. The high levels of LH and FSH indicate that testosterone alone is less effective in suppressing LHRH than is the combination of testosterone and dehydrotestosterone.

OVARIES

PHYSIOLOGY

Follicle Development

The human ovaries are nodular bodies whose morphology and function are dynamically interwoven. Each weighs about 4 grams and measures 4 cm. long by 2 cm. wide. The adult ovary is estimated to contain 400,000 primordial follicles: oocytes encased in an avascular envelope of granulosa cells. At the onset of each menstrual cycle, several follicles migrate from the periphery of the ovary toward its center; concomitantly, there is proliferation of both the granulosa cells to form a multilayer band and the cells of the theca, which develops as an outer vascular mantle. As these processes progress, indentation of each follicle occurs, producing a cavity or antrum. Although these early events apparently do not require gonadotropins, FSH is required for the subsequent development of the mature graafian follicle. Of the several follicles that have undergone the changes just described, only one continues to develop; the remaining follicles regress into atretic forms. Under FSH stimulation, the chosen follicle accumulates fluid in its antrum, the cells of the granulosa and theca proliferate, and the whole mass migrates to the periphery. The ripened follicle comes to lie just beneath the outer covering of the ovary, creating a detectable bulge in its surface. As the follicle matures, the theca differentiates into the vascular theca interna and a theca externa, made up of stroma-like cells. The theca interna is composed of large glandular cells which under FSH stimulation elaborate estrogen. Their secretory activity accelerates throughout the preovulatory stage, reaching a peak just before ovulation.

Ovulation

There is evidence that the rising level of estrogen (estradiol) triggers the release of LH — a positive feedback phenomenon — and that the high concentration of plasma LH acts on the theca cells to effect the release of the ovum from the ripened follicle. Following the extrusion of the ovum, the graafian follicle is transformed into the corpus luteum under the continued influence of LH. This complex process of luteinization includes cellular hypertrophy of both the granulosa and theca interna and their development into tissues which are capable of steroid hormone synthesis. If pregnancy does not occur, the corpus luteum continues to secrete progesterone and estrogen for two weeks, and as this function ceases, the levels of plasma estrogen and progesterone fall abruptly and menstruation occurs. The morphologic and functional changes that the ovary undergoes during the menstrual cycle have been lucidly described in a review by Franchi.

Endometrial Changes

During the preovulatory or follicular phase of the cycle, proliferation of the endometrium occurs under the stimulation of estrogen. During the postovulatory or luteal phase of the cycle, both progesterone and estrogen act to slow down endometrial growth and to so alter its structure that it is prepared for the nidation of a fertilized ovum. Glandular elements become engorged with secretions and there is a substantial increase in vascularization. These uterine phases, corresponding to the follicular and luteal periods of ovarian function, are termed proliferative and secretory, respectively.

Pregnancy

There is evidence that the ovum is susceptible to fertilization for only a brief time following its release. When spermatozoa are present, fertilization usually occurs within six hours of ovulation in the distal third of the fallopian tube. The fertilized ovum then slowly migrates to the uterine cavity and becomes implanted in the secretory endometrium about eight days after conception. Almost immediately, the implanted blastocyst or trophoblast begins to secrete chorionic gonadotropin which stimulates the continued secretion of progesterone and estrogen by the corpus luteum. The latter hormones cause a continuing buildup of the endometrium, forming the decidua. Very early in pregnancy, the ovaries are the principal source of the necessary sex steroids; later, the fetal placental unit assumes this responsibility, and pregnancy proceeds without further assistance from the ovaries. It should be noted that the function of the corpus luteum becomes nearly autonomous following ovulation, secreting estrogen and progesterone with but little stimulation from pituitary gonadotropins. Thus, the pituitary is not necessary for the maintenance of pregnancy, and only a very low level of circulating gonadotropins is required for corpus luteum function. This conclusion was recently substantiated by a report describing the induction of ovulation by the administration of human menopausal and chorionic gonadotropins in a woman who had undergone hypophysectomy. The patient conceived, and the pregnancy proceeded uneventfully to a normal spontaneous delivery at term. Plasma levels of estrogen, pregnanediol (a metabolite of progesterone), and chorionic gonadotropin were normal throughout the pregnancy.

Hypothalamic-Pituitary-Ovarian Interactions

Current evidence, albeit incomplete, indicates that the secretion of FSH and LH by the anterior pituitary is subservient to regulation by hypothalamic releasing factors, as mentioned earlier in this chapter. These, in turn, are influenced by plasma levels of estrogen, progesterone, and, undoubtedly, neural signals from higher centers. An understanding of the interactions among hypothalamic, pituitary, and ovarian factors in regulating the complex sequence of events of the menstrual cycle is gradually emerging. FSH stimulates follicle growth during the first (follicular) phase of the cycle; ovulation has been attributed to a rapid increase in plasma LH. Actually, both FSH and LH increase sharply just before ovulation. As mentioned above, most investigators believe that the surge in LH is stimulated by the rapidly rising concentration of estrogen. Odell and co-workers believe that 17-

hydroxyprogesterone, possibly in conjunction with estradiol, may be involved. Although FSH appears to be the principal factor which stimulates estrogen formation by the follicle, it is probable that both FSH and LH are necessary for optimal estrogen synthesis and release. Little if any progesterone is secreted by the developing follicle, a finding inconsistent with the thesis that progesterone stimulates the preovulatory surge of LH. It is generally agreed that following ovulation, the corpus luteum secretes the sex steroids with relatively little stimulation from the pituitary for about 14 days. The abrupt fall in plasma estrogen and progesterone at the end of this time is responsible not only for initiating menstruation but, in all likelihood, for the re-institution of FSH secretion. Thus, the first day of menstruation signifies both the end and the beginning of the cycle.

Biosynthesis, Transport, Mechanism of Action, and Disposal of Estrogen and Progesterone

The formation of both estrogens and progesterone follows the basic pathway already described for cortisol synthesis (see Figure 32–6). In this sequence, cholesterol is converted to pregnenolone, the intermediate common to all the steroid hormones. Conversion of pregnenolone to progesterone requires two enzymes: an isomerase to shift the double bond in ring B to ring A, and a dehydrogenase to oxidize the hydroxy- at the 3 position to a keto- structure. Cleavage of the $C_{20, 21}$ side chain yields an androgen, androstenedione, the major precursor of estrogen. Removal of C_{19} and aromatization of ring A yields estrone. Estrone and 17-beta-estradiol, the most potent estrogen, are interconvertible.

The ovarian hormones circulate bound to carrier proteins. The plasma levels of estrone and estradiol in normal females range from 10 to 100 ng. per 100 ml. of plasma, depending on the time of the cycle. Plasma progesterone concentrations average about 140 ng. per 100 ml. during the follicular phase and about 1000 ng. per 100 ml. during the luteal phase. These steroid hormones are inactivated primarily in the liver by conversion to water-soluble glucuronide and sulfate derivatives. Pregnanediol is the chief excretory metabolite of progesterone, and its content in a 24-hour urine colletion provides a reasonable index of progesterone activity.

The principal functions of the ovarian hormones are to interact with both the hypothalamic-pituitary unit and the uterus to orchestrate the tightly integrated sequence of follicular development, ovulation, corpus luteum formation, and either menstruation or pregnancy. Beyond their direct effects on reproduction, the ovarian hormones, especially estrogen, are necessary for the development and maintenance of secondary sexual characteristics in the female. Estrogens also appear to promote epiphyseal closure and thus the termination of longitudinal growth, a role comparable to that of testosterone in the male. Estrogen deficiency in the adult female is associated with osteoporosis.

CLINICAL ENTITIES

Gonadal Aplasia (Turner's Syndrome)

In 1938, Turner described seven females with distinctive phenotypic abnormalities, including sexual infantilism, short stature, webbed neck, and an increased carrying angle of the upper extremities. Surgical explorations revealed gonadal tissue consisting only of a primitive streak in the broad ligaments. On histologic examination, this tissue was sufficiently undifferentiated that it could not definitely be identified as ovarian. Because of the scanty amount and primitive nature of the gonadal tissue, the term "gonadal aplasia" was introduced and is currently the accepted, non-eponymic designation of the syndrome.

Although uncommon, the syndrome has been a focal point for the elucidation of sex determination. The determination of nuclear chromatin revealed that the majority of patients with Turner's syndrome have negative patterns. This finding, coupled with the high incidence of color blindness by Polani et al led to the hypothesis that a deficient X chromosome was a basic factor in the pathogenesis of the syndrome. When it became possible to characterize the chromosomal constitution of individuals, the validity of the hypothesis was borne out. Patients with gonadal aplasia and a negative nuclear chromatin pattern were found to have a karyotype of 44 + XO. Without the protection of a normal X chromosome, these individuals are subject to color blindness, a sex-linked recessive defect, with the same frequency as males. The 44 + XO karyotype can be explained on the basis of nondisjunction occurring during gametogenesis in either parent. It is of academic interest that the site of abnormal meiosis can be determined in some instances by the pattern of red-green color blindness in the patient and her family. For instance, if both the patient and her father were color blind, one would suspect that nondisjunction occurred in oogenesis, depriving the patient of a maternal X chromosome.

The principal clinical features of Turner's syndrome are (1) primary amenorrhea, underdevelopment of secondary sexual characteristics, and infantile female internal genitalia; (2) short stature, usually less than 5 feet; (3) increased carrying angle of the arm (cubitus valgus); (4) webbed neck (pterygium colli); (5) shield chest; (6) coarctation of the aorta; (7) unexplained hypertension; and (8)

TABLE 32–13   DIFFERENTIAL DIAGNOSIS—PITUITARY INFANTILISM AND GONADAL APLASIA
(TURNER'S SYNDROME)
In the Adolescent or Young Adult Female

	Turner's Syndrome	*Pituitary Infantilism*
Stature	Usually < 5 feet	< 5 feet
Bone age	Delayed-Normal*	Marked delay
Secondary sexual characteristics		
Breasts, vagina, uterus, tubes	Infantile	Infantile
Sexual hair	Delayed	Absent
Axillary hair	Delayed	Absent
Urinary findings		
Gonadotropins	High titer, usually	0 titer
17-OHC (mg./24-hr.)	1 to 2	0.5 or less
17-KS (mg./24 hr.)	1 to 3	1.0 or less
Mental status	Normal or defective	Normal
Nuclear chromatin pattern	Negative	Positive
Chromosomal constitution	44 + XO, XX/XO, or XX	44 + XX
Hypertension	Frequent (even in absence of coarctation)	Absent
Other findings	Webbed neck, cubitus valgus, coarctation of aorta, skeletal defects	Headaches, visual field defects

*Because of delay in epiphyseal closures, bone age appears retarded in the adolescent. By early adulthood (e.g., 25 years) bone age is normal, adult.

skeletal defects. Of these, the first two are most consistently seen. As with Klinefelter's syndrome, a spectrum of variants has been reported. Some of these result from mosaicism, in which some clonal lines have the deficiency of a sex chromosome (XO) while others are normal. Partial forms of the syndrome may also be due to deletion of a portion of an X chromosome, the karyotype being expressed as Xx. If the deletion is of the short arm of the X chromosome, the patient has short stature and the somatic features of the syndrome but may experience normal sexual development. If the deletion is of the long arm, the patient manifests sexual infantilism but is of normal stature and has few if any of the somatic anomalies.

The disorder does not seem to be familial. Only a few instances have been reported in which more than one member of a family has been affected. Neither does maternal age seem to be a causal factor; in a series of 27 cases, the mean maternal age was 24 years, the same as in a control group. Although theoretically one might expect Turner's syndrome to occur with the same frequency as Klinefelter's syndrome, this is not the case. The determination of nuclear sex chromatin patterns in 1800 consecutive newborn females failed to

demonstrate a single instance of the negative pattern. In contrast, comparable studies suggest an incidence of the positive pattern in about 1 of 500 newborn males.

The occurrence of short stature in an individual with severe gonadal deficiency is at first glance inconsistent with the observation that castration in the prepubescent youth leads to a tall eunuchoid individual. The latter event is presumably related to delayed closure of epiphyses of long bones due to the absence of the gonadal hormones. If the basic abnormality in Turner's syndrome was limited to gonadal aplasia, i.e., equivalent to castration in infancy or youth, one would not expect short stature. Actually, Turner's is a multiple system disease, and short stature is but one of several defects that are associated with, but not caused by, gonadal aplasia.

The typical patient with Turner's syndrome seeks medical advice during early adolescent years because of a delay in menarche and in the development of secondary sexual characteristics. The differential diagnosis of the triad of short stature, sexual infantilism, and primary amenorrhea involves Turner's syndrome and hypopituitarism. Often, additional clinical findings point to the correct diagnosis with near certainty. A webbed neck, coarctation of the aorta, or other stigmata of Turner's syndrome in a patient with this triad would be virtually diagnostic. On the other hand, findings such as bitemporal hemianopsia would implicate a primary disease of the pituitary. When such features are absent or equivocal, the diagnosis can be established by appropriate laboratory studies. Examination of buccal mucosal scrapings reveals a negative chromatin pattern in 80 per cent of cases of Turner's syndrome. Karyotypes prepared from leukocytes reveal a modal chromosomal constitution of 44 + XO in the majority of cases. Determination of urinary 24-hour gonadotropins usually provides a clear separation between the two entities, the amount being very low or absent in hypopituitarism and higher than normal in Turner's syndrome. The latter finding reflects the absence of feedback inhibition of the anterior pituitary by sex steroids.

Another test of pituitary function, determination of growth hormone secretory capacity, is nearly always abnormal in pituitary infantilism. The clinical and laboratory findings in these two conditions are contrasted in Table 32–13.

In the past, physicians have occasionally erred in considering patients with Turner's syndrome as being "genetically male." This attitude probably arises from equating a *negative* chromatin pattern with genetic maleness. When the karyotype is 44 + XO, as in Turner's syndrome, such an interpretation is illogical. Without deliberate investigation, one has no way of knowing the nature of the missing chromosome. Maleness is determined by the presence of a Y chromosome, not by the presence of a single X. Thus, the physician has scientific reasons, as well as those dictated by tact, to use great caution in discussing the genetic basis of Turner's syndrome with the patient and *her* family.

REFERENCES

GENERAL

Bondy, P. K., and Rosenberg, L. E. (eds.): Duncan's Diseases of Metabolism, 7th ed. W. B. Saunders Co., Philadelphia, 1974.
Catt K. J.: An ABC Of Endocrinology. Little, Brown & Co., Boston, 1971.
Stanbury, J. B., Wyngaarden, J. B., and Fredrickson, D. S. (eds.): The Metabolic Basis of Inherited Disease, 3rd ed. McGraw-Hill Book Co., New York, 1972.
Williams, R. H. (ed.): Textbook of Endocrinology, 5th ed. W. B. Saunders Co., Philadelphia, 1974.

INTRODUCTION, PATHOPHYSIOLOGY OF ENDOCRINE DISEASE

Flier, T. S., Kahn, C. R., Roth, J., and Bar, R. S.: Antibodies that impair receptor binding in an unusual diabetic syndrome with secure insulin resistance. Science, 190:63, 1975.
Huxley, J. S.: Chemical regulation and the hormone concept. Biol. Rev., 10:427, 1935.
Kahn, C. R. (Moderator): NIH Conference. Receptors for peptide hormones; new insights into the pathophysiology of disease states in man. Ann. Int. Med., 86:205, 1977.
Lefkowitz, R. J.: Isolated hormone receptors: physiological and clinical implications. N. Engl. J. Med. 288:1061, 1973.
Liddle, G. W., et al.: Clinical and laboratory studies of ectopic humoral syndromes. Recent Progr. Horm. Res., 25:283, 1969.
McEven, B. S.: Interactions between hormones and nervous tissue. Sci. Am., July, 1976.
Odell, W. D., and Moyer, D. L.: Hormone Measurement. In Physiology of Reproduction. The C. V. Mosby Co., St. Louis, 1971, pp. 1–13.
O'Malley, B. W., and Schrader, W. T.: The receptors of steroid hormones. Sci. Am., 234:32–43, 1976.
O'Malley, B. W.: Mechanisms of action of steroid hormones. N. Engl. J. Med., 284:370, 1971.
Pastan, I., and Perlaman, R. L.: Regulation of Gene Transcription in Escherichia Coli by Cyclic AMP. In Greengard, P., Paoletti, R., and Robison, G. A.: Advances in Cyclic Nucleotide Research, Vol. 1. Raven Press, New York, 1972.
Robison, G. A., Butcher, R. W., and Sutherland, E. W.: Cyclic AMP. Academic Press, New York, 1971.
Roth, J., Neville, D. M., Kahn, C. R., and Gorden, P.: Hormone resistance and hormone sensitivity. N. Engl. J. Med., 296:277, 1977.

HYPOTHALAMUS

Anderson, M. S., et al.: Synthetic thyrotropin-releasing hormone. N. Engl. J. Med., 285:1279, 1971.
Besser, G. M.: Hypothalamus as an endocrine organ — I. Br. Med. J., 3:560, 613, 1974.
Fleischer, N., et al.: Synthetic thyrotropin-releasing factor as a test of pituitary thyrotropin reserve. J. Clin. Endocrinol. Metab., 34:617, 1972.
Frohman, L. A.: Clinical neuropharmacology of hypothalamic releasing factors. N. Engl. J. Med., 286:1391, 1972.
Goldstein, A.: Opioid peptides (endorphins) in pituitary and brain. Science, 193:1081–1086, 1976.
Hall, R., et al.: The thyrotrophin-releasing hormone test in diseases of the pituitary and hypothalamus. Lancet, 1:759, 1972.
Heuser, G. (Moderator): Trends in clinical neuroendocrinology: clinical case conference. Ann. Intern. Med., 73:783, 1970.
Kastin, A. J., et al.: Release of LH and FSH after Administration of Synthetic LH-releasing hormone. J. Clin. Endocrinol. Metab., 34:735, 1972.
McCann, S. M.: Luteinizing hormone-releasing hormone. N. Engl. J. Med. 296:797–802, 1977.
Pittman, J. A., Jr., Haigler, E. D., Jr., Herhsman, J. M., and Pittman, C. S.: Hypothalamic hypothyroidism. N. Engl. J. Med., 285:844, 1971.
Redding, T. W., Schally, A. V., Arimura, A., and Matsuo, H.: Stimulation of release and synthesis of luteinizing hormone (LH) and follicle stimulating hormone (FSH) in tissue cultures of rat pituitaries in response to natural and synthetic LH and FSH releasing hormone. Endocrinology, 90:764, 1972.

ANTERIOR PITUITARY

Archer, D. E.: Current concepts of prolactin physiology in normal and abnormal conditions. Fertil. Steril., 28:125–134, 1977.
Bardin, C. W., et al.: Studies of the pituitary-Leydig cell axis in young men with hypogonadotropic hypogonadism and hyposemia: comparison with normal men, prepubertal boys, and hypopituitary patients. J. Clin. Invest., 48:2046, 1969.
Daughaday, W. H.: Sulfation factor regulation of skeletal growth: a stable mechanism dependent on intermittent growth hormone secretion Am. J. Med., 50:277, 1971.

Frantz, A. G., et al.: Studies on prolactin in man. Recent Progr. Horm. Res., *28*:527, 1972.

Ganguly, A., et al.: Cushing's syndrome in a patient with an empty sella turcica and a microadenoma of the adenohypophysis. Am. J. Med., *60*:306, 1976.

Gill, G. N.: Mechanism of ACTH action. Metabolism, *21*:571, 1972.

Goodman, H. G., Grumbach, M. M., and Kaplan, S. L.: Growth and growth hormone II. A comparison of isolated growth-hormone deficiency and multiple pituitary-hormone deficiencies in 35 patients with idiopathic hypopituitary dwarfism. N. Engl. J. Med., *278*:57, 1968.

Laron, Z., Pertzelan, A., and Mannheimer, S.: Genetic pituitary dwarfism with high serum concentration of growth hormone. A new inborn error of metabolism? Isr. J. Med. Sci., *2*:162, 1966.

McKusick, V. A., and Rimoin, D. L.: General Tom Thumb and other midgets. Sci. Am., *217*:102, July, 1967.

Merimee, T. J., Hall, J. D., Rimoin, D. L., and McKusick, V. A.: A metabolic and hormonal basis for classifying ateliotic dwarfs. Lancet, *1*:963, 1969.

Merimee, T. J., et al.: Glucose and lipid homeostasis in the absence of human growth hormones. J. Clin. Invest., *50*:574, 1971.

Neelon, F. A., Goree, J. A., and Lebovitz, H. E.: The primary empty sella: clinical and radiographic characteristics and endocrine function. Medicine, *52*:73, 1973.

Nelson, D. H., Meakin, J. W., and Thorn, G. W.: ACTH-producing pituitary tumors following adrenalectomy for Cushing's syndrome. Ann. Intern. Med., *52*:560, 1960.

Purnell, D. C., Randall, R. V., and Ryncarson, E. H.: Postpartum pituitary insufficiency (Sheehan's syndrome): review of 18 cases. Mayo Clin. Proc., *39*:321, 1964.

Rabkin, M. T., and Frantz, A. G.: Hypopituitarism: a study of growth hormone and other endocrine functions. Ann. Intern. Med., *64*:1197–1207, June, 1966.

Rimoin, D. L., Merimee, T. J., Rabinowitz, D., Cavalli-Sforza, L. L., and McKusick, V. A.: Peripheral subresponsiveness to human growth hormone in the african pygmies. N. Engl. J. Med., *281*:1383, 1969.

Sheehan, H. L., and Summers, V. K.: The syndrome of hypopituitarism. Q. J. Med., *18*:319, 1949.

VanWyke, J. J., et al.: The somatomedins: a family of insulin-like under growth hormone control. Recent Progr. Horm. Res., *30*:259, 1974.

POSTERIOR PITUITARY

Bartter, F. C.: The syndrome of inappropriate anti-diuretic hormone secretion (SIADH). D. M., November, 1973.

Coggins, C. H., and Leaf, A.: Diabetes inspidus. Am. J. Med., *42*:807, 1967.

Lauson, H. D.: Metabolism of antidiuretic hormones. Am. J. Med., *42*:713, 1967.

Martin, F. I. R.: Familial diabetes insipidus. Q. J. Med., *28*:573, 1959.

Moses, A. M.: Diabetes insipidus and ADH regulation. Hosp. Prac. July, 1977.

Robison, G. A.: Isolation, assay, and secretion of individual human neurophysins. J. Clin. Invest., *55*:360–367, 1975.

Robertson, G. L.: Vasopressin in osmotic regulation in man. Ann. Rev. Med., *25*:315, 1974.

Sachs, H., et al.: Biosynthesis and release of vasopressin and neurophysine. Recent Progr. Horm. Res., *25*:447, 1969.

Schwartz, I. L., and Schwartz, W. B.: Symposium on anti-diuretic hormones: dedication to Vincent du Vigneaud. Am. J. Med., *42*:651, 1967.

Thomas, W. C.: Diabetes insipidus (teaching clinic). J. Clin. Endocrinol., *17*:565, 1957.

THYROID

Adams, D. D., and Purves, H. D.: Abnormal responses in the assay of thyrotrophin. Proc. Otago Med. Sch., *34*:11, 1956.

Burke, G.: The triiodothyronine suppression test. Am. J. Med., *42*:600, 1967.

Chopra, I.: An assessment of daily production and significance of thyroidal secretion of reverse triiodothyronine (rT3) in man. J. Clin. Endocrinol., *58*:32, 1976.

Favus, M. J., et al.: Thyroid cancer occurring as a late consequence of head-and-neck irradiation: evaluation of 1056 patients. N. Engl. J. Med., *294*:1019, 1976.

Gavin, L., et al.: Extrathyroidal conversion of thyroxine to triiodothyronine and reverse triiodothyronine in humans. J. Clin. Endocrinol. Metab., *44*:733, 1977.

Hershman, J. M., and Pittmann, J. A., Jr.: Control of thyrotrophin secretion in man. N. Engl. J. Med., *285*:997, 1971.

Ivy, H. K., Wahner, H. W., and Gorman C. A.: "Triiodothyronine (T3) toxicosis." Its role in Graves' disease. Arch. Intern. Med., *128*:529, 1971.

Larsen, P. R.: Test of thyroid function. Med. Clin North Am., *59*:1063, 1975.

Larsen, P. R.: Hyperthyroidism. D. M., *22*:3, 1976.

Means, J. H., DeGroot, L. H., and Stanbury, J. B.: The Thyroid and Its Diseases, 3rd ed. McGraw-Hill Book Co., New York, 1963.

Melvin, K. E. W., et al.: Studies in familial (medullary) thyroid carcinoma. Recent Progr. Horm. Res., *28*:399, 1972.

Mitsuma, T., Nihei, N., Gershengom, M. C., and Hollander, C. S.: Serum triiodothyronine: measurements in human serum by radioimmunoassay with correboration by gas-liquid chromatography. J. Clin. Invest., *50*:2679, 1971.

Schimmel, M., and Utiger, R. D.: Thyroid and peripheral production of thyroid hormones. Ann. Intern. Med., *87*:760–68, 1977.

Selenkow, H. A., and Hoffman, F. (eds.): Symposium On The Diagnosis And Treatment of Common Thyroid Diseases, San Francisco, 1970. Excerpta Medica, Amsterdam, 1971.

Sterling, K.: The significance of circulating triiodothyronine. Recent Progr. Horm. Res., *26*:249, 1970.

Werner, S. C., and Ingbar, S. H. (eds.): The Thyroid, 4th ed. Harper and Row, New York, 1978.

ADRENAL CORTEX

Besser, G. M. and Edwards, C. R. W.: Cushing's syndrome. Clinics In Endocrinology and Metabolism., *1*:45, 1972.

Burke, C. W. and Beardriell, C. G.: Cushing's syndrome. Q. J. Med., *42*:175, 1973.

Conn, J. W.: Primary aldosteronism, a new clinical syndrome. J. Lab. Clin. Med., *45*:6, 1955.

Eisenstein, A. B.: Addison's disease: etiology and relationship to other endocrine disorders. Med. Clin. North Am., *52*:327, 1968.

Frawley, T. F.: Adrenal Cortical Insufficiency. In Eisenstein, A. B. (ed.): The Adrenal Cortex. Little, Brown & Co., Boston, 1967, p. 439.

Horton, R.: Aldosterone: a review of its physiology and diagnostic aspects of primary aldosteronism. Metabolism, *22*:1525, 1973.

Laragh, J. H.: Modern system for treating high blood pressure based on renin profiling and vasoconstriction-volume analysis. Am. J. Med., *61*:797, 1976.

Lee, P. A., et al.: Congenital Adrenal Hyperplasia. University Park Press, Baltimore, 1977.

Liddle, G. W.: Cushing's Syndrome. In Eisenstein, A. B. (ed.): The Adrenal Cortex. Little, Brown & Co., Boston, 1967, p. 523.

Melby, J. C.: Assessment of adrenocortical function. N. Engl. J. Med., *285*:735, 1971.

Nerup, J.: Addison's disease. Acta Endocrinol., *76*:127, 1974.

Ross, E. J., Marshall-Jones, P., and Friedman, M.: Cushing's syndrome: diagnostic criteria. Q. J. Med., *35*:149, 1966.

Thorn, G. W.: The adrenal cortex. I. Historical aspects. II. Clinical considerations. Johns Hopkins Med. J., *123*:49, 1968.

PARATHYROIDS

Albright, F., Burnett, C. H., Smith, P. H., and Parson, W.: Pseudohypoparathyroidism: an example of the "Seabright-Bantam syndrome." Report of three cases. Endocrinology, *30*:922, 1942.

Albright, F., and Reifenstein, E. C., Jr.: The Parathyroid Glands And Metabolic Bone Disease. Williams & Wilkins, Baltimore, 1948.

Auerbach, G. D., et al.: Structure, synthesis and mechanisms of action of PTH. Recent Progr. Horm. Res., 28:353, 1972.

Bachelot, I., Wolfsen, A. R., and O'Dell, W.: Pituitary and plasma lipotropins: demonstration of the artifactual nature of β MSH. J. Clin. Endocrinol. Metab., 44:939, 1977.

Condon, O., et al.: Osteoporosis. Lancet, 1:180, 1970.

Copp, D. H.: Endocrine regulation of calcium metabolism. Ann. Rev. Physiol., 32:61, 1970.

Copp, D. H., et al.: Evidence for calcitonin—a new hormone from the parathyroid that lowers blood calcium. Endocrinology, 70:638, 1962.

DeLuca, H. R., and Schnoes, H. K.: Metabolism and mechanism of action of vitamin D. Ann. Rev. Biochem., 45:631–666, 1976.

Greenberg, S. R., Karabell, S., and Saade, G. A.: Pseudohypoparathyroidism: a disease of the second messenger (3'5'-cyclic AMP). Arch. Intern. Med., 129:633, 1972.

Habener, J. E., and Schillor, A. L.: Pathogenesis of renal osteodystrophy — a role for calcitonin? N. Engl. J. Med., 296:1112–3, 1977.

Harris, W. H., and Heaney, R. P.: Skeletal renewal and metabolic bone disease. N. Engl. J. Med., 280:193, 1969.

Hermans, P. E., Gorman, C. A., Martin, W. J., and Kelly, P. J.: Pseudopseudohypoparathyroidism (Albright's hereditary osteodystrophy): a family study. Mayo Clin. Proc., 39:81, 1964.

Kleeman, C. R., Massry, S. G., Coburn, J. W., and Popostzer, M. M.: The problem and unanswered questions: renal osteodystrophy, soft tissue calcification and disturbed divalent ion metabolism in chronic renal failure. Arch. Intern. Med., 124:262, 1969.

Krane, S. M.: Selected features of the clinical course of hypoparathyroidism. J.A.M.A., 178:472, 1961.

Lafferty, F. W.: Pseudohyperparathyroidism. Medicine, 45:247, 1966.

Lee, J. B., Tashyian, A. H., Streato, J. A., and Frantz, A. G.: Familial pseudohypoparathyroidism. N. Engl. J. Med., 279:1179, 1968.

Norman, A. G., and Henry, H.: 1,25 Dihydroxycholecalciferol — a hormonally active form of vitamin D. Recent Progr. Horm. Res., 30:431, 1974.

Pyrah, L. N., Hodgkinson, A., and Anderson, C. K.: Primary hyperparathyroidism. Br. J. Surg., 53:245, 1966.

Rasmussen, H.: Ionic and hormonal control of calcium homeostasis. Am. J. Med., 50:567, 1971.

Ridgway, C. E., et al.: Thyrotropin and prolactin pituitary reserve in the "empty sella syndrome." J. Clin. Endocrinol. Metab., 41:968, 1975.

Sinha, T. K., Deluce, H. G., and Bell, N. H.: Evidence for a defect of 1,25 dihydroxy vitamin D in pseudohypoparathyroidism. Metabolism, 26:731, 1977.

Stanbury, S. W., Lumb, G. A., and Mawer, E. B.: Osteodystrophy developing spontaneously in the course of chronic renal failure. Arch. Intern. Med., 124:274, 1969.

ADRENAL MEDULLA

Hermann, H., and Mornex, R.: Human Tumors Secreting Catecholamines. The Macmillan Co., New York, 1964.

Odell, W. D., et al.: Catecholamines: a symposium. Calif. Med., 117:32, 1972.

Page, L. B., and Copeland, R. B.: Pheochromocytoma. D. M., 1:1, 1968.

Sjoerdsma, A.: Pheochromocytoma: current concepts of diagnosis and treatment. Clinical Staff Conference, National Institutes of Health. Ann. Intern. Med., 65:1302, 1966.

PANCREAS

Arieff, A. I., and Carroll, H. J.: Nonketotic hyperosmolar coma with hyperglycemia: clinical features, pathophysiology, renal function, acid-base balance, plasma-cerebrospinal fluid equilibria and the effects of therapy in 37 cases. Medicine, 51:73, 1972.

Arky, R. A., and Knopp, R. H.: Evaluation of islet-cell function in man. N. Engl. J. Med., 285:1130, 1971.

Cahill, G. F.: The physiology of insulin in man. Diabetes, 20:785, 1971.

Clinicopathological Conference: Diabetes mellitus with hyperosmotic coma. Am. J. Med., 52:115, 1972.

Ellenberg, M., and Rifkin, H. (eds.): Diabetes Mellitus: Theory and Practice. McGraw-Hill Book Co., New York, 1970.

Fajans, S. S., et al.: The various faces of diabetes in the young. Arch. Intern. Med., 136:144, 1976.

Flatt, J. P.: On the maximal possible rate of ketogenesis. Diabetes, 21:50, 1972.

Ganda, D. P., et al.: Somatostatinoma: a somatostatin-containing tumor of the endocrine pancreas. N. Engl. J. Med., 296:963–969, 1977.

Gerich, J. E., Martin, M. M., and Recant, L.: Clinical and metabolic characteristics of hyperosmolar nonketotic coma. Diabetes, 20:228, 1971.

Gorman, C. K.: Hypoglycemia. Med. Clin. North Am., 49:947, 1965.

McGarry, J. D.: Ketogenesis and its regulation. Am. J. Med., 61:9, 1976.

Schein, P. S.: Islet cell tumors: current concepts and management. Ann. Intern. Med., 79:239–257, 1973.

Siperstein, M. D., Unger, R. H., and Madison, L. L.: Studies of muscle capillary basement membranes in normal subjects, diabetic, and pre-diabetic patients. J. Clin. Invest., 47:1973, 1968.

Somogyi, M.: Exacerbation of diabetes by excess insulin action. Am. J. Med., 26:169, 1959.

Steiner, D. F., et al.: Proinsulin and the biosynthesis of insulin. Recent Progr. Horm. Res., 25:207, 1969.

Sussman, K. E., and Metz, R. J. S. (eds.): Diabetes Mellitus: Diagnosis and Treatment, Volume IV. American Diabetes Association, New York, 1975.

Unger, R. H., and Orci, C.: The essential role of glucagon in the pathogenesis of diabetes mellitus. Lancet 14, 1976.

Unger, R. H.: Glucagon physiology and pathophysiology. N. Engl. J. Med., 285:443, 1971.

Yalow, R. S., and Berson, S. A.: Dynamics of insulin secretion in hypoglycemia. Diabetes, 14:341, 1965.

TESTES

Barr, M. L., and Bertram, E. G.: A morphological distinction between neurons of the male and female, and the behavior of the nucleolar satellite during accelerated nucleoprotein synthesis. Nature, 163:676, 1949.

Davidson, W. M., and Smith, D. R.: A morphological sex difference in the polymorphonuclear neutrophil leukocytes. Br. Med. J., 2:6, 1954.

Federman, D. D.: Disorders of sexual development. N. Engl. J. Med., 277:351, 1967.

Griffin, J. E., Punyashthiti, K., and Wilson, J. P.: Dihydrotestosterone binding by cultured fibroblasts. J. Clin. Invest., 57:1342–51, 1976.

Hecht, F., Wyandt, H. E., and Erbe, R. W.: Revolutionary cytogenetics. N. Engl. J. Med., 285:1482, 1971.

Kallman, F. J., Schoenfeld, W. A., and Barrera, S. E.: The genetic aspects of primary eunuchoidism. Am. J. Ment. Defic., 48:203, 1944.

Kastin, A. J., et al.: Stimulation of LH release in men and women by LH-releasing hormone purified from porcine hypothalami. J. Clin. Endocrinol., 29:1046, 1969.

Klinefelter, H. F., Jr., Reifenstein, E. C., Jr., and Albright, F.: Syndrome characterized by gynecomastia aspermatogenesis without A-Leydigism, and increased excretion of follicle stimulating hormone. J. Clin. Endocrinol., 2:615, 1942.

Park, I. J., et al.: An etiologic and pathogenic classification of male hermaphroditism. Am. J. Obstet. Gynecol., 123:505–518, 1975.

Paulsen, C. A., et al.: Klinefelter's syndrome and its variants: a hormonal and chromosomal study. Recent Progr. Horm. Res., 24:321, 1968.

Peterson, R. E., et al.: Male pseudohermaphroditism due to steroid 5 α reductase deficiency. Am. J. Med., *62*:170–191, 1977.

Plunkett, E. R., and Barr, M. L.: Cytologic test of sex in congenital testicular hypoplasia. J. Clin. Endocrinol. Metab., *16*:829, 1956.

Tjio, J. H., and Levan, A.: The chromosome number of man. Hereditas, *42*:1, 1956.

Wilson, J. D. (ed.): Roosters' Reifenstein's syndrome and hormone resistance. N. Engl. J. Med., *297*:386, 1977.

OVARIES

Corral, J., Calderon, J., and Goldzieher, J. W.: Induction of ovulation and term pregnancy in a hypophysectomized woman. Obstet. Gynecol., *39*:397, 1972.

Franchi, L. L.: The Ovary. *In* Philipp, E. E., Barnes, J., and Newton, M. (eds.): Scientitific Foundations of Obstetrics and Gynaecology. F. A. Davis Co., Philadelphia, 1970.

Gemzell, C. A.: Ovulation. *In* Philipp, E. E., Barnes, J., and Newton, M. (eds.): Scientific Foundations of Obstetrics and Gynaecology. F. A. Davis Co., Philadelphia, 1970.

Israel, S. L.: Menstruation. *In* Philipp, E. E., Barnes, J., and Newton, M. (eds.): Scientific Foundations of Obstetrics and Gynaecology. F. A. Davis Co., Philadelphia, 1970.

Lipsett, M. B., Cargille, C. M., and Ross, G. T.: Methodologic advances and clinical studies. National Institutes of Health Conference on Reproductive Endocrinology. Ann. Intern. Med., *72*:933, 1970.

Means, A. R., and O'Malley, B. W.: Mechanism of estrogen action: early transcriptional and translational events. Metabolism, *21*:357, 1972.

Odell, W. D., and Swerdloff, R. S.: Progestogen-induced luteinizing and follicle-stimulating hormone surge in post-menopausal women: simulated ovulatory peak. Proc. Natl. Acad. Sci., *61*:529, 1968.

Penny, R., et al.: Correlation of serum follicular stimulating hormone (FSH) and luteinizing hormone (LH) as measured by radioimmunoassay in disorders of sexual development. J. Clin. Invest., *49*:1847, 1970.

Penny, R., Foley, T. P., Jr., and Blizzard, R. M.: Serum follicular-stimulating hormone and luteinizing hormone as measured by radioimmunoassay correlated with sexual development in hypopituitary subjects. J. Clin. Invest., *51*:74, 1972.

Polani, P. E., Lessof, M. H., and Bishop, P. M. F.: Color blindness in "ovarian agenesis" (gonadal dysplasia). Lancet, *271*:118, 1956.

Prunty, E. T. G.: Hirsutism, virilism and apparent virilism and their gonadal relationship. J. Endocrinol., *38*:85, 1967.

Ross, G. T., et al.: Pituitary and gonadal hormones in women during spontaneous and induced ovulatory cycles. Rec. Progr. Horm. Res., *26*:1, 1970.

Turner, H. H.: A syndrome of infantilism, congenital webbed neck and cubitus valgus. Endocrinology, *23*:566, 1938.

TOXIC PHYSICAL AND CHEMICAL AGENTS

33

Effects of Physical Agents

Charles E. Billings*

INTRODUCTION

There exist within man's physical environment a great number of stressors or stimuli, nearly all of which in some dose over some time period are capable of causing dysfunction, disease, or death. These agents, however, are unique in that nearly all are essential to life and in that too little, as well as too much, of many of them may be injurious. It is the intent of this chapter to outline the tolerance envelope for each of these agents and to indicate what physiologic alterations occur when man encounters unusual environments.

We may consider the physical environment as being made up of three parts, each necessary to life. One is the *gaseous* environment: the atmospheric envelope which surrounds our planet, exerting a pressure upon every living thing on its surface and containing the oxygen, carbon dioxide, and nitrogen without which life, either animal or plant, could not have come to be.

Another facet of the environment is what we may call the *electromagnetic* environment: the sum of the electromagnetic waves and energetic particles which constantly bathe the earth. The infrared radiation upon which we depend for warmth, the light which allows us to visualize our surroundings and which triggers the photosynthetic reactions upon which we depend for food, the ultraviolet rays which produce vitamin D within our skin — all are necessary to life, yet each in insufficient or excessive amounts is harmful.

We may call the third part of our surroundings the *kinetic* environment — the accelerative forces which act upon us. Although many of the accelerations which we encounter are a consequence of our technology, gravity subjects us all to a constant acceleration toward the earth's center of mass. With our present dependence upon machines for transportation, we must consider other linear and radial accelerations as well, and also the effects of rapid deceleration or impact. Vibration and noise are other products of our technology which evoke physiopathologic responses.

Life has been characterized as "the struggle of an organism to remain distinct from its environment." The attribute of biologic systems which allows them to carry on this struggle is adaptability — the ability to respond *actively* to imposed stresses. The sum of these responses is what we know as the physiology of man; it is this which allows him, for a time, to withstand the universe's inexorable march toward greater entropy. Man cannot avoid his physical environment as he can toxic chemicals or microorganisms; indeed, he depends upon his environment for the oxygen, food, and energy necessary for survival. He must therefore learn to cope with naturally occurring alterations in the physical environment. It is the mechanisms of this coping behavior which we shall examine here.

THE GASEOUS ENVIRONMENT

Under this heading, we must consider man's tolerance envelope for barometric pressure, his ability to withstand changes in pressure, and his tolerance limits for each of the gases found in his environment: oxygen, carbon dioxide, nitrogen, and the noble gases, argon, neon, helium, kryp-

*The author wishes to thank Dr. Paul Webb, who read the manuscript and offered helpful criticisms.

ton, and xenon. In general, we shall examine the lower end of the tolerance spectrum first, then attempt to define optimal levels for productive existence, and finally define the upper limits of tolerance as a time-dependent phenomenon.

First a word about units of measurement: Although the Système Internationale (S.I.) has been recommended for universal adoption, its unit of pressure being the Newton per square meter, nearly all texts on physiology still define pressures in millimeters of mercury. In order not to burden the reader unduly, we shall use mm. Hg as our primary unit here, although we shall sometimes include in parentheses the equivalent in N/m.² or in the more commonly used equivalent, millibars (mb.). One additional pressure unit will also be used in discussing life at high pressures — atmospheres absolute (ATA). Since several systems of pressure measurement are in common use in Western countries, Figure 33–1 is

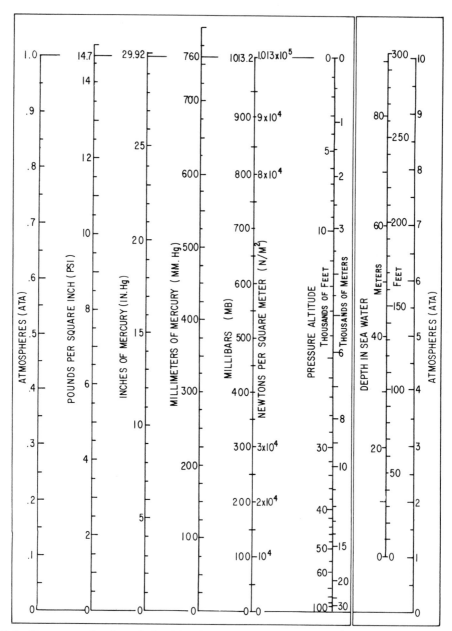

Figure 33–1 Nomogram showing relationship of barometric pressure, altitude or elevation, and depth in sea water. Several equivalent systems of pressure measurement are shown.

provided as a convenient reference. It is a nomogram which shows the quantitative relationships among the various systems. It also shows barometric pressure as a function of pressure, altitude above mean sea level in meters and feet, and depth in sea water.

1 atmosphere absolute (ATA)
= 1.013×10^5 Newtons per square meter (N/m.²)
= 1013.6 millibars (mb.)
= 760.0 millimeters of mercury (mm. Hg)
= 29.92 inches of mercury (in. Hg)
= 14.70 pounds per square inch (psi)
= 33.0 feet of sea water
= 34.2 feet of fresh water

Barometric Pressure

Normal Range. While 760 mm. Hg (1.013×10^5 N/m.², 29.92 in. Hg) is the "standard" pressure exerted by the weight of the atmosphere upon the surface of the earth at mean sea level, the actual barometric pressure at any point on the earth's surface at a given time fluctuates with weather phenomena, with elevation, and with the acceleration due to gravity, which varies with latitude. Fluctuations caused by weather are generally in the range 745 to 785 mm. Hg (980 to 1045 mb.), though pressures at the center of severe thunderstorms or hurricanes may be as low as 956 and occasional readings as high as 1062 mb. are reported. Pressures through the range of terrestrial elevations are shown in Figure 33–1.

Tolerance Limits for Low Barometric Pressure. The lowest barometric pressure at which a sea-level equivalent alveolar gas composition can be maintained if 100 per cent oxygen is breathed is about 187 mm. Hg ($PA_{O_2} = 100$, $PA_{CO_2} = 40$, $P_{H_2O} = 47$). This pressure is encountered at an altitude of 34,000 feet. At pressures below this, alveolar and therefore arterial oxygen tension decreases. A modest degree of hyperventilation occurs when the carotid sinus chemoreceptors sense a drop in arterial oxygen tension. The limit for continued consciousness occurs at an alveolar P_{O_2} of about 30 mm. Hg, thus, at barometric pressures below about 100 mm. Hg ($P_{O_2} = 30$, $P_{CO_2} = 25$, $P_{H_2O} = 47$), volitional human function ceases.

The ultimate limit for human tolerance of low barometric pressure is roughly 47 mm. Hg (63,000 feet), the vapor pressure of water at body temperature. Sudden exposure to lower pressures causes rapid evolution of water vapor bubbles within the blood and tissues, the condition known as *ebullism*. Central venous pressure rises as bubbles form in the more distensible venous reservoir and soon meets or exceeds mean arterial

pressure. Circulation then ceases. Ventricular fibrillation may ensue within 90 seconds, although animals (dogs, primates) have sometimes recovered after exposure at 2 mm. Hg absolute for as long as 180 seconds.

Humans breathing 100 per cent oxygen have survived and functioned for long periods of time at barometric pressures in the range 187 to 285 mm. Hg (250 to 380 mb.). The pressure suits used in lunar exploratory missions provided a total pressure of 187 mm. Hg, 3.5 psi, and the Apollo spacecraft were pressurized at 285 mm. Hg, 5.5 psi. There have been problems at these pressures (see Inert Gases) but they do not appear to have been caused by pressure as such.

For men breathing air, tolerance limits for low barometric pressures are related to hypoxia and will be discussed under that heading.

Effects of Pressure Fluctuations on Earth. A number of investigators have inferred from epidemiologic studies that psychological depression and suicide rates are more common during periods of weather which involve very low barometric pressures. Conclusive evidence is lacking. Patients with various forms of arthropathy commonly state that they can predict weather changes by observing changes in the pain and stiffness of their diseased joints. We are not aware of controlled studies of this phenomenon, but neither are we inclined to reject it out of hand.

Effects of High Barometric Pressure. We do not know what the ultimate tolerance limit for high pressures will be. Leaving aside the effects of high partial pressures of the various gases in man's breathing medium and the effects of relatively rapid changes in pressure, we know that normal men can live and work at pressures of 37 to 50 ATA (equivalent to 1200 to 1600 feet depth in sea water) for substantial periods of time; briefer exposures at over 60 ATA have been successfully tolerated, and studies at higher pressures are in the offing. Fenn has suggested that the limits will occur at the point at which oxidative biochemical reactions, many of which involve increases in molecular volume, are inhibited by hydrostatic pressures. It seems more likely that limits will be imposed by impairment of distribution and mixing of inspired with alveolar air, and by limitations in the ability to perform the work involved in breathing extremely dense gas mixtures, although Lambertson has demonstrated that fit young men can perform moderate work while breathing gas the density of which approximates that which will be encountered at 150 ATA (5000 feet depth in sea water).

Effects of Rapid Changes in Barometric Pressure. Under this heading, we must consider the effects of both increases and decreases in total pressure as they act on gases within the various gas-containing cavities of the body (middle ear, paranasal sinuses, lungs, gut) and on gases dissolved in body fluids according to Henry's law. Dissolved gases can only evolve as bubbles when the total pressure on them is decreased, whereas trapped gas in body cavities will attempt to obey Boyle's law as the pressure on the body changes in either direction.

Increasing Barometric Pressures. Any increase in barometric pressure will cause a decrease in the volume of a given quantity of gas. If the gas is in free communication with a gaseous environment, more gas will flow into a rigid cavity of a given size. If such gas is not available from the environment (as in underwater swimming or breath-hold diving), a relative negative pressure will occur within the cavity.

The human middle ear is a cavity of relatively fixed volume which is ventilated only through the eustachian tube. The mucosal lining of the eustachian tube is so constructed that air within the middle ear can leave the cavity passively. Reentry of air, however, is impeded and in most people requires voluntary action (yawning, swallowing) to contract the pharyngeal muscles and open the tubal orifices. Attempts to ventilate the middle ear during a descent from altitude or a dive in shallow water may be impeded by swelling of the nasopharyngeal mucosa or lymphoid hypertrophy (as found in upper respiratory infections, allergic rhinitis, and so on).

If a substantial negative pressure differential is allowed to build up within the ear, voluntary attempts to reopen the eustachian tubes may become difficult or impossible. The Valsalva maneuver may help by forcing air into the ear. If the relative vacuum persists, however, fluid is drawn into the middle ear; it may be serous or hemorrhagic in character. Rarely, the tympanic membrane may rupture. Treatment of this condition, known as aerotitis or barotitis, is physiologic: air is introduced into the middle ear by myringotomy or eustachian tube catheterization to neutralize the pressure differential across the eardrum.

If the paranasal sinus ostia are occluded by mucosal swelling, a similar condition may arise in these cavities. This condition is called aero- or barosinusitis. Unlike the middle ear, however, sinus pain may occur during either ascent or descent. The pain may be intense and incapacitating. It is caused by either a positive or negative differential pressure in the sinus cavities.

The lungs, unlike the middle ears and sinuses, are contained in a cavity of variable volume. The thoracic cavity is thus free to contract, within limits, even when air is not available from the environment (e.g., breath-hold diving). Limits are imposed on the contraction in volume, however; once the residual volume of the lungs is reached, further increases in barometric pressure

cause a relative negative pressure to occur within the thorax (thoracic squeeze). This is compensated for in part by an increase in the volume of blood in the lesser circulation and the intrathoracic portion of the venous reservoir, but at high negative pressures, pulmonary parenchymal injury results. The world's record for a breath-hold dive is 231 feet, 760 to 6080 mm. Hg.

If gas is available outside the body, very rapid increases in pressure are tolerated. Some people appear able to ventilate their eustachian tubes continuously; such subjects can tolerate pressure increases on the order of 60 mm. Hg per sec. (1 psi per sec.) without difficulty. Entry of air into the lungs is not a limiting factor in these circumstances.

Blast waves in free air, however, may be a problem, since very high overpressures with very short rise times may occur. In these circumstances, air does not have time to enter the lungs and very considerable differential pressures may occur across the chest wall, followed by marked underpressures in the environment during the rarefaction wave which follows the initial overpressure. These events occur so rapidly that the lung-chest system does not have time to adapt; it acts as a rigid system in which shear forces may cause tearing of delicate structures.

Decreasing Barometric Pressures. Relatively rapid decreases in barometric pressure occur during an ascent from depth to the surface in water, during decompression of a caisson, and during ascent to altitude in aircraft. The effects of such decreases in pressure are expansion of trapped gas and, when a substantial decrease in pressure is involved, evolution of gases from solution in the blood and body fluids.

Because of the peculiar structure of the eustachian tube, ear discomfort is almost never a problem when barometric pressure decreases. Barosinusitis or barodontalgia, however, may occur owing to expansion of trapped gas. The latter disorder is due to pockets of gas in improperly filled or infected teeth.

Under normal circumstances, the gastrointestinal tract contains relatively small amounts of gas. As this gas expands, stretch receptors in the wall of the gut are stimulated and peristalsis becomes more active. Relief from cramps is obtained by belching or passing flatus. During an extremely rapid decompression, however, massive expansion may occur before a muscular response is possible; the result may be vagovagal syncope. Rapid decompressions can occur in the event of a window, door seal, or wall failure in pressurized jet aircraft.

The foregoing comments suggest that the physician should be careful about allowing patients with hypomotile gut disorders to fly at high altitudes in unpressurized aircraft. Modern passenger aircraft are pressurized to keep cabin altitude at or below 8000 feet (564 mm. Hg). Even at this moderate pressure, however, relative gas volume (saturated) is 38 per cent over sea-level values. In unpressurized light aircraft, altitudes of 12,000 feet ($P_B = 483$ mm. Hg) are common.

The human lung-airway system at resting expiratory level has a time constant in the neighborhood of 0.05 to 0.10 seconds. During rapid decompression of an aircraft, if the time constant of the cabin (a function of its volume and the orifice through which air is escaping) is appreciably longer than that of the lungs and airway, no substantial overpressure will occur within the chest. If the reverse is true, however, overpressures will occur within the lungs. If the magnitude of the pressure drop is great enough, the lungs can become distended: a further buildup of differential pressure within the lungs can cause parenchymal tears and possibly air embolism. Such rapid decompressions are very rare in civil aircraft but can occur in military jets which have small cabin volumes and large canopies.

It should be noted that during ascent from deep water to the surface, pressure decreases at the rate of 1 ATA per 33 feet. If a diver inspires from a breathing apparatus at depth, then attempts breath-holding during an ascent, he is in grave danger of lung rupture. It is necessary to expire actively throughout this maneuver and to limit the ascent rate. Naval divers are warned to "follow their bubbles" during such ascents, which gives them an ascent rate of about 60 feet per minute. This same precaution is necessary during emergency escape from submarines, which is accomplished through pressurized air locks.

Decompression Sickness. When the total pressure on a fluid containing dissolved gas is sharply decreased, the gases emerge from solution as bubbles (the phenomenon of effervescence observed when a bottle of soda or beer is uncapped). In the body, inert gas as well as oxygen and carbon dioxide are dissolved, both in water and in fat. The amount of inert gas in solution is a function of the alveolar partial pressure of the gas and its solubility coefficients in water and in oil.

Once bubbles of gas form in the tissues or the blood, they obey Boyle's law. If the pressure on the body is reduced further, they expand; if the pressure is increased, they contract, but they do not disappear until the pressure is increased considerably above the pressure at which they were formed.

During any ascent to high altitude or from depth, the amount of inert gas in solution in blood and various tissues is the limiting factor, since decompression at too rapid a rate will favor formation of bubbles. The rate at which inert gas is eliminated from any tissue is a function of the perfusion of that tissue and the partial pressure of inert gas in the perfusing blood. Since different tissues contain different proportions of lipid and water and have different rates of perfusion, some (such as depot fat) give up inert gas very slowly, whereas diffusion proceeds rapidly in muscle and liver.

The symptoms which occur when man is decompressed too rapidly are known collectively as *decompression sickness*. Although it is not certain that all the manifestations of decompression sickness are due to evolved gas, this is the most consistent explanation which has been offered to date. Regardless of the cause, however, the symptoms of decompression sickness are consistent. They fall into five distinct categories.

The most common and least ominous form of this disorder is called the bends, after the grotesque postures effected in an effort to minimize the often excruciating joint and periarticular pain which characterizes the syndrome. Bends may come on suddenly or insidiously. Pain in or around a joint is the first symptom. It often afflicts a joint in use, or one which has previously been injured. The pain may remain localized, may migrate, or may affect several joints sequentially. A relatively small increase in barometric pressure may produce complete relief. If decompression continues, however, the pain may become incapacitating, or other forms of decompression sickness may supervene.

Localized paresthesias, itching, and rashes may also occur, presumably owing to bubbles in the skin or subcutaneous tissues. They are not dangerous. Much more ominous is a painless mottling of the skin which resembles patchy cyanosis. Its precise etiology is uncertain, but it is often seen in combination with or preceding the onset of the more severe forms of decompression sickness listed below.

A more serious form of decompression sickness is the symptom complex known as the chokes. This form is characterized by tachypnea, burning substernal pain that worsens on deep inspiration, and dry cough. It is believed that these symptoms, together with pulmonary hypertension, are caused by showers of bubbles arising in the venous circulation, which lodge in pulmonary arterioles and capillaries. The chokes are a grave development, for they often precede the most serious forms of decompression sickness.

Central nervous system decompression sickness may occur in isolation or in combination with other forms of the disease. The symptoms may mimic virtually any acute discrete or disseminated CNS lesion. Hemianopsia, hemiparesis, aphasia, confusion, delirium, and other equally frightening symptoms and signs may be observed. These are thought to be caused by gas bubbles which either block or evoke severe spasm in cerebral arterioles. Despite the serious nature of this syndrome, dramatic relief is usually produced by immediate recompression to a pressure well above that at which the symptoms appeared. With effective treatment, permanent sequelae are rare though not unknown.

Syncope may be the first or a secondary symptom of decompression sickness. Particularly when recompression is prompt, the patient will usually return to consciousness rapidly. After some time, however, such a patient may quite suddenly begin to show signs of shock, which can progress rapidly to severe levels, with anuria, refractory peripheral vascular collapse, coma and death.

The treatment of decompression sickness is relatively simple if, and only if, adequate facilities are at hand. Recompression is the specific treatment for this disorder. In the case of decompression sickness occurring at high altitude, and persisting after return to sea level, overcompression in hyperbaric chambers has been remarkably successful. Although such treatment does not make gas bubbles dissolve immediately, it does make them smaller and probably promotes more rapid dissolution. Details as to the compression treatment of this disorder may be found in the U.S. Navy Diving Manual, the basic source document for anyone involved in situations in which decompression sickness can occur.

A late finding in caisson workers and divers who are repeatedly exposed to compression and marginally adequate decompressions is aseptic bone necrosis, which often occurs in the heads of the long bones but may be seen elsewhere as well. This disorder may be serious and disabling. Once present, it does not differ appreciably from aseptic necrosis caused by other agents. It is probably due to compromise of the circulation to these areas.

Oxygen

The oxygen concentration in the lower atmosphere (below 50,000 feet) is remarkedly constant at about 20.9 per cent. Since barometric pressure changes geometrically with altitude (Fig. 33–1), the partial pressure of oxygen in air changes in the same manner. The reader will recall that humidification of air in the upper airways causes a decrease in the partial pressure of oxygen in the inspirate; another more marked drop in oxygen pressure or tension occurs in the alveoli due to continuous extraction of oxygen from and addition of carbon dioxide to the alveolar air. A further drop is seen when pulmonary venous blood is examined (the alveolar-arterial gradient); there is another slight decrease in arterial oxygen tension due to admixture of venous with arterial blood. The relatively long diffusion pathway for oxygen in the tissues means that the oxygen tension at the mitochondria is usually remarkably low. This entire pathway must be considered when we deal with alterations in oxygen partial pressures in the environment or in the human.

Absence of Oxygen; Anoxia. True tissue anoxia probably occurs only when circulation ceases. With the exceptions of oxygen dissolved in tissue fluids and oxygen bound to myoglobin and hemoglobin, the body has no storage capacity for this vital substance. When circulation to the brain ceases completely, as in ventricular fibrillation or rapid decompressions to near-vacuum conditions, consciousness is lost within 5 to 10 seconds; in animals, anoxic brain damage is seen after 90 to 180 seconds. It is interesting that even after such extreme exposures, if consciousness is regained at all, signs of cerebral dysfunction may be transitory and usually an apparently complete recovery follows. This may also be true following accidental electrocution.

Decreases in Oxygen; Hypoxia. As noted earlier, man's ultimate tolerance for hypoxia of a duration longer than a few minutes is governed by his ability to maintain a state of consciousness. Consciousness is usually lost within 10 to 15 seconds after alveolar oxygen tension drops below 30 mm. Hg. The arterial oxygen tension under these circumstances is generally below 20 mm. Hg. The retina and brain have the highest oxygen uptakes per unit mass of any tissues in the body, and thus are the tissues most rapidly and severely affected by hypoxia.

In persons breathing air, time of useful consciousness varies from hours at a barometric pressure of 350 to 380 mm. Hg to about 10 to 20 seconds at a barometric pressure of 120 to 140 mm. Hg.

At pressures greater than 380 mm. Hg, indefinite survival on air is possible, although not without severe dysfunction. Impaired mentation and coordination are common during acute exposures to hypoxia of this degree. The symptoms of moderate hypoxia include dyspnea, difficulty in concentrating, and altered judgment and mood; euphoria or depression may be noted. The symptoms may be similar to those of intoxication with ethanol and are due to impaired cerebral oxygenation, magnified by hypocapnia, which causes a degree of cerebral ischemia.

If exposure to alveolar oxygen tensions below about 50 mm. Hg is prolonged for more than 6 to 12 hours, as in mountain climbing, symptoms of acute altitude sickness begin to appear. These symptoms include malaise, headaches (which may be severe), nausea, anorexia, and insomnia. They are made worse by strenuous physical activity or exposure to cold. Breathlessness and dyspnea may be extreme. The incidence of this syndrome reaches its height between 24 and 48 hours and usually subsides thereafter.

The cause of the disorder is not known, though it occurs during a period of multiple physiologic changes. In response to hyperventilation and hypocapnia, fixed base is excreted in the urine. Plasma and extracellular water decrease; the intracellular fluid space increases. A generalized stress response is observed. Roy and others have observed that diuresis usually occurs on the second or third day at altitude, and that symptoms usually decline in severity at this time.

Nearly all persons going to high altitudes experience symptoms of acute altitude sickness. The severity of the symptoms may be lessened by taking acetazolamide for 24 hours prior to ascent.

A few people, instead of feeling better after an initial period of discomfort at altitude, may continue to have difficulty. If hypoxic exposure is continued, some will develop one or more symptoms of a more serious disorder known as chronic altitude sickness. The most ominous forms of this condition involve either cerebral edema or acute pulmonary edema or both. These are life-threatening if hypoxic exposure is not terminated.

Again, the ultimate cause is not known. Hultgren has performed cardiac catheterization studies at altitude on persons susceptible to high altitude pulmonary edema and has found grossly elevated pulmonary arterial pressures; wedge pressures were normal. Some persons can endure repeated hypoxic exposures without showing these signs; others appear inordinately susceptible. The young are more affected; physical activity by susceptible persons hastens the onset of symptoms.

As exposure to hypoxia is prolonged past three to five days, hematologic changes begin to be evident. The hemoglobin, red cell count, and hematocrit all rise. The latter reaches values of 60 per cent or so after a month of exposure. Concomitant with these changes, heart rates at rest and during work decline; work tolerance increases, though not to sea-level values. Appetite improves and fluid intake increases.

The changes noted here, and others beyond the scope of this review, gradually revert toward sea-level values following cessation of exposure to hypoxia. Normal sea-level values are reached within two to three weeks after return from altitude.

Exposure to hypoxia in the range of barometric pressures 640 to 520 mm. Hg (5000 to 10,000 feet) normally evokes only mild to moderate exertional dyspnea, mild fatigue for a few days, and subtle psychomotor defects, though scotopic visual thresholds are moderately to markedly elevated.

Oxygen Tensions at Sea Level; Normoxia. It can be shown that the oxygen tension of arterial blood at sea level (95 to 105 mm. Hg) is still low enough to cause a mild tonic ventilatory stimulus in the carotid chemoreceptors. Nonetheless, persons with normal oxygen transport systems appear to have no other symptoms of hypoxia at rest at barometric pressures in the neighborhood of 760 mm. Hg. During severe physical exercise, the administration of high concentrations of oxygen produces substantial reductions in minute ventilation and increases endurance and work capacity.

Increases in Oxygen; Hyperoxia. Since the arterial blood is virtually fully saturated with oxygen at an alveolar partial pressure of 100 mm. Hg, an increase in alveolar oxygen tension above its normal sea-level value of 100 to 110 mm. Hg results in an increase only in the quantity of oxygen dissolved in plasma, normally about 0.3 ml. per 100 ml. at an oxygen tension of 100 mm. Hg. It is possible to attain alveolar oxygen tensions as high as 670 mm. Hg by breathing 100 per cent oxygen at sea level for several hours. The gain in oxygen content of whole blood is only about 2 ml. per 100 ml., however, in a normal person. If arterial desaturation is present owing to an increased A:a gradient, of course, the use of increased concentrations of oxygen can have much more substantial results. It should be emphasized, however, that the prolonged use of oxygen in persons who do not have either a ventilation or diffusion defect is not physiologic and may be harmful.

Oxygen at pressures above 200 to 250 mm. Hg is toxic to man. The toxicity is a time-dependent phenomenon. The most important manifestations of this toxicity at oxygen pressures up to 1 ATA are pulmonary–inflammatory changes, and later pulmonary edema. It also appears that high oxygen tensions interfere with surfactant formation or excretion, with the result that small areas of atelectasis are observed. One should note that all these pulmonary changes interfere with oxygenation of the blood, which is the reason oxygen is being administered. Such administration, therefore, is a two-edged sword. There is considerable evidence that intermittent administration of oxygen delays or prevents the appearance of pulmonary oxygen toxicity; this should be kept in mind when the gas is to be used for long periods of time.

At pressures of 2 to 3 ATA, oxygen begins to cause central nervous system dysfunction. Tremors, anxiety, and grand mal convulsions are seen. Again, the effects are time- and pressure-dependent, an increase in either causing more severe signs. Oxygen at these pressures is used in the initial treatment of carbon monoxide poisoning, in treatment of gas gangrene and clostridial sepsis, and to enhance the radiosensitivity of certain tumors. It has been useful in cardiac surgery, though hyperbaric oxygen causes coronary and cerebral vasoconstriction; one study has shown as much as a 40 per cent decrease in cerebral oxygen uptake. Again, oxygen administration is clearly a two-edged sword.

Nitrogen

There is no evidence that the human organism is able to "fix" or incorporate molecular nitrogen into chemical compounds. In the absence of such evidence, we are unable to state with finality that gaseous nitrogen is an essential substance. It is necessary, in any discussion of this gas, to distinguish between its role as a unique element and its role as a diluent gas for oxygen, in which latter role any physiologically inert gas will serve as well.

The Role of Nitrogen. As we have said, there is no clear evidence that gaseous nitrogen is essential to human survival, though Allen has shown that chick embryos fail to develop in environments free of the gas. Adult males have functioned effectively for up to two weeks in atmospheres virtually devoid of nitrogen in Gemini and some Apollo space flights.

There is absolutely no evidence that nitrogen at sea-level pressures of roughly 600 mm. Hg is toxic. At substantially higher pressures, however, gaseous nitrogen begins to exert a narcotic effect. This effect limits the depth to which divers can descend breathing air. Nitrogen narcosis is pronounced at total pressures of 10 ATA (P_{N_2} of 6000 mm. Hg), equivalent to a depth of about 270 feet of sea water.

This effect is not unique; we shall see that virtually all physiologically inert gases are narcotic at some pressure. The narcotic effect of nitrogen is enhanced by physical activity; it appears to be lessened by repeated exposure to narcotic pressures.

The Role of Inert Gases. While nitrogen as such has not been shown to be essential, it has been shown that the absence of inert diluent gases has specific and predictable effects. Pure oxygen is absorbed rapidly in the lung, and even at pressures below toxic levels, patchy atelectasis has been demonstrated in subjects breathing 100 per cent oxygen. A similar phenomenon occurs in the middle ear if that cavity, after depressurization, is ventilated with pure oxygen. The gas is absorbed slowly, and the resulting pressure decrease within the ear causes symptoms of barotitis.

Inert diluent gases are necessary at sea level and higher barometric pressures, if only to prevent oxygen pressures from reaching toxic levels. At considerable depth, other inert gases must be substituted for nitrogen to avoid nitrogen narcosis. The most commonly used substitute is helium; neon is also used under special circumstances, though it is extremely expensive.

Helium

Effects of High Pressures of Helium. Helium is not an essential element and is normally present in air only in minute amounts. Helium-oxygen mixtures may be substituted for the usual nitrogen-oxygen mixture at sea level with predictable effects but without causing harm, even over extended periods of exposure.

Helium is much less dense than nitrogen, although its viscosity is slightly higher than that of nitrogen. The work of breathing at rest at sea level is largely expended in producing laminar air flow and is a function of the viscosity of the gas mixture. Turbulent air flow, however, is a function of density; when the proportion of turbulent air flow is increased, either during intense work or in the presence of significant airway narrowing (as in bronchial asthma), the use of helium-oxygen mixtures appreciably reduces the work of breathing.

Also, helium has a very high thermal conductivity. Comfort temperatures in a helium-oxygen environment are several degrees higher than in air, as a result. The convective heat loss in helium environments is a serious problem in deep diving, particularly when hard work is being performed; respiratory heat loss under these circumstances may exceed the capacity of the diver to produce heat.

Only minimal narcotic effects of helium are seen even at the highest barometric pressures to which man has thus far been exposed. The narcotic potency of all the noble gases is proportional to molecular weight, however; there is no reason to believe that helium will not be narcotic at some pressure, as yet undefined.

The relative insolubility of helium in body fluids, its low density, and its low narcotic potential have made it the diluent of choice in diving. Its disadvantages are its high thermal conductivity and its effects on speech; in the latter, the fundamental frequency is shifted upward and the harmonic structure is sharply modified by altered gas density. At high helium pressure, human speech may become virtually unintelligible.

Other Inert Gases

Neon has been used in diving and in experimental sojourns at moderate depths. It is less narcotic than nitrogen and more dense than helium, so that speech is less altered; heat loss is sharply reduced compared to helium. Its major disadvantages are its expense and its narcotic action at pressures above 10 ATA, although research in this range is inadequate.

Argon is more soluble in fat than nitrogen. Its use in diving therefore prolongs decompression time. *Krypton* and *xenon* are both potent narcotics at pressures near atmospheric. For these reasons, these gases have not been used in diving, or as other than tracer gases at sea level.

THE ELECTROMAGNETIC ENVIRONMENT

Figure 33–2 is a schematic representation of the electromagnetic environment. It serves to remind us of the reciprocal relation of frequency and wavelength, of the increasing energy of radiation as frequency increases, and of a few of the important effects of electromagnetic waves: molecular excitation at low frequencies, molecular interactions at higher frequencies, and molecular ionization and disruption at the highest frequencies.

In this section, we shall also consider briefly the effects of electric currents which may pass through the body, and we shall mention certain questions which have been raised about the effects of continuous and alternating magnetic fields on the human organism.

The reader will recall that electromagnetic waves are propagated at the speed of light. Since the speed of light varies in different materials, these waves, upon encountering matter, may be reflected, refracted, transmitted, or absorbed. When matter is truly transparent to waves, they transfer none of their energy to that matter. Only if matter is opaque or translucent to waves can energy transfer take place. The student interested in pursuing this area in more detail should review briefly the thermodynamics of heat transfer.

Magnetism

Almost since the discovery of the lodestone, man has speculated about the possible effects of magnetic fields upon physiologic function. Much medical quackery has been based on the supposed beneficial effects of magnetic fields. More recently, with the advent of manned space flight, there has been genuine concern about the possible detrimental effects of prolonged existence in environments virtually free of such fields. Beischer and others have devoted several years to animal and human studies.

Exposure to high-intensity magnetic fields causes the appearance of visual phosphenes, though whether these are due to the magnetic or to an induced electrical field in the retina is uncertain. Growth disturbances have been observed in very high, non-uniform magnetic fields. Behavioral effects have also been reported. In theory, very high field strengths can cause migration of cell substances, though it should be noted that fields of several thousand gauss are not strong enough to overshadow the normal thermal movement of such molecules.

Electricity

Electricity is so much a part of our lives, and is so easily kept under our control, that we tend to overlook its considerable dangers. Nearly everyone in a technologic society has been "bitten" by an electric current at some time; the overwhelming majority of such incidents cause nothing more than momentary annoyance. Yet electrical deaths are daily occurrences, and the difference between mere annoyance and a fatal outcome may be nothing more than fortuitous: a matter of whether one's hands are dry, whether shoes are being worn, and the like.

In medicine, where biomedical sensors and monitors are increasingly useful, the hazards of inadvertent electrocution are compounded, since these devices are attached to the body in ways which minimize resistance to the passage of stray currents.

When the body is exposed to an electrical current, the electrical characteristics of the exposed part will determine how much current enters the body. Within the body, the conductivity of tissues between the entrance and exit points will determine the path taken by the current and the proportion of the total energy dissipated within the body as heat. Wide variations in individual responses are the rule.

In general, the threshold of perception for current entering the hand is about 5 milliamperes (mA) for direct current, and less than 1 mA for 60 Hz alternating current. Little more than these amounts is generally reported as painful by some investigators; others report the range of 3 to 10 mA as the pain threshold.

With direct current, involuntary muscular contractions sufficient to prevent the exposed person from removing his hand from the source of current are produced by less than 60 mA in men, 40 mA in women. With alternating currents, corresponding values are 9 and 6 mA.

The most serious hazard in accidental contacts with electricity is ventricular fibrillation, since currents passing from a hand to any other extremity must traverse the chest. The heart is absolutely refractory to the induction of ventricular fibrillation except during a short period during the repolarization phase of the ventricles; thus, the timing of brief shocks is important.

Speaking generally, a 60 Hz alternating current of 100 mA crossing the chest for 1 second or more will often induce fibrillation. About five times this current, delivered during the sensitive phase of the cardiac cycle, is required with direct current. Much smaller currents are sufficient when they are delivered directly to the heart.

Electrical currents are used in electroconvulsive therapy of neurotic and psychotic depressive reactions. Currents of several hundred mA (60 Hz AC) passed transversely across the cerebrum produce momentary respiratory arrest and tonic,

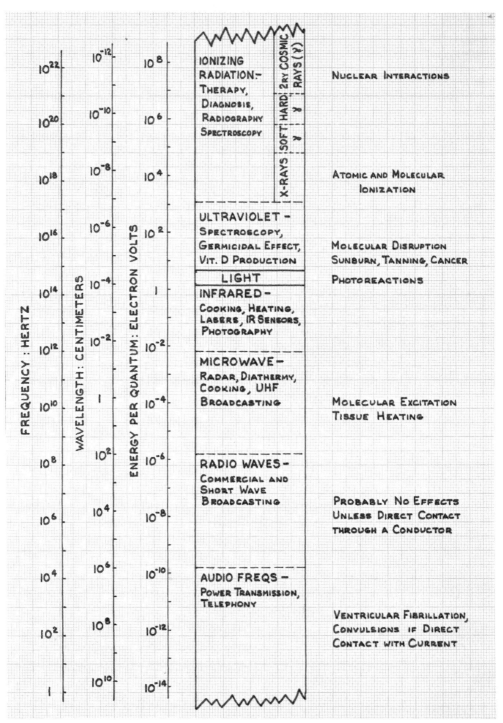

Figure 33–2 This chart shows the relationship between frequency, wavelength, and energy of electromagnetic waves, together with the commonly used division of the spectrum and comments on biologic effects.

then clonic, convulsions, unconsciousness, and amnesia. Much smaller currents passed longitudinally through the brain stem produce severe physiologic respiratory arrest, often without other dysfunction or injury. It may be for this reason that recovery from accidental electrocution may occur after even protracted assisted ventilation. More severe shocks, as in legal electrocution, cause gross disruption of brain tissues and hemorrhage.

Electrical defibrillation of the heart can be lifesaving in cases of "spontaneous" ventricular fibrillation. It is generally agreed that direct currents are safer than alternating currents for this purpose. Most defibrillators make use of a condenser discharge at controlled levels. The energy delivered to the chest wall can be varied from 25 to several hundred watt-seconds (joules).

When an electric current is delivered to a tissue the resistance of which is high, a considerable proportion of the energy appears as heat. The resistance of the skin is usually much higher than that of the interior of the body; this is the reason for the often serious electrical burns at entrance and exit points, even when the current through the body has not caused permanent injury. Use is made of this in electrocautery, which is also used to coagulate small blood vessels during surgery. Controlled electrical coagulation of portions of the central nervous system has also been used, both experimentally and therapeutically.

It should be noted that both the rate at which heat energy is generated in a tissue and the rate at which it can be dissipated by conduction or by convective transfer in blood are equally important in determining whether irreversible denaturation of tissue proteins will occur. Poorly vascularized tissues in the body, such as the lens of the eye, are particularly susceptible to injury by electricity or other radiation which can cause rapid energy transfer. Lenticular cataracts have been produced by electrical currents as well as by infrared and microwave radiation.

Electromagnetic Waves; Radio Frequencies

The human body is essentially transparent to low-frequency electromagnetic waves. Waves of frequencies above 200 megahertz (MHz), however, are absorbed to an increasing degree by biologic tissues. The energy thus absorbed appears as heat (molecular excitation). Such waves are encountered in ultra-high-frequency radio and television broadcasting, in which they are usually propagated omnidirectionally, and in Radar (*ra*dio *d*etection *a*nd *r*anging), in which they are usually focused into a narrow beam by a parabolic antenna and reflector. Transmission may be continuous (CW) in broadcasting or pulsed (PW) in most radar applications. Microwave diathermy units, operating at about 2500 MHz, and microwave ovens, at similar frequencies, are usually CW devices, though some recent studies have suggested that PW devices may be more effective in diathermy.

A detailed description of this exceedingly broad band of radiation is beyond the scope of this review. Certain general principles can be stated, however. As frequency increases, penetration of these waves decreases in water or biologic tissues; the radiation is absorbed, therefore, by a smaller cone of tissue and the local heating increases. For example, 1 joule transferred through 1 cm.^{2} of skin and absorbed in a depth of 1 cm. would yield the heat equivalent of 1 joule per cm.^{3}, whereas the same energy transfer at a higher frequency absorbed in the top 1 mm. of skin, would yield the heat equivalent of 10 joules per cm.^{3}.

Since the body has temperature receptors only at its surface, it has no way of sensing the presence of low-frequency microwave energy, which passes into the body core. High-intensity fields at high frequencies, however, may be sensed as warmth or a burning sensation.

Microwave radiation is reflected by metals and to a lesser extent by earth. Metal screens can be used to protect persons working in microwave fields.

Some investigators in this area have reported effects of microwave radiation other than thermogenic effects. The most consistent findings have been in the hematopoietic system, though these reports are disputed by others. Interference with nerve conduction has also been reported.

There is little question that microwave radiation in large doses can cause cataracts. Reports of such lesions in industry have been rare, however, as have authentic reports of systemic injury caused by microwave radiation in general. Nonetheless, the introduction of microwave heating and cooking equipment into homes, with the attendant possibilities for misuse, warrant a degree of caution on the part of physicians. Microwave transmitters may also interfere with the function of cardiac pacemakers.

Infrared or Thermal Radiation

It is not possible to set a clear boundary between microwave and thermal, or infrared, radiation. As we have seen, tissue heating is produced by electromagnetic waves of much lower than infrared frequencies. Most authors place the boundary in the neighborhood of 10^6 MHz, or a wavelength of 3×10^7 Ångström units (A.U.).

Since thermal radiation is effectively absorbed by the body, and since metabolism results in endogenous heat production, we must consider in some detail the physiopathology evoked by both excessive and insufficient heat.

It will be recalled that the human must maintain rather precise internal temperature control in the face of widely varying environmental temperatures and levels of heat production. Thermal inputs to the body come by radiation, convection, or conduction from the environment, and from metabolic heat production. Man can lose heat to his environment by radiation, convection, conduction, and evaporation of water or sweat. His range of tolerance for heat is remarkably narrow: if we consider him purely as a container of heat, his total heat content is in the neighborhood of 9000 kilocalories (kcal.) but his tolerance for alterations in heat content is only about ± 150 kcal.

We shall look first at the systemic effects of heat, then its local effects. Cold, or insufficient heat, will be considered in the same way.

Heat. ACUTE SYSTEMIC EFFECTS. Whenever man is exposed to heat stress, a number of systems respond in an effort to rid the body of the thermal load. Peripheral vasodilatation occurs; as peripheral resistance falls, heart rate and cardiac output increase. If temperature gradients between the skin and the surrounding air are adequate, convective heat dissipation increases enough to restore balance. If not, or if the thermal load is large, sweating occurs. Evaporation is an extremely effective method of heat dissipation because of the high latent heat of vaporization of water. For evaporation to occur, however, the air surrounding the body must have a vapor pressure below the saturation vapor pressure at skin temperature.

If these mechanisms for heat loss are not adequate to keep pace with the rate of heat input to the body, heat storage must occur; the core temperature will rise. A number of symptom complexes are seen when man encounters heat stress beyond his capacities.

Heat stroke is the most serious of these syndromes. Its presence is made known by anxiety, irritability, visual disturbances, delirium, collapse, coma, and death if treatment is inadequate. The skin is dry, hot, and flushed. The rectal temperature is very high (40 to 43° C.). Cessation of sweating in the presence of continued thermal stress, probably owing to failure of central thermoregulatory centers, allows a very rapid increase in the rate of heat storage.

Heat stroke constitutes a true medical emergency. Removal of the patient from the source of heat stress followed by vigorous attempts to cool the body are the first measures to be instituted. Rapid cooling should be used, although it must be realized that skin cooling induces peripheral vas-

oconstriction, which inhibits conduction of core heat to the surface.

As the rectal and core temperature begin to fall, it becomes necessary to moderate treatment so that one does not induce hypothermia, for it must be realized that the thermoregulatory failure which allows heat to be retained will also fail to protect against excessive heat loss. In essence, the therapist must take over the task of maintaining thermal homeostasis until the patient recovers that capacity. Persons who have had heat stroke may tolerate intense heat poorly thereafter, because of permanent damage in the thermoregulatory centers.

Heat exhaustion is characterized by weakness, hypotension and elevated temperature. The skin is not dry, however; often the patient has been sweating vigorously. The condition is probably caused by moderate dehydration and salt imbalance. Removal from heat and treatment with fluid and electrolytes (the intravenous route may be necessary if the patient is nauseated) usually produce prompt recovery. There are no sequelae.

Heat cramps are seen in unacclimatized subjects doing strenuous work in hot environments. These cramps are attributed to salt depletion. The oral administration of dilute salt solution, or intravenous administration of physiologic saline, produces dramatic relief. These symptoms can be prevented by acclimatization (see later).

Thermogenic anhidrosis has been observed in healthy, acclimatized subjects after a considerable period of heat exposure. Profuse sweating for a prolonged period suddenly terminates except on the face and neck. Patients complain of malaise, warmth, fatigue, shakiness, and lightheadedness. The rectal temperature is usually normal. The skin is dry. Severe prickly heat is invariably present. The cause of the disorder appears to be either physical obstruction or physiologic exhaustion of sweat glands. Treatment consists of rest and return to a cooler environment.

CHRONIC SYSTEMIC EFFECTS. Even physically fit men cannot work long or strenuously when they are first exposed to a very hot environment. If, however, they are allowed to perform work of gradually increasing intensity during the first one to two weeks of exposure, their work tolerance increases markedly. A number of physiologic changes are observed in the course of this acclimatization process. The volume of sweat increases; its electrolyte concentration decreases. Heart rates at given work loads decrease sharply. Postural hypotension no longer occurs. Work tolerance approaches values previously obtained in cool environments. Water intake increases sharply, although thirst still is not an adequate guide for fluid replacement.

Acclimatization is impeded or reversed, once present, by fatigue, ingestion of alcohol, restriction of water, systemic illness, or temporary removal from exposure.

Tolerance for work in hot environments has been studied by many authors. The data shown in Figure 33–3 are representative.

LOCAL EFFECTS.   It has been noted repeatedly here that the radiant energy transferred to a volume of tissue, relative to the capacity of that tissue and its perfusing blood to remove heat, will determine whether heat storage and a temperature rise will occur. Most human proteins are easily denatured by heat; thus, the thermal capacity of living tissue is rather small.

If the rate of heat input to the skin is high, local heating occurs. Histamine and other vasodilator substances are released, producing erythema. If the temperature rises further, local vesiculation occurs. If the temperature continues to rise, coagulation necrosis of the germinal epithelium results and the skin will slough. At still higher temperatures, charring is observed. This, in brief, is the sequence seen when the skin is burned. The relationship between the rate of energy input and duration of input is logarithmic.

The secondary and tertiary adjustments in fluid and electrolyte balance which occur following burns of considerable extent are beyond the scope of this survey. References to recent reviews of the topic will be found at the end of this chapter.

There is evidence that increases in the temperature of the testes in man inhibit spermatogenesis. This is thought to be one of the reasons why spermatogenesis is inhibited in an undescended testicle. Increases in testicular temperature may also increase the rate of "spontaneous" mutations in the germinal cells, though the quantum energies in this portion of the electromagnetic spectrum are very low.

Infrared Radiation: Effects on the Eye.   The cornea is virtually transparent to the highest portion of the IR spectrum (wavelengths shorter than 19,000 A.U.). The crystalline lens has a similar but not identical transmissibility characteristic; it becomes increasingly transparent at wavelengths shorter than 15,000 A.U.

There is, therefore, a range of wavelengths in the high infrared portion of the spectrum for which the cornea and aqueous are more transparent than the lens. As a result, heating of the lens occurs, both directly and secondarily as a result of absorption of the same wavelengths by the iris.

The industrial phenomenon now known as "glass-blower's cataract" was described in the 18th century. Since that time, many workers have studied these lesions and have established

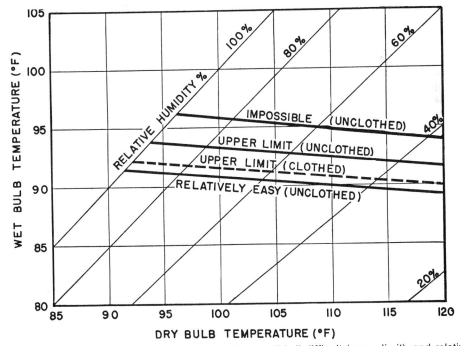

Figure 33–3   Diagram indicating equivalent zones of "impossible," difficult (upper limit), and relatively easy combinations of dry and wet bulb temperatures; the effect of relative humidity and of clothing on acclimatized men working for 4 hours at an energy expenditure of about 300 kcal./hr. (From Largent and Ashe, 1958.)

conclusively that they are caused by thermal radiation rather than by light, as was first thought. The cataracts typically begin to form at the posterior pole of the lens and develop slowly after months or years of exposure to intense thermal radiation from industrial furnaces or other similar sources. Similar lesions would likely be produced by lasers radiating at appropriate wavelengths.

Normal Thermal Environments for Man. Much research has been done on the limits of environmental comfort for man under various conditions of activity. Since comfort is a subjective phenomenon, most of this research has necessarily made use of subjective indices. A unit of thermal insulation has been developed, the clo, which is "the amount of insulation necessary to maintain comfort in a seated, resting subject in a normally ventilated room (air movement 20 ft. per min. or 10 cm. per sec.) at a temperature of 70° F. (21° C.) and a relative humidity of the air of less than 50 per cent." For American men and women wearing 1 clo of insulation, thermal comfort ranges are 70 to 85° F. (21 to 29° C.).

As environmental temperature falls, man's thermal environment begins to require him to cope with an inadequate thermal input. We call this *cold*.

Cold. SYSTEMIC EFFECTS. In general, where man faces, lives with, and can acclimatize to heat, he tends to avoid or circumvent the effects of cold. Man has only a limited number of ways of coping with the lack of environmental heat; in the course of evolution, he has lost many of the mechanisms available to other mammals.

Man can increase his insulation somewhat by peripheral vasocontriction: skin temperature drops and skin-environment gradients decrease. If cold air is flowing by the skin, however, convective losses are still considerable. The thick blanket of hair and the piloerector mechanisms of our mammalian cousins have long since been lost to man, as has the ability to vasoconstrict the rich blanket of scalp vessels in response to cold.

We do retain the ability to increase our rate of heat production, either by moving muscles in doing work or by shivering. We can also increase our effective insulation blanket by wearing clothing. The disadvantage of clothing is that the amount of insulation necessary to maintain comfort at rest is entirely too much when strenuous work is performed. Also, the insulating value of clothing is considerably reduced as it becomes wetted by sweat. It is thus necessary to maintain air flow over the skin to aid in evaporation while such work is being performed.

When man is unable to maintain thermal balance, his core temperature begins to drop. Severe shivering and exhaustion induced by voluntary work give way to profound feelings of lassitude and an overwhelming desire to sleep. More prolonged exposure causes continued body cooling and usually death by ventricular fibrillation when the cardiac temperature reaches 27° C., though survival has been reported after rapid rewarming of humans whose core temperature was as low as 18° C.

Just as rapidly moving air removes heat from a warm object more rapidly than still air, so water, with its high specific heat, removes heat from the body very much more rapidly than air. Immersion in water at near-freezing temperature renders a man incapable of helping himself within a very few minutes and is usually fatal in less than an hour, whereas he will survive in still air at this temperature for many hours.

LOCAL EFFECTS. When an extremity or other body part with the exception of the scalp is exposed to cold, piloerection ("goose pimples") and vasoconstriction occur. As the skin temperature approaches 0° C., metabolic needs are maintained for a time; pain in the area gives way to numbness. Thereafter, edema and blistering may appear. Gangrene, with or without infection, will occur if the part is allowed to remain cold; if rapid rewarming is instituted, permanent injury is minimized, though the part may be painful for a considerable time. If cell disruption due to formation of ice crystals has occurred, permanent disability of some degree is likely. This is the picture of *frostbite*.

Exposure of extremities (most often the feet) to cold, wet environments gives rise to a related disorder known as *trench foot* or shelter foot. In this condition, actual tissue freezing is rare, but tissue maceration may be extreme, and permanent disability is not uncommon.

There is some evidence that local adaptation to cold may occur, especially in the hands. Massey's data suggest that such adaptation proceeds over a period of perhaps seven weeks. Other studies indicate that there may be seasonal fluctuations in hand blood flow in cold climates, larger flows being observed in the coldest seasons.

Visible Radiation: Light

The narrow band of electromagnetic waves lying between 7.7 and 3.8×10^8 MHz (wavelengths between about 3900 and 7700 A.U.) has an importance to man out of all proportion to its miniscule contribution to the total energy flux within the universe. It is important because our eyes can sense this band; visible radiation illuminates our world and thus gives us the mobility which has made us what we are. No less important, it is a portion of this band which provides the specific energy levels required for photosynthesis, the basic source of all our nutritive needs.

The physiology of the eye is adequately described in textbooks; it will be alluded to only briefly here. More important in terms of pathologic physiology are the tolerable range of light intensities and man's efforts to adapt to levels outside this range.

The human retina has two types of sensors: rods, or scotopic sensors, and cones, or photopic sensors. The rods are found in greatest numbers at distances of about 10 degrees from the center of the fovea; their numbers remain relatively constant for a considerable distance toward the periphery. There are no rods at the center of the fovea, however, where cone cells are found in greatest density.

The rod cells in the completely dark-adapted eye have a threshold on the order of 5×10^{-6} millilamberts (mL.). Cones reach their maximum acuity at illumination intensities above 10^5 mL. The retina's visual range is thus at least 10 orders of magnitude.

After prolonged exposure to bright light, the retinal sensors require a finite time to become maximally adapted to low levels of light. It is presumed that this adaptation time reflects the time necessary for complete regeneration of the photosensitive pigments within the sensors. Cone cells reach maximum sensitivity (0.001 to 0.01 mL.) within 6 to 8 minutes, whereas the more sensitive rods require about 30 minutes of darkness (or dim red light, to which they are insensitive) to reach maximum sensitivity (less than 0.00001 mL.). Many environmental and endogenous factors influence these values; the effect of hypoxia has been mentioned, as an instance.

The eye and brain can perceive, though not in fine detail, objects illuminated by starlight. Given this incredible sensitivity, it is fair to ask whether this sensing mechanism is damaged by complete darkness: by the total absence of light.

If one eye of certain mammals is covered for even a few days or weeks during early postnatal development, there is an almost complete shift of ocular dominance to the contralateral eye. These effects appear to be permanent. Although comparable data are not available for man, Weisel suggests that a child whose eye is covered for a short period during the critical phase of postnatal central nervous system development may well end up with a permanent visual defect in that eye. The initial period in monkeys is the first six weeks of life; it may well be longer in man.

At the other end of the range of light intensities, we must consider the effects of exceedingly intense levels of illumination. The luminance of a nuclear fireball viewed from 4 miles away may exceed 10^8 mL.; the sun, viewed from earth, has a luminance of 4×10^8 mL. In evaluating the effects of those intensities, we must consider two factors peculiar to visible radiation and the eye. First, the cornea, aqueous, lens, and vitreous are all relatively transparent to electromagnetic waves in the visible band. Second, and perhaps more important, the eye is not merely a sensing system; it focuses a point source of light on the retina. For this reason, very intense light sources concentrate their energy on a very small area of the retina and choroid, where pigment absorbs nearly all visible radiation which reaches it. Thus, nearly all the energy incident upon this small area is converted to heat, in amounts which very rapidly produce irreversible changes in the affected cells.

Retinal burns from solar, nuclear, or laser radiation produce permanent visual field defects or blind spots. If these are in the periphery, they represent no great problem. Unfortunately, it is also "only human" to look directly toward the source of intense light, which focuses the radiation directly on the fovea. The central field defect thus produced severely limits the visual acuity of the eye — or of both eyes — thereafter, because acuity rapidly declines at angular distances of even a few degrees from the fovea. Eclipse blindness, caused by viewing solar eclipses through inadequate filters, is a form of this lesion. Even the image of the solar corona, still visible at the moment of total eclipse, is bright enough to cause such burns.

Lasers (*L*ight *a*mplification by *s*timulated *e*mission of *r*adiation) represent a special hazard. Because the energy emitted by these devices is coherent (all of one frequency), there is almost no beam divergence, and unbelievably energetic pulses of radiation can be generated. These can literally vaporize any matter not transparent to them. The increasing use of such devices in science, industry, and military applications multiplies the hazards to which workers, or troops, may be subjected.

Ultraviolet Radiation

Visible radiation is energetic enough to trigger photosynthesis, as well as a variety of oxidative reactions in inorganic chemicals. Since the energy content of radiation is directly proportional to its frequency, the ultraviolet band (wavelengths from roughly 3900 to 1000 A.U.) contains increasingly energetic radiation, whose energies are powerful enough to disrupt various types of intramolecular chemical bonds. Indeed, the considerable germicidal effectiveness of UV is due to its ability to disrupt the helical structure of DNA.

Fortunately, earth's atmosphere absorbs nearly all the very considerable flux of ultraviolet radiation which reaches it. Wavelengths shorter than 2400 A.U. are strongly absorbed by molecular oxygen, with the production of ozone in the upper atmosphere. Ozone itself absorbs all UV radiation shorter than 2900 A.U. and some of that between 2900 and 3200 A.U. Water vapor and dust in the troposphere absorb more, so that the flux of ultraviolet light at the earth's surface is very small. Nonetheless, enough reaches us to cause a variety of physiologic and pathologic effects. In the former category, we may place the conversion of provitamin D to vitamin D; in the latter, the production of sunburn and tanning.

Vitamin D is produced in the human epidermis from 7-dehydrocholesterol by ultraviolet radiation in the 2900 to 3200 A.U. band. Since little UV reaches the surface of the earth when the sun is less than 20 degrees above the horizon (owing to atmospheric scattering), it is clear that people living in the high north latitudes may be at risk of vitamin D deficiency for a substantial part of each year. This is especially true in industrial urban areas, where air pollution by dust is considerable and where people may have little exposure to sunlight. In these days of vitamin D-supplemented milk, one seldom recalls how serious a problem rickets was and for how long.

Sunburn is produced by ultraviolet light in the band of 2900 to 3200 A.U., though large doses of radiation longer than 3200 A.U. do produce erythema. After a latent period of up to several hours following exposure, cutaneous blood vessels dilate, with resultant erythema over the exposed area, and discomfort and pain. The erythema reaches a peak between 8 and 24 hours following exposure and then gradually fades. If the burn is severe, vesiculation may occur, followed after a variable time by desquamation. A suntan of variable degree replaces the burn. Adaptation of the skin to repeated UV exposure occurs, manifested by deposition of melanin in the skin, though other adaptive mechanisms may be involved as well.

It should be emphasized that these signs are manifestations of injury to the dermis. Increases in mitotic activity are seen as desquamation takes place, together with marked thickening of the Malpighian layer of the epidermis. The relationship between such changes and the eventual development of cancers is not known, though it is clear that repeated sunburn causes degenerative changes in both dermis and epidermis. It has also been shown, both experimentally in animals and by epidemiologic studies in man, that ultraviolet radiation in the 2800 to 3150 A.U. band does produce skin cancer.

Ionizing Radiation*

The Nature of Ionizing Radiation. Figure 33–2 shows a dotted line separating ultraviolet from ionizing radiation. There is no clear boundary; we

*This section was originally prepared by Dr. Bertram D. Dinman, to whom the author is grateful for his conceptualization of the problem. He also acknowledges the helpful contributions of Dr. William R. Carpentier, who reviewed the manuscript.

shall see that some of the effects of ionizing radiation differ only in magnitude from those of less energetic forms of radiation. Electromagnetic waves of comparatively low energy can disrupt intramolecular chemical bonds; such disruption is one of the characteristic — and most harmful — effects of waves or particles of higher energy. As with all electromagnetic radiation, the effect of ionizing radiation depends on its absorption within the body. The absorption of ionizing radiation depends in great part on its physical characteristics: whether it is particulate or photon radiation; if particulate, whether it carries a charge; and its energy content.

All radioactive isotopes, or radionuclides, decay at a characteristic rate, which is expressed in terms of the time required for one-half of a given quantity to decay. This is the *physical half-life* of the isotope. The decay may involve the emission of a photon, a beta particle, or portions of the nucleus.

It is important to remember that an atom of any element behaves chemically in a characteristic fashion, regardless of whether it is a stable or unstable isotope. The human body has no way to differentiate between isotopes. It turns over each element and compound at a characteristic rate, however; this is the *biologic half-life* of the substance. The *effective half-life* of a radionuclide within the body is a function of how rapidly it decays and of how rapidly it is excreted by the body.

Forms of Ionizing Radiation. An understanding of certain of the physical properties of the various forms of ionizing radiation is a necessary prerequisite to an understanding of the biologic effects of such radiation. The most important forms are:

X-Rays. These are photons, or quanta, or energy which have no mass or charge and travel at the speed of light. They are produced by transformations of extranuclear orbital electrons or by sudden deceleration of high-speed electrons, as in an x-ray tube. They may have virtually any energy content from very low (a few hundred electron volts) to extremely high. Because they have no mass or charge, their ability to penetrate matter is considerable.

GAMMA RAYS. These, like x-rays, are photons, but they are produced in the process of radioactive decay. Their energy content is a characteristic of the isotope undergoing decay, and ranges from low to several million electron volts.

BETA PARTICLES AND HIGH-ENERGY ELECTRONS. Beta particles are energetic electrons carrying either a negative or positive charge. Both are produced by nuclear transformations; negatively charged high-energy electrons can also be produced in accelerating devices. They may have a wide spectrum of energies, although the average energy level of beta particles produced in nuclear transformations is characteristic. Because they are particles, they have momentum; ionization is produced when this momentum is transferred to another particle. Beta particles may also lose energy when decelerated; an x-ray is emitted.

PROTONS.   These are nuclear constituents having a positive charge and a mass of one. Because of their charge, they can produce ionization by interacting with other charged particles; they can also produce ionization by transferring momentum to other particles. They are rarely a problem on earth but exist in great numbers in the Van Allen radiation belts surrounding our planet and are produced in enormous numbers during solar flares. They therefore pose a hazard for space travelers and to a lesser extent for persons flying in supersonic transport aircraft at very high altitudes. These aircraft carry warning systems to alert their pilots to the presence of excessive radiation levels.

ALPHA PARTICLES.   The alpha particle is identical to the nucleus of the helium atom; it consists of two protons and two neutrons. Because of its large mass and charge, it has enormous ionizing potential but relatively short range in any sort of matter, including air. Alpha particles are produced spontaneously in radioactive decay of heavy elements.

NEUTRONS.   These are particles with a mass of one, like protons, but they carry no electrical charge. Their energy is entirely a function of their velocity. Because they carry no charge, they interact with other matter only when they collide with it; ionization occurs indirectly as a result of the energy transfer during such collisions.

It is obvious from the foregoing that the relative effect of these forms of ionizing radiation in biologic tissues will vary considerably. Those forms which have relatively large mass and charge have short ranges in tissues but produce enormous damage within that range; the most penetrating forms of radiation have a much lower likelihood of interacting with tissues. Because of this variation in biologic effect, quantities of radiation are measured in terms which take account only of the number of quanta actually absorbed in the body. The generally accepted radiation dose unit is the *rad*, an acronym for "radiation absorbed dose." One rad equals 100 ergs of energy absorbed per gram of tissue. The biologic effect of the energy transfer is a function of the type of radiation, its energy content, and the density of the tissue into which it is directed.

Biologic Effects of Ionizing Radiation.   The most sensitive structural and chemical component of the cell appears to be the deoxyribonucleic acid molecule. This is not surprising; we have already noted that even thermal radiation may increase the rate of mutations in germinal cells, and that ultraviolet radiation's germicidal effectiveness is due to its ability to disrupt the helical structure of DNA.

Although nucleoproteins are at highest risk of alteration from ionizing radiation, lipids and carbohydrates may also be altered by such radiation. At the atomic level, ionizing radiation can result in excitation of an orbital electron or ejection of the electron from its orbit. An ion pair is created when an electron is ejected: an energetic, negatively charged electron and the positively charged residual atom or molecule. These pairs survive only a short time, but they are extremely reactive and ultimately cause molecular damage by reacting with other cellular components. Because approximately 80 per cent of biologic systems are aqueous, the free radicals formed in water are $-OH$ and $-H$, in addition to H^+ and OH^- ions. The free radicals react to form H_2, H_2O and H_2O_2, an active oxidizing agent. It is the latter which is believed to produce physiochemical changes. Organic peroxides may be formed in the same fashion by free radical action.

Pathologic Physiology of Radiation Injury.   The susceptibility of body tissues to injury by ionizing radiation is in general directly proportional to their rate of cell division, or growth rate, and inversely proportional to their degree of differentiation. By this criterion, the hematopoietic system should be highly vulnerable to radiation, the rapidly-replaced gastrointestinal mucosal cells somewhat less, and the central nervous system cellular elements least sensitive. Within the hematopoietic system, leukocytes and especially lymphocytes are highly susceptible; platelet formation is even more severely affected.

The manifestations of acute radiation injury are predictable. Infection and hemorrhage, particularly in the gastrointestinal tract, are the rule. Platelet deficiencies result in altered coagulation. Multiple tissue and gastrointestinal hemorrhages follow; these phenomena are aggravated by alterations in vascular permeability.

By contrast, although severe exposure and early death may be accompanied by marked central nervous system signs and symptoms, neuronal structural changes are minimal. The predominant changes in central nervous system function are due to altered vascular permeability, resulting in both perivascular and generalized cerebral edema.

Clinical Manifestations of Radiation Injury.   The acute syndrome that follows radiation exposure is not unlike other inflammatory or toxic events. The damage depends on the dose of radiation and the period of time over which it is administered. The stages of illness parallel those of viral infections, with a prodrome, a latent period, then manifest illness, and finally death or convalescence and recovery. The periods between the stages are dose-dependent. Cautious predictions as to outcome sometimes can be made within the first 24–48 hours.

Since the degree of injury is dependent on the

absorbed dose of radiation, a dose-related classification of responses can be described. This may be divided into five groups:

GROUP I. Dose, less than 150 rads. Most patients are asymptomatic; a few will have prodromal symptoms but not later signs of illness.

GROUP II. Dose, 200 to 400 rads. Most patients will have a mild form of the acute radiation syndrome with transient prodromal nausea and vomiting and subsequent evidence of hematopoietic alterations (Figure 33–4 illustrates these alterations). Most will recover; if death occurs it will be due to sequelae of the hematologic depression.

GROUP III. Dose, 400 to 600 rads. The dose which causes 50 per cent mortality in untreated cases is 450 to 500 rads. Persons in group III will exhibit serious effects associated with severe hematopoietic damage and variable degrees of gastrointestinal damage.

GROUP IV. Dose, 600 to 1400 rads. An accelerated version of the acute syndrome is seen, dominated by the effects of gastrointestinal injury. The length of survival depends on the severity of the gastrointestinal damage.

GROUP V. Dose, greater than 2000 rads. The course is fulminating, with severe central system manifestations.

Stages of Illness. As noted above, the course of acute radiation sickness can be divided into four stages.

STAGE 1 — PRODROMAL STAGE. Regardless of dose, the psychologic concomitants of a known exposure may dominate and obscure the physio-pathology of this stage. In general, however, the earlier the onset of symptoms, the higher the likely dose. If no nausea and vomiting occur within the first few hours, the patient has probably received a Group I exposure. In Groups II and III, these symptoms are usually seen within an hour or so after exposure. In Groups IV and V, there is a rapid onset of diarrhea, ataxia, disorientation, coma, and shock.

Prodromal symptoms reach a maximum within 6 to 8 hours. During this time, patients in Groups III–V have weakness and fatigue, sweating, and paresthesias. Within 24 to 48 hours, the symptoms subside in Groups I and II, become less severe in Group III, and progress without a latent period into the manifest illness in Groups IV and especially V.

STAGE 2 — LATENT PERIOD. In Group I patients, the illness usually ends with the prodromal period. In the other groups, the length of the latent period is inversely proportional to dose. Weakness and fatigue may continue through this period.

STAGE 3 — MANIFEST ILLNESS. Group II patients may exhibit chills, fever, weight loss, fatigue, and epilation (if the dose was greater than 350 rads). Pharyngitis, upper respiratory infections, melena, hematuria, gingival hemorrhages, and mild purpura reflect the hematopoietic damage. Various combinations of these symptoms may persist for 40 to 50 days, becoming gradually less thereafter.

In Group III patients, similar but more severe symptoms and signs appear earlier. Within a

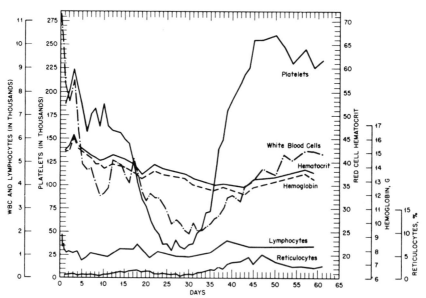

Figure 33–4 Average values of blood elements of five individuals exposed to estimated doses of 200 to 350 rads. (From Saenger, E. L. (ed.): Medical Aspects of Radiation Accidents: A Handbook for Physicians, Health Physicists and Industrial Hygienists. United States Atomic Energy Commission, 1963).

month of exposure gastrointestinal damage becomes manifest by severe, bloody diarrhea, abdominal pain, and hematemesis. Hematuria and oliguria may appear. Coma and profound shock may be followed by death in 25 to 40 days.

Group IV patients usually run an abbreviated course and die within 15 to 30 days after exhibiting more severe signs of gastrointestinal damage.

Group V patients do not live long enough to manifest hematologic signs. Ataxia, incoherence, disorientation, vomiting, diarrhea, and abdominal cramps occur within an hour or two after exposure. Although there may be a brief period of mental clarity, the usual course is inexorably downward, regardless of treatment.

It should be noted that this narrative describes the effect of a single dose of ionizing radiation. The effect of fractional doses delivered over a period of time is much less severe.

STAGE 4 — RECOVERY. In Group II patients, convalescence ordinarily begins between two and three months after exposure. Clinical recovery usually is apparent within six months, although some weakness may persist thereafter. Those patients in Groups III and IV who do not die follow a generally similar course, though weakness persists for many months.

Therapeutic Principles. It is obvious that doses in the range above 400 to 500 rads pose severe or insuperable problems. Although measures to replace blood elements are available, there is no way to correct the gastrointestinal defects seen in these groups. Death is probably inevitable after doses of 800 to 1000 rads.

Group I patients may be followed as outpatients. Other patients require hospitalization. Therapy should be directed toward protection against the effects of thrombocytopenia and leukopenia. Hemorrhages may require blood, enriched plasma, or platelet transfusions. Antibiotics, strict antisepsis, and isolation are necessary to protect against infection. Careful maintenance of fluid balance and proper nutrition are essential.

Effects of Surface Irradiation. Irradiation of the skin by low energy x-rays or beta radiation may produce damage restricted to the skin. The effect of such radiation is similar in appearance and course to a thermal burn, although some features of the acute radiation syndrome may appear.

Internal Deposition of Radionuclides. The naturally radioactive elements (uranium, thorium, actinium, plutonium, etc.) decay by emission of alpha particles. Because these particles have such a limited range, they represent only a slight hazard outside the body. Within the body, however, serious damage may be caused because of the intensely ionizing nature of these particles. Inhalation of these substances presents a special risk, because even insoluble forms of the elements may be trapped in the lungs. Discussion of this problem is beyond the scope of this review, but all cases of suspected inhalation or ingestion of radionuclides should be referred to appropriate specialists immediately for treatment designed to remove as much of the substances as possible prior to their fixation or distribution within the body.

Effects of Local Irradiation. There is suggestive evidence that whole-body irradiation may shorten life span more than local radiation. Local radiation also causes serious effects, however. Such radiation in the range of 600 to 1000 rads to the eye may produce clinically significant cataracts. Elsewhere, degenerative changes in vascular beds may occur, associated with late parenchymal cell destruction. Atrophy of epithelial cells and dermal appendages in the skin is seen, though local areas of hypertrophy may also appear. Progressive fibrosis of the lungs with vascular sclerosis is reported. Arterionephrosclerosis with hypertension may follow local irradiation of the kidneys.

Late Effects of Whole-Body Radiation. The longevity of radiologists in the years prior to 1945 strongly suggests a life-shortening effect from prolonged exposure to relatively small doses of radiation, although this is difficult to establish conclusively. It appears likely, however, that the effects of even small doses of ionizing radiation may be expressed either in the individual, in the form of degenerative lesions or malignancies, or in future generations through the production of inheritable defects. Although germ cells are especially vulnerable to radiation, effects in somatic cells are also possible.

Radiation Carcinogenesis. Among early radiologists, skin cancers were an obvious hazard; the demonstration that leukemia was a late consequence of radiation exposure came much later. Osteosarcomas due to absorption and bone deposition of radium have been well documented, as have been thyroid adenocarcinomas following irradiation of the neck in childhood and lung tumors in uranium miners exposed to radium daughter products.

Whether a threshold dose for carcinogenic effects exists is open to question — a question which cannot, unfortunately, be answered unequivocally. It does seem clear, however, that unlike electromagnetic radiation of longer wavelengths and lower energies, ionizing radiation has no beneficial physiologic effects. For this reason, any preventable exposure to such radiation must be considered from the standpoint of the secondary benefits to be gained compared with the possible costs in terms of later physiopathology.

THE KINETIC ENVIRONMENT

In a previous section, we referred to man's mobility as one of the attributes that has made him what he is. In his constant attempts to master and control his environment, man has found mobility to be an absolute essential since earliest times. He cannot synthesize glucose from readily available simpler compounds; he must therefore search out plants which do so. He is puny, compared to some of the animal predators (including his fellow man), so he must be able to flee from them. He reproduces rapidly; crowding and his own desire to know the unknown have led him to explore his entire planet, and recently to go even beyond its confines.

Movement requires work — kinetic energy. To understand man with respect to his physical environment, we must understand how he is affected by force fields, either natural or of his own making. That is the purpose of this section. We shall first consider the effects of gravity and its absence, together with the effects of activity and inactivity. The effects of supragravitational force fields will be discussed. Thereafter, vibration and noise will be considered, for they are inevitable concomitants of an industrial society. Finally, we must discuss briefly man's responses to combinations of stresses, since he rarely encounters environmental stress in isolation.

Gravity

Man, and every other biologic organism on earth, has evolved under the constant influence of the acceleration of gravity, a force field which pulls us toward the earth's center of mass at roughly 32 ft. per sec.^{2} Each time man rises from the supine to the erect position, the column of blood within him is accelerated toward his feet; each time he raises his arms, the action is resisted. When he climbs a hill, he gains potential energy at the cost of an expenditure of roughly five times as much energy, for the human organism works at only about 20 per cent efficiency.

The constant pull of gravity has profound effects on a motile organism, and especially on one which normally extends itself to its full height. The column of blood in the venous reservoir is 5 to 6 feet high; there is, therefore, a gradient in pressure from the top to the bottom of that column of 5 to 6 feet of water, or about 120 mm. Hg. Were it not for the valves in our veins, this entire pressure would be exerted on the vessels in our lower legs whenever we are erect. The heart must supply the brain with blood at adequate perfusion pressures both when the body is supine and the hydrostatic column is horizontal, and when it is upright, with a hydrostatic column over a foot high.

Man has learned to cope with this situation, although not without cost to himself. One instance of this cost is varicose veins in the lower extremities, a serious and disfiguring problem for many. Stasis ulcers of the skin over the legs are another probably allied problem. More serious for some is postural hypotension, an inability to maintain adequate cardiac output and peripheral resistance in the upright position.

Even in those of us who can cope with sudden changes in position, fairly major physiologic responses are involved. When we assume the recumbent position for any period of time, venous return is improved. The volume receptors in the right atrium sense this, and a water diuresis results. Over a longer period of time, calcium mobilization and excretion lead to demineralization of bone. The muscles, especially the antigravity muscles, lose strength and mass. The smooth muscle in the walls of blood vessels may also lose tone and the capacity to respond to changes in posture.

All these changes make little difference — as long as we remain supine. If, however, we return to the erect posture, we find ourselves unable to cope with gravitational stress. Bed rest for prolonged periods robs man of many of his normal modes of coping with his environment.

Weightlessness. Bed rest is *not* weightlessness, although it is tempting to consider them together. As man began to explore the space above our atmosphere, medical support personnel began to worry about whether the deadaptive changes seen in prolonged recumbency would appear in astronauts, when the centrifugal accelerations involved in orbital flight exactly balanced the centripedal acceleration due to gravity. It has been found that many of the changes observed are indeed similar, though the data are far from conclusive. Man has thus far experienced weightlessness for over seven weeks. Bone densitometry has suggested that a degree of demineralization occurs; physical deconditioning with diminished exercise tolerance has been observed. Intolerance to upright tilt has in some cases been profound, though short-lived. Decreases in circulating red cell mass and plasma volume have been noted.

The importance of these and other related findings is still disputed. Some believe that prolonged weightlessness will have profound and dangerous effects on man; others feel that by two weeks of exposure, man begins to readapt despite his altered environment. One of the principal purposes of NASA's Skylab program, involving 28- and 56-day exposures, was to explore this matter further.

Little research has been done on man in supragravity force fields, in part because of the very elaborate equipment required. Smith and others have exposed animals, notably fowl, to long periods in strong gravitational fields. They find evidence of adaptation, notably in bone structure, antigravity muscle mass, and postural reflexes.

One of the major factors inhibiting research in this area is that weightlessness cannot be simulated on earth for more than a few seconds. To date, the best tool for such research has been suspension under water at neutral buoyancy in a pressurized space suit. This technique, however well it simulates the difficulties of moving and working in a zero-G field, has severe drawbacks for physiologic experimentation.

Physical Activity. It was noted above that prolonged bed rest causes a variety of deadaptive changes in the human organism. The fullest development of heat acclimatization requires both heat and physical work. The importance of physical activity in maintaining the adaptability of the human organism has become a popular topic of discussion in recent years; many easily available scientific and popular texts consider this topic in detail. It is necessary, however, that it receive at least brief consideration here as well.

Just as musculoskeletal inactivity causes disuse atrophy and skeletal demineralization, so the performance of musculoskeletal work produces, over a period of time, hypertrophy and increased capillarity of skeletal muscles, optimal mineralization of long bones, and a number of adaptive alterations in the heart and cardiovascular system, including greater cardiac volume and output per stroke, lower resting heart rates, greater work capacity, higher oxygen uptake during work (with consequent sparing of the less efficient anaerobic energy sources), and often an increased sense of well-being.

The induction of these changes requires that the organism be stressed repeatedly by the performance of strenuous physical work. A number of carefully controlled studies indicate that optimal cardiorespiratory fitness can better be achieved and maintained by relatively brief spurts of fairly intense exercise than by much longer periods of less intense exercise. It seems certain, however, that the maintenance of man's reserve capacity to deal with physiologic stress requires that man be stressed on a continuing basis; this truism is nowhere more clear than with respect to man's capacity to perform muscular work.

Prolonged Acceleration. Aircraft have freedom of motion in all spatial axes. As a result of this freedom, they are capable of accelerations, especially angular, which significantly displace or alter the magnitude of the apparent normal G vector. Detailed consideration of this field, in which much research has been done, is beyond the scope of this review. It will simply be said here that, as an instance, in a 60-degree banked turn in level flight an acceleration of twice normal gravity (2G) is imparted to the occupants of an aircraft. The acceleration in this case is parallel to the long axis of the body. Exactly the same acceleration may occur when an airplane pulls out of a dive into level flight or into a climb.

Since the net G vector is the same in both instances, the pilot or occupant may be unable to differentiate those two quite dissimilar situations unless he is provided with gyroscopic instruments to tell him what is occurring. The result is spatial disorientation, a common and dangerous problem in flight. If the natural horizon is not visible, the pilot must use instruments, which are not affected as are his semicircular canals and otoliths by angular and linear accelerations.

With respect to both orientation and cardiovascular physiology, prolonged linear and radial accelerations induce changes which may be adaptive or deadaptive. Several references are provided; standard texts cover these topics in detail.

Abrupt Accelerations; Impact

Whenever a body acquires momentum, it must dissipate that momentum to return to rest. Since momentum is the product of mass times velocity, the faster we go the more dangerous it becomes to stop abruptly.

Any consideration of the effects of impact upon man must take into account the rate of onset of the decelerative impulse, the peak magnitude of the deceleration, its duration, the orientation of the man with respect to the force field, and the nature of any protective equipment and of the environment around him.

The average magnitude of an impact may be simply estimated in terms of the initial velocity, the final velocity (usually zero), and the distance over which the vehicle or man came to rest. The deceleration thus derived is usually expressed as a ratio, the denominator of which is the acceleration due to gravity. Figure 33–5 shows a variety of deceleration and impact experiences in terms of initial velocity and stopping distance. Body orientation differs in these experiences; the approximate survival limits shown must be interpreted cautiously.

Tolerance limits depend to a considerable extent on the peak acceleration during an impact. Peak transverse accelerations of 100 to 200 G for 0.01 second are tolerated without injury, whereas only 20 to 30 G can be tolerated for 1 second. The duration of an applied acceleration determines whether the body acts as a rigid, or a viscoelastic, object. During accelerations or decelerations longer than 0.05 to 0.10 sec., the internal organs and blood are significantly affected; physiologic adaptations begin to occur.

Tolerance for vertical or longitudinal impact is substantially less than for transverse (anteroposterior) forces. The outcome of such an impact depends to a considerable extent on whether one's knees are locked or are allowed to flex (thus increasing the distance over which the trunk is decelerated).

Following moderate transverse impacts (15 to 25 G with onset rates from 400 to 1000 G per sec.), a number of transient physiologic changes are seen

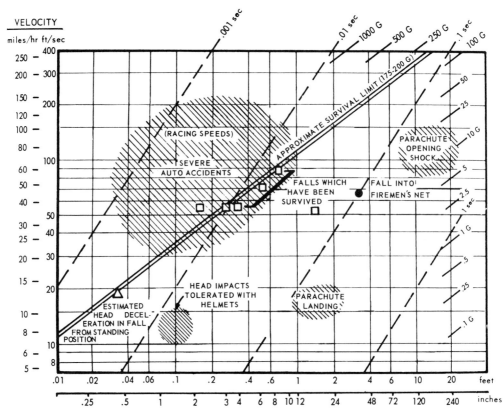

Figure 33–5 This figure brings together a variety of impact and deceleration experiences by plotting the data from a number of sources on the common axes of deceleration distance and velocity. Stopping time and impact force in G units are shown as secondary scales. The data points with hollow squares are for free falls of 50 to 150 ft. with survival. The line labeled "approximate survival limit" must be used with caution, since many biophysical factors influence the injury due to deceleration (From Parker, J. F., and West, V. R. (eds.): Bioastronautics Data Book, 2nd ed. U. S. Government Printing Office, Washington, D.C., 1973.)

in subjects who are free from structural damage. These include hypotension, bradycardia (a vagal effect which is blocked by atropine), transient neurologic changes, changes in blood platelets, psychologic changes, and generalized stress reactions. These effects must be taken into account when evaluating the condition of persons involved in auto accidents.

It should be pointed out here that in auto crashes, the most serious injuries are usually caused by a secondary impact of occupants with steering wheel, interior structure, windshield, or objects in the vicinity, if the occupants are ejected from the vehicle. Adequate restraint systems are now available in new automobiles; the decline in fatalities and in the number and severity of injuries which would result from their universal use would be startling. While auto manufacturers, prodded by new federal standards, have made considerable strides in delethalizing interiors, the simplest way to avoid injury from impacting vehicle parts is not to contact them; there is no substitute for an adequate restraint system in this regard.

Vibration

Vibration may be thought of as repeated brief accelerations; these may be sinusoidal or random in character and may be applied to a part of the body (as when vibrating hand tools are used) or to the whole body.

Human responses to vibration depend to a considerable extent upon the frequency of the vibration with respect to the resonant frequencies of various body organs. All studies of whole-body vibration show a sharp decrease in voluntary tolerance at frequencies of 4 to 7 cycles per sec. owing to resonance of the abdominal organs, as an instance.

G forces during vibration are a function of frequency and amplitude of the applied acceleration. The amplitude of the seat or platform, however, is usually damped considerably by the body. Head movement, for instance, is usually very much less than seat movement.

Limits of voluntary tolerance for longitudinal vibration in the seated position are from 0.1 to 0.4 G at frequencies of 1 to 40 cycles per sec. Minor injury begins to occur at levels of 2 to 5 G, depending on exposure time. Such injuries are the result of mechanical deformation and shear forces upon adjacent tissues of differing densities and masses.

A different sort of injury pattern is seen in some workers whose jobs involve prolonged contact with vibrating hand tools. After a variable period of exposure, usually in cold environments, a proportion of these workers will begin to show vascular changes in the hands, with vascular spasm typical of Raynaud's phenomenon. It is not certain whether the changes seen in the arteries are primary or secondary to nerve injury, but considerable thickening of arterial walls has been demonstrated. The disorder is disabling, since once present, it is exacerbated by exposure of the individual or of his hand to cold, as well as to vibration.

Noise

The human ear, like the eye, has an enormous tolerance for cyclic pressure changes which reach the eardrum through the air. The auditory threshold in normal young persons is in the neighborhood of 10^{-4} dynes per cm.^{2}; the ear can tolerate sound pressure levels as high as 10^3 dynes per cm.^{2} In contemporary society, however, much louder sound pressure levels are produced by certain machines and by explosives; these sounds and others of lesser magnitude for longer periods of exposure can cause harm. Both acute dysfunction and chronic damage of the very sensitive auditory mechanism result from exposure to high sound pressure levels.

Because of the very wide range of pressures to which the ear can respond, it is conventional to express sound pressure levels in decibels (dB) relative to the threshold of hearing. Figure 33–6 shows the overall SPLs of a variety of common environmental sources of sound.

The frequency spectrum to which the normal ear responds is roughly 30 to 12,000 cycles per second (hertz). Since sounds containing substantial proportions of high-frequency energy are somewhat more injurious than predominantly low-frequency sounds, it is necessary to evaluate the sound environment in terms of its frequency components as well as its overall sound pressure levels.

Noise has been defined as "unwanted sound." It has become common practice, therefore, to talk of "noisy environments" and of "the effects of noise." It will be immediately obvious to those who have been exposed to rock-and-roll music in close quarters that one man's sound may be another's noise. However, the damage caused by sound, or noise, is a function of its energy content, not its information content.

Intense sound (SPL greater than 85 to 95 dB) causes, after a period of exposure, an upward shift in auditory thresholds for pure tones. If sound exposure is terminated or interrupted, this "temporary threshold shift" disappears over a period of hours or a few days and auditory acuity again becomes normal. The exact physiologic nature of this phenomenon is not known, though it appears to be an end-organ rather than a central response. Regardless of the frequency content of the sound which induces the temporary shift, the shift itself is seen earliest and to the greatest degrees in range of frequencies between 1500 and 4000 Hz.

If exposures to sound pressure levels of this magnitude are continued over a long time period, a gradual permanent threshold shift occurs. The rate of onset and magnitude of this shift vary considerably, but they are roughly proportional to the intensity of the sound to which persons are exposed. Fairly good normative data are available for continuous noise exposure; the effects of exposure to impulse noise are less well understood.

The permanent threshold shift (which may have a further temporary shift superimposed upon it) represents true neural deafness and is irreversible. It results from degeneration of the sensory cells in the organ of Corti. Deafness from noise exposure may be difficult to differentiate from presbycusis, the usual decrease in auditory acuity seen in older people, since both forms cause greater deficits in acuity for tones of high frequencies (4000 to 12,000 Hz). Indeed, some have argued that presbycusis itself is induced by exposure to high sound pressures over a lifetime. (This may be true in part, but it is probably not a full explanation; genetic factors are certainly involved).

Temporary deafness of a different sort results from obstruction in the external ear canal (water or cerumen), from fluid in the middle ear due to barotitis, or from a ruptured tympanic membrane. Although the human tympanum is very resistant to rupture, an explosive blast or very high pressure differential across the drum may cause traumatic rupture. The lesion is self-limiting, and spontaneous healing ordinarily occurs within a

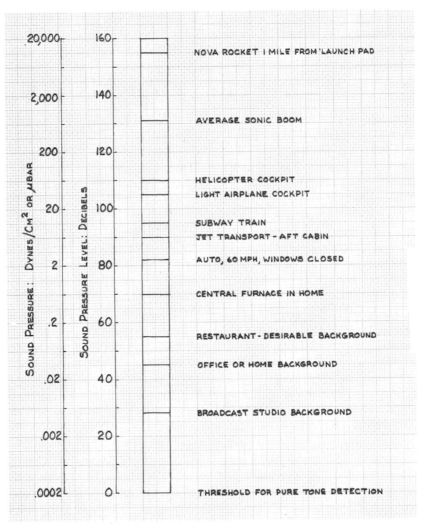

Figure 33–6 Range of auditory sensitivity showing sound pressure levels generated by various sources.

few days. Repeated episodes of serous otitis media, however, may cause thickening of the eardrum, with damping of its motion and loss of elasticity. The threshold shift seen in such cases tends to be roughly uniform across low and high frequencies. A similar picture is seen in otosclerosis. Such hearing losses are characteristic of conductive, as opposed to neural, or perceptive, deafness and are sometimes amenable to medical or surgical treatment.

Ultrasound

Mechanical vibrations with frequencies above about 15,000 Hz are not detected by the human ear; such waves therefore are called ultrasonic. As frequency increases, propagation through air de-

creases; extremely high ultrasonic vibrations are readily transmitted only by relatively incompressible (liquid or solid) materials. The energy contained in such waves can, however, be converted to thermal energy in the tissues; this is the basis of continuous output ultrasonic diathermy units. Alternatively, again by proper selection of frequencies and with use of a pulsed wave transmitter and receiver, ultrasound can be used to visualize tissue discontinuities within the body. It is used, for instance, to determine the location of the placenta prior to amniocentesis. The power outputs used in such studies are not hazardous. It has also been suggested that changes in cell membrane permeability can be induced by ultrasound without destruction or denaturation of cell proteins.

COMBINED STRESSES

In this brief review of man's responses to his physical environment, most of our discussion has dealt with the effects of single stressors. No such discussion can be complete, however, if it does not emphasize that man rarely encounters these stressors in isolation. We normally live and work and play in the presence of a great variety of physical, chemical, biologic, and sociocultural stressors, some antagonistic, others additive or synergistic. Indeed, we know from sensory deprivation experiments that too little stress may be at least as damaging to man as too much stress, that man functions best in a fairly rich environment.

The aluminum foundry worker must perform strenuous work in the face of often severe thermal stress; the mountain climber must exert himself while affected by both hypoxia and cold. Operators of heavy equipment are exposed to high levels of noise and vibration under a wide range of climatic conditions. Each of these persons is working under the influence as well of biologic and socioeconomic factors which may or may not impose additional stress upon him.

In dealing with disorders caused by environmental stresses, the physician must keep in mind the pathologic physiology of these disorders if his therapeutic efforts are to be effective. The person who performs muscular work in a hot environment must share his cardiac output between his working muscles, which depend on the blood for oxygen, and his skin, to which heat is carried from the core by blood. These two stresses therefore are additive with respect to their physiologic demands. Their combined effects are multiplied when fluid must be expended for evaporative cooling, reducing the plasma volume.

Many other examples could be cited; the important point is simply that such problems as these are amenable to rational treatment aimed at restoring the body to its normal homeostatic condition, or at supporting the patient until he can again adapt to stress. This is the essence of environmental medicine once injury has occurred. The same reasoning, however, based on knowledge of physiology, can as easily be applied to the prevention of such injuries. Herein lie our most stimulating challenges in the field of environmental health.

REFERENCES

Literature concerning this broad area of study is widely spread among journals devoted to medicine, physiology, psychology, and engineering. There are a few publications in which reports relating to a variety of environmental stressors are gathered together. Because of their particular value, they are listed here; individual reports follow in alphabetical order.

Bedwell, T. C., and Strughold, H. (Eds.): Bioastronautics and the Exploration of Space. Available from Clearinghouse for Federal Scientific and Technical Information, Springfield, Virginia, 1965.

Bennett, P. B., and Elliott, D. H.: The Physiology and Medicine of Diving and Compressed Air Work. Williams and Wilkins Co., Baltimore, 1969.

Dill, D. B. (Ed.): Handbook of Physiology. Section 4, Adaptation to the Environment. American Physiological Society, Washington, D.C., 1964.

Lambertsen, C. J. (Ed.): Proceedings of the Third Symposium on Underwater Physiology. Williams and Wilkins Co., Baltimore, 1967.

Lambertsen, C. J. (Ed.): Proceedings of the Fourth Symposium on Underwater Physiology. Academic Press, New York, 1971.

Lambertson, C. J., (Ed.): Proceedings of the Fifth Symposium on Underwater Physiology. Bethesda, Md.: Federated American Societies for Experimental Biology, 1975.

Leithead, C. S., and Lind, A. R.: Heat Stress and Heat Disorders. F. A. Davis Co., Philadelphia, 1964.

McFarland, A.: Human Factors in Air Transportation. New York, McGraw-Hill Book Co., 1953.

Randel, H. W. (ed.): Aerospace Medicine, 2nd ed. Williams and Wilkins Co., Baltimore, 1971.

Parker, J. F., Jr., and West, V. R. (Eds.): Bioastronautics Data Book. 2nd ed. NASA SP–3006. U.S. Government Printing Office, Washington, D.C., 1973.

Allen, S. C.: A comparison of the effects of nitrogen lack and hyperoxia on the vascular development of the chick embryo. Aerospace Med. 34:897, 1963.

Anonymous: Radiation Induced Cancer. Proceedings Series. International Atomic Energy Agency, Vienna, Austria, 1969.

Bartleson, C. J.: Retinal burns from intense light sources. Am. Industr. Hyg. Assoc. J., 29:415, 1968.

Bass, D. E., Kleeman, R., Quinn, M., Henschel, A., and Hegnauer, H.: Mechanisms of acclimatization to heat in man. Medicine, 34:323, 1955.

Billings, C. E., Brashear, R. E., Bason, R., and Mathews, D. K.: Medical observations during 20 days at 3800 meters. Arch. Environ. Health, 18:987, 1969.

Boerema, I., et al. (Eds.): Clinical Applications of Hyperbaric Oxygen. Elsevier Publishing Co., Amsterdam, 1964.

Burton, A. C. and Edholm, O. G.: Man in a Cold Environment. Edward Arnold, London, 1955.

Clark, J. M., and Lambertsen, C. J.: Pulmonary oxygen toxicity: A review. Pharmacol. Rev., 23:37, 1971.

Cogan, D. G.: Lesions of the eye from radiant energy. J.A.M.A., 142:145, 1950.

DiGiovanni, C., Jr., and Chambers, R. M.: Physiologic and psychologic aspects of the gravity spectrum. N. Engl. J. Med., 270:35, 88, 134; 1964.

Fenn, W. O.: Possible role of hydrostatic pressure in diving. In Lambertsen, C. J. (Ed.): Underwater Physiology. Williams and Wilkins Co., Baltimore, 1967.

Folk, G. E., Jr.: Introduction to Environmental Physiology: Environmental Extremes and Mammalian Survival. Lea and Febiger, Philadelphia, 1966.

Fox, R. H., Goldsmith, R., Hampton, I. F. G., and Hunt, J. J.: Heat acclimatization by controlled hyperthermia in hot-dry and hot-wet climates. J. Appl. Physiol., 22:39, 1967.

Fox, R. H., Goldsmith, R., Kidd, D. J., and Lewis, H. E.: Acclimatization to heat in man by controlled elevation of body temperature. J. Physiol., 166:530, 1963.

Fryer, D. I.: Subatmospheric Decompression Sickness in Man. Slough, England, Technivision Services, 1969.

Gauer, O. H. and Zuidema, G. D.: Gravitational Stress in Aerospace Medicine. Little, Brown & Co., Boston, 1961.

Glorig, A., Ward, W. D., and Nixon, J.: Damage risk criteria and noise-induced hearing loss. Arch. Otolaryngol., *74*:413, 1961.

Hopps, J. A.: The electric shock hazard in hospitals. Canad. Med. Assoc. J., *98*:1002, 1968.

Howath, S. M. (Ed.): Cold Injury. Transactions of the Sixth Conference, Josiah Macy, Jr., Foundation, New York, 1960.

Hultgren, H. N., Spickard, W., and Lopez, C.: Further studies of high-altitude pulmonary oedema. Brit. Heart J., *24*:95, 1962.

International Commission on Radiological Protection: The Evaluation of Risks from Radiation. ICRP Publication No. 8. Pergamon Press, Oxford, 1966.

Kryter, K. D.: The Effects of Noise on Man. Academic Press, New York, 1970.

Largent, E. J. and Ashe, W. F.: Upper limits of thermal stress for workmen. Am. Industr. Hyg. Assoc. J., *19*:246, 1958.

Levi, L. (Ed.): Emotional Stress. American Elsevier Publishing Co., New York, 1967.

Lichter, I., Borrie, J., and Miller, W. M.: Radio-frequency hazards with cardiac pacemakers. Br. Med. J., *1*:1513, 1965.

Linder, G. S.: Mechanical vibration effects on human beings. Aerospace Med., *33*:939, 1962.

Margaria, R.: Exercise at Altitude. Excerpta Medica Foundation, New York, 1967.

Mathews, D. K., Stacy, R. W., and Hoover, G. N.: Physiology of Muscular Activity and Exercise. Ronald Press, New York, 1964.

McCally, M., and Graveline, D. E.: Physiologic aspects of prolonged weightlessness. N. Engl. J. Med., *269*:508, 1963.

Menon, N. D.: High-altitude edema. N. Engl. J. Med., *273*:66, 1965.

Peyton, M. F. (Ed.): Biological Effects of Microwave Radiation, Vol. I. Plenum Press, New York, 1961.

Roy, S.: Acute mountain sickness in Himalayan terrain. *In* Hegnauer, A. H. (ed.): Biomedicine of High Terrestrial Elevations. U.S. Army Medical Research and Development Command, Washington, D.C., January, 1969.

Sacq, Z. M., and Alexander, P. A.: Fundamentals of Radiobiology. Pergamon Press, Oxford, 1961.

Schaefer, K. E., et al.: Pulmonary and circulatory adjustments determining the limits of depth in breathhold diving. Science, *162*:1020, 1968.

Saenger, E. L. (Ed.): Medical Aspects of Radiation Accidents. A Handbook for Physicians, Health Physicists and Industrial Hygienists. U.S. Atomic Energy Commission, 1963.

Sugimoto, T., Schall, S. F., and Wallace, A. G.: Factors determining vulnerability to ventricular fibrillation induced by 60–CPS alternating current. Circ. Res., *21*:601, 1967.

Webb, P.: Body heat loss in undersea gaseous environment. Aerospace Med., *41*:1283, 1970.

Weisel, T. N.: Effects of monocular deprivation on the cat's visual cortex. Trans. Am. Acad. Ophthal. Otolaryng., *75*:1186, 1971.

Wood, J. E. and Bass, D. E.: Thermoregulatory and circulatory adjustments during acclimatization to heat in man. J. Clin. Invest., *39*:825, 1960.

34

Chemical Agents and Disease

EDMUND B. FLINK, AND ANANDA S. PRASAD

INTRODUCTION

All biologic processes are dependent on chemical reactions. All living cells contain bundles of innumerable enzymes supported in an orderly arrangement by a chemical skeleton appropriate for the function of an organelle or of the whole cell. For optimal function of all the enzymes in the cells, the physical and chemical architecture must be correct. If one enzyme system is disturbed by a toxic substance, its reaction may be blocked or its equilibrium accelerated or delayed. Such disturbance can cripple or destroy the cell and organism. Many toxic chemicals have profound effects which are grossly evident, but the precise metabolic targets (enzyme or enzyme sequence) may not be known. Adverse effects can be classified in five groups: (1) irritant, caustic or corrosive, e.g., $HgCl_2$ or "corrosive sublimate" on oral and gastrointestinal mucosa; (2) specific toxicologic reactions, e.g., botulinus toxin on nerve terminals in muscle; (3) mutagenic reactions, e.g., x-ray and radioactive nuclides; (4) carcinogenic reactions, e.g., B-naphtylamine, 1,2 benzanthracene, cresols, butter yellow, methyl cholanthrene, arsenic and thorium dioxide; and (5) teratogenic reactions, e.g., thalidomide causing phocomelia and alcohol causing the fetal alcohol syndrome.

ROUTE OF ADMINISTRATION OR EXPOSURE

Unique properties of chemicals as well as the anatomic site of exposure determine the reaction to a given chemical. The chemical agent may gain access to the internal milieu by various routes. Most agents must penetrate the cells to do damage; however, they may affect the cell membrane so that its protective action is disrupted. The cell wall has a double-layered lipoprotein structure with each layer 35 to 50 Å units in thickness. Interaction with the cell membrane depends on both physical and chemical properties, whereas penetration of the cell membrane may be dependent on diffusion, e.g., gases, pinocytosis or phagocytosis of liquid and particulate matter.

The Percutaneous Route

Percutaneous absorption through intact skin depends on the lipid solubility of the chemical. The skin acts as a natural barrier to water-soluble (polar) compounds. This barrier is changed by lipid solvents such as methanol, ethanol, hexane, acetone, or a mixture of chloroform-methanol (2:1), which cause a marked alteration in skin permeability. DDT, carbon tetrachloride, analine, phenol and its derivatives, gasoline, kerosene, tetraethyl lead, steroid hormones, and vitamins D and K can be absorbed through the skin. Petroleum products and especially tetraethyl lead can cause serious chronic toxicity by absorption through the skin. Denuded surfaces such as burns or open wounds bypass the lipid skin barrier and permit absorption of polar compounds, so that an extensive burn can be the portal of entry for drugs applied to the area, e.g., sulfonamides and antibiotics.

The Respiratory Route

The lungs serve as the route of absorption of many important drugs such as inhalation anesthetics. For some compounds, such as the two odorless gases, carbon monoxide and nitrous oxide, lethal intoxication occurs only via the lungs. Water soluble chemicals such as NH_3, chlorine and HCl (gas) can be tolerated in small concentration by the "scrubbing" action of the upper respiratory passages, but, in large concentrations, these penetrate to cause severe irritation of the lungs with serious or fatal pulmonary edema. Under ordinary urban conditions, air pollution with carbon monoxide, sulfur dioxide, oxides of nitrogen, and fly ash is no real threat to human life. Under abnormal atmospheric conditions, such as has occurred in several well-publicized disasters at Donora, Pennsylvania, and London, England, concentration of pollutants has resulted in many deaths, particularly among the elderly and those with pulmonary or cardiovascular disease.

Pneumoconioses emphasize the specificity and uniqueness of reactions to noxious stimuli. Particulate matter of appropriate size and physical state carried in the air in industrial situations of mining, sand blasting, stone polishing, and cotton milling can cause serious damage to lungs. Particles from 0.5 to 5.0 μ in diameter are capable of reaching alveoli and may be deposited in phagocytes. Reactions vary with both the physical and chemical nature of the particle. Crystalline silicon dioxide is fibrogenic, but amorphous silicates are not. Asbestos fibers are inelastic and produce serious fibrotic changes, but Fiberglas particles of same size are elastic and deformable and do not cause a parenchymal reaction. Asbestos is also a serious carcinogen in the respiratory tract. Silicosis provides an excellent example that the severity of a chronic illness depends on time and intensity of exposure. Massive exposure can cause fatal pulmonary insufficiency in a few months, as in the Gaulley Bridge (West Virginia) disaster in 1931, whereas minor exposure over many years will produce some silicotic lung reaction but no pulmonary insufficiency.

The Oral Route

Toxic reactions may result from ingestion of appropriate drugs in excessive dose, allergic or hypersensitive responses to accepted dose levels, and the ingestion of chemicals not intended for human consumption, such as accidental ingestion of heavy metals. Foods and beverages may be contaminated with organic mercury compounds, arsenic, cadmium, and lead. Ingestion of lead oxide paint chips (pica) from old houses by young children in urban areas poses one of the more important environmental hazards in our society. In New York City alone, there were 4000 new cases of lead poisoning in 1970 and 1971.

Most ingested chemicals are absorbed by the small intestine, but some, such as alcohol and nitroglycerin, are absorbed also from the mouth and stomach. Slowing of small intestinal motility, particularly after hypnotic drugs, may result in sequestration and extended absorption with prolonged and fluctuating coma (e.g., glutethimide). Many chemicals are fat-soluble and may be stored in fat, permitting cumulative toxicity. This concentration effect can be a source of human intoxication by the ingestion of meat (fat) of animals chronically exposed to DDT, for instance.

Many ingested chemicals are detoxified by the liver. Detoxification begins with oxidation or reduction on the first passage. Certain chemicals are made more toxic by biotransformation. Nevertheless, most chemicals which are completely absorbed are less toxic after an oral dose than those given by the parenteral route in similar doses.

Parenteral Route

Toxic reactions can occur following subcutaneous, intramuscular, intravenous, and intraperitoneal administration. Increase in illicit drug use has broadened the opportunities for exposure. Reactions may take many forms. There may be an unexpected sensitivity to an accepted dose or deliberate or accidental overdose. Intravenously administered medication may result in achieving peak blood levels almost instantaneously. Unless there is an antidote, the only way of ameliorating toxic reactions after parenteral administration is by elimination of the chemical via renal excretion, hepatic detoxification, or dialysis.

BIOLOGIC COMPLEXITY OF TOXIC REACTIONS

The toxicity of chemical agents is multifaceted. Some agents are tremendously useful therapeutically at appropriate dosage levels but can cause serious toxic and lethal effects with small increases. An excellent example is digitalis and its derivatives. Digitalis affects both the contractibility and rhythmicity of the failing heart in a very beneficial way at appropriate doses, but just twice this ideal dose can cause serious and often fatal arrhythmia. Many drugs share this kind of critical dosage consideration. Even glucose can be rendered toxic by causing hyperglycemia, polyuria, dehydration, and ketoacidosis in a totally insulin-deficient person.

This complexity is also illustrated by the importance of dose in relation to time. An example is lead poisoning. A relatively large single dose is tolerated without serious or fatal result, but a much smaller dose repeated over months accumulates and *can* cause serious or fatal intoxication.

Certain toxic chemicals produce reactions that are unique and highly specific. Two examples are cyanide and carbon monoxide. Cyanide poisons heme-containing enzymes, particularly cytochrome A_3, in all cells and causes death quickly by blocking the electron transport system. Carbon monoxide causes tissue anoxia by displacing oxygen from the hemoglobin molecules and also by shifting the oxygen dissociation curve for remaining oxygenated hemoglobin so oxygen is not released normally. Carbon monoxide has an affinity for hemoglobin 240 times greater than that of oxygen.

Some chemicals have a high degree of affinity for certain organs such as carbon tetrachloride (CCl_4) and dichloromethane for the liver. Many combinations of chemicals are not only additive but actually synergistic. Moderate doses of CCl_4 inhaled or ingested, particularly by a person also taking alcohol, result in serious renal insufficiency as well as liver damage.

GENETIC FACTORS AND CHEMICAL TOXICITY

Genetically determined serious toxic reactions to usual doses of commonly used drugs (e.g., sulfonamide) or usual servings of a food (e.g., fava bean) are examples of the exquisite sensitivity and specificity of toxic reactions. Four genetically determined sensitivities are illustrated below.

Glucose 6 Phosphate Dehydrogenase (G6PD) Deficiency: An X-Linked Phenomenon

Aging red cells are hemolyzed first. G6PD is involved at the beginning of the hexose monophosphate shunt (HMP) and results in an increase in nicotine adenine dinucleotide phosphate (NADP) and consequently in reduced glutathione (GSH) (see Fig. 34–1). This sequence helps resist oxidant stresses of fava beans, primaquine, quinine, aspirin, and phenacetin in large doses, the nitrofurans, sulfones, many sulfonamides, para-aminosalicylic acid, probenecid, quinidine, phenylhydrazine, water-soluble analogues of vitamin K, and naphthalene. The severity of the stress varies with the drug and the dose as well as genetic state, whether homozygous or heterozygous. G6PD deficiency occurs in 10 per cent of American blacks and 8 to 20 per cent of West African blacks, but in only 2 per cent of South African Bantus and virtually no Caucasians other than

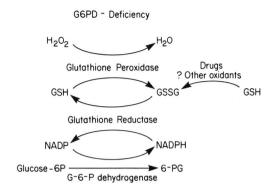

Wintrobe, M.M., Clinical Hematology, 7th Edition, Lea & Febiger, Phil, 1974, P. 104

Figure 34–1 The biochemical interactions of G6PD and glutathione metabolism are shown here. (From Wintrobe, M. M.: Clinical Hematology, 7th ed. Lea & Febiger, Philadelphia, 1974, p. 104.)

some of Mediterranean descent who suffer from favism. Eating the bean or inhaling pollen of the broad bean *Vicia fava* causes *favism* — an acute hemolytic anemia due to G6PD deficiency. This occurs in Caucasians only, mostly in Greeks, Italians, Kurdish Jews, and Sardinians. G6PD deficiency may be beneficial in blacks in affording some protection against falciparum malaria.

The unstable hemoglobins Zurich, Shepherd's Bush, and Torino spontaneously form methemoglobin, and hemolysis can be produced by all the drugs listed under G6PD deficiency. There is a defect in the hemoglobin molecule which then resists oxidant stresses poorly.

Isoniazid (INH) and Deficiency of N-Acetyltransferase

Toxicity of INH, a drug of great importance in control of tuberculosis, is related to rate of inactivation by acetylation and excretion. "Rapid inactivators" have an enzyme in the liver which acetylates INH and, therefore, hastens formation of acetyl INH. "Slow inactivators" will form acetyl INH but do so slowly. Toxicity of INH occurs primarily in the rapid inactivators. Ability to acetylate is inherited as an autosomal recessive trait. Adjustment of dose and careful surveillance are indicated in patients treated with INH to avoid toxic accumulation.

Succinylcholine Susceptibility

Succinylcholine is a tremendously useful short-acting muscle relaxant employed during anesthesia. Acetylcholinesterase rapidly inactivates the drug. About 1 in 3000 persons is affected with the trait of acetylcholinesterase deficiency. With failure of inactivation of the muscle relaxant, prolonged apnea results. The setting of anesthesia permits appropriate ventilatory assistance and the apnea is rarely fatal. Nevertheless, family members should be warned to inform their doctor about this defect so that this drug will not be used during anesthesia for any operation.

Malignant Hyperthermia

Approximately 1 in 20,000 persons reacts to the anesthetics, halothane, Fluothane, methoxyflurane, and the relaxant succinylcholine with fatal hyperthermia. This is familial, and other family members must be warned. Treatment of the patient after the reaction is initiated is totally ineffective, and the mortality rate is high.

The above genetic variants illustrate the spectacular success of science in defining precise chemical reactions. Obviously none of these defects (with the possible exception of favism) could have been found if reactions had not occurred to potent and very useful drugs introduced in the last 40 years. Undoubtedly there are many other similar enzyme deficits which are causing adverse reactions. The only way further discoveries can be made is to carry on a careful surveillance with information about family, race, grouping of unusual or unexpected reactions, etc. Many reactions now considered to be "idiosyncratic" may well have a genetic basis. Hypersensitivity reactions of allergic nature are dealt with elsewhere in Chapter 18.

ENVIRONMENT

During the past century the environment has become contaminated by a large number of pollutants as a result of the industrial growth. Emissions from chimneys and automobile exhausts pollute the air with sulfur dioxide, oxides of nitrogen, carbon monoxide, chlorides, ammonia, and dust. Sewage from industrial plants has killed aquatic life and made many rivers not fit sources for water for domestic use. Industrial accidents result in massive spills of chemicals, such as carbon tetrachloride into streams. Transportation of toxic chemicals by truck or train may result in serious acute local air pollution with lethal or serious concentrations of gases, such as chlorine. Chemical additives to food represent a threat to all of us. Butter yellow is a classic example which was removed years ago. The U.S. Food and Drug Adminstration maintains a constant surveillance of such problems.

The home environment poses many serious hazards. Children under five are victims of careless storage and failure to seal containers of toxic chemicals, such as caustic soda, liquid drain cleaner, cleaning fluids such as ammonia and carbon tetrachloride, and drugs such as aspirin, acetaminophen, and a whole spectrum of prescription drugs from ferrous sulfate to tricyclic antidepressants. Adults may deliberately take an overdose of any drug. Alcohol is universally available and is the single most important lethal chemical in our society. Its acute effects can cause violent behavior, coma and death, or fatal automobile accidents (50 per cent of fatal automobile accidents are alcohol-related). Its chronic effects result in prolonged serious illnesses and ultimately death. Cigarette smoking causes contamination of one's personal environment by inhaled nicotine, carbon monoxide, and tars, resulting in accelerated atherosclerosis of all arteries, pulmonary insufficiency, and cancer of the respiratory tract. Cigarette smoking is an excellent example of the equation, dose $\times$ time = cumulative toxicity.

Important toxic chemical reactions will be discussed in the remainder of the chapter to illustrate the pathophysiology of specific intoxications. The importance of accidental or deliberate poisoning is clearly apparent from the data for 1972 reported to the National Clearinghouse for Poison Information Center. There were 105,018 incidents in children under five and a total of 160,824 in all ages. Medicines alone accounted for 47,625 incidents and of these 8146 were due to aspirin in the under-five age group. An overwhelming preponderance of accidental ingestion of cleaning and polishing agents, petroleum products, cosmetics, pesticides, turpentine and paints, plants, and miscellaneous agents is recorded in the under-five age group. The mortality rate is high. These deaths are preventable.

In the New York Hospital during a four-year period (1969–1973) the order of frequency of severe drug overdose was as follows: alcohol, barbiturates or glutethimide, heroin or methadone, methaqualone, meprobamate, scopolamine, amphetamine, imipramine, lithium, salicylates, phenothiazines, diphenylhydantoin, dicumarol, coumadin, tolbutamide, phenformin, and insulin. This order does not apply to the fatality rate.

In the United States, 80 to 90 per cent of chemical-induced deaths in adults involved only four groups of agents: barbiturates and narcotics, carbon monoxide, salicylates, and alcohol. In 1968, in New York City alone, there were 1205 deaths from narcotic abuse. Because of these data, the pathophysiology and possible antidotes for common intoxications will be discussed. Prevention of deaths and injuries of innocent children must have a high priority in medicine. Prevention of accidents by proper labeling and storage also has a high priority.

All favorable and unfavorable chemical reactions are specific, time-related, dose-related from undetectable to toxic and lethal, and often genetically modified or variable depending on host factors not clearly genetic.

In the clinical setting, it is important to have available an up-to-date detailed data base on all known toxic substances in a retrievable form at the Poison Control Center for the geographic area. For quick reference, the current Physicians' Desk Reference is useful. A different set of rules applies to each chemical agent. It is necessary that each physician know how to have access to the information. A corollary of this is the absolute need to get precise information about the chemical agents taken, the amount, and the route. The label on the bottle of drug or chemical is the most reliable source of information, so it is vitally important to obtain the container. Because of their overwhelming importance, certain of the toxins (alcohol, aspirin, barbiturates, opiates, carbon monoxide, and acetaminophen) will be discussed in some detail, emphasizing the features of early toxic reaction. Table 34–1 at the end of this chapter gives some basic information about a number of toxic chemicals and naturally occurring poisons.

Salicylates

Salicylate intoxication is a leading cause of death in children under five. Aspirin or methyl salicylate are ingested because "children's" aspirin tastes like candy or because the odor of methyl salicylate is enticing if these compounds are left in unsafe containers within reach of young children. Infants can be intoxicated by inadvertent therapeutic overdosage because of unfamiliarity with the appropriate dose. Suicide attempts in adolescents or young adults also account for a number of serious or fatal poisonings.

Hyperventilation is the most characteristic manifestation, but delirium, hallucinations, convulsions, coma, and profound shock are also signs of severe intoxication. Chemically, there is, at first, a marked respiratory alkalosis because of stimulation of the respiratory center by salicylates. This changes imperceptibly to metabolic acidosis after a few hours. Arterial blood pH must be determined at regular intervals, since clinical differentiation of respiratory alkalosis and metabolic acidosis is difficult without pH determination. Salicylates act as a general metabolic stimulant capable of uncoupling oxidative phosphorylation with an increase of CO_2 production. There is interference with normal metabolism of carbohydrates and lipids such that ketone bodies and other organic acids accumulate. Toxic levels of salicylate lower brain glucose concentration in the face of normal plasma glucose. Brain edema can occur because of depletion of brain glucose, causing uncal herniation and sudden death. Furthermore, salicylates interfere with normal renal handling of ketones and other metabolic acids. Salicylate excretion is accelerated by alkalizing the urine by administration of acetazolamide and sodium bicarbonate. Giving sodium bicarbonate alone may not adequately increase the pH of the urine.

The determination of salicylate level is of great importance because a level over 100 mg./dl. at zero time (levels can be projected to zero time from a nomogram by Done) is a very serious prognostic sign. Semiquantitative determination of salicylates in the blood can be made by using "Phenstix" and referring to a color chart with a "small reaction" indicating 25 to 50 mg./dl. or a "large reaction" indicating 150 mg./dl. or more. Ferric chloride (10 per cent) solution is useful in detecting the presence of salicylate in the urine. $FeCl_3$ reacts with salicylates, resulting in a burgundy red color which is not changed by boiling the urine (acetoacetic acid also gives this color, but acetoacetic acid is volatile and disappears on boiling the urine).

In summary, salicylates have a striking and characteristic effect on metabolism, beginning with respiratory alkalosis and changing to metabolic acidosis. Severe intoxication results in serious cerebral and systemic effects, coma, and death. Treatment includes hydration, induction of vomiting, or intubation and lavage (if seen within four hours), potassium administration, monitoring of salicylate level and arterial pH, and alkalinizing urine using acetazolamide and sodium bicarbonate. General supportive measures for circulation and respiration are obviously needed, as in any serious intoxication. Vitamin K is needed to counteract the prothrombin deficiency regularly produced by salicylates. Exchange transfusion for infants, peritoneal dialysis with albumin-containing fluid, or hemodialysis are sometimes needed when the patient is very ill with very high salicylate level. Prevention should have high priority.

Acetaminophen

Acetaminophen or N-acetyl para-aminophenol (Tylenol, Tempra) has become an important and serious poison in the United States. It has been a serious toxin in England for a number of years. When compared with aspirin, the drug is free of some distressing side-effects at modest doses, but in large doses it is toxic to the liver, causing centrilobular necrosis. Renal damage due to tubule necrosis is common in patients surviving more than two days.

Acetaminophen is rapidly absorbed from the intestinal tract, and peak plasma concentrations are achieved in one to two hours. Acetaminophen can cause sudden death before the patient can be admitted to the hospital. Early deaths probably occur from vomiting and aspiration. The concentration in the plasma is the principal predictor of the occurrence of hepatic toxicity. Plasma half-life has been reported to be from one to three hours in normal subjects to a mean of four hours in mild intoxication and a mean of ten hours in fatal instances. Plasma levels below 150 mg. per liter at four hours or 50 mg. per liter at 12 hours are unlikely to result in severe hepatic toxicity. At four hours, a level above 300 mg. per liter results in hepatic necrosis. About 80 per cent of a therapeutic dose of acetaminophen is cleared from the blood by biotransformation by microsomal enzymes to a conjugate with glucuronic acid and sulfate. These metabolic products are inactive and excreted. Minor metabolites of acetaminophen are formed by hydroxylation and deacetylation. Production of hydroxylated metabolites involves oxidation by cytochrome P450 and mixed-function oxidases. This minor metabolite is a highly reactive arylating agent. The hydroxylated metabolite is conjugated with hepatic glutathione, further conjugated with cysteine and mercapturic acid, and is excreted in the urine. When a large dose is taken, large amounts of the toxic intermediates accumulate and hepatic glutathione is depleted. It is important to note that drugs such as phenobarbital induce the cytochrome P450 enzyme system and that consequently there is an acceleration of the formation of hydroxylated intermediates which are active arylating compounds. Glutathione depletion is hastened, with expected toxic consequences. Vital hepatocellular macromolecules bind covalently with these toxic intermediates, causing hepatic necrosis.

A key metabolic feature is depletion of hepatic cellular glutathione, and this has resulted in the suggestion and use of sulfhydryl donors in treatment of patients with plasma levels high enough to indicate moderate to severe hepatic injury. Cysteamine and n-acetyl cysteine have been effective, and one of these agents should be used when plasma levels indicate the probability of hepatic toxicity. Survivors apparently do not have residual liver damage.

Chronic excessive use can cause toxic hepatitis when the drug dose has been in the range of 5 to 8 grams. This dose is just slightly less than the amount which can cause acute toxicity. It is likely that the incidence of liver damage from chronic therapeutic use of large doses will increase.

Barbiturates, Related Compounds, and Narcotics

Hypnotics and opiates have similar depressive actions on respiratory and circulatory centers and on cerebral function. It is not unusual for a subject to take multiple hypnotic drugs in a suicide attempt. Barbiturates are generally divided into short-acting barbiturates (represented by pentobarbital, secobarbital, and amobarbital) and the long-acting barbiturates (represented by phenobarbital, barbital, and mephobarbital). The long-acting barbiturates are mainly excreted by the kidneys but are also detoxified by the liver. The drug concentration is important for determining prognosis, and it also is important for consideration of hemodialysis in patients with phenobarbital, barbital, or mephobarbital intoxication. Urea- or mannitol-induced diuresis and alkalinization of the urine is helpful in treatment of severe intoxication with both kinds of barbiturates, but particularly the long-acting ones.

Glutethimide intoxication has special problems. Forced diuresis is of little value. Hemodialysis, either aqueous or lipid, does not remove very much drug. Glutethimide is lipid-soluble, and blood levels are not closely correlated with severity of depression. There may be a fluctuating level of consciousness and, particularly, deepening coma, even after starting treatment. Treatment consists of eliminating drug sequestered in the intestine and supporting the respiratory and circulatory systems.

Opiates and synthetic narcotics may cause serious intoxication characterized by coma, severe respiratory slowing or arrest, and shock. Intoxication results from accidental overdose from the use of "street" heroin of uncertain strength or from intentional or suicidal overdose. A competitive inhibitor of narcotics in general, naloxone (Narcan), is very useful therapeutically and diagnostically in an opiate overdose. It should be injected repeatedly as needed, particularly for respiratory depression. It has one undesirable side-effect, namely, it will cause acute withdrawal reaction in an addicted individual. Support of circulation and respiration is, of course, essential.

In all vertebrate studies, the cell membranes of some of the neurons of the central nervous system have synaptosomal receptors. These areas correspond to well-characterized anatomic pathways involved in pain perception. Crude extracts of brain will displace labeled opium derivatives and an opium antagonist like naloxone from synaptosomal preparations. The opiate-like substances are pentapeptides, Leu[5]-enkephalin and Met[5]-enkephalin. The compounds are present in larger molecules derived from an extract of hypothalamus-neurohypophysis with Met[5]-enkephalin as their n-terminal. These latter compounds are called endorphins. In synaptosomal opiate binding assays, alpha and gamma endorphins are as active as morphine, and beta endorphin is five to ten times as active. Naloxone can inhibit the action of endorphins. In the intact animal, alpha, beta, and gamma endorphins have quite different effects. Naloxone blocks stimulation-produced analgesia and acupuncture analgesia. Endorphins probably will have an enormous impact on future understanding of neurophysiology and neuropharmacology.

The social problems of addiction to heroin and other opium compounds, cocaine, and the sedative and hypnotic drugs are enormous. The effects on the person are shattering. An incidental but very serious effect is the frequent association of systemic bacterial and fungal infections, often with bacterial endocarditis, as a result of "main line" administration. Physical and psychologic dependence is a threat from the use of any of the above agents. Withdrawal reactions are similar in many respects, but each group of agents has certain unique and potentially lethal features.

Ethanol

Ethanol (ethyl alcohol, beverage alcohol) is the most important toxic material in our society today. It accounts for more deaths than any other toxic substance when one considers sudden death from acute overdose, deaths from auto accidents, and deaths from chronic alcohol-related diseases such as hepatic cirrhosis, chronic brain syndrome, and alcoholic cardiomyopathy.

Ethanol diffuses readily across all biologic membranes except the skin, and so it is absorbed from all parts of the gastrointestinal tract, lungs, urinary bladder, peritoneum, pleura, and from subcutaneous sites. Alcohol distributes uniformly in the total body water by rapidly diffusing across capillary, cell, and organelle membranes. Alcohols interact with the lipid phase of cell membranes. Very high concentration disrupts the membranes. Ethanol changes membrane permeability to Na^+ and K^+. It depresses the functional activity of nerve cells by a direct effect on the excitable membranes of neuronal tissue. A typical reaction to ethanol ingestion is euphoria and exhilaration, followed by mental slowing and, finally, coma as the alcohol level increases progressively.

Ethanol is converted to acetaldehyde by the enzyme alcohol dehydrogenase; the acetaldehyde is converted to acetate by aldehyde oxidizing enzymes (see Fig. 34-2). Alcohol dehydrogenase, 90 per cent of which is located in the cytosol, attaches to a molecule of oxidized coenzyme, nicotine-adenine dinucleotide (NAD). The hydrogen of alcohol is accepted by NAD, which is converted to the reduced form, NADH. This is the rate-limiting step. Accumulation of NADH accounts for some of ethanol's effects on carbohydrate metabolism and on the production of fatty liver. Conversion of NADH or NAD is accomplished by electron transfer along the respiratory chain located in the mitochondria. A large number of alcohols and aldehydes have considerable affinity for alcohol dehydrogenase.

Ethanol has significant effects on the metabolism of carbohydrate. The oxidation of alcohol results in the increase in NADH/NAD in liver

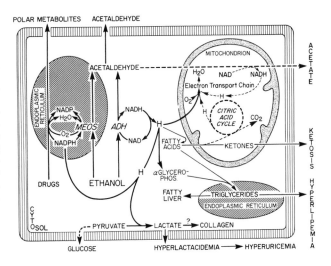

Figure 34–2 Metabolism of ethanol in the hepatocyte and schematic representation of its link to fatty liver, hyperlipemia, hyperuricemia, hyperlactacidemia, and ketosis. Pathways that are decreased by ethanol are represented by dashed lines. ADH, alcohol dehydrogenase; MEOS, microsomal ethanol oxidizing system; NAD, nicotinamide adenine dinucleotide; NADH, nicotinamide adenine dinucleotide, reduced form; NADP, nicotinamide adenine dinucleotide phosphate; NADPH, nicotinamide adenine dinucleotide phosphate, reduced form. (From Lieber, C. M., Teschke, R., Hasumura, Y., and Decarli, L. M.: Fed. Proc., 34:2061, 1975.)

cytosol. This increase in NADH/NAD ratio alters the equilibrium between the trioses, dihydroxyacetone phosphate and alpha glycerophosphate, favoring the latter. This shift in ratio results in more glycerol and, hence, the formation of hepatic triglycerides. Ethanol inhibits the utilization of galactose metabolism so that galactose is excreted in the urine. When fructose is administered with alcohol, fructose doubles the splanchnic uptake of alcohol and the production of acetate. Alcohol diverts some fructose to sorbitol via sorbitol dehydrogenase and NADH. This results in a higher proportion of glycerol formation from fructose and more glycerophosphate.

Ethanol can cause hypoglycemia in a fasting subject by slowing down gluconeogenesis. Alanine is the prime regulator of gluconeogenesis. Ethanol lowers circulating levels of alanine and other important glucogenic amino acids and, hence, impairs gluconeogenesis. The high NADH/NAD concentration ratio as a result of oxidation of ethanol to acetate impairs the conversion of glutamic acid to alpha ketoglutarate by interfering with the activity of glutamic dehydrogenase. Metabolism of ethanol increases the lactate-pyruvate ratio in the setting of an increased NADH/NAD ratio. In summary, ethanol impairs gluconeogenesis because it preempts mitochondrial cofactors, inhibits enzymes, channels precursors away from gluconeogenic pathways, and blocks uptake of precursors.

The velocity of the reaction of alcohol dehydrogenase (ADH) and ethanol is approximately seven times that for ADH and methanol, and the affinity of ethanol and ADH is twice that of methanol and ADH. For these reasons, ethanol can be given to a person poisoned with methanol, thus preventing the oxidation of methanol to the very toxic products, formaldehyde and formic acid. Unchanged methanol can then be excreted by the kidney. Methanol is easily oxidized by catalase, but ethanol is also a good competitive inhibitor of this reaction. Therefore, at this step also, ethanol prevents oxidation of methanol to toxic products so that methanol can be excreted. Similarly, ethylene glycol has a slow velocity of reaction and affinity for ADH compared with ethanol. Ethanol in a large dose competitively inhibits the oxidation of ethylene glycol to the highly toxic oxalic acid and is of considerable practical value in treatment of ethylene glycol poisoning.

Inhibitors of the metabolism of ethanol to acetaldehyde to acetate are useful in treating alcoholism. Disulfiram (Antabuse, tetraethylthiuram disulfide) is converted to diethylthiocarbamate. This compound chelates zinc and the metals of the aldehyde oxidizing system. Disulfiram can inactivate dehydrogenases by formation of disulfide linkages with active sulfhydryl groups of enzymes. The inhibition of alcohol and aldehyde metabolizing enzymes causes the disulfiram–alcohol syndrome when the two drugs are taken together. Other compounds, butyraldoxime, sulfonylurea compounds, and metronidazole, produce disulfiram-like reactions.

Catalase found in most animal tissues forms H_2O_2, which reacts with a hydrogen donor. Considerable turnover rates are observed in vitro with methanol, ethanol, and formate. Catalase, however, does not have a major role in normal ethanol metabolism.

Acetate enters the two-carbon pool through acetyl coenzyme A. Two dehydrogenases using NAD as coenzyme, two oxidases producing H_2O_2, and a third group of enzymes, the lyases, are responsible for acetaldehyde oxidation to acetate. Free acetate activation to acetyl coenzyme A is diminished when ethanol is actively being metabolized. Acetate is a central metabolic product and can be oxidized to CO_2 and water or used in the synthesis of fatty acids, steroids, and ketone bodies.

The level of alcohol dehydrogenase is decreased in the livers of animals pretreated with alcohol. The liver shows damage in the form of steatosis. Intolerance to ethanol has been observed in patients with an abnormal liver. A microsomal ethanol oxidizing system (MEOS) of the smooth endoplasmic reticulum has been found by a number of investigators. Chronic ethanol ingestion causes proliferation of the smooth endoplasmic reticulum, which could account for the induction of drug-metabolizing enzymes that results in the increased resistance of alcoholic subjects to the action of sedative drugs. Significant tolerance to ethanol is built up by chronic ingestion of ethanol in persons who do not have overt liver damage.

Ethanol has a direct etiologic role in the pathogenesis of alcoholic fatty liver and cirrhosis. Ethanol fed to normal volunteer men and alcoholic men caused fatty infiltration of the liver in each group, despite a well-balanced standard diet and even massive supplementation with protein and choline. The amount and duration of ethanol intake rather than malnutrition account for fatty liver in adult humans. After ethanol administration, phospholipids are increased in the liver, whereas fatty liver produced by choline deficiency has decreased phospholipids.

Fatty liver induced by moderate amounts of ethanol is reversible and benign. However, a florid kind of fatty metamorphosis called alcoholic hepatitis occurs, with extensive cellular degeneration, appearance of alcoholic hyaline of Mallory, hepatic cell necrosis, and inflammatory cells. Ultrastructural cell changes in ordinary fatty liver and alcoholic hepatitis are the same, namely, striking alterations in mitochondria and endoplasmic reticulum and focal cytoplasmic degradation with formation of autophagic vacuoles containing clumps and whorls of osmophilic material. The cisternae and vacuoles of the Golgi apparatus are dilated and filled with osmophilic material, probably lipoprotein particles. The similarity of ultrastructural changes in simple alcoholic fatty liver and in alcoholic hepatitis suggests that the process is a continuum. The pathogenesis of alcoholic cirrhosis clearly is related to fatty metamorphosis, but the exact mechanism is still unclear.

Ethanol intoxication is a phenomenon recognizable by everyone. The blood level of ethanol and, therefore, the dose ingested is related directly to the severity of intoxication. A person unaccustomed to ethanol exhibits intoxication at ethanol levels of 50 to 100 mg./dl., whereas a person who drinks alcohol regularly exhibits intoxication at levels above 150 mg./dl. At 200 mg./dl., most individuals are unmistakably drunk. Intoxication is severe at 350 mg./dl. and over. Levels as low as 350 mg./dl. have caused death, and levels above 550 mg./dl. are usually fatal. By extrapolation of blood levels at time of death to zero time, the levels usually are 500 to 600 mg./dl. This level will kill in a short time or will cause sufficient brain damage to cause death after several hours. The median LD_{50} in terms of blood ethanol has been estimated to be 400 mg./dl. These data emphasize the very serious acute toxic effect of ethanol on the brain.

A very common and serious effect of chronic ethanol abuse is the acute withdrawal reaction manifested as alcoholic hallucinosis and delirium tremens. One of the biochemical phenomena associated with these disturbances is a large increase of free fatty acids in the blood. Another feature is the occurrence of hypomagnesemia and total body magnesium deficit. By careful management, the mortality rate from delirium tremens has been reduced greatly over the past two decades; nevertheless, it is a serious, acute medical emergency.

The most common nervous system lesion is alcoholic neuropathy with all the signs of neuropathy. Thiamine particularly but also pyridoxine and pantothenic acid are useful therapeutically, but only if ethanol is stopped.

The mechanism of production of chronic alcoholic encephalopathy is not clear, but certain facts are relevant. Chronic dementia of the Korsakoff type frequently is preceded by acute Wernicke's encephalopathy due to thiamine deficiency. Simple dementia, however, occurs with alcohol-induced brain atrophy. Rare specific localized encephalopathies, such as central pontine myelinolysis, toxic amblyopia, and Marchiafava-Bignami disease, depend on the specific area of the brain affected. Since alcohol causes acute cerebral effects which can be profound and, if repetitive, could have direct degenerative effects on the brain, it is understandable that ethanol can cause chronic encephalopathy. Chronic alcohol dementia accounts for a large number of patients in mental hospitals. Cerebellar degeneration is a common result of alcoholism and may occur with cerebral lesions or may be the only residual lesion.

Ethanol is a direct and frequent cause of gastritis, with serious and sometimes fatal gastric hemorrhage. Ethanol also is the most frequent cause of pancreatitis and all its complications, including a high mortality rate. Ethanol is the usual cause of chronic relapsing pancreatitis.

Alcoholic cardiomyopathy is a serious and often fatal condition caused by continuous high ethanol ingestion. The cause of the cardiomyopathy is not clear, but there is some evidence that acetaldehyde has deleterious effects on both the electrical and mechanical parameters of myocardial function.

Although the relationship between maternal ethanol abuse and undesirable outcomes of pregnancy has been recognized since ancient times, it has gained scientific validation only recently. Infants and children born to alcoholic mothers exhibit characteristic clinical features. *Fetal alcohol syndrome* refers to these clinical characteristics. Major features of fetal alcohol syndrome are prenatal and postnatal growth retardation, mental deficiency, small head size relative to height, and minor anomalies of the face, eyes, heart, joints, and external genitalia. Mental retardation is the most serious defect. Ocular anomalies include epicanthal folds, convergence defects, ptosis, and palpebral fissures that are below average in length. Minimal diagnostic criteria are physical and mental retardation with associated minor birth defects and a history of chronic maternal alcoholism.

The pathogenesis of the teratogenic effects of ethanol remains unknown. In rats, a deficiency of zinc during crucial stages of gestation is known to be teratogenic. Many enzymes required for DNA synthesis are zinc-dependent, and an adverse effect of zinc deficiency on the activity of deoxythymidine kinase has been reported. Inasmuch as ethanol ingestion may affect zinc balance adversely, one may speculate that the teratogenic effect of alcohol is mediated through zinc enzymes involved in DNA synthesis. Further studies must be carried out in order to understand fully the pathogenetic mechanisms of fetal alcohol syndrome so that proper therapeutic measures may be undertaken.

In summary, ethanol is the most serious chemical toxin in modern society because of its

TABLE 34–1 TOXIC CHEMICALS AND POISONS

Toxin	Special Features of Exposure	Target Tissue or Organ	Enzymes Affected; Physiologic or Pharmacologic Features	Clinical or Pathologic Results	Antidote, Special Form of Treatment, or Prevention
Antimony (Sb^{3+}) Stilbine (SbH_3)	Tartar emetic Metallurgy; mining and smelting; rubber manufacture; exposure to nascent H to Sb_2O_3	CNS, skin, bone	Sulfhydryl group of enzymes	Vomiting, dermatitis and conjunctivitis, acute encephalopathy, acute hemolysis due to stilbine	BAL as in arsenic poisoning; avoid generation of stilbine
Arsenic (As^{3+}) As_2O_3 Arsine (AsH_3)	Deliberate—homicide Fowler's solution as medicine; industrial exposure nascent H to As_2O_3	CNS and peripheral nerves, bone marrow kidney, skin and fingernails	Sulfhydryl groups of many enzymes; carcinogenesis	Shock and death, acute hemolytic anemia, hemoglobinuria, nephropathy, encephalopathy, cardiomyopathy; hyperkeratoses and basal cell cancers (Bowen's disease), Mee's lines	Acute: BAL (dimercaprol or British antiLewisite); hemodialysis for acute renal failure; stop use of Fowler's solution
Cadmium (Cd^{2+})	Industrial waste of battery factories in water supply (Japan); inhalation	Kidneys, lungs, bone	Necrosis of respiratory epithelium, renal glucosuria, phosphaturia, hypophosphatemia, and low molecular weight proteinuria; cadmium interferes with metabolism and utilization of zinc	Pulmonary edema and interstitial pneumonitis; osteomalacia (Itai-Itai or "ouch-ouch" disease) in Japan	Stop water pollution with cadmium (battery industry); treat osteomalacia, $CaNa_2$ EDTA therapy
Iron ferrous salts	Accidental in children under 5 years; suicidal	CNS, liver, heart	High level of plasma free iron with transferrin fully saturated	Hypotension, progressive shock, dyspnea, coma	Desferoxamine (Desfera) IV and orally; prevent
Lead (Pb^{2+}) and tetraethyl lead	Pica (eating of paint chips by young children), paint dust in building repair, "moonshine" whiskey, leaded gasoline auto exhaust	CNS, bone marrow, joints, kidneys	(1) Delta amino levulinic acid (ALA) synthetase (probable) (2) ALA dehydratase (Zn dependent) (3) Heme synthetase	Encephalopathy, neuropathy of motor nerves, abdominal crises, anemia; nephropathy, hyperuricemia and "Saturnine" gout; possible mental retardation	Ethylene diamine tetraacetic acid ($CaNa_2$ EDTA) and penicillamine; eliminate lead in paint and gasoline; excess dietary zinc is protective against lead toxicity in rats and horses
Mercury, (Hg^{2+}) mercury bichloride ($HgCl_2$) Calomel (HgCl) (Hg^{1+})	Suicidal intent, industrial use, medicine use	All tissues, kidney, CNS	Sulfhydryl groups, denaturation of all proteins (corrosive action) and cell death, acute renal tubule cell injury	Corrosion of mucosa and skin, acute renal failure, personality disorder or "erethism" ("mad as a hatter"); acrodynia (calomel)	BAL hemodialysis nacetyl, d.l. penicillamine; eliminate calomel as medication; dietary selenium may be protective against toxic effects of methylmercury compounds in rats
Methyl and Ethyl mercury	Hg contamination of water, biotransformation by bacteria to organic Hg, then ingested by fish (tuna and swordfish) (Minamata Bay and Niigata, Japan, epidemic	CNS; fetal intoxication of CNS	Volatile, penetrate mucosa readily; concentrate in CNS	Serious CNS injury including newborns born to mothers who have ingested alkyl mercury	Surveillance of Hg concentration in fish; clean up streams and stop Hg contamination of water; n acetyl d.l. penicillamine
Thallium (Tl^{1+})	Rodent poison; depilatory	CNS, hair follicles, liver, kidney	Degenerative changes in all cells, especially of hair follicles	Alopecia is pathognomonic; encephalopathy with ataxia, choreiform movement and delirium and coma; central lobular necrosis of liver and renal tubule injury	Prussian blue by mouth as a chelator of Tl in exchange for K^+. Eliminate use of thallium as domestic rodent poison

Barbiturates, Opiates, Sedatives and Antidepressants

Agent	Circumstances	Site	Mechanism	Effects	Treatment
Barbiturates: short-acting—amobarbital, pentobarbital secobarbital; long-acting—phenobarbital, barbital, mephobarbital	Suicide attempts, chronic dependence	CNS	Renal and hepatic elimination of long-acting barbiturates; hepatic detoxification of short acting barbiturates; physiologic dependence or addiction	Sedation, convulsions, stupor, coma, shock, apnea and death; withdrawal reaction with delirium; intact pupillary reflexes	Support vital functions; diuresis and alkalinization of urine; hemodialysis for long-acting barbiturates
Benzodiazepines: diazepam, chlordiazepoxide, flurazepam	Often taken with alcohol or other drugs	CNS	Minor tranquilizer; sedation; physiologic dependence or addiction	Coma, rarely fatal unless other drugs; withdrawal reaction	Support of vital functions
Ethchlorvinyl	Storage in fat	CNS	Sedation; physiologic dependence; fat soluble	Withdrawal reaction, coma, often prolonged because of storage in fat	Support of vital functions
Glutethimide (Doriden)	Short-acting like secobarbital	CNS	Sequestered in bowel with fluctuating coma, physiologic dependence, pupillary reflexes lost	Coma, often severe, tends to produce hypotension	Support of vital functions
Meprobamate (Equanil)		CNS	Minor tranquilizer, physiologic dependence	Coma, withdrawal seizures common	Support of vital functions; treat seizures
Methaqualone (Quaalude)	Abuse common	CNS; blood coagulation	Sedation; physiologic dependence quickly; dangerous dose relatively small	Coma, hallucinations, motor hyperactivity, myoclonus, convulsions, heart failure	Support of vital functions; treat seizures
Opium and related compounds / Cocaine	Addiction from therapeutic use and deliberate abuse; impurity of street drugs and uncertain dose	CNS	Narcosis; euphoria; physiologic dependence; endorphins are brain receptors; cocaine—excitement, mania	Special effects on respiratory and circulatory control; altering of pupil reflexes—constricted; stupor, coma, apnea, shock and death	Support of vital functions; naloxone (Narcan) as often as necessary—opiates
Tricyclic antidepressants	Often taken with other agents (and prescribed for already depressed patients)	CNS, cardiac conduction	Anticholinergic action	Dry mouth, bladder retention, ileus, blurred vision, sinus tachycardia, agitation, coma	Support of vital functions; physostigmin salicylate; well adsorbed by charcoal

Solvents and Alcohols

Agent	Circumstances	Site	Mechanism	Effects	Treatment
Carbon tetrachloride	Particularly bad in a person also exposed to alcohols	Liver, kidney	Disruption of lipid membranes	Fatty liver and necrosis; acute tubule necrosis with acute renal failure	Supportive; dialysis as needed (peritoneal or hemodialysis); eliminate as domestic dry cleaner
Ethanol	Generally available, most widely used toxin	Liver, CNS, all tissues	Alcohol dehydrogenase; physiologic and psychologic dependence	Drunkenness and belligerence, coma and death, hepatic cirrhosis, anemia, acute and chronic brain syndromes	Support of vital functions in profound intoxication; prevention of alcoholism
Ethylene glycol	Sweet taste, careless storage	Kidney	(1) Oxidase converts it to oxalic acid; (2) Ethanol competes favorably for oxidase-preventing reaction 1.	Calcium oxalate injury to kidney causing acute renal failure and death	Ethanol permits ethylene glycol excretion; hemodialysis or peritoneal dialysis as needed for acute renal failure
Methanol	Careless storage, suicide attempt	Optic nerve, whole body, CNS	(1) Oxidase catalyses it to formaldehyde and formic acid (2) Ethanol competes favorably for oxidase preventing reaction 1	Blindness, severe acidosis, death	Dialysis immediately; ethanol competes for methanol oxidation permitting methanol excretion

Table continued on following page

TABLE 34–1 TOXIC CHEMICALS AND POISONS (Continued)

Toxin	Special Features of Exposure	Target Tissue or Organ	Enzymes Affected; Physiologic or Pharmacologic Features	Clinical or Pathologic Results	Antidote, Special Form of Treatment, or Prevention
Miscellaneous Toxins					
Acetylsalicylic acid and salicylates	Careless storage	CNS, respiration center	Stimulate respiration; stimulate metabolism; uncouple oxidative phosphorylation	Respiratory alkalosis, metabolism acidosis, coma and death	Dialysis if severe; sodium bicarbonate and acetazolamide to increase excretion of salicylates in alkaline urine
Acetaminophen	Suicidal intent	Liver, kidney, CNS	Hydroxylated intermediate by glutathione under influence of cytochrome P450	Liver necrosis, renal tubule necrosis; toxic metabolites from covalent bonds with macromolecules; deplete glutathione	Cysteamine or n, acetylcyseine (Mucormyst) act as sulfhydryl donors
Atropa belladonna	Attractive berries	Many organs (parasympathetic nerves)	Block cholinergic impulses (atropine poisoning)	Dry mouth, wide pupils tachycardia, delirium, fever, death	Pilocarpine; support
Datura stramonium (Jimson weed)	Attractive plant	Many organs	Block cholinergic impulse (stramonium poisoning)	Same as atropine, belladonna	Pilocarpine; support
Cyanide (CN⁻)	Homicide and suicide; very small dose	Respiratory enzymes (heme-containing) of all cells	Inactivates cytochrome A_3; paralyzes electron transfer	Tissue anoxia and death	Na thiosulfate and Na nitrite →cyanmethemoglobin thus neutralizing CN⁻
Botulinus toxin (Clostridium botulinum)	Contaminated canned food not cooked or stored in open container	Motor end-plate	Toxin is heat labile; blocks nerve impulse at motor end-plate	Paralysis of skeletal muscle	Antitoxin (type-specific; prevent by cooking canned food thoroughly (to boiling)
Cholera toxin (Vibrio cholera)	Epidemic; contaminated water supply	Mucosa of small intestine (no inflammation)	Activates adenyl cyclase → cyclic AMP	Massive secretion of salt and water with circulatory collapse and death	Replace H_2O and electrolytes quantitatively
Clostridium perfringens toxin	Picnics, contaminated food; toxin is heat labile	Small intestine mucosa		Massive diarrhea; rarely fatal	Replace losses of H_2O and electrolytes; cook canned or stored food; refrigerate properly
Staphylococcus enterotoxin A, B, C, D	Picnics, contaminated food, improperly refrigerated, e.g., cream pies, etc.	Probably CNS	Toxin is heat and trypsin stable	Abdominal cramping pain, vomiting, diarrhea variable	Careful food handling and refrigeration; replace fluids and electrolytes
Phosphate ester insecticides (parathion, malathion, etc.)	Industrial; insecticide sprays, dusting; penetrates skin; careless storage—accidental ingestion	Parasympathetic nervous system, skeletal muscles, erythrocytes	Cholinergic action (powerful anticholinesterases), muscle paralysis; decrease RBC cholinesterase	Muscarine effects plus muscle paralysis cause respiratory failure	Atropine (2–3 mg.) repeated at 5–10 minutes; pralidoxime chloride –1 gm. IV in 2 minutes and repeat in 1 hour as needed for adults. Prevent: careful bathing, handling of clothes, proper equipment, monitor RBC cholinesterase

widespread use. It causes serious chronic social and physical disturbances that probably exceed the devastation of alcohol-induced death.

Carbon Monoxide

Carbon monoxide (CO) is a serious environmental poison. Although CO is used as a highly successful vehicle for suicide, most deaths and morbidity result from accidental poisoning, such as occurs in fires in an unventilated room, from leaks in smoke ducts, and from destructive fires in a building. CO is odorless and, therefore, doubly hazardous.

The biochemistry of CO in the body is straightforward, and its toxicity has been known since Claude Bernard reported on it in 1857. J. S. Haldane (1895) was a pioneering investigator of the physiology and toxicology of CO. Hemoglobin has an affinity for CO that is 240 times that for O_2. CO readily displaces O_2 from hemoglobin at partial pressures only 1/240 that of O_2, forming carbon monoxide hemoglobin (COHG). Furthermore, the O_2 dissociation curve is "shifted to the left," so the oxyhemoglobin present in blood does not dissociate at usual oxygen tensions. Other heme-containing enzymes also react with CO. Generalized tissue anoxia results in a response curve dependent on atmospheric CO. At 0.01 per cent CO, the COHG is 44 per cent; at 0.1 per cent CO, the COHG is 62 per cent. All COHG concentrations above 20 per cent produce cerebral symptoms.

The tissues most easily injured by CO are the brain and myocardium because these tissues have greatest O_2 consumption. A pre-existing cerebral or myocardial abnormality predisposes the patient to adverse effects of levels not injurious to normals. Late sequelae include late fatal demyelinization, permanent cerebral dysfunction, peripheral neuropathy, and effects on the conduction system of the heart.

Laboratory tests are of obvious diagnostic value, but treatment should be instituted on the basis of history and findings before results are obtained. Arterial blood gases reveal a normal paO_2 since the plasma equilibrates with alveolar blood gases, but the blood content of O_2 is seriously decreased.

Treatment is simply administration of 100 per cent oxygen by mask. Two volumes per cent of O_2 are attained by this maneuver. CO excretion is enhanced by O_2 by shifting the equilibrium toward oxyhemoglobin. Brain edema occurs in most severe instances, and dexamethasone treatment is indicated.

Chronic exposure to CO concentrations insufficient to cause clinical (cerebral) symptoms but sufficient to elevate COHG concentrations occurs in our urban society because of the CO output of internal combustion engines and all fossil fuel-using machines. The COHG level in cigarette smokers is directly correlated with the number of cigarettes smoked each day. The COHG can be as high as 5 to 8 per cent in smokers who inhale.

CO may have an etiologic role in atherosclerosis. The deposit of cholesterol in the aorta in rabbits is enhanced by anoxia induced by decreasing partial pressure of O_2 or by slight excess of CO in the atmosphere. Anoxia increases the permeability of artery walls to serum proteins as measured by isotope-labeled protein. It has been postulated that chronic low-grade exposure to CO can result in significant effects on arteries by low-grade hypoxia. Patients who already have coronary artery disease with angina pectoris have such a small margin of safety that an increase in COHG can precipitate ischemic pain. The effects of chronic exposure to increased CO are just now being fully appreciated.

REFERENCES

Arena, J. M.: Salicylates (Poisoning). In Davison's Compleat Pediatrician. Lea & Febiger, Philadelphia, 1969.

Arky, R. A.: Carbohydrate Metabolism in Alcoholics. In Kissin, B., and Begleiter, H. (eds.): The Biology of Alcoholism, Vol. I. Plenum Press, New York, London, 1971, pp. 197–227.

Astrup, P.: Some physiological and pathological effects of moderate carbon monoxide exposure. Br. Med. J., 1:12, 1973.

Beutler, E.: Abnormalities of the hexose monophosphate shunt. Seminars Hematol., 8:311, 1971.

Done, A. K.: Salicylate intoxication. Significance of salicylate in blood in cases of acute ingestion. Pediatrics, 26:800, 1960.

Dreosti, I. E., and Harley, L. S.: Depressed thymidine kinase activity in zinc deficient rat embryos. Proc. Soc. Exp. Biol. Med., 150:161–165, 1975.

Flink, E. B.: Heavy Metal Poisoning. In Beeson, P., and McDermott, W. (eds.): Textbook of Medicine, 14th ed. W. B. Saunders Co., Philadelphia, 1975.

Flink, E. B.: Mineral Metabolism in Alcoholism. In Kissin, B., and Begleiter, H. (eds.): The Biology of Alcoholism, Vol. I. Plenum Press, New York, London, 1971, pp. 377–396.

French, S. W.: Acute and Chronic Toxicity of Alcohol. In Kissin, B., and Begleiter, H. (eds.): The Biology of Alcoholism, Vol. I. Plenum Press, New York, London, 1971, pp. 437–511.

Gleason, M., Gosselin, R., Hodge, H., and Smith, R.: Clinical Toxicology of Commercial Products, 4th ed. Baltimore, Williams & Wilkins Co., 1973.

Guillemin, R.: Endorphins: brain peptides that act like opiates. N. Engl. J. Med., 296:226–228, 1977.

Goldsmith, J. R., and Landaw, S. A.: Carbon monoxide and human health. Science, 162:1352, 1968.

Henderson, F., Vietti, T. J., and Brown, E. B.: Desferrioxamine in the treatment of acute toxic reaction to ferrous gluconate. J.A.M.A., *186*:1139, 1963.

Henderson, L. W., and Merrill, J. P.: Treatment of barbiturate intoxication. Ann. Int. Med., *64*:876, 1966.

Jones, K. L., Smith, D. W., Ulleland, C. N., and Streissguth, A. P.: Pattern of malformation in offspring of chronic alcoholic mothers. Lancet, *1*:1267–1271, 1973.

Kalant, H.: Effects of Biological Membranes. *In* Kissin, B., and Begleiter, H. (eds.): The Biology of Alcoholism, Vol. I. Plenum Press, New York, London, 1971, pp. 1–62.

Koch-Weser, J.: Acetaminophen. N. Engl. J. Med., *295*:1297, 1976.

Kvenzolok, E. P., Best, L., and Manoguerra, A. S.: Acetaminophen toxicity. Am. J. Hosp. Pharmacy, *34*:391, 1977.

Lieber, C. S., and De Carli, L. M.: Effects of Ethanol on Lipid, Uric Acid, Intermediary and Drug Metabolism including Pathogenesis of the Alcoholic Fatty Liver. *In* Kissin, B., and Begleiter, H.: The Biology of Alcoholism, Vol. I. Plenum Press, New York, London, 1971, pp. 264–305.

Loomis, Ted A.: Essentials of Toxicology, 2nd ed. Lea & Febiger, Philadelphia, 1974.

Milby, T. H.: Prevention and management of organophosphate poisoning. J.A.M.A., *216*:2131, 1971.

Morgan W. K. C., and Seaton, A.: Occupational Lung Diseases. W. B. Saunders Co., Philadelphia, 1975.

Myschetzky, A., and Lassen, N. A.: Forced Diuresis in Treatment of Acute Barbiturate Poisoning. *In* Matthew, H. (ed.): Acute Barbiturate Poisoning, Excerpta Medica, Amsterdam, 1971, pp. 95–204.

Peterson, R. G., and Rumack, B. H.: Treating acute acetaminophen poisoning with acetylcysteine. J.A.M.A., *237*:2406, 1977.

Plum, Fred.: Acute Drug Poisoning. *In* Beeson, P., and McDermott, W. (eds.): Textbook of Medicine, 14th ed. W. B. Saunders Co., Philadelphia, 1975.

Prasad, A. S., and Oberleas, D.: Thymidine kinase activity and incorporation of thymidine into DNA in zinc-deficient tissue. J. Lab. Clin. Med., *83*:634–639, 1974.

Prasad, A. S. (ed.): Trace Elements in Human Health and Disease. Academic Press, New York, pp. 1–20, 401–416, 443–476, 1976.

Prescott, L. F., Park, J., Sutherland, G. R., Smith, I. J., and Proudfoot, A. T.: Cysteamine, methionine, and penicillamine in the treatment of paracetomol poisoning. Lancet, *2*:109, 1976.

Thurston, J. H., Pollock, P. G., and Warren, S. K.: Reduced brain glucose with normal plasma glucose in salicylate poisoning. J. Clin. Invest., *49*:2139, 1970.

Tobis, J.: Cardiac complications in amitriptyline poisoning: successful treatment with physostigmine. J.A.M.A., *235*:1474, 1976.

Truitt, J. B., Jr., and Walsh, M. J.: The Role of Acetaldehyde in the Action of·Ethanol. *In* Kissin, B., and Begleiter, H. (eds.): The Biology of Alcoholism, Vol. I. Plenum Press, New York, London, 1971, pp. 186–187.

Von Wartburg, J. P.: The Metabolism of Alcohol in Normals and Alcoholics: Enzymes. *In* Kissin, B., and Begleiter, H. (eds.): The Biology of Alcoholism, Vol. I. Plenum Press, New York, London, 1971, pp. 63–102.

Wallgren, H.: Effect of Ethanol on Intracellular Respiration and Cerebral Function. *In* Kissin, B., and Begleiter, H. (eds.): The Biology of Alcoholism, Vol. I. Plenum Press, New York, London, 1971, pp. 117–119.

INDEX

Note: Page numbers in *italics* refer to illustrations. Page numbers followed by (t) refer to tables.